SURGICAL ONCOLOGY

SURGICAL ONCOLOGY

Yosef H. Pilch, M.D.

Professor of Surgery
Head, Surgical Oncology Service
University of California, San Diego
School of Medicine

McGraw-Hill Book Company

New York   St. Louis   San Francisco   Auckland   Bogotá   Guatemala   Hamburg   Johannesburg
Lisbon   London   Madrid   Mexico   Montreal   New Delhi   Panama   Paris
San Juan   São Paulo   Singapore   Sydney
Tokyo   Toronto

NOTICE

Medicine is an ever-changing science. As new research and clinical experience broaden our knowledge, changes in treatment and drug therapy are required. The editors and the publisher of this work have made every effort to ensure that the drug dosage schedules herein are accurate and in accord with the standards accepted at the time of publication. Readers are advised, however, to check the product information sheet included in the package of each drug they plan to administer to be certain that changes have not been made in the recommended dose or in the contraindications for administration. This recommendation is of particular importance in regard to new or infrequently used drugs.

SURGICAL ONCOLOGY

Copyright © 1984 by McGraw-Hill, Inc. All rights reserved. Printed in the United States of America. Except as permitted under the United States Copyright Act of 1976, no part of this publication may be reproduced or distributed in any form or by any means, or stored in a data base or retrieval system, without the prior written permission of the publisher.

1 2 3 4 5 6 7 8 9 0   HALHAL   8 9 8 7 6 5 4 3

ISBN 0-07-049997-7

This book was set in Baskerville by Monotype Composition Company, Inc; the editing supervisor was Maggie Schwarz; the production supervisors were Jeanne Skahan and Avé McCracken; the designer was Elliot Epstein. Halliday Lithograph Corporation was printer and binder.

Library of Congress Cataloging in Publication Data

Main entry under title:

Surgical oncology.

    Bibliography: p.
    Includes index.
    1. Cancer—Surgery.   I. Pilch, Yosef H.   [DNLM:
1. Neoplasms—Surgery.   QZ 268 S9612]
RD651.S932   1984   616.99′4059   83-7983
ISBN 0-07-049997-7

לאבי מורי ר׳ יהודה
בן יוסף חיים אשר
קים את המצוה "ושננתם
לבניך"

To my father and teacher, Dr. Judah Pilch, who fulfilled the commandment "and thou shall teach them diligently unto thy children."

CONTENTS

List of Contributors xi

Preface xvii

Part One BASIC CONCEPTS IN ONCOLOGY

Chapter 1 Introduction *Yosef H. Pilch, M.D.* 3

Chapter 2 Environmental Carcinogenesis *Michael B. Shimkin, M.D.* 7

Chapter 3 Cancer Epidemiology: Methods and Applications *Jonathan Amsel, Sc.D.* 23

Chapter 4 Genetic and Familial Aspects of Cancer
Louise A. Paquin, Ph.D., David T. Purtilo, M.D. 46

Chapter 5 Tumor Viruses—Vectors of Carcinogenesis at the Molecular Level
Fred Rapp, Ph.D., Mary K. Howett, Ph.D. 65

Chapter 6 The Molecular Virology of Breast Cancer and Its Clinical Implications
Sol Spiegelman, Ph.D., Ricardo Mesa-Tejada, M.D., Tsuneya Ohno, M.D., Ph.D. 88

Chapter 7 Tumor Cell Biology and Kinetics *Robert B. Livingston, M.D.* 108

Chapter 8 Principles of Cancer Chemotherapy *Robert B. Livingston, M.D.* 124

Chapter 9 Tumor Immunology *Yosef H. Pilch, M.D.* 142

Chapter 10 Monoclonal Antibodies: Current and Potential Application in Cancer Diagnosis and Therapy *Robert O. Dillman, M.D.* 163

Chapter 11 Basic Principles of Radiation Biology and Radiation Oncology
Ralph R. Weichselbaum, M.D., Samuel Hellman, M.D. 176

Chapter 12 Mechanisms of Metastasis Formation
Everett V. Sugarbaker, M.D., Daniel N. Weingrad, M.D., James M. Roseman, M.D. 198

Chapter 13 Psychological Aspects of Cancer *Claus B. Bahnson, Ph.D.* 231

Chapter 14 Design of the Controlled Clinical Trial
Carol Redmond, Sc.D., Bernard Fisher, M.D. 254

Part Two **TUMORS OF THE HEAD AND NECK**

Chapter 15 Tumors of the Tongue, Lips, and Oral Cavity
Elliot W. Strong, M.D., Ronald H. Spiro, M.D. 275

Chapter 16 Tumors of the Nasopharynx, Nasal Cavity, and Paranasal Sinuses
José J. Terz, M.D., Walter J. Lawrence, Jr., M.D. 309

Chapter 17 Tumors of the Oropharynx, Hypopharynx, and Cervical Esophagus
Terence M. Davidson, M.D. 335

Chapter 18 Tumors of the Laryngeal Apparatus
Leslie M. Greenberg, M.D., Donald G. Sessions, M.D. 361

Chapter 19 Tumors of the Major and Minor Salivary Glands *Harvey W. Baker, M.D.* 388

Chapter 20 Tumors of the Thyroid and Parathyroid
Arthur G. James, M.D., William B. Farrar, M.D., Marc Cooperman, M.D. 405

Part Three **INTRATHORACIC NEOPLASMS**

Chapter 21 Pulmonary Neoplasms *E. Carmack Holmes, M.D.* 433

Chapter 22 Malignant Tumors of the Esophagus
Samuel E. Wilson, M.D., John R. Benfield, M.D. 448

Chapter 23 Tumors of the Mediastinum
John R. Benfield, M.D., Robert M. Bearman, M.D., John L. Werner, M.D. 470

Part Four   TUMORS OF THE BREAST

Chapter 24   Breast Cancer   *Yosef H. Pilch, M.D.*   491

Part Five   INTRAABDOMINAL NEOPLASMS

Chapter 25   Carcinoma of the Stomach
E. Douglas Holyoke, M.D., Harold O. Douglass, Jr., M.D.   543

Chapter 26   Hepatobiliary and Periampullary Neoplasms   *Joseph G. Fortner, M.D.*   559

Chapter 27   Tumors of the Pancreas   *Bimal C. Ghosh, M.D.*   580

Chapter 28   Cancer of the Colon and Rectum
E. Douglas Holyoke, M.D., Arnold Mittelman, M.D.   596

Chapter 29   Adrenal Tumors   *Glenn W. Geelhoed, M.D.*   610

Chapter 30   The Carcinoid Cell, Tumors, and Syndromes   *Glenn W. Geelhoed, M.D.*   630

Part Six   UROLOGIC NEOPLASMS

Chapter 31   Malignant Tumors of the Kidney   *Jean B. deKernion, M.D.*   645

Chapter 32   Tumors of the Renal Pelvis and Ureter   *Jerome P. Richie, M.D.*   664

Chapter 33   Bladder Carcinoma   *George R. Prout, Jr., M.D.*   679

Chapter 34   Tumors of the Prostate   *Jeffrey J. Pollen, M.D., Joseph D. Schmidt, M.D.*   698

Chapter 35   Testicular Cancer   *Nasser Javadpour, M.D., Ph.D.*   729

Chapter 36   Tumors of the Penis and Urethra   *David F. Paulson, M.D.*   741

Part Seven   GYNECOLOGIC NEOPLASMS

Chapter 37   Cervical Cancer   *John R. van Nagell, Jr., M.D.*   751

Chapter 38 Cancers of the Uterine Corpus *William E. Lucas, M.D.* 780

Chapter 39 Tumors of the Ovary *Philip J. DiSaia, M.D., William M. Rich, M.D.* 807

Chapter 40 Tumors of the Vulva, Vagina, and Female Urethra *Samuel C. Ballon, M.D.* 826

Chapter 41 Diagnosis and Treatment of Gestational Trophoblastic Neoplasia
Charles B. Hammond, M.D., John L. Currie, M.D. 844

Part Eight MELANOMA, SARCOMAS, AND LYMPHOMAS

Chapter 42 Malignant Melanoma *Yosef H. Pilch, M.D.* 861

Chapter 43 Sarcomas of Bone and Soft Tissue *Frederick R. Eilber, M.D.* 888

Chapter 44 Hodgkin's Disease and the Non-Hodgkin's Lymphomas
Mark R. Green, M.D., Joan F. Kroener, M.D. 904

Part Nine NEUROSURGICAL ONCOLOGY

Chapter 45 Primary Tumors of the Central Nervous System
Mark Rosenblum, M.D., Lawrence F. Marshall, M.D. 929

Chapter 46 The Treatment of Metastatic Disease to the Central Nervous System and Spine *Lawrence F. Marshall, M.D.* 965

Part Ten MISCELLANEOUS ASPECTS

Chapter 47 Management of Pain in Cancer
Ronald J. Ignelzi, M.D., J. Hampton Atkinson, Jr., M.D. 983

Chapter 48 Paraneoplastic Syndromes *Charles M. Haskell, M.D.* 1025

Chapter 49 Rehabilitation and Reconstruction for the Cancer Patient
J. Herbert Dietz, Jr., M.D. 1041

Index 1077

LIST OF CONTRIBUTORS

Jonathan Amsel, Sc.D.

Associate Professor, Program for Epidemiologic Research and Training, University of Pennsylvania, Philadelphia.

J. Hampton Atkinson, Jr., M.D.

Assistant Professor of Psychiatry, University of California, San Diego, School of Medicine.

Claus B. Bahnson, Ph.D.

Professor of Psychosomatics and Psychotherapy, University of California, San Francisco; Director of Behavioral Sciences, Department of Family Practice, Valley Medical Center, Fresno, California.

Harvey W. Baker, M.D.

Professor of Surgery, School of Medicine, The Oregon Health Sciences University, Portland.

Samuel C. Ballon, M.D.

Associate Professor, Department of Gynecology and Obstetrics, Stanford University School of Medicine; Director, Section of Gynecologic Oncology, Stanford University Medical Center, Palo Alto, California.

Robert M. Bearman, M.D.

Department of Pathology, City of Hope Medical Center, Duarte, California.

John R. Benfield, M.D.

Chairman, Division of Surgery, City of Hope Medical Center, Duarte, California.

Marc Cooperman, M.D.

Assistant Professor of Surgery, Ohio State University College of Medicine, Columbus.

John L. Currie, M.D.

Assistant Professor, Department of Obstetrics and Gynecology, Duke University School of Medicine, Durham, North Carolina.

Terence M. Davidson, M.D.

Assistant Professor of Surgery, University of California, San Diego, School of Medicine.

Jean B. deKernion, M.D.

Associate Professor of Surgery, Head, Urologic Oncology, University of California, Los Angeles, School of Medicine; Director for Clinical Programs, UCLA-Jonsson Cancer Center, Los Angeles.

J. Herbert Dietz, Jr., M.D.

Professor Emeritus of Surgery, Cornell University Medical College; Attending Surgeon and Chief, Rehabilitation Service, Memorial Hospital for Cancer and Allied Diseases, New York.

Philip J. DiSaia, M.D.

Professor and Chairman, Division of Gynecologic Oncology, California College of Medicine, University of California, Irvine.

Harold O. Douglass, Jr., M.D.

Associate Chief, Department of Surgical Oncology, Roswell Park Memorial Institute, Buffalo.

Frederick R. Eilber, M.D.

Professor of Surgery, University of California, Los Angeles, School of Medicine.

Bernard Fisher, M.D.

Professor of Surgery, University of Pittsburgh School of Medicine; Project Chairman, National Surgical Adjuvant Project for Breast and Bowel Cancers, Pittsburgh.

Joseph G. Fortner, M.D.

Professor of Surgery, Cornell University Medical College; Attending Surgeon, Memorial Sloan-Kettering Cancer Center, New York.

Glenn W. Geelhoed, M.D.

Associate Professor of Surgery, School of Medicine and Health Sciences, George Washington University, Washington, D.C.

Bimal C. Ghosh, M.D.

Head, Surgical Section, Clinical Investigations Branch, Division of Cancer Treatment, Cancer Therapy Evaluation Program, National Cancer Institute, National Institutes of Health, Bethesda, Maryland.

Mark R. Green, M.D.

Associate Professor of Medicine, University of California, San Diego, School of Medicine.

Leslie M. Greenburg, M.D.

Resident in Surgery, Washington University Medical School, St. Louis.

Charles B. Hammond, M.D.

Professor and Chairman, Department of Obstetrics and Gynecology, Duke University School of Medicine, Durham, North Carolina.

Charles M. Haskell, M.D.

Associate Professor of Medicine and Surgery, University of California, Los Angeles, School of Medicine; Director, Wadsworth Cancer Center; Chief, Hematology and Oncology Section, Wadsworth Division Veterans Administration Medical Center, Los Angeles.

Samuel Hellman, M.D.

Alvan T. and Viola D. Fuller American Cancer Society Professor and Chairman, Department of Radiation Therapy, Harvard Medical School; Director, Joint Center for Radiation Therapy, Boston.

E. Carmack Holmes, M.D.

Professor of Surgery, University of California, Los Angeles, School of Medicine; Chief, Surgical Service, Sepulveda Veterans Administration Hospital, Sepulveda, California.

E. Douglas Holyoke, M.D.

Chief, Department of Surgical Oncology, Roswell Park Memorial Institute, Buffalo.

Mary K. Howett, Ph.D.

Assistant Professor of Microbiology, The Pennsylvania State University College of Medicine, Hershey.

Ronald J. Ignelzi, M.D.

Assistant Professor of Surgery, University of California, San Diego, School of Medicine.

Arthur G. James, M.D.

Professor of Surgery and Chief, Division of Oncology, Ohio State University College of Medicine, Columbus.

Nasser Javadpour, M.D., Ph.D.

Urologist in Charge and Senior Investigator, Surgery Branch, National Cancer Institute, National Institutes of Health, Bethesda, Maryland.

Joan F. Kroener, M.D.

Clinical Instructor of Medicine, University of California, San Diego, School of Medicine.

Walter Lawrence, M.D.

Professor of Surgery, Medical College of Virginia, Richmond.

Robert B. Livingston, M.D.

Professor of Medicine and Chairman, Department of Medical Oncology, University of Washington School of Medicine, Seattle.

William E. Lucas, M.D.

Professor of Reproductive Medicine, Head, Division of Gynecologic Oncology, University of California, San Diego, School of Medicine.

Lawrence F. Marshall, M.D.

Associate Professor of Surgery, University of California, San Diego, School of Medicine.

Ricardo Mesa-Tejada, M.D.

Assistant Professor of Pathology, College of Physicians and Surgeons, Columbia University; Senior Research Associate, Institute of Cancer Research, College of Physicians and Surgeons, Columbia University, New York.

Arnold Mittelman, M.D.

Department of Surgical Oncology, Roswell Park Memorial Institute, Buffalo.

Tsuneya Ohno, M.D., Ph.D.

Assistant Professor of Pathology, College of Physicians and Surgeons, Columbia University; Senior Research Associate, Institute of Cancer Research, College of Physicians and Surgeons, Columbia University, New York.

Louise A. Paquin, Ph.D.

Assistant Professor of Biology, Western Maryland College, Westminster.

David F. Paulson, M.D.

Professor and Chairman, Department of Urology, Duke University School of Medicine, Durham, North Carolina.

Jeffrey J. Pollen, M.D.

Assistant Professor of Surgery, University of California, San Diego, School of Medicine.

Yosef H. Pilch, M.D.

Professor of Surgery, Head, Surgical Oncology Service, University of California, San Diego, School of Medicine.

George R. Prout, Jr., M.D.

Professor of Surgery, Harvard Medical School; Chief, Urological Service, Massachusetts General Hospital, Boston.

David T. Purtilo, M.D.

Professor and Chairman, Department of Pathology and Laboratory Medicine, University of Nebraska College of Medicine, Omaha.

Fred Rapp, Ph.D.

Professor and Chairman, Department of Microbiology, The Pennsylvania State University College of Medicine, Hershey.

Carol Redmond, Sc.D.

Director, Statistical Unit, National Surgical Adjuvant Project for Breast and Bowel Cancers, Pittsburgh.

William M. Rich, M.D.

Assistant Professor, Department of Obstetrics and Gynecology, California College of Medicine, University of California, Irvine.

Jerome P. Richie, M.D.

Assistant Professor of Surgery, Harvard Medical School; Chief of Urologic Oncology, Brigham and Women's Hospital, Boston.

Mark Rosenblum, M.D.

Assistant Professor of Neurosurgery, University of California, San Francisco, School of Medicine.

Joseph D. Schmidt, M.D.

Professor of Surgery, Head, Division of Urology, University of California, San Diego, School of Medicine.

Donald G. Sessions, M.D.

Professor of Otolaryngology, Washington University Medical School, St. Louis.

Michael B. Shimkin, M.D.

Professor Emeritus of Community Medicine and Oncology, University of California, San Diego, School of Medicine.

Sol Spiegelman, Ph.D.

Late Professor, Columbia University; Late Director, Comprehensive Cancer Center, Institute of Cancer Research, College of Physicians and Surgeons, Columbia University, New York.

Ronald H. Spiro, M.D.

Associate Clinical Professor of Surgery, Cornell University; Attending Surgeon, Memorial Sloan-Kettering Cancer Center, New York.

Elliot W. Strong, M.D.

Professor of Surgery, Cornell University Medical College; Attending Surgeon and Chief, Head and Neck Service, Department of Surgery, Memorial Sloan-Kettering Cancer Center, New York.

Everett V. Sugarbaker, M.D.

Director, Surgical Oncology Division, Miami Cancer Institute, Miami.

José J. Terz, M.D.

Director, Department of General and Oncologic Surgery, City of Hope Medical Center, Duarte, California.

John R. van Nagell, Jr., M.D.

Professor and Director, Division of Gynecologic Oncology, American Cancer Society Professor of Clinical Oncology, University of Kentucky College of Medicine, Lexington.

Ralph R. Weichselbaum, M.D.

Associate Professor of Radiation Therapy, Harvard Medical School; Head, Sidney Farber Cancer Institute Division, Joint Center for Radiation Therapy, Boston.

John L. Werner, M.D.

Department of Radiology, City of Hope Medical Center, Duarte, California.

Samuel E. Wilson, M.D.

Professor of Surgery, University of California, Los Angeles, School of Medicine; Chairman, Department of Surgery, Harbor-UCLA Medical Center, Torrance.

The following names were inadvertently omitted from the list of contributors:

Robert O. Dillman, M.D.

Assistant Professor of Medicine, University of California, San Diego, School of Medicine.

William B. Farrar, M.D.

Clinical Instructor of Surgery, Ohio State University College of Medicine, Columbus.

James M. Roseman, M.D.

Surgical Oncology Division, Miami Cancer Institute, Miami.

Daniel N. Weingrad, M.D.

Surgical Oncology Division, Miami Cancer Institute, Miami.

PREFACE

Surgery is the most frequently applied modality of cancer treatment, although it is no longer the sole treatment. Bernard Fisher wrote in 1977 that "surgery makes its contribution to cancer treatment in concert with other modalities." Advances in the treatment of cancer will derive from the improved orchestration of surgery, radiotherapy, chemotherapy, and immunotherapy rather than from improved operative technique alone.

This book is the complete reference to all neoplasms that can be surgically treated. It discusses the rationale for care and management and their alternatives. In addition, it specifically details selection of operative procedures and adjuvant therapies.

The book has been organized by organ system and the tumor types found in that organ. Part 1 deals with the general concepts of oncology that underline the material covered in succeeding parts. Parts 2 through 10 deal with specific tumor types and their diagnosis, staging, and treatment.

The editor has chosen to make this a reference book directed primarily toward surgeons and has, therefore, eliminated those neoplasms for which surgery plays little or no role. Hence hematologic malignancies such as leukemia are not discussed. Malignant lymphomas, however, are included because surgery is often important in their management.

I wish to acknowledge a few of the people who have been instrumental in bringing this tremendous project to fruition. They have been responsible individually and collectively for supporting and advising me throughout the preparation of *Surgical Oncology*. I must thank J. Dereck Jeffers, Richard Laufer, Ellen Warren, and the staff at McGraw-Hill, particularly Maggie Schwarz and Robert E. McGrath, for their professionalism. I wish to thank my secretary, Ms. Mary Sooy for her invaluable and indispensable contributions, which far exceeded the typing of letters and manuscripts. Lastly, I thank my wife, Patricia, for her constant and unfailing support and encouragement, and for putting up with the disruptions and pressures that this project frequently caused.

Yosef H. Pilch

SURGICAL ONCOLOGY

PART ONE

BASIC CONCEPTS IN ONCOLOGY

1
INTRODUCTION

Yosef H. Pilch

I have tried all other measures,
The knife must cut the cancer out,
Infection, averted while it can be,
From our numbers.

Ovid, *Metamorphoses*
Book I, "Jove's Intervention"

SURGICAL ONCOLOGY

Surgery was the first technique to be applied to cancer therapy and, until only several decades ago, was the only effective method of treatment. Today surgery remains one of the most important modalities in cancer diagnosis and therapy. A surgical procedure is frequently required to obtain tissue for diagnosis and/or staging. Exploratory surgical procedures are often utilized to determine the extent of disease, even under circumstances where surgical resection is not feasible or desirable. Surgery remains the most frequently applied therapeutic modality in cancer treatment and is important both for its curative potential and for its frequent palliative value.

Most patients who are cured of cancer are cured by surgery. More cancer patients are cured by surgery than by any other therapeutic modality. According to National Cancer Institute statistics, 785,000 patients were diagnosed as having cancers (nonmelanoma skin cancers were excluded) in 1980. Of those, 356,000, or 45 percent, were potentially curable. Of the 356,000 curable patients, 220,000 were treated with surgery alone, and 90,000 with surgery combined with radiation therapy.

Surgery is a regional modality usually affecting only the tissues directly removed. (A notable exception to the above is the cytotoxic effects of ischemia when the arterial blood supply to a tumor, or to an organ harboring a tumor, is interrupted surgically.) There are no systemic therapeutic effects. Surgery operates by zero-order kinetics in that 100 percent of the cells at risk, i.e., surgically extirpated, are killed with a single treatment, whereas radiotherapy and chemotherapy operate by first-order kinetics. Only a certain percentage of the cells at risk are killed during a given exposure to treatment, and regrowth usually follows. However, surgery is totally nonspecific, being as injurious to normal cells as to cancer cells. Since normal tissue is usually removed along with tumor tissue, surgery often is ablative of normal structure and function. The "dose-limiting toxicity" of surgical treatment then becomes the nature and degree of deformity and/or disability produced by the extent of normal tissue removed. Fortunately, most of the toxic effects of surgery are fairly immediate and "late toxicity" is not usually a serious problem.

Chemotherapy and radiation therapy are partially, but incompletely, specific. They are preferentially toxic to cancer cells as opposed to normal cells. However, because this specificity is incomplete, these modalities of therapy are also toxic to normal cells. Toxicity is usually related to dose and to the susceptibility of particular normal tissues (e.g., bone marrow, bowel mucosa, cardiac muscle, neural tissue, and renal parenchyma). Toxicity often limits dose, and dose-limiting toxicity often limits clinical efficacy.

Whereas radiation therapy, like surgery, is a regional modality, chemotherapy is a systemic modality. Many recent advances in cancer treatment have been brought about by combining two or three treatment modalities either sequentially or concomitantly. This "combined modality" approach exploits the marked regional cytoreductive effects of surgery and radiation therapy with the systemic effects of chemotherapy.

What, then, is surgical oncology? Ronald Raven has defined oncology as "a multidisciplinary subject where different arts and sciences are synthesized for the study of neoplastic diseases."[1] Surgical oncology emphasizes the application of surgical techniques in the diagnosis, staging, and treatment of neoplasms. This extends far beyond the mere technical conduct of surgical procedures into regions of etiology, pathology, pharmacology, endocrinology, immunology, biochemistry, and others. A profound understanding of the roles of chemotherapy and radiation therapy, particularly when combined with surgery, is essential to surgical oncology.

DEVELOPMENT OF SURGICAL ONCOLOGY

Although Hippocrates described many forms of cancer and originated the term *carcinoma*, he did not record any recommendations for treatment. In the second century A.D., Galen published an extensive classification of tumors. He considered cancer a systemic disease related to an excess of "black bile" and therefore not amenable to cure by surgery. His teachings held sway for 1600 years. Then, in the eighteenth century, a number of surgeons promulgated the hypothesis that cancer, at its outset, is a local, and therefore curable, disease. Valsalva, in 1704, theorized that cancer is at first a local lesion curable by operation, that it spreads via the lymphatics, and that it is prone to recur. Le Dran of France, in 1757, and Morgagne of Italy, in 1769, were strong supporters of this view of the disease.[2] They originated the theory that cancer begins as a local disease which can be cured by surgery if discovered sufficiently early.

Although the first modern cancer operation was probably the subtotal gastrectomy first performed by Billroth in 1881, the principles upon which most modern surgical procedures for cancer are based were formulated around 1890 by William Stuart Halsted of the Johns Hopkins Hospital in Baltimore. He developed the concept that effective therapy for tumors with a propensity to spread to regional lymph nodes (and this was thought to include the majority of solid tumors) is to extirpate the organ harboring the tumor, or a substantial portion thereof, together with the draining lymph nodes and the intervening lymphatics, in one continuous specimen. This principle of the "en bloc" resection, first enunciated in the Halsted radical mastectomy which he performed for the first time in 1890, formed the basis for most of the operations of modern cancer surgery.[3] Moreover, when applied to women with clinically negative axillary lymph nodes, the radical mastectomy constituted the first and prime example of the elective or "prophylactic" dissection of clinically uninvolved regional lymph nodes.

Halsted believed that cancer spread circumfugally to contiguous tissues via tissue planes and lymphatics, and disseminated lymphagenously to regional lymph nodes. It was only later in the course of the disease that dissemination to distant organs occurred. Distant dissemination occurred when regional lymph nodes were so extensively involved by tumor deposits as to become "saturated" and no longer capable of containing additional tumor cells. Tumor cells could then traverse or leave the nodes via the efferent lymphatics rather like particles through a leaky sieve. Hematogenous dissemination was not considered to be an important or common event, at least during early stages of tumor growth.

Two other concepts arose in the late nineteenth century which had an impact on the work of Halsted and participated in giving rise to "modern" cancer surgery. The first was the view that cancers progressed in temporally distant and consecutive stages. Initially, a growing tumor remained localized at its site of origin. Then, after a period of time, invasion of lymphatics and metastases to regional lymph nodes took place, giving rise to "regional" disease. Then, after an additional interval of time, systemic dissemination to distant organs occurred. A corollary of this concept was the theory, first advanced by Virchow in 1860, that lymph nodes constitute an effective barrier to the passage of tumor cells, at least temporarily.[4]

From these beliefs, it was logical to assume that operations which encompassed progressively larger regions about the primary tumor site would result in progressive increments in cure, especially if applied "in time," i.e., while the disease was still locoregional and distant dissemination had not yet occurred. The principle of the en bloc resection, i.e., the removal of the primary tumor together with the regional lymphatics and regional lymph nodes, was applied to surgical procedures for cancers of many organs. The combined operations for cancers of the head and neck, and the radical hysterectomy for carcinoma of the cervix are but two examples.

In the years following World War II, with the advent of better supportive measures—e.g., blood transfusions, improved anesthesia, and antibiotics—and the development of greater technical skills, superradical operations were developed, including the extended radical mastectomy, pelvic exenteration, hemipelvectomy, and forequarter amputation. When surgical extirpation of all regional tissues was not feasible, and/or in order to manage foci of residual tumor cells which escaped surgical excision, postoperative radiotherapy was often administered in the belief that better control of locoregional disease could be equated with increased cure. Most important, these radical operations were performed on all patients with technically resectable tumors who had no evidence of distant metastases, regardless of tumor size and usually regardless of whether regional lymph nodes were clinically involved or not. There was no attempt to individualize therapy based on staging parameters or prognostic factors.

To a degree, these approaches did improve results in several cancers, primarily those wherein local disease in the absence of distant dissemination is a significant contributing factor in mortality, e.g., head and neck cancer and cancer of the rectum. In these, and a number of other cancers, such as breast cancer and sarcomas of bone and soft tissue, local control was certainly improved. For most cancers, however, disease-free and overall survival did not ensue (lung cancer and cancer of the pancreas, to name just two).

During the past two decades, basic changes have occurred in our understanding of cancer biology. Now most, if not all, cancers are viewed as *systemic* diseases from their inception, or at least from the moment they are clinically detectable. Have we returned to the concepts of Galen without the invocation of "black bile"? We understand that hematogenous dissemination is a frequent and possibly inevitable consequence of malignancy. Micrometastases may be present in many or most cancer patients at the time of diagnosis. Whether these give rise to clinically significant metastatic disease depends upon the biology of the tumor cell and the tumor-host interaction. More extensive regional surgery and/or the superimposition of the two regional modalities, surgery and radiotherapy, cannot hope to affect systemic disease. Only systemic therapy can affect metastatic disease and provide further advances in cancer treatment.

With this new understanding, the past two decades have witnessed the apogee of radical cancer surgery and the beginning of attempts to reduce the scope of surgical procedures by relying more heavily on the adjunctive use of chemotherapy and/or radiation therapy. Of equal importance is the trend toward better patient selection based on staging of individual patients for extent of disease and/or other prognostic factors. Rather than a single treatment for all resectable cancers of each type, different treatments are being applied. The hallowed concept of elective or prophylactic node dissection is gradually yielding to therapeutic node dissections reserved for subsets of patients with proven nodal disease. In other settings, node dissections are now performed primarily for staging the disease rather than exclusively for curing it. Finally, the technical wizardry of the surgeon is increasingly focusing on techniques *preserving* structure and function, and on methods for reconstructing defects created by cancer surgery.

THE SURGICAL ONCOLOGIST

What, or rather who, is a surgical oncologist? There are recognized specialty boards who certify practitioners of both medical oncology and radiation oncology. Almost every medical school and every large general hospital has a division or department of medical oncology and radiation oncology. Divisions or departments of surgical oncology are much less common. If surgery is such an important modality for cancer treatment, and if surgical therapy preceded medical and radiation therapy by decades, even centuries, why is surgical oncology such an obscure entity?

The answer may be found in the devolpment of surgery as a discipline. Until the late nineteenth and early twentieth centuries, practitioners of surgery rarely specialized, and what surgery was done (in the preanesthetic era) was usually performed by individuals with little or no specialized training. A possible exception to this rule is the military surgeons who tended those wounded in battle. Initially, surgeons were truly "general." They operated on all parts of the body and treated all types of diseases amenable to surgery. With the advent of anesthesia and the progress of medical science in general, surgery became more specialized, and "surgical specialties" have emerged one by one. These specialties have evolved primarily along anatomic, rather than disease-oriented, lines, as has been the case with most developing medical specialties. Anatomy is perhaps the single basic science most vital to surgery, whereas physiology, biochemistry, and pharmacology are more important to practitioners of medicine. Therefore, while many medical specialties evolved as *disease-oriented* disciplines (e.g., rheumatology, allergy, endocrinology, and hematology), surgical specialties evolved as *region-oriented* disciplines, or as disciplines oriented to organ systems (e.g., neurosurgery, ophthalmology, urology, otorhinolaryngology, and thoracic surgery). Since tumors arise in all these regions, surgical specialists became involved in the surgical treatment of the neoplasms of the regions of their specialty. All surgeons were part-time surgical oncologists, but very few surgeons were *full-time* surgical oncologists, and there are still few full-time surgical oncologists today.

It is trite to define a surgical oncologist as "an oncologist possessing surgical skills and trained in the technical conduct of operative procedures," or as "an oncologist who is trained as a surgeon and therefore treats certain tumors operatively." The best definition of a surgical oncologist is "a surgeon who specializes in the treatment of tumors." He or she is primarily a surgical oncologist, whether a urologist, neurosurgeon, gynecologist, general surgeon, or head and neck surgeon by designation or board certification. In any case, the emphasis is on the dedication to oncology as a *disease-oriented* discipline. Certainly, the surgical oncologist must possess knowledge relating to tumors whose diagnosis, staging, and treatment often require surgical intervention of some kind. But this knowledge must extend far beyond cancer surgery. It must encompass detection, diagnosis, staging, alternative options for therapy, adjuvant therapies, follow-up care, and detection and treatment and/or metastases. A surgical oncologist is more than simply a surgeon who occasionally operates on cancer patients. He or she possesses a deep knowledge of oncology and maintains central involvement in the overall care of the cancer patient.

REFERENCES

1. Raven RW: *Principles of Surgical Oncology,* Plenum Medical, New York, 1977.
2. Hayward OS: The history of oncology. I. Early oncology and the literature of discovery. *Surgery* 58:460, 1965.
3. Halsted WS: The results of radical operations for the cure of carcinoma of the breast. *Ann Surg* 46:1, 1907.
4. Fisher B: The changing role of surgery in the treatment of cancer. In *Cancer,* Becker FF (ed), vol 6. Plenum Press, New York, 1977.

2
ENVIRONMENTAL CARCINOGENESIS

Michael B. Shimkin

HISTORICAL INTRODUCTION

In 1775, Percivall Pott, the prestigious surgeon of St. Bartholomew's Hospital in London, broke his leg. During his recovery he wrote a book on his surgical experiences which included a few pages on cancer of the scrotum among chimney sweeps, a condition long known by the workers as the "soot wart." This was the first clear medical description of an occupational environmental cancer.

During the industrial revolution, additional examples of occupational skin cancer among workers exposed to various oils, shales, and petroleum products were recorded. In 1879, an analysis of deaths among the miners of Germany's Black Forest region revealed that three-fourths were due to malignant neoplasms of the lung. This was perhaps the first record of an internal cancer attributable to exposure to environmental factors, eventually identified as ore dusts, including radioactive uranium, which the miners inhaled. Detection of urinary bladder cancers among workers in the aniline dye industry, reported by Rehn in 1895, added to the picture an example of a distant carcinogenic effect involving transport and metabolism of the culprit chemical.

At the turn of the century, when the sun could never set on the British flag, medical missionaries in India described the Kangri and the Chutta cancers among the natives. Kangri cancer of the abdominal wall was the consequence of the custom of wearing wicker baskets with live coals under clothes as a source of heat; repeated burns to the abdominal area were sustained. Chutta cancer of the mouth occurred in women who smoked cheroots with the lighted end held inside their mouths. In Egypt, British pathologists reported the association of urinary bladder cancer with fluke infestation in peasants who toiled in the waters of the Nile.

These examples of environmental cancer were considered by European and American authorities as unusual, limited to poor, dirty industrial classes and to even poorer and dirtier natives of distant lands. Cancer as they defined it on the basis of their experience was a disease of unknown etiology, perhaps an inevitable consequence of advancing age, somatic mutation, and a touch of predestination. The concept that viruses could be causative agents of cancer, demonstrated in chickens by 1911, was dismissed as being limited to chickens.

In 1915, two patient Japanese investigators experimentally reproduced Pott's observations by painting tar repeatedly on ears of rabbits and eliciting invasive, metastasizing epitheliomas. The active carcinogenic ingredient in tar, benzo[a]pyrene, a polycyclic hydrocarbon that fluoresced prettily under ultraviolet light, was identified during the early 1930s by a London research group. At the same time, the female sex hormone steroids were identified and were found to produce breast cancers in male mice. Organic chemists synthesized many analogues of both classes of compounds, which structurally resembled cholesterol. A powerful carcinogen, 3-methylcholanthrene, was synthesized from bile acids, adding credence to the postulation that chemical carcinogens could arise endogenously, and that cancer could be an inborn error of metabolism. Attention in the laboratories was turned toward intriguing studies on metabolism and dwindled in the area of identifying exogenous sources of cancer-producing chemicals.

The list of unrelated chemicals that induced cancers in laboratory animals became ever longer, and the search for endogenous carcinogens, more elusive. The number of virus-induced cancers also grew to include examples among rabbits, mice, and even frogs, in addition to several varieties in chickens. Viruses became less abstract to research workers when they could be photographed under the new electron microscope.

The victory over poliomyelitis during the 1950s threatened unemployment for virologists as well as an end for the voluntary agency that supported their activities. Virus research on cancer was an attractive alternate area, and viral oncology became a heavily subsidized field. Work during a fertile decade expanded knowledge about viruses and cell-virus interactions but fell short of demonstrating a central role for viruses in human cancer. A feeling of disappointment in the viral approach was voiced even by cancer research luminaries whose forays were rewarded by Nobel prizes.

Cancer research turned again to the environmental, exogenous factors that now loomed more visible and more attractive as areas for exploration. This shift was stimulated by the development of epidemiology as an accepted scientific discipline, and by the contributions epidemiology was making.

Studies of cancer in human populations became increasingly more feasible and reliable with improvements in national censuses, in mortality and disease reporting and registries, and in the diagnosis of cancer in many parts of the world. All human and animal populations that were studied carefully into older ages were shown to develop neoplastic diseases, but there were striking differences in the incidence of many cancers specified by site and type. These differences were related, for some cancers, to geographic locale, social class, and other characteristics considered to be primarily environmental rather than inherent. Some cancers displayed temporal changes, increasing or decreasing with time, and others appeared to remain more constant. The incidence of some cancers changed when the population migrated to new habitations, thus connoting the importance of environmental factors.

Epidemiology also elicited and substantiated what was probably the major "breakthrough" concerning cancer in European populations that has been achieved during the past half-century. This was the elucidation of the causative role of tobacco smoking in the smoldering pandemic of lung cancer, and its participatory role in several other cancers, including those of the urinary bladder.

Analytic studies of cancer death rates by geographic area made unavoidable the suspicion that the so-called occupational cancers were not limited to employees. Maps of bladder cancer rates in areas around plants that use identified carcinogens and observations of the relatives of asbestos workers demonstrated that the effects of such carcinogens extended well beyond the gates of the manufacturing plants. Furthermore, cancers resulting from peculiar habits were not limited to exotic tribes in Asia and Africa but occurred in all of us. Laboratories well supported by public funds ground out data on insecticides, food additives, cosmetics, and other chemicals that are the pride of our industrial civilization. Alas, a large proportion of such chemicals was demonstrated to increase one type of neoplastic reaction or another in mice or rats exposed to maximum tolerated doses over their entire life-span. These were deemed carcinogens by presumed experts in the field, and immediately came under the regulatory provisions stimulated by politically active environmentalists and enforced by the expanding authority of the government. Data on rodents took a minimum of 3 years to obtain, so use of more rapid and less direct sources of information, such as mutations of bacteria or of mammalian cells grown in glass dishes, developed influential proponents.

Epidemiologists, flushed with their promotion to the more classical academies of science, proffered statistical estimates of the importance of environmental factors in human cancer. One approach was to compare cancer rates in different parts of the world and to assume that all rates above the lowest reported from anywhere were attributable to exogenous factors. Thus, if the incidence of endometrial cancer among the South African Bantus was 0.2 per 100,000, and among Hawaiians it was 24 per 100,000, 23.8 per 100,000, or 99 percent, of endometrial cancers among Hawaiians were due to exogenous factors. This led to suggestions, soon emphasized as claims, that 80 to 90 percent of all human cancers were due to environmental factors and thus "theoretically preventable"; the adverb was soon dropped.

No cancer has ever arisen in the absence of a multicellular organism reacting to exogenous or endogenous factors, so it would be correct, and redundant, to claim that 100 percent of all cancers are due to inherent intracellular mechanisms. The importance of environmental causes of cancer does not require exaggeration. In examining the information we have in this area, it will soon become obvious that facts are few and suggestions and expectations are many. If any rough estimate can be more helpful than otherwise, it is that there is some knowledge of causation for perhaps 20 percent of the neoplasms and that 80 percent still lie in that unexplored bourne from which research travelers some day *will* return.

CARCINOGENESIS

Cancer, like all pathological processes, is the result of exogenous or endogenous stimuli interacting with a genetically susceptible host. The interaction is influenced by a myriad of factors related to the stimulus (e.g., dose, concentration, schedule of exposure, vehicle, route, temperature, etc.), and by as many factors involving the host (age, sex, nutritional and immunologic status, etc.). The balance between the stimulus and the host determines the proportion and rate of the process.

The response to stimuli leading to the cancer is, as is true in other biological reactions, dose dependent. The greater or more prolonged such stimulation is, the more cancers will arise, and the shorter will be the latent period. The range over which this relationship exists is, of course, limited and is not necessarily linear. At higher doses, toxic effects on the host or the cell population may inhibit the neoplastic reaction. At very low doses, the reaction may be obscured by the "background noise" of the spontaneous rate of neoplasia for the population. "Spontaneous" tumors must be due to undefined reactions between stimuli and the host, also, so that the adjective represents simply an admission of ignorance regarding the causative factors involved.

There has been considerable discussion regarding the "no threshold" response to carcinogens, meaning that there is no absolutely safe dose. This mathematical abstraction is hard to relate to the real world, not only for carcinogens but for any chemical or physical agents that evoke a response. As a basis for legislation such as the Delaney clause, which prohibits the addition of any amount of carcinogens to food, it has the clarity of the Ten Commandments. In reality, however, it requires human interpretation, including definition of *carcinogen*. Some exposure to carcinogens is unavoidable, and attempting to reach absolute avoidance is probably of greater risk than simply trying to diminish exposure if indeed, that can be accomplished. For instance, the growth of vegetables in soil incorporates into food some concentrations of arsenic, lead, and other heavy-metal salts that are carcinogenic. Food regulations acknowledge the impossibility of avoiding the metals by requiring that no more than 5 ppm of such metals be present, a value far short of absolute zero. It is also now established that some chemicals, defined as carcinogens because high-dose exposure increases the hepatoma rate in rodents, are nutritionally *essential* and may even be cancer-inhibiting in very low doses. An example of this is selenium. Furthermore, some carcinogens may be synthesized by the body itself, such as nitrosamines from nitrites and amines and, of course, estrogenic steroids.

The Stimuli

Lists of chemical and physical agents that have been defined as carcinogens in humans or by tests in laboratory animals are available in many recent publications. There are now literally thousands, although many are analogues of parent carcinogens. A sample is shown in Fig. 2-1.

For agents established as, or strongly suspected to be, carcinogenic for humans, one traditional presentation in such lists is an array by the situational exposure: occupational, iatrogenic, or general. There is obvious overlap between such categories. Another attempt at systematization is to list the agents by route of entry, such as contact, ingestion, or inhalation; here, too, distinct differences are an exception rather than the rule. Chemical structure also can be used as the organizing framework. For human populations, however, there are few situations in which only one chemical can be incriminated. People are usually exposed to complex mixtures under a variety of conditions that impose further modifications.

A simple alphabetical listing, as in Table 2-1, may be

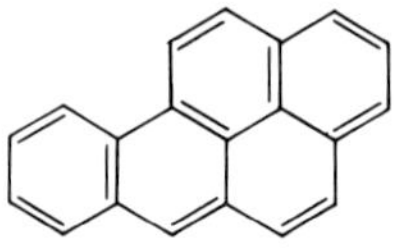

Benzo[a]pyrene
(3.4-benzpyrene)

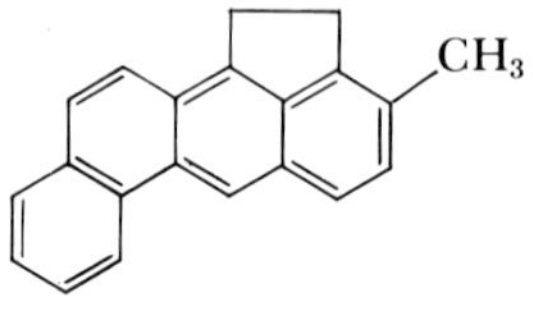

3-Methylcholanthrene

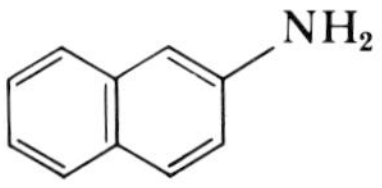

2-Naphthylamine

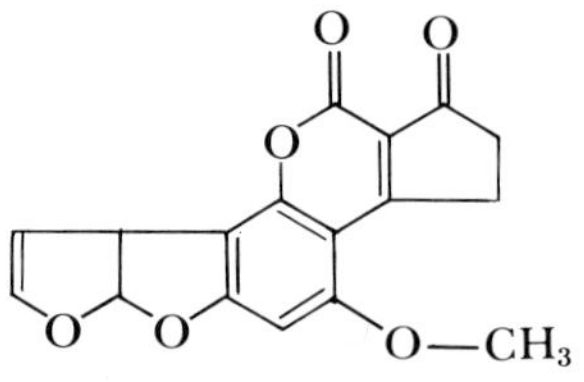

Aflatoxin B_1

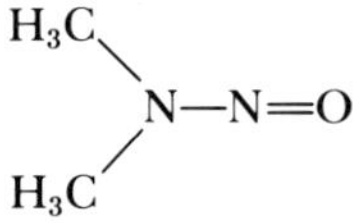

Dimethylnitrosamine

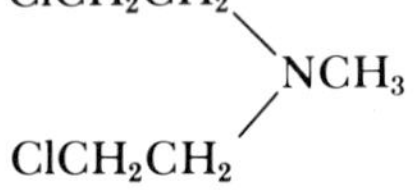

Nitrogen mustard (HN_2)

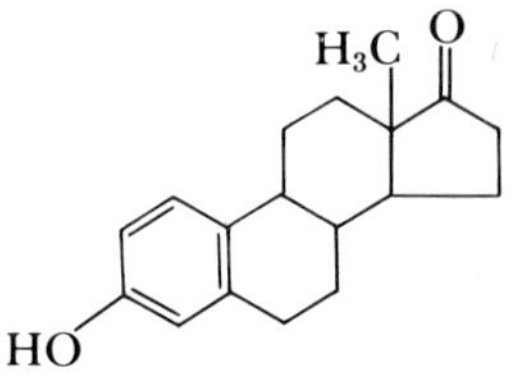

Estrone

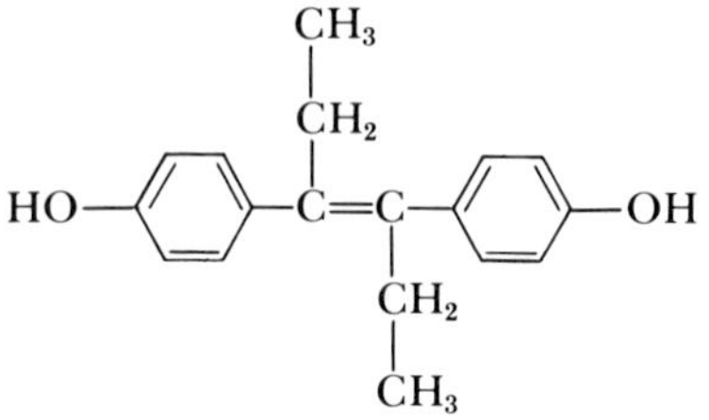

Diethylstilbestrol

FIGURE 2-1 The chemical structures of some important carcinogens.

as informative as any other, as long as it is accepted as a checklist that does not attempt either to be exhaustive or to assign equal weight and validity to its individual items. Thus, an important carcinogen mixture of tobacco smoke, affecting millions of people, occupies the same space as some alkylating agents restricted to the chemotherapy of advanced cancer.

There is, of course, no basic difference between human and animal carcinogens, although animals can be exposed to single chemicals under controlled conditions. Chemicals found to be carcinogens in animals certainly must be considered as potential human carcinogens. The problems of defining carcinogens and of dose and route extrapolations will be discussed later in this chapter.

PHYSICAL AGENTS

Among the physical environmental agents clearly established as carcinogenic in human beings and in animals are ionizing radiation and ultraviolet radiation in the range of 3000 Å. Ultraviolet radiation is limited to the induction of skin cancer, and is most carcinogenic in fair-skinned races. Albinos, human or animal, are particularly susceptible, and the DNA-repair genetic aberration xeroderma pigmentosum is exquisitely sensitive to carcinogenic transformation. It is probable that most skin cancers of the exposed areas in so-called white races are evoked by solar radiation. The risk of melanoma of the skin is also increased.

Ionizing radiation induces a wide variety of neoplastic reactions in human beings as well as in animals. The

TABLE 2-1 Human Carcinogens

Agent	Main type of exposure	Main route of exposure	Site of cancer
Aflatoxins	Dietary, environmental	Oral	Liver
4-Aminobiphenyl	Occupational	Inhalation, skin, oral	Bladder
Androgens	Medicinal	Oral	Liver
Arsenic compounds	Occupational, medicinal, environmental	Inhalation, skin, oral	Skin, lung
Asbestos	Occupational	Inhalation, oral	Lung, pleural and peritoneal serosa, gastrointestinal tract
Auramine	Occupational	Inhalation, skin, oral	Bladder
Benzene	Occupational	Inhalation, skin	Hemopoietic system
Benzidine	Occupational	Inhalation, skin, oral	Bladder
N,N-Bis(2-chloroethyl)-2-naphthylamine	Medicinal	Oral	Bladder
Bis(chloromethyl)ether and chloromethyl methyl ether	Occupational	Inhalation	Lung
Cadium-using industries (possibly cadmium oxide)	Occupational	Inhalation, oral	Prostate
Chloramphenicol	Medicinal	Oral, injection	Hemopoietic system
Chromium (chromate-producing industries)	Occupational	Inhalation	Lung
Cyclophosphamide	Medicinal	Oral, injection	Bladder
Diethylstilbestrol	Medicinal	Oral	Uterus, vagina
Estrogens	Medicinal	Oral, injection	Endometrium
Hematite mining (? radon)	Occupational	Inhalation	Lung
Immunosuppressants	Medicinal	Oral, injection	Lymphatic system
Isopropyl oils	Occupational	Inhalation	Nasal cavity, larynx
Melphalan	Medicinal	Oral, injection	Hemopoietic system
Mustard gas	Occupational	Inhalation	Lung, larynx
2-Naphthylamine	Occupational	Inhalation, skin, oral	Bladder
Nickel ore	Occupational	Inhalation	Nasal cavity, lung
Phenacetin	Medicinal	Oral	Kidney
Phenytoin	Medicinal	Oral, injection	Lymphoreticular tissues
Radiation, ionizing	Occupational, environmental, medicinal	Externally, injection	Various
Radiation, ultraviolet	Occupational, environmental	Skin	Skin
Schistosoma haematobium	Occupational, environmental	Skin	Urinary bladder
Soot, tars, and oils	Occupational, environmental	Inhalation skin	Lung, skin
Tobacco smoke	Habit	Inhalation	Lung, oral cavity, larynx, bladder
Vinyl chloride	Occupational	Inhalation, skin	Liver

tragedy of Hiroshima proved that acute myelocytic leukemia and cancer of the thyroid are two results, with increased rates of breast and lung cancer also now being recorded. However, only a small proportion of leukemias in the general population are attributable to ionizing radiation, and even smaller proportions of breast and lung cancers.

Sources of ionizing radiation retained by the body and deposited in various sites lead to neoplasms at the impingement site: inhaled radon daughters from uranium, in the lung; from plutonium, in bone; and from thorotrast, in the liver and spleen. The contribution of radiation-induced neoplasms to the total of even the rarer entities is also small. The thorotrast neoplasms are, it is hoped, now of historical interest only.

In the above situations, either the doses of radiation are large or the exposure is continuous over protracted periods. However, there are data that indicate an increase in acute leukemia among children exposed while in utero to x-rays in the diagnostic dose range of 1 R. Since radiation is also incriminated in mutagenesis and teratogenesis, care is mandatory to reduce exposure of pregnant women. Radiation exposure in utero less than doubles the risk of leukemia, however, and cannot account for more than a small proportion of the total occurrences.

POLYCYCLIC AROMATIC HYDROCARBONS

Of the many chemicals of interest regarding cancer in human beings, the polycyclic aromatic hydrocarbons (PAH), in complex mixtures of soot, tar, creosote, shale, and petroleum and in the complex smokes of gasoline, coal, and incomplete combustion products of vegetable materials such as tobacco, probably represent the most common, ubiquitous sources of hazard. These are essentially contact carcinogens, exerting their effects on the skin, or on the respiratory tract if inhaled. Cigarette smoke fits into the latter category.

The complex nature of this class of carcinogens must be emphasized since the content of the actual hydrocarbons, especially benzo[a]pyrene, is too low to account for the carcinogenic activity of, say, tar. The mixtures must contain other chemicals that act as promoters or in some way accelerate the action of the more specific constituents. In fact, it is this discrepancy between the content of benzo[a]pyrene and the carcinogenic effect of tar fractions that led to the supposition of cocarcinogens. Tobacco smoke condensates also contain concentrations of polycyclic hydrocarbons too low to account for carcinogenic activity demonstrable on skin of mice, and also must contain cocarcinogens, perhaps phenolic compounds.

The blame for the pandemic of lung cancer, the top neoplastic killer of men and vying for second position among women in the United States, can be laid squarely on tobacco smoking, especially of cigarettes. Yet not all lung cancers are due to smoking alone, though smoking accounts for some three-fourths of the total. When cancer of the mouth, larynx, esophagus, and even the urinary bladder are related to the smoking habit, it can be calculated that one-sixth of the total cancer burden can be attributed to this one carcinogenic habit. It is by far the most prominent single cause of cancer in our population that has been clearly defined, and for which the preventive methodology is so obvious, and so neglected.

Polycyclic aromatic hydrocarbons do not seem to have an important role in gastrointestinal cancer. In animal experiments, long-term ingestion of large amounts is necessary to induce cancer. Even in the lung, particulate impingement of the chemicals is required for the elicitation of bronchogenic cancer. Perhaps asbestos particles provide this impingement for the synergistic effect of asbestos and tobacco smoking.

AROMATIC AMINES

Historically, the next group of compounds found to be carcinogenic for human beings were the aromatic amines, many of which are involved in various steps of the dye and rubber industries. The primary end organ is the urinary bladder.

The classical compound of the group is 2-naphthylamine, shown to produce bladder cancer in dogs over 40 years after it was described as an occupational carcinogen. Human beings are quite sensitive to this chemical, which is required in larger concentrations for carcinogenesis in animals. Benzidine and its derivatives and other phenyls, Aramine, and related compounds are also represented. In long-term tests on mice and on rats, these compounds primarily induce liver tumors rather than tumors of the urinary system.

In animal experiments, the related azo dyes and fluorenamines have been used extensively, especially for the clarification of their metabolic conversions. The first step is N-hydroxylation, and since this reaction does not occur in the guinea pig, the parent compound is not carcinogenic in this species although the converted product is. The investigations served to demonstrate that many carcinogens require metabolic conversions in which the original chemical is metabolized (usually in the liver) to more proximal carcinogens.

A significant proportion of cancers of the urinary bladder in the industrial areas of the United States are suspected to be related to chemical contamination of water, food, and air by aromatic amines. Cigarette smoking is also associated with an increased risk to bladder cancer, due to unidentified metabolites probably not of the PAH type.

In Egypt, the wide occurrence of urinary bladder cancer secondary to infestation with *Schistosoma haematobium* and its encystment in the bladder wall has continued for thousands of years. The solution awaits a scientific attack upon the snail intermediary of the fluke found in the waters of Africa.

ALKYLATING AGENTS

The alkylating agents, with sulfur and nitrogen mustard war gases as the starting points for chemotherapeutic agents against cancer, represent another group of carcinogenic agents. Exposure to the gases does increase the frequency of subsequent lung cancer, but presumably war gases are no longer being manufactured. Instead, there are a wide variety of analogues, such as melphalan, and related compounds such as busulfan, that are still found useful against lymphomas, leukemias, and some advanced neoplasms in human beings. The chemicals are definitely carcinogenic in many animals, and are mutagenic.

Carcinogenic activity of these chemicals in human beings was first evinced with an analogue (chlornaphazin) that combined 2-naphthylamine with an alkylating reactive site. Not unexpectedly, it produced cancers of the urinary bladder. It is no longer used. The other alkylating drugs are associated with an increased occurrence of leukemia in patients cured of Hodgkin's disease and other lymphomas by radiation combined with a regimen of chemotherapy. Thus, these drugs cause iatrogenic cancer, and, as such, should be restricted in use to advanced neoplastic disease. Certainly their use in reversible, nonfatal conditions such as arthritis must be questioned. However, even with protracted courses of large doses, the occurrence of leukemia is an infrequent event and does not contribute a measurable number of instances to the total incidence of leukemia. Alkylating agents used as drugs and otherwise available in the environment cannot be considered as serious general carcinogenic hazards.

INORGANIC CHEMICALS

Inorganic chemicals, such as salts of metals, have attracted relatively little attention in the laboratory but represent an important class of carcinogens for human beings. The inhalation of chromate ores, for example, yields increased hazard of bronchogenic cancer among the workers, and nickel carbamyl induces cancer of the nasal sinuses. Workers in iron mines exposed to hematite dust also experience an increase, of about twofold, in lung cancer.

One of the anomalies between animal and human data is seen with inorganic arsenic, accepted as being carcinogenic in human beings but never having been so demonstrated in animals. During the Victorian era, the universal tonic was Fowler's solution, which is potassium arsenite. Cases of skin keratoses and cancer, including some on the palms and soles of the feet, were described by 1888. Cancer of the lungs was later attributed to arsenical sprays in vineyards. Arsenical cancers are now becoming one of the problems of the past.

Of great contemporary importance and concern is asbestos, a mixture of silicates that is useful as fire-resistant material for insulation. Some 30 years ago cases of mesothelioma of the pleura and the peritoneum were described among asbestos workers in South Africa. The wide distribution of the material, however, has spread the hazard to a large general population. Of greatest importance is the synergism of asbestosis with tobacco smoking; the combination increases the risk of bronchogenic carcinoma by over 50-fold. Thus, since nothing can be done for asbestos already in the body, prohibition of smoking among those who have been exposed to asbestos is essential.

Asbestos carcinogenesis is an important current problem to which all the usual questions apply. Are there levels of exposure that are relatively safe? Is the surveillance of individuals already exposed useful in terms of "earlier" detection and treatment? How can we reconcile the usefulness, perhaps irreplaceability of a material with its health hazards? Is ingested asbestos as hazardous as inhaled material? Are there "safer" forms of asbestos particles, or possible combinations with other materials?

NITROSAMINES

This reactive, mutagenic class of compounds represents a recent addition to the list of carcinogens. The implications of this group of carcinogens, especially for human beings, remain to be clarified, but the animal data firmly suggest that such implications will be important.

Nitrosamines are powerful carcinogens, producing cancers at many sites and of many types with low-dose exposure to several species of experimental animals, including subhuman primates. Nitrosamine analogues demonstrate specific organotropisms. The nitrosoguanine compound, for example, easily induces adenocarcinoma of the stomach in rodents and dogs; before the discovery of this compound by Sugimura, this neoplasm was very difficult to induce. Nitrosamines are readily absorbed, and they diffuse in the body, including transplacentally. Perhaps most significant, nitrosamines arise by biosynthesis, in saliva, the gastric contents, and the intestine, by combinations of nitrates and amines. Since nitrosamines demonstrate carcinogenic action in susceptible-strain mice at concentrations encountered under biosynthetic circumstances (perhaps as low as parts per billion), and since the constituents from which they are synthesized are unavoidable components of foods and tissues, the possibilities that they may be involved in human carcinogenesis are obviously high.

Yet the expectations as well as the alarums need to be kept in check. The use of nitrates as a meat preservative may or may not represent a hazard, for example. Alternate methods of preservation certainly should be sought. Announcements of mutagenic activity induced by overcooked hamburger, however, should not be a signal to embrace vegetarianism.

AFLATOXIN AND OTHER NATURAL CARCINOGENS

Another group of powerful carcinogens with primary effects on the liver are the products of the mold *Aspergillus flavus,* lactones that fluoresce green or blue under ultraviolet light. Aflatoxin was first encountered as a hepatotoxin lethal to newly hatched poultry and was soon related to hepatocarcinoma in rainbow trout raised on food contaminated with the mold. Epidemiologic studies in Indochina relate the occurrence of hepatocarcinoma to aflatoxin content of food.

Peanut products and other proteinaceous foods in the United States are now monitored for aflatoxin. No relationship of hepatoma and aflatoxin is adduced in this country.

Among the "natural" sources of carcinogens are cycasin, from the cycas nut, and bracken fern. The latter produces hemorrhagic cystitis and cancer in cows ingesting the plant. Cycasin, discovered to produce hepatocarcinomas in rats, is of interest because the natural glycone in the plant has to be broken down by intestinal bacteria to the absorbable aglycone. The glycone will not produce tumors in bacteria-free rats. Analogous participation of intestinal flora in carcinogenic transformations is now again an area for research, resurrecting similar postulations of 40 years ago. It is said that bracken fern is used as a food herb in Japan, but neither cycasin nor bracken fern have an established or strongly suspected role in human carcinogenesis. Obviously, they serve as instructive models for the further search for and identification of similar agents.

VINYL CHLORIDE AND OTHER INDUSTRIAL CHEMICALS

The definition of vinyl chloride as a carcinogen for human beings was predictable, in retrospect, from animal studies that showed the material to be a hepatocarcinogen. This has encouraged the idea of considering all chemicals given to rodents at maximum doses as potential carcinogens for human beings. The problem of dose-response relationships, however, looms large.

Vinyl chloride cancers in human beings, occurring among workers heavily exposed in the process of its manufacture, have been limited in number and appear to be restricted to hemangiosarcomas of the liver. Obviously, better occupational safety standards had to be evolved, and better surveillance of more general contamination of the surrounding areas by atmospheric fumes containing vinyl chloride were accepted in regulatory provisions. Even with this weak carcinogen, however, the assumption that any dose level is a hazard and cannot be metabolized deserves query and research.

Epidemiologically, there is a relationship between exposures to benzene and an increase in leukemia and the occurrence of cancer of the nasal fossa among furniture workers, perhaps due to exposure to varnishing agents as well as to wood dust.

HORMONES

Hormonal carcinogenesis, in human beings as well as in animals, represents a topic with unusual, if not unique, features. One of the earliest observations about experimental cancer, at the turn of the century, was that breast cancer in mice, which occurs almost exclusively in females, could be inhibited by the removal of the ovaries. In 1932, Lacassagne reported that exogenous estrogens given to male mice evoked breast cancer.

A galaxy of tumors in rodents can be produced by long-continued exposure to the natural or synthetic female sex hormones, chiefly cancers of the hormonally regulated end organs such as the breast, testes, pituitary, and uterus, but not excluding leukemia. Until the 1970s, however, there was no evidence that hormones were carcinogenic in human beings, although this certainly could have been inferred from animal data.

A rude awakening followed the report of adenocarcinomas of the vagina in daughters of mothers who had received diethylstilbestrol (DES) in large doses during their pregnancy. Purportedly this was to avert threatened abortion. It adjusted some laboratory values, but the treatment was shown to be useless for threatened abortion in formal clinical trials. Instead, a carcinogenic, transplacental, in utero simulant of the thalidomide tragedy had been induced iatrogenically. This also established that estrogens, at least DES, were indeed carcinogenic for human beings. For every vaginal cancer in the treated female offspring, estimated to be 1 per 1000, there are less serious adenoses and vaginal abnormalities, and the full effects in male offspring remain to be recorded.

Later observations on the significant, albeit small, increase in endometrial carcinoma among women who strove to be "forever feminine" by "natural" exogenous estrogen replacement extended knowledge of the carcinogenic effects of estrogens beyond the fetal stage to adult females. There is also suspicion that contraceptive steroids may be associated with a mild increase in breast cancer among younger women.

The use of the contraceptive steroids, usually containing estrogens as well as progestins, and of anabolic androgens taken by athletes to increase muscle mass has resulted in the appearance of liver tumors, usually adenomas. The risk of hemorrhage from such tumors is greater than the possibility of malignancy. It certainly suggests that these hepatomas are not in the identical class with the usual hepatocellular carcinomas. Relationships beween dose and length of exposure here also are not identical with, say, aflatoxin.

Restrictions on the addition of diethylstilbestrol to the feed of steers to yield a more tender and more lucrative product is still being resisted by the meat industry. Of course, modern methods of detection of DES now permit determination of a countable number of molecules, so that dose-effect relationships loom large in the considerations. All things considered, it does seem good public policy not to dose the feed of animals used in human nutrition with sex steroids, antibiotics, fungicides, and preservatives.

VIRUSES

With several dozen well-established viral cancers defined in several species, ranging from frogs to nonhuman primates, it is inevitable that human viral cancers also will be identified. Indeed, several are close to such identification, although the crucial tests for certitude remain to be performed.

Among the most promising current candidates for a human oncovirus is a DNA, herpes-type entity, the EB (Epstein-Barr) virus, first recovered from the African lymphoma of Burkitt, and also involved in the Chinese nasopharyngeal cancer. EB virus is the causative agent in infectious mononucleosis, a benign, self-limiting disease. With the involvement of environmental factors such as malaria, a sequence of latency and cellular hybridization apparently can lead to carcinogenesis. Since direct experimentation that would prove the causal role of EB virus is not possible, field trials of vaccination are being considered in high-risk populations as an indirect approach. The animal models already available are the successful attenuated and avirulent vaccines against Marek's disease of chickens, a herpes-type virus–induced lymphoma.

More inferentially, using serologic evidence, a role of herpes hominis 2 virus in cancer of the uterine cervix is a possibility.

The key disputation regarding oncoviruses is no longer whether some can induce some types of neoplasia, but whether viruses are a necessary component of all neoplastic processes. The latter view, presented as the oncogene theory, proposes a RNA virus that is a component of the cellular genome, and that can be activated by DNA viruses as well as other environmental stimuli. RNA virus cancers are prominently represented among chickens and mice, but up to now the evidence regarding human beings has not been convincing. If RNA viruses are eventually demonstrated to be carcinogenic in the human species, they probably would be added to a long list of exogenous or endogenous stimuli that can trigger the neoplastic sequence rather than being considered essential for all such transformations.

Evidence in support of the view that among viruses are carcinogenic entities distinct from the more casual chemical agents is the immunologic identicality of tumors induced by viruses; tumors resultant from chemical stimuli vary widely immunologically. This suggests that the viral genetic information becomes incorporated in the tumor-transformed cell, but that chemical carcinogenic effects on the cellular genome are more variable and are not mediated through a limited set of genes of a latent viral component.

The Host

It is obvious that the divisions between stimuli and host could be rearranged and would overlap. Thus, hormones could have been placed in the category of host factors, whereas nutrition could be considered exogenous. It merely demonstrates that both participate in the reactions that eventuate in neoplasia.

HEREDITY

Almost a century of observations throughout the world and work on mammalian genetics have shown that no human or animal population is "immune" to neoplastic diseases. Different inbred strains of mice and rats, maintained under identical environmental conditions, display different spectra of tumors. Genetic factors are intimately involved in neoplastic as well as all other reactions of all animals, including human beings. It is more than probable that there are as many genetic differences between, say, Bantus and Icelanders as there are between mice of strains A and C_{57} black.

No "cancer gene" has been found, and the development of tumors appears to be a phenotype reflecting complexes of genotypes. There are, however, some genetic traits in human beings that are related to increased risk of specific types of cancer. The examples of retinoblastoma, multiple polyposis of the colon, and xeroderma pigmentosum are well known. There are also a group of autosomal recessive syndromes in which the risk to cancer is increased; these include Fanconi's anemia and ataxia telangiectasia. Determinations of occurrence of cancer among relatives of patients with these rare syndromes show that they also experience significantly increased cancer rates, indicating that the susceptibility extends to the more frequent heterozygotes.

Studies of familial distribution of cancer indicate aggregations, particularly of breast and colon cancers, and of melanoma. Refinements in analysis can to some degree separate the hereditary components from the sharing of common environments. For whatever reason, individuals from families with multiple cancer histories are more prone to develop cancer than individuals of families in which records of cancer are rare. This information has obvious implications for cancer control.

AGE

Of all the determinants for cancer, advancing age is the most obvious and striking. There are examples of childhood cancer, of course, such as Wilms's tumor of the kidney and rhabdomyosarcoma. The higher incidence among older people of most cancers represents accumulation of exposures or progression of factors, rather than progressively greater susceptibility. Experimentally, younger animals, especially the newborn, are more susceptible to carcinogenic agents than older animals. In transplacental carcinogenesis, the stage of fetal development is related to the neoplastic response. Thus, the adenocarcinomas of the vagina induced by diethylstilbestrol connote that the carcinogenic transformation occurs during the müllerian-duct stage of vaginal differentiation.

In general, therefore, cancer susceptibility is highest among younger, healthier, better-fed animals than among old, sick, and undernourished ones. It is more than probable that the same facts appertain to human populations as well.

SEX

The most obvious influence of sex in neoplastic reactions is evident in cancers of target organs related to gender. Breast cancer is rare in males of all species, simply because the breast is vestigal in males. With estrogenic stimulation, male mice of strains in which females develop breast cancer can develop as many breast cancers as the females. Human males who undergo surgical and hormonal conversion to female appearance also develop breast cancer.

In organs and tissues possessed by both sexes, the human female develops fewer cancers than the male. There are two exceptions: cancer of the thyroid and cancer of the gallbladder, in which there is slight female preponderance. Experimentally, several types of cancer of nongonadal tissues have been shown to be influenced by sex, by exogenously administered sex hormones, and by the ablation of the gonads. Spontaneous hepatomas are more frequent in male mice than in females, but females are somewhat more responsive than males to hepatomagenesis with azo dyes. Castration or exogenous steroids obliterate or change the differences.

The seeming greater "resistance" to carcinogenesis in the human female (who also usually has a better prognosis with neoplastic disease) may be due to lesser exposure to exogenous carcinogens, to better self-awareness, or to undefined metabolic and genetic factors. Analyses of cigarette-induced lung cancer, for example, show a "sex factor" of a lower incidence among women that is not attributable to the amount and length of exposure. However, such analyses lack data on the possible differences in inhalation patterns in the two sexes.

NUTRITION

During the 1940s Tannenbaum clearly recorded that mice kept on restricted diets developed less cancers than mice on an ad libitum diet. The one-third restriction in unlimited food available to the pampered laboratory rodents produced slimmer but healthy animals that outlived their obese relatives. They also developed only one-third as many breast cancers, which in mice involve a RNA virus; furthermore, fewer skin cancers could be induced by applications of benzo[a]pyrene.

Investigations of specific vitamins in relation to carcinogenesis also showed that deficiencies resulted in inhibition of many neoplastic reactions, but at levels that impaired the growth or nutritional stability of the host. Cancer growth also could be inhibited by such draconian measures, demonstrating that cancer cells require the same nutrients as normal cells, albeit they are rather successful parasitic competitors.

Research on dietary aspects of carcinogenesis practically disappeared for almost two decades. It has been resurrected by epidemiologists who compared international cancer incidence rates and related them to the food intake. Religious groups in the United States who are abstemious in their use of tobacco, alcohol, and meat have 30 percent less cancer than the general population. Burkitt, the discoverer of the African lymphoma that bears his name, stressed the absence of colorectal cancer and other colorectal diseases among the African natives as compared with their American descendants, who have a high incidence of such diseases. The role of diet was invoked, with roughage and the transport time of the intestinal contents being offered as the explanations for the difference. Comparisons were extended to estimates of total caloric intake, and thence to consumption of fats and saturated fats. Significant relationships were elicited, especially for breast and for colorectal cancer. Relationships were also evident between the content of selenium in the diets of people living in various geographic areas and their cancer rates; here the relationships were inverse, suggesting a protective role for selenium. At high doses, producing cirrhosis, selenium *increases* hepatomas on rats, however.

Some of these epidemiologic relationships were supportable by experimental data. Mice on diets with larger proportions of fats developed more intestinal tumors following exposure to nitrosamines than animals with less fat in the food. Selenium supplementation inhibited the appearance of breast cancers and other tumors in mice; other antioxidants, such as vitamin E, demonstrated similar effects.

The role of diet in cancer has again returned to a prominent position in research. There seems to be little question that the most dangerous components in food are excess calories, which accelerate atherosclerosis as well as neoplasia. Fats, of course, are an important source of calories. Fats also may facilitate absorption of unknown carcinogens in the food, or the elaboration of carcinogens from food elements by intestinal flora, in turn also influenced by diet. In these relationships, the role of diet is visualized as being an indirect one, and is a behavioral as well as a biochemical problem, but that does not reduce its potential importance.

A more direct carcinogenic effect of diet may be through the intentional or accidental introduction of carcinogens. In the former category, as possibilities, are the chemicals added by the food industry that preserve, color, and otherwise modify food preparations. In the latter, aflatoxin contamination is always a possibility under humid conditions.

The most common drug abused by Western European peoples is alcohol. It is not considered to be a carcinogen, although satisfactorily complete tests on animals are lacking. Alcohol is known to be involved in cancer of the mouth and the esophagus, as a promoting agent in association with tobacco smoking, poor hygiene, and inadequate nutrition. Perhaps alcohol solubilizes carcinogens and allows better absorption, or the damaged cells become less resistant.

Alcohol in our culture is also associated with portal cirrhosis of the liver. In autopsy series of hepatocellular carcinoma, cirrhosis is an almost universal concomitant. Thus, alcoholic cirrhosis is associated with hepatic carcinoma considerably more convincingly than with DDT. The mechanism of the association is not clear, and may be truncated rather than sequential.

Alcohol consumption, as excessive food ingestion, is a problem of behavior. It is another example where the carcinogenic process can be aborted by strategies other than defining and eliminating carcinogens.

IMMUNE STATUS

One of the attractive discoveries in oncology of the last decade was that some tumors contain antigens that are sufficiently foreign to the host to elicit immune response. A theory was propounded of immune surveillance, in which transformed cells are destroyed by alerted lymphocytes before they can progress to overt cancer. Immunologic measures were explored against experimental and clinical cancers, with effects too modest for the expectations.

It has been demonstrated that rodents made immunologically incompetent by chemicals, radiation, and thymectomy will accept foreign tissue grafts, including heterologous tumors, and will develop more tumors following injection of carcinogens such as urethane. Clinical observations on patients in whom immune response was inhibited in order to protect transplanted kidneys against rejection were shown to have high rates of neoplasms of the lymphatic apparatus. Genetic deficiencies of immune response, such as agammaglobulinemia, also were associated with high risk of lymphomas. Thus, depression of the cellular immune apparatus definitely has neoplastic import.

Claims have been made that nonspecific enhancement of the immune system, such as BCG vaccination, protects against leukemia. The data are retrospective and not convincing, but certainly deserve further study.

Immunologic processes are, of course, not the only protective mechanisms the body has for the elimination and neutralization of noxious materials, carcinogenic or otherwise. The liver is the primary organ for enzymatic binding and alteration of chemicals, and one system of protection is the induction of such enzymes. Phenobarbital, for example, induces enzymes that detoxify polycyclic aromatic hydrocarbons, and fewer tumors are obtained in experimental animals so pretreated.

Among the reasons that neonatal rodents are more susceptible to carcinogens than adult animals is that both their immune system and the hepatic detoxification enzymes are not fully developed. As a result, urethane and chemicals of the PAH type are retained longer in the body of younger animals, in effect exposing them to higher doses over longer periods than mature animals with fully developed protective systems. It is not clear how these data apply to species with more complete development at birth, such as the ungulates or human beings. Special protection of the young is empirically sound nevertheless, if for no other reason than the expectation of a longer period of survival, during which neoplasms could develop to clinical exteriorization. Thus, radiation therapy or the use of carcinogenic chemotherapeutic drugs are to be avoided, if at all possible, in children, and the contraindications become less compelling among the aged patients with more limited actuarial expectations.

DISCUSSION

Other Chemical Carcinogens

The discussion up to now has centered on stimuli and responses of established importance to human beings, including experimental animal data when these were considered relevant. There are available thick tomes listing thousands of chemical compounds that have been administered to various species of animals under a variety of conditions, and reporting that several hundred of these produced, increased, or accelerated one type of tumor or another. The list of these "carcinogens" grows apace. Are all to be considered hazardous for human beings, especially if the no-threshold theory for carcinogens is accepted so that no safe exposure level can be proposed? This question requires consideration of the questions What is cancer? What is a carcinogen? and of the subsidiary topics of whether these represent a single entity or multiple entities, leading to the unavoidable discussion of risk-benefit balances.

Cancers, or the neoplastic diseases, are characterized by permanent, progressive changes in somatic cells, which acquire properties of relatively unrestricted growth, producing invasion and metastasis. The single most important attribute of cancer is that it kills, inexorably, unless it is totally obliterated.

The diagnosis of cancer is made by pathologists examining stained, thin sections of relevant tissues under a microscope. This pictorial recognition is related to a century of experience of what happens to patients with lesions demonstrating such appearances. Lesions resembling cancer that do not progress are reclassified as nonmalignant, whereas lesions that progress despite their benign appearance are recognized as having malignant import. The classification of neoplasms is limited to the primary organ or tissue of origin, and to the cellular appearance. As useful and irreplaceable as is histopathology (in the absence of alternate methods), it must be admitted that it resembles the classification of fevers before the bacteriological era. Think where the diagnosis of infectious diseases would be if diagnoses were limited to the morphological features of microorganisms.

The interpretation of animal tumors by criteria evolved in human pathology can be questioned. Many tests for carcinogenic activity are designed to expose mice and rats to maximal levels of a chemical over the life-span of the animals. When the surviving animals are sacrificed at 2 or 3 years, advanced age for small rodents, is the finding of a statistically significant increase in hepatomas, or thyroid tumors, or nonmetastasizing bladder carcinomas, none of which influenced survival or were tested for transplantability, to be considered as evidence of carcinogenic activity? For reasons of economy, maximal exposures in biological tests are reasonable. But can such levels be extrapolated to any level as producing cancer, and thus being potentially hazardous? Hepatotoxins such as chloroform produce hepatomas in rats. Are the levels of chloroform synthesized from chlorine in water supplies, at parts per billion, of biological significance to human beings or to animals?

It should be pointed out that many studies on carcinogenesis in rodents are single investigations, so that replication is often not available. But a more fundamentally important issue is whether all lesions morphologically called neoplasms in rats and mice are biologically cancer. At present there are no answers to the question, and resolution is arrived at by judgment of presumably knowledgeable committees. Committees assembled by the bureaucracies of the government usually accept the safest interpretation, and prudently declare that all chemicals that increase neoplasms in rodents are potential carcinogens for human beings. Such committees also shy away from designating carcinogens by some quantitative scale, since the necessary information is seldom available. Yet N-nitrosamine is obviously a powerful carcinogen, and safrol is obviously a weak one.

No one would want to expose people to carcinogens, and legislators are hardly likely to pass regulations that would allow such exposure. Nor would one wish to affirm a chemical as an actual carcinogen in human beings after it had been shown to be a carcinogen for rats. All human carcinogens, with the exception of arsenic, are replicated as carcinogens in animals. The reverse may not be also true, but the reason tests on animals are performed is to spare human beings the experience. The question is really what compounds are "true" carcinogens in test animals. There can be assumed reasonable levels of safety for carcinogens, as are assumed for drugs in regard to lethality and other toxic effects. It is a challenge to research to provide information on the basis of which a reasonable balance between absolutes and the relative real world can be achieved.

The Carcinogenic Process

There is considerable evidence that cancer is a group of diseases rather than one disease, and that several different processes can eventuate in cancer. Similar differences are also evident in the many substances that can trigger the carcinogenic process.

Some carcinogens act directly at point of contact; of course, even these must be absorbed, penetrate into cells, and gain attachment at specific sites of the cell.

Other carcinogens require extensive metabolic conversion, either in the tissue affected or at distant sites such as the liver, to proximate carcinogens, which then are transported to the target organ. The proximate carcinogens then can bind covalently with nucleic acids or proteins in the cells. The organotropic nature of many carcinogens is best explained by the presence of specific attachment sites within the cell. The model of estrogen receptors is undoubtedly applicable to carcinogens as well.

The current conception of the carcinogenic process is that it is a somatic mutation, a change in the genetic mechanism of the cell that is then transmitted to the daughter cells. It is not established whether one or more mutations have to occur, or whether an identical DNA lesion has to be affected in all cases. Most theories favor two to five mutations rather than single ones.

Alternate epigenetic explanations can and have been proposed, suggesting that cancer is a defect in differentiation, or that it is due to the activation of a latent virus. These postulates also necessarily involve an alteration in the functional genome expression that is maintained in the descendant generations of the altered cells.

For most human and animal cancers, the long latent period, as well as other experimental evidence, demonstrates that carcinogenesis involves at least two phases, one of rapid initiation, followed by one of slower promotion. The latter phase is epigenetic, probably reducing the host resistance factors rather than having direct action on the latent cancer cells.

It has been pointed out by Berenblum that inconsistencies in our current concepts of carcinogenesis may be more informative than generalizations. Hormone carcinogenesis does not fit well into the schemes proposed for direct or indirect chemical carcinogens, and the occurrence of sarcomas following subcutaneous implantation of plastic or metal films in rats ("solid-state" carcinogenesis) is an enigma within the neoplastic mystery.

Some Applications

The practical reason for being interested in carcinogenesis is that knowledge regarding causes and processes provides entry points that can be exploited toward prevention of the overt diseases. The shortest approach to such knowledge is research on mechanisms into how and why the intriguing caricature of the typical cancer arises. This is also known as basic research.

The occurrence of disease can be prevented by avoidance of the stimulus, or the protection of the organism against the stimulus. This is *primary* prevention, the goal of the topic here discussed.

Table 2-2 summarizes some of the known or suspected causative factors in some of the major sites or types of neoplasia. Some of these factors suggest possible preventive measures.

In the United States, the most important of the identified carcinogenic stimuli are the habits of tobacco smoking and of heavy alcohol consumption. Self-indulgent excessive nutritional habits may be added to make a triad. Except for limited populations exposed occupationally, these three factors are by far the most important, on the basis of present knowledge.

It is very human to ignore the uncomfortably obvious and exaggerate the less likely. Little has been accomplished in changing the tobacco habits of our population, a real, important cause of cancer. Alcohol consumption, accelerating several cancers if not causing them, remains as high as ever. Excessive indulgence in food is a mark of our prosperous economy. Much more attention is directed by newspapers and communication media to alarms raised by finding that some rats fed inordinate amounts of saccharin developed nonmetastasizing lesions of the urinary bladder or that chloroform in parts per billon is present in some water sources or that there are mutagenic and carcinogenic hair dyes. The public soon loses interest in this surfeit of information no one can interpret, which does not keep the bureaucratic apparatus of the government from grinding out more protective regulations.

The identification of subpopulations of particular susceptibility to cancer appears to be useful for special surveillance of the individuals in order that their treatable cancers may be detected as "early" as possible. Without knowledge of the nature of the susceptibility, no primary preventive measures can be suggested. It has been proposed that susceptibles should be excluded from occupations exposing them to carcinogens. This is, of course, accepted in established cases; for example, albinos are excluded from outdoor exposure to sunlight. An important current care is not to expose tobacco smokers to asbestos, or, vice versa, to prevent (somehow) workers unavoidably exposed to asbestos from smoking. Experimentally, however, susceptibility to spontaneous forms of cancer does not necessarily parallel susceptibility to the induction of the same forms of cancer. Thus, the high occurrence of leukemia among patients with Down's syndrome does not necessarily mean that they have a greater likelihood of leukemogenesis following exposure to ionizing radiation.

Life, of course, cannot be without hazard, and what is sought is a reasonable balance. Despite environmental Jeremiahs, the life-span in the United States has risen steadily, so that now it is 75 years for men from birth and 81 years for women. We must have been doing something right!

The current return to emphasis on environmental carcinogenesis stems from the realization that prevention may be a more rewarding approach to cancer than some of the more popular fields of the recent past, such as chemotherapy and viral oncology. This view, of course, represents in part disappointment at not having achieved rapid payoffs in research on chemotherapy and viral oncology, as well as a manifestation of the environmentalist outlook so popular these days.

It should be emphasized that the choices are not either-or; no contradictions exist in not limiting our options. Prevention of cancer should be pursued avidly in circumstances and situations where important dangers have been defined. Such conditions exist in the case of

TABLE 2-2 Factors Related to Occurrence of Cancers

Site	Causative or predisposing factors	
	Exogenous	*Endogenous*
Mouth and pharynx	Tobacco, alcohol, nutritional deficiency	Plummer-Vinson syndrome (sideropenia)
Nasopharynx	? EB virus	?
Esophagus	Alcohol, tobacco, nutritional deficiency, stricture (lye)	Sideropenia, tylosis
Stomach	? Nitrosamines	Achlorhydria, pernicious anemia
Colorectum	Nutritional excess	Familial (multiple) polyposis, ulcerative colitis, Gardner's syndrome
Liver	Alcohol, ? nutritional deficiency, aflatoxin, hepatitis B virus	Hemochromatosis, cirrhosis
Larynx	Tobacco, alcohol	?
Lung	Tobacco; air pollution; occupational inhalation of chromate, asbestos, nickel, uranium, etc.	?
Urinary bladder	Tobacco; *Schistosoma haematobium;* occupational: aniline dye products	? Tryptophan metabolism abnormality
Testis	? Mumps virus	Cryptorchidism
Uterine cervix	Early intercourse, promiscuity, ? uncircumcised partner, ? *herpes hominis 2* virus	?
Endometrium	Estrogens	Endocrine: obesity, infertility, diabetes ? Ovarian hyperfunction
Breast	Nutritional excess, ionizing radiation	Nulliparity; family history; endocrine: obesity, diabetes
Skin (including genitalia)	Actinic radiation, ionizing radiation, arsenic, petroleum, tar products, burn scars	Fair complexion, xeroderma pigmentosum
Leukemia (myelocytic)	Ionizing radiation, phenylbutazone, benzol	Mongolism, Bloom's syndrome, Fanconi syndrome
Lymphoma	Immunosuppression	Agammaglobulinemia, Aldrich syndrome
Thyroid	Ionizing radiation, iodine deficiency	?
Bone	Ionizing radiation (radium)	Paget's disease

tobacco smoking or occupational exposure to asbestos, and prevention here is the only way to go. But we cannot prevent all possible or implied hazards, and such prevention carries its own risks—social and economical as well as biological costs and risks. In this connection the century-old counsel of Bagehot remains valid: "In nine cases out of ten cure is better than prevention. By looking forward to all possible evils we waste the strength that had best be concentrated in curing the one evil which happens."

Prevention and cure are not antithetical, of course. The choice and balance between the two options depend on the efficacy and ease of each.

The battle of the human intellect against the riddle of cancer must proceed on many fronts. Grouping too great a proportion of resources on a few popular topics is not wise, and certainly premature. Most of the field of cancer research still lies in the area of exploration and unpredictable outcome. The strategy, therefore, should be to mount many teams of different training and ideas, rather than to organize disciplined armies pursuing a few programs under a limited number of commanders.

Environmental carcinogens and the role of nutrition should be an important area of research, but this in no way should deemphasize research on cure by systemic agents, or on viral causation of some human cancers. These areas are just as promising as they were 20 years ago, and just as worth pursuing, with an ever-increasing fund of knowledge.

We can repeat, with confidence, that cancer is a solvable problem, solvable by the human thought-and-action methods of scientific research. Through research, some cancers will be prevented not only by avoidance of causative agents but by protection with vaccination and metabolic neutralization. Through research, some cancers will be cured by systemic chemical and biological treatments. And, one day, the hot x-ray tube and the cold surgical knife as the approach to cancer will be retired to museums to rest among other medical curiosities of the past.

BIBLIOGRAPHY*

Fraumeni JF (ed): *Persons at High Risk of Cancer,* Academic, New York, 1975.

Hiatt HH et al (eds): *Origins of Cancer,* Cold Spring Harbor Laboratory, 1977.

Holland JF, Frei E (eds): *Cancer Medicine,* Laurel, Philadelphia, 1973.

Schottenfeld D (ed): *Cancer Epidemiology and Prevention,* Charles C Thomas, Springfield, Ill, 1974.

Shimkin, MB: *Contrary to Nature: An Illustrated History of Cancer,* GPO, Washington, DC, 1977.

* This essay represents an attempt at a synthesis. It raises more questions than it answers, and depends upon an extensive literature, which in turn has been synthesized and summarized previously by many authors, including myself. The primary references are not given here, as they are to be found in several recent books. Books of special relevance are listed here. Support of specific statements will be found in them. Interpretations, right or wrong, alas, are mine.

SELECTED BIBLIOGRAPHY

DeVita VT Jr et al (eds): *Cancer: Principles and Practice of Oncology,* Lippincott, Philadelphia, 1982.

Fraumeni JF (ed): *Persons at High Risk of Cancer,* Academic Press, New York, 1975.

Hiatt HH et al (eds): *Origins of Cancer,* Cold Spring Harbor Laboratory of Quantitative Biology, 1977.

Holland JF, Frei E (eds): *Cancer Medicine,* 2nd ed, Lea and Febiger, Philadelphia, 1982.

Schottenfeld D (ed): *Cancer Epidemiology and Prevention,* Charles C Thomas, Springfield, Ill., 1974.

Shimkin MB: *Contrary to Nature: An Illustrated History of Cancer,* Government Printing Office, Washington, D.C., 1977.

3
CANCER EPIDEMIOLOGY: METHODS AND APPLICATIONS

Jonathan Amsel

Epidemiology is the study of the distribution and determinants of disease frequency in human beings.[1] It is a method of reasoning about disease that deals with deriving biologic inferences from observations of disease phenomena in defined populations.[2] Epidemiology effectively integrates the biomedical disciplines of biochemistry, pathology, microbiology, and physiology with the mathematical and statistical sciences.

The primary considerations of epidemiology in discerning the causation and prevention of disease are summarized by Lilienfeld et al.[3] as follows:

1. To formulate etiologic hypotheses by using descriptive techniques which correlate variations in disease incidence over time with differences in the biologic (or genetic) and environmental characteristics of study populations
2. To test whether a "causal relationship" exists between a putative etiologic factor(s) and the disease of interest, such that exposure to the hypothesized etiologic factor increases the probability of developing the disease
3. To determine whether the putative etiologic factor can be manipulated experimentally, using laboratory methods, to include the disease of interest
4. To demonstrate a change in the incidence of the disease of interest following a reduction in exposure to the putative etiologic factor(s)

In this chapter the principal methods in current use in cancer epidemiology will be described in detail. The advantages of these methods in studying the natural history of cancer in order to provide clues to etiology will be stressed.

Although epidemiologic techniques were not systematically used in the study of cancer until after World War II, much of the knowledge of carcinogenesis has stemmed directly from isolated observations which were essentially epidemiologic in character. Table 3-1 summarizes some historic landmarks in cancer epidemiology, starting with the seminal observation by Percival Pott (1775) that cancer of the scrotum was particularly prevalent and occurred at an unusually early age among chimney sweeps.[4,5] While the observations of Pott remained neglected for 150 years, they eventually provided the catalyst for the preparation of the first pure chemical carcinogen, 1,2:5,6-dibenzanthracene, in 1932.[6] This

---

The author wishes to express his gratitude to Eileen Lynch for her considerable contribution to this chapter.

24 BASIC CONCEPTS IN ONCOLOGY

TABLE 3-1 Some Historic Landmarks in Cancer Epidemiology

Type of cancer	Population at risk	Putative etiologic factor	Reference
Breast cancer	Nuns	Celibacy (association later related to nulliparity)	Ramazzini (1713)
Cancer of nose	Snuff users	?	Hill (1766)
Scrotal cancer	Chimney sweeps	Chronic exposure to soot	Pott[4]
Cancer of lower lip	Pipe smokers	?	Soemmering (1975)
Bronchogenic carcinoma	Uranium miners	Exact nature of carcinogen debated for many years. (Radioactivity from uranium, Wagoner, et al., 1964)	Harting and Hesse (1879)
Bladder cancer	Workers in aniline dye industry	Naphthylamines and benzidine	Rehn (1895)
Bladder cancer	Agricultural workers	*Schistosoma haematobium*	Ferguson (1911)
Osteogenic sarcoma	Radium dial painters	Ionizing radiation	Martland and Humphries (1929)

SOURCE: Adapted from Shimkin MB: Some Historical Landmarks in Cancer Epidemiology. *Cancer Epidemiology and Prevention,* David Schottenfeld (ed), Springfield, Ill.: Charles C Thomas, 60–75, 1975.

development in turn led to the identification of 3,4-benzpyrene, the first substance commonly found in the environment to be identified as a carcinogen.[7]

DEFINITION OF CANCER

A neoplasm, or tumor, is characterized by the growth of tissue which has escaped the body's normal regulation of growth. Cancer, or malignant neoplasm, is further characterized by invasion into surrounding normal tissue and/or distant spread of the disease (metastases). Cytologic differences between benign and malignant tumors are presented in Table 3-2.

Cancer is not a single disease but rather a collection of diseases which differ widely in etiology—in frequency, in pattern of occurrence, and in clinical manifestations. Additional differences are characterized by anatomic site and histology.

CLASSIFICATIONS OF TUMORS

Classification by Anatomic Site of Primary Tumor

One of the principal anatomic classifications used for neoplastic diseases is the nosology provided by the World Health Organization's *International Classification of Diseases: Clinical Modification*(ICD-9-CM).[8] The major advantages of a nosologic classification such as the ICD-9-CM are

1. International usage
2. Uniform rules for coding diseases
3. Comparability of data from different geographic areas
4. Comparability of data from different time periods

The broad groups of neoplastic diseases contained in ICD-9-CM are shown in Table 3-3.

The International Classification of Diseases for Oncology (ICD-0) is a more detailed version of the ICD-9-CM.[9] The ICD-0, however, provides specific topographic codes to resolve ambiguities related to coding diagnoses referring to ill-defined anatomic sites.

Classification by Histologic Type of Tumor

ICD-0, unlike ICD-9-CM, also includes a morphology or histology section, preferred terms being those used in the *International Classification of Tumors*.[10] The justification for coding the morphology of a tumor is that neoplasms developing at the same anatomic site may differ widely in biologic properties as well as in etiology.

Gastric cancer is an example where comparative histologic differences have been used successfully in epidemiologic investigations. Jarvi and Lauren[11] and

TABLE 3-2 Cytologic Features of Benign and Malignant Tumors

Nuclei	Benign tumors	Malignant tumors	
Size	Uniform	Various sizes; large and small nuclei }	Pleomorphism
Shape	Round, oval, spindle	Irregular	
Chromatin	Finely granular, evenly divided	Coarsely lumpy, unevenly divided, increased }	Hyperchromasin
Chromosome number	Euploid	Abnormal as a rule	
Chromosome shape	Uniform	(Noneuploid); enlarged or shrunken; e.g., V-form chromosomes	
DNA content	Normal euploid	Deviating, noneuploid, great scattering	
Number of mitoses	Few	Increased, atypical mitoses	

SOURCE: Reproduced with permission from W Sandritter, WB Wartman: *Color Atlas and Textbook of Tissue and Cellular Pathology*, 5th ed., Year Book, Chicago, 1976. Copyright © 1976 by Year Book Medical Publishers, Inc.

Lauren[12] have described two types of gastric cancer which differ both structurally and histochemically: intestinal gastric carcinoma and diffuse gastric carcinoma. The intestinal type, so called because it is formed by intestinal rather than gastric cells, appears to be related etiologically more to environmental factors than the diffuse type. Individuals residing in geographic areas characterized as "high risk" for gastric cancer are more likely to have the intestinal type.[13]

Thyroid cancer is another example of histologic subtypes differing in their respective etiologies: follicular and anaplastic cancers seem to be associated with iodine deficiency, while papillary carcinomas are characteristic of individuals consuming too much iodine.[14]

Kreyberg[15] classified bronchial carcinomas according to distinct histologic categories as shown in Table 3-4. The observed increase in the frequency of group I tumors, particularly among cigarette smokers, provided substantial evidence for an etiologic relationship between smoking and bronchogenic carcinomas.

Further discussion of the important role of histology in cancer epidemiology may be found in the review papers by Berg[16] and Peto.[17]

A major difficulty with histologic typing is the lack of standardization in microscopic diagnoses. Also, pathologists tend to classify tumors by broad rather than by specific histologic type. This tendency was observed in histologic data collected during the *Third National Cancer Survey* (TNCS). Of the 180 possible histologic types, 101 types had fewer than 100 cases reported and 34 types fewer than 10 cases.[18] Consequently, whenever an epidemiologic study requires histologic typing, the effect of observer variation must be reduced to a minimum. This requires a well-written pathology protocol that standardizes the diagnostic criteria and laboratory procedures to be used in the preparation of tissue samples.

TABLE 3-3 ICD-9-CM Classification of Neoplastic Diseases

Code Number	Category
149–195	Malignant neoplasms, stated or presumed to be primary, or specified sites, except of lymphatic and hematopoietic tissue
196–198	Malignant neoplasms, stated or presumed to be secondary, of specified sites
199	Malignant neoplasms, without specification of site
200–208	Malignant neoplasms, stated or presumed to be primary, of lymphatic and hematopietic tissue
210–229	Benign neoplasms
230–234	Carcinoma in situ
235–238	Neoplasms of uncertain behavior
239	Neoplasms of unspecified nature

TABLE 3-4 Histologic Types of Lung Cancer

Group	Type of tumor
I	Epidermoid carcinomas
	Small-cell anaplastic carcinomas
II	Adrenocarcinomas
	Bronchiolas alveolar-cell carcinomas
	Carcinoids
	Mucous gland tumors

SOURCE: Adapted from Kreyberg.[15]

The use of histologic grading and differentiation also varies among pathologists throughout the world, and in many instances malignant tumors are not routinely graded. The use of terms designating degrees of differentiation is also inconsistent.

Classification by Stage of Disease

Currently, a number of different staging systems are being used for the classification of malignant diseases.[19,20] The extent to which these systems are being used varies from hospital to hospital, and even between departments within a hospital. However, each system that is used is based on a careful documentation of the extent of disease—a detailed description of how far the tumor has spread from the primary site.

The staging of malignant disease can be based solely on clinical findings or on a combination of clinical findings together with observations made during surgery and the results of histopathologic examination of excised tissue. Staging of diseases is a valuable procedure for evaluating the prognosis of a patient; nevertheless it is an imperfect one. Observer variation and lack of standardization in the system which is used can be considerable. Still, even with these shortcomings, staging of disease remains a useful procedure in evaluating a patient's prognosis as well as the natural history of specific tumors.

Latency Period

The concept of a latency period for cancer is analogous to that of the incubation period for infectious diseases. The latency period is the span of time required for the initial malignant transformation and tumor growth to a size that permits recognition and diagnosis. Its overall importance is that it provides an approximate time frame for determining relevant etiologic exposure. Latency periods have been shown to vary with the specific site and with the particular carcinogenic stimulus.[21]

The biologic activity of the target tissue and its inherent susceptibility to neoplastic transformation must also be considered, e.g., the incidence of breast cancer among atomic bomb survivors. McGregor et al.[22] have observed that the radiogenic tumor response of breast tissue was greater for women 10 to 19 years of age at the time of the bomb (ATB) than among older groups. Presumably the differential age response was due to increased mitotic activity related to pubescence.

Related to the concept of latency period is the use of mathematical models to describe multistage processes which are presumed to underlie the induction of a large majority of human cancers. Simply stated, the multistage hypothesis is "that a few distinct changes (each heritable when cells carrying them divide) are necessary to alter a normal cell into a malignant cell, and that human cancer usually arises from the proliferation of a clone derived from a single cell that suffered all the necessary changes and then started to proliferate malignantly."[17] There are different variants of the multistage model but all are stochastic in approach (i.e., a probabilistic model used to investigate random phenomena dependent on time). A more complete discussion of epidemiology and multistage models of carcinogenesis is presented by Peto in *Origins of Human Cancer*.[17]

Because latency periods of malignant diseases may exceed 35 years, e.g., bronchogenic carcinomas,[21] the clinical manifestation of the disease is often far removed in time from the original carcinogenic stimulus. Consequently, the ability to identify and evaluate antecedent risk factors involved in the etiology of malignant diseases may be inversely related to the length of the latent interval. This is due to an increased likelihood of some factor intervening to modify or eliminate the exposure variable of interest.

DESCRIPTIVE EPIDEMIOLOGY

Measurement of Frequency of Occurrence

Descriptive epidemiology is the study of patterns of disease occurrence in human populations. Most epidemiologic methods of study relate individuals with the disease of interest (cases) to the population from which they came. In order to make comparisons, rates (quantitative descriptions of the relationships between case and population) must be computed.

According to Lilienfeld,[23] rates have three essential elements:

1. A population group exposed to the risk of disease
2. A time factor
3. The number of cases of disease or deaths occurring in the exposed population during or at a certain time period

Specifically, descriptive epidemiologic studies use three types of rates: incidence, mortality, and prevalence. These rates can be calculated separately for site-specific cancers, sex and/or age groups, occupations, and urban or rural populations.

INCIDENCE AND PREVALENCE

Incidence and prevalence are the two major measurements of morbidity. *Incidence* measures the rate at which new events, e.g., new cases of a disease, are occurring in a population. *Prevalence* measures the number of cases observed in a population at a designated time. Incidence provides a direct estimate of the probability of developing a disease, while prevalence provides an estimate of disease burden* within a specified community or population. These rates are defined as follows:

$$\text{Incidence} = \frac{\text{number of new cases of a disease}}{\text{population at risk}} \text{ over a specified period of time}$$

$$\text{Prevalence} = \frac{\text{number of existing cases of a disease}}{\text{total population}}$$

Lilienfeld et al.[3] specify two types of prevalence rates: point prevalence and period prevalence. Point prevalence refers to the frequency of the number of cases at a given moment of time, whereas period prevalence refers to the frequency of the number of cases observed during (rather than at) a specified period of time—for example, during a year. Period prevalence, therefore, consists of the point prevalence at the beginning of a specified period of time plus all cases that arose during the period.

An important relationship exists between incidence and prevalence. A change in the prevalence rate of a disease may be the result of changes either in the incidence or duration of that disease. For example, an improvement in the chemotherapeutic treatment of chronic leukemia could result in improved 5-year survival rates, thereby increasing the prevalence of chronic leukemia.

MORTALITY

A mortality, or death, rate expresses the frequency with which members of a population die of a disease. Like incidence, a mortality rate is also an estimate of the probability of an event occurring, i.e., death. A crude mortality rate is defined as follows:

$$\text{Mortality} = \frac{\text{number of deaths among area residents in calendar year}}{\text{midyear population in area in that year}}$$

A relationship exists between mortality rate and incidence. For some malignant diseases—such as pancreatic cancer, in which the median survival time for all ages is 3.0 months for whites—mortality rate is a valid index of incidence. Conversely, for bladder cancer, in which the median survival time is approximately 4.0 years for whites, mortality rate correlates poorly with incidence.

EXAMPLES OF RATE CALCULATIONS

Calculation of the three principal types of rates can be illustrated using data from Table 3-5. The assumption is made that Table 3-5 includes all the cases of chronic leukemia in the white population of Brooklyn at risk of developing chronic leukemia, which in 1950 (the midpoint for the 5-year period 1948 to 1952) numbered 2,525,000.

Prevalence (Point) The numerator consists of individuals with chronic leukemia who are alive at the beginning of the year, i.e., 1948, 1949 ... 1952 (column 1). The denominator is the population at risk for developing chronic leukemia; in this example the size of the population at risk is equal to 2,525,000. The point prevalence of chronic leukemia numerically is

$$\frac{708}{2,525,000} \times 100,000 = 28.03$$

The population unit in which the rate is expressed (per 100,000 in this example) is arbitrary but should be specified. In the event an average annual point preva-

---

* *Burden* is defined as the balance between the addition of new cases of a disease developing in the population and the withdrawal of cases because of death or cure.

TABLE 3-5 Data on Patients with Chronic Leukemia, Brooklyn, New York, Whites, 1948 to 1952

Year	Patients alive at beginning of year	New cases diagnosed in year	Deaths in year
1948	129	79	50
1949	150	83	71
1950	157	90	90
1951	151	61	84
1952	121	53	89
Total	708	366	384

SOURCE: MacMahon and Clark, *Blood* 11:871–881, 1956.

lence rate is desired, simply divide the 5-year rate by 5 (28.03 ÷ 5 = 5.61).

Incidence The time period during which new cases of chronic leukemia are diagnosed is the basis for deriving incidence (column 2). Similar to prevalence, the incidence rates are usually expressed per annum.

$$\frac{366}{5} \times \frac{100,000}{2,525,000} = 2.90$$

Mortality The annual mortality rate for chronic leukemia is derived from column 3:

$$\frac{384}{5} \times \frac{100,000}{2,525,000} = 3.04$$

USE OF RATES

The choice of incidence, prevalence, or mortality rates as a measure of disease frequency in a population is dependent upon the nature of the specific problem under study. Whenever the elucidation of etiologic factors is of primary interest, incidence data are more appropriate in searching for variation in the frequency of cancer by time, place, person. Prevalence rates are most useful in the planning of selected administrative activities, e.g., planning medical services. As stated previously, mortality rates can be used, under certain circumstances, as valid indices of incidence. Because of routine death registration together with the specification of cause of death, mortality data are generally available even when morbidity data are not.

Time, Place, and Person

A concept underlying most epidemiologic research is that *disease does not occur randomly*, and that identifying and describing these nonrandom occurrences is fundamental to the formulation of specific hypotheses concerning etiologic relationships. Time, place, and person are the major descriptive variables used in epidemiologic research.

TIME

Study of disease occurrence by time is a basic aspect of epidemiologic analysis. Changes by time may be long-term variations called *secular trends,* periodic fluctuations called *cyclic changes,* or short-term fluctuations such as are found in infectious disease epidemics.

In cancer epidemiology, time trends in cancer incidence or mortality rates often give clues to either the introduction or withdrawal of some particular etiologic factor. The data shown in Table 3-6 illustrate time trends in incidence for lung and stomach cancer by race and sex.

Data from this table indicate a decreasing incidence of stomach cancer since 1937—a trend believed to be due to dietary changes. Trend data showing an increasing incidence of lung cancer led to an extensive series of studies which ultimately demonstrated an association with cigarette smoking. Allowing for a relatively long latency period, the dramatic increase in lung cancer incidence (particularly of the epidermoid type) coincided with the increased use of tobacco among males during World War II. For women, the widespread use of tobacco did not start until many years later, thereby explaining their relatively lower risk of developing lung cancer.

TABLE 3-6 Time Trends in Cancer Incidence Rates for Stomach and Lung

Site	Race and Sex	1937	1947	1969
Stomach	White Male	44.0	34.1	14.0
	White Female	26.1	18.3	6.1
	Black Male	38.3	39.6	20.5
	Black Female	22.2	22.8	10.0
Lung	White Male	13.7	29.5	68.9
	White Female	4.0	6.5	13.5
	Black Male	8.4	25.4	84.7
	Black Female	3.4	5.8	18.2

From three surveys conducted by NCI: 1937, 1947, and 1969.
SOURCE: Levin et al.[76]

Another form of time-trend analysis having considerable relevance in forming etiologic hypotheses is birth-cohort analysis (i.e., persons born within a particular period of time). Birth-cohort analysis is useful for generating etiologic hypotheses and in predicting trends in disease occurrence, when age and generational effects are indistinguishable. An example where cross-sectional (or current age) and birth-cohort or generational curves for lung cancer are compared is shown in Fig. 3-1. It is observed that for birth cohorts (solid lines) the risk of developing lung cancer continues to increase throughout life, but that at any given age rates are higher for later rather than earlier cohorts. These differential rates can be explained on the basis of increased cigarette smoking with successive generations.

PLACE

Frequency of disease can be related to place of occurrence in terms of areas set off either by natural geographic barriers or by political boundaries.

The variable of place has been useful in identifying major international differences in both cancer morbidity and mortality rates. For example, the geographic distribution of stomach cancer morbidity is varied, as shown in Table 3-7.

Several possible explanations have been offered for the extreme variation observed for stomach cancer: genetic background, social and cultural habits (e.g., diet), geographic factors (e.g., nitrate deposits).

Studies which take advantage of international differences in cancer risk are migrant studies. These studies are intended to discriminate between genetic and environmental factors as determinants of cancer risk by investigating population migration. One of the best-known migrant cancer studies is that by Haenszel et al.[24] concerning stomach cancer among Japanese in Hawaii.

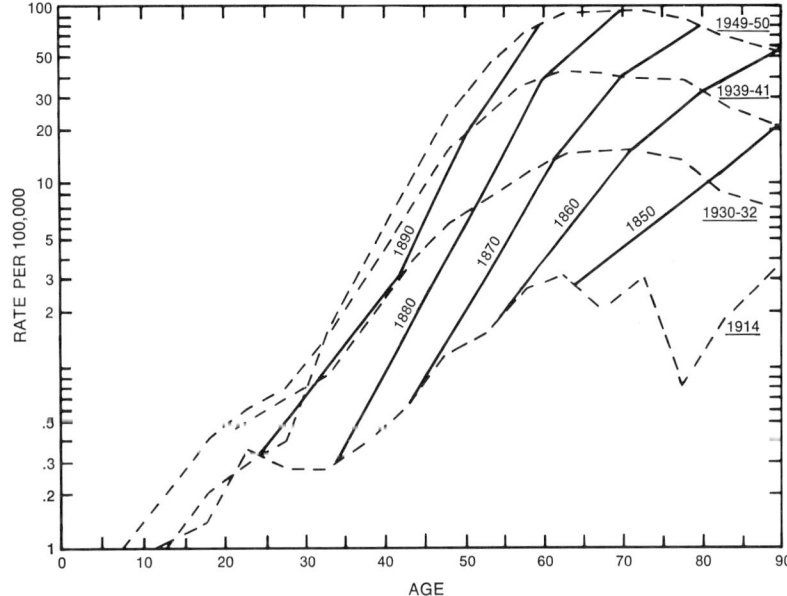

FIGURE 3-1 Mortality rates for cancer of the lung, United States, 1914 to 1950. Solid lines are birth-cohort curves, broken lines are cross-sectional or current-age curves. (From HF Dorn, SJ Cutler: Morbidity from cancer in the United States. Public Health Monograph N. 56, U.S. Government Printing Office, 1959.)

TABLE 3-7 Age-Adjusted Incidence Rates (per 100,000) for Stomach Cancer among Males by Country, 1976

Country	Age-adjusted incidence rates
Japan:	123.6
Miyage	
Okayama	128.2
Osaka	134.6
Singapore, Chinese	63.5
Finland	56.8
Connecticut	20.7
Iowa	14.3

SOURCE: Adapted from *Cancer Incidence in Five Continents*. International Agency for Research on Cancer.[41]

PERSON

In epidemiologic study, usually three characteristics of person are specified: age, sex, and ethnic group or race. In cancer epidemiology especially, the variable of person may also include genetic determinants.

When considering the role genetic predisposition plays in the etiology of cancer, Knudson[25] distinguishes between those instances where tumors segregate as simple Mendelian traits, and where tumors are the product of the interaction between genetic and environmental factors. The embryonic tumors of early childhood are the best-known examples of mendelizing tumors. Regarding the latter, xeroderma pigmentosum and ataxia-telangiectasia are both conditions involving defective repair of damage to DNA; consequently, affected individuals experience an increased risk for certain types of malignancies. Mulvihill[26] presents a detailed compendium of neoplastic diseases which are single-gene traits or the complication of other Mendelian disorders.

In addition to the repository of cancer genes an individual may carry, descriptive variables such as age and sex also serve to characterize patterns of cancer morbidity and mortality. Cancer epidemiologists traditionally have been interested in age-specific incidence patterns, particularly as an aid to understanding the mechanisms of carcinogenesis. In a discussion of various age patterns of cancer incidence, Doll[27] summarizes their epidemiologic significance:

1. A peak incidence in childhood, adolescence, or early adult life can be related to a period of heightened mitotic activity in the tissue, or to a brief exposure to a carcinogenic agent.
2. A rapid and progressive increase in the incidence of cancer with age suggests that the tissue is regularly exposed to a carcinogenic agent over a long period.
3. For those cancers that increase rapidly in incidence with age, the relationship between incidence and age can be described by the equation $I = b(t - w)^k$, where I is the incidence of the cancer, t is the age of the subjects at risk, w is the sum of the pre-exposure period and the length of time needed for the pathological development of the tumor before clinical recognition, b is proportional to the mean daily dose of the agents, and k is approximately 4. With this notation, $t - w$ can also be described as the duration of effective exposure and b may perhaps be more properly defined as the mean dose per mitotic cycle.
4. An unusually rapid increase in incidence with age is due to a long pre-exposure period, a prolonged development time, or a reduction in the exposure of successive cohorts to environmental carcinogens.
5. A reversal of the trend in old age, leading to a peak followed by a decline in incidence, can be a cohort effect due to increasing exposure of successive cohorts to environmental carcinogens. Alternatively, it may be spurious, due to inadequate diagnosis and incomplete use of medical services by old people.
6. A break in the progressive increase in incidence with age, followed by a slower rate of increase or a steady incidence—as in cancer of the breast and cancer of the cervix uteri—may be due to reduction in, or complete cessation of, exposure to carcinogenic agents.

These conclusions, I would stress, are put forward tentatively. They are derived from a few epidemiological data that enable cancer incidence in man to be related quantitatively to exposure to carcinogenic agents and have been supported by an even smaller number of experimental observations in animals. Insofar as they are not trivial much more evidence is needed before they can be regarded as established.

Another well-documented epidemiologic feature of many site-specific cancers is the sex differential. For example, an increased male-female ratio may reflect an increased exposure of the male to some environmental carcinogen in the workplace. Whatever the relationship, male-female differences can be important in specifying etiologic hypotheses.

SOURCES OF DATA

Unique sources of data are available for epidemiologic investigation of malignant diseases. Certain compilations of cancer incidence and mortality data have no counterpart in other disease areas (e.g., cardiovascular disease) and make feasible studies that could not be implemented without these data. Sources of morbidity and mortality data which relate to a defined population will be described briefly.

Mortality Data

U.S. COUNTY MORTALITY DATA

These are mortality data from 1950 to 1969 for all U.S. counties.[28] These data were used to prepare computer-generated maps for 35 cancer sites for males and females. Cancer atlases have been prepared for both white[29] and nonwhite[30] populations. These data have shown a variety of site-specific geographic patterns and clusters. Much of the geographic variation being investigated uses correlational analyses linking county mortality rates with demographic, industrial, and environmental data available at the county level.[31] These correlational studies have proved very useful in formulating specific etiologic hypotheses.

INTERNATIONAL MORTALITY STUDIES

Segi et al.[32-37] have used national death statistics for selected cancer sites in 24 counties from 1950 through 1967 to provide international comparative mortality data. These data are both age- and sex-specific and age-adjusted to a single standard population age distribution. The effects of using vital statistics on the interpretation of international patterns of cancer mortality rates are discussed by Reid.[38]

Morbidity Data

POPULATION-BASED CANCER REGISTRIES

The three volumes of *Cancer Incidence in Five Continents*[39-45] use international incidence data from 62 cancer registers. The most recent volume[41] provides a compilation of international comparative incidence data for selected cancer sites, 1968 to 1972. The main consideration for inclusion of registry data has been the reliability of both numerator and denominator information. This includes examining the adequacy and completeness of reporting to each participating registry. Finally, because geographic variation plays such an important role in identifying populations at high and low risk for cancer, tumor registries were selected on the basis of adequate geographic representation.

NATIONAL CANCER SURVEYS FOR SELECTED U.S. STATES OR CITIES

Since 1937 there have been three national cancer incidence surveys: the *Third National Cancer Survey* (1969–1971),[42] which was a sequel to two earlier surveys, commonly referred to as the *Ten Cities Survey* of 1937[43] and 1947,[44] and the Iowa study of 1950.[49] Detailed information is provided for cancer incidence classified according to sex, race, and age of the patient; anatomic site; and histologic type of the cancer. With some exceptions, the survey data permit trend analysis in cancer morbidity rates from 1937 to 1971. Also, the data are useful for studying variation in incidence among different population groups living in the major geographic regions of the United States.

SURVEILLANCE, EPIDEMIOLOGY, AND END RESULTS (SEER) PROGRAM

The SEER program[46] is an outgrowth of the end results program[47] and the National Cancer Surveys[42-44] of the National Cancer Institute. Among the objectives of SEER is the provision of detailed information on cancer incidence and survivors. Data are collected on demographics, anatomic site, histologic cell type, staging, type of treatment, and follow-up status. The 11 population-based tumor registries participating in the program represent the major geographic regions of the United States.

CENTRALIZED CANCER PATIENT DATA SYSTEM (CCPDS) FOR COMPREHENSIVE CANCER CENTERS

The primary purpose of CCPDS[48] is to provide a statistical base for evaluating the 21 comprehensive cancer centers located throughout the United States. Because CCPDS and SEER are intended to complement each other, both collect and maintain compatible diagnostic treatment and survival rate data.

The tumor registries forming CCPDS, unlike those of the SEER program, do not have referable population bases. Consequently, cancer incidence data are not available from CCPDS.

ANALYTIC EPIDEMIOLOGY

While descriptive epidemiology focuses on the amount and distribution of disease within a population, analytic epidemiology studies the determinants of disease or

TABLE 3-8 Comparison of Retrospective and Prospective Studies

	Retrospective	Prospective
Starting population defined by	Disease	Exposure
Rates computed	Exposure frequency	Disease frequency
Difference in ratio	Excess exposure	Attributable risk
Ratio of rates	Relative exposure	Relative risk
Odds computed	Odds of exposure	Odds of disease
Ratio of odds	Relative odds	Relative odds
Principal determinant of required sample size	Exposure frequency	Disease frequency
Principal bias	Influence of disease on recall of exposure	Influence of exposure on diagnosis of disease
Focus of study	One disease	Multiple disease outcomes

SOURCE: D Schottenfeld: *Cancer Epidemiology and Prevention,* Thomas, Springfield, Ill., 1975. Courtesy of Charles C Thomas, Publisher.

reasons for relatively high or low frequency in specific population groups.

The two principal types of analytic study are retrospective (or case-control) and prospective (or cohort) studies. In a retrospective study, the intent is to measure the frequency of some putative antecedent etiologic factor or characteristic in individuals who have the disease in comparison with those who do not have the disease. Conversely, in a prospective study the investigator starts with a group of individuals with and without the hypothesized etiologic exposure or characteristic. The main distinctions between the two types of study are shown in Table 3-8.

Retrospective Studies

Generally, in a retrospective, or case-control, study a specific hypothesis is being tested, for example, that an association exists between bronchogenic carcinoma and antecedent smoking habits, or between prior occupational exposure to vinyl chloride and angiosarcoma of the liver. It is because the focus of attention is on antecedent exposure to possible etiologic factors that the term *retrospective* was coined. The principal interest in retrospective epidemiologic study is to determine whether among cases there is a greater proportion of individuals with the hypothesized risk factor compared with controls.

The basic design of a retrospective study is shown in the accompanying table. If $a/(a + c)$ is statistically significantly greater than $b/(b + d)$, then a statistical association is said to exist between the disease and the hypothesized etiologic factor. Procedures for determining statistical significance will not be discussed in this chapter. The reader is referred to any one of several elementary biostatistical textbooks.[49,50]

A basic assumption underlying the analysis of retrospective data is that cases selected for study are representative of all persons with the disease. This implies that either all cases with the disease or a representative sample thereof has been ascertained. Other analogous premises are that the control or comparison group is

Framework of a Retrospective Study

Hypothesized etiologic factor	Number of individuals		
	With disease (cases)	Without disease (controls)	
With	a	b	$a + b$
Without	c	d	$c + d$
Total	$a + c$	$b + d$	N

representative of the nondiseased population, or that the prevalence of the characteristic under study is the same in the control group as in the general population.[1] Because the inferential quality of retrospective data is dependent on the extent to which these assumptions are met, the methods used for selecting the cases and controls become very important.

SELECTION OF CASES AND CONTROLS

Various methods have been used to select cases and controls for retrospective studies; frequently they are obtained from hospital patient populations, as in the case-control studies examining the relationship between smoking and lung cancer.[51,52] Case-control studies of this sort are popular because data can usually be collected easily and inexpensively.

A major disadvantage in using hospital patients concerns the introduction of what is commonly called *selection bias*. Berkson[53] was the first to demonstrate that a false association could be obtained between diseases or between a characteristic and a disease because of differential probabilities of admission to a hospital for those with the disease, without the disease, and with the characteristic of interest. Selection bias may be controlled by obtaining controls from more than one source, permitting comparisons between cases and different control groups. For example, an investigator can select a hospital control and a nonhospitalized control (e.g., an individual who resides in the same neighborhood as the case). Consistency of findings based on such multiple comparisons will increase the strength of the inferences derived from case-control studies. For those interested in a more detailed discussion of the different sources available for selecting cases and controls in retrospective studies, either MacMahon and Pugh[54] or Lilienfeld[1] should be consulted.

CONFOUNDING VARIABLES

Confounding variables are defined by MacMahon and Pugh[54] as variables which may introduce differences between cases and controls that do not reflect differences in the variables of primary interest.

In retrospective studies, matching is one of the most common techniques used to ensure that the controls are similar to the cases with respect to certain confounding variables. The procedure requires that the individuals selected from the control population match the corresponding case with respect to specified criteria. Examples of these criteria include age, sex, and race. In retrospective studies involving collaboration with other institutions, *institution* is used frequently as a matching criterion to control for bias arising from interinstitutional variability, both with respect to diagnostic acumen and methods as well as procedures for data collection and handling. In addition, it is often necessary to control for the heterogeneous distribution of demographic characteristics for patients by institution. An alternate method for controlling confounding is to use statistical techniques in adjusting the data during the analytic phase of the study.[55,56] Choice of the appropriate method to be used for controlling confounding should be made in consultation with a biostatistician.

Prospective Studies

Because of limitations of inferences derived from retrospective studies, it is desirable to confirm any association observed in a retrospective study by using prospective (or cohort) methodology. According to Lilienfeld[1] the concept of a prospective study is a relatively simple one:

A sample of the population is selected and information is obtained to determine if they have the characteristic, whether a particular living habit, exposure to a possible etiological agent, or a physiological trait, that may be related to the development of the disease being investigated. These people are then followed for several years to observe which ones develop and/or die from that disease.

Morbidity or mortality rates are then calculated, and the rates for those exposed and not exposed are compared. An association is said to exist between an exposure variable and the disease of interest when these rates differ. Just as it is important to control confounding in retrospective studies, it is equally important to do so in prospective studies. It is necessary, therefore, to collect data regarding the comparability of the exposed and nonexposed populations. Such data would routinely include age, sex, race, or any other variable known to be related to the disease of interest. Statistical methods are available for examining the "statistical effect" of confounding on the outcome measure (disease, no disease) and for adjusting the outcome measure for those effects.[56] At present, there are two generally recognized types of prospective studies: concurrent and nonconcurrent studies. A diagrammatic representation contrasting these two different approaches is shown in Fig. 3-2.

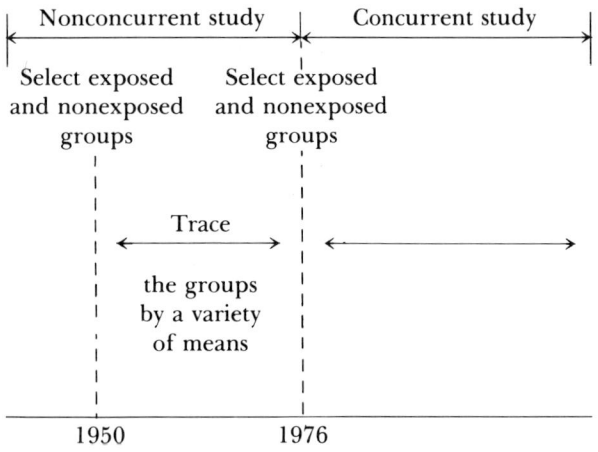

FIGURE 3-2 Diagrammatic representation of concurrent and nonconcurrent prospective studies. (*From A Lilienfeld: Foundations of Epidemiology, Oxford University Press, New York, 1976.*)

The distinction between concurrent and nonconcurrent study is a particularly important one in the epidemiologic study of cancer. The long latency periods associated with most malignant diseases make it desirable to have an available method for combining the "retrospective" identification of special exposure groups with the "prospective" ability of determining the risk (or probability) of developing the disease of interest in the presence or absence of the hypothesized risk factor(s).

Many examples of concurrent prospective studies of cancer can be found in the literature. Several well-known examples include (1) the American Cancer Society study of approximately 190,000 white males,[57] (2) the study of smoking and mortality rate in 293,658 veterans who held U.S. government life insurance policies in 1953.[58,59]

Examples illustrating the use of nonconcurrent methodology include (1) cancer mortality rate following radiation therapy for ankylosing spondylitis,[60] (2) risk of leukemia in individuals receiving Thorotrast in Portugal between 1930 and 1955,[61] (3) leukemogenic effect of radiation among atomic bomb survivors in Hiroshima and Nagasaki.[62–64]

At present, nonconcurrent studies are particularly popular in the study of occupationally related neoplastic diseases. Examples of special occupation groups which have been studied include radiologists,[65] radium dial painters,[66] and asbestos workers.[67]

One of the major difficulties in conducting both concurrent and nonconcurrent prospective studies concerns the possible introduction of biases due to the differential follow-up of exposed and nonexposed persons. Methods should be developed from the beginning of the study to reduce, to the extent possible, the number of individuals lost to follow-up. Nonconcurrent studies pose the additional problem of having to go back in time, perhaps 20 to 30 years, and trace individuals forward in time from their initial exposure to the etiologic factor of interest.

Because of difficulties related to follow-up and unequal periods of observation, two closely related methods of analyzing prospective studies are available: (1) life tables and (2) calculation of person-years (or -months) of observation as the denominator for the computation of incidence or mortality rates.

Some consider life-table analysis the preferred method of examining the probability of developing or dying from a particular disease.[68,69] Person-years of observation of patients are frequently used as denominators in the computation of rates in prospective studies, particularly when it is not possible to use life-table analysis because of varying periods of observation as a result of individuals entering and leaving the study at different ages and times.

Measures for Comparing Risks

The basic difference between prospective and retrospective studies concerns the outcome measure being investigated: prospective studies, whether concurrent or nonconcurrent, are concerned with estimating the risk of disease among exposed and nonexposed; while retrospective studies are concerned with determining whether exposure rates differ among diseased and nondiseased individuals. Ultimately, the epidemiologist needs to evaluate whether an association exists between a suspected etiologic factor and a disease. There are three measures used for making this evaluation: relative risk, odds ratio, and attributable risk. These measures are defined as follows.

Relative risk is the ratio of the incidence (or death) rates in the population exposed to the putative etiologic factor to the incidence (or death) rates in the population not exposed to the putative etiologic factor.

Odds ratio (or *cross-product ratio*) is the ratio of the probability that disease will occur when the putative etiologic factor is present to the probability that disease will occur when the putative etiologic factor is absent.

Attributable risk is the absolute difference in incidence (or death) rates between the population exposed and not exposed to the putative etiologic factor. In case-control studies only the odds ratio can be meaningfully calculated. This is owing to the fact that both the relative and attributable risk estimates are dependent upon knowing the population distribution of both the disease and the characteristic or etiologic factor of interest. Under certain circumstances the odds ratio is a good approximation of relative risk. For a complete discussion of the statistical properties of relative risk, odds ratio, and attributable risk, the reader is urged to consult Fleiss.[70]

Causal Inferences from Epidemiologic Studies

Direct evidence of a causal relationship between an etiologic agent and a disease can be provided only by experimentation and elucidation of the biologic mechanism. Although inferences drawn from epidemiologic studies may take into account all of the known and relevant biologic knowledge concerning the disease at hand, data from which these inferences are drawn are still several steps removed from the actual disease process. Even though a causal relationship between cigarette smoking and lung cancer is highly probable, based on available epidemiologic evidence, knowledge regarding the biologic mechanism of either the particulate or gaseous phase of cigarette smoking in the pathogenesis of lung cancer remains incomplete. As a framework within which to evaluate causal inferences drawn from epidemiologic data, Lilienfeld[1] presents a series of postulates paralleling those of Koch:

1. Prevalence of the disease should be significantly higher in those exposed to the hypothesized cause than in controls not so exposed.
2. Exposure to the hypothesized cause should be more frequent among those with the disease than in controls without the disease—when all other risk factors are held constant.
3. Incidence of the disease should be significantly higher in those exposed to the cause than in those not so exposed, as shown by prospective studies.
4. Temporally, the disease should follow exposure to the hypothesized causative agent with a distribution of incubation periods on a bell-shaped curve.
5. A spectrum of host responses should follow exposure to the hypothesized agent along a logical biological gradient from mild to severe.
6. A measurable host response following exposure to the hypothesized cause should have a high probability of appearing in those lacking this before exposure (e.g., antibody, cancer cells), or should increase in magnitude if present before exposure; this response pattern should occur infrequently in persons not so exposed.
7. Experimental reproduction of the disease should occur frequently in animals or man appropriately exposed to hypothesized cause than in those not so exposed; this exposure may be deliberate in volunteers, experimentally induced in the laboratory, or may represent a regulation of natural exposure.
8. Elimination or modification of the hypothesized cause should decrease the incidence of the disease (i.e., attenuation of a virus, removal of tar from cigarettes).
9. Prevention or modification of the host's response on exposure to the hypothesized cause should decrease or eliminate the disease (i.e., immunization, drugs to lower cholesterol, specific lymphocyte transfer factor in cancer).
10. All of the relationships and findings should make biologic and epidemiologic sense.

EPIDEMIOLOGIC FEATURES OF SELECTED SITE-SPECIFIC CANCERS

Cancer is a group of diseases that differ in occurrence, by anatomic site and within human populations. Epidemiologic observations about cancer in human populations have demonstrated that the distribution and occurrence of specific forms of malignant neoplasms are associated with a variety of factors such as age, sex, race, socioeconomic status, and occupational exposures. For epidemiologic purposes, therefore, it is better to think of cancer as a collection of diseases, with cancer of each site considered separately. Several of the more interesting differences in the distribution of site-specific cancers and hypothesized risk factors are presented below.

Nasopharynx

Cancer of the nasopharynx (ICD-CM-9:147) is rare in the United States, and incidence rates have remained fairly constant over the past 30 years. Rates are higher for males in almost every age group. Nonwhites show higher rates than whites.

While relatively rare in most countries, cancer of the nasopharynx is found frequently in southern China and is fairly common in other populations of Southeast Asia. An increased frequency has also been reported in North Africa, Malta, and in Eskimo populations. Chinese migrants to the United States show rates much higher than do native-born whites. There is some evidence of a decreased risk of nasopharyngeal cancer for Chinese born in the United States.

Risk factors associated with nasopharyngeal carcinoma include opium smoking, exposures to smoke and fumes, and history of prior ear, nose, or throat disease. Circumstantial evidence has associated Epstein-Barr virus (EBV) with this cancer since virtually every patient with nasopharyngeal cancer has anti-EBV antibodies with mean titers substantially higher than among controls.[71]

Occupational exposures are associated with increased risk of cancer of the mouth and pharynx for printing press operators and textile workers. Workers exposed to chromium, isopropyl oil, nickel, and wood dust are at increased risk for cancer of the nasal cavity and sinuses.

Digestive System

ESOPHAGUS

Cancer of the esophagus (ICD-9-CM: 150), a relatively rare cancer in the United States, is increasing markedly in incidence in black males but not in white males or in females. At present, in black males cancer of the esophagus ranks sixth among the 10 most frequent cancer sites. In the other sex-color groups, the esophagus does not rank among the first 10 sites. The age-adjusted death rate for esophageal cancer accounts for 5 percent of the combined rate for all sites in nonwhite males.[72]

Cancer of the esophagus shows wide geographic variation in incidence. High frequencies are reported from France, Switzerland, South Africa, Iran, the Caribbean and northern China.[73] A feature of this cancer is the widely contrasting incidence within relatively limited geographic areas, e.g., around Lake Victoria and in the Iranian Caspian provinces of Mazanderan and Gilan, where a 30-fold gradient in incidence exists in females.[74] Age-adjusted death rates for esophageal cancer for all migrant groups, except Hungarian and Italian females, were higher than in the United States.[75]

Genetically similar groups that are geographically widely separated show differences in incidence. For instance, the Indians of Natal, South Africa, have a lower rate than Indians in Bombay; blacks of west Africa have a lower rate than U.S. blacks (75 percent of American blacks are descended from west Africans). Environmental factors are probably responsible for such differences in risk.[76]

Epidemiologic studies have suggested that alcohol consumption and tobacco smoking may be of etiologic significance.[77] Because alcohol consumption is nearly ubiquitous and varies geographically less than esophageal cancer rates, it is suggested that the carcinogenic agent elevating the risk in alcohol drinkers is not alcohol but a contaminant. Esophageal cancer may also be related to the nitrosamine content of some beverages.[78] Other suggested etiologic factors are chewing betel nuts, contamination of food with silica particles, consumption of tannin-rich foods, and Plummer-Vinson syndrome.

STOMACH

Incidence and mortality rates for stomach cancer (ICD-9-CM:151) have shown a substantial secular decline in the United States for the past several decades,[58,79] although nonwhites and the foreign-born continue to be at greater risk. Since it is fairly certain that changes in the genetic structure of the population could not produce this effect in so short a time, such a marked change may indicate a decrease in exposure of the population to etiologic agents in the environment.[27]

Internationally, age-adjusted mortality rates for stomach cancer are high for Japan, Chile, Austria, and several Eastern European countries.[80] Relatively low risks are reported for some parts of Latin America, Mozambique, Java, and among South African Bantus, but the data for the non-Western populations are fragmentary.[81] Within the United States, mortality rates from stomach cancer are highest in the northeastern states and lowest in the southern states for both whites and nonwhites.[82]

Migrants from high-risk to low-risk areas show a large excess risk of stomach cancer over time compared with the rates of the population in the low-risk host country.[28] This excess risk decreases in the descendants of the migrants, but the risk still may exceed that of the native-born population, which suggests an environmental factor in the pathogenesis of this neoplasm.

Of the two major histologic types of adenocarcinoma of the stomach, an "intestinal type" of stomach cancer predominates in high-risk areas while a "diffuse type" is seen most frequently in low-risk areas.[13,83] The risk of the intestinal type rises in males, after age 40, causing a rise in the male-female ratio from close to 1 at young ages to almost 2 at ages 55 to 60; the ratio thereafter declines as rates for females begin to rise. Intestinal metaplasia of the stomach may represent a precursor of the intestinal type of cancer; this metaplasia may be irreversibly established at an early age by an environmental agent. This could account for the continued high liability of gastric cancer observed in migrants from high- to low-risk countries.[24,76]

Many countries report higher incidence rates of stomach cancer among lower socioeconomic classes and in certain occupational groups, e.g., heavily exposed asbestos workers, textile workers, and coal miners.[84] Several studies have shown that close relatives of stomach cancer patients are at increased risk of the disease, but this may be due more to a shared environment than to any inherited susceptibility.

An apparent association between diet and stomach cancer has suggested that consumption of foods prepared or preserved by certain methods—e.g., smoked, pickled, or salted foods—and lack of fresh fruits and green leafy vegetables may be significant etiologic factors. International, regional, and cultural differences in food habits may also explain the geographic and ethnic variation in incidence. Other associations include pernicious anemia, achlorhydria, gastritis, and n-nitroso compounds. No significant relationships have been found between stomach cancer and the use of alcohol, tobacco, and spices, or the temperature of foods and beverages.

LARGE BOWEL

Large-bowel cancer [colon (ICD-9-CM:153) and rectal cancer (ICD-9-CM:154) combined] is the most frequent type of cancer and the second leading cause of cancer deaths in the United States. More than 90 percent of the patients are age 40 years or older. For purposes of reporting, large-bowel cancer is usually separated into colon cancer and cancer of the rectum.

For colon cancer, white male incidence rates have been increasing slightly over the past 30 years, whereas rates for white females have been leveling off for the same period. Mortality rates for colon cancer have increased for white males and decreased slightly for white females. Incidence and mortality rates have risen for blacks for the past three decades and are now approaching the rates for whites of the same sex.

For cancer of the rectum, incidence and mortality rates have been decreasing except in black males, who show a reverse trend. For both sexes, white rates are generally higher than those for blacks, although this difference is gradually diminishing. The recent decrease in rectal cancer rates may be due to changes in specifying the anatomic site of the cancer.

Internationally, Scotland and Denmark have relatively high mortality rates for cancer of both colon and rectum. Africa, China, and Japan rank low for both sites. Since cancers of the large intestine and rectum arise in similar tissue, populations with differing colon-rectum ratios are of epidemiologic interest. For example, Austria and Germany rank significantly lower for colon cancer than for rectal cancer, while the reverse is true for Australia and U.S. whites. The apparent differences in tumor localization may be artifactual due to anatomic classification practices and quality of death certifications. The international differences, however, may be due to different etiologies for cancer of the rectum and of the colon. High-risk populations show an excess of tumors in the upper sigmoid, descending colon, and upper rectum–rectosigmoid areas.[85]

Observations on migrants to the United States from Japan, Norway, and Poland, countries where much lower risks of the colon and/or rectum prevail, suggest a role for environmental agent(s) since the changes in risk have occurred in too short a time to be ascribed to genetic changes. Colon cancer mortality among these migrants has tended to rise to the U.S. level, with the displacement being more complete for men than for women.[75,86,87] The offspring of migrants born in the United States appear to experience the colon and rectum risks typical of the communities in which they reside.

Within the United States, the highest rates for colorectal cancer are found in the northeastern states. There is also some increase in bowel cancer rates in urban as opposed to rural populations, although this gradient is small. Colon cancer risk increases slightly with higher socioeconomic status, while for rectal cancer a small trend in the opposite direction is seen. Slight increased risk of bowel cancer has been found in males occupationally exposed to asbestos.

Two main hypotheses have been suggested in carcinogenesis of the large bowel. The first, advocated initially by Burkitt,[88] concerns protection from bowel cancer risk by high dietary fiber content. While international differences in large-bowel cancer rates support this, direct dietary studies within populations have not consistently found decreased risk with increased dietary fiber content.

The second hypothesis centers on increased bowel cancer risk due to the frequent ingestion of meat, particularly animal fats. This hypothesis is supported by studies of international dietary differences, case-control studies of diet and colon cancer,[89] and laboratory studies of animals and humans, suggesting that meat or fat ingestion could enhance carcinogenic activity in the bowel. Some studies have also attempted to link these dietary factors to changes in the bile acid content of the colon or to the bacterial flora. A recent dietary study of colon cancer cases has found a protective effect from the ingestion of crucifers (cabbage, brussel sprouts, and broccoli). Animal research has shown that the high indole content of these vegetables blocks the carcinogenic activity of some intestinal carcinogens. It has been suggested that rectal cancer in particular may be related to beer consumption, but data from several studies are conflicting.

The other major etiologic risk factor for colorectal cancer is the presence of adenomatous polyps. A high risk for large-bowel cancer has been found in patients with familial polyposis (Gardner's syndrome and Peutz-Jeghers syndrome) and with colorectal polyposis. Populations at high risk for colon cancer have been found to have a higher incidence of polyps in the anatomic location most frequently affected by colorectal cancer. Patients who have had ulcerative colitis for 2 years or more and immediate relatives of patients with large-bowel cancer are also at increased risk for colon cancer.

PANCREAS

The pancreas (ICD-9-CM:157) is among the 10 most frequent sites of cancer in the United States. In the industrialized countries of North America and Europe, an increase in incidence has been reported, but this may be due to improved diagnosis. In the United States, the age-adjusted mortality rates are highest for nonwhite males and lowest for white females. Age-adjusted mortality rates for pancreatic cancer show an increasing trend after age 45 for both sexes among whites.[82] Some of the nonwhite excess in age-adjusted mortality rates (14 percent for males; 15 percent for females) may be due to the differential over- and undernumeration in the census of the nonwhite population at older and younger ages respectively[90]; it is almost certain however, that the black-white differential in mortality from pancreatic cancer is real.

In most countries, incidence rates for pancreatic cancer are low, especially in Italy,[91] but a high frequency of this cancer has been reported among Maoris in New Zealand. Worldwide, the highest rates are found among nonwhites in the United States.

The increased risk of cancer of the pancreas in cigarette smokers is supported by histologic evidence. Atypical changes have been observed in the nuclei of pancreatic duct cells among smokers coming to autopsy, with the extent of such changes increasing with the amount of smoking.[92]

A study of diabetics showed a statistically significant excessive cancer mortality rate only for malignancies of the pancreas.[93] This suggests the possible role of exogeneous insulin—a substance with known teratogenic and antigenic activity—in pancreatic carcinogenesis. Chronic pancreatitis is frequently mentioned as a causal factor, but it is difficult to separate its effects from those of chronic alcoholism, with which it is frequently associated.[94] Industrial agents have been repeatedly suspected, particularly since chemicals can induce pancreatic cancer in laboratory animals. Yet the evidence so far is fragmentary.

Lung

Cancer of the lung (ICD-9-CM:162), a rare disease 50 years ago, is now the most common cause of death from cancer among males in the United States. While part of the increased incidence rate may be due to improved diagnosis, the upward trend reflects a true increase in risk. There is little difference in the age-adjusted mortality rates between whites and blacks. Incidence rates for blacks are showing a slightly greater increase than rates for whites. Although mortality rates for females are only one-sixth of the total lung cancer deaths, recent increases in smoking by women have led to a decline in the male-female mortality ratio.[95]

Internationally, the highest rates for lung cancer are found in Scotland, England and Wales, and Finland. The lowest rates are observed in Portugal. Age-adjusted death rates among migrant groups of both sexes are higher than among U.S. native whites, although rates in most countries of origin are lower than those in U.S. whites. This confirms the strong influence of environmental factors in the pathogenesis of this neoplasm.

Extensive data from studies of lung cancer have confirmed the association of cigarette smoking with excess risks in mortality and morbidity.[96] Cigarette smoking is the chief epidemiologic factor in epidermoid carcinoma of the lung. Pulmonary adenocarcinoma does not appear to be significantly affected by smoking. There is some evidence of an interaction between smoking and occupational exposure to asbestos or uranium so that the relative risk is greater than expected.

Factors associated with increased risk include air pollution, low socioeconomic status, and urbanization. Occupational groups at high risk are uranium miners, painters, carpenters, and handlers of chromate, nickel, and asbestos.

Breast

Cancer of the breast (ICD-9-CM:174) is the most frequent cancer and the leading cause of cancer mortality in black and white females in the United States. This cancer rarely occurs in males. Although incidence has increased, mortality rates have remained relatively unchanged since 1940 because of increased survival rates. Incidence rates tend to be higher for white females than those for black females.

A bimodal age distribution of breast cancer incidence, with one pre- and one postmenopausal peak and a slight dip around the age of menopause, suggests that etiologic factors in breast cancer may differ for pre- and postmenopausal females.[97,98]

International data show the highest incidence rates occur in North America and in Western Europe. Much lower rates are observed in developing nations and in Asia, especially Japan. Polish and Irish migrants to the United States show an increased risk of breast cancer, whereas Japanese migrants maintain the low rates characteristic of Japan. Cancer of the breast is relatively uncommon among Chinese Americans and among American Indians. These data support the importance of genetic factors but do not rule out environmental factors.

Epidemiologic research suggests that environmental, reproductive, and demographic variables as well as heredity (familial predisposition) may influence the risk of breast cancer (Table 3-9).

In high-risk areas, breast cancer rates generally increase with higher socioeconomic levels. Early age at first full pregnancy seems to exert a protective effect from breast cancer. Early age at menarche and late age at natural menopause, however, are factors which appear to increase risk. Increased risk has also been associated with higher estrogen/androgen ratios, and estriol/estrone-estradial ratios.[99] Other risk factors include obesity, history of benign breast disease, ionizing radiation, and a high fat and animal protein diet. Research to date has not indicated that oral contraceptives increase the risk of breast cancer.

Type B virus particles structurally similar to mouse mammary tumor virus have been observed in human milk and breast cancer tissue, but the evidence for a viral etiology is not conclusive.

TABLE 3-9 Summary of Risk Factors for Breast Cancer

Variable	Risk of breast cancer	
	Lower	Higher
Race	Oriental	Caucasian
Caucasian admixture in Negroes	Lesser	Greater
Ethnic group	Gentiles	Jews
Marital status	Married	Single
Age at first pregnancy	Younger	Older
Number of pregnancies	More	Fewer
Age at menarche	Later	Earlier
Artificial menopause	Present	Absent
Benign breast disease	Absent	Present
Family history of breast cancer	Absent	Present
Socioeconomic status	Lower	Higher
Blood group phenotype ss in S antigen system	Absent	Present
Obesity; high intake of butter, cheese, milk, green vegetables, sugar, fat	Absent	Present

SOURCE: C Zippen, NL Petrakis: Identification of high risk groups in breast cancer. *Cancer* 28:1381–1387, 1971.

Genitourinary System

CERVIX OF THE UTERUS

Incidence and mortality rates for invasive carcinomas of the cervix (ICD-9-CM:180) have been declining rapidly in the United States. Incidence among nonwhite females is twice that among white females, although the rates for nonwhites are also declining. There were twice as many in situ carcinomas as there were invasive carcinomas for whites and nonwhites. Incidence and mortality rates for cervical cancer increase gradually with age after the age of 20.

Worldwide, cervical cancer shows marked variations in frequency. It is the most common cancer in women in Latin America and in Africa, whereas the incidence is much lower in the United States and Israel.

This neoplasm has been shown to have strong associations with sexual activity, but the nature of the mechanism is not yet understood. Cervical cancer is rare in nuns, very frequent among prostitutes, and more frequent among married women than single women and among women having multiple marriages and multiple sexual partners.[100] Although a low rate has been observed in Jewish women, circumcision of male partners is no longer considered the cause of this phenomenon. An excess number of cervical cancer patients with previous herpes simplex type 2 virus have been reported, but no etiologic link has as yet been established.[101]

Some cases of clear-cell adenocarcinoma of the cervix have been reported for maternal exposure during pregnancy to stilbestrol and related compounds.[102]

The role of the Papanicolaou smear in the declining incidence of cervical cancer is also controversial. Prior to the widespread use of cytological screening, the incidence of this disease was already declining. Studies of the usual time course of histopathologic changes in the development of cervical cancer and the effectiveness of frequent use of this screening technique indicate its usefulness is more beneficial in females at high risk.[103] Studies of high-risk populations in other countries indicate a more rapid histopathologic transition from in situ lesions to invasive cervical cancer.

PROSTATE

Cancer of the prostate (ICD-9-CM:185) is the second most common form of malignant neoplasm among U.S. males. Over the past four decades, incidence rates have risen slightly for U.S. whites, whereas incidence and mortality rates have risen sharply for U.S. blacks.[104] Mortality from prostatic cancer ranks second among all cancer sites for U.S. blacks; the third most frequent in U.S. whites. A comparison of age-adjusted mortality rates for prostatic cancer in various countries shows the highest mortality rate for U.S. nonwhites, although an overall increase in mortality has been reported in many countries. Worldwide, the highest rates are found in the United States, Canada, New Zealand, and Western Europe, with the lowest rates in Japan and Israel. Among Japanese migrants to the United States, the incidence of prostatic cancer has been increasing.[105] Irish migrants exhibited the greatest excess in mortality from this neoplasm.[75] Mortality rates for cancer of the prostate do not begin to rise until about age 40, when the mortality rate increases almost linearly and continuously throughout life, with nonwhite rates remaining higher than those for whites.

Relatively little is known about the etiology of prostatic cancer. Researchers have been unable to induce an analogue to human prostate cancer in experimental animals. Some epidemiologic studies of this cancer suggest increased frequency among male relatives of prostatic cancer patients. No urban-rural differences are observed in mortality rates from cancer of the prostate among whites. The major demographic features include a higher frequency among married than single men (in contrast to other neoplasms) and a higher frequency among blacks.[106] Increased risk may also be associated with male sexual activity.[107] Viral and hormonal etiologies have also been suggested. An excess frequency of viral and gram-negative bacterial infections of the prostate has been noted in patients with cancer of the prostate, although this may be a manifestation of the disease process itself rather than an etiologic factor.

BLADDER

Cancer of the bladder (ICD-90-CM:188) is the eighth most common cancer in the United States. The incidence is highest among white males and lowest among black females. In both races, 80 percent of the cancer of the bladder occurs among males. The trend of bladder cancer incidence in males and females differs markedly.[108] Among both white and black men the incidence has been increasing, in contrast to a decrease in incidence among women.

Internationally, the highest rates for bladder cancer are found in the United States, Israel, Canada, and parts of Africa. The lowest rates are found in Eastern Europe. No discernible difference is apparent in the mortality for the various migrant groups and countries of origin. Within the United States, the highest bladder cancer rates are found in urban areas such as in the northeast, especially New Jersey.

Demographic factors associated with bladder cancer are urbanization and a higher frequency in males. A known risk factor is occupational exposure to β-naphthylamine and other aromatic amines in the aniline dye industry. Cigarette smoking is also considered important as an etiologic factor.[109] The causal role of coffee is equivocal. Schistosomiasis, a parasitic infection, has been associated, both clinically and geographically, with bladder cancer in Egypt.[150] More recent controversy has centered on the role of saccharin in the etiology of bladder cancer. However, human studies to date have given conflicting results.

At present, the National Cancer Institute is conducting a national study of bladder cancer. One objective of the study is designed to investigate the relation between drinking water quality and bladder cancer. Specifically, trihalomethane exposure is being examined closely.

Lymphomas

Lymphomas (ICD-9-CM:200), including multiple myeloma, are presently the sixth most frequent type of cancer in the United States. The major lymphomas are Hodgkin's disease, lymphosarcoma, and reticulum-cell sarcoma. Incidence and mortality rates for these cancers have generally been increasing in the United States since 1950. There is a pronounced black-white differential in both morbidity and mortality rates for multiple myeloma. Male rates are about 50 percent higher than female rates.

Over 20 percent of all lymphomas are diagnosed as Hodgkin's disease, the most common neoplasms in the young adult group and later at ages 65 to 74. The male-female ratio is higher in the younger age groups and gradually declines with time. The age-specific rates for other lymphomas show a more stable rise with increasing age.

Internationally, the highest rates for lymphomas and Hodgkin's disease are found in the United States and Western Europe, with lower rates in Japan, Asia, and developing countries. Burkitt's lymphoma is an unusual sarcoma occurring virtually only in children in Africa and New Guinea. Burkitt's lymphoma shows an association with Epstein-Barr virus, with a possible synergistic role for malaria infection.

The clinical symptoms of Hodgkin's disease (fever and sweats) that are particularly common in young adults are suggestive of a response to an infectious agent. This hypothesis is supported by evidence that the risk for family associates of Hodgkin's disease cases in contracting the disease is three times that of the general population, that case clustering has been noted with apparent spread via cases and contacts,[111] and that some mononucleosis patients may subsequently develop the disease.[112] Epstein-Barr virus has been suggested as an etiologic agent since elevated antibody titers to this virus have been reported in some individuals with Hodgkin's disease. Similarities of Hodgkin's disease are noted, however, with infectious mononucleosis and Burkitt's lymphoma, both of which are associated with Epstein-Barr viruses. The etiologic role of EBV in Hodgkin's disease is still equivocal. Tonsillectomy has also been reported as a risk factor in Hodgkin's disease, but data are conflicting.

Increased incidence of reticulum-cell sarcoma is found in persons taking immunosuppressive drugs.

Occupational exposures may be of importance in the etiology of lymphomas. Increased risk has been found in chemists and arsenic workers.

MULTIPLE PRIMARY NEOPLASMS

The occurrence of multiple cancers in the same person (two or more primary malignant tumors in different locations) has demonstrated that with certain sites, there is a substantial excess risk of a second cancer in the same or different organ or in a paired organ. The development of the second primary tumor may be due to the same etiologic factor(s) responsible for the first primary or to the carcinogenic action of radiation or chemotherapy used for treating the first primary.

Although the number of individuals who develop second primary tumors is small compared with the number of those who develop first tumors, certain site pairs seem to occur with unusually high frequency. By comparing the observed and expected number of second primary tumors, it is possible to show that the site pairs occur more frequently than expected on the basis of chance. In order to be meaningful, the observed associations need not only statistically significant results but also biologically plausible mechanisms. Grouping of certain tumor complexes according to possible etiologic explanations is presented in Table 3-10.

The establishment of tumor registries and good follow-up procedures of well-defined population groups will permit the accumulation of data necessary to define the risk of subsequent primary cancer with more precision. Findings from such studies are of immediate value to the clinician concerned with detecting the second malignancy at the earliest possible stage. These analyses are also useful in identifying the high-risk cancer patients, and these individuals warrant further study for possible etiologic factors.

FAMILIAL SUSCEPTIBILITY

The aggregation of cancer in families is a well-documented phenomenon. Data accumulated during the first half of this century[113] indicate that a family history of a neoplasm can double a person's risk for developing that neoplasm. The excess risk of developing cancer of the same site for relatives of cancer patients does not appear to be due solely to chance.

Available data suggest increased familial risk of cancer of the same site for cancers of the breast (in women), stomach, lung, large intestine, endometrium, prostate, and possibly ovary.[76] The etiologic significance of familial aggregation of tumors is still undecided. The risk factors

TABLE 3-10 Examples of Site-Group Pairs with Excess of Observed or Expected Second Primary Malignancies

Suggested etiologic factors	Complexes of multiple primary neoplasms
1. Common etiologic factors	
a. Same or paired organs	Multicentric colorectal carcinoma
	Bilateral breast carcinoma
b. Chemical carcinogens	
(1) Tobacco	Carcinomas of upper respiratory and gastrointestinal tracts
	Carcinomas of lung and bladder
(2) Mineral oil	Carcinomas of scrotum and lung
c. Endocrine and nutritional	Carcinomas of breast, uterine corpus, ovary, and colon
	Meningioma and carcinoma of breast (?)
d. Genetic	Carcinomas of colon and uterine corpus
	Retinoblastoma and lower extremity osteosarcoma
	Multiple endocrine adenomatosis: Tumors of anterior pituitary; parathyroid; pancreatic islet cells; and, less frequently, neoplasms of the thyroid, adrenal cortex, and carcinoid tumors of the intestine and bronchus
	Hippel-Lindau disease: Hemangiomas of the retina and cerebellum with an excessive frequency of hypernephroma, pheochromocytoma, and ependymoma
	Von Recklinghausen's disease: Multiple neurofibromas, glioma, meningioma, acoustic neuroma, and pheochromocytoma
	Pheochromocytoma, medullary thyroid carcinoma, multiple neuromas, and parathyroid tumors
	Turcot's syndrome: Polyposis of colon and brain tumors
	Gardner's syndrome: Polyposis of colon with osteomas, fibromas, lipomas, and epidermal cysts
2. Treatment	
a. Radiation	Rectal cancer following cancer of the uterine corpus or cervix
	Osteosarcoma, soft-tissue sarcoma, or skin cancer of the orbit following retinoblastoma
b. Chemotherapy	Other neoplasms following Hodgkin's disease
	Acute myeloblastic or acute myelomonoblastic leukemia following multiple myeloma
c. Surgery	Lymphangiosarcoma following breast cancer
3. Immune defects	Thymoma and other primary neoplasms
	Chronic lymphatic leukemia and skin cancer
4. Unknown etiologic significance	
a. Confirmed by other studies	Breast and salivary gland cancers
b. Unconfirmed by other studies	Prostate or testis cancers with leukemia

SOURCE: BS Schoenberg: Multiple primary neoplasms, in JF Fraumini, Jr (ed): *Persons at High Risk of Cancer*, Academic Press, New York, 1975.

involved may be inherited susceptibility or common exposure to known or unknown environmental carcinogenic agents. The possible interaction between genetic and environmental factors has only recently become an area for more detailed investigation.

Some relatively rare neoplasms are inherited, in whole or in part, in a definite Mendelian manner, such as Gardner's syndrome.[114] There are also a number of relatively rare genetically determined disorders that increase the risk of developing specific types of cancer, such as multiple polyposis and cancer of the colon, Fanconi's and Bloom's syndrome and leukemia, xeroderma pigmentosum and skin cancer. In addition, there are some associations between chromosome structure and malignancy, such as Down's syndrome and acute lymphoblastic leukemia.

Several cancer syndromes within families have also been reported in which family members present excess numbers of specific combinations of tumors that are similar to those experienced by individuals with multiple primary neoplasms.

REFERENCES

1. Lilienfeld AM: *Foundations of Epidemiology*, Oxford University Press, New York, 1976.
2. Lilienfeld D: Definitions of epidemiology. *Am J Epidemiol* 107:87–90, 1978.
3. Lilienfeld AM et al: *Cancer Epidemiology: Methods of Study*, Johns Hopkins Press, Baltimore, 1967.
4. Pott P: *The Chirurgical Works of Percival Pott—1775*, W Clarke, R Collins (eds), Hawes, London, 1775.
5. Shimkin MB, Triolo VA: History of chemical carcinogenesis: Some prospective remarks. *Prog Exp Tumor Res* 11:1–20, 1967.
6. Cook JW et al: Production of cancer by pure hydrocarbons: Part I. *Proc Roy Soc* 3:455–484, 1932.
7. Cook JW, Hewett CL: The isolation of a cancer producing hydrocarbon from coal tar. *J Chem Soc* 1:395–405, 1933.
8. World Health Organization: *International Classification of Diseases: Clinical Modification*, 9th rev., Commission on Professional and Hospital Activities, Ann Arbor, Mich.; 1978.
9. World Health Organization: *International Classification of Diseases for Oncology*, Geneva, 1976.
10. World Health Organization: *International Histological Classification of Tumours*, Geneva, 1900.
11. Jarvi O, Lauren P: On the role of heteropias of the intestinal epithelium in the pathogenesis of gastric cancer. *Acta Pathol Microbiol Scand* 29:26–45, 1951.
12. Lauren P: The two histological main types of gastric carcinoma: Diffuse and so-called intestinal type carcinoma. An attempt at a histo-clinical classification. *Acta Pathol Microbiol Scand* 64:31–49, 1965.
13. Correa P et al: Carcinoma and intestinal metaplasia of the stomach in Colombian migrants. *J Nat Cancer Inst* 44:297–306, 1970.
14. Correa P et al: *Epidemiology of Different Types of Thyroid Cancer*, UICC Conference on Thyroid Cancer, Lausanne, 1968.
15. Kreyberg L: Non-smokers and geographical pathology of lung cancer, in AA Liebow et al (eds): *The Lung*, Williams & Wilkins, Baltimore, 1968.
16. Berg JW: Some intercountry and intergroup differences in histological types of cancer. *J Chronic Dis* 23:325–334, 1970.
17. Peto R: Epidemiology, multistage models and short-term mutagenicity tests, in HH Hiatt et al (eds): *Origins of Human Cancer*, vol. 4, Cold Spring Harbor Conferences on Cell Proliferation, Cold Spring Harbor Laboratory, New York, 1977.
18. Third National Cancer Survey: *Incidence Data*, S Cutler et al (eds), Biometry Branch Division of Cancer Cause and Prevention, National Cancer Institute, NCI Monograph 41, DHEW Publication (NIH) 75-787, 1975.
19. SEER Program: *Classification for Extent of Disease*, EM Shambaugh (ed), Biometry Branch, National Cancer Institute, DHEW Publication (NIH) 77-1448, 1977.
20. American Joint Committee for Cancer Staging: *Manual for Staging of Cancer*, 1977.
21. Armenian H, Lilienfeld AM: The distribution of incubation periods of neoplastic diseases. *Am J Epidemiol* 99:92–100, 1974.
22. McGregor DH et al: Breast cancer incidence among atomic bomb survivors, Hiroshima and Nagasaki, 1950–1969. Atomic Bomb Casualty Commission Technical Report 32, 1971.
23. Lilienfeld AM: The distribution of disease in the population. *J Chronic Dis* 11:471–483, 1960.
24. Haenszel W et al: Stomach cancer among Japanese in Hawaii. *J Nat Cancer Inst* 49:969–988, 1972.
25. Knudson AG: Genetic predisposition to cancer, in HH Hiatt et al (eds): *Origins of Human Cancer*, vol. A, Cold Spring Harbor Laboratory, New York, 1977.
26. Mulvihill JJ: Congenital and genetic diseases, in JJ Fraumeni (ed): *Persons at High Risk of Cancer: An Approach to Cancer Etiology and Control*, Academic Press, New York, 1975.
27. Doll R: *The Age Distribution of Cancer in Man*, A Engel, T Larson (eds), Thule International Symposia, Nordiska Bokhondelns Förlag, Stockholm, 1968.
28. Mason TJ, McKay FW: *U.S. Cancer Mortality by County: 1950–1969*, DHEW Publication (NIH) 74-615, 1974.
29. Mason TJ et al: *Atlas of Cancer Mortality for U.S. Counties: 1950–1969*, U.S Government Printing Office, 1975.
30. Mason TJ et al: *Atlas of Cancer Mortality Among U.S. Nonwhites: 1950–1969*, U.S. Government Printing Office, 1976.
31. Blot WJ et al: 1977 Cancer by county: Etiologic implications, in HH Hiatt et al (eds): *Origins of Human Cancer*, vol. A, Cold Spring Harbor Laboratory, New York, 1977.
32. Segi M: *Cancer Mortality for Selected Sites in 24 Countries (1950–1957)*, Tohoku University School of Medicine, Sendai, Japan, 1960.
33. Segi M, Kurihara M: *Cancer Mortality for Selected Sites in 24 Countries (1958–1959)*, no. 2, Tohoku University School of Medicine, Sendai, Japan, 1962.

34. Segi M: *Cancer Mortality for Selected Sites in 24 Countries (1960–1961)*, no. 3, Tohoku University School of Medicine, Sendai, Japan, 1964.
35. Segi M: *Cancer Mortality for Selected Sites in 24 Countries (1962–1963)*, no. 4, Tohoku University School of Medicine, Sendai, Japan, 1966.
36. Segi M et al: *Cancer Mortality for Selected Sites in 24 Countries, (1964–1965)*, no. 5, Tohoku University School of Medicine, Sendai, Japan, 1969.
37. Segi M, Kurihara M: *Cancer Mortality for Selected Sites in 24 Countries (1966–1967), no. 6, Japan Cancer Society, 1972.*
38. Reid DD: International studies in epidemiology. *Amer J Epidemiol* 102:469–484, 1975.
39. Union Internationale contre le Cancer: *Cancer Incidence in Five Continents*, vol. I: *A Technical Report*, R Doll et al (eds), Geneva, 1966.
40. Union Internationale contre le Cancer: *Cancer Incidence in Five Continents*, vol. II, R Doll et al (eds), Geneva, 1970.
41. International Agency for Research on Cancer: *Cancer Incidence in Five Continents*, vol. III, J Waterhouse et al (eds), Lyon, 1976.
42. Third National Cancer Survey: National Cancer Institute Monograph 41, DHEW Publication (NIH) 75-787, 1975.
43. Dorn HF: *Illness from Cancer in the United States*, Public Health Reports 59:33–48, 65–77, 97–115, 1944.
44. Dorn HF, Cutler SJ: *Morbidity from Cancer in the United States: Parts I and II*, DHEW Public Health Monograph 56, 1959.
45. Haenszel W et al: *Cancer Morbidity in Urban and Rural Iowa*, DHEW Public Health Monograph 37, 1956.
46. SEER Program: *Cancer Incidence and Mortality in the United States 1973–1976*, DHEW Publication (NIH) 78-1837, 1978.
47. Axtell LM et al (eds): *Cancer Patient Survival*, Report 5, DHEW Publication (NIH) 77-992, 1977.
48. Feigl P et al: The U.S. centralized cancer patient data system for uniform communication among cancer centers. *J Nat Cancer Inst* (in press).
49. Colton T: *Statistics in Medicine*, Little, Brown, Boston, 1974.
50. Snedecor GW, Cochran WH: *Statistical Methods*, 6th ed, Iowa State University Press, Ames, Iowa, 1967.
51. Wynder EL, Graham EA: Tobacco smoking as a possible etiologic factor in bronchiogenic carcinoma. A study of six hundred and eighty-four proved cases. *JAMA* 143:329, 1950.
52. Levin ML et al: Cancer and tobacco smoke: A preliminary report. *JAMA* 143:336, 1950.
53. Berkson J: Limitations of the application of fourfold table analysis to hospital data. *Biometrics* 2:47–53, 1946.
54. MacMahon B, Pugh TF: *Epidemiology: Principles and Methods*, Little, Brown, Boston, 1970.
55. Mantel N, Haenszel W: Statistical aspects of the analysis of data from retrospective studies of disease. *J Nat Cancer Inst* 22:719–748, 1959.
56. Anderson S et al: *Statistical Methods for Comparative Studies*, Wiley, New York, 1980.
57. Hammond EC, Horn D: Smoking and death rates—Report on forty-four months of follow-up of 187,783 men. *JAMA* 166:1159–1172, 1294–1308, 1958.
58. Dorn HF: Tobacco consumption and mortality from cancer and other diseases. *Public Health Rep* 74:581–593, 1959.
59. Kahn HA: The Dorn study of smoking and mortality among U.S. veterans: Report on eight and one-half years of observation, in W Haenszel (ed): *Epidemiological Approaches to the Study of Cancer and Other Chronic Diseases*, National Cancer Institute Monograph 19, 1966.
60. Court-Brown WM, Doll R: Mortality from cancer and other causes after radiotherapy for ankylosing spondylitis. *Br Med J* 2:1327–1332, 1965.
61. Abbatt JD: Human leukemic risk data derived from Portuguese thorotrast experience, in *Radionuclide Carcinogenesis, Proceedings of the 12th Annual Hanford Biology Symposium*, U.S. Atomic Energy Commission, 1973.
62. Ishimaru T et al: Leukemia in atomic bomb survivors: Hiroshima and Nagasaki, 1 October 1950–30 September 1966. *Radiat Res* 45:216–233, 1971.
63. Jablon S, Kato H: Studies of the mortality of A-bomb survivors, 5: Radiation dose and mortality, 1950–1970. *Radiat Res* 50:649–698, 1972.
64. Jablon S et al: Cancer in Japanese exposed as children to atomic bombs. *Lancet* 1:927–932, 1971.
65. Seltser R, Sartwell PE: The influence of occupation exposure to radiation on the mortality of American radiologists and other medical specialists. *Am J Epidemiol* 81:2–22, 1965.
66. United Nations Scientific Committee on the Effects of Atomic Radiation: *Ionizing Radiation: Levels and Effects*, vol. II: *Effects*, United Nations, New York, 1972.
67. Selikoff IJ: Cancer Risk of Asbestos Exposure, in HH Hiatt et al (eds): *Origins of Human Cancer*, Cold Spring Harbor Laboratory, New York, 1977.
68. Zdeb MS: The probability of developing cancer. *Am J Epidemiol* 106:6–16, 1977.
69. Goldberg ID et al: The probability of developing cancer. *J Nat Cancer Survey* 17:155–173, 1956.
70. Fleiss JL: *Statistical Methods for Rates and Proportions*, Wiley, New York, 1981.
71. Henle W et al: Antibodies to Epstein-Barr virus in nasopharyngeal carcinoma, other head and neck neoplasms and control groups. *J Nat Cancer Inst* 44:225–231, 1970.
72. Petrakis NL: Some preliminary observations on the influence of genetic admixture on cancer incidence in American Negroes. *Int J Cancer* 7:256–258, 1971.
73. Higginson J et al: Environmental carcinogenesis—A global problem. *Curr Prob Cancer* 7:1–43, 1981.
74. Mahboubi E et al: Oesophageal cancer study in Caspian

littoral of Iran: The Caspian Center Registry. *Br J Cancer* 28:197–214, 1973.
75. Haenszel W: Cancer mortality among the foreign-born in the United States. *J Nat Cancer Inst* 26:37–132, 1961.
76. Levin DL et al: *Cancer Rates and Risks*, 2d ed, DHEW Publication (NIH) 76–691, 1974.
77. Wynder EL, Mabuchi K: Etiological and preventive aspects of human cancer. *Prev Med* 1:300–334, 1972.
78. Cook P: Cancer of the esophagus in Africa. *Br J Cancer* 25:853–880, 1971.
79. Axtell LM et al (eds): *End Results in Cancer*, Report 4, DHEW Publication (NIH) 73-272, 1972.
80. Segi M et al: *Age-adjusted Death Rates for Cancer for Selected Sites in 51 Countries in 1974*, Segi Institute of Cancer Epidemiology, Nagoya, Japan, 1979.
81. Wynder EL et al: An epidemiological investigation of gastric cancer. *Cancer* 16:1461–1496, 1963.
82. Gordon T et al: Cancer mortality trends in the U.S. 1930–1955, in *End Results and Mortality Trends in Cancer*, *Nat Cancer Inst* Monograph 6, 162–169, 1961.
83. Correa P et al: Pathology of gastric carcinoma in Japanese populations: Comparisons between Miyagi Prefecture, Japan, and Hawaii. *J Nat Cancer Inst* 5:1449–1457, 1973.
84. Matolo NM et al: High incidence of gastric cancer in a coal mining region. *Cancer* 29:733–737, 1972.
85. Haenszel W, Correa P: Cancer of the large intestine: Epidemiologic findings. *Dis Colon Rectum* 16:371–377, 1973.
86. Haenszel W, Kurihara M; Mortality from cancer and other disease among Japanese in the United States. *J Nat Cancer Inst* 40:43–68, 1968.
87. Staszewski J, Haenszel W: Cancer mortality among the Polish-born in the United States. *J Nat Cancer Inst* 35:291–297, 1965.
88. Burkitt DP: Some diseases characteristic of modern Western civilization. *Br Med J* 1:274–278, 1973.
89. Haenszel W et al: Large-bowel cancer in Hawaiian Japanese. *J Nat Cancer Inst* 51:1765–1779, 1973.
90. Siegel JS, Zelnik M: An evaluation of coverage in the 1960 census of population by techniques of demographic analysis and by composite methods, in *Proc Am Stat Assoc*, Soc Stat section, 1966.
91. World Health Organization: *Annual Epidemiological and Vital Statistics 1960*, Geneva, 1963.
92. Hammond EC: Tobacco, in JF Fraumeni Jr (ed): *Persons at High Risk of Cancer*, Academic Press, New York, 1975.
93. Kessler II: Cancer Mortality among diabetics. *J Nat Cancer Inst* 44:673–686, 1970.
94. Burch GE, Ansoni A: Chronic alcoholism and carcinoma of the pancreas. *Arch Intern Med* 122:273–275, 1968.
95. Burbank F: United States lung cancer death rates begin to rise proportionately more rapidly for females than for males: A dose-response effect? *J Chronic Dis* 25:473–479, 1972.
96. *The Health Consequences of Smoking. A Report of the Surgeon General*, DHEW Publication (HSM) 71-7513, 1971.
97. DeWaard F: The epidemiology of breast cancer: Reviews and prospects. *Int J Cancer* 4:577–586, 1969.
98. Anderson DE: Familial Susceptibility, in JF Fraumeni Jr (ed): *Persons at High Risk of Cancer*, Academic Press, New York, 1975.
99. MacMahon B et al: Oestrogen profiles of Asian and North American women. *Lancet* 2:900–902, 1971.
100. Martin CE: Marital and coital factors in cervical cancer. *Am J Public Health* 57:803–814, 1967.
101. Naib ZM et al: Genital herpetic infection and cervical dysplasia and cancer. *Cancer* 23:940–945, 1969.
102. Herbst AL et al: Clear cell adenocarcinoma of the genital tract in young females. *N Eng J Med* 287:1259–1264, 1972.
103. Christopherson WM et al: Cervix death rates and mass cytologic screening. *Cancer* 26:808–811, 1970.
104. Henschke UK et al: Alarming increase of the cancer mortality in the U.S. black population (1950–1967). *Cancer* 31:763–768, 1973.
105. Akazaki K, Stemmerman GN: Comparative study of latent carcinoma of the prostate among Japanese in Japan and Hawaii. *J Nat Cancer Inst* 50:1137–1144, 1973.
106. King H et al: Some epidemiological aspects of cancer of the prostate. *J Chron Dis* 16:117–153, 1963.
107. Wynder El et al: Epidemiology of cancer of the prostate. *Cancer* 28:344–360, 1971.
108. Cutler SJ: Report of the Third National Cancer Survey, in *Proceedings of the Seventh National Cancer Conference*, Lippincott, Philadelphia, 1972.
109. King H, Bailar JC III: Epidemiology of urinary bladder cancer: A review of selected literature. *J Chron Dis* 19:735–772, 1966.
110. Hashem M: The aetiology and pathogenesis of the bilharzial bladder cancer. *J Egypt Med Assoc* 44:857–966, 1961.
111. Vianna NJ et al: Extended epidemic of Hodgkin's disease in high school students. *Lancet* 1:1209–1211, 1971.
112. Connelly RR, Christine BW: A cohort study of cancer following infectious mononucleosis. *Cancer Res* 44:1172–1178, 1974.
113. Clemmesen J: Statistical studies in the aetiology of malignant neoplasms, I: Review and results. *Acta Pathol Microbiol Scand Suppl* 174:1–543, 1965.
114. Mulvihill JJ et al (eds): *Genetics of Human Cancer*, vol. 3: *Progress in Cancer Research and Therapy*, Raven Press, New York, 1977.

4
GENETIC AND FAMILIAL ASPECTS OF CANCER

Louise A. Paquin   *David T. Purtilo*

A recent review by Purtilo et al. has provided an extensive listing of more than 240 inherited neoplastic syndromes showing simple Mendelian inheritance patterns.[1] Also, the recent publication of five books on genetics of cancer illustrates the renewed interest in genetic factors.[2-6] In recent years a phenomenal acquisition of new knowledge of inherited traits in humans has occurred: Victor McKusick's catalog now lists nearly 3000 separate traits.[7] No longer can physicians restrict themselves simply to thinking of one patient at a time. All clinicians, especially those working with cancer patients, must become "family" doctors. The presentation in this chapter provides both conceptual and practical information about the pathogenesis of inherited cancer and stresses methods for recognition and investigation of familial cancer.

First, the focus is on chromosomal abnormalities associated with cancer; methods of ascertainment of cancer by pedigree analysis are sketched, cardinal clinical features of inherited cancer syndromes are noted, and specific laboratory studies which can be done to detect cancer early in families at high risk are discussed.

This investigation was supported by Grant CA 23561 from the National Institutes of Health.

Common familial cancer syndromes likely to be encountered by practicing clinicians—carcinomas of the colon, breast, and skin; inherited endocrine tumors; and familial tumors of the peripheral and central nervous system—are considered, using examples from the authors' experience. The X-linked lymphoproliferative syndrome (XLP), which is under intense investigation in our laboratory, will be presented as a model for studying immunogenetic factors in the pathogenesis of inherited cancers. The discussion begins with childhood malignancies which have provided provocative insights into the pathogenesis of inherited cancer.

HEREDITARY CHILDHOOD CANCERS

The prototype of inherited childhood malignancy is retinoblastoma, the most common intraocular tumor in children.[8] It strikes 1 in 20,000 children in sporadic and hereditary forms.

Based on characteristic early age at onset of retinoblastoma, occurrence of bilateral and multiple primary tumors, and familial involvement (cf. Table 4-1), Knudson and colleagues have developed a pathogenetic model

TABLE 4-1 Characteristics of Familial Cancer

Early age of onset of malignancy

Multiple primary tumors

Multicentric tumor origin

Family history of malignancy beyond the general population

Mendelian pattern of inheritance

Chromosomal abnormalities

Birth defects, recurrent spontaneous abortions, and cancer in the family

Pigmentation and vascular anomalies

---

which involves at least two mutational steps.[4,9,10] The first mutation occurs either in germ cells (in hereditary cases) or in somatic cells (in nonhereditary cases); the second mutation is somatic in either case. Knudson's calculations indicate that hereditary cases account for approximately 40 percent of tumors. Children with this defective gene have a 95 percent chance of developing at least unilateral retinoblastoma; typically three to four tumors ensue, most often bilaterally. Diagnoses occur at less than 18 months in 73 percent of bilateral and 29 percent of unilateral inherited cases. Nonhereditary cases occur later, often after 4 years of age.[11] Several of the hereditary cases are due to a new dominant mutation, occurring at a rate of approximately five mutations per million genes at the locus per generation. No family history is ascertained in the latter children.[12]

Retinoblastoma exemplifies the two-mutation model; the first mutation in all cells increases the probability of a second mutation in somatic retinal cells at an early age, of frequent bilaterality, and of multicentric origin. A germ cell mutation correlates with the increased frequency of second primary cancers. For example, osteogenic sarcoma[13] commonly occurs in children with retinoblastoma, and independent primary gliomas have also been reported,[14] especially following irradiation.[15] This phenomenon is true also for other childhood cancers; survivors of childhood cancer[16] showed a 20 percent higher risk for a second cancer than previously unaffected children. While Li's study involved children treated with radiotherapy, another study[17] found that 33 of 102 children not associated with such treatment developed second malignancies. Purtilo and associates have likewise described individuals with familial cancer syndromes who developed multiple primary tumors.[18,19]

occurring during a period of a decade or more. An increased frequency of a second primary tumor in children with retinoblastoma has occurred in recent years because of improved survival rates. Another by-product of improved survival rates is the resulting increase in progeny with the gene. This increase may also be from an apparent increase in the spontaneous mutation rate in the population at large and in susceptible persons.[8] Strong[20] has cautioned afflicted families about the possible deleterious impact of environmental carcinogens and treatment-related mutagenic agents such as irradiation and chemotherapy.

Childhood hereditary neoplasia is frequently associated with various congenital malformations (Fig. 4-1). For example, 41 percent of children with malignancy also show evidence of congenital malformation.[4] Wilms's tumor is frequently associated with aniridia, hemihypertrophy, genitourinary tract malformations, and numerous pigmented nevi.

Most known carcinogens are also teratogens. The time at which an injury strikes the organism probably determines whether the effect is teratogenic or oncogenic (cf. Ref. 21). Maurer et al.[22] described two pairs of monozygotic twins discordant for Wilms's tumor. Both members of one pair had aniridia and psychomotor retardation, and one had bilateral Wilms's tumor. In contrast, only one of the second pair, with unilateral Wilms's tumor, also had hemihypertrophy. The former cases were probably hereditary, while the latter Wilms's tumor was sporadic, that is, the mutation occurred in the postzygotic period. A problem in hereditary bilateral Wilms's tumor is that detection of minute tumors in the contralateral kidney preoperatively is difficult.[23] Li and associates (in personal communications) have detected a chromosomal translocation (3;8) associated with bilateral renal cancer in a family. Screening of the family with karyotyping and intravenous pyelogram has led to the early detection of bilateral renal cancers.

The features described for retinoblastoma and Wilms's tumor can be generalized to many other childhood cancers. For example, irradiation of persons with nevoid basal cell carcinoma syndrome can lead to rapid onset of multiple cancers.[4] Similarly, neuroblastoma can be familial and is characterized by multiple primary tumors.[24] In this case the first mutation, or disposing factor, can be von Recklinghausen's disease (neurofibromatosis),[25] suggesting a disruption of a particular developmental function. Similar disturbance of embryonic development has also been suggested as the cause of an

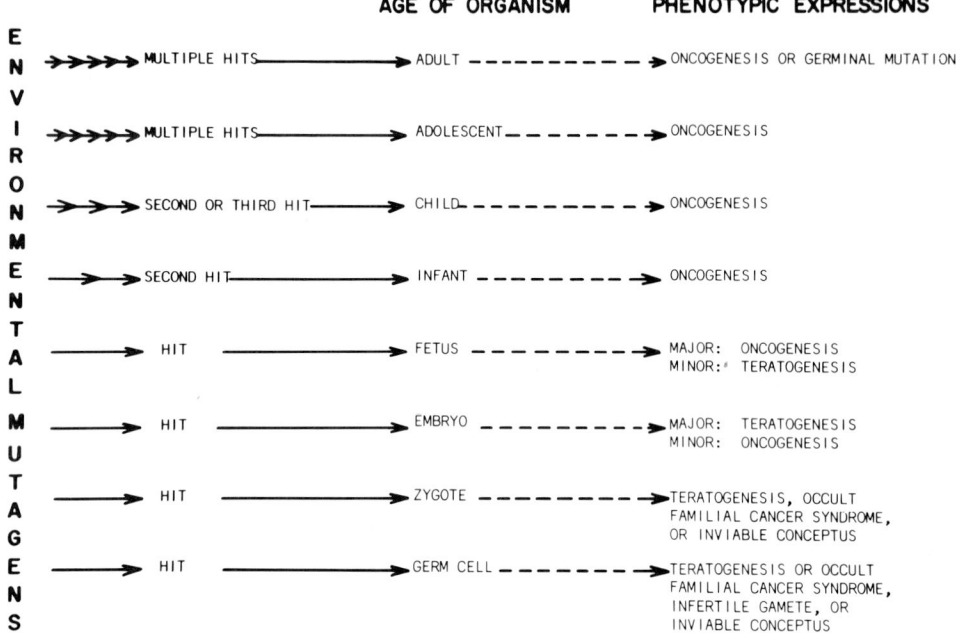

FIGURE 4-1 Hypothesis regarding the variable phenotypic expression of mutational hits at various periods in the life of the organism. (*From DT Purtilo, LA Paquin, T Gindhart: Genetics of neoplasia: Impact of ecogenetics on oncogenesis. Amer J Path 91:609–688, 1978.*)

unusual dysplasia—malformation—cancer syndrome involving gross malformation of the lower limb, followed by malignant transformation, metastasis, and death.[26]

CHROMOSOMES AND CANCER

In assessing the relationship between chromosomal abnormalities and cancer, one must distinguish between two different phenomena: constitutional chromosomal anomalies, in all of an individual's somatic cells, which predispose to cancer; and chromosomal abnormalities found in tumor cells. Both of these categories can and should be informative to the clinician.

Of the constitutional somatic karyotypic abnormalities predisposing to malignancy, Down's syndrome occurs most frequently. An increase in leukemia in persons with trisomy 21 is about 18 times above predicted levels.[27] This occurrence, as well as an increase in other forms of cancer, is also related to immunodeficiency in Down's syndrome.[28] Risk of breast cancer is increased in persons with Klinefelter's syndrome.[29] In Turner's syndrome, especially in individuals with mosaic karyotypes (e.g., 45,X/46,XY), gonadoblastoma often develops in the dysgenetic ovary.[30]

In patients with retinoblastoma, chromosomal abnormalities have also been found. Although most persons with the disease have normal karyotypes, some have deletions in chromosome 13 (Fig. 4-2), especially occurring in the area of 13q14; these may be hereditary. Cases of retinoblastoma with 13q deletions often show other anomalies as well,[31] consistent with the deletion or disturbance of more than one set of genes.

Specific chromosome imbalance may or may not be the primary event in tumorigenesis, but such imbalance can involve loss or duplication of controlling genes, genes affecting virus-cell interactions, or other molecular events (cf. Ref. 32). In any case, the advent of chromosome-banding techniques (cf. Ref. 33) has led to increased knowledge about the associations between chromosome aberration and malignancy.

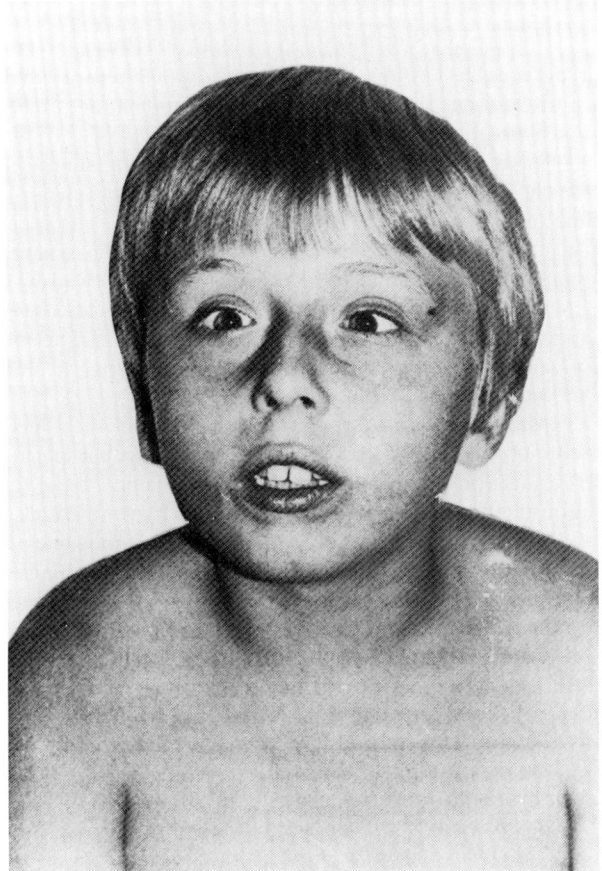

FIGURE 4-2 Aniridia in Wilms's tumor patient. (*From V Ricciardi, E Sujansky, A Smith, V Francke: Chromosomal imbalance in the Aniridia-Wilms's tumor association: 11 p Interstitial deletion, Pediatrics 61(4), 1978, p 606.*)

CLASTOGENIC SYNDROMES PREDISPOSING TO CANCER

Several autosomal recessive clastogenic syndromes show excessive chromsome breakage (cf. Ref. 34). Although rare, they provide a model for studying chromosomes and oncogenesis. Classically, they include Bloom's syndrome, Fanconi's anemia, and ataxia-telangiectasia. Recent additions to the list include dyskeratosis congenita, porokeratosis of Mibelli, nevoid basal cell carcinoma, and incontinentia pigmenti. Others will likely be discovered.

Bloom's syndrome (BS) usually presents with growth retardation, telangiectatic lesions, and immunodeficiency in fair-haired, blue-eyed individuals, although phenotypes are highly variable. Chromosomal aberrations include breaks, gaps, and tetraradial configurations, indicating defective homologous chromatid exchange.[35] The latter is also confirmed by the demonstration of increased rates of sister chromatid exchange (SCE). Malignancy occurs in about 20 percent of BS patients, predominantly lymphocytic leukemias.[36]

Fanconi's anemia (FA), another autosomal recessive clastogenic disorder, is characterized by pancytopenia, marrow hypoplasia, and congenital anomalies. Chromosomes show frequent chromatid gaps and breaks and nonhomologous interchange, but no increase in SCE and no change in DNA chain elongation.[37] Acute myelocytic leukemia and squamous cell carcinoma have been found, and 10 in 11 cases show acute nonlymphocytic leukemia.[38] Not only homozygotes, but also heterozygotes are at increased risk for malignancy.[32] The genetic defect in FA seems to be the impairment of chromosome condensation during mitosis.[39] There is also a significant decrease in DNA ligase activity.[40]

Ataxia-telangiectasia (AT) is characterized by cerebellar ataxia, telangiectatic lesions, depressed lymphocyte function, recurrent infections, decreased lymphoid tissue, and other immunodeficiencies. Approximately 10 to 14 percent of AT patients develop lymphocytic leukemia or lymphoma.[41] All hematologic malignancies have affected the lymphoid cells.[42]

Increased breakage is seen in AT chromosomes in general, but a particularly consistent abnormality of chromosome 14, with breakpoint at position 14q12, has been identified.[43,44] This same abnormality is found in fibroblasts as well as lymphocytes and is also found in heterozygotes. AT patients show increased serum antibody response to the early antigen (EA) of Epstein-Barr virus (EBV) and the viral capsid antigen (VCA). B cells of these patients, as well as of those with African Burkitt's lymphoma (BL) may be genetically defective.[45] Fukuhara[46] has suggested that chromosome 14 is the single most important marker in malignant lymphoma. DNA repair errors are also prominent in AT. Slow excision of x-ray damage bases[47] makes cells of these patients especially sensitive to irradiation.[48]

In *dyskeratosis congenita*, the evidence of chromosomal instability is still minimal, probably because immunodeficiency in these cases is such that karyotyping is especially difficult.[49] There is, however, an increase in SCE and increased breakage.[50] There is also a marked increase in solid tumors[50,51] especially of the tongue, buccal mucosa, rectum, cervix, etc.

The constitutional chromosomal abnormalities correlated with an increased frequency of malignancy having been considered, karyotypic abnormalities in malignant tissues, especially the limited number associated with specific karyotypic changes, will now be examined. Other cancers show random increased karyotypic abnormalities which lack specificity.

The specific chromosomal abnormality of a tumor already mentioned is the 14q+ anomaly in African BL. This marker is found in virtually all cases of African BL, which are EBV-positive; as well as in most cases of American BL, whether EBV-positive or -negative.[52,53] The same karyotypic change occurs when such cell lines are transplanted into nude mice.[54] Most of the markers represent 14q+ chromosomes whose extra material originates from a translocation from chromosome 8, although several other sources have frequently been described as well.[46] Other tumors have also shown 14q+ abnormalities. These include a retinoblastoma in a patient whose constitutional karyotype was normal,[55] several non-Hodgkin's lymphomas,[46] multiple myeloma and plasma cell leukemia,[56] and B-cell lymphoblastic leukemias.[57] The latter cases suggest that the marker, while of various translocation sources, especially chromosome 11, may be useful in defining acute lymphoblastic leukemia subtypes, the B cells seem predisposed to 14q+ abnormalities when involved in malignancy. In the case of BL, it is probable that EBV, 14q+, and immunodeficiency are all required.[58] Further chromosomal abnormalities in lymphoma include elevated SCE frequency, which is markedly increased by certain chemotherapeutic regimens.[59]

Chronic myelogenous leukemia (CML) and the Philadelphia chromosome (Ph^1) is the chromosome defect most extensively studied. Ph^1 is an abnormal 22q−.[60] The Ph^1 chromosome occurs in almost 85 percent of CMLs and is most often a result of a translocation of chromosome-22 material to chromosome 9.[61] Approximately 8 percent of Ph^1-positive CML results from other complex chromosomal rearrangements. In blast crisis, other chromosomal abnormalities are found, often several months in advance of acute clinical symptoms. The most common changes are a second Ph^1, an extra 8, or an isochromosome 17q. Since the latter is especially rare in the chronic phase, its appearance is probably the best indicator of an acute crisis. Hypodiploidy is extremely rare (less than 1 percent).[62] The number of hyperdiploid cells is small in the chronic stage, and they presumably clone during the blast phase.

Ph^1 probably originates in a pluripotent stem cell which becomes excessively proliferative because this aneuploid type grows best. Moreover, these cells seem resistant to chemotherapy.[63] In two cases of Ph^1 in acute lymphocytic leukemia (ALL), for example, Ph^1-positive CML developed during ALL remission. This also suggests aberration in the pluripotential stem cell.[64] The Ph^1 in ALL frequently seems to disappear with remission and reappear at blastic relapse.[65]

Other leukemias also have marker chromosomes: acute promyelocytic leukemia is correlated with a specific translocation (15;17) (q22;q21) and seems now to be diagnostic for this disease. Rowley's research group has also indicated the relative consistency of a chromosome-12 abnormality in rapidly progressive hairy cell leukemia.[67]

Acute lymphocytic leukemia and acute nonlymphocytic leukemia (ANLL) both show frequency of aneuploidy of approximately 50 percent in marrow cells. In ALL the tendency is to hyperdiploidy, while in ANLL it is to hypodiploidy. In ALL the losses and gains most frequently involve numbers 14, 15, X, and 21; rearrangements involve the numbers 6, 9, 17, and 22. In ANLL, the loss of a 7 and gain of 8 or 21 are seen, and rearrangements involve 5, 8, 12, and 17. Median survival time is longer when normal karyotypes are found in ANLL.[68] This can be predicted to some extent on the basis of the abnormality; for example, patients with monosomy 7 have complete remission frequency of 13 percent, while those with 8;21 translocation have complete remission in 50 percent.[69] Familial leukemias can also be associated with chromosomal breakage.[70]

Chromosomal aberrations are likewise found in human malignant solid tumors. Most frequently, such tumor material contains multiple abnormalities, and attempts are being made to find patterns of these abnormalities in order to assess if possible the earlier stem-line karyotypes. A group from Czechoslovakia,[71] for example, has been examining cell lines from different phases of progression of cervical carcinoma. In these, as in studies of gastric polyps and cancers,[72] the most common findings are pseudodiploid cells with multiple rearrangements. In the polyps, there are fewer chromosomal abnormalities. Henry and colleagues[73] have attempted direct karyotyping of tumor material in malignant melanoma, but the problems of necrosis and location of metaphases are vast. Other studies have been restricted to the study of a particular chromosome, notably chromosome 1. In 9 of 10 solid tumors studied by Kovacs,[74] mostly colon and breast malignancies, particular areas of the long arm of this chromosome were especially involved, although the tumors showed multiple anomalies.

Studies of peripheral blood of persons with solid tumors or with hematologic malignancies, unless there are blasts in the peripheral blood, usually show no abnormalities, presumably since these tumors are somatic in origin. However, some of the so-called cancer families have been shown to have some irregularities. In a family of four children with various malignancies, peripheral blood samples showed a high level of aneuploidy (14 to 26 percent), 2 to 8 percent cells with chromatid breaks, and, in some family members, "fragile" 16q chromosomes.[75] Similarly, in several CML and cancer families Cheng et al.[76] showed excessive breaks (5 to 10 percent) and/or fragments in 22 of 32 abnormal individuals. Aneuploidy was also found, mostly random losses. In the tumor patients this could be attributable to radiotherapy, but abnormalities were also found among relatives. In two of the families, spouses were also found to have karyotypic abnormalities, implying possible environmental causation.

Approximately 85 percent of cancers of human beings are thought to be caused by environmental agents such as chemicals, irradiation, and viruses.[4] But simply identifying potential environmental carcinogens seems too limited an approach to explain oncogenesis. After all, cancer occurs in only a fraction of persons exposed equally to a given carcinogen. Hence, it seems more plausible that environmental carcinogens cause cancer in a few individuals who show genetic susceptibility to carcinogenesis. Numerous histopathologic types of tumors afflicting virtually every organ of the body can emerge from simple Mendelian inheritance. As mentioned earlier, more than 240 familial neoplastic syndromes are transmitted on a Mendelian basis;[1] or nearly 8 percent of all known inherited traits can result in neoplasia. Space prohibits a detailed discussion of these myriad neoplastic syndromes. Remarks will be confined to selected inherited malignancies: carcinoma of the colon, breast, and skin; familial endocrine tumors; neoplasms of the peripheral and central nervous system; and selected inherited hematologic cancers, especially the X-linked lymphoproliferative syndrome.

FAMILIAL CANCER SYNDROMES

Recognition

Inherited neoplastic syndromes reveal cardinal features (Table 4-1). Recognition of one or more of these features should increase suspicion that an individual patient exhibiting one of the signs has an inherited neoplasia. Clinicians should seek extensive pedigree information and documentation of suspected familial neoplasms. For example, inherited cancers develop at a younger age than do noninherited tumors of the same pathologic type. Inherited cancer is often seen in children or in young adults rather than in elderly persons. Bilateral or multiple tumors of the same or of different histopathologic types regularly signal inherited predisposition to cancer. Evaluation of a person whose family is known to have inherited cancer should compel the physician to pursue detection of two or more tumors and not just one. Conversely, patients presenting with multiple lesions must be suspected of having a heritable cancer. Congenital defects, hamartomas, hyperplasias, and immune deficiency syndromes can be hallmarks of inherited predisposition to cancer. Generally, the inherited neoplasms show dominant autosomal inheritance. Pedigree information permits documentation and ascertainment of Mendelian inheritance predisposing to cancer.

The occurrence of a malignancy in multiple siblings suggests, but does not definitely demonstrate, Mendelian inheritance. Common exposure to an environmental carcinogen is a possibility as well. Confidence grows when the trait is also demonstrated in other relatives. History should be able to rule out a common environmental agent causing the cancer in a family. Thorough histopathological reevaluation is mandatory to clearly document the specific types of cancer occurring in a family. The authors' experience has revealed that vague and inaccurate diagnoses often mislead the physician. Generic terms such as "cancer of the kidney" or of the liver, and cancer of the intestine, for example, are misleading, for all have been demonstrated upon reexamination of the surgical biopsy or autopsy specimens to be lymphomas which had occurred in these anatomic sites.

Familial cancer syndromes selected for discussion are grouped by anatomic site. They have been selected because they are common or illustrate special aspects of inherited cancer syndromes. The need for accurate pedigree, and histopathological documentation, the need

TABLE 4-2 Selected Inherited Syndromes Predisposing to Colon Cancer

	Mode of inheritance*	Reference†
Familial polyposis coli	AD	17510
		15700
Gardner's syndrome	AD	17530
Peutz-Jeghers syndrome (intestinal polyps, ovarian tumors in 5 percent females)	AD	17520
Colorectal carcinoma	AD	131
Turcot's syndrome	AR	27630
Familial polyposis IV with discrete polyps	AD	17540
Juvenile polyposis	AD	15835
Diffuse GI polyposis	AD	17500
Colon cancer	AD	11450
Colon cancer; adenocarcinoma	AD	11440

*AR = autosomal recessive, XR = X-linked recessive, AD = autosomal dominant, XD = X-linked dominant.
†Five-digit numbers indicate listings in McKusick's catalogs.[7] Other numbers indicate end-of-chapter references.

for continuing surveillance of persons at high risk of cancers, and the need to develop testable hypotheses which might explain the pathogenetic mechanisms of increased susceptibility to cancer all should be emphasized.

Familial Colon Carcinoma Syndromes

Colon cancer, the leading visceral malignancy in the United States, is estimated to occur on a genetic basis in from 12 to 25 percent of all patients.[77] Colon cancer is determined also by environmental associations: populations at high risk, in general, consume a diet low in vegetable fiber and high in animal fat and refined carbohydrates.[78,79] Colon cancer, carcinoma of the breast, and lymphoma are frequent where much beef is consumed.[80]

Familial colon cancer syndromes show autosomal dominant inheritance (Table 4-2), except for Turcot's syndrome, which probably occurs on an autosomal recessive basis. Studies of one family have revealed numerous cardinal features of inherited cancer, probably due to Turcot's syndrome, which consists of adenomatous polyps and adenocarcinoma of the colon with brain tumor. Four of five brothers, 8 to 18 years of age, died during a 10-year period. Three died of glioblastoma multiforme and the fourth of colon cancer.[81] Such families require continuing surveillance for cancer. For example, a boy developed lymphoma in the colon at age 6, had selective IgA deficiency at 14, malignant lymphoma in his jaw at 15, and died 6 months later of glioblastoma multiforme. Multiple adenomatous colonic polyps, in addition to the brain tumor, were found at autopsy. Laboratory studies implicated EBV as the etiologic agent of the submandibular lymphoma.[81] The etiology of the brain tumor and the adenomatous polyps in the colon remain a mystery.

Another family illustrative of the need of continuing surveillance for the emergence of cancer is depicted in Fig. 4-3; 17 individuals in this black kindred have developed malignancy.[19] This family has been studied during the past 4 years and has the autosomal dominant familial cancer syndrome. Early onset of adenocarcinoma involved the colon, endometrium, and breast and less common other cancers; multiple tumors have occurred in two individuals. During the summer of 1976, the authors embarked on a screening program to detect

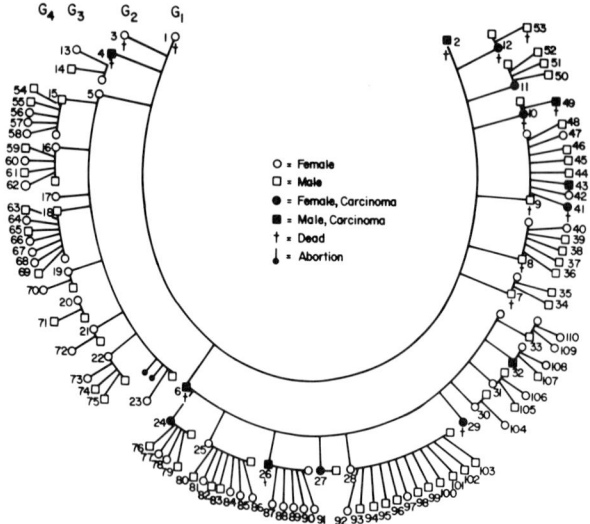

FIGURE 4-3 Autosomal dominant transmission of cancer in a kindred. (*From DT Purtilo, LA Paquin, T Gindhart: Genetics of neoplasia: Impact of ecogenetics on oncogenesis, Amer J Path 91:609–688, 1978.*)

cancer in family members. Plasma and urinary carcinoembryonic antigen (CEA) were measured; and complete blood counts and proctoscopic and cytological evaluations were performed. The 44-year-old woman depicted in the pedigree figure as G3-24 developed endometrial adenocarcinoma at age 36. The evaluation by Purtilo et al.* revealed elevated plasma CEA to 8.1 ng/dL, but the physical examination and proctoscopic and other studies were normal. Carcinoma of the breast was diagnosed in August 1978 and glioblastoma multiforme in November, and she succumbed in January, evidencing autosomal dominant cancer syndrome. In addition, during March 1979, an evaluation was made regarding adenocarcinoma of the colon in a 27-year-old woman (G4-78) who had not been previously evaluated. Her CEA declined postoperatively from its preoperative higher level, indicating probable total removal of the cancer. Given her family history and early phenotypic expressions of the syndrome, she should be monitored every 3 to 6 months for additional colon, endometrial, breast, or other malignancies, using selected screening measures of CEA, cytology, colonoscopy, and mammography.

Others have developed screening protocols for colon cancer which are applicable to families with familial cancer syndromes.[82] For example, Miller et al.[83] detected colon carcinoma in a 61-year-old man by CEA, barium enema, and proctoscopic examination. The colon cancer syndromes are usually inherited as autosomal dominant traits, and adenomatous polyps involving the colon or other portions of the gastrointestinal tract precede cancer (Fig. 4-2). The adenomatous polyps which precede adenocarcinoma imply that two or more mutational events lead to malignancy. For example, multihit mutational events seem to occur in familial colorectal polyposis syndrome (FCPS).[84] Multiple family members can be involved by FCPS, or sporadic cases, individuals with polyps and cancer, may be encountered with germinal mutations, in which event there is no family history. In persons with FCPS, adenomatous polyps emerge at approximately 20 years of age; colorectal adenocarcinoma usually develops by age 50.[85] Such observations suggest that adenomatous polyps result from a second or delayed mutation in a somatic cell; another mutation in mucosal cells culminates in cancer in the fourth to sixth decade.[84] Colon cancer could arise as a consequence of any one of at least 10 different known mutations (Table 4-2).[77]

* Purtilo DT, Geelhoed C, Li F (unpublished)

Persons with FCPS and another polyposis syndrome, Gardner's syndrome (GS), show abnormalities in their fibroblasts. In FCPS, cultured skin fibroblasts show increased susceptibility to transformation by murine sarcoma virus compared with normal controls.[86] Skin cultures derived from patients with GS containing both epithelioid and fibroblastic cells reveal increased tetraploid mitotic figures,[87] a finding which may help to identify asymptomatic individuals with the defective gene.[88]

Invariably, individuals with FCPS develop cancer by the ninth decade if a prophylactic total colectomy is not performed. The penetrance of the mutation and thus the occurrence of polyps and cancer in this syndrome is extremely high. In contrast, malignant tumors associated with Peutz-Jeghers syndrome are rare (Table 4-2). Additional remarks regarding the methods of screening and approach to study of families having inherited colon cancer syndromes and other neoplastic syndromes are summarized at the conclusion of this chapter.

Inherited Breast Cancer Syndromes

Carcinoma of the breast is the most common cause of death from cancer in women. Breast cancer has a multifactorial basis involving environmental, hormonal, and genetic factors.[77,89] A noteworthy environmental factor is diet: countries showing low consumption of beef are typified by low incidence of carcinoma of the breast. Conversely, countries with high consumption of beef show high incidence.[90] For example, Japanese women follow this rule; however, when Japanese women migrate to the United States they become at an increased risk for breast cancer presumably from exposure to an American diet or other environmental factors. Hormones are a second important factor in breast oncogenesis: a 100-fold greater risk of breast cancer is seen in females compared with males.[91] Moreover, dysgenetic males with XXY Klinefelter's syndrome, have a 20-fold increased risk of developing breast cancer as compared to normal males.[92]

The exact contribution of inherited predisposition to breast carcinogenesis is unknown. Lynch et al. have estimated that approximately 13 percent of carcinomas of the breast are familial.[93] Anderson[77] found a two- to threefold increase in breast cancer in relatives of breast cancer patients. Diagnosis in the premenopausal period resulted in a 3.1-fold risk, whereas postmenopausal diagnosis resulted in a 1.5-fold risk compared with

TABLE 4-3 Selected Inherited Syndromes Predisposing to Breast Cancer

	Mode of inheritance*	Reference*
Breast cancer in males	XR	107, 108
Breast cancer in females	AR	21200
Klinefelter's syndrome	Nondisjunction	50
Familial cancer syndrome	AD	131

*See footnotes to Table 4-2.

controls. Bilaterality increased the risk to 8.8-fold in sisters. In contrast, relatives of patients with the usual breast cancer occurring postmenopausally and unilaterally, exhibited only a 1.2-fold higher risk. Anderson has surmised that any one of several mutations, inherited in an autosomal dominant fashion, predispose to breast cancer (Table 4-3). The phenotypic expression of these inherited breast cancers includes the expression solely as breast carcinoma. But in other families, breast cancer is associated with gastrointestinal cancers. A third syndrome, the familial cancer syndrome, manifests as a group of estrogen-sensitive tumors of breast, ovary, and endometrium. An unusual association of breast cancer in mothers and sarcoma, leukemia, or brain tumors in their children, is a rare genetic syndrome.[94] Familial male breast cancer has also been described.[95]

Lynch et al.[93] have found that mothers with breast cancer averaged age 57 and daughters age 45 in 33 kindreds investigated. Early onset of carcinoma in daughters was thought to result from changing lifestyles of women in the twentieth century. But fallacies of numerical reasoning could produce artifactual statistical evidence of earlier onset. As for other inherited neoplastic syndromes, the clinician should look for cardinal manifestations of inherited breast cancer and be attuned to the greater possibility of bilateral tumors or involvement of other estrogen-dependent organs or cancers in other members of the family. In summary, women predisposed to breast cancer seem to be exquisitely sensitive to carcinogens, not only in the breast, but also in other estrogen-sensitive organs.

Genodermatoses

The old cliché that "the skin mirrors many systemic diseases" is extremely important in the recognition of familial cancer syndromes. Lynch and Frichot[96] have identified approximately 50 genetic disorders wherein cutaneous signs signal cutaneous or internal malignancy. The ease of visual inspection of skin as an aid to diagnosis cannot be overemphasized. The interaction between environmental agents and genetic susceptibility to carcinogenesis is often portrayed in the skin (Fig. 4-4).

Selected genodermatoses with associated cancers are shown in Table 4-4. They reflect the variety of pathogenetic mechanisms involved. For example, individuals with *albinism* have a total or partial lack of pigmentation, are not shielded from actinic carcinogenic rays, and thus, basal and squamous cell carcinomas emerge in sun-exposed skin at an alarming rate. Individuals with epidermodysplasia verruciformis have an increased oncogenic susceptibility to human papilloma virus, type 4, associated with squamous cell carcinoma,[97] another example of ecogenetics. Xeroderma pigmentosum is due to failure to repair chromosomes. In these individuals, DNA of keratinocytes is readily damaged by ultraviolet light and the cells lack enzymes necessary for specific

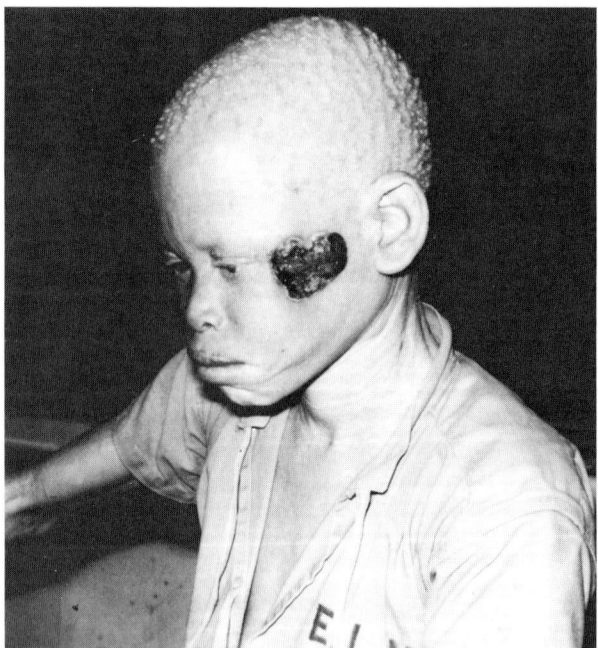

FIGURE 4-4 This albino boy has developed squamous cell carcinoma from exposure to sunlight. (*From DT Purtilo, A Survey of Human Diseases. Addison-Wesley, Reading. Mass., 1978.*)

TABLE 4-4 Selected Genodermatoses and Phacomatoses with Associated Neoplasia

	Mode of inheritance*	Reference*
Malignant melanoma	AD	15560
Malignant melanoma, intracellular		15570
Neurocutaneous melanosis	AR	24940
Universal melanosis	AD	15580
Nevi (pigmented and halo)	AD AR	16290 16300 16310
Giant pigmented hairy nevi	AD	13755
Albinism	AR	20310
Xeroderma pigmentosum; xerodermoid pigmentosum (including DeSanctis-Cacchione syndrome)	AR AD	27870 27880 19550
Epidermolysis bullosa dystrophica	AD	13170 22660
Disseminated superficial actinic porokeratosis	AR	17590
Acrokeratosis verruciformis, van den Bosch's syndrome	AD XR	10190 31450
Darier-White disease	AD	12420
Scleroatrophy and keratosis of limbs	AD	18160
Pachyonychia congenita	AD	12760
Multiple trichoepithelioma (Spiegler-Brooke tumors; cylindromatosis)	AD XD AD	13270 31310 12385
Self-healing squamous epithelioma	AD	13280
Hyperkeratosis lenticularis perstans	AD	14415
Steatocystoma multiplex ± pachyonychia congenita	AD AD	18450 16720
Epidermodysplasia verruciformis	AR	22640
Epithelioma calcificans of Malherbe (pilomatricoma)	AD	13260
Multiple syringoma	AD	18660
Cheilitis glandularis	AD	132
Hidrotic ectodermal dysplasia	AD	12950

TABLE 4-4 Selected Genodermatoses and Phacomatoses with Associated Neoplasia (con't)

	Mode of inheritance*	Reference*
Familial atypical multiple mole, melanoma syndrome	AD	102
Piebald trait	AD	17280
Parakeratosis of Mibelli	AD	17580
Blue rubber bleb nevus	AD	11220
Porphyria cutanea tarda	AD	17610

*See footnotes to Table 4-2.

kinds of DNA repair;[98] thus, skin carcinoma frequently occurs.

Hereditary melanoma is estimated to be responsible for from 3 to 10 percent of all melanomas, and 80 percent of patients with melanoma have pigmented nevi antedating the tumor.[99] As is the case with other familial cancers, inherited melanoma occurs at an early age.[100] Thus, melanoma in children is thought to be due predominantly to endogenous (genetic) causes, whereas environment is more likely the predominant cause in older individuals.[100,101] This view is supported by the generalized distribution of melanoma in inherited forms as opposed to the predominant occurrence in sun-exposed areas of nonhereditary cases. Multiple melanomas are frequently encountered among members of afflicted families, and persons of Celtic origin are more frequently affected.[100,102] Melanoma-prone families are also at excess risk for breast, gastrointestinal, and lymphoid malignancies. Several other genodermatoses, including XLP, von Recklinghausen's neurofibromatosis, and congenital pigmented hairy nevus predispose to malignant melanoma.[103]

Neurofibromatosis (von Recklinghausen's Syndrome)

This autosomal dominant genodermatosis is phenotypically expressed as café au lait spots and fibromatous skin tumors.[2] Occasional features include scoliosis, pseudoarthrosis of tibia, mental retardation, hypertension, hypoglycemia, malignant tumors in the peripheral nerves and brain, and pheochromocytoma. Common cellular expressions are seen in a group of diseases arising from abnormalities of neural crest embryogenesis which are called *neurocristopathies*.[104] These inherited genodermatoses include Sipple's syndrome, the multiple mucosal neuroma syndrome, von Recklinghausen's neurofibromatosis, and others with neural crest association. Confusion in diagnosis of neurofibromatosis is widespread. The cutaneous manifestations of neurofibromatosis appear at varying times during childhood, but generally they do so by the end of the second decade. Like other familial neoplastic syndromes, there are also sporadic occurrences as well. Approximately 13 to 39 percent of patients with neurofibromatosis develop malignant schwannomas of peripheral nerves, and uncommonly, a pheochromocytoma or glioma may develop.[2]

Accurate histopathologic diagnosis is mandatory. The family depicted in Fig. 4-5 was diagnosed as having von Recklinghausen's syndrome. The clinical diagnosis was correct, but the pathological diagnosis of neurofibromas was incorrect: schwannomas had occurred throughout the family. This tumor has a much more favorable prognosis than neurofibromas, which are more apt to become malignant. Incorrect diagnosis of von Recklinghausen's syndrome has also occurred in patients with "Leopard" syndrome.[105]

Other phacomatoses or neurocutaneous syndromes requiring differential diagnoses are tuberous sclerosis (Bourneville's disease), retinocerebral angiomatosis (von Hippel-Lindau disease), encephalofacial angiomatosis (Sturge-Weber disease), neurocutaneous melanosis (giant pigmented hairy nevus), neuroblastoma, multiple lentigines (Leopard syndrome), multiple endocrine adenomatoses, Albright's syndrome, and lichen striatus.[106]

Multiple Endocrine Neoplastic Syndromes

Pierce[104] formulated a unifying hypothesis of common embryologic development of cells in many organs which originate from the neural crest. These cells can give rise to multiple endocrine neoplasia (MEN) syndromes, which are often inherited as autosomal dominant traits (Table 4-5). The acronym APUD is derived from the biochemical function of the cells as follows: A = amines, PU = precursor uptake, D = L-aromatic amino acid decarboxylase. In short, APUD cells can take up precursors of biogenic amines and convert them to amine neurotransmitters by the decarboxylase. The cells synthesize and secrete specific peptide hormones; characteristic neurosecretory granules can be seen in the cytoplasm in electron micrographs or by immunofluorescence. Bolande has coined the term *neurocristopathy*, which is synonymous with *apudomas*.[107]

Penetrance of the MEN syndromes is high, but variable expression is seen. For example, Baylin[108] has observed a man with MEN I beta-cell islet tumors with a brother who had a non-beta-cell tumor secreting another hormone. The variable effect of this gene expressed as different islet tumors suggested to Baylin that the inherited defect had occurred in a totopotential precursor cell of the islets and that a subsequent mutation (second hit) became responsible for tumor progression from one of several different, but related, cells. Differences of immune competence or an exposure to different carcinogens could explain the phenotypic variance.

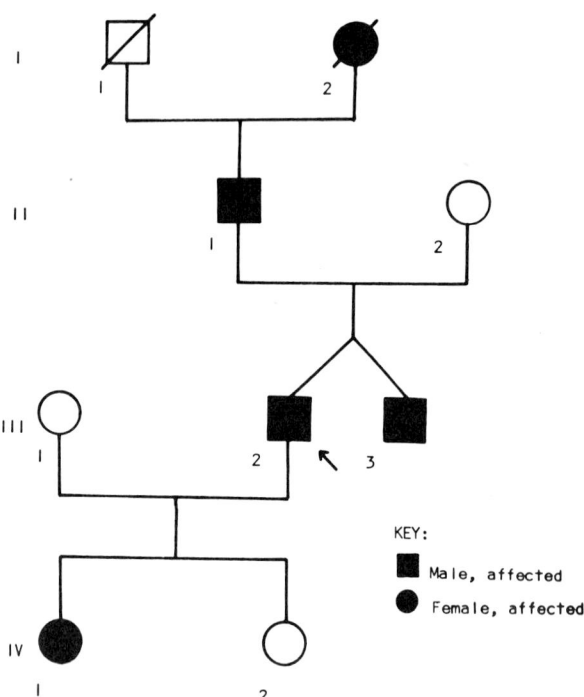

FIGURE 4-5 Autosomal dominant neurofibromatosis in a family. (*Pedigree prepared by Janet K. Hamilton, M.S.*)

TABLE 4-5 Multiple Endocrine Neoplasias

	Mode of Inheritance*	Reference*
MEN I (Werner's syndrome)	AD	13110
MEN IIa (Sipple's syndrome)	AD	17140
MEN IIb	AD	16230
Zollinger-Ellison syndrome	AD	13110

*See footnotes to Table 4-2.

In Table 4-5 the three major types of MEN syndromes are outlined: MEN I, or Sipple's syndrome (or IIa), differs from MEN III by the addition of parathyroid abnormalities. The MEN III (IIb) syndrome is characterized by medullary thyroid carcinoma, frequent bilateral pheochromocytomas, and multiple mucosal neuromata of lips and tongue. MEN III is sometimes not familial.[108]

Screening of family members for excessive secretion of neuroamines or other hormones involved in the APUD system is of proven value in the early detection of tumors. Variously, pancreatic tumors can produce insulin, glucagon, or gastrin. Parathyroid gland involvement can result in hyperparathyroidism, and medullary thyroid carcinomas can promote chronic hypocalcemia due to the production of thyrocalcitonin. Involvement by pheochromocytomas can result in characteristic flushing, hypertension, and the excessive production of norepinephrine and related compounds. Baylin has demonstrated increased concentrations of histaminase (diamine oxydase) in the enzyme produced by medullary thyroid carcinoma.[108,109] However, only one-half of patients with the tumor have elevations of this enzyme and these patients have advanced disease. Screening tests which provoke the release of hormones from tumors can aid in detecting occult neoplasia.[110,111] Provocative challenge for hereditary medullary carcinoma of the thyroid includes induction of calcitonin release by pentagastrin, cholecystokinin-pancreozymin, or ethanol.[110] Also, infusion of calcium gluconate may induce thyrocalcitonin release by the tumor. A group of Boston investigators, for a period of 7 years, have been screening a kindred now numbering 107 individuals for medullary carcinoma.[111] Provoking calcitonin secretion by infusion of calcium or pentagastrin or both has resulted in the identification of 21 persons in the kindred who have converted from normal to abnormal responses to the infusion. Moreover, 20 of 21 thyroid glands surgically removed showed C-cell hyperplasia, and 8 of the 20 also showed small foci of carcinoma. During recent years the tumors detected have become smaller, often unilateral, and without detectable metastases. Thus, this comprehensive screening program has resulted in detection and elimination of this potential life-threatening carcinoma in a family.

Inherited CNS Tumors

Familial CNS tumors occur more frequently than is generally appreciated. Twenty-nine separate reports of two or more siblings having brain tumors or neuroblastoma have been reported.[2] Familial CNS tumors include well-differentiated gliomas as occurring in tuberous sclerosis, lymphomas, meningiomas, and glioblastoma multiforme. These CNS tumors (Table 4-6) can be classified into three major catagories of association with other phenotypes: neurocutaneous or phacomatosis syndromes, those unassociated with cutaneous markers, and those associated with neuroblastoma. Neurocutaneous defects are associated with brain tumors such as disturbances in melanin and blood vessel formation (phacomatosis syndromes). Thus intrinsic dysmorphogenesis antedates and possibly predisposes to certain tumors.[112]

Brain tumors can be an expression of the autosomal dominant cancer familial syndrome.[2] Li and Fraumeni[113] have reported CNS tumors associated with rhabdomyosarcoma in a child and other primary relatives with brain tumors or adrenocortical carcinoma. The association of CNS and colon tumors in Turcot's syndrome was discussed earlier.

XLP as a Model

Our studies of XLP demonstrate the interaction between genetic predisposition to oncogenesis triggered by an environmental agent (EBV). Prior to a discussion of the comprehensive program for studying XLP, the immunopathogenesis of Burkitt's lymphoma (BL) and infectious mononucleosis (IM) will be considered.

The results of studies done by numerous investigators during the past two decades substantiate the view that

TABLE 4-6 Selected Inherited Syndromes with CNS Cancers*

	Mode of Inheritance†	*Reference*†
Retinoblastoma, bilateral	AD	18020
Acoustic neuroma, bilateral	AD	10100
Neuroblastoma	AR	25670
	AD	133
Megalencephaly	AD	15535
Megalencephaly	AR	24800
Glioma of brain	AD	13780
Meningioma	AD	15610

*See also Table 4-4, Phacomatoses.
†See footnotes to Table 4-2.

EBV can be an oncogenic agent in immunodeficient individuals. A brief historical review follows which provides background information for the discussion of EBV-induced oncogenesis in immune-deficient persons. The keen epidemiological observations of Denis Burkitt in tropical Africa delineated a new malignant lymphoma which often involves the jaws or abdominal organs.[114] Endemic African BL is present in areas of hyperendemic malaria. A hematopathology committee of the World Health Organization has defined BL as having a characteristic starry-sky pattern and specific cytochemical findings of oil red O and methyl green pyronin positivity and PAS (periodic acid-Schiff) negativity.[115]

William Damashek observed that IM is a lymphoma-like illness which, though often serious, is rarely fatal.[116] Diagnosis of IM requires fulfillment of a triad of clinical, hematologic, and serologic criteria. Werner and Gertrude Henle, in 1968, demonstrated that EBV was the etiologic agent of IM.[117] Specific antibody responses to EBV form against early antigen and are transient, whereas VCA and EB nuclear-associated antigen (EBNA) persist throughout life. Approximately 90 percent of adults have EBV antibodies to EBV, indicating past infection.

In 1964, Epstein and Barr identified a unique herpesvirus in a BL-derived lymphoblastoid cell line.[118] EBNA was identified in EBV-transformed B cells by Reedman and Klein in 1973 by immunofluorescence.[119] Many investigators have attempted to determine whether EBV is an oncogenic virus in human beings. Three major EBV-associated diseases occur: IM in adolescents in Western countries, BL in the tropics, and nasopharyngeal carcinoma (NPC) in Southeast Asia. Although EBV has been demonstrated in tumor tissue derived from BL and NPC, absolute proof that EBV is an oncogenic virus is lacking.[120]

Zeigler and associates[12] have summarized several hypotheses associating EBV with malignancy. Two hypotheses seem plausible based on experimental observations. The passenger hypothesis proposes that EBV secondarily infects malignantly transformed B cells or, alternatively, that latent virus in B cells becomes activated following malignant transformation by some other agent. A second major hypothesis is that inherited or acquired immune deficiency may allow EBV to become an oncogenic virus. Results of studies of the X-linked recessive lymphoproliferative syndrome (XLP) support the hypothesis that inherited immune deficiency can render susceptible individuals to oncogenesis by EBV.

In 1969, an 8-year-old boy in the Duncan kindred died of IM. Purtilo performed the autopsy. During the ensuing 6 years it was noted that five maternally related males in the Duncan family had succumbed to IM, agammaglobulinemia following IM, or malignant lymphoma. Thus, two common biological threads in the Duncan family were identified: X-linked recessive inheritance of B-cell disorders.[122-127] Since the association of EBV with IM was known, it was postulated that males affected by XLP had an immune deficiency, especially to EBV, which, following infection, triggered proliferation of B cells, leading to fatal IM or malignant lymphoma.[123]

Subsequently, we have found a large kindred in which approximately 20 males have succumbed to a variety of B-cell disorders including IM, American BL, and other B-cell malignancies and deficiencies[124] (Table 4-7).

The laboratories are conducting comprehensive studies on XLP involving genetic, pathologic, immunologic, virologic, and biochemical techniques. A central organizational focus of the program is the registry of XLP. Employing the diagnostic criteria of phenotypic expression of two or more maternally related males, the authors have identified in the medical literature and by referrals from collaborative clinicians and pathologists more than 20 families including approximately 105 affected males. Examples of families affected by the syndrome include those reported by Maurer et al., Falletta et al., Bar et al., and Provisor et al.[125]

Hematopathologic features of XLP include the ap-

TABLE 4-7 Pleiotropic Effects of the X-Linked Recessive Lymphoproliferative Syndrome

Aproliferative phenotypes:
  Acquired agammaglobulinemia
  Aplastic anemia
  Agranulocytosis

Proliferative phenotypes:
  American Burkitt's lymphoma
  Immunoblastic sarcoma of B cells
  "Histiocytic" lymphoma
  Fatal infectious mononucleosis
  Plasmacytoma
  Immunodeficiency with hyper-IgM
  Other

Birth defect phenotypes:
  Cardiac defects
  Neurological defects
  Other

pearance of atypical lymphocytes in the peripheral blood of males showing the IM phenotype. These individuals lack capacity to stop the proliferation of EBV-infected B cells because they often lack antibodies against EBV. Their lymphocytes grow spontaneously in culture and contain EBV.[126,127] Often, Monospot and heterophile determinations are positive.

The patients with XLP succumb from complications of IM: extensive visceral organ and CNS infiltration by lymphocytes can lead to dysfunction of vital organs, or infections ensue secondary to suppression of bone marrow with aplastic anemia, or agammaglobulinemia ensues leading to opportunistic infections. Occasionally malignant lymphomas emerge in the males who survive for a month or longer with IM. Possibly, the polyclonal proliferation of IM switches to a monoclonal malignant lymphoma, in some patients with XLP, because of a karyotypic abnormality in a transformed B cell. Thus, the cell bearing the defective chromosome may escape host defenses.

Hematopathologic lesions are widespread involving all hematopoietic organs. Thymus gland changes vary depending on the interval following infection by EBV. During the first 2 weeks of illness the gland often shows increased numbers of proliferating immunoblasts. The following week depletion of thymocytes and a replacement by plasma cells occurs. A loss of corticomedullary demarcation is noted and then Hassall's corpuscles become depleted. Males surviving 1 month or longer show a marked depletion of thymocytes, and Hassall's corpuscles may be totally absent or calcified; connective tissue stroma with a few plasma cells and lymphocytes remain. Rarely, malignant lymphomas occur in the thymus gland.

Thymus-dependent areas in the lymph nodes and spleen often show necrosis, and T cells are replaced by immunoblasts and plasmacytoid cells. Eventually, depletion of paracortical regions is seen and these areas are replaced by plasmacytoid cells, or a reticular stromal skeleton is seen with severe lymphoid depletion. The immunological battle that occurs with IM is most dramatically seen in the periarterial sheath of the spleen where nuclear debris is evident; plasmacytoid cells infiltrate the T-cell sheath.

Bone marrow appears normal prior to the onset of profound polyclonal B-cell proliferation of IM. Later in the disease, one of two processes may occur: either aplastic anemia or replacement of marrow by plasmacytoid and plasma cells appears.

The skin shows infiltration reminiscent of graft-vs.-host disease in boys with IM. Periportal infiltrate in the liver with hepatocellular necrosis is often intense. The heart and other visceral organs may become infiltrated. The brain often shows a perivascular plasma cell and lymphoid infiltrate.

The malignant lymphomas which have appeared in XLP have spanned the spectrum of B-cell tumors ranging from classical American BL to immunoblastic sarcoma of B cells with plasma cell differentiation or so-called histocytic lymphoma.[126,127] We have observed many cases wherein the IM and immunoblastic sarcoma phenotype have occurred concurrently. Therefore, in patients with XLP it has been demonstrated that IM can progress to malignant lymphoma. It has been hypothesized that for the polyclonal proliferation characteristic of IM to become a monoclonal proliferation, a karyotypic abnormality appears which leads to a malignant monoclonal tumor cell. For example, the 14q+ marker chromosome of BL may be present.[127] This hypothesis is being tested by periodically testing affected males. Remarkable similarities between graft-vs.-host disease and XLP are seen.[128,129]

In summary, we have developed a registry and laboratory of XLP dedicated to conducting multidisciplinary studies to provide the following:

1. Consultation to clinicians, families, and pathologists seeking diagnosis, treatment, evaluation, and genetic counseling
2. Collection of data to define diagnostic criteria
3. Further delineation of the diverse immune deficiencies and the basic genetic-immunologic defects responsible for the various phenotypic expressions
4. The establishment of lymphoblastoid cell lines from patients with XLP and related lymphoproliferative disorders which occur on genetic or sporadic bases for comparative studies
5. Testing of the hypothesis that the common, ubiquitous EBV can produce lethal lymphoproliferative disorders in individuals with inherited or acquired immunodeficiency
6. Development of rational immunoprophylaxis and therapy against virus-induced oncogenesis.

SCREENING FOR INHERITED PREDISPOSITION TO CANCER

Many benefits can be derived from evaluating individuals and families for inherited cancer syndromes. For example, early diagnosis and intervention becomes possible. Secondly, pathogenetic mechanisms predisposing to cancer can be investigated and the interaction with environmental carcinogens assessed. Thirdly, the families should receive counseling from the physician or other qualified individuals to explain inheritance and risks in offspring. A pessimistic or nihilistic attitude need not pervade. Positive action can be taken to relieve the tremendous burden carried by family members at high risk of cancer.

A thorough family history with pedigree is mandatory for the recognition of genetic disease. This inexpensive but invaluable technique permits ascertainment of familial cancer patterns and possible modes of inheritance. Enlistment of a highly motivated family member who will document the names, dates, and addresses, and locate clinical and pathological records, facilitates data gathering. Documentation of histopathologic types of tumors is necessary.

Clinical history and physical examination is aimed at identifying cardinal features of inherited cancer (Table 4-1) such as early onset of cancer, bilateral and multiple tumors in the same individual, associated congenital defects, occurrence of a similar malignancy in multiple siblings, and so on. Following ascertainment of pedigree and review of the clinical and pathological data on a family, a screening program should be tailor-made for each syndrome and family. Guides to the evaluation of three groups of patients genetically predisposed to cancer follow. In children, many of the inherited cancers are autosomal dominant. They involve the eye (retinoblastoma), kidney (Wilms's tumor), adrenals (neuroblastoma), and connective tissue (rhabdomyosarcoma). Physical examination for associated birth defects such as aniridia and palpation for abdominal masses is required.

Routine laboratory screening includes complete blood count, urinalysis, and x-rays. Special studies include intravenous pyelogram for renal and adrenal tumors and measurement of various markers in blood and urine. Carcinoembryonic antigen (CEA) has been elevated in Wilms's tumor and in other inherited cancer.[130] Specific diagnoses invariably require a biopsy with pathological confirmation. On obtaining the tumor biopsy specimen, a karyotype should be performed on cultured cells of the tumor tissue itself, as well as of peripheral blood. In so doing, abnormal chromosomes such as the 13q− of retinoblastoma and various other marker chromosomes may be detected.

The clastogenic syndromes, which often show autosomal recessive inheritance, can also be evaluated by karyotyping cutaneous fibroblasts and peripheral blood. Inspection of the skin for unusually fair complexion and telangiectatic abnormalities is of great value. Since leukemia is a major complication in individuals with ataxia-telangiectasia and Bloom's syndrome, the blood should be evaluated morphologically for leukemic cells and a bone marrow aspiration performed for definitive diagnosis. Since the clastogenic syndromes are characterized by susceptibility to cutaneous malignancies, suspicious lesions ought to be biopsied and studied microscopically. Enlistment of specialists capable of studying the rare clastogenic syndromes can be obtained to ascertain the impact of ultraviolet light or irradiation in inducing chromosomal damage in vitro or monitoring sister chromatid exchange.

The families found to show inheritance of the more common cancer syndromes such as familial colon carcinoma, breast carcinoma, or the less commonly occurring MEN syndromes, can also be evaluated by tailoring screening programs. For example, inherited colon cancer generally shows autosomal dominant inheritance. Often colonoscopy and barium-contrast enema x-ray studies reveal numerous polyps. The evaluation of blood for elevated CEA and stool for occult blood can be of value for the early detection of cancer. Biopsy of suspicious lesions with histopathologic evaluation is necessary. Important preventive surgical prophylactic colectomies can be performed in individuals with specific colorectal polyposis syndromes.

Families showing inherited breast cancer syndromes should be instructed on breast self-examination, and receive periodic breast examination and mammography by the clinician. Biopsy of suspicious lesions is also indicated. Special effort for detection of cancer in the bilateral contralateral breast and in other estrogen-dependent organs is urged.

Screening for the MEN syndromes can be challenging and rewarding. Noting specific cutaneous and oral abnormalities such as neuromata may provide clues to diagnosis. Measurement of excessive secretion of neuroamines or other hormones produced by the APUD endocrine system is valuable for early detection of tumors. For example, parathyroid tumors can result in hyperparathyroidism and thyroid by medullary carcinoma which cause excessive production of parathormone and thyrocalcitonin, respectively. Baylin has demonstrated increased concentrations of histaminase in blood of patients with medullary thyroid carcinoma.[108] Provocative challenge with pentagastrin, ethanol, or calcium gluconate can provoke release of thyrocalcitonin by a tumor. Following documentation of excessive release of thyrocalcitonin, surgical exploration with prophylactic thyroidectomy has led to the early recognition of medullary thyroid carcinoma and the precursor lesion, hyperplastic C cells.[111]

Children with inherited immune deficiency syndromes are at high risk for developing lymphoproliferative malignancies. The various immune deficiency syndromes can be recognized by characteristic increased susceptibility to infectious agents, cutaneous and ocular telangiectasia, and lymph node enlargement; and abdominal tumor masses should be searched for. Careful evaluation of the peripheral blood smear and bone marrow for lymphocytic leukemia, if necessary, may be indicated. An immune profile consisting of T and B lymphocytes and responsiveness to phytomitogens is indicated, as is quantification of immunoglobulin levels. This screening protocol can be modified according to the specific syndrome diagnosed. For example, we have been evaluating families with XLP by obtaining immune profiles and noting the presence of EBV and lack of antibody response to the virus.

Benefits derived from screening of families showing inherited immune deficiency syndromes include improved health of individuals with previously undetected immune deficiency. Such children may be placed on long-term antibiotic prophylaxis and gamma globulin can be administered. They can be periodically monitored for the emergence of malignancies.

Finally, the clinician who discovers a family with inherited cancer syndrome is under moral obligation to provide genetic counseling for the family. If he or she does not feel equipped to provide counseling, then a referral to a genetic counseling center, which is usually available at major medical centers, is indicated. The purpose of counseling is to explain to the families the inheritance pattern of the cancer, to dispel misconceptions about what has occurred in the family, and to provide accurate information. This information should also be conveyed to them in a written narrative. Opportunities for follow-up discussions with the family members should also be made available. The authors' experiences in providing genetic counseling and attempts at comprehensive screening programs and investigation of inherited neoplastic syndromes have been rewarded by early diagnosis of premalignant or malignant conditions and have provided excellent opportunities for definitive intervention.

REFERENCES

1. Purtilo DT et al: Genetics of neoplasia: Impact of ecogenetics on oncogenesis. *Am J Pathol* 91:609–688, 1978.
2. Fraumeni JF Jr (ed): *Persons at High Risk of Cancer: An Approach to Cancer Etiology and Control,* Academic, New York, 1975.
3. Lynch HT (ed): *Cancer Genetics,* Thomas, Springfield, Ill., 1976.
4. Mulvihill JJ et al (eds): *Genetics of Human Cancer,* Raven, New York 1977.
5. German J (ed): *Chromosomes and Cancer,* Wiley, New York 1974.
6. Schimke RN: *Genetics and Cancer in Man,* Churchill Livingstone, New York, 1978.
7. McKusick VA: *Mendelian Inheritance in Man,* 5th ed, Johns Hopkins, Baltimore, 1978.
8. Sang D, Alber D: Recent advances in the study of retinoblastoma, in G Peyman et al (eds): *Intraocular Tumors,* Appleton Century Crofts, New York, 1977.
9. Knudson A: Genetics and etiology of human cancer. *Adv Hum Genet* 8:1–66, 1977.
10. Knudson A: Retinoblastoma: A prototype hereditary neoplasm. *Semin Oncol* 5:57–60, 1978.
11. Matsunaga E: Hereditary retinoblastoma: Penetrance, expressivity, and age of onset. *Hum Genet* 33:1–15, 1976.
12. Hethcote H, Knudson, A: Model for the incidence of embryonal cancers: Application to retinoblastoma. *Proc Nat Acad Sci* 75:2453–2457, 1978.
13. Kitchen F, Ellsworth R: Pleiotropic effects of the gene for retinoblastoma. *J Med Genet* 11:244–246, 1974.
14. Jakobiec F et al: Retinoblastoma and intracranial malignancy. *Cancer* 39:2048–2058, 1977.
15. Chan H, Pratt C: A new familian cancer syndrome? A spectrum of malignant and benign tumors including retinoblastoma, carcinoma of the bladder and other genitourinary tumors, thyroid adenoma, and a probable case of multifocal osteosarcoma. *J Nat Cancer Inst* 58:205–207, 1977.
16. Li, F: Second malignant tumors after cancer in childhood. *Cancer* 40:1899–1902, 1977.
17. Meadows A et al: Patterns of second malignant neoplasms in children. *Cancer* 40:1903–1911, 1977.
18. Purtilo DT et al: Autosomal dominant colon adenocarcinoma syndrome. *Lab Invest* 36:349, 1977.

19. Purtilo DT et al: Malignancies and immunological abnormalities in five brothers. *Arch Dis Child* 52:310–313, 1977.
20. Strong L: Genetic and environmental interactions. *Cancer* 40 (suppl):1861–1866, 1977.
21. Pendergrass TW: Congenital anomalies in children with Wilm's tumor. *Cancer* 37:403–409, 1976.
22. Maurer H et al: The role of genetic factors in the etiology of Wilm's tumor. *Cancer* 43:205–208, 1979.
23. Bishop H et al: Survival in bilateral Wilm's tumor—Review of 30 national Wilm's tumor study cases. *J Pediatr Surg* 12:631–638, 1977.
24. Roberts F, Lee K: Familial neuroblastoma presenting as multiple tumors. *Radiology* 116:133–136, 1975.
25. Wander J, Das Gupta T: Neurofibromatosis. *Curr Prob Surg* 14:1–81, 1977.
26. Durkin-Stamm MV et al: An unusual dysplasia-malformation cancer syndrome in two patients. *Am J Med Genet* 1:279–289, 1978.
27. Gericke GS et al: Leukaemogenesis in Down's syndrome. *S Afr Med J* 51:158–162, 1977.
28. Levin S et al: Thymic deficiency in Down's syndrome. *Pediatrics* 63:80–87, 1979.
29. Fujita K, Fujita H: Klinefelter's syndrome and bladder cancer. *J Urol* 116:836–837, 1976.
30. Hart WR, Burkons DM: Germ cell neoplasms arising in gonadoblastomas. *Cancer* 43:669–678, 1979.
31. Walbaum R et al: Un cas de retinoblastome bilateral avec monosomie 13 partielle (q12–q14). *Hum Genet* 44:219–226, 1978.
32. Hirschorn K: Chromosomes and cancer. *Birth Defects Original Article Series* 12:113–121, 1976.
33. Comings DE: Mechanisms of chromosome banding and implications for chromosome structure. *Ann Rev Genet* 12:25–46, 1978.
34. Arlett C, Lehmann A: Human disorders showing increased sensitivity to the induction of genetic damage. *Ann Rev Genet* 12:95–115, 1978.
35. German J: Oncogenic implications of chromosomal instability, in V McKusick, R Claiborne (eds): *Medical Genetics,* HP Publishing, New York, 1973.
36. German J et al: Bloom's syndrome; V: Surveillance for cancer in affected families. *Clin Genet* 12:162–168, 1977.
37. Hand R, German J: Bloom's syndrome: DNA replication in cultured fibroblasts and lymphocytes. *Hum Genet* 38:297–306, 1977.
38. Bourgeois CA, Hill FC: Fanconi anemia leading to acute myelomonocytic leukemia: Cytogenetic studies. *Cancer* 39:1163–1167, 1977.
39. Schmid W, Fanconi G: Fragility and spiralization anomalies of the chromosomes in the cases including fraternal twins, with Fanconi's anemia, type Estren-Dameshek. *Cytogenet Cell Genet* 20:141–149, 1978.
40. Hirsch-Kauffman M et al: Deficiency of DNA ligase activity in Fanconi's anemia. *Hum Genet* 45:25–32, 1978.
41. Spector B et al: Genetically determined immunodeficiency diseases (GDID) and malignancy: Report from the immunodeficiency-cancer registry. *Clin Immunol Immunopathol* 11:12–29, 1978.
42. Levin S et al: Ataxia telangiectasia. *Paediatrician* 6:135–146, 1977.
43. McCaw B et al: Somatic rearrangement of chromosome 14 in human lymphocytes. *Proc Nat Acad Sci USA* 72:2071–2075, 1975.
44. Nelson M et al: Chromosomes in ataxia telangiectasia. *Lancet* 1:518–519, 1975.
45. Joncas J et al: Unusual prevalence of antibodies to Epstein-Barr virus early antigen in ataxia telangiectasia. *Lancet* 1:1160, 1977.
46. Fukuhara S: Significance of 14q translocations in non-Hodgkin lymphomas. *Virchows Arch B* 29:99–106, 1978.
47. Cleaver J: Human diseases with in vitro manifestations of altered repair and replication of DNA, in JJ Mulvihill et al (eds): *Genetics of Human Cancer,* Raven, New York, 1977.
48. Taylor AMR et al: Ataxia telangiectasia: A human mutation with abnormal radiation sensitivity. *Nature* 258:427–429, 1975.
49. Sirinavin C, Trowbridge A: Dyskeratosis congenita: Clinical features and genetic aspects. *J Med Genet* 12:339–354, 1975.
50. Burgdorf W et al: Sister chromatid exchange in dyskeratosis congenita lymphocytes. *J Med Genet* 14:256–257, 1977.
51. Trowbridge A et al: Dyskeratosis congenita: Hematologic evaluation of a sibship and review of the literature. *Am J Hematol* 3:143–152, 1977.
52. Hillman E et al: Biological characterization of an Epstein-Barr nuclear antigen positive American Burkitt's tumor-derived cell line. *Cancer Res* 37:4546–4558, 1977.
53. Kaiser-McCaw B et al: Chromosome 14 translocations in African and North American Burkitt's lymphoma. *Int J Cancer* 19:482–486, 1977.
54. Kaplan H et al: Biology and virology of the human malignant lymphomas. *Cancer* 43:1–24, 1979.
55. Hassfeld, D: Chromosome 14q+ in a retinoblastoma. *Int J Cancer* 21:720–723, 1978.
56. Liang W, Rowley J: 14q+ marker chromosomes in multiple myeloma and plasma cell leukemia. *Lancet* 1:96, 1978.
57. Roth DG et a1: B cell acute lymphoblastic leukemia with a 14q+ chromosome abnormality. *Blood* 53:235–243, 1979.
58. Temple M: The cytogenetics of human lymphoma and lymphoblastoid cell lines, Ph.D. thesis. Georgetown University Department of Biology, 1977.
59. Kurvink K et al: Sister chromatid exchange in lymphocytes from patients with malignant lymphoma. *Hum Genet* 44:137–144, 1978.
60. Nowell PC, Hungerford DA: A minute chromosome in human chronic granulocytic leukemia. *Science* 132:1497, 1960.
61. Rowley J: A new consistent chromosomal abnormality in

61. chronic myelogenous leukemia identified by quinacrine fluorescence and Giemsa staining. *Nature* 243:290, 1973.
62. First International Workshop on Chromosomes in Leukemia: Chromosomes in Ph¹-positive chronic granulocytic leukemia. *Br J Haematol* 39:305-309, 1978.
63. Pederson B: Pathogenesis and blastic transformation of chronic myeloid leukemia as consequences of Ph¹ positive stem cell hyperplasia: A unifying concept. *Blood Cells* 3:535-551, 1977.
64. Gibbs T et al: The significance of Ph¹ in acute lymphoblastic leukemia: A report of two cases. *Br J Haematol* 37:447-453, 1977.
65. Forman E et al: Ph¹ positive childhood leukemias: Spectrum of lymphoid-myeloid expressions. *Blood* 49:549-558, 1977.
66. Rowley J et al: Further evidence for a non-random chromosomal abnormality in acute promyelocytic leukemia. *Int J Cancer* 20:869-872, 1977.
67. Golomb H et al: Correlation of clinical finding with quinacrine-banded chromosomes in 90 adults with acute nonlymphocytic leukemia. *N Engl J Med* 299:613-619, 1978.
68. Cimino MC et al: Banding studies of chromosomal abnormalities in patients with acute lymphocytic leukemia. *Cancer Res* 39:227-238, 1979.
69. First International Workshop on Chromosomes in Leukemia: Chromosomes in acute non-lymphocytic leukemia. *Br J Haematol* 39:311-316, 1978.
70. Cervenka J et al: Familial leukemia and inherited chromosomal aberration. *Int J Cancer* 19:783-788, 1977.
71. Petrakova A et al: (abstract) *XIV Int Cong Genet* II:640, 1978.
72. Ganina K, Gritzenko A: USSR karyotype study in human gastric cancers and polyps. *XIV Int Cong Genet* II:448, 1978.
73. Henry WM et al: Tumor cell karyotypes in malignant melanoma. *J Surg Oncol* 11:31-38, 1979.
74. Kovacs G: Abnormalities of chromosome no. 1 in human solid malignant tumors. *Int J Cancer* 21:688-694, 1978.
75. Meisner L et al: Genetic mechanisms in cancer predisposition. *Cancer* 43:679-689, 1979.
76. Cheng W et al: Sister chromatid exchanges and chromosomes in chronic myelogenous leukemia and cancer families. *Int J Cancer* 23:8-13, 1979.
77. Anderson DE: Familial cancer in families. *Semin Oncol* 5:11-16, 1978.
78. Burkitt DP: Large-bowel cancer: An epidemiologic jigsaw puzzle. *J Nat Cancer Inst* 54:3-6, 1975.
79. Enstrom JE: Colorectal cancer and consumption of beef and fat. *Br J Cancer* 32:432-439, 1975.
80. Cunningham AS: Lymphomas and animal-protein consumption. *Lancet* 2:1184-1186, 1976.
81. Purtilo DT et al: Teratogenesis and oncogenesis in a family: Variable phenotypic expression of Turcot's syndrome. Unpublished observations.
82. Winawer SJ, Sherlock P: Approach to screening and diagnosis in colorectal cancer. *Semin Oncol* 3:387-397, 1976.
83. Miller MS et al: Familial colon cancer. *Cancer* 37:946-948, 1976.
84. Knudson AG et al: Heredity and cancer in man, in AG Steinberg, AG Bearn (eds): *Progress in Medical Genetics*, vol 9, Grune & Stratton, New York, 1973.
85. DeCosse JJ et al: Familial polyposis. *Cancer* 39:267-273, 1977.
86. Kopelovich L et al: Recent studies on the identification of proliferative abnormalities and of oncogenic potential of cutaneous cells in individuals at increased risk of colon cancer. *Semin Oncol* 3:369-372, 1972.
87. Danes BS: The Gardner syndrome: A study in cell culture. *Cancer* 36:2327-2333, 1975.
88. Danes BS, Krush AJ: The Gardner syndrome: A family study in cell culture. *J Nat Cancer Inst* 58:771-775, 1977.
89. Armstrong A, Davies J: Familial breast cancer: Report of a family pedigree. *Br J Cancer* 37:294-307, 1978.
90. Miller AB et al: A study of diet and breast cancer. *Am J Epidemiol* 107:499-509, 1978.
91. Moore D, Charney J: Breast Cancer: Etiology and possible prevention. *Am Sci* 63:160-168, 1975.
92. Scheike O: Male breast cancer. *Acta Pathol Microbiol Scand A Suppl* 251:13-35, 1975.
93. Lynch HT et al: Genetic heterogeneity and familial carcinoma of the breast. *Surg Gynecol Obstet* 142:693-699, 1976.
94. Li FP, Fraumeni JF Jr: Familial breast cancer, soft-tissue sarcomas, and other neoplasms. *Ann Intern Med* 83:833-834, 1975.
95. Everson RB et al: Familial male breast cancer. *Lancet* 1:9-12, 1976.
96. Lynch H, Frichot B: Skin, heredity and cancer. *Semin Oncol* 5:67-84, 1978.
97. Orth G et al: Characteristics of the lesions and risk of malignant conversion associated with the type of human papillomavirus involved in Epidermodysplasia verruciformis. *Cancer Res* 39:1074-1082, 1979.
98. Cleaver JE: Human diseases with in vitro manifestations of altered repair and replication of DNA, in JJ Mulvihill et al (eds): *Genetics of Human Cancer*, Raven, New York, 1977.
99. McGovern VJ: Epidemiology aspects of melanoma: A review. *Pathology* 9:233-241, 1977.
100. Magnus K: Incidence of malignant melanoma of the skin in 5 Nordic countries: Significance of solar radiation. *Int J Cancer* 20:477-485, 1977.
101. Wallace DC, Exton LA: Genetic predisposition to the development of malignant melanoma, in WH McCarthy, VNC Blight (eds): *Melanoma and Skin Cancer*, Proceedings of the International Cancer Conference, Australia Government Printers, Sidney, 1972.

102. Frichot BC et al: New cutaneous phenotype in familial malignant melanoma. *Lancet* 1:864–865, 1977.
103. Lynch HJ, Frichot BC: Skin, heredity, and cancer. *Semin Oncol* 5:67–84, 1978.
104. Pierce AGE: Cell migration in the alimentary system: Endocrine contributions of the neurocrist to the gut and its derivatives. *Digestion* 8:372–385, 1973.
105. Bhawan J et al: Giant and "granular melanosomes" in LEOPARD syndrome: An ultrastructural study. *J Cutan Pathol* 3:207–216, 1976.
106. Solomon IM, Esterly NB: Epidermal and other congenital organoid nevi. *Curr Probl Pediatr* 6:1–56, 1975.
107. Bolande RP: The neurocristopathies: A unifying concept of disease arising in neural crest maldevelopment. *Hum Biol* 5:409–429, 1974.
108. Baylin SB: The multiple endocrine neoplasia syndromes: Implications for the study of inherited tumors. *Semin Oncol* 5:35–46, 1978.
109. Baylin S et al: Inherited medullary thyroid carcinoma: A final monoclonal mutation in one of multiple clones of susceptible cells. *Science* 199:429–431, 1978.
110. Telenius-Berg M et al: Screening for medullary carcinoma of the thyroid in families with Sipple syndrome. *Eur J Clin Invest* 7:7–16, 1977.
111. Graze K et al: Natural history of familial medullary carcinoma. *N Engl J Med* 299:980–985, 1978.
112. Miller RW: Deaths from childhood cancer in sibs. *N Engl J Med* 279:122–126, 1968.
113. Li FP, Fraumeni JF: Soft-tissue sarcomas, breast cancer, and other neoplasms: A familial syndrome? *Ann Intern Med* 71:747–752, 1969.
114. Burkitt DP: A sarcoma involving the jaws in African children. *Br J Surg* 46:218–223, 1958.
115. Berard C et al: Histopathological definition of Burkitt's tumour. *Bull WHO* 40:601–607, 1969.
116. Damashek W, Gunz F: *Leukemia*, New York, 1964, p 556.
117. Henle G et al: Relation of Burkitt's tumor-associated Herpes-type virus to infectious mononucleosis. *Proc Nat Acad Sci* 59:94, 1968.
118. Epstein MA et al: Virus particles in cultured lymphoblasts from Burkitt's lymphoma. *Lancet* 1:702–703, 1964.
119. Reedman BM, Klein G: Cellular localizations of an Epstein-Barr virus (EBV)-associated complement-fixing antigen in producer and non-producer lymphoblastoid cell lines. *Int J Cancer* 11:499–520, 1973.
120. Klein G: The Epstein-Barr virus and neoplasia. *N Engl J Med* 293:1353–1357, 1975.
121. Ziegler JL et al: Epstein-Barr virus in human malignancy. *Ann Intern Med* 86:323, 1978.
122. Purtilo DT et al: X-linked recessive progressive combined variable immunodeficiency (Duncan's disease). *Lancet* 1:935–941, 1975.
123. Purtilo DT: Hypothesis: Pathogenesis and phenotypes of an X-linked lymphoproliferative syndrome. *Lancet* 2:882–885, 1976.
124. Purtilo DT et al: Variable phenotypic expression of an X-linked recessive lymphoproliferative syndrome. *N Engl J Med* 297:1077–1081, 1977.
125. Hamilton JK et al: X-linked lymphoproliferative syndrome registry report. *J Pediatr* 96:669–673, 1980.
126. Purtilo DT et al: Diagnosis and immunopathogenesis of the X-linked recessive lymphoproliferative syndrome. *Semin Hematol* (in press).
127. Purtilo DT et al: Biomakers in immunodeficiency syndromes predisposing to cancer, in H Lynch, H Guirgis (eds): Van Nostrand-Reinhold, New York (in press).
128. Kersey H et al: Graft vs. host reactions following transplantation of allogenic hematopoietic cells. *Hum Pathol* 2:389–402, 1974.
129. Seemayer T et al: Thymic epithelial injury in graft vs. host reactions following adrenalectomy. *Am J Pathol* 93:325–331, 1978.
130. Mann JR et al: Clinical applications of serum carcinoembryonic antigen and alpha-fetoprotein levels in children with solid tumours. *Arch Dis Child* 53:366–374, 1978.
131. Wennstrom J et al: Hereditary benign and malignant lesions of the large bowel. *Cancer* 34:850–857, 1974.
132. Schweich L: Cheilitis glandularis simplex. *Arch Dermatol* 89:301–302, 1964.
133. Knudson AG, Strong LC: Mutation and cancer: Neuroblastoma and pheochromocytoma. *Am J Hum Genet* 24:541–532, 1972.

SELECTED BIBLIOGRAPHY

Fraumeni JF Jr: Genetic factors, in JF Holland, E Frei (eds): *Cancer Medicine,* Lea & Febiger, Philadephia, 1982, pp 5–12.

Meisner LF: Genetic factors in human cancer, in SB Kahn et al (eds): *Concepts in Cancer Medicine,* Grune & Stratton, New York, 1983, pp 165–176.

Miller G: On the nature of susceptibility to cancer. *Cancer* 96:1307–1318, 1980.

5
TUMOR VIRUSES—VECTORS OF CARCINOGENESIS AT THE MOLECULAR LEVEL

Fred Rapp   *Mary K. Howett*

A tumor, as it is seen by the eyes of a practicing oncologist, represents the propagation of a successful renegade cell into a multicellular mass capable of commanding its own blood supply and space, often at the expense of the body organs. Demands of the tumor-bearing patient require measures that are not immediately concerned with the initial causes of the mass, but these causes have ultimately occupied the intellectual and scientific curiosities of biomedical workers involved in every aspect of the cancer problem.

Clinicians and basic researchers have studied a number of factors that appear to be capable of inducing the abnormal growth of that initial renegade cell. The persistent reader will find whole areas of investigation devoted to chemical carcinogens, to radiation, to tumor viruses, to the genetic predisposition to cancer, literally to every possible cause of neoplasia.[1] In this chapter, we will explore one such factor, tumor viruses. Evidence will be presented that these infectious agents have, as a life-cycle option, the ability to alter the growth regulation of the infected cell as a consequence of the expression of virus gene products. Because of the extensive literature on this subject, we will not attempt to specifically reference individual work. The reader is, therefore, referred to several excellent reviews that are cited at the end of this chapter.

The first demonstration of a virus association with malignancy occurred in 1908 when Ellermann and Bang demonstrated that filtrates of chicken leukemic cells, known to be free of bacteria, could transmit the disease when reinoculated into disease-free chickens. Because leukemia was then not yet recognized by physicians as a malignancy, the importance of this finding was overshadowed in 1911 when Peyton Rous demonstrated that a solid tumor (a transplantable sarcoma of chickens) could also be transmitted by a cell-free filtrate.

These early observations, while of recognized importance, were largely ignored for decades because the technology to exploit them remained to be developed. In recent years, with the advent of molecular biology, new inroads associating viruses with the etiology of cancer have been made. In general, the progress in this area has depended on several major approaches including (1) development of in vitro models to study virus replication and the ability of viruses to alter normal cellular growth regulation; (2) development of in vivo models to study tumorigenesis by viruses; (3) isolation of viruses from naturally occurring tumors; (4) development of specific and sensitive methods to probe transformed cells and tumors for virus nucleic acids and antigens; and finally (5) epidemiologic studies, especially in human populations, to associate viruses with certain tumor types. As a result of these efforts, several groups of viruses (DNA and RNA) have been implicated in both animal and human tumors. These groups include, among the DNA viruses, the adenoviruses, the papovaviruses (both the papilloma and polyoma subgroups), the herpesviruses, and hepatitis B virus. One major group of RNA viruses, the retroviruses, has also been extensively associated with tumors in animals. We will present in vitro and in vivo evidence for tumorigenesis by viruses and discuss the current understanding of molecular events that lead to carcinogenesis.

PROPERTIES OF CELLS TRANSFORMED BY VIRUSES

To discuss in vitro models for virus carcinogenesis, it is important to acquire a framework of knowledge concerning the *transformed* state of abnormally growing cells. The term *transformation* can be best defined in this context as the acquisition of a new and inheritable trait by a cell.

The interaction of viruses with cells or a multicellular organism will usually result in a productive or lytic infection but occasionally, especially if the infected cell type will not support virus replication, will result in stable acquisition by the cell of a subset or an entire complement of virus genetic information. In carcinogenesis this heritable change is usually one that results in the immortalization of the cell. The transformed cell is now removed from normal growth regulation. The consequence in vitro is the establishment of a continuous cell line with new growth properties; in vivo the cell may be capable of tumorigenesis. In many cases continued expression of virus gene products is required for immortalization of the cell, but it is not presently known whether this is always true.

A well-studied example of cell transformation is the interaction of the papovavirus simian virus 40 (SV40) with hamster cells. After infection with SV40, a culture of hamster cells will appear transiently stimulated for growth, will demonstrate increased DNA synthesis, and will contain virus-specific antigens, coded by the "early" region of the SV40 DNA. This infection is "abortive" because the cells will not replicate virus, i.e., the "late" region of SV40 DNA, the region coding for virus structural proteins, is not transcribed into messenger RNA, and there is no synthesis of virus DNA. The transient stimulation of cell macromolecular synthesis that occurs early after infection is referred to as *abortive transformation* because most of the cells in the culture will revert to a normal phenotype after some time in culture. However, a small number of the cells will become stably transformed; they continue to express virus-specific antigens, can be demonstrated to contain SV40 DNA, and they assume certain properties of malignant transformants (see below). If the original infected culture was from a primary tissue explant, the abortive transformants will die after a limited life-span. The stable transformants will grow for an indefinite number of passages in culture. In certain cell lines derived after SV40 transformation, it is possible to "rescue" the virus by fusing the transformed cell with a "permissive" cell (one that will support virus growth) and subsequently to demonstrate synthesis of virus progeny. Rescue of virus demonstrates the continued presence of virus genetic information in the transformed cells.

The study of such transformed cells in culture, including tumor cells excised and placed in culture, has clearly defined a set of "abnormal" growth characteristics associated with the transformed state. These characteristics are summarized in Table 5-1 and will be discussed in some detail. It should be clear, however, that not all of these characteristics are associated with any given transformed cell or cell line and that the presence of one or more of these traits in a cell line does not ensure tumorigenicity of that cell line in an appropriate host.

It is possible to view transformed cells as being more vigorous than their normal counterparts. This vigor is reflected in several characteristics. For example, rodent cells transformed by papovaviruses routinely grow more rapidly than normal cells. These transformed cells will grow quite efficiently in cell culture medium containing 1% bovine serum, whereas normal cells routinely require higher serum concentrations (5 to 10%). When certain rodent cells that are nonpermissive for the replication of SV40 are infected with this virus, stable transformation will occur at a predictable frequency, and an investigator can observe areas (foci) where transformation has occurred because one stably transformed cell will give rise to a clump (focus) of cells. The focus of cells is discernible because these cells, by virtue of their loss of contact inhibition, will grow over one another to form multilayers of cell growth. Normal cells generally respect territorial boundaries much more strictly. The multilayered growth

TABLE 5-1 Properties of Cells Transformed by Virus

Altered morphology

Decreased contact inhibition in culture

Increased saturation density in culture

Decreased length of cell cycle

Growth without attachment to a physical substrate

Chromosomal aberrations

Abnormal chromosome numbers

Ability of cells to divide in low serum medium

Decreased actin filaments

Increased synthesis of the protease plasminogen activator

Acquisition of virus nucleic acids

Acquisition of new cell surface antigens and, often, of intranuclear antigens

Decrease in the ratio of cytoplasmic to nuclear volume

Ability to form tumors in immunologically compromised or syngeneic hosts

---

of the transformed cells results in an increased number of cells per given area (saturation density) in a culture flask. Growth without attachment to a solid substrate will also frequently take place. This latter quality will allow one transformed cell to form a focus by growing after suspension in medium containing soft (sloppy) agar (3%) or 0.5% methylcellulose.

Certain cell structures are also altered in cells transformed by viruses or carcinogens or in cells that become otherwise transformed. Chromosomal aberrations and abnormal chromosome numbers are common, and structural actin filaments (the cell cytoskeleton) are decreased in number. It is possible to demonstrate an abnormal but stable karyotype in cells transformed by certain herpesviruses. By using fluorescently labeled antiactin antibody, it has been shown that transformation of rodent cells by papovaviruses leads to a disruption of the cell cytoskeleton.

Macromolecular changes in cells also accompany transformation. These include acquisition of a variety of newly synthesized antigens, both virus-specific and cell-induced. Papovavirus- and retrovirus-transformed cells demonstrate about 50 new cell proteins, in addition to antigens that are specific to the transforming virus. These new cell proteins include molecules involved in membrane changes and in mechanisms of proteolysis.

One can conclude from this list of transformed cell properties that multicomponent mechanisms are involved in the establishment and maintenance of the transformed state. Regardless of the criterion selected by the research investigator, the biologically significant characteristic of transformation is tumor formation. Thus, in vitro measurements of transformation merely indicate possible success for malignant transformation of cells.

RETROVIRUSES

The retroviruses represent a group of RNA-containing viruses that have been isolated over several decades from an enormous number of naturally occurring animal tumors as well as from tumors that have been experimentally induced by chemical carcinogens, radiation, or by genetic breeding of high-tumor-incidence animal strains.[2,3] These viruses can be transmitted both vertically and horizontally. In the past these viruses have been called *leukoviruses, C-type RNA viruses, oncornaviruses,* and *RNA tumor viruses,* but all of these names have been put aside, since they describe characteristics that do not apply to every member of this group. For example, not every member of the group has been shown to be oncogenic. The new name, *retrovirus,* refers to their distinguishing characteristic: the fact that they carry in the virion (virus particle) the enzyme *reverse transcriptase,* an RNA-dependent DNA polymerase. This enzyme allows the RNA genome of these viruses to replicate through a DNA intermediate (see below).

As mentioned in the beginning of this chapter, the first association of viruses with neoplasia was made at the beginning of the twentieth century for avian leukemias and sarcomas. It is now known that these tumors are caused by retroviruses, but progress was slow until the 1950s, when a retrovirus was linked with leukemias in certain high-incidence strains of mice. This virus group is now known to cause a large variety of tumors of connective tissue and of tissues of the hemopoietic and reticuloendothelial systems. A certain subgroup of the viruses has also been shown to be involved in mammary tumor formation since Bittner, in 1936, discovered the mouse mammary tumor virus in the milk of certain high-incidence mouse strains. These observations sparked a huge research effort based on the hope that retroviruses would be found in human tumors. This

BASIC CONCEPTS IN ONCOLOGY

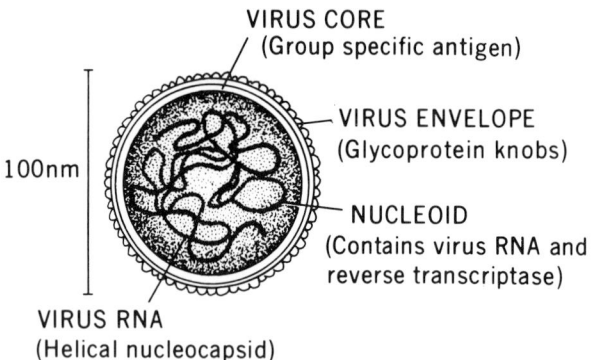

FIGURE 5-1 Structure of a typical retrovirus. The virus particle is enveloped with glycoprotein knobs on the surface. The nucleoid contains the virus RNA, helically complexed to protein. The nucleoid also contains the virion enzyme reverse transcriptase. C-type particles have centric nucleoid structures; B-type particles contain acentric nucleoids.

hope has been frustrated by the relative ease of detection of these agents in animal tissues coupled with failure to readily isolate comparable viruses from human tissues. The limited evidence for human retroviruses will be discussed later in this chapter. In addition to neoplasia, the widespread appearance of these viruses in animal tissues has led to hypotheses that retroviruses may be involved in normal biologic processes such as evolution, gene regulation, somatic cell mutation, and embryonic differentiation. These topics are outside the scope of this review, but the reader should be aware of their existence.

The structure of a typical retrovirus is depicted in Fig. 5-1. The viruses are enveloped, with the envelope derived from host plasma membrane as well as virus-specific proteins, often glycoproteins. There is a *core shell* within the envelope composed of virion-specific protein, and the core itself contains a helical RNA genome, more virus-specific protein, and the virion enzyme reverse transcriptase. The RNA of the virus is in the form of a 70 S dimer composed of two identical 35 S subunits. The 35 S RNA subunit is single stranded and has all the characteristics of a messenger RNA such as a 5′ terminal cap structure and a polyadenylated 3′ end.

During the course of virus replication, the single-stranded RNA of this virus replicates through a double-stranded DNA intermediate (Fig. 5-2). Briefly, the genome RNA is copied into a double-stranded complementary DNA molecule (provirus DNA) that integrates into the cell DNA after host cell division. The provirus DNA serves as the template for synthesis of new virion RNA and virus messenger RNA by host cell RNA polymerase. During synthesis of new virus RNA, the virus mRNA directs concomitant synthesis of virus proteins in the cytoplasm of the cell. Subsequently the nucleocapsid leaves the cell by budding through the cytoplasmic membrane. The name *C-type virus* was, in fact, derived from the appearance of the budding nucleocapsid (Fig. 5-3). In addition to *C-type particles,* containing a centric nucleocapsid structure, there are also *B-type particles,* containing an acentric nucleocapsid. The mouse mammary tumor viruses are the prototype of B-type particles. *A-type particles* have also been described and represent intracellular structures with "hollow," possibly immature, nucleocapsids.

In addition to their unique mode of RNA replication, there are several other biologic properties of the retroviruses that make them unique. Two of these properties are (1) a predominant tendency to occur in paired groupings, i.e., leukemia/sarcoma virus complexes, and (2) derivation of genomes from sequences carried in the DNA of normal cells. These two properties will be discussed in detail.

Leukemia/Sarcoma Virus Complexes

A great deal of the molecular biology of the avian retroviruses is known, so they will serve as a model for the rest of the group. Variances from the model that occur in the mammalian retroviruses will be discussed when appropriate. Avian sarcoma virus (ASV) is epitomized by the Rous sarcoma virus (RSV), a "nondefective" virus capable of replicating by itself in chicken cells. Infected chicken cells in vitro will shed newly produced virus and will also undergo transformation. The virus agent will cause sarcomas in inoculated chickens. Figure 5-4 illustrates the organization of the ASV genome. Essentially, four genes are coded within one subunit of the dimeric virus RNA. Traveling in a 5′-to-3′ direction, there are four genes associated with the ASV RNA: (1) the *gag* gene, coding for the core protein of the virion, the group-specific antigen; (2) the *pol* gene, coding for the reverse transcriptase enzyme; (3) the *env* gene, coding for the envelope proteins; and (4) the *src* gene coding for the products responsible for transformation of fibroblast cells in vitro. In addition to these defined structural genes there is a region (termed *c*) common to

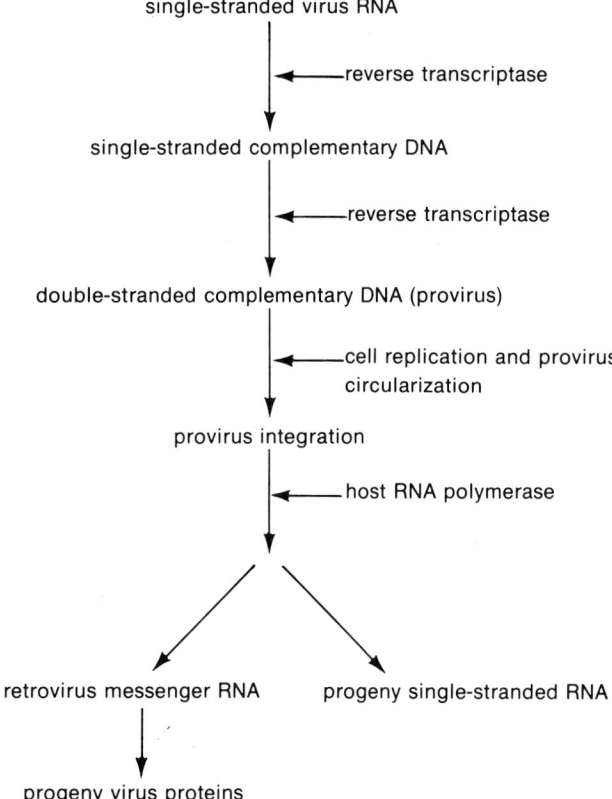

FIGURE 5-2 Schematic representation of the replication of retrovirus RNA. The integrated provirus serves as a template for progeny virion RNA and also for synthesis of retrovirus RNA. (*Adapted from JM Bishop².*)

several retroviruses on the 3' end of the *src* gene. The coding capacity of c is uncertain, although there is tentative evidence that a virus mRNA is transcribed from this region. The single-stranded virion RNA also has a 5' methylated cap and a 3' polyadenylated tail.

The organization of the avian leukosis virus (ALV) is identical except that the region of the genome that codes for the *src* gene is missing. ALV is also a nondefective virus, but the virus shedding that occurs subsequent to infection of chicken cells with this virus is not accompanied by transformation of the cells. This virus is leukemogenic in chickens, but very little is known about virus gene products involved in the oncogenic process.

As described for ALVs, the mammalian leukemia viruses are also nondefective. They contain the *gag*, *pol*, and *env* genes, lack *src*, and are capable of replication in cell culture. They do not transform cells in culture and, as with ALV, very little is known about how they interact with their host target cells to cause leukemia. The first mammalian leukemia virus was isolated by Gross from the AKR strain of mice, a high-incidence leukemic strain. Many other mammalian species, including rat, cat, cow, and baboon, also have leukemia retroviruses. Multiple leukemia virus isolates have been isolated in many cases from a single species.

The mammalian sarcoma viruses, however, differ from the avian sarcoma viruses in one critical detail. The mammalian sarcoma viruses are all defective for growth. For example, murine sarcoma virus (MSV) is capable of transforming murine cells and is known to carry the *src* gene; however, the virus cannot replicate when murine cells are infected in culture. In order for replication of the sarcoma virus to occur, the concomitant presence of a replicating leukemia virus is required. It is now understood that the mammalian sarcoma viruses are defective in one or more portions of the *gag*, *pol*, or *env* genes and that this defectiveness renders them incapable of autonomous replication. Concomitant synthesis of the missing

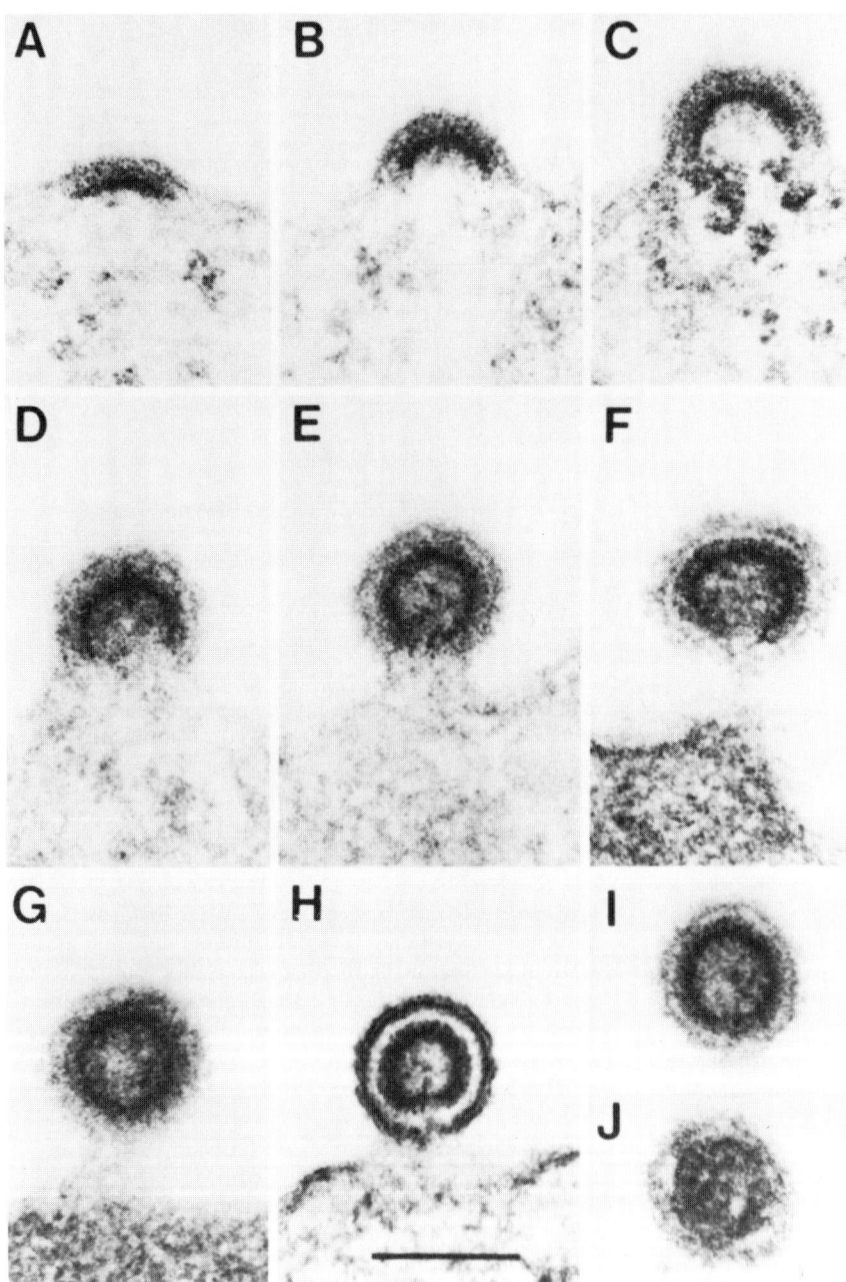

FIGURE 5-3 The budding nucleocapsid of murine leukemia virus. Panels A to J represent the sequential steps of budding as the core of the virus particle leaves the cell and acquires the virus envelope. (*From PH Yuen, PKY Wong: A morphological study on the ultrastructure and assembly of murine leukemia virus using a temperature-sensitive mutant restricted in assembly, Virology 80:260, 1977.*)

gene products by the coinfecting leukemia virus serves to complement the sarcoma virus genome.

Elegant studies in the avian system by Bishop et al. and in the mouse system by Scolnick et al. utilizing wild-type and transformation-deficient mutants of sarcoma viruses have implicated *src* as the single gene required for transformation of fibroblast cells in culture. Nucleic acid probes specific for the *src* gene of ASV and MSV

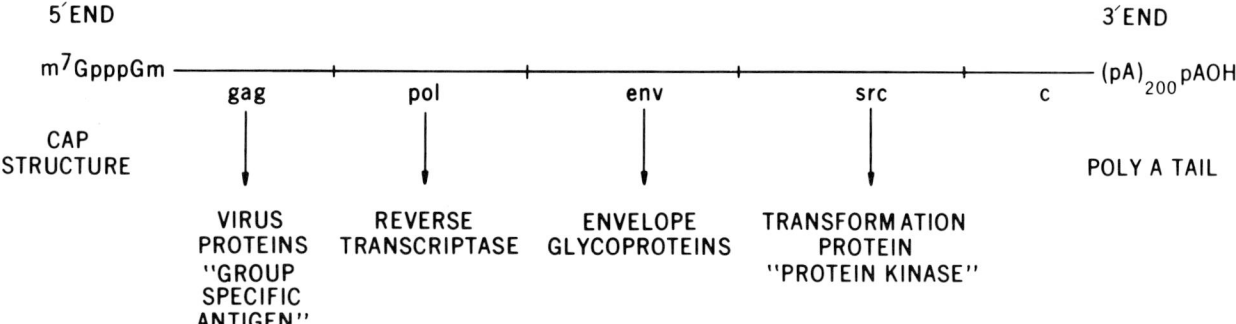

FIGURE 5-4 A schematic representation of one 35 S subunit of a typical sarcoma virus. The four genes of the virus are represented by genes coding for *gag*, the group-specific antigen; *pol*, the reverse transcriptase; *env*, the envelope glycoproteins; and *src*, the sarcoma virus transforming protein. The virion RNA has the characteristics of an RNA, a methylated 5′ cap and a polyadenylated 3′ end. Leukemia viruses, as a general rule, lack the *src* gene region. (*Adapted from JM Bishop*[2].)

have been produced and used to confirm this observation. It is now known that the *src* portion of the genome codes for a protein with a molecular weight of about 60,000 and that has, as at least one of its functions, protein kinase activity. It is not difficult to imagine that an enzyme capable of modulating phosphorylation of host cell protein could regulate cell growth. In addition, the enzyme appears to phosphorylate tyrosine rather than serine (the usual substrate). The significance of this difference remains obscure.

Endogenous Retrovirus Sequences

Nucleic acid homology studies to detect retrovirus genes integrated as provirus DNA in transformed cells soon led to the discovery that sequences homologous to retrovirus RNA (both the leukemia virus genes and the *src* gene) are present in the cell DNA of some normal cells. It is now apparent that sequences such as these are carried through the germ line of certain species. These provirus sequences do not ordinarily result in the formation of virus particles, although some of the sequences can be induced to do so. It has been hypothesized by Huebner that these sequences have oncogenic potential and that their derepression leads to tumor formation (the oncogene hypothesis). Temin, however, feels that these sequences serve some normal cell function and that a mutational event is required to lead to acquisition of oncogenic potential (the protovirus hypothesis).

It appears likely, however, that the viruses originally detected as tumor-bearing agents arose sometime in the past, perhaps millions of years ago, from endogenous virus sequences that escaped host control and established themselves as *exogenous viruses*. Extensive studies by Todaro have shown that many of the exogenous viruses infect species different than those from which they arose. To illustrate the point, the RD-114 virus was isolated from domestic cats in 1973 (see Fig. 5-5). Domestic cat DNA contains retrovirus sequences (referred to as *virogenes*) that are transmitted in the germ line from parent to progeny and can subsequently produce endogenous RD-114 viruses. The RD-114 genome has been shown by serology, host range, and partial nucleic acid homology to be partially homologous to endogenous retrovirus sequences found as provirus DNA sequences in baboons. Related sequences are not found in the DNAs of other mammals. These observations suggest that endogenous baboon retrovirus sequences escaped cell control and formed a virus that was able to infect cats and incorporate as a provirus sequence into cat DNA. From that time the introduced provirus DNA could be carried in the germ line of the cat. In addition, this cat provirus can yield a virus particle in cats. This example points to viruses as vectors for transferring genes from one species to another. The evolutionary implication of such interspecies transfer of genetic information is not yet clear.

Human and Primate Retroviruses

Despite the isolation of retroviruses from tissues of many different animal species, the search for retroviruses and/or endogenous retrovirus sequences in tissues of

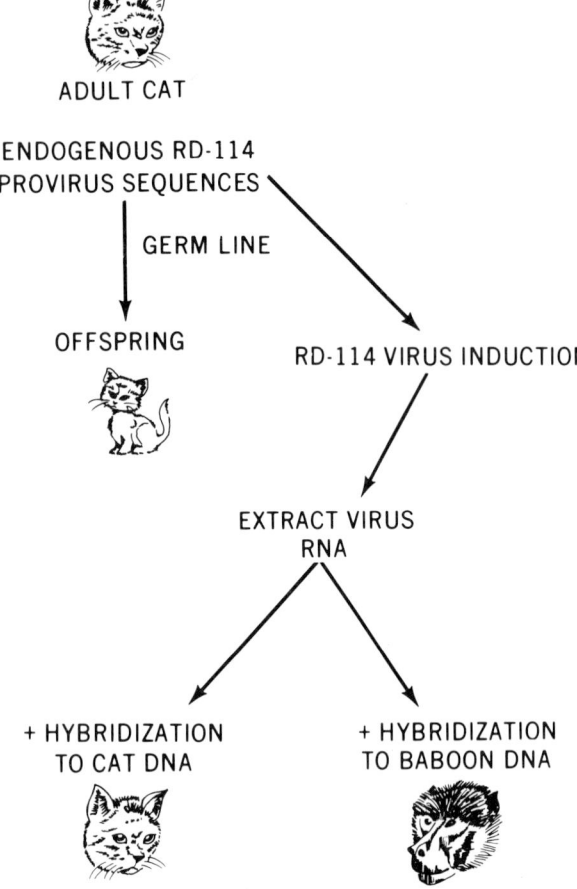

FIGURE 5-5 Sequences of the RD-114 provirus in the domestic cat. RD-114 virus sequences exist integrated in cat DNA and are passed in the germ line to offspring. Virus induction yields a virus that shows sequence homology to both cat and baboon DNA but not to DNA of other mammals. It has been theorized that an endogenous baboon retrovirus sequence escaped host control and formed a virus that subsequently infected cats and became a provirus. The provirus at that point began to be vertically transmitted in cats.

humans and higher primates has been difficult and frought with frustration. There has not been a consistent report of exogenous natural infection of human tissues with known retroviruses of animal origin, and it has not been possible to reliably detect endogenous human virus. Huebner et al. have also been unable to detect specific mammalian retrovirus antigens or antibodies in over 100 humans using a sensitive radioimmunoassay.

It has been possible to isolate baboon leukemia viruses from normal and leukemic baboon tissues and, in addition, gibbon ape leukemia viruses from normal and leukemic tissues. A virus termed *simiansarcoma virus* was isolated from a rhabdomyosarcoma on the neck of a pet woolly monkey, but this represents a single isolate. This virus has a leukemia virus associated with it (woolly monkey leukemia virus). The simian sarcoma–woolly monkey leukemia virus complex and the gibbon ape leukemia virus seem to have arisen from rodent-derived viruses that were able to exogenously infect primates. The baboon leukemia virus, however, represents expression of endogenous baboon sequences.

One problem with the isolation of putative human retroviruses is that isolations are frequently shown to be laboratory contaminants of human cell lines by animal retroviruses. Despite extensive searching, the only human tissue that is consistently shown to contain particles resembling C-type particles is the human placenta. It has not been possible, however, to transfer these particles in culture, and they are presently thought to be noninfectious.

Robert Gallo et al. have isolated two putative human retroviruses from malignant cells of a patient with acute myeloblastic leukemia. Two separate isolations, one from blood and one from bone marrow, yielded virus-containing cultures. It is suspicious, however, that these cultures both contain a mixture of two viruses, one that cross-reacts immunologically with baboon leukemia virus and one that cross-reacts with simian sarcoma virus. Efforts by these same researchers have shown, however, that cells from 10 to 20 percent of patients with myelogenous leukemia contain provirus sequences that hybridize with a baboon leukemia virus probe. Because the conditions of hybridization were not stringent, these data reflect approximate rather than strict homology. Definite confirmation of these two agents as human retroviruses is elusive at this time.

PAPOVAVIRUSES

The papovaviruses can be divided into the polyoma and the papilloma virus subgroups. The name *papova-* is derived from three principal members of the group: *pa*pilloma viruses, *po*lyoma virus, and SV40, a *va*cuolating virus. These viruses are unenveloped and contain a double-stranded, circular, covalently closed, and supercoiled DNA. Considerable evidence that members of this group affect cell proliferative control has been obtained.[4-6] The papilloma viruses play an etiologic role in human warts, but study of these viruses has been hampered by lack of an appropriate in vitro system for virus growth. The polyoma subgroup, however, has been extensively researched, and SV40 DNA has been completely sequenced. SV40, originally isolated from monkey cell cultures used to prepare poliovirus vaccine, forced study of the possible role of this virus in human oncogenesis. Although a significant role in human tumor formation has not been established for SV40, this virus has become a model for the study of tumor viruses and transforming genes. SV40 will be primarily discussed as a prototype virus of the polyoma subgroup since polyoma virus has many properties similar to SV40.

Polyoma Subgroup

SV40 was discovered by Sweet and Hilleman in 1960 in cultures of monkey kidney cells. This virus has the ability to lyse permissive (e.g., African green monkey kidney) cells, and Girardi et al. first showed it could transform a variety of nonpermissive (e.g., hamster or other rodent) cells in culture. Rabson et al. in 1962 showed that injection of SV40 into some newborn hosts (e.g., hamsters) will directly result in the formation of tumors.

The DNA of the virus is a supercoiled, circular, double-stranded molecule with an approximate molecular weight of 3.5×10^6 daltons. When permissive or nonpermissive cells are infected by SV40, the virus adsorbs to and is engulfed by the cell membrane (viropexis) and then traverses the cytoplasm within a vesicle formed by the cell membrane. This vesicle coalesces with the nuclear membrane, and virus is released into the nucleus, where uncoating and replication occur. During lytic infection by SV40, the events that occur are generally divided into "early" and "late" events. *Early* refers to the period prior to replication of virus DNA. Immediately after uncoating, early virus RNA is transcribed, and cellular RNA and DNA synthesis are stimulated. Early in infection a 19-S RNA appears in the cytoplasm which is identical to the SV40-specific RNAs found in transformed cell lines. Subsequent to viral DNA synthesis, both 19-S and 16-S (late RNA) species are present in the cytoplasm. The 19-S RNA made late is different from that transcribed at early times, but continued synthesis of early 19-S mRNA occurs (see Fig. 5-6).

Prior to DNA synthesis, the induction of several distinct enzymes occurs in infected cells. These include DNA polymerase, DNA ligase, thymidine kinase, dTMP

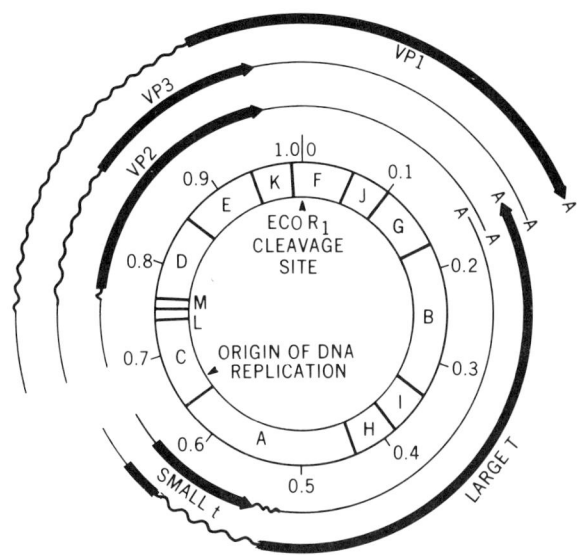

FIGURE 5-6 The restriction enzyme cleavage map of SV40 DNA after double digestion with the restriction enzymes *Hind* II and *Hind* III. SV40 DNA is a circular molecule, and map coordinates have been established using arbitrary units (0 to 1.0) with the single cleavage site of the restriction enzyme *Eco* RI as the starting point on the map. The *Hind* II- and *Hind* III-generated fragments are lettered (A to M, in order of decreasing size) and are placed on the map relative to this *Eco* RI site. For purposes of illustration, the RNA molecules generated during SV40 infection have also been drawn. Large T and small t are coded by the two classes of 19 S early mRNA. The darkened areas represent the actual coding regions of the messages. The virus structural proteins (virion protein 1, VP1, VP2, and VP3) are coded by the 19 S and 16 S mRNA classes made late after infection. (*From W Fiers et al: Complete nucleotide sequence of SV40 DNA, Nature 273:113, 1978.*)

kinase, dTDP kinase, cytidine kinase, dCMP deaminase, CDP reductase, dTMP synthetase, dihydrofolate reductase, and probably others. Following early RNA and antigen synthesis, cellular DNA synthesis is induced. This induction occurs synchronously when contact-inhibited cells are infected, since all of the cells in resting cultures are accumulated in the G_1 phase of the cell cycle. Pretreatment of cells early in infection with fluorodeoxyuridine can synchronize the onset of DNA synthesis even further. Histones and nuclear acidic proteins are induced at this time, as is the replication of mitochondrial DNA. Only one cell line (a permanent monkey kidney cell line) has been found in which SV40 can replicate with minimal cellular DNA induction; the meaning of this is not clear. The mechanism of the induction is not fully understood, but it seems to depend at least in part on the early region of the virus genome. Tegtmeyer in 1972 showed that induction is a gene A (early gene) function since a functional gene A product is required for initiation of virus DNA synthesis.

At the same time, or shortly after the induction of cellular DNA synthesis, the replication of virus DNA begins. Replication occurs in the nuclei of permissive cells. Concurrent with or shortly after viral DNA synthesis, the structural proteins of the virus are synthesized in the infected cells. After synthesis of SV40 progeny DNA and structural proteins, assembly and maturation of new virions occur in the nuclei.

When nonpermissive (i.e., hamster or mouse) cells, are infected by SV40, the virus is adsorbed to the cell and enters the nucleus just as in permissive cell–virus interactions. The virus infection is capable of altering the growth pattern of the cells, which causes them to behave like transformed cells (see Table 5-1). This transformation is abortive, however, since the cells regain their normal somatic cell properties after several mitoses. No virus DNA synthesis occurs under these conditions. Abortive transformation of 3T3 cells infected with SV40 was first observed by Smith and her colleagues in 1970. The abortively transformed cells have the ability to grow in low concentrations of serum. The altered growth patterns of these cells seem to depend on the expression of early virus genes, because it is blocked by interferon. Abortive transformation also induces the same spectrum of cellular enzymes (especially those involved with DNA synthesis) that is seen in infected permissive cells; cellular DNA synthesis is also induced. Attempts to demonstrate synthesis of virus DNA or structural antigens in infected nonpermissive cells have consistently failed.

A small percentage of abortively transformed cells becomes stably transformed. The "fixation" of transformation is dependent on at least one round of mitosis in infected cells. In synchronized cells which are abortively transformed, the addition of interferon before the S period of the cell cycle prevents the fixation of transformation, therefore implying that fixation occurs either in the S or G_2 phase of the cell cycle. Stably transformed cells permanently possess all of the properties described for the abortive transformants, and several techniques have demonstrated that these cells possess stably integrated virus DNA.

Many transformed lines must contain the equivalent of one complete SV40 genome since the virus can be rescued as a result of cell hybrids formed between these lines and permissive cells either by cocultivation or fusion of the two cells in the presence of inactivated Sendai virus. Transformed cell lines from which virus cannot be rescued by this technique are presumed to contain SV40 DNA lacking complete virus genetic information. Knowles et al. in 1968 were able to rescue two different nonrescuable transformed lines by fusion with a third permissive cell. This phenomenon is evidently dependent on complementation between the SV40 DNAs of the two transformed cells. Some transformed lines still exist, however, from which virus has not been rescued.

The state of the viral DNA in the transformed cells was examined by Sambrook et al. in 1968. Since the high molecular weight portion of cellular DNA was found to contain SV40-specific gene sequences and since the association was alkali stable, he concluded that the SV40 DNA is covalently integrated into the DNA of the host. These results were confirmed by several other laboratories. SV40 DNA has also been demonstrated in various transformed lines by measuring the nucleic acid hybridization between virus-specific RNA and the total DNA extracted from the cells. Radioactively labeled viral RNA for use in hybridization experiments can be synthesized by transcription in vitro of SV40 DNA by *Escherichia coli* RNA polymerase. Similar measurements have also been performed by hybridizing small amounts of denatured, labeled SV40 DNA with the total DNA extracted from the transformed cells. Transformed lines containing up to 60 integrated SV40 genomes have been examined.

Because of the limited coding capacity of SV40 DNA, a great deal of attention was paid to identification of the transforming genes and gene products. An antigen synthesized early after virus infection and also in transformed cells was first identified using serum from tumor-bearing hamsters. This was named the tumor (T) antigen and can be detected by immunofluorescence or complement fixation assays. Accurate purification of the T antigen took a long time with Del Villano and Defendi in 1973 giving the first molecular weight estimate as 100,000 for this protein. Prives et al. were able to show in 1975 in vitro synthesis of T antigen could be directed by the early 19S SV40 messenger RNA. Since that time, careful studies have clearly defined two proteins whose synthesis can be directed in vitro by the 19S early mRNA, a 94,000-molecular-weight protein, now termed *large T* (*T*), and a 17,000-molecular-weight protein, referred to as *small t* (*t*). Thus, in the 19S early mRNA, there must be two species of mRNAs. These mRNAs have now been mapped both for large T and small t antigens. The coding sequences for these messages can be seen on the SV40 map (Fig. 5-6).

Considerable evidence has implicated both of these antigens in malignant cell transformation. Large T antigen has been shown to bind to DNA, and Stark et al. showed specific binding to the origin of SV40 DNA replication. It is now known that large T antigen, the virus gene A product, is required for SV40 DNA synthesis, controls transcription of the late region of the virus, and self-regulates transcription of the early strand.

The question of a human polyoma subgroup of papovaviruses has become an issue due to the isolation of several papovaviruses from human patients. One group (typified by the JC isolate) has been obtained from biopsies of progressive multifocal leukoencephalopathy (PML), a progressive, degenerative disease of the central nervous system. JC virus has a very limited host range in culture, growing only in fetal human glial cells; however, this virus has been shown to cause transplantable brain tumors in hamsters.

A second human papovavirus, BK virus, was isolated from the urine of an immunosuppressed renal allograft patient. BK virus is very similar to SV40 and is capable of in vitro transformation. BK virus has been the subject of intensive molecular studies, and in fact, the entire genome of this virus has been sequenced just as has SV40 DNA.

The human population has a high prevalence of antibodies to the human papovavirus isolates, but so far they have not been associated with human cancer. Research is underway to try to establish an etiologic role for the JC virus in the pathogenesis of PML. Virtually every PML biopsy shows evidence of papovaviruses, and JC virus has been used to produce a PML syndrome in macaques. It must be remembered that SV40 fails to cause any known disease in its natural host, the cynomolgus monkey. The possibility of a similar relationship between human beings and the human papovavirus isolates must be considered.

Papilloma Virus Subgroup

The papilloma viruses are also members of the papovaviridae family, but they comprise a second subgroup of these unenveloped, icosahedral, DNA viruses because their double-stranded, circular, covalently closed virion DNAs are larger (about 5×10^6 daltons) than those found in the polyoma subgroup. The human isolates of papilloma viruses appear to constitute several subtypes that naturally cause a variety of benign epithelial warts. The group contains a variety of animal viruses with many members being highly host and tissue specific. Even though most human warts are benign, a few animal papilloma viruses can cause benign lesions that progress, under both natural and experimental conditions, to malignancy. The most notable examples of such animal viruses are the Shope papilloma virus of cottontail rabbits, bovine fibropapilloma virus, and bovine alimentary tract papilloma virus.

The Shope papilloma virus is the most well studied, and the disease was first described by Shope in 1933. Kidd and Rous in 1940 and Syverton in 1952 observed that papillomas caused by this virus on rabbit skin frequently progressed to invasive, metastatic squamous-cell carcinoma. In domestic rabbits inoculated with the cottontail virus, 75 percent of the skin papillomas will progress after the sixth month of life. The establishment of these carcinomas can be experimentally augmented by application of certain aromatic hydrocarbons to the rabbit skin. These data suggest that a cocarcinogenic phenomenon may be naturally involved in progression of the benign lesion to a carcinoma. The idea is supported by the fact that feeding of carcinogenic bracken fern to cattle with alimentary tract papillomas will also hasten malignant changes.

Papilloma viruses are generally species specific and infect only the epithelium of their natural host or closely related species. The animal viruses, therefore, do not infect human beings. The viruses that use fibroblast cells as their host target (e.g., bovine fibropapilloma virus) show a wider host and tissue range. The study of this virus group has been greatly hindered because most have not been grown in cell culture; however, the fibropapilloma viruses have been used to transform cells in vitro in experiments similar to transformation by the polyoma subgroup.

The presence and persistence of virus in Shope papillomas have been extensively studied since early work demonstrated large amounts of virus in most cottontail rabbit papillomas; virus was generally not observed in the benign lesions of domestic rabbits. It is now known that this latter observation was caused by limitations in detection techniques. It is of interest that the domestic rabbit, containing a decreased amount of infectious virus, develops carcinoma about three times more often than the wild cottontail rabbit. It remains difficult, however, to recover virus from either primary or metastatic carcinomas in either strain, and virus has been recovered in low amounts from the malignant tumors only after transplantation to new animals.

By analogy with other transforming DNA viruses, the Shope papilloma virus can presumably abortively infect and transform one or more epithelial cells of the rabbit epidermis. If followed by integration of virus DNA, the cell will exhibit altered growth characteristics. Virus DNA synthesis and virus capsid antigens cannot be detected in these cells, and a "T-like" intranuclear antigen has not been demonstrated. The altered growth characteristics of these epidermal cells are accompanied by the fact that injection of killed papilloma cells confers tumor immunity. This suggests the existence of a tumor-specific transplantation antigen (TSTA) which may be virus specific. Virus replication in the papillomas occurs as the epidermal epithelial cells progress to the surface during keratinization, and virus capsid antigens and virus particles are only detected in the keratinizing cells.

Numerous epithelial papillomas have been described in humans, and when such experiments were considered fashionable and ethical, many were transmitted to human volunteers using filtered cell extracts. The major papillomas of human beings are briefly described in Table 5-2. With the exception of epidermodysplasia verruciformis, a genetic disorder, most of the lesions are benign and rarely progress to carcinomas. Electron microscopy and biochemical studies have shown virus particles in many of these warts, and analogy to the Shope papilloma system is assumed. The extensive work of Orth and separately that of zur Hausen demonstrated that human warts contain, and may be caused by, a fairly large number of papilloma virus subtypes. As in rabbits, virus replication appears to be confined to the keratinizing epithelium.

In summary, the papilloma viruses constitute a fairly ubiquitous group of transforming DNA viruses. The natural etiology of warts suggests that these viruses usually cause benign lesions in the naturally infected host, but one must consider evidence from animal and human systems that these agents can be directly oncogenic. Molecular biology studies with the papilloma viruses are scarce due to the lack of cell culture systems, and the question of whether continued papilloma virus information is required in a wart-derived carcinoma remains to be answered.

ADENOVIRUSES

After the demonstration of the oncogenicity of papovaviruses in newborn rodents, Trentin et al. demonstrated in 1962 that adenovirus type 12 (Ad-12) produces tumors when inoculated into newborn hamsters. The adenoviruses comprise a large group of unenveloped DNA viruses that contain a double-stranded DNA ge-

TABLE 5-2 Common Human Warts

Type	Description	Virus presence	Malignant potential
Verruca vulgaris	Finger wart	+	Rare
Verruca plantaris	Skin wart	+	Rare
Verruca plana	Flat wart	+	Rare
Epidermodysplasia verruciformis	Diffuse skin warts—genetically predisposed	+	Common, especially after exposure to sunlight
Condyloma acuminatum	Anal or genital wart	Low frequency	Rare
Oral papilloma	Oral wart	Low frequency	Rare
Oral focal epithelial hyperplasia	Oral hyperplasia	+	Rare
Juvenile laryngeal papillomatosis	Laryngeal wart	Rare	Rare

nome of about 30×10^6 daltons. These viruses frequent the upper respiratory tract and can cause human respiratory disease and other infections, especially in crowded or institutional situations. There are 31 serotypes of human adenovirus isolates. Three serotypes are highly oncogenic and five are moderately oncogenic (fewer tumors are produced, and they occur later in life) when inoculated into newborn hamsters. Most of the isolates can transform rodent cells in vitro, and studies performed on these transformants have described many of the same properties that can be found in papovavirus-transformed cell lines.[7]

Cells transformed by adenoviruses or cells derived from adenovirus-induced tumors have at least a part of the virus genome integrated, transcribe mRNA specific for adenovirus, and express an intranuclear tumor (T) antigen specific for transformation by the virus group; this antigen is not identical serologically to the T antigen of the polyoma virus subgroup and is specified by the left-hand end of the adenovirus DNA. Sambrook et al. in 1975 showed that Ad-2–transformed cells contain as a minimum portion of the virus DNA a segment from the left 14 percent of the virus genome. Sharp et al. have since estimated that transcription of only 7 percent of the Ad-2 genome (a DNA fragment of about 1.6×10^6 daltons) is responsible for the virus-transformed phenotype of cells in culture. Graham and van der Eb have used the left-hand end of the Ad-2 genome to transform cells in vitro, but the oncogenicity of such transformants is not always certain. Even when comparing adenovirus-transformed cell lines that contain more than the left 14 percent of the virus DNA, the common transcriptional product in the cells is an mRNA from the left-hand portion of the genome.

Because of the ubiquitous nature of human adenovirus and because humans may be infected early in life by several subtypes, concern has arisen that these viruses may mediate oncogenesis in the human population. To date, it has not been possible to detect sequences homologous to the human adenoviruses in several types of human tumors. The most extensive study by Green et al. failed to find such sequences in a large number of both lung and gastrointestinal tumors. These workers used very sensitive adenovirus DNA probes radioactively labeled to high specific activity to search for DNA sequences in human tumors that would be specific for adenovirus DNA. Both whole virus DNA and DNA restriction endonuclease fragments were used. Even with carefully controlled hybridization conditions these workers failed to find evidence of Ad-12 or Ad-2 DNA in these two human tumors.

HEPATITIS B VIRUS

Hepatitis can be defined as "inflammation of the liver." This inflammation can be caused by virus agents and also by chemical agents that are toxic to liver components. One of the virus agents, hepatitis B virus (HBV) has been implicated in the development of primary hepatocellular carcinoma (PHC), a carcinoma derived from the parenchymal cells of the liver (see Table 5-3).

It has been suggested for many years that damage due to chronic liver disease may result in the development of PHC. Such cancers represent a small percentage (1 to 2 percent) of all malignancies found in the Americas and Europe but may constitute 20 to 30 percent of African and Asian tumors. The incidence of primary liver cancer in men is substantially higher (two- to fourfold) than in women with a peak incidence between 50 and 70 years of age. Clinical observations have associated about 75 percent of liver cell cancers (hepatomas) and about 20 to 50 percent of duct cell cancers (cholangiomas) with cirrhosis. Hepatomas often occur

TABLE 5-3 Evidence for the Association of Hepatitis B Virus (HBV) Infection with Primary Hepatocellular Carcinoma (PHC)

1. High frequency of PHC in areas where hepatitis B carrier rate is high
2. A close association of hepatitis B infection and also the carrier state with subsequent development of PHC, both in high PHC and low PHC incidence areas
3. Superimposition of PHC on posthepatic cirrhosis
4. HBsAg* and HBcAg in cells of PHC biopsies
5. Identification of integrated HBV DNA in hepatoma cell lines derived from PHC patients
6. Familial clustering of HBV carrier state, chronic liver disease, posthepatic cirrhosis, and PHC
7. High rate of maternal transmission of the HBV carrier state to newborns in areas where PHC rate is high
8. Evidence that a similar virus or disease complex leads to PHC development in the Pennsylvania woodchuck

* HBsAg, hepatitis B surface antigen; HBcAg, hepatitis B core antigen.

(10 to 15 percent of cases) subsequent to postnecrotic cirrhosis and hemochromatosis but do not commonly occur in patients with Laennec's cirrhosis. In areas of the world with high endogenous HBV infection rates or in areas with a high incidence of aflatoxin (a carcinogen) contamination in the diet, there is a coincident increase in the per capita incidence of liver carcinoma.

A large number of individuals infected with HBV develop the carrier state (i.e., chronic infection that may or may not be accompanied by active liver disease), and chronically infected women can transmit the disease to newborn infants. Third world countries often have a dramatically increased chronic infection rate. The role of such carriers in development of PHC will be discussed later in this review.

Acute liver infections can be caused by at least three different viruses, and the diseases are commonly referred to as hepatitis A (infectious hepatitis), hepatitis B (serum hepatitis), and hepatitis C (non-A, non-B hepatitis).[8] Hepatitis A infections are characterized by a short incubation period (about 30 days), and the virus is shed into the feces of infected individuals. The primary route of infection is the oral/fecal route. These infections are acute and do not result in the development of chronic infections. This disease is presently thought to be transmitted by a small RNA-containing virus. The pathology of non-A, non-B hepatitis is similar to that of hepatitis B, but its etiology is not well understood. These agents will not be further discussed in detail here.

HBV causes serum hepatitis, a disease characterized by a longer incubation than hepatitis A. The primary route of spread of this agent is via infected blood or blood components, but the virus can also be transmitted by other routes. In the 1960s Krugman and his coworkers demonstrated that serum from patients with long incubation hepatitis could transmit a similar disease to human volunteers, a hepatitis with an incubation period of about 60 days. If this serum was boiled prior to administration, it was capable of immunizing patients and no longer transmitted disease.

In 1963, Baruch Blumberg, in screening thousands of blood samples to examine genetic variation of serum proteins, found an antigen in a serum from an Australian aborigine that reacted with antibodies in serum of an American hemophilia patient. Further studies demonstrated that this antigen was rare in North America and Western Europe and more common in Africa and Asia. It is now known that this antigen is indicative of serum hepatitis and the nature of the *Australia antigen* as well as the structure of HBV has been worked out in detail.

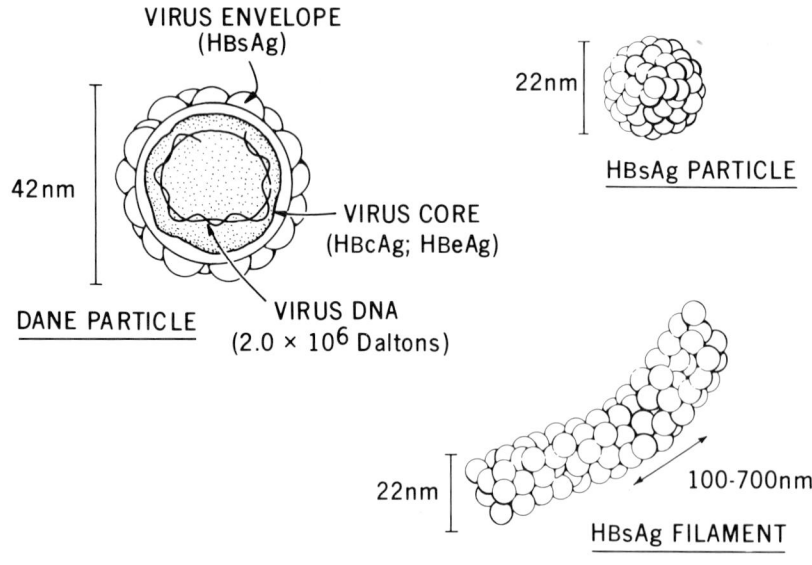

FIGURE 5-7 The major structural elements found in the blood of hepatitis B patients. The Dane particle represents the infectious virion and is an enveloped DNA virus containing a circular double-stranded DNA molecule with a large gap in one strand and a nick in the other. The nucleocapsid contains a core antigen (HBcAg), HBeAg, and a DNA polymerase. The relative frequency of Dane particles is low when compared to the presence of hepatitis B surface antigen (HBsAg) particles and filaments. HBsAg is present in large amounts in the blood of acutely infected individuals and of HBV carriers. HBsAg-containing human blood serves as a source for preparation of a formalin-inactivated vaccine against HBV infection. (*Adapted from JL Melnick et al: Viral hepatitis, Sci Am 237:44, 1977.*)

HBV, as an infectious entity, appears to be composed of a virus particle (average diameter of 42 nm) commonly referred to as the *Dane particle* (see Fig. 5-7) and essentially is an enveloped virus with an internal core structure that contains a double-stranded circular DNA (with a gap in one strand and a nick in the opposite strand) and a virus-specific DNA polymerase.[9] Dane particles are found in the blood of acutely and chronically infected individuals and also in sections of infected liver.

The concentration of infectious particles in blood is low compared to the presence of circulating subunits of virus particles, the HBV surface antigen (HBsAg). This surface antigen is identical to the Australia antigen and is made up of spheres (22 nm) or filaments (22 nm wide, 100 to 700 nm long) in blood or other body fluids of infected individuals. These particles can be present in blood of carriers at a concentration of 10^{12} per milliliter of blood. Antibody to HBsAg will agglutinate both these subunit structures and the Dane particles. Naked cores, however, can be prepared by treating Dane particles with lipid solvents. The core structure is not agglutinated by antibody to HBsAg but possesses its own antigenic specificity, the core antigen, HBcAg.

In infected liver cells HBsAg is found in the cytoplasm, whereas HBcAg is found only in the nucleus. As mentioned previously, the core contains a double-stranded DNA and a virus-specific DNA polymerase. The core contains about three proteins, and the polymerase possesses its own antigenicity, commonly referred to as HBeAg. Serologically, HBeAg is found only in patients with HBsAg and is accompanied by increased numbers of Dane particles and increased HBV polymerase activity. A carrier who is HBeAg positive is more likely to have active liver disease. Transmission to newborn infants is more likely when the mother is HBeAg positive, and HBeAg-positive blood is more likely to transmit disease.

The development of the carrier state seems heavily implicated in the development of PHC. High frequencies of PHC occur in areas with high frequencies of HBV carriers. Familial clustering of chronic liver disease, cirrhosis, and PHC has been noted in areas where the HBV carrier rate is high. Since maternal virus transmission to offspring occurs at a high frequency, these areas have large numbers of individuals who are essentially lifelong carriers of HBV. In controlled studies in these areas, there was an association of cancer with active HBV infection. It is interesting that PHC patients show a high incidence of HBV infection even in areas where HBV and PHC rates are low. HBV structures, proteins, and virus DNA can frequently be demonstrated in PHC biopsies.

It is not known, however, whether PHC develops directly because of gene expression by HBV or whether the development of carcinoma is coincidental to the tissue trauma caused by chronic liver disease. The latter possibility is supported by the fact that PHC, in high-incidence HBV areas, is usually superimposed on chronic liver damage and also by the fact that certain dietary carcinogens such as aflatoxin, a fungal contaminant of grain, appear to independently cause chronic liver damage and a high incidence of PHC.

Presently, a cell culture system for growing HBV is not available, slowing work aimed at detailing virus gene expression. The exact role of virus gene products in transformation of liver cells is therefore unknown. The recent discovery of a woodchuck hepatitis virus will undoubtedly aid study of this disease complex since this virus (similar physically to HBV) can also cause a spectrum of diseases including acute and chronic hepatitis, cirrhosis, and PHC in the Pennsylvania woodchuck.

Recent advances in the prevention of HBV infection may yield long-range information proving the relationship of this virus to carcinoma. Early studies showed that antibody to HBsAg is protective against serum hepatitis. Clinical trials are now in progress to vaccinate humans with a surface antigen (free of nucleic acid) vaccine prepared from the blood of human HBV carriers. If used successfully in Africa and Asia to prevent HBV infection, this vaccine may eventually reduce the endogenous incidence of PHC and prove to be the first effective human cancer vaccine.

HERPESVIRUSES

The herpesviruses are a large group of double-stranded DNA-containing viruses that can be identified by their morphology in the electron microscope, their sensitivity to ether, the characteristic size of their genome, and their antigenic constitution. Herpesviruses have been identified as common virus agents in a large number of species, and all members of the group have essentially the same structure: an icosahedral nucleocapsid that contains the DNA and is surrounded by one or more lipid bilayer envelopes (Fig. 5-8).

These virus agents are particularly well adapted to survival, since acute infection frequently results in establishment of latency. Virus persists in the infected host,

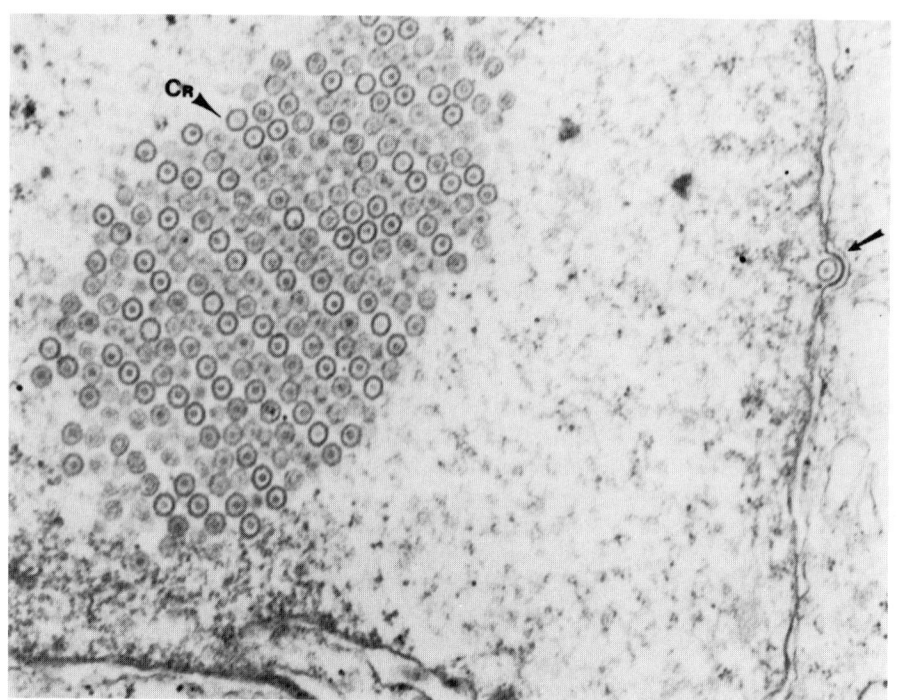

FIGURE 5-8 An electron micrograph of a cell infected by herpes simplex virus. Virus crystals (Cr) accumulate in the nucleus of the cell. The virion envelope is acquired as the virus buds through the nuclear membrane. Virus can also be seen budding through the cytoplasmic membrane.

commonly in nervous tissue, in an unknown but apparently noninfectious state. Latent herpesviruses can be reactivated and repeatedly establish active infections that may or may not be similar in pathology to the primary infection. Primary and recurrent disease are often accompanied by virus shedding and even latently infected hosts that lack overt disease can shed virus intermittently. Transmission and propagation of the herpesviruses are, therefore, highly efficient.

This group of viruses is also interesting because they have been implicated in a number of naturally occurring neoplastic diseases.[4,6,10] Many of the animal herpesviruses cause tumors and four of the five human herpesviruses are suspected to varying degrees in the etiology of human neoplasia.

Because of limitations in the scope of this chapter, we will not discuss in detail all of the animal models that are established for oncogenesis by this virus group but will concentrate instead on the five human agents. The reader should be briefly informed, however, of two classic animal systems for herpesvirus-induced neoplasia, the Lucké renal tumor of frogs and Marek's lymphoma of chickens.

Lucké Frog Virus

Lucké frog virus was discovered when Lucké observed Cowdry type A inclusion bodies in cells from some renal carcinomas of the leopard frog (*Rana pipiens*). Subsequent examination of these frog tumors revealed that the tumor cells only contain virus particles when derived from tumor-bearing frogs that have been captured in the winter or maintained in the laboratory at 4 to 9°C. "Summer" tumors do not contain virus particles so that it would appear that synthesis of the causative agent of this tumor is temperature sensitive. Cell-free extracts from tumors can induce carcinomas in inoculated animals held at 4 to 9°C, but the exact relationship between virus growth and tumor formation is not understood. It is known that maintenance of summer tumors in vitro at low temperature will induce virus. Study of the Lucké frog virus has been greatly hampered by lack of a cell culture system for growth of this agent. An additional problem is that procurement of animals carrying this virus in the wild is becoming extremely difficult for some unknown reason. Because of these problems there is a paucity of information regarding the molecular processes involved in tumor formation by this virus, but its role in the etiology of the leopard frog renal carcinoma is firmly established.

Marek's Disease Virus

Marek's disease is a highly malignant lymphoma of chickens and is efficiently spread from animal to animal. The disease is caused by a herpesvirus (Marek's disease virus, MDV) that replicates only in feather follicle epithelium, and infectious virus is transmitted via skin dander to the respiratory tract of susceptible birds. Because of the economic consequences of this disease, a large research effort eventually resulted in an effective virus vaccine against Marek's disease. Inoculation of newborn chickens with a suspension of a nonpathogenic herpesvirus of turkeys (HVT) protects against malignant lymphoma associated with MDV infection, but leaves the animals susceptible to infection with MDV. This "cancer" vaccine apparently interferes with tumorigenesis by preventing spread of virus to the target cell leading to malignancy. HVT cross-reacts serologically with MDV, and this cross-reactivity is probably responsible for the efficacy of the vaccine. It has been reported that these two viruses share only a 9 percent nucleic acid homology, but this is apparently sufficient to account for common antigenic determinants.

Herpes Simplex Viruses

Although herpesviruses have also been shown to produce tumors in rabbits, cattle, guinea pigs, and monkeys, we will go on to discuss the human herpesviruses and their suspected role in human neoplasia. There are five known human herpesviruses; four have been associated with various types of human tumors by either epidemiologic studies or by direct virological techniques. In addition, these same four have been shown to transform normal cells in vitro to a malignant phenotype. These four viruses are herpes simplex virus types 1 and 2 (HSV-1, HSV-2), Epstein-Barr virus (EBV), and cytomegalovirus (CMV). These agents all cause primary, latent, and recurrent diseases (see Table 5-4). The fifth human herpesvirus, varicella-zoster virus (VZV) causes chickenpox at primary infection and can recur as shingles later in life. To date VZV has not been associated with malignancy in vivo or transformation in vitro, and its oncogenic potential is unknown; however, it is suspected by analogy with the other members of this group.

The two human herpes simplex virus subgroups, HSV-1 and HSV-2, were originally distinguished by serological procedures. These two viruses are similar in composition, and both viruses are capable of causing the same disease syndromes in humans, although HSV-1 generally is associated with oral or facial infections, whereas HSV-2 is generally found in sexually transmitted herpetic infections. The genomes of these two viruses vary in base composition by 2 percent, with HSV-1 (69 percent guanine plus cytosine) sharing about 50 percent DNA homology with HSV-2 (71 percent guanine plus cytosine). The DNA of HSV is large (100×10^6 daltons) and extremely complex in structure and function. The reader is referred to a comprehensive review for information concerning the molecular biology of HSV DNA.[11]

In 1971, the observation was made in this laboratory that HSV-2 rendered nonlytic by ultraviolet irradiation was capable of transforming hamster embryo fibroblasts to tumorigenicity. Subsequently, HSV-1 was also used to transform hamster cells and several other laboratories have demonstrated formation of morphologically transformed foci after HSV infection of mouse, rat, chicken, and human cells. In most cases the lytic capacity of the transforming virus is hampered, often by inactivation by ultraviolet light, in order to enable transformation. Temperature-sensitive (ts) mutants of HSV have also been used for transformation. By infecting cells with ts mutants and holding cultures at a nonpermissive temperature, virus fails to replicate lytically, and transformed foci of cells can be established. In the absence of inactivation, most susceptible cells are killed by HSV and therefore no longer serve as targets for transformation. It is possible that in the body, defective or incapacitated HSV particles may initiate the transforming event. The possibility that host defenses dampen virus replication should also be considered.

Both serotypes of HSV have been associated with human cancer. HSV-1 has been suggested as a factor in squamous-cell carcinoma of the lip. The tumor is rare, however, and additional studies are necessary before a strong etiologic role for HSV-1 can be established for this disease. More substantial evidence has linked HSV-2 with cervical carcinoma. Table 5-5 summarizes data indicating a causal role for HSV-2 in cancer of the cervix. The majority of data has involved epidemiologic studies; direct biologic observations have been more difficult to obtain.

It appears that the occurrence of cervical cancer is linked to sexual contact and depends at least in part on

TABLE 5-4 Diseases Due to Human Herpesviruses

Herpes simplex virus type 1	Acute herpetic gingivostomatitis Recurrent herpes labialis Keratoconjunctivitis Herpes genitalis Neonatal encephalitis Neonatal herpetic septicemia Primary herpetic dermatitis Eczema varicelliform herpeticum Kaposi Traumatic herpes Herpetic encephalitis in adults Trigeminal neuralgia Carcinoma of lip* Cervical carcinoma*
Herpes simplex virus type 2	Herpes genitalis Neonatal encephalitis Neonatal herpetic septicemia Acute herpetic gingivostomatitis Recurrent herpes labialis Keratoconjunctivitis Primary herpetic dermatitis Eczema varicelliform herpeticum Kaposi Traumatic herpes Herpetic encephalitis in adults Trigeminal neuralgia Cervical carcinoma* Carcinoma of lip*
Cytomegalovirus	Cytomegalic inclusion disease Mononucleosis-like syndrome Pneumonia in immunosuppressed patients Cancer of the prostate* Kaposi's sarcoma*
Epstein-Barr virus	Infectious mononucleosis Burkitt's lymphoma* Nasopharyngeal carcinoma*
Varicella-zoster virus	Chicken pox Shingles Ophthalmic zoster Varicella pneumonia Congenital abnormalities Hemorrhagic varicella Encephalitis

* Neoplastic diseases associated with virus agent.

low socioeconomic status, sexual promiscuity, and early first intercourse. A number of epidemiologic studies illustrate that women with cervical carcinoma have a higher incidence and generally higher titers of anti-HSV-2 antibodies. This information prompted researchers to look for virus nucleic acids and virus proteins in tumor cells. These studies are limited due to the fact that only small (milligram) amounts of tissue are usually available from cervical biopsy materials.

HSV-2 antigens have been observed at increased frequencies in cells from cervical lesions. Royston and Aurelian observed increased staining of exfoliated neo-

TABLE 5-5 Evidence for the Association of Herpes Simplex Virus Type 2 (HSV-2) with Cervical Cancer

1. Epidemiology of virus isolation and anti-HSV-2 antibodies
2. Detection of virus antigens in cultured tumor cells
3. Detection of HSV-2 DNA in one cervical carcinoma biopsy
4. Transformation in culture of normal cells to malignancy by HSV-2
5. Detection of HSV-2 messenger RNA in carcinoma in situ and dysplasia of the cervix
6. Induction of cervical carcinoma in mice by intravaginal administration of inactivated HSV-2

plastic cervical cells by anti-HSV-2 antibody using an indirect immunofluorescence assay. Attempts to stain sections of cervical biopsy using this assay were unsuccessful when attempted by these same investigators as well as others. Nahmias and his coworkers showed antigens in some cervical biopsies using the more sensitive anticomplement immunofluorescence assay.

Only one report, by Frenkel et al., has been published to date indicating the presence of HSV-2 DNA in a cervical carcinoma biopsy. These investigators used DNA-DNA hybridization to measure reassociation of cervical biopsy DNA with a radioactively labeled HSV-2 DNA probe. Attempts to repeat these findings have been unsuccessful in several laboratories, including Dr. Frenkel's, but several valid reasons may contribute to the lack of detection. Data already discussed for the papovaviruses and adenoviruses indicate that as little as 1 to 1.5 $\times 10^6$ daltons of DNA is sufficient for a transforming gene. This would only represent 1 to 1.5 percent of the HSV genome and DNA-DNA hybridization techniques in the HSV system are not presently sensitive enough to detect such a small piece of DNA, even if it were present in every cell.

Because of these problems, recent studies have turned to the detection of HSV-specific messenger RNA in biopsy material. The rationale for these experiments is based on the assumption that any biologically relevant HSV-2 DNA sequences would exert their control in the tumor cell by transcription into messenger RNA and subsequent translation into protein gene products. If more than one copy of messenger RNA is transcribed, the DNA sequence will be amplified. Using in situ hybridization of radioactively labeled HSV-2 DNA probe to messenger RNA in cryostat sections of biopsy material,

McDougall and his colleagues have reported a fairly high incidence (about 70 percent) of positive hybridization of their HSV-2 DNA probe to sections from dysplasia and carcinoma in situ of the cervix. Control cervical tissues only rarely hybridized the HSV-2 probe. Additionally, radioactively labeled λ bacteriophage and SV40 DNA probes failed to hybridize to the experimental sections. These investigators, however, inexplicably failed to detect HSV-2–specific sequences in invasive cervical carcinoma. The possibility of detection limitations may again be relevant, or it is possible that the continued presence of virus genetic information is not required. Observations in a number of other laboratories have recently suggested that HSV-2 mRNA sequences can be detected in biopsies of invasive carcinoma of the cervix. Only a small number (less than 100) of patient tissues have been studied, but intensive efforts are necessary to confirm this interesting and promising observation.

Attempts to define a subset of HSV sequences that might effect transformation in vitro are also actively underway. These experiments are based on the assumption that the same sequences will potentiate tumor formation in vivo. It has been previously shown by several investigators that not only inactivated virus preparations can transform but that transfection with intact HSV DNA can potentiate transformation. Random and fairly extensive shearing of the virus DNA prior to transfection or treatment of the DNA with certain, but not all, restriction endonucleases abolishes the transforming potential. This last piece of information indicates that extensive shearing and certain restriction endonucleases can introduce cuts into essential transforming genes. Because certain restriction enzymes do not appear to cut essential transforming genes, the possibility arises that one can transform by transfection of cells with purified DNA fragments (i.e., subsets of the virus genome). HSV DNA has the capacity to code for 50 to 100 proteins, so that dealing with a subset of the virus DNA narrows the number of potentially transforming virus gene products. The approach for such an experiment is briefly outlined in Fig. 5-9.

Using transfection of hamster cells by DNA fragments, Camacho and Spear reported morphological transformation using the XbaI F restriction fragment of HSV-1. This fragment maps in the region between 0.30 and 0.45 from the left-hand side of the HSV DNA genome and corresponds to the region coding for two virus glycoproteins. To date, however, no tumors have been obtained by inoculation of these cells into syngeneic

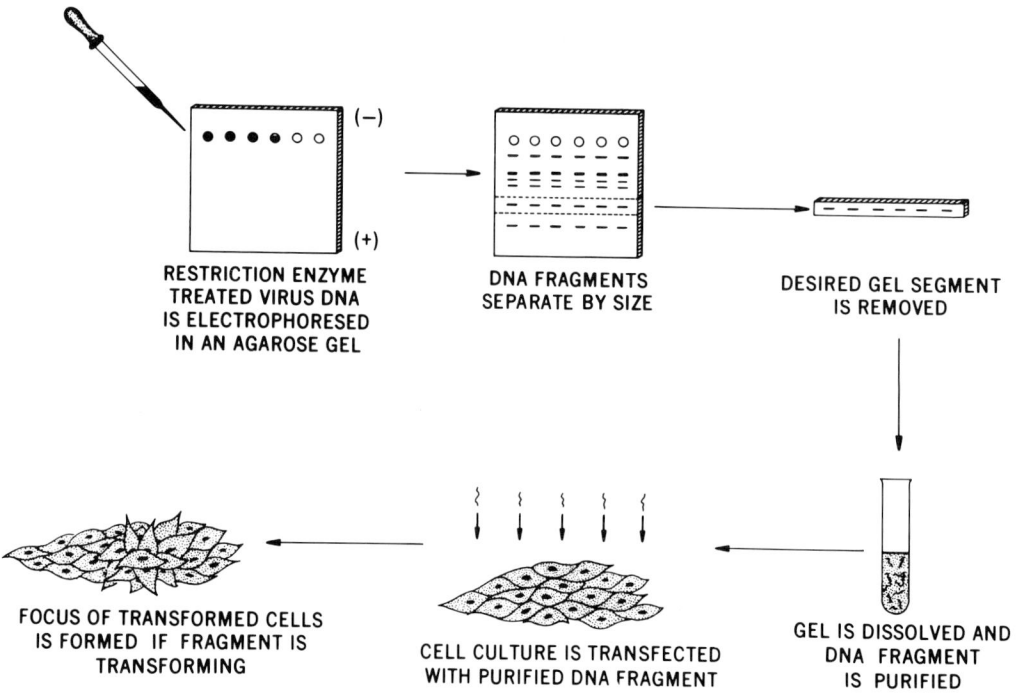

FIGURE 5-9 Idealized protocol for the in vitro transformation of cells by subfragments of tumor virus DNA. Virion DNA is cleaved by specific restriction endonucleases and separated by electrophoresis on agarose gel slabs. After visualization of the DNA fragments (usually by staining with ethidium bromide) the desired gel segment is cut out of the gel with a razor blade, dissolved, and a particular DNA fragment purified (usually by differential adsorption of the DNA to hydroxyapatite). The purified DNA fragment can be transfected into a cell culture, and a focus of transformed cells will form if that fragment is transforming.

newborn hamsters, and a search for HSV-1 glycoproteins in the cells proved negative. Whether these cells represent true HSV-1 transformants remains to be determined. Hayward et al. have also reported morphological transformation of hamster cells by the BglII N fragment of HSV-2 DNA. This fragment maps between 0.582 and 0.682 on the HSV-2 DNA map. Support for this suggestion has come from Galloway et al. who have detected retained HSV-2 sequences mapping between 0.60 and 0.65 in a number of subclones of 333-8-9, a cell line originally transformed to oncogenicity by ultraviolet-irradiated HSV-2 in 1971.

The case is therefore building for transformation in vitro by HSV and explanation of the mechanism of such transformation. Circumstantial evidence strongly suggests the presence of virus, not necessarily as the sole agent of oncogenesis, but at least as a cofactor, in cancer of the cervix. One additional report by Herbert et al. in 1976 has also suggested that patients with benign hyperplasia of the prostate or prostatic carcinoma may have a higher than normal incidence of HSV-2 infection. This report requires further investigation. As additional data become available, it may be possible to unequivocally establish oncogenicity by this agent in the human population.

Epstein-Barr Virus

In 1958, Denis Burkitt, an English surgeon in Uganda, reported a prevalence of a particular, connective tissue jaw tumor in African children. Malignant jaw lymphomas with a similar pathology are seen only rarely in other parts of the world. In addition to a high rate of Burkitt's lymphoma in native Ugandan children, children of foreign missionaries stationed in equatorial Africa were also at increased risk for the disease. In his original report, Dr. Burkitt noted that clustering of the disease occurred in areas where climate and environment allow the occurrence of endemic malaria. Burkitt's lymphoma (BL) is most often found in the lower jaw but can also arise at other locations including the upper jaw, the thyroid, the ovaries, the liver, and the kidneys.

Attempts to grow tumor tissue in culture yielded lymphoblastoid cell lines that could be grown indefinitely in suspension culture. A subsequent search for a virus etiology of the tumor resulted in the discovery by Epstein and Barr of herpesviruslike particles in the cells of the tumor. In addition, some of the cell lines derived from the lymphomas released virus particles (EBV), and it was possible to show that cell-free supernatants from these cultures were capable of transforming normal human lymphocytes to immortalized lymphoblastoid lines. It is now known that only a few of the cells in the culture shed virus. To date, normal lymphocytes that have been transformed by EBV include those from human umbilical cord, human adults and infants, marmosets, gibbons and owl, squirrel, and cebus monkeys.

In response to the association of BL with EBV, a large research effort was mounted to examine the relationship of the virus to tumor formation.[4,6,12] As a serendipitous by-product of this effort, Drs. Gertrude and Werner Henle discovered that EBV is the causative agent of infectious mononucleosis (IM) and is, in fact, a ubiquitous virus in the human population. This association was made when a research technician in the Henle laboratory contracted IM and simultaneously seroconverted with antibody specific for EBV. The epidemiology of EBV infection is now more clearly understood. The virus is ubiquitous, and children in lower socioeconomic areas are commonly infected before adolescence. In higher socioeconomic backgrounds, infection usually occurs during mid- to late adolescence and results in the disease syndrome known as IM. The occurrence of IM results in a nonmalignant proliferative response in certain types of lymphocytes, and the clinical course of disease can vary from subclinical to prolonged disease characterized by sporadic fever and fatigue. Peripheral blood smears from IM patients sometimes contain white blood cells suggestive of acute lymphocytic leukemia, but this response is limited and disappears as the patient recovers. Infectious EBV is shed into the oropharyngeal secretions of infected individuals, and infection is usually transmitted by salivary contact, i.e., kissing. Limited studies have not been able to demonstrate any increased cancer incidence in patients with IM, although blood samples from IM patients can also be used to establish immortalized lymphoblastoid lines, and it has been shown that EBV DNA is present in infected lymphocytes and in the IM-derived lymphoblastoid lines.

Antisera from IM and BL patients allow one to distinguish three antigens: early antigens (EA), corresponding to those proteins made soon after EBV infection, virus structural or capsid antigens (VCA), and a nuclear antigen (EBNA) associated with EBV infection and transformation. An analogy between EBNA and the papovavirus T antigen can be made since all of the cells in a lymphoblastoid culture will be EBNA positive, but only a small number of cells will be EA or VCA positive. These VCA-positive cells seem to be associated with the ability to shed virus. A translocation in chromosome 14 of human lymphoblasts carrying EBV was observed by Zech in 1976.

There are apparently two types of EBV. One variety, P3J-HR-1, isolated from a BL patient, can superinfect EBV lymphoblastoid cell lines and induce virus antigen synthesis, but cannot transform cord blood leukocytes. The other strain, B95-8, was isolated from marmoset lymphoblastoid cells transformed by an IM isolate of EBV. George Miller et al. have shown that this strain does not induce EA but readily transforms cord leukocytes. Kieff et al. have identified a region of virus DNA (about 15 percent of the genome) that is present in P3J-HR-1 but missing in B95-8. The effect of this difference on the transforming potential of this virus is presently being investigated by these workers.

The link between EBV and human cancer has been considerably strengthened since the first association was made. Table 5-6 lists the cumulative evidence pointing to an etiologic role for EBV in BL.

A second geographically restricted tumor, nasopharyngeal carcinoma (NPC), has also been strongly linked to EBV, and evidence that has accumulated is similar to that listed in Table 5-6. NPC is associated with the southern Chinese population and recent studies suggest that genetic factors may predispose an individual for development of the disease. Epidemiologic and direct biologic studies, however, have again strongly implicated EBV in the causation of this disease. Simons et al. in 1975 found that the presence of two HLA-related antigens (A2 and B Sin2) increased an individual's risk for

TABLE 5-6 Evidence for the Etiologic Role of Epstein-Barr Virus (EBV) in Burkitt's Lymphoma (BL)

1. Association of virus particles, antigens, and nucleic acids with tumor tissues
2. Presence of the virus in BL-afflicted regions
3. Increased anti-EBV antibody in BL patients
4. Transformation in vitro to immortality of human lymphocytes by EBV shed from BL tumor tissue
5. Proliferative response of infectious mononucleosis (IM) patient lymphocytes
6. Transformation in vitro to immortality of human B lymphocytes by EBV
7. Induction of malignant lymphoma in nonhuman New World primates by EBV infection

the development of NPC. This correlation has only held up for the southern Chinese population and not for NPC patients of non-Chinese heritage. The exact role of HLA antigens in determining NPC risk is not clear.

Cytomegalovirus

Another human herpesvirus thought to have oncogenic potential is human cytomegalovirus (CMV). CMV possesses properties commonly associated with known oncogenic DNA viruses, i.e., it can stimulate the DNA synthesis of host cells infected in culture. Albrecht and Rapp were the first to establish a continuous line of hamster cells transformed to malignancy by CMV. Indirect immunofluorescence tests established the presence of virus antigens in the cytoplasm and membranes of cells from this line. This line of cells is tumorigenic when inoculated into newborn hamsters. Work by Geder et al. has also demonstrated that infection of human embryo lung cells with a prostatic isolate of CMV (Major strain) can lead to a long-term persistent infection and that occasional cell transformants can arise in the culture. These transformants do not shed infectious virus but contain virus-specific membrane and intracellular antigens. These human cell transformants share common antigens with the CMV-transformed hamster cells and can induce nondifferentiated tumors when injected into athymic nude mice.

CMV infection is very common with close to 90 percent of the human population infected at some time in life. Infection of a healthy adult is clinically inapparent, but serious problems arise when congenital CMV infection occurs. Infected infants can have mild to severe central nervous system involvement as well as virus growth in other organs. This virus is also a problem in immunosuppressed patients who may develop CMV pneumonia.

The involvement of CMV in human neoplasia has been suggested but not extensively studied. Several reports have suggested that CMV may play a role in genital cancers. CMV can spread transplacentally and venereally as well as by parenteral, respiratory, and urinary routes. Lang et al. detected the presence of CMV in human semen, and there are many examples of CMV isolates from prostatic tissue.

CMV has been implicated in malignancies of humans, especially Kaposi's sarcoma and cancer of the prostate. Giraldo et al. reported increased anti-CMV antibody titers in European Kaposi's sarcoma patients. This correlation did not hold true, however, in African patients with this same tumor. In addition, Huang et al. have detected CMV DNA by nucleic acid hybridization in a small number of colon carcinomas. These exciting results require confirmation.

The fact that human embryo cells can be transformed to malignancy by prostatic CMV isolates supports the idea that CMV may play a role in the etiology of prostatic carcinoma. Geder et al. have been able to extend the life in culture of normal prostatic fibroblasts, and these cells were shown to contain CMV DNA sequences by nucleic acid hybridization. To date, however, these prostatic cell lines have not induced tumors. Patients with prostatic cancer have significantly increased anti-CMV antibody titers and, in addition, it has been possible to demonstrate by immunofluorescence that two cultures established in vitro from biopsies of prostatic carcinoma contain CMV antigens.

SUMMARY

Several groups of viruses have been discussed that are known to transform cells in culture and to cause tumor formation in animals. Some of these virus groups have been strongly associated with malignant tumors in humans, most notably several of the human herpesviruses and HBV. The case is overwhelming that EBV and HBV are involved in BL and PHC respectively. Even if the concession is made that the viruses fulfill only one of a number of causal roles, the evidence for involvement of these two viruses in human neoplasia has fulfilled all of the necessary requirements short of showing that removal of the virus prevents the tumor. The role of HSV-2 in cervical cancer is also very strong. The most recent evidence that HSV-2–specific RNA sequences can be found in biopsies of dysplasia, carcinoma in situ, and invasive carcinoma of the cervix lends strong support to the accumulated evidence that this virus has oncogenic potential.

The papilloma viruses definitely can cause benign warts. It has been much more difficult, however, to associate the papovaviruses, adenoviruses, and retroviruses with neoplasia in the human population despite abundant examples of tumor formation by these agents in the animal kingdom. Especially disturbing is the paucity of data indicating the existence of naturally occurring human retroviruses. The ease with which the retroviruses can be obtained from animals would seem to indicate a fundamental oversight by biologists in their approach to isolation of retroviruses from human tissue. The real possibility that these agents do not exist at high frequency in human tissue must, however, be considered.

The failure to detect genomes of tumorigenic viruses in tumor samples can only be considered valid if the detection limit of the method used is sufficiently sensitive to pick up as little as one foreign gene per tumor cell. Even this approach is not proof positive since, despite evidence in animal models, persistence of virus genes in the tumor cell is not necessarily required.

The reader should also realize that association of an infectious agent with a tumor is not definite proof of a causal relationship. It is only by removing the infectious agent (for example, by virus vaccination) and demonstrating concurrent cessation of tumor incidence that an exact etiologic role for a virus in neoplasia can be defined. Attempts presently in progress to obliterate HBV infection in Third World countries by use of an HBsAg vaccine should yield data over the next 50 years that will definitely resolve whether this one putative tumor virus causes liver cancer. Preparation of vaccines against other virus agents, especially herpesvirus vaccines, is a subject of ongoing research. Only effective prevention of virus infection will ultimately define their true role in oncogenic disease.

ACKNOWLEDGMENTS

Investigations carried out in this laboratory were supported by contract NO1 CP 53516 within the Virus Cancer Program of the National Cancer Institute and by grants CA 18450 and CA 25305 awarded by the National Cancer Institute. M. K. Howett is the recipient of a special fellowship from the Leukemia Society of America, Incorporated.

The authors would like to thank Melissa C. Reese for helpful editorial assistance.

REFERENCES

1. Hiatt HH et al: Origins of human cancer, in *Cold Spring Harbor Conferences on Cell Proliferation,* Vol 4, Cold Spring Harbor, NY, 1977.
2. Bishop JM: Retroviruses. *Annu Rev Biochem* 47:35, 1978.
3. Coffin JM: Structure, replication and recombination of retrovirus genomes: Some unifying hypotheses. *J Gen Virol* 42:1, 1979.
4. Rapp F, Westmoreland D: Cell transformation by DNA-containing viruses. *Biochim Biophys Acta* 458:167, 1976.
5. Fareed GC, Davoli D: Molecular biology of papovaviruses. *Annu Rev Biochem* 46:471, 1977.
6. Rapp F: Transformation *in vitro* by DNA tumor viruses, in RC Gallo (ed): *Recent Advances in Cancer Research Cell Biology, Molecular Biology and Tumor Virology,* Vol 1, CRC Press, Cleveland, 1977.
7. Flint J: The topography and transcription of the adenovirus genome. *Cell* 10:153, 1977.
8. WHO Expert Committee on Viral Hepatitis: Advances in viral hepatitis. *WHO Tech Rep* ser 602, Geneva, 1977.
9. Robinson WS: The genome of hepatitis B virus. *Annu Rev Microbiol* 31:357, 1977.
10. de-Thé G et al (eds): *Oncogenesis and Herpesviruses III,* Vols 1 and 2, International Agency for Research on Cancer, Lyon, France, 1978.
11. Roizman B: The structure and isomerization of herpes simplex virus genomes. *Cell* 16:481, 1979.
12. Epstein MA, Achong BG (eds): *The Epstein Barr Virus,* Springer Verlag, New York, 1979.

6

THE MOLECULAR VIROLOGY OF BREAST CANCER AND ITS CLINICAL IMPLICATIONS

Sol Spiegelman   *Ricardo Mesa-Tejada*   *Tsuneya Ohno*

This chapter summarizes our investigations exploring the possible association of RNA tumor viruses with human neoplasia and the exploitation of any leads which could be of conceivable use in the prevention, diagnosis, or therapy of human cancer.

The hope and intent was that a parallel study of the animal in the human disease by the newer methodologies of molecular biology would yield clinically useful information. The underlying belief was that assessment of the applicability to human cancer of the information derived from experimental models would more likely emerge if the same laboratory that operated at the basic level would commit itself to the examination of human material.

It is important to emphasize at the outset that the primary purpose of the investigations did not center on proving that viruses cause human cancer either in general or in particular. The "multihit" nature of the carcinogenic process discourages any simplistic approach designed to find the single cause. It is unlikely that cancer is a puzzle with a unique solution. It is probable that cancer is a collection of problems and therefore more likely to be resolved by a set of compatible alternatives.

We were attracted to the possibility of viral involvement in at least certain human cancers because of the following two facts: (1) it is a testable hypothesis by the technology of molecular biology; and (2) the accumulated information in comparable animal disease supports the existence of this mechanism. The credible assumption was made that human biology would not be so unique as to make animal studies completely irrelevant to the human disease. It seemed plausible, therefore, to entertain the working hypothesis that at least some human neoplasias would have a biologic basis similar to that observed in comparable animal models.

Since the major objective was to generate information that would be clinically relevant, our effort with experimental models has always been paralleled by extensive investigations with human material. The aim was to identify which of the observations made with the laboratory models could be confirmed in the human disease.

Much of this chapter focuses on the problem of human breast cancer. The leukemias could equally well have been chosen as the major effort. However, the decision to focus on breast cancer was conditioned by a number of factors. First, an excellent experimental animal model existed in the form of the murine mammary tumor. Second, compared to the leukemias, breast cancer represents a quantitatively more important problem in clinical oncology. Third, and perhaps most important, was the recognition that in the case of the leukemias, clinicians do have available excellent systemic indicators of the disease status from examinations of peripheral blood cells and of bone marrow aspirates. The situation is much more difficult in breast cancers and other solid tumors. Here systemic indicators are virtually nonexistent, and the problems of diagnosis and of monitoring of the disease status during therapy remain unresolved. It was clear that providing usable information in this area could have profound effects on the effectiveness of even the existing modes of treatment. One need but point to the dramatic effect on the success rate in the treatment of choriocarcinoma that followed from the discovery of the indicator hormone subunit HCGβ in the urine of women with this tumor.

The search for a tumor-specific antigen and its possible use both as a diagnostic and monitoring signal is hardly a unique idea. Whatever novelty exists in the approach we employed lies in the adoption of the working assumption that the tumor-specific antigen is likely to be virus-related. As will be seen below, the discovery of a tumor-specific antigen in the case of the human breast cancer was certainly catalyzed, if not made possible, by this working assumption. Again, it will also be seen that the continual interplay between the animal model and the human material guided us in designing the experiments which led to the detection of the tumor-specific antigen in the human. Indeed the animal model provided the reagents which in fact made this possible.

GENETIC ASPECTS OF THE CANCER PROBLEM

For molecular geneticists one of the most striking characteristics of the cancer cell is that the malignant state is transmissible to its progeny. Over the years a number of explanations (Table 6-1) have been proposed to explain the cellular heritability of the cancerous state. The first involves somatic mutations in either a structural or a regulatory gene, induced by either chemicals or radiation. The second depends on chromosomal inversions or translocation, as is indicated, for example, by the existence of the Philadelphia chromosome in some patients with chronic myelogenous leukemia. The third mechanism is one proposed long ago by the German biologist Boveri, who suggested that imbalances resulting from the loss or duplication of one or more chromosomes lead to the malignant state. The fourth has emerged

TABLE 6-1 Hypotheses of Cancer Etiology and Their DNA-Sequence Consequences

Hypothesis	Mechanism	Sequence change detectable by hybridization
1. Mutation	Individual base changes in structural or regulatory genes	None
2. Chromosomal rearrangement	Translocation, inversion, etc.	None
3. Chromosomal imbalance	Loss or duplication	Loss or gain of old sequences
4. Transduction	Insertion of viral genes	Gain of new sequences
5. Phenotypic modification	Self-reinforcing derepression of silent genes	None

from advances in molecular biology through the use of bacteria and their "transducing" viruses. Here one has a phenomenon in which the virus inserts its genetic information into the genome of the host cell. If the virus is a DNA agent, no chemical problems are posed and the mechanism of insertion is quite well understood. If, however, the virus involved contains RNA, a transcription of the RNA into a DNA strand is required via a suitable enzyme (reverse transcriptase) as postulated some time ago by the provirus hypothesis of Temin.[1] The fifth hypothesis involves a heritable phenotypic modification unaccompanied by any change in the genetic information. Here we assume the preexistence of a silent malignant segment of genetic information that is repressed but can undergo a self-reinforcing derepression.

It is important to recognize that the five mechanisms listed in Table 6-1 do not constitute an exhaustive list of all possibilities, nor are they mutually exclusive. Various forms of cancer in the same animal might be mediated by different mechanisms, and similarly for the same cancer in different animals. Further, more than one of the mechanisms listed might be implicated in the occurrence of one and the same neoplasia. For example, a mutation might predispose to the insertion of a virus, or vice versa. In effect, all one can experimentally hope to decide is whether one of the mechanisms is involved in a specific neoplasia in a particular animal. Experimental support for one mechanism in a particular instance does not eliminate the others. The strongest statement one can logically make is that none of the others can be the sole cause of the disease.

From the viewpoint of the authors' biases as molecular geneticists with experience in virology, the fourth mechanism was particularly attractive. It made the kinds of predictions that we were technically competent to challenge experimentally. It was the only hypothesis that demanded the active participation of a viral agent at some point in the carcinogenic process. It was also the only one that predicted the acquisition by the malignant cell of virus-related information that would not be found in its complete form in a normal cell.

Any attempt to examine human cancer from this point of view must start with a search for evidence of viral agents in the human disease. Animal viral oncology has amassed a considerable fund of information in the last 50 years concerning the so-called RNA tumor viruses, i.e., oncornaviruses. These agents have been implicated in a wide spectrum of cancers, both in the laboratory and in the field. As we have already noted, it seemed improbable to us that cancer in human beings is so different that the information provided by animal experiments would not be relevant to at least some of the corresponding human diseases.

ONCORNAVIRUSES AND HUMAN CANCER: SEQUENCE HOMOLOGY

Ten years ago there were five animal-model systems available which were used in our initial experiments. Four of these were causative agents of leukemias and sarcomas: the avian myeloblastosis virus (AMV) and Rous sarcoma virus (RSV) in chickens, and the Rauscher leukemia virus (RLV) and murine sarcoma virus (MSV) in mice. Finally, there was also the murine mammary tumor virus (MMTV), originally known as the Bittner milk factor, which is an etiologic agent for mammary tumors.

When these viruses are examined for sequence homologies among their nucleic acids, a rather informative pattern emerges. The two chicken agents share sequences in common. For the murine viruses, the nucleic acids of the agents that cause the mesenchymal neoplasias (leukemia, lymphomas, and sarcomas) show homology to one another, but not to either of the two avian agents or to the mammary tumor virus. Finally, the mouse mammary tumor virus has a singular sequence that is homologous only to itself.

If analogous virus particles are associated with the corresponding human diseases, certain predictions might be hazarded on the basis of the specificities observed with the animal viruses:

1. In view of the lack of homology between the avian and murine agents, it is unlikely that human agents, should they exist, would show homology to the avian group.
2. It follows from this and evolutionary considerations that the murine viruses would represent a more hopeful source of the molecular probes to search for similar information in the analogous human cancers.
3. If particles are found to be associated with the human leukemias, sarcomas, and lymphomas, their RNAs would show homology to one another, and possibly to that of the murine leukemia virus.
4. If RNA particles are identified in human breast cancer, they should not exhibit homology to the RNA of viruslike particles associated with the human mesenchymal neoplasias or to the RNA of Rauscher leukemia virus; they might, however exhibit detectable homology to the RNA of MMTV.

Molecular Hybridization with Viral Sequences

Because of their availability and the considerations outlined above, the murine agents were initially chosen for the production of the molecular probes needed to look for corresponding information in the human diseases. Probes were of course also made with the avian agents to serve as suitable controls. Further, in order to monitor the biological consistency of the findings and its comparability to the animal system, the human neoplasias for which there are suitable animal models — the mesenchymal tumors and human breast cancer — were examined in parallel. The data obtained would help determine quickly whether the findings in humans mirrored biologically what was known from the animal experimental models.

The technology and experimental design used in these series of experiments are illustrated in Fig. 6-1. A highly radioactive DNA copy of a viral RNA was synthesized using the reverse transcriptase and the 70-S RNA of the appropriate animal virus. This DNA, which consists of small pieces, is used as a probe in annealing experiments to test for homologous virus-specific sequences in the RNA of the two major human neoplasias examined. The presence of a viral sequence is assessed by cesium sulfate equilibrium density-gradient centrif-

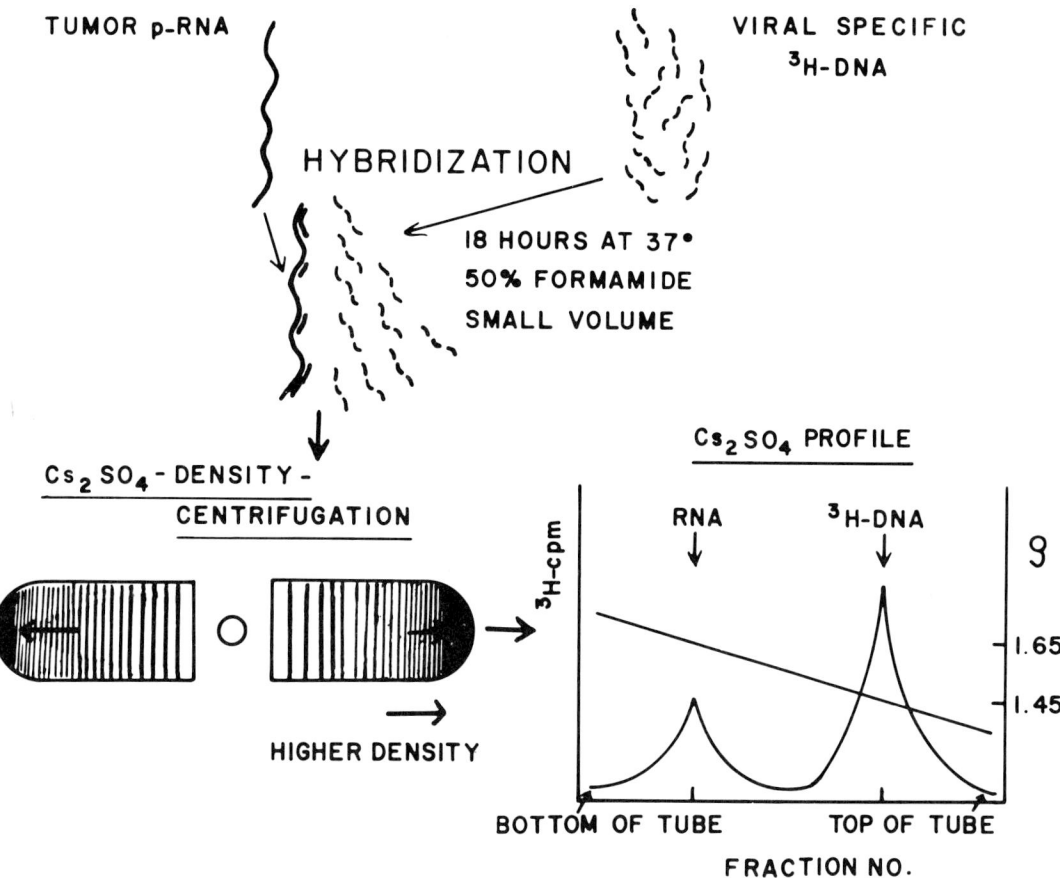

FIGURE 6-1 Molecular hybridization and detection with viral-specific [³H]DNA and tumor RNA.

ugation. The movement of the tritiated DNA region of the density gradient is the signal that the DNA probe has found complementary sequences in the tumor RNA with which it is being challenged.

Table 6-2 summarizes in diagrammatic form the outcome of this survey. The proportion of positives ranged from 67 percent for breast cancer to 92 percent for the leukemias. No normal or nonmalignant samples from breast tissue gave positive responses, and similarly, no normal nonmalignant leukocytes ever yielded a positive response.

The most noteworthy feature about the pattern exhibited in Table 6-2 is its concordance with the prediction that is deducible from the avian and murine models. Thus, human breast cancer would appear to contain RNA homologous only to that of the MMTV of RNA. Human leukemias, sarcomas, and lymphomas all contain

TABLE 6-2 Homologies among Human Neoplastic RNAs and Animal Tumor Viral RNAs*

	Human neoplastic RNAs			
Viral RNAs†	Breast cancer	Leukemia	Sarcoma	Lymphoma
MMTV	+	−	−	−
RLV	−	+	+	+
AMV	−	−	−	−

*The results of molecular hybridization between [³H]DNA complementary to the various viral RNAs and pRNA preparations from the indicated neoplastic tissues. The plus sign indicates that hybridizations were positive and the negative sign that none could be detected.
†MMTV = murine mammary tumor virus; RLV = murine Rauscher leukemia virus; AMV = avian myeloblastosis virus.

RNA that shows some homology to that of the murine leukemia virus (RLV), but these neoplasias contain no RNA homologous to the RNA of MMTV. Finally, none of the human tumors contain RNA detectably related to that of the avian myeloblastosis virus. In summary, the specificity pattern of the unique RNA found in the human neoplasias is in complete agreement with what has been described for the corresponding virus-induced malignancies in the mouse.

Simultaneous Detection Test for Reverse Transcriptase and High-Molecular-Weight RNA

Needless to say, the existence of the remarkable concordance exhibited in Table 6-2 did not establish a viral etiology for these diseases in human beings. The next step required performance of experiments designed to answer questions about the size of the RNA being detected, and about whether this RNA is associated with a reverse transcriptase in a particle that possesses other features of complete or incomplete virus particles. This required a method for detecting in human material the presence of particles similar to the RNA tumor viruses.

The oncornaviruses exhibit two identifying characteristics. They contain a large single-stranded RNA molecule having a sedimentation coefficient of 60-S to 70-S (or 35-S if it has dissociated into its subunits), and they also possess a reverse transcriptase complexed to the RNA which can be used as a template to make a complementary DNA copy. The possibility of a concomitant test for both the enzyme and its template was suggested by our earlier experience with RNA polymerization. If a template-directed polymerization is interrupted and the protein is removed by the usual phenol treatment, the nascent product complexes to its template in a Watson-Crick structure. Examination of the intermediates of reverse transcriptase reactions revealed that under such conditions the nascent DNA product is in fact found complexed to the large 70-S RNA template.[2] These structures can be detected by the unusual position of the newly synthesized, small tritiated DNA products in cesium sulfate density gradients, in glycerol velocity gradients, and electrophoretically in acrylamide gels.[3] The most informative assay is to subject the isotopically labeled product to sedimentation analysis before the removal of the RNA. If the labeled DNA product behaves as if it is a 70-S molecule, and if it can be shown that it does so because it is complexed to a 70-S RNA molecule, then evidence is provided for the presence of a reverse transcriptase that uses a 70-S RNA template. One may then tentatively conclude that the material examined contains particles similar to the RNA tumor virus. On this basis Schlom and Spiegelman[4] developed the simultaneous detection test that was used to demonstrate the presence in human milk of particles containing 70-S RNA and reverse transcriptase.[5] The test was modified[6] to be applicable to tumor tissue using the murine mammary tumor as the experimental model.

The procedure is diagramed in Fig. 6-2. Tumor cells are disrupted and then fractionated by differential centrifugation. A high-speed cytoplasmic pellet is isolated; if virus is present, it is most likely to be found in this fraction. A brief endogenous reverse transcriptase reaction is then performed with this pellet. The product of the reaction with its RNA template is freed of protein and then analyzed both in a glycerol velocity gradient to determine the sedimentation coefficient of the tritiated DNA and in a cesium sulfate equilibrium gradient to determine its density.

The presence of particles encapsulating 70-S RNA and reverse transcriptase is indicated by the appearance of a peak of newly synthesized DNA traveling at a speed corresponding to a 70-S (or 35-S) RNA molecule. That its apparent large size is due to its being complexed to an RNA molecule can be readily verified by subjecting the purified nucleic acid to ribonuclease before analysis with the velocity gradient, which should result in the disappearance of the 70-S "tritiated DNA." Similarly, if the reaction is positive, newly synthesized DNA should appear in the RNA and hybrid regions of the cesium sulfate density gradient, and these also should be eliminated by prior treatment with ribonuclease.

The simultaneous detection test was first applied to human breast cancer.[7] Figure 6-3 demonstrates a positive reaction with the material obtained from a malignant adenocarcinoma of the breast that was treated as outlined in Fig. 6-2, in which the 70-S DNA complex can be observed with the fraction examined. It is evident that this complex involves RNA because prior treatment with ribonuclease eliminates the tritiated DNA from the 70-S region of the velocity gradient. In this series of patients, 38 adenocarcinomas and 10 nonmalignant controls were examined in this manner; 79 percent of the malignant breast samples were positive for the simultaneous detection reaction, whereas all of the control samples from either normal or benign tissues were negative.

We further demonstrated that the breast carcinoma

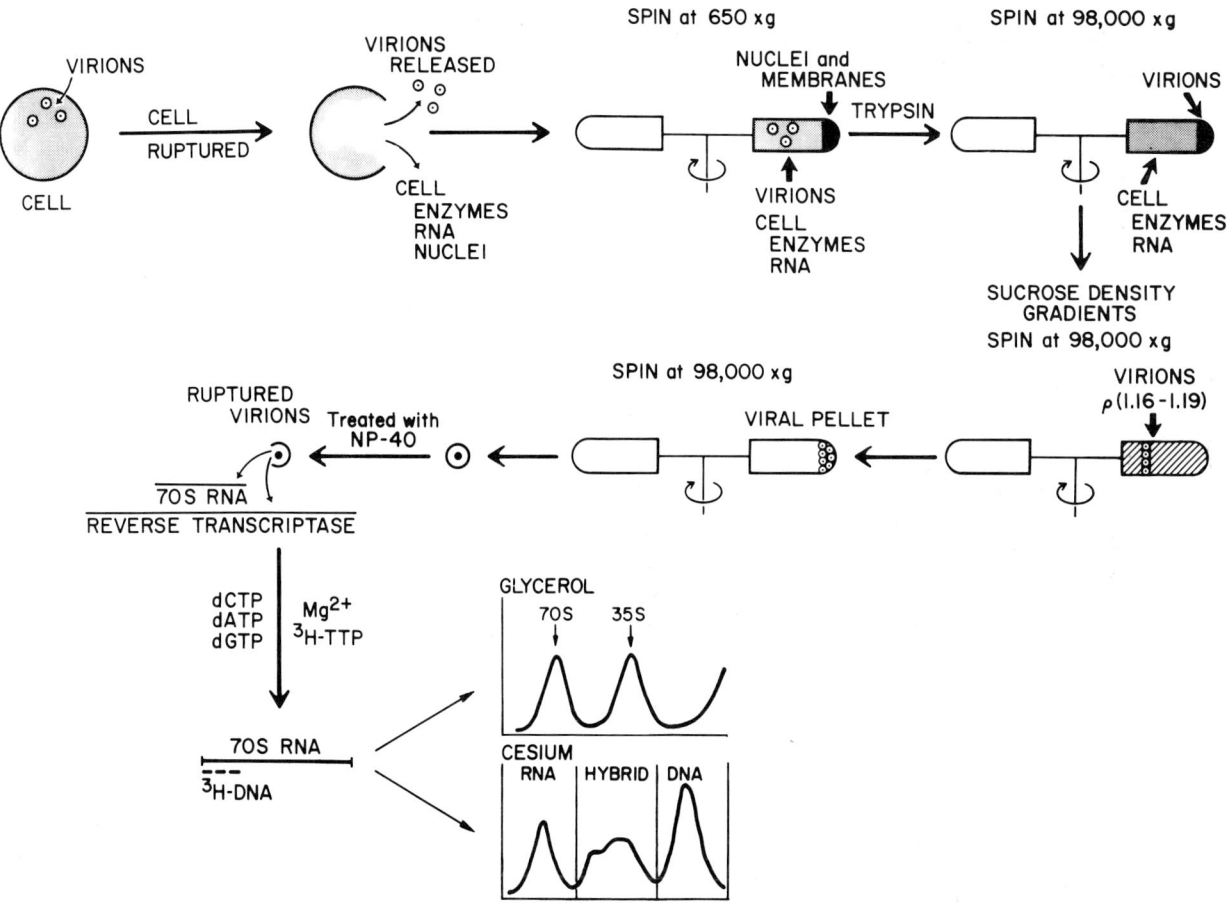

FIGURE 6-2 Simultaneous detection test for 70-S RNA and reverse transcriptase in neoplastic tissue.

particles encapsulating the 70-S RNA and reverse transcriptase had a density of between 1.16 and 1.19 g/mL, the density characteristic of the oncogenic viruses. Identical experiments were undertaken with human leukemias, lymphomas, and sarcomas;[8] these results were briefly summarized in Table 6-3. Note that positive outcomes were observed in more than 95 percent of the leukemia patients, whether they were acute or chronic, lymphoblastic or myelogenous. Thus, despite their disparate clinical pictures and differing cellular pathologies, these various types of leukemias behave similarly with respect to this test.

These experiments on human breast cancer and the mesenchymal malignancies were designed to probe the significance of our exploratory investigations, which identified by molecular hybridization the presence in these neoplasias of RNA that was homologous to those of the corresponding murine oncornaviruses. The data obtained with the simultaneous detection tests established that at least a portion of the tumor-specific, virus-related RNA being detected was in the form of a 70-S RNA template physically associated with the reverse transcriptase in a particle possessing a density between 1.16 and 1.19 g/mL—three of the diagnostic features of the animal RNA tumor viruses.

Subsequent application of the simultaneous detection test to other human tumors revealed that positive reactions could be detected with very high frequency in virtually every major tumor site, including melanomas, colon, stomach, rectum, lung, brain, and ovary.[9,10,11]

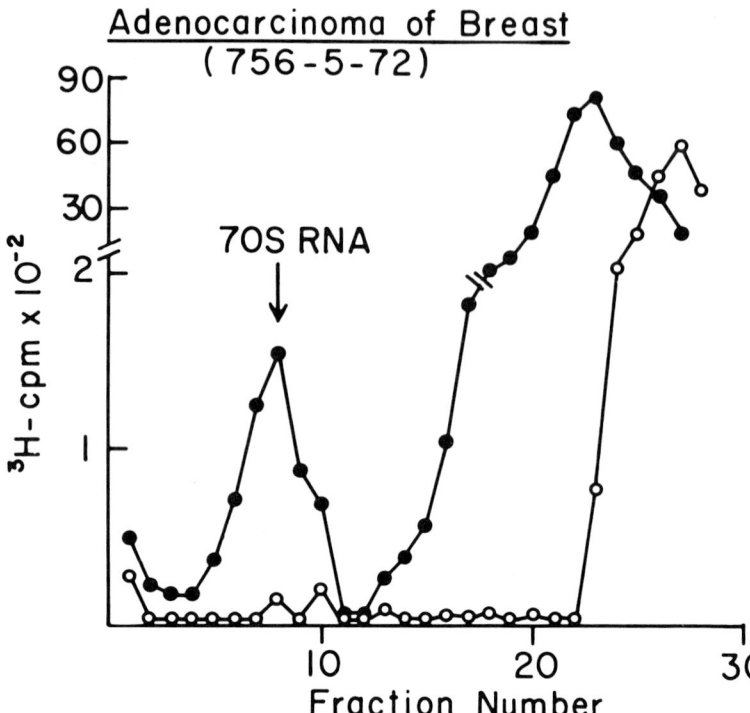

FIGURE 6-3 Effect of ribonuclease on the detection of the high molecular-weight RNA-[^{3}H]DNA complex. The viral pellet (P-100) was suspended in buffer and divided into two equal parts. A standard RNA-instructed DNA polymerase reaction was performed on one part of the P-100 fraction; after incubation the nucleic acid complex was extracted and was sized on a linear glycerol gradient (0——0). After disruption with detergent, the other half of the P-100 fraction was incubated in the presence of RNase A and RNase T$_1$. A standard RNA-instructed DNA polymerase reaction was then performed (0——0).

Implications of the Presence of Tumor-Specific Particles

One of the remarkable features of the particles found in the various tumors is that they obeyed the sequence dissimilarity rule already noted between the particles found in the breast carcinomas compared with those in the mesenchymal tumors. Each particular organ site had associated with its tumor a uniquely identifiable viruslike particle readily distinguishable in terms of sequence differences.

Once the presence of unique particles in the various types of human carcinomas has been established, the natural tendency is to try to design and perform experiments that could decide whether these particles are the etiologic agents of the corresponding neoplasias. However, there are unfortunately formidable difficulties with extending the effort in this direction. For example, although awareness of MMTV has existed for more than 40 years, no one has succeeded in producing a mammary tumor in any other animal but the mouse with this agent. It is likely that any human particles of a similar kind would face the same kind of species barriers. An attempt to overcome this difficulty might well consume the lifetimes of numerous investigators, perhaps for several generations to come. It seemed futile to dwell on the etiologic implications of these particles because no hard conclusions could in fact be drawn until more definitive experiments became possible.

Another approach offered potentially more immediate and useful consequences. Whether the cause or the consequence of human malignancy, the presence of these tumor-related particles and their uniqueness provided a novel opportunity to generate information of potentially practical importance for the diagnosis and management of the disease. What was needed was a systemic signal of the presence of these particles, which could then serve to alert the observer that a particular tumor was present. One possibility would perhaps be to explore whether bits and pieces of the particle nucleic acid might not be found in the circulation; this could be done by the use of molecular hybridization, a relatively sensitive technique. However, this pathway presents a number of difficulties. One is the expense involved in synthesizing the necessary radioactive probes to the specific activities required to perform the tests. Another is the necessity of introducing this rather sophisticated and laborious technology into clinical pathology laboratories. Finally, it is not unreasonable to suppose that complete particles may not always be present in a tumor; thus protein coded for by the viral genome, previously incorporated to the host DNA, may be the only component available for detection.

A more practical approach, therefore, would be one that depended on detecting a protein rather than a nucleic acid. This seemed plausible because the unique sequences in the various particles should code for very different proteins. Once these divergences are transferred from the nucleic acids to the level of proteins, the extensive armamentarium of immunology becomes available for their detection. Further, this approach involves procedures and methodologies that are both comparatively inexpensive and readily performed in pathology laboratories. Thus, if one or more of the particle proteins appear in the circulation, they could easily serve as systemic signals for the presence of the corresponding tumor.

The feasibility of this approach was explored and established with the mouse mammary tumor model. Radioimmunoassays showed that the plasma level of gp52, a viral protein, is an excellent diagnostic device for both primary and metastatic mammary tumors. It also provides a reliable prognostic indication of the ultimate effectiveness of surgical and adjuvant chemotherapy.[12]

Any attempt at an extension of this approach to the human disease must begin by answering the following questions: (1) What kind of antigen should be sought in the human disease? (2) Where and how should one look for this antigen?

Before embarking on a blind quest for an antigen specific for a human tumor, it would seem prudent to take advantage of the clues supplied by the information gained from the animal model. The human breast cancer problem became the focus because there was an excellent animal model available. Further, from a quantitative clinical point of view, it was one of the more frequent solid tumors affecting humans; any advance in monitoring or diagnosing this disease would have a detectable clinical impact. It was also felt that success with one solid tumor could pave the way to solving common technological problems applicable to other solid tumors. In any event, virtually all that follows will focus on human breast cancer.

ONCORNAVIRUSES AND HUMAN BREAST CANCER: ANTIGENIC RELATIONSHIP

The fact that some homology has existed between the RNAs of the human and the murine particles suggested that an antigenic relationship might also conceivably exist between one or another of the proteins of these particles. The plausibility of this expectation is supported by serological investigations with sera from breast cancer patients, in which antibodies interacting with MMTV components have been identified.[13] In addition, migration-inhibition studies of leukocytes from breast cancer

TABLE 6-3 Simultaneous Detection Tests with Human Tumors and Controls*

Tissue	Number of positive reactions	Average (70 S), cycles/min	Number of negative reactions	Average (70 S), cycles/min	Positive reaction, %
Carcinoma of the breast	28	668	10	20	74
Control (nonmalignant breast tissue)	0	0	10	8	0
Leukemia	22	481	1	0	95
Hodgkin's disease	22	379	6	14	79
Burkitt's lymphoma	9	369	2	14	82
Other lymphomas	7	347	1	24	88
Control (spleens)	0	0	14	14	0

*Results of simultaneous detection assays with human tumors and controls. The average of the cycles per minute in the 70-S position monitored by external size markers is summarized. The reactions were designated as positive if the cycles per minute exceeded 30 above background (*Kufe et al., 1973*).

patients have provided immunological evidence of cross reactivity with the gp52 of MMTV.[14] Cross-reactive components have also been detected in an established human breast carcinoma cell line.[15]

In considering the question of where to look for such antigens in humans, it must be recognized that there are logistical and quantitative limitations in transferring certain technologies from mice to humans. Thus the temptation to set up radioimmunoassays for cross-reacting proteins in human plasmas is likely to meet with disappointment because of the 1000-fold difference in blood volume between mice and humans. Even if a human tumor is every bit as effective, per gram, as a mouse tumor in producing protein antigens in the blood, there is still the fact that the signal would be diluted 1000-fold in the human compared with the mouse. Indeed, two recently reported studies attempting to detect MMTV-related proteins by radioimmunoassay in the sera of breast cancer patients were not successful.[16,17] For this and other reasons, we decided to first center our efforts on the tumor itself as the most plausible site to initiate the search for a cross-reactive protein in humans. Once an antigen was identified, it could possibly be isolated and the necessary reagents required for a sensitive assay could be prepared.

The murine model again helped to develop a convenient, reliable, and sensitive microscopic method for identifying such an agent in the cells.

Immunohistochemical Localization of MMTV in Mouse Mammary Tumors

Most previous investigators have used immunofluorescence as a detecting device in the localization of MMTV proteins in mouse mammary tumor tissues.[13] The numerous limitations and disadvantages inherent in the routine use of this particular technique led us to explore the applicability of the immunoperoxidase method which appeared more suitable to the immediate purpose and future needs.

Aside from its applicability to immunoelectromicroscopy, the immunoperoxidase procedure has three major advantages that make it an exceedingly attractive method for antigen localization with conventional bright-field microscopy.[18] Briefly, these are as follows:

1. The positive staining reaction appears as a brown precipitate that, in combination with an appropriate counterstain, provides sufficient histologic detail to permit precise cytological identification and localization.
2. The preparations do not fade and thus can be filed as permanent records for future comparison.
3. Paraffin sections can be used if the antigenic determinants of the substance being localized withstand the routine fixation and embedding procedures required.

In view of the ultimate goal to transfer this technology

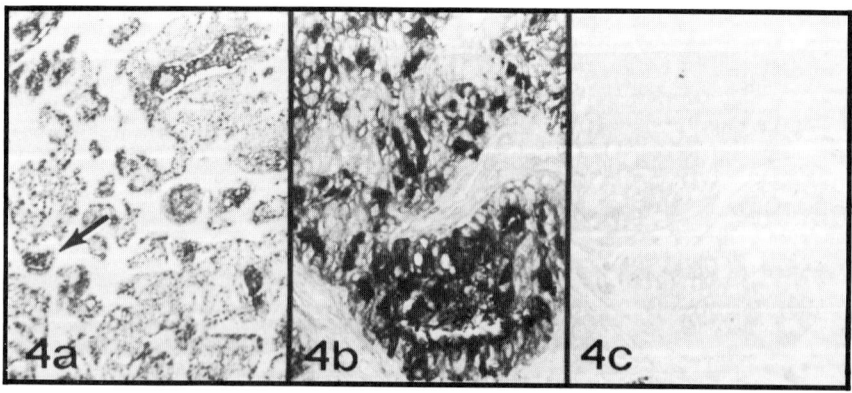

FIGURE 6-4 (a) Immunoperoxidase stain of mammary adenocarcinoma from Paris RIII mouse using anti-MMTV as primary antibody.

(b) High magnification of small field (a) (arrow) illustrates differences in intensity and pattern of stain in tumor glands as compared to adjacent cluster of cells.

(c) Identical field in adjacent serial section stained with anti-MMTV previously absorbed with MMTV. (Methylene blue counterstain; a, 40 ×; b and c, 250 ×)

to human material, the possibility of using paraffin sections was particularly intriguing. Therefore, the immunohistochemical localization of MMTV antigens in parallel paraffin and frozen sections cut from the same tumor were compared using the indirect immunoperoxidase method and rabbit anti-MMTV immunoglobulin G. In agreement with previous experience with other antigens,[18] it was found that localization of MMTV antigens in the mammary tumor is visualized with greater precision and sensitivity in the paraffin sections than in frozen sections.[19] This may be attributed to the superior fixation and preservation of cytologic integrity that results from paraffin embedding compared with use of frozen sections in which diffusion of antigen and cellular destruction occurs readily.

A representative example of the type of staining observed in the mouse mammary tumors is illustrated in Fig. 6-4. In this typical mammary adenocarcinoma, localization of MMTV antigen can be seen in most cells and within the lumina of tumor glands. The intracellular staining varies from coarsely granular to diffuse, and in the case of cells lining the tumor glands, staining is most common along the apical, intraluminal border of the cells (Fig. 6-4b). In agreement with previously reported immunofluorescent studies,[20] the staining pattern varies according to the degree of histologic differentiation of the tumor. Thus, in areas of poor differentiation, as in the nest of cells in Fig. 6-4b, the staining is sparse to absent; wherever the tumor forms glands, however, a greater amount of reaction product is noted in the cells and in secretions within these glands. Similar reactions, varying somewhat in intensity, were noted in all of the mammary tumors tested in these studies. The specificity of the reaction was determined by its complete absence after absorption of the anti-MMTV with whole disrupted MMTV (Fig. 6-4c).

In eight tumor-bearing mice examined for metastatic lesions, three pulmonary and one hepatic metastases were found. Examples of the staining reaction of these lesions are illustrated in Figs. 6-5 and 6-6. It does not differ substantially from the primary tumor in its staining characteristics. The ability to detect even microscopic metastatic lesions by this specific staining procedure was particularly satisfying, in that it augured well for the potential usefulness of the procedure in diagnosing the origin of metastatic lesions.

Before the discussion of the mouse tumors is concluded, it should be noted that highly infected mouse strains were deliberately chosen to optimize the chances

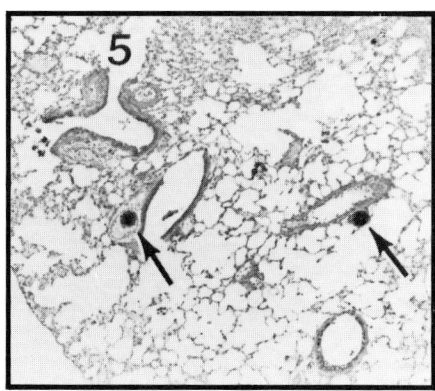

FIGURE 6-5 Mammary tumor metastasis in lung of CD8F1 mouse stained with anti-MMTV. Note the microscopic metastasis in peribronchiolar vessel (left arrow). (Methylene blue counterstain; 35 ×)

of observing a reaction and perfecting the method of localizing MMTV antigens. Nevertheless, even in these mouse mammary tumors, MMTV antigens could not be detected in numerous cells that were obviously malignant. This cellular heterogeneity of antigen expression is frequently observed in human tumors with respect to other tumor-associated antigens.[21]

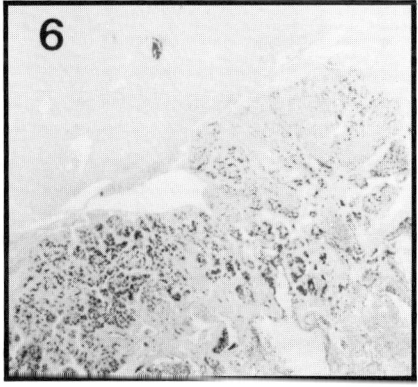

FIGURE 6-6 Mammary tumor metastasis in liver of CD8F1 mouse stained with anti-MMTV. Note unstained liver tissue surrounding tumor. (Methylene blue counterstain; 23 ×)

TABLE 6-4 Immunoperoxidase Staining of Carcinoma of the Breast

Source	Number of cases	Positive	Positive, %
Columbia Presbyterian	274	133	48.5
Memorial Sloan-Kettering	69	31	44.9
Michigan Cancer Foundation	104	48	46.2
Total	447	212	47.4

Immunohistochemical Detection of MMTV-Related Components in Human Breast Cancer

The successful application of the immunoperoxidase technique to the localization of MMTV antigens in sections of paraffin-embedded mouse mammary tissues made possible extensive, primarily retrospective, studies of human breast cancer tissues. Once the need for fresh tissues in the search for a cross-reacting human antigen had been eliminated, it became possible to use the same tissues received by the pathology laboratory, which could be tested without interfering with the diagnostic function of the surgical pathologist. Serial sections for immunohistochemical staining were cut from paraffin blocks of tissues used for diagnostic purposes from several sources. The methods and reagents used on the human tissues were essentially the same as those used in the mouse mammary tumor studies with minor modifications.*

* The preparation, purification, and characterization of the immunologic and other reagents used in these studies are described by Mesa-Tejada et al.[22]

MALIGNANT BREAST TISSUE

Up to the present time a positive staining reaction has been observed in 212 (47.4 percent) of 447 randomly selected cases of human breast carcinoma tested, including those received from other institutions (Table 6-4). The results observed in the Columbia Presbyterian breast cancer case subdivided with respect to histopathologic types are summarized in Table 6-5. A significantly larger percentage of positive cases in the mixed intraductal and invasive group (64.4 percent) reflects a trend noted in our original report of 131 cases and suggests a definite correlation in this enlarged series. It appears, therefore, that an invasive carcinoma associated with an intraductal component is more likely to contain the cross-reacting antigen than either a purely intraductal or purely invasive tumor. The pattern of immunohistochemical staining in the human breast carcinomas tends to be focal, intracellular, and cytoplasmic, with considerable variability even within the same tumor (Figs. 6-7 to 6-10). For example, in the intraductal and invasive carcinoma illustrated in Fig. 6-7, only some of the cells within intraductal lesions are stained, while most of the surrounding invasive cells contain reaction product. In other sections of tumor from this same case, however, staining was completely absent in some intraductal lesions surrounded by strongly reactive invasive cells; the reverse situation was also occasionally seen. The invasive tumor illustrated in Fig. 6-8 represents the strongest staining reaction we have yet observed in a human tumor and compares in intensity with that observed in a mouse mammary tumor with the same reagents. As can be seen at the higher magnification (Fig. 6-8b), essentially every tumor cell contains reaction product in varying amounts. In another microscopic field of the same section (Fig. 6-9), the staining reaction is observed only in the small

TABLE 6-5 Immunoperoxidase Staining of Carcinoma of the Breast*

Classification	Number of cases	Positive	Positive, %
Intraductal	25	10	40.0
Intraductal and invasive	73	47	64.4
Invasive	109	53	48.6
Medullary	18	7	38.9
Metastatic	49	16	32.7
Total	274	133	48.5

* Histopathologic classification of Columbia Presbyterian cases.

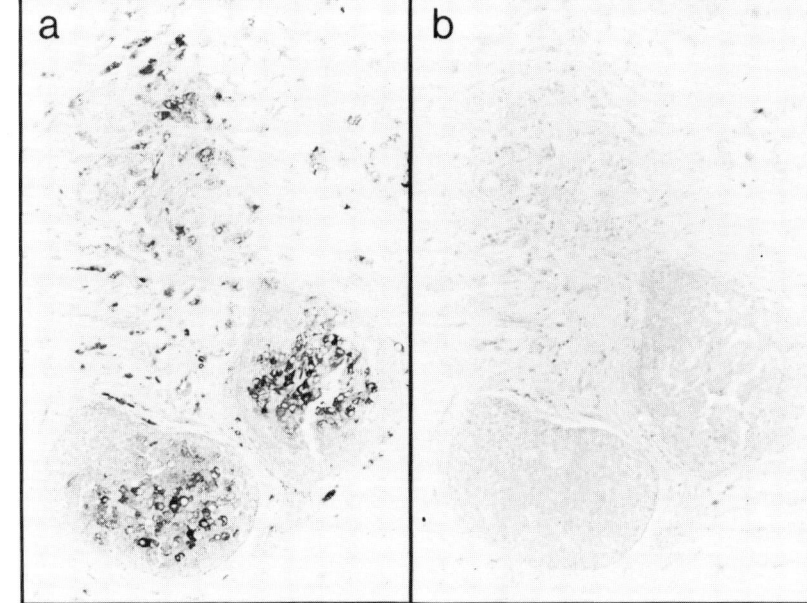

FIGURE 6-7 Immunoperoxidase stain of intraductal and small cell invasive human breast carcinoma with anti-gp52 before (*a*) and after (*b*) absorption with gp52. Some of the cells in the intraductal lesion and most of the invasive cells contain reaction product. (Methylene blue counterstain; 45 ×)

focus of invasive carcinoma, whereas no reaction product is noted in either the surrounding dense fibrous tissue or in the neighboring morphologically benign epithelial tissue such as the adjacent hyperplastic lobules.

Figures 6-10 and 6-11 illustrate a positive reaction seen in an invasive tumor and in a microscopic metastatic lesion in the peripheral sinus of an axillary lymph node from the same case. Although in this case more or less the same degree of reactivity is seen in both the primary and metastatic malignant cells, we have noted that both regional (axillary) and distant metastatic lesions present more or less the same degree of variability in the expression of detectable antigen as the primary tumors themselves. However, a sufficient number of cases of primary and corresponding metastatic carcinomas have not as yet been tested to be able to establish the existence of a correlation in antigen expression between the primary carcinoma and its regional or distant metastases.

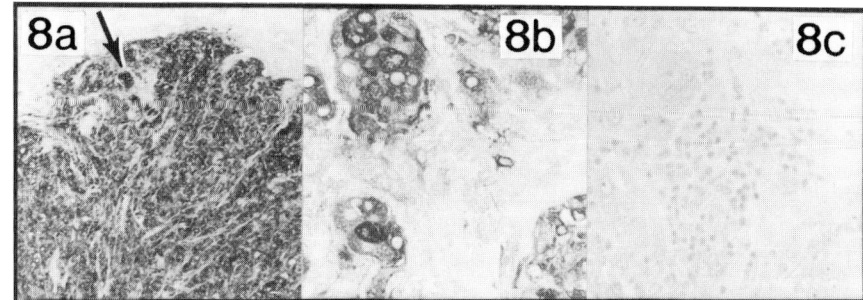

FIGURE 6-8 Immunoperoxidase stain of invasive breast carcinoma with anti-MMTV before (*a, b*) and after (*c*) absorption with gp52. Note in (*b*) (detail of area indicated by arrow in [*a*]) strong reaction in practically all tumor cells, and absence of stain in central area consisting mostly of lymphocytic infiltrate. Sparse extracellular reaction product may be due to antigen diffusion before fixation. (Methylene blue counterstain; *a*, 27 ×; *b* and *c*, 167 ×)

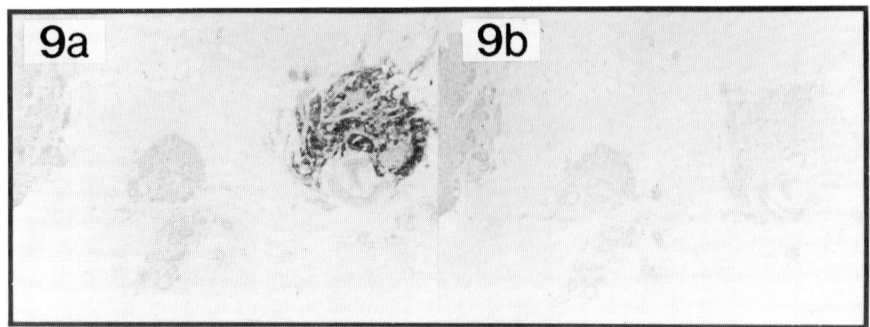

FIGURE 6-9 Another field in same section as Figure 6-8 showing staining of small focus of invasive carcinoma and lack of reaction in nearby hyperplastic lobule (*a*) as well as complete elimination of the former reaction after absorption with gp52 (*b*). (Methylene blue counterstain; 27 ×.)

In evaluating the results illustrated above, it is important to realize that there is considerable sampling error inherent in the testing procedure, and therefore the percentages given in Table 6-4 represent, at best, minimal values. This conclusion is based on the following facts:

1. Diagnostic tissue blocks of a given case are usually representative of, but seldom include, the entire tumor.
2. These studies were limited to an average of less than three (one, in cases from other institutions) representative blocks per case, and as previously noted, there was a considerable variability in antigen localization among and within sections of positive cases.
3. In contrast to in vitro methods, where a given tissue can be analyzed in bulk, this test is limited to 5-μm sections, which represent only a minute fraction of the entire tumor (approximately one one-thousandth of a 0.5-cm tumor).

NORMAL AND BENIGN BREAST TISSUE

Normal (resting and lactating) and benign (cystic disease, fibroadenoma, intraductal papilloma, and gynecomastia)

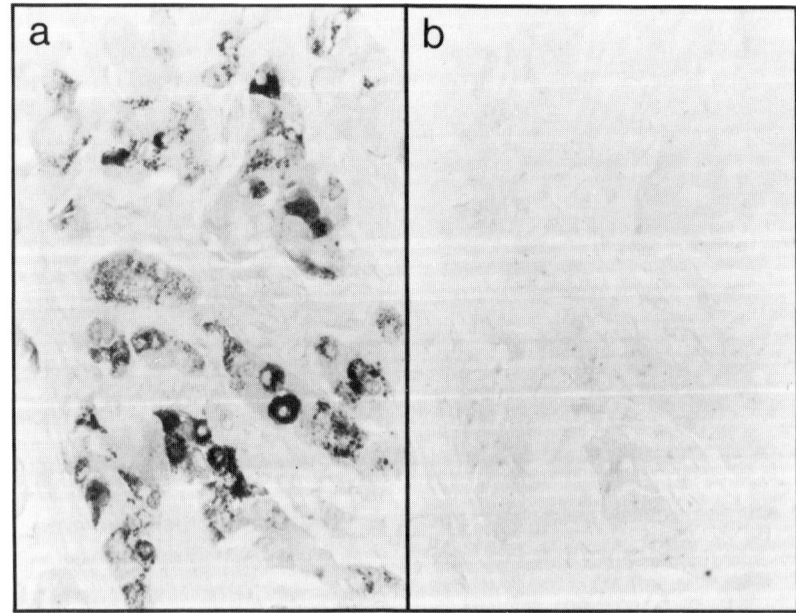

FIGURE 6-10 Adjacent sections of invasive breast carcinoma stained with anti-gp52 before (*a*) and after (*b*) absorption with gp52; many malignant cells contain reaction product. (Methylene blue counterstain; 178 ×)

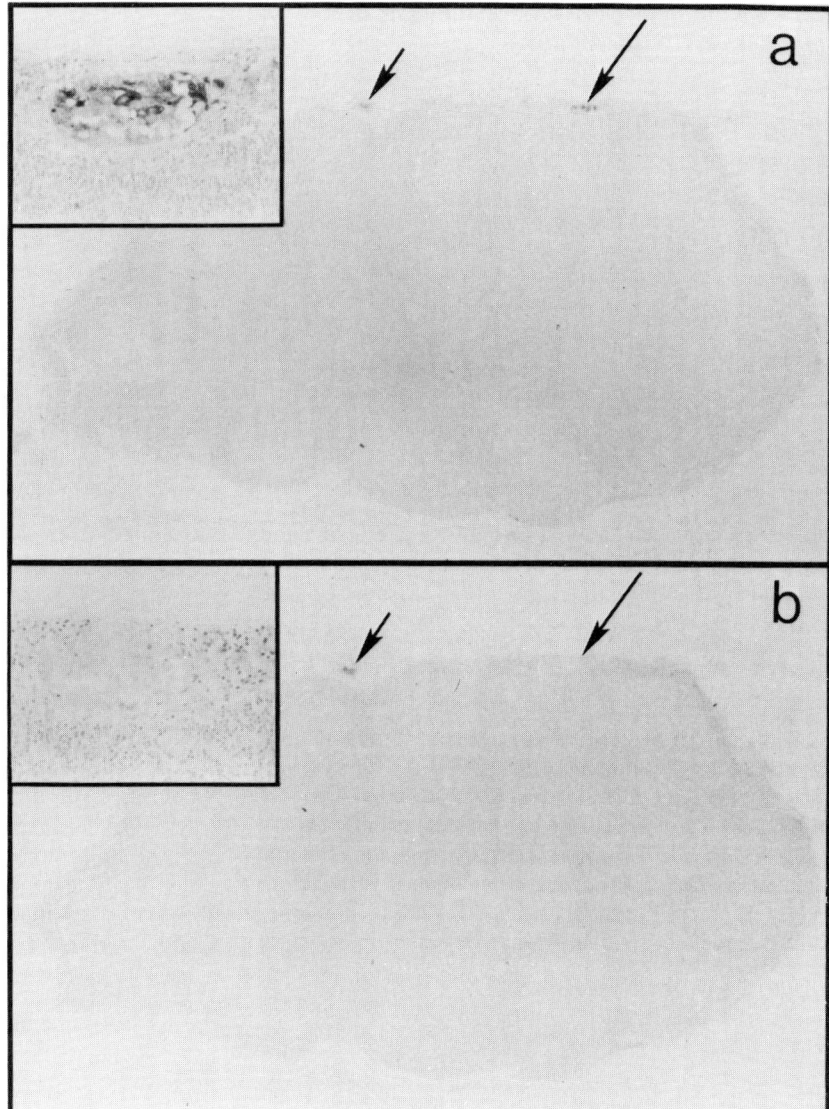

FIGURE 6-11 Axillary lymph node from same patient with tumor shown in Figure 6-10 showing microscopic metastatic lesion in marginal sinus (long arrow, insets). Most of the neoplastic cells stain with anti-gp52 (*a*); this reaction is eliminated by absorption with gp52 (*b*). Note that stain seen in erythrocytes in small blood vessel (short arrow) is unaffected by the absorption indicating endogenous peroxidase activity or nonspecific reaction. (Methylene blue counterstain; 16 ×; inset 80 ×)

breast tissue from 137 patients were examined with negative results (Table 6-6, Figs. 6-12 and 6-13). It should be noted that 74 of these negatively staining benign lesions coincided with the presence of carcinoma, in the same breast, that gave a positive staining reaction, frequently in the same tissue section.

APOCRINE METAPLASIA

The only exception to the absence of staining reaction in nonmalignant breast tissue was the focal staining observed in apocrine metaplasia, one of the microscopic features of cystic disease. This reaction, which is shared by the morphologically and histochemically indistin-

TABLE 6-6 Immunoperoxidase Staining of Benign and Normal Breast Tissues

Type	Number of cases	Associated with breast carcinoma*	Positive
Cystic disease†	81	60	0
Fibroadenoma	19	4	0
Intraductal papilloma	10	10	0
Gynecomastia	9	0	0
Resting gland (normal)	9	0	0
Lactating gland (normal)	9	0	0
Total	137	74	0

* In the same breast.
† Excluding foci of apocrine metaplasia.

guishable epithelium of apocrine glands of the axilla and perineum, differs in specificity from the reaction observed in the carcinomas (Fig. 6-14) as explained in the next section.

MALIGNANCIES OTHER THAN BREAST CARCINOMAS

Table 6-7 summarizes the results observed in 99 primary carcinomas from other organs and 8 cases of cystosarcoma phyllodes. Only 1 of these 107 tumors, a mucoepidermoid carcinoma of the parotid gland, gave a positive reaction. Two other parotid carcinomas of the same histopathologic type were negative. It is therefore evident that the antigen being detected by the anti-MMTV and anti-gp52 in human breast carcinomas is confined principally to malignant epithelial cells of mammary gland origin.

The Specificity of the Immunoperoxidase Reaction in Human Breast Carcinomas

The tissue specificity of the staining reaction was discussed in the preceding paragraphs, and it appears that a positive specific reaction is confined principally to the cytoplasm of breast carcinoma cells. A precise evaluation of the immunologic specificity in immunohistochemical staining reactions demands meticulous specific absorptions of the primary antibodies not only with homologous antigens but also with related antigens that might be

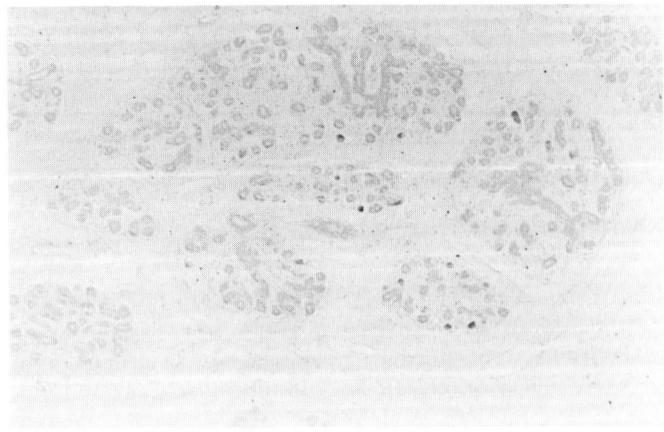

FIGURE 6-12 Complete absence of reaction product in normal breast lobules stained with anti-MMTV. Dark spots are due to counterstain (methylene blue). (40 ×)

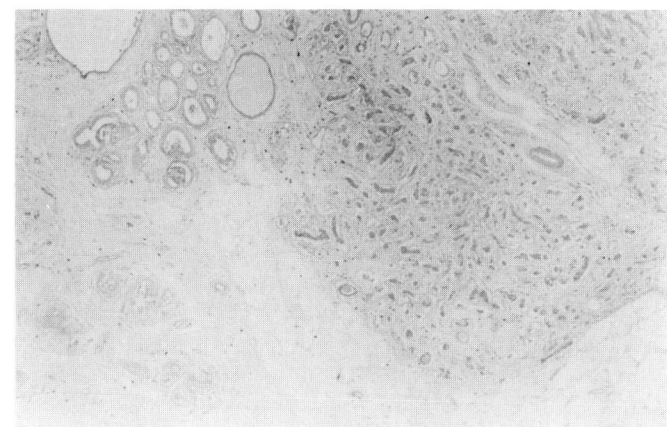

FIGURE 6-13 Complete absence of reaction product in area of cystic disease stained with anti-MMTV. (Methylene blue counterstain; 25 ×)

responsible for undesirable or irrelevant cross-reactive phenomena. Therefore, numerous immunoabsorbents (Table 6-8) were used for this purpose.*

The outstanding difference between mouse and human tumors with respect to antigen localization with anti-MMTV is readily apparent. In contrast with mouse tumors where only absorptions with whole disrupted MMTV completely eliminated the staining reaction (Fig. 6-4c), absorption with gp52 alone was sufficient to obliterate the reaction in positive-staining human tumors (Figs. 6-7b, 6-8c, 6-9b, 6-10b, and 6-11c). A reaction in human tissues, therefore, was considered positive only when (1) definite staining was seen, and (2) the staining was completely absent in an adjacent serial section stained with the same antibody preparation previously absorbed with gp52. The specificity of the staining reaction was further explored by absorption with the various preparations of MMTV and gp52 listed in Table 6-8. The fact that all eliminated the staining reaction indicates that the species differences previously reported for gp52 of the C_3H and RIII strain of MMTV[13] do not play a role in this reaction. On the other hand, absorptions with unrelated preparations (Rauscher leukemia virus, simian sarcoma virus, Mason-Pfizer monkey virus, and baboon endogenous virus) and with several possible cross-reacting substances, also listed in Table 6-8, failed to eliminate the staining reaction. Further, the source of gp52 and the host cell of the virus (murine cells or feline cells), had no influence on the ability to eliminate the activity of the antibodies tested.

* Their preparation and the conditions of absorption are described by Mesa-Tejada et al.[22]

These absorptions also led to the suspicion that the staining reaction observed in the apocrine epithelium (Fig. 6-14) differs in specificity from the reaction observed in the carcinomas, for the following reasons:

TABLE 6-7 Immunoperoxidase Staining of Malignancies Other than Breast Carcinomas

Malignancy*	Number of cases	Positive
Colon	12	0
Stomach	3	0
Pancreas	3	0
Liver	4	0
Lung	9	0
Endometrium	22	0
Ovary	20	0
Prostate	8	0
Kidney	5	0
Urinary bladder	4	0
Skin	2	0
Thyroid gland	4	0
Parotid gland	3	1
Cystosarcoma phyllodes	8	0
Total	107	1

* Primary sites of nonbreast carcinomas stained with α-MMTV. Cystosarcoma phyllodes is also listed because it is the most common noncarcinomatous malignancy of the breast.

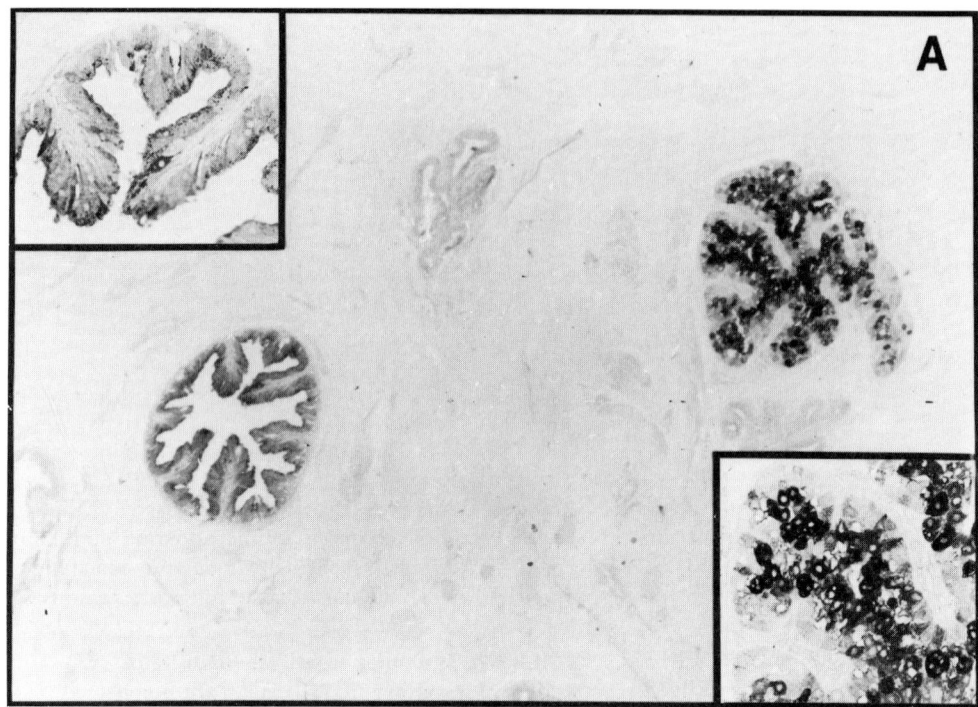

FIGURE 6-14 (*a*) Immunoperoxidase stain with anti-MMTV of cross section of nipple duct from a case of intraductal and invasive carcinoma of the breast showing one duct involved by in situ carcinoma (right) and another with apocrine metaplasia (left). (Insets) Details of the above, showing considerable intracellular reaction product in the neoplastic cells and characteristic intracellular granular staining in the apocrine epithelium. (*b*) Immunoperoxidase stain

1. Absorption with gp52 blocks only part of the reaction in the apocrine glands and metaplasia while completely eliminating the reaction in the carcinomas. If this absorption is carried out with gp52 that has not previously been extraced with ether, both reactions are completely blocked.
2. Absorption with mucin almost completely eliminates the reaction of the apocrine epithelium but does not interfere with the staining of the carcinoma, indicating that the reaction in the apocrine material is due, at least in part, to a carbohydrate moiety.

The Role of the Sugar Residues in the Cross Reactivity of gp52

It was of obvious importance to establish whether the sugar or the protein moiety of the gp52 glycoprotein was responsible for its ability to block the immunologic cross reaction with the antigen found in the breast cancer cells, so this problem was systematically investigated.[23] Sugar-free gp52 was prepared by deglycosylation with a mixture of glycosidases, and the resulting polypeptide was used in absorption studies. Figure 6-14 is a cross section of the nipple ducts from a case with intraductal and invasive breast carcinoma; one nipple duct contains lobular carcinoma in situ, and a nearby duct exhibits apocrine metaplasia. Both the neoplastic cells and the apocrine epithelium give a positive staining reaction with anti-MMTV (Fig. 6-14*a*). After absorption of the antibodies with deglycosylated gp52, however, the staining reaction is completely eliminated in the neoplastic cells, although it is virtually unchanged in the apocrine epithelium (Fig. 6-14*b*). Conversely, absorption of the anti-MMTV IgG with the polysaccharide isolated from the

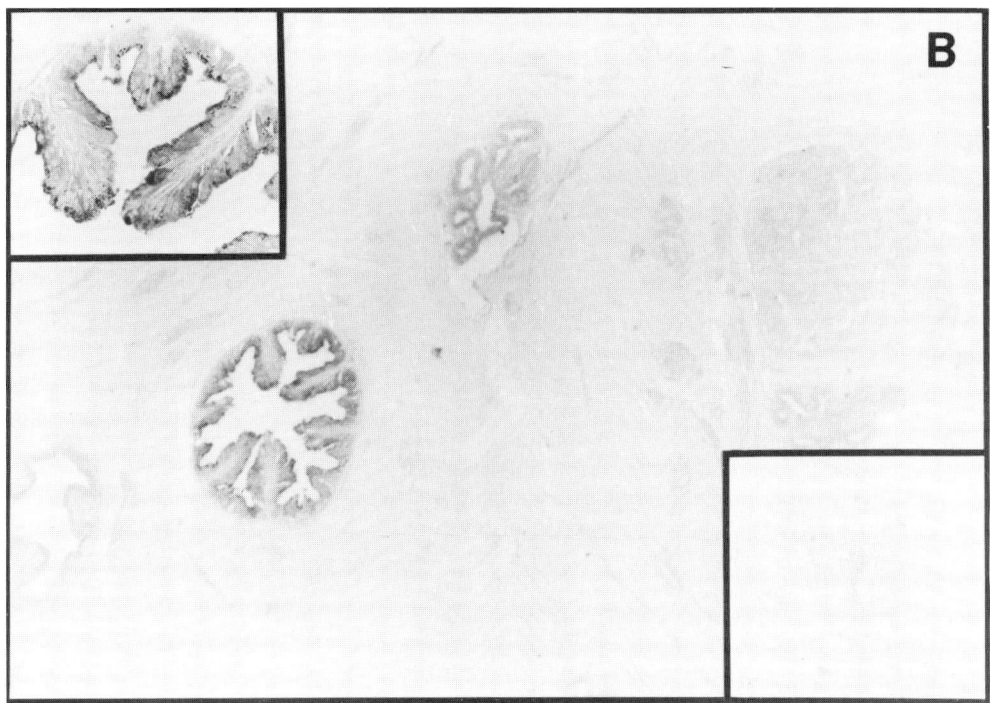

of adjacent serial section using anti-MMTV previously absorbed with sugar-free gp52. Note complete absence of reaction product in the neoplastic cells, whereas the intensity of the staining reaction in the apocrine epithelium is essentially the same as in (a). (Methylene blue counterstain, 58 ×; Insets, 144 ×.)

proteinase K–treated gp52 failed to affect the staining of the tumor cells but decreased the intensity of the reaction observed in the apocrine metaplasia. It is evident that the antibodies responsible for the staining reaction in the human breast carcinoma are those specifically directed at the polypeptide moiety of gp52.

Conclusions

The fact that it is the polypeptide rather than the polysaccharide portion of the gp52 that is responsible for the immunological reactivity between the human antigen and antibody against gp52 adds additional weight to the biological implications of the similarities that exist between the human and the murine mammary neoplasias. At the very least, these results indicate that the immunological interrelationship between the human tumor antigen and gp52 is more than a chance correspondence of polysaccharide complexes.

It is of course gratifying to have extended to the protein level a relation between human breast cancer and the mouse mammary tumor virus that was initially discovered in terms of nucleic acid sequence homology. However, the etiologic implications of this finding are not the immediate concern, but rather the possibility that such experimental data can be used to generate clinically useful information. With this purpose in mind, the resolution of the following issues assumes priority:

1. Can any clinically useful correlations be drawn between antigen localization in tissue and the natural history of the disease in terms of definable and identifiable clinical parameters?
2. What is the biochemical nature of the gp52 cross-reacting antigen found in human breast cancer cells?

3. Can additional specific antigens be detected by using other types of antibodies to other oncornaviruses with suspected cross reactivities?

An answer to the first question is being actively pursued both in the Institute of Cancer Research (Columbia University) and in collaboration with a number of other institutions (Michigan Cancer Foundation, Sloan-Kettering Cancer Center, Duke University Medical Center). We have already noted in our local cases that a significantly greater number of patients with a family history of breast cancer expressed the gp52 cross-reactive antigen in the tumor compared with patients with no such family history.

A resolution of the second question will require purification to homogeneity of the relevant human breast cancer antigen. The possibility of realizing this task has been greatly enhanced by the establishment of a cell line[24] from the cells of a malignant pleural effusion from a patient with intraductal and invasive breast carcinoma. This cell line, T47D, also expresses immunohistochemically detectable gp52-related antigen. It seems likely, therefore, that this tissue culture will be the ultimate source of this antigen. Its availability will also facilitate the production of the immunologic reagents needed to develop the heterologous radioimmunoassays that can hope to attain the sensitivities required for the measurement of the systemic signal in the human disease.

TABLE 6-8 Absorption Specificity Tests of Immunoperoxidase Staining of Human Breast Carcinomas with α-MMTV

Completely eliminated by	Not eliminated by
MMTV (RIII)	Viruses:
MMTV (C_3H)	Rauscher leukemia virus
	Simian sarcoma virus
gp52 (RIII)	Mason-Pfizer monkey virus
gp52 (C_3H)	Baboon endogenous virus
	Human:
	Normal plasma
	Normal leukocytes
	Collagen
	Actin
	Hyaluronic acid
	Milk
	Normal breast tissue
	Bovine:
	Mucin
	Fetal calf serum
	Sheep erythrocytes

REFERENCES

1. Temin HM: Homology between RNA from Rous sarcoma virus and DNA from Rous sarcoma virus-infected cells. *Proc Nat Acad Sci USA* 52:323, 1964.
2. Spiegelman S et al: DNA-directed DNA polymerase activity in oncogenic RNA viruses. *Nature* 227:1029, 1970.
3. Bishop DHL et al: Deoxyribonucleic acid polymerase of Rous sarcoma virus: Reaction conditions and analysis of the reaction product nucleic acids. *J Virol* 8:730, 1971.
4. Schlom J, Spiegelman S: Simultaneous detection of reverse transcriptase and high molecular weight RNA unique to oncogenic RNA viruses. *Science* 174:840, 1971.
5. Schlom J et al: Detection of high molecular weight RNA in particles from human milk. *Science* 175:542, 1972.
6. Gulati SC et al: Detection of RNA-instructed DNA polymerase and high molecular weight RNA in malignant tissue. *Proc Nat Acad Sci USA* 69:2020, 1972.
7. Axel R et al: Particles containing RNA-instructed DNA polymerase and virus-related RNA in human breast cancers. *Proc Nat Acad Sci USA* 69:3133, 1972.
8. Spiegelman S: Molecular evidence for the association of RNA tumor viruses with human mesenchymal malignancies, in R Neth et al (eds): *Modern Trends in Human Leukemia*, vol. 2, JF Lehmanns, Munich, 1976.
9. Cuatico W et al: Particles with RNA of high molecular weight and RNA-directed DNA polymerase in human brain tumors. *Proc Nat Acad Sci USA* 70:2789, 1973.
10. Cuatico W et al: Evidence of particle-associated RNA-directed DNA polymerase and high molecular weight RNA in human gastrointestinal and lung malignancies. *Proc Nat Acad Sci USA* 71:3304, 1974.
11. Hehlmann R et al: Murine and human melanomas containing a high molecular weight RNA associated with an RNA-instructed DNA polymerase. *Int J Dermatol* 17(2):114, 1978.
12. Ritzi E et al: Plasma levels of a viral protein as a diagnostic signal for the presence of mammary tumor: The effect of tumor removal. *J Exp Med* 145:999, 1977.
13. Moore DH et al: Mammary tumor viruses, in G Klein, S Weinhouse (eds): *Advances in Cancer Research*, Academic, New York, 1979.

14. Black MM et al: Cellular hypersensitivity to gp55 of RIII-murine mammary tumor virus and gp55-like protein of human breast cancers. *Cancer Res* 36:4137, 1976.
15. Yang NS et al: Expression of murine tumor virus-related antigens in human breast carcinoma (MCF-7) cells. *J Nat Cancer Inst* 59:1357, 1977.
16. Zangerle PF et al: Radioimmunoassay for glycoprotein gp47 of murine mammary tumor virus in organs and serum of mice and search for related antigens in human sera. *Cancer Res* 37:4326, 1977.
17. Hendrick J-C et al: Radioimmunoassay for protein p28 of murine mammary tumor virus in organs and serum of mice and search for related antigens in human sera and breast cancer extracts. *Cancer Res* 38:1826, 1978.
18. Mesa-Tejada R et al: Immunoperoxidase: A sensitive immunohistochemical technique as a "special stain" in the diagnostic pathology laboratory. *Hum Pathol* 8:313, 1977.
19. Keydar I et al: Detection of viral proteins in mouse mammary tumors by immunoperoxidase staining of paraffin sections. *Proc Nat Acad Sci USA* 75:1524, 1978.
20. Zotter S et al: Korrelation zwischen der Produktion reifer Virus-Partikel und der histo-morphologischen Differenzierung virusinduzierter muriner Mammakarzinome. *Arch Geschwulstforsch* 44:212, 1974.
21. Wolfe HJ: Tumor-cell markers: A biologic shell game? *N Engl J Med* 299:146, 1979.
22. Mesa-Tejada R et al: Immunohistochemical detection of a cross-reacting virus antigen in mouse mammary tumors and human breast carcinomas. *J Histochem Cytochem* 26:532, 1978.
23. Ohno T et al: The human breast carcinoma antigen is immunologically related to the polypeptide of the group-specific glycoprotein of the mouse mammary tumor virus. *Proc Nat Acad Sci USA* 76:2460, 1979.
24. Keydar I et al: Establishment and characterization of a cell line of human breast carcinoma origin. *Eur J Cancer* 15:659, 1979.

SELECTED BIBLIOGRAPHY

Barbacid M et al: Humans have antibodies capable of recognizing oncoviral glycoproteins: Demonstration that these are formed in response to cellular modification of glycoproteins rather than as a consequence of exposure to virus. *Proc Natl Acad Sci [USA]* 77:1617–1621, 1980.

Holder WD Jr, Wells SA Jr: Antibody reacting with mammary tumor virus in the serum of patients with carcinoma: A possible serological detection method for breast carcinoma. *Cancer Res* 43:239–244, 1983.

Snyder HW Jr, Fleissner E: Specificity of human antibodies to oncovirus glycoproteins: Recognition of antigen by natural antibodies directed against carbohydrate structures. *Proc Natl Acad Sci [USA]* 77:1622–1626, 1980.

Tomana M et al: Antibodies to mouse mammary tumor versus related antigen in sera of patients with breast carcinoma. *Cancer* 47:2696–2703, 1981.

7
TUMOR CELL BIOLOGY AND KINETICS

Robert B. Livingston

DEFINITIONS AND BASIC CONCEPTS

The cell proliferation cycle and its compartments, as currently recognized and understood, are shown in Fig. 7-1. Using light microscopy alone, only mitosis (M phase) can be identified; hence, the former use of the term *interphase* to describe the remainder of the cycle. With the advent of autoradiography and an understanding of the mechanisms of DNA synthesis, it became possible to identify the S phase, during which the DNA molecule replicates itself entirely, preparatory to cell reproduction.

This definition of the S phase is based on the fact that thymidine, a specific pyrimidine base in the DNA molecule, is incorporated into cells in large quantities only during the S phase. When a cell which is actively synthesizing DNA is exposed to radioactive thymidine (^{3}HTdR), it emits β particles which, when they bombard a photographic emulsion, produce a characteristic pattern of black dots (developed silver grains) over the cell's nucleus (see Fig. 7-1). If one counts the number of cells in a given population which are so "labeled," and expresses the result as a percent, the calculated fraction is the *thymidine labeling index* (LI). The LI provides an estimate of the fraction of cells which are actually synthesizing DNA for reproductive purposes ("semicon- servative" DNA synthesis) at a given point in time, and a crude estimate, by extrapolation, of the *growth fraction*.

The growth fraction (G_F) may be considered as that proportion of an entire cell population which is actively committed to proliferation, or is "in the cycle." The remainder of the cell population may be considered as "end-stage" from the standpoint of proliferative capacity, and, in terms of tumors, it will ultimately form the *cell-loss fraction*. Cells which appear to be in G_1 are actually made up of two subpopulations: those which have the

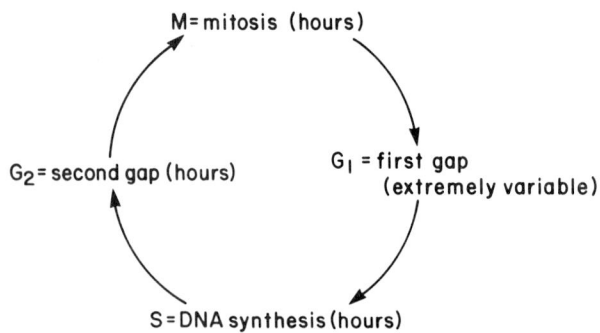

FIGURE 7-1 The cell cycle.

potential to initiate cell division and those which have lost it. Thus, in the clinical situation, it is impossible to measure accurately the growth and cell-loss fractions. In fact, if the cell population being studied is markedly heterogeneous (e.g., contains tumor cells as well as normal host cells), only those methods of measuring which are tied to morphology (the mitotic and labeling indexes) can be applied, and only the M and S fractions can therefore be estimated. This is the usual clinical setting. In homogeneous samples, the fraction of cells synthesizing DNA may be estimated by the simpler technique of scintillation counting;[1] using semiautomated flow microfluorometry, $G_2 + M$ and S may be estimated directly, and G_1 estimated by subtraction.[2] Barring the development of reliable, efficient techniques for separation of normal from tumor cells, the LI as determined by autoradiography remains the single most useful cell kinetic measurement.

Most animal tumor systems follow a pattern of growth over time which can be represented as a Gompertzian curve. This pattern, characterized by rapid early growth and progressively decreasing rates of growth toward the end of a tumor's natural history, appears to fit the general behavior of most human solid tumors.[3] The working assumption of most experimental and human cancer therapists until recently was that very small tumors had the highest fraction of proliferating cells (as in the "adjuvant" chemotherapy setting, after surgical resection of all apparent disease). Since there is evidence that most, if not all, available antineoplastic drugs preferentially kill proliferating cells, this logically leads to the hypothesis that chemotherapy should be relatively most effective in the adjuvant setting of minimal residual disease. A second logical assumption was that if chemotherapy resulted in a marked reduction in the size of an advanced tumor, there would be a corresponding increase in the growth fraction, and greater sensitivity to S phase–active agents.[4] This led to the design of many protocols in which *cell cycle–nonspecific* drugs were followed by *cell cycle–specific* ones.

A modification in the clinical interpretation of the Gompertzian curve (rather than its abandonment) has been suggested by Norton and Simon,[5] based on several theoretical considerations and clinical observations (see Fig. 7-2). The implications of their model may be summarized as follows: (1) the maximum growth rate is achieved when the tumor is at point 3 (already 37 percent of its maximum size), the clinical correlate of which may be regional spread (e.g., positive nodes); (2) small numbers (up to 10^7 or more) of tumor cells may have a low growth rate, the clinical correlate of which may be "microscopic" disease; and (3) the most intensive chemotherapy may be required at the time of "complete remission," rather than in the beginning.

This model appears to have clinical relevance: it could explain the relative lack of efficacy for effective combination chemotherapy in postmenopausal breast cancer patients with minimal residual disease,[6] the appearance of "late" relapses in acute leukemia and Hodgkin's disease, and the apparently greater efficacy of 5-fluorouracil (5-FU) in the adjuvant treatment of colorectal cancer for Duke's C versus Duke's B patients.[7] However, the model may be a more accurate approximation of a tumor's natural history than of its perturbed behavior. For example, reductions in tumor cell mass by 75 percent

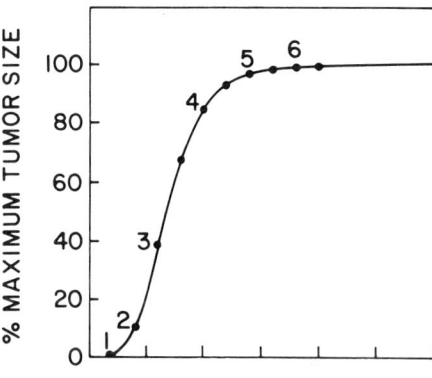

Point	Maximum size, %	Maximum growth, fraction, %	Maximum growth, rate, %	Tumor weight	Number tumor cells
1	0.5	50	7	50 mg	5×10^7
2	10	20	64	100 g	1×10^{11}
3	37	8	100	370 g	3.7×10^{11}
4	85	1	38	850 g	8.5×10^{11}
5	97	0.3	8	970 g	9.7×10^{11}
6	99	0.05	1	1 kg	1×10^{12}

FIGURE 7-2 A growth model for human solid tumors. (*From L Norton, R Simon: Tumor size, sensitivity to therapy, and design of treatment schedules. Cancer Treat Rep 61:1307, 1977.*)

or more (but rarely by 99 percent or more) are common in the treatment of multiple myeloma. Yet patients with myeloma who respond to alkylating agents (cell cycle–nonspecific) are *not* rendered further responsive to cell cycle–specific chemotherapy,[8] and, in fact, the labeling index of patients with multiple myeloma[9,10] and solid tumors[11,12] appears to be depressed for extended periods of time in responders. This suggests that selective killing of proliferating cells indeed occurs with chemotherapy (and radiation therapy), but is not followed by a rapid expansion of the growth fraction until clinical relapse occurs.[9] This would dictate an opposite tack in advanced disease, namely to put the most intensive therapy at first, as *induction,* and to use cell cycle–nonspecific modalities in *maintenance.*

The general implications of the debate concerning the interpretation of Gompertzian growth are highly relevant to concepts of chemotherapy in the surgical adjuvant setting. If Norton and Simon are correct, such treatment is likely to produce the greatest fractional cell kill in a setting of regional spread (e.g., nodal involvement), where the total tumor weight is 100 to 500 g (see Fig. 7-2), rather than in a setting of localized tumor, where the total weight is 1 to 10 g. If more classical interpretations are correct, the smaller a tumor is, the more sensitive it should be to chemotherapy.

What we are really referring to in the adjuvant situation, of course, is chemotherapy of micrometastases which have been left behind after resection of all grossly apparent tumor. Whether these microaggregates have growth kinetics similar to those of the resected primary lesion is a separate question. Simpson-Herren has reported that removal of bulk tumor mass in the Lewis lung system leads to an increase in the LI of micrometastases which are present in the lungs.[13] Schabel has summarized the results of surgical adjuvant chemotherapy for murine tumors, which demonstrates unequivocally the greater efficacy of chemotherapy against minimal residual disease in the experimental setting.[14]

CELL-CYCLE SPECIFICITY AND CELL-KILL MECHANISM

Table 7-1 lists the relationship of the cell cycle to drug sensitivity for the common antineoplastic chemotherapeutic agents. It should be noted that a number of drugs listed as cell cycle–nonspecific actually exert preferential killing effects on cycling cells, and that several cell cycle–specific drugs have multiple sites of action within the cycle. Most of the drugs useful against human solid tumors are cell cycle–nonspecific, the exceptions being methotrexate and methylglyoxel bis-guanylhydrazone (MGBG).

The term *kinetics of cell kill by chemotherapeutic agents* does not refer to the kinetics of tumor cell growth but to the fraction of cells which are destroyed per course of therapy. Theoretical considerations and observations in experimental systems imply that this *fraction* is a constant, i.e., that the same percentage of cells is killed by a given dose regardless of the absolute number of tumor cells. Thus, cytotoxic chemotherapy is classically said to follow first-order kinetics, as opposed to other modalities (see Table 7-2). This means that it takes as much treatment to go from 10^{12} cells (about 1 kg of tumor) to 10^9 (about 1 g) as it does to go from 10^6 (about 1 mg) to 10^3. And residual tumor burdens of 10^3 are fully capable of producing fatal relapse,[15] at least in experimental systems. This forms the rationale for *maintenance chemotherapy* against disseminated disease in remission, and for prolonged, intermittent chemotherapy against presumed residual disease in the adjuvant setting.

The mechanism of cell kill by surgery is zero order in the sense that, in terms of the *ultimate* result, a tumor is either eradicated completely or regrows (from occult metastatic spread) as though the operation had never been performed.

Radiation therapy produces fractional kill per unit dose, but the fraction is not constant. The size of this fraction depends on such factors as oxygenation, reassortment, and repair. Like surgery, the effectiveness of radiation therapy is limited by tumor extent and the relationship of tumor tissue to critical, normal vital structures.

Immunotherapy, at least in those animal models where it is effective, also appears to follow zero-order or all-or-none kinetics. It specifically does not seem to depend on the proliferative state of the cell. Hormone therapy produces fractional cell kill which is dependent on the proportion of hormone-dependent cells in a tumor population. There appears to be no dependence of the efficacy of hormone therapy on the proliferative state of a tumor.[16]

The interrelationships of the various antitumor modalities suggest immediately the virtues of a combined approach. This is so not only because surgery and radiation can be used to eradicate local disease, and the systemic modalities to eradicate micrometastases elsewhere. The following proven or potential interactions

TABLE 7-1 Cell Cycle Loci of Drug Activity

Agent(s)	Cell cycle–nonspecific	Cell cycle-specific sensitive phases				Reference(s)
		M	G_1	S	G_2	
Nitrogen mustard	√*					125
Cyclophosphamide	√†					126
Adriamycin	√†					127–129
Mitomycin C	√†					130, 131
Nitrosoureas	√*					125
Busulfan	√					125
Actinomycin D	√					126, 132
Bleomycin	√‡	√	?		√	125, 133, 134
Vincristine		√	√	√		135–137
Vinblastine		√		√		134
5-FU	√‡			√		126, 138–140
Methotrexate				√		139, 140
Cytosine arabinoside				√		138
Thiopurines			√(?)	√		139, 141
L-Asparaginase	√(?)					
VP-16				√(?)	√	142
cis-Platinum(II)	√					143, 144
DTIC	√					145, 146
Hydroxyurea				√		132
MGBG			√(?)	√(?)		147

* Preferential kill of cycling cells, with M and G_1 most sensitive.
† Preferential kill of cycling cells, with S phase most sensitive.
‡ Available information contradictory.

also exist: (1) surgical debulking may increase the growth fraction of residual disease and make it more sensitive to subsequent chemotherapy[13]; (2) chemotherapeutic agents may potentiate radiation effects on tumor tissue by inhibiting the repair of single-strand breaks in DNA,[17] by increasing the fraction of cells in G_2 and M, where cell-cycle sensitivity to irradiation is greatest,[18] or by reducing tumor bulk and improving oxygenation; (3) hormonal and immunotherapy may produce cell kill complementary to chemotherapy by their lack of proliferation dependence.

TABLE 7-2 Kinetics of Cell Kill—Various Modalities

Modality	Kinetics
Surgery	Zero-order (all-or-none)
Radiation therapy	Complex fractional but varying
Chemotherapy	First-order (constant fraction)
Immunotherapy	Zero-order (<10^5 cells)
Hormone therapy	Affects receptor-positive population

TUMOR CELL BIOLOGY—CHEMOTHERAPEUTIC EXPLOITABILITY

It was once thought that cell kinetic differences might be fundamental in distinguishing between tumor and normal host tissues: that tumor cells might have a longer S phase, or more cells in the growth fraction, than the most sensitive vital normal tissue. Except that cancer cells in general show some prolongation of G_2, major differences in the length of phases in the cell cycle have not been demonstrated.[19] Although a few human tumors have a very high growth fraction, most solid neoplasms have a relatively low growth fraction compared to normal sensitive tissues like the bone marrow or gastrointestinal mucosa. This fact has also some favorable implications, since the recovery process in sensitive host renewal tissues occurs much more quickly than the recovery process in sensitive tumors.[20] Thus, by proper timing of chemotherapy, antitumor effects can be maximized and host toxicity minimized.

A variety of characteristics have now been identified which seem to distinguish malignant (or virally transformed) cells from their normal counterparts. As shown in Table 7-3, some of these may be related to the efficacy of available antitumor agents, although many of these relationships are not proven.

Increased biosynthesis of the polyamines, especially putrescine and spermidine, may be a ubiquitous feature of the neoplastic state.[21,22] These simple molecules may play a role in catalyzing the initiation of DNA synthesis,[23] the synthesis of microtubules,[24] and the synthesis of transfer RNA,[25] each of which is in turn a subject of possible tumor-specific differences.

Although quantitative levels of DNA synthesis may be low in most clinically apparent tumors, data from minimal deviation hepatomas in the rat suggests that there is increased activity of certain "key enzymes" which can provide tumors with a marked advantage in terms of the *potential* to initiate reproduction of the genome. This data has been summarized eloquently by Weber.[26] It remains to be seen whether such *key enzyme hypertrophy* is a common characteristic of human tumors.

Microtubules, which are complex, submicroscopic, cylindrical structures made up of tubulin subunits, play a number of roles in vital cellular processes, among them (1) maintenance of the structural integrity of the cytoskeleton, which determines a variety of cell membrane properties;[27] (2) formation of the mitotic spindle;[28] and (3) axonal transport.[29] Microtubular dysfunction may be related to alterations in membrane permeability, fluidity, and even antigenicity associated with the transformed state.[30]

TABLE 7-3 Potentially Exploitable Differences between Tumor and Normal Cells—Possible Relationships to Drug Efficacy

Characteristic (tumor or transformed cell vs. normal)	*Drug(s) with related action mechanism postulated*
Increased polyamine biosynthesis[21,22]	MGBG,[151] DTIC,[152] bleomycin,[153] vinca alkaloids,[154,155]
Increased activity of "key enzymes"[26]	5-FU, 6MP, methotrexate, hydroxyurea, PALA, Ara-C, glutamine analogues[26]
Microtubular dysfunction with altered cell membrane permeability[148,149]	Vinca alkaloids,[149,158,159] neocarzinostatin[160]
Increased activity of tRNA methylases[31,32]	Procarbazine,[156] inhibitors of protein synthesis, hexamethylmelamine[157]
Increased alkylation susceptibility[33]	Alkylating agents, nitrosoureas, mitomycin C, *cis*-platinum(II)
Altered DNA polymerase activity[35]	Ara-C[161]
Decreased or absent asparaginase synthetase[36]	Asparaginase
Hormone receptors present[150] or absent[38]	Sex steroids, glucocorticoids[113,150] Cytotoxic chemotherapy

Increased activity of enzymes which methylate newly formed RNA may be another ubiquitous characteristic of tumor cells,[31,32] in some way related to the production of increased amounts of certain enzymes or structural proteins which are critical to maintenance (or initiation) of the neoplastic state.

Increased susceptibility to alkylation of DNA,[33,34] altered DNA polymerase activity,[35] decreased or absent asparagine synthetase activity,[36] and the presence or absence of hormone receptors[37,38] in tumor tissue have all been reported to play a role in response of tumors to chemotherapy.

CLINICAL OBSERVATIONS AND CELL KINETIC CORRELATIONS

As already cited, the theoretical interpretations of Gompertzian growth are in a state of flux. Available clinical data about tumor size and growth fraction (as approximated by the LI) are also inconsistent. On the other hand, it has been reported that axillary nodal metastases in breast cancer in general have a higher LI than do primary tumors.[39] This fits well with the Gompertzian growth concept. However, larger primary breast cancers (greater than 3 cm) have been reported to have a higher LI than smaller, but still clinically evident, tumors (less than 1.5 cm in diameter).[40] Crude mathematical extrapolation suggests that the difference in tumor weight involved here is on the order of 10 to 15 versus 1 to 2 g, and reference to Fig. 7-2 in turn suggests that this difference in sizes could reflect the zone of inflection between points 1 and 2 on the graph. This would support the Norton-Simon hypothesis. More recent observations from the same laboratory, however, have not borne out the difference in LI as related to primary tumor size.[41] Finally, the LI in multiple myeloma is highest at the time of clinical relapse from remission and lowest during clinical response, with the expected somewhat higher values for patients presenting with intermediate tumor mass compared to very high tumor burdens.[9,10] These observations again strongly suggest that the natural history of tumors obeys Gompertzian kinetics, but not their perturbed history, at least until there is a loss of drug sensitivity.

Of perhaps more practical importance is the question, Does the height of the LI predict for response to chemotherapy? In animal tumors, a direct correlation exists for both solid neoplasms and leukemias.[42] The situation is much more complex with human cancers.

Hart et al.[43] reported that a direct relationship exists between height of the pretreatment LI and the likelihood of complete response for patients with acute leukemia, studying a population composed largely of adults with acute myelocytic leukemia. This analysis was carried out for treatment with regimens in which the cell cycle–specific agent cytosine arabinoside was the core of induction therapy. Hillen[44] and Vogler[45] reported a similar correlation between pretreatment LI and response, also with regimens which relied primarily on cytosine arabinoside or methotrexate, another cycle-specific agent.

When the backbone of induction therapy is cytosine arabinoside (Ara-C) plus thioguanine given simultaneously on a twice-daily schedule, the relationship of pretreatment LI to response may disappear: Vogler found no difference in LI between 45 responders and 27 nonresponders on such a regimen,[46] nor did Raich[47] or Arlin.[48] This suggests that thioguanine, designed as an antimetabolite but known to be incorporated into the DNA of non-S cells,[49] may play a role in the induction of response among patients with a low LI, while Ara-C is most important for those with a higher LI. However, Crowther also reported no correlation between pretreatment LI and response[50] in adult patients with acute myelogenous leukemia who received a combination of daunorubicin and Ara-C; moreover, in these 58 patients a positive correlation was reported for LI with length of remission, as well as with survival among those who achieved remission. In children with acute lymphocytic leukemia, Mauer[51] has observed no relationship between pretreatment LI and response; here, of course, a major component of remission induction is the cell cycle–nonspecific agent prednisone.

Among patients with solid tumors, an increasing body of data suggests that there is a direct relationship between pretreatment LI and the likelihood of response to a variety of cytotoxic drug regimens. Sulkes et al.[52] determined the LI pretreatment in 25 patients with disseminated breast carcinoma who then received a combination of adriamycin, cyclophosphamide, and fluorinated pyrimidine chemotherapy. The LI was significantly higher in responders to chemotherapy versus the nonresponders (mean of 15 versus 7.1, $p < .01$). Furthermore, 0 of 9 patients with LI less than 9 responded, compared to 11 of 16 responses if the initial LI was greater or equal to 9. Thirlwell et al.[53] reported similar results in a series of patients with melanoma on regimens containing DTIC: 8 responders had a median LI of 8, compared to 3.2 for the nonresponders. The fact that small-cell (oat-cell) carcinoma has a much higher response rate to both chemotherapy and radiation therapy than do non-small-cell lung tumors, is well known. The median LI of small-cell tumors is in the 15 to 25 percent range, while that of squamous and adenocarcinomas is 2.5 to 4.0 percent.[54] Recent information about the large-cell undifferentiated variant of lung cancer indicates that both the LI[55] and the response to chemotherapy[56] are higher than for the more differentiated squamous and adenocarcinomas. Among urologic neoplasms, those tumors with high LIs like Wilms's and embryonal carcinoma are quite sensitive to chemotherapy, while prostate and renal cancer, with lower growth fractions, are much more resistant.

Clearly, other factors than LI are important in determining whether a tumor responds to chemotherapy. Both multiple myeloma and chronic lymphocytic leukemia are relatively chemoresponsive diseases, in spite of a typically low LI. But the pretreatment LI may be an important index of response likelihood for the common solid tumors. Whether LI determination of the primary tumor will also be predictive for success of adjuvant chemotherapy is a provocative but unproven possibility.

HORMONE STIMULATION, SUPPRESSION, AND RESPONSE

Weichselbaum et al.[57] have shown that, in a hormone-responsive, estrogen receptor–positive human breast cancer cell line, estradiol at physiologic concentrations causes stimulation of cell proliferation, while estradiol at pharmacologic concentrations reduces the fraction of cells in S phase. These results suggest that it might be better to administer cytotoxic chemotherapy, in hormone receptor–positive tumors, after a period of physiologic stimulation with hormones, then to administer suppressive doses of hormone therapy in pharmacologic amounts. They also suggest that coadministration of hormone therapy in pharmacologic doses with cytotoxic chemotherapy could diminish the effect of the chemotherapy.

There appears to be a relationship between estrogen receptor status and LI in breast cancer. Two investigators have reported that higher LI and estrogen receptor negativity are directly correlated.[58,59] Lippmann et al. have reported a significantly higher response rate to cytotoxic chemotherapy in patients with estrogen receptor negativity. These observations, if confirmed, seem to fit a pattern when taken together with the report of Sulkes et al.: receptor positivity would imply more sensitivity to hormones and less to chemotherapy, with the opposite being true for receptor negativity. It should be emphasized that most breast cancers (and presumably, by inference, other tumors with hormone dependence) are in fact heterogeneous with respect to receptor positivity.[60,61] Thus, a patient with an initially receptor-positive lesion who receives long-term suppressive hormone therapy might be expected to develop receptor-negative, hormone-insensitive recurrent disease from an originally small number of such cells. No direct evidence exists as yet to support this hypothesis.

The effect of glucocorticoids on tumor cell kinetics is a potentially fertile area which has been little explored. Marshall et al.[62] reported results of LI determination after a single intravenous dose of prednisone in 10 patients with normal bone marrows and 11 with acute leukemia: 8 of 10 normals had a significant increase at 6 h with a return to baseline levels at 24 and 48 h; the leukemic marrows demonstrated peak DNA synthesis at 24 h, with a return to baseline at over 48 h. This provocative observation requires confirmation. That steroids produce a G_1-S block in many systems in tissue culture is well established,[63,64] and this also appears to be the case for indomethacin.[65] Braunschweiger et al. have recently suggested that pretreatment with glucocorticoids leads to increased responsiveness of an experimental mammary tumor to chemotherapy.[66]

RECRUITMENT AND SYNCHRONIZATION ATTEMPTS

Experimental Tumors

Dethlefsen et al.[67] recently reviewed the use of the S phase–specific inhibitors cytosine arabinoside and hydroxyurea in attempts to block cell populations in S with subsequent release of a synchronized cohort. In a variety of rodent systems, they conclude that "the published data strongly suggest that the drug . . . which can cause good synchronization in vitro, can exert only a mild synchronizing effect in vivo and then only in tissues that have a relatively high growth fraction and short cell cycle–transit time." However the work of Gibson and Bertalanffy[68] suggested that repeated injections of cytosine arabinoside (about 40 mg/m² every 2 h for a total of eight injections, or 16 h: roughly twice the mean duration of S) results in marked synchronization of the B16 melanoma, a solid murine tumor with an intermediate baseline LI (19 percent) and growth fraction (53 percent).

Vinca alkaloids have been shown to arrest both tumor and normal cells in mitosis.[69] Klein et al.[70] demonstrated that Ehrlich ascites tumor cells in vivo could escape from the mitotic arrest produced by vincristine and travel as a synchronized cohort through at least two successive waves of mitosis. As demonstrated by labeling experiments, the second peak consisted almost entirely of cells that had been arrested by vincristine in the first peak. Thus, vincristine here produced synchronization and not recruitment of cells from a nonproliferating pool.

Work by Capizzi[71] and by Chlopkiewicz et al.[72] demonstrated an apparent increase in the therapeutic index of methotrexate when it was preceded by L-asparaginase given several days before. This may be due to shutting-off of protein-dependent initiation of DNA synthesis secondary to asparaginase, with a resultant piling up at the G_1-S interface of cells which are then released when intracellular drug levels decline to a point sufficient to allow renewed DNA synthesis, resulting in progression of a temporarily synchronized cohort of tumor cells through S.

All work with drugs in synchronizing schedules, in which a second, systemically administered agent serves as the "executor," shares one problem: synchrony of normal cell populations may occur as well, resulting in increased host toxicity. Further work is greatly needed to delineate the time sequence of synchronization and loss of synchrony in tumor versus sensitive host tissues; it may be that sufficient differential exists to allow for therapeutic exploitation with appropriate scheduling. A different approach involves administration of a synchronizing agent followed by local therapy aimed at the tumor that kills the synchronized cohort cells most efficiently; an example is administration of radiation (most effective at killing cells in G_2 and M) after synchronization with 5-FU, as reported by Ganzer and Nitze.[73] Vincristine or colchicine pretreatment might be effective as well in this setting.

Human Tumors

Lampkin et al. were among the first to suggest that cell synchronization techniques could increase therapeutic efficacy in acute leukemia.[74] They reported that partial synchronization could be achieved with pulse doses of cytosine arabinoside in acute lymphocytic leukemia (ALL), and that "a greater therapeutic advantage can be achieved by a second cycle-dependent drug after synchronization than after the second drug alone." The time between administration of cytosine arabinoside and the peak in LI varied from 24 to 96 h, with no synchronization observed in 4 of 20 serial studies. Lampkin et al.[75] then reported their results in 21 patients with acute myelogenous leukemia (AML) who received Ara-C as an IV push injection of 5 mg/kg (100 to 180 mg/m²). Of 14 patients in whom consecutive LI and MI determinations were performed, 7 showed a significant increase in LI and 12 in MI at 19 to 24 h after the Ara-C. The patients then received 12-h continuous infusion with Ara-C 5 mg/kg every 12 h, started at the time of maximal S-phase accumulation (usually 18–24 h after the initial Ara-C), and continued until complete remission, with escalations in Ara-C dose if the patient failed to respond to lower doses. A complete remission was achieved in 12 out of 16 children and in all 5 adults (81 percent).

Other investigators have not found evidence of synchronization after push doses of Ara-C in AML,[76] possibly because of lower doses, or differences in sampling time or patient population. Kremer et al.[77] found an increase in LI in 11 out of 14 patients with remission or "antileukemic effect" who received either one or three daily push doses of Ara-C, followed 48 h after the last Ara-C dose by LI determination and treatment with vincristine and methotrexate, while only 3 out of 9 patients with no response or early death demonstrated such an increase (5 out of 10 responders sampled at 24 h and 4 out of 11 nonresponders had a similar increase). MacKinney et al.[78] used the Lampkin AML schedule in 23 adults with acute leukemia: they achieved complete marrow remissions in only 6.

Buchner et al.[79] reported a continuous infusion schedule of Ara-C in patients with acute leukemia: 100 mg/m² per day for 48 h. They found in 8 out of 11 patients a 1.3- to 4.0-fold increase in cells in the S-phase range, by DNA histogram, at the conclusion of the infusion. They employed ifosfamide as the executor drug.

More work is needed to clarify the role of Ara-C as a synchronizing agent in acute leukemia, both in clinical studies and experimental models. In a homogeneous tumor cell population, the use of pulse cytophotometry to provide rapid DNA histogram analysis should allow the clinician to determine more accurately at what point synchronization is (or is not) achieved and allow for more precise timing of executor agents.

Capizzi has extended his work with asparaginase and methotrexate to clinical studies in ALL;[80] in several patients studied sequentially after asparaginase (dose of 40,000 units/m²), he found evidence of initial depression in leukemic cell DNA synthesis, followed by recovery and "overshoot" at days 7 to 10; a similar decline in LI of normal bone marrow precursors was followed by more rapid recovery, overshoot, and return to baseline. He observed complete remission in 9 out of 11 adults with ALL, all of whom were refractory to prior methotrexate, with a median response duration of 6 months.

In solid tumors, clinical protocols have been designed along synchronization lines using a variety of drugs and concepts. Based on the observation that continuous infusion of bleomycin for 48 h produced an increase in LI in the nodules of patients with melanoma[81] (presumably as a result of S-G_2 arrest and subsequent release), Costanzi designed a regimen[82] in which 17 patients with disseminated carcinoma of the head and neck were treated with bleomycin as in IV infusion at 7.5 units/m² per 24 h for 48 h. Methotrexate (30 mg/m²) and hydroxyurea (2000 mg/m²) were administered in a single dose after a 24-h rest period to allow the synchronized cohort to traverse G_2, M, and G_1 and reach the G_1-S interface. Tumor response was seen in 10 out of 17 (59 percent), not better than what one might achieve with methotrexate alone. Costanzi then adopted a 96-h bleomycin infusion (to allow for S-G_2 trapping of more cells) and changed the rest period to 48 h and the executor to methotrexate, 250 mg/m² with citrovorum factor rescue. The clinical outcome was not improved.

Samuels[83] has compared a program in which bleomycin was given on a standard twice weekly schedule, with intermittent high-dose vinblastine (VB-1), to one in which bleomycin was given as a 96-h continuous infusion followed by vinblastine. Patients with metastatic embryonal carcinoma of the testis appeared to fare better on VB-3, while those with teratocarcinomas responded better to VB-1. Unique toxicity (hypertension, jaundice, and hemolysis) was observed with bleomycin as a continuous infusion.

The observation that vincristine reliably produces stathmokinetic arrest (i.e., in G_2 and M) in human tissues 6 to 24 h after injection, coupled with the apparent cell-kill specificity of bleomycin for cells in G_2 and M, led Livingston et al. to design a two-drug combination in which the former was given 6 h earlier.[84] An encouraging response rate in this pilot study was seen in patients with lung carcinoma (4 of 15) and led to its inclusion in more complex combination regimens designed primarily for patients with lung tumors.[85,86] Unfortunately, kinetic data were never obtained to support this hypothesis, and the most recent trial involving this combination indicates that vincristine and "staggered" bleomycin added nothing to the antitumor efficacy of a simpler, three-drug regimen.[87] Encouraging results were obtained with a similar staggered schedule in carcinoma of the cervix[88]; in a study of Adriamycin, vincristine, and bleomycin in testicular cancer[89]; and in Einhorn's initial study of vinblastine, bleomycin, and platinum in testicular cancer.[90] It is conceivable that this combination may produce an increase in the therapeutic index of bleomycin, given (1) some degree of inherent efficacy for bleomycin against the tumor cells involved, and (2) a sufficiently large growth fraction that arrest of cells in G_2 and M by vincristine becomes meaningful, in terms of subsequent mitotic cell kill of a synchronized cohort. The lack of a suitable experimental model has prevented testing of the concept to date at a basic level. More recently, Einhorn has discontinued the staggering of vinblastine and bleomycin administration, with no apparent therapeutic effect on results in testicular cancer.[91]

Only one published clinical study has looked at Ara-C in solid tumors as a potential synchronizing agent.[92] In this study, a push dose of Ara-C (200 mg/m²) was followed by methotrexate 24 h later, in a variety of patients who were already refractory to first-line chemotherapy. No striking evidence of synergy was seen, possibly because the empiric schedule was too imprecise or simply wrong in its timing. This study again points up the need for serial measurements of kinetic effects if meaningful clinical studies, seeking to demonstrate efficacy of kinetic manipulations, are to be conducted.

A number of investigators have explored "kinetically oriented" approaches in which a cell cycle–nonspecific agent was followed by a cell cycle–specific one, with varying results. Burke and Owens[93] employed in acute leukemia a sequence of cyclophosphamide followed by vincristine at 24 h and Ara-C, as a 48-h IV infusion begun 12 h after vincristine. No consistent effect of cyclophosphamide was seen on LI prior to vincristine and Ara-C, but it could be argued that the cyclophosphamide dose was too low and the time interval too short. The other clinical study which offers laboratory support for an increase in growth fraction after alkylator therapy was reported by Hayes and Mauer.[94] Cyclophosphamide was administered to children with disseminated neuroblastoma at a dose of 150 mg/m² per day for 7 days. The patients received Adriamycin 25 mg/m² on day 8. Among nine patients whose tumor cells could be selectively studied from bone marrow aspirates, seven had an increase in LI after the cyclophosphamide, and six responded with a decrease in LI and remission after Adriamycin. Furthermore, if the LI and MI decreased immediately after the 7 days of cyclophosphamide, the clinical response to the sequential regimen was poor.

Other studies with encouraging clinical results, but no kinetic measurements, have been carried out in oat-cell carcinoma of the lung[95] and non-oat-cell lung tumors[96] with the sequential combination of cyclophosphamide and methotrexate. However, equally encouraging results have been obtained in these tumor categories using simultaneous combinations of drugs without any kinetic rationale.

Klein's work with vincristine in Ehrlich ascites tumor led him to do clinical trials with two doses of vincristine followed at various, empirically chosen intervals by cyclophosphamide.[70] He treated 55 patients, of whom 39 had lymphomas, 7 had oat-cell lung carcinoma, 7 had acute leukemia, and 2 had unknown primary sites. He observed a 60 percent complete and 90 percent complete plus partial response rate; although these are good results, they are not extraordinary, particularly since all but two of the complete remissions were in leukemia or lymphoma. Pouillart et al.[97,98] have also treated patients with lymphoma, lung carcinoma, and other malignancies with vincristine given twice, followed by other executor compounds, with good results but not kinetic data. As Pouillart himself has emphasized,[99] some of the heightened effectiveness of the combinations may be due to pharmacodynamic interactions, rather than to kinetic effects.

The ability of bleomycin to produce arrest in the G_2 and M phases of the cell cycle and its property of inducing single-strand breaks in DNA led Miyamoto et al.[100] to explore a regimen of sequential administration of bleomycin followed by mitomycin C.[101] Their rationale was that (1) an increased number of cells might be placed in the phase of the cell cycle most sensitive to mitomycin, and (2) mitomycin might render irreversible much of the "potentially lethal" damage to DNA induced by bleomycin. Initial results of this regimen in cervical cancer were very encouraging, and have led to similar scheduling of bleomycin and mitomycin C in other cell types. Kinetic data in which the LI was measured serially would greatly strengthen their argument.

IN VITRO PREDICTIVE TESTS AND CELL KINETICS

Changes in LI and Response

Sky-Peck[102] reported that a decrease in LI after a course of therapy correlated highly with the likelihood of subsequent clinical response to that therapy. Using a technique[103] that allowed for rapid autoradiography on representative samples of viable tumor cells, Murphy et al.[104] confirmed this observation; in 63 patients with a variety of solid tumors and on numerous different chemotherapeutic regimens, clinical response was observed in 12 out of 16 patients with a significant decrease in LI after therapy, and in only 2 of 47 who failed to show such a decrease.[54] Data from experimental tumors[105] also demonstrate that tumor regression after chemotherapy is accompanied by a decrease in LI; however, decreases of LI (though of lesser magnitude) have also been reported in tumors resistant to the agent employed.[106,107] Given that suppression of DNA synthesis in a tumor does not guarantee response, clinical and experimental data strongly suggest that it is a sine qua non for response to occur, at least with agents that preferentially kill proliferating cells. This appears to be true as well for radiation; in studies reported by Tubiana,[108] among patients with head and neck tumors who underwent weekly LI determination during continuous radiation treatment, a greater than 50 percent decrease in LI correlated with clinical radiosensitivity, and a less than 50 percent decrease with nonresponse. Breitenecker et al.[109] made a similar observation with radiation in carcinoma of the cervix. Elequin et al.[110] determined the LI of fine-needle aspirates from 38 patients before, during, and after radiotherapy. Whenever postradiation therapy LIs showed at least a two-thirds decrease from the pretherapy levels, significant tumor regression was observed. The posttreatment samples were usually obtained on the last day of radiation therapy.

As a clinically useful predictor of response, the study of LI pre- and posttherapy has two serious drawbacks: (1) the tumor must be accessible to repeated biopsy, and (2) the patient must be committed to a course of treatment before its effect can be evaluated. Several investigators have reported preliminary studies to test a more useful hypothesis (if correct): that drug therapy in vitro may predictably suppress DNA synthesis in sensitive cells. Cline[111] has summarized the conditions that should be met to test such a hypothesis: (1) the drug(s) must be in active form (or converted to it) in the in vitro system; (2) the drug(s) must be present in concentrations approximating those achieved in vivo; (3) the rate and other characteristics of DNA synthesis of the malignant cells in vivo and in vitro must be sufficiently similar so that drug effects under the two conditions are comparable; and (4) there must be sufficient time for drug action to become manifest. Zittoun et al.[112] used a test system in which drugs were directly added to leukemic cells, at concentrations that produced a 50 percent decrease in [^{14}C]thymidine incorporation of control nonleukemic marrows after 2 h; in vitro depression of labeled thymidine incorporation was more marked in those who responded to therapy than in the nonresponders. The mean decrease in 16 responders was 52 percent compared to 24 percent in 26 nonresponders ($p < .001$). No difference was observed in depression of [^{3}H]uridine incorporation between responders and nonresponders. Lippmann et al.[113] found that, when leukemic blasts from ALL patients were incubated 18 h with dexamethasone directly added in vitro, ^{3}HTdR incorporation was significantly inhibited in glucocorticoid-sensitive, but not in glucocorticoid-resistant, cells. Furthermore, the minimal concentration necessary to achieve this effect approximated that necessary to saturate steroid-binding protein receptor sites.

Problems associated with direct addition of drugs to in vitro systems include the following: (1) the drug may not be present in its active form in the in vitro system, and (2) the drug (or metabolite) concentration achievable in vivo may not be approximated under in vitro conditions, either through oversight or (commonly) lack of pharmacologic data. An attempt to circumvent these difficulties involves the use of *treated serum,* defined as serum obtained from the patient shortly after drug administration, at a time when pharmacologic concentration of active metabolites may be nearly maximal. Such a technique has precedent in the use of various dilutions of host serum containing antibiotics to determine whether adequate bactericidal concentrations have been reached.[114] The determination of antineoplastic activity of treated sera, for the purpose of determining duration of antitumor effect after a single dose, also has precedent in experimental systems.[115]

Burns et al.[116] measured ^{3}HTdR incorporation by scintillography of leukemic cells incubated with pretreatment (control) serum versus serum from the same patient obtained after 2 days of therapy with Ara-C. The period of incubation with treated serum was 4 h. All patients who had depression of thymidine uptake by 65 percent or more showed response, while depression by less than 50 percent was not associated with clinical response.

It is probable that 4 h of incubation is not, in many instances, a sufficient period of time for drug effect on DNA synthesis to become manifest. This is suggested by experimental tumor work with alkylating agents[106] which shows that maximal inhibition of DNA synthesis occurs 24 to 72 h after their administration in vivo, and by the failure of systems using short-term exposure conditions to demonstrate consistent, good correlation between changes in DNA synthesis and response.[117,118] Using a 24-h period of incubation with treated serum versus fresh and 24-h control serum, Thirlwell et al.[119] found the following: (1) the LI of tumor cells remained constant over 24 h in 90 percent of controls, with no evidence of a nonspecific effect from serum itself; (2) treated serums did, in some cases, produce significant decreases in LI after 24 h relative to controls; and (3) these decreases correlated with the subsequent observed clinical response. In 6 patients with objective clinical response, 5 had a significant decrease in LI in vitro; in 12 without a decrease, none had response, 1 improved, and 11 had progressive disease. Further work by Livingston (unpublished data) demonstrated that 24 h was not a sufficient period of exposure to see consistent correlation of in vitro with in vivo results. By extending the period of in vitro exposure to 96 h, and comparing the LI of treated versus untreated cells at 24, 48, 72, and 96 h, it appears to be possible to predict response (in the case of tumors) or myelosuppression (in the case of normal bone marrow) in a high percentage of instances.[120]

Direct Cloning Assays

In many ways, the most appealing in vitro test for response to chemotherapy would be one in which the actual ability of tumor cells to reproduce (clone) themselves were the parameter being assayed, rather than an indirect measure of reproductive capability like the LI. Until recently, efforts to grow most human tumors in culture had met with frustrating failure.[121] Salmon et al.,[122] using a soft agar system in which growth is induced by a medium conditioned by the adherent spleen cells of mineral oil–primed BALB/c mice, appear to have succeeded in developing a clonogenic assay system with consistent successful growth, at least for certain tumor types. Of greatest interest is the correlation between drug-induced suppression of the growth of tumor cell colonies in vitro and in vivo success of the same chemotherapeutic agents. It appears that the cells being assayed are primarily those which were in S-phase initially, since tritiated thymidine suicide incubation (exposure to a lethal concentration of ^{3}HTdR) reduced colony formation to as little as 35 percent of control.[123]

Even a successful in vitro cloning assay system may not be reflective of in vivo events, as shown by the experience of Twentyman, who found little correlation between drug effects on colony formation of the EMT 6 tumor in vitro and the in vivo results with the same chemotherapy.[124] It is undoubtedly naive to presume that an in vitro test system can ever completely mimic the vivo situation. However, recent results with assays based on changes in LI and clonogenicity (which may be measuring similar phenomena) are encouraging. They may at least allow the clinician to decide which drugs *not* to use for an individual patient's therapy.

REFERENCES

1. Godwin HA et al: Peripheral leukocyte studies of acute leukemia in relapse and remission and chronic myelocytic leukemia in blast crisis. *Blood* 31:686, 1968.
2. Barlogie B et al: Pulse cytophotometric analysis of synchronized cells in vitro. *Cancer Res* 36:1176, 1976.
3. Laird AK: Dynamics of growth in tumors and normal organisms. *Natl Cancer Inst Monogr* 30:15, 1969.
4. Griswold DP Jr et al: Altered sensitivity of a hamster plasmacytoma to cytosine arabinoside. *Cancer Chemother Rep* 54:337, 1970.
5. Norton L, Simon R: Tumor size, sensitivity to therapy, and design of treatment schedules. *Cancer Treat Rep* 61:1307, 1977.
6. Bonadonna G et al: The CMF program for operable breast cancer with positive axillary nodes. *Cancer* 39:2904, 1977.
7. Grage TB et al: The role of 5-fluorouracil as an adjuvant to the surgical treatment of large bowel cancer, in S Salmon, SE Jones (eds): *Adjuvant Therapy of Cancer*, Elsevier-North Holland, New York, p. 259, 1977.
8. Alberts DS et al: Treatment of multiple myeloma in remission with anticancer drugs having cell cycle specific characteristics. *Cancer Treat Rep* 61:381, 1977.
9. Durie BGM et al: Polyamines as markers of response and disease activity in cancer chemotherapy. *Cancer Res* 37:214, 1977.
10. Durie BGM et al: Prognostic significance of tritiated thymidine labeling index in multiple myeloma and acute myeloid leukemia. *Proc AACR-ASCO* 18:80, 1977.
11. Murphy W et al: Serial labeling index determination as a predictor of response in human solid tumors. *Cancer Res* 35:1438, 1975.
12. Livingston RB, Hart JS: The clinical applications of cell kinetics in cancer therapy. *Annu Rev Pharmacol Toxicol* 17:529, 1977.
13. Simpson-Herren L et al: Effects of surgery on the cell kinetics of residual tumor. *Cancer Treat Rep* 60:1749, 1976.
14. Schabel FM Jr: Surgical adjuvant chemotherapy of metastatic murine tumors. *Cancer* 40:558, 1977.
15. Schabel FM Jr, Simpson-Herren L: Some variables in experimental tumor systems which complicate interpretation of data from in vivo kinetic and pharmacologic studies with anticancer drugs, in H Schonfeld et al (eds): *Antibiotics and Chemotherapy,* Karger, Basel, 1978.
16. Kofman S et al: A correlation between the incorporation of formate-C^{14} in tumors and the clinical course of patients with disseminated breast cancer. *Cancer* 13:425, 1960.
17. Erickson LC et al: Differential inhibition of the rejoining of x-ray–induced DNA strand breaks in normal and transformed human fibroblasts treated with 1,3-bis(2-chloroethyl)-1-nitrosourea in vitro. *Cancer Res* 38:672, 1978.
18. Little JB: Cellular effects of ionizing radiation. *N Engl J Med* 278:308, 1968.
19. Mendelsohn ML: The cell cycle in malignant and normal tissues, in *The Cell Cycle in Malignancy and Immunity,* Natl Tech Inf Serv, US Dep Commerce, Springfield, Va., 1975.
20. Young RC: Kinetic aids to proper chemotherapeutic scheduling: Labeled nucleoside incorporation studies in vivo. *Cancer Treat Rep* 60:1947, 1976.
21. Russell DH: The roles of the polyamines, putrescine, spermidine, and spermine in normal and malignant tissues. *Life Sci* 13:1635, 1973.
22. Russell DH: Clinical relevance of polyamines as biochemical markers of tumor kinetics. *Clin Chem* 23:11, 1977.
23. Andersson G, Heby O: Kinetics of cell proliferation and polyamine synthesis during Ehrlich ascites tumor growth. *Cancer Res* 37:4361, 1977.
24. Chen KC et al: Studies of the regulation of ornithine decarboxylase activity by the microtubules: The effect of colchicine and vinblastine. *Biochem Biophys Res Commun* 68:401, 1976.
25. Sakai T, Cohen S: Effects of polyamines on the structure and reactivity of tRNA. *Prog Nucleic Acid Res Mol Biol* 17:15, 1976.
26. Weber G: Enzymology of cancer cells. *N Engl J Med* 296:486, 1977.
27. Berlin RD et al: The cell surface. *N Engl J Med* 299:515, 1975.
28. Tucker RW et al: Correlation of cytotoxicity and mitotic spindle dissolution by vinblastine in mammalian cells. *Cancer Res* 37:4346, 1977.
29. Paulson JC, McClure WO: Microtubules and axoplasmic transport. Inhibition of transport by podophyllotoxin: An

29. interaction with microtubule protein. *J Cell Biol* 67:461, 1975.
30. Wilson L, Bryan J: Biochemical and pharmacological properties of microtubules. *Adv Cell Mol Biol* 3:21, 1974.
31. Hacker B: Modulation of transfer RNA–methylating enzyme activities in murine leukemic cells. *Cancer Res* 32:1143, 1972.
32. Borek E et al: High turnover rate of transfer RNA in tumor tissue. *Cancer Res* 37:3362, 1977.
33. Erickson LC et al: Differential repair of 1-(2-chloroethyl)-3-(4-methylcyclohexyl)-1-nitrosourea–induced DNA damage to two human colon tumor cell lines. *Cancer Res* 38:802, 1978.
34. Schmidt LH et al: Comparative pharmacology of alkylating agents. *Cancer Chemother Rep* [suppl 2] parts 1, 2, and 3, p 1, 1965.
35. Gerard GF et al: Detection in human ovary and prostate tumors of DNA polymerase activity that copies poly(2'-O-methylcytidylate · oligodeoxyguanylate. *Cancer Res* 38:1008, 1978.
36. Cooney DA, Handschumacher RE: L-Asparaginase and s-asparagine metabolism. *Annu Rev Pharmacol* 10:421, 1970.
37. Allegra JC et al: An association between steroid hormone receptors and response to cytotoxic chemotherapy in patients with metastatic breast cancer. *Cancer Res* 38:4299, 1978.
38. Lippman ME, Allegra JC: Estrogen receptor and endocrine therapy of breast cancer. *N Engl J Med* 299:930, 1978.
39. Schiffer LM et al: Studies on the cell kinetics of human solid tumors, in B Drewinko, RM Humphrey (eds): *Growth Kinetics and Biochemical Regulation of Normal and Malignant Cells*, Williams & Wilkins, Baltimore, p 663, 1977.
40. Meyer JS, Bauer WC: In vitro determination of tritiated thymidine labeling index (LI). *Cancer* 36:1374, 1975.
41. Meyer JS, Facher R: Thymidine labeling index of human breast carcinoma. *Cancer* 39:2524, 1977.
42. Skipper HE: Kinetic behavior versus response to chemotherapy. Presented at CCIRC Symposium, Cascades Conf, Williamsburg, Va, 1970.
43. Hart JS et al: Prognostic significance of pretreatment proliferative activity in adult acute leukemia. *Cancer* 39:1603, 1977.
44. Hillen H et al: Bone marrow proliferation patterns in acute lyeloblastic leukemia determined by pulse cytophotometry. *Lancet* 1:609, 1975.
45. Volger W et al: Correlation of cytosine arabinoside–induced increment in growth fraction of leukemia cells with clinical response. *Cancer* 33:603, 1971.
46. Volger W et al: Cell kinetics in acute leukemia. *Arch Intern Med* 135:950, 1975.
47. Raich P: In vitro prediction of therapeutic response in acute leukemia. *Proc AACR-ASCO* 17:182, 1976.
48. Arlin Z et al: Significance of pulse ³H-thymidine labeling index in adult acute myeloid leukemia. *Proc AACR-ASCO* 17:296, 1976.
49. Nelson JA et al: Mechanisms of action of 6-thioguanine, 6-mercaptopurine, and 8-azaguanine. *Cancer Res* 35:2872, 1975.
50. Crowther D et al: Factors influencing prognosis in adults with acute myelogenous leukaemia. *Br J Cancer* 32:456, 1975.
51. Mauer A et al: Scheduling and recruitment in leukemic populations, in B Drewinko, RM Humphrey (eds): *Growth Kinetics and Biochemical Regulation of Normal and Malignant Cells*, Williams & Wilkins, Baltimore, p 855, 1977.
52. Sulkes A et al: Tritiated thymidine labeling index and response in human breast cancer. *J Natl Cancer Inst* 62:513–515, 1979.
53. Thirlwell M, Mansell P: A correlation of clinical response with in vitro pre-chemotherapy labeling index in human solid tumors. *Proc AACR-ASCO* 17:307, 1976.
54. Livingston RB et al: Cell kinetic parameters: Correlation with clinical response, in B Drewinko, RM Humphrey (eds): *Growth Kinetics and Biochemical Regulation of Normal and Malignant Cells*, Williams & Wilkins, Baltimore, p 767, 1977.
55. Hainau B et al: Cell proliferation and histologic classification of bronchogenic carcinoma. *J Natl Cancer Inst* 59:1113, 1977.
56. Livingston, RB: Combination chemotherapy of bronchogenic carcinoma: I. Non-oat cell. *Cancer Treat Rev* 4:153, 1977.
57. Weichselbaum RR et al: Proliferation kinetics of a human breast cancer line in vitro following treatment with 17beta-estradiol and 1-beta-D-arabinosuranosylcytosine. *Cancer Res* 38:2339, 1978.
58. Meyer JS et al: Low incidence of estrogen receptor in breast carcinomas with rapid rates of cellular replication. *Cancer* 40:2290, 1977.
59. Moran RE et al: Variation in labeling index and estrogen receptor protein in human breast cancer. *Proc AACR-ASCO* 19:72, 1978.
60. Pertschuk LP et al: Immunofluorescent detection of estrogen receptors in breast cancer. *Cancer* 41:907, 1978.
61. Lee SH: Cytochemical study of estrogen receptor in human mammary cancer. *Am J Clin Pathol* 70:197, 1978.
62. Marshall GJ et al: The effect of pulse intravenous prednisolone on marrow cell incorporation of thymidine-C-14 and deoxyuridine-C-14. *Proc AACR-ASCO* 8:38, 1971.
63. Rosen F, Milholland RJ: Mechanism of action of glucocorticoids, in *Handbuch fuer Experimentelle Pharmakologie: Antineoplastic and Immunosuppressive Agents*, Springer, New York, vol 38, p 85, 1974–1975.
64. Sato S: Effect of prednisolone on tumor cells. *Kitakanto Med J* 27:41, 1977.
65. Bayer BM, Veaven MA: Evidence that indomethacin inhibits growth of cells in the G_1 phase of the cell cycle. *Fed Proc* 37:896, 1978.
66. Braunschweiger PG et al: Glucocorticosteroid-induced cell synchronization in C3H spontaneous mammary tumors: Therapeutic implications. *Proc AACR-ASCO* 19:19, 1978.

67. Dethlefsen LA et al: Cell synchronization in vivo: Fact or fancy? in B Drewinko, RM Humphrey (eds): *Growth Kinetics and Biochemical Regulation of Normal and Malignant Cells*, Williams & Wilkins, Baltimore, p 491, 1977.
68. Gibson MH, Bertalanffy FD: In vivo synchrony of solid B_{16} melanoma by cytosine arabinoside, an inhibitor of DNA synthesis. *J Natl Cancer Inst* 49:1007, 1972.
69. Frei E III et al: The stathmokinetic effect of vincristine. *Cancer Res* 24:1918, 1964.
70. Klein HO et al: In vivo and in vitro studies on cell kinetics and synchronization of human tumor: Their significance in tumor chemotherapy. *Dtsch Med Wochenschr* 97:1273, 1972.
71. Capizzi R et al: L-Asparaginase–induced alternation of amethopterin (methotrexate) activity in mouse leukemia L5178Y. *Ann NY Acad Sci* 186:302, 1971.
72. Chlopkiewicz B, Koziorowska J: Role of amino acid depletion in combined treatment of neoplastic cells with methotrexate and L-asparaginase. *Cancer Res* 35:1524, 1975.
73. Ganzer U, Nitze H: Die strahlenbehandlung synchronissierter hauttumoren der maus. *Strahlentherapie* 140:711, 1970.
74. Lampkin B et al: Synchronization and recruitment in acute leukemia. *J Clin Invest* 50:2204, 1971.
75. Lampkin B et al: Manipulation of the mitotic cycle in treatment of acute myeloblastic leukemia. *Abstr 17th Ann Meet Am Soc Hematol*, p 70, 1974.
76. Ernst P et al: Perturbation of cell cycle of human leukaemic myeloblast in vivo by cytosine arabinoside. *Scand J Haematol* 10:209, 1973.
77. Kremer W et al: An attempt at synchronization of marrow cells in acute leukemia. *Cancer* 37:390, 1976.
78. MacKinney A, Flynn B: Synchronization and recruitment in the treatment of adult acute leukemia. *Clin Res* 24:378, 1976.
79. Buchner T et al: Accumulation of S-phase cells in the bone marrow of patients with acute leukemia by cytosine arabinoside. *Blut* 28:299, 1974.
80. Capizzi R: Biochemical interaction between asparaginase and methotrexate in leukemia cells. *Proc AACR-ASCO* 15:77, 1974.
81. Barranco S et al: Bleomycin as a possible synchronizing agent for human tumor cells in vivo. *Cancer Res* 33:882, 1973.
82. Costanzi J: Bleomycin infusion as a potential synchronizing agent in carcinoma of the head and neck. *Proc AACR-ASCO* 17:11, 1976.
83. Samuels ML et al: Continuous intravenous bleomycin therapy with vinblastine in stage III testicular neoplasia. *Cancer Chemother Rep* 59:563, 1975.
84. Livingston R et al: Kinetic scheduling of vincristine and bleomycin in patients with lung cancer and other malignant tumors. *Cancer Chemother Rep* 57:219, 1973.
85. Livingston R et al: COMB: A four-drug combination in solid tumors. *Cancer* 36:327, 1975.
86. Livingston R et al: BACON (bleomycin, Adriamycin, CCNU, oncovin, and nitrogen mustard) in squamous lung cancer. *Cancer* 37:1237, 1976.
87. Livingston RB et al: Comparative trial of combination chemotherapy in extensive squamous carcinoma of the lung: A Southwest Oncology Group study. *Cancer Treat Rep* 61:1623, 1977.
88. Baker LH et al: Phase II study of mitomycin-C, vincristine, and bleomycin in advanced squamous cell carcinoma of the uterine cervix. *Cancer* 38:2222, 1976.
89. Burgess M et al: Treatment of metastatic germ cell tumors with adriamycin, vincristine, and bleomycin. *Proc AACR-ASCO* 16:244, 1975.
90. Einhorn L, Donohue J: cis-Diamminedichloroplatinum, vinblastine, and bleomycin combination chemotherapy in disseminated testicular cancer. *Ann Intern Med* 87:293, 1977.
91. Einhorn L: Personal communication.
92. Wheeler W, Thirlwell M: Sequential cytosine arabinoside and methotrexate in solid tumors. *Proc AACR-ASCO* 16:237, 1975.
93. Burke P, Woens A: Attempted recruitment of leukemic myeloblasts to proliferative activity by sequential drug treatment. *Cancer* 28:830, 1971.
94. Hayes FA, Mauer AM: Cell kinetics and chemotherapy in neuroblastoma. *J Natl Cancer Inst* 57:697, 1976.
95. Eagan R et al: Combination chemotherapy and radiation therapy in small cell carcinoma of the lung. *Cancer* 32:371, 1973.
96. Straus MJ: Combination chemotherapy in advanced lung cancer with increased survival. *Cancer* 38:2232, 1976.
97. Pouillart P et al: Essai de recrutement cellulaire par synchronisation partielle pour l'établissement d'une combinaison chimiothérapique. *Bull Cancer* 60:187, 1973.
98. Pouillart P et al: Combinaisons chimiothérapiques de drogues se potentialisant. *Nouv Presse Med* 4:10, 717, 1975.
99. Pouillart P et al: Sequential administration of two oncostatic drugs: Study of modalities for pharmacodynamic potentiation. *Biomedicine* 21:471, 1974.
100. Iqbal ZM et al: Single-strand scission and repair of DNA in mammalian cells by bleomycin. *Cancer Res* 36:3834, 1976.
101. Miyamoti T et al: Effectiveness of a sequential combination of bleomycin and mitomycin-C on an advanced cervical cancer. *Cancer* 41:403, 1978.
102. Sky-Peck HH: Effects of chemotherapy on the incorporation of ^{3}H-thymidine into DNA of human neoplastic tissue. *Natl Cancer Inst Monogr* 34:197, 1971.
103. Livingston RB et al: In vitro determination of thymidine-^{3}H labeling index in human solid tumors. *Cancer Res* 34:1376, 1974.
104. Murphy W et al: Serial labeling index determination as a predictor of response in human solid tumors. *Cancer Res* 35:1438, 1975.
105. Wheeler G, Alexander J: Studies with mustards: IV. Effects

106. Wheeler G, Alexander J: Effects of nitrogen mustard and cyclophosphamide upon the synthesis of DNA in vivo and in cell-free preparations. *Cancer Res* 29:98, 1969.
107. Brereton H et al: Inhibition and recovery of DNA synthesis in host tissues and sensitive and resistant B_{16} melanoma after 1-(2-chloroethyl)-3-(trans-4-methylcyclohexyl)-1-nitrosourea, a predictor of therapeutic efficacy. *Cancer Res* 35:2420, 1975.
108. Tubiana M et al: Determinants of cellular kinetics in radiotherapy, in B Drewinko, RM Humphrey (eds): *Growth Kinetics and Biochemical Regulation of Normal and Malignant Cells,* Williams & Wilkins, Baltimore, p 826, 1977.
109. Breitenecker G, Tatra G: Histological and autoradiographical investigations during radiotherapy of carcinoma of the cervix. *Strahlentherapie* 146:664, 1973.
110. Elequin FT et al: Correlation between in vitro labeling indices and tumor regression following radiotherapy. *Int J Radiat Oncol Biol Phys* 4:207, 1978.
111. Cline M: In vitro test systems for anticancer drugs. *N Engl J Med* 280:955, 1969.
112. Zittoun R et al: Prediction of the response to chemotherapy in acute leukemia. *Cancer* 35:507, 1975.
113. Lippmann M et al: Glucocorticoid-binding proteins in human acute lymphoblastic leukemic cells. *J Clin Invest* 52:1715, 1973.
114. Dunlap SG: The serum dilution bactericidal test for antibiotic effectiveness. *Am J Med Technol* 31:69, 1965.
115. Kline K et al: Duration of drug levels in mice as indicated by residual antileukemic efficacy. *Chemotherapy* 13:28, 1968.
116. Burns C et al: Prediction of the response of patients with acute nonlymphocytic leukemia to cytosine arabinoside therapy. *Cancer Chemother Rep* 56:527, 1972.
117. Volm M et al: The effects of cytostatic drugs on transplanted tumors: An investigation of the correlation between in vivo and in vitro results. *Arch Geschwulstforsch* 43:137, 1974.
118. Wayss K et al: Correlation of in vitro testing and therapeutic results after cytostatic treatment of animals with transplanted tumors. *Arzneim Forsch* 25:77, 1975.
119. Thirlwell MP et al: A rapid in vitro labeling index method for predicting response of human solid tumors to chemotherapy. *Cancer Res* 36:3279, 1976.
120. Livingston RB: In vitro prediction of chemotherapy response. *Clin Res* 26:776a, 1978.
121. Ioachim HL: Tissue culture of human tumors: Its use and prospects. *Pathol Annu* 5:217, 1970.
122. Salmon SE et al: Quantitation of differential sensitivity of human-tumor stem cells to anticancer drugs. *N Engl J Med* 298:1321, 1978.
123. Hamburger AW et al: Direct cloning of human ovarian carcinoma cells in agar. *Cancer Res* 38:3438, 1978.
124. Twentyman PR: Sensitivity to 1,3-bis(2-chloroethyl)-1-nitrosourea and 1-(2-chloroethyl)-3-(4-methylcyclohexyl)-1-nitrosourea of the EMT6 tumor in vivo as determined by both tumor volume response and in vitro plating assay. *Cancer Res* 38:2395, 1978.
125. Bhuyan BK, Fraser TJ: Cytotoxicity of antitumor agents in a synchronous mammalian cell system. *Cancer Chemother Rep* 58:149, 1974.
126. Skipper HE et al: Implications of biochemical, cytokinetic, pharmacologic, and toxicologic relationships in the design of optimal therapeutic schedules. *Cancer Chemother Rep* 54:431, 1970.
127. Barranco SC et al: Survival and cell kinetics effects of adriamycin on mammalian cells. *Cancer Res* 33:11, 1973.
128. Barranco SC: Review of the survival and cell kinetics effects of adriamycin on mammalian cells. *Cancer Chemother Rep* 6:147, 1975.
129. Krishan A, Frei E III: Effect of adriamycin on the cell cycle traverse and kinetics of cultured human lymphoblasts. *Cancer Res* 36:143, 1976.
130. Crooke ST, Bradner WT: Mitomycin C: A review. *Cancer Treat Rev* 3:121, 1976.
131. Lahiri SK: Response of mouse bone marrow colony forming units in different stages of the cell cycle to in vitro incubation with mitomycin-C. *Cell Tissue Kinet* 6:509, 1973.
132. Hart JS et al: Neoplasia, kinetics, and chemotherapy. *Semin Oncol* 3:259, 1976.
133. Barranco SC, Humphrey RM: The effects of bleomycin on survival and cell progression in Chinese hamster cells in vitro. *Cancer Res* 28:2437, 1968.
134. Twentyman PR: Comparative chemosensitivity of exponential versus plateau-phase cells in both in vitro and in vivo model systems. *Cancer Treat Rep* 60:1719, 1976.
135. Madoc-Jones H, Mauro F: Interphase action of vinblastine and vincristine: Differences in their lethal action through the mitotic cycle of cultured mammalian cells. *J Cell Physiol* 72:185, 1968.
136. Schrek R: Cytotoxicity of vincristine to normal leukemic cells. *Am J Clin Pathol* 62:3, 1974.
137. Rosner F et al: In vitro combination chemotherapy demonstrating potentiation of vincristine cytotoxicity by prednisolone. *Cancer Res* 35:700, 1975.
138. Bhuyan BK et al: Cell cycle phase specificity of antitumor agents. *Cancer Res* 32:398, 1972.
139. Wheeler GP et al: Comparison of the effects of several inhibitors of the synthesis of nucleic acids upon the viability and progression through the cell cycle of cultured H. Ep. no. 2 cells. *Cancer Res* 32:2661, 1972.
140. Madoc-Jones H, Mauro F: Site of action of cytotoxic agents in the cell life cycle, in Antineoplastic and Immunosuppressive Agents, Springer-Verlag, Berlin, p 205, vol 1, 1974.
141. Barranco SC, Humphrey RM: The effects of B-2′-deoxythioguanosine on survival and progression in mammalian cells. *Cancer Res* 31:583, 1971.

142. Rozencweig M et al: VM 26 and VP 16-213: A comparative analysis. *Cancer* 40:334, 1977.
143. Heinen E, Bassleer R: Mode of action of *cis*-dichlorodiamine platinum (II) on mouse Ehrlich ascites tumor cells. *Biochem Pharmacol* 25:1871, 1976.
144. Drewinko B, Gottlieb JA: Action of *cis*-dichlorodiamineplatinum (II) at the cellular level. *Cancer Chemother Rep* 59:665, 1975.
145. Bono VH Jr: Studies on the mechanism of action of DTIC. *Cancer Treat Rep* 60:141, 1976.
146. Gerulath AH et al: The effects of treatments with 5 (3,3 dimethyl-1-triazeno) imidazole-4-carboxamide in darkness and in light on survival and progression in Chinese hamster ovary cells in vitro. *Cancer Res* 34:1921, 1974.
147. Andersson G, Heby O: Population kinetics of an Ehrlich ascites tumor following treatment with methylglyoxal bis (guanylhydrazone), a polyamine synthesis inhibitor. *Cancer Lett* 2:59, 1977.
148. DeBrabander MJ et al: The effects of methyl (5-(2-thienylcarbonyl)-1H-benzimidazole-2-yl)carbamate, (R 17934; NSC 238159), a new synthetic antitumoral drug interfering with microtubules, on mammalian cells cultured in vitro. *Cancer Res* 36:905, 1976.
149. Frucht LT, Scott RE: Effect of vinblastine sulfate, colchicine, and lumicolchicine on membrane organization of normal and transformed cells. *Exp Cell Res* 96:271, 1975.
150. McGuire WL: Hormone receptors: Their role in predicting prognosis and response to endocrine therapy. *Semin Oncol* 5:428–433, 1978.
151. Corti A, Dave C: Specific inhibition of the enzymatic decarboxylation of S-adenosylmethionine by methylglyoxal bis (guanylhydrazone) and related substances. *Biochem J* 139:351, 1974.
152. Bachrach U: Polyamines as chemical markers of malignancy. *Ital J Biochem* 25:77, 1976.
153. Lapi L, Cohen SS: Inhibition of the lethality of bleomycin A_5 in the L-cells by Hirudonine. *Cancer Res* 37:1384, 1977.
154. Beck WT: Partial reversal of vinca alkaloid cytotoxicity by spermine in cultured mammalian cells. *Proc AACR-ASCO* 18:72, 1977.
155. Chen K: Studies on the regulation of ornithine decarboxylase activity by the microtubules: The effect of colchicine and vinblastine. *Biochem Biophys Res Commun* 68:401, 1976.
156. Miller E: Development of procarbazine, in SK Carter (ed): *Proceedings of the Chemotherapy Conference on Procarbazine (Matulane: DNS-77213): Development and Application*, GPO, p. 3, Washington, DC, 1971.
157. Lake LM et al: Toxicity and antitumor activity of hexamethylmelamine and its *N*-demethylated metabolites in mice with transplantable tumors. *Cancer Res* 35:2858, 1975.
158. Himes RH et al: Action of the vinca alkaloids vincristine, vinblastine, and desacetyl vinblastine amide on microtubules in vitro. *Cancer Res* 36:3798, 1976.
159. Tucker RW et al: Correlation of cytotoxicity and mitotic spindle dissolution by vinblastine in mammalian cells. *Cancer Res* 37:4346, 1977.
160. Ebina T et al: Inhibition of surface immunoglobulin central capping of daudi cells and cell spreading of HeLa-S3 cells by neocarzinostatin. *Cancer Res* 37:4423, 1977.
161. Roberts D, Loehr EV: Depression of thymidylate synthetase activity in response to cytosine arabinoside. *Cancer Res* 32:1160, 1972.

8
PRINCIPLES OF CANCER CHEMOTHERAPY

Robert B. Livingston

The surgical oncologist needs an understanding of the basic principles of cancer chemotherapy for the same reason that the medical oncologist needs to understand the elements of surgical approach and results in a given malignant disease: decisions about what is best for a patient increasingly depend on an understanding of modalities in concert and planned sequences, rather than competition and unplanned sequential therapy. There are at least two other reasons: (1) the surgeon may be called upon to administer chemotherapy, especially in the adjuvant situation; and (2) the surgeon is often asked to see cancer patients with disseminated disease who are on (or have received) chemotherapy. This chapter will consider, first, those principles of drug treatment that are established and apply especially to management of patients with disseminated disease and, second, principles of adjuvant treatment, which are far less certain. Basic features of the major drug classes, and management of acute toxicity from these agents, are also considered. For a discussion of kinetic principles and those which are related to tumor cell biology, please see Chap. 7.

Regardless of the mechanism whereby it comes about, the basis for effective chemotherapy is selective antitumor effect relative to sensitive normal target tissues, which may be graphically depicted as in Fig. 8-1. This result may come about through any of several mechanisms: (1) a greater fraction of the tumor cell population may be destroyed by proliferation-dependent chemotherapy, because it has a higher growth fraction than other host target tissues; (2) the tumor cell population may have slower recovery, and take longer to repopulate; (3) tumor cells may have selective uptake and retention characteristics; or (4) vital intracellular mechanisms may be affected which are qualitatively different between tumor and normal cell targets. These mechanisms are strongly interrelated. For instance, it is true that higher growth fraction tumors are, in general, more sensitive to chemotherapy.[1,2] However, the growth fraction of continuous renewal systems which are vital to life, such as the bone marrow and intestinal mucosa, is also high: generally higher than that in human tumors. Young and his coworkers have elegantly demonstrated the importance of delayed tumor recovery relative to host tissues in several experimental systems, measuring rate of DNA synthesis as a parameter.[3,4] This, in turn, may be related to selective or longer retention of the active drug metabolites in tumor cells.[5] Several proven or apparent differences exist between tumor and normal cells, to which the effectiveness of certain chemotherapeutic agents may be related (see Chap. 7).

FACTORS AFFECTING CHOICE OF CHEMOTHERAPY

Factors to be considered in the choice of chemotherapy include (1) general sensitivity of the tumor to chemotherapy; (2) specific sensitivity of an individual's tumor to individual agents; (3) the likelihood of response and clinical improvement versus serious toxicity (assessment of therapeutic index); and (4) whether chemotherapy is to be used in the setting of advanced disease as a single modality, in a combined modality setting (e.g., with radiation therapy for regional disease), or in the adjuvant setting after potentially curative surgery.

Since acute leukemia, lymphomas, pediatric solid tumors, breast and ovarian cancer, and small-cell lung cancer are generally sensitive to chemotherapy, the choice of antineoplastic drug treatment is generally an appropriate one, even if the patient is bedfast from the disease. On the other hand, the relative chemoinsensitivity of renal, pancreatic, esophageal, colorectal, non-small-cell lung cancer, and melanoma, coupled with the negative effect of adverse performance status on the likelihood of a meaningful response, is such that most medical oncologists prefer to avoid the toxicity of presently available chemotherapy in nonambulatory patients with these diagnoses. Whether to treat the ambulatory patient with dissemination of one of these cancers depends on several factors, including the patient's own informed desire for treatment, the availability of adequate facilities, and the possibility of contributing toward an eventual solution through involvement in a therapeutic research protocol.

To be able to determine the specific sensitivity (or lack of it) of an individual patient's tumor to chemotherapeutic agents is a long-sought but frustratingly distant goal. The importance of the estrogen receptor content of a mammary tumor in determining whether endocrine therapy should be employed is the most significant advance yet made.[6] Recent work with effects of chemotherapeutic agents on clonability of human tumor cells in vitro,[7] and on the labeling index of tumor cells in vitro[8] is promising, but still short of routine clinical usefulness (see Chap. 7).

Assessment of therapeutic index may be vastly different, depending on the patient. For example, a 60-year-old, debilitated man with head and neck cancer is a less suitable candidate for *cis*-platinum(II) than a relatively healthy, 30-year-old woman with ovarian cancer: although the likelihood of a partial response may be the same, the latter individual is much less likely to have disastrous side effects.

The setting in which chemotherapy is to be used is an extremely important variable. In disseminated breast cancer, many oncologists would choose Adriamycin as a component of initial treatment. Its use in simultaneous combination with radiation therapy to the chest wall in a patient with stage III disease can produce severe local toxicity as a result of their interaction, and militates toward at least a reduction in dosage. In the treatment of patients with disease which may have been eradicated by surgery the majority of surgeons are unwilling to expose the patient to the risks of even a "little bit" of Adriamycin in many communities.

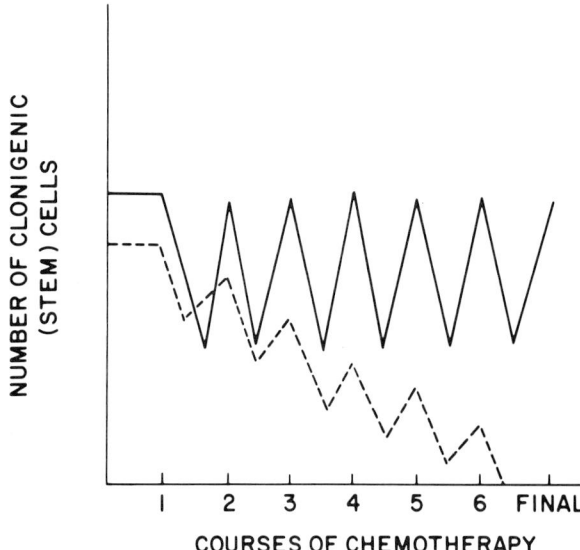

FIGURE 8-1 The basis of effective chemotherapy. ———, normal cell target population (e.g., bone marrow, gastrointestinal mucosa); – – –, tumor cell population.

PHARMACOLOGY

As with antibiotic therapy for bacterial infection, it is necessary to obtain a certain minimal inhibitory concentration (MIC) for a critical length of time (concentration

× time) to achieve tumor cell destruction. Table 8-1 demonstrates the relationship between schedule, duration of biologic effect after a single dose, peak concentration, MIC, and the concentration obtained with continuous infusion (where known) for some of the antineoplastic agents. Although the optimal schedule remains unknown or controversial for most of them, there is a clear relationship of very short biologic effect after a single dose to the efficacy of a continuous infusion, especially for agents which are S phase–specific, like Ara-C. Agents with long durations of biologic effect from a single dose, like vincristine and MGBG, are probably least effective and most dangerous on a schedule which achieves peak (potentially cumulative) concentrations on a daily basis.[9,10] Drugs with a peak concentration which is very high relative to their MIC and prolonged circulation in plasma, like methotrexate, are much more dependent on time (duration of exposure) than on concentration (at usual doses) for their toxic effects.[11] Ara-C has so short a duration of biologic effect that it is without any toxicity (except nausea) administered as a single bolus, regardless of the dose (concentration achieved).[12] The pharmacologic data suggest that there may be a clinically important threshold for concentration achieved (i.e., dose may be a crucial variable) in the case of Adriamycin. This is supported by clinical observations in sarcomas,[13] but not in all human tumors. The relationship of pharmacology to cell kinetics is more complex than might be at first supposed. For example, the apparent antitumor efficacy of high-dose, intermittent therapy with single doses of 5-FU[14] or methotrexate[15] (though these are probably not the optimal schedules for either drug) would seem to belie their cell-cycle specificity, until one takes into account that long-term intracellular binding of these agents to tumor tissue takes place. As noted, the duration of intracellular drug levels after a single dose may be a critical variable determining tumor sensitivity versus resistance.[5]

Table 8-1 refers to sites of activation, degradation, and excretion for some of the more common agents. It bears emphasis here that (1) with respect to antitumor effect peak concentration is usually less important than that achieved during the second (or third) half-life of a drug; (2) the toxicities of drugs can be profoundly influenced by the site of metabolism and excretion (e.g., the liver and Adriamycin), or the site of excretion of drug which is largely not metabolized (e.g., the kidney and methotrexate); (3) plasma concentrations (though they are what we can usually measure) are, at best, crude reflections of concentration in the critical tissues of interest; and (4) many drugs are excluded from certain parts of the body, especially the central nervous system (*pharmacologic sanctuaries*).

RESISTANCE

Resistance which develops in a few weeks or months in a tumor which was originally sensitive to chemotherapy is a problem almost as big as that of primary insensitivity. When it occurs, there is rarely any usefulness to further treatment with the agent(s) involved, and new therapy must be initiated. There are at least five potential mechanisms for drug resistance, each of which has been described in experimental systems: (1) decreased uptake of the drug;[16,17] (1) increased catabolism;[18] (3) decreased or absent activation (e.g., phosphorylation);[19] (4) increases in the level of the affected substrate or enzyme, overcoming the metabolic block;[20] and (5) increased activity of DNA repair mechanisms.[21] In clinical practice, the mechanism of resistance is almost never something which can be determined, although this could be theoretically of great utility.

Cross-resistance implies that if a tumor is resistant to one agent, it will be resistant to another, usually related in structure or mechanism of action. It is commonly believed that cross-resistance exists among the classical alkylating agents like nitrogen mustard, cyclophosphamide, and melphalan. However, some clinical[22] and experimental evidence[23] contradicts this belief. Cross-resistance is probably solid among the various thiopurines and fluorinated pyrimidines, but does not exist between streptozotocin and the other nitrosoureas.[24] Although Adriamycin and actinomycin D are cross-resistant in experimental systems, a number of the responses first seen to Adriamycin were in patients with sarcomas resistant to actinomycin D.[25] The nitrosoureas and platinum, although commonly believed to act by alkylation of DNA, are not cross-resistant with the classical alkylating agents.

PRINCIPLES OF COMBINATION CHEMOTHERAPY

The first principle of combination chemotherapy, which has been occasionally but never convincingly violated, is to select for use in combination only agents which have some evidence of activity as single drugs against the tumor to be treated. In experimental tumor systems, it is possible to define those which have antagonistic,

TABLE 8-1 Pharmacologic Interactions of Chemotherapeutic Agents

Drug	Optimal schedule in human beings*	Duration of biologic effect (single dose) in plasma	Peak concentration (single dose)	Minimal inhibitory concentration (most sensitive system)	Concentrations with continuous infusion	Activation-degradation	Excretion
Cytoxan[123–125]	NE	Minutes to hours	1×10^{-8} mol/mL; $50–100 \times 10^{-9}$ mol/mL†	$30–80 \times 10^{-9}$ mol/mL†	?	Hepatic	Renal
5-FU[126–131]	CI(?)	~30 min‡	$1–5 \times 10^{-7}$ mol/mL	10^{-9} mol/mL	1.5×10^{-9} mol/mL (variable)	Hepatic (major)	Renal (minor)
ADR[132–134]	NE	12–24‡	0.4×10^{-9} mol/mL	0.05×10^{-9} mol/mL	?	Hepatic	Hepatic, renal
MTX[135,136]	NE	24–36 h or more	$1–2 \times 10^{-9}$ mol/mL	1×10^{-11} mol/mL (L1210)	10^{-5} mol/mL§	Minimal, hepatic	Renal (major)
VCR (VBL)[137–140]	LDI(?)	Hours	4×10^{-10} mol/mL	1×10^{-11} mol/mL (L1210)	?	Hepatic (?)	Hepatic (major), renal (minor)
BLM[141,144]	LDI or CI	12–24 h‡	1–3 µg/mL	0.1 µg/mL	0.2 µg/mL = 100 mU/mL	Tissue	Renal
Ara-C[131,145]	CI	~30 min	—	0.05 µg/mL	0.1 µg/mL	Tissue (major)	Renal
Nitrosoureas[146]	HDI (?)	~90 min (mice)	¶	¶	¶	Spontaneous : liver	Renal
Thiopurines[147]	NE	~90 min‡	—	—	—	Tissue	Renal
MGBG[147–149]	LDI	>6 h	3×10^{-8} mol/mL	2×10^{-9} mol/mL	—	Minimal	Renal (major), hepatic (minor)
VP-16[150–152]	NE	>6 h	0.26 µg/mL	0.05 µg/mL	—	Uncertain	Renal; hepatic (?)
Actinomycin D[153,154]	HDI (?)	Short‡	0.1 µg/mL	0.07 µg/mL	—	Minimal	Hepatic
Mitomycin C[102,155]	HDI (?)	15–30 min	0.5–2.0 µg/mL	<1 µg/mL	—	Liver and other tissues	Renal

* HDI = high-dose intermittent; NE = not established; CI = continuous infusion; LDI = low-dose intermittent.
† Phosphoramide mustard; much lower values reported for "activated cyclophosphamide" precursors.[156]
‡ Persists in tissues.
§ Followed by citrovorum factor "rescue."
¶ Parent compounds not identified.

subadditive, additive, and synergistic effects. This is not often possible in clinical experience, although a few probable examples exist (Table 8-2).

The second principle is to minimize overlapping toxicity. Examples are the successful, synergistic combination of vincristine and prednisone in acute lymphocytic

TABLE 8-2 Clinical Drug Interactions

Type*	Example	Tumor
Synergistic	Vincristine + prednisone	ALL[157]
Additive	Vinblastine + bleomycin	Testicular[158]
Subadditive	Cyclophosphamide + methotrexate + 5-FU	Breast[159]
Antagonistic	Adriamycin + 6MP	[160]

* Synergistic: efficacy greater than expected by adding the expected single-drug effects independently. Additive: efficacy equals that of the single-drug effects, added independently (e.g., 50% response = 25% + 25%). Subadditive: efficacy greater than either alone, but less than additive. Antagonistic: efficacy less than either drug used alone (usually implies toxic interaction).

leukemia, and the additive combination of vinblastine and bleomycin in testicular cancer. Where there is significant overlapping toxicity (e.g., myelosuppression), the resultant effect is usually subadditive, as in cyclophosphamide plus methotrexate plus 5-FU (CMF) for breast cancer. This may still result in a combination which is importantly better than any of its components used singly, especially if the frequency of complete responses is increased.

A third principle, and one of relatively new origin, is the utilization of mutually non-cross-resistant combinations in intentional, alternating fashion, before development of any clinical evidence of resistance. This approach has become feasible for certain tumors (breast cancer, lymphomas, small-cell lung cancer) in which a variety of agents with different mechanisms of action now exist which have single-drug activity, with encouraging preliminary results.[26] The rationale is that this approach offers the greatest chance of eradicating cells which are potentially resistant to one combination or the other by exposing them to all possible effective agents while their number is still too small to be clinically detectable. The possible drawback is that this principle assumes collateral sensitivity to both combinations. If the tumor cell population is, in fact, sensitive to one and resistant to the other, the result could be earlier tumor regrowth than would otherwise occur.

Other ideas in combination chemotherapy with important, but controversial, status currently include (1) the use of cell kinetic manipulations to achieve "cycling" of cells into a more sensitive phase for the action of subsequently administered, "executor" agents (see Chap. 7); (2) the use of reinduction[27] or *intensification*; (3) maintenance chemotherapy; and (4) alteration of cell membrane permeability by one agent to increase the efficacy of another one subsequently administered.[28,29] The future role of these concepts remains to be determined.

DOSE RESPONSE AND THERAPEUTIC INDEX

In most experimental systems studied, there is a predictable, direct relationship between response (and curability) and the dose of effective drug(s) which is administered until doses producing appreciable lethality from toxicity are reached.[30] This is not necessarily the case in human tumors. It is possible to see responses without toxicity,[31] especially when chronic, low-dose regimens are employed, even with combination chemotherapy.[32] The prevalent view holds that high-dose, intermittent scheduling is best, both because of an assumed dose-response relationship and because it is this schedule which allows for recovery of host immunologic mechanisms to baseline levels between courses of chemotherapy. That high-dose intermittent treatment is really best is not yet proven, and may be reasonably questioned, especially in patients who have relatively resistant tumor types and are unwilling (or unable) to undergo intensive chemotherapy. Tattersall et al.[34] have reviewed this topic, with emphasis on the (current) minority view.

ADJUVANT CHEMOTHERAPY—THEORY, EXPERIMENT, AND PRACTICE

"Most cancer patients not curable by surgery or radiation (about two-thirds of all patients) are those with systemic disease when their tumor is first detected. The systemic disease in these patients is the proper target for chemotherapy and immunotherapy, because it is vulnerable to both."[35] Schabel, in a paper from which this quote is taken, summarized the results of surgical adjuvant chemotherapy in murine tumor systems. These include a number of transplantable tumors (lung, breast, colon, and melanoma), which, in the absence of therapy, are universally fatal following subcutaneous implantation. Several observations are generally applicable in all these systems: (1) Surgical cure is possible, but surgical cure rates drop as primary tumor mass at the time of surgery increases; (2) grossly evident "primary" tumors are generally not curable by drug treatment alone; (3) surgical adjuvant chemotherapy, with appropriately selected agents, can reproducibly increase the surgical cure rate, and increase the life-span of curative failures; (4) the effectiveness of drug therapy was directly related to dose and inversely related to the body burden of metastatic tumor at the time of drug treatment. The most effective drugs in the adjuvant setting were those which were effective in producing tumor regression or prolonging life-span of animals with gross metastatic disease, but lack of response to a drug of grossly apparent tumor did not preclude the efficacy of the same agent in the adjuvant setting.

These results in experimental tumor systems have furnished tremendous impetus to the design of clinical trials of adjuvant chemotherapy, and rightly so. It is important, however, to recognize that these are some fundamental differences between the experimental adjuvant therapy situation and that which obtains clinically. First, most of the tumor systems studied were high-growth fraction, transplanted tumors,[36] rather than spontaneous, low-growth fraction tumors (the usual human situation). Second, the degree of effectiveness of the antitumor agents used in the setting of far-advanced *murine* disease was often (but not always) greater than the degree of effectiveness of the antitumor agents used in the setting of far-advanced human disease. Third, many of the most striking results in the experimental systems studied involved nitrosoureas. These agents appear to be much more effective against murine than against human neoplasms, as a general rule.

Theoretically, a number of factors favor the use of chemotherapy in the surgical adjuvant setting: (1) the tumor growth fraction may be higher (a controversial concept—see Chap. 7); (2) the vascular supply and tissue oxygenation of micrometastases should be better than those of advanced lesions, which are often necrotic in some areas; and (3) the likelihood of achieving fractional reduction of the relatively small total-body tumor burden to a level with which host defenses can successfully cope, prior to development of clinical drug resistance, should be greater.

Information is still very preliminary from which to draw conclusions about the clinical practice of adjuvant chemotherapy. A few things have, however, been demonstrated. Bonadonna et al. have shown,[37] in a prospective, controlled comparison to surgery alone, that adjuvant chemotherapy improves the overall survival of women with breast cancer. This advantage, however, was confined to premenopausal patients: some kinetic reasons why this might be so are cited in Chap. 7. Disease-free survival of patients with Ewing's sarcoma[38] and osteogenic sarcoma[39,40] have almost certainly been improved by the use of adjuvant chemotherapy, although these conclusions are not quite as firm, since they depend on a comparison to historical control results. The use of single agents with a partial response rate of 20 to 30 percent in the advanced disease setting, on the other hand, has led to inconclusive results in the attempt to improve results of primary treatment for colorectal cancer and brain tumors with chemotherapy.[41,42] In lung cancer use of single agents with 10 to 15 percent rates has been a total failure.[43] There seems little doubt that the prolonged, chronic use of alkylating agents in the adjuvant setting is associated with an increased risk of carcinogenesis, especially with respect to the development of acute leukemia.[44]

A few general guidelines seem applicable to the present use of adjuvant chemotherapy. First, the patient to be treated must be in a high-risk category: it is probably not indicated to expose someone to the short-term and potential long-term side effects of presently available drugs if the odds are already 4 in 5 that he or she has been cured by local therapy. Second, there should be evidence of significant antitumor effects by the agents to be employed, in a setting of disseminated gross disease. It appears likely that this means partial response rates greater than or equal to 40 percent and complete response rates of at least 10 to 15 percent. Third (and perhaps most important), the indiscriminate use of unproven agents or combinations, in the private practice setting as adjuvant therapy, is ethically and scientifically unjustified. The place to find out whether adjuvant therapy is of value is in clinical trials, and the use of randomized controls (patients receiving standard therapy only) is much more likely to yield persuasive results than the use of historical controls. It should be remembered that the patient who fails on adjuvant therapy has failed doubly, because the treatment which would ordinarily have been chosen for any recurrent disease is one to which the tumor will be in all likelihood, already resistant.

The use of adjuvant immunotherapy is discussed elsewhere in this book (Chap. 9). With this modality, and probably also with adjuvant hormone therapy, the relative lack of toxicity of the agents being employed may lead to their justifiable use in a clinical setting where the high probability of surgical cure contraindicates chemotherapy. Previous trials of hormonal ablation in women with breast cancer on a "prophylactic" basis had negative[45] or marginally positive[46] results. However, since these trials were carried out in premenopausal women, a large proportion of whom are now known to be estrogen receptor–negative,[47] and responses to hormonal manipulation occur primarily in receptor-positive patients,[48] this is an area which deserves reevaluation.

MAJOR DRUG CLASSES— GENERAL FEATURES

Table 8-3 summarizes general features of the commonly employed cancer chemotherapeutic agents, including general class, side effects, common indications, and interactions with other drugs. Mechanisms of action are considered here briefly.

Cyclophosphamide and the other classical alkylating agents all contain electrophilic alkyl groups which can react with a variety of nucleophilic molecules within the cell, the most important of which is probably the N7 group in guanine, with resultant potential for irreversible cross-linking of the DNA molecule.[49] Internal cyclization of a bis (β-chlorethyl) grouping is essential to the biologic activity of the mustard derivatives. This takes place through formation of the highly reactive, electrophilic ethylenimonium derivative from the tertiary amine in solution, according to the following general reaction:

$$\begin{array}{c} CH_2 CH_2 Cl \\ | \\ R{-}N \\ | \\ CH_2 CH_2 Cl \end{array} \quad \longrightarrow \quad R{-}{}^+N\begin{array}{c} CH_2 \\ \diagdown \\ {-}CH_2 \\ | \\ CH_2 CH_2 Cl \end{array} + Cl^-$$

Among the nonclassical alkylating agents, the nitrosoureas have the ability to cross-link DNA,[50] to carbamylate intracellular protein,[51] and to block thymidine uptake.[52] Currently, cross-linking appears to be the most important mechanism.

Mitomycin C has alkylating potential through the presence of both a quinone and an aziridine ring.[53] An additional mechanism of action via free-radical formation (analogous to ionizing radiation) has recently been proposed for mitomycin C and Adriamycin.[54]

cis-Platinum(II) can cross-link DNA[55] but, like the nitrosoureas and mitomycin C, has a somewhat different spectrum of activity and clear activity against tumors which are resistant to the classical alkylating agents.

The mechanisms of action of DTIC and procarbazine are poorly defined, although both are tentatively listed as alkylating agents.

The DNA binders probably all sterically inhibit DNA-template replication, either of DNA and RNA (anthracyclines) or of DNA-directed RNA synthesis (actinomycin D). Other possible mechanisms of action suggested for Adriamycin include a cell membrane–specific effect.[56]

The vinca alkaloids are commonly referred to as *mitotic spindle poisons*. This is really a misnomer; a more appropriate name would be *antitubulins*, since some of their biologic effects (e.g., peripheral neuropathy, rapid lowering of peripheral blast counts) are clearly not related to antimitotic action.

VP-16 and the related podophyllotoxin derivative, VM-26, have a poorly understood mechanism of action. They inhibit entry into mitosis[57] and are probably cell-cycle specific.

All of the antimetabolites inhibit key enzymes in the synthesis of DNA, although only cytosine arabinoside and hydroxyurea are totally specific for DNA synthesis. In the clinical setting, all are probably S phase–specific, but both 5-FU and methotrexate have the potential for prolonged intracellular retention, and 6-thioguanine can be incorporated into DNA.

Bleomycin produces single-strand breaks in DNA[58] and seems to exert preferential kill against cells in G_2 and M phases of the cell cycle,[59] although, in some systems, it appears to be more effective against nonproliferating cells.[60]

MGBG may act as an inhibitor of polyamine biosynthesis.[61] L-Asparaginase acts by hydrolyzing asparagine, leading to cell death in tumor populations which lack the enzyme asparagine synthetase.[62] Unfortunately, this enzyme is present in most tumor, as well as normal, cells. The mechanism of action of hexamethylmelamine is unknown.

MANAGEMENT OF ACUTE TOXICITY OF CHEMOTHERAPEUTIC AGENTS

Myelosuppression

Several different patterns of bone marrow suppression are produced, depending on the nature of the chemotherapeutic agent. These are shown in Table 8-3. Approaches to the treatment of anemia, thrombocytopenia, and leukopenia are considered separately.

Most malignant diseases are themselves associated with "the anemia of chronic disease," a poorly understood entity for which there is no specific treatment. Those

TABLE 8-3 Cancer Chemotherapeutic Agents—General Features

		Side effects							
		Myelosuppression		Gastrointestinal toxicity					
Class	Group (agent)	Granulocytes	Platelets	Stomatitis	Nausea and vomiting	Alopecia	Other side effects	Tumors commonly treated	Interaction with other drugs
Alkylating agents	Classical: Cyclophosphamide (Cytoxan)	+	±	−	++	+	Pulmonary fibrosis,* SIADH,* hemorrhagic cystitis	Breast, lung, ovary hematologic	Synergism with Adriamycin (?)
	Melphalan (L-PAM, Alkeran)	+	+	−	+	−		Breast, ovary, myeloma	
	Chlorambucil (Leukeran)	+	+	−	±	−		Chronic lymphocytic leukemia	
	Mechlorethamine (Mustargen, nitrogen mustard)	+	+	−	+++	±	CNS,* extravasation necrosis	Hodgkin's disease, malignant effusions	
	Thiotepa	+	+	−	+	±		Breast, malignant effusions	
	Busulfan (Myleran)	+	++	−	+	−	Addison's disease*	Chronic myelocytic leukemia	
	Nonclassical: BCNU, CCNU, MeCCNU	+(delayed)	+(delayed)	−	++	−	Pulmonary fibrosis*	Brain, Hodgkin's	Antagonism with streptozotocin
Nitrosoureas	Streptozotocin	−	−	−	++	−	Renal damage	Islet-cell, carcinoid	Antagonism with other nitrosoureas
	cis-Platinum(II) (DDP, platinum)	+	+	−	+++	−	Anaphylaxis,* renal damage, hearing loss, peripheral neuropathy	Testicular (germ-cell), lung, ovary, prostate, bladder	Synergism with Adriamycin, other alkylating agents (?)
	Mitomycin C	+	++	−	+	−	Glomerulonephritis,* extravasation necrosis	Lung, gastric, breast, colorectal	May potentiate Adriamycin cardiac toxicity
	DTIC (dimethyltriazeno imidazole carboxamide, DIC)	+(20%)	++(20%)	−	+++	−	Flulike syndrome	Melanoma, sarcoma	Synergism with Adriamycin (sarcomas)
	Procarbazine	+	+	−	+	−		Hodgkin's, brain	Toxicity potentiated by MAO inhibitors
DNA-binders (intercalators)	Anthracyclines: Adriamycin (Doxorubicin)	+	±	±(schedule-dependent)	++	+++	Cardiomyopathy (dose-related),* extravasation necrosis	Lung, breast, hematologic, sarcomas, ovary, bladder, prostate	Synergism with several; antagonism with thiopurines
	Daunorubicin	+	±	±	++	+++	Same as for Adriamycin	Acute leukemia	
	Rubidazone	+	±	±	++	+++	Same as for Adriamycin	Acute leukemia	
	Actinomycin D	+	+	+	++	+	Extravasation necrosis, dermatitis	Wilms's testicular, melanoma	May potentiate Adriamycin cardiac toxicity

TABLE 8-3 Cancer Chemotherapeutic Agents—General Features (cont.)

Class	Group (agent)	Myelosuppression		Gastrointestinal toxicity		Alopecia	Other side effects	Tumors commonly treated	Interaction with other drugs
		Granulocytes	Platelets	Stomatitis	Nausea and vomiting				
	Mithramycin	+	+ +	±	+ +	+	Hemorrhagic diathesis	Testicular, Paget's disease (bone)	
	AMSA (Cain's acridine)	+	+	–	–	–	?	?	
Plant products	Vinca alkaloids:						Extravasation necrosis		
	Vincristine	–	–	Rare	–	+	Peripheral neuropathy, constipation, SIADH*	Lung, breast, hematologic, childhood solid tumors	Synergism with prednisone (ALL)
	Vinblastine	+	+	+	+	+	Myalgias, glossitis, neuropathy, constipation	Testicular, renal, Hodgkin's, histiocytosis X	Additive with bleomycin (testicular cancer)
	VP-16	+	+	–	±	±	Hypotension	Lung, testicular	
Antimetabolites	5-FU, FUdR	+	+	+ (Especially with continuous infusion)	+	–	Cerebellar ataxia, diarrhea	Colorectal, gastric, ovary, bladder; other adenocarcinoma	
	Ftorafur	±	±	+	+	–	Confusion, ataxia	Colorectal, other adenocarcinomas	
	Methotrexate (Amethopterin, MTX)	+	+	+ +	±	–	Cirrhosis* (chronic), pulmonary fibrosis,* hepatitis, dermatitis, conjunctivitis, renal damage (high dose)	Head and neck, ALL, lung (oat-cell), breast, sarcoma, bladder	

tumors in which there is replacement of normal marrow by tumor cells may cause anemia on a *myelophthisic* basis. Thus, the evaluation of anemia as drug-induced is complicated. Regardless of the cause, the treatment is the same: transfusion, usually with packed red cells. Patients who have been chronically anemic will frequently tolerate a hemoglobin in the 7 range without significant symptomatology. Those who have an acute drop in hemoglobin to less than 9, particularly in the older age group where underlying cardiovascular diseases may be unmasked, should in general be transfused as required to maintain a hemoglobin of 9 to 10. Unless a specific cause can be demonstrated, the use of hematinics or anabolic steroids is not indicated.

As with anemia, the patient who is chronically thrombocytopenic (e.g., with acute leukemia) may tolerate a modest further decrease in platelets without significant bleeding problems. On the other hand, the patient with a solid tumor who has a daily halving of the platelet count as a result of chemotherapy should be hospitalized for observation and possible transfusion at a level of 50,000 per milliliter or so, until one can be certain that the nadir has been reached and the danger is past. As a general rule, prophylactic transfusion of platelets is indicated below levels of 20,000 per milliliter. Therapeutic platelet transfusion is indicated in the presence of bleeding, even at somewhat higher levels.[63] However, bleeding is unlikely to be due to thrombocytopenia per se at levels of 50,000 per milliliter or higher; disseminated intravascular coagulation or some other reason should

TABLE 8-3 Cancer Chemotherapeutic Agents—General Features (cont.)

		Side effects							
		Myelosuppression		Gastrointestinal toxicity					
Class	Group (agent)	Granulocytes	Platelets	Stomatitis	Nausea and vomiting	Alopecia	Other side effects	Tumors commonly treated	Interaction with other drugs
	Cytosine arabinoside (Ara-C)	+	+	−	+	−	Fever (rare)	AML	
	Hydroxyurea	+	+	−	−	−		Chronic myelocytic leukemia	
	PALA	−	−	+	+	?		?	
	6MP, 6TG (6-mercaptopurine, 6-thioguanine)	+	+	−	±	−	Hepatitis	Acute leukemia	Potentiated by allopurinol
Other compounds	Bleomycin	−	−	+	−	−	Hemolysis (continuous infusion), pulmonary fibrosis (dose-related), dermatosis, Bullous dermatitis*	Testicular, Hodgkin's, head and neck, lung	Additive with vinblastine (testicular cancer)
	MGBG (methyl GAG)	±	±	+	−	−	Esophagitis, hypoglycemia, vasculitis	Bladder, esophagus, colorectal	
	L-Asparaginase	−	−	−	+	−	Hemorrhagic pancreatitis, coma,* hemorrhage, hyperglycemia, anaphylaxis	ALL	Allows increased dosage of sequenced methotrexate
	Hexamethylmelamine	+	+	−	++	−	Peripheral neuropathy	Lung (oat-cell), ovary	

* Rare but potentially fatal.
Note: ALL = acute lymphocytic leukemia. AML = acute myelocytic leukemia. SiADH = syndrome of inappropriate ADH secretion.

be considered instead. The use of agents like vincristine to stimulate platelet production has been suggested, and appears to be of proven value in idiopathic thrombocytopenic purpura.[64] Whether it will have any role in management of drug-induced thrombocytopenia remains to be determined, but seems less likely.

Lymphocytes are depressed earlier, and reappear sooner in the peripheral blood, than granulocytes.[65] Many patients with cancer have lymphopenia as part of their underlying disease process, apart from any effects of specific treatment.[66] It does not appear at present that the infections related to leukopenia are related to suppression of lymphocyte function, but rather, in most cases, to suppression of granulocyte function. In patients with underlying solid tumors, the infections associated with leukopenia are usually bacterial, and granulocyte transfusions are seldom necessary, although with more intensive approaches to certain diseases (e.g., ovary, breast, small-cell lung cancer) their role may increase. Recent work by Stein et al.[67] and others[68,69] suggests that lithium may be a useful agent in the amelioration of chemotherapy-induced granulocytopenia, apparently through a direct stimulatory effect on bone marrow stem cells. Current trials in several research centers should resolve the question of whether lithium use can actually prevent infections in some patients who would otherwise develop them. It must be emphasized that lithium is an experimental drug for this use, and has its own protean side effects: patients receiving the drug should have blood levels of lithium monitored on a regular basis.[70] Although the glucocorticoids produce an increase in circulating white blood cells, this is not the result of bone marrow stimulation, but of release from the marginating pool.[71] They are not indicated in the treatment of drug-induced leukopenia, and may even be harmful due to their immunosuppressive and other side effects.

In any patient with persistent "myelosuppression" after chemotherapy, the physician must reevaluate the possibility that the depressed counts have another basis, like bone marrow infiltration by tumor, splenomegaly, or disseminated intravascular coagulation.

Experimental approaches to the treatment and even prevention of the complications of drug-induced myelosuppression include "prophylactic" white blood cell transfusions[72] and autologous marrow reinfusion.[73] The latter approach may have special utility in the setting where drugs producing delayed onset of myelosuppression are employed.[74]

Gastrointestinal Side Effects

Anorexia and, less commonly, nausea or vomiting are general concomitants of the malignant process itself in many patients, again making the assessment of drug-induced effects of this type complicated. Sedation before and during chemotherapy administration may be useful with some patients, particularly those who have developed vomiting as a conditioned response to the sight of the offending drug. The use of intravenous hyperalimentation has, among other things, been reported to reduce the frequency and severity of nausea and vomiting.[75] This requires further evaluation, as does the possible use of enteral alimentation with a continuous infusion, rather than bolus, approach.[76] Although as a general rule glucocorticoids should be avoided, they can reverse anorexia and produce appetite stimulation in some terminal patients, and many oncologists employ them judiciously in this setting.

Stomatitis is frequently the dose-limiting toxicity of methotrexate. It is also common with 5-FU, bleomycin, high-dose vinblastine (with which painful glossitis may predominate), and Adriamycin, especially if the latter drug is given on a schedule of daily administration for 3 to 5 days.[77] If due to methotrexate, early oral ulceration may be responsive to the administration of citrovorum factor (calcium leukovorin) as a mouthwash, without compromise of systemic drug effectiveness,[78] at least with high methotrexate doses. Due to other causes, it is best treated by (1) discontinuation of the offending agent(s) until the ulcerations have cleared completely; (2) good oral hygiene; and (3) the liberal use of viscous xylocaine. If the lips are the major site of involvement, it is better to apply the viscous xylocaine as an ointment; if the oral pharynx, to use a mouthwash containing viscous xylocaine, with or without other ingredients such as diphenhydramine (Benadryl) and magnesium—aluminum hydroxide antacids.

Esophagitis is rarely seen with any drug used alone unless generalized mucositis is present, or there is concomitant radiation therapy to a field involving the esophagus. Under these circumstances, Adriamycin may be a particular offender.[79] Methylgloyoxal bisguanylhydrazone (MGBG, methyl GAG) is an exception: esophagitis may be the only manifestation of drug toxicity.[80] The treatment of esophagitis is similar to that of stomatitis involving the oral pharynx. It is well to remember that pain on swallowing can also be due to candidal esophagitis, especially in the leukemic patient: a barium swallow and/or esophagoscopy may be indicated to rule out this possibility.

Like esophagitis, symptomatic proctitis is rarely seen in the absence of generalized mucositis or concomitant local radiation therapy with the exception of 5-FU and the other fluorinated pyrimidines. There is no useful local therapy, other than stool softeners and good anal care.

Under some conditions, mucositis is an indication for hospitalization, especially if there is associated leukopenia: the combination of the two increases the likelihood of sepsis from the patient's own gut flora. The conditions include (1) confluent oral ulceration, with or without oral bleeding or fever; (2) inability to swallow liquids (in general, these patients also handle their secretions poorly), and (3) loose stools in a frequency of six or more per day, and/or bloody diarrhea or prolapsed hemorrhoids associated with proctitis. Intravenous fluids and close monitoring of vital signs and electrolytes are indicated in all such patients.

One drug, vincristine (and occasionally its relative, vinblastine), produces constipation, really by effects on the autonomic nervous system rather than the gastrointestinal tract directly. This is best treated by prophylaxis with stool softeners, a bulk laxative such as methyl cellulose (Metamucil) or milk of magnesia at bedtime. If high colonic impaction develops associated with obstipation, the patient may require hospitalization and supportive care.

L-Asparaginase is the only chemotherapeutic agent which produces pancreatitis. When it occurs, the pancreatitis is usually symptomatic and frequently hemorrhagic; it may be fatal.[81] Routine monitoring of serum amylase is indicated in all patients receiving L-asparaginase. The drug should be discontinued if the amylase become abnormal or the patient develops symptoms suggesting pancreatitis. Immediate hospitalization and care as for any other form of acute pancreatitis is indicated.

Cyclocytidine, an analogue of cytosine arabinoside, produces transient jaw pain associated with sialadenitis. The same symptom (though probably not from the same cause) is occasionally seen with the vinca alkaloids. No specific therapy is indicated.

Hepatitis of clinical significance is, fortunately, an unusual complication of chemotherapy for cancer, although many of the agents will produce transient, mild elevation of liver enzymes shortly after administration. In patients with preexisting serious liver disease, methotrexate can rarely produce fatal hepatitis. The cirrhosis which develops in some patients on long-term, daily methotrexate is a complication of chronic use.[82] Thiopurines and the sex steroids may produce jaundice, usually of the self-limited, "cholestatic" type. Although Adriamycin itself is not hepatotoxic, its use in combination with thiopurines like 6-mercaptopurine (6MP) may produce serious hepatic damage.[83] The same observation has been made for the combination of two nitrosoureas which normally produce only "chemical" hepatitis, streptozotocin, and BCNU.[84]

Pulmonary Damage

Bleomycin produces at least two pathologically different forms of lung damage, either of which may present acutely as dyspnea, hypoxia, and diffuse interstitial disease.[85] One form, an acute hypersensitivity pneumonitis, is usually steroid responsive, and may be characterized by eosinophilia, while the other, with a pattern characterized by early fibrotic changes, is not. Because it is clinically difficult to determine which type is involved, short of a lung biopsy, a therapeutic trial of steroids is indicated in most patients who develop this potentially fatal complication. Patients who receive a total dose in excess of 200 units/m^2, and/or are in excess of 70 years of age, are more likely to develop it.[86]

Other chemotherapeutic agents, especially busulfan,[87] nitrosoureas,[88] and methotrexate, occasionally produce idiosyncratic, diffuse interstitial fibrosis. Although usually seen after repeated administration of the drug, this is not a clearly dose-related phenomenon. With the alkylating agents, it is rarely reversible. In the case of methotrexate, the lesion may be primarily cellular and reversible, or fibrous and irreversible: its responsiveness to steriods is controversial.[89]

Cardiac Damage

Adriamycin and the related anthracycline antibiotics are the agents in common clinical use which produce heart damage. This usually presents as the acute onset of congestive heart failure, and is almost universally confined to patients who have received a total Adriamycin dose greater than or equal to 450 mg/m^2 (or its equivalent). It may be more likely to occur in patients with concomitant chest irradiation,[90] or coadministration of other DNA-binding drugs like actinomycin D[91] and mitomycin C.[92] Although the original cases observed were almost always fatal, many cases which develop in patients who receive a total dose of less than 600 mg/m^2 are clinically reversible with vigorous therapy for congestive heart failure. The incidence of cardiomyopathy may be reduced by giving the drug on a weekly schedule, rather than as higher doses less frequently.[93]

Intense current interest centers on the possibility of preventing Adriamycin heart damage. One British study suggests the usefulness of prophylactic digitalis glycosides,[94] although experimentally these did not look promising in animals. The use of vitamin E derivatives also appears of interest,[95] although commercially available preparations of this vitamin are definitely ineffective and may be dangerous if taken in large doses.

Sangivamycin, ethidium chloride, and the interferon inducer poly IC are other chemotherapeutic agents with potential cardiac toxicity in human beings. None is in common clinical use.

Renal Damage

cis-Platinum(II) is, like other heavy metals, a nephrotoxin. A variety of approaches have been taken in attempts to prevent or decrease this side effect, including (1) prehydration for 12 to 24 h with intravenous saline and no diuresis[96]; (2) similar prehydration with the use of mannitol and/or furosemide diuresis at the time of platinum administration[97,98]; and (3) the weekly administration of low doses without specific measures except outpatient hydration. At present, it is not clear which of these methods will ultimately find greatest favor in the oncologic community. But, regardless of the measures employed, some degree of renal damage seems inevitable. The typical patient will tolerate three or four courses of induction therapy for testicular carcinoma before renal damage becomes dose-limiting. Gentamicin-cephalothin therapy potentiates the nephrotoxicity of *cis*-platinum and should be avoided in patients receiving this drug.

Streptozotocin is the other chemotherapeutic agent in common use which produces direct, predictable renal damage.[100,101] It is related to both glomerular and tubular effects and appears to be unaffected by the use of any diuretic or hydration techniques.

Mitomycin C rarely produces glomerulonephritis, sometimes in a clinical setting which suggests Goodpasture's syndrome. This should be treated by permanent discontinuation of the drug. It may be related to the administration of higher total doses.[102] Methotrexate in very high concentrations, such as those achieved by the high-dose programs with citrovorum rescue, can be directly nephrotoxic: this complication can be at least partially prevented by alkalinization of the urine.[103]

Hemorrhagic cystitis is a relatively uncommon complication of cyclophosphamide administration, but occurs much more frequently with its congener, ifosfamide.[104] It can be minimized by adequate hydration of the patient during and immediately after chemotherapy. Many oncologists will switch to another alkylating agent after one episode of hemorrhagic cystitis from cyclophosphamide, since it is a complication with life-threatening potential.

Nervous System Toxicity

Several chemotherapeutic agents can produce a metabolic encephalopathy manifesting as obtundation or even coma. These include L-asparaginase, methotrexate (especially when given intrathecally in a setting of prior systemic methotrexate and cranial irradiation),[105] 6-azauracil, and high-dose intravenous procarbazine.[106] In each case, as with the rare steroid or asparaginase-induced psychosis, the abnormality is entirely reversible upon discontinuation of the drug. In the case of L-asparaginase, however, this may take several days.

Peripheral neuropathy is regularly produced by vincristine and occasionally by vinblastine.[107] It is slowly reversible upon discontinuation of the drug, often incompletely. Exercise has been suggested as a possible factor in lessening this side effect.[108] *cis*-Platinum(II) and hexamethylmelamine also can cause peripheral neuropathy. It is relatively rare with the former,[109] and common with the latter.[110] Whether the administration of pyridoxine affects the action of hexamethylmelamine remains unproven, but it does not seem to have any effect on the drug's antitumor properties. Rarely, vincristine can produce other effects, such as the syndrome of inappropriate ADH secretion[107] or cranial nerve palsies. Other causes should be ruled out before one of these phenomena is attributed to the drug.

Cerebellar ataxia accompanies the administration of 5-FU in less than 5 percent of cases. Central nervous system toxicity with the analogue, ftorafur, is much more common, with lethargy and confusion prominent.[111] Improvement is prompt when the drug is discontinued.

Skin and Integument

Several agents can produce severe local tissue necrosis if they are extravasated, including Adriamycin, vincristine, vinblastine, actinomycin D, mitomycin C, and nitrogen mustard. An ounce of prevention is truly worth a pound of cure for this complication. Care should be taken to inject the agent only into a freshly started, freely running infusion, or to use the two-syringe technique if this is preferred. If possible, the dorsa of the hands and feet should be avoided, since these areas are in close proximity to superficial tendons. Under no circumstances should one of these drugs be left to infuse slowly from an IV bag or bottle without personal supervision by the nurse or physician. Any of these agents, and some which do not produce soft tissue necrosis (e.g., 5-FU), may also produce local phlebitis along the course of the injected vein. This is especially true of 5-FU given by continuous infusion. In the latter case, the addition of heparin or a small amount of hydrocortisone may reduce the associated phlebitis. Routine flushing of the IV line with saline or D5W is the most helpful measure that can be taken after drug administration to minimize venous irritation.

Bleomycin routinely produces a dose-related form of generalized skin damage,[112] clinically manifest as hyperpigmentation, induration, and erythema (especially over extensor surfaces and pressure points), and sometimes progressing to the formation of vesicles or bullae. The latter complication may be more common in black individuals. Early signs of bleomycin skin toxicity are often tenderness, induration, and erythema of the fingertips and toes. If progression to vesicles or bullae occurs, the drug should be at least temporarily discontinued. Steroids do not seem to be helpful. There is no clear-cut relationship between severity of skin toxicity and the likelihood of lung damage. Nail changes, including thickening and longitudinal banding, may be seen with several agents, including bleomycin, Adriamycin, and 5-FU.

Dermatitis, usually a generalized erythroderma but sometimes progressing to frank exfoliation, can occur as a "hypersensitivity" or radiation recall phenomenon related to the administration of several drugs, notably methotrexate. It is usually quickly reversible when the drug is discontinued. Less commonly a serositis involving the pleura or pericardium may complicate the use of methotrexate, actinomycin D,[113] or Adriamycin, in a patient with prior mediastinal irradiation. Actinomycin D causes a peculiar acneiform eruption resembling that seen with therapeutic iodide administration; this is also self-limiting. If pustular, it may require the usual measures directed at acne for control.

Methylglyoxal bis-guanylhydrazone has a variety of side effects involving the skin, apparently the result of vasculitis, when administered in relatively high doses on a 5-day schedule.[114] These include furuncles, pyoderma gangrenosum, ulceration, and even autoamputation of the fingertips, toes, and penis. Such complications have not been observed with weekly administration of the drug at a lower dose.[115] There is no effective treatment known.

Miscellaneous Toxicities

Lacrimal gland irritation, producing a sensation of burning and dry eyes, has been reported with 5-FU.[116] Conjunctivitis may be seen with methotrexate.[117] Neither requires specific therapy, but the use of methylcellulose drops ("artificial tears") may give temporary relief.

Weakness is a frequent complaint of the patient with cancer, often seeming to be made worse by the therapy. It is a particularly common complaint after Adriamycin, and may be related to the drug's ability to damage skeletal as well as cardiac muscle.[118]

Hyperglycemia, and occasionally acidosis, can be produced in some patients by the administration of L-asparaginase. Streptozotocin can produce the same effects by its inhibitory action on the pancreatic β cells. If hyperglycemia develops with one of these drugs, or in association with glucocorticoid administration, the diabetic syndrome should be managed accordingly. It is not usually severe and generally reversible when the drug is stopped. Only one chemotherapeutic agent, MGBG, produces hypoglycemia as a complication.[114] With current modes of administration, this complication is unusual; but special care must be taken to monitor blood sugar if the patient is receiving concomitant insulin, sulfonylurea, or propranolol therapy.

The administration of L-asparaginase produces a profoundly hypofibrinogenemic state, which occasionally results in bleeding, although the drug is not myelosuppressive. This is usually not of clinical significance.[119] The hemorrhagic diathesis produced by mithramycin, especially on the older daily schedule used in testicular cancer, can be disastrous. There is no specific or effective treatment. It can, however, be largely prevented by use of an alternate-day schedule of administration, careful attention to prodromal symptoms such as facial flushing after the drug is administered, and monitoring of the SGOT and LDH prior to each dose.[120]

Anaphylaxis can occur after administration of L-asparaginase and should be treated accordingly. This means having epinephrine, diphenhydramine, steroids, and the necessary facilities for intubation available whenever the drug is given. If anaphylaxis occurs, the same preparation of asparaginase should not be given again; one derived from a different bacterial source may be utilized.[121] Very rarely, anaphylactic reactions have been reported after the administration of other antineoplastic agents, especially *cis*-platinum(II)[122] and bleomycin (in lymphoma patients).

Reversible orthostatic hypotension can occur with rapid administration of VP-16 (epipodophyllotoxin derivative) or MGBG. It may be prevented by prolonging the period of infusion to at least 30 min.

Fever is very common in the evening after bleomycin administration, rarely accompanied by a chilling sensation. It may be effectively treated by aspirin, acetaminophen, or prednisone. Methotrexate and cytosine arabinoside rarely cause fever as a reproducible, idiosyncratic reaction. This, too, should be treated conservatively after ruling out an infectious cause.

REFERENCES

1. Livingston RB, Hart JS: The clinical applications of cell kinetics in cancer therapy. *Annu Rev Pharmacol Toxicol* 17: 529, 1977.

2. Livingston, RB et al: Cell kinetic parameters: Correlation with clinical response, in B Drewinko, RM Humphrey (eds): *Growth Kinetics and Biochemical Regulation of Normal and Malignant Cells (The University of Texas System Cancer Center M.D. Anderson Hospital and Tumor Institute 29th Annual Symposium on Fundamental Cancer Research, 1976)*, Williams & Wilkins, Baltimore, pp 767–785, 1977.
3. Rosenoff et al: The effect of chemotherapy on the kinetics and proliferative capacity of normal and tumorous tissues in vivo. *Blood* 45:107, 1975.
4. Rosenoff S et al: Recovery of normal hematopoietic tissue and tumor following chemotherapeutic injury from cyclophosphamide.. *Blood* 45:465, 1975.
5. Klubes P et al: Effects of 5-fluorouracil on 5-fluorodeoxyuridine 5'-monophosphate and 2-deoxyuridine 5'-monophosphate pools, and DNA synthesis in solid mouse L1210 and rat Walker 256 tumors. *Cancer Res* 38:235, 1978.
6. McGuire WL: Hormone receptors: Their role in predicting prognosis and response to endocrine therapy. *Semin Oncol* 5:428–433, 1978.
7. Salmon SE et al: Quantitation of differential sensitivity of human-tumor stem cells to anticancer drugs. *N Engl J Med* 298:1321, 1978.
8. Livingston, RB: In vitro prediction of chemotherapy response. *Clin Res* 26:776a, 1978.
9. Carey RW et al. A comparison of two dosage regimens for vincristine. *Cancer Chemother Rep* 27:91, 1963.
10. Regelson W, Holland JF: Clinical experience with methylglyoxal bis(guanylhydrazone) dihydrochloride: A new agent with clinical activity in acute myelocytic leukemia and the lymphomas. *Cancer Chemother Rep* 27:15, 1963.
11. Vogler WR et al: Toxicity and antitumor effect of divided doses of methotrexate. *Arch Intern Med* 115:285, 1965.
12. Frei E III et al: Dose schedule and antitumor studies of arabinosyl cytosine. *Cancer Res* 19:1325, 1969.
13. O'Bryan RM et al: Dose response evaluation of Adriamycin in human neoplasia. *Cancer* 39:1940, 1977.
14. Ahmann DL et al: A controlled evaluation of 5-fluorouracil utilizing a single injection technique. *Oncology* 29:166, 1974.
15. Condit PT et al: Studies on the folic acid vitamins mVH: —The effects of large doses of amethopterin in patients with cancer. *Cancer Res* 22:706, 1962.
16. Bertino JR, Skeel RT: Resistance to folic acid antagonists: Clinical aspects. *Biochem Pharmacol [Suppl] #2*:101, 1974.
17. Klatt O et al: The effect of nitrogen mustard treatment on the deoxyribonucleic acid of sensitive and resistant Ehrlich tumor cells. *Cancer Res* 29:286, 1969.
18. Steuart CD, Burke PJ: Cytidine deaminase and the development of resistance to arabinosyl cytosine. *Nature [New Biol]* 233:109, 1971.
19. Kreis W et al: Characterization of protein and DNA in P815 cells sensitive and resistant to 1-β-D-arabinofuranosylcytosine. *Cancer Res* 32:696, 1972.
20. Hanggi UJ, Littlefield JW: Altered regulation of the rate of synthesis of dihydrofolate reductase in methotrexate-resistant hamster cells. *J. Biol Chem* 251:3075, 1976.
21. Fox BW: DNA repair and tumour resistance. *Br J Cancer* 29:410, 1974.
22. Benjamin RS et al: A comparison of cyclophosphamide, vincristine, and prednisone with nitrogen mustard, vincristine, procarbazine, and prednisone in the treatment of nodular, poorly differentiated, lymphocytic lymphoma. *Cancer* 38:1896, 1976.
23. Schabel FM Jr et al: Patterns of resistance and therapeutic synergism among alkylating agents. *Antibiot Chem* 23: 200–215, 1978.
24. Schein PS et al: Clinical antitumor activity and toxicity of streptozotocin. *Cancer* 34:993, 1974.
25. Gottlieb J: Personal communication.
26. Cohen MH et al: Cyclic alternating complication chemotherapy of small cell bronchogenic carcinoma. *Proc AACR-ASCO* 10:359, 1978.
27. Bodey GP et al: Late intensification therapy for acute leukemia in remission. *JAMA* 235:1021, 1976.
28. Pouillart P et al: Sequential administration of two oncostatic drugs: Study of modalities for pharmacodynamic potentiation. *Biomedicine* 21:471, 1974.
29. Medoff J et al: Amphotericin B–induced sensitivity to actinomycin D in drug-resistant HeLa cella. *Cancer Res* 35: 2548, 1975
30. Skipper HE et al: Implications of biochemical, cytokinetic, pharmacologic, and toxicologic relationships in the design of optimal therapeutic schedules. *Cancer Chemother Rep* 54: 431, 1970.
31. Bross LDJ et al: Is toxicity really necessary? II. Source and analysis of data. *Cancer* 19:1785, 1966.
32. Foley JF et al: Low dosage methotrexate and cyclophosphamide for solid tumors. *Cancer Chemother Rep* 54:41, 1970.
33. Hersh EM et al: Host defense, chemical immunosuppression, and the transplant recipient. Relative effects of intermittent versus continuous immunosuppressive therapy with reference to the objects of treatment. *Transplant Proc* 5:1191–95, 1973.
34. Tattersall MHN, Tobias JS: How strong is the case for intensive cancer chemotherapy? *Lancet* 2:1071, 1976.
35. Schabel FM Jr: Surgical adjuvant chemotherapy of metastatic murine tumors. *Cancer* 40:558–568, 1977.
36. Hart JS et al: Neoplasia, kinetics, and chemotherapy. *Semin Oncol* 3:259, 1976.
37. Bonadonna G et al: Improvement of disease-free and overall survival by adjuvant CMF in operable breast cancer. *Proc AACR-ASCO* 19:215, 1978.
38. Rosen et al: Curability of Wring's sarcoma and considerations for future therapeutic trials. *Cancer* 41:888, 1978.
39. Frei et al: Adjuvant chemotherapy of osteogenic sarcoma: Progress and perspectives. *J. Natl Cancer Inst* 60:3, 1978.
40. Sutow WW et al: Adjuvant chemotherapy in primary treatment of osteogenic sarcoma. *Cancer* 36:1598, 1975.

41. Higgins GA et al: The case for adjuvant 5-fluorouracil in colorectal cancer. *Cancer Clin Trials* 1:35, 1978.
42. Brisman R et al: Adjuvant nitrosourea therapy for glioblastoma. *Arch Neurol* 33:745, 1976.
43. Livingston RB: Combined modality approaches in lung cancer, in SE Salmon, SE Jones (eds): *Adjuvant Therapy of Cancer*, Elsevier/North Holland, Amsterdam, pp. 191–205, 1977.
44. Lerner HJ.: Acute myelogenous leukemia in patients receiving chlorambucil as long-term adjuvant chemotherapy for stage II breast cancer. *Cancer Treat Rep* 62:1135, 1978.
45. Radvin RG et al: Results of a clinical trial concerning the worth of prophylactic oophorectomy for breast cancer. *Surg Gynecol Obstet* 131:1055, 1970.
46. Meakin JW et al: Ovarian irradiation and prednisone following surgery for carcinoma of the breast, in SE Salmon, SE Jones (eds): *Adjuvant Therapy of Cancer*, Elsevier/North Holland, Amsterdam, 95, 1977.
47. McGuire WL et al: Estrogen receptors in human breast cancer: An overview in WL McGuire et al (eds): *Estrogen Receptors in Human Breast Cancer*, Raven Press, New York, pp 1–7, 1975.
48. McGuire WL et al: Current status of estrogen and progesterone receptors in breast cancer. *Cancer* 39:2934, 1977.
49. Kohn KW et al: Interstrand cross-linking of DNA by nitrogen mustard. *J Mol Biol* 19:266, 1966.
50. Thomas CB et al: DNA cross-linking by in vivo treatment with 1-(2-chloroethyl)-3-(4-methylcyclohexyl)-1-nitrosourea of sensitive and resistant human colon carcinoma xenografts in nude mice. *Cancer Res* 38:2448, 1978.
51. Wheeler GP et al: Carbamylation of amino acids, peptides, and proteins by nitrosoureas. *Cancer Res* 35:2974, 1975.
52. Connors TA, Hare JR: Studies of the mechanism of action of the tumour-inhibitory nitrosoureas. *Biochem Pharmacol* 24:2133, 1975.
53. Tomasz M et al: The mode of interaction of mitomycin C with deoxyribonucleic acid and other polynucleotides in vitro. *Biochemistry* 13:4878, 1974.
54. Bachur NR et al: A general mechanism for microsomal activation of quinone anticancer agents to free radicals. *Cancer Res* 38:1745, 1978.
55. Roberts JJ, Pascoe JM: Cross-linking of complementary strands of DNA in mammalian cells by antitumour platinum compounds (letter). *Nature* 235:282, 1972.
56. Murphree SA et al: Effects of Adriamycin on surface properties of sarcoma 180 ascites cells. *Biochem Pharmacol* 25:1227, 1976.
57. Krishan A *et al*: Cytofluorometric studies on the action of podophyllotoxin and epipodophyllotoxins (VM 26, VP 16-213) on the cell cycle traverse of human lymphoblasts. *J Cell Biol* 66:521, 1975.
58. Haide CW: Fragmentation of deoxyribonucleic acid by bleomycin. *Mol Pharmacol* 7:645, 1971.
59. Barranco SC, Humphrey RM: The effects of bleomycin survival and cell progression in Chinese hamster cells in vitro. *Cancer Res* 31:1218, 1971.
60. Fujimoto M et al: Intracellular distribution of [^{14}C]bleomycin and the cytokinetic effects of bleomycin in the mouse tumor. *Cancer Res* 36:2248, 1976.
61. Corti A, Dave C: Specific inhibition of the enzymatic decarboxylation of 5-adenosylmethionine by methylglyoxal bis(guanylhydrazone) and related substances. *Biochem J* 139:351, 1974.
62. Cooney DA, Handschumacher RE: L-Asparaginase and L-asparagine metabolism. *Annu Rev Pharmacol* 10:421, 1970.
63. Platelet Transfusion Subcommittee of the Acute Leukemia Task Force: Platelet transfusion procedures. *Cancer Chemother Rep* (part 3) 1:1, 1968.
64. Ahn YS et al: Vincristine therapy of idiopathic and secondary thrombocytopenias. *N Engl J Med* 291:376, 1974.
65. Hersh EM et al: Chemotherapy, immunocompetence, immunosuppression, and prognosis in acute leukemia. *N Engl J Med* 285:1211, 1971.
66. Herberman RB: Immunologic approaches to the diagnosis of cancer. *Cancer* 37:549, 1976.
67. Stein RS et al: Lithium carbonate attenuation of chemotherapy-induced neutropenia. *N Engl J Med* 297:430, 1977.
68. Greco FA, Brereton HD: Effect of lithium carbonate on the neutropenia caused by chemotherapy: A preliminary clinical trial. *Oncology* 34:153, 1977.
69. Rothstein G et al: Effect of lithium on neutrophil mass and production. *New Engl J Med* 298:178–180, 1978.
70. Baldessarini RJ, Lipinski Jf: Lithium salts: 1970–1975. *Ann Intern Med* 83:527, 1975.
71. Bishop CR et al: The mechanism of cortisol-induced granulocytosis. *Clin Res* 15: 1967.
72. Tobias JS et al: Prophylactic granulocyte support in experimental septicemia. *Blood* 47:473, 1976.
73. Tobias JS, Tattersall HN: Perspectives in cancer research: Autologous marrow support and intensive chemotherapy in cancer patients. *Eur J Cancer* 12:1, 1976.
74. Stevens EE, Dicke KA: Bone marrow transfusion in mice treated with BCNU. *Proc AACR-ASCO* 17:57, 1976.
75. Issell BF et al: Protection of chemotherapy toxicities by intravenous hyperalimentation. *Proc AACR-ASCO* 19:149, 1978.
76. Page CP et al: Continual catheter administration of an elemental diet. *Surg Gynecol Obstet* 142:184, 1976.
77. Middleman E et al: Clinical trials with Adriamycin. *Cancer* 28:844, 1971.
78. Bruckner HW, Bertino JR: Absorption of leucovorin from a "mouthwash." *Cancer Chemother Rep* 59:575, 1975.
79. Greco FA et al: Adriamycin and enhanced radiation reaction in normal esophagus and skin. *Ann Intern Med* 85:294, 1976.
80. Knight WA et al: Phase I–II trial of methyl/GAG: A South West Oncology Group pilot study. *Cancer Treat Rep* 63: 1933–1937, 1979.

81. Whitecar JP et al: L-Asparaginase. *N Engl J Med* 282:732, 1970.
82. Roenigk HH et al: Hepatoxicity of methotrexate in treatment of psoriasis. *Arch Dermatol* 103:205, 1971.
83. Minow RA et al: Clinicopathologic correlation of liver damage in patients treated with 6-mercaptopurine and Adriamycin. *Cancer* 38:1524, 1976.
84. Lokich JJ et al: Hepatic toxicity of nitrosourea analogues. *Clin Pharmacol Ther* 16:363, 1974.
85. Holoye PY et al: Bleomycin hypersensitivity pneumonitis. *Ann Intern Med* 88:47, 1978.
86. Blum RH et al: A clinical review of bleomycin, a new antineoplastic agent. *Cancer* 31:903, 1973.
87. Leake E et al: Diffuse interstitial pulmonary fibrosis after busulphan therapy. *Lancet* 2:432, 1963.
88. Holoye PY et al: Pulmonary toxicity in long-term administration of BCNU. *Cancer Treat Rep* 60:1691, 1976.
89. Sostman HD et al: Methotrexate-induced pneumonitis. *Medicine* 55:371, 1976.
90. Minow RA et al: Adriamycin cardiomyopathy: An overview with determination of risk factors. *Cancer Chemother Rep* 6:195, 1975.
91. Buzdar AU et al: Adriamycin and mitomycin-C: Possible synergistic cardiotoxicity. *Cancer Treat Rep* 62:1005, 1978.
92. Pacciarini MA et al: Distribution and antitumor activity of Adriamycin given in a high dose and a repeated low-dose schedule to mice. *Cancer Treat Rep* 62:791, 1978.
93. Weiss AJ et al: Studies on Adriamycin using a weekly regimen demonstrating its clinical effectiveness and lack of cardiac toxicity. *Cancer Treat Rep* 60:813, 1976.
94. Guthrie D, Gibson AL: Doxorubicin cardiotoxicity: Possible role of digoxin in its prevention. *Br Med J* 2:1447, 1977.
95. Myers C et al: Adriamycin: The role of lipid peroxidation in cardiac toxicity and tumor response. *Science* 197:165, 1977.
96. Einhorn LH, Donohue J: Cis-Diamminedichloroplatinum, vinblastine, and bleomycin combination chemotherapy in disseminated testicular cancer. *Ann Intern Med* 87:293, 1977.
97. Ward JM et al: Prevention of renal failure in rats receiving *cis*-diamminedichloroplatinum (II) by administration of furosemide. *Cancer Res* 37:1238, 1977.
98. Hayes DM et al: High dose *cis*-platinum diammine dichloride. *Cancer* 39:1372, 1977.
99. Gonzalez-Vitale JC et al: Acute renal failure after *cis*-dichlorodiammineplatinum (II) and gentamicin-cephalothin therapies. *Cancer Treat Rep* 62:693, 1978.
100. Sadoff L: Nephrotoxicity of streptozotocin. *Cancer Chemother Rep* 54:457, 1970.
101. Myerowitz RL et al: Nephrotoxic and cytoproliferative effects of streptozotocin. *Cancer* 38:1550, 1976.
102. Crooke ST, Bradner WT: Mitomycin C: A review. *Cancer Treat Rev* 3:121, 1976.
103. Pitman S, Frei E III: Weekly methotrexate citrovorum with alkalinization: Tumor response in a phase II study. *Proc AACR-ASCO* 18:124, 1977.
104. Bremmer DN et al: Clinical trial of isophosphamide: Results and side effects. *Cancer Chemother Rep* 58:889, 1974.
105. Bleyer WA: Methotrexate clinical pharmacology: Current status and therapeutic guidelines. *Cancer Treat Rev* 4:87, 1977.
106. Chabner BA et al: High-dose intermittent intravenous infusion of procarbazine. *Cancer Chemother Rep* 57:361, 1973.
107. Rosenthal S, Kaufman S: Vincristine neurotoxicity. *Ann Intern Med* 80:733, 1974.
108. Sakamoto A: Physical activity: A possible determinant of vincristine neuropathy. *Cancer Chemother Rep* 58:413, 1974.
109. Kedar A et al: Peripheral neuropathy as a complication of *cis*-dichlorodiammineplatinum(II) treatment: A case report. *Cancer Treat Rep* 62:819, 1978.
110. Legha SS et al: Hexamethylmelamine. *Cancer* 38:27, 1976.
111. Buroker T et al: Phase II trial of ftorafur with mitomycin C versus ftorafur with methyl-CCNU in untreated colorectal cancer. *Cancer Treat Rep* 62:689, 1978.
112. Ohnuma T et al: Clinical study with bleomycin tolerance to twice weekly dosage. *Cancer* 30:914, 1972.
113. Corder MP, Flannery EP: Possible radiation pericarditis precipitated by actinomycin D. *Oncology* 30:81, 1974.
114. Levin RH et al: Treatment of acute leukemia with methylglyoxal-bis-guanylhydrazone (methyl GAG). *Clin Pharmacol Ther* 6:31, 1964.
115. Shnider B, Colsky J: Effectiveness of methyl GAG administered intramuscularly. *Cancer Chemother Rep* 58:689, 1974.
116. Haidak DJ et al: Tear-duct fibrosis due to 5-fluorouracil. *Ann Intern Med* 88:657, 1978.
117. Hansen HH et al: The variability of individual tolerance to methotrexate in cancer patients. *Br J Cancer* 25:298, 1971.
118. Lefrak EA et al: Adriamycin cardiomyopathy. *Cancer Chemother Rep* 6:203, 1975.
119. Gralnick HR, Henderson E: Hypofibrinogenemia and coagulation factor deficiencies with L-asparaginase treatment. *Cancer* 27:1313, 1971.
120. Kennedy BJ: Mithramycin therapy in advanced testicular neoplasms. *Cancer* 26:755, 1970.
121. Dellinger CT, Miale TD: Comparison of anaphylactic reactions to asparaginase derived from *Escherichia coli* and from *Erwinia* cultures. *Cancer* 38:1834, 1976.
122. Von Hogg DD, Slavik M: Allergic reactions to *cis*-platinum. *Lancet* 1:90, 1976.
123. Bagley CM Jr et al: Clinical pharmacology of cyclophosphamide. *Cancer Res* 33:226, 1973.
124. Jardine I et al: Quantitation by gas chromatography–chemical ionization mass spectrometry of cyclophosphamide, phosphoramide mustard, and nornitrogen mustard in the plasma and urine of patients receiving cyclophosphamide therapy. *Cancer Res* 38:408, 1978.

125. Maddock SL et al: Primary evaluation of alkylating agent cyclohexylamine salt of N,N-bis(2-chloroethyl)phosphorodiamidic acid (NSC 69945, OMF 59) in experimental antitumor assay systems. *Cancer Chemother Rep* 50:629, 1966.
126. Hartman HA Jr et al: Five-day continuous infusion of 5-FU for advanced colorectal adenocarcinoma. *Proc AACR-ASCO* 19:368, 1978.
127. Grillo-Lopez AJ et al: Survival of patients with advanced gastrointestinal cancer treatment with 5-fluorouracil drip. *Proc AACR-ASCO* 18:331, 1977.
128. Andersson G, Heby O: Population kinetics of an Ehrlich ascites tumor following treatment with methylglyoxal bis (guanylhydrazone), a polyamine synthesis inhibitor. *Cancer Lett* 3:59, 1977.
129. Chaudhuri NK et al: Studies on fluorinated pyrimidines: III. The metabolism of 5-fluorouracil-2-C^{14} and 5-fluoroorotic-2-C^{14} acid in vivo. *Cancer Res* 18:318, 1958.
130. Finn C, Sadee W: Determination of 5-fluorouracil plasma levels in rats and man by isotope dilution–mass fragmentography. *Cancer Chemother Rep* 59:279, 1975.
131. Hunt DE, Pittillo RF: Determination of certain antitumor agents in mouse blood by microbiologic assay. *Cancer Res* 28:1095, 1968.
132. Benjamin RS et al: Plasma pharmacokinetics of Adriamycin and its metabolites in humans with normal hepatic and renal function. *Cancer Res* 37:1416, 1977.
133. Meriwether WD, Bachur NR: Inhibition of DNA and RNA metabolism by daunorubicin and Adriamycin in L1210 mouse leukemia. *Cancer Res* 32:1137, 1972.
134. Drewinko B, Gottlieb JA: Survival kinetics of cultured human lymphoma cells exposed to Adriamycin. *Cancer Res* 33:1141, 1973.
135. Freeman-Narrod M et al: Comparison of serum concentrations of methotrexate after various routes of administration. *Cancer* 36:1619, 1975.
136. Chabner BA et al: The clinical pharmacology of antineoplastic agents. *N Engl J Med* 292:1107, 1975.
137. Owellen RJ et al: Pharmacokinetics of vindesine and vincristine in humans. *Cancer Res* 37:2603, 1977.
138. Morasca L et al: Duration of cytotoxic activity of vincristine in the blood of leukemic children. *Eur J Cancer* 5:79, 1969.
139. Castle MC et al: Distribution and excretion of [^{3}H]vincristine in the rat and the dog. *Cancer Res* 36:3684, 1976.
140. Jackson DV, Bender RA: Cytotoxic thresholds of vincristine in L1210 murine leukemia and a human lymphoblastic leukemia cell line in vitro. *Clin Res* 26:437A, 1978.
141. Fujita H, Kimura K: Blood levels, tissue distribution, excretion, and inactivation of bleomycin, in progress in antimicrobial and anticancer chemotherapy, in *Proceedings of the 6th International Congress of Chemotherapy,* University Park Press, Baltimore, vol 2, p 309, 1970.
142. Ohnuma T et al: Microbiological assay of bleomycin: Inactivation, tissue distribution, and clearance. *Cancer* 33:1230, 1974.
143. Crooke ST et al: Bleomycin serum pharmacokinetics as determined by a radioimmunoassay and a microbiologic assay in a patient with compromised renal function. *Cancer* 39:1430, 1977.
144. Broughton A: Bleomycin pharmacokinetics. *Cancer* 40:2773, 1977.
145. Wan SH et al: Pharmacokinetics of 1-β-D-arabinofuranosylcytosine in humans. *Cancer Res* 34:392, 1974.
146. Kline I et al: Duration of drug levels in mice as indicated by residual antileukemic efficacy. *Chemotherapy* 13:28, 1968.
147. Oliverio T, Zubrod CG: Clinical pharmacology of the effective antitumor drugs. *Annu Rev Pharmacol* 5:335, 1965.
148. Mihich E: Current studies with methylglyoxal bis(guanylhydrazone). *Cancer Res* 23:1375, 1963.
149. Krokan H, Eriksen A: DNA synthesis in HeLa cells and isolated nuclei after treatment with an inhibitor of spermidine synthesis, methylglyoxal bis(guanylhydrazone). *Eur J Biochem* 2:501, 1977.
150. Rozencweig M et al: VM-26 and VP-16-213: A comparative analysis. *Cancer* 40:334, 1977.
151. Krishan A et al: Cytofluorometric studies on the action of podophyllotoxin and epipodophyllotoxins (VM-26 VP-16-213) on the cell cycle transverse of human lymphoblasts. *J Cell Biol* 66:521, 1975.
152. Allen LM, Creaven PJ: Comparison of the human pharmacokinetic of VM-26 and VP-16, two antineoplastic epipodophyllotoxin glucopyranoside derivatives. *Eur J Cancer* 11:697, 1975.
153. Benjamin RS et al: A pharmacokinetically based phase I-II study of single-dose actinomycin D *Cancer Treat Rep* 60:289, 1976.
154. Tattersall MHN et al: Pharmacokinetics of actinomycin D in patients with malignant melanoma. *Clin Pharmacol Ther* 17:701, 1975.
155. Lahiri SK: Response of mouse bone marrow colony forming units in different stages of the cell cycle to in vitro incubation with mitomycin-C. *Cell Tissue Kinet* 6:509, 1973.
156. Wagner T et al: Characterization and quantitative estimation of activated cyclophosphamide in blood and urine. *Cancer Res* 37:2592, 1977.
157. Frei E III, Freireich EJ: Progress and perspectives in the chemotherapy of acute leukemia, in *Advances in Chemotherapy,* Academic, New York, vol 2, p 269, 1965.
158. Samuels ML et al: Bleomycin combination chemotherapy in the management of testicular neoplasia. *Cancer* 3:318, 1975.
159. Canellos GP et al: Combination chemotherapy for advanced breast cancer: Response and effect on survival. *Ann Intern Med* 84:389, 1976.
160. Minow RA et al: Clinicopathologic correlation of liver damage in patients treated with 6-mercaptopurine and Adriamycin. *Cancer* 38:1524, 1976.

9
TUMOR IMMUNOLOGY

Yosef H. Pilch

> *When we think of cancer in general terms we are apt to conjure up a process characterized by a steady, remorseless and inexorable progress in which the disease is all-conquering and none of the immunological and other defense forces which help us to survive the onslaught of bacterial and viral infections can serve to arrest the faltering footsteps to the grave.*
>
> William Boyd[1]

William Boyd, the great Canadian pathologist whose wonderful Thoreauvian prose opens this chapter, introduced the chapter on tumors in the sixth edition of his *Textbook of Pathology* with the observation that "No single sentence definition of a tumor can be satisfactory . . . but for most purposes a tumor or neoplasm may be defined as a local growth of new cells which proliferate without control and which serve no useful function."[2] There is now abundant evidence to suggest that host defense mechanisms (i.e., immunity in its broadest sense) probably play a significant, although incompletely understood, role in controlling the development, growth, metastasis, regression, and recurrence of tumors in animals and in humans.

Stimulated by the great advances made in the immunology of microbial infections, the hope was widely held at the beginning of this century that dissimilarities between neoplastic cells and normal cells could be demonstrated by immunologic methods and exploited in order to vaccinate against cancer. This idea stimulated intense experimentation with so-called transplantable tumors originating in, carried in, and tested in noninbred mice and rats. Animals were immunized with attenuated or subthreshold tumor inocula and challenged later with a graft of viable tumor tissue or tumor cells. These experiments were usually successful in inducing partial or complete resistance to tumor transplantation. However, it soon became evident that the rejection of these tumor grafts was largely due to sensitization of the recipient to the normal alloantigens (histocompatibility antigens) present in the animal in which the tumor originated (and therefore in the tumor) but not in the recipient.[3-6] Moreover, similar resistance could be induced by immunization with normal tissue from the tumor donor.

When inbred strains of rodents became available, tumors arising in these strains were readily transplanted into other members of that same strain (syngeneic recipients) with no evidence of rejection whatsoever. Until the 1950s experiments to produce tumor rejection performed with tumors originating in and carried in such strains all yielded negative results. In retrospect, these negative results were largely due to errors in methodology. Often, inappropriate methods of immunization were used, including the use of subcellular preparations in which tumor-associated antigens were destroyed or degraded. But most important, recipient animals were challenged with overwhelmingly large doses of tumor cells. These doses of tumor cells were based on the old experiments with early "transplantable" tumors wherein it was possible to immunize animals effectively against huge tumor inocula. It is now known that immunity to tumor-specific antigens can protect the host against only a relatively small number of tumor cells (10^6 to 10^7 at most).

Tumor immunology fell into disrepute. Tumor cells, it was felt by many, could not possibly contain tumor-specific antigens because this would inevitably lead to immune elimination by the host; yet when a tumor develops, it almost invariably grows and eventually kills the host. Moreover, tumor cells are indigenous to the host of origin, and all their antigens must, therefore, be recognized as "self" by the immune system. The fact that neoplasms commonly metastasize to lymph nodes was viewed as an additional indication that immunologic mechanisms did not play a role in resisting the growth and spread of tumors.

Although Gross, in 1943,[7] demonstrated active immunization of inbred mice to transplants of a methylcholanthrene-induced sarcoma, his findings were received with skepticism since immunity to only a single tumor did not obviate the possibility that the tumor arose in a mouse with a mutant gene at some histocompatibility locus. The first clear demonstration of tumor-specific immunogenicity in syngeneic hosts was reported by Foley in 1953.[8] His experiments included the use of tumors recently induced by methylcholanthrene (MCA) in syngeneic mice. Removal of a growing transplant of the MCA-induced sarcoma was followed by resistance to subsequent challenge with the same tumor. These results were confirmed by Baldwin in 1955.[9] Then, in 1957, Prehn and Main[10] showed that mice from which growing transplants of a MCA-induced sarcoma had been excised were resistant to subsequent transplants of the same tumor. Moreover, immunization with normal tissues did not protect mice against tumor isografts, and mice rendered resistant to tumors still accepted skin grafts from the primary hosts of these tumors. In 1960, Klein et al.[11] extended these observations when they demonstrated the induction of tumor-specific immunity against MCA-induced sarcomas in primary autochthonous hosts. The existence of tumor-specific antigens (at least in chemically induced murine sarcomas) had been established. Since these antigens were detected by transplantation techniques and induced transplantation resistance, they were referred to as tumor-specific transplantation antigens (TSTAs).

These observations were soon extended, as the existence of TSTAs was demonstrated in tumors induced in inbred rodents by a variety of other polycyclic hydrocarbons,[12,13] other types of chemical carcinogens,[14,15] and a number of physical agents, including irradiation, radioactive isotopes, implanted cellophane films,[16] and millipore filters. A distinguishing feature of the chemically induced tumors and tumors induced by physical agents was found to be, with few exceptions, that their tumor-specific transplantation antigens were unique to each particular tumor.[13,17,18] (See Table 9-1.) This was true even when the tumors were produced by the same chemical agent in the same highly inbred strain, had nearly identical morphologic characteristics, and were highly immunogenic against themselves.

Individual chemically induced tumors were also found to vary with respect to the strength of their immunogenicity as measured by the number of viable tumor cells which a recipient could reject following a standard immunization procedure. An animal immunized with a "weakly antigenic" tumor would reject only 10^2 to 10^4 tumor cells, whereas an animal immunized with a "highly antigenic tumor" could reject 10^6 or even 10^7 tumor cells. However, in every case the degree of immunity was finite, and if greater numbers of tumor cells were inoculated, the immunity was overcome and progressive tumor growth ensued. It was discovered, moreover, that strongly antigenic tumors tended to arise earlier (i.e., after shorter latency periods) than the weakly antigenic tumors. It appeared that highly antigenic tumors could be rejected by the host unless the immune response was outpaced by a very rapidly growing tumor. Slowly growing tumors, therefore, would grow out only if they were weakly antigenic (assuming a normally immunocompetent host—more on this subject later in this chapter). Moreover, highly antigenic tumors recurred and metastasized less frequently after excision than did weakly antigenic tumors.

In subsequent experiments, it was shown by a number of investigators that tumor-specific transplantation immunity could be adoptively transferred to previously untreated syngeneic recipients by immunocompetent cells from immunized donors, e.g., spleen cells[19] and peritoneal exudate cells.[20,21] It has also been possible to detect evidence of circulating antitumor antibodies in mice from which MCA-induced tumors had been excised.[22,23]

In 1961, Habel[24] and Sjörgren et al.[25] independently demonstrated that mice which had been infected as adults with polyoma virus (an oncogenic DNA virus) became resistant to transplants of tumors induced by that virus. Since attenuated virus or passively transferred antibodies had no effect, it was presumed that polyoma-specific TSTA was induced by the virus in some of the infected cells. Immunization with virus-free tumor cells transformed by polyoma virus was also effective.[26] The

TABLE 9-1 Tumor-Specific Transplantation Antigens in Tumors of Experimental Animals

Tumor	Predominant antigens
Chemically induced tumors (polycyclic hydrocarbons)	Transplantation antigens specific for each tumor
Tumors induced by DNA viruses (polyoma, SV 40, adenovirus)	Transplantation antigens and neoantigens common to tumors induced by the same virus; tumor cells usually lack virion antigens and do not release infective virus
Tumors and leukemias induced by RNA viruses (avian and murine leukemia-sarcoma viruses, mammary tumor virus)	Transplantation antigens and viral antigens common to cells transformed by the same virus; tumor cells release infective virus

polyoma TSTA was found to be shared by all tumors induced by the polyoma virus (even tumors induced in different rodent species) but did not cross-react with the TSTA of tumors induced by other viruses.

In subsequent years, TSTAs were demonstrated in tumors induced by a number of oncogenic viruses. In contrast to the specificity of the TSTAs of chemically induced tumors for each particular tumor, the TSTAs of virus-induced tumors were generally the same for all tumors induced by a single virus, but differed in tumors induced by different viruses (see Table 9-1). This was true for tumors induced by both DNA and RNA viruses. While it appeared at first that these phenomena delineated a sharp distinction between chemically and virally induced tumors, it has since been found that this distinction is not absolute. Some virally induced tumors have been shown to contain unique tumor-associated antigens, and some chemically induced tumors have been shown to share cross-reacting antigens.[27]

BIOLOGICAL SIGNIFICANCE OF TUMOR-ASSOCIATED ANTIGENS

Although tumor-associated antigens (TAAs) have been demonstrated, their relationship to the process of oncogenesis and subsequent tumor progression remains undefined. Whether such antigens are an integral structural part of neoplastic cells or are simply associated with products of viral genomes remains to be seen. The evidence is far from conclusive, but it does suggest that the acquisition of tumor-specific antigens is a sine qua non of malignant transformation. Such a conclusion is based on the almost ubiquitous occurrence of TAAs, their persistence despite immunoselection within the host, as well as their early appearance in neoplastic transformation. In addition, it has been shown that cell-surface antigens of the transplantation type (TSTAs), specified by the polyoma virus, are major determinants in the behavior of neoplastic cells in the primary host.[28] Such TSTAs are able to evoke an immune response that can check or eliminate foci of neoplastic cells.

The demonstration of tumor-associated antigens has raised another important question. Are these antigens dependent on new genetic information which results from mutation or viral infection, or do they represent a fetal gene which has become derepressed or an aberrant gene expression without actual gene alteration? The specificity of the tumor antigens of tumors induced by viruses for each particular species of oncogenic virus, the cross-reactivity between tumors induced by the same virus, and the fact that rescued viral genomes will induce specific transplantation resistance suggest that integrated viral genomes may, directly or indirectly, be responsible for the coding of at least some TAAs.

The possibility has not been excluded that a brief exposure to an oncogenic agent might produce some heritable derepression within a cellular genome. Certain gene groups, which were active during fetal life but later repressed, may be derepressed by an oncogenic virus or chemical carcinogen and code for the synthesis of antigenic substances recognized experimentally as tumor-specific antigens (see below for discussion of oncofetal antigens). Experimental data to support the concept that TSTAs may be oncofetal antigens are sparse and must be interpreted with caution. In most systems wherein fetal antigens and TSTAs can both be demonstrated, the TSTAs bear no obvious relationship to the fetal antigens.

However, Prehn was able to induce some resistance to transplants of syngeneic methylcholanthrene-induced sarcomas by the prior treatment of the recipient mice with fragments of syngeneic embryo.[29] Another example may be the TL (T-lymphocyte) antigen of thymus cells in certain mouse strains which is expressed only after viral leukemogenesis.[30] Since this antigen is known to be coded for by the genome of the host cell, its expression only after infection with a leukemogenic virus suggests that it is a product of a gene derepressed during the process of leukemogenesis. Antigens phenotypically expressed in normal embryonic cells but not in differentiated cells have also been known to reappear after neoplastic transformation with the polyoma virus.[31]

Regardless of the exact nature of TAAs and the mechanism by which they are generated, the fact remains that TAAs have been demonstrated in most (and may exist in all) tumors. Several critical questions then arise: (1) How do antigenic tumors develop in apparently immunocompetent hosts despite their antigenicity? (2) If it were not for the immune response, would the incidence of tumor development actually be much greater than that normally observed? (3) Once tumors arise, why are they not rejected, but rather continue to grow and frequently metastasize? (4) Are defects in host immunity necessary in order for tumors to develop?

Immunologic Surveillance

There is considerable evidence to support the theory that the immune response tends to suppress and/or control the incidence of tumor development. Such lines of evidence include the following.

1. Measures which suppress immunoreactivity, such as neonatal thymectomy, total-body irradiation, and the administration of antilymphocyte serum or immunosuppressive drugs, increase the susceptibility of animals to the induction of neoplasia. Animals so treated manifest an increased incidence of tumor development when exposed to oncogenic viruses.[32-35] However, it has generally been difficult to facilitate the induction of tumors by chemical carcinogens by these methods. The effects are minor and this subject remains controversial.[36,37]
2. Stimulation of the immune response results in a decreased incidence of tumor development in animals infected with certain tumor viruses and a prolongation of the latency period of spontaneous mammary carcinomas and chemically induced tumors. This may be achieved by specific immunization to tumor antigens or to oncogenic viruses, or by nonspecific immunization with immunoadjuvants such as bacillus Calmette-Guérin (BCG). However, all attempts to prevent *chemical* carcinogenesis by immunologic means have failed.
3. Aging, with its accompanying decline in immunocompetence, is associated with an increasing incidence of tumor formation.[38]
4. Caloric intake restriction can reduce the incidence of neoplasia. It also increases the efficacy of cellular immunity.
5. Very early neoplasms, especially in the skin where these lesions can be readily examined, are usually associated with a dense lymphocytic infiltration.
6. The fact that overt malignancies sometimes regress suggests the existence of immunologic resistance. If this can occur in the case of large lesions, it may be that regression is the virtual rule in the case of microscopic, nascent tumors.
7. Tumors, as we know them, do not occur in invertebrates, and invertebrates do not manifest an allograft type of immune response. It may be that allograft immunity that evolved during phylogeny parallels neoplasia's need to develop, under selection pressures, a new specific defense mechanism for controlling tumor development. This bit of teleological reasoning is interesting but highly speculative.
8. Human patients, such as renal allograft recipients, who have undergone immunosuppressive therapy, have a greatly increased frequency of various types of neoplasms.[38,39]

Mechanisms of Escape and the Problem of Concomitant Immunity

The fact remains that tumors do develop in animals and in humans and that these tumors grow progressively and kill the host. If immunologic surveillance exists, there must be loopholes or escape mechanisms by which tumors evade the controlling influences of the immune response. Evidence exists for several possible mechanisms of escape from immunologic surveillance.

In the case of chemically induced tumors, it is possible that tumors develop because the chemical carcinogens are themselves immunosuppressive. Lymphocytes from mice injected with chemical carcinogens have diminished capacity to produce antibody,[40] and such mice show decreased ability to reject skin allografts and tumor grafts.[41,42]

At early stages of tumor development, small foci of tumor cells may elaborate too small a quantity of tumor antigens to provide sufficient antigenic stimulation to elicit a strong antitumor immune response. These cells may then "sneak through" host immune responses. By the time the host is fully sensitized, the tumor may be too large and fast-growing to be rejected.

It has been suggested that tumor-bearing animals possess "factors" that nonspecifically depress their immunocompetence, or lack factors requisite for normal immunologic reactivity. Perhaps tumors themselves elaborate immunosuppressive factors. This is suggested by the fact that both nonspecific and antitumor immune responses appear to be depressed in animals bearing large tumors. This suppression seems to be reversible since good immunity is often restored if the tumor is removed or otherwise successfully treated. Similar findings have been noted in humans bearing large tumor burdens.

Perhaps tumors develop in hosts rendered specifically tolerant to the TAAs of their own tumors. An example of this is the tolerance to MTV-induced mammary carcinomas exhibited by mice that carry the mammary tumor virus.[44] However, it appears that, in most instances, tumor-bearing animals are sensitized to the antigens of their tumors and do mount an active antitumor immune response, at least until their tumors become fairly large.

The development and continued growth of antigenic neoplasms in the face of active host immunologic responses directed against tumor-specific antigens of the tumor is an important paradox of tumor immunobiology referred to as *concomitant immunity*. This implies that the tumor-bearing host's immune response to the tumor-specific antigens is either quantitatively inadequate to prevent continued growth, or that a potentially adequate immune response is evaded or "blocked" in some way. Possibly, the problem is simply one of logistics—the quantity of tumor cells and the tumor doubling time exceeding the cytolytic and cytostatic capacity of a finite immune response. There is considerable evidence to suggest that the presence of a growing tumor mass may, in some way, impede or interfere with certain aspects of the host's immune response, and there is evidence to support the theory that the extent of immunologic suppression is related to the size of the tumor burden of the host.

It may be that the immune responses of the host are intact and vigorous, but the tumor cell itself is rendered nonantigenic or is protected from destruction by the immune responses of the host. TSTA on tumor cell surfaces may be coated with substances such as sialomucin, and may not be recognized unless the coating is removed. Experimental evidence suggests that such coatings exist and may be removed by treating tumor cells with certain enzymes, e.g., trypsin or neuraminidase.[45–47] Tumor cells themselves appear to be capable of altering their antigenicity and/or their antigen expression, thereby reducing their vulnerability to immunologic attack. An example of *adaptive antigenic alteration* is the "antigenic modulation" which occurs in one particular murine tumor system.[48] In this system, when mouse lymphoma cells bearing the TL (thymus-lymphocyte) antigen are exposed to anti-TL antibody, there is suppression of antigen synthesis and the TL antigen disappears. This change is maintained as long as antibody is present. When the tumor cells are passed in the absence of antibody, the TL antigen reappears.

True "immunoselection" may also occur, whereby, under selection pressures of host immune responses, genetic variants of reduced or altered antigenicity may emerge.[49,50] Immunoselection may be important in determining whether or not metastases occur. Available evidence strongly suggests that most circulating tumor cells do not form clinically significant metastases, presumably, in part, because of host immune defenses. Certainly, tumor cells of altered or diminished antigenicity would have a better chance of establishing a metastasis. In a recent study, Sugarbaker et al. have demonstrated, in a mouse tumor model, antigenic differences between pulmonary metastases and the primary tumor.[51] Not only did pulmonary metastases differ antigenically from the primary tumor, but different pulmonary metastases within the same mouse were found to be antigenically different from one another. Both "antigen deletion" (loss of antigenicity) and "antigen shift" were noted in the metastatic deposits. This phenomenon may explain, in part, the frequent lack of success in treating metastatic tumors by immunotherapy.

HUMAN TUMOR IMMUNOLOGY

The proper study of mankind is man.

Alexander Pope

There is a wide variety of well-documented clinical observations which have long suggested the existence of host defenses against cancer in humans. Although there has been little direct evidence to support an immunologic basis for these observations, they are most consistent with the hypothesis that immune defenses play a significant role in controlling the development and growth of cancer in humans.

The following clinical observations suggest the existence of host immunity against human cancer.

1. Spontaneous prolonged or permanent regression of established tumors is an infrequent but well-documented phenomenon (1:300). Everson and Cole have collected 72 well-documented cases from the literature, and Boyd has reviewed several others.[52] Spontaneous remissions are particularly frequent in neuroblastomas of children, malignant melanomas, choriocarcinomas, adenocarcinomas of the kidney, and soft-tissue sarcomas, and have been observed in other tumors as well.
2. Spontaneous regression of metastatic lesions following removal of the primary tumor is also well documented and occurs most frequently in hypernephromas and neuroblastomas.
3. Prolonged survival or "cure" of patients following incomplete removal of their cancers is not uncommon.[53]
4. Delayed recurrences, 10 or 20 years after apparently successful treatment of the primary tumor, occur fairly commonly, especially in carcinomas of the breast and cervix, and in melanoma.
5. The cellular infiltration of tumors by histiocytes, plasma cells, lymphocytes, and eosinophils, commonly seen in certain tumors, implies the activity of cellular immune mechanisms. This histologic picture often can be correlated with a more favorable prognosis in may neoplasms, such as carcinoma of the breast and malignant melanoma.
6. The incidence and number of cancer cells found in operative wound washings or in postoperative wound drainages do not correlate with the subsequent development of local recurrence. Obviously, these cells are destroyed by the host.
7. The incidence and number of circulating tumor cells found in the blood or lymphatics of cancer patients do not correlate with the subsequent development of metastases. Obviously, most of these cells are destroyed by host defense mechanisms.
8. It is exceedingly difficult to autotransplant human cancer. The incidence of successful autotransplantation varies between 10 and 25 percent, even in patients with advanced malignancies. Southam's studies suggest that this resistance is relative rather than absolute since tumor inocula of greater than 100 million tumor cells usually resulted in tumor growth.[54] Evidence that humoral and cellular immune factors are responsible for the inhibition of tumor autotransplants was provided by Southam's observations that the mixture of tumor cells with autologous leukocytes or plasma inhibited growth in almost half of the patients studied.
9. Immunocompetence declines with increasing age, and the incidence of cancer increases in a directly inverse correlation with declining immunocompetence.
10. The incidence of malignancy in patients with immunologic deficiency diseases such as Wiskott-Aldrich syndrome, ataxia-telangiectasia, and Bruton's agammaglobulinemia is approximately 500 to 1000 times that observed in normal children and young adults.[55] Interestingly, the majority of these tumors involve the lymphoreticular system.
11. The incidence of tumor development in renal allograft recipients maintained on chronic immunosuppressive therapy is 50 times that of normal young adults. Again, most of these tumors are lymphoreticular neoplasms.[55,56]

THE RELATIONSHIP BETWEEN IMMUNODEFICIENCY AND MALIGNANCY

Much discussion has already been devoted to the theory of immunologic surveillance and the mechanisms by which tumors may "escape" from surveillance. Although it is likely that some tumors, by virtue of weak antigenicity, rapid growth rate, or other factors, may develop and grow to become clinically manifest, it is possible that many cancers develop because of an "immunologic accident"—a temporary immunosuppressive incident.

There is, moreover, considerable evidence to suggest that aberrations of immunocompetence (particularly cellular immunoreactivity) correlate with the prognosis and clinical course of human cancer. Therefore, much effort has been devoted to the study of the general immunocompetence of cancer patients. (Another application of such tests of immunocompetence may be to influence the selection of the immunotherapeutic modality most appropriate for each patient. Active immunization is probably not a suitable approach for an anergic cancer patient. Anergic patients may be better served by passive or adoptive forms of immunotherapy.) Such studies can be grouped into two categories—those concerned with humoral antibody production and those dealing with cell-mediated immunity.

Antibody formation by cancer patients to standard test antigens has been studied by a number of investigators, who have concluded that antibody formation is generally not impaired, even in patients with advanced disease. Thus, there is no evidence to implicate a defect in humoral antibody production as a factor in the progression of neoplastic disease.

Cell-mediated immune reactions in cancer patients have also been assessed by a variety of techniques. Perhaps no single reaction of cellular immunity is so simple and so readily estimated as the delayed cutaneous hypersensitivity responses. Because of their simplicity, safety, and ease and rapidity of elicitation, delayed cutaneous hypersensitivity responses in cancer patients have been more extensively studied than any other immunologic parameter. The vast majority of these studies have dealt with the evaluation of skin test reactivity to nonspecific antigens. Two general groups of antigens have been employed. The first group are common "recall" antigens—antigens to which all or most adults may be expected to have been sensitized. These include tuberculin (PPD), *Monilia,* mumps, trichophyton, and the streptococcal antigens streptokinase and streptodornase (Varidase). The second group consists of organic chemical haptens which do not exist in nature but which are potent sensitizing haptens when applied to human skin. Sensitization occurs when the hapten combines with proteins in the skin. When a challenging dose of the same hapten is applied 2 weeks later, a delayed cutaneous hypersensitivity response results in most immunocompetent subjects. On the assumption that exposure of the host to the tumor-associated antigens of a newly established tumor constitutes a primary stimulus to a new antigen, it has been widely held that testing with such haptenic antigens may have special relevance in immunocompetence testing of cancer patients. In addition, these haptens have the unquestioned advantage of testing antigen recognition and processing (the afferent arc of the immune response) as well as effector responses. The most widely employed haptenic agent for such testing has been dinitrochlorobenzene (DNCB).

Pioneering studies by Eilber and Morton suggested that there was a significant correlation between the cellular immunologic reactivity as measured by the ability to manifest delayed cutaneous hypersensitivity (DCH) reactions following sensitization to DNCB and the clinical course of cancer patients.[57,58] It was found that over 95 percent of normal adults, patients with benign neoplasms, and cancer patients free of disease 5 years or more following treatment could be effectively sensitized to DNCB. However, only 72 percent of all cancer patients who presented themselves as candidates for definitive operation were able to be sensitized. The remaining 28 percent exhibited cutaneous anergy to this chemical. The anergic patients had a uniformly poor prognosis following operation. Over 95 percent of these patients were found to be inoperable, or, if their tumors were resectable, the patient developed recurrent disease and/or distant metastases within 6 months. On the other hand, patients who were immunocompetent, as evidenced by their ability to be sensitized to DNCB, had a much better prognosis. Eighty-four percent of these patients were found to have localized tumors that could be resected and were free of disease for at least 6 months after operation. However, there appeared to be differences in the significance of positive DNCB reactivity in patients with different histologic types of tumors. Patients with epidermoid carcinomas of the cervix or head and neck showed a strong correlation between a positive DNCB response and a good prognosis following operation. In contrast, there appeared to be little correlation between positive DNCB tests and prognosis following operation for carcinomas of the breast and colon, melanomas, and sarcomas. Most sarcoma patients were immunocompetent regardless of their clinical course. However, it appeared that patients with severe impairment of their cell-mediated immune reaction, as indicated by cutaneous anergy to DNCB, had a uniformly poor prognosis after surgical therapy regardless of the histologic type of their neoplasm.

Several other investigators then correlated cellular immunologic reactivity with the stage of Hodgkin's disease,[59,60] leukemia,[61–63] and bronchogenic carcinoma.[64] However, at least two subsequent studies, although confirming the fact that many cancer patients fail to mount delayed cutaneous hypersensitivity reactions to DNCB, failed to confirm the prognostic value of the DNCB test.[64,65]

A number of sophisticated tests of lymphocyte stimulation in vitro have been applied to the study of cellular immunocompetence in cancer patients; and attempts are being made to correlate the results of these tests with stage of disease and prognosis and with cutaneous reactivity to recall antigens and DNCB. Early results suggested that lymphocytes from cancer patients exhibited a depressed response in blastogenic lymphocyte function tests.[66] These deficiencies were most pronounced in blastogenesis to concanavalin A and in the mixed lymphocyte culture reaction. Moreover, it was shown that serum from some cancer patients suppressed lymphocyte blastogenesis to phytohemagglutinin in vitro,[67] and that serum from cancer patients contained a peptide factor which was immunosuppressive.[68]

The clinical usefulness (i.e., prognostic value) of these tests remains to be established, and many conflicting reports have appeared in the literature. In general, early studies reporting significant signs of immunosuppression in cancer patients and indicating substantial correlation between depressed cellular immune responses and clinical course (i.e., prognosis) have not been substantiated by more recent, more rigorous; and better-controlled studies. Such studies have been performed in patients bearing a variety of different tumor types. An exhaustive review of the literature is inappropriate here. However, investigations performed on breast cancer patients will be described in detail in order to illustrate the dilemma.

Delayed Cutaneous Hypersensitivity (DCH) Reactions

Eilber and Morton's original study[57] of patients undergoing definite surgery for cancer reported that of those who had complete resection of their tumor and remained free of disease for 6 months, over 90 percent had positive DNCB tests preoperatively; whereas, of those who had nonresectable disease or who developed recurrence and/or metastases within 6 months, over 90 percent had negative DNCB skin tests. Although their study involved patients with a variety of malignancies, a sizable number of patients with breast cancer were included. These observations were confirmed by Pinsky et al. in 1974.[69] Pinsky's group later reported that DNCB reactivity at the time of definitive surgery correlated not only with 6-month recurrence rates, but also with long-term recurrence rates and survival times.[70] Again, their studies involved patients with many types of cancer but included a significant number of patients with breast cancer. They reported that 90 percent of 21 patients with localized breast cancer had positive DNCB tests, whereas no patient with metastatic breast cancer had a positive test.[24] Cunningham et al.[71] reported in 1976 that patients with recurrent breast cancer who exhibited strong DNCB reactivity had a statistically superior survival rate as opposed to patients with weak or absent DNCB responses.

Similar results have been obtained from studies of DCH reactivity to recall antigens. Mitchell reported depressed DCH responses to Varidase in breast cancer patients.[72] A suggestion of greater depression in patients with poorly differentiated tumors was noted. Roberts and Jones-Williams also found reduced DCH reactivity to Varidase.[73] They reported that women with stage I breast cancer exhibited less reactivity to Varidase than controls, and that women with advanced breast cancer were significantly less reactive than patients with localized disease. Nemoto et al.[74] reported anergic responses to recall antigens in only 1 of 8 patients with benign breast disease and 0 of 13 patients with localized breast cancer, whereas 11 of 34 patients with metastatic breast cancer had negative skin tests.

Many investigators have utilized combined testing with one or more recall antigens and DNCB. Most of these studies suggest that DNCB testing is more useful or at least more discriminating than recall antigen tests. Bolton et al.,[75] using both DNCB and recall antigen skin tests, confirmed the tendency of breast cancer patients with metastatic disease to have depressed skin test reactivity, but noted that anergy occurred later and to a less severe degree than in comparable patients with advanced colon cancer. These authors found that "the DNCB test [was] the most discriminating of the five tests of immune function studied."[76] Responses to DNCB were significantly depressed in patients with early breast cancer compared with controls, and patients with disseminated breast cancer showed greater depression than patients with early stages of disease. Surprisingly, patients with locally advanced tumors, despite a poor prognosis, had good DNCB responses. Depressed DCH reactivity in such patients may result from poor nutritional status and/or some specific but uncharacterized effect of the tumor itself.

However, in a more recent study by Wanebo et al.,[77] again using both DNCB and recall antigen testing, the authors failed to demonstrate impairment of DCH reactivity in patients with stages I, II, and III breast cancer, and noted no significant difference in reactivity between patients with nodal metastases and patients with negative nodes. DCH reactivity was measured at the time of breast surgery in 134 patients with "primary operable breast cancer" and 63 patients with benign breast disease. They found that DNCB reactivity was normal in breast cancer patients with negative nodes (89 percent were DNCB-positive) and only slightly but not significantly depressed in patients with positive nodes (80 percent were DNCB-positive).

In general, it can be concluded that DCH reactivity is generally depressed in patients with advanced breast cancer but may be normal or only minimally depressed in patients with early breast cancer. Reactivity may be less depressed in breast cancer patients than in patients with other cancers of comparable stage. It is unclear whether depressed cellular immunity as evidenced by diminished DCH reactivity bears a causal relationship in the genesis of advanced disease, results from it, or simply correlates with it. It does seem that DNCB testing is more discriminating than testing with recall antigens. At the University of California Medical Center, San Diego, studies of DNCB reactivity in breast cancer patients[78] also indicate that DNCB reactivity tends to correlate with the extent of tumor burden. Loss of DNCB reactivity did not occur until patients had large recurrences and/or metastases and/or were receiving combination chemotherapy, which in and of itself may be immunosuppressive. The available data does not support the clinical usefulness of skin testing in predicting prognosis or as a guide to therapy. These conclusions are confirmed by a very recent report by Krown et al.[79] They tested (with recall antigens and DNCB) 202 women with breast cancer at all stages of disease. A significant linear trend of decreasing DNCB reactivity was seen with increasing extent of disease. Recall antigen tests were unchanged. No significant difference in recurrence distributions was noted between patients with primary operable breast cancer who were DNCB-positive and those who were DNCB-negative. Surprisingly, there was a slight trend toward early recurrence for DNCB-positive patients with operable breast cancer when presence or absence of nodal involvement was taken into account. Although the survival rate of all DNCB-positive patients was better than all DNCB-negative patients, when patients with different stages of disease were analyzed separately, no significant differences in survival times were seen. These authors concluded that "although DNCB reactivity is progressively impaired in patients with increasing tumor burden and correlates with survival in breast cancer patients in general, ... such tests do not provide prognostically important information above that given by careful clinical and pathologic staging."

In Vitro Tests Employing Peripheral Blood Lymphocytes (PBL)

These tests may be divided into three groups: (1) total PBL counts, (2) enumeration of T- and B-cell subpopulations, and (3) in vitro tests of lymphocyte function, usually blastogenic responses to mitogens or recall antigens.

Certainly, the simplest in vitro test for cellular immunocompetence is enumeration of circulating lymphocytes. Riesco in 1969,[80] and Papatestas and Kark in 1974,[81] retrospectively examined PBL counts in breast cancer patients and found that patients fated to develop recurrence seemed to have lower pretreatment lymphocyte counts than individuals who experienced long disease-free survival time or cure. A slight trend toward lower PBL counts with increasing extent of disease at the time of presentation was also noted. In a later report, Papatestas et al.[82] found that patients with less extensive disease at the time of diagnosis had higher pretreatment PBL counts than patients with more advanced disease. They then compared survival within each stage (stages I, II, and III) for patients whose PBL counts were greater than or less than 200 per cubic millimeter. Five-year survival rates were significantly different for stages II and III, with patients whose PBL counts were less than 200 per cubic millimeter having a poorer survival rate than those whose lymphocyte counts were greater than 200 per cubic millimeter. No difference in survival rates was noted in stage I patients. Stein et al.[83] determined PBL counts in patients with various stages of breast cancer and compared them with counts in a control population of healthy volunteers (not a population of patients with benign breast disease). They found depressed PBL counts only in patients with metastatic disease. Patients with less extensive disease, including those with "inoperable" local disease, evidenced no diminution in PBL numbers. Several other investigators, however, have failed to confirm these trends. Wanebo et al.,[77,84] Krown et al.,[79] and Nemoto et al.[74] found no significant differences in PBL counts between breast cancer patients at various stages of disease, and/or between breast cancer patients and patients with benign breast disease. Bolton et al.[76] also found no significant difference in PBL counts between control and breast cancer patients. As did Stein et al.,[83] they noted a lower lymphocyte count in patients with metastatic disease, but when the data was adjusted for the older age of the patients with metastatic disease, the difference was no longer significant.

A more interesting and more sophisticated measure of cells involved in cellular immune reactions is the enumeration of PBL subpopulations of T cells and B cells. It would be expected that depression of T-cell numbers might result in or be correlated with impairment of cellular immunocompetence. T cells are almost always enumerated by the so-called E rosette technique, which is based on the empirical observation that sheep red blood cells adhere to the surface of T lymphocytes to form rosettes. B lymphocytes may be counted by two methods, which may or may not, in fact, measure identical lymphocyte subpopulations. One technique, the so-called EAC rosette technique, counts lymphocytes which have membrane receptors for C3, the third component of complement. The second technique, which utilizes indirect immunofluorescence, detects lymphocytes bearing surface immunoglobulins. The former method has been more extensively utilized than the latter. A few studies, such as those of Wanebo et al.,[77,84] have used both. For the purposes of this review, the method employed for determining numbers of B cells will not be specified unless particularly germane to the matter under discussion.

Whitehead et al.[85] measured T and B lymphocytes in 71 patients with breast cancer at various stages of disease and 99 controls (healthy women or women with benign breast disease). They reported that T-cell percentages were significantly depressed in all stages of breast cancer except stage III. B-cell percentages were similar in all groups. (A significant problem with this study is the fact that only the percentage of T cells, B cells, and null cells are reported, and the *absolute numbers* of T cells are not provided.) The most interesting finding of this study was that low T-cell levels returned to normal after incubation with papain (a proteolytic enzyme) in vitro, but fell again after resuspending the treated lymphocytes in autologous (cancer patient) serum. These results suggested that a "masking" factor was present in the serum of cancer patients which bound to the surface of some T lymphocytes and was removable by digestion with proteolytic enzymes.

Stein et al.,[83] who measured T-cell numbers and percentage of T cells but not B cells, found a trend toward lower T-cell numbers in breast cancer patients, but the differences were not statistically significant. In two later reports from the same group,[86,86] T-cell percentage values were found to be significantly lower in breast cancer patients at all stages of disease than in a control group of healthy women. However, the degree of depression did not correlate with the extent of disease and was of no prognostic significance. Wanebo et al.[77,84] measured T cells and B cells in 134 patients with operable breast cancer and in 63 patients with benign breast disease. Lymphocytes bearing C3 receptors and lymphocytes bearing surface immunoglobulins were determined separately. No depression of T cells was found in the breast cancer patients, whereas B cells bearing C3 receptors were slightly decreased and B cells bearing surface immunoglobulins were slightly increased. The latter findings would seem to be of questionable significance. There were no distinctive correlations of lymphocyte subpopulations with prognostic categories of risk. Both Nemoto et al.,[74] who measured only T cells, and Krown et al.,[79] who measured both T and B cells, found no evidence for depression of T-cell counts in breast cancer patients and found no correlation between numbers of T and B cells and stage of disease.

In vitro tests of the function of lymphocytes from breast cancer patients usually involve measurement of lymphocyte blastogenesis following stimulation with mitogens or microbial recall antigens. By far the most commonly used mitogen is phytohemagglutinin (PHA), although conconavalin A and pokeweed mitogen have also been used. The recall antigens used for testing have included PPD, *Escherichia coli, Staphylococcus aureus,* and *Candida albicans.* Of all these tests, PHA stimulation has aroused the greatest interest.

In 1971, Whittaker and Clark[88] reported that lymphocytes from patients with breast cancer evidenced reduced ability to undergo blast transformation in response to PHA. The greatest depression of response was found in patients with advanced or recurrent disease.

Lymphocytes from patients who were clinically free of disease a year or more after treatment responded normally to PHA stimulation. Of great interest was the finding that the inhibition of PHA response appeared to be due, at least in large part, to a factor in the serum of breast cancer patients. Lymphocytes from healthy individuals, which responded normally in autologous serum, evidenced depressed responses in "cancer" serum, and lymphocytes from breast cancer patients, which evidenced depressed responses in autologous serum, responded normally in "normal" serum. These investigators postulated "that the reduced immunological reactivity in these [breast cancer] patients is a secondary rather than a primary event and is possibly related to the extent . . . of the disease." Stein et al.[83] also measured lymphocyte responses to PHA in breast cancer patients at varying stages of disease and compared them with the responses of 100 normal controls. They found impaired PHA responses in all groups of patients. This depressed responsiveness was greatest in patients with metastatic disease, but was similar in patients with operable and inoperable primary tumors. Unfortunately, these investigators did not examine the serum of their patients for the presence of inhibitory serum factors.

However, Bolton et al.[76] could find no significant differences in lymphocyte response to PHA between "early" breast cancer patients and control patients with benign breast disease or between breast cancer patients of varying stages of disease. Krown et al.[78] also found that lymphocyte proliferative responses to several mitogens (including PHA) and microbial antigens in patients with advanced breast cancer did not change significantly with increasing extent of disease and appeared to be of no prognostic significance.

Wanebo et al.[77,84] measured lymphocyte responses to three mitogens (including PHA) and several microbial recall antigens in 134 patients with operable breast cancer (stages I, II, and III) and 63 patients with benign breast disease. They found that only lymphocyte stimulation with PHA showed a continued decrease with increasing extent of disease. Lymphocyte stimulation with other mitogens and antigens showed a paradoxical increase with increasing pathologic stage. They concluded that "PHA response is markedly influenced by the primary tumor burden and thus indirectly reflects the risk of recurrence." Again, the serum of the cancer patients was not tested for the presence of inhibitory serum factors. Adler et al.[86,87] studied lymphocyte stimulation by PHA and PPD at the time of diagnosis in 158 patients with operable (stages I and II) breast cancer who were then followed for 3 to 6 years. They attempted to correlate these results with incidence of recurrence and disease-free period. They also studied 52 patients with metastatic disease and attempted to correlate results of lymphocyte stimulation tests with duration of survival. They found that, within each stage, patients with operable breast cancer who were "suboptimal responders" at the time of diagnosis had a much higher probability of developing recurrent disease within 4 years than patients who were "optimal responders." Lymphocyte responses were found to be of little value in predicting survival rates of patients with metastatic disease.

In summary, total PBL counts and enumeration of T cells and B cells have failed to demonstrate a consistent defect of the cellular immunocompetence of breast cancer patients, nor have these tests proved to be useful as prognostic indicators. Some breast cancer patients with sizable tumor burdens may have reduced T-cell numbers, possibly related to a serum factor. Lymphocyte transformation following stimulation with PHA has been found to be depressed in breast cancer patients, although the results of different studies are conflicting. Depression may be greater in patients with advanced disease. Again a suppressive serum factor related to tumor burden may be, at least in large part, responsible for this finding.

TUMOR-SPECIFIC ANTIGENS IN HUMAN NEOPLASMS

For obvious reasons, it has not been possible to demonstrate the existence of tumor-specific antigens in human tumors by transplantation techniques. Even if ethical considerations did not preclude this type of experimentation, human transplantation studies would be of little value since human beings are obstinately heterozygous—there are no inbred strains. One must demonstrate the existence of tumor-associated antigens in human neoplasms by other means, usually by detecting evidence of a tumor-specific immune response in a tumor-bearing host. One must demonstrate either a cell-mediated or humoral immune response directed against tumor cells or extracts of tumor cells and provide evidence of the specificity of the reaction for a particular tumor. Tumor-associated antigens have been demonstrated in most human tumors which have been adequately studied by suitable techniques and may exist in all human tumors.

Burkitt's Lymphoma and Nasopharyngeal Carcinoma

The first human tumor that was clearly shown to contain tumor-associated antigens and to be immunogenic in the primary autochthonous host was Burkitt's lymphoma.[89,90]

The participation of host immune factors in the course of this malignant disease was suggested by the observation of spontaneous regressions of these neoplasms, and by the high incidence of cures occurring in patients receiving an amount of chemotherapy which would appear to be inadequate for the treatment of a tumor of the extent of that present. Often a single dose of cyclophosphamide would totally eradicate the disease.[91] Experimental evidence supporting the role of host immune responses was provided when, by immunofluorescent techniques, specific antibodies were found in the sera of patients with Burkitt's lymphoma. Moreover these sera reacted not only with autologous lymphoma cells, but with tumor cells from other patients with similar tumors and with tissue culture cells derived from these tumors. A variety of different immunologic studies, including these, suggested that Burkitt's lymphoma was antigenic in its host of origin and that cells from all (or most) Burkitt's lymphomas shared common tumor antigens.

The peculiar geographic distribution of this tumor led Burkitt to suspect that the disease might be caused by an infectious agent carried by an arthropodal vector. The immunologic evidence that Burkitt's tumor cells from different patients shared common antigens supported this view. A DNA virus of the herpes group was soon isolated from cultured Burkitt's cells and named the Epstein-Barr (EB) virus after the EB-1 Burkitt cell line from which it was first isolated.[92,93] Whether the EB virus is the etiologic agent in Burkitt's lymphoma or merely a passenger virus is uncertain. Thus far all attempts have failed to induce tumors with this virus in animals. The EB virus is either the same or antigenically very similar to the virus responsible for infectious mononucleosis,[93] and is present in all or most lymphoblastoid cell lines established in tissue culture. Moreover, the same antigens are found in both Burkitt's tumor and nasopharyngeal carcinoma.

At least four types of antigens have been detected in Burkitt's cells by serologic methods:[94]

1. Viral capsid antigens induced by the EB virus are located in the cytoplasm and are detected by immunofluorescence on fixed smears of Burkitt's cells. Antibodies to this antigen have no correlation with clinical course and can be found in normal sera.
2. Membrane antigens are located on the cell surface and detected by membrane immunofluorescence on living cells. The clinical course of patients with Burkitt's lymphoma appears to correlate with antibody titers to membrane antigens. Titers are high with remission of Burkitt's lymphoma and fall when the disease recurs.
3. Early antigens induced by the EB virus may be demonstrated by immunofluorescence on acetone-fixed cells shortly after infection with EB virus. Antibodies to these antigens are found in the sera of patients with Burkitt's lymphoma, nasopharyngeal carcinoma, and infectious mononucleosis.
4. The so-called precipitating antigens are detected by immunodiffusion reactions with an antigen prepared from concentrates of cells derived from Burkitt's lymphoma. Antibodies to these antigens are found in sera from patients with active disease, may disappear when regression of Burkitt's lymphoma occurs, and may reappear when the disease relapses.

In addition, cell-mediated immune responses to Burkitt's lymphoma have been demonstrated by delayed cutaneous hypersensitivity reactions to extracts of autologous tumor cells and by lymphocyte-mediated cytotoxic reactions of lymphocytes from tumor-bearing patients.

Neuroblastoma

Neuroblastoma, like Burkitt's lymphoma, has a clinical course which suggests that immunologic mechanisms may be active. Regression of metastases has been observed following resection of primary tumors, and "cures" have been observed following incomplete removal of primary tumors.

Neuroblastoma was the first human tumor in which tumor-associated antigens were detected by assessing lymphocyte-mediated reactions against tumor cells. By measuring the capacity of lymphoid cells from neuroblastoma cells in tissue culture, Hellström et al. demonstrated that neuroblastoma patients manifested cellular immunity to their own tumors.[96,97] Moreover, lymphocytes from one neuroblastoma patient were shown to react with neuroblastoma cells from other patients as well as with autologous tumor cells. Furthermore, the lymphocytes from mothers of children with neuroblastomas reacted with neuroblastoma cells in tissue culture regardless of whether the explanted tumor cells were obtained from their own offspring or from other neuroblastoma patients. These results suggest the possibility that neuroblastomas are induced by a virus which infects both mother and fetus during pregnancy, but which is oncogenic only in the infant. Alternatively, mothers may be immunized during pregnancy by antigens released from tumors borne by the fetus.

It was later shown that lymphocytes from neuroblastoma patients inhibited neuroblastoma cells regardless of whether the lymphocytes were obtained from patients with progressive disease or from those who were ostensibly cured. However, serum from patients with active disease specifically blocked the inhibitory effect of the lymphocytes upon the neuroblastoma cells. This blocking effect was not found in sera of the patients who were free of disease. Moreover, serum from patients who were "cured" not only failed to block but was sometimes directly cytotxic to neuroblastoma cells. Furthermore, when such sera were mixed with known blocking sera, they would abrogate the blocking effect and were therefore termed "unblocking sera."

Colon Carcinoma

Findings similar to those just described in the studies of neuroblastoma have been obtained in studies of human colon carcinoma. Lymphocytes from patients with colon cancer have been shown to be toxic to autochthonous and allogenic colon cancer cells in vitro, but not to normal colonic mucosa cells or skin fibroblasts obtained from the same patients.[98,99] The degree of toxicity was comparable in the colony inhibition assay and the lymphocyte cytotoxicity test. Lymphocytes from patients with progressive colon cancer were approximately as inhibitory (cytotoxic) as lymphocytes from patients who were clinically free of disease after therapy. Sera from the former group of patients, but not from the latter, blocked the lymphocyte effect.[100] One patient, whose colon cancer had undergone spontaneous regression, was of particular interest. His lymphocytes were strongly toxic for colon cancer cells. His serum not only lacked blocking activity but was strongly "unblocking," i.e., it abrogated the blocking activity of sera from patients with growing colon cancer,[101] similar to the "unblocking" sera previously found in neuroblastoma patients.

Another point of interest is that lymphocytes from patients with colon cancer were found to be cytotoxic for cultured epithelial cells derived from fetal gut liver and pancreas, while they had no effect on kidney cells from the same fetus (or on adult colonic mucosa cells), a specificity that parallels that of carcinoembryonic antigen (CEA—see below), but does not imply that CEA is the target.[98]

Malignant Melanoma

Malignant melanoma also has clinical features suggesting active host defense mechanisms. Spontaneous regressions are more frequent in malignant melanoma than in any other human neoplasm, and long-term survival of patients with residual disease is not uncommon.

Characteristic antigens associated with malignant melanoma were first described independently by Morton et al.[102] and Lewis et al.[103] in 1968 and 1969, respectively. Both investigations utilized immunofluorescent techniques to detect in vitro in the sera of melanoma patients antibodies which reacted with melanoma cells. Morton et al. demonstrated common melanoma antigens shared by all or most melanoma cells. Sera from melanoma patients usually reacted with their autologous melanoma cells but in addition often reacted with melanoma cells from other patients. Lewis et al. presented evidence of another group of melanoma antigens which were individually distinct from each melanoma. Both Lewis and Morton noted that sera from patients with localized disease usually contained antibodies, whereas antibodies often could not be detected in sera from patients with disseminated disease,[58,103] indicating a correlation between the clinical stage of the disease and the presence of antimelanoma antibodies in the serum. (One wonders if antibodies could not be detected in the serum of patients with advanced disease because they are bound to tumor antigen elaborated by the tumor in the form of immune complexes.)

The existence of melanoma-specific antigens was then confirmed by a variety of additional techniques, including colony inhibition,[104] complement fixation,[58,105] antibody-mediated cytotoxicity,[103] and lymphocyte-mediated cytotoxicity. Moreover, serum factors which block lymphocyte-mediated cytotoxicity were detected in the serum of melanoma patients with active disease.[106,107] When clinical improvement occurred, this blocking activity disappeared from the serum.

Two types of melanoma-associated antigens have been

detected in melanoma cells and in body fluids: cytoplasmic antigens and membrane-bound antigens.[108] Cytoplasmic antigens have been reported to be common to all melanoma cells,[109–111] although allotypic specificities have been reported.[112,113] Thus a patient's antiserum may react in a serologic test preferentially with autologous melanoma cells in contrast to melanoma cells from other patients. When xenoantisera specific to melanoma cells were used in cross absorption experiments with homogenates from melanoma cells of a given patient, either the reactivity of the xenoantisera with some cells from other melanoma patients was not affected or the reactivity of the xenoantisera with some of the panel of melanoma cells was completely removed.[113] Humoral immune responsiveness to cytoplasmic antigens occurs later than that to membrane-associated antigens, does not appear to have a relationship to the stage of the disease, and may often be detected in advanced stages and metastatic phases of the disease.[108,114]

Although cytoplasmic melanoma-associated antigens are of interest in studies of immunodiagnosis, membrane-bound antigens, because of their location, probably elicit the reaction which most influences tumor growth, since both cell-mediated and humoral immune reactions can kill tumor cells only by interacting with cell-surface antigens. Membrane-bound melanoma-associated antigens display alloantigenic specificities.[109,118] Thus, melanoma cells will display different and distinct patterns of reactivity when tested against a panel of sera from melanoma patients, and sera from certain melanoma patients will react only with autologous tumor cells. Some melanoma cells used to absorb the sera from melanoma patients only partially remove those sera's reactivity to certain melanoma cells.[115,119,120] Similarly, sera from individual melanoma patients display different and distinct patterns of reactivity when tested against a panel of melanoma cells.[117–119,121,125] Some sera react with all the allogenic melanoma cells tested. At present it is not known whether such sera contain antibodies to common melanoma-specific antigens or multiple antibodies with various specificities. The answer to this question is crucial in the design of effective immunodiagnosis, and in defining whether antigens to be utilized as targets in a serologic assay for a melanoma patient should be derived from each patient's own autochthonous tumor cells or may be taken from another allogenic source such as a continuous line of melanoma cells in culture. The answer to this question is also of critical importance in the design of agents for active specific immunotherapy, in defining whether a "tumor cell vaccine" should be derived from each patient's own tumor cells or whether allogenic melanoma cells may be utilized.

A new dimension has been added to the serologic analysis of tumor antigens in general, and of melanoma antigens in particular, owing to the development of hybridoma methodology.[17] Hybridomas secreting monoclonal antibodies to melanoma cell–surface antigens have been produced by immunizing mice with human melanoma cells and fusing their spleen cells with mouse myeloma cell lines. Several investigators have utilized monoclonal antibodies to define various surface antigens on melanoma cells and some other human cancers. Murine monoclonal antibodies can only tell us, of course, what the mouse recognizes on human cancer cells. As human myelomas are now becoming available for fusion with human lymphocytes, we will be able to produce human monoclonal antibodies and more precisely define the cancer cell–surface antigens that can be detected by the human immune system. Once correlations of certain clinical features with the presence or absence of cell-surface antigens detected by these antibodies have been established, this work may eventually lead to new applications of monoclonal antibodies in diagnosis and in therapy.

Sarcomas

In 1969, Morton and Malmgren, utilizing immunofluorescence, demonstrated antibodies in the sera of patients with osteogenic sarcomas which reacted with their own tumor cells and also with cells from other human sarcomas.[126] Further studies revealed that such sera would react with sarcomas of various histologic types, and an antigen was identified which was common to all sarcomas regardless of histologic type. The existence of one or more common sarcoma-specific antigens was then confirmed in studies utilizing complement fixation,[58] antibody-mediated cytotoxicity,[127] colony inhibition,[128] lymphocyte transformation,[129] and lymphocyte-mediated cytotoxicity.[130] Morton et al. suggested that immune responses to sarcoma antigens correlated with the clinical state of the patient. They obtained sera from sarcoma patients who had remained free of disease for several years. These sera were assayed for antisarcoma antibodies by complement fixation. High titers of antibody were detected, and the antibodies persisted with little variation up to 3 and 4 years following removal of the primary tumor.[58] Analysis of serum obtained from patients before and after operation for removal of primary sarcomas revealed that, in those who remained free of disease, antisarcoma antibody titers rose and remained elevated. On the other hand, in patients who subsequently developed metastases, antibody titers either failed to rise or rose initially but later declined. The titer of antisarcoma antibody, in all cases, declined to zero or near zero as the disease became widespread. Furthermore, antisarcoma antibody titers were noted to rise and remain elevated in patients who had pulmonary resections for metastatic sarcomas and subsequently remained free of disease. However, in those patients who had resections and subsequently developed additional pulmonary metastasis, titers declined to undetectable levels when additional metastases appeared. It is unclear whether the antisarcoma antibody titer fell before or subsequent to the development of metastases. Did the fall in titer allow the development of metastases or did the increasing tumor burden suppress the immune response? Perhaps antigen released from the growing tumor masses complexed with the antibody and prevented its detection. Serum blocking factors have also been detected in the sera of sarcoma patients with active disease.[130]

Other Tumors

Tumor-associated antigens have been detected in virtually every human neoplasm which has been adequately studied. These antigens are detected by demonstrating serologic or cell-mediated immune reactions between serum or lymphoid cells from tumor-bearing patients and autologous tumor cells or allogenic tumor cells of the same histologic type, utilizing methods identical or very similar to those described above. Tumors in which tumor-associated antigens have been detected include: carcinoma of the urinary bladder,[131-135] renal cell carcinoma,[136,137] testicular tumors,[136] Wilms's tumor,[138,139] gliomas,[140] meningiomas,[141] leukemias,[142,143] and carcinomas of the breast,[144] lung, endometrium, and ovary.[136]

As a general rule human tumors have been shown to contain common antigens which are shared by all or most tumors of the same histologic type. Cross-reactivity between tumors of different histologic types is not usually found. This pattern of antigenic specificity is the same as that observed for tumors of experimental animals which are induced by oncogenic viruses. This certainly is suggestive evidence for a viral etiology for most human tumors. However, it also suggests that different viruses are responsible for the inducton of tumors of different histologic types. Certain human tumors have also been shown to contain individually unique antigens as well as common antigens, a situation similar to that observed in murine mammary carcinomas induced by the mouse mammary tumor virus. Thus, in some tumors (such as melanoma, which has just been discussed in detail) both "private" and common tumor antigens have been found. This may suggest a dual role of both viruses and chemicals in carcinogenesis—at least in the case of some cancers. Perhaps the chemicals act as "cocarcinogens" on cells already possessing a latent viral genome. Recently this pattern of antigenic specificities has been found in leukemia,[145] brain tumors,[146] and renal cell carcinoma,[147] in addition to melanoma.

Oncofetal Antigens

The concept that neoplastic transformation is accompanied by dedifferentiation and reversion to an embryonic state has been expressed by many investigators during the past century, but it is only during the past decade and a half that antigens specific for fetal tissues have been described in various human neoplasms. These carcinoembryonic or oncofetal antigens are antigenic substances produced during fetal life. Production of these fetal antigens is repressed shortly after birth, and they are not normally found in normal adult tissues. However, when adult cells undergo malignant transformation, the production of these primitive embryonic constituents is derepressed. The role of fetal antigens as host resistance to cancer is unclear at the present time. These antigens have their greatest importance as tumor markers since the antigens circulate and can be measured in the serum by a variety of techniques. When present, the quantitative levels of these antigens detected in the blood is usually proportional to the body burden of tumor and can often be used to follow response to therapy and/or monitor patients who are in remission for relapse of their disease. Only the two principal oncofetal antigens of human tumors will be discussed here.

CARCINOEMBRYONIC ANTIGEN

The carcinoembryonic antigen (CEA) is a fetal antigen first described by Gold and Freedman in 1965.[148] It was found in adenocarcinomas of the human digestive system (structures derived from the epithelium of the entodermal gut), particularly carcinomas of the colon and rectum. Cancers of the colon and rectum were found to contain a higher concentration of the antigen than did cancers of the stomach, esophagus, duodenum, and pancreas. Benign tumors of the pancreas, colon, and rectum, as well as all tumors originating outside of the digestive system, lacked the antigen. In addition, metastases to the colon, pancreas, or liver from ovarian or prostatic malignancies did not contain the antigen. It was concluded that the antigen's presence was dependent upon the tumor's site or origin rather than its site of growth. A similar antigen was found in embryonal and fetal gut, pancreas, and liver during the first two trimesters of gestation.

CEA is a protein-polysaccharide molecule, found in the glycocalyx adjacent to the cell membrane. Radioimmunoassays have been developed which are capable of detecting minute quantities of CEA in the circulation. The amount of CEA in the serum is proportional to the total tumor mass. The presence of very high levels of CEA is strongly suggestive of digestive system cancer. Total removal of tumor tissue usually results in the disappearance of CEA from the circulation. The presence of residual tumor is indicated by persistence of circulating CEA. When the serum concentration of CEA falls to an undetectable level following operation, subsequent reappearance of antigen in the serum suggests recurrence or metastasis. CEA appears to be antigenic in humans, since antibody to CEA can be detected in a large proportion of patients with localized cancers of the digestive tract and in sera of pregnant women. However, antibodies to CEA are never detectable in patients with metastatic disease.

Unfortunately, since the development of sensitive radioimmunoassays, increased levels of CEA or a similar substance have been found in the plasma of patients with cancers of several other organs (especially lung), and in patients with chronic liver disease, chronic renal disease, and inflammatory diseases of the colon, particularly ulcerative colitis.[149,150] Therefore, CEA appears to lack sufficient specificity to be useful as a screening test for colorectal cancer. However, CEA remains of great value as an adjunctive test for the presence of colon cancer in high-risk or highly suspect patients and as a tumor marker in following patients who have undergone resection or other treatment for colorectal cancer.

α-FETOPROTEIN

This antigen appears in the blood of patients with hepatomas and germinal teratocarcinomas. It is a second example of a characteristically fetal product synthesized by cancer cells.[151,152] Tests with sera from several thousand individuals gave positive results only in cases of malignant hepatoma or embryonal carcinoma of the ovary or testis. The test was negative with sera from healthy donors and from patients with bile duct carcinoma, liver metastases from tumors of other primary sites, and nonneoplastic liver disease. The incidence of positive tests with sera from patients with malignant hepatoma is as high as 85 percent.

The protein is a 70,000-molecular-weight protein with an α-electrophoretic motility that is synthesized by parenchymal cells of the liver, yolk sac, and gastrointestinal tract of the fetus. Although the synthesis of α-fetoprotein is a specific feature of hepatocellular carcinomas and germinal teratocarcinomas, elevated levels of α-fetoprotein have also been observed, at a lower frequency, in the serum of patients with other types of neoplasms, especially those derived from fetal entoderm.[153] In one study, elevated levels were noted in 23 percent of 44 patients with pancreatic cancer, 18 percent of 91 patients with gastric cancer, 5 percent of 193 patients with colon cancer, and 7 percent of 150 patients with lung cancer.[153,154] Elevated α-fetoprotein levels have also been noted in patients with certain forms of liver disease, including viral hepatitis, alcoholic hepatitis, and cirrhosis.[155] It should be noted that virtually all patients with benign liver disease (other than those with subacute hepatic necrosis) have α-fetoprotein levels below 500 ng/mL, whereas the majority of patients with hepatomas have levels above 500 ng/mL. Therefore, like CEA, α-fetoprotein is of inadequate specificity to permit its utilization as a screening test for any specific tumor but is of great value as a tumor marker in following the clinical course of patients known to have tumors that synthesize and secrete this protein.

CONCLUSION

There is excellent evidence that most human tumors contain tumor-specific or, at least, tumor-associated antigens. There is also excellent evidence that most cancer patients are relatively immunocompetent, at least during the early stages of their disease. Yet, at the time of this writing, immunotherapy is still an unproven modality in the treatment of cancer and has not been conclusively demonstrated to be of definite value in the treatment of any tumor at any stage of disease. Immunotherapy has been a disappointment to many investigators who exhibited great hope and enthusiasm only a decade ago. There are several explanations for this: (1) Tumor antigens may be too weak. (2) Although human tumor-associated antigens exist, they do not function effectively as "transplantation-type" antigens. (3) Tumor antigens may induce tolerance. (4) Tumor immunity is an important biological force, but tumor growth is so rapid that the immune responses responsible for killing tumor cells can never effectively "catch up." (5) Cancer patients have serious defects in immunocompetence which are not as yet understood. (6) Tumors elaborate specific immunosuppressive factors.

Great progress has been made in the science of tumor immunology over the past 20 years. It may be unreasonable to expect prompt success in the application of these advances to clinical cancer therapy. Certainly, the oncofetal antigens have proved clinically useful as tumor markers. Perhaps effective immunotherapy must await further progress in our basic understanding of tumor immunology, the nature of the immune response in general, and the biology of the neoplastic process.

REFERENCES

1. Boyd W: Spontaneous regression of cancer. Thomas, Springfield, Ill., 1966, p 3.
2. Boyd W, *Textbook of Pathology*, 6th ed, Lea and Febiger, Philadelphia, 1953, p 220.
3. Hauschka TS: Immunologic aspects of cancer: A review. *Cancer Res* 12:615, 1962.
4. Klein G: Usefulness and limitation of tumor transplantation in cancer research: A review. *Cancer Res* 19:343, 1959.
5. Snell GD: Homograft reaction. *Annu Rev Microbiol* 11:439, 1957.
6. Woglom WH: Immunity to transplantable tumors. *Cancer Res* 4:129, 1929.
7. Gross L: Intradermal immunization of C_3H mice against a sarcoma that originated in an animal of the same line. *Cancer Res* 3:326, 1943.
8. Foley EJ: Antigeneic properties of methylcholanthrene-induced tumors in mice of the strain of origin. *Cancer Res* 13:835, 1953.
9. Baldwin RW: Immunity to methylcholanthrene-induced tumors in inbred rats following implantation and regression of implanted tumors. *Br J Cancer* 9:652, 1955.
10. Prehn RT, Main JM: Immunity to methylcholanthrene-induced sarcomas. *J Natl Cancer Inst* 18:769, 1957.
11. Klein G et al: Demonstration of resistance against methylcholanthrene-induced sarcomas in the primary autochthonous host. *Cancer Res* 20:1561, 1960.
12. Baldwin RW: Antigeneic modifications in malignancy, in HN Green et al (eds): *An Immunological Approach to Cancer*, Butterworth, London, 1967, p 165.
13. Old LJ et al: Antigenic properties of chemically induced tumors. *Ann NY Acad Sci* 101:80, 1962.
14. Baldwin RW: Tumour specific antigens associated with chemically induced tumours. *Eur J Clin Biol Res* 15:593, 1970.
15. Rapp HJ et al: Antigenicity of a new diethylnitrosamine-induced transplantable guinea pig hepatoma: Pathology and formation of ascites variant. *J Natl Cancer Inst* 41:1, 1968.
16. Klein G et al: Demonstration of host resistance against sarcomas induced by implantation of cellophane films in isologous (syngeneic) recipients. *Cancer Res* 23:84, 1963.
17. Old LJ: Cancer immunology: The search for specificity. *Cancer Res* 41:361, 1981.
18. Prehn RT: Specific isoantigenicities among chemically induced tumors. *Ann NY Acad Sci* 101:107, 1962.
19. Bard DS, Pilch YH: The role of the spleen in the immunity to a chemically induced sarcoma in C_3H mice. *Cancer Res* 29:1125, 1969.
20. Wepsic HT, Rapp HJ: Systemic transfer of tumor immunity delayed hypersensitivity and suppression of tumor growth. *J Natl Cancer Inst* 44:955, 1970.
21. Zbar B et al: Tumor-graft rejection in syngeneic guinea pigs: Evidence of two-step mechanism. *J Natl Cancer Inst* 44:473, 1970.
22. Bloom ET: Quantitative detection of cytotoxic antibodies against tumor specific antigens of murine sarcomas induced by 3-methylcholanthrene. *J Natl Cancer Inst* 42:443, 1970.
23. Pilch YH, Riggins RS: Antibodies to spontaneous methylcholanthrene-induced tumors in inbred mice. *Cancer Res* 26:871, 1966.
24. Habel K: Resistance of polyoma virus immune animals to transplanted polyoma tumors. *Proc Soc Exp Biol Med* 106:772, 1961.
25. Sjögren HO et al: Resistance of polyoma virus immunized mice to transplantation of established polyoma tumor. *Exp Cell Res* 23:204, 1961.
26. Sjögren HO: Studies on the specific transplantation resistance against polyoma virus-induced tumors; III: Transplantation resistance against genetically compatible polyoma tumors induced by polyoma tumor homografts. *J Natl Cancer Inst* 32:645, 1964.
27. Cleveland PH et al: Tumor associated antigens of chemically-induced murine tumors: The emergence of MuLV and fetal antigens after serial passage in culture. *Int J Cancer* 23:380, 1979.
28. Law LW et al: Prevention of virus-induced neoplasms in mice through passive transfer of immunity by sensitized syngeneic lymphoid cells. *Proc Natl Acad Sci USA* 57:1068, 1967.
29. Prehn RT: The significance of tumor-specific histocom-

29. patibility antigens, in JJ Trentin (ed): *Cross-Reacting Antigens and Neoantigens,* Williams & Wilkins, Baltimore, 1967, p 111.
30. Boyse EA, Old LJ: Some aspects of normal and abnormal cell surface genetics. *Annu Rev Genet* 3:269, 1969.
31. Defendi V: The significance of tumor-distinctive histocompatibility antigens; in JJ Trentin (ed): *Cross-Reacting Antigens and Neoantigens,* Williams & Wilkins, Baltimore, 1967, p 117.
32. Allison AC, Taylor RB: Observations on thymectomy and carcinogenesis. *Cancer Res* 27:703, 1967.
33. Law LW: Studies of thymic function with emphasis on the role of the thymus oncogenesis. *Cancer Res* 26:551, 1966.
34. Ting RC; Law LW: Thymic junction and carcinogenesis. *Prog Exp Tumor Res* 9:165, 1967.
35. Vandeputte M: Antilymphocyte serum and polyoma oncogenesis in rats. *Transplant Proc* 1:100, 1969.
36. Balner H; Dersjant H: Neonatal thymectomy and tumor induction with methylcholanthrene in mice. *J Natl Cancer Inst* 36:513, 1966.
37. Wagner JL, Haughton G: Immunosuppression by antilymphocyte serum and its effect on tumors induced by 3-methylcholanthrene in mice. *J Natl Cancer Inst* 46:1, 1971.
38. Good RA, Finstad J: *Essential Relationship between the Lymphoid System, Immunity, and Malignancy,* National Cancer Institute Monograph 31, 1969, p 41.
39. Penn IH et al: De novo malignant tumors in organ transplant recipients. *Transplantation Proc* 3:773, 1971.
40. Stjernsward J: Age-dependent tumor-host barrier and effect of carcinogen-induced immunodepression or rejection of isografted methylcholanthrene-induced sarcoma cells. *J Natl Cancer Inst* 37:505, 1966.
41. Stjernsward J: Further immunologic studies on chemical carcinogenesis. *J Natl Cancer Inst* 38:515, 1967.
42. Prehn RT: Function of depressed immunologic reactivity during carcinogenesis. *J Natl Cancer Inst* 31:797, 1963.
43. Linder OEA: Survival of skin homografts in methylcholanthrene-treated mice and in mice with spontaneous mammary cancers. *Cancer Res* 22:380, 1962.
44. Weiss DW et al: Studies on the immunology of spontaneous mammary carcinomas of mice; in WJ Burdette (ed): *Viruses Inducing Cancer,* University of Utah Press, Salt Lake City, 1966, p 138.
45. Currie GA, Bagsharve KD: The role of sialic acid in antigenic expressions: Further studies of the Landshiitz ascites tumor. *Br J Cancer* 22:843, 1968.
46. Sanford BH: An alteration in tumor histocompatability induced by neuraminidase. *Transplantation* 4:1273, 1967.
47. Simmons RL et al: Effect of neuraminidase on the growth of methylcholanthrene fibrosarcoma in normal and immunosuppressed syngeneic mice. *J Natl Cancer Inst* 47:1087, 1971.
48. Old LJ et al: Antigenic modulation: Loss of TL antigen from cells exposed to TL antibody: Study of the phenomenon in-vitro. *J Exp Med* 127:523, 1968.
49. Fenyo EM et al: Selection of an immunoresistant Moloney lymphoma subline with decreased concentration of tumor-specific surface antigens. *J Natl Cancer Inst* 40:69, 1968.
50. Hauschka TS et al: Immunoselection of polypoid from predominantly diploid cell populations. *Ann NY Acad Sci* 63:683, 1956.
51. Sugarbaker EV et al: Altered antigenicity in spontaneous pulmonary metastases from an antigeneic murine sarcoma. *Surgery* 72:155, 1972.
52. Everson TC, Cole WH: *Spontaneous Regression of Cancer,* Saunders, Philadelphia, 1966.
53. Solomon HA, Kreps SI: Twenty-six years of survival following cancer of sigmoid with prolonged liver metastases. *JAMA* 144:221, 1950.
54. Southam CM: Applications of immunology to clinical cancer: Past attempts and future possibilities. *Cancer Res* 21:1302, 1961.
55. McKhann CF: Immunobiology of cancer, in JS Najarian, RL Simmons (eds): *Transplantation,* Lea and Febiger, Philadelphia, 1972, p 297.
56. Penn I: Malignant tumors in organ transplant recipients, in *Recent Results in Cancer Research,* vol 35, Springer-Verlag, New York, 1970.
57. Eilber FR, Morton DL: Impaired immunologic reactivity and recurrence following cancer surgery. *Cancer,* 25:362, 1970.
58. Morton DL et al: Immunological aspects of neoplasia: A national basis for immunotherapy. *Ann Intern Med* 74:587, 1971.
59. Aisenberg AC: Studies on delayed hypersensitivity in Hodgkin's disease. *J Clin Invest* 41:1964, 1962.
60. Brown R et al: Hodgkin's disease: Immunologic, clinical and histologic features of 50 untreated patients. *Ann Intern Med* 67:291, 1967.
61. Cone L, Uhr JW: Immunological deficiency disorders associated with chronic lymphocytic leukemia and multiple myeloma. *J Clin Invest* 43:2241, 1964.
62. Epstein WL: Induction of allergic contact dermatitis in patients with lymphoma-leukemia complex. *J Invest Dermatol* 30:39, 1958.
63. Hersh EM et al: Chemotherapy immunocompetence, immunosuppression and prognosis in acute leukemia. *N Engl J Med* 285:1211, 1971.
64. Catalona WJ, Chretien PB: Abnormalities of quantitative dinitrochlorobenzene sensitization in cancer patients: Correlation with tumor stage and histology. *Cancer* 31:353, 1973.
65. Chakravorty RC et al: The delayed hypersensitivity reaction in the cancer patient: Observations on sensitization to DNCB. *Surgery* 73:730, 1973.
66. O'Connell TX et al: Lymphocyte stimulation tests in cancer patients. *Surg Forum* 24:107, 1973.

67. Catalona WJ, Chretien PJ: Personal communication.
68. Glasgow AH et al: An immonosuppressive peptide fraction in the serum of cancer patients. *Surgery* 76:35, 1974.
69. Pinsky CM et al: Delayed hypersensitivity reactions in patients with cancer: Recent Results. *Cancer Res* 47:37, 1974.
70. Pinsky CM et al: Delayed cutaneous hypersensitivity reactions and prognosis in patients with cancer. *Ann NY Acad Sci* 276:407, 1976.
71. Cunningham TJ et al: Aconelation of DNCB-induced delayed cutaneous hypersensitivity reactions and the course of disease in patients with recurrent breast cancer. *Cancer* 37:1696, 1976.
72. Mitchell RJ: The delayed hypersensitivity response in primary breast carcinoma as an index of host resistance. *Br J Surg* 59:505, 1972.
73. Roberts MM, Jones-Williams W: The delayed hypersensitivity reaction in breast cancer. *Br J Surg* 61:549, 1974.
74. Nemoto et al: Cell-mediated immune status of breast cancer patients: Evaluation by skin tests, lymphocyte stimulation and counts of rosette-forming cells. *J Natl Cancer Inst* 53:641, 1974
75. Bolton PM et al: Cellular immunity in cancer: Comparison of delayed hypersensitivity skin tests in the common cancers. *Br Med J* 3:18, 1975.
76. Bolton PM et al: Immune competence in breast cancer—Relationship of pretreatment immunologic tests to diagnosis and tumor stage. *Cancer Immunol Immunother* 1:251, 1976.
77. Wanebo, HJ et al: Immunologic reactivity in patients with primary operable breast cancer. *Cancer* 41:84, 1978.
78. Schick PM et al: Local delayed cutaneous hypersensitivity reactions in breast cancer patients with and without removal of axillary lymph nodes. *Am J Surg* 132:40, 1976.
79. Krown SE et al: Immunologic reactivity and prognosis in breast cancer. *Cancer* 46:1746, 1980.
80. Riesco A: Five year cancer cure: Relation to total amount of peripheral lymphocytes and neutrophils. *Cancer* 25:135, 1969.
81. Papatestas AE, Kark AE: Peripheral lymphocyte counts in breast carcinoma: An index of immune competence. *Cancer* 34:2014, 1974.
82. Papatestas AE et al: The prognostic significance of peripheral lymphocyte counts in patients with breast carcinoma. *Cancer* 37:164, 1976.
83. Stein JA et al: Immunocompetence, immunosuppression and human breast cancer, I: An analysis of their relationship by known parameters of cell-mediated immunity in well-defined clinical stages of disease. *Cancer* 38:1171, 1976.
84. Wanebo HJ et al: Immunobiology of operable breast cancer: An assessment of biologic risk by immunoparameters. *Ann Surg* 184:258, 1976.
85. Whitehead RH et al: T and B lymphocytes in breast cancer: Stage relationship and abrogation of T-lymphocyte depression by enzyme treatment in vitro. *Lancet* 1:330, 1976.
86. Adler A et al: Immunocompetence, immunosuppression and human breast cancer, II: Further evidence of initial immune impairment by integrated assessment effect of nodal involvement (N) and primary tumor size (T). *Cancer* 45:2061, 1980.
87. Adler A et al: Immunocompetence, immunosuppression and human breast cancer, III: Prognostic significance of initial level of immunocompetence in early and advanced disease. *Cancer* 45:2074, 1980.
88. Whittaker MG, Clark CG: Depressed lymphocyte function in carcinoma of the breast. *Br J Surg* 58:717, 1971.
89. Klein E, Clifford P: Search for host defenses in Burkitt's lymphoma: Membrane immunofluorescence tests on biopsies and tissue culture lines. *Cancer Res* 27:2510, 1967.
90. Klein G et al: Membrane immunofluorescence reactions of Burkitt's lymphoma cells from biopsy specimens and tissue cultures. *J Natl Cancer Inst* 39:1027, 1967.
91. Clifford P et al: Long term survival of patients with Burkitt's lymphoma: An assessment of treatment and other factors which may relate to survival. *Cancer Res* 27:2578, 1967.
92. Ellman L, Green G: L2C guinea pig leukemia: Immunoprotection and immunotherapy. *Cancer* 28:647, 1971.
93. Minowada J et al: Studies of Burkitt lymphoma cells. *Cancer* 20:1430, 1967.
94. Henle G et al: Relation of Burkitt's tumor-associated herpes-type virus to infectious mononucleosis. *Proc Natl Acad Sci USA* 54:97, 1968.
95. Pearson G et al: Relation between neutralization of Epstein-Barr virus and antibodies to cell membrane antigens induced by the virus. *J Natl Cancer Inst* 45:989, 1970.
96. Hellstrom I et al: Studies on cellular immunity to human neuroblastoma cells. *Int J Cancer* 6:172, 1970.
97. Hellstrom I et al: Demonstration of cell-bound and humoral immunity against neuroblastoma cells. *Proc Natl Acad Sci USA* 60:1231, 1968.
98. Hellstrom I et al: Cellular immunity to colonic carcinomas in man, in WJ Burdette (ed): *Carcinomas of Colon and Antecedent Epithelium*, Thomas, Springfield, Ill., 1970, p 176.
99. Hellstrom I et al: Demonstration of cell mediated immunity to human neoplasms of various histological types. *Int J Cancer* 7:1, 1971.
100. Hellstrom I et al: Blocking of cell-mediated tumor immunity by sera from patients with growing neoplasms. *Int J Cancer* 7:226, 1971.
101. Hellstrom I et al: Serum factors in tumor-free patients cancelling the blocking of cell-mediated tumor immunity. *Int J Cancer* 8:185, 1971.
102. Morton DL et al: Demonstration of antibodies against

103. Lewis MG et al: Tumour-specific antibodies in human malignant melanoma and their relationship to the extent of the disease. *Br Med J* 1:547, 1969
104. Hellstrom KE, Hellstrom I: Immunity to neuroblastoma and melanomas. *Annu Rev Med* 23:19, 1972.
105. Morton DL et al: Immunological factors which influence response to immunotherapy in malignant melanoma. *Surgery* 68:158, 1970.
106. Hellstrom I et al: Sequential studies on cell-mediated tumor immunity and blocking serum activity in ten patients with malignant melanoma. *Int J Cancer* 11:280, 1973.
107. Heppner GH et al: Cell mediated immunity and serum blocking reactivity to tumor antigens in patients with malignant melanoma. *Int J Cancer* 11:245, 1973.
108. Lewis MG et al: Tumor-associated antigens in human malignant melanoma. *Yale J Biol Med* 46:661, 1973.
109. Lewis MG et al: Tumour-specific antibodies in human malignant melanoma and their relationshp to the extent of the disease. *Br Med J* 3:547, 1969.
110. Nairn RC et al: Anti-tumor immunoreactivity in patients with malignant melanoma. *Med J Aust* 1:397, 1969.
111. Federman JL et al: Tumor-associated antibodies to ocular and cutaneous malignant melanomas: Negative interaction with normal choroidal melanocytes. *J Natl Cancer Inst* 52:587, 1974.
112. Wood GW, Barth RF: Immunofluorescent studies of the serologic reactivity of patients with malignant melanoma against tumor-associated cytoplasmic antigens. *J Natl Cancer Inst* 53:309, 1974.
113. Ghose T et al: Tumor localization of ^{131}I-labeled antibodies by radionuclide imaging. *Radiology* 116:445, 1975.
114. Lewis MG et al: Antibodies and anti-antibodies in human malignancy: An expression of deranged immune regulation. *Ann NY Acad Sci* 276:316, 1976.
115. Lewis MG, Phillips TM: The specificity of surface membrane immunofluoresence in human malignant melanoma. *Int J Cancer* 10:105, 1972.
116. The TH et al: Surface antigens on cultured malignant melanoma cells as detected by a membrane immunofluorescence method with human sera: Lack of tumor-specific reaction on melanoma lines. *Ann NY Acad Sci* 254:528, 1975.
117. Carey TE et al: Cell surface antigens of human malignant melanoma: Mixed hemadsorption assays for humoral immunity to cultured autologous melanoma cells. *Proc Natl Acad Sci USA* 73:3278, 1976.
118. Ferrone S, Pellegrino MA: Cytotoxic antibodies to cultured melanoma cells in the sera of melanoma patients. *J Natl Cancer Inst* 58:1201, 1977.
119. Shiku H et al: Cell surface antigens of human malignant melanoma; II: Serological typing with immune adherence assays and definition of two new surface antigens. *J Exp Med* 144:873, 1976.
120. Hersey P et al: Antigens on melanoma cells detected by leukocyte-dependent antibody assays of human melanoma antigens. *Int J Cancer* 18:564, 1976.
121. Morton DL et al: Demonstration of antibodies against human malignant melanoma by immunofluorescence. *Surgery* 64:233, 1968.
122. Rhomsdahl MM, Cox IS: Human malignant melanoma antibodies demonstrated by immunofluorescence. *Arch Surg* 100:291, 1970.
123. Fossati G et al: Cellular and humoral immunity against human melanoma. *Int J Cancer* 8:344, 1971.
124. Macher E et al: Evidence for cross-reacting membrane-associated specific melanoma antigens as detected by immunofluorescence and immune adherence. *Behring Inst Mitt* 56:86, 1975.
125. Irie RF et al: Membrane antigens common to human cancer and fetal brain tissue. *Cancer Res* 36:3510, 1976.
126. Morton DL, Malmgren RA: Human osteosarcomas: Immunologic evidence suggesting an associated infectious agent. *Science* 162:1279, 1969.
127. Wood WC, Morton D: Microcytotoxicity test: Detection in sarcoma patients of antibody cytotoxic to human sarcoma cells. *Science* 170:1318, 1970.
128. Morton DL et al: Immunologic and virus studies with human sarcomas. *Surgery* 66:152, 1969.
129. Morton DL et al: Immunological factors in human sarcomas and melanomas: A rational basis for immunotherapy. *Ann Surg* 172:740, 1970.
130. Cohen AM et al: Specific inhibition of sarcoma-specific cellular immunity by sera from patients with growing sarcomas. *Int J Cancer* 11:273, 1973.
131. Bibemol J et al: Cellular and humoral immune responses to human urinary bladder carcinomas. *Int J Cancer* 5:310, 1970.
132. Bubenik J et al: Immune response to urinary bladder tumors in man. *Int J Cancer* 5:39, 1970.
133. O'Toole C et al: Cellular immunity to human urinary bladder carcinoma, II: Effect of surgery and preoperative irradiation. *Int J Cancer* 10:92, 1972.
134. O'Toole C et al: Cellular immunity to human urinary bladder carcinoma, I: Correlation to clinical stage and radiotherapy. *Int J Cancer* 10:77, 1972.
135. O'Toole C et al: The cellular immune response to carcinoma of the urinary bladder: Correlation to clinical stage and treatment. *Br J Cancer* 28 (suppl 1):266, 1973.
136. Bubenik JJ et al: Cellular immunity to renal carcinoma in man. *Int J Cancer* 8:503, 1971.
137. Hellstrom I et al: Demonstration of cell-mediated immunity to human neoplasms of various histological types. *Int J Cancer* 7:1, 1971.

138. Diehl V et al: Cellular immunity to nephroblastoma. *Int J Cancer* 7:277, 1971.
139. Kumar S et al: Cellular immunity in Wilms' tumor and neuroblastoma. *Int J Cancer* 10:36, 1972.
140. Wahlstrom T et al: Cell-bound immunity in patients with malignant tumors of the brain. *Cell Immunol* 5:161, 1973.
141. Catalona WJ et al: Common antigen in meningioma-derived cell cultures. *Science* 175:180, 1972.
142. Hersh EM et al: Chemotherapy immunocompetence, immunosuppression and prognosis in acute leukemia. *N Engl J Med* 285:1211, 1971.
143. Rosenberg EB et al: Lymphocyte cytotoxicity reactions to leukemia associated antigens in identical twins. *Int J Cancer* 9:648, 1972.
144. Herberman RB: Assessment of cellular immune response to cancers of the breast. *Ann Clin Lab Sci* 9:467, 1979.
145. Garrett TJ et al: Detection of antibody to autologous human leukemia cells by immune adherence assays. *Proc Natl Acad Sci* 74:4587, 1977.
146. Pfreundschuh M et al: Serological analysis of cell surface antigens of human malignant brain tumors. *Proc Am Assoc Cancer Res* 19:198, 1978.
147. Ueda R et al: Serological analysis of cell-surface antigens of human renal cancer. *Proc Am Assoc Cancer Res* 19:198, 1978.
148. Gold P, Freedman SO: Specific carcinoembryonic antigens of the human digestive system. *J Exp Med* 122:467, 1965.
149. LoGerfo P et al: Demonstration of an antigen common to several varieties of neoplasia. *N Engl J Med* 285:138, 1971.
150. Moore TL et al: Carcinoembryonic antigen assay in cancer of the colon and pancreas and other digestive tract disorders. *Am J Dig Dis* 16:1, 1971.
151. Alpert ME et al: Alphafetoglobulins in the diagnosis of human hepatoma. *N Engl J Med* 278:984, 1968.
152. Purves LR et al: Serum alpha-fetoprotein and primary cancer of the liver in man. *Cancer* 25:1261, 1970.
153. Waldmann TA, McIntire KR: The use of a radioimmunoassay for alpha-fetoprotein in the diagnosis of malignancy. *Cancer* 34:1510, 1974.
154. McIntire KR et al: Serum alpha-fetoprotein in patients with neoplasms of the gastrointestinal tract. *Cancer Res* 35:991, 1975.
155. Waldmann TA, McIntire KR: The use of sensitive assays for alpha-fetoprotein in monitoring the treatment of malignancy, in RB Herberman, KR McIntire (eds): *Immunodiagnosis of Cancer*, vol 1, Dekker, New York, 1979, p 130.

SELECTED BIBLIOGRAPHY

Howard RJ: Nonspecific host defenses in surgical cancer patients, in *Current Problems in Cancer,* vol 7, no 8, Yearbook Medical, Chicago, 1983.

10

MONOCLONAL ANTIBODIES: CURRENT AND POTENTIAL APPLICATION IN CANCER DIAGNOSIS AND THERAPY

Robert O. Dillman

PRODUCTION AND CHARACTERIZATION

The era of monoclonal antibodies was ushered in by Kohler and Milstein in 1975.[1] The technique they reported has been reproduced and refined in laboratories around the world, and the procedure itself has been standardized in research institutions and industry. The hybridoma technology offers several advantages over classic schemes of antisera production (see Table 10-1). Understanding these advantages is critical for appreciation of the revolutionary impact this technology has had on medical research and will have on medical care in the future.[2–4]

The main source in antisera production was the guinea pig, rabbit, horse, or other animal which was "immunized" by repeated inoculation with an antigenic substance. This antigenic substance might be tissue extracts, cells, or, ideally, a purified substance. After allowing time for an immune response to develop, the animal underwent phlebotomy and the serum was isolated. This serum contained various antibodies which reacted with myriad antigens from the immunogen. Some of these antibodies were relatively specific for a target antigen, and were therefore desirable. Others reacted with a variety of other tissues or cells. In order to restrict the reactivity of the serum, one could absorb the serum with a variety of tissues, cells, or other substances which would remove any material, including antibodies, which bound to them. The remaining serum was continually tested for reactivity within the target

TABLE 10-1 Contrast of Antisera and Monoclonal Antibodies

Antisera	*Monoclonal*
Heterogeneous	Homogenous
Variable specificity	Unique specificity
Variable affinity	Unique affinity
Limited production	Unlimited production
Variable lots	Reproducible lots
Purified antigen optimal	Impure antigen satisfactory
Absorptions for specificity	Screening for specificity

Supported by American Cancer Society Grant JFCF-602, the University of California San Diego Cancer Center Grant CA-23100, and the Veterans Administration.

antigen. After an adequate number of absorptions, one was left with an antiserum which was relatively specific for the target antigen. It consisted of various classes of antibodies with a variety of affinities for the target antigen. In general, the more pure the initial immunogenic antigen, the fewer purification and absorption steps required to obtain a useful antiserum. This final antiserum usually contained a variety of other biochemical products which had not been absorbed out. The final product was difficult to reproduce, even from the same animal, and production of large quantities was restricted by the blood supply of the antibody-producing mammal.

In monoclonal antibody (MoAb) production one can start with either a purified antigen or a crude material such as whole cells or tissue extracts. To produce murine MoAbs, a mouse is inoculated with the immunogen, and then splenectomized. This spleen contains numerous activated B cells, each of which has been primed to produce heavy and light chains of a specific antibody. These cells are fused with a B-cell line, which can be sustained continuously in culture medium, and which also has the capacity to produce antibody. A variant B-cell line is chosen typically because of its inability to secrete the antibody it produces. A typical example of such a line is the NS-1 murine myeloma cell line. Use of such a "nonsecretor" avoids the problem of production of more than one antibody type. The fusion of spleen cells and myeloma cells occurs with a low frequency, and several techniques have evolved to enhance this fusion. Polyethylene glycol (PEG) has been widely used to increase fusion frequency.

After the fusion, cells are grown in "HAT" (hypoxanthine-Aminopterin-thymidine) medium. The variant mouse myeloma cells chosen for fusion lack the enzyme hypoxanthine phosphoribosyl transferase ($HPRT^-$) and therefore cannot utilize exogenous hypoxanthine to synthesize purines. Aminopterin blocks the endogenous synthesis of both purines and pyrimidines; so, when $HPRT^-$ cells are grown in its presence, they die. However, the hybrid cells are able to use the HPRT enzyme system provided by the spleen cells; so they survive by utilizing the exogenous hypoxanthine and thymidine. Normal spleen cells can survive in HAT medium, but they do not grow well in tissue culture. Thus, the HAT medium selects for the hybridomas only, since the unfused spleen cells and myeloma cells die out.

Within 2 to 4 weeks after fusion, the hybrid clones become visible microscopically in the wells of tissue culture plates. Typically, radioimmunoassays (RIA) or enzyme-linked immunosorbent assays (ELISA) are utilized to screen the media from the hybrid wells for reactivity with the immunogen or other specific target antigens. Dilution techniques are utilized to ensure a high probability that any hybrid clones produced are monoclonal. However, subcloning techniques can ensure monoclonality when more than one clone is present, either initially or after the appearance of variants. The resulting hybridomas can be frozen and stored to preserve the hybrid line. The combination of these variables—the nonsecreting $HPRT^-$ B-cell line, the HAT medium selection for hybrids, the diluting techniques for selecting single cells, the analyses for immunoreactivity, and subcloning techniques—ensures the production and isolation of antibodies of a single heavy-chain and light-chain type that are produced by the daughters of a single hybrid cell; hence the term *monoclonal antibody*.

Although the methodology described above has become routine in innumerable laboratories, several problems continually arise. These include the relatively low frequency of fusion, the need for variant B-cell lines that are nonsecretors and $HPRT^-$, and the instability of many hybrids. Extensive screening and characterization is required to select high-affinity antibodies with the appropriate selective immunoreactivity. Finally, there is the problem of quantity. In tissue culture, hybrids produce antibody on the order of 10 to 100 $\mu g/mL$. However, it turns out that the hybrids grow well in the peritoneal cavity of mice of the same strain. In that site they produce tumors and ascites that are rich in MoAb, with concentrations of 10 to 20 mg/mL. Various purification techniques can subsequently yield a large quantity of a reagent-grade MoAb.

Clearly, the advantages of monoclonal antibodies over heterologous antisera are numerous. While antiserum consists of a mixture of antibodies, monoclonal preparation consists of only the monoclonal antibody. Antisera typically have low concentrations of the desired antibody, while ascitic sources contain very high concentrations of antibody. There is great variability in antisera lots, while MoAb lots are relatively uniform as long as the hybridoma is stable. Antisera are available in small volumes, while MoAb production is virtually unlimited. Antiserum lots vary in terms of binding, while MoAbs have homogenous binding. In general, the more pure the immunogen, the better the yield of antibody when antiserum is produced, while because of screening techniques, impure immunogens can be used with equivalent results in the production of monoclonal antibodies. Of the above, probably the greatest advantage of MoAbs over antisera in the arena of oncology is the potential unlimited availability. This ensures that all of the research needed to test the potential utility of monoclonal antibodies for specific immunodiagnosis and therapy can be readily conducted.

MONOCLONAL ANTIBODIES TO TUMOR-ASSOCIATED ANTIGENS

Since Ehrlich first proposed the "magic bullet" concept of antibody therapy, a major goal of tumor immunology has been identification of *tumor-specific antigens*. Antibodies directed against such antigens would be invaluable tools for histologic diagnosis, measurement of free tumor antigen in serum and, theoretically, for in vivo diagnosis and therapy. Unfortunately, no one has been able to prove the existence of a truly tumor-specific antigen, and for the present we must be content with *tumor-associated antigens* (TAA) which are relatively tumor-specific. Numerous murine MoAbs have been produced against a variety of normal and neoplastic tissues. Some of them do satisfy the conditions of being relatively tumor-specific tumor-associated antigens.

As circulating cells are readily available for study, the majority of reports of monoclonal antibody production have dealt with MoAbs which react with antigens on hematopoietic cells. Large-scale screening can be performed on established hematopoietic cell lines as well as on human peripheral blood samples using radioimmunoassays, enzyme-linked immunosorbent assays (ELISA), and immunofluorescence tests. Rapid advances in the cytofluorometric field have greatly facilitated the analysis of MoAb reactivity with single-cell suspensions. Table 10-2 lists a number of MoAbs which react rather specifically with various hematopoietic cells, all of which have the potential to proliferate in a malignant process. However, few of these have been extensively studied for reactivity with fresh human tissue because of problems outlined below. The so-called common acute lymphoblastic leukemia antigen (CALLA) was thought to be a tumor-specific antigen for acute lymphoblastic leukemia. Monoclonal antibody J5 was developed for its specific reactivity with CALLA.[26] However, subsequent work disclosed that CALLA was also present on a small proportion of normal marrow cells, and analysis of fresh tissue led to the discovery of CALLA on renal tubular cells.[30]

The study of MoAb reactivity with normal human tissue and the characterization of MoAbs directed against solid tumor antigens have been hampered by technical problems related to tissue collection and preparation. Normal, fresh, adult, human tissues are not available in large quantities from pathology laboratories, and one must utilize immunofluorescence or immunohistochemical staining of thin tissue sections to determine the distribution of antigen reactivity.[31] Frozen sections work best for the former, while immunoperoxidase techniques have made it possible to detect many antigens in fixed tissue. However, there is always concern that fixation may alter an antigen, and the requirement for fresh rather than autopsy material persists because of the potential antigenic alteration by autolysis. Another technique used has been immunoprecipitation and determination of the molecular weight of the antigen. Unfortunately, this procedure is much more complex and less readily applicable to extensive screening of MoAbs. Human solid tumor cell lines have been used in screening antibodies, but they are of little value in excluding reactivity with normal tissue.

In spite of these problems, a number of anti-solid tumor MoAbs have been produced. A representative summary of these is presented in Table 10-3. Obviously, there is tremendous interest in antilung, anticolorectal, antibreast, and antiprostate cancer antigens because of the prevalence of these malignancies and the limitations of current diagnostic techniques and therapy. However, the antibodies which have been best characterized to date are the antimelanoma MoAbs. Brown, at Seattle, has performed extensive immunoprecipitation experiments to establish the relative specificity of the P97 antigen for melanoma as opposed to normal tissue.[43,53] This antigen is also present in certain other tumors as well. Melanoma antibodies produced at Wistar Insti-

TABLE 10-2 Monoclonal Antibodies to Hematopoietic Tissues

Lymphocytes
  T cells[5-11]
  B cells[12-14]
	Burkitt's lymphomas[25]

	Lymphoblastic leukemia[26]
Monocytes[15,16]	Myeloblastic leukemia[27]
Myeloid cells[17,18]	Chronic lymphocytic leukemia[9,28]
Ia antigens[19-21]	Natural killer cells[29]
Transferrin receptors[22-24]	

TABLE 10-3 Monoclonal Antibodies to Solid Tumor Antigens

Breast[32,33]	Melanoma[43–46]
Carcinoembryonic antigen[34,35]	Osteosarcoma[47,48]
Colorectal (non-CEA)[36]	Ovary[49]
Glioma[37]	Pancreas[50]
Leiomyosarcoma[38]	Prostate[51]
Lung[39–42]	Renal cell[52]

tute,[44] Memorial Sloan-Kettering,[45] and Scripps Clinic[46] also have been well studied, and are strongly tumor-associated and relatively tumor-specific. These MoAbs react with known melanomas but not with benign nevi.

Several laboratories and companies have produced anti-CEA (carcinoembryonic antigen) MoAbs.[34,35] The potential utility of anti-CEA antibodies has been hampered by the large number of anti-CEA MoAbs which cross-react with granulocytes.[54] This reactivity appears to include determinants in addition to the normal cross-reacting antigen (NCA) previously reported.[55] These antibodies should have good in vitro application in serum CEA determination and histochemical studies of tissues (malignant versus benign polyps, for example). Their in vivo utility will depend on their true in vivo specificity. Minna et al.[39,42] have produced some relatively specific anti-small-cell carcinoma of the lung antibodies, but most of the antilung cancer antibodies reported have lacked definitive testing to ensure an adequate degree of specificity.[40,41]

PRESENT AND FUTURE ANTICANCER APPLICATIONS

At the present time the only established application of murine monoclonal antibodies is in laboratory diagnostic work and monitoring of certain diseases. The extensive battery of antilymphocyte surface antigens available has enabled detailed phenotypic characterization of normal and proliferating lymphocytes.[9,57–60] This has led to appreciation of a much greater heterogeneity of disease phenotype than had been previously expected and has been particularly applicable to lymphoproliferative diseases. Studies which are now underway may prove a clinical utility for this extensive phenotyping.[61,62]

The proportion and number of B cells, T cells, and subtypes of each can be readily measured from a sample of peripheral blood. Much larger numbers of cells can be sampled to determine the composition of the complete blood count (CBC) than can be assessed under a microscope. Thus, we can anticipate that MoAb reagents will replace many of the antisera currently used in diagnostic laboratories. In addition, their use in combination with advances in mechanical technology should lead to new equipment for routine sophisticated analysis and monitoring of peripheral blood for CBCs and circulating antigen detection. There is already a competitive market for MoAbs which detect various lymphocyte subtypes, α-fetoprotein, carcinoembryonic antigen, human chorionic gonadotropin, acid phosphatase, etc. Such MoAbs are of great help to pathologists in the precise classification of certain diseases. Thus, a lymph node which is called "undifferentiated malignancy" may be classified as a T-cell lymphoma if the vast majority of cells share identical antigens defined by a battery of monoclonal antibodies.

Future oncologic application of MoAbs may include in vivo diagnostic imaging, in vivo passive anticancer immunotherapy, in vivo MoAb conjugate anticancer therapy, and in vitro purification of bone marrow for autologous transplantation. Each of these areas is being actively researched at the present time.

Before reviewing the status of anticancer therapy with MoAbs, it would be useful to review certain aspects of antibody therapy which have emerged from antisera trials. During the past 40 years there have been many reports of inhibition of malignant cell growth using heterologous antisera.[63,64] In summary, in laboratory animals such therapy has been most successful against inducible lymphoid tumors and when given shortly after the tumor cell inoculation. Except for certain viral-induced animal tumors, established cancer has been generally unresponsive to passive serotherapy. The mechanism of an antitumor response in such animal models is not entirely clear. However, Lanier et al.[65] were able to eliminate growth of the CH1 murine B-cell lymphoma by passively administering the xenogenic anti-idiotype serum in mice who were genetically C5-deficient or cobra venom factor–treated to deplete complement; so they felt complement-mediated lysis was not necessary for a clinical effect. In addition, they found that splenectomy, thymectomy, sublethal irradiation, elimination of suppressor cells, and cyclophosphamide therapy also failed to abrogate the benefit of such therapy. Thus, immunosuppression by a variety of mechanisms did not stop the therapeutic effect. However, F(ab')$_2$ was ineffective in preventing tumor growth, suggesting the importance of the Fc receptor in the mechanism of tumor cell kill.

The antitumor potential of MoAb therapy directed against tumor-associated antigens has been confirmed in animal studies. Bernstein et al.[66,67] conducted a series of elaborate trials in AKR/J mice injected with a transplantable soft-tissue leukemia/lymphoma. They showed that an IgG$_{2a}$ anti-Thy 1.1 monoclonal antibody was useful in prolonging survival while an IgG$_1$ and IgM anti-Thy 1.1 were no more effective than placebo. This was accomplished even though the antibody also reacted with normal T cells and thymocytes. In vitro experiments showed that the IgM was cytolytic in the presence of rabbit complement but did not mediate antibody-dependent cellular cytotoxicity (ADCC) in the presence of normal effector cells. For this reason, the authors suggested the in vivo effect was probably not complement-dependent, although they were able to augment the antitumor effect by infusing rabbit complement.

Other investigators have also reported therapeutic success in transplantable murine tumor models by using MoAbs directed against T-lymphocyte differentiation antigens[68] and the transferrin receptor.[69] Again, the beneficial effects varied according to Ig subclass of the MoAbs and the timing of serotherapy related to tumor implantation. These studies also concluded that complement-mediated cytolysis was unlikely to be the mechanism of tumor cell removal.

Antitumor responses have also been observed in solid tumor animal models. Herlyn et al.[70] obtained encouraging results using MoAb treatment in nude mice with human colorectal carcinomas. Anticolorectal antibodies inhibited or retarded tumor growth following inoculation with tumor cells. In vitro studies showed that the antibody mediated ADCC in the presence of CBA/J effector cells. Similar success was achieved in retarding the development of human melanoma in athymic mice treated with antimelanoma monoclonal antibody.[44] The mechanism of tumor inhibition in such animal models is not entirely clear. However, these studies and others with heterologous antiserum suggest that complement-mediated lysis is probably not an important mechanism of tumor cell lysis in vivo. The clinical efficacy of passive MoAb therapy in a spontaneous animal solid tumor model has not been reported.

Human studies with MoAbs reactive with lymphocyte antigens have already been initiated and were recently reviewed.[71] Nadler et al.[72] reported treatment of a lymphoma patient with MoAb AB89. On successive days, 25 mg, 75 mg, and 150 mg of the MoAb were given by slow infusion, and 1 month later 1.5 g was given. The patient had very high levels of circulating antigen, and the investigators had great difficulty demonstrating binding to tumor cells in vivo, presumably because of antigen blocking the MoAb. However, they were able to demonstrate a transient decrease in white blood cells (WBC) after each treatment. Analysis of circulating cells suggested that up to 30 percent of tumor cells were damaged by the antibody infusion. Infusion of ^{51}Cr-labeled tumor cells, which had been incubated with AB89 in vitro, resulted in marked hepatic uptake of the radiolabel. In vitro tests demonstrated cytolysis by complement-mediated cytotoxicity (CMC) using the patient's serum or animal sources of complement, but AB89 failed to affect ADCC. Transient diminution of creatinine clearance was the only toxicity described. This report emphasizes the potential problems created by high levels of antigen in the circulation.

Ritz et al.[73] treated four patients with acute lymphoblastic leukemia with MoAb J-5, which was thought to be specific for the common acute lymphoblastic antigen (CALLA). In one patient, 4-h infusions of 85 mg, 170 mg, and 170 mg were given on 3 successive days. Blast counts were diminished during the infusion, but returned to normal levels by completion of the treatment. The cellularity of bone marrow specimens was unchanged. In spite of the drop in WBC, a high proportion of lymphoblasts persisted in the circulation even though CALLA$^+$ cells dropped to 1 percent. Bone marrow blasts also stopped expressing CALLA after the MoAb infusion. J-5 binding to lymphoblasts in vivo could not be demonstrated, although J-5 serum levels were detectable for at least 2 days following the last infusion. A second patient received 3 mg of J-5 on days 1 and 2, and 7.5 mg on day 4 of a treatment schedule. These treatments were given over 2 h on days 1 and 2, and over only 15 min on day 4. At these lower doses, J-5 antibody was detectable in the serum for only 1 to 2 h after each infusion. Again there was a decrease in circulating CALLA$^+$ cells, but a high proportion of lymphoblasts persisted which had become CALLA$^-$. Once J-5 antibody was no longer detectable in the patient's serum, the lymphoblasts reexpressed CALLA. A third patient who lacked circulating lymphoblasts but had a packed marrow received 1 mg of J-5 on day 1, 10 mg on day 2, and 20 mg on day 4.

All three of these treatments were given over 10 to 15 min. Not surprisingly, there was no effect on the circulating WBC level. Bone marrow studies done before and after treatments showed no change in lymphoblast cellularity. J-5 binding to marrow lymphoblasts was demonstrated, but the cells did not appear to be lysed. A fourth patient received multiple infusions of J-5 for 4 days in doses ranging from 8 to 25 mg. As in the first two patients, there was a rapid decrease in circulating lymphoblasts with a nadir in WBC occurring 1 to 2 hours after the infusion followed by a rapid return of circulating lymphoblasts to pretreatment levels in 4 to 6 h. In this case the investigators were able to demonstrate J-5 on the circulating cells prior to the disappearance of these cells from the circulation. During the course of therapy the phenotype of the leukemic cells changed with eventual loss of expression of CALLA. As in the first patient, once J-5 antibody had disappeared from the serum, there ensued a reexpression of CALLA by the circulating lymphoblasts. The eventual resistance to therapy which was noted in each of these patients, and the changes in lymphoblast phenotype with loss of CALLA, were attributed to modulation of the antigen. This was a problem the investigators had previously demonstrated in vitro.[74] Other in vitro studies with J-5 showed that it could mediate complement-mediated cytotoxicity in the presence of rabbit complement, but not human complement. However, in one patient the investigators were able to demonstrate deposition of C3 on antibody-coated cells. There was no significant toxicity noted in these patients, although three had temperature elevations following therapy. This work emphasizes the therapeutic difficulties created by antigenic modulation.

Miller and Levy have also reported decreasing circulating malignant cells by infusing MoAbs.[75,76] They administered MoAb L17F12 (Leu 1) to patients with T-cell leukemias and cutaneous T-cell lymphomas (CTCL). They have now treated at least 10 patients with from 1 to 92 mg of the anti-T-cell MoAb for up to 10 weeks. Two cases have been reported in the literature. One patient with T-cell leukemia received doses of 1 mg and 5 mg on successive days, and several weeks later received an additional 1-mg dose. The MoAb was delivered over a 6-h time period and was not associated with any toxicity. A marked drop in WBC was seen which was maximal at the end of the infusion but was followed by a rapid increase in the WBC level by the following day. The investigators were unable to demonstrate free L17F12 in serum samples during treatment, and were also unable to demonstrate the antibody on circulating tumor cells. Prior to antibody therapy they infused the patient with indium-111-labeled autologous tumor cells in order to see the effect of antibody administration. The radioactivity in the blood markedly decreased during therapy and did not return even as the WBC increased to normal levels. This was compatible with the hypothesis that cell destruction rather than sequestration accounted for the drop in WBC, and that cells from other tumor depots were entering the circulation to account for the increase in WBC. Radionuclide scans showed increased uptake in the liver and spleen, suggesting that the reticuloendothelial system was responsible for cell removal. Serum C3 and C4 complement levels were unchanged during treatment, and the investigators also showed that although L17F12 was lytic in the presence of rabbit complement, it was not lytic in the presence of the patient's serum as a source of complement. Also of note in this study was the finding that the 5-mg dose given on the second day of treatment had no effect on the WBC. Further study showed that the circulating cells at that time had a decreased reactivity with L17F12, suggesting that antigenic modulation had taken place. In addition, although circulating free antigen was not demonstrable prior to treatment, it did become detectable following therapy, and was associated with a slight decrease in creatinine clearance during therapy. This study suggests that the timing of antibody administration may be critical, because of the release of antigen by treated tumor cells and the induction of antigenic modulation. The investigators also found small levels of IgM antimouse antibody suggesting that endogenous antimouse immunoglobulin production could be a potential problem in therapy.

Miller et al.[75] reported a remarkable therapeutic success using L17F12 in a patient with CTCL. This patient recieved 1 to 20 mg in 17 courses over a 10-week period without any toxic symptoms. Antigenic modulation was seen with each treatment but reversed within 3 to 4 days. An impressive partial remission was obtained in lymph nodes, skin lesions, and a neck mass. As in other patients, the WBC fell after each dose of treatment but returned to pretreatment levels within 24 to 48 h. It was bothersome that the investigators also saw a decrease in both monocytes and granulocytes, and not just lymphocytes bearing the tumor-associated antigen. In spite of the dramatic clinical improvement in this patient with mycosis fungoides, he eventually relapsed in lymph nodes with cells which continued to express the tumor antigen. The mechanism of tumor resistance was not clear, but the investigators reported no evidence of an antimouse immune response throughout the duration of treatment. This study is particularly noteworthy because of the clinical response which was achieved, suggesting that MoAb therapy could be at least as effective as serotherapy.[77,78]

More recently, these same investigators have reported a dramatic complete remission in a patient with a B-cell lymphoma who was treated with a monoclonal anti-idiotype antibody.[79] In that case increasing doses of the MoAb finally led to disappearance of circulating antigen and resolution of all disease. The patient has remained in remission over 10 months even though therapy was discontinued.

Another clinical use of an anti-T-cell antibody has been reported in the treatment of two patients who were experiencing acute rejection of renal allografts.[80] Therapy with OKT3, an anti-T-cell antibody,[6] was associated with disappearance of OKT3$^+$ cells from the circulation and a reversal of the rejection. The only toxicity encountered was a brief episode of chills and fever after the first treatment, but subsequent daily therapy for 9 successive days was unassociated with any complication.

Dillman et al.[54,81–84] have initiated preliminary trials with murine MoAbs in chronic lymphocytic leukemia (CLL), CTCL, colorectal carcinoma, and melanoma. They have treated three CLL patients with IV infusions of T101, an IgG$_{2a}$ murine monoclonal antibody which detects a 65,000-dalton antigen (T65) and reacts with malignant and normal T cells, thymocytes, and CLL cells.[9,19,85] Based on immunofluorescence techniques, it does not react with any other tissues or hematopoietic cells, nor does it react with myeloid or erythroid bone marrow progenitor cells.[86]

One CLL patient received T101 infusions of 1 and 3 mg on 2 successive days, and 12 mg 2 weeks later. A second patient received one infusion of 10 mg. In both of these patients infusions were given rapidly over 10 to 15 min. A third patient has received 5 separate infusions of 10 mg of T101 over 1½ to 2 h. The lymphocyte count dropped with each infusion, but returned at the conclusion of each treatment. The third patient, who had had progressive disease for several months prior to treatment, appeared to have a stabilization of his disease for another 2-month period following therapy. There was no evidence of antigenic modulation in spite of the repeated therapy in this patient. The major observations made in these studies were as follows: (1) T101 murine monoclonal antibody bound to cells with T65 surface antigen in vivo. (2) T101 serotherapy produced a rapid but relatively transient decrease in cells bearing T65. The decrease in leukemic cells was maximal 2 h following a rapid infusion, or at the end of a 2-h infusion. (3) Saturation of T101 binding sites and presence of free serum T101 were demonstrable. (4) Free serum T65 antigen was not demonstrable either before, during, or after therapy. (5) Cells which bound T101 disappeared from the circulation by 2 to 3 h after treatment. (6) Free serum T101 disappeared by 2 to 4 h after infusion. (7) T101 did not appear to induce significant modulation, i.e., lymphocytes which were present expressed T65 throughout the observation periods. (8) T101 serotherapy resulted in some intravascular cell injury, but the decrease in circulating cells appeared to be due primarily to sequestration and destruction in the liver and lung, based on work using ^{111}In-labeled autologous tumor cells. (9) Rapid infusion of greater than 10 mg of T101 was associated with untoward systemic reactions. The systemic complications included dyspnea and hypotension in both patients, and extensive urticaria in one. These problems were readily managed with hydration and epinephrine, and there were no long-term consequences of the therapy. The 2-h infusions have been unassociated with any complication other than low-grade fever. (10) T101 is lytic to normal and CLL cells in the presence of rabbit complement, but not in the presence of normal serum or patient serum as sources of complement. (11) T101 is not lytic for T cells or CLL cells in the presence of normal human lymphocyte effector cells. (12) The density of T65 antigen on the surface cells is related to the rapidity with which such cells are cleared following T101 therapy. (13) Levels of C3, C4, and CH50 were unaffected by the T101 therapy.

One patient with CTCL received 14 different courses of T101: one 5-mg, eight 10-mg, three 20-mg, and two 40-mg infusion(s). These infusions were administered over 1½ h and were unassociated with complications. In contrast to the experience with CLL, modulation was observed during the 1½-h infusion. There was a marked drop in circulating Sézary cells with most treatments, but this effect was maximum 45 min into the infusion, and by the end of infusion the lymphocyte count was actually increasing. Some of the later infusions of T101 were ineffective in eliminating T65$^+$ cells. Subsequent work confirmed that in CTCL repeated therapy led to formation of endogenous antimouse antibodies which served as blocking factors. In spite of the failure to decrease the lymphocyte count in treatments 6, 7, and 8 in this patient, treatment 9 with 10 mg, and treatment 10 with 20 mg did not result in a marked drop in WBC as before. Clinically, this patient had some improvement in his pruritis and erythroderma, but his total malignant lymphocyte count was relatively unaffected during the course of therapy, and he had no lymph node or visceral disease to follow for a response. There were no acute or long-term complications noted in this patient, who has now been treated and followed for 6 months.

In summary, clinical use of MoAbs to hematopoietic cells has been reproducibly associated with transient decreases in circulating target cells, and encouraging clinical responses in certain patients. Toxicity has been tolerable, and similar to that seen with antisera in the past. Additional trials to determine optimum therapeutic doses and clinical efficacy in diseases with human T-cell antigens are in progress.

Reports of use of MoAbs in the treatment of nonhematopoietic tissues has been extremely limited to date. Sobol et al.[84] reported treatment of two melanoma patients with an IgG_{2a} murine monoclonal antibody which detects a 240,000-dalton antigen.[46] These two patients had no complications associated with a 10-mg infusion over 2 h. A third melanoma patient received two infusions of 10 to 50 mg of an antimelanoma antibody which detects a 97,000-dalton antigen.[43] These infusions were also unassociated with toxicity. Biopsies failed to confirm uptake of antibody into superficial tumors. No tumor responses were seen with this limited therapy.

Dillman et al.[54] have treated seven patients with colorectal carcinoma who have received 1 to 6 mg of an anti-CEA MoAb. These treatments were given as 10-min infusions in saline in four patients and as 2-h infusions in three patients. Three patients had fever and chills 1 to 3 h after treatment, and two patients had low-grade fever without chills. Unfortunately, these acute toxicities appeared to be related to cross-reactivity with an antigen on the surface of granulocytes and were unrelated to dose or rate of infusion. Other work suggests that this granulocyte antigen is different from the normal cross-reacting antigen.

Sears et al.[87] treated four patients with 15 to 200 mg of an MoAb directed against gastrointestinal malignancies. No complications were reported, but three patients developed antimouse antibodies. One patient who also received an hepatic artery infusion of autologous mononuclear cells mixed with antibody may have had regression of liver metastases. In other work, the same group studied ex vivo profusion of surgically resected colon segments containing colorectal carcinoma.[88] These studies suggest that cross-reactivity of anticolorectal antibodies with normal mucosa may be a problem in some patients. No long-term toxicities were seen in any of these patients.

Based on the clinical trials reported to date, it appears reasonably safe to infuse murine MoAbs over a 1- to 2-h period at a rate of less than 1 mg/min. Rapid infusions in the setting of circulating antigen bearing cells can result in significant toxicity. Murine MoAbs may have potential as passive serotherapy in the treatment of cancer and clearly can bind and eliminate circulating tumor cells. In certain situations, however, this treatment is hampered by antigen secretion, modulation, or induction of antimouse antibodies. The bulk of evidence to date suggests that complement-mediated cell lysis is not critical to removal of these cells but rather that cells appear to be removed in the reticuloendothelial system. Efficacy of passive intravenous MoAb therapy in nonhematopoietic solid tumors has not yet appeared, but sufficient data now exists on the specificity of various antimelanoma MoAbs to justify such studies with that tumor.

Many investigators feel the best future utility of MoAbs will be as conjugates to radioisotopes, chemotherapeutic drugs, or cellular toxins. In each case the MoAb would serve as a carrier which would target the antitumor agent rather than relying on the antibody itself or the host immune system for an antitumor effect. Radioisotope conjugates may be useful either as diagnostic imaging agents or as radiation-delivering therapeutic agents. The potential for radioisotope-antibody conjugate imaging has been demonstrated in various tumors using antisera in the past.[89-92] Some investigators have even claimed therapeutic efficacy from administration of radiolabeled antibody.[93,94] Athymic mouse models with animal tumors and a variety of human tumor xenografts have been successfully imaged using ^{131}I-conjugates of MoAbs,[95-98] but subtraction techniques have been required, and the relatively increased tumor uptake may be due to a decreased rate of dehalogenation in tumor tissue, since the vast majority of the isotope is excreted in the urine.[99] Chelated conjugates of MoAbs using indium 111 appear much more promising, with greater specific tumor uptake in animal models.[99-101] Successful imaging in humans with ^{131}I-antimelanoma and ^{131}I-anti-CEA MoAbs have been reported as abstracts, but the very low uptake of the iodine isotope suggests the chelated MoAbs with other isotopes will be superior. Such chelation products appear to be stable in vivo, and specificity looks promising in animal models.

Once the stability and specificity of radioisotope targeting has been confirmed, other isotopes, probably α or β emitters, can be conjugated for delivering therapeutic radiation to tumor sites. This is especially attractive as a potential therapy because of inherent problems caused by tumor vascularity and variability of antigen expression in a given tumor. The very low tumor incorporation of ^{131}I from such conjugates suggests that that isotope will not be suitable for therapeutic purposes.

Cellular toxins, such as diphtheria toxin and ricin, have been successfully conjugated to MoAbs. Such toxins consist of the active A chain and a binding B chain which are linked by a disulphide bond. This bond can be split and the A chain directly conjugated to the MoAb. This provides great specificity and a wide therapeutic index compared to A chain alone in vitro.[102–105] High concentrations of lactose also provide a wide therapeutic index when whole-toxin conjugates are compared to toxin alone in killing cell suspensions in vitro.[106] Unfortunately, the applicability of such toxin conjugates has not been verified in vivo. Stability of such conjugates in vivo and nonspecific uptake by the reticuloendothelial system may limit such application. However, several investigators have demonstrated the in vitro specificity and efficacy of such conjugates, and they may be superior to using MoAb plus complement in eliminating residual tumor cells from bone marrows of patients undergoing intensive therapy followed by autologous bone marrow transplantation.[102,104]

Application of MoAb-chemotherapy conjugates may have similar limitations. Prior experience with antisera-chemotherapy resulted in limited success.[107,108] New chemotherapy agents, the advent of MoAbs, and advances in biochemistry have rekindled enthusiasm for these conjugates.[109] However, few in vivo studies have been published.

Another future development one can anticipate in this area is the production of human-human hybridomas, i.e., human B-cell lines fused with human tissues with the nucleic acid information for the desired antibody. This would be most desirable from the standpoint of in vivo MoAb applications since antimouse antibodies are certain to limit the efficacy of murine MoAb in most cases. Human-human hybridomas have been reported for irrelevant antigens, demonstrating that the basic mouse technology is applicable to human MoAb production.[110,111] The major difficulty has been in identification and establishment of satisfactory human myeloma or lymphoblastoid cell lines. Kaplan and Olsson[110] obtained human-human anti-dinitrochlorobenzene (DNCB) MoAbs by fusing spleen cells from patients with Hodgkin's disease with a B-cell line. These patients were immunized prior to diagnostic splenectomy with DNCB. Unfortunately, the B-cell line used in these studies subsequently became contaminated with *Mycoplasma*.

Handley and Royston "rescued" the immunoglobulin secretory capacity of human chronic lymphocytic leukemia cells by fusing them with lymphoblastoid cells.[111] MoAbs were produced, but no significant antigen was identified with the antibodies. The suitability of such lymphoblastoid cell lines has been confirmed by others as well.

The potential application of this technology to relevant human MoAb production was shown by Schlom et al.[112] They fused human lymph nodes draining breast cancer to mouse myeloma cells and were able to produce human-murine MoAbs with relative specificity for breast cancer rather than normal breast tissue. Thus, one can visualize the successful production of human-human antitumor antibodies by fusing cells from draining lymphoid tissue with an appropriate B-cell line. Similar success has been achieved by taking hilar and bronchial lymph nodes from patients with lung cancer and fusing these with mouse and rat cell lines.[113] Thus, one can visualize the successful production of human-human antitumor antibodies by fusing cells from draining lymphoid tissue with an appropriate B-cell line. Sikora[114] has reported such success in raising human hybridomas to gliomas. Lymphocytes from resected gliomas were fused with a human myeloma cell line and glioma-binding activity was present in supernatants from several hybridomas. The tumor specificity of the antigens identified by these antibodies was not established.

SUMMARY

Monoclonal antibody technology will potentially have great impact in a variety of areas involved with cancer research and clinical care. The technology itself is well established and widespread throughout laboratories around the world. There is already a large market for in vitro diagnostic application of these agents, where it seems likely they will replace many, if not all, diagnostic antisera in use today. There are some encouraging animal models for the in vivo diagnostic and therapeutic use of murine MoAbs, but additional research is needed with spontaneous animal tumors. Human studies have already begun in certain hematopoietic diseases. These studies have demonstrated the ability of the mouse antibodies to bind to circulating target cells, and dramatic clinical efficacy has been obtained in some diseases, even in the absence of a truly tumor-specific antigen. Much basic and animal research in the coming years will deal with conjugates of monoclonal antibodies, including radioisotopes, chemotherapeutic agents, and toxins. Perhaps the best potential application for in vivo use is radioisotope-MoAb conjugates because of the potential for diagnostic imaging as well as relatively specific therapy. Wide-scale production of human-human antitumor antibodies can be anticipated, and this may obviate some of the demonstrated and potential problems inherent in the murine proteins.

REFERENCES

1. Kohler G, Milstein C: Continuous cultures of fused cells secreting antibody of predetermined specificity. *Nature* 256:495–497, 1975.
2. Diamond BA et al: Monoclonal antibodies: A new technology for producing serologic reagents. *N Engl J Med* 304:1344–1349, 1981.
3. Lampson SA, Levy R: A role for clonal antigens in cancer diagnosis and therapy. *J Natl Cancer Inst* 62:217–219, 1979.
4. Boman BM, Fathman CG: Monoclonal antibodies: The next attempt at tumor immunotherapy. *Mayo Clin Proc* 56(10):641–644, 1981.
5. Reinherz EL et al: A monoclonal antibody with selective reactivity with functionally mature human thymocytes and all peripheral human T cells. *J Immunol* 123:1312–1317, 1979.
6. Kung PC et al: Monoclonal antibodies defining distinctive human T cell surface antigens. *Science* 206:347–349, 1979.
7. Engleman EG et al: Studies of a human T lymphocyte antigen recognized by a monoclonal antibody. *Proc Natl Acad Sci USA* 78:1791–1795, 1981.
8. Ledbetter JA et al: Human Leu T cell differentiation antigens, quantitative expression on normal lymphoid cells and cell lines, in Hammerling et al (eds): *Monoclonal Antibodies and T Cell Hybridomas*, Elsevier/North Holland, New York, 1981, pp 16–22.
9. Royston I et al: Human T cell antigens defined by monoclonal antibodies. The 65,000-dalton antigen of T cells (T65) is also found on chronic lymphocytic leukemia cells bearing surface immunoglobulin. *J Immunol* 125:725–731, 1980.
10. Haynes BF: Human T lymphocytes antigens as defined by monoclonal antibodies. *Immunol Rev* 57:127–161, 1981.
11. Kamoun M et al: Identification of a human T lymphocyte surface protein associated with the E-rosette receptor. *J Exp Med* 153:207–212, 1981.
12. Stashenko P et al: Characterization of a human B lymphocyte-specific antigen. *J Immunol* 125:1678–1685, 1980.
13. Nadler LM et al: Characterization of a human B cell-specific antigen (B2) distinct from B1. *Blood* 57:1105–1110, 1981.
14. Abramson CS et al: A monoclonal antibody (BA-1) reactive with cells of human B lymphocyte lineage. *J Immunol* 126:83–88, 1981.
15. Todd RF et al: Antigens on human monocytes identified by monoclonal antibodies. *J Immunol* 126(4):1435–1442, 1981.
16. Ugolini V et al: Initial characterization of monoclonal antibodies against human monocytes. *Proc Natl Acad Sci USA* 77:6764–6768, 1980.
17. Griffin JD et al: Expression of myeloid differentiation antigens on normal and malignant myeloid cells. *J Clin Invest* 68(4):932–941, 1981.
18. Bernstein ID et al: Normal and malignant human myelocytic and monocytic cells identified by monoclonal antibodies. *J Immunol* 128(2):876–881, 1982.
19. Royston I et al: Monoclonal antibodies to a human T-cell antigen and Ia-like antigen in the characterization of lymphoid leukemia. *Transplant Proc* 13:761–766, 1981.
20. Quaranta V et al: Serological, functional, and immunochemical characterization of a monoclonal antibody (MoAb Q2170) to human Ia-like antigens. *Human Immunol* 3:211–223, 1980.
21. Reinherz EL et al: Ia determinants on human T-cell subsets defined by monoclonal antibody. Activation stimuli required for expression. *J Exp Med* 150:1472–1482, 1979.
22. Trowbridge IS, Omary MB: Human cell surface glycoprotein related to cell proliferation is the receptor for transferrin. *Proc Natl Acad Sci USA* 78(5):3039–3043, 1981.
23. Haynes BF et al: Characterization of a monoclonal antibody (5E9) that defines a human cell surface antigen of cell activation. *J Immunol* 127(1):347–351, 1981.
24. Goding JW, Burns GF: Monoclonal antibody OKT-9 recognizes the receptor for transferrin on human acute lymphocytic leukemia cells. *J Immunol* 127(3):1256–1258, 1981.
25. Wiels J et al: Monoclonal antibody against a Burkitt lymphoma–associated antigen. *Proc Natl Acad Sci USA* 78(10):6485–6488, 1981.
26. Ritz J et al: A monoclonal antibody to human acute lymphoblastic leukemia antigen. *Nature* 1:10–11, 1982.
27. Deng CT et al: Monoclonal antibody specific for human T acute lymphoblastic leukemia. *Lancet* 1:10–11, 1982.

28. Martin PJ et al: A new human T-cell differentiation antigen. Unexpected expression on chronic lymphocytic leukemia cells. *Immunogen* 11:429–439, 1980.
29. Abo T, Balch CM: A differentiation antigen of human NK and K cells identified by a monoclonal antibody (HNK-1). *J Immunol* 127:1024–1029, 1981.
30. Metzgar RS et al: Distribution of common acute lymphoblastic leukemia antigen in nonhematopoietic tissues. *J Exp Med* 154:1249–1254, 1981.
31. Wood GS, Warnke RA: The immunologic phenotyping of bone marrow biopsies and aspirates. Frozen section techniques. *Blood* 59:913–921, 1982.
32. Colcher D et al: A spectrum of monoclonal antibodies reactive with human mammary tumor cells. *Proc Natl Acad Sci USA* 78(5):3199–3203, 1981.
33. Arklie J et al: Differentiation antigens expressed by epithelial cells in the lactating breast are also detectable in breast cancers. *Int J Cancer* 28(1):23–29, 1981.
34. Rogers GT et al: Somatic-cell hybrids producing antibodies against CEA. *Br J Cancer* 43(1):1–4, 1981.
35. Acolla RS et al: Monoclonal antibodies specific for carcinoembryonic antigen and produced by two hybrid cell lines. *Proc Natl Acad Sci USA* 77:563–566, 1980.
36. Steplewski Z, Koprowski H: Anti-colorectal carcinoma monoclonal antibodies, in MS Mitchell, HF Oettgen (eds): *Hybridomas in Cancer Diagnosis and Treatment,* Raven, New York, 1982, pp 207–211.
37. Schnegg HF et al: Human glioma-associated antigens detected by monoclonal antibodies. *Cancer Res* 41(3):1209–1213, 1981.
38. Deng C et al: Cytotoxic monoclonal antibody to a human leiomyosarcoma. *Lancet* 1(8217):403–405, 1981.
39. Cuttitta F et al: Monoclonal antibodies that demonstrate specificity for several types of human lung cancer. *Proc Natl Acad Sci USA* 78:4581–4595, 1981.
40. Kasai M et al: Hybridoma monoclonal antibody. Use in defining surface antigens on human lung carcinoma cells. *Transplant Proc* 23(4):1942–1946, 1981.
41. Mazauric T et al: Monoclonal antibody-defined human lung cell surface protein antigens. *Cancer Res* 42(1):150–154, 1982.
42. Minna JD et al: Methods for production of monoclonal antibodies with specificity for human lung cancer cells. *In Vitro* 17(12):1058–1070, 1982.
43. Brown JP et al: Structural characterization of human melanoma-associated antigen P97 with monoclonal antibodies. *J Immunol* 127(2):539–546, 1981.
44. Koprowski H et al: Studies of antibodies against human melanoma cells produced by somatic cell hybrids. *Proc Natl Acad Sci USA* 75:3405–3409, 1978.
45. Dippold WG et al: Cell surface antigens of human malignant melanoma, Definition of six antigenic systems with mouse monoclonal antibodies. *Proc Natl Acad Sci USA* 77(10):6114–6118, 1980.
46. Imai K et al: Monoclonal antibodies to human melanoma-associated antigens. *Transplant Proc* 12:380–383, 1980.
47. Embleton MJ et al: Antitumor reactins of monoclonal antibody against a human osteogenic-sarcoma cell line. *Br J Cancer* 43(5):582–587, 1981.
48. Hosoi S et al: Detection of human osteosarcoma-associated antigens by monoclonal antibodies. *Cancer Res* 42:654–659, 1982.
49. Bast RC, Jr, et al: Reactivity of a monoclonal antibody with human ovarian carcinoma *J Clin Invest* 68(5):1331–1337, 1981.
50. Metzgar RS et al: Antigens of human pancreatic adenocarcinoma cells defined by murine monoclonal antibodies. *Cancer Res* 42(2):601–608, 1982.
51. Ware JL et al: Production of monoclonal antibody alpha pro3 recognizing a human prostatic carcinoma antigen. *Cancer Res* 42(2):1215–1222, 1982.
52. Ueda R et al: Cell surface antigens of human renal cancer defined by mouse monoclonal antibodies: identification of tissue-specific kidney glycoproteins. *Proc Natl Acad Sci USA* 78(8):5122–5126, 1981.
53. Brown JP et al: Qualitative analysis of melanoma-associated antigen P97 in normal and neoplastic tissue. *Proc Natl Acad Sci USA* 78:539–543, 1981.
54. Dillman RO et al: Results of early trials using murine monoclonal antibodies as anti-cancer therapy, in H Peeters (ed): *Protides of the Biological Fluids,* vol 30, Pergamon, New York (in press).
55. Bordes M et al: Carcinoembryonic antigen (CEA) and related antigens in blood cells and hematopoietic tissues. *Eur J Cancer* 11:703–786, 1975.
56. Rogers GT et al: Application of monoclonal antibodies to purified CEA in clinical radioimmunoassay of human serum. *Br J Cancer* 44(3):371–380, 1981.
57. Haynes BF et al: Phenotypic characterization of cutaneous T-cell lymphoma. *N Engl J Med* 304:1319–1323, 1981.
58. LeBien TW et al: Use of monoclonal antibodies, morphology and cytochemistry to probe the cellular heterogeneity of acute leukemia and lymphoma. *Cancer Res* 41:4776–4780, 1981.
59. Kung PC et al: Cutaneous T cell lymphoma: Characterization by monoclonal antibodies. *Blood* 57(2):261–266, 1981.
60. Martin PJ et al: Monoclonal antibodies recognizing normal human T-lymphocytes and malignant human B-lymphocytes: A comparative study. *J Immunol* 127:1920–1923, 1981.
61. Yu AL et al: Utility of monoclonal antibodies in the immunologic phenotyping of acute lymphoblastic leukemia. *Hybridoma* 1:91–98, 1982.
62. Dillman RO et al: Chronic lymphocytic leukemia and other chronic lymphoid proliferations: Surface marker phenotypes and clinical correlations. *J Clin Oncol* (in press).
63. Currie GA: Eighty years of immunotherapy. A review of

immunobiological methods used in the treatment of cancer. *Int J Cancer* 26:141–153, 1972.
64. Rosenberg SA, Terry WD: Passive immunotherapy of cancer in animals and man. *Adv Cancer Res* 23:323–388, 1977.
65. Lanier LL et al: Mechanism of B cell lymphoma immunotherapy with passive xenogenic anti-idiotype serum. *J Immunol* 125:1730–1736, 1980.
66. Bernstein ID et al: Mouse leukemia. Therapy with monoclonal antibodies against a thymus differentiation antigen. *Science* 207:68–71, 1980.
67. Bernstein ID et al: Monoclonal antibody therapy of mouse leukemia, in RH Kennet et al (eds): *Monoclonal Antibodies*, Plenum, New York, 1980, pp 275–291.
68. Kirch ME, Hammerling U: Immunotherapy of murine leukemias by monoclonal antibody, Effect of passively administered antibody on growth of transplanted tumor cells. *J Immunol* 127:805–810, 1981.
69. Trowbridge IS, Domingo DL: Anti-transferrin receptor monoclonal antibody and toxin-antibody conjugates affect growth of human tumor cells. *Nature* 294(5837):171–173, 1981.
70. Herlyn DM et al: Inhibition of growth of colorectal carcinoma in nude mice by monoclonal antibody. *Cancer Res* 40:717–721, 1980.
71. Ritz J, Schlossman SF: Utilization of monoclonal antibodies in the treatment of leukemia and lymphoma. *Blood* 59:1–11, 1982.
72. Nadler LM et al: Serotherapy of a patient with a monoclonal antibody directed against a human lymphoma-associated antigen. *Cancer Res* 40:3147–3154, 1980.
73. Ritz J et al: Serotherapy of acute lymphoblastic leukemias with monoclonal antibody. *Blood* 58:141–152, 1981.
74. Ritz J et al: Modulation of human acute lymphoblastic leukemia antigen induced by monoclonal antibody *in vitro*. *J Immunol* 125:1506–1513, 1980.
75. Miller RA, Levy R: Response of cutaneous T cell lymphoma to therapy with hybridoma monoclonal antibody. *Lancet* 2:226–230.
76. Miller RA et al: *In vivo* effects of murine hybridoma monoclonal antibody in a patient with T-cell leukemia. *Blood* 58:78–86, 1981.
77. Fisher RI et al: Regression of a T-cell lymphoma after administration of anti-thymocyte globulin. *Ann Intern Med* 88:799–800, 1978.
78. Edelson RL et al: Anti-thymocyte globulin in the management of cutaneous T cell lymphoma. *Cancer Treat Rep* 63:675–680, 1979.
79. Miller RA et al: Treatment of B-cell lymphoma with monoclonal anti-idiotype antibody. *N Engl J Med* 306:517–522, 1981.
80. Cosimi AB et al: Use of monoclonal antibodies to T-cell subsets for immunological monitoring and treatment in recipients of renal allografts. *N Engl J Med* 305:308–314, 1981.
81. Dillman RO et al: T101 monoclonal antibody therapy in chronic lymphocytic leukemia, in M Mitchell, HF Oettgen (eds): *Hybridomas in Cancer Diagnosis and Treatment*, Raven, New York, 1981, pp 151–172.
82. Dillman RO et al: Murine monoclonal antibody therapy in two patients with chronic lymphocytic leukemia. *Blood* 59:1036–1045, 1982.
83. Dillman RO et al: Phase I trials of murine monoclonal antibodies to tumor associated antigens, Preliminary observations, in H Peeters (ed): *Protides of the Biological Fluids*, vol 29, Pergamon, New York, 1982, pp 915–920.
84. Sobol RE et al: Phase I evaluation of murine monoclonal anti-melanoma antibody in man, Preliminary observations, in M Mitchell, HF Oettgen (eds): *Hybridomas in Cancer Diagnosis and Treatment*, Raven, New York, 1981, pp 199–206.
85. Wormsley SB et al: Comparative density of the human T-cell antigen T65 on normal peripheral blood T cells and chronic lymphocytic leukemia cells. *Blood* 4:657–662, 1981.
86. Taetle R, Royston I: Human T-cell antigens defined by monoclonal antibodies, Absence of T65 on committed myeloid and erythroid progenitors. *Blood* 56:943–946, 1980.
87. Sears HF et al: Phase I clinical trial of monoclonal antibody in treatment of gastrointestinal tumors. *Lancet* 1(8275):762–765, 1982.
88. Sears HF et al: Ex vivo perfusion of human colon with monoclonal anticolorectal cancer antibodies. *Cancer* 49(6):1231–1235, 1982.
89. Bagshawe KD et al: Preliminary therapeutic and localization studies with human chronic gonadotrophia. *Cancer Res* 40:3016–3017, 1980.
90. Goldenberg DM et al: Clinical studies on the radioimmunodetection of tumors containing alpha-fetoprotein. *Cancer* 45:2500–2505, 1980.
91. Van Nagell JR et al: Radioimmunodetection of primary and metastatic ovarian cancer using radiolabeled antibodies to carcinoembryonic antigen. *Cancer Res* 40:502–506, 1980.
92. Mach JP et al: Tumor localization of radiolabeled antibodies against carcinoembryonic antigen in patients with carcinoma. *N Engl J Med* 303:5–10, 1980.
93. Order SE et al: Use of isotopic immunoglobulin in therapy. *Cancer Res* 40:3001–3007, 1980.
94. Ettinger DS et al: Phase I-II study of isotopic immunoglobulin therapy for primary liver cancer. *Cancer Treat Rep* 66:289–296, 1982.
95. Houston LL et al: Specific *in vivo* localization of monoclonal antibodies directed against the thy 1.1 antigen. *J Immunol* 125:837–843, 1980.
96. Warenius HM et al: Attempted targeting of a monoclonal antibody in a human tumor xenograft system. *Eur J Cancer Clin Oncol* 17(9):1009–1015, 1981.
97. Solter D et al: Radioimmunodetection of tumors using monoclonal antibodies, in M Mitchell, HF Oettgen (eds):

Hybridomas in Cancer Diagnosis and Treatment, Raven, New York, 1981, pp 241–244.
98. Moshakis V et al: Localization of human tumor xenografts after IV administration of radiolabeled monoclonal antibodies. *Br J Cancer* 44:(1):91–99, 1981.
99. Stern P et al: The effect of the radiolabel on the kinetics of monoclonal anti-CEA in a nude mouse-human colon tumor model, in M Mitchell, HF Oettgen (eds): *Hybridomas in Cancer Diagnosis and Treatment*, Raven, New York, 1981, pp 245–253.
100. Schienberg DA, Strand M: Leukemic cell targeting and therapy by monoclonal antibody in a mouse model system. *Cancer Res* 42:44–49, 1982.
101. Scheinberg DA et al: Tumor imaging with radioactive metal chelate conjugated to monoclonal antibodies. *Science* 215:1511–1513, 1982.
102. Blythman HE et al: Immunotoxins hybrid molecules of monoclonal antibodies and a toxin subunit specifically kill tumor cells. *Nature* 290:145–146, 1981.
103. Gilliland DG et al: Antibody-directed cytotoxic agents, Use of monoclonal antibody to direct the action of toxin A chains to colorectal carcinoma cells. *Proc Natl Acad Sci USA* 77:4539–4543, 1980.
104. Krolick KA et al: Selective killing of leukemia cells by antibody-toxin conjugates, Implications for autologous bone marrow transplantation. *Nature* 295:604–605, 1982.
105. Raso V et al: Monoclonal antibody-ricin A chain conjugate selectively cytotoxic for cells bearing the common acute lymphoblastic leukemia antigen. *Cancer Res* 42(2):457–464, 1982.
106. Youle RJ, Neville DM: Anti-thy 1.2 monoclonal antibody linked to ricin is a potent cell-type specific toxin. *Proc Natl Acad Sci USA* 77:5483–5485, 1980.
107. Ghose T: Antibody-linked cytotoxic agents in the treatment of cancer. Current status and future prospects. *J Natl Cancer Inst* 61:657–674, 1978.
108. Tai J et al: Tumor inhibition by chlorambucil linked to antitumor globulin. *Eur J Cancer* 15:1357–1363, 1979.
109. Rowland GF et al: The potential use of monoclonal antibodies in drug targeting, in H Peeters (ed): *Protides of the Biological Fluids*, vol 29, Pergamon, New York, 1982, pp 221–226.
110. Olsson L, Kaplan HS: Human-human hybridomas producing monoclonal antibodies of predefined antigenic specificity. *Proc Natl Acad Sci USA* 77(9):5429–5431, 1980.
111. Handley HH, Royston I: A human lymphoblastoid B cell line useful for generating immunoglobulin secreting human hybridomas, in M Mitchell, HF Oettgen (eds): *Hybridomas in Cancer Diagnosis and Treatment*, Raven, New York, 1981, pp 125–132.
112. Schlom J et al: Generation of human monoclonal antibodies reactive with human mammary carcinoma cells. *Proc Natl Acad Sci USA* 77:6841–6845, 1980.
113. Sikora K, Wright R: Human monoclonal antibodies to lung-cancer antigens. *Br J Cancer* 43(5):696–700, 1981.
114. Sikora K et al: Human hybridomas from malignant gliomas. *Lancet* 1(8262):11–14, 1982.

SELECTED BIBLIOGRAPHY

Farrands PA et al: Radioimmunodetection of human colorectal cancers by an anti-tumor monoclonal antibody. *Lancet* 2: 8295, 1982.
Foon KA et al: Monoclonal antibody therapy: Assessment by animal tumor models. *J Biol Resp Mod* 1:277, 1982.
Goldenberg DM, Leland FH: History and status of tumor imaging with radiolabeled antibodies. *J Biol Resp Mod* 1:121, 1982.
Krolick KA et al: In vivo therapy of a murine B cell tumor (BCL_1) using antibody-ricin A chain immunotoxins. *J Exp Med* 155:1797, 1982.
Larson SM et al: Diagnostic imaging of malignant melanoma with radiolabeled antibodies. *J Biol Resp Mod* 1:121, 1982.
Stratte PT et al: In vivo effects of murine monoclonal antihuman T cell antibodies in subhuman primates. *J Biol Resp Mod* 1: 137, 1982.

11
BASIC PRINCIPLES OF RADIATION BIOLOGY AND RADIATION ONCOLOGY

Ralph Weichselbaum *Samuel Hellman*

The clinical uses of ionizing radiation were initiated shortly after the discovery of x-rays by Roentgen and of natural radioactivity by the Curies and Becquerel. Coolidge developed an effective x-ray tube, establishing the physical foundation for external radiation therapy. In 1922, Regaud and Coutard developed a specific regimen of protracted fractionation (administering the total dose in small daily doses as compared to a large single dose) which became the basis of modern radiation treatment schedules. Radiation therapists, surgeons, and gynecologists in France, Scandinavia, and England developed techniques for the treatment of carcinoma of the cervix and defined guidelines for local radium application. Thus, modern radiation oncology has origins in surgery and gynecology as well as biology and physics.

With the development of supervoltage radiation equipment, it became possible to deliver larger doses of radiation to deep-seated tumors and, therefore, to produce an effective therapeutic ratio. From this technological advance modern radiotherapy has emerged, and, combined with improved interstitial techniques, has permitted improved cure rates in the past 20 years of a variety of categories of malignant disease, including head and neck cancer, hematologic malignancies, cancer of the female reproductive system, and other tumors. In many circumstances this is accomplished without major loss of form or function. We will attempt to delineate general principles of radiation therapy, including those of radiation biology and radiation physics, and highlight their importance and applicability to specific neoplastic diseases.

RADIATION PHYSICS AND BIOLOGY

The energy and penetrating power of ionizing radiation increases as the photon wavelength decreases. Differences in physical characteristics are, therefore, of major importance. External radiation is divided into superficial, orthovoltage, and supervoltage radiation. Clinically important advantages are seen when radiation is above 500 kV. For example, above 500 kV there is (1) decreased absorption in bone, (2) less damage to the skin at portal entry, and (3) better treatment characteristics, such as reduced lateral scatter of radiation into other tissues. Ionizing radiation over 500 kV is generally referred to as *supervoltage*. Ionizing radiation generated at the 200 to 400 kV range is termed *orthovoltage*. The lower energy radiation range is designated as *superficial* (50 to 140 kV).

Supervoltage radiation has been of great importance in treating tumors deep in the body because in these situations skin tolerance no longer limits doses delivered (maximum ionization occurs below the level of the epidermis). Also, the percent of radiation at any specific depth compared with the surface dose increases as energy increases and produces a therapeutic advantage. Another method of achieving greater dose delivered to a tumor is to employ multiple fields or to rotate the machine so that normal tissue surrounding the tumor receives less dose while the tumor receives the maximum dose. An advantage of orthovoltage and superficial radiation may be seen in the treatment of skin tumors without excessive irradiation of underlying normal tissues (Figure 11-1).

Local irradiation may be applied by sources closely applied to tumors, as in the uterus, vagina, and maxillary antrum. This may be accomplished with hollow containers which are loaded with radioactive isotopes after placement. This is referred to as *intracavitary irradiation*. *Interstitial irradiation* refers to the application of removable sources, such as radium 226, cobalt 60, or iridium 192, or nonremovable sources, such as radon or radioactive gold, inserted directly into the tumor. Radioactive isotopes in solution or colloidal form such as ^{32}P and ^{131}I, may be administered systemically or directly into body cavities. A combination of intelligent application of physical concepts and consideration of the natural history of malignant disease is essential for optimal therapeutic results.

Radiation therapy, like surgery, has a technical aspect, and this must be handled artfully for maximal effectiveness. *Treatment planning* is essential for delivery of radiotherapy. Guidelines for the anatomic localization of the tumor may be necessary, using, for example, computer tomography, radionuclide scanning, or ultrasound scanning in association with contrast radiography. Treatment planning is designed to ensure that a tumor receives an optimal dose and that the normal tissues receive as little radiation as possible. The concept includes not only maximizing tumor dose while minimizing normal tissue dose but also meticulous attention to reproducibility of clinical treatment. This treatment may involve immobilization by casting, etc., as well as obtaining frequent check or portal films to compare with original planning films to ascertain errors in daily delivery of therapy.[1–3]

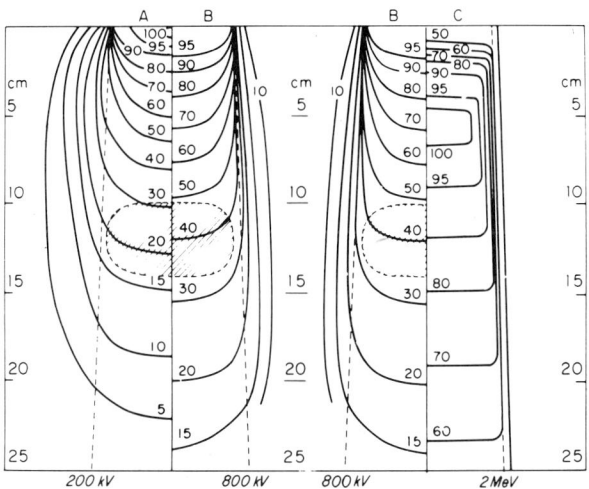

FIGURE 11-1 Comparison of isodose curves in a large volume of tissues with 200-kV (a), 800-kV (b), and 31-MeV (c) radiation. Field size = 7.5-cm diameter. Focus to skin distance = 100 cm. Note the reduction of lateral scattering with 800-kV and 31-MeV compared to 200-kV radiation. Dotted line indicates the geometrical beams. Additional advantage of supervoltage radiation is that maximum dosage is not at skin, and therefore the epidermis is no longer the limiting tissue. (*From F. Buscke and R. Parker.*[1])

Interaction with Matter

X-rays and γ rays are forms of electromagnetic radiation and do not differ from one another in nature or properties. X-rays are produced in an electrical device which accelerates electrons to a high energy and then stops them abruptly at a target. Part of the kinetic energy, or energy of motion, of the electrons is converted into x-rays. On the other hand γ rays are spontaneously emitted by radioactive isotopes and represent excess energy given off as the unstable nucleus breaks up and decays in its effort to reach a stable form.

Ionizing radiations include high-energy (shortwave) electromagnetic radiation and high-speed subatomic particles. These interact with atoms by two mechanisms: excitation and ionization. In excited atoms electrons are shifted to different orbits and become more reactive chemically. In ionized atoms the orbiting electrons are completely ejected from atoms, leaving free radicals which are highly reactive because of the presence of unpaired electrons in the outer shell. Thus, radiation may be *direct* (dominant among high-LET [linear energy transfer, see next section] radiation) or *indirect*, the result of interactions between molecules which produce free radicals. Particulate types of radiation (electrons, protons) are directly ionizing, with sufficient kinetic energy to break chemical bonds. Forms of electromagnetic radiation (gamma and x-rays as well as neutrons) are indirectly ionizing, that is, they do not disrupt chemical bonds directly but produce charged particles with high kinetic energy which then break these bonds.

For the indirect chain of events the final observed effects may be as follows:

Incident x-ray photon
↓
Fast electron
↓
Ion radical pairs
↓
Free radical
↓
Chemical changes due to the breakage of bonds
↓
Biologic effects[2-4]

Linear Energy Transfer

Linear energy transfer (LET) refers to energy transferred per unit length of radiation beam track in the absorbing material. The unit used for this quality is kiloelectronvolts (keV) per micron (μm) of unit density material. Differences in LET can account for the fact that although different radiation may produce qualitatively similar effects (initially, ionization), there are marked differences in biologic effects. For example, photons or x-rays give rise to fast electrons; however, neutrons give rise to recoil protons, particles also carry an electric charge but which have a mass nearly 2000 times greater than that of the electrons. Thus, a greater biologic effect will be produced with more densely ionizing radiation. Typical LET values are as follows:

cobalt 60 gamma rays	0.3 keV/μm
250-keV x-rays	2 keV/μm
14-MeV neutrons	12 keV/μm

The possible applications of high-LET radiation to clinical radiotherapy will be described.[3-5]

Relative Biologic Effect

Equal doses of different types of ionizing radiation do not produce equal biologic effects. It is customary to regard 250-keV x-rays as the standard. This level was chosen because its effects were well documented at the time the convention was adopted. The relative biologic effect (RBE) of some test radiation compared with the 250-keV x-ray is defined by the ratio of D_{250}/D_r, where D_{250} and D_r are the doses of 250-keV x-rays and the radiation r respectively required for an equal effect. This ratio varies with the biologic system and the level of damage produced in that system. In general, up to a certain LET value, RBE increases as LET increases. However, sufficiently densely ionizing radiation may be inefficient because it deposits more energy than necessary in critical sites within the cell, and energy is wasted. These concepts will become important when the oxygen effect and clinical determinants of radiocurability are considered (Fig. 11-2).[2-5]

Survival Curve Reproductive Integrity

A cell may be physically present, morphologically viable, and able to synthesize DNA but have lost the capacity to divide infinitely and produce progeny. Loss of reproductive integrity is the radiobiologic definition of death. A survivor which has retained its reproductive integrity and is able to proliferate indefinitely is said to be *clonogenic*. This is of optimal importance to the clinical cancer therapist, who is concerned with the elimination of the last clonogenic cancer cell. In general, radiation produces a *reproductive* death; that is, cells must divide to express irradiation lethality. Exceptions to this are the small lymphocyte and type A spermatogonia which die an *intermitotic* death.

Data derived from in vitro studies of the relationship between a lethal cellular response and radiation dose was first demonstrated by Puck and Marcus.[6] Their investigations emphasized reproductive integrity, and cells were scored as nonviable unless they demonstrated an ability to sustain proliferation. Cell death need not be closely related in time with cell lysis. Several studies have shown that nonviable cells may survive in a metabolic sense for prolonged periods and may pass through several divisions before lysis. Thompson and Suit in an elegant study demonstrated by cinephotographic observations that mammalian cells irradiated in vitro produced progeny which underwent as many as nine divisions along

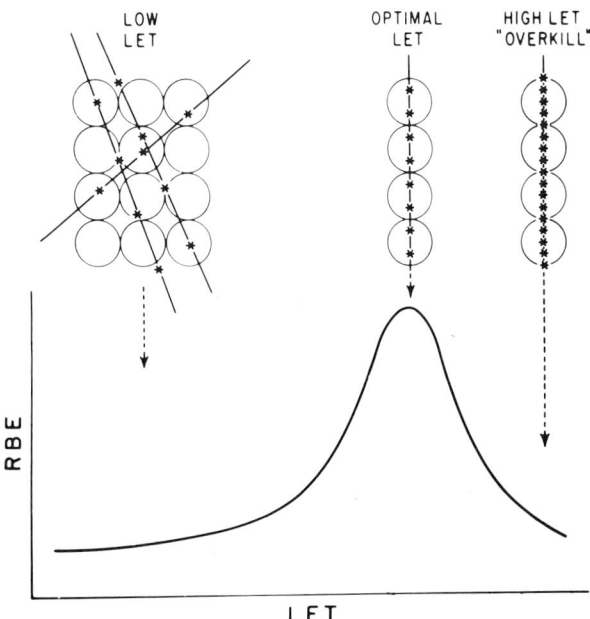

FIGURE 11-2 For a cell to be killed, energy must be deposited in a number of critical sites within the cell. Sparsely ionizing radiation is inefficient because more than one particle must pass through the cell in order to kill it. Densely ionizing radiation is also inefficient because it deposits more than enough energy in the critical sites within the cell; energy is wasted, the cells are "overkilled." Radiation of optimum LET deposits just enough energy to inactivate the critical targets. (*From E. J. Hall.*[3])

The cell cycle can be represented into four stages beginning with M (mitosis), G_1 (gap 1), S (DNA synthesis), and G_2 (gap 2) (see Fig. 11-4). Effects of irradiation at different stages in the cell's life cycle can be studied by using a synchronized population of cells in vitro. This varies from cell line to cell line; however, there are some generalizations.

1. Cells are generally most sensitive near or at mitosis.
2. If G_1 is of appreciable length, a resistant period is usually evident early followed by a decline in survival toward S. The end of G_1 may be as sensitive as S.
3. In most cell lines resistance rises during S to a maximum in the latter part of S. This is usually the most resistant part of the cycle.
4. In most cell lines the G_2 period is sensitive, perhaps as sensitive as the mitosis period in some cells[3,6] (see Fig. 11-5).

branches of the pedigree before cells underwent lysis.[7] This has important clinical implications, since it is obvious that morphological criteria should not be strictly applied to determine clinical radiocurability.

Figure 11-3 shows a typical mammalian radiation survival curve. The inverse of the slope of the straight-line portion of the survival curve is expressed as the dose required to reduce the clonogenic cells by a factor of 0.63 in this portion of the curve and is referred to as the D_0, or the *radiosensitivity* (as distinguished from radiocurability). The extrapolation number $\bar{n}$ is determined by extrapolating the straight-line portion of the curve until it intersects the ordinate (surviving fraction axis). The extrapolation number is significant because it is the measure of the extent of the initial shoulder and the ability to accumulate sublethal damage.[3]

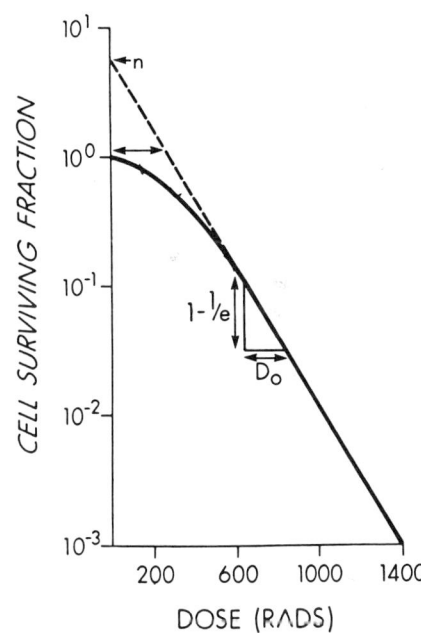

FIGURE 11-3 D_0 is the radiosensitivity, or slope of straight-line portion of the survival curve; $\bar{n}$ is the back extrapolate of the slope to the ordinate and represents the ability to accumulate sublethal damage. (*Adapted from E. J. Hall.*[3])

180 BASIC CONCEPTS IN ONCOLOGY

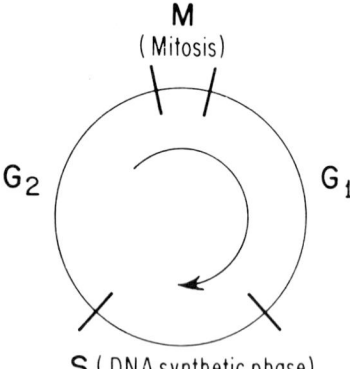

FIGURE 11-4 Diagrammatic representation of the different phases of the mammalian cell growth cycle. (*From E. J. Hall.*[3])

Oxygen and Radiosensitivity

Many of the ionization and excitation properties of radiation depend on molecular oxygen, and it was noted by early workers in radiation biology that cells were relatively resistant to radiation in the absence of oxygen. The exact mechanism of oxygen as a dose-modifying agent is not completely agreed upon; however, it is generally thought to act at the level of free radical formation. As discussed earlier, the absorption of radiation leads to the production of fast charged particles passing through biologic material to produce ion pairs. These ion pairs produce free radicals that are highly reactive molecules because they have unpaired valance electrons. It is these free radicals which break chemical bonds and produce chemical changes and initiate the chain of events which result in the expression of biologic damage. If oxygen is present, it reacts with the free radical R and the reaction produces RO_2: an organic peroxide which is a nonrestorable form of the target material; that is, it is assumed to change in chemical composition. When no oxygen is present, this reaction does not take place, and many of the ionized target molecules can repair or recover from the inability to function normally. The shape of the radiation survival curve is the same under aerated and hypoxic conditions, and the difference is the magnitude of the dose required to produce a given degree of biologic damage, measured as survival (Fig. 11-6). The ratio of hypoxic to aerated doses needed to achieve the same biologic effect is the same at all survival levels because oxygen is said to be a dose-modifying agent. This ratio is called the *oxygen enhancement ratio,* or OER.[3,9,10]

Importance of Hypoxic Cells in Radiotherapy

Thomlinson and Gray studied thin transverse sections of human lung tumors which showed necrotic areas surrounded by intact tumor cells. They found that no tumor cord which had a radius in excess of 200 μm was without a necrotic center. The thickness of the sheaths of actively growing tumor cells was never in excess of 180 μm. Thus, as the necrotic area increased, the sheath of tumor cells remained relatively constant to 100 to 280 μm. Tumor cells could grow only if they were in close proximity to a supply of oxygen. Thomlinson and Gray concluded that the O_2 concentration would fall off sharply with increasing distance from the capillaries, and thus a group of radioresistant hypoxic cells might exist

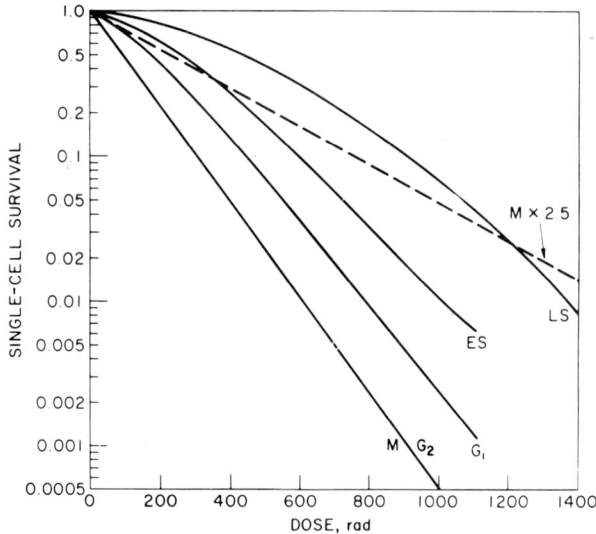

FIGURE 11-5 Representative cell-survival curves for Chinese hamster cells at various stages of the cell cycle. At mitosis, the survival curve is steep and has no shoulder. For cells late in S, the curve is less steep and has a large initial shoulder. G_1 and early S are intermediate in sensitivity. The broken line is a calculated curve expected to apply to mitotic cells under hypoxia. (*From W. K. Sinclair.*[8])

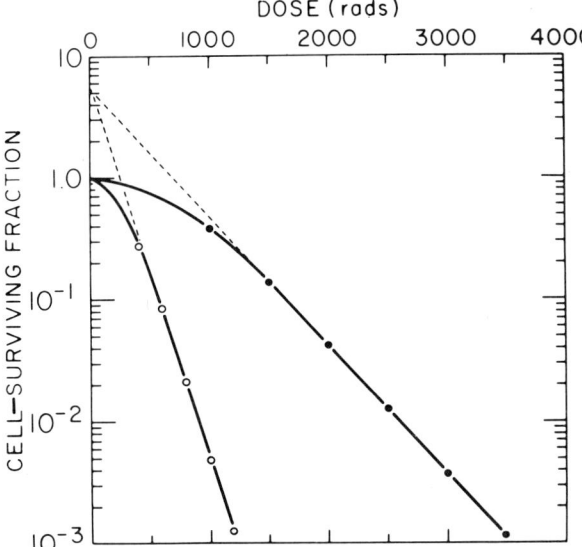

FIGURE 11-6 Typical data of survival curves of mammalian cells exposed to x-rays under aerobic and hypoxic conditions illustrating an oxygen enhancement ratio (OER) of 3.0. The hypoxic cells are more radioresistant. Aerated D_0 = 150 rads; hypoxic D_0 = 450 rads; OER = 3.0. (*Courtesy of E. J. Hall.*[3])

and these hypoxic cells might render a tumor radioincurable (see Fig. 11-7).[10–12]

Reoxygenation

Van Putten[12] determined the portion of hypoxic cells in a transplantable mouse sarcoma. This tumor was transplanted from one generation of animals to the next by subcutaneous inoculation with a known number of tumor cells and was allowed to grow for a period of 2 weeks. The tumor was irradiated in vivo, excised, and the proportion of hypoxic cells determined. Van Putten found that the proportion of hypoxic cells in the untreated tumor was 14 percent. He then determined the proportion of hypoxic cells following various fractionated radiation treatments and determined that the proportion of hypoxic cells in the tumor was approximately the same at the end of fractionated radiotherapy as in the untreated tumor. This was interpreted as evidence that during the course of treatment cells move from the hypoxic to the well-oxygenated compartment of the tumor. If this were not the case, the proportion of hypoxic cells would increase during the course of fractionated treatment because radiation would depopulate the aerated compartment more than the hypoxic compartment, since aerated cells are more sensitive to ionizing radiation. This phenomenon, whereby hypoxic cells became oxygenated after doses of radiation, has been termed *reoxygenation*.[12–14]

Repair of Radiation Damage

Cells in an irradiated population fall into one of four categories: An ionizing event may not have occurred in

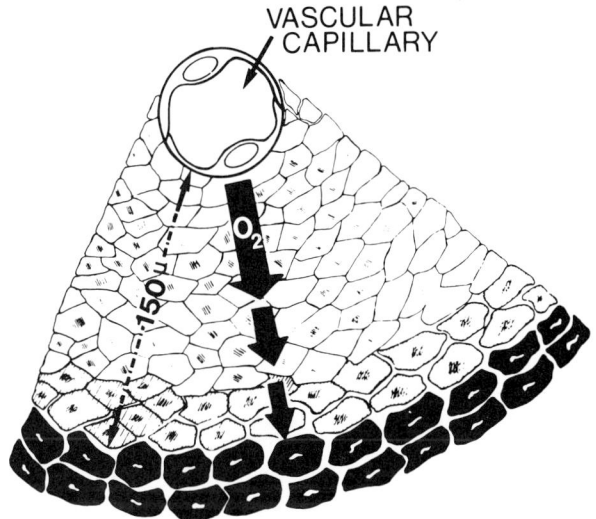

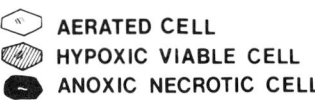

FIGURE 11-7 Diffusion of oxygen from a capillary through tumor tissue. The diffusion distance of oxygen is limited largely by the rapid rate at which it is metabolized by respiring tumor cells. Up to about 150 μm from a capillary, cells are well-oxygenated. At greater distances, oxygen is depleted, and tumor cells become necrotic. Hypoxic tumor cells form a layer in between, and the oxygen concentration is high enough for the cells to be viable but low enough for them to be relatively protected from the effects of x-rays. These cells may limit the radiocurability of the tumor. (*Courtesy of E. J. Hall.*[3])

any of the critical targets, and therefore the cell is unchanged. An ionizing event may have occurred in all of the critical targets sites, in which case the cell is killed, i.e., has lost its reproductive integrity. A cell may have received an ionizing event at some but not all of its critical sites. The cell is then said to have suffered sublethal damage, and, given time, it may be able to repair and recover from the effects of this damage. Finally, a cell may have suffered an ionizing event which is lethal under normal circumstances but which may be repaired sufficiently to permit survival if exposed to appropriate posttreatment conditions. This is referred to as potentially lethal radiation damage.

REPAIR OF SUBLETHAL DAMAGE

When the surviving fraction is plotted against dose on a semilogarithmic plot, there is a shoulder followed by a steeper portion. The threshold of response implies that damage must be accumulated in a cell before it loses reproductive integrity. This multiplicity of target sites accounts for the initial shoulder of survival curve. A cell may have received an ionizing event at some but not in all of its critical sites and may be said to have suffered sublethal damage; it has been damaged but not killed. Given time, the cell may repair the effects of sublethal damage and completely recover from it. The time period required for repair of sublethal damage is approximately 1 h.

Repair of sublethal damage (SLDR) was extensively studied by Elkind and his collaborators.[15–17] They introduced a technique by which the effect of exposure to a single dose of radiation was compared with the effect of exposure to the total dose divided into equal fractions. Figure 11-8 shows an increase in survival between fractions. However, this is a complex function, as the figure shows, with an enhancement, decrement, and second enhancement in survival. This is because radiation lethality and repair are cell cycle–specific. For example, in the case of Chinese hamster cells shown in Fig. 11-8, the majority of the survivors are located in the S phase of the cycle. If a period of time is allowed to elapse before a second dose is given, this group of initially exposed cells may progress around the period of the cell cycle, which in the case of Chinese hamster cells would be late G_2 or M. If the increase in radiosensitivity moving from S to late G_2 exceeds the effect of repair of sublethal damage, the surviving fraction falls. The pattern is shown in Fig. 11-8 and is a combination of two processes

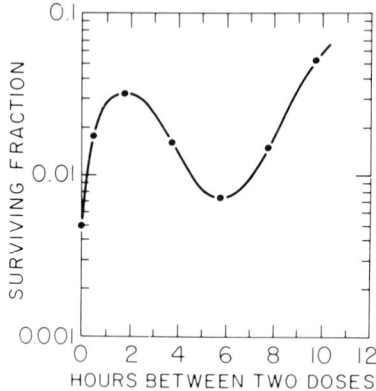

FIGURE 11-8 Survival of Chinese hamster cells exposed to two fractions of x-rays and incubated at 37°C for various time intervals between the two doses (707 and 804 rads). (*From M. M. Elkind et al.*[17])

taking place: first, the repair of sublethal damage and second, progression of the cell cycle. Enhancement in ultimate survival due to sublethal damage repair over a 30-fraction treatment scheme even with a very small $\bar{n}$ might be quite important clinically.

REPAIR OF POTENTIALLY LETHAL DAMAGE

Environmental conditions after exposure to x-ray can influence cells that survive a given dose. Initial studies were performed with culture cells in vitro. The fraction of cells surviving a given dose could be increased above or decreased below the normal level, depending on the nature of the perturbed postirradiation condition. If survival after a given dose is increased above the normal level, this can be interpreted to mean that potentially lethal damage has been repaired. If survival is decreased below normal levels, this can be interpreted to mean that more potentially lethal damage has been expressed. Initally some investigators studied cells incubated in balanced salt solution. This condition did not closely mimic conditions seen in vivo, however, and density-inhibited plateau-phase cells are now employed and are a considerably better in vitro model for tumor cells in vivo.

Weichselbaum and Little have shown that cells from some human tumors considered nonradiocurable do considerably more potentially lethal damage repair (PLDR) in vitro than cells derived from tumors considered radiocurable, with a large heterogeneous intermediate group.[20,21] PLDR may be a major determinant of poor radiocurability since human tumors of varying radiocurability have been shown to have relatively similar radiosensitivity in vitro. Exceptions to this may be human melanoma and glioblastoma cell lines, which some investigators have shown to be resistant to ionizing radiation in vitro (Table 11-1). Even small amounts of PLDR may be deleterious to clinical radiocurability, especially if this is added to sublethal damage repair (SLDR) (Figs. 11-9 and 11-10). SLDR and PLDR may be the major cellular determinants of radiocurability in vitro.

Molecular DNA Repair

Repair of ultraviolet (UV) light damage in mammalian cells DNA is better characterized than damage induced by x-rays. The autosomal recessive disease xeroderma pigmentosum, which has a deficiency in excision repair, has greatly aided in the study of both UV mammalian damage repair and carcinogenesis. Some bacterial model systems for the investigation of x-ray damage include the study of repair of breaks in single and/or double strands of DNA. After the introduction of the alkaline-sucrose gradient centrification technique in bacteria, this method was quickly adapted to the use of mammalian cells. There is general agreement that under physiolog-

TABLE 11-1 Radiosensitivity of Exponentially Growing Human Tumor Cell Lines in Vitro*

Cell line	Tumor type	D_0 (exp.)	$\bar{n}$ (exp.)
TX-4	Osteosarcoma	145±7	1.8±0.3
SAOS	Osteosarcoma	135±9	2.2±0.5
TX-7	Medulloblastoma	135±14	1.5±0.3
TX-14	Medulloblastoma	131±8	1.6±0.9
TX-13	Glioblastoma	143±10	1.4±0.5
MCF-7	Breast carcinoma	134±13	1.3±0.3
LAN-1	Neuroblastoma	149±7	1.2±0.2
MEL-H	Melanoma	150±5	2.5±0.4
PAS	Hypernephroma	131±11	1.2±0.4

* Relatively similar radiosensitivities of human tumor cells in vivo. Exceptions may be some radioresistant melanoma and glioma lines (D_0 220–250).
SOURCE: Courtesy of R. Weichselbaum.

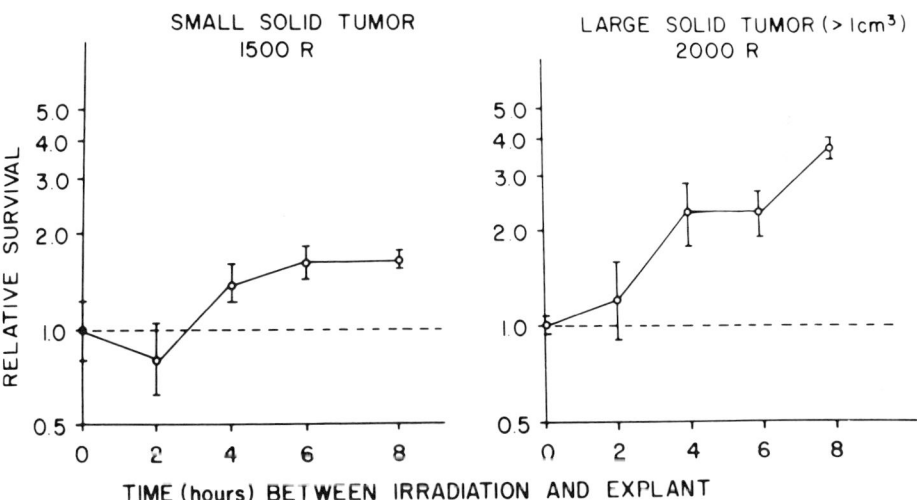

FIGURE 11-9 Repair of potentially lethal damage (PLD) in mouse fibrosarcomas. The tumors were irradiated in situ, then removed and prepared into single-cell suspensions. The number of survivors was then determined by their ability to form colonies in vitro when plated into petri dishes. The fraction of cells surviving a given dose increases if a time interval is allowed between irradiation and removal of the tumor because during this interval PD is repaired. (From J. B. Little et al.[18])

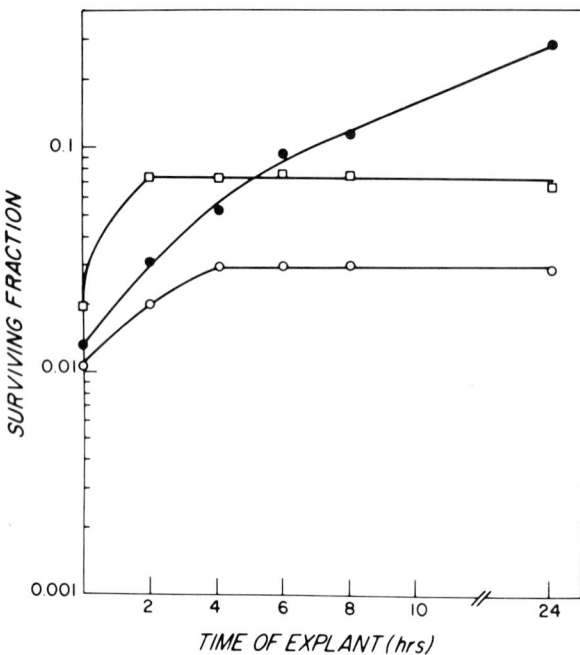

FIGURE 11-10 Darkened circles indicate repair of potentially lethal x-ray damage of a human osteosarcoma compared to a normal human diploid cell strain (open circles) and LICH cells (squares). (*Courtesy of R. Weichselbaum.*)

ical conditions most single-band breaks are repaired. However, the relevance of the single-stranded breaks to reproductive integrity in mammalian cells has been severely challenged, since most doses which induce a high degree of strand breaks are not physiological i.e., 20,000 rads. It may be that there is a critical portion of unrejoined strands which may lead to the loss of reproductive integrity of the cell.

Another type of DNA lesion produced by ionizing radiation is base damage. The role of base damage in cell killing is unknown, and some investigators feel that this may be more important for radiation-induced mutagenesis and perhaps carcinogenesis than actual cell killing.[7] Hopefully techniques will be developed better to study gamma-ray induced molecular DNA damage in mammalian cells.

Normal Tissue Reactions

Normal tissue reactions to radiation therapy are related to the volume of tissue irradiated, the time of administration of treatment, and the total dose of radiation administered. Acute reactions develop as a consequence of radiation damage to proliferating cell renewal systems and are, therefore, most noticeable in tissues with rapidly proliferating cell renewal systems. This includes, for example, the mucosal lining of the oral cavity and pharynx and the lining of the gastrointestinal tract. Interruption of treatment for a variable period during a planned course or a decrease in fraction size (if this is not too great, i.e., from 200 to 180 rads/day) may be necessary to complete a treatment course. There seems to be individual patient variation, which must be considered, but this appears related to patient age and general condition.

A specific example of an acute reaction is the mucositis of oral irradiation that occurs because the destruction of cells in the basal layers exceeds their production. The patient notices pain in the mouth and has difficulty in swallowing. The acute effects are generally reversible by decreasing the killing or allowing more time for cell proliferation.

In contrast to acute reactions, the chronic effects of irradiation are observed from months to years following irradiation. The mechanism of chronic radiation complications is not generally thought to be related to acute interruption of normal cell renewal systems but rather to the effects of radiation on the vascular supply (vascular endothelial damage) although the exact mechanism(s) are unclear (for example, the effect of radiation on postmitotic cells is not well studied). Recently Withers has hypothesized that the late effects of radiation are strongly dependent on damage to somatic cells of the organ at risk and not on the vascular supply alone.[22,23] Each organ has a unique radiation tolerance, and thus compromises of the vascular supply may not entirely explain all long-term effects of radiation. These late radiation therapy complications are very important and frequently are the most critical limitation in treatment. Even though tolerance doses may be exceeded, not all patients will develop problems, since the likelihood of complications is a probability event. In practice, this probability is balanced against a probability of tumor control, and allowing the radiation therapist to decide the dose that will be likely to control the tumor while having at the same time an estimate of the risk of normal tissue damage produced by this dose.

Time/Dose Relationships in Radiotherapy

The pioneers in radiation therapy found that radiation was more effective in curing tumors and decreasing damage to the normal tissues when small doses were given each day as opposed to one single large dose. The final effect of radiation on both the normal and malignant tissue is dependent on (1) final overall dose, (2) fraction size or the dose given per treatment session, (3) the total number of days over which the radiation is delivered, and (4) the volume of tissue irradiated. Although sophisticated formulas have been developed to equate different fractionation schemes, experience plays the most important role in the clinical development of this concept.[24] It must be pointed out that the ultimate limiting factors in normal tissue tolerance are generally not the acute effects of radiation (e.g., mucositis) but the long-term effects (necrosis).

Clinical Radiocurability

The term *radiocurability* refers to whether a tumor is cured by the maximum tolerable dose of radiation; *radioresponsive* refers to the rate of regression after irradiation but not to whether a tumor is radiocurable; and *radiosensitivity* refers to the D_0 (see earlier discussion). Carcinoma of the prostate, for example, is characterized by a relatively slow cell renewal system but is controlled locally by radiotherapy in a high percentage of cases, and rates of regression are meaningless. The surgeon must not be misled by positive biopsies obtained at inappropriate time intervals, or by slow regression rates. Thus, prostate cancer is radiocurable but not radioresponsive. On the other hand, oat-cell carcinoma of the lung regresses rapidly after delivery of relatively low doses (3000 to 3500 rads) yet one-third to one-half of these lesions may fail locally, even with relatively high doses (5500 to 6000 rads). Therefore, oat-cell carcinoma is extremely radioresponsive but not necessarily radiocurable. It is essential that these concepts be sharply distinguished when therapies are employed in malignant disease and end results are evaluated.

As should be understood from previous discussion, repair, reoxygenation, repopulation, and possibly redistribution of tumor cells may be determinants of radiocurability. The rate of tumor regression is related not only to cell kill but to cell loss. The cell loss factor may be defined as the ratio of cell loss to the rate of new tumor cell production. Thus, the overall growth or regression of a tumor is the result of an equilibrium achieved by clonogenic cell production (or destruction) and various types of cell loss. Many cells lost from a tumor may be dead from treatment or inadequate nutrition, or they may be viable cells with metastatic potential.[25]

Control of Subclinical Disease

An important concept in modern radiation therapy is that subclinical (microscopic) disease is controlled with lower doses than grossly detectable cancer. The probability of local control for a variety of carcinomas (subclinical disease) as a function of dose is seen in Table 11-2. Most patients with microscopic disease are controlled with doses of 5000 rads in five weeks, and in general this has been shown to be relatively independent of disease type or site (neck nodes, breast cancer, soft-tissue sarcomas, etc.).[26] This clinical concept is supported by biologic data discussed previously; for example, small tumors (microscopic) are much less likely to have hypoxic and/or necrotic centers, and, in any case, since radiation kills a fixed proportion of cells, the fewer cells present, the higher the probability of control. Furthermore, less potentially lethal radiation damage may be repaired by smaller tumors as compared to larger tumors. This concept may be extended to gross clinical disease and supported by the fact that T_1 lesions in general, regardless of site of histology, are more radiocurable than T_3 or T_4 lesions (see "Tumors Cured Primarily with Radiotherapy," below). These clinical and biologic observations have led to consideration of conservative surgery and combined with moderate doses of irradiation.[26] The advantage of such an approach is to employ nonmutilating surgery with doses of radiation that do not have a high likelihood of long-term complications.

TABLE 11-2 Percent of Control of Subclinical Disease in Function of Dose*

Adenocarcinoma of the breast		Squamous cell carcinoma of the upper respiratory and digestive tracts	
3000–3500 rads (89 patients)	60–70%	3000–4000 rads (50 patients)	60–70%
4000 rads (121 patients)	80–90%	5000 rads (356 patients)	>90%
5000 rads (273 patients)	>90%	6000 rads (65 patients)	>90%

* 1000 rads/week, 5 days a week.
SOURCE: From Fletcher.[26]

TREATMENT PHILOSOPHY

In terms of the therapeutic role for radiation therapy in the management of patients with malignant disease, two broad categories are established: Therapy for patients treated for cure by the application of any modality is generally termed *radical,* and, with few exceptions, this involves aggressive therapy. The second category of therapy applies to patients who are treated for relief of specific symptoms and is termed *palliative.* The dose of radiation in this instance is often less than what would be employed for cure, since the production of side effects is undesirable, and complete tumor eradication is frequently unnecessary. The specific role for radiation therapy in a curative or palliative posture is related to the stage of the tumor, and the goals of therapy must be clearly delineated.

Risk versus Gain

The concept of risk versus gain has been shown to be valuable in the formulation of treatment of malignant disease at many sites. When making this determination, the clinical oncologist must bear in mind not only the probability of cure but the consequences of the treatment modality. For example, patients might select a therapeutic modality which produces a lesser cure rate (radiation therapy in advanced bladder cancer) but preserves function (sexual function, urinary function, etc.). Certainly, when cure rates are equal or close to equal, nonmutilating therapy must be given preference. End results in neoplastic disease are not only analyzed by survival but by a detailed analysis of failure, e.g., local, regional, or distant. In some diseases (most head and neck cancer) local control is tantamount to cure. In other diseases (breast cancer), survival is largely determined by control of distant metastasis.

It is useful for our discussion to classify tumors as (1) curative primarily with radiotherapy; (2) curative with combinations of radiotherapy and surgery with radiotherapy delivered pre- or postoperatively (this does not necessarily imply that a full cancer operation must be performed and, as we will explain, intermediate doses of radiation may be combined with conservative surgery; chemotherapy may be added as well, although its role is evolving); and (3) having a very low probability of cure (lung, esophagus).

Several representative diseases in each of the curative categories have been selected for examination of the role of radiotherapy in each class of disease. Biologic principles are integrated in the clinical discussion, but to cover all diseases in each category is impossible. The detailed role of radiotherapy is elaborated upon in each individual disease–oriented chapter.

TUMORS CURED PRIMARILY WITH RADIOTHERAPY

Local control is associated with cure in head and neck cancer although many patients die of intercurrent disease. Second primary tumors of the aerodigestive tract may also take their toll. Bone invasion connotes an ominous prognosis for patients treated with radiation alone, and in general these patients require radiation therapy and surgery together.

Carcinoma of the palatine arch, retromolar trigone, and tonsil are successfully managed with external radiation and implantation (to boost local doses). Results of preoperative radiation therapy and composite resection are comparable to radiation therapy alone, but cosmetic results with radiation therapy as the sole therapeutic modality are much superior to combination therapy.[26-28]

Carcinoma of the base of the tongue has a much graver prognosis than cancer of the anterior two-thirds of the tongue and floor of the mouth and/or other oropharyngeal lesions. These are frequently deeply infiltrating, and 70 percent of such patients may present with lymph node metastasis. These patients are generally treated with radiotherapy since a total glossectomy is mutilating and a therapeutically unsatisfactory procedure. The base of tongue is an extremely difficult region in which to obtain an adequate geometric implant. The overall survival is approximately 20 percent, but it should be noted that many patients present with advanced disease.

Radiotherapy plays a major role in the treatment of oral cavity cancer. Tumors are classified using the TNM system of either the American Joint Committee or UICC. T refers to primary tumor size, N to regional node involvement, and M to distant metastasis. Although these staging systems undergo constant modifications, T_1 lesions are obviously smaller and more favorable than advanced T_4 lesions. External irradiation and implantation is the treatment of choice for carcinoma of the anterior two-thirds of the tongue and floor of the mouth. Furthermore, cosmetic results with radiotherapy are usually superior to those achieved by surgical procedures.

The exceptions are very small (less than 2 cm) lesions of the tongue which may be excised. Very large lesions or lesions which involve the mandible or other alveolar bone are managed with preoperative radiotherapy and surgical resection. Excellent results obtained with radiotherapy in carcinoma of the floor of the mouth are shown in Table 11-3.[26,28,29] It should be noted that good surgical salvage is noted for the radiation failures in these lesions. The advantages of prophylactic neck irradiation will be discussed. Results from carcinoma of the anterior two-thirds of the tongue are similar.

Carcinoma of the tongue and oropharynx illustrate several interesting biologic principles. First, for reasons unknown, bony invasion confers poor radiocurability upon lesions which might be otherwise controlled. Second, if an adequate geometric implant can be performed, local control rates are extremely high. This may be due to high dose delivery to tumor relative to normal tissue and/or the fact that the *dose rate* from interstitial implant is approximately 40 rads/h, and this may confer a special therapeutic advantage with regard to tumor control versus normal tissue tolerance. The effects of low dose rates on normal and malignant tissues are presently under investigation.

Larynx

Tumors of the true vocal cord are treated by curative radiotherapy. Final functional and tumor control results, as in other parts of the body, are dependent upon the total dose, number of fractions given, volume of irradiation, and fraction size per day. In general, the mobility of the cords is used to stage lesions: in T_1 both cords have normal mobility; in T_2 there is partial mobility; in T_3 there is complete fixation; and in T_4 there has been invasion of the cartilage. The cure rates with radiotherapy alone for T_1 and T_2 lesions are approximately 90 percent and 80 percent, respectively. Salvage surgery adds another 5 to 10 percent to the ultimate cure rate in early lesions.

Carcinoma of the Uterine Cervix

Radiation therapy plays a major role in the treatment of carcinoma of the uterine cervix, with the exception of cancer in stage IA (usually managed with a conservative surgical procedure) and stage IB, where radical surgery is an alternative offering equal survival. Radiotherapy is preferred in all other stages. A combination of intracavitary and external irradiation is used. Early-stage disease is treated with intracavitary radiation which supplies the majority or all of the radiation to central disease, and with supplemental parametrial external radiation. In advanced disease, however, increasing increments of external radiation become necessary, and decreasing amounts of central radium are possible.

The technique currently employed in most of the United States generally includes two radium applications

TABLE 11-3 Results of Primary Irradiation of Carcinoma of the Floor of the Mouth, M. D. Anderson Hospital, 1948–1968

Stage	Percentage of patients by stages and modality of treatment		Local results in patients treated with irradiation		
	Surgical excision, %	Irrad., %	Failures following irradiation, %	Patients salvaged by surgical excision†	Ultimate local failures, %
T_1	35	23	2 (1/49)	1/1	0
T_2	24	36	11.5 (9/77)	4/9	6.5
T_3	28	30	23 (14/60)	11/14	5
T_4	13	11	79 (19/24)	0/19	79
Total number of patients	68	210	20.5 (43/210)		13 (27/210)

* Squamous cell carcinoma developing at any time in the follow-up in the vicinity of the initial lesion is counted as recurrence.
† NED at 2 years after treatment of failure.
SOURCE: Adapted from Fletcher.[26]

for a total of approximately 7000 rads to central disease in early-stage cervix cancer. As stated before, the amount of central radium used in late-stage disease decreases as the amount of external irradiation that is necessary increases. The most important aspect of this therapy is that it is highly effective, with cure rates in stage IB of between 80 and 90 percent; IIA between 75 and 80 percent; IIB, between 60 and 65 percent; IIIA, 50 percent; IIIB, 30 to 40 percent. Patients with IVA disease have a poor prognosis unless only bladder is involved, in which case the survival is approximately 30 percent. Technique plays a large role in good results, and geometric application of the ovoids (colpostats) and tandem must be adequate to ensure a uniform dose to the entire lesion. Important in the radiation therapy is the blending of intracavitary and external radiation to ensure adequate doses to the sites at risk for tumor. With early disease, the emphasis is on central and parametrial doses. With advanced disease, effective radiation of the pelvic lymph nodes causes greater need for external irradiation.

Adenocarcinoma of the cervix is treated exactly like epidermoid carcinoma of the cervix. A myth has arisen that this is radioresistant; however, the results are comparable for both cell types within each state.[34,35]

TREATMENT OF SUBCLINICAL DISEASE BY RADIATION ALONE

Prophylactic Irradiation of the Neck

The presence of subclinical disease (disease present but not clinically detectable) in cervical lymph nodes has been documented by elective radical neck dissection. The incidence of neck metastasis in clinically negative patients with carcinoma of the mobile tongue has been reported from 40 to 60 percent and is even as high as 20 percent in patients with early lesions.[36,37] Historically, controversy arose over the advisability of elective neck dissections. At the M. D. Anderson Hospital, most patients with squamous carcinoma of the nasopharynx, palatine arch, tonsillar fossa, and base of the tongue were treated by irradiation to both sides of the neck.[26] The dose to the upper neck was never less than 5000 rads and often 6000 rads. Although the lower neck was occasionally omitted from treatment, patients with palatine arch lesions have been treated by variable approaches, some involving only ipsilateral or bilateral subdigastric areas rather than the entire neck. In the above groups, new neck disease appeared in 12 percent of patients whose necks were *partially* irradiated (much lower than the expected rate of metastasis). Only 1.7 percent of patients in whom the *entire* neck was irradiated (their primaries usually in the nasopharynx, tonsil, and base of the tongue) showed metastasis in areas which were initially clinically negative. More than one-third of these patients were initially staged N_3 and had a high risk for occult disease.

Table 11-4 shows a marked decrease in metastasis (all head and neck sites) in the opposite side of the neck in patients who were prophylactically irradiated as part of an overall treatment plan. Fewer metastases developed as dose increased. For example, when no irradiation was delivered, 46 of 187 (24 percent) developed metastasis in the contralateral neck. When modest (3000 to 4000 rads) doses were employed 5 of 50 (10 percent) patients developed new metastatic disease. When 5000 to 6000 rads were employed, only 1 of 137 patients developed metastatic nodes. Both of the above examples clearly show that as *volume* and *dose* increase, the number of new metastatic sites drop far below their expected frequency. Between 4500 and 5000 rads will sterilize microscopic lymph nodes in the neck, which is consistent with the previously elucidated biologic principles. The treatment of occult metastasis has been a major advance in the treatment of head and neck cancer, and a prophylactic neck dissection may be avoided.[26,36-41]

These are examples of disease managed with radiotherapy alone. Others include Hodgkin's disease and non-Hodgkin's lymphomas, seminoma, all varieties of nasopharynx cancer, gliomas, carcinoma of the prostate, and a variety of pediatric tumors (usually managed with chemotherapy and minimal surgery).

DISEASES MANAGED WITH PRE- OR POSTOPERATIVE RADIOTHERAPY AND SURGERY

The rationale for preoperative radiotherapy is to sterilize the well-oxygenated peripheral cells in a tumor and to remove the central nidus with a surgical excision. This may not only increase local control but decrease the shedding of cells at the time of surgery and decrease the incidence of distant metastasis. Postoperative radiotherapy may decrease local recurrences by eradicating microscopic disease left in the surgical bed. Both pre- and postoperative radiotherapy have been combined with radical surgical approaches. A new concept is emerging of delivering intermediate doses of radiation combined with conservative surgical procedures to maximize local control while preserving cosmesis and function.

TABLE 11-4 Control of Subclinical Disease in Squamous Cell Carcinoma of the Floor of Mouth, Oral Tongue, Faucial Arch, Supraglottic Larynx, and Pyriform Sinus—Primary Lesion and Initial Neck Disease Controlled*

	Without irradiation				With irradiation	
Floor of mouth (N_1 and N_2)†	47.5%	(9/19)	10.5%	(3/28)	3000 rads/3 weeks to 4000 rads/4 weeks	To opposite subdigastric & submaxillary triangle nodes
Oral tongue (N_1 and N_2)†	27.0%	(8/30)	9.0%	(2/22)		
Faucial Arch (N_1 & N_2)†	30.0%		0%	(0/72)	5000 rads/5 weeks	To opposite subdigastric nodes
Supraglottic larynx and pyriform sinus†	20.0%	(26/128)	1.5%	(1/65)	6000 rads/6 weeks upper neck 5000 rads/5 weeks given dose to lower neck	
Total	24.0%	(46/187)	3.0%	(6/187)		

* All treatments 1000 rads/week 5 days a week. New disease in opposite side of neck initially clinically negative. Control of subclinical disease is consistent with previously elucidated biologic principles.
† N_1: single clinically positive node ≤ 3 cm; N_2: single clinically positive node > 3 cm not fixed or multiple clinically positive ipsilateral nodes.
SOURCE: From Fletcher.[26]

Metastatic Neck Nodes

The treatment of carcinoma metastatic to neck nodes has evolved into a multidisciplinary problem. Previously, radical neck dissection alone was considered adequate treatment. However, the incidence of recurrent cancer in the neck after radical neck dissection is between 26.5 and 36.5 percent.[36,37] When the operative specimen is positive, 54 percent of patients with positive nodes and 71 percent of patients with positive nodes in multiple levels develop recurrent disease. This is likely to be due to microscopic cancer in lymphatic channels which are not totally removed. In both randomized and nonrandomized trials, pre- or postoperative irradiation has dramatically diminished the incidence of recurrences. The policy at the M. D. Anderson Hospital is to combine moderate doses of radiation with radical or modified radical neck dissection. The results are clearly superior to those for patients treated with surgery alone (local failure in combination treatment group is 8.8 percent).[20,30–40] It should be pointed out that small, movable nodes can be treated by external radiotherapy and implantation or irradiation and electron beam. Studies from the University of Maryland and Stanford University show very good local control rates, even in the face of gross disease. In general, we agree with Jesse and Fletcher that high doses to the neck or whole-neck implant should be avoided, and that moderate-dose radiotherapy (5000 rads) with modified neck dissection of gross disease is a reasonable choice for treatment of multiple nodes. Single nodes can be managed with radiation and surgery or radiation and small volume implant. It must be emphasized that carcinoma in neck nodes is not radioresistant.[36–42]

Salivary Gland Tumors

Malignant tumors arise in both major and minor salivary glands. Of these tumors 70 to 80 percent occur in the parotid, and most are benign. Tumors in the minor salivary glands are more likely to be malignant than parotid tumors and are scattered within the mucosal lining of the hypopharynx, larynx, oral cavity, oropharynx, and paranasal sinuses. The accepted classification of salivary gland tumors is that of Foote and Frazel, which divides malignant salivary gland tumors into malignant mixed tumors, mucoepidermoid tumors (low- and high-grade), squamous carcinoma, unclassified tumors, and the adenocarcinoma group, which includes adenoidcystic carcinoma, acinic cell carcinoma, and a miscellaneous group.[44] The traditional treatment of malignant salivary gland tumors has been radical surgery, based on the assumption that these tumors are radioresistant. A review of Beahrs' study from the Mayo Clinic demonstrated a local recurrence rate of 37.5 percent in moderately malignant tumors of the parotid gland and 72.5 percent in highly malignant tumors.[42] An attempt at preservation of facial nerve function was embarked upon by Guillamondegui and Fletcher.[45] They have shown radiation is an effective adjunct to local excision when gross cancer is removed, even when disease is present at the surgical margin. Only 2 of 30 patients treated in this fashion, i.e., by removal of gross tumor and radiation, had local recurrence. Radiation is generally delivered in a homogeneous treatment volume to the ipsilateral parotid and frequently includes the stylomastoid foramen. In general, the policy of conservative surgery and postoperative radiotherapy may be applied to minor salivary gland tumors. Low-grade tumors that are completely excised are generally not followed with postoperative radiotherapy; however, a major exception to this is the adenoidcystic group. These tumors have an extremely long natural history and invade perineural spaces. Local recurrence distal even to a large surgical resection is frequent, and these patients should always have postoperative radiotherapy to include the base of the skull.

Rectum-Rectosigmoid Tumors

Following abdominoperineal resection, local recurrence rates of between 25 and 50 percent in B_2-C_2 lesions may be anticipated. Preoperative radiotherapy has been shown to significantly reduce the number of local recurrences and to decrease the expected surgical state of lesions. Furthermore, the only randomized trial to date shows a survival advantage in patients treated with relatively low dose preoperative radiotherapy for rectal cancer. Recently, the concept of postoperative radiotherapy in carcinoma of the rectum has emerged. Theoretically, this is appealing since the radiation oncologist, in general, would not recommend treatment for A, B_1, or D lesions, thereby eliminating many patients who might be treated with preoperative radiotherapy. Selection, therefore, highlights the group to be benefited. These principles may also apply to the low sigmoid colon. Local recurrence for the rest of the colon is less of a problem and patients must be individualized regarding pre- or postoperative radiotherapy.[26]

Bladder

Of all patients with carcinoma of the bladder 40 to 50 percent fail to show extrapelvic extension of tumor, and therefore local treatment is of great importance. Staging is generally based on infiltration into the muscle and perivesicle fat. In Europe the TNM system is employed, whereas designations A through D (connoting muscle and fat invasion) are employed in the United States. Patients are staged B_2 and/or C with deep muscle invasion and/or perivesicle fat extension. Optimum therapeutic results are obtained with preoperative radiotherapy to a total dose of 4000 to 5000 rads and cystectomy. Approximately 20 percent of all patients with B_2-C lesions as well as an additional 10 percent (total of 30 percent) may be cured with radical radiotherapy and salvage surgery. Results in B_2-C lesions with preoperative radiotherapy and surgery are approximately 45 percent 5-year NED survival. Risk versus gain arguments may be employed since loss of urinary and sexual function accompanies cystectomy. Some patients may opt for lower survival probability to continue these functions. Alternative treatment in B_1 lesions is external beam followed by implantation (or implantation alone) with radioactive material directly into the bladder. This must be done in cooperation with the urologist with direct intravesicle implantation. Good results (60 percent 5-year survival) have been reported.

In the previous sections we have discussed pre- and postoperative radiotherapy in combination with radical cancer operations (except in salivary gland tumors). We will now discuss treatment strategies which include radiotherapy employed in higher doses than in the previous section and with conservative surgery permitting optimum cosmesis and function.

Breast

Radical surgery has been standard treatment for breast carcinoma in the United States for many years. Primary radiation therapy has been more commonly employed in Europe and Canada.

Most oncologists agree that long-term survival in breast carcinoma depends upon prevention of distant metastasis although adequate local control must be obtained for cure. Therefore, efficiency of local treatment should be judged by local control as well as cosmetic and functional results after treatment. Radical mastectomy may achieve local control in approximately 90 percent of patients with early carcinoma of the breast. However, the cosmetic results following the surgery are unacceptable to many women. Radiation therapy following excisional biopsy offers a possibility of local control and

TABLE 11-5 Patients with Stages I and II Breast Cancer Treated between July, 1968, and December, 1976, by the Joint Center for Radiation Therapy

TNM category	Stage	No. of patients	Bilateral tumors	Range of follow-up
T_1, N_0	I	45	2	11–89 months
T_2, N_0	II	52	2	12–97 months
T_1, N_1	II	14	1	
T_2, N_1	II	18	1	
Total		129	6	11–97 months

SOURCE: Courtesy of J. R. Harris.

cosmetic preservation. At the Harvard Joint Center for Radiation Therapy 98 percent of patients with stage I breast cancer and 88 percent of patients with stage II carcinoma have been locally controlled. Figure 11-11 shows the cumulative incidence of local failure. This is a valid indicator since most local recurrences occur within 2 years after treatment.

The extent of surgery can be adjusted by the amount of tissue resected; similarly, radiation therapy can be varied by dose, time, and volume of normal tissues and tumor irradiated. The concept of dose-response as previously discussed is essential to the current practice of radiation therapy. Increasing doses give increased likelihood of tumor control but also of complications; 4500 to 5000 rads have been effective in eradicating microscopic disease. The general plan at the Harvard Joint Center is for a combination of total excisional biopsy of primary tumor mass followed by external radiation to a total dose of 5000 rads at 200 rads per fraction, 5 days a week, with an additional 1500 to 2000 rads interstitial implantation. Although most microscopic disease is controlled at 4500 to 5000 rads, almost all can be controlled when additional interstitial radiation is given. Since the volume is small, this does not appear to affect cosmetic results. These were reviewed by the Joint Center group and found to be excellent (Figs. 11-12 and 11-13).[46,47]

Requirements for radiation therapy for breast cancer include supervoltage equipment, sufficient treatment planning to ensure coverage of all potentially involved areas, and compensation for missing tissue and to reduce dose inhomogeneity. Similar experience in breast carcinoma has been demonstrated at Yale and at Jefferson Universities. Even more extensive experience has been reported from France. The high local control rates in breast carcinoma as well as excellent cosmetic results are consistent[46,47] with biologic principles previously elucidated.

The role of postoperative therapy is more controversial. There is significant evidence that local control is enhanced by postoperative radiotherapy, especially when medial lesions with positive axillary nodes and/or large lesions are selected. Results regarding the effect of postoperative radiotherapy on survival are conflicting, and analysis of failure from adjuvant chemotherapy studies may help to define the role of postoperative radiotherapy.

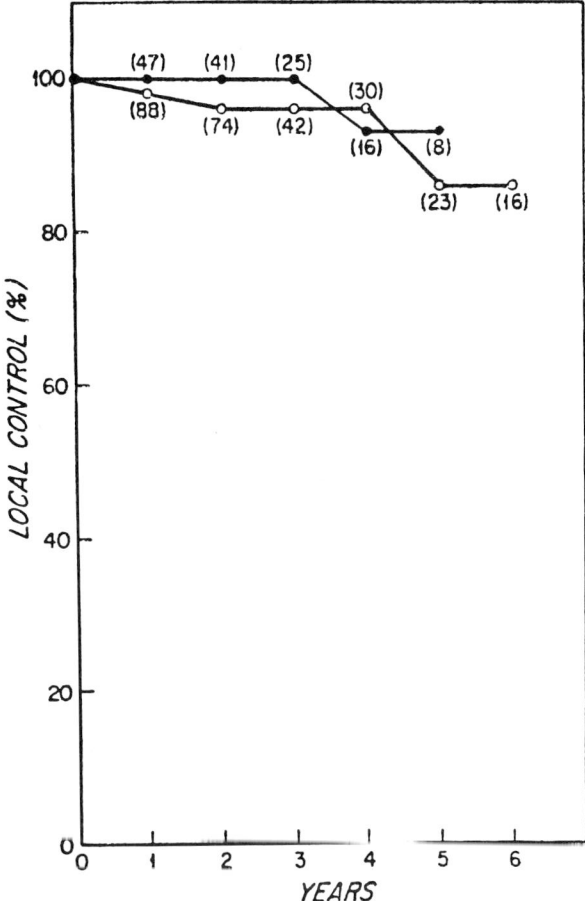

FIGURE 11-11 Cumulative probability of local control of stages I and II breast cancer is shown, after definitive radiotherapy. Closed circles = stage I; open circles = stage II. (Courtesy of J. R. Harris.)

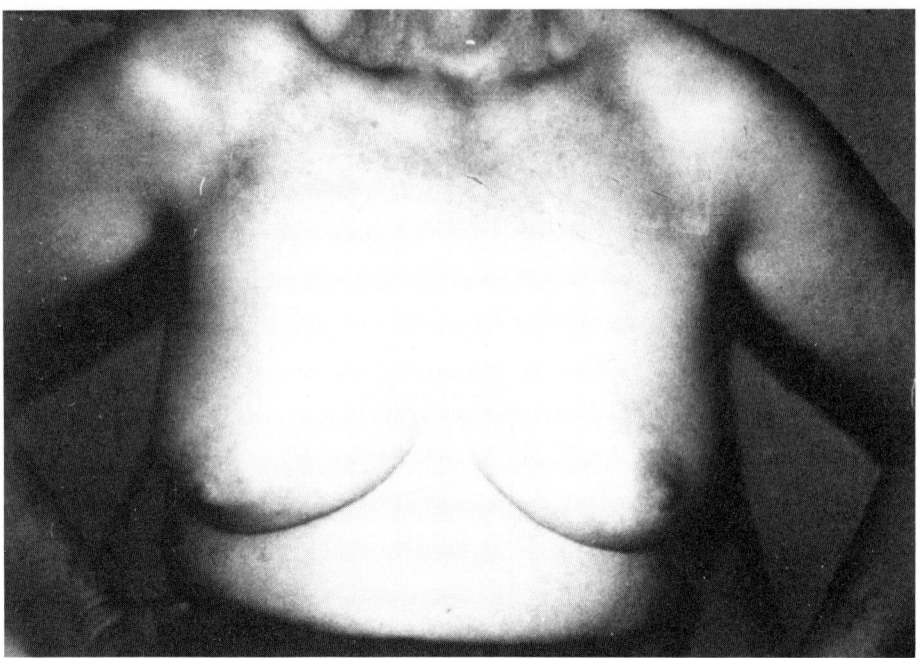

FIGURE 11-12 Patient with stage I carcinoma of the right breast treated 33 months before photograph. (*Courtesy of J. R. Harris.*)

SELECTED FUTURE DEVELOPMENTS IN RADIOTHERAPY

Biologic Modifiers: Radiation Protectors

Some substances do not affect the radiosensitivity of cells but protect whole animals because they result in vasoconstriction or upset the normal process of metabolism to an extent that the oxygen concentration of critical organs is reduced. Examples of this are sodium cyanide, epinephrine, histamine, and serotonin. These are not true protectors, and we mention them only to avoid confusion. The sulfhydryl compounds of which cysteine, a sulfhydryl containing amino acid, has been shown to protect small rodents from the effects of total-body gamma radiation when the drug is ingested in large amounts before x-ray exposure and has been proven to be effective in the protection of mammalian cells in culture.

Cysteamine is a much more potent protector and is a decarboxylated cysteine. Animals injected with cysteamine to a concentration of approximately 150 mg/kg body weight require a dose of x-rays 1.8 times as large as control animals to produce the same level of mortality. The mechanism by which these compounds exert their protective effect is not completely understood, and there are several proposed mechanisms of action. The most favored is the "radical scavenger" hypothesis. According to this hypothesis as an intermediate step between the ion pairs and the breaking of chemical bonds, free radicals are formed, and sulfhydryl compounds block this process by reacting with free radicals in competition with oxygen.[3]

This hypothesis tends to parallel the oxygen effect, being maximal for sparsely ionizing x-rays and minimal for densely ionizing radiation. Yuhas has proposed that the thiophosphate derivative of cysteamine (WR 2721) could be used as a protector in clinical radiotherapy. Kligerman and Yuhas showed that WR 2721 applied topically reduced the mucositis resulting from radiotherapy in the oral cavity. At present Yuhas is investigating the systemic administration of WR 2721 before radiotherapy treatment. He hypothesizes that this pro-

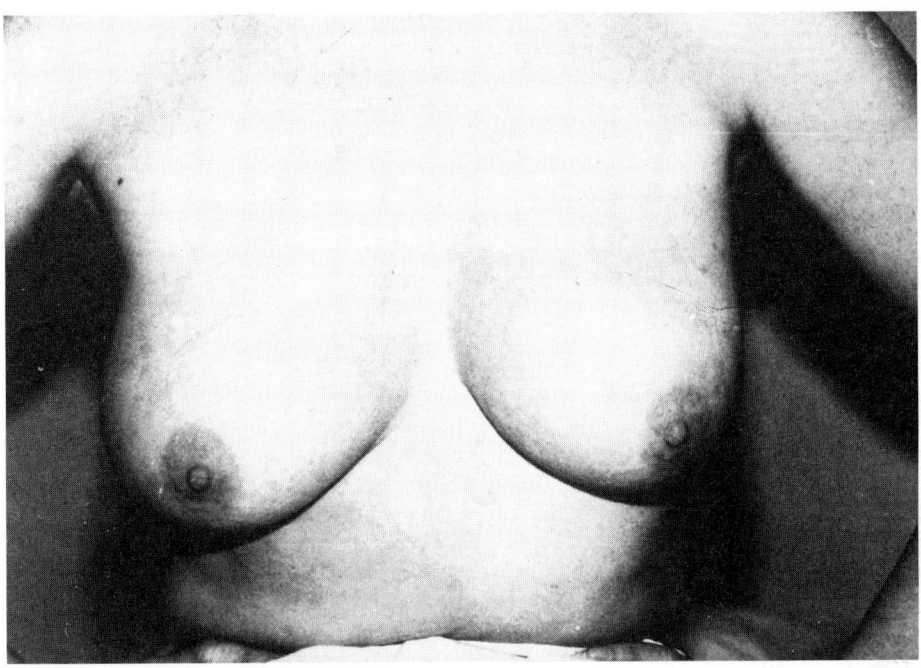

FIGURE 11-13 Patient with stage I carcinoma of the left breast treated 48 months before photograph. (*Courtesy of J. R. Harris.*)

tects normal tissues that have a good blood supply and take the drug up quickly while having a lesser effect on poorly vascularized tumor.[3]

Sensitizers

Sensitizers are chemical agents which when administered in conjunction with radiation therapy increase the lethal effects of radiation.

The combining size (van der Waals radius) of an atom of chlorine, bromine, or iodine is very similar to that of the methyl group, CH_3. Thus, the halogenated pyrimidines (IUDR, BUDR, etc.) are very similar to the normal DNA precursor thymidine, having a halogen substituted in place of a methyl group. The similarity is so close that these agents may actually be incorporated into the DNA side chain in place of thymidine. They appear to "weaken" the DNA chain, and consequently cells are more susceptible to x-ray damage. These agents are only effective sensitizers if they are made available to cells for several generations in order that an appreciable quantity of analogue may be actually incorporated into DNA.

The effectiveness of the halogenated pyrimidines as x-ray sensitizers has been demonstrated in bacteria and mammalian cells. However, these agents have not proved clinically effective because the liver rapidly dehalogenates these circulating halogenated pyrimidines.

Infusion of these analogues into the main vessel supplying the neoplasm has been attempted; however, clinical trials have not proved effective. This is likely due to poor understanding of the optimum way to administer these compounds. Perhaps a better biologic understanding of the mechanism of action of the halogenated pyrimidines will make clinical investigation more fruitful.

Apparent sensitizers include a variety of different compounds such as antibiotics, alkylating agents, and antimetabolites that have been tested in experimental systems and appear to potentiate the effects of x-rays although the effects of such agents may be additive and therefore not "true" sensitizers. Actinomycin D is an antibiotic known to depress DNA-dependent RNA synthesis; it intercalates in the ribose DNA backbone. In concentrations which produce some cell death the drug potentiates the effects of x-rays in that it steepens the x-ray survival curve and has been shown to alter the pattern of repair of sublethal damage between split doses of x-ray. Actinomycin D has proved widely applicable in combination with other drugs and x-rays in pediatric tumors, and a clinically interesting phenomenon known as "recall" has been demonstrated with combinations of x-rays and actinomycin D. Radiation given at a time far after the administration of actinomycin D may produce a brisk reaction just as actinomycin D given at a time after radiation administration may also produce a brisk reaction.[48-50]

Methotrexate is a folate antagonist that inhibits the enzyme dihydrofolate reductase. Methotrexate (MTX) appears to be additive rather than synergistic and is not a radiosensitizing agent in the true sense. Adriamycin, an anthracycline antibiotic which also intercalates in the DNA ribose backbone, appears to enhance radiation effects; however, it is not clear that this represents true sensitization rather than an additive effect. However, a recall reaction similar to that seen with actinomycin D occurs with Adriamycin, and Adriamycin is an important drug employed in clinical oncology. Fundamental investigation of drug/x-ray interaction is important for the future of combined modality therapy.[3,48-51]

Sensitizers of Hypoxic Cells

In the early 1960s compounds were found to sensitize hypoxic microorganisms and helped establish the hypothesis that the efficiency of sensitization is directly related to the electron affinity of these compounds. The largest group studied was the nitrofurans; however, their applicability to animals was limited by their toxicity and chemical and pharmacological instability. Ideally a hypoxic sensitizer should sensitize hypoxic cells at a concentration which results in acceptable toxicity in normal tissues, and be stable and soluble in water or lipids as well as capable of reaching the nonvascularized mass of hypoxic cells. Also, a sensitizer must be effective throughout most of the cell cycle or at least in the early part of G_1, and should be effective at relatively low doses, i.e., a few hundred rads used in conventional fractions in radiotherapy.[3,52-54]

Metronidazole, marketed as Flagyl, was the first drug to possess some of these properties and to be employed in clinical trials. Figure 11-14 shows hypoxic cell radiosensitizer survival curves in air and under hypoxic conditions with and without Flagyl. Urtason et al. did a clinical trial treating patients with glioblastoma with

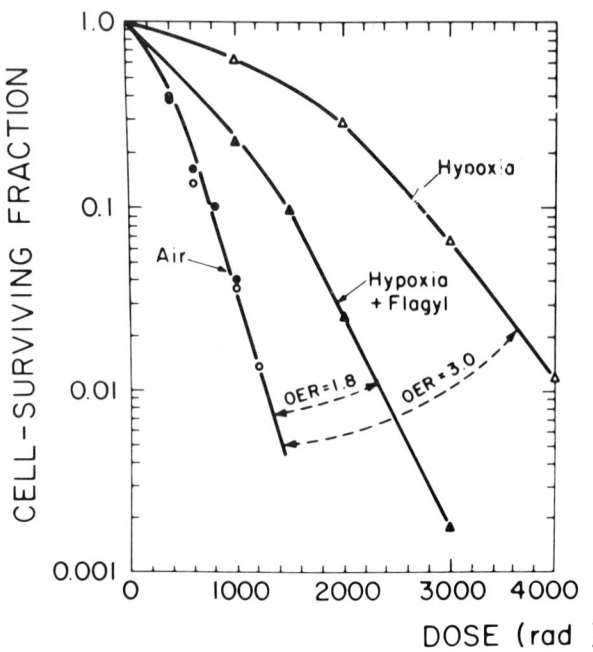

FIGURE 11-14 This illustrates the effect of the hypoxic cell radiosensitizer metronidazole. The figure shows survival curves for Chinese hamster cells irradiated with cobalt (^{60}Co γ rays) under aerated and hypoxic conditions. The sensitivity of the cells under hypoxia is substantially enhanced by the presence of metronidazole at a high concentration (10 mM). This is reflected by a reduction of the oxygen enhancement ratio (OER) from 3.0 to 1.8. Open circle = air; closed circle = air + 10 mM Flagyl; open triangle = hypoxia; closed triangle = hypoxia + 10 mM Flagyl. (*Adapted from E. J. Hall et al.*[55])

radiation alone and radiation combined with metronidazole.[52] A criticism of the study was that patients were not treated with ideal fractionated radiotherapy, but this was the first clinical evidence that sensitizers might be of some use.

A new compound, misonidazole RO-07-0582, has electron affinities even higher than metronidazole and may be effective at lower concentrations, thus giving lower toxicity. Effort is being made in Great Britain and the United States to synthesize and test new drugs that may be superior, since misonidazole may give considerable neurotoxicity.

Particle Therapy: Fast Neutrons

Neutrons have been suggested as an alternative or as treatment in addition to x-rays for radiation therapy on the basis of their biologic properties. Neutrons are particles with a mass similar to that of a proton but they carry no electrical charge. Since neutrons are uncharged, they are highly penetrating compared with charged particles of the same mass and energy, and set in motion fast-recoil protons, alpha particles, and heavier nuclear fragments by interaction with the nuclei of atoms of the absorbing material. The potential advantages of neutrons over more conventional radiation modalities are a lower oxygen enhancement ratio, little or no repair of sublethal or potentially lethal damage, and the lesser variation of cell cycle sensitivity with phases of the mitotic cycle for neutrons than for x-rays. Neutrons are considered high-LET (linear energy transfer) radiation because of the dense secondary ionization produced by the nuclear reaction. Clinical trials are presently underway at centers in the United States and Britain employing neutrons alone and in combination with photon radiation for a variety of malignant tumors.[55-58]

Negative Pi Mesons

Pions behave like heavy electrons in the first few centimeters of absorbing material but then produce densely ionizing fragments in a localized area at the end of their tract (Fig. 11-15). Pions come to rest at the end of their range and may be captured by one of the constituent atoms of tissue. Other constituent atoms such as oxygen or nitrogen explode to produce different combinations of heavy fragments, and this constitutes "star" production which is a unique feature of negative pions (Fig. 11-15).

Pions have two potential advantages for radiotherapy: (1) they have a superior depth-dose pattern because of the "star" effect and (2) the peak region contains a high-LET component which reduces the oxygen enhancement ratio. Clinical trials are being carried out at Los Alamos in the United States as well as at Triumf in Vancouver and at Zurich, Switzerland.[58-60]

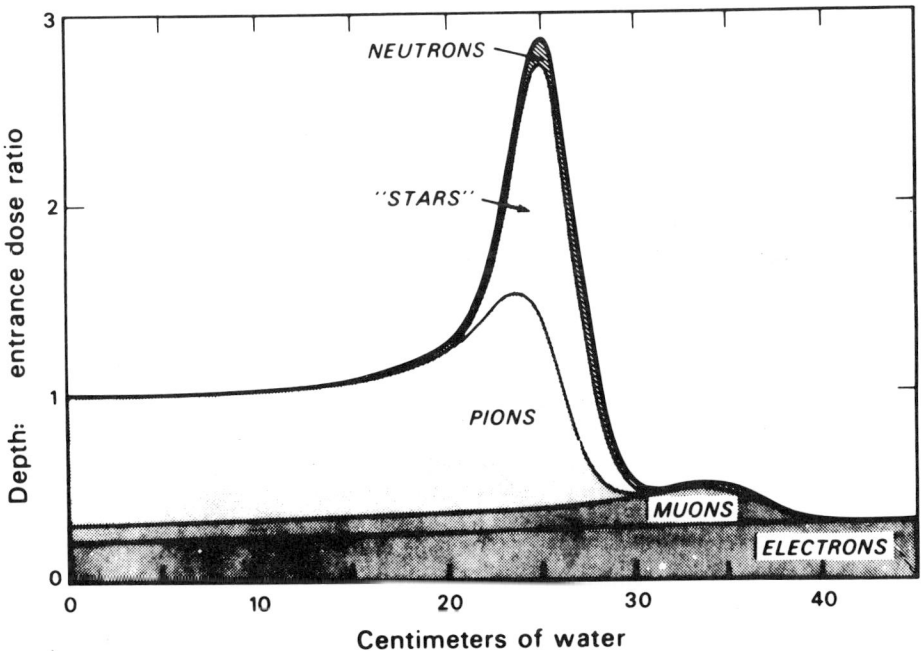

FIGURE 11-15 Depth-dose profile for a beam of negative pi mesons. The dose reaches a maximum near the end of the particles range. Proportions of dose due to primary and secondary particles are 65 percent pions, 25 percent electrons, and 10 percent muons. $P_0 = 190 \pm 5$ MeV/c. (*From J. B. Curtis and M. R. Raju.*[60])

Protons

Protons are not considered high-LET radiation and have an RBE which is approximately the same as 250-keV x-ray. Protons are attractive for radiotherapy because of their physical dose distribution. The dose deposited by a beam of a monoenergetic proton increases slowly with depth but reaches a sharp peak maximum near the end of the particle's range referred to as the Bragg peak.

The beam has sharp edges with little side scatter, and the dose falls to essentially zero after the peak of the particle stop. Thus, protons have selected uses in radiotherapy; for example, ocular melanomas and certain types of pituitary tumors lend themselves to treatment with protons.

REFERENCES

1. Buschke F, Parker R: *Radiation Therapy in Cancer Management*, Grune Stratton, New York and London, 1972.
2. Johns HE, Cunningham JR: *The Physics of Radiology*, Charles C Thomas, Springfield, Ill, 1969.
3. Hall EJ: *Radiobiology for the Radiologist*, 2d ed, Harper & Row, Hagerstown, Md, 1978.
4. Zirkle RE: The radiobiological importance of linear energy transfer, in Hollander A (ed): *Radiation Biology*, vol 1, McGraw-Hill, New York, 1954, pp 315–350.
5. Field SB: The relative biological effectiveness of fast neutrons for mammalian tissue. *Radiology* 93:915–920, 1969.
6. Puck TT, Marcus PI: Action of x-rays on mammalian cells. *J Exp Med* 103:653–666, 1956.
7. Thompson LH, Suit HD: Proliferation kinetics of x-irradiated mouse L cells studied with time lapse photography. *Int J Radiat Biol* 15:347, 1966.
8. Sinclair WK, Morton, RA: X-ray sensitivity during the cell generation cycle of cultured Chinese hamster cells. *Radiat Res* 450–474, 1966.
9. Crabtree HG, Kramer W: Action of radium on cancer cells. Some factors affecting susceptibility of cancer cells to radium. *Proc R Soc Lon [Biol]* 113:238, 1933.
10. Wright EA, Howard-Flanders P: The influence of oxygen on the radiosensitivity of mammalian tissues. *Acta Radiol* 48:26–32, 1957.
11. Thomlinson RH, Gray LH: The histologic structure of some human lung cancers and the possible implications for radiotherapy. *Br J Cancer* 9:539–549, 1955.
12. Van Putten LM: Tumor reoxygenation during fractionated radiotherapy: Studies with a transplantable osteosarcoma. *Eur J Cancer* 4:173–182, 1968.
13. Kallman RF et al: Effects of different schedules of dose fractionation on the oxygenation status of a transplantable mouse sarcoma. *J Natl Cancer Inst* 44:369–377, 1970.
14. Thomlinson RH: Reoxygenation as a function of tumor size and histopathological type, in *Proceedings of the Carmel Conference on Time/Dose Relationships and Radiation Biology as Applied to Radiotherapy*, BNL Report 50203 C-57, 1969.
15. Elkind MM, Sutton H: Radiation response of mammalian cells grown in culture: 1. Repair of x-ray damage in surviving Chinese hamster cells. *Radiat Res* 13:556–593, 1960.
16. Belli JA et al: Radiation response of mammalian tumor cells: 1. Repair of sublethal damage in vivo. *J Natl Cancer Inst* 38:673–682, 1967.
17. Elkind MM et al: Radiation response of mammalian cells in culture: V. Temperature dependence of the repair of x-ray damage in surviving cells (aerobic and hypoxic). *Radia Res* 25:359–376, 1965.
18. Little JB et al: Repair of potentially lethal radiation damage in vitro and in vivo. *Radiology* 106:689–694, 1973.
19. Little JB: Repair of sublethal and potentially lethal radiation damage in plateau phase cultures of human cells. *Nature* 224:804–806, 1969.
20. Weichselbaum RR et al: Response of human osteosarcoma *in vitro* to x-irradiation: Evidence for unusual cellular repair activity. *Int J Radiat Biol* 31:295–299, 1977.
21. Weichselbaum RR et al: Radiation response of human tumor cells *in vitro*, in Meyn RE, Withers HR (eds): *Radiation Biology in Cancer Research*, Raven Press, New York, 1980, pp 345–351.
22. Withers HR et al: The pathobiology of late effects of radiation, in Meyn RE, Withers, HR (eds): *Radiation Biology in Cancer Research*, Raven Press, New York, 1980, pp 439–448.
23. Hopell JW: The importance of vascular damage in the development of late radiation effects in normal tissue, in Meyn RE, Withers HR (eds): *Radiation Biology in Cancer Research*, Raven Press, New York, 1980, pp 449–459.
24. Ellis F: Dose, time and fractionation: A clinical hypothesis. *Clin Radiol* 20:1–7, 1969.
25. Steele GG, Lamberton LF: The growth rate of human tumors. *Br J Cancer* 20:74–86, 1966.
26. Fletcher GH (ed): *Textbook of Radiotherapy*, Lea Febiger, Philadelphia, 1973.
27. Fletcher GH, Lindberg RD: Squamous cell carcinomas of the tonsillar area and pallatine arch. *Am J Roentgenol Radium Ther Nucl Med* 96:574, 1966.
28. Crews OE Fletcher GH: Comparative evaluation of the sequential use of radiation and surgery in primary tumors of the oral cavity, oropharynx, larynx and the hypopharynx. *Am J Roentgenol Radium Ther Nucl Med* 11:73, 1971.
29. Chu AM, Fletcher GH: Incidence and causes of failure to control by irradiation the primary lesions in squamous cell carcinoma of the anterior two-thirds of the tongue and floor of mouth. *Am J Roentgenol Radium Ther Nucl Med* 11:502, 1973.
30. Fletcher GH et al: The place of radiotherapy in the man-

agement of squamous cell carcinoma of the supraglottic larynx. *Am J Roentgenol Radium Ther Nucl Med* 108:19, 1970.
31. Fletcher GH, Jesse RH: Interaction of surgery and irradiation in head and neck cancers, in Mosely RD (ed): *Current Problems in Radiology*, Year Book, Chicago, 1971, pp 1,3.
32. Shukovsky LJ: Dose, time, volume relationships in squamous carcinoma of the supraglottic larynx. *Am J Roentgenol Radium Ther Nucl Med* 108:27, 1980.
33. Von Essen CF: in Fletcher, GH (ed): *Textbook of Radiotherapy*, Lea Febiger, Philadelphia, 1973, pp. 197–211.
34. Fletcher GH, Rutledge F: Carcinoma of the uterine cervix, in Deely TJ (ed) *Modern Radiotherapy*, Butterworth, London 1971, p 11.
35. Fletcher GH et al: in: *Carcinoma of the Cervix, Endometrium, and Ovary*, Year Book, Chicago, 1962, p 69.
36. Beahrs OH, Barber KW: The value of radical neck dissection of the structures of the neck and the management of carcinomas of the lip, mouth and larynx. *Arch Surg* 85:49, 1962.
37. Strong EW: Preoperative radiation and radical neck dissection. *Surg Clin North Am* 49:271, 1969.
38. Lindberg RD, Jesse RH: Treatment of cervical lymph node metastasis from primary lesions of the oropharynx, supraglottic larynx and hypopharynx. *Am J Roentgenol* 102:132, 1968.
39. Jesse RH et al: Cancer of the oral cavity: Is elective neck dissection beneficial? *Am J Surg* 125:05, 1970.
40. Berger DS et al: Elective irradiation of the neck lymphatics for squamous cell carcinoma of the nasopharynx and oropharynx. *Am J Roentgenol* 111:66, 1971.
41. Fletcher GH: Elective irradiation of subclinical disease in cancer of the head and neck. *Cancer* 29:1450, 1972.
42. Votava C et al: Management of cervical nodes either fixed or bilateral from primary squamous carcinoma of the oral cavity and faucial arch. *Radiology* 105:417, 1972.
43. Beahrs OH et al: Surgical management of parotid lesions. *Arch Surg* 80:890, 1960.
44. Foote FW Jr, Frazel EL: *Tumors of the Major Salivary Glands*. Armed Forces Institute of Pathology, Washington, D.C., 1954.
45. Gullamondegui O et al: Malignant tumors of the salivary glands, in Fletcher GH (ed): *Textbook of Radiotherapy*, Lea Febiger, Philadelphia, 1973, pp 348–365.
46. Levene MB et al: Primary radiation therapy for operable carcinoma of the breast. *Surg Clin North Am* 58: 767–776, 1978.
47. Hellman S et al: Radiation therapy of early carcinoma of the breast without mastectomy. *Cancer* 46:988–994, 1980.
48. Elkind MM et al: Actinomycin-D: Suppression of recovery in x-irradiated mammalian cells. *Science* 143:1454–1457, 1964.
49. Bagshaw, MA: Possible role of potentiators in radiation therapy. *Am J Roentgenol* 85:822, 1961.
50. Bagshaw MA et al: Intra-arterial 5-bromodeoxyuridine and x-ray therapy. *Am J Roentgenol* 99:889–894, 1967.
51. Kriss JP, Revez L: The distribution and fate of bromodeoxyuridine and bromodeoxycytosine in the mouse and rat. *Cancer Res* 22:254–265, 1962.
52. Urtason RC et al: Radiation and high dose metronidazole (Flagyl) in supratentorial glioblastoma. *N Engl J Med* 294: 1364–1367, 1976.
53. Adams GE: Chemical radiosensitization of hypoxic cells. *Br Med Bull* 29:48–53, 1973.
54. Adams GE et al: Hypoxic cells in radiotherapy. *Lancet* 186–188, 1976.
55. Hall EJ, Roizin-Towle L: Hypoxic sensitizers: Radiobiological studies at the cellular level. *Radiology* 117:453, 1975.
56. Catterall M: The treatment of advanced cancer by fast neutrons from the Medical Research Council cyclotron at Hammersmith Hospital, London. *Eur J Cancer* 10:343, 1974.
57. Broerse JJ, Barendsen GW: Relative biological effectiveness of fast neutrons for effects on normal tissues. *Curr Top Radiat Res* 8:305–350, 1973.
58. Hall EJ: Radiobiology of heavy particle radiation therapy. *Cell Stud Radiol* 108:119–129, 1973.
59. Field SB: A historical survey of radiobiology and radiotherapy of fast neutrons. *Curr Top Radiat Res* 11:1–86, 1976.
60. Curtis SB, Raju MR: A calculation of the physical characteristics of negative pion beams. *Radiat Res* 239–255, 1968.

SELECTED BIBLIOGRAPHY

Markoe AM: Practical clinical radiation therapy, in Kahn SB et al (eds): *Concepts in Cancer Medicine*, Grune & Stratton, New York, 1983, pp 323–335.
Raju MR et al: OER and RBE for negative pion beams of different peak widths. *Br J Radiol* 52(618):494–498, 1979.

Siemann DW, Sutherland RM: A comparison of the pharmacokinetics of multiple and single administrations of Adriamycin. Vol 5(8):1971–1974, 1979.
Wasserman TW et al: Initial United States clinical and pharmacologic evaluation of misonidazole (RO-07-0582), a hypoxic cell radiosensitizer. Vol 5(6):775–786, 1979.

12
MECHANISMS OF METASTASIS FORMATION

Everett V. Sugarbaker   *Daniel N. Weingrad*   *James M. Roseman*

From the surgical viewpoint the greatest risk to the patient with apparently localized malignancy is the risk that incurable metastases are present at diagnosis or that they will develop after effective treatment of the primary malignancy. *Metastasis* is defined in most dictionaries as a shifting of disease from one part or organ of the body to another, as by transfer of cells of a malignant tumor. This distant transfer of malignant cells is the nemesis of often successful surgical resection and results in the eventual death of about 50 percent of patients with resectable primary tumors. Paradoxically, when the technical abilities of the surgical oncologist have been maximally deployed, as in the successful execution of a pancreaticoduodenal resection, a total pelvic exenteration, a craniofacial exenteration, major hepatic resections, extensive head and neck resections and reconstructions, and a myriad of other specific procedures for major or recurrent malignant disease problems, the even greater risk for metastasis often causes deep disappointment and/or death in approximately 70 to 90 percent of patients who have had such successful anatomic engineering feats performed. Thus the impact of the problem of metastasis has fostered extensive laboratory investigation, and much has been elucidated regarding the biology of this event. This chapter develops a current working model for experimental metastasis formation, emphasizing some variability in the many experimental models used.

HISTORICAL PERSPECTIVE; THE EVOLUTION OF THE CELLULAR-EMBOLIC THEORY OF CANCER METASTASIS

A perspective on the evolution of the cellular theory of cancer metastasis and the translation of this concept into surgical therapeutic procedures in the late nineteenth century is pertinent to the objectives of this chapter of providing a better understanding of the currently employed experimental and therapeutic concepts of cancer metastasis.

Metastasis Interpreted as Black Bile or a Diffusing Humor

One of the first organized attempts to understand cancer dissemination was made by Galen (A.D. 131–203). According to Galen the black bile (one of the humors) was responsible for malignancy. In autopsy studies distant foci of breast cancer were interpreted as pools of black bile. Only a minor modification of this theory occurred in the ensuing 1400 years. Paracelsus (1493–1541) reinterpreted Galen's black bile as representing mineral salts. Distant foci of malignancy were precipitates of mineral salts. This interpretation may have been related to the finding of calcifications in many malignancies. For both these theories the primary tumor was not conceptually separated from secondary deposits, or metastases.[1]

Development of the Cellular Theory of Metastasis

The cellular theory of cancer metastasis awaited the work of Johannes Peter Müller, who in 1828 established that cells were basic components of malignant diseases. In the next year Joseph Claude Récamier demonstrated the presence of secondary deposits of carcinoma of the breast in the brain of a patient. He also noted invasion of the disease into the veins at the primary site in the breast, and coined the term *metastasis* to describe the secondary tumor growths.[1] Rudolph Virchow (1821–1902) expanded Müller's views and in his famous *Cellular Pathology*[2] expounded the doctrine of "all cells from cells." Yet, paradoxically, despite his conviction of the basic cellular composition of primary malignant tumors, Virchow retained the humoral theory for development of metastases.

The manner in which metastatic diffusion takes place is by means of certain fluids and these possess the power of producing an infection which disposes different parts to a reproduction of a mass of the same nature as the one which originally existed.[2]

Sir James Paget (1814–1899), an influential surgeon of the same era, likewise maintained:

We need not assume that corpuscles of pus or cancer, or any kind of germs already formed, must be thus carried for multiplication or dissemination of disease. A rudimentary liquid, an unformed cancerous blastema, mingled with blood, may be as effectual as any germs; and must almost necessarily be assumed, in the explanation of cures in which dissemination takes place ... in organs beyond.[3]

Solid evidence was needed in order to refute this concept of metastasis. Karl Thiersch (1822–1895) studied metastasizing epithelial tumors of the skin by using histological serial sectioning techniques. He reasoned that the malignant epithelial cells found in lymph nodes reached this position by cellular embolism. He also stated that although toxic fluids are released from malignant growths, it is the cancer cells themselves that produce metastases. He supported his conclusions with many clinical observations, including autopsy studies of a woman with carcinoma of the uterus. Metastases were present in pelvic lymph nodes, ovary and external iliac veins, and other organs. Also, clusters of identical tumor cells were present in the thoracic duct. The entire pattern could be explained by the known anatomy of the circulation, further supporting the cellular theory of metastasis.[1] Langenbeck[4] showed in 1841 that cancer cells could be microscopically identified in the blood of patients dying with metastases. In 1878 Waldeyer extended Thiersch's proof by studies of metastases of gastrointestinal carcinomas, tracing their origins to the epithelial primary tumors. Hoggan (1878) wrote a persuasive treatise supporting this concept, "On Cancer and Its Relationship to Lymphatic Vessels."[5] Von Recklinghausen (1885) showed that neoplastic obstruction of lymphatics can cause rerouting and opening of collateral lymphatic channels, thus explaining some unusual sites of metastasis.[6] Thus in the late nineteenth century the cellular theory of metastasis became solidly established.[1,7]

The Cellular-Embolic Theory Translated into Surgical Therapy

Clearly the conceptualization of how cancer spreads is important in determining therapeutic approaches in cancer management. If tumor cells embolized to regional nodes as the first stations of dissemination, shouldn't these sites be extirpated along with the primary tumor? Translating this hypothesis into treatment, surgical procedures were designed to encompass both the local primary tumor and the regional lymph nodes. In 1867, in reference to breast carcinoma, surgeon Charles H. Moore of Middlesex Hospital, England, wrote:

No morbid structure should be exposed ... be set free and lodge in the wound. Diseased axillary glands should be taken away *by the same* dissection as the breast itself without dividing the intervening lymphatics. ... The practice of removing successive portions [of the tumor] should be abandoned.[8]

The en bloc resection of the primary tumor and its regional lymphatics thus became soundly based conceptually with uniform acceptance of the cellular-embolic theory of metastasis. Some final elements of proof of this concept came in 1906 to 1907 with publication of the classic clinicopathological studies of malignant melanoma and breast carcinoma by W. Sampson Handley.[9,10] These studies histologically traced the routes of metastasis through the lymphatics to regional lymph nodes in patients who had succumbed to their diseases (Fig. 12-1). These clinicopathological correlations substantiated the concept that regional nodes were filter barriers which trapped tumor cells at least for a time. The necessity of surgical extirpation of regional nodes in addition to wide removal of the primary lesion was an obvious extension of logic and became widely accepted.

Precise definitions of the anatomic routes for regional metastasis were provided by Sappey[11] and other anatomists and allowed for the design of surgical procedures which would extirpate regional lymph nodes. Between 1890 and 1908 en bloc procedures of radical mastectomy (Halstead[12]), in continuity node dissections for melanoma (Pringle),[13] abdominal perineal resection (Miles),[14] and radical neck dissection (Crile)[15] were designed around the cellular-embolic concept of regional cancer dissemination and immediately began to save the lives of many patients who otherwise would have succumbed to their diseases. The enthusiasm of these early authors in their publications is obvious, and a major advance was thought to have been made by application of this concept of metastasis.

Extensions of the Surgical Perimeter Based on Cellular-Embolic Theory

When recurrences and metastases were noted in some patients despite en bloc resection, a major direction in cancer therapy—from 1910 to the 1960s—was to extend the surgical perimeter to include more tissue about the primary tumor. During this period, with major advances in surgical techniques, blood replacement, antibiotics, and intensive care, superradical extirpation became feasible. The Whipple procedure (pancreaticoduodenectomy),[16] extended radical gastrectomy,[17] superradical mastectomy,[18] and hemicorporectomy were all devised within this conceptual framework and remain as tributes to the ingenuity and daring of their surgical innovators, as well as to their concern for the survival of their patients at whatever cost. However, this was an era of diminishing return, for most patients so treated succumbed to the problems of distant metastatic disease.

Revisions of Cellular-Embolic Theory to Include Systemic Dissemination

Despite these extensions of the surgical perimeter to their anatomic limits, many patients still died from systemic metastasis. Surgery alone, although successful in eradicating the primary tumor, often failed to "trap" the disease in the regionalized state. The regional cellular theory of metastasis, which initially established the concept of en bloc resection, thus had to be expanded to include the frequently systemic nature of metastatic dissemination. Not to be forgotten, however, is the fact that many patients with regional lymph node metastases are still apparently cured by surgical extirpation of the primary tumor and the involved regional lymph nodes. This fact indicates at least the partial validity of the regional-embolic conceptualization of cancer spread. This concept is still employed in most current cancer operations and in the design of ports for radiation

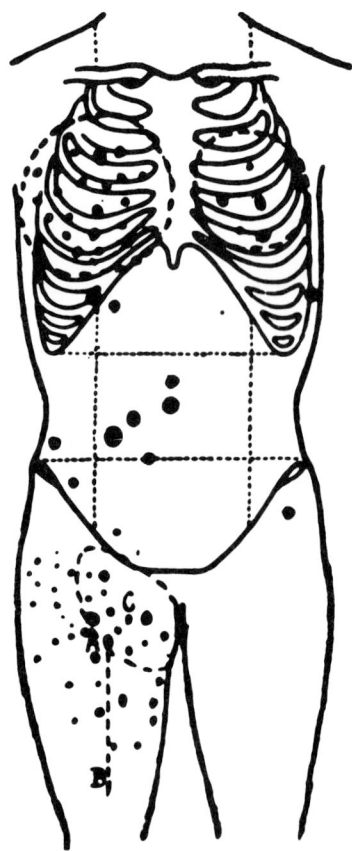

FIGURE 12-1 W. S. Handley published one of the classical histopathologic studies of metastasis in malignant melanoma.

therapy. Realization of the systemic nature of malignancy has provided stimulus for the extensive clinical and laboratory investigations discussed in subsequent portions of this chapter.

THE THREE PHASES OF METASTASIS

The establishment of a single successful metastasis requires three major steps (Fig. 12-2). First a malignant cell (or small clump) must gain access to a vascular conduit. Second, this conduit must safely transport these cells to a distant organ site. Third, the cell(s) must be able to proliferate in the distant organ. It is convenient to compartmentalize metastases into these three stages for purposes of discussion, and much of the research on mechanisms involved has been oriented toward one of these three phases. However, despite the convenience of this three-phase concept in the organization of thought about metastasis, it must be stressed that organization is of necessity a gross oversimplification of the process. Host interaction with the malignancy probably begins with the initial transformation of the original malignant cell at the primary site. Likewise, the tumor is perfused with host blood and cells. The progressive tumor growth modulates the host by as yet incompletely understood mechanisms. Malignant cells entering the circulation at early phases of tumor growth could well face an environment far different from that faced by a tumor cell entering the circulation after a prolonged period of tumor host-interaction and modulation. The interactions between tumor and host are particularly pertinent to observations on clinical metastasis, for frequently the primary tumor is thought to have been present in the host for a prolonged period of time before a metastasis becomes apparent. Thus, although three phases of metastasis occur, the metastasizing tumor cell is affected by the host, the properties of the primary tumor, and by a less well defined product of complex tumor-host interactions.

EXPERIMENTAL STUDIES OF METASTASIS

Early Experimental Data

As discussed, the earliest studies of metastasis were histopathological observations made at autopsy and of surgical specimens of humans in the nineteenth century. However, around the turn of the century techniques for transplantation of murine tumors were developed. Rapidly thereafter, experimental oncology blossomed and many studies of experimental metastasis were performed. The studies of Goldman,[19] Levin,[20] Takahashi,[21] and Tyzzer,[22] document widespread interest in experimental metastasis in the early twentieth century. The

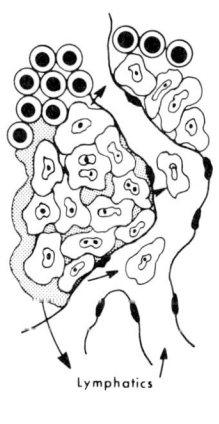
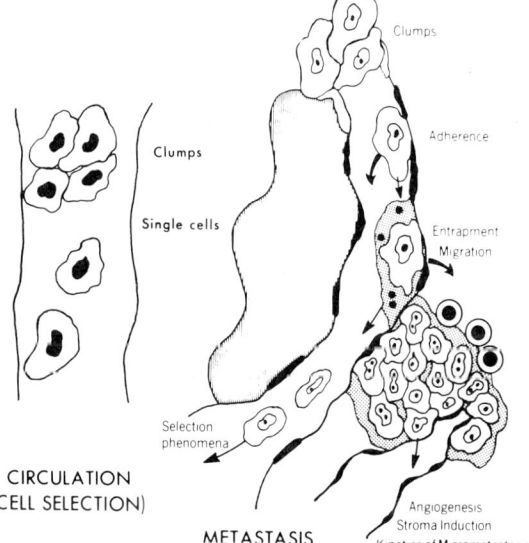

FIGURE 12-2 Metastasis occurs in three phases: entrance of cells into the circulation, transport to a distant organ site, and arrest and eventual formation of a true metastasis.

central hypotheses explored by these early investigators remain currently of interest and include the mechanisms of tumor arrest, fibrin precipitation in tumor cell arrest, an inhibitory effect of a primary tumor on metastasis, and other related studies. Then, except for sporadic reports,[23] laboratory interest in metastases waned until the 1950s. The development of isogenic strains of mice by Snell et al. was a major contribution, overcoming histocompatibility differences that had been present between transplantable tumors and genetically dissimilar hosts. This important development had obscured meaningful studies. Over the last 30 years many studies of experimental metastasis have been published. Many important mechanisms for metastasis have been well defined, and much more rigorously than would have been possible in the human model.

Entrance of Tumor Cells into the Circulation

Tumor cells have been shown to enter the perfusing and/or surrounding circulation of the host, either passively (termed *intravasation*) or by active tumor cell–initiated mechanisms (termed *invasion*) (Fig. 12-3).

INTRAVASATION: PRIMARY TUMOR CHARACTERISTICS FACILITATING VASCULAR ENTRY OF TUMOR CELLS

Tumor Vascularization The nature of tumor vascularization is one of the unique features of neoplastic growth. Warren et al.[24–26] have classified *tumor vessels* as (1) arteries and arterioles; (2) capillaries with basement membranes; (3) capillary sprouts, particularly at the neovascularization of the tumor periphery; (4) sinusoidal vessels; (5) blood channels lined only by tumor cells, and *without endothelium;* (6) giant marginal capillaries; (7) capillaries with *large fenestrations* in the endothelium; (8) venules and veins; and (9) arteriovenous anastomoses. The relationship of tumor cells to the important class 5 nonendothelialized tumor sinusoid is seen in Fig. 12-4. For both class 5 and class 7 tumor vessels, tumor cells have direct access to the effluent venous circulation. These class 5 vessels tend to occur in or near areas of tumor necrosis.[26] Pertinent to the ease of detachment of these tumor cells, Weiss[27] showed that more tumor cells could be readily detached from the Walker 256 tumor adjacent to areas of necrosis than in peripheral locations. Additionally, the detachability of both normal liver cells and tumor cells was increased by incubation of these

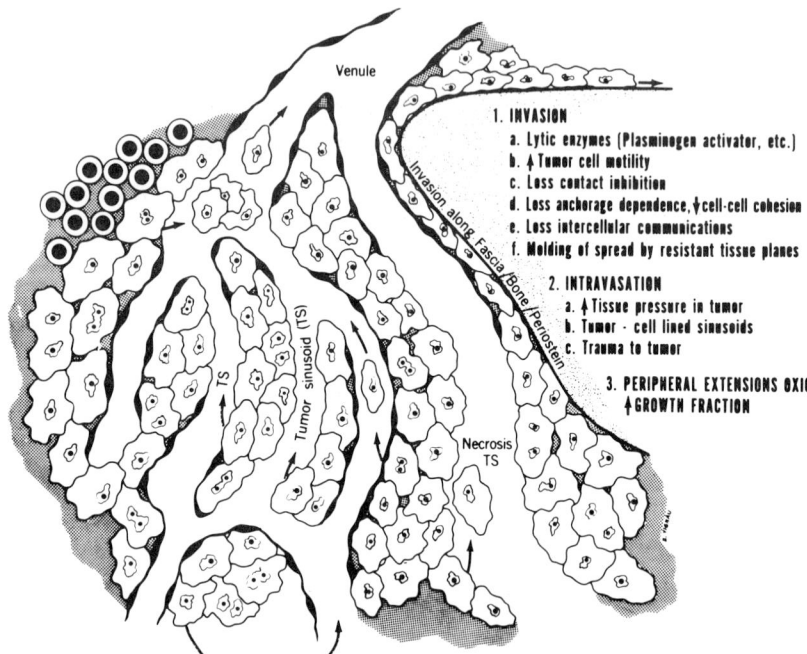

FIGURE 12-3 Invasion and entrance of cells into the vascular system. The processes of invasion and intravasation are both thought important to the entrance of cells into the circulation.

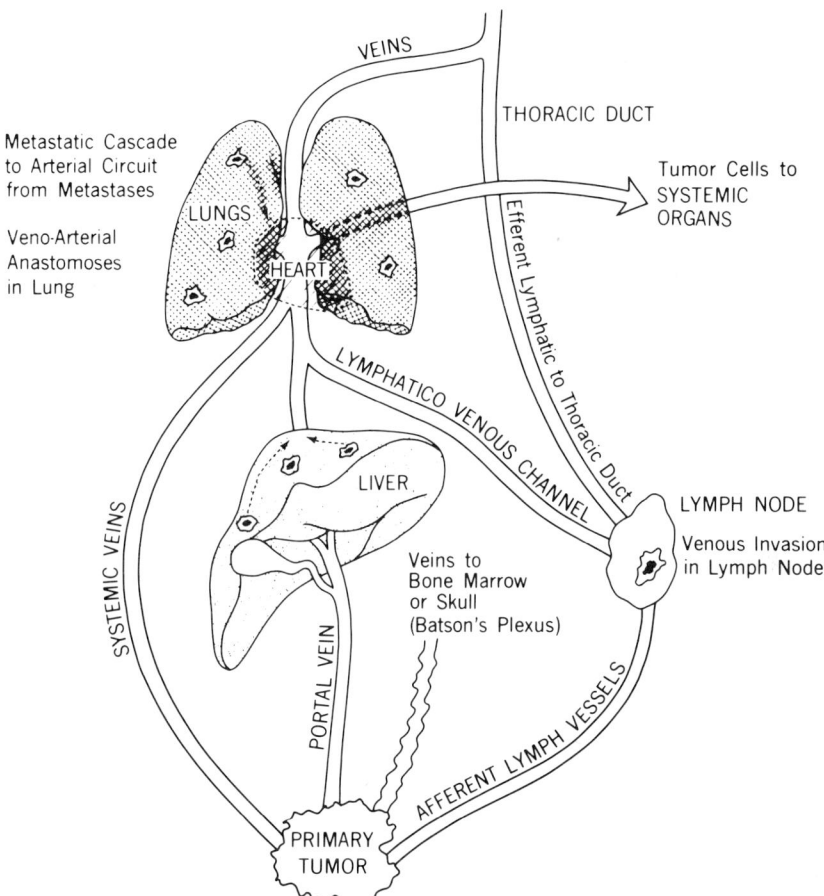

FIGURE 12-4 The primary tumor, by virtue of its pattern of vascularization, is both a kinetic and metabolic mosaic. Importantly, from the viewpoint of entry of cells into the vasculature, areas of near necrosis develop "lakes," or sinusoids, which are actually lined by tumor cells themselves. Such sinusoids near areas of necrosis give ready access of tumor cells and/or cell clumps to the efferent circulation.

tissues with extracts of necrotic tissues. He concluded that necrosis facilitated the release of viable tumor cells, and this observation, coupled with the regionalization of class 5 and to a lesser degree class 7 vessels near the necrotic areas, would clearly facilitate intravasation of tumor cells. These findings are consistent with those of Post,[28] who demonstrated that increased detachability of tumor cells occurs with sublethal immune autolysis due to necrotic release of lysosomal enzymes. Logically, even minute changes in tissue pressure resulting from muscle contraction, minor trauma, or other causes could allow the release of cancer cells into the circulation from those areas in direct contact with the blood supply and greatly diminished intercellular attachments. The fact that *clumps* of tumor cells could easily be released from the lining of these vascular lakes and sinusoids might also be important in view of the greater potential for metastasis by tumor cell clumps.[29]

Increased Interstitial Tumor Tissue Pressures A primary tumor represents uncontrolled growth, and the mass produced is limited by the confines of the surrounding tissues. Likewise, the blood supply, as discussed previously, is not subject to the normal arteriolar pressure regulations on entry into the tumor, and higher than normal perfusion pressures could result. Additionally, malignancies originating in the muscle or other contractile organs are subject to pressures physiologically applied to the tumor where it normally resides in the host. These mechanisms and perhaps others are thought to contribute to the increased tissue pressure that has been measured in malignant tumors.[30-33] It has been hypothesized that this increased intratumoral pressure forces microscopic extensions of tumor cells along tissue planes of least resistance, analogous to the roots of a plant being forced into the earth, powered by cell division of the advancing rootlet.[33] In testing this hypothesis Eaves[34] injected a quick-setting gel into animal tissues and was able to mimic some of the patterns of invasion in malignant tumors. These increased intratumoral pressures would certainly contribute to the entry of tumor cells into the circulation, and would correlate with the clinical observation that the most rapidly dividing (anaplastic) tumors tend also to be highly invasive.[35]

The Central-to-Peripheral Interstitial Fluid Flow in Malignant Tumors Malignant tumors have no definable lymphatics; however, about the tumor periphery lymphatic channels are large in size and widely fenestrated, and can be seen to gape open.[36,37] These anatomic findings are thought to be related to the tumor interstitial fluid dynamics.

Gullino et al.[31,36,38] have studied the interstitial fluid dynamics of experimental tumors. Their basic technique was to use micropore chambers (0.45-μm pore size), which were embedded into tumors and normal tissues. This chamber allows free passage of fluid, and neoplastic cells can grow only around the chamber. A small catheter exits from this chamber and can measure fluid flow and/or interstitial fluid pressure within the chamber. Using this technique, Gullino found high pressures to 8 to 30 cmH$_2$O in the tumor core. Pressure in normal regional subcutaneous tissues was atmospheric. The rate of fluid drainage from the tumor micropore chamber was 4 to 6 mL compared with only 1 mL per 24-h period from normal tissues. Quantitative measurements thus established the presence of a *high pressure gradient from tumor core to periphery and a significant stream of interstitial fluid traveling from the center to the periphery of the tumor.* The halo of edema seen frequently around primary tumors is a direct result of this convective current. Such fluid currents may favor the flushing of tumor cells into the open pores of the lymphatic channels as has been hypothesized by Gullino[36] and other authors.[37] For cells not entering lymphatic channels the interstitial pressure transmitted to peripheral fingers of invasion may facilitate the opening of tissue spaces for extensions of tumor radiating under the pressure head developed within the central tumor mass.

Location of the Primary Tumor in the Host The pressures of muscle contraction such as for soft-tissue sarcomas, confinement by regional fascial planes such as occurs in the testicular tunic, and a frequently traumatized extremity location, for example, could all be factors that influence the rate of entry of tumor cells by this passive mechanism of tumor pressure and intravasation. Showers of tumor cells are also seen in the effluent blood during and after surgical resection, indicating that the mobilization of a malignancy for resection can also cause this type of intravasation.[39]

INVASION: ACTIVE ENTRANCE OF TUMOR CELLS INTO THE CIRCULATION

Although the aforementioned characteristics of primary tumor vasculature, interstitial pressure, and fluid dynamics all favor the passive intravasation of tumor cells into the circulation, active tumor cell participation in this process is thought more important and is clearly demonstrated by experiments showing active invasion of organ explants in tissue culture tumor cells added to the culture fluid.[40] Likewise, tumor cell deposits can frequently be seen in tissues dissociated from the primary tumor, indicating an active tumor cell locomotion.[41] Thus a great deal of experimental work has focused on the mechanisms of active tumor cell invasion of host tissues and regional vasculature.

Tumor Cell Locomotion in Invasion Tumor cell translocational movements would also aid penetration into surrounding tissues and would facilitate crawling of tumor cells into vascular conduits. As recently reviewed by Strauli and Weiss,[41] significant evidence supports the concept of tumor cell locomotion. The cytoskeleton of many tumor cells possesses the actin-myosin fibrils needed for such cell movement.[42,43] The potential relevance to metastasis formation is suggested by studies showing increased metastasis from hamster melanomas with the greatest ameboid activity in vitro.[44] Tumor lysosomal enzymes—discussed subsequently—could also be effective in destroying the cell junctions between tumor cells, enabling them to "crawl away," perhaps into a vascular conduit from which they can be swept away into the circulation.[41] Despite these intriguing and suggestive aspects of tumor cell locomotion in invasion and metastasis, the relative role of each of these tumor cell properties remains controversial.[44]

Tumor Cell Lytic Enzymes Facilitating Invasion Sylven[45,40] has shown that proteases are present in experimental murine tumors and hypothesized that these enzymes facilitate invasion. Collagenase activity has been found in human cancer.[47–50] Lytic enzymes clearly facilitate tumor invasion in vitro.[45] Liotta et al. have shown that tumor cells possessing intense lytic enzyme activity may be predisposed to entrance into the bloodstream.[51] The cells found in the circulation degraded basement membrane to a much greater degree than did cells taken from the primary tumor itself in these experiments. Likewise these intravascular migrating tumor cells had a much higher collagenase activity. The type of collagenase present has subsequently been shown to be type IV, which is specific for the degradation of the basement membrane–type collagen found in endothelium.[49,50]

Wood[52] has suggested that fibrinolysis is important in invasion and metastasis. Interestingly, many malignant cell lines contain serine protease, which is a potent plasminogen activator. This enzyme specifically activates the potent fibrinolytic protease plasmin. When tumor cells release serine protease, the host fibrinolytic system could be activated, lysing possible fibrin barriers to invasion. Importantly, plasmin can also hydrolyze *fibronectin*, an important structural component of the basement membrane of the endothelium, that is thought to maintain the tight contact between the basement membrane and the endothelial cell.[53] Within this conceptual framework, Wang et al.[54] have demonstrated correlation between the level of fibrinolytic activity in vitro and metastatic capability in vivo. Thus malignant tumors possess the necessary enzymatic machinery for degradation of several of components of the capillary endothelial barriers that would interfere with their entry into the circulation. These experimental data certainly support the concept of active participation of tumor cell lytic enzymes in the invasion of tumor cells into the circulation. The effect of these same enzyme systems in facilitating the egress of tumor cells out of the capillary bed at a distant site of metastasis is subsequently discussed.

Increased detachment of tumor cells from each other. Even after gaining access to a vascular conduit, the tumor cell must detach itself from other tumor cells. Using micromanipulation experiments, Coman[55] showed that tumor cells can be more readily pulled away from an adjacent tumor cell than can cells of normal tissues. He hypothesized that an increased ease of detachability could contribute to metastasis.

More recently Weiss et al.[56,57,60] have studied tumor cell detachment, using methods that apply precise shear stresses to tumor surfaces. Their initial observations indicated that elevated rates of tumor cell division in tissue culture favor increased detachment of cells from the solid surface of the tissue culture plate.[57] High rates of cell detachment were found in the Walker 256 tumor implanted in the liver. Interestingly, it was also found that normal liver cells detached more readily from normal regenerating rat liver than from intact liver.[56] Additionally, the portion of a normal liver closely adjacent to the Walker 256 implant showed a marked increase in cell detachment. Therefore, easy detachment—a characteristic of tumor cells—was also associated with rapid rates of cell division in the adjacent normal regenerating liver; yet the tumor could also convey the increased detachability to adjacent normal liver. Thus, although not a unique property of tumor cells (it is also a property of benign, rapidly dividing cell populations), increased cell detachment can be correlated with metastasis. Implications of these results for an interaction of detachability with tumor cell kinetics in metastasis is subsequently discussed.

Possible role of lytic enzymes and diminished tumor fibronectin in detachability. Poste[59] has hypothesized that "sublethal autolysis" by released lysosomal enzymes can facilitate tumor cell detachment. His demonstration that vitamin A—a lysosomal activator—enhanced in vitro detachability and in vivo spontaneous metastasis from a mouse mammary carcinoma supports this concept.[60,61] The tumor cell populations also have been shown to have a diminished fibronectin content, which, as discussed, is thought to have an important role in cell-to-cell or cell-to-surface adhesion,[62] and tumor cells also possess a plasmin activator which enables the enzymatic degradation of fibronectin.[53]

QUANTITATION OF THE ENTRANCE OF TUMOR CELLS INTO THE CIRCULATION

Through the mechanism of *intravasation* and *invasion* tumor cells can enter the circulation. The extent to which either of these two mechanisms is active in a given tumor situation remains unresolved. However, several investigators have studied the "net effect" by quantitating the number of tumor cells or tumor cell clumps which enter the venous effluent draining an implanted experimental tumor. Also it has been conclusively demonstrated that cell shedding from malignant tumors occurs frequently. Based on kinetic calculations, Steele[63] estimated that up to 10 percent of cells undergoing division in human lung cancer may be shed into the circulation. Gullino et al.[36,64]

directly measured total tumor cell release from a murine mammary carcinoma transplanted into the ovary. They isolated artery and efferent draining vein and precisely measured the number of cells released. In seven experiments the mean number of released tumor cells was $3.2 \pm 1.4 \times 10^6$ cells per 24-h period per gram of tumor in a tumor size range of 1 to 8 g. Results could also be expressed as 16.83 ± 7.59 neoplastic cells released in each milliliter of blood draining the tumor. Liotta et al.[65,66] similarly quantitated cell release from an experimental sarcoma implanted in the thigh, and found that more than 100 tumor cells per milliliter of perfusate are released from the larger tumors. Also, the number of circulating tumor cells increased with the size of the malignancy.

Other investigators[67,68] have used experiments employing quantitative bioassay methodology to quantitate large numbers of released tumor cells, and have noted that the number of cells released increases with the tumor size. The studies of Hewitt and Blake[69] indicate that many cells also enter the lymphatics. These studies thus indicate that in these experimental tumors, a large number of tumor cells are continuously being released into the circulation. Cells are observed in the effluent circulation immediately after tumor vascularization occurs and before it becomes palpable.[65,66]

These experimental findings would seem to correlate with the clinical findings of human tumor cells in the peripheral blood of 20 percent of patients considered curable, and in 30 percent of those with disseminated disease.[70,71] In studies of resected surgical specimens of breast and colon cancer, malignant cells can be readily detected in effluent venous blood.[39,71,72] At least on occasion active DNA synthesis of these malignant cells has been confirmed by in vitro ^{3}HTdR uptake.[73] Furthermore, a human neuroblastoma tissue culture line has been established from cells found in a patient's circulation,[74] documenting the viability of at least some of the cells morphologically identified.

Thus entry of tumor cells into the circulation is a frequent event. However, as will be subsequently discussed, there is a definite dose-response relationship between the number of tumor cells entering the circulation and the probability of formation of metastasis. In clinical management this definite dose-response relationship mandates minimizing the effects of surgical trauma in increasing the showers of tumor cells released at the time of surgical manipulation.

Tumor Cell Circulation and the Inefficiency of Metastasis Formation

Through mechanisms of invasion and/or intravasation many tumor cells enter the circulation by either venous effluent or lymphatics (lymphatic metastasis is discussed subsequently). Once released into the circulation the tumor cell undergoes passive transport to the first capillary bed encountered, and then moves on subsequently to many organs. Earlier studies used bioassays of blood and organs in animals with inoculated primary tumors.[67,68,75] Soon after inoculation of the primary tumor growth, clonogenic tumor cells could be identified in the blood and in many organs. Additionally, a close correlation has been found between the primary tumor size and the dose or number of tumor cells released.[64,65] Other experiments using quantitative inoculations of viable tumor cells intravenously clearly establish the *dose-response* relationship between the number of tumor cells injected above a set threshold and the incidence of metastases.[29,65,76] In studies of the B-16 melanoma only 0.1 percent of cells injected intravenously actually developed into pulmonary metastases.[77] Although the dose-response characteristics are dependent on the tumor system employed, it is clear that *most tumor cells* are destroyed or die during the phase of tumor cell circulation. Since many experimental and human tumors are of epithelial origin, it is possible that very primitive recognition mechanisms eliminate most of these foreign elements in the circulation; or it is possible that depending on their tissue of origin most of these cells, being partially differentiated, simply cannot survive in the strange environment of the bloodstream or lymphatics. The turbulence of the bloodstream also has been hypothesized to cause traumatic tumor cell death within the vascular circulation. Regardless of the destructive mechanisms only a very small percentage of "selected" viable cells entering the bloodstream actually survive to become a metastasis.

TUMOR CELLS IN THE CIRCULATION: ORGAN ARREST PATTERN BY RADIOACTIVE LABELING

Quantitative studies of the timing of circulation, arrest, and recirculation of tumor cells using radioactively labeled tumor cells has been performed by several investigators.[77-80] Radioactive iododeoxyuridine (^{165}IUdR) is an excellent label for such studies because it is incorporated into the nucleus and does not diminish tumor cell viability; it is liberated only after tumor lysis and then promptly excreted into the urine without reutilization in other tissues. In studies of the B-16 melanoma that were serially performed 10 min to 14 days after injection of 200,000 viable ^{125}IUdR-tagged cells, tumor cells were found dominantly arrested in the lungs and less so in the liver.[77,80] Specifically the number of viable labeled cells in the lungs dropped to 136,000 in 1 min, 108,000 in 1 h, 5500 after 12 h, and 355 after 14 days.[81] The measurable radioactivity peaks in the liver and spleen before the label is excreted in the urine in these experiments, but these organs never become the sites of metastasis. This suggests that the reticuloendothelial capabilities of liver and spleen are engulfing nonviable tumor cells in these locations. An almost identical early pattern of labeled tumor cell arrest occurs in other murine fibrosarcomas.[79,80] In a murine lymphoma, however, liver and lung tumor cell (and radioactivity) after intravenous injection were equal, demonstrating the variability of the arrest pattern and metastasis formation based on the histologic type of tumor under study.[79] Because of this major attrition of cancer cells in the circulation, the circulation has been termed a "hostile" environment, causing the very short survival time of most tumor cell emboli.

TRANSORGAN PASSAGE OF VIABLE TUMOR CELLS

In studies using radioactively labeled tumor cells, pulmonary localization of the label as well as the eventual site of metastasis was predominant after intravenous injection. Nevertheless, viable tumor cells do reach all points of the circulation. Pulmonary arteriovenous shunts are known to be present in many animal systems and can serve as conduits for transorgan passage. By use of graded sizes of microspheres these arteriovenous shunts have been identified in many organs. Despite these physiologic shunts, labeled tumor cells are, in fact, trapped largely in *target* organs regardless of the route of inoculation.[82]

The Arrest of Tumor Cells and Growth of a Metastasis

As has been discussed, considerable evidence demonstrates that large numbers of tumor cells are released into the circulation. The studies of radioactively labeled tumor cells indicate that nearly all of them reach target organs for metastasis that is peculiar to the experimental system under study. Nevertheless it is also clear that after this initial encounter with the target organ most cells die and only a few develop as eventual gross metastases. A number of factors favoring the arrest, growth, and/or destruction of tumor cells have been elucidated experimentally and contribute significantly to the understanding of the mechanisms of metastasis.

THE MORPHOLOGY AND DYNAMICS OF THE ARREST AND GROWTH OF TUMOR CELLS

The arrest and eventual growth of metastases in a capillary bed have been observed and photographed by Wood[52] in the rabbit ear chamber and by Sato in the rat omentum,[83] using phase cinemicroscopy (Fig. 12-5). The observed events are (1) adherence of tumor cells to the capillary endothelium; (2) entrapment of the tumor cells by a fibrin-platelet microthrombus; (3) tumor cell penetration of the endothelium, either through insinuation between endothelial cells or by apparent dissolution of the capillary wall; (4) migration through the underlying basement membrane (not seen in phase cinemicroscopy) with entrance into the extravascular space; (5) cell division and proliferation with the inducement of a new capillary blood flow and stroma. Failure at any of these steps in the arrest aborts the development of a true metastasis. In these experiments the target organs studied (of necessity for technical reasons) are not the expected sites of metastasis for the tumor systems under study. Also the relatively invasive methods required for the phase-cinemicroscopic observations performed in these studies could well alter the capillary bed or propensity for local clot formation. Therefore there remains some justifiable doubt as to whether these observed events are generally typical of the actual process of metastasis in vivo. Nevertheless, these observations have provided a framework for reviewing this process, and much of the research performed has been organized along these lines.

CLUMPING OF TUMOR CELLS INCREASES METASTATIC EFFICIENCY

Cells released in optimally sized *clumps* have an advantage in metastasis because they can wedge into capillary vessels, propagate, and "burst" the walls and initiate true metastasis.[21] Larger clumps (depending on the system) may perish, wedged in impenetrable muscular arterioles.[84] The rate of release for clumps vs. single cells has been studied in one model, and about 40 percent of the cells released in this isolation-perfusion study of a tumor-

208 BASIC CONCEPTS IN ONCOLOGY

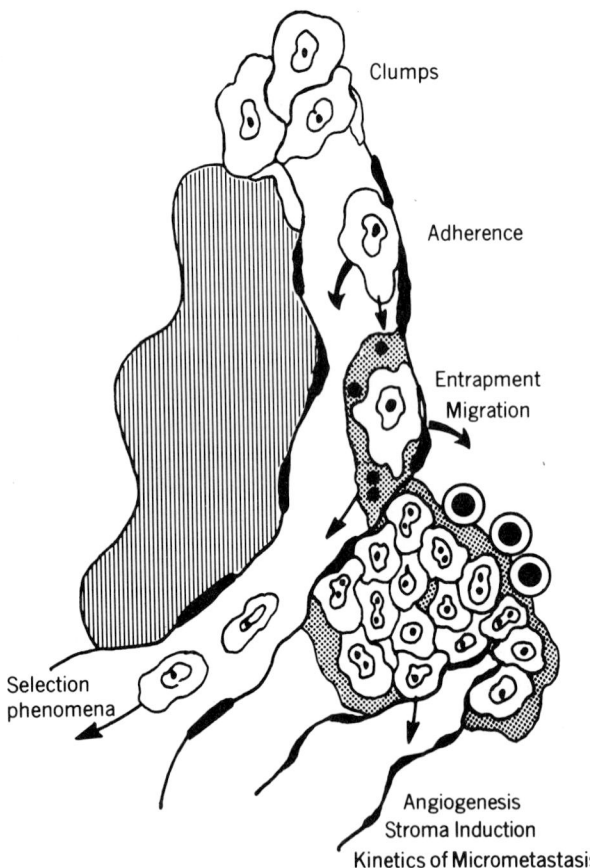

FIGURE 12-5 In a different organ, tumor cells must undergo arrest if they are to be successful as a metastasis. A number of steps are involved in becoming a successful metastasis.

bearing limb were released as cell clumps.[66] Interestingly, the ratio of cell clumps to single cells was relatively constant for all primary tumor sizes, rising in parallel with the total number of cells released and with the increase in the percentage of grossly observed metastatic lesions in the lungs. Fidler[29] has also shown that cell clumps in B-16 melanoma are favored for metastasis formation. It remains possible that the tendency to release tumor clumps rather than single cells is an important determinant in the process of metastasis. As discussed earlier this propensity may be related to the pattern of tumor vascularization.

TUMOR CELL MEMBRANE AND TUMOR CELL ARREST

It is thought that the relationship of the tumor cell membrane to the lining of the distant capillary bed is critical to determining the outcome of the metastatic process. This hypothesis has stimulated a great deal of work focusing on various membrane characteristics in metastasis. It has been emphasized that even at the level of the tumor cell membrane, current concepts of membrane fluidity[28] dictate that specific membrane characteristics must be understood as a mosaic pattern distributed over the cell's surface. This means that studies that try to define a "net" cell membrane property may miss an important mobile membrane determinant responsible for an important aspect of cell behavior. Nevertheless, despite the complexity of this aspect of metastasis, considerable efforts have been made in attempting to identify surface properties of tumor cells capable of influencing their ability to arrest and therefore metastasize.

Recent evidence firmly establishes the critical nature of the plasma cell membrane in determining the arrest of cells for metastasis formation. These series of experiments[85,86] utilize the fact that both high and low metastatic B-16 melanoma cells shed intact plasma membrane vesicles that can be collected, isolated, purified, and then re-fused to tumor cells using polyethylene glycol. *Membrane vesicles* collected from the highly metastatic B-16, F-10 cell line were fused to the intact B-16, F-1 cell line, which is poorly metastatic. The resulting cells showed an increased incidence of arrest and, most importantly, a greatly increased production of pulmonary metastases similar to the highly metastatic strain from which the membrane vesicles had been harvested. Surface labeling of vesicles with ferritin or ^{125}I showed that the new vesicles persist in the cell membrane for only about 18 to 24 h after polyethylene glycol fusion. Since the proliferation of extravasated tumor cells does not begin for 24 to 48 h after tumor cell injection intravenously, the effect of these critical, short-lived membrane components must be to act on the early phase of tumor cell arrests in the capillary bed. What then is the nature of these membrane components seemingly critical to the earliest, and probably most important, phases of metastasis?

A number of tumor cell properties either directly or indirectly associated with the plasma cell membrane have been studied in relationship to tumor cell arrest and metastasis. It should be emphasized that no holistic and unifying relationship has yet been developed, and many cell properties would seem to influence the propensity for metastasis. The tumor cell properties that have been extensively studied and which will be discussed in this section include (1) tumor cell deformability or rigidity, (2) stickiness or adherence, (3) cell surface charge and mobility of cell surface charge, (4) biochemical-enzymatic properties, and (5) other characteristics.

Tumor Cell Deformability or Rigidity For the single circulating cancer cell, the property of tumor cell deformability has been correlated with the propensity for metastasis. The hypothesis based on morphologic observations has been that the rigid cell is subject to mechanical arrest in the capillary bed and should have a greater propensity for metastasis, while the more deformable cell can "squeeze through" to an eventual death in the circulation or to possible metastasis in other organs. With the use of phase-cinemicroscopic techniques, Zeidman[87] compared the relative deformability of the Brown-Pearce (BP) carcinoma cells with that of VX2 tumor cells. The VX2 tumor cells were more rigid and became lodged in the lungs, which are also the dominant site of the metastasis. The BP cells were more deformable and passed through the lungs so that the tumor produced a more widespread pattern of organ metastasis. Sato et al. have extensively studied the relative deformabilities of several strains of rat hepatoma.[83,88,89] They found that the rigid-cell strains were arrested in the lungs after intravenous injection and that the lung was the dominant site of development of metastasis. The deformable strains readily passed through the lungs and also exhibited a diffuse pattern of gross organ metastasis. These studies suggested that the *rigid* cell is favored for metastasis in the first capillary bed encountered. The more deformable cell passes on and can produce a more diffuse organ pattern of metastasis after intravenous injection. Whether mechanical impaction in a capillary is the critical event, or whether other cell surface characteristics that could be associated with such rigidity or deformability are most important remains to be determined.[90]

Tumor Cell Stickiness or Adherence Tumor cell stickiness refers to the propensity of cells to stick to glass or other foreign substances. Kojima and Sakai[91] showed that "sticky" hepatoma tumor cell lines metastasize readily, suggesting that after release from the primary tumor they are more easily lodged in distant organs. Additionally, stickiness to glass correlated inversely with the adherence of tumor cells to each other (cohesion), indicating that the cells that are most likely to stick to a foreign surface are those most easily detached from other tumor cells in the primary tumor (see previous studies of cell detachment by Weiss[56]). Other studies[92,93] quantitatively assessed the stickiness of the high and low metastatic B-16 melanoma cell lines. They found that the highly metastatic cell lines most rapidly stick to endothelial cells in tissue culture. Additionally, and seemingly at variance with the results of Kojima and Sakai, these studies showed that the "selected" highly metastatic B-16 cells most rapidly adhere to each other, apparently manifesting an increased tendency to tumor cell clumping. In other studies investigating organ specificity of the stickiness of B-16 melanoma strains, the high and low metastatic cell lines were incubated with syngeneic cell suspensions prepared from mouse lung, liver, kidney, and spleen.[92] Stickiness of the highly metastatic cell line to the lung tissues was pronounced and was much greater than with the normal or low metastatic B-16 cell line. Additionally, since tumor cells need an "anchor" in order to initiate translocational movements, stickiness could well be partly responsible for the tumor cells' "crawling out" of the capillary bed. Hagmar and Ryd[94] have reported that when cell locomotion is paralyzed, as with the compound cytochalasin B, more cells seem to be passively transported through the capillary circulation, leading to an enhanced postpulmonary pattern of metastasis.

Some work has been done pertaining to specific biochemical or biophysical determinants that influence cell rigidity or deformability, and stickiness or adhesion. Some evidence suggests that these cell properties may be correlated with net cell surface charge. Purdom and Ambrose[95] demonstrated that the propensity for metastasis correlated directly with net cell negativity. In other studies by Weiss,[90] cell rigidity has been associated with surface anion concentrations, particularly in sialic acids. Cleavage of the 2,3- and 2,6-glycosidic linkages between these anions (sialic acids) and the underlying mucopolysaccharides of the cell periphery decreases negative surface charge and greatly increases deformability, associated with diminished metastasis formation.

The highest negative charge related to greater rigidity, however, would seemingly interfere with the sticking of the cell to the endothelium, also charged negatively. Despite this paradoxical situation, the *great mobility* of malignant cell membrane constituents may be important in cell arrest for metastasis. Despite the mutually negative charges between the tumor cell periphery and the capillary endothelium, small islands of positive charge could develop by the lateral rotation of anionic components.[28] Conceivably, platelets adhering to tumor cells could stimulate capillary endothelial contraction, thereby exposing basement membrane in the capillary, and promote stickiness. This hypothesis is consistent with the work of Gasic,[96] who demonstrated that tumor cell stickiness to platelets increases metastasis formation.

Biochemical Characteristics With the availability of the high (F-10) and low (F-1) metastatic cell lines of the B-16 melanoma, a number of biochemical features of these variant lines have been compared in search of possible biochemical mechanisms active in tumor cell arrest and metastasis. As recently reviewed by Fidler and Nicholson,[97] comparative studies of lectin agglutinability, surface labeling by lactoperoxidase-catalyzed iodination, surface-bound and secreted enzymes, and some antigens and glycopeptides released by trypsin or pronase have been studied comparatively in these variants. So far, no major clues to the biochemistry of the cell membrane properties essential for metastasis have been identified, with the possible exception of a decreased sialoglycoprotein labeling of the highly metastatic B-16, F-10 line.[98]

Thus, although a definitive statement on the biophysical and biochemical nature of tumor cell arrest and subsequent metastasis cannot be made, the tumor cell membrane itself has been demonstrated a critical element in metastasis, and many hypotheses continue to be explored in this regard.

INVASIVE PROPERTIES AND TRANSCAPILLARY MIGRATION OF TUMOR CELLS

Although tumor cell clumps have been observed to burst the walls of small vessels in which they become mechanically impacted, an equally important event is the arrest of single cells or small clumps of cells in a distant capillary bed. For this type of arrest a different series of events has been demonstrated.[99] Single tumor cells have been observed morphologically to migrate to the extravascular space by a process which is morphologically similar to the migration of leukocytes, which indeed may precede tumor cells on their way to the extravascular space.[52] The site of penetration of capillary endothelium is difficult to visualize by phase-microscopic techniques, but electron microscopic studies of this event by Dingemans,[100] Warren et al.,[101] Sindelar et al.,[102] and Nakamura et al.[99] suggest that the migration primarily occurs between endothelial cells. Although cell rigidity may favor tumor cell arrest, the migration by extensions of pseudopodia and squeezing of these pseudopodia between existing capillary cells requires significant deformability.

After the cells have passed the endothelium, the basement membrane remains a theoretical barrier to invasion.

Two important models for the study of invasion and for the selection of highly invasive variants of overall tumor cell populations have recently been described. Models of both a mouse bladder and a chick chorioallantoic membrane have been used for selecting and studying the most highly invasive variants of the B-16 melanoma, as recently described by Hart[103] and Poste et al.[104] Importantly, the cells selected in vitro for maximal invasiveness formed more spontaneous metastases in vivo than the parent cells.[103,104] Additionally, the highly invasive and metastatic cell lines degrade type IV collagen (a critical component of capillary endothelial basement cell membrane) to a much greater degree, and such collagenolytic activity facilitates basement membrane penetration by a tumor cell which has reached this depth of the capillary barrier.[50] Other factors important for invasion at the primary tumor location could facilitate metastasis by enhancing invasion at the site of arrest in the distant capillary bed.

HOST FACTORS INVOLVED IN TUMOR CELL ARREST AND METASTASIS

Capillary Physiology The data presented above indicate that the arrest of tumor cells is critical to the eventual formation of metastasis. For example, when tumor cells are layered over somatic cells in tissue, in some models they are repelled from the top surface and cannot stick unless bare areas develop, exposing an underlying fibrin plate.[105] It would seem, therefore, that endothelial cells do a good job of repelling circulating cells (including tumor cells) and preventing sludging in the microcirculation. Much data suggests that several aspects of the normal capillary cell physiology could influence tumor cell arrest. Studies of the physiology of capillary and mesothelial cells (lining the peritoneum) indicate that these cells can dynamically contract and expand their periphery, utilizing contractile cytoskeletal elements (the actin-myosin fibrils).[41] Histamine[106] and thrombin[107] have been shown to be potent mediators of endothelial cell contractility. Therefore, it is reasonable to hypothesize that contraction of endothelial cells could bare the underlying basement membrane, thus facilitating the adherence of circulating tumor cells. Other data indicate that endothelial cells may be periodically shed into the circulation and then replaced.[101] Before these cells are replaced, small gaps remain that expose the basement membrane as a favored site of tumor cell adherence. The importance of these aspects of capillary endothelial cell physiology in the implantation of tumor cells is demonstrated by the scanning electron microscopic studies of Warren and Vales.[101,107] They studied the lodging of lymphomas and carcinoma cells onto the vena cava in a model system. Firm and permanent implantation of tumor cells occurred in the damaged or denuded areas of the endothelium. In areas where the endothelium was intact temporary arrest of tumor cells by a loose thrombus could be seen, but this tumor cell fibrin thrombus was rapidly dissolved by the endogenous fibrinolytic activity of the endothelial cells. Similar observations have been made in relationship to the peritoneal cavity. In these experiments tumor cells selectively adhered to areas of raw collagen created by periodic mesothelial cell retraction and/or direct trauma.[108]

These data support the hypothesis that capillary physiology (including the specific dynamics of capillary cell shedding and replacement, contractility, and fibrinolytic activity) interacts with the arrest of tumor cells in the process of metastasis. It is obvious that the dynamics of capillary physiology may vary from organ to organ, which could at least in part explain the various patterns of tumor metastasis discussed subsequently. Notably, when the barrier has been disrupted by acute injury, metastasis can reach organs that otherwise would never become sites of metastasis in control animals.[109,110]

Coman[84] showed that tumor cells or cell clumps trapped in arterioles failed to penetrate these muscular walls and became surrounded in a dense fibrinous process and perished. Organs with numerous arteriolar structures could cause the very large clumps of tumor cells to perish by this mechanism. This property of the circulatory anatomy could be relevant for the destruction of large tumor cell clumps which otherwise (as noted above) would be favored for metastasis formation.

Entrapment of Arrested Cells: The Role of Fibrin, Platelets, and Anticoagulation The morphologic demonstration of fibrin deposition around adherent tumor cells[52] stimulated many studies of the effect of anticoagulation (warfarin, heparin, fibrinolysis),[111] defibrination,[112] thrombocytopenia,[96] and inhibitors of platelet aggregation (aspirin, dipyridamole),[96,113,114] on metastatic spread. Brown[78] demonstrated diminished implantation of ^{125}IUdR-tagged tumor cells in the lungs in warfarin-treated mice. No direct tumor cell cytotoxicity due to warfarin was demonstrable in this tumor system, and he concluded that tumor cell implantation was diminished by anticoagulation treatment. Similarly, thrombocytopenia or aspirin decreased implantation of ^{125}IUdR-tagged tumor cells and reduced metastasis formation.[96,113] Tanaka et al.[115] have shown that tumor cells with the highest thromboplastic activity may have an advantage for metastasis by initiating the clotting sequence that leads to the entrapment of these cells in the capillary bed. Nevertheless, since capillary endothelial cells are capable of intense fibrinolytic activity, they would also seem to be able to lyse such thrombi, as demonstrated by Warren et al.[107] However, an imbalance of the thrombotic-fibrinolytic process could create conditions favorable for entrapment and therefore metastasis formation.

The Neovascularization and Growth of Tumor Cells in the Extravascular Space As observed morphologically, tumor cells that still have potential to succeed as metastases reach the extravascular space within about 24 h of their arrest, and mitotic cell division can be observed. Passive diffusion of nutrients supports the growth of the metastatic nidus up to 1 mm in diameter, but continued growth requires the ingrowth of host capillaries—the process of neovascularization. Inhibition of growth at such a small tumor size could result in a state of dormancy. Extracts of some tumors (as opposed to tumor cells), however, have been shown to produce a tumor angiogenic factor which stimulates capillary ingrowth. Host lymphocytes and macrophages also produce angiogenic factors such that this effect may not always be tumor-specific but could be augmented by host-passenger cells.[116] Additionally, epithelial growth factor (EGF) and other stimulants of cell growth[117] can be found in platelets and may also participate in stimulating the growth of tumor cells in the extravascular space. Similarly, epithelial tumor cells optimally require a substrate for growth and probably induce an architectural stroma from host substances. Having achieved these final phases of metastatic growth, the metastasis undergoes progressive enlargement.

KINETICS OF THE GROWTH OF MICROMETASTASES

Schabel[118] and Simpson-Herren et al.[119] have shown that the transplantation of small bits of tissue from a large primary tumor causes a prompt increase in their growth fraction. The same phenomenon occurs in small metastatic foci; i.e., despite the fact that a large primary tumor has a small growth fraction, micrometastases may be growing maximally. An important question is, To what extent does the high growth fraction of the micrometastases reflect better vascularization? Do metastases maintain a kinetic advantage through all sizes of growth, suggesting that cell selection for superior "growth" characteristics occur during metastasis?

Metastasis to Regional Lymph Nodes

ENTRANCE INTO LYMPHATICS

The process of invasion facilitates entry into lymphatics as well as venules. Since tumors are thought not to contain any lymphatics, entry into lymphatics must occur at the invasive tumor periphery. The interstitial fluid convection currents described by Gullino et al.[31,35] drain into lymphatics and are hypothesized to transport tumor cells into them. Lunscken and Strauli[37] demonstrated the existence of widely patent intercellular junctions in the lymphatics of the diaphragm and showed that tumor cells are passively transported into lymphatics through these large openings. In other studies, Carr et al. found that tumor cells enter through gaps between endothelial cells of the lymphatic vessel in a manner indistinguishable from that of macrophages[120]; and it seemed that cytoplasmic processes of tumor cells probed the endothelial surface for the best route for the cell to take.[121] In some of these studies, trypsinization, which removes surface anions and presumably enhances cell deformability, increased the rate of lymphatic metastases.[121]

LYMPHATIC TRANSPORT, ENTRAPMENT, AND TRANSNODAL PASSAGE OF TUMOR CELLS

Cells entering lymphatics are transported to lymph nodes, and the afferent vessels deposit cells in the peripheral subcapsular sinuses of the nodes. In relation to subsequent phenomena there is significant variability in experimental results and in their interpretation from one model to another. Several animal models indicate significant tumor cell destruction in the lymph nodes, and at least temporary entrapment. This is the filter-barrier concept of lymphatic metastasis. Ludwig and Titus[122] injected labeled Walker 256 tumor cells into rat footpads. Most of the cells reaching subcapsular sinuses of lymph nodes were killed, and only 0.2 percent reached the medullary sinuses of lymph nodes within 24 h. Zeidman and Buss[123] compared the take of equal doses of V2 carcinoma injected either intravenously or intralymphatically in rabbits. More metastases developed after intravenous injection, and it was concluded that more cells were killed in the lymph nodes. Additionally, V2 cancer cells were retained in the regional lymph nodes for approximately 3 weeks. Carr et al.[120] also observed temporary arrest of cells in lymph nodes. These data, in addition to those reviewed by Strauli,[124] indicate that in appropriate models the lymph nodes serve as temporary "functional filters" for cancer cells, an experimental concept consistent with many clinical observations.

For the cells that *lodge* in nodes, proliferation takes place first peripherally and then, with time, involves the medullary regions of the node, presumably thereafter shedding cells into the efferent vessels. Carr et al.[120] showed that the dose of cells needed for successful growth in the lymph node (using an anaplastic carcinogen-induced tumor) was far lower than the dose required for "take" in the footpad, and he suggested that some degree of "immunologic" privilege for tumor growth existed in the node in this system.

INTERRELATED LYMPHATICOVENOUS CIRCULATION OF TUMOR CELLS IN SOME SYSTEMS

Although the data described previously imply that the lymph node is a temporary barrier, other data in different model systems indicate that the lymph node does *not* significantly impair or retard tumor dissemination. (See Fig. 12-6.) These experiments led to the conclusion that most cells reaching the lymph nodes rapidly enter efferent channels or the systemic circulation through lymphaticovenous anastomoses.[125,126] Cells passing through lymph nodes retain the capacity for metastasis to other organs, and the few cells lodging in lymph nodes develop into metastases. Using quantitative bioassay methods, Hewitt and Blake[69] studied the dynamics of spontaneous lymphatic metastasis from a nonimmunogenic spontaneous squamous cell carcinoma in mice, in which spontaneous nodal metastases only rarely occurred. Regional nodes contained viable tumor cells detected by bioassay, but gross metastases rarely developed. As the primary tumor increased in size, the numbers of cells in the nodes remained constant. Therefore, these authors concluded that the nodes have a

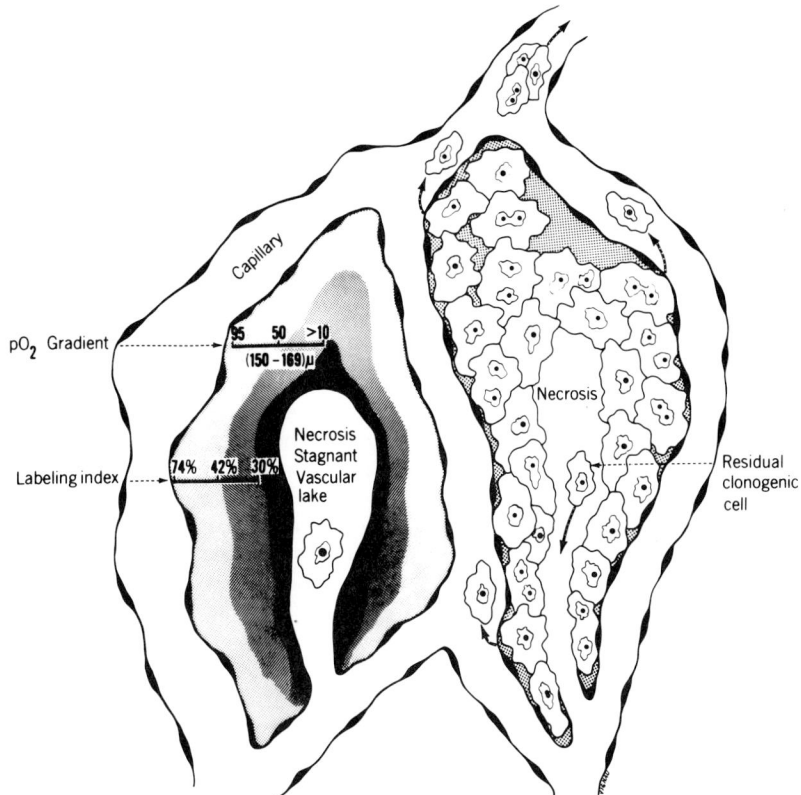

FIGURE 12-6 Interrelated distribution of tumor cells in the lymphatic and vascular systems. Tumor cells released from a primary tumor can gain access to either lymphatic or venous systems. In lymph nodes, some cells pass directly into the efferent system, gaining access to the general circulation through the thoracic duct. Also lymphaticovenous channels have been demonstrated in lymph nodes, interrelating these circulations. Many cells, depending on the tumor system, seem to bypass lymph nodes and reach the general circulation.

reasonably constant "holding capacity" and that above such a threshold, all other tumor cells passed on into efferent channels and into the general circulation.

In summary, different model systems for studies of lymphatic metastasis have given conflicting results, as have the various models of hematogenous metastasis. Nevertheless, in models in which lymphatic metastasis occurs the sequence of events is not remarkably dissimilar from that described for hematogenous metastasis; most cells are killed or pass on into the efferent lymphatic or venous circulation, and a "selected" few remain to generate the true metastasis.

TUMOR-HOST FACTORS MODULATING METASTASIS

In the previous discussions the various phases in metastasis have been viewed relatively mechanistically. Cells are released, circulate, and dynamically interact with the distant capillary bed, and a few form metastases. Although the complexity of these interactions is far from being completely understood, these events must be eventually interpreted in a much broader context.

The host responds to tumor growth and dissemination with a reaction that varies with the stage of neoplastic growth. The intensity of any one of several host reactions may, in the short time frame, vary chronobiologically, and in a longer time frame may be influenced by nutritional factors, varying growth conditions, and other variables. Similarly, when spontaneous metastasis occurs in a host with a growing tumor, that tumor has further modified the environment in which cancer cells attempt to metastasize. In most common solid tumors in humans there is a long, preclinical period during which tumor or host factors can modulate metastasis formation. This chapter cannot accommodate an intensive review of all possible tumor-host factors that may modulate the process of metastasis; however, these aspects of neoplastic dissemination are intuitively of great importance in the metastatic process in humans. Several aspects of tumor and host interactions that have been shown experimentally to influence this phenomenon will therefore be discussed.

Primary Tumor Factors That Modulate Metastasis

ORGAN SITE OF THE PRIMARY TUMOR

Obviously the site of experimental tumor implantation determines, by proximity, the first organ or lymph nodes encountered by cells released from that site. The influence of primary site, however, exceeds pure anatomic considerations. The methylcholanthrene-induced (MCA-induced) sarcoma, currently under study in the laboratory at the Miami Cancer Institute, metastasizes to the lung when growing in muscle but does not metastasize at all after subcutaneous inoculation. It has also been observed that the usually widely metastasizing Lewis lung carcinoma does not metastasize after implantation in the peritoneal cavity. Furthermore the growth rate of many experimental tumors varies depending on the organ into which they are transplanted.

SIZE OF THE PRIMARY TUMOR AND METASTATIC POTENTIAL

As has been reviewed in relation to clinical cancer metastases[126a] size of primary tumor variably affects the propensity for spontaneous metastasis. Since primary tumor size has a definite and quantifiable effect on tumor metastasis in many experimental systems and in humans, it can be used to assess the metastatic potential of various experimental tumors.

If *metastatic potential* is defined as *the propensity for metastasis in relation to primary tumor size,* then it is possible to classify many experimental and clinical cancers by their metastatic potential. For instance, the Lewis lung carcinoma usually metastasizes in several days from intramuscular transplantation in mice, before the primary tumor is even palpable in the hind limb. Since metastasis occurs from a very small tumor, the Lewis lung is judged to have very high metastatic potential. An even greater extreme in metastatic potential is found in the L1210 leukemia, which disseminates after transplantation of only a single cell. On the other hand, the MCA-induced sarcoma does not metastasize before reaching more than 1.5 cm in diameter. Other MCA-induced sarcomas do not metastasize at all, regardless of the size they achieve before local growth causes death.

Thus, according to this definition, in tumors of high metastatic potential, tumor size does not significantly influence metastasis. Tumors of moderate metastatic potential resemble the common clinical cancers in which increasing size correlates with metastasis. Tumors of low metastatic potential metastasize only after attaining large proportions in relation to the size of the host, and some invasive malignant tumors do not metastasize at all. This concept is summarized in Fig. 12-7.

For tumors of moderate or low metastatic potential *why does increasing size increase metastases?* One obvious cause is the increasing *doses of cells* released from larger tumors. The aforementioned studies of Liotta[65] and Gullino et al.[64] clearly show that increasing numbers of tumor cells are shed into the circulation as the tumor increases in size. Other data, however, suggest that other agents released from the primary tumor may also influence metastasis.

Products of cell necrosis released from or diffusing about the periphery of the primary tumor can be implicated.

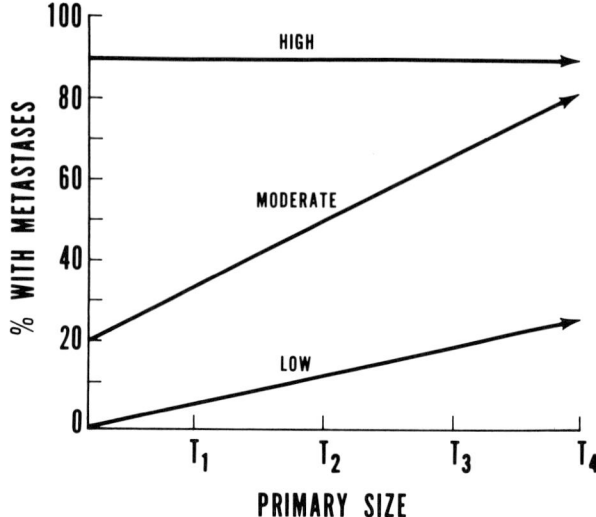

FIGURE 12-7 Metastatic potential of primary tumors. Metastatic potential can be defined as the statistical risk for metastasis in relationship to the size of the primary tumor. (*Reproduced with permission from EV Sugarbaker: Cancer metastasis: A product of tumor-host interactions, in RC Hickey et al (eds): Current Problems in Cancer, Year Book, Chicago, 1979.*)

Weiss et al.[58] have shown that water-soluble extracts from the necrotic core of large Walker 256 tumors growing subcutaneously increase the ease of cell detachment from viable parts of the same tumor. The sublethal autolysis by tumor lysozymes that occurs in tumor zones adjacent to areas of necrosis has been suggested as the mechanism that facilitates this increased ease of cell detachment.[59] The *feeder effect* of necrotic products which decrease the threshold for the take of increasing numbers of viable cells released is another hypothesis. As shown by Revesz,[127] the dose of cells required for the successful subcutaneous implantation of a tumor is greatly reduced by adding lethally irradiated tumor cells to viable cell suspensions. Moreover, the sensitivity of lung colony bioassay for quantitating the numbers of viable cells is greatly increased by adding "feeder" dead tumor cells before intravenous inoculation.[128] With larger tumor size, extensive necrosis can be expected to occur, along with a large flow of tumor interstitial fluid (containing proteins, antigens, and other materials) from the tumor core to periphery.[64] Recent studies[129] show that inoculation of extracts from large primary tumors into mice with smaller tumors increases spontaneous metastasis. Whether this effect is due to the release of free tumor antigen, as suggested by Vaage,[130] or to other products of tumor necrosis is not clear. The potential flood of bioactive materials from areas of tumor necrosis would include polyamines, lysozymes, and other toxic products that could modulate the host milieu for either increased or diminished metastasis formation from the cells released into the circulation.

INTERRELATIONSHIP OF GROWTH RATE OF PRIMARY TUMORS AND METASTASES

A significant body of literature[131] substantiates the hypothesis that primary tumors can suppress the growth rate of distant metastases. It has been shown experimentally that surgical removal or irradiation of a primary tumor is followed by growth of larger metastases than that which occurs when the primary tumor is left intact, even though experimental animals survive for equal times.

A most convincing demonstration of this phenomenon is found in the studies of Schatten,[132] later confirmed by Ketcham et al.[133] In multiple experimental tumor systems, they consistently noted an increased size of metastases after amputation of the primary tumor. Schatten also demonstrated progressive growth of pulmonary metastases after tumor amputation, while the metastatic size in tumor-bearing animals remained unchanged, apparently inhibited by the presence of the primary tumor. DeWys[128] provided insight into the mechanisms involved. He demonstrated a nearly synchronous slowing of the growth rate of a primary tumor and its spontaneous metastases after the primary tumor reached a critical size. Amputation of the primary tumor resulted in renewed proliferation in lung metastases. Since DeWys's tumor system was not immunogenic and since pulmonary metastases were well vascularized (therefore excluding poor oxygenation and nutrition as likely reasons for growth retardation), he hypothesized the existence of a "tumor-related systemic growth retarding factor." The relevance of this type of modulation of metastases by the primary tumor to the rapid clinical growth of metastases that occurs occasionally after surgery has been studied by Simpson-Herren et al.[134] They demonstrated that in mice whose primary tumor is amputated just *after* metastases occur, survival time can actually be diminished compared with that in mice with intact primary tumors and "inhibited" pulmonary metastases. This hypothesis is diagramed in Fig. 12-8.

INFLUENCE OF THE KINETICS OF PRIMARY TUMOR GROWTH ON METASTASIS

It has been stated that, clinically, the most rapidly growing tumors are those that metastasize most readily.[135] Nevertheless, it can be questioned whether the short survival time after resection (or other treatment) of rapidly

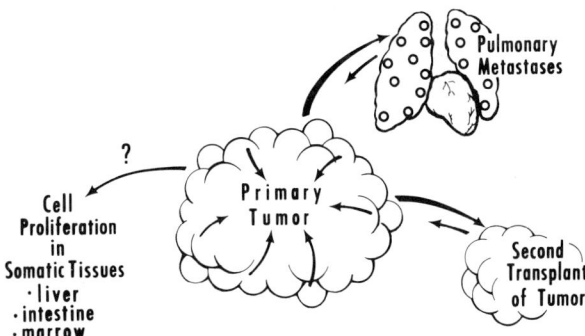

FIGURE 12-8 The inhibitory effects of a primary tumor on metastatic disease. Significant experimental evidence indicates an interrelationship of the kinetics of a primary tumor and distant metastases. (*Reproduced with permission from EV Sugarbaker: Cancer metastasis: A product of tumor-host interactions, in RC Hickey et al (eds): Current Problems in Cancer, Year Book, Chicago, 1979.*)

growing primary cancers is due to the rapid growth in the mass of established metastases (reflecting their origin from a rapidly growing primary) or whether more numerous metastases actually develop from rapidly growing tumors. Several pieces of experimental evidence suggest the latter answer. As previously discussed, Weiss[56,57] noted increased cell detachability from rapidly dividing tumors. Thus, by increasing the dose of cells entering the circulation, metastasis from the most rapidly dividing tumors might be enhanced. Suzuki et al.[136] studied the clonogenicity of cell populations in various phases of the cell cycle, using a lung colony assay. Since cell size and buoyant density characteristics change as cells move through the cell cycle, these populations can be separated in preparative quantitites by centrifugal elutriation techniques. Interestingly, S-, G_2- and M-phase cells produced significantly more metastases (lung colonies) than G_1-phase cells. Control studies showed that in vitro tissue culture clonogenicity was the same for all populations. Although the larger size of S-, G_2-, and M-phase cells or tumor cell membrane alterations such as surface stickiness or deformability could explain these results, it can be reasonably hypothesized that rapidly dividing primary tumors would shed not only greater numbers of but also more clonogenic cells. These observations may also be relevant to the selection of cells for metastasis, as is subsequently discussed.

CELLULAR AND ZONAL HETEROGENEITY OF THE PRIMARY TUMOR

The heterogeneity of primary neoplasia has long been recognized, but implications of this fact and the relevance to the mechanisms of metastasis, as well as the recent data documenting the profound therapeutic implications of such heterogeneity, have been emphasized in the last several years.

The Tumor Vasculature and Intrinsic Metabolic Heterogeneity By virtue of the pattern of vascularization that is seemingly intrinsic to neoplastic growth, the primary tumor is heterogeneous. It has been shown that, as tumor cells divide, cords of cells are "pushed" farther and farther away from capillary blood supply.[32,137] When this distance reaches approximately 150 to 169 μm, morphologic necrosis is observed histologically.[137,138] Using microelectrodes, other investigators have detected a Po_2 gradient over a similar distance (Fig. 12-9).[139] Thus, cells vary from viable and well-oxygenated to necrotic and nonviable. The environment of borderline oxygenation might prove a stimulus for genetic errors and therefore mutagenesis as a further stimulus to tumor cell heterogeneity within the primary tumor.

Partial Retention of a Maturation Gradient in Primary Epithelial Malignancies Many experimental and clinical ma-

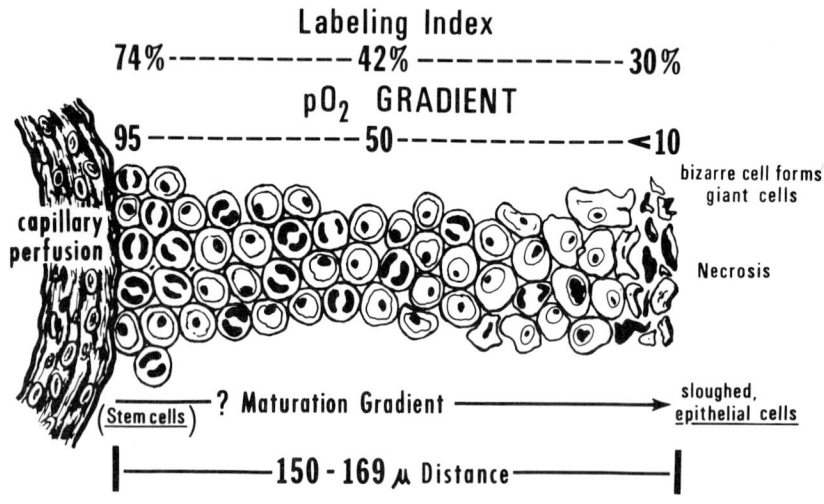

FIGURE 12-9 Metabolic and kinetic heterogeneity within a primary tumor. The properties of tumor vasculature intrinsically create metabolic heterogeneity, and epithelial malignancies may maintain a maturation gradient, adding a further element of heterogeneity. (*Reproduced with permission from EV Sugarbaker, Cancer metastasis: A product of tumor-host interactions, in RC Hickey et al (eds): Current Problems in Cancer, Year Book, Chicago, 1979.*)

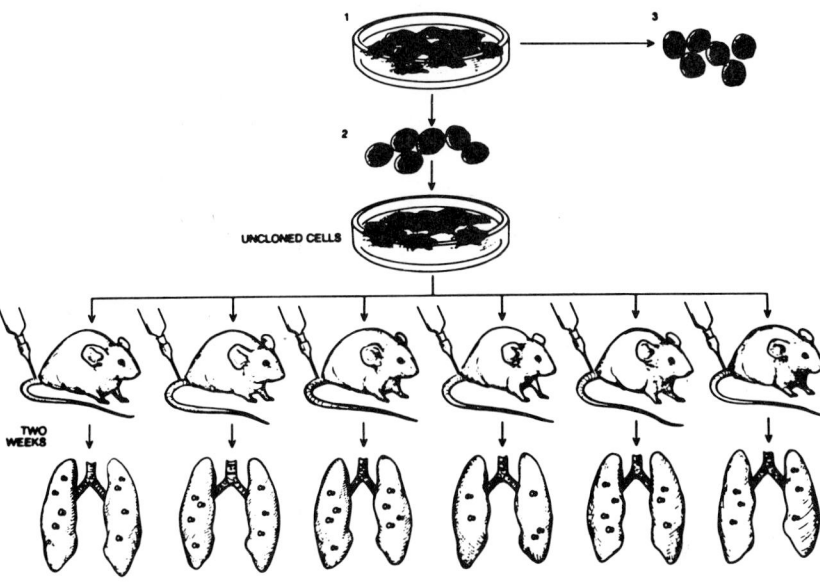

FIGURE 12-10 Classic experiments demonstrating heterogeneity for metastasis formation in the B-16 melanoma and an early generation ultraviolet radiation—induced sarcoma. (Continued in Fig. 12-11.)

lignancies originate from epithelial surfaces, and despite the uncontrolled growth characteristic of neoplasia, these tumors often retain to some degree a differentiation gradient from proliferating stem cells. Thus, to some extent, retention of an embryologically derived maturation gradient produces cellular heterogeneity in malignant neoplasms.

Demonstration of Tumor Cell Heterogeneity Heterogeneity of the cell populations has been demonstrated in many direct studies of the primary tumor and also by looking at the properties of *clones* derived from single cells separated from the primary tumor using soft-agar tissue culture techniques. Alternatively other investigators have looked at the characteristics of metastases themselves, since these can be interpreted as representing an in vivo clone developing from a single cell or small clump derived from the primary tumor.[140–144] Many studies in human and experimental neoplasms document the primary tumor to be heterogeneous with respect to immunogenicity,[145] ploidy,[146] histology,[146] estrogen receptor content,[148] enzyme content,[149] and myriad other properties.[85] Importantly, Fidler and Hart[150] have shown that heterogeneity can be *zonal* within a primary tumor rather than on a individual cellular basis. In fact, as shown by these studies, in order to maintain the zonal heterogeneity for pigment production, in an experimental melanoma cellular suspensions must be inoculated rather than tumor fragments. This observation has significant impact on the design of experimental models and indicates optimal methods for transfer of tumor materials in serial transplantation.[150]

Heterogeneity for Metastasis Formation in Primary Tumors Particularly relevant to the mechanisms of metastasis is the finding that primary malignant tumors contain cells with differing metastatic capabilities. In an initial series of experiments Fidler[142] enriched the metastatic subpopulation of a primary B-16 melanoma by repeated in vivo–in vitro cloning experiments. The F-10 (10 such passages), B-16 melanoma variant population was obtained and exhibited a very high (and stable) metastatic potential for pulmonary metastasis. Other studies by Nicholson et al.[151] showed that B-16 strains could be specifically selected for other sites of organ metastasis by identical in vivo–in vitro enrichment of the metastasing subpopulation of cells. Conceptually similar enrichment-selection experiments have identified highly invasive (as opposed to metastatic) subpopulations, as previously described.[103,104] Other tumor cell properties can also be selected by an appropriate enrichment procedure and/or selection procedure.[85]

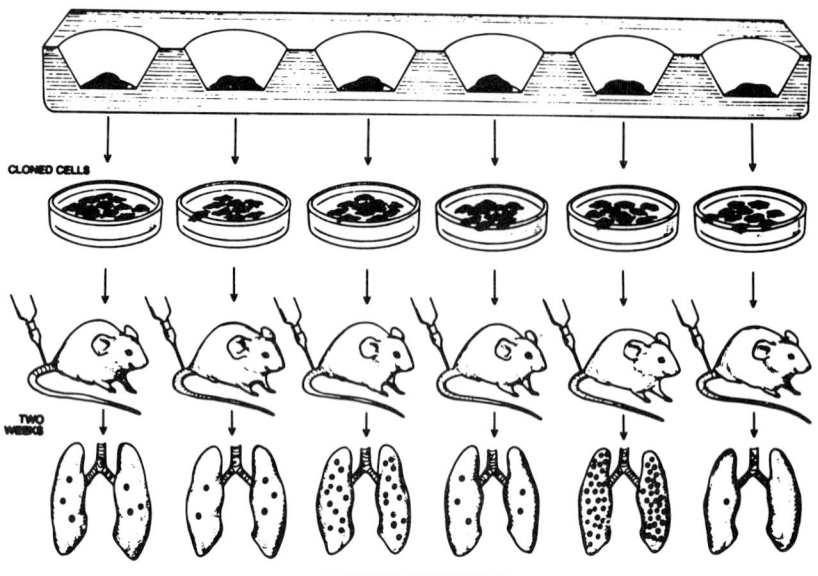

FIGURE 12-11 (Continued from Figure 12-10.)

Definitive evidence for preexisting metastatic subpopulations in primary tumors has been more recently provided by classic experiments, reproduced in Fig. 12-10. In these experiments Fidler and Kripke[143] prepared a cell suspension from a single B-16 primary tumor and divided the cell suspension into two equal aliquots. One part was cloned in soft agar, and 17 different cell lines were isolated. Each of these separate cell lines was then injected intravenously and assayed for the production of metastases in the lungs. The second aliquot was directly injected into tail veins of mice and assayed for pulmonary metastases. As seen in Fig. 12-10, the cell suspension prepared from the primary tumor produced equal numbers of metastases, as was expected. Strikingly, however, the 17 clones isolated from the primary tumor showed vast differences in metastatic capability (Fig. 12-11). These experiments indicated that the parent B-16 tumor is heterogeneous for metastases, and that highly metastatic variants are preexistent in the primary tumor cell population. Kripke and Fidler[144] extended these observations to a newly induced ultraviolet fibrosarcoma, indicating that the observed preexisting heterogeneity for metastases seen in the B-16 melanoma was not the result of its long-term in vitro–in vivo passage since its spontaneous origin in 1954.[144]

Stability of Selected High and Low Metastatic Cell Lines (F-1 and F-10) vs. Clonal Instability of Isolated Subpopulations   As recently reviewed by Fidler and Nicholson[97] and reported by Poste,[140] the in vivo–in vitro selected (or enriched) high (F-10) and low (F-1) metastatic cell lines have retained quantitatively similar metastatic capabilities after many weeks of tissue culture and up to 35 subcutaneous transplantations. Therefore, these selected high and low metastatic cell lines remain stable with regard to their metastatic potential.

Such is not the case, however, for clonal populations of cells separated from the primary tumor, or, importantly, from metastases themselves. In recent studies, Poste et al.[140] showed that individual clones isolated from the B-16 melanoma showed a highly unstable metastatic phenotype and rapidly generated subclones with widely differing metastatic properties. When all clones from the parent population were mixed and cocultivated, this instability could not be identified, suggesting that there is evidence for an "interaction" in polyclonal populations that stabilizes the relative proportion of each of the subpopulations within the population as a whole.

Such a mechanism would be analogous to growth control mechanisms seen in normal organs which are composed of many classes of cells. Similarly, results have been obtained in studies of mouse mammary tumors in which five isolated subpopulations showed a wide range of phenotypic stability.[141,142] A growth interaction in vivo between these clonal subpopulations has also been demonstrated.[146] The interaction pattern in these experiments is complex with a uni- and bidirectional growth regulatory effects and complex cytotoxic drug sensitivities—resistance depending on the clonal mixture being tested. Sugarbaker et al.[145] have shown that there can be transient changes in tumor cell phenotype during the process of metastasis perhaps related to these observations.

EXPERIMENTAL AND THERAPEUTIC IMPLICATIONS OF THE INSTABILITY OF CLONES SEPARATED FROM PRIMARY TUMORS

As indicated by Poste et al.[140] these observations have highly significant implications for continued research and for treatment rationale. First, these data indicate that research focusing on the properties of single clonal populations may indeed be misleading. Rather, biologic interactions of subpopulations of tumor cells is an important aspect of tumor cell heterogeneity and must be considered in interpretation of experimental results.

Secondly, polyclonal interactions maintain the "stability" of that metastatic phenotype. Therapies or other selection pressures (such as chemotherapy or host resistance) that eliminate or reduce a given subpopulation effect a disturbance of this balanced internal milieu of the tumor and promote phenotypic instability. If a therapy such as chemotherapy were also mutagenic, it could theoretically further increase the emergence of new and resistant phenotypes as a result. Reports of major differences in drug sensitivities among cells from primary tumors and metastases[152] seem consistent with this hypothesis. Likewise, UV radiation (which is a mutagenic agent) greatly increased the metastatic potential of isolated clones from a primary fibrosarcoma.[153]

ORIGIN OF HETEROGENEITY IN PRIMARY TUMORS

Thus, significant evidence substantiates the heterogeneity of primary tumor cell populations with regard to metastatic potential. Nowell[154] hypothesized that neoplastic progression occurred because of the selection of mutant variants with increased malignant characteristics. As host selection pressures are applied, perhaps irradicating or diminishing a given population of tumor cells, the resultant mutational instability could result in cells with increased metastatic potential, heightening the malignancy of the tumor.

Host Factors and Modulation of Metastases

HOST IMMUNORESISTANCE/IMMUNOSTIMULATION OF METASTASIS

Many experimental tumor cells (particularly those of carcinogen-induced tumors) have been shown to possess tumor-associated antigens that can elicit host reactions potentially lethal for the offending tumor cells. It is now realized that this original concept of the eradication of foreign tumor cells by an avenging host is much oversimplified.

As reviewed by Balch,[155] the immune system is now known to have many morphologic (and a much greater number of morphologically indistinguishable) functional components with often opposing capabilities that are balanced by a large number of interrelating polypeptides akin to the endocrine system. The basic morphologically identifiable components are the macrophage (including the phagocytic monocyte), the neutrophil, and the lymphocyte. Within the lymphocyte population are antibody-producing cells (B lymphocytes) and thymus-dependent lymphocytes (T lymphocytes). Some lymphocyte cells *suppress* the cytotoxic reactions of other lymphoid populations. These are termed suppressor cells and have been shown to enhance tumor growth. Similarly, in macrophage populations, some cells "eat" other cells, in their confirmed role of scavengers. Others, however, activate or suppress the actions of lymphocytes. Nevertheless, the phylogenetically primitive macrophage can remain "armed" and kill without the delay of sensitization through the afferent arc of the immune system. If into this complex reactive immunologic mechanism is injected a primary tumor—with heterogeneous antigenicities and releasing variable numbers of circulating tumor cells and other subcellular debris—it is little wonder that widely varying results are obtained in experiments using many different model systems and methods.

Some experiments support immune resistance to metastasis. Kim[156] demonstrated that highly immunogenic carcinogen-induced tumors had the least tendency for spontaneous metastasis. Poorly immunogenic or nonimmunogenic tumors had the highest incidence of spontaneous metastasis formation. Additionally, the administration of antilymphocyte serum increased metastasis formation.[157] Similarly, total-body irradiation increased metastatic formation, which could be reversed by administration of nonspecific immunostimulants, such as *Corynebacterium granulosum* or BCG.[158]

Currie and Alexander[159] correlated the metastatic behavior of two methylcholanthrene-induced tumors with their ability to shed soluble tumor-specific transplantation antigen (TSTA) in vitro. One metastasizing sarcoma shed large amounts of TSTA, the other, which did not metastasize, did not shed antigen. In tumors that shed antigen rapidly, little antigen persisted in the tumor plasma membranes so that they were weakly immunogenic tumors. Simultaneously, the large amount of antigen "paralyzed" the immune response, allowing the growth of metastases. They have hypothesized that the rate of antigen shedding is a factor in determining both immunogenicity of the primary tumor and its ability to metastasize.

Data from other experimental tumor systems suggest another mechanism for metastatic spread in the face of active concomitant immunity to the primary tumor. Comparative studies of the antigenicity of primary tumors and metastases using transplantation methods have shown some metastases to be antigenically dissimilar from the primary tumor.[160] Other findings[161] likewise suggest that metastases have an altered antigenicity and may thereby escape activated immune surveillance by the host. Some of these mechanisms are diagrammed in Fig. 12-12.

Many other observations cast considerable doubt on the presence of an effective immune surveillance mechanism in combating metastasis, and, under appropriate conditions, apparent immunostimulation of metastatic growth has been observed. Based on extensive documentation Prehn[162] has hypothesized that, in fact, immunostimulation may occur during a lymphodependent

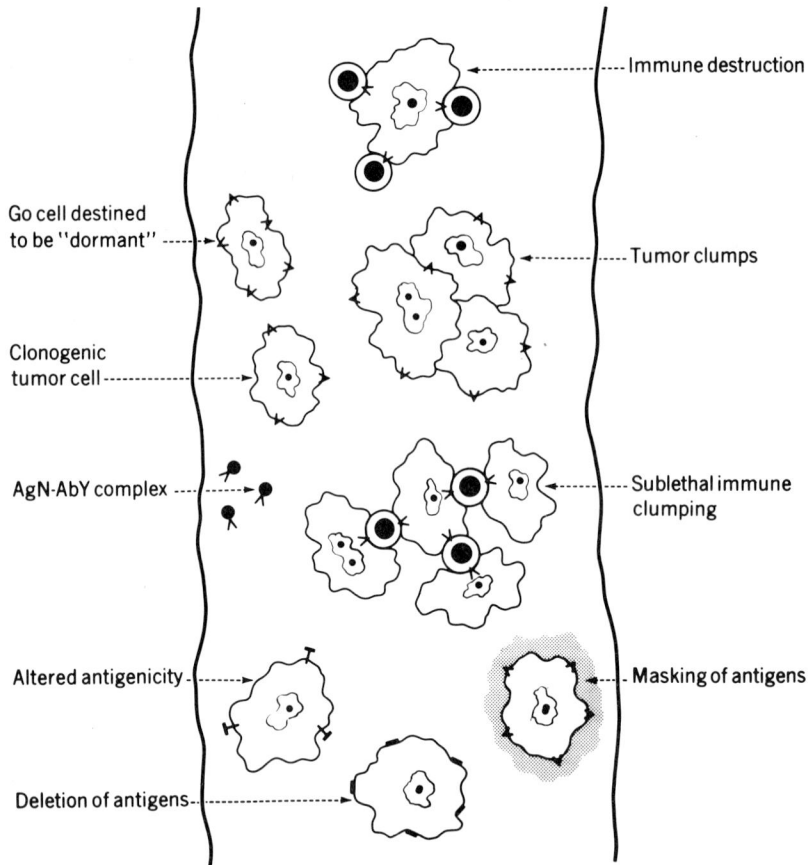

FIGURE 12-12 Immune reactions to tumor cells may take many forms and are prominent during cell circulation. Many hypothetical mechanisms are illustrated.

phase of tumor growth. The dependency of metastasis on immune stimulation by the T-cell lymphocyte is suggested by the dramatic lack of metastasis from aggressive human cancers transplanted into athymic (nude) mice[163,164]; however, other features of the model should also be considered, such as the recently demonstrated presence of large numbers of natural killer (NK) cells.[164] Fewer metastases result when the B-16 melanoma is injected into thymectomized mice.[165] Furthermore, Fidler demonstrated that sublethal clumping of lymphocytes to B-16 melanoma cells increased the metastatic potential of cells injected intravenously. Other immunostimulatory effects on tumor metastasis may be caused by antigen-antibody complexes.[130,166]

NATURAL RESISTANCE AND THE ACTIVATED MACROPHAGE

It is of great interest that vast numbers of tumor cells injected into the bloodstream, or occurring naturally as spontaneous metastasis, rapidly undergo sudden death.[77,167] To the extent that this massive cell destruction is not a spontaneous event due to intrinsic nonviability of cells in the circulation, actively armed host defenses must participate. Since cell-mediated immune destruction of tumors requires 5 to 7 days for even first-set rejection, other killer-cell mechanisms must be involved. Macrophages are activated by a wide variety of environmental stimuli and could accomplish such acute destruction. This surmise is particularly relevant to models using intravenous injection into the pulmonary bed. Alveolar macrophages are thought to be constantly "angry" by virtue of constant interaction with environmental stimuli. Also, macrophages are highly discriminatory, being able to distinguish senescent red cells from young ones. When a large population of cells of foreign epithelial origin reaches the pulmonary bed and lodges there, it is easy to visualize this destruction by the angry yet "discriminating" population of scavenging cells. Some additional support for this concept is found in the fact that appropriately timed macrophage treatments (injections of activated syngeneic macrophages) can protect against metastases after intravenous injection of B-16 melanoma cells,[168] and injection of liposome-packaged macrophage-activating lymphokines can diminish spontaneous metastasis formation.[169] Search for organ-specific or -selective liposomes for the delivery of macrophage-activating substances is vigorously underway.[170]

EFFECT OF THERAPEUTIC MANEUVERS AND HOST INJURY–REPAIR MECHANISM IN METASTASIS

Therapy of clinical malignant tumors can cause increased showers of tumor cells into the circulation just at the time when host injury–repair mechanisms have been maximally activated. Many experimental models have shown that forceful manipulations of the primary tumor increase metastases,[171] although clinical evidence for a definite detrimental effect is equivocal. A question remains concerning the extent to which the trauma of surgery or the immunosuppressive effects of radiation therapy are iatrogenic contributions to cancer metastasis.[172]

Many experiments have shown that the trauma of experimental laparotomy, anesthesia, and acute or chronic tissue injury increase metastasis if a certain amount of manipulation of the model system occurs. As previously discussed, acute tissue injury clearly can localize circulating tumor cells (Fig. 12-13), but the systematic effects are more difficult to demonstrate conclusively. Trauma-induced unilateral activation of the blood coagulation mechanism out of balance with fibrinolytic mechanisms has been implicated as a cause of metastasis.[172]

ENDOCRINE MODULATION OF METASTASIS

The partial retention of the hormone responsiveness of the parent somatic tissue after neoplastic transformation has emphasized the potential of manipulations of the endocrine system in control of metastasis. In experimental and clinical mammary cancer, the presence of estrogen receptor indicates a poorly metastasizing tumor and the possibility of temporarily controlling metastases by ablation of estrogen-producing organs. Metastatically differentiated carcinoma of the thyroid also is often dependent on thyroid-stimulating hormone for growth. Suppression of pituitary TSH by exogenous thyroxine arrests metastatic growth in clinical and experimental models. Prostate cancer can be cited as an additional example.

Metastatic Phenomena Produced by Complex Tumor-Host Interactions

ORGAN REJECTION OR SELECTION OF METASTASIS

It is a confirmed clinical and experimental observation that metastasizing cells prefer some organs over others

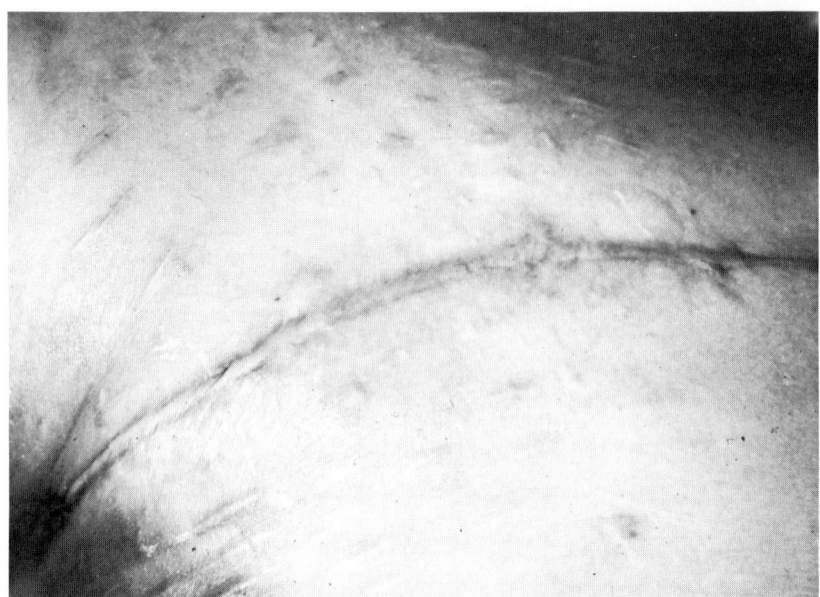

FIGURE 12-13 Localization of metastases at sites of tissue trauma. This woman underwent mastectomy and had positive nodes. Her referring surgeon performed multiple small cutaneous incisions to reduce the tension on the skin closure. Almost all these incisional sites became the sites of cutaneous metastasis. (*Reproduced with permission of EV Sugarbaker: Patterns of metastasis in human malignancies, in J Marchalonis et al (eds): Cancer Biology Reviews, Dekker, New York, 1981.*)

for metastatic growth. The "seed-soil" hypothesis of Paget[173] states that some cancers find certain organs more fertile ground for metastatic growth. This propensity for "homing in" on preferential organs has been demonstrated in the extreme by the organ-specific metastasis from an experimental sarcoma to the lung (in situ) or to small subcutaneous transplants of lung tissue, but to no other organs.[174–176] The strength of this organ preference in some tumor systems is likewise documented by organ-specific metastasis across a parabiotic union.[135,167,175]

Studies using tagged tumor cells [69,77,78] and bioassay techniques [67,68,75] demonstrate that an ubiquitous pattern of distribution of tumor cells coexists with organ-specific growth of metastases. Hart et al. [175,176] recently demonstrated increased *cell arrest* is not necessary for organ-specific metastasis and hypothesized that the presence of complex tumor cell, organ, and host interactions are important in organ-specific metastasis.

A significant question remains as to why certain organs are selected for metastasis and, of equal importance, why most organs that receive viable tumor cells reject them.[177] Little is known about the specific mechanisms involved in organ rejection or selection of metastases. Nicholson and Winkelhake,[92] however, have shown that when pulmonophilic B-16 melanoma cells are suspended with partially purified organ cells, specific aggregation of tumor and lung cells occurs. The affinity of these B-16 melanoma cells for lung organ cells is much greater than aggregation to the liver, kidney, spleen, or red cells, in that order. These data suggest that factors at the tumor cell membrane–organ capillary cell interface are important. This demonstration seems to substantiate the hypothesis of Green and Harvey[67] about the important role of the tumor cell–endothelial cell "bond" in organ selection of metastases. Pilgrim[68] hypothesized that organ specificity could be a remnant of the embryonic phenotypic homing to the cell's site for terminal differentiation. As recently reviewed, some evidence exists for embryologic homing in human malignant melanoma.[177]

Further evidence for the importance of cell surface properties is found in experiments which alter the pattern of distribution of labeled tumor cells with trypsin and neuraminidase.[58,178] Immunologic factors may also affect the pattern of metastasis. Immunosuppression by cortisone of high doses of cyclophosphamide can cause a wider distribution of spontaneous metastatic patterns,[179] and host immunization alters the distribution of labeled tumor cells after intravenous injection.[180]

Nicholson has recently shown that when organ pattern of metastasis is subject to vigorous selective pressures it can be altered to include many other organs.[151] A number of parameters related to the implantation of tumor cells could alone or in combination influence this aspect of metastasis formation. Characteristics of tumor cells themselves and of the organs they enter could both be important. A list of hypothetical tumor cell–organ interactions is seen on Table 12-1.

TUMOR CELL DORMANCY

Metastatic tumor growth may reappear many years after effective and permanent control of the primary tumor. This intriguing characteristic of malignant cell growth implies that poorly proliferating or nonproliferating cells have persisted for long periods of time, existing in symbiosis with the host. Several experimental models for tumor cell dormancy have been described, each emphasizing different possible mechanisms for stimulating resurgent growth of dormant cells. No data, however, pertain clearly to the anatomic location, kinetic status, or other aspects of this intriguing type of metastasizing cell. The clinical importance of "dormant" cells is demonstrated by the late time course of distant metastasis sometimes seen in patients with hypernephroma, malignant melanoma, and carcinoma of the breast.

Fisher et al.[181] and Sugarbaker et al.[182] have shown that trauma can cause growth of dormant Walker 256 cancer cells in the liver. Growth-stimulating factors from regenerating liver or traumatic dislodgement of these intravascular cells to an extrasinusoidal position are possible explanations for the findings in this model.

TABLE 12-1 Hypothetical Mechanisms for Tumor-Organ Interactions in Metastasis *

Mechanism	Tumor cell characteristics	Variable organ characteristics
Enzyme digestion	Plasmirogen activator Collagenase type IV	Basement membrane exposure/characteristics/collagen IV Fibronectin characteristics
Blood coagulation	↑ Thromboplastic properties ↑ Adherence of platelets	"Gaps" in endothelium (size/frequency/endothelial cell renewal rate) Endothelial fibrinolytic capacity Endothelial cell retractility

Mechanical cell arrest	↑ Clump formation
	   Tumor cell/tumor cell
	   Tumor cell/platelet
	   Tumor cell/lymphocytes
	Cell rigidity or deformability
		Arteriolar diameter
		Flexibility of capillary diameter
		
		Capillary vasoactivity

Embryologic homing	Residual of normal somatic cell property Cell surface receptor	Determined embryologically Organ cell receptors
Tumor immune stimulation or resistance	↑↓ Antigenicity ↑ Detachability ↓ Clonogeneity of cells	Organ-variable tumor immunity
Tumor cell kinetics	↑ Growth rate when arrested	Organ site-specific growth rates
Tumor cell–capillary cell "bond"	↑ Stickiness to organ cells Cell membrane characteristics ↑ Mobility of cell membrane components	Type of endothelial cell Cell surface characteristics

* ↑ = increased; ↓ = decreased; ↑↓ = variable data have been published.

Eccles and Alexander[183] have demonstrated dormant pulmonary metastases on rats. Nevertheless, when these rats were immunosuppressed by whole-body irradiation or by thoracic duct lymph drainage, macroscopic metastases developed. These experiments suggest possible immunologically mediated restraint of dormant tumor metastases. In an estrogen-dependent experimental tumor system, Noble and Hoover[184] have achieved estrogen stimulation of dormant cells after 10 months of dormancy. Dormancy has also been shown to characterize some micrometastases which were isolated from tumor angiogenesis factor.[116] Intuitively, one assumes that these dormant cells are in a nonproliferating (G_0) state. Nevertheless, a controlled balance between cell proliferation and cell destruction may just as possibly be maintained by host defenses. Events that tip this hypothetical balance in favor of the dormant cells would cause the appearance of gross metastases at delayed intervals.

SELECTION OF A METASTASIS: A DECATHLON WINNER IN NEOPLASTIC PROGRESSION

As we reexamine the model of metastases, it is clear that many tumor cell characteristics (Table 12-2); primary tumor characteristics, host characteristics, and complex tumor-host interactions all interact with a tumor cell attempting to run the gauntlet to become a successful metastasis. As noted, the primary tumor cell population is heterogeneous, and a sequence of events, each requiring special cell attributes, must be accomplished before a metastasis is formed. Does the development of a metastasis reflect a selection process, or are metastases a random, arbitrary choice of some cells for metastasis? If a selection process occurs, which of these many host, tumor, and/or cellular parameters are important determinants?

Teleologically it can be reasoned that the living cancer cell possesses the basic drive for survival. This might be accomplished by its acquisition of special properties or by favorable modulation of environment by tumor-host factors for growth of a cell. For selection to be an important mechanism in metastasis, the environment for the cancer cell must challenge it and the cancer cell population must be heterogeneous. This means that cells with the special properties required for metastasis are actually present. Since many more cells enter the circulation than form metastases, the developing metastasis seems analogous to a clone developing in tissue culture, and may manifest only selected characteristics appropriate to the dynamic status of the tumor-host environment. Immunologic, metabolic, genetic, and kinetic selection pressures may singly or in combination influence this process. The definitive demonstration of heterogeneity in tumor cell populations indicates that the metastatic cell may be analogous to the clonal selection of mutant subpopulations derived from a common progenitor for neoplastic progression.[154] The poor prognosis associated with recurrent tumors, even when clinically localized, may relate to such selection of "super cells" for metastasis or recurrence. The cells that survive in a hostile environment may need to possess a combination of the cell characteristics listed in Table 12-2. Therefore, much like a decathlon winner in an athletic contest, a surviving tumor cell has to perform well in more than one event. Since zonal heterogeneity has also been demonstrated in primary tumors,[150] cell clumps from an appropriate zone could also have the special characteristics needed to facilitate the metastatic process. Moreover, if the tumor-host environment is modulated to such a degree that host conditions become highly favorable to metastasis from cells released in the circulation, selection would not seem important. The complete collapse of all mechanisms for host resistance with the terminal phase of cancer dissemination could be an example of metastasis enhanced by such modulation.

TABLE 12-2 Cell Characteristics Favoring Metastasis *

? Anaerobic metabolism
↑ Detachability
↑ Kinetics (rate of cell division)
↑ Lytic enzyme production/collagenase IV
↑ Translocational capabilities
↑ Cell rigidity, deformability
↑ Stickiness (to platelets, endothelium)
↑ Mobility of membrane components
↑ Cell size
↑ Clump formation (adherence)
↑ Thromboplastin, plasminogen activator
↑ Ploidy (hyperdiploid, aneuploid)
↑↓ Antigenicity
↑ Glycoprotein coating
↓ Hormone responsiveness
↑ Production of tumor angiogenesis factor
? Biochemical factors membrane

* ↑ = increased; ↓ = decreased

CONCLUSIONS AND THERAPEUTIC IMPLICATIONS OF EXPERIMENTAL STUDIES IN METASTASIS

As has been reviewed, the process of metastasis is a complex, multifaceted event involving tumor characteristics, host characteristics, and a complex, interrelated tumor-host modulation, over a prolonged period of time, particularly as observed in human beings. Certain practical aspects of this event with therapeutic implications, however, should be emphasized.

First, as observed in humans, metastases, if present, have occurred at the time the diagnosis is made. Therefore, therapeutic experimental models should focus on the eradication of established micrometastatic disease with emphasis on treating varying tumor burdens between 10^2 and 10^9 cells in each possible metastatic focus, as in this range they are beneath the current resolution of diagnostic methods.

Secondly, the current state of the art is insufficient in its ability to accurately diagnose the presence of metastatic disease. The currently available scanning and radiographic techniques are fraught with considerable error. Hopefully, monoclonal antibody techniques and immunoimaging will help to ameliorate this current deficiency.

Thirdly, the risk of a given patient for metastatic disease can only be predicted with a statistical probability. Since medicine is practiced one-on-one, individualized treatment decisions must be made, and population statistics are often insufficient as applied to the individual patient. This major deficiency in the current state of the art creates many clinical dilemmas and controversies regarding appropriate treatment of individual patients. The young nude mouse model for metastasis reported by Hanna and Fidler[164] may help with more appropriate individualized predictions of metastatic potential for human malignancies.

Fourthly, currently available adjuvant therapies used in addition to primary tumor eradication are, in general, inadequate. Better adjuvant therapies must be devised.

Fifthly, as discussed, the fact that tumors are heterogeneous for metastasis formation has emphasized the need for studies directed toward this small but critical metastatic subpopulation of cells within many primary tumors. Such studies of the metastatic subpopulation could be more fruitful in defining more appropriate and specific adjuvant therapies for the eradication of metastatic disease. Indeed, it is possible that all drug screening procedures should focus specifically on these critical subpopulations of cells which cause the deaths of many patients. It is hoped that continued laboratory research in models relevant to the clinical problem of metastasis, as well as careful study of human tumor specimens, will continue to improve therapies for this most extreme expression of the malignant cell phenotype.

REFERENCES

1. Wilder RJ: The historical development of the concept of metastasis. *J Mt Sinai Hosp NY* 23:728, 1956.
2. Virchow R: *Cellular Pathology,* F Chance (trans), Lippincott, Philadelphia, 1863, p 219.
3. Paget J: *Lectures on Surgical Pathology* Longman, Brown, Green and Longmans, London, 1863, p 580.
4. Langenbeck A: On the development of cancer in the veins, and the transmission of cancer from man to the lower animals. *Edinburgh Med Surg J* 55:251, 1841.
5. Hoggan G: On cancer and its relationship to the lymphatic vessels. *Trans Pathol Soc Lond* 29:384, 1878.
6. Von Recklinghausen F: *Virchows Arch Pathol Anat* 100:503, 1885.
7. Onuigbo WIB: A history of hematogenous metastasis. *Cancer Res* 30:2821, 1970.
8. Moore H: On the influence of inadequate operations on the theory of cancer. *R Med Chir Soc London* 1:245, 1867.
9. Handley WS: The Hunterian lectures on the pathology of melanotic growths in relation to their operative treatment. *Lancet* 1:927, 1907.
10. Handley WS: *Cancer of the Breast.* Murray, London, 1906.
11. Sappey MPC: *Anatomie, Physiologie, Pathologie des Vaisseaux Lymphatiques.* DeLayaye, Lacrosnier, Paris, 1874.
12. Halstead WS: The results of operations for the cure of cancer of the breast performed at the Johns Hopkins Hospital from June 1889 to January 1894. *Johns Hopkins Hosp Rep* 4:297, 1894.
13. Pringle JH: A method of operation in cases of melanotic tumors of the skin. *Edinburgh Med J* 23:496, 1908.
14. Miles W: Abdominoperineal operation. *Cancer* 2:1812, 1908.
15. Crile G: Excision of cancer of the head and neck with special reference to plan of dissection based on 132 operations. *JAMA* 57:1780, 1906.
16. Whipple AO et al: Treatment of carcinoma of the ampulla of Vater. *Ann Surg* 102:763, 1935.
17. McNeer G et al: A more thorough operation for gastric cancer: Anatomical basis and description of technique. *Cancer* 4:957, 1951.
18. Wangensteen OH et al: The extended or super-radical mastectomy for carcinoma of the breast. *Surg Clin North Am* 36:1051, 1956.

19. Goldman LI et al: Immune surveillance and tumor dissemination: In vitro comparison of the B16 melanoma in primary and metastatic form. *Surgery* 76:50, 1974.
20. Levin I: The mechanisms of metastasis formation in experimental cancer. *J Exp Med* 18:397, 1913.
21. Takahashi M: An experimental study of metastasis. *J Pathol Bacteriol* 20:1, 1915.
22. Tyzzer EE: Factors in the production and growth of tumor metastases. *J Med Res* 28:309, 1913.
23. Warren S, Gates O: The fate of intravenously infected tumor cells. *Am J Cancer* 27:485, 1936.
24. Warren BA: The vascular morphology of tumors, in HI Peterson (ed): *Tumor Blood Circulation: Angiogenesis, Vascular Morphology, and Blood Flow of Experimental and Human Tumors*, CRC Press, West Palm Beach, Fla, 1979, chap 1.
25. Warren BA et al: Metastasis via the blood stream: The method of intravasation of tumor cells in a transplantable melanoma of the hamster. *Cancer Lett* 4:245–251, 1978.
26. Warren BA, Shubik, P: The growth of the blood supply to melanoma transplants in the hamster cheek pouch. *Lab Invest* 15:464, 1966.
27. Weiss L: Tumor necrosis and cell detachment. *Int J Cancer* 20:87–92, 1977.
28. Poste, G: The cell surface and metastasis, in SB Day (ed): *Cancer Invasion and Metastases: Biologic Mechanisms and Therapy*, Raven Press, New York, 1977, p 19.
29. Fidler IJ: The relationship of embolic homogeneity, number, size and viability to the incidence of experimental metastasis. *Eur J Cancer* 9:223, 1973.
30. Young JS et al: The significance of the "tissue pressure" of normal testicular and of neoplastic (Brown-Pearce carcinoma) tissue in the rabbit. *J Pathol Bacteriol* 62:313–333, 1950.
31. Butler TP, Gullino PM: Bulk transfer of fluid in the interstitial compartment of mammary tumors. *Cancer Res* 35:3084, 1975.
32. Tannock IF, Steele GG: Quantitative techniques for the study of the anatomy and function of small blood vessels in tumors. *J Nat Cancer Inst* 42:771, 1969.
33. Easty DM, Easty, GC: Measurement of the ability of cells to infiltrate normal tissues in vitro. *Br J Cancer*, 29:36–49, 1974.
34. Eaves G: The invasive growth of malignant tumors as a purely mechanical process. *J Pathol* 109:233–237, 1973.
35. Franks LM: Structure and biological malignancy of tumors, in S Garattin, G Franchi (eds): *Chemotherapy of Cancer Dissemination and Metastasis*, Raven Press, NY, 1973, pp 71–78.
36. Gullino PM: In vivo release of neoplastic cells by mammary tumors. *Gann* 20:49, 1977.
37. Lunscken C, Strauli P: Penetration of an ascitic reticulum cell sarcoma of the golden hamster into the body wall and through the diaphragm. *Virchows Arch Cell Pathol* 34:997, 1974.
38. Swabb EA et al: Diffusion and convection in normal and neoplastic tissues. *Cancer Res* 34:2814, 1974.
39. Griffiths JD et al: Carcinoma of the colon and rectum: Circulating malignant cells and 5-year survival. *Cancer* 31:226, 1973.
40. Noguchi PD et al: Chick embryonic skin as a rapid organ culture assay for cellular neoplasia. *Science* 199:980–983, 1978.
41. Strauli P: The barrier function of lymph nodes, in F Saegesser, J Petavel (eds): *Surgical Oncology*, Williams Wilkins, Baltimore, 1970, p 161.
42. Felix H, Strauli P: Different distribution pattern of 100-A filaments resting and locomotive leukemia cells. *Nature* 261:604, 1976.
43. Dingemans KP et al: Invasion of liver tissue by tumor cells and leukocytes: Comparative ultrastructure. *J Nat Cancer Inst* 60:583–598, 1978.
44. Hart IR: Mechanisms of tumor cell invasion, in JJ Marchalonis et al (eds): *Cancer Biology Reviews*, vol 2, Dekker, New York, 1981, pp 29–58.
45. Sylven B: Biochemical factors accompanying growth and invasion, in RW Wissler et al (eds): *Endogenous Factors Influencing Host-Tumor Balance*, University of Chicago Press, Chicago, 1976, p 267.
46. Sylven B: Lysosomal enzyme activity in the interstitial fluid of solid mouse tumour transplants. *Eur J Cancer* 4:463, 1968.
47. Dresden MH et al: Collagenolytic enzymes in human neoplasms. *Cancer Res* 32:993, 1972.
48. Yamanishi Y et al: Collagenolytic activity in malignant melanoma: Physiochemical studies, *Cancer Res* 33:2507, 1973.
49. Liotta LA et al: Preferential digestion of basement membrane collagen by an enzyme derived from a metastatic murine tumor. *Proc Nat Acad Sci USA* 76:2268–2272, 1979.
50. Liotta LA et al: Metastatic potential correlates with enzymatic degradation of basement membrane collagen. *Nature* 284:67–68, 1980.
51. Kleinerman J, Liotta L: Release of tumor cells, in S Day (ed): *Progress in Cancer Research and Therapy*, Raven Press, New York, p 135.
52. Wood S Jr: Experimental studies of the intravascular dissemination of ascitic V2 carcinoma cells in the rabbit, with special reference to fibrinogen and fibrinolytic agents. *Bull Schwiez Akad Med Wiss* 20:92, 1964.
53. Zetter BR et al: The isolation of vascular endothelial cell lines with altered cell surface and platelet-binding properties. *Cell* 14: 501–509, 1978.
54. Wang BS et al: Correlation of the production of plasminogen activator with tumor metastasis in B16 mouse melanoma cell lines. *Cancer Res* 40:288–292, 1980.
55. Coman DR: Decreased mutual adhesiveness, a property of cells from squamous cell carcinomas. *Cancer Res* 4:625, 1944.

56. Weiss L: Cell detachment and metastasis, in PG Stansly, H Sato (eds): *Cancer Metastasis, Approaches to the Mechanism, Prevention, and Treatment,* University of Tokyo Press, Tokyo, 1977, p 25.
57. Weiss L: Studies on cellular adhesion in tissue culture, VII: Surface activity and cell detachment. *Exp Cell Res* 33:277, 1964.
58. Weiss L et al: The influence of host immunity on the arrest of circulating cancer cells, and its modification by neuraminidase. *Int J Cancer,* 13:850, 1974.
59. Poste G: Sub-lethal autolysis: Modification of the cell periphery by lysosomal enzymes. *Exp Cell Res* 67:11–16, 1971.
60. Weiss L: Tumor necrosis and cell detachment. *Int J Cancer* 20:87–92, 1977.
61. Weiss L, Holyoke D: Some effects of hypervitaminosis A on metastasis of spontaneous breast cancer in mice. *J Nat Cancer Inst* 43:1045–1054, 1969.
62. Yamada KM, Olden K: Fibronectins Adhesive glycoproteins of cell surface and blood. *Nature* 275:179–184, 1978.
63. Steele GG: The cell cycle in tumours: An examination of data gained by the technique of labelled mitoses. *Cell Tissue Kinet* 5:87, 1972.
64. Butler, TP, Gullino, PM: Quantitation of cell shedding into efferent blood of mammary adenocarcinoma. *Cancer Res* 35:512, 1975.
65. Liotta LA et al: Quantitative relationships of intravascular tumor cells, tumor vessels and pulmonary metastases following tumor implantation. *Cancer Res* 34:997–1004, 1974.
66. Liotta LA et al: The significance of hematogenous tumor cell clumps in the metastatic process. *Cancer Res* 36:889–894, 1976.
67. Greene HSN, Harvey EK: The relationship between the dissemination of tumor cells and the distribution of metastases. *Cancer Res* 24:799, 1964.
68. Pilgrim HI: The metastatic behavior of a splenotropic reticulum cell sarcoma in splenectomized mice. *Proc Soc Exp Biol Med* 138:178, 1971.
69. Hewitt HB, Blake E: Quantitative studies of translymphoidal passage of tumour cells naturally disseminated from a nonimmunogenic murine squamous carcinoma. *Br J Cancer* 31:25, 1975.
70. Goldblatt SA, Nadel EM: Cancer cells in the circulating blood: A critical review, II. *Acta Cytol.* 9:6–20, 1965.
71. Salsbury AJ: The significance of the circulating cancer cell. *Cancer Treat Rev* 2:55, 1975.
72. Golinger RC et al.: Tumor cells in venous blood draining mammary carcinomas. *Arch Surg* 112:707, 1977.
73. Sato K, Marchetta FA: Radioautography of in vitro labeled tumor cells in postoperative wound drainage. *Cancer* 19:735, 1966.
74. Gerson JM et al.: Isolation and characterization of a neuroblastoma cell line from peripheral blood in a patient with disseminated disease. *Cancer* 29:2508, 1977.
75. Parks RC: Increased tumor metastasis after in vitro alteration of the cell surface. *J Nat Cancer Inst* 54:1473, 1975.
76. Baserga R et al: The dose-response relationship between the number of embolic tumor cells and the incidence of blood-borne metastases. *Br J Cancer* 24:173, 1960.
77. Fidler IJ: Metastasis: Quantitative analysis of distribution and fate of tumor emboli labeled with ^{125}I-5-iodo-2'-deoxyuridine. *J Nat Cancer Inst* 45:775, 1970.
78. Brown JM: A study of the mechanism by which anticoagulation with warfarin inhibits blood-borne metastases. *Cancer Res* 33:1217, 1973.
79. Glaves D, Weiss L: Early arrest of circulating tumor cells in tumor-bearing mice, in SB Day et al (eds): *Cancer Invasion and Metastasis: Biologic Mechanisms and Therapy,* Raven Press, New York, 1977, p 175.
80. Proctor JW, et al: The distribution and fate of blood-borne IUdR-labelled tumor cells in immune syngeneic rats. *Int J Cancer* 18:255–262, 1976.
81. Fidler IJ: Patterns of tumor cell arrest and development. L Weiss (ed): in *Fundamental Aspects of Metastasis,* North-Holland, Amsterdam, 1976, pp 275–290.
82. Proctor JW: Rat sarcoma mode supports both "soil seed" and "mechanical" theories of metastatic spread. *Br J Cancer* 34:651, 1976.
83. Sato H, Suzuki M: Experimental studies on metastasis formation, microcirculation, in T Shimamoto et al (eds): *Atherogenesis, II: Thrombogenesis and Pyridinol-Carbamate Treatment, Proc 2d Int Symp Atherogenesis, Tokyo,* Excerpta Medica, Amsterdam, 1972), p 168.
84. Coman DR: Mechanisms responsible for the origin and distribution of blood-borne tumor metastases—A review. *Cancer Res* 13:397, 1953.
85. Poste G, Fidler IJ: The pathogenesis of cancer metastasis. *Nature* 283:139–146, 1980.
86. Poste G, Nicholson GL: Arrest and metastasis of bloodbourne tumor cells are modified by fusion of plasma membrane vesicles from highly metastatic cells. *Proc Nat Acad Sci USA* 77:399–403, 1980.
87. Zeidman I: The fate of circulating tumor cells, I: Passage of cell through capillaries. *Cancer Res* 21:38, 1961.
88. Sato H, Suzuki M: Deformability and viability of tumor cells by transcapillary passage with reference to organ affinity of metastasis in cancer, in L Weiss (ed): *Fundamental Aspects of Metastasis,* North-Holland, Amsterdam, 1976, p 311.
89. Sato H et al: Deformability and filterability of tumor cells through "nucleopore" filter, with reference to viability and metastatic spread, in PG Stansly, H Sato (eds): *Cancer Metastasis: Approaches to the Mechanism, Prevention, and Treatment,* University of Tokyo Press, Tokyo, 1977, p 53.
90. Weiss L: Cell deformability: Some general considerations, in L Weiss (ed): *Fundamental Aspects of Metastasis,* North-Holland, New York, 1976, p 305.

91. Kojima K, Sakai I: On the role of stickiness of tumor cells in the formation of metastases. *Cancer Res* 24:1887, 1964.
92. Nicholson GL, Winkelhake JL: Organ specificity of blood-borne tumour metastasis determined by cell adhesion. *Nature* 255:230, 1975.
93. Winkelhake JL, Nicholson GL: Determination of adhesive properties of variant metastatic melanoma cells to BLAB/3T3 cells and their virus-transformed derivatives by a monolayer attachment assay. *J Nat Cancer Inst* 56:285, 1976.
94. Hagmar B, Ryd W: Tumor cell locomotion—A factor in metastasis formation? Influence of cytochalasin B on a tumor dissemination pattern. *Int J Cancer,* 19:576, 1977.
95. Purdom L, Ambrose EJ: A correlation between electrical surface charge and some biological characteristics during the stepwise progression of a mouse sarcoma. *Nature* 181:1586, 1958.
96. Gasic GJ et al: Platelet-tumor cell interaction in mice: The role of platelets in the spread of malignant disease. *Int J Cancer* 11:704, 1973.
97. Fidler IJ, Nicholson GL: Immunobiology of experimental metastatic melanoma, in JJ Marchalonis et al (eds): *Cancer Biology Reviews,* vol 2, Dekker, New York, 1981, pp 171–234.
98. Raz a et al: Cell surface properties of B16 melanoma variants with differing metastatic potential. *Cancer Res* 40:1645–1651, 1980.
99. Nakamura K et al: Electron-microscopic studies on extravasation or tumor cells and early foci of hematogeneous metastases, in PG Stansly, H Sato (eds): *Cancer Metastasis: Approaches to the Mechanism, Prevention, and Treatment,* University of Tokyo Press, Tokyo, 1977, p 57.
100. Dingemans KP: Invasion of liver tissue by blood-borne mammary carcinoma cells. *J Nat Cancer Inst* 53:1813, 1974.
101. Warren BA, Vales O: The adhesion of thromboplastic tumour emboli to vessel walls in vivo. *Br J Exp Pathol* 53:301, 1972.
102. Sindelar WF et al: Electron microscopic observations on formation of pulmonary metastases. *J Surg Res* 18:137, 1975.
103. Hart IR: The selection and characterization of an invasive variant of the B15 melanoma. *Am J Pathol* 97:587–600, 1979.
104. Poste G et al: In vitro selection of murine B16 melanoma variants with enhanced tissue invasive properties. *Cancer Res* 40:1636–1644, 1980.
105. De Ridder L et al: Adhesion of malignant and nonmalignant cells to cultured embryonic substrates. *Cancer Res* 35:3167, 1975.
106. Majno G et al: Endothelial contraction induced by histamine-type mediators. *J Cell Biol* 42:646, 1969.
107. Warren BA: Environment of the blood-borne tumor embolus adherent to vessel wall. *J Med* 4:150, 1973.
108. Buck RC: Walker 256 tumor implantation in normal and injured peritoneum studied by electron microscopy, scanning electron microscopy, and autoradiography. *Cancer Res* 33:3181, 1973.
109. Agostino D, Clifton EE: Trauma as a cause of localization of blood-borne metastases: Preventive effect of heparin and fibrinolysin. *Ann Surg* 161:97, 1965.
110. Alexander JW, Altermeier WA: Susceptibility of injured tissues to hematogenous metastases: An experimental study. *Ann Surg* 159:933, 1964.
111. Ketcham AS et al: Clotting factors and metastasis formation. *Am J Roengenol* 111:42, 1971.
112. Jagelman DG: Inhibition of experimental metastases by defibrination. *Ann R Coll Surg Engl* 54:271, 1974.
113. Gasic GJ et al: Antimetastatic effect of aspirin. *Lancet* 2:932, 1972.
114. Gastpar H: Platelet-cancer cell interaction in metastasis formation: A possible therapeutic approach to metastasis prophylaxis. *J Med* 8:103, 1977.
115. Tanaka K et al: Tumor metastasis and thrombosis, with special reference to thromboplastic and fibrinolytic activities of tumor cells, in PG Stansly, H Sato (eds): *Cancer Metastasis: Approaches to the Mechanism, Prevention, and Treatment,* University of Tokyo Press, Tokyo, 1977, p 97.
116. Folkman J: Tumor angiogenesis: A possible control point in tumor growth. *Ann Int Med* 82:96–100, 1975.
117. Gospodarowicz D et al: Factors involved in the modulation of cell proliferation in vivo and in vitro: The role of fibroblast and epidermal growth factors in the proliferative response of mammalian cells. *In Vitro* 14:85–118, 1978.
118. Schabel FM Jr: Concepts for systemic treatment of micrometastases. *Cancer* 35:15, 1975.
119. Simpson-Herren L et al: Further studies of the population kinetics of primary and metastatic Lewis lung carcinoma in BDF mice. *Proc Am Assoc Cancer Res* 14:27, 1973.
120. Carr I et al: The fine structure of neoplastic invasion: Invasion of liver, skeletal muscle and lymphatic vessels by the Rd/3 tumour. *J Pathol* 118:91, 1976.
121. Freedman H (ed): *The Reticuloendothelial System in Health and Disease,* Plenum Press, New York, 1976, p 319.
122. Ludwig J, Titus JL: Experimental tumor cell emboli in lymph nodes. *Arch Pathol* 84:304, 1967.
123. Zeidmen I, Buss JM: Experimental studies on the spread of cancer in the lymphatic system. *Cancer Res* 14:402, 1954.
124. Strauli P: The barrier function of lymph nodes, in F Saegesser, J Petavel (eds): *Surgical Oncology,* Williams & Wilkins, Baltimore, 1970, p 161.
125. Fisher B, Fisher ER: Barrier function of lymph node to tumor cells and erythrocytes. *Cancer* 20:1907, 1967.
126. Madden RE, Gyure L: Translymphonodal passage of tumor cells. *Oncology* 22:281, 1968.
126a. Sugarbaker EV: Cancer metastasis: A product of tumor-host interactions, in RC Hickey et al (eds): *Current Problems in Cancer,* Year Book, Chicago, 1979, p 7.
127. Revesz L: Development of tumors from inocula containing

a mixed population of viable and lethally damaged tumor cells. *Acta Uni Int Cancer,* 15:893, 1959.
128. Dewys WD: Studies correlating the growth rate of a tumor and its metastases and providing evidence for tumor-related systemic growth-retarding factors. *Cancer Res* 32:374, 1972.
129. Temple WJ et al: The effect of tumor-associated antigen on spontaneous metastasis and concomitant immunity (in preparation).
130. Vaage J: Humoral and cellular immune factors in the systemic control of artificially induced metastases in C3Hf mice. *Cancer Res* 33:1957, 1973.
131. Sugarbaker EV et al: Inhibitory effect of a primary tumor on metastasis, in SB Day, et al (eds): *Cancer Invasion and Metastasis: Biologic Mechanisms and Therapy,* Raven Press, New York, 1977, p 227.
132. Schatten WE: An experimental study of postoperative tumor metastases. *Cancer* 11:455, 1958.
133. Ketcham AS et al: The development of spontaneous metastases after the removal of a primary tumor. *Cancer* 14:875, 1961.
134. Simpson-Herren L et al: Kinetics of metastases in experimental tumors, in SB Day, et al (eds): *Cancer Invasion and Metastasis: Biologic Mechanisms and Therapy,* Raven Press, New York, 1977, p 117.
135. Glucksmann A: The relation of radiosensitivity and radiocurability to the histology of tumor tissue. *Br J Radiol* 21:559, 1948.
136. Suzuki N et al: Cell cycle dependency of metastatic lung colony formation. *Cancer Res* 37:3690, 1977.
137. Tannock IF: The relation between cell proliferation and the vascular system in a transplanted mouse mammary tumor. *Br J Cancer* 22:258, 1968.
138. Thomlinson RH, Gray LH: The histological structure of some human lung cancers and the possible implications for radiotherapy. *Br J Cancer* 9:538, 1955.
139. Goldacre RJ, Sylven B: On the access of blood-borne dyes to various tumor regions. *Br J Cancer* 16:306, 1962.
140. Poste G et al: Interactions between clonal subpopulations affect the stability of the metastatic phenotype in polyclonal populations of B16 melanoma cells (cancer/cellular interactions/phenotypic regulation/growth control), *Proceedings of the National Academy of Science* 78:6226–6230, 1981.
141. Hager JC et al: Epithelial characteristics of five subpopulations of a heterogeneous strain BALB/cfC$_3$H mouse mammary tumor. *Cancer Res* 41: May 1981.
142. Miller BE et al: Growth interaction in vivo between tumor subpopulations derived from a single mouse mammary tumor. *Cancer Res* 40:3977–3981, November 1980.
143. Fidler IJ, Kripke ML: Metastasis resulting from preexisting variant cells within a malignant tumor. *Science* 197:893, 1977.
144. Kripke IJ et al: Heterogeneity of metastatic potential in cells from a murine UV-induced fibrosarcoma. *Proc Am Assoc Cancer Res* 19:213, 1978.
145. Sugarbaker EV et al: Transient changes in tumor-cell characteristics during spontaneous pulmonary metastasis formation. *Surg Forum* 30:134–136, 1979.
146. Vindelov LL et al: Clonal heterogeneity of small-cell anaplastic carcinoma of the lung demonstrated by flow-cytometric DNA analysis. *Cancer Res* 40:4295–4300, November 1980.
147. Brattain MG et al: Heterogeneity of malignant cells from a human colonic carcinoma. *Cancer Res* 41:1751–1756, May 1981.
148. Rosen PP et al: Estrogen receptor protein (ERP) in multiple tumor specimens from individual patients with breast cancer. *Cancer* 39:2194, 1977.
149. Beaven MA et al: Variable content of histaminase, L-dopa decarboxylase and calcitonin in small-cell carcinoma of the lung. *N Engl J Med* 299:105, 1978.
150. Fidler IJ, Hart IR: Biological and experimental consequences of the zonal composition of solid tumors. *Cancer Res* 41:3266–3267, August 1981.
151. Nicholson GL et al: An approach to studying the cellular properties associated with metastases: Some in vitro properties of tumor variants selected in vivo for enhanced metastasis, in L Weiss (ed): *Fundamental Aspects of Metastasis,* North-Holland, Amsterdam, 1976, p 291.
152. Tsuruo T, Fidler IJ: Differences in drug sensitivity among tumor cells from parental tumors, selected variants, and spontaneous metastases. *Cancer Res* 41:3058–3064, August 1981.
153. Fisher MS, Cifone MA: Enhanced metastatic potential of murine fibrosarcomas treated in vitro with ultraviolet radiation. *Cancer Res* 41:3018–2023, August 1981.
154. Nowell PC: The clonal evolution of tumor cell populations. *Science* 194:23, 1976.
155. Balch CM: Recent advances in human cellular immunobiology, in RL Simmons (ed): *Surgical Aspects of Immunology,* Saunders, Philadelphia, (in press).
156. Kim U: Metastasizing mammary carcinomas in rats: Induction and study of their immunogenicity. *Science* 167:72, 1970.
157. James SE, Salsbury AJ: Facilitation of metastasis by antithymocyte globulin. *Cancer Res* 34:357, 1974.
158. Milas, L et al: *Corynebacterium granulosum*–induced protection against artificial pulmonary metastases of a syngeneic fibrosarcoma in mice. *Cancer Res* 34:613, 1971.
159. Currie GA, Alexander P: Spontaneous shedding of TSTA by viable sarcoma cells: Its possible role in facilitating metastatic spread. *Br J Cancer* 29:72, 1974.
160. Sugarbaker EV, Cohen AM: Altered antigenicity in spontaneous pulmonary metastases from an antigenic murine sarcoma. *Surgery* 72:155, 1972.
161. Goldman LI et al: Immune surveillance and tumor dis-

semination: In vitro comparison of the B15 melanoma in primary and metastatic form. *Surgery* 76:50, 1974.
162. Prehn RT: Immunostimulation of the lymphodependent phase of neoplastic growth. *J Nat Cancer Inst* 59:1043, 1977.
163. Maguire H et al: Brief communication: Invasion and metastasis of a xenogeneic tumor in nude mice. *J Nat Cancer Inst* 57:439, 1976.
164. Hanna N, Fidler IJ: Expression of metastatic potential of allogeneic and xenogeneic neoplasms in young nude mice. *Cancer Res* 41:438–444, 1981.
165. Fidler IJ: Immune stimulation-inhibition of experimental cancer metastasis. *Cancer Res* 34:491, 1974.
166. Vaage J: Host serum factors in immune resistance to metastases, in SB Day et al (eds): *Biologic Mechanisms and Therapy,* Raven Press, New York, 1977, p 305.
167. Fidler IJ, Nicholson, GL: Fate of recirculating B16 melanoma metastatic variant cells in parabiotic syngeneic recipients. *J Nat Cancer Inst* 58:1867, 1977.
168. Fidler IJ: Inhibition of pulmonary metastasis by intravenous injection of specifically activated macrophages. *Cancer Res* 34:1074, 1974.
169. Fidler IJ: Therapy of spontaneous metastases by intravenous injection of liposomes containing lymphokines. *Science* 208:1469–1471, 1980.
170. Fidler IJ et al: Design of liposomes to improve delivery of macrophage-augmenting agents to alveolar macrophages. *Cancer Res* 40:4460–4466, 1980.
171. Foss OP et al: Invasion of tumor cells into the bloodstream caused by palpation or biopsy of the tumor. *Surgery* 59:691, 1966.
172. Sugarbaker EV, Ketcham AS: Mechanism and prevention of cancer dissemination: An overview. *Semin Oncol* 4:19, 1977.
173. Paget S: The distribution of secondary growths in cancer of the breast. *Lancet* 1:571, 1889.
174. Sugarbaker, EV et al: Do metastases metastasize? *Ann Surg* 174:151, 1971.
175. Hart IR, Fidler IJ: Role of organ selectivity in the determination of metastatic patterns of B15 melanoma. *Cancer Res* 40:2281–2287, 1980.
176. Hart IR et al: Metastatic behavior of a murine reticulum cell sarcoma exhibiting organ specific growth. *Cancer Res* 41:1281–1287, 1981.
177. Sugarbaker EV: Patterns of metastasis in human malignancies, in JJ Marchalonis et al (eds): *Cancer Biology Reviews, vol 2,* Dekker, New York, 1981, pp 235–278.
178. Sinha BK, Goldenberg, GHL: The effect of trypsin and neuraminidase on the circulation of organ distribution of tumor cells. *Cancer* 34:1956, 1974.
179. Sugarbaker EV et al: Facilitated metastatic distribution of the Walker 256 tumor and Sprague-Dawley rats with hydrocortisone and/or cyclophosphamide. *J Surg Oncol* 2:227, 1970.
180. Glaves D, Weiss L: Effect of host sensitization on patterns of metastasis. *Transplant Proc* 7:253, 1975.
181. Fisher B, Fisher ER: Experimental evidence in support of the dormant tumor cell. *Science* 130:918, 1959.
182. Sugarbaker EV et al: Studies of dormant tumor cells. *Cancer* 28:545, 1971.
183. Eccles SA, Alexander P: Immunologically mediated restraint of latent tumour metastases. *Nature* 257:52, 1975.
184. Noble RL, Hoover L: A classification of transplantable tumors in Nb rats controlled by estrogen from dormancy to automony. *Cancer Res* 35:2935, 1975.

13
PSYCHOLOGICAL ASPECTS OF CANCER

Claus Bahne Bahnson

HISTORICAL BACKGROUND

In considering the psychosocial factors operating in the development of cancer, it should be noted that such factors have been addressed in the literature since the times of Galen, who in 200 A.D. stated that melancholy (depressed) women more often develop breast cancer than do sanguine (happy and spirited) women. Similar ideas have reappeared frequently in the literature, particularly during the eighteenth and nineteenth centuries. A number of clinicians, such as Gendron,[1] Guy,[2] Walshe,[3] and Amussat,[4] have remarked on the obvious effect of depression and melancholy, sadness and dullness, and stress and grief on the development of cancer. Many clinicians making similar statements in the literature during the nineteenth century have been reviewed elsewhere.[5] A number of psychoanalytic studies followed in the 1920s, e.g., Hoffman,[6] Evans,[7] and Meyer,[8] giving greater detail of observation. Evans stated that her patients had lost or had disrupted a major emotional relationship prior to the development of disease, thus expressing for the first time a psychodynamic predisposition to cancer.

After the Second World War a new wave of psychosomatic research into malignant disease appeared and sponsored two new main approaches to cancer: one related to loss and depression as an antecedent; the other emphasized that a particular personality configuration, characterized by denial and repression as well as strong internalized controls and commitment to social norms, facilitates a malignant development. These two approaches will be surveyed in the following paragraphs, and subsequently some of the possible mediating mechanisms that might explain "the mysterious leap" (Deutsch[9]) from the environment, via the mind, to the body will be discussed. However, first it seems helpful to consider some of the main conceptual problems inherent in the study of the psychophysiological aspects of the development of cancer, since these are reflected in the strengths and weaknesses of study methods and research design.

THE EPISTEMOLOGICAL PROBLEM

Critics of psychosomatic studies of cancer often have alluded to "the hen and egg problem," suggesting that the obtained results may reflect the *effect* of the disease on mood, object relationships, and lifestyle rather than the preexisting conditions that may have facilitated the development of the disease. On a simple-minded level there is some truth to this thought, and it must be responded to (as it now has been) with prospective studies utilizing psychosocial data that far precede the occurrence of the disease. However, the simplistic dichotomizing of psyche and soma, which characterizes such thinking, certainly has been put in question, not only by classical philosophers such as Spinoza, Leibniz, and Hegel, but by more present-day conceptualizations as represented in system theory (von Bertalanffy[10]) and in psychosomatic holistic concepts, which consider the interfacing of psyche and soma not as a tennis game between independent opponents but as an arbitrary epistemological representation on different conceptual levels of one central and multidimensional process.

Since cancer may take many decades to develop and since selected individuals may be brought into this world with specific propensities for developing malignancies, the problem of "what causes what" becomes quite elusive and obscure. Therefore, it may become necessary to redefine the problem in terms of triggering or releasing factors instead of causal factors. On the physiological level it is well known that a tumor is not diagnosable before it reaches a certain size and that microscopic lesions may exist undiagnosed in the body for many years. In this case it appears to be a meaningless question whether a personality factor is a cause of, or is caused by, a microscopic lesion or its endocrinologic correlates. All that is known is that certain psychological and physiological conditions seem to occur simultaneously, and that these processes possibly can be conceptually integrated in a supraordinate theoretical construct including both chains of events.

If one assumes that changes in personal experience go hand in hand with nonobservable physiological (endocrinologic) events that in some individuals are related to carcinogenesis, then it may seem obvious that attention ought to be given to these observable psychological events, whether they be conceptualized as cause, concurrent events, or effects of physiological change. The very fact that psychological events and overt behavior produce readily observable data favors the psychological approach to the study of cancer, particularly *before* the malignant process has become clinically manifest. This approach may assist in identifying a beginning malignant process years before it is possible to diagnose a tumor clinically, irrespective of whether the psychological state is seen as a causal or an index variable. The most likely "truth" is that the psychological state is a *concurrent* manifestation of a total, psychobiological, multilevel process related to vulnerability to clinical cancer but assessable long before the process can be identified physiologically.

DEPRESSION AND HOPELESSNESS AS ANTECEDENT STATES

With these introductory thoughts in mind, let us first move to the current theories and studies relating loss and depressive states to the clinical occurrence of cancer. In a series of studies Greene et al.[11-13] and Schmale and Iker[14,15] evaluated personality factors in patients with lymphomas and leukemias, and uterine malignancies, respectively, and found repeatedly that severe loss or separation, with concomitant depression, helplessness, and hopelessness, were characteristic antecedents to the development of both types of malignancies. Greene reported that separation from a significant person or the loss of a major goal, with ensuing depression, was a key factor gleaned from carefully analyzed clinical and test studies of patients with lymphomas and leukemias. Greene[16] also reported that in monozygotic twin pairs discordant for leukemia it was the unfortunate twin who had been subject to individual frustration or misfortune that developed leukemia, whereas the more fortunate twin remained well. Schmale and Iker[15] used a predictive technique, selecting from a group of women at higher risk (Papanicolaou III smears) those who might develop cervical cancer, based on a recent history of loss and hopelessness. Their predictions were correct beyond the .02 level of significance. Schmale's work has been reproduced in a more objective way in a recent study by Spence,[17] who used a computer technique to count words referring to depression and hopelessness in the speech of a sample of patients who were to be screened for cervical cancer by cone biopsy. Spence found that he could predict outcome of the biopsy by means of "lexical leakage" reflecting depression and hopelessness, so that he blindly could pick out the cancer patients at a significance level of $p < .01$. Thus, using automated computer counts of predetermined "depressive words," Spence was well able to predict the diagnosis of his subjects.

Using clinical studies and a number of tests, LeShan et al.,[18-20] after working with more than 500 cancer patients, reached a similar conclusion. LeShan emphasized that serious and incapacitating depletion and depression (or, as he prefers to call it, "despair" in the sense of the Danish philosopher Kierkegaard) earmarked these patients who were experiencing insolvable life problems prior to the onset of cancer. He found that cancer patients (1) had suffered a loss of an important relationship before the diagnosis; (2) had no ability to express hostile feelings; and (3) showed tension over the death of a parent, usually an event which had occurred many years previously.

Hagnell,[21] in an impressive prospective population study of 2550 persons in Sweden in which Sjöbring's personality test was given some 20 years prior to the assessment of disease in this population, found that cancer patients, particularly female cancer patients, compared with controls, more often were of the substable and depressive personality type, again indicating that a depressive mood or attitude was present in these patients scores of years prior to the clinical onset of a malignancy. In a more recent study, Bieliauskas et al.[22] carried out another predictive study of cancer on the basis of Minnesota Multiphasic Personality Inventory (MMPI) data collected 17 years previously on 2107 subjects in the Western Electric Health Study. Of these subjects, 83 had contracted, and died of, cancer at this time, and for these subjects a significant association ($p < .01$) existed between their elevated depression scales 17 years previously and their later development of cancer. Using the relative peak of the depression scale over other scales of the MMPI as a discriminator, the significance raised even higher: $p < .001$. The particular aspect of depression that contributed most heavily to the prediction of a future malignancy was a vegetative expression of depression, i.e., observable behavioral indications of depression rather than self-reported sadness. It should be noted, again, that findings produced by smaller-scale cross-sectional and clinical studies are corroborated by large-scale prospective studies, even when the instruments for assessment do not focus precisely on the hypothesized dimensions.

This author's investigations showed why loss and despair would be particularly crucial to future cancer patients. Many people experience loss and separation, but seldom with the concomitant development of a malignancy. In cancer patients the traumatic loss or separation during adulthood gains its particularly devastating effect on the basis of a particular biographical background.

CHILDHOOD EXPERIENCES OF CANCER PATIENTS

It appears that cancer patients have had an unsatisfying and difficult relationship with one or both of their parents, particularly with the mother, characterized by excessive, but unsatisfied, dependency needs, leading to ample ambivalence and underlying anger and rage. Clinically, these patients report very poor parenting so that, as children, they could maintain only an uncertain and brittle relationship with the significant parent, who seemed cold and indifferent to the child. With this background, the adolescent separation from the parents became particularly painful and was perceived as a renewed deprivation against which they struggled in their adult years by attempting to establish close emotional relationships with a mate or spouse, or frequently through substitute investments in creativity or work. They had difficulties establishing an emotional relationship as adults, and when a precariously established relationship or investment broke down in adulthood, the original despair and hopelessness of the deprived and longing child reemerged, isolating the individual, who was left with little hope that any real warmth and support could ever be obtained from others. This idiosyncratic interpretation of loss and closeness may be the basis for the future cancer patient turning toward himself, often giving up all efforts to interact emotionally with other people.

In investigations of the relationship between cancer patients and their parents, using the Roe-Siegelman parent-child relationship questionnaire,[23] it was found that cancer patients remember their parents as more neglecting and colder than do other physically ill patients and normal control subjects. The parents of future cancer patients were less loving, protective, and rewarding, and more rigid than the parents of all control groups. These observations are in agreement with those of Booth,[24] and Thomas and Duszynski,[25] and have an affinity with those of Spitz,[26] Harlow and Harlow,[27] Ader and Friedman,[28] and Wrye.[29] In comparative studies using animal models, Riley[30] and Henry[31] have indicated the importance of early conditions of nurturance and security for effective coping with later stresses. Riley subjected various groups of mice to environmental stresses and compared them with groups growing up in protected environments. The strain carried the Bittner oncogenic virus, which usually leads to the development of mammary tumors within 8 to 18 months after birth. Incidence rates at 400 days were studies, with the result that 92 percent of the "stress" mice and 7 percent of the "protected" mice had developed tumors. These observations suggest that the importance of the parent-child situation is not specific to human beings, but represents a special human elaboration of a much more widely generalized phenomenon.

The preponderance of perception of inner control in cancer patients and their loneliness, rigidity, and depressive leanings, all may result from their experiences of isolation and inhibition during childhood. Also, the excessive use of secondary repression and denial, so frequently reported in cancer patients (Kissen,[32] Bahnson,[33] Henderson,[34] and others) may be understood as sequelae of the "centrifugal" childhood family pattern of the cancer patient. In the family of orientation of the cancer patient, the emphasis was not on personal closeness, social adaptation, and social success (as is the case, for example, in families of coronary patients) but on full inner personal control and on narcissistic gratification. Thus, the reliance on inner resources and the preference for personal fulfillment rather than social affiliation were created for the cancer-prone individual, who must regress to childish self-isolation when failing to produce in the image of the self. Selye[35] has suggested that cancer cells grow to destroy themselves by their uncontrolled "egotistic" development, violating the adaptations necessary for the "socialization" of the cell. The cell regresses to behavior characteristic of the archaic unicellular organism. This statement is isomorphic with the hypothesis concerning psychobiologic, narcissistic regression in cancer patients.

REPRESSIVE PERSONALITY IN CANCER PATIENTS

The other main approach to psychological factors in cancer, dealing with secondary repression,* denial, "poor emotional outlet," and lack of self-communication as predisposing antecedents to cancer will now be reviewed briefly. Several of those authors who have emphasized depression and the perception of loss also have reported striking observations of denial and "blandness" in their patients. Although a survey of the literature indicates

---
* A psychoanalytic concept referring to intense rejection and repression of a thought, need, or feeling, when it returns after a primary and initial repression.

that these observations "creep into" nearly all reports, only a few groups have emphasized the importance of these long-term psychodynamic aspects of the patients' personalities. Kissen et al.[32,36,37] have pursued this particular approach, starting with clinical observations and later moving into objective research, making use of the Maudsley personality inventory (MPI) developed by Eysenck, in order to validate on a quantitative and statistical basis their clinical impressions. Using well-validated scales such as the extraversion-introversion and neuroticism scales of the MPI, Kissen's group found that cancer patients had marked difficulty with emotional discharge and tended to be inhibited and repressive subjects compared with control patients with other serious diseases of similar sites.

Blumberg et al.[38] reported MMPI findings from cancer vs. control patients, and described the cancer patients as defensive, anxious, overcontrolled subjects, with no ability to release tension through motor or verbal discharge or any kind of "acting out." Their MMPI and Rorschach results suggested that cancer patients with fast-developing disease were more defensive and overcontrolled than patients with slowly developing disease. Patients with rapidly progressing cancers also showed lack of ability to decrease anxiety, and presented a polite, apologetic, almost painful acquiescence. This was contrasted with the more expressive, and sometimes bizarre, personalities of those who responded well to therapy with long remissions and long survival times. Klopfer (in the Gengerelli symposium[39]), related ego defense and ego strength to the differential development of fast- and slow-growing cancers. Using a theoretical model with two axes—(1) investment in ego defense and (2) impairment of reality testing—Klopfer found that fast-growing cancers correlated significantly with high investment, and slow-growing cancers with low investment, in ego defenses. Several other authors have contributed to the overall picture of constriction and repression in cancer patients, deduced either from clinical interviews or psychological testing, including Reznikoff,[40] Perrin and Pierce,[41] Cobb,[42] Tarlau and Smalheiser,[43] and several others.

Bahnson et al. have pursued the study of ego defenses, using a psychoanalytic model and applying questionnaire methods, a variety of projective techniques, adjective checklists of mood (both conscious and preconscious), clinical interviews, and therapy sessions. The results are reported in a number of publications[44-50] and can be summarized as presenting general support for and confirmation of the hypothesis that cancer patients, compared with other patient populations and normal samples, make heavy use of denial and repression, and have lost awareness of their own covert needs and wishes. Although they present a realistic and alert, as well as an acquiescent and pleasant interpersonal attitude, they seem to live a rather constricted, boring, and repetitive life. On the basis of studies of the childhood of these patients, it was concluded that the rigid defensiveness and lack of awareness of inner feelings may be related to early interactions with their parents, not allowing these patients (as children) to develop affective communications with the parents, and thus impairing later affective expression, as so many researchers have observed and stated.

Cutler,[51] working with terminal cancer patients, described them as individuals who fail to express themselves and who repress hostility. Jacobs[52] similarly remarked on the pronounced self-destructive forces and rigid armoring of the cancer patient. Greer and Morris,[53] basically following Kissen's methodology, found in 160 women admitted to the hospital for breast tumor biopsy that a significant association existed between the diagnosis of breast cancer and a behavior pattern, persisting throughout adult life, of abnormal release of emotions. This abnormality was, in most cases, extreme suppression of anger, and in patients over 40 years old, extreme suppression of other feelings as well. Extreme expression of emotions, though much less common, also occurred in a higher proportion of cancer patients than controls. It is of interest to note that although most cancer patients by far were extreme *suppressors* of emotion, there was a subgroup whose members lost control and suffered from temper outbursts. This observation is consistent with the basic dynamic concept of repressive defenses that are strong and rigid. Such defenses seldom are flexible and do not allow for alternative coping methods when the basic coping strategy fails. In other words, people who rely on heavy repression do not develop alternative coping styles but blurt out or explode with emotion when the usual repressive strategy fails. Thus, conceptually, Greer and Morris's findings are consistent with the results of previous research emphasizing a repressive cancer personality, e.g., Brown et al.,[54] Goldfarb et al.,[55] Bahnson,[47] and several others.

Thus, it is not loss and depression alone that usher in clinical onset of cancer, but a very special dynamic interpretation of loss and stress based on early traumatic life experiences that may make some individuals vulnerable to clinical manifestations of cancer. Since both ego-defensive patterns and sensitivity to certain traumata are conditions "learned" in the family from early childhood, the interrelated and complex multifactorial biographical conditions become obvious antecedents. In other words, we are concerned not with short-term stresses that can be clearly delineated without reference to the particular life history and personality of the person but with long-term conditions of stress and adaptation, which carry roots far back into an individual's early life history.

GENERAL AND SPECIFIC FACTORS

So far, cancer has been discussed as a general condition, without considering the particular site or the particular type or histology of the disease. Some studies are of an experimental population with mixed cancer sites and types, whereas others have utilized patient populations with a specific cancer site, e.g., lung cancer or cancer of the cervix. That similar personality and life history constructs have emerged from such disparate patient populations suggests that we are dealing with what may be called a *G factor*, or general factor, which cuts across specific types and sites of the disease. However, it is also of interest to define an *S factor*, which delineates the specific conditions characterizing the psychosocial aspects of cancer of a specific site or type. In this chapter, gynecologic cancers, including cancer of the cervix and cancer of the breast, will be briefly reviewed. Only a few studies, disparate in methodology, have been selected in order to gain a perspective on current knowledge of these cancers.

Stephenson and Grace,[56] in their classic study of cancer of the cervix, used a personal interview technique including a number of background variables, relevant physiological information, and a history of sexual and marital function as well as personality function. Their study indicated that personality features and behavior play an important role in the development of cervical cancer. Prominent in this study was a dislike of sexual intercourse, amounting to an actual aversion to it, in a high proportion of the patients. The failure to achieve orgasmic satisfaction in intercourse; the high incidence of divorce, desertion, and unfaithful husbands; separation; and frequent sexual intercourse with multiple extramarital partners are probable indicators of poor sexual adjustment. Schmale[15] and Spence,[17] as discussed previously, emphasized the depression and hopelessness factors in their studies of cervical cancer patients, thus focusing in on what seems to be a G rather than an S factor. However, Schmale et al. also mention the frequently observed early losses and hardships of cervical cancer patients, particularly the early loss of their fathers, necessitating that they leave home or terminate school early to go to work.

Tarlau and Smalheiser,[43] Wheeler and Caldwell,[57] Jones et al.,[58] Graham,[59] and Terris and Oalman[60] are among the other psychosocial researchers who have studied cervical cancer patients. In addition to the repeatedly mentioned disturbed sexual orientation and gender confusion, these researchers also noted that the patients' mothers frequently were described as overly dominant, although they frequently died before the patients were 12 years old. Most often the young girls had very negative and angry feelings about parental discipline. These studies also indicate that the socioeconomic conditions for the cervical patients-to-be were relatively poor compared with, for example, those of breast cancer patients, a fact that may explain several of the psychosocial earmarks of the early family health problems, and the childhood emotional and hardship variables. Finally, the peculiar combination of aversion to intercourse and infrequent orgasm, coupled with early and extensive sexual activity and involvement leading to early pregnancy, also was repeatedly observed by the different study groups.

Reznikoff[40] studied psychological factors in breast cancer patients and found that these patients more frequently were a middle child (compared to controls with benign disorders, or well controls); had more frequently experienced deaths of siblings at birth or in infancy; and reported more frequently that both parents were dead, that they had many responsibilities as a child, that they were less frequently a favorite child of one or both parents, that they more frequently had two or more siblings, that they carried heavy responsibilities for caring for siblings or other younger children when they were children, and that as adults they expressed negative feelings toward pregnancy and birth. They were dissatisfied with their home situation, but rarely were sufficiently independent and assertive to depart from the family setting. They infrequently perceived maternal figures as consoling, protective, or abetting, and male figures were seen as rejecting and unresponsive to women's needs for love and attention. Only a few cancer patients expressed basic contentment with interpersonal contacts, and most manifested profound sexual confusion associated with their self-image and specific disturbances in gender identification. Other results indicated that breast cancer patients, more often than controls, were ashamed, confused, and surprised by the onset of menstruation; that they "mother" their husbands or men in general; and that they had negative or ambivalent feelings about heterosexual love.

With a completely different methodology, Fraumeni et al.[61] studied the cancer mortality rate among nuns, and observed that nuns project a striking increase of the incidence of breast cancer, in line with the observation that single women, in general, experience substantially higher rates than do married women. However, although nuns do not differ significantly from the normal population with regard to cancer of most other sites, the breast cancer incidence rate shows a significant excess for the age spans over 40 years of age and with increasing differentiation, not only from the normal, but also from the single population. Nuns also develop breast cancer earlier than the control group, showing a typical upward trend in the increase between ages 45 to 49, five years earlier than the accelerated increase for digestive cancers. The higher incidence rate of breast cancer in nuns is consistent with the psychodynamic hypotheses relating this incidence to avoidance or dislike of the motherly and female sexual role, with ensuing rejection of reproductive and sexual behaviors.

Katz et al.[62] studied the relationship between psychoendocrine, ego-defensive, and prognostic variables in a group of women hospitalized for breast biopsy. They found that in women with breast cancer, the effectivity of the ego-defensive processes against depression and anxiety were predictive of hydrocortisone production, in the sense that women with a breakdown in their defensive system had much higher hydrocortisone outputs *as well as a poorer general prognosis* than had women with a more flexible and more effective style of coping. Possibly, the increased hydrocortisone production in the women with the breakdown in their defenses may have served as an inhibitor of their optional immunologic reactions. Again, where the defensive system is flexible and makes possible a containment of overwhelming emotion, the hydrocortisone production is moderate and the prognosis positive. Where the defenses are rigid and repressive, and break down under the impact of the trauma of (pending) diagnosis, the hydrocortisone production is increased and the prognosis is poor. These observations dovetail with those reported previously by

Greer and Morris[53] that breast cancer patients compared with patients with benign tumors have long-standing difficulties with the release of emotions, either through extreme suppression or explosive expression. Schonfield[63] also studied women with suspicious lesions of the breast on the day prior to biopsy. He used the Holmes-Rahe SRE (schedule of recent experience) and the MMPI; and although he did not find significant results with the Holmes-Rahe, the MMPI indicated that the "young" cancer patients (under 42 years of age) had significantly higher covert anxiety scores than the benign patients, and even more importantly, that the MMPI "lie scale" scores were significantly higher for women with malignant tumors of the breast. This scale measures denial of aggression, weakness of character, and poor self-control. Schonfield writes: "Thus the finding of such denial among cancer patients of European or American origin would extend the findings of Huggan and Bahnson of greater denial among patients with known cancers back to their premorbid condition, before they had any knowledge of their disease status." Here then, we see a breast cancer predictive study that focuses on the G rather than the S factor, but which supports the hypotheses outlined previously.

Wrye[64] studied breast cancer patients vs. controls by means of a written journal which they had produced in response to a number of key research questions such as "dialogues with their mother" or "reflections about my breasts." A careful study of the extensive responses indicated that breast cancer patients perceived their own mothers to have been unable or unprepared to fully assume the mothering role for them. Their mothers had not focused on them, had been distracted, and had provided insufficient mothering. The cancer patients characterized their relationships with their fathers as stressed or lacking—a strong and independent support of our own previous study using the Roe-Spiegelman parent-child questionnaire, in which father's protectiveness and "presence" also was lacking. Each cancer patient described a belief in her own inadequacy, felt that other siblings were preferred over her, and expressed a sense of being different from others as well as feelings of loneliness and neglect. Wrye's patients also described a fear of loss of control and reported periods of marked depression long prior to the occurrence of the breast cancer, associated with the pattern of "turning anger inward" rather than comfortably expressing it outward. A study by Cramer et al.[65] of 40 female cancer patients of whom 30 were breast cancer patients, using a German adaptation of the psychosocial questionnaire developed by Bahnson et al., again gave general support to the hypotheses developed in the United States, and earmarked the dimensions specific for breast cancer. Breast cancer patients, again, compared with the matched-pair control group showed the following characteristics: fewer (or no) children, difficulties with release of aggression along with containment of anger; commitment to social norms and, especially, the church; and difficulty in making a decision. The cancer patients cannot take things lightly and are easily irritated over minor problems of no importance, but, as was the case in Kissen's study and other American studies, they denied emotional problems during their childhood, as manifested by nightmares or phobias. In this study it may be observed again, as with a preceding study using this screening questionnaire in Philadelphia, that the difficulties with control of affect and a tendency to repress and turn anger inward, coupled with authoritarian, conformistic, and religious orientation, characterized the breast cancer patients.

In clinical studies of breast cancer patients, as presented in a recent publication,[49] it was found again that rather severe childhood trauma—e.g., loss of a parental figure—and lack of a protected and loving childhood, coupled with parental coldness, characterized the early lives of these breast cancer patients. Also, a main underlying depression and hopelessness seemed to color all the experiences since early childhood in these patients, associated with the certainty that everything is doomed to go wrong and simultaneous guilt feelings that they cannot live up to the expectancies of their parents. A further observation from these clinical investigations is that the breast-cancer-patient-to-be develops a "double life" or a "double self" (also called "schizophasia" by the French researcher R. Fresco), which allows realistic and adaptive ego operations to operate, but which is separated from and independent of a parallel "shadow self" that feels isolated, unloved, hurt, and deserted. In psychiatric "borderline" personalities similar splits occur, and the manifestations of these splits are sometimes observable as different roles or personalities within the patient (as in multiple personalities), appearing sequentially and often as defenses against other threatening aspects of the personality represented by controlled, "unacceptable" behaviors. In breast cancer patients a similar split has been observed—the schizophasia—but the alternative self is not expressed or reacted against, but is silent and covert and seems associated only with the somatization, with the disease process itself. This observation leads back to the theory of complementarity developed several years ago,[31,33] which conceptualizes the development of a chronic somatic disease as an alternative to a serious emotional regression, when such a process is halted and contained.

Thus, a brief review of cervical and breast cancer from both epidemiologic and clinical studies indicates that these patients not only exhibit a G factor of repressive, overcontrolled, authoritarian, committted, and religious attitudes, but also show inner conflict over the gender role, including both aspects of sexuality and of the generative role through childbearing and child-rearing. Apparently, something went seriously wrong in the patient's relationship with her mother, and possibly also with her father, in the sense that she dislikes or is ambivalent about her own female identity. The breast cancer patient is unhappy with heterosexual sexuality, which she often finds objectionable, even disgusting, and she shows diminished interest for bearing and rearing children. This may be because she was overtaxed as a child taking care of smaller siblings and now has negative memories of that taxing role, or perhaps because she anticipates experiencing similar negative feelings about motherhood as those that she remembers from her own mother. The cervical cancer patient frequently starts from a similar base to that of the breast cancer patient, but often she takes another and more stormy route, trying to overcome her ambivalence and uncertainty about her own image by throwing herself into early and multiple relationships in order to seek satisfaction and a relieving solution. The repeated disappointments may lead to a frantic search for sexual meaning that is doomed to repeated frustration, often sending the patient on a prolonged search for new solutions in her life. She often is tempted to become cynical and hard, because her innocent longings repeatedly are ignored or even chastised. The tendency to what used to be called promiscuity thus serves as a defense against the emotional disappointment experienced by these women, who then develop cervical cancer when failing to control their lives.

The breast cancer and the cervical cancer patient seem to start with similar psychosexual problems; but while the breast cancer patient delays or avoids sexuality, the cervical cancer patient throws herself into the sexual field to try to overcome her own frigidity, conflict, and anxiety about her gender.

What is repressed, denied, and pushed aside, then, is *site-specific*, or an S factor. The general propensity for potential cancer patients to deny, repress, and contain holds true also for cervical and breast cancer patients, but the *content* of the repression is specific and relates to basic instincts or needs of a sexual and procreative nature.

This brief survey of etiologic psychological studies shows that oncology does not encompass a random group of patients, but that many cancer patients share some difficult life experiences that predispose them to specific reactions to their disease and its sequelae. Obviously, there are frequent exceptions to the general picture that has emerged of the cancer patient from the previous studies, and one must be cautious not to overgeneralize unduly or to approach patients with rigid preconceived ideas. However, it may be helpful to be aware of the life histories and attitudes shared by many cancer patients before entering into a therapeutic or supportive relationship with them.

It may be particularly important to know that although cancer patients often seem self-sufficient and in good control of the situation, they often long for a supportive and helping hand but cannot express this need. It may also be important to know that although most cancer patients are self-contained, realistic, and socially appropriate, they often struggle with deep inner worries with which they need help, even when they cannot ask. They have been accustomed to taking care of things themselves and feel too embarrassed or ashamed to open up. Often they are not even aware of this inner trouble that has been so deeply repressed for years. Most have not been lucky enough to have good emotional communication at home so that they expect little help. It is on the basis of this emotional background that free communication and emotional openness become such important aspects of relating to cancer patients, especially at critical points in their illness.

THE CANCER PATIENT AND THE FAMILY

A family is not simply a conglomeration of individuals who happen to live together. It is an intricate emotional and communicational, as well as cognitive, system in which changes in one part of the system immediately dictate changes or reorganization in the remainder of the system. Whenever an individual falls seriously ill, all close relationships with other family members change, and the total family system will reestablish balance by redistributing roles and responsibilities among other family members, who become "delegates" of the ailing person. Loving and hostile feelings become "homeless" when an individual develops a serious illness and is no longer fully available to the family. The family members who gave or took affection from the sick family member now must look for other family members toward whom to discharge, or from whom to receive, these emotions. That often creates serious psychological problems, because it is usually not safe, for example, for a daughter to receive unbridled affection from the father, or the son from the mother, when the other parent is seriously ill; and, on the other hand, these new figures who have to supply emotional support in lieu of the sick member may not be able to fill the void. The rearrangement of affective bonds can seldom be accepted without guilt and defensive retaliation toward self, or projected to others, leading to family hostilities of one type or another. Similarly, the hostile and aggressive urges that always are ambivalently tied in with the affective ones, also have become homeless, except that some family members perceive their own hostility and anger as being discharged when another in the family falls ill. They are responsible, they have "made her ill," or they have "destroyed him." This is one of the reasons why the seriously ill person always is described with so much affection and glorification—the hostile part of the ambivalence has been discharged and only the positive part of the ambivalence remains. However, remaining unresolved hostility may be directed to other family members, so that a sibling or parent suddenly may experience rage or anger from other family members for which they cannot account.

The family often perceives the serious illness (or death) of another family member either as an expulsion or a rejection of this sick member from the family system, or, alternatively, as if the sick (or departing) member had angrily rejected or destroyed the family system. This depends on whether the patient is a child or a parent, a spouse or a dependent figure. Children often perceive the terminal illness of one of their parents as a cop-out, as if the parent was disappointed and angry with them and wanted to desert them. Similarly, parents often have tremendous guilt when a child falls seriously ill, as if their own neglect of, or lack of investment in, the child had resulted in the disease (or death).

One way in which the family can try to reestablish equilibrium is to replace the sick or lost child by investing in another child; or, in families where a parent is ill or lost, by reintroducing a new figure to fill the gap. In active families, that is, two-generational families in which parents and children still form a strong functional unit, such a reestablishment of equilibrium nearly always takes place. A less desirable resolution of the equilibrium is expressed in the frequent illness of other family members during the stress of serious illness of the primary patient, or after the terminal patient has died. Other members of the family fall ill, often with a similar disease; surviving spouses statistically have a manifold increase of risk during the first years after their spouse's death. This is another destructive way of recreating equilibrium and combating the guilt that is associated with loss of the sick family member. One other rather unfortunate resolution is often seen in a narcissistic reinvestment of the affectionate charges that were previously placed with the sick or dying family member. The remaining individual or individuals become more self-absorbed as they are separating from the sick patient, and thus reverse their own development back to the original narcissistic position. Of course, the mourning process so carefully described by Freud consists in part of such narcissistic reinvestment for a period, which is then reversed with the end of mourning. This phenomenon is difficult to treat because it counteracts the efforts of the therapist to reestablish a new equilibrium of emotional communication in the family, particularly inhibiting the important relationships with the terminal patient. The "psychological death" often takes place when the patient receives a malignant diagnosis, so that the interpersonal separation is initiated long before the patient dies. The patient needs increased communication and emotional openness with other family members, and the therapeutic doctor will try to facilitate such communication for the reasons mentioned previously. However, both the narcissistic withdrawal and the attempts at reinvestment of "homeless affects" in other family members frequently work against efforts at increased communication and participation with the patient.

THE AGE CONTINUUM

Both individual and family reactions to serious illness and death differ with the age of the patient. If we consider the cathectic arc (Fig. 13-1), in which the baby begins life with self-investment and narcissism, moves toward increasing interest in other persons and symbolic endeavors during adulthood, and then slowly returns to a transcendental self-investment again in old age, then it becomes obvious that from the point of view of both

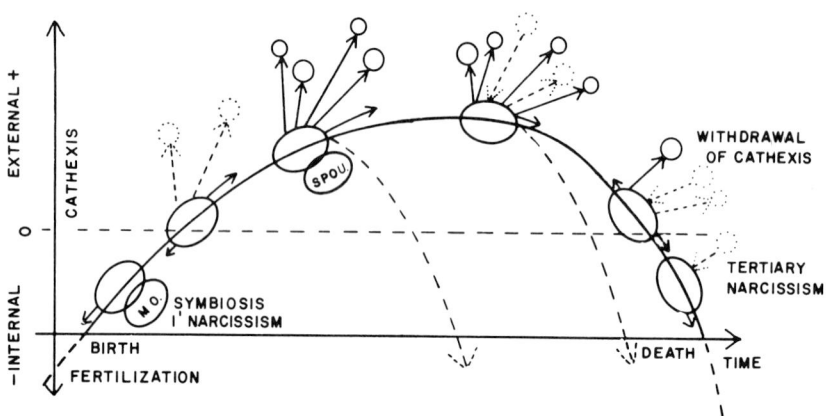

FIGURE 13-1 The developmental arc of cathexis related to reactions to death. X axis = a dimension from internal to external cathexis; MO. = mother; SPOU. = spouse; loop = person; arrows extending from loop = cathexes, or investments in other persons, object, or tasks; reversed arrows = withdrawal of cathexis; arrows attached to "the person," but without targets = trends of movement under stress, early regression versus later progression in development; solid arc = total healthy life span; dotted descending lines = premature disease and death; figure = different problems arising for individuals when they fall ill very early, during young adulthood, or during middle or old age.

patient and family, the greatest difficulties ensue when the patient is maximally involved and engaged with others. The system disturbance caused by cancer is much greater in the procreative family than when parents are old and have already withdrawn. Not only the quantity but also the quality of problems differs. For the young or middle-aged adult the projected course of life is directed ahead, from the top of the cathectic arc, toward creativity, enhanced self-expression, and continued responsibility for others. The interruption and premature diversion of this projection creates rage, helplessness, and despair. Similarly, for the family it often implies a perception of this parent's "failure" of completing his or her task and responsibility in life, and the perception of the illness as desertion. It goes without saying that strong feelings of empathy, sorrow, and pity also are mobilized, but the basic disappointments nonetheless emerge. Such family problems can be resolved in a variety of ways. Among the negative and unfortunate solutions are the patient's withdrawal, anger, and retaliatory bitterness, or the helpless and sorrowful regression to an overly dependent and succorant adaptation—the "hurt child" syndrome. Among the more positive solutions, found in families that have emotional resources and often can utilize therapeutic help, are increased communication and mutual caring support, which allow the patient to remain emotionally important to the other family members, because he or she has found new ways of remaining supportive to the others and has found ways to accept a new level of support from them. Frequently, a cancer patient may become a significant source of advice and emotional support for the younger family members, who then learn to perceive the sick person as mentally wise and well. In these happier instances, the cohesion of the family is retained, and the illness is easier to bear for all.

For the old person, the pending shift from involvement with others to a moving inward and to "other shores" simply is hastened, the curvature of the cathectic arc dipping deeper and faster than expected. Here the most frequent reaction of the family is to experience guilt for not having held on to the terminally ill family member intensely or long enough. The old person, however, often perceives illness and impending death as a rebirth, as Theodor Fechner so beautifully described in his little-known treatise on the "life hereafter."

The terminally ill child has a different job to do. Being on the ascending portion of the cathectic arc, he or she sees fulfillment of the coming familial function as the one who invests in others, who cares for others more than for the self. These young cancer patients collapse within a few months or years all the personal investments they may (will) not be able to complete leisurely and over time. They often become the protectors of their parents, the family therapists in their families, and often at their death leave their parents bewildered and disoriented when they find out that they lost a "parent," not a child. The three-generational guilt is magnified, and the parents must reconcile the ledger by paying their debts to others in the family. The dead child becomes the saint who died for all.

THE PATIENT'S RESPONSE TO DIAGNOSIS AND TREATMENT

Although a patient's response to the diagnosis and treatment of cancer varies widely with background and view of life, some reactions to the different phases of disease and treatment tend to recur. Among the important background factors determining the reactions are age; gender; educational level; ethnic, religious, and socioeconomic background; family and work status; and previous experience in the family or among friends, with the process and outcome of cancer. Frequently, a patient's response to the diagnosis of cancer is colored by previous experiences in the family, e.g., as in a case where a cancer patient recently has nurtured and cared for a parent or an aunt or uncle with a similar disease until they passed away. In these cases, the meaning of the diagnosis is quite different from that in a person who has had no, or only a fleeting, relationship to cancer in the family or among friends.

Patients vary widely in their reactions to the stress of cancer. One good predictor of a patient's capacity to adapt optimally to illness is a previous history of adaptation to difficult and stressful events in life—e.g., to serious losses of close persons or frustration of main career or life hopes—or adaptation in response to previous illnesses. One way to gauge this capacity for adaptation is to discuss such previous experiences with the patients and their significant others, both in order to gain this information and to alert the patient to potential strengths and coping capacity. Another general predictor is the availability of support from family and friends on which the patient can draw in this difficult life situation, although not all patients are alike with regard to their need for emotional "togetherness" in such situations. However, even if a patient seems to prefer isolation and a more stoic lonely withdrawal, it is still true that the awareness of available support makes a great deal of difference. At the other extreme are patients who like to be embedded in a group of people, the *Homo familias*, for whom the possible isolation and lack of the usual embeddedness seems to pose a great threat. For this type of patient it is of even greater importance to mobilize the necessary emotional family support, particularly since all patients have an unconscious fear of being abandoned in this situation. The lonely fighter, the stoic patient, is usually recruited from the Protestant ethic population, from the New England type "WASP", and from other middle class and upper class professionals and managers, who are accustomed to direct more than share, and who may be uncomfortable about too much sentimentality. In contrast, and varying by class, patients of a Mediterranean ethnic background are more accustomed to a sharing and communicating type of family life, and need continued reaffirmation that they still belong in their group. They do best when the family is visibly around during the hospitalization. These, of course, are rough generalizations and do not cover several other ethnic groups, each with their own characteristics. Further, as shall be seen, individual emotional needs often may cut across ethnically and socially defined reaction patterns and prevail for any patient, whatever the background.

Another basic determinant for a patient's general reactions is intellectual and scientific knowledge about cancer, and the degree to which the patient is aware of sensations and processes within the body. The awareness of interoceptive cues and pain varies widely among patients. Obviously, it is easier for the medical staff to support a patient's intellectualizing defenses if the patient can understand and participate in the reading of the diagnostic material, and is sufficiently acquainted with medicine to understand the different diagnostic and treatment processes. However, underlying this intellectual adaptation to the disease, an emotional and irrational response often coexists that may relate the illness to expiation of guilt, or cause a perception of it as a retaliation for omissions or commissions in the patient's life. Patients often complain and moan, speaking to no one and to everyone, "What have I done that I deserve this terrible pain?" Obviously, such an exclamation reflects the underlying mystical belief of many patients that the disease is an affliction determined by their own previous sins or mistakes. One should remember that such beliefs and feelings can also exist in patients who otherwise may be highly intellectual and who in other moments can talk about their disease with their doctors as if it were an impersonal objective and medical process.

The patient's reactions to the different phases of the disease and the specific reactions to cancer of a number of common sites will now be discussed.

PATIENT, FAMILY, AND PROFESSIONAL PROBLEMS AROUND DIAGNOSIS

The emotional problems that emerge at the time of diagnosis are quite different from those that characterize recurrence, or the terminal phase. The emotional adaptation to having cancer is a process with many phases and is also deeply interwoven with the family's reactions and the family's total situation. The diagnosis can be conveyed in many ways. Sometimes diagnosis is made at a routine examination without premonitions on the part of the patient; at other times it follows an escalation of minor problems and symptoms that often may have been minimized, both by patient and family doctor. However, in most cases the patient is aware, on some level of experience, that something is going awry with his or her health. This marginal awareness often may emerge in dreams, in "flashbacks," and in fantasies, at times when the patient's psychic apparatus is off guard, less occupied or organized, and more open to "leakage." Spence's study,[17] referred to previously, indicates that, indeed, patients who were *later* diagnosed as having a malignancy, compared with control patients, gave evidence of a "leakage" into their language of words with a somber or depressive connotation even before conscious awareness could be possible. Different types of catastrophic dreams often antecede the diagnosis, indicating that, on some level, the patient may be vaguely aware of the disease.

Although the concept of cancer is changing rapidly because of the increase in treatment possibilities and demystification of the disease, it may still be true that the very diagnosis of cancer is most often perceived as a deadly blow that produces a sinking feeling of anxiety and hopelessness in most patients, irrespective of the rational medical hope that the situation can be successfully treated and controlled. For the adult, there is often an experience of life closing in and of the end of the otherwise open-ended and not so clearly defined future. Although we all know that our time is limited, there is somehow a hopeful coloring associated with the possibility that many good things still may happen, and that there may be many years during which to catch up with unfulfilled dreams. When a cancer diagnosis is made, the patient and the patient's family are deprived of this open-ended dream to come. Fate is denying the patient "leisure hours." For young adults, the diagnosis also triggers a fear that they will not be able to see their children grow up, and they may then feel great anxiety about what might happen to their families without them.

Patients, of course, vary considerably with regard to their first reactions to diagnosis, spanning from anxiety and panic, through depression and helplessness, to denial and efforts at ignoring the situation, sometimes coupled with hypomanic reactions resembling gallows humor. A frequent response is "Why me," in which the patient sees the disease as a punishment for something, or by somebody, for past omissions or commissions. This attitude is often associated with feelings of injustice, expressed something like this: "Why should not my irresponsible and psychopathic neighbor, who never does anything for anybody, get this dreaded disease instead of me, who has tried so hard to be a good spouse, parent, and citizen, to the very best of my ability?"

The most helpful therapeutic response is to explore in greater depth the patient's perceptions of the injustice in his or her life, and to allow expression of affect, thus establishing a therapeutic alliance with the patient that allows for a full expression of concerns otherwise held back and repressed. In patients with excessive denial, it may be helpful to go along with such a denial for awhile, but also question why it is necessary for the patient to be so certain about his or her own complete health, and why the doctors and the medical diagnosis may be all wrong. Again, this has to be done gently and supportively, since any effort at broadening the patient's experience might otherwise backfire and lead to further constriction, denial, and unreachability.

Often the diagnosis is made in such an ambiguous or euphemistic way that the medical staff plays into the common need for denial, thus making it even more difficult for the patient to know what to believe. Using ambiguous terms such as a *lesion* in order to avoid calling the disease a malignancy or a malignant tumor, may invite denial by the patient, who may not dare to ask the next question, thus letting the diagnostic implications hang in the air. Although it is not pleasant to give a difficult diagnosis to a patient, it still is much preferable to do so, albeit gently and with empathy and compassion, rather than produce a climate which may trigger further patient confusion and denial. If the patient "doesn't hear the diagnosis," it simply means that the patient is not yet ready to take in and deal with the information, and that the diagnosis must be discussed in several subsequent sessions or visits, after the immediate defensive posture has subsided somewhat.

Another grave error frequently committed in good faith by the physician is either to inform the family without informing the patient, or to inform the patient without informing the family. It appears that a closer proximity in age, profession, and social status between patient and doctor often results in a greater openness between them, but then often with the family kept out of the picture; whereas a greater discrepancy between the age and social parameters of the doctor and patient often results in information being given to the family but not to the patient. In either case, trouble is being built into the patient's relationships with the family in the sense that there now is a secret that cannot be approached, and which serves as a screen or barrier between the patient and the family. This one-sided or mutual denial in the family serves to obstruct good communication, and serves as a "crystal" around which many other "silences" are being deposited. Silence about the disease pulls with it silence about many other important family matters, and all too often families end up as strangers vis-à-vis their sick family member under such circumstances. In contrast, the mutual information given to both patient and family, and the joint response of the whole family to the situation, consolidates the emotional cohesiveness of the family and also facilitates the resolution of the many problems secondary to the family member's disease.

SPECIFIC EMOTIONAL STATES EARLY IN THE DISEASE

Anxiety is the predominant reaction to the diagnosis of cancer, both in the patient and in the family. The patient may feel panic about what is ahead. The minotaur is charging. To alleviate panic and unbridled emotion about what is ahead, a "treatment alliance" should be established early between the treating doctor and the patient. The diagnosis of cancer sometimes makes "the bottom of the world fall out from under the feet of the patient." Any constructive treatment procedure that provides hope for a cure, or at least prolonged control of the disease, can help the patient and the patient's family to master the initial anxiety and reduce the stress of the situation. The treatment plan, therefore, serves not only a medical and physiological purpose, but also has marked beneficial psychological effects on the patient and family; thus, the way in which the treatment plan is first presented to the patient is of utmost importance for the patient's further emotional coping. It is also important to enlist the patient's own activity in the treatment plan. Whenever the patient instead of the nurse or family member can carry out an aspect of the treatment, this should be the preferred modality because it mobilizes the patient in the fight against the disease. Being able to do something constructive about your own situation reduces anxiety, and so far as is known, also may increase the body's psychophysiological defenses.

Many patients may regress under the impact of the initial anxiety in response to a cancer diagnosis and may begin to behave irrationally or childishly, often irritating the doctors, either with a clinging dependency that makes the attending doctor uncomfortable, or through a pollyannish, childish denial of the situation, which also is counterproductive to the development of a doctor-patient relationship and to an effective treatment plan. The oncologist must understand that these reactions are in response to rampant anxiety, and they represent defensive coping strategies on the part of the patient. Therefore, staff irritation or the doctor admonishing the patient for inappropriate behavior are very counterproductive. Instead, the medical staff should provide emotional support, understanding, and care of the patient. Therapeutic support will accelerate the patient's return to a more mature and calm equilibrium, whereas punitive or rejecting responses actually may enhance the patient's regression and disorganization.

Some patients respond to the first diagnosis not with anxiety but with anger, hostility, and paranoid feelings. This is a defensive way of trying to cope. Often patients complain about their families, who minimized the symptoms, or the referring doctors, who "missed" the diagnosis and brought the patient in danger. Instead of feeling rage and anger against the disease process, these patients will direct the anger toward the medical staff, the hospital, or even against family members who may have "done something wrong," or "mistreated" the patient, thus causing the disease. It is difficult for the attending doctor to respond with kindness when being attacked by the patient, or when the patient attacks the doctor's colleagues, whom he must ethically defend. However, the oncologist's understanding of the emotional process is particularly important in this case. Asking cancer patients to ventilate and express their anger and explain in detail how they see the situation easily alleviates the anger, and a positive relationship can be built up, both supportive of patients and facilitating the future treatment process. The medical staff must understand patients' reactions during early diagnostic phases of cancer as symptoms rather than taking them at face value or, even worse, taking them personally.

Perhaps the most difficult response to cope with is deep depression, helplessness, and withdrawal in patients in response to their diagnosis. A hopeless withdrawal and feelings that treatment efforts may be of no use are reactions that may reduce motivation for medical efforts if doctors are not aware that this response also is a situational emotional reaction and does not represent the true interest or attitude of the patient. When a patient withdraws with a hurt and pessimistic outlook, the oncologist's own underlying negative attitude may be reinforced, resulting in decreased efforts on his or her part. It is important to understand that depression often is the result of self-punitive and self-defeating, inwardly directed hostility, which is associated with guilt feelings or thoughts of one's own shortcomings and "sins." Therefore, again, doctors should not take such responses at face value but understand them as a variety of situational responses to the stress of a cancer diagnosis. The best way to help the patient with a depressive reaction is to give emotional support and let the patient talk about this depression without stopping him or her, and to share some of the depressive views with the patient so that the patient may let the therapeutic person grieve as well, thus freeing the patient from part of the depressive charge. Superficial efforts at cheering up the patient, using brusque humor and boy scout attitudes to try to make the patient come around, always fail. With depressed patients, a willingness to hear the patient out and emphatic sharing in their sadness are the best approaches.

The fear of being abandoned and forgotten triggers some of the most difficult reactions. This fear obviously relates back to early childhood and the unreliability of the parent as a supplier of safety, and has roots in reality. It is well known that the terminally ill "leper" is often abandoned by family and staff alike in situations where resources, emotional maturity, and compassion are at low levels. The therapeutic goal here is to help both patient and family to experience that the patient, though in a dependent state, has something valuable to give the family—so that the fear of abandonment as an undesirable "dirty" person can be counteracted. The capacities of a seriously ill person can always be of help to other family members, whether the patient is a child or an old person. To be able to deliver something of importance and to help the others allows the patient to accept protection and affection and to feel less abandoned and lost.

The diagnosis should never be given to the patient and family without qualifications, without hope, and without clear information that treatment—and, as a matter of fact, several types of treatment—are available for this condition and will be followed up to the hilt in order to assist the patient in fighting the disease. Hope is a peculiar thing. None of us can hope to live forever, although many magically hold the belief that the self indeed cannot disappear or die. Hope means rather that one will be helped, assisted, loved, and not abandoned by the significant others and by the "medical magic" which has to save one from the premature death, pain, or infirmity. To hope, therefore, is to know that all the support systems, both medical and humanistic, are in place, and that one is not dealing alone with the fight against the disease but has a true group of friends at the round table. Not to tell the patient and family what is going on is a desertion in fear on the staff's part, since it begs the question, increases uncertainty and anxiety, leaves the patient and the family alone to cope without any immediate assistance, and deteriorates the doctor-patient relationship from the very beginning.

THE STRESS OF RECURRENCE OF METASTASES

The initial treatment in most cases leads to a period free of disease, and very often the patient is either told, or believes, that he or she is cured, because the initial disease process was halted or removed, and because the medical team may have talked with optimism about having cured the original disease. Of course, cure takes place in some cases, and it is therefore easy to understand that both physician and patient lean toward the most optimistic outcome of the first encounter. Further, it is probably important to instill a hope where a true cure seems possible, because the very anxiety and depression associated with beliefs of incurability may accelerate the recurrence of the disease, and may adversely modify a patient's life to become more hesitant and constricted—a condition that probably would accelerate rather than halt a covert disease process.

In many cases there may have been a period of years, often 3 to 6 years, during which no symptoms or problems have recurred. When suddenly a new tumor occurs or an old, dormant site flares up, this is a terrible blow to the patient, who may have thought that he or she was disease-free. Bitterness and hopelessness often set in, and increased anxiety may take over because the patient, on the basis of previous surgical or treatment experience, has become more aware of what is ahead, and what the recurrence or metastases means. If the recurrence comes soon after the primary event, and the patient has not yet had the possibility for fully reestablishing his or her life pattern or progress, the recurrence may be even more depressing because it seems that fate is draining and depriving the patient faster and more relentlessly than he or she can tolerate.

Usually, the denial that colored the responses to the initial episode has faded, and more often an open depressive response to recurrence is seen. However, anxiety is usually somewhat blunted, because the worst did not happen at the time of the initial onset of the malignancy, and the patient has been "conditioned" to view the treatment procedures as unpleasant but tolerable. Thus, some of the drama has been played out, and the recurrence much more often triggers general hopelessness with feelings of fatigue, helplessness, hopelessness, and sometimes despair. It is at this point that many oncologists emphasize the other avenues of treatment that are available, thus trying to instill some hope into the patient.

The family often perceives the recurrence, whether in adult or child, as an ill omen, and as a wrecking of the hopes that had unfolded for a total cure. The family often starts to regroup, and (if psychological treatment is not handled correctly), without the patient's knowledge, begins to assign responsibility away from the patient to other family members, or in other ways develops new alliances that may exclude the patient from their midst. In other words, recurrence signals to the family members that the patient is on the way out and that they should regroup to prepare for getting along without the patient. Therapeutically, it is important at this stage to make an extra effort to include the patient in the family's considerations. The mother or father certainly can remain an important resource person, even when physically absent, for decision making, guidance, instruction and explanation, and emotional support; and even a child can be very important to parents as a "redeemer of sins," and as a saint who helps and forgives. Therefore, the therapeutic thrust must be to reengage the patient within the family, even at this stage where so many get disappointed and give up.

NO-MAN'S-LAND

Modern chemotherapy has produced a new "phase" in cancer illness, after the metastatic phase and prior to the terminal phase, constituted by the often long period of time during which the patient is being treated, not palliatively or curatively, but in order to retard the malignant process, to prevent or slow down further metastases, stabilizing or even temporarily regressing the extent of malignant expansiveness—all in all giving the patient more time. Emotionally, this is a very difficult period for both patient and family, often most difficult for the family. At this stage of disease the patient often has acquiesced to the situation and has gained a certain equanimity and calmness vis-à-vis the disease and the future. This period usually comes after several stormy events in the disease history, and at this time the patient often relates well to the oncologist and often nearly has become a member of the medical team. This is not to say that the patient is happy, because very often he or she is despondent and pessimistic; but the wild panic, anger, and paranoid attitudes are gone, and a new existence in a no-man's-land has started. Some call these patients "the living dead," a very unkind and biased way of looking at this newly won time span wrestled from fate by modern medicine. However, there is some truth to this description in the sense that the patients usually are not so vital and engaged anymore, and, at the same time, often are somewhat philosophical, not only about treatment but also about life and their families. They often feel unreal, suspended between a pragmatic world left behind and anticipation of not being, at the same time that some aspects of life continue as if nothing had happened. From a psychotherapist's point of view, these patients often have gained tremendous insight compared with their previous adaptations, and they may serve as the soothsayers in their families. The families have the most trouble with these patients because there exists in the unconscious of the family a natural separation mechanism that triggers an emotional withdrawal from members who are about to die and who are no longer practically functional within the family structure. In more primitive societies we see how older people are expelled from the family; for example, the aged person in Greenland's Eskimo society is sent away—or walks away—from the igloo to die by the cold or the bear when he or she is no longer socially functional. Traces of the same attitudes still remain in our modern society where we see a tendency to isolate and remove the nonfunctional, "dying" family member. However, in this case the death has been forestalled—delayed—and the patient has entered an often long period of half-life, during which life functions are waxing and waning and the family must say goodby and then again receive the patient in an emotional embrace, a process that slowly wears down the family's capacity to have the patient reenter or stay in their midst. The patient has "overstayed his welcome." It is difficult, for example, for parents of children with malignant disease to go through the mourning process of losing the child and then have the lost child come back as a "Lazarus." The family's capacity for repeatedly restructuring loss, and then negation of loss, is probably limited, and a certain apathy and affectlessness develops in which the fatigue of the system is expressed through the lessened intensity of emotional relationships among its members.

The therapist can help the family come to terms with this problem through allowing ventilation of anger, anxiety, guilt, and disappointment among family members around the problem of entry and reentry, and by assisting the family in developing a modus vivendi by which the positive aspects of the interpersonal relationships can be boosted, and by the help of which the family can develop other constellations to support it and prevent the "exhaustion syndrome."

THE TERMINAL PHASE

The terminal patient is nearly always either consciously or unconsciously aware that death is close. The patient does not arrive there suddenly, but has lived through periods of varying medical and psychological stages of waxing and waning hope, physical trauma (surgery), improvement, and recurrence; and changing emotional adaptations spanning from anger and paranoid feelings, through depression, to inner acceptance of impending death. Kübler-Ross[66] has mapped these different stages in context and detail, and has pointed out that the emotional reactions usually unfold with a certain regularity.

When a patient has much unfinished emotional business—is not ready to die—we see both anger and depression, sometimes alternating, sometimes combined, the anger often directed toward both medical staff and family. It is of great importance for the patient to be allowed to discuss and to resolve these problems in order to be able to fully accept impending death. The treating oncologist or psychotherapist must be able to accept the patient's anger toward him or her as an expression of the patient's pain, and not be defensive or retaliatory about it. When the treating person understands why the patient shows so much anger and suspicion, the patient usually is able to move ahead to greater acceptance of the inevitable. Only when the oncologist accepts the concept of a limited existence can the patient be helped to come to terms with dying.

The depression in some patients over lost illusions, or lost hope of being able to arrive at some of the most desired experiences in life, often is too difficult for the oncologist to bear, and a neuropsychiatrist is called in or antidepressive medication is prescribed in order to avoid the contact with such difficult material, shared by all who partake in human existence. The patient also taxes the tolerance of the caretaking staff, who often try to use euphoria, kidding, or humor as antidotes to the threatening despair in their patients, a despair which they unknowingly share. Again, it is desirable that the treating staff member share and partake in the patient's suffering, so that the support stemming from this participation can allow the patient to accept death without feeling abandoned or rejected.

Denial of nonexistence often takes the form of religion or religious beliefs of a continued life after death. This form of denial can be either helpful or destructive, depending on whether it constitutes a flight from the solution of urgent interpersonal problems, or whether it becomes part of the mosaic of security characterizing the final stage of acceptance of death. In the former case, the treating therapist should help the patient come to grips with the unfinished business rather than flee into a compensatory belief system. In the latter case, the patient must be supported in acceptance of the transition of death within the parameters of his or her own belief system.

Terminal stages of life have different subjective meanings depending on where a patient is located on the historical and developmental arc (see Fig. 12-1). A person's developmental path can be conceptualized as starting with a phase of narcissism, symbiosis with the mother, and extreme dependence during early childhood; moving toward greater degrees of independence and emphasis on relationships outside of self during adolescence; reaching full investment in humanity, society, and concrete or theoretical creative acts, coupled with high levels of activity and thrust during adulthood; only to return slowly to more introverted and self-oriented activities during old age, ending up with a rather dependent and narcissistic position during the last stages when close to death. If the projected course of an individual's life without disease is considered as being tangential to this arc at any given point of development, a geometric metaphor then emerges for the specific problems that arise when terminal disease occurs at premature stages of development.

If the terminal disease occurs very early in life, the problems that are activated still revolve around increased needs for protection, nurturance, and care from the mother or the mother substitute, and the disease process is often perceived (nonconsciously) by the very young patient as an indication that the parents reject or have withdrawn love from him or her. If terminal disease sets in near the arc's peak, in young adulthood, the patient still expects psychologically to project him- or herself through significant activities to higher levels of expression in educational, creative, or other outwardly directed activities, a projection now thwarted by the inhibiting illness. The frustration that these activities cannot be maintained and continued creates anger and resentment, and most of the psychological problems associated with impending death are associated with the inability to complete self-fulfillment and self-projection in the arena of active life pursuits. The patient is often enraged that projected activities have to be given up, and feels that fate is robbing and cheating him or her from goals and pursuits that are nearly within grasp, but which now are receding out of reach due to the illness. For the mature person who is somewhat older and has established a family and accepted the responsibilities of active adulthood, the completion of these responsibilties and the continued projection of self through family, children, and work become the most significant area of concern. The patient often feels that he or she has failed and that it is shameful not to be able to complete effective guidance and shielding of the family as well as the chosen creative course of life. Alternatively, many patients also feel cheated and feel pity for themselves that they will not any longer be a part of a family or of a work group. A mother may weep because she will not see her children graduate, and a father may bemoan that he did not save enough to see his family through. Here the turn of the arc is being accelerated downward toward the zero point, and the natural process of aging and disengagement collapses within a much briefer time period because the patient has to arrive at a point of disengagement prematurely.

For the aged person, the needs for nurturance, security, and care become more urgent because the person now has moved toward emotional adaptations similar to those of the young child, except that the members of the next generation now have become "the parents" and are the caretakers for the older patient. Thus, for the older patient the problems of safety and protection become as paramount as they were for the young child. All patients, not only the very young or the very old, have needs for nurturance and care owing to the inhibiting and regressive effects of serious illness, and may adopt childish and dependent attitudes side by side with whatever other projections of their life goals they otherwise pursue.

By keeping these developmental differences in mind, it becomes clear that the needs of terminal patients differ, depending on their stage of development when they become terminal. The very old or very young patient will respond to simple measures of protection, love, and care, whereas patients at the apex of their developmental arc need to get help, preferably professional help, finding substitutes and alternatives for their creative and societal responsibilities in ways other than those they now must give up. The psychological treatment of the terminal patient is more than goodwill and love, and must be geared to covering the particular needs of the patient with regard to his or her life situation. This does not negate the need for openness, communication, empathy, and support that holds true whatever the patient's problem may be.

THE FAMILY'S PROBLEMS IN TERMINAL DISEASE

Not only the patient but also the family has difficulty in coming to terms with premature death. Impending death mobilizes massive anxieties, fears, uncertainties, and depression in other family members. Frequently, very practical and mundane problems of an economic or organizational nature become the manifest targets for the underlying anxiety about losing a husband or father, a wife or mother. The fact that the terminal patient functionally moves out from the family and leaves a void creates immediate problems for the rest of the family. The family may not wish to give up the terminally ill family member as the significant other or, alternatively, they may have already excluded the "leper" and, in spite of their guilt, have functionally separated from the dying person. Where family members have not given up the affective contact with the terminal patient, they usually become overly protective and loving because the patient's illness represents a "binding" of their previous hostile feelings toward the terminal family member, with the result that all the positive and affectionate emotions are released and become available for the terminal patient. In contrast, where a high level of anger and bitterness has existed prior to the terminal situation, the patient's illness may not have "drained off" a sufficient amount of the hostility directed toward him or her by the other family members, and the family still feels unable to give support to the dying patient due to covert anger. In such situations, it is best to develop alternative support systems for the patient, e.g., psychological and social work staff, side by side with an effort to activate existing resources within the family.

Other family members often have the fantasy that they are somehow responsible for the illness. There are innumerable examples of how family members express guilt (over their covert hostility) for having delayed or not encouraged the terminal patient's appointment with the physician; for having given him or her unhealthy or carcinogenic food or cigarettes; for having induced life stress or hardships for the terminal patient; and so on. This guilt in other family members may spur extensive demonstrations of love and care, often of an unreal or artificial character. At other times family members try to avoid contact with the terminally ill because this contact increases their feelings of guilt and concern, and they attempt to avoid the guilt by running away ("out of sight, out of mind"). The loss of the terminal patient often releases new affects among the rest of the family so that a sibling or parent may suddenly experience rage or anger from other family members for which they cannot account and with which they cannot deal.

Therapeutically, the family needs help in understanding that many manifestations of anger, regression, and disturbance, although not obviously related to the terminal disease in a family member, nonetheless are a displaced expression of despair and should be understood and responded to as such. School phobias in the children, resulting in distraction and failure in class; acting out in adolescents with a sick parent; or psychosomatic disease in other family members, all are symptoms of family members' reactions to the terminal stage of their sick parent or spouse. They are observable in every family experiencing this stress, but often are treated and responded to piecemeal and out of context by family, authorities, or other medical personnel. The terminal patient needs increased communication and openness with other family members, and such contact and communication should be fostered and facilitated. However, both the narcissistic withdrawal of the patient and the attempts of other family members to find some gratification from others in or outside the family often work against the effort at increased communication and participation with the patient. Particularly when the patient has "overstayed his welcome," or when the family already has separated from and found new life solutions not including the terminal patient, it becomes increasingly difficult to reengage the family as suppliers of support and feeling during the patient's terminal days. When this situation occurs, alternate support systems provided by the hospital and the therapeutic staff must be activated in order to ensure that the patient has the proper support and communication during this most difficult period in most patients' lives.

THE USE OF IMAGERY AND ALTERED STATES IN THERAPEUTIC GUIDANCE OF THE SERIOUSLY ILL AND DYING PERSON

The use of imagery and induced altered states of consciousness in terminal patients can signifcantly help them overcome pain, depression, and a variety of worries. The imagery with which it is helpful to work always derives from the patient's own associations, images, and dreams, and never from a preconceived, generalized, or typified imagery projected onto the patient. Imagery produced originally by the patient is preferable because it most often represents crucial isomorphic, metaphorical statements on the patient's central concerns and conflicts and about the disease, rather than reflecting external concepts inserted into the patient's experiential world during therapy. Some patients present, spontaneously and without fail, such basic material to be expanded and explored in further imagery interchange. They will tell you about one or more dreams they have had, or where they would like to be, or which experiences in their lives are of greatest import to them (peak experience). Where this does not happen, the therapist can facilitate the personal generation of imagery by discussing favorite places, activities, or surroundings with the patient, thus eliciting the concrete counterpart to an underlying fantasy.

When such material has been found, the therapist's task then is to mobilize this fantasy material as an organizing and ameliorating dimension which will allow the patient to supersede the immediate threats and concerns, and in a constructive fashion to resolve needs and aspirations within a process of guided altered states. Use of guided imagery and altered states in the terminally ill can drastically reduce pain, can relieve depression and anxiety, and can assist the patient in modifying the response to pain and disease. Some patients will remain within naturalistic and time-limited awareness, when close to death. Others, often of a religious faith, prefer to think of death as a transition and will produce extensive imagery about afterlife, including the reunion with lost and loved ones.

Images Frequently Helpful in the Therapy of Terminal Patients

One of the images that appears most frequently in terminal patients is "the beach," usually at the seashore, often in the proximity of trees or palms, and frequently close to the outlet of a beautiful river. This image of a blissful place to be is so universal that about half of our patients produce this as a significant element in their favorite imagery. Obviously, it relates to the age-old metaphor about the water as a vehicle for transcendence to other worlds, and to the psychoanalytic concepts of water as related to mother, birth, and rebirth. One patient, crippled by bony metastases and with intractable pain, wished to be on a beach, particularly if he could be close to his daughter whom he loved so much, in order to feel relief and peace. During light hypnosis this wish was fulfilled and suggestions were made that he would be free of pain and feel mobile and agile when dwelling on this ideal beach. Indeed, the pain did subside in spite of the physiological unlikeliness thereof, and the patient lived much longer and better than was expected, even being able to dance at the wedding of his beloved daughter after his disease previously had immobilized him with intense pain for long periods of time.

The beach sometimes appears as a single image, but at other times it is combined with the imagery of dolphins, in particular—dolphins that are friendly and helpful and can transport the patient through a fluidum of gentle relief. The dolphin seems to appear to many terminally ill patients as the rescuer and reliever, and sometimes in combination with the color yellow, either in the sense that the dolphin itself is yellow, or that the sun produces a yellow halo around it. Yellow seems to represent life, warmth, and creativity. A middle-aged breast cancer patient, who was late in her disease with metastases to the bone and was in considerable pain, produced just such an image of a dolphin, this time swimming in the clear waters of southern Italy, and inviting her to join it in the green and blue gentle waters for a swim. During altered states, the dolphin became more than a companion, actually carrying the patient, in her fantasy, through mystical waters and finally toward a dark, sunken castle with beautifully adorned entrances deep down under the surface of the sea. By going deeper and deeper with the dolphin and feeling better and better each time, she was able to accept metaphorically the transition to "the sunken cathedral" actually longing for the final swim during which she would be transported passively by holding on to the back fin of the dolphin. Another patient, who was not so close to death but who produced similar imagery in a dreamlike state, saw a yellow dolphin in an enclosed pool near the sea so that she could inspect and playfully engage with it when it was still in captivity. This might be understood as a partial resolution of the fear of going into open waters with the dolphin, and as expressing the need to become more familiar with it. This dolphin was yellow and "shone like the sunset."

Another patient, also suffering from metastatic breast cancer and in severe pain, started with imagery from her summer residence, with pictures of a beautiful, old surviving fruit tree and a large flock of birds at the sea who prepared to migrate south. This imagery was supplemented by nearly biblical imagery of a snake living under the tree and some unpleasant rats that were destroying her house. Working with guided imagery, this patient let the birds return from the south for another season and thus survived longer, after which she finally imagined that she herself flew south, joining the birds in their transition. This imagery is reminiscent of archaic Chinese mythology describing how the enormous fish "Kun" arose from the northern waters, became a dragon, and flew to rest at a lake in the warm southern mountains. The imagery of the transition from north to south as the metaphor of a life span is age-old. The work with this imagery made it possible for the patient to better handle her disease and pain and to resolve most anxieties and interpersonal problems in a beautiful and genuine way. She died suddenly of a stroke on a sunny morning while visiting her daughter, before her disease got too advanced and impossibly painful.

Another image frequently appearing spontaneously for the seriously ill is the tall mountain and the mountain stream, often combined with images of clouds that may become solid and scalable. High mountains are places where one is above it all, and where contact with the cosmos and the beyond is at arms' length. A small mountain stream high up in the mountains above the clouds, among scattered wildflowers and heather, and with a grand view past other mountain peaks is a nearly ideal image for assisting the patient to achieve a calm and resolved state of mind, leaving pain and fear behind.

SPECIAL REACTIONS RELATED TO SITE OF CANCER

Each part of the body has its special symbolic meanings—some parts more obvious than others—as, for example, the breast for a woman, or the eye for all. The damage to a body part not only brings objective functional disturbance, but also implies changes in the psychological makeup of a person. Classical myths showed that millennia ago damage to the eyes or legs, or to the sexual organs, had far-reaching impacts on the lives of the victims. Therefore, it is shortsighted not to seriously consider the psychological impact of any cancer over and above the general level of stress induced by the disease. Each site has its own special effects on the psychology of the patient and of the family.

Since the face is one of our primary means of communicating with others, and is an uncovered part of the body, any disfiguration—e.g., removal of the jaw, tongue, or eye, or absence of the neck muscles—will be noticed by all and serves as a visual social clue that the patient is seriously ill and maimed. This often results in serious self-conscious feelings of shame and ugliness and also in beliefs (partly realistic beliefs) that one will be rejected as socially unacceptable. The patient should be informed *before* surgery about the expected amount of disfiguration, the plan for rehabilitation, and the probability of cure or long-term control to be gained. If possible, a previously treated patient should see the patient preoperatively to reassure him or her of the beneficial, long-term effects of the intended surgery.

A great number of head and neck cancer patients are chronic alcoholics and have severe underlying emotional problems which have to be dealt with in addition to the more evident questions of disfiguration, disability, and probability of cure. In these cases family resources should be mobilized to support the patient's adaptation process in order to secure a tolerable postoperative existence. The loss of the jaw or the lower part of the face, aside from being an obvious disfiguration, also is associated with a special horror of a prehuman inability to communicate. Some of these patients feel like mute animals and withdraw to hide. It is imperative that prosthesis be offered and that the treating team show full acceptance and support to these patients.

Blindness is often perceived as a punishment for "sins," particularly those of a sexual nature, that are associated with seeing the forbidden. One interesting aspect of the emotional reactions to blindness is that both patient and family also consider the patient wiser and more knowledgeable as a function of the loss of eyesight. Perhaps the classic myth of the wise person's "inner eye" replacing the outer eye still prevails.

Externalization of the intestinal tract is very difficult to accept because of the fear of smelling, and of being incontinent, conditions which are both personally and socially regressive and embarrassing. Although patients often can be reassured that modern technical appliances can control these problems, such assurances often do not alleviate underlying fears and fantasies. It may help to have other colostomy patients visit prior to surgery and to have the patient join an "ostomy" club postoperatively in order to reduce the fears of social unacceptability. However, most often, more intensive psychotherapeutic work reaching the unconscious correlates of the externalization of the intestinal tract is effective and can make the difference between a "cosmetic denial" with ample emotional disturbance and a deeper acceptance of this physical damage.

Damage to sexual organs and functions presents another area of fear and panic. Mastectomies are the most common cause of this problem, although not the only one. Women naturally fear that they will be sexually unattractive after their mastectomy. There is some reality to this fear, considering the attitudes of most men, and that has to be understood and not denied by the medical team. However, the patient can be reassured by the oncological surgeon that she can overcome these setbacks and will be able to continue her sexual relationships by emphasing other body areas, and that prostheses are available which cannot be distinguished easily from the natural breast and thus will prevent gross changes in a patient's usual social interrelationships. The therapist can discuss with the mate the feelings of shame and insecurity that the patient may have regarding her own attractiveness. The patient and her mate should openly discuss this problem both alone and with a therapist present. It should also be explained to the mate that his wife or partner will be extremely sensitive to his reaction at the first unveiling of the scar. Even if he is not usually supportive of his mate, this could be the time to begin, as long as the response is prompted by genuine feelings of care and concern. This encounter, if handled sympathetically and gently, may greatly bolster the patient's security and development of her later sexual relationship.

Hysterectomy and oophorectomy should not necessarily interfere with the patient's sexuality, but often do. The body image associated with being modified or "desexualized" can, in turn, have profound effects on both the patient and her sexual partner. The mere thought of being sterile can profoundly change sexual and interpersonal behavior, and, most often, leads to personality changes in the patient as well as in the spouse.

Although hormonal therapy and prostheses can modify and mask these severe reactions, there can be no doubt that the realities of life will be molded by these surgical procedures, and that only shortsighted denial on the part of the staff can explain the usual expectancy that nothing ought to change in the patient's sexual life. On the other hand, all efforts must be mounted to help the patient accept the new limitations, and learn new and modified ways of obtaining sexual satisfaction for both herself and her mate. Prudishness is not appropriate here; rather, frank and knowledgeable sexual counseling are needed.

Although less is written about male cancer surgery, problems are not different for men, possibly worse, because so many aspects of male effectiveness and success are linked with fantasies of sexual potency and performance. What was said about surgery of female sexual organs most certainly holds for prostatectomy, orchiectomy, and other male cancer surgery. Psychotherapeutic help with feelings of shame and depression are often required, and realistic sexual counseling is always necessary.

These are only a few of the possible sites, each having its specific emotional correlates. One general response is a regressive one: The patient feels messy, dirty, and uncouth, and that triggers unconscious feelings of being like a helpless child who cannot even keep him or herself clean and presentable. It is highly recommended that the medical staff understand these emotional reactions to major surgery and mutilation, as well as to full-scale chemotherapy and radiotherapy. The patients do not react pragmatically or logically, but on the basis of deeply buried attitudes toward major malfunctions in their bodies, often associated with shame and tragic feelings of failure. Gentle and emphatic participation and support on the part of the medical team can help the patient to go a long way toward a meaningful acceptance and a successful rehabilitation. Where cure is not possible, the oncologist can at least ensure that the patient has a protected and emotionally supported existence with feelings of dignity and acceptance. Thus, the formerly abandoned and neglected cancer patient should become a phenomenon of the past.

REFERENCES

1. Gendron D: *Enquiries into the Nature, Knowledge and Cure of Cancer,* Smithson and Greene, London, 1701.
2. Guy R: *An essay on Schirrhous Tumours and Cancer,* Owen, London, 1759.
3. Walshe WH: *Nature and Treatment of Cancer,* Taylor and Walton, London, 1846.
4. Amussat JZ: *Quelques Réflexions sur la Curabilité du Cancer,* Thunot et CIE, Paris, 1854.
5. Bahnson CB: Emotional and personality characteristics of cancer patients; in A. Sutnick (ed): *Recent Developments in Medical Oncology,* University Park Press, Baltimore, Md, 1976.
6. Hoffman FC: *Some Cancer Facts and Fallacies,* Prudential, Newark, NJ, 1925.
7. Evans E: *A Psychological Study of Cancer,* Dodd Mead, New York, 1926.
8. Meyer, W: *Cancer,* Hoeber, New York, 1931.
9. Deutsch F: On the formation of the conversion symptom, in F. Deutsch (ed): On the Mysterious Leap from the Mind to the Body, 1959, pp 59–72.
10. Bertalanffy L von: *General System Theory,* George Braziller, New York, 1968.
11. Greene WA: Psychological factors and reticuloendothelial disease, I: Preliminary observations of a group of males with lymphomas and leukemias. *Psychosom Med* 16:220–230, 1954.
12. Greene W et al: Psychological factors and reticuloendothelial disease; II: Observations on a group of women with lymphomas and leukemias. *Psychosom Med* 18:282–303, 1956.
13. Greene W: The psychosocial setting of the development of leukemia and lymphoma. *Ann NY Acad Sci* 125(3):794–801, 1966.
14. Schmale AH Jr, Iker HP: The affect of hopelessness in the development of cancer, I: The prediction of uterine cervical cancer in women with atypical cytology. *Psychosom Med* 26: 634–635, 1964.
15. Schmale AH Jr, Iker HP: The psychological setting of uterine cervical cancer. *Ann NY Acad Sci* 125(3):807–813, 1966.
16. Greene WA, Swisher SN: Psychological and somatic variables associated with the development and course of monozygotic twins discordant for leukemia. *Ann NY Acad Sci* 164: 394–408, 1969.
17. Spence D: Somato-psychic signs of cervical cancer. Paper presented at 87th Annual APA Convention, New York, September 1979.
18. LeShan LL, Worthington RE: Some recurrent life history patterns observed in patients with malignant disease. *J Nerv Ment Dis* 124:460–465, 1956.
19. LeShan LL, Reznikoff M: A psychological factor apparently associated with neoplastic disease. *J Abnorm Soc Psychol* 60: 439–440, 1960.
20. LeShan LL: An emotional life-history pattern associated

with neoplastic disease. *Ann NY Acad Sci* 125:(3)780–793, 1966.
21. Hagnell O: The premorbid personality of persons who develop cancer in a total population investigated in 1947 and 1957. *Ann NY Acad Sci* 125(3):846–855, 1966.
22. Bieliauskas L et al: Prospective studies of psychological depression and cancer. Paper presented at meeting of APA, New York, September 1979.
23. Roe A, Siegelman M: A parent-child relations questionnaire. *Child Dev* 34:355–369, 1963.
24. Booth G: Cancer and humanism: Psychosomatic aspects of evolution, in D Kissen, LL LeShan (eds): *Psychosomatic Aspects of Neoplastic Disease* Pitman, London, 1964, pp 159–169.
25. Thomas CB, Duszynski KR: Closeness to parents and the family constellation in a prospective study of five disease states: Suicide, mental illness, malignant tumor, hypertension and coronary heart disease. *Johns Hopkins Med J* 134: 251–270, 1974.
26. Spitz RA: Hospitalism: An inquiry into the genesis of psychiatric conditions in early childhood, in *The Psychoanalytic Study of the Child*, vol. 1, University Press, New York, 1945.
27. Harlow HF, Harlow MK: The effect of rearing conditions on behavior. *Bull Menninger Clin* 26:213–224, 1962.
28. Ader R, Friedman SB: Social factors affecting emotionality and resistance to disease in animals, IV: Differential housing, emotionality and Walker—256 carcinosarcoma in the rat. *Psychol Rep* 15:535–541, 1964.
29. Wrye H: The crisis of cancer: Intervention perspectives: Journal writing with women with breast cancer. Paper presented at 87th APA Convention, New York, September 1979.
30. Riley V: Mouse mammary tumors: Alteration of incidence as apparent function of stress. *Science* 189:465–467, August 8, 1975.
31. Henry JP, Stephens PM: *Stress, Health and the Social Environment: A Sociobiologic Approach to Medicine*, Springer-Verlag, New York, 1977.
32. Kissen DM: The significance of personality in lung cancer in men. *Ann NY Acad Sci* 125(3):820–826, 1966.
33. Bahnson CB: Psychophysiological complementarity in malignancies: Past work and future vistas, in CB Bahnson (ed): Second conference on Psychophysiological aspects of cancer. *Ann NY Acad Sci* 164(2):319–334, 1969.
34. Henderson JG: Denial and repression as factors in the delay of patients with cancer presenting themselves to the physician. *Ann NY Acad Sci* 125(3):856–869, 1966.
35. Selye H: *Stress without Distress*, McClelland, Steward, Toronto, 1974.
36. Kissen DM: Personality characteristics in males conducive to lung cancer, *Br J Med Psychol* 36:27–36, 1963.
37. Kissen DM: Psychosocial factors, personality and lung cancer in men aged 55–64. *Br J Med Psychol* 40:29–43, 1967.
38. Blumberg EM et al: MMPI findings in human cancer; in *Basic Readings on the MMPI in Psychology and Medicine;* Minnesota University Press, Minneapolis, Minn, 1956, pp 452–460.
39. Gengerelli JA, Kirkner FJ (eds): *The Psychological Variables, in Human Cancer: A Symposium;* University of California Press, Berkeley, 1954.
40. Reznikoff M: Psychological factors in breast cancer: A preliminary study of some personality trends in patients with cancer of the breast. *Psychosom Med* 17:96–108, 1955.
41. Perrin GM, Pierce IR: Psychosomatic aspects of cancer: A review. *Psychosom Med* 21:397–421, 1959.
42. Cobb B: Emotional problems of adult cancer patients. *J Amer Geriat Soc*, 1:274–285, 1959.
43. Tarlau M, Smalheiser I: Personality patterns in patients with malignant tumors of the breast and cervix: An exploratory study. *Psychosom Med* 13:117–121, 1951.
44. Bahnson CB, Bahnson MB: Cancer as an alternative to psychosis: A theoretical model of somatic and psychological regression in DM Kissen, LL LeShan (eds): *Psychosomatic Aspects of Neoplastic Disease*, Pitman London, 1964, pp 184–202.
45. Bahnson CB, Kissen DM (eds): Psychophysiological aspects of cancer. *Ann NY Acad Sci* 125:773–1055, 1966.
46. Bahnson CB: Psychodynamische Prozesse und Persönlichkeits-faktoren bei Krebskranken, *Prophylaxe Intern J Prophylac Med Soc Hygiene,* 6(2):17–26, 1967.
47. Bahnson CB: Psychophysiological complementarity in malignancies: Past work and future vistas, in CB Bahnson (ed): Second conference on psychophysiological aspects of cancer. *Ann NY Acad Sci,* 164(2):319–334, 1969.
48. Bahnson CB: Psychosomatische Dimensionen in Krebs. In Th von Uexküll (ed): *Lehrbuch der Psychosomatischen Medizin*, Urban and Schwarzenberg, München-Wien-Baltimore, 1978.
49. Bahnson CB: An historical family systems approach to coronary heart disease and cancer, in Schaefer KE et al. (eds): *A New Image of Man in Medicine*, vol. III: *Individuation Process and Biographical Aspects of Disease*, Futura; Mount Kisco, New York, 1979.
50. Bahnson CB: Psychosomatic approach to cancer. Paper delivered at the 6th International Congress of Psychosomatic Obstetrics and Gynecology, Berlin, West Germany, September 1980.
51. Cutler M: Behavioral characteristics of 40 women with cancer of the breast, in JA Gengerelli, FJ Kirkner (eds): *The Psychological Variables in Human Cancer;* University of California Press, Berkeley, 1954.
52. Jacobs JSL: Cancer: Host-resistance and host-acquiescence, in JA Gengerelli, FJ Kirkner (eds): *The Psychological Variable in Human Cancer,* University of California Press, Berkeley, 1954.
53. Greer S, Morris T: Psychological attributes of women who develop breast cancer: A controlled study. *J Psychosom Res* 19:147–153, 1975.

54. Brown F et al: The patient under study for cancer: A personality evaluation. *Psychosom Med* 23:166–171, 1961.
55. Goldfarb C et al: Psychophysiologic aspects of malignancy. *Amer J Psychiatr* 123:1545–1552, 1967.
56. Stephenson J, Grace WJ: Life stress and cancer of the cervix. *Psychosom Med* 16:287–294, 1954.
57. Wheeler JI, Caldwell BM: Psychological evaluation of women with cancer of the breast and of the cervix. *Psychosom Med* 17:256–268, 1955.
58. Jones EG et al: A Study of epidemiologic factors in carcinoma of the uterine cervix. *Amer J Obstetr Gynecol* 76:1, 1958.
59. Graham JB: *Carcinoma of the Cervix,* Saunders, Philadelphia, 1962.
60. Terris M, Oalmann M: Carcinoma of the cervix. *JAMA* 174:155, 1960.
61. Fraumeni JF et al: Cancer mortality among nuns: Role of marital status in etiology of neoplastic disease in women. *J Nat Cancer Inst* 42:455–468, 1969.
62. Katz J et al: Psychoendocrine considerations in cancer of the breast. *Ann NY Acad Sci* 164(2):509–516, 1969.
63. Schonfield J: Psychological and life-experience differences between Israeli women with benign and cancerous breast lesions. *J Psychosom Res* 19:299–234, 1975.
64. Wrye H: Belief systems of women with breast cancer. Doctoral thesis, Wright Institute, Los Angeles, 1978.
65. Cramer I et al: Psychosoziale Faktoren und Krebs: Untersuchung von 80 Frauen mit einem psychosozialen Fragebogen. *Münch med Wschr* 119, no. 43:1387–1392, 1977.
66. Kübler-Ross E: *On Death and Dying,* Macmillan, New York, 1969.

14

DESIGN OF THE CONTROLLED CLINICAL TRIAL

Carol Redmond *Bernard Fisher*

> From here on, as far ahead as one can see, medicine must be building, as a central part of its scientific base, a solid underpinning of statistical knowledge. Hunches and intuitive impressions are essential for getting the work started, but it is only through the quality of the numbers at the end that the truth can be told.
>
> *Lewis Thomas, M.D.*

One of the greatest advances of the last 50 years has been the introduction of prospective, randomized controlled trials into clinical medicine. Those efforts apply the scientific method to clinical problem solving and provide the mechanism for obtaining answers to important clinical and biological questions which can be obtained in no other way. When properly employed, clinical trials supply definitive information about the worth of therapies prior to their widespread use on populations as a whole. They afford an alternative to the haphazard fashion by which treatment regimens too often slip in and out of popularity. Despite their importance and increasing use, there is a lack of appreciation by most practicing physicians of the fact that clinical trials are highly sophisticated endeavors requiring the interactions of clinicians, investigators, and statisticians as equal partners in a common effort that requires discipline as rigid as a laboratory experiment. Medical schools must be held accountable for this deficit. Few, indeed, provide their students with even the rudiments of information concerning the importance and structure of clinical trials; in fact, the entire philosophy behind the clinical training of medical students is antithetical to the process. They are taught to be individual decision makers and to treat patients according to their "clinical judgment." Thus, they are unprepared to accept the clinical trial concept, which requires that they treat their patients according to a predefined protocol; and since therapies in the clinical trial are selected randomly, they have no chance to exercise their own decision making. Such a conflict is easily resolved by ignoring that in which they have not been instructed, i.e., the clinical trial. Just as sterile technique is automatically followed by the trained surgeon entering the operating theater, so must every physician be so thoroughly indoctrinated with the clinical trial mechanism that it too becomes an integral part of daily activities.

There are three types, or phases, of clinical trial conducted on cancer patients, and each is directed toward supplying answers to different questions. In phase I trials, studies are carried out to determine safe dose levels and/or schedules of drugs in humans. They may be aimed at using known drugs in combinations heretofore not tried or at determining the tolerably toxic dose of drugs that has shown benefit in animal models. Efficacy is not a defined goal of phase I trials, but such observations are usually made along with those about toxicity. Such trials are usually carried out in patients with advanced or progressive disease which has been inadequately controlled by conventional treatment methods.

Utilizing schedules, dosages, and incorporating limitations discovered in phase I trials, studies are next conducted that are aimed at determining therapeutic efficacy, i.e., phase II trials. They are performed on patients with the same tumor type and measurable disease (usually stage IV). In neither phase I nor II trials is randomization a feature. With demonstration of at least some efficacy in a phase II trial, a therapy becomes a candidate for full-scale testing and comparison with a currently "standard" therapy in a phase III trial.

The purpose of this report is to present an overview of some of the more salient aspects and components of phase III trials, particularly as employed for evaluation of therapy of stages I and II cancer. Comments will be made relative to their design, conduction, and statistical requirements with the hope that the current younger generation of surgeons will become aware of their importance and will be stimulated to participate in such endeavors. This overview is not meant for the statistician or for the sophisticate who is well-versed in the vast literature which is accumulating in this area. Comments are primarily based upon experiences derived from the conduct of clinical trials by the National Surgical Adjuvant Breast and Bowel Project (NSABP) for a quarter of a century. Where appropriate, breast cancer will serve as the model for discussion.

HISTORICAL BACKGROUND OF CLINICAL TRIALS

Exactly what study constituted the first clinical trial and by whom it was carried out is a subject of uncertainty. The purist may point to the Book of Daniel, chapter 1, in the Old Testament. When the king of Babylon besieged Jerusalem he demanded that certain of the children of Israel be brought before him. They were to be apportioned a daily provision of the king's meat and wine so that they would be properly nourished and become free of blemishes prior to standing before him. Daniel did not wish for his children to be defiled by the king's meat or wine and requested of the prince of the eunuchs who was in charge that they instead be given, unknown to the king, pulse and water. The children belonging to the others received the meat and wine. It is written in verse 15, "and at the end of 10 days their countenance appeared fairer and fatter in flesh than all of the children which did eat of the portion of the king's meat." Seeing this the prince of the eunuchs took away the meat and wine from the others and gave them all pulse and water.

Those forces which led to development of the scientifically based clinical trial as we know it are difficult to precisely document.[1,2] Over the last few centuries several trends took place which ultimately converged to create the present mechanism. Of particular importance was the treatise of P. C. A. Louis, who in 1834 laid down rules for the use of his "numerical method" in the assessment of therapy.[3] Some of his comments made almost 150 years ago are still so appropriate that they are worthy of quotation.

As to different methods of treatment, if it is possible for us to assure ourselves of the superiority of one or other among them in any disease whatever, having regard to the different circumstances of age, sex, and temperament, of strength and weakness, it is doubtless to be done by enquiring if under those circumstances a greater number of individuals have been cured by one means or another. Here again it is necessary to count. And it is, in great part at least, because hitherto this method has been not at all, or rarely employed, that the science of therapeutics is still so uncertain.

He stated then what is so often emphasized today,

in order that the calculations may lead to useful or true results it is not sufficient to take account of the modifying powers of the individual; it is also necessary to know with precision at what period of the disease the treatment has been commenced; and especially we ought to know the natural progress of the disease, in all degrees, when it is abandoned to itself, and whether the subjects have or have not committed errors of regimen; with other particulars.

Louis was certainly au courant when he stated that

the only reproach which can be made to the Numerical Method ... is that it offers real difficulties in its execution. It neither can, nor ought to be applied to any other than exact observations, and these are not common; and on the other hand, this method requires much more labour and time than the most distinguished members of our profession can dedicate to it.

Another important trend was the greater application of statistical techniques.[4] Although they were used in other fields during the nineteenth century, they were not introduced into clinical research until Pearson devised the chi-square test in 1900 and Gosset and Fisher developed techniques for the treatment of small samples during the next two decades. Those methods found their way into the clinic only after they had been used in the laboratory. Finally, the new sciences of pharmacology and bacteriology produced new remedies which required evaluation. Out of those three factors—the tabulation of clinical data, the use of statistical procedures, and the development of new therapeutic agents which coalesced about 1920—emerged the clinical trial. Although the general statistical principles of experimental design continued to be espoused by R. A. Fisher in the 1920s and 1930s,[5,6] prior to World War II the controlled clinical trial was virtually unknown in medicine. While there were several investigations that might fulfill requirements for what today may be considered a controlled clinical trial, any of which could be acclaimed as the "first," the British Medical Research Council (MRC) trial of streptomycin in the treatment of tuberculosis (1946) is most frequently recognized as having demonstrated by sound scientific investigation the therapeutic worth of a new agent and consequently has been elevated to that position.[7]

Why, it may be asked, if the principles upon which clinical trials are based were implied in classical writings of the past, has it been such a long and hard struggle to reach their present posture of acceptance, which is as yet distressingly far from common, by the medical profession? Until modern times "facts" were deduced by arguments from premises approved by tradition and authority without appeal to experimental validation. Even when observation ran counter to facts, it was still felt that in some mysterious way authority must still be correct, particularly at a time in history when the fabric of society tended to frown upon the challenge of authority. The modern therapeutic trial offers an alternative in that it places reliance upon impartial observance without regard for authoritarianism. Such an approach provides the foundation of scientific medicine.

In earlier times, as today, certain factors which were thought to impinge upon the doctor-patient relationship were likely to have hindered participation in clinical trials by physicians. To do so was and is still considered by many to be an admission of a lack of superior capability and a display of ambivalence regarding how best to treat a patient. Such a position is antithetical to the authoritarian attitude which has been considered to be most appropriate for a proper doctor-patient relationship. Finally, in former times as today, the carrying out of careful comparative study was inconvenient in a busy practice.

Other factors, such as the lack of recording and publishing of scientific information, lack of facilities for investigation, lack of active remedies to be tested, and the use of polypharmacy, inhibited the implementation of clinical trials. Polypharmacy in particular implied that the effect of each of the ingredients in a mixture and of their interaction in combination were known when indeed they were not. Consequently, as still happens today, no rational evaluation of a mixture could be made.

Failure to use clinical trials in surgery requires special comment. Surgery in contrast to medicine made great progress in ancient times. It dealt with lesions of simple etiology and diagnosis, and with the application of simple mechanical principles producing immediate spectacular results. Perhaps, as a consequence, surgeons have continued to believe that similar methods can be employed to evaluate the outcome of more complicated surgical undertakings. They have been less appreciative of the fact that methods of trial and error have been repeatedly misleading and that without controls, adequate patient follow-up, and statistical analyses the worth of such operations, particularly those for cancer, cannot be properly assessed.

THE RATIONALE FOR THE CONDUCT OF A PROSPECTIVE, RANDOMIZED CONTROLLED CLINICAL TRIAL

The reason for such a trial is to ensure that the progress of patients receiving a particular therapy, the worth of which is being evaluated, is as comparable as possible to the progress of those who do not receive the therapy. Every known parameter which might conceivably affect the natural history of the disease must be considered, and there must be assurance that those variables occur with equal frequency in the group of patients receiving the therapy in question as in the group which serves as the control group, i.e., those patients receiving "standard" therapy. Thus, should a difference in the outcome of the two groups be noted, it is likely to be a result of the therapy rather than of patient or tumor "factors" unrelated to the treatment which are found more often in one group than the other. In every study, unfortunately, there are undefined factors which can affect the result. Every effort must be made to ensure that there is an equal distribution between the groups of patients possessing those variables so as to minimize their effect on the outcome. Thus, the primary aim of a trial is to eliminate all biases—overt, covert, or otherwise—which might influence the findings. The process of randomization is the technique used in clinical trials to accomplish this goal.

CONSIDERATIONS RELATIVE TO PROTOCOL PLANNING AND EXPERIMENTAL DESIGN

There is general agreement that the only source of reliable evidence about the usefulness of any therapy or surgical intervention is that obtained from *well-planned*, *well-designed* and *carefully conducted* randomized clinical trials. The components of a well-planned and well-designed study are more difficult to find in the literature than is the statement of their necessity. Involvement with the design and implementation of 14 successive NSABP breast cancer trials and two colorectal trials over the past two decades has been a learning experience that has led to the following general and specific considerations which may be taken into account by those planning a large-scale clinical trial for the evaluation of cancer therapy.

Defining the Specific Aim(s)

First and foremost, it is imperative that the question(s) that stimulates consideration of a clinical trial be capable of being answered. It must be framed so that it is as lucid and specific as possible. The mentally fertile clinician and investigator has no dearth of questions needing answers. They are of various degrees of importance. Since large-scale trials commit for many years substantial numbers of patients, great sums of money, large cadres of medical, paramedical, and nonmedical personnel, statisticians and their support systems, it is vital that only questions whose answers are apt to have the greatest impact on the cure and understanding of a disease be given first priority. Since the commitment in resources is so great and the questions so many, it has been the view of those participating in the NSABP that the decision as to what the specific aims of a trial should be are too important to leave entirely to an individual or a small committee of persons with limited or biased points of view. Input must be obtained from those representing a variety of disciplines whose expertise may be helpful. Every NSABP protocol has been so synthesized, and it is thought that the best and most meaningful questions are those which can lead to answers having biological as well as clinical importance—answers which add credence to or refute present hypotheses and concepts of therapy or which give rise to new principles.

Finally, the major aims of the trial must be stated in a specific enough fashion to enable in collaboration with the statistician the development of sample size and other study design criteria to ensure that the study will provide reasonable answers to the hypotheses of interest.

The present NSABP trial evaluating lumpectomy, for example, is not only seeking to determine the clinical merit of the operation but also is designed to provide information regarding the biological significance of breast cancer multicentricity. NSABP trials of adjuvant chemotherapy have been carried out in sequential fashion utilizing progressively greater numbers of chemotherapeutic agents. Their aim has not been to test "toothpaste A vs. toothpaste B," but to provide information regarding patient subset heterogeneity and to add confirmation or to refute current biological concepts upon which the use of adjuvant chemotherapy is based.

One of the commonest errors that has been observed to occur in the planning of oncologic trials over the years is that which results from attempting to accommodate the disparate desires of potential participants; the so-called appeasement protocol. In such protocols the specific aims are so many that the protocol design becomes complex to the point of incomprehension, and the trial is unlikely to be completed. Thus, the primary aims of any study should be few. This does not preclude trials from providing information to resolve ancillary issues. Those who are familiar with research know that often the original goals became displaced as a result of unanticipated findings which are of greater importance than those which were originally sought.

Estimating Available Resources

The objectives of the trial having been determined, it becomes important to ascertain prior to proceeding further with planning whether they can realistically be met or are unattainable. Are the required resources available?

RELATIVE TO NUMBERS OF PATIENTS AND LENGTH OF FOLLOW-UP

Obviously, the first and most important requirement is to know the number of patients that will be necessary in order to answer the questions asked. Over the years a question most frequently posed to statisticians by clinicians is, "How many patients will we need to do the study?" While to the average clinician that would seem to be a fairly straightforward question, obtaining the answer is much more complicated and usually requires the application of a combination of statistical, scientific, and practical considerations.[8,9]

Before the statistician can determine the number of patients needed to detect gains or losses with a high degree of probability, it must be known what differences in therapies are to be considered clinically significant, i.e., the magnitude of differences in the results between therapies which will justify accepting or rejecting a therapy. For example, if prior to beginning a trial to compare radical with total mastectomy it is considered by surgeons (or patients) that a 10 percent or better survival rate of radical mastectomy patients would continue to justify use of that operation, then the trial would be designed to ensure that the detection of that difference, if present, would be accomplished with a high probability. That probability is referred to as the *power*. The larger the sample size and/or the difference specified, the greater will be the power, i.e., the probability of identifying a difference when there is a real difference between the two therapies. Other factors, such as the significance level chosen, the technique of statistical analysis to be employed, and the study design, influence power. The significance level chosen, i.e., the probability of accepting a difference which is not real (α, or Type I error) is influential. If one is willing to take the chance that the difference accepted is apt to be wrong only one time out of a hundred ($\alpha = .01$), the power is less for a given sample size than if one is willing to accept a 5 percent chance of error ($\alpha = .05$).

One method of estimating sample size requirements which is used frequently for clinical trials involving recurrence of disease or survival of cancer patients as the outcome of interest is based on the assumption that time to recurrence is approximately exponential. In practical terms this assumption means that the rate of recurrence is constant, that is, the recurrence rate does not change with time, or a plot of the disease-free survival rate on a log scale will be linear.

If an exponential recurrence rate is assumed, the number of patients needed in each treatment group will depend upon how small a difference between treatments would be considered clinically meaningful. For a fixed significance level (*p* value) and fixed probability of detecting a significant difference, the number of patients required increases as the difference considered clinically important decreases between treatments. The difference between the treatments can be expressed in terms of the median time to recurrence or in terms of average recurrence rates. If the time to recurrence is exponential, then the median is a function of the recurrence rate. If the new treatment reduces the recurrence rate by 50 percent (say, from 20 to 10 percent), then the median time to recurrence for patients receiving the new treatment will be double the median for the standard treatment. When treatments are compared in terms of the percent decrease (based on the ratio of the two rates), the same number of patients would be required to detect a 50 percent decrease in the recurrence rate regardless of whether the standard recurrence rate was 20 percent or 50 percent. On the other hand, if the comparison is based on the *difference* between two recurrence rates, then a larger sample size is required to detect the difference between 50 and 40 percent than the number required to detect the difference between 20 and 10 percent. This is because 50 to 40 percent represents only a 20 percent decrease, whereas reducing a recurrence rate from 20 to 10 percent is a 50 percent decrease.

In this discussion, the required sample size refers to the number of *recurrences* needed in order to have the desired probability of detecting a specified decrease. That is, the chances of detecting the 50 percent decrease will not be as high as specified until all patients have shown recurrence. However, for patient groups with a relatively low rate of recurrence it may not be practical to wait for recurrence in all patients. For example, if the recurrence rate is 10 percent per year, the median time to recurrence is approximately 7 years. If the numbers of patients are available, one could enter more patients on the trial in order to reduce the time needed to observe the required number of recurrences. If 25 recurrences were needed and the recurrence rate was 10 percent per year, then it would take approximately 2.5 years to observe 25 recurrences in 100 patients, but with 250 patients, it would take just 1 year. However, this latter study also has its drawbacks; that is, although the additional accrual makes possible an earlier evaluation of the treatments, namely after 1 year instead of 2.5 years, it should be emphasized that with only 1 year of follow-up there is no information available to project what the differences might be at 2 or 5 years. On the other hand, the study which requires more follow-up time would also provide some information from which to check the assumption of constant recurrence rates.

To relate these concepts to a specific situation, consider the subgroup of stage II breast cancer patients who are 50 to 70 years of age and have four or more pathologically positive axillary nodes. Using current data from NSABP protocol B-07, the estimated yearly recurrence rate for these patients treated with L-PAM (melphalan) 5-FU (5-fluorouracil) is approximately 15 percent. If time to recurrence is exponential, this 15 percent recurrence rate corresponds to a median of over 4.5 years. To estimate the number of patients required to compare L-PAM + 5-FU with a new regimen, for example, L-PAM + 5-FU + tamoxifen, it is necessary to decide the smallest reduction in recurrence rates which would be considered clinically meaningful. With enough

TABLE 14-1 Probability of Detecting a 25 Percent Decrease in Yearly Recurrence Rates (from 15 to 11.3 Percent)*

Years of accrual	Number of patients per arm	Years of follow-up after accrual period									
		1	2	3	4	5	6	7	8	9	10
2	120	0.26	0.32	0.37	0.42	0.46	0.49	0.52	0.55	0.57	0.59
3	180	0.38	0.46	0.52	0.58	0.62	0.65	0.68	0.71	0.73	0.75
3	210	0.42	0.51	0.58	0.63	0.68	0.71	0.74	0.77	0.79	0.80
3	240	0.46	0.55	0.63	0.68	0.73	0.76	0.79	0.81	0.83	0.85
3	270	0.50	0.59	0.67	0.73	0.77	0.81	0.83	0.85	0.87	0.88

* Using a one-tailed test with $\alpha = .05$.

patients, it would be possible to have a very good chance of identifying a reduction from 15 to 14 percent, but is that reduction large enough to justify the commitment of so many patients?

The calculations shown in Table 14-1 were based on a 25 percent reduction from 15 to 11.3 percent. While this difference in recurrence rates may appear negligible, a decrease of 25 percent would mean an increase in the median time to recurrence from 4.5 years to over 6 years. A $33\frac{1}{3}$ percent decrease (Table 14-2) in recurrence rates (from 15 to 10 percent) would increase the median to 7 years, while a 50 percent decrease in recurrence rates (from 15 to 7.5 percent) would double the median time to recurrence (from 4.5 to 9 years).

The entries in these tables show how the chances of detecting the specified reduction in recurrence rate increases as follow-up time increases for different sample sizes. The first sample size shown is 120 evaluable patients entered over a 2-year accrual period. Examination of the entries in Table 14-1 for this sample size shows that if accrual is terminated at 2 years, then even with 10 years of additional follow-up, there would be less than a 60 percent chance of detecting a 25 percent decrease in the recurrence rate. Inspection of Table 14-2 shows that with this number of patients it would take an additional 7 to 8 years of follow-up in order to have a 75 to 80 percent chance of detecting a $33\frac{1}{3}$ percent decrease (from 15 to 10 percent). As can be seen in Table 14-3 only 2 to 3 years of additional follow-up would be needed in order to have a 75 percent chance of identifying a reduction of 50 percent in recurrence rate.

From this it may be seen that if the identification of a 25 percent reduction in the recurrence rate for this subgroup is considered important, then accrual would need to be continued beyond 2 years. The remaining sample sizes show the expected results of patients accrued in the third year (60, 90, 120, 150). Thus, if 60 additional patients were entered during the third year, the total of 180 patients would need to be followed for an additional 10 years in order to have a 75 percent chance of identifying a 25 percent reduction in the recurrence

TABLE 14-2 Probability of Detecting a $33\frac{1}{3}$ Percent Decrease in Yearly Recurrence Rates (from 15 to 10 Percent)*

Years of accrual	Number of patients per arm	Years of follow-up after accrual period									
		1	2	3	4	5	6	7	8	9	10
2	120	0.37	0.48	0.56	0.62	0.67	0.72	0.75	0.78	0.80	0.82
3	180	0.56	0.66	0.74	0.80	0.84	0.87	0.89	0.91	0.92	0.93
3	210	0.61	0.72	0.80	0.85	0.88	0.91	0.93	0.94	0.95	0.96
3	240	0.66	0.77	0.84	0.89	0.92	0.94	0.95	0.96	0.97	0.97
3	270	0.71	0.82	0.88	0.92	0.94	0.96	0.97	0.98	0.98	0.98

* Using a one-tailed test with $\alpha = .05$.

TABLE 14-3 Probability of Detecting a 50 Percent Decrease in Recurrence Rates (from 15 to 7.5 Percent)*

Years of accrual	Number of patients per arm	Years of follow-up after accrual period									
		1	2	3	4	5	6	7	8	9	10
2	120	0.63	0.77	0.86	0.91	0.94	0.96	0.97	0.98	0.98	0.99
3	180	0.85	0.93	0.96	0.98	0.99	0.99	0.99	0.99	0.99	0.99
3	210	0.89	0.96	0.98	0.99	0.99	0.99	0.99	0.99	0.99	1.00
3	240	0.93	0.97	0.99	0.99	0.99	0.99	0.99	1.00	1.00	1.00
3	270	0.95	0.98	0.99	0.99	0.99	1.00	1.00	1.00	1.00	1.00

* Using a one-tailed test with $\alpha = .05$.

rate; whereas if a total of 270 patients were entered over a 3-year period, only 5 additional years of follow-up would be needed in order to have the same probability of identifying this reduction in the recurrence rate. Since the logistics of following patients for extended time periods are difficult, if not impossible, one must question the soundness of a study design for which one could not expect to have conclusive findings within a maximum of 5 years after completion of accrual. Thus, recommendations for patient accrual are based on the need to have sufficient patients to provide answers to study questions within a reasonable follow-up time without serious dwindling in patient accrual as investigators' interests diffuse.

Recent improvements in the disease-free interval of stage II patients on adjuvant chemotherapy have led to the use of chemotherapy in the control arm for all NSABP stage II protocols. Consequently, since the capability to detect differences between control and treated groups is dependent upon the number of observed treatment failures, the number of patients accrued and/or the length of follow-up time required before these protocols can be analyzed has increased. The differential effects of chemotherapy within various age-node strata have also increased sample size requirements owing to a need to consider results separately within subgroups of interest. An additional difficulty in designing the recent NSABP protocols is the lack of information on the long-term effectiveness of the chemotherapeutic regimen (L-PAM + 5-FU) used for the control arm. For example, at the time the protocol (B-09) comparing L-PAM + 5-FU vs. L-PAM + 5-FU + tamoxifen was planned, approximately 1 year of follow-up was available on patients in the protocol (B-07) comparing L-PAM with L-PAM + 5-FU for use as baseline data. Therefore, we have found it necessary to reevaluate periodically the sample size requirements for protocol B-09 in the light of more recent updates of protocol B-07 results.

It may be seen from the preceding that the entry of patients into clinical trials should be terminated as rapidly as possible for many reasons. Obviously, when patients are entered as a "bolus," meaningful findings become available earlier. When they are accrued at a lethargic pace, the results of other trials may become known which force changes in the study or even make it unethical to continue. New findings, such as impact of estrogen receptor (ER) status not only on stratification but also on treatment, may make a study obsolete before patient accrual is even complete. The questions which originally inspired the trial and seemed so compelling no longer have relevance when the answers are obtained. The findings may make the effort seem redundant or, even worse, a nonsequitur.

It is also obvious that clinical trials relative to stages I and II cancer require large numbers of patients and lengthy follow-up in order to fulfill the requirements for subset analysis. To begin such trials without having reasonable assurance that such patient populations are likely to be available is a tragedy since that resource could have been utilized in other trials. Unfortunately, the competition which exists between cooperative groups for similar patients, the increasing prominence of consumerism affecting the willingness of patients to participate in such studies; and the continued indifference or biases of clinicians all are making it more difficult to complete protocols with adequate numbers of patients to attain the study objectives.

COST OF CONDUCTING A CLINICAL TRIAL

Any form of clinical trial is expensive. Not only is there a long-term commitment of human resources to the kinds of trials being discussed here, but there must be a long-term financial commitment as well. It would be unethical to commit a large number of patients to a study and 5, 10, or even 15 years later find that there are no funds available to allow for collection and processing of data, which are apt to be most meaningful at those times.

The largest financier of cooperative clinical trials in the United States is the National Cancer Institute (NCI). Of a total NCI budget of almost $1 billion in 1980, $35 million was allocated to the entire Clinical Cooperative Group Program, which accounts for the vast majority of trials carried out utilizing all stages of all malignancies. The projected funding for the next few years indicates a minuscule increase overall. It has been estimated that on the average it costs about $2000 per patient in a trial. Such a figure is, of course, variable. Patients on long-term follow-up, such as those on NSABP B-04, which is now in its tenth year, are more expensive than those who are on an advanced disease protocol and who live only 1 or 2 years. On the other hand, surgical protocols are cheaper to carry out than are those evaluating chemotherapy. Until recently, noninvestigational drugs employed in trials were furnished by the NCI at no cost to the patient. Recent fiscal retrenchment will change that policy. Since most clinical trials do not include the use of treatment procedures which are outside of the framework of good medical care, there is ample reason for third-party coverage to defray the patient costs for most of the laboratory tests and commercially available medication. The greatest expense in carrying out a trial is related to the cost of data collection and processing; this is particularly true for a multicenter trial. At each location there must be a staff of well-trained people to procure and transmit data to the central headquarters, where it is collated with that from all of the contributors, reviewed at all levels by trained personnel, and is ultimately analyzed by the statisticians of the project.

The results of a trial are no better than the data collected and analyzed. That function is intimately related to the quality of personnel charged with that responsibility. Such people command greater reimbursement than less highly skilled personnel. Thus, this aspect of the trial requires sufficient funds for doing the job well or not at all. Despite the most noble intent there really is little point to carrying out a trial without sufficient financial support.

Preparation of the Protocol

Once the aims of the trial, the experimental design, and the availability of adequate resources have been decided upon, the next and most vital step is the preparation of a protocol. That document details every aspect of the conduct of the trial. It serves as the reference manual for the investigator. Consequently, in preparing the protocol an attempt is made to anticipate in advance all questions and aspects of the study which will require clarification. From years of experience in protocol preparation it may be stated with assurance that there will always be situations arising during the conduct of a trial which have not been anticipated. Nonetheless, with each successive protocol there are fewer such incidents.

Information contained in a typical NSABP protocol is summarized as follows. The background presents the rationale for the study, with pertinent literature references. In the specific aims there appears the hypothesis which is being tested. Operative procedures and other key terms employed in the study, such as estrogen receptor status, additional therapy (prophylactic, for primary treatment failure or for recurrence) permitted or not permitted, are carefully defined. The primary end points to be used for statistical studies—i.e., treatment failure, and survival and morbidity rates, are listed. Strict documentation of patient eligibility and ineligibility is listed. The material necessary for pathologic studies is described. How and on what basis patients are allocated to treatment groups is carefully described. The parameters required at every phase of the study are listed, and a detailed description of drug administration, duration of treatment, and dose modification appear. Records to be kept, statistical considerations, and a sample consent form are included, as are descriptions of any special studies to be carried out. An example of the contents of a recent NSABP protocol is provided to illustrate the organization of a protocol (Fig. 14-1).

The Randomization Process

Prior to beginning a trial, patients who are eligible for participation are carefully defined. They are then allocated to the treatment and control groups entirely by chance, i.e., by randomization.[10-13] That process is not to be misconstrued as meaning that patients are assigned in a haphazard fashion or that randomization is a simplistic procedure that can be carried out without planning. There are a variety of techniques available for randomizing patients. Some are unacceptable because of the actual or potential bias which they may introduce, whereas others are satisfactory in that they ensure that the treatment allocation is not subjected to the personal

FIGURE 14-1 Table of contents of a clinical trial protocol

Background	1
Plan of Investigation	3
Summary of Study	3
Specific Aims	3
Definitions	4
Endpoints	4
Conduct of Study	5
Selection of Patients	5
Pathologic Studies	7
Allocation of Patients to Treatment Groups	8
Study Parameters	8
Follow-up Studies	10
Postmortem Examination	13
Drug Administration, Duration of Treatment, and Dose Modification	14
Records to be Kept	17
Randomization and Statistical Consideration	17
Patient Consent	17
Proposed Clinical Trials Involving Patients with Pathologically Positive Nodes	18
Table A (Estimated Sample Sizes for Patients with Pathologically Positive Nodes)	18
Drug Information	18A
Bibliography	19
Schema	20
Summary of Study Parameters	22
Patient Consent Form	24
Appendix I: Procedure for ER and PR Assay Collection	26
Appendix II: Collections of Blood Samples for Determination of Ovarian Function	30
Appendix III: Body Surface Area of Adults	36

judgment and prejudices of the investigator and of the patient. Those unfamiliar with the process must realize that for the process to be acceptable neither the physician nor the patient can play a role in determining which of the therapeutic options will be employed. Despite this seeming lack of involvement, the physician plays a key role in the process. It is the physician who, following careful evaluation, determines whether the patient is or is not eligible for participation in the trial and is thus an appropriate candidate for submission to randomization.

That action by the physician is of fundamental importance. It could be a source of bias that would affect the credibility of a trial relative to the population to which the findings relate, or it may influence the trial's ability to identify important differences. If, for example, breast cancer patients of a certain predetermined type were to be allocated (1) according to the day of the month they were admitted to the hospital, (2) by assigning alternative cases to each of the groups, (3) by utilizing the last digit of the hospital number or the first letter of the surname, or the month of birth, there would be the possibility that concealed differences could occur between the treatment groups. By using those methods the treatment allocation could be determined before the decision to enter the patient to the study was made. Thus, with this a priori knowledge regarding the treatment the physician would have the opportunity by using clinical judgment to determine that a particular patient was not a candidate for the study because the treatment group to which the patient would be assigned was inappropriate for that particular individual. The physician could withhold admission until the "right day," or until the patient was assured of receiving the "right" treatment by noting the treatment received by the previous patient, or by not entering the patient in the study at all.

Other possibilities for randomization include the flipping of a coin, the drawing of a slip of paper from a container, or other less elegant means which are not in the best interest of good doctor-patient relationships and which could afford physicians with opportunity for bias. In early NSABP trials the use of sealed, serially numbered opaque envelopes was effectively employed. As each patient was deemed eligible, the next envelope in the stack was opened and the card inside indicated the treatment to be used. The sequencing of the cards was determined from a table of random numbers. While this method may be satisfactory, it is not ideal. If the stack of cards is available to the investigator who is delivering the therapy, the possibility exists that the contents of an envelope may become known *prior* to patient entry on a trial. The use of such a procedure in a multicenter trial causes procedural problems. Attempting to keep track of individual series of envelopes at 50 or more institutions is not easily accomplished.

The randomization procedure found to be preferable by the NSABP in its recent generation of clinical trials involving about 70 institutions and many thousands of patients is that which is carried out entirely by telephone contact by an investigator or a designate with the Headquarters Statistical Center, i.e., "central" randomization. When a patient is deemed eligible, telephone contact is made and the treatment assignment is carried out. A computer-generated, random treatment assignment is used for that purpose. Prior to making the assignment, however, the randomizer reviews a checklist of major eligibility requirements with the individual entering the patient to ensure that they have been met. While in the long run sequences based on random numbers will result in approximately equal numbers in the groups, there may by chance be a fairly large imbalance. To prevent this, the statistician may introduce methods for correction by restoring balance after the entry of each block of a fixed number of patients.

Another approach to achieving balance of the groups is to decide prior to beginning the study which factors it is most important that there be equivalence in. In a breast cancer trial, for example, it is known that patient age, number of axillary nodes involved with tumor, and estrogen receptor status of tumors may all affect prognosis. Consequently, in order to establish equality of the groups, patients are *stratified* according to those variables. Thus, a similar proportion of patients in each of the groups will be apt to contain, for example, patients 49 years of age or less and 50 years of age or more, or patients with 1 to 3 positive axillary nodes and 4 or more positive nodes. By employing a separate randomization sequence for each prognostic stratum, such balance may be achieved. There obviously comes a point where stratification by too many prognostic variables results in a loss of power as well as in procedural difficulties. In order to overcome this limitation, methods have been developed to adapt the randomization of patients while the trial is accruing patients to compensate for imbalance in prognostic factors within treatment groups. Such approaches are becoming increasingly used, especially for small-sized trials where stratification to ensure balance is not feasible. In addition, heterogeneity in prognostic factors not accounted for a priori can be considered at the time of analysis in order to avoid either false-positive or false-negative findings attributable to imbalance. Stratification a priori or at analysis also serves to improve the efficiency of comparisons by identifying those patients most or least likely to have recurrences.

Despite the convincing justification for having simultaneous control groups when conducting trials, as well as for ensuring that neither the investigator nor the patient is aware at the time of initial registration of the specific treatment to be administered, there are times when practical considerations make such efforts almost impossible. Nowhere is this better demonstrated than in the current NSABP protocol (B-06) evaluating the worth of lumpectomy. In that protocol patients are randomized to receive either total mastectomy plus axillary dissection, segmental mastectomy (lumpectomy) plus axillary dissection, or segmental mastectomy plus axillary dissection plus breast radiation. For a time patient accrual into the protocol was so low that there was serious question regarding the likelihood of ever accruing a sufficient number of patients. Physicians were reluctant to ask women to participate in a trial which *following* patient consent would result in chance assignment to surgical therapies as diverse as having a breast removed or merely having a lumpectomy. Needless to say, patients also had difficulty in dealing with such a presentation. In some instances, neither patients nor physicians were certain that a breast cancer was present, yet they were asked to consider participation in a trial in which if cancer was found at operation they could wake up with or without a breast. Since it was deemed that this trial was one of the most important ever conducted relative to breast cancer and should be carried to completion, several alternative approaches to the conventional randomization procedure were considered. It was finally decided that "prerandomization" afforded a satisfactory compromise.[14]

In the usual randomization procedure, the physician will, after determining the patient's eligibility, explain the protocol, including all treatment possibilities, and obtain the patient's consent to be randomized. After the patient signs the consent form, the physician contacts the randomization office and receives the treatment assignment. The prerandomization procedure differs in that after verifying patient eligibility for the trial, the physician will telephone the randomization office and receive a treatment assignment *before* presenting the protocol to the patient. The trial is then explained to the patient. All treatment options are made known just as in the more conventional presentation. The patient is informed, however, that if participation is agreed upon the treatment to be received is the one which has already been randomly selected. Just as in the conventionally randomized trial, the patient is told that the therapy was determined by randomization. It is only at this point that the informed consent is obtained. If the patient does not wish to receive the assigned therapy, that patient is considered a "refusal" in the assigned treatment arm. Even should the patient refuse the assigned therapy, it is crucial that data relative to patient characteristics, subsequent treatment, and follow-up be submitted to permit evaluation. Further, for analysis the patient must be kept in the group to which she or he was randomized.

In order for the prerandomization procedure to be credible several conditions must be met. Refusals must be kept to a very low rate within each treatment if the final groups are to be considered as "randomized" for treatment comparisons. Total estimated sample sizes require inflation to allow for the additional "losses" due to the anticipated refusals, since a decrease in the ability to detect differences among the randomized treatment groups occurs as a result of the refusals. As a result of the implementation of prerandomization, patient accrual has increased. It is strongly emphasized, however, that prerandomization is a compromise procedure instituted to cope with an unusual circumstance. It is not a mechanism recommended for replacement of conventional methods of randomization.

Another proposal aimed at resolving the dilemma for those clinical investigators who decline to participate in randomized studies because they believe that patient-physician relationships become compromised by such involvement has been described by Zelen.[15] This method is especially suited for comparison of a best standard or control treatment with an experimental treatment. It does not, however, eliminate randomization since eligible patients are initially allocated into two groups by this mechanism. Those assigned by randomization to group A receive standard treatment and, according to Zelen, are not approached for consent to enter the trial. Those in group B are asked if they will participate in the trial and if they will accept the experimental therapy. If they decline the "new" therapy, they receive the standard therapy. A modification that might be introduced is that those randomized to group B, rather than being presented with the opportunity to receive an experimental therapy, are presented with the two therapies and are asked to make a choice, i.e., between the standard and the new therapy. It is Zelen's opinion that such a design represents a valid randomized trial. There are obviously certain ethical issues raised by this approach which do not exist in the prerandomization procedure as carried out by the NSABP. In analyzing the results obtained by these new approaches, findings from patients in group A are compared with the overall results obtained in group B which represent a compilation of findings from those receiving both the standard and the experimental therapies. Only by including *all* patients in group B is the comparison valid, even though it dilutes the measurable effect of the new treatment. Other analytic problems are addressed by Zelen.

Zelen has pointed out that at least three ethical issues arise from his method. Should patients assigned to group A without their knowledge be informed as to why they are getting the standard treatment? Should permission be obtained to use the data from patients in this group? Is it proper to offer the experimental treatment to only one-half of the patients in group B?

As far as is known Zelen's technique has not yet been used to conduct a clinical trial. Whether it will take its place as a viable alternative for the more conventional randomization procedure or for the prerandomization approach is speculative.

The Control Group

For a variety of reasons patients and/or physicians remain reluctant to participate in randomized clinical trials. There are those who believe that a patient entered into the control arm of a randomized clinical trial are essentially "wasted" since patients who are comparable in prognosis can be selected retrospectively for the control, thus achieving the same end.[16] The entire issue of the value of such retrospective studies and the use of retrospectively acquired controls has been one of the most contentious in the entire clinical trial process. Arguments relative to the pros and cons of such procedures have been harmful to the acceptance of clinical trials in that they have focused on process rather than on the substantive positive aspects of such undertakings. Be that as it may, it is necessary that a proper control group be employed.

RETROSPECTIVE STUDIES AND HISTORICAL CONTROLS

There are many in positions of leadership in medicine and surgery who still fail to understand the reasons for lack of complete endorsement and full acceptance of findings obtained retrospectively. They are convinced that such actions represent a plot by those who don't *understand* clinical medicine! In 1970 it was emphasized that there is nothing inherently wrong with retrospective studies but that the trouble is with those who ascribe more validity to their findings than they deserve by failing to recognize their purpose and limitations.[17] Just as the prime purpose of laboratory investigation is to provide guidelines and clues as to what might be expected to occur when such studies are applied to the human, so may the results of retrospective clinical analyses supply hints for future definitive evaluation. No better is this exemplified than when one considers the worth of lumpectomy for breast cancer. The reports of Crile,[17a] Peters,[17b] Mustakallio,[17c] and others describing experience with the procedure following a retrospective examination of their records are of such a nature. They are directly akin to findings obtained from phase II trials of chemotherapy. They have made available "suggestive evidence" that such a procedure could be of value, at least in some subsets of patients, and thus have provided the justification for carrying out a properly conceived, prospective clinical trial with randomization of similar patients so that one group receive the lumpectomy and the other the present standard therapy. Until information is so obtained, there will always be doubt regarding the merits of the procedure.

There is little argument that conclusions derived by comparing two separate retrospectively accumulated studies are apt to be meaningless because one cannot be sure of the comparability of the patients being compared. A perusal of the literature of a decade or two ago regarding the surgical treatment of breast cancer makes the point. There is absolutely no way that a comparison of, for example, findings by Haagensen[17d] relative to radical mastectomy can be compared with, for example, those of Crile[17a] or Peters[17b] regarding lumpectomy or simple mastectomy. The equivalence of the patients being compared cannot possibly be completely ascertained, whereas randomization allows one to compute a probability that two groups are comparable both on known and unknown factors.

Is a conclusion derived following the comparison of end results from a prospectively accumulated data set with those from a nonconcurrent (historical) control valid, or must the control always be simultaneous? There are situations in which nonrandomized studies are appropriate. In phase I studies, where the aim is to explore the feasibility of administering a new therapy and where toxicity and dose of drug are being assessed, there is no need for a randomized study. A similar situation prevails in phase II trials, which are preliminary studies of therapeutic effectiveness. In a disease in which the prognosis is so predictably poor that any improvement could only be ascribed to the treatment, no control group would be required. For trials of adjuvant therapy or surgery in stages I and II breast cancer, on the other hand, a simultaneous control is not only appropriate but mandatory. There can be no guarantee that historical controls are so similar that increments of gain—e.g., 10 percent, 15 percent, or even 20 percent—are the results of the therapy and not due to some difference in patients or even the nature of the disease. Pocock[18] collated results from 19 studies where consecutive trials at the same institutions with a common arm from one trial to the next had been done. In comparing the same arm from earlier to later trials, he found 10 of the 19 had two-sided p values $< .2$ and 3 of 19 $< .02$. Only four p values $<.2$ would have been expected by chance alone. The argument relative to simultaneous vs. historical controls in trials evaluating primary operable breast cancer patients had almost precipitously become a moot point. With recent evidence indicating the importance of tumor estrogen receptor (ER) status as an important prognostic factor, it is now necessary that randomization procedures and data evaluation take that variable into account. Since in no historical control group is such information yet available that has been accumulated over a prolonged time period, it would be impossible to use such patients as controls and hope that the qualitative and quantitative ER values are similar to those which are known to be present in the current group being evaluated. The major problem with retrospective controls is that during the time information was collected on such patients it was never anticipated that it would be used for such a purpose. Consequently, it is apt to be incomplete and unreliable.

BLINDING AND THE USE OF PLACEBOS

After treatments have been randomly assigned to patients, it is necessary that steps be taken to ensure that biases do not occur as the trial progresses, i.e., during the treatment of patients and at the time of evaluation of the outcome of therapy. So that those treating a patient do not subconsciously or consciously influence the results by subtly managing patients on one therapy arm differently from those on another, and in order to ensure that patients do not introduce biases, clinical trials are conducted in a single- or double-blind fashion when possible. In the former the patient is unaware of whether she or he is in the treatment or control group, but the physician is knowledgeable. In the latter neither the physician nor the patient is aware of which treatment the patient has received. In certain drug trials this can be accomplished by administration of a tablet identical to that under test except that it does not contain the active ingredient. Such a preparation is called a *placebo,* from the Latin word meaning "I will please." In the 1947 edition of *Dorland's Illustrated Dictionary* it was defined as "a makebelieve medicine given to please or gratify the patient." In the 1965 edition it was considered to be "an inactive substance or preparation, formerly given to please or gratify a patient, now also used in controlled studies to determine the efficacy of medicinal substances." For obvious reasons, in most trials with cancer patients such double-blind techniques are not feasible or relevant. It is rarely suitable to have patients with advanced cancer receive no treatment. In early disease, placebo injections or sham operations can rarely be justified. Consequently, its use is appropriate only when oral medication is being employed. Even under such circumstances rarely will the study remain blind for very long. With more or less effort both the physician and the patient are apt to be able to recognize which treatment is being employed. The side effects which are characteristic of the drug give it away. Thus, only drugs with minimal toxicity may be appropriate for use in such a way. Obviously, surgical trials defy the use of blinding. The comparison of radical mastectomy with lumpectomy, for example, could never be carried out in such fashion!

A current NSABP protocol evaluating the effectiveness of tamoxifen in axillary node-negative breast cancer patients who are estrogen-receptor-positive is being carried out in attempt to maintain double-blindedness. This trial is a two-arm study. Patients are randomized to receive either a placebo or tamoxifen. There is a special rationale for doing this. Because of the expected low rate of recurrence in node-negative patients with ER-positive tumors, it is essential that both patient groups be managed according to their assigned treatment. If only a relatively few more patients who are assigned to receive no medication are switched to tamoxifen or to some other nonprotocol therapy because of physician bias, the likelihood of determining differences in results between the groups is diminished to a point where the trial becomes "no contest." The double-blind methodology is not expected to reduce the overall incidence of crossovers with respect to nonprotocol therapy, but it will eliminate the potential for bias and obscuring treatment differences which would exist if noncompliance with protocol therapy occurred selectively in one of the groups.

In general, only where the assessment of the course of a disease is highly subjective is it likely that the advantages to be gained by a double-blind trial are apt to be substantial. In patients with solid tumors the difficulties and associated impossibilities will, as already mentioned, preclude the use of blinding techniques very often. In one of the early trials of adjuvant chemotherapy conducted by the NSABP its use led to interesting findings. Patients were randomized to placebo or oral L-PAM therapy. It was surprising that a substantial proportion of patients receiving the placebo displayed toxicity similar to that displayed by L-PAM–treated patients.[19]

Since knowledge of a treatment program can subconsciously affect a clinician's assessment of a patient, it would be ideal, but not practical, for a patient's assessment to be carried out by an observer unassociated with the therapy administered. In a trial, for example, evaluating radical mastectomy with a lesser procedure or a chemotherapy regimen with another, a participant who favors one type of treatment over another could quite possibly be less stringent about the criteria employed for documenting a recurrence in those patients receiving the less-favored therapy. Such patients may be more rapidly designated as treatment failures and started on other therapy than are patients in the group receiving the favored therapy.

Ethical and Related Considerations

As Moore so aptly put it more than a decade ago, "If a teaching hospital or a university medical school is doing its job and carrying out its responsibility to the public, it must be involved with initial trials and therapeutic innovations that raise ethical problems."[20] Rutstein carries this further: "If the question under study is an ethical one, and if the design of study is sound, taking both the ethical and scientific constraints into consideration, controlled studies when indicated impose fewer ethical problems than uncontrolled human experiments."[21] By the same token he suggests, "It may be accepted as a maxim that a poorly or improperly designed study involving human subjects ... is by definition unethical. Moreover when a study is in itself scientifically invalid, all other ethical considerations become irrelevant. There is no point in obtaining informed consent to perform a useless study." In this era of consumerism and the dominance of a legalistic society there is ample opportunity to debate every aspect of a clinical trial from the beginning of its planning through its termination and ultimate analysis. Such opportunities of course multiply the chances for veto and the attendant risks of stalemate and paralysis. Obviously, the latter must not be permitted to occur since the "winners will be the losers."

What are some of the major issues created by clinical trials which are perceived to be ethical problems?

RELATIVE TO CONTROL GROUPS

There are those who question the ethics of there being a control group in a trial, and are concerned as to how a potentially beneficial treatment can be withheld from a proportion of the patients. In trials of therapy it is customary to use the current "standard" therapy as the control. Thus, control patients are being denied nothing. They are receiving that which is considered to be the best available therapy at the time. Those in the test group are receiving a therapy which is considered to be *potentially* better than the standard therapy but which has not yet been proved to be so. Insofar as therapy for solid tumors is concerned, prior to instituting a full-scale trial, the systemic treatment to be evaluated has or should have undergone animal testing and preliminary testing in humans to determine its effectiveness in a limited setting, e.g., in advanced disease, and should have a biologic (pharmacologic) rationale for its use. The premise prior to testing the new regimen must be that if it is not better it at least is not likely to be worse. It must be acknowledged, however, that in any trial, which *is* a clinical experiment, there exists the possibility that the contemplated better therapy may indeed be less effective. This cannot and should not be denied, nor should such an admission be employed to summarily dismiss clinical trials as unethical. As long as it is not known whether the regimen being evaluated is better than the standard, there can be no charge that a better treatment is being withheld.

Obviously, if the investigator believes that the treatment *is* of more value, then it is unethical for that investigator to participate in a randomized controlled trial evaluating that agent. When a treatment has begun to be used with more regularity than would seem justified by the limited data to support its use, and yet an investigator can honestly state that it is not known whether such a treatment is or is not of value, it is much more ethical for that investigator to participate in a clinical trial to resolve the issue than to submit to peer and/or patient pressure to use the treatment or, equally as bad, to completely turn a deaf ear to the possible benefits of the new therapy.

Over the years, multifaceted trials of the NSABP have forced its members to face such issues many times. When in 1971 a trial to compare radical mastectomy with total mastectomy with and without radiation was instituted, radical mastectomy patients served as the control group since at that time the operation was standard treatment for breast cancer.[22] There were many surgeons who truly believed that anything less than that operation would be harmful to patients; there were others who were convinced beyond a shadow of a doubt that the lesser treatments were absolutely as good. It would have been unethical for surgeons possessing either of those convictions to have participated in that trial and to have randomized their patients so that some received what they thought of as an "inferior" treatment.

A similar situation exists at present relative to the NSABP trial comparing lumpectomy (with or without radiation) with the present standard operation, total mastectomy plus axillary dissection. Despite the emotional fervor surrounding the use of lumpectomy, there remains a question regarding the equivalence of mastectomy and lumpectomy in all patients, and there are no data to indicate whether all lumpectomy patients do or do not need to receive breast radiation. Consequently, there can be no ethical breach by carrying out lumpectomy and radiation on only a proportion of patients. To do otherwise could as reasonably be considered such a violation.

These issues have become even more compelling of consideration in trials of systemic adjuvant chemotherapy. Is it still possible at the present time to randomize[22] patients following operation so that one-half, for example, receive adjuvant chemotherapy and the other half no systemic therapy? The no-therapy group serves as the control. Obviously, it is easier for the physician and for the patient if both groups receive a treatment. It is almost incomprehensible to a patient to be asked to participate in a study in which "something or nothing" is prescribed. The physician, with justification, does not appreciate being placed in that position vis-à-vis the patient. If, however, it is not established beyond a doubt that the therapy to be given to the control group has demonstrated a benefit, justification for its use is tenuous and it is better to remain with the standard therapy, which is "nothing."

CONCERNING PATIENT CONSENT

In the United States, the National Institutes of Health (NIH) require that every patient in every clinical trial carried out under NIH financing give informed consent prior to participation. Moreover, the NIH has further required (1971) that there be an Institutional Review Board (IRB) in every medical facility carrying out clinical investigation that must examine and approve every protocol to ensure that the rights and welfare of patients are protected. The committee is made up of persons knowledgeable in "institutional commitments and regulations, applicable law, standards of professional conduct and practice and community attitudes." These mandates arose in the Nuremberg Code in 1947[23] and were given further impetus by the World Health Organization (WHO) in the Declaration of Helsinki adopted by the Eighteenth World Medical Assembly in 1964.[24] In the decade following the Helsinki Declaration the WHO continued to refine safeguards to human subjects. In addition to advocating freedom of choice without coercion, consent of patient participation was related to an explanation of the risks involved as well as the possible benefits. It was established that it was the obligation of the investigator to see that the study be continually monitored for unexpected risks.

The approval of protocols by such committees, together with the informed consent of patients, are protective not only of the patient but of the physician as well since he or she has shared the burden of deciding whether the experiment is justified and how best to protect the rights of patients. Overall, the mechanism has been highly effective and has helped to uplift human dignity and in all probability has improved the quality of scientific thought. In the United States there would be little support for those who would argue against the principle of patient consent and protocol review by an "impartial" panel. Such has not always been the case in the rest of the world. The philosophy in Great Britain has until the present been as summarized by the following comments by Hill:[25]

Having made up your mind that you are not in any way subjecting either patient to a recognized and unjustifiable danger, pain or discomfort can anything be gained by endeavoring to explain to them your own state of ignorance and to describe the attempts you are making to remove it? . . . Once you have decided that either treatment *for all you know* may be equally well exhibited to the patient's benefit, and without detriment, is there any real basis for seeking consent or refusal?

and by Atkins:[26]

From the point of view of ethics a problem arises of whether patients should be informed that they are taking part in a trial. Often this is desirable, and may in many instances be helpful and encouraging the patient to attend for the frequent examinations that may be demanded in the interests of the trial rather than the patient. Nevertheless, it is not always desirable, and at a meeting of the Medical Research Council which was attended by the Treasury Solicitors, and where the legal and ethical aspects of this matter were considered, it was decided that there was no obligation on the part of an investigator to inform a patient that he was participating in a trial. Particularly is this so in the trial of methods of treatment for desperate cases or advanced disease. If the trial is ethical by the criteria outlined, and if therefore the choice of treatment is really being made by the "toss of a coin," it is not considered to be the best part of doctoring to inform a patient so gravely ill that we do not know how to treat her, and that the choice of treatment is being so determined.

Despite the above comments, there is increasing agreement for having the patient consent. There is less agreement about the process. What should be in the consent form? How can one be sure that the patient understands what he or she is agreeing to? What constitutes "informed"? By 1975 in the United States the ethics of informed consent required that six conditions be met under the surveillance of institutional committees. Patients need to be advised of (1) the procedure to be followed in the study, (2) the anticipated benefits for the individual, (3) the discomforts and risks that are to be "reasonably expected," (4) the alternative methods of therapy, (5) the willingness of the investigator to answer inquiries, and (6) the right to refuse or withdraw from the study without prejudices.

One must fervently hope that these monumental gains do not become so analyzed, politicized, and bureaucratized by those with self-serving interests or causes that they destroy their very purpose, i.e., to protect human rights without impeding the obtaining of knowledge which can be of benefit to humanity. There is no dichotomy of purpose between preservation of human rights and dignity and freedom of inquiry. There must be strict vigilance to ensure that there is no serious conflict between the forces defending subjects' rights and those defending freedom of inquiry. In such a confrontation, once again, "winners may become losers."

DATA INTEGRITY AND CLINICAL TRIALS

It is redundant to emphasize that the results of a trial are only as credible as the data collected. As is so often true in any facet of human activity, exceptions attract attention. Recent publicity has suggested that falsification of information had occurred in the data submitted to the collection center of a group conducting trials.[27] Admittedly one instance is one too many, but when one considers the thousands of physicians participating in hundreds of trials utilizing tens of thousands of patients, even if such an accusation were found true (which has not yet been the case) the incidence of such deception is apt to be very small indeed. To classify what is falsification and what is careless data collection, which is apt to be more prevalent, may be extremely difficult and constitutes another issue. In either instance the consequences for the trial are apt to be the same. They impinge upon the credibility of the trial. The vigilance necessary to ensure reliable data is especially important since the normal rule of science requires replication before a result can be accepted. Independent replication of trials that have taken years and millions of dollars to carry out may be impossible to repeat. Consequently, they must be done right the first time. It is easy to enter patients into clinical trials. It is infinitely more difficult to maintain a level of investigator enthusiasm year after year so that data is collected as meticulously and as thoroughly at the fifth year of study, for example, as at the fifth week. It is the obligation of those who institute and carry out a trial, as well as of those who participate, to develop and cooperate in mechanisms to ensure the integrity of the data. Such efforts should not be considered by the investigator as adversary or demonstrating lack of trust. Rather, they are to achieve impeccability.

ADVANTAGES IN CLINICAL TRIAL PARTICIPATION

There are certain advantages to both patients and physicians who participate in clinical trials. Since, as previously pointed out, the clinical trial is almost always the product of a multiplicity of expert physicians, the patient is in effect, by participating, receiving the synthesis of multiple consultations or "second opinions." In addition, patients on trials can be assured of a most careful pretherapy evaluation and follow-up carried out in a logical, organized fashion.

When patients are provided with appropriate information about a study to aid them in making an intelligent decision, there is created an opportunity for enhancement of the doctor-patient relationship. Increased respect and confidence in the doctor by the patient is apt to occur. It becomes more firm than that resulting when authoritarianism is responsible for the interaction. At a time when uncertainty exists relative to what should be done, clinical trials afford the physician with a mechanism for rational therapeutic management. Finally, not inconsequential to some patients, is the satisfaction they derive from participation in trials by knowing that they could be making a contribution to knowledge which may be of help to others.

DATA EVALUATION

The outcome of interest in cancer clinical trials frequently involves analysis of an event, such as recurrence or death, that is time-related. Appropriate analysis of the data must take into account the time at which the event occurred. Statistical theory dealing with these issues is sometimes referred to as *failure time* or *life-table analysis*. Although a detailed discussion of this topic is beyond the present scope, some understanding of the methods is useful for reading and interpreting the literature. A brief summary of basic points is presented here, while for more comprehensive treatment of the basic methodology the reader is referred to the articles by Cutler and Ederer[28] and Petro et al.[29]

In calculating survival rates to some point in time after entry to the study, the basic data consist of times. For those who die, it is the time of death. Since, generally, not everyone has been followed to death, the times for some individuals are the known survival (follow-up) times. If all patients were followed to death, it would be a simple matter to plot survival vs. time on study. Even where not all patients have died but have been followed for at least some minimum time since entry on study, it is possible to obtain a direct estimate of the probability of surviving to that minimum time, say 5 years. For example, if among N patients who have all been followed for at least 5 years since entry to the study the number of deaths occurring within the first 5 years is D, the proportion surviving 5 or more years (P_5) is equal to $(N - D)/N$.

However, not all patients enter on study at the same time; hence, some of the N patients will attain 5 years of observation sooner than others. One could calculate a 5-year survival rate similar to that shown above, but based only upon those patients who have been under observation for 5 or more years (N_5). In calculating this survival proportion, only those deaths occurring in patients who had been under observation for at least 5 years (P_5) would be included, or

$$P_5 = \frac{N_5 - D_5}{N_5}$$

From a statistical standpoint this method of calculation is wasteful, since it ignores the information on those patients who have been on study for less than 5 years but who could have contributed to a 1-year, 2-year, etc., estimate of survival if these had been calculated. Since P_5 is based on only a subgroup of all patients followed, its standard error will be larger than if one were able to take into account the partial information supplied by those patients who have been observed less than 5 years.

In order to use this additional data, the chance of surviving for 5 years must be visualized in the following way. Let us consider that P_1 is the proportion surviving the first year for patients followed 1 year or more, P_2 is the proportion surviving the second year for patients who did not die in the first year and who were followed the second year, P_3 is the proportion surviving the third year for patients who did not die in the preceding 2 years and who were followed the third year, and so on.

Surviving for 5 years implies surviving the first year *and* the second year *and* the third year *and* the fourth year *and* the fifth year after entry to the study, or translated into a formula,

$$P_5 = P_1 \times P_2 \times P_3 \times P_4 \times P_5$$

since the use of *and* means multiplication of appropriate probabilities. (If the multiplication is not obvious, consider tossing two coins. The chance is one-half of getting heads on the first coin *and* one-half of getting heads on the second; the chance of getting two heads is one-fourth, or $\frac{1}{2} \times \frac{1}{2}$. This can be considered analogous to survival over two time periods, where if the chance of surviving the first interval is P_1, the chance of surviving the second is $P_1 \times P_2$.) When the times to death are grouped into intervals, as in the preceding illustration, the resulting survival distribution is referred to as an *actuarial life table*. On the other hand, one may present the data in an ungrouped fashion so that the distinct time of each death is apparent. The latter are usually referred to as Kaplan-Meier life tables.

Several comments on this method of expressing survival for 5 or more years are as follows:

1. We can now use times for patients who have less than 5 full years of observation. Follow-up times may be expressed in any time unit, such as months *or* days, and the same logic will apply. Since the method assumes that those who have not been observed for the full observation period will have the same survival experience as those who have been observed, there is a need to assure that follow-up is up to date and that no biases exist in reporting of information in the treatment groups.
2. In the situation where all patients have at least 5 years of observation, this formula will give results identical to the direct method first shown.
3. Certain other complexities enter into interpretation of life tables, such as consideration of patients lost to follow-up, whose experience may not be the same as that of patients who are followed. If the losses are substantial, then uncertainty relative to the extent of bias that may be associated with the life-table estimates detracts from the firmness of any treatment comparisons.
4. The number of patients under observation at various points in the survival curve is useful information for evaluating the reliability of any plateaus or sudden drops in the curves. More often than not, the life-table curves shown in the literature have too few observations to draw conclusions about the longest intervals shown.
5. Methods have been developed that allow adjustment for other prognostic factors when comparing life-table curves of treatment groups. The use of such techniques, particularly in randomized trials where an imbalance is present or in trials utilizing nonrandomized controls, is important to ascertain the extent to which observed treatment differences may be ascribable to the other known risk factors.

Simple graphical display of the life-table curve with percentage of patients disease-free on a *logarithmic scale* can provide a useful display of how patients fail with time. If the plot is approximately linear on a logarithmic scale, then the patients on that therapy are failing at a constant rate. If such a trend continues, one can infer that eventually all patients will show recurrence, i.e., therapy has not cured anyone. If the life-table plot has a steeper slope early in follow-up and becomes less steep later in follow-up, then the failure rate is slowing down with time. Conversely, if the life-table plot exhibits a less steep slope in the initial period with a steeper slope later on, the failure rates are increasing with time. A particular life table may have patterns indicative of several increasing or decreasing trends over time. Therefore, one can consider from the logarithmic life-table graphs whether there is an increase in the failure rate of patients when they go off chemotherapy at 2 years. By comparing life tables of placebo- with drug-treated patients, one can infer how the pattern in failure rates has been altered by chemotherapy. Another point of interest in comparing two or more curves is whether the failure rates are the same for certain time intervals. A period of time where the life-table plots appear parallel on a logarithmic scale indicates that the patients in the groups compared have similar failure rates for that time interval. Interpretations from the *arithmetic plots* of the life tables that are frequently presented in the literature are limited to the absolute value of the survival time and differences in survival rates over time.

Probability Values and Statistical Tests of Life Tables

All probability values depend upon carrying out a test of a hypothesis. The hypothesis is generally framed negatively for statistical analysis, e.g., the null hypothesis of no difference between two treatment regimens. Prior to actual testing of the data, it is necessary for the statistician in conjunction with the clinical investigator to determine how large the differences should be to be considered clinically important. There is little reason to test differences that are too small to be clinically significant. There is also a need to decide upon what p value would be sufficiently small to provide reasonable evidence for concluding that a difference exists. Conventional levels are .05 and .01, but these are arbitrary and may be too conservative or too extreme depending upon the particular situation.

The probability values quoted may be either the exact probability level resulting from the test or whether the test result is above or below some predetermined cutoff, say $p < .05$. The value reported is the smallest level at which the observations are significant in a particular direction. *This probability denotes the chance that the observed results are attributable solely to random fluctuations.* The p value does *not* denote the probability that the treatments are equivalent. If exact values are stated, individual investigators can use these probability values when deciding whether or not to reject the null hypothesis, i.e., when they are deciding whether or not they have a "statistically significant" result.

Since a test is either one-sided or two-sided, one must decide which deviations are of concern. For instance, a two-sided test might be used to look for significant beneficial *or* detrimental effects of an experimental therapy, while a one-sided test might be desired if one wants to examine whether or not a new therapy is equivalent to or better than the old therapy.

There is disagreement among statisticians concerning the use of one-sided vs. two-sided tests. For example, a two-sided test acknowledges that a drug might have a detrimental effect and is a more conservative test, while a one-sided test may be more descriptive. (Note that the p value for a two-sided test can be obtained by doubling the p value from a one-sided test.)

Another reason for regarding probability levels with conservatism is that occasional preliminary examination of data prior to final analysis leads to the computed p value being an underestimate of the actual p value because of multiplicity of comparisons. Thus, if an investigator makes a large number of comparisons, the probability that at least one chance significance will occur becomes greater than the actual computed p value.[30] An exact p value cannot be given for these preliminary examinations. A rule of thumb recommended by some statisticians is to mentally double or triple the quoted p value associated with preliminary reports.[31]

The data of most interest for statistical purposes are the times to failure or death, since two groups might have for statistical purposes identical total numbers of failures at the end of observation but quite dissimilar times to failure, if treatment results in *delaying* progression of disease rather than preventing recurrence. There are several methods for testing the times to failure. Two common approaches are the log rank test[32] and the Wilcoxon test as generalized by Gehan.[33] These tests are usually preferred by statisticians to t tests of the differences between the life-table curves at specific points in time, since the entire pattern of the curves is considered.

One final caution about probability values is that it is very easy to rely too heavily on them and ignore other relevant aspects of the data. The probability values should be viewed as only one important piece of information in an analysis.

REFERENCES

1. Dowling HF: The emergence of the cooperative clinical trial. *Trans Stud Coll Physicians Phila* 43:20, 1975.
2. Bull JP: The historical development of clinical therapeutic trials. *J Chronic Dis* 10:218, 1959.
3. Louis PCA: *Essay on Clinical Instruction*, P Martin (trans), Highley, London, 1834, pp 26–28.
4. Mainland D: The rise of experimental statistics and the problems of a medical statistician. *Yale J Biol Med* 27:1, 1954.

5. Fisher RA: *Statistical Methods for Research Workers,* 1st ed, Oliver and Boyd, Edinburgh, London, 1925.
6. Fisher RA: *The Design of Experiments,* 1st ed, Oliver and Boyd, Edinburgh, London, 1935.
7. Medical Research Council: Streptomycin treatment of pulmonary tuberculosis. *Br Med J* 2:769, 1948.
8. George S, Desu MM: Planning the size and duration of a clinical trial: Studying the time to some critical event. *J Chronic Dis* 27:15, 1974.
9. Pasternak BS, Gilbert HS: Planning the duration of long-term survival time studies designed for accrual by cohorts. *J Chronic Dis* 24:681, 1971.
10. Byar DP et al: Randomized clinical trials: Perspectives on some recent ideas. *N Engl J Med* 295:74, 1976.
11. Chalmers TC: Symposium on diseases of the liver: Randomization of the first patient. *Med Clin North Am* 59:1035, 1975.
12. Ederer F: The randomized controlled clinical trial. *Am J Ophthalmol* 79:752, 1975.
13. Lasagna L: The controlled clinical trial: Theory and practice. *J Chronic Dis* 1:353, 1955.
14. Redmond CK, Bauer M: Statisticians report, in *NSABP Progress Report,* May 1980, pp. 69–72.
15. Zelen M: A new design for randomized clinical trials. *N Engl J Med* 300:1242, 1979.
16. Gehan EA, Freireich EJ: Non-randomized controls in cancer clinical trials. *N Engl J Med* 290:198, 1974.
17. Fisher B: The surgical dilemma in the primary therapy of invasive breast cancer: A critical appraisal. *Curr Prob Surg,* October 1970.
17a. Crile G Jr: Treatment of breast cancer by local excision. *Am J Surg* 109:400, 1965.
17b. Peters MV: Wedge resection and irradiation, an effective treatment in early breast cancer. *J Am Med Assoc* 200:134, 1967.
17c. Mustakallio S: Treatment of breast cancer by tumor extirpation and roentgen therapy instead of radical operation. *J Fac Radiologists* 6:23, 1954.
17d. Haagensen CD, Cooley E: Radical mastectomy for mammary carcinoma. *Ann Surg* 170:884, 1969.
18. Peto R et al: Design and analysis of randomized clinical trials requiring prolonged observation of each patient, I: Introduction and design. *Br J Cancer* 34:585, 1976.
19. Glass A et al: Acute toxicity during adjuvant chemotherapy for breast cancer: The National Surgical Adjuvant Breast and Bowel Project (NSABP) experience from 1717 patients receiving single and multiple agents. *Cancer Treat Rep* 65:363, 1981.
20. Moore FD: Ethical aspects of human experimentation. *Daedalus J Am Acad Arts Sci* Spring, 502, 1969.
21. Rutstein DR: ibid, p 523.
22. Fisher B et al: The contribution of recent NSABP clinical trials of primary breast cancer therapy to an understanding of tumor biology—An overview of findings. *Cancer* 46:1009, 1980.
23. *Trials of War Criminals Before the Nuerenberg Military Tribunals,* vol. 2, United States Government Printing Office, 1949.
24. World Medical Association: The significance of the declaration of Helsinki: An interpretive commentary. *World Med J* 25:58, 1978.
25. Hill AB: Medical ethics and controlled trials. *Br Med J* 1:1043, 1963.
26. Atkins H: Conduct of a controlled clinical trial. *Br Med J* 2:377, 1966.
27. Meinert CL: Clinical trials and data integrity. *Controlled Clin Trials* 1:189, 1980.
28. Cutler SJ, Ederer F: Maximum utilizing of the life table method in analyzing survival. *J Chronic Dis* 8:699, 1958.
29. Peto R et al: Design and analysis of randomized clinical trials requiring prolonged observation of each patient, II: Analysis and examples. *Br J Cancer* 35:1, 1977.
30. Tukey JW: Some thoughts on clinical trials, especially on problems of multiplicity. *Science* 198:679, 1977.
31. McPherson K: Statistics: The problem of examining accumulating data more than once. *N Engl J Med* 290:591, 1974.
32. Peto R, Peto J: Asymptotically efficient rank invariant test procedures. *J R Statist Soc* A135:185, 1972.
33. Gehan EA: A generalized Wilcoxon test for comparing arbitrarily single-censored samples. *Biometrika* 42:203, 1965.

PART TWO

TUMORS OF THE HEAD AND NECK

15
CANCER OF THE TONGUE, LIPS, AND ORAL CAVITY

Elliot Strong   *Ronald H. Spiro*

Cancer of the head and neck is an uncommon disease. According to American Cancer Society estimates,[1] the oral cavity gives rise to 5 percent of all cancers in men and 2 percent of all cancers in women. The overall incidence has remained relatively constant, but the proportion of women with oral and laryngeal cancer seems to be increasing.[2] In an anatomic area so readily accessible for examination without special and expensive diagnostic equipment, it is unfortunate that many patients still present with advanced cancer. Since the prognosis is so intimately related to stage of disease,[2] it seems mandatory to encourage patients to present for evaluation at the earliest stage of abnormality and to encourage their medical and dental advisors to perform a complete head and neck examination. The detection, diagnosis, and prompt treatment of early cancers will result in improved survival.

Treatment must be directed to effective disease eradication with preservation of as near normal cosmetic and functional status as possible. Patients with one head and neck cancer run a significant risk of incurring a second cancer, either in the head and neck or elsewhere[2] and must be carefully followed for the remainder of their lives at sufficiently frequent intervals that such neoplasms can be detected early and treated appropriately. Head and neck cancer is in large part a preventable disease,[3] but given the social habits and mores of our population, its eradication is unlikely. Those patients at high risk must be encouraged to submit to periodic examination. Only by such efforts can the morbidity and mortality of oral cancer be reduced.

HISTORY

Oral cancer has been recognized for centuries. The Ebers Papyrus (approximately 1500 B.C.) refers to "eating ulcers" of the gums and of "illness of the tongue," and Hippocrates (460–370 B.C.) described "chronic ulcers at the borders of the tongue—often related to sharp teeth" which were probably malignant. Alexander Reade published the first definitive case report of tongue cancer in England in 1635. With the prevalence of syphilis and the increasing consumption of alcohol and of tobacco after its introduction in England in 1586, the incidence of tongue cancer, and presumably other oral cancers, increased in Europe during the eighteenth and nineteenth centuries. What role the consumption of hot tea and coffee and the increasing use of spices had is uncertain. With relative increase in life expectancy the incidence of oral cancer also rose.[4]

Prior to the seventeenth century most oral cancer was untreated. Amputation of the tongue as punishment for blasphemy was practiced by certain early religious fanatics, who were astonished at the ability of victims to rehabilitate their speech and deglutition. By the eighteenth century there were many references to extirpative procedures on the tongue using cautery, strangulating ligatures, ecraseurs, and caustics. Langenbeck introduced the scalpel "V" excision of the tongue with closure in 1819. Other authors described other surgical approaches to the oral cavity. Bilroth, Kocher, and Langenbeck introduced approaches through the submandibular and suprahyoid areas for more adequate excision. By 1908, Butlin could describe his personal series of 197 patients operated for cancer of the tongue of whom 55 lived for 3 to 22 years without recurrence. Subsequent reports described refinement in case selection and treatment methods while accumulating large series of patients.[4] In his classic paper in 1906, George Crile described his personal series of 132 patients who underwent systematic excision of cervical lymph nodes for head and neck cancer, thus establishing radical neck dissection as a standard surgical procedure.[5]

Roentgen discovered x-rays in 1895 and the Curies discovered radium in 1897. By 1902, Beck suggested tongue cancer could be suitably treated with radiation. Dominicci, in 1908, described the radium pack, and Stevenson, in 1914, reported the interstitial use of radioactive sources. Thus, the foundations for the treatment of oral cancer by radiation were established.[4] The use of combinations of radiation and surgery soon followed, and the twentieth century has seen the increasing use of multidisciplinary efforts to attempt control of the scourge of oral cancer.

INCIDENCE, ETIOLOGY, AND EPIDEMIOLOGY

The geographic variations in the incidence of oral cancer are great. Many of these seem to be related to social habits and customs, with a lesser influence of environment, diet, and nutrition. Although the precise etiology of mouth cancer is unknown, the observed variations seem to be related to certain factors.[3,6–8]

Tobacco

The incidence of oral squamous cancer appears to be directly related to the use of tobacco in any form. In the United States, the relative risk of mouth cancer in both sexes increases with the amount smoked and the duration of the exposure.[3,8,9] The incidence of oral carcinoma among cigarette smokers is estimated to be six times that of nonsmokers.[8–10] Further evidence of the influence of smoking comes from Moore's report[11] of patients "cured" of their first oral cancer. In those who continued to smoke, a second cancer developed in tobacco-contact tissues in 40 percent, while in those who stopped smoking similar cancers developed in only 6 percent. Moreover, the overall survival rates were significantly higher in those who stopped smoking compared to those who did not.

More intimate mucosal contact with tobacco is seen in certain regions. In parts of India, the Philippines, Venezuela, and Panama reverse smoking is practiced, wherein the lighted end of the cigarette is inserted into the mouth. The incidence of cancer of the hard palate seems to be significantly higher in these patients.[7] The use of snuff, raw tobacco, held against the oral mucous membranes, particularly by women in the southern United States, produces a characteristic type of verrucous carcinoma typically involving the buccal mucosa.[6] In India and other areas of southern Asia, the high incidence of oral carcinoma, particularly of the buccal mucosa, appears to be related to the use of a compound of dried and cured tobacco leaf with pan (powdered betal and betal leaves coated with slaked lime). These cancers, almost uniformly of low histologic grade, occur in the oral cavity adjacent to the retained quid, most prominently in the buccal mucosa but also in the oral tongue.[7,12] The quid is kept in these areas for hours, producing intimate and prolonged mucosal contact.

Alcohol

The relationship of alcohol consumption to oral squamous carcinoma has been long recognized.[3,8,13,14] The increased incidence of oral cancer with increasing alcohol consumption has been documented.[13–16] The combination of tobacco and alcohol exposure increases the risk of oral cancer for an individual over that of nonsmoking teetotallers by as much as 20 times.[14,15] Mashberg and associates[16] have recently concluded that heavy drinkers may be at greater risk of oral cancer than heavy smokers and that beer and wine may be greater risk factors than whiskey in the development of oral cancer. The precise mechanism(s) by which the risks are increased is unknown.[14]

Nutrition

Nutritional deficiencies, from either undernutrition and/or as a direct result of alcohol intake producing impaired absorption or enhanced elimination, may play a role in the etiology of head and neck cancer. In Scandinavia a high incidence of cancer of the upper alimentary track associated with sideropenia and anemia—Plummer-Vinson syndrome—was noted in the absence of exposure to other recognized carcinogens. Deficiencies of iron and vitamins were recognized, and appropriate public health measures have significantly lessened the incidence of the syndrome and its associated cancers.[4] Degenerative mucosal changes occur in riboflavin-deficient rats similar to those seen with Plummer-Vinson syndrome. As the epithelial deficiency increases, the pathologic changes progress from atrophy to hyperkeratosis and, in some instances, to hyperplasia. Vitamin A has been shown to be important in the maturation of epithelial tissues, and its deficiency may predispose to neoplastic epithelial changes. Dietary zinc deficiency in laboratory animals has rendered them more susceptible to carcinogenic stimuli, particularly with respect to cancer of the esophagus.[14] Further research may better identify the role of nutritional deficiencies in the genesis of oral cancer.

Sunlight

The lower lip is the only "oral" site significantly exposed to sunlight. Evidence for the etiologic influence of actinic exposure is derived from the degenerative pathologic changes seen in the heavily sun-exposed lip and the striking predominance in incidence of lower over upper lip cancer. Differences in geographic and occupational exposure also attest to the importance of sunlight in the etiology of lip cancer.[17,18]

Other

Poor oral hygiene and neglected dentition have been implicated in the etiology of oral cancer. Graham et al.[13] found a synergistic relationship between poor dentition, tobacco and alcohol abuse, and cancer. It is well known that heavy users of tobacco and alcohol have less regard for their personal health and will often have poor oral hygiene and poor or absent dentition.

The older reports implicating syphilitic glossitis in the etiology of mouth cancer are outdated. The direct relationship was uncertain, and the atrophic glossitis of advanced syphilis is now rare. However, clinical experience has identified a small group, usually consisting of elderly women, who report neither tobacco nor alcohol exposure but who show significant abnormalities of tongue mucosa. Atrophy is common, and many eventually develop multifocal tongue cancer. No obvious etiologic factors have been identified, but nutritional deficiencies may be involved.

The increased incidence of oral cancer in males in those U.S. counties with leather, paper, and chemical manufacturing industries and in females in counties with apparel and textile manufacturing has been described.[6] An increased incidence of mouth cancer in males in urban over rural areas throughout the United States has been reported. This fact may be explained, in part, by the increased alcohol and tobacco usage in urban as opposed to rural areas.

PATHOLOGY

More than 90 percent of malignant oral tumors are squamous cell or epidermoid carcinoma of mucosal origin.[19] Most of the remainder are adenocarcinomas arising from minor salivary glands. These glands are extensively distributed throughout the upper aerodigestive tract but are particularly abundant in the submucosa of the palate, cheeks, and lips. These tumors are similar pathologically to their counterparts in the major or paired salivary glands but differ in their frequency of occurrence and biologic behavior.[19] Other pathologic entities which may involve the oral mucosa include melanoma, lymphoma, and sarcoma. Metastatic lesions to the oral mucosa are exceedingly rare. History and formal biopsy are required to accurately identify the nature of the oral mucosal abnormality.

Premalignant Lesions

The concept of precancerous lesions of the oral mucosa has evoked considerable debate. Normally oral mucosal epithelial cells progress in an orderly fashion from their origin in the basal cell layer to the surface without significant keratin accumulation. A white patch, clinically called *leukoplakia*, is a cornified, opaque zone on the surface and may represent one of several pathologic processes. *Hyperkeratosis* is a simple thickening of the superficial mucosal layer—the stratum corneum. *Parakeratosis* is the abnormal accumulation of increased numbers of nucleated cells near the epithelial surface. *Acanthosis* represents the accentuation of the basal cell layer, the stratum granulosum, and may be accompanied by extension of the rete ridges into the submucosa. *Dyskeratosis* indicates a variable degree of abnormal orientation and proliferation of epithelial cells. Various combinations of these abnormalities may occur, with or without accompanying inflammatory reaction. All are benign changes presumably resulting from abnormal mucosal stimuli.[19]

Among the white mucosal oral lesions are "premalignant" atypical hyperplasia, hyperkeratosis, papillary hyperplasia, white sponge nevus, lichen planus, discoid lupus, leukoplakia, and erythroplakia. Simple hyperplasias usually represent a response to injury and should not be confused with epidermoid carcinoma. The most common of these is the papillary hyperplasia of the palatal mucosa commonly seen beneath an ill-fitting denture. Pseudoepitheliomatous hyperplasia usually overlies the margin of an inflammatory lesion and commonly accompanies the so-called granular cell myoblastoma. White sponge nevus is a rare, entirely benign, familial ectodermal disorder diffusely involving the oral mucosa. Lichen planus, a common dermatologic lesion, may present several appearances on the oral mucosa, but only rarely has the erosive variety been reported to precede oral cancer.[20] The oral lesions of discoid lupus may be accompanied by epithelial dysplasia but are rarely, if ever, precancerous. Leukoplakia, defined as a white patch or plaque not less than 5 mm in diameter which cannot be removed by rubbing and which cannot be attributed to any specific disorder, has been considered a premalignant lesion, with subsequent malignant "transformation" recorded in 1.4 to 36.4 percent of patients after observation periods from 1 month to 15 or more years.[20] In their study of 248 patients with histologically benign leukoplakias followed for up to 10 years, Pindborg et al.[21] found that 37.4 percent of the lesions disappeared spontaneously, 45.3 percent were unchanged, and 3.3 percent enlarged, while only 4.4 percent showed carcinoma in the area of previous leukoplakia. In another study[22] of 782 patients with leukoplakia, oral cancer developed in 2.4 percent after 10 and 4 percent after 20 years' observation. Oral leukoplakia was more common in tobacco users than nonusers, but the frequency of subsequent cancer was eight times greater among tobacco *non*users than users! Also the removal of the original leukoplakia by excision of electrodesiccation did *not* reduce the subsequent appearance of oral cancer.

Oral leukoplakia is more common in older men than in women and occurs predominantly on the lower gingiva and buccal mucosa.[23] Prediction of the histology on clinical examination is unreliable, and formal biopsy is necessary. In their large series of clinical leukoplakias Waldron and Shafer[23] found mild to moderate epithelial dysplasia in 12.2 percent, severe epithelial dysplasia or carcinoma in situ in 4.5 percent, and infiltrating squamous carcinoma in 3.1 percent. Epithelial alterations from dysplasia to carcinoma were most common in lesions on the floor of the mouth, less common in lesions of the tongue and lip. Thus, it is apparent that relatively few white lesions will be malignant.

The earliest sign of an asymptomatic in situ or infiltrating carcinoma may be a red lesion.[24] The erythroplastic (red) lesion is usually flat or slightly elevated, homogeneously or speckled red to deep-blood red, velvety or slightly granular, often glistening, and rather well circumscribed. While white lesions are much more common than red ones, the likelihood of dysplasia, carcinoma in situ, or infiltrating cancer is much higher in the red erythroplastic than in the white leukoplakial lesion.[25]

GROSS APPEARANCE

While the early infiltrating oral cancer may be indistinguishable from innocuous-appearing leukoplakia or erythroplakia without biopsy, the typical more-advanced lesion has a much more characteristic appearance. The usual lesion shows a rolled, indurated border with a shaggy central ulceration with some degree of necrosis. The tumor may, however, assume other appearances and be exophytic, extending significantly above the surrounding normal mucosal surface; endophytic, infiltrating deeply with minimal external elevation; or frequently combinations of both. Occasionally ulceration may be minimal, with the lesion presenting as a firm, indurated, seemingly submucosal mass, usually with ill-defined margins best appreciated by palpation. The most superficial lesions may have no palpable induration whatsoever but present as flat, erythroplastic plaques.

The term *verrucous carcinoma* refers to certain tumors which are typically white, exophytic, micronodular, and papillary in appearance, histologically composed of highly differentiated epithelial cells covered by a thick keratinized layer arranged in deeply invaginated folds proliferating from a well-formed, essentially intact basement membrane. There is a distinct tendency to invade by pushing club-shaped projections deeply, with free groups of invading cancer cells unusual. Lymph node metastases are probably very rare and distant metastases unknown. Verrucous carcinoma may occur in the mouth, larynx, or nasal cavity, but also appears on the skin, genitalia, and rectum, among other sites.[26] The prognosis following total excision is generally good because of the distinct tendency to remain localized.[19,26]

MICROSCOPIC APPEARANCE

A detailed description of the microscopic appearance of epidermoid carcinoma is beyond the scope of this chapter. Formal attempts to grade the microscopic appearance began with Broders in 1926[27] and have continued by others, most notably recently Jakobsson,[28] attempting to predict clinical behavior on the basis of the histologic appearance of the cancer *and* the cellular response of the host tissues. The presence of epithelial pearls and keratinization with minimal pleomorphism and few mitoses suggest the tumor is of low histologic grade. Cellular pleomorphism, many mitoses, and negligible keratinization characterize high-grade tumors.

The role of histologic grading is currently uncertain. Standardization of grading has not been achieved, which explains why interpretation by different pathologists may vary. Most patients have intermediate-grade tumors, and experience suggests that stage of disease is more important prognostically than histologic grade. The histologic diagnosis of verrucous cancer may be difficult to obtain unless a large representative sample of the basal portion of the lesion is examined.

REGIONAL METASTASES

Head and neck cancers have a distinct propensity to spread via regional lymphatics to cervical lymph nodes. Depending upon the site and size of the primary cancer, generalizations about the distribution of lymph node metastases can be made.[29,30] Lesions of the lip, anterior floor of mouth, anterior gingiva, and tip of tongue typically metastasize initially to submandibular and submental lymph nodes. More posteriorly situated floor-of-mouth, lateral and posterior gingival, and lateral tongue lesions commonly spread initially to subdigastric and upper deep-jugular lymph nodes. Primary tumors of the hard palate and buccal mucosa may initially involve the lymph nodes over or just beneath the mandible in the submandibular triangle. With more advanced cancers there tends to be progressive involvement from upper to lower jugular lymph nodes. However, the progression of cervical metastatic involvement is not always predictable, and the first manifestation of cervical nodal metastases may be a lower-neck or even contralateral lymph node enlargement.

Cervical lymph node involvement is initially seen in about one-third of our patients with squamous carcinoma of the tongue, floor of mouth, gingiva, or buccal mucosa on initial examination. The incidence is usually related to the size of the primary cancer. Cervical lymph node metastases from small, clinically occult oral cancers do occur but much less frequently than from pharyngeal primaries. The lower incidence from cancers of the lip and hard palate may relate to less extensive lymphatic drainage or to the fact that the primary lesions tend to be detected early when small and well differentiated.

The presence of regional lymphatic metastases from oral cancer is an ominous prognostic finding.[2,31,34] The extent of such involvement is of vital importance. Few patients are salvaged when they have multiple extensively involved nodes. Metastatic tumor which has extensively breached the capsule of the lymph node(s) with soft-tissue invasion or in-transit lymphatic involvement or perineural or vascular invasion is particularly ominous.[32-34]

DISTANT METASTASES

Oral squamous cancer tends to remain localized to the primary site of origin and regional lymph nodes until relatively late in the course of the disease. Original reports suggested that oral cancer rarely metastasized to distant sites, but with more effective local tumor control it is apparent that distant metastases are common. Recent reports of distant metastases from head and neck cancer based on clinical data cite incidence from 5.3 to 23.9 percent whereas autopsy series report distant metastases in 17 to 46.5 percent of such patients studied.[35] In one large clinical series the overall incidence of distant metastases was 10.9 percent; varying from 3.1 percent for vocal cord cancers to 28.1 percent from cancers of the nasopharynx; 7.5 percent of oral cavity primary cancers were ultimately accompanied by distant metastases. The lungs and bones were the most common first sites for metastases, with liver and mediastinum unusual initial sites. Almost one-half of the metastases were detected within 9 months of treatment and 80 percent within 2 years. The incidence of distant metastases was influenced more by the stage of the cervical lymphatic metastases (N) than by the stage of the primary cancer (T). Recurrence above the clavicle more than doubled the likelihood of distant metastases.[35]

MULTIPLE PRIMARIES

Patients afflicted with one oral cancer have significant risk of one or more synchronous or metachronous cancers at other sites. In our experience 24 percent of 1034 patients with oral and pharyngeal cancers had multiple primaries.[2] Among these patients 15 percent had second cancers in the upper aerodigestive tract, approximately one-half of which were in the oral cavity, with the remainder in the lung, larynx, pharynx, and esophagus in decreasing frequency. Approximately 10 percent of these had three separate regional primary cancers. Slaughter et al.[36] documented the multifocal nature of most oral cancers and coined the term *field cancerization*. The wonder is, perhaps, that more patients with oral cancer do not have multiple primary tumors. The deleterious effects of continued tobacco and alcohol abuse on the incidence of secondary primary cancers have been amply documented.[10,11]

CLINICAL STAGING

The staging of cancer represents an attempt to group patients according to the extent of the neoplastic process. Proper staging will permit the physician to select treatment most appropriately, to evaluate the results of treatment more reliably, to predict prognosis more accurately, and to facilitate comparison of treatment results with those of others more objectively. Proper staging demands a careful clinical assessment of the extent of the tumor. The anatomic margins of the oral cavity are defined and illustrated in Fig. 15-1. Tumors of the oral cavity can generally be adequately staged on clinical grounds, carefully assessing the three dimensions of the tumor. Additional diagnostic studies may be required for adequate staging of tumors of certain sites.

Staging may be done at several points in the natural history of the cancer. Staging is done on initial presentation (clinical-diagnostic staging); after surgical exploration (surgical-evaluative staging); after examination of the resected specimen (postsurgical treatment–pathologic staging); at the time of recurrence (retreatment staging); or, finally, at autopsy (autopsy staging). Staging is most commonly done at initial evaluation prior to any treatment. Pathologic examination and staging is always more accurate than clinical staging. Obviously, pathologic confirmation of the nature of the tumor by

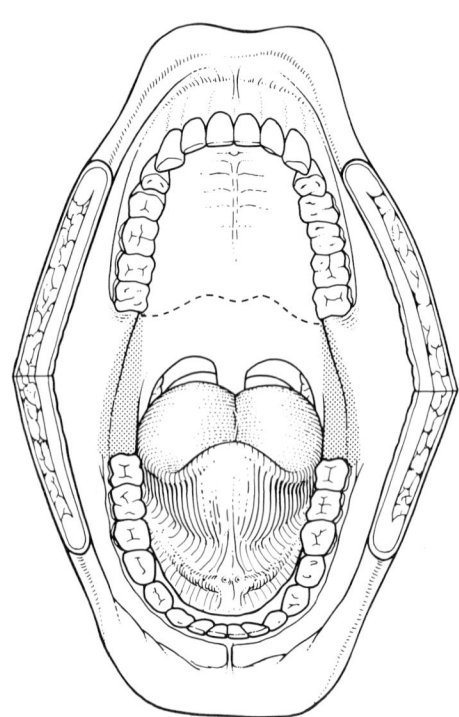

FIGURE 15-1 The oral cavity extends from the vermillion border of the lips anteriorly to the junction of the hard and soft palate and the line of the circumvallate papillae of the tongue posteriorly. The stippled areas represent the retromolar gingiva. The soft palate and base of tongue are oropharyngeal structures.

TABLE 15-1 TNM staging system for oral squamous cancer

	PRIMARY TUMOR (T)
T_0	No evidence of primary tumor
T_{IS}	Carcinoma in situ
T_1	Tumor 2 cm. or less in greatest diameter
T_2	Tumor more than 2 cm. but less than 4 cm. in greatest diameter
T_3	Tumor more than 4 cm. in greatest diameter
T_4	Massive tumor more than 4 cm. in diameter with deep invasion to involve antrum, pterygoid muscles, base of tongue or skin of neck

	CERVICAL LYMPH NODES (N)
N_0	No clinically positive node
N_1	Single clinically positive homolateral node 3 cm. or less in diameter
N_2	Single clinically positive homolateral node more than 3 cm. but less than 6 cm. in diameter or multiple clinically positive homolateral nodes, none more than 6 cm. in diameter
N_{2a}	single clinically positive homolateral node more than 3 cm. but less than 6 cm. in diameter
N_{2b}	multiple clinically positive homolateral nodes, none more than 6 cm. in diameter
N_3	Massive homolateral node(s), bilateral, or contralateral node(s)
N_{3a}	clinically positive homolateral node(s), one more than 6 cm. in diameter
N_{3b}	bilateral clinically positive nodes (each side staged separately)
N_{3c}	contralateral positive node(s) only

	DISTANT METASTASES (M)
M_0	No (known) distant metastases
M_1	Distant metastases present

The detailed scheme is illustrated in Table 15-1. Increasing subscript indicates increasing tumor burden. The T category is defined by the greatest dimension of the primary tumor, except for the "massive" lesion, T_4, which indicates extensive involvement outside the oral cavity. The N status is purely clinical and is based upon assessment of the size, number, and laterality of suspicious lymph nodes. M status refers to the presence or absence of distant metastases and is based upon largely clinical or radiographic assessment. A summary of stage groupings is illustrated in Fig. 15-2.

Despite the obvious value of the concept of clinical staging, there are inherent limitations in the system. Although most oral tumors are relatively accessible for measurement, actual tumor size may be grossly underestimated if only the visible extent of the lesion is measured rather than its palpable mass. Furthermore, clinical estimates of primary tumor size are based upon two rather than three dimensions—area as opposed to volume. There is usually a relationship between the two, but the 4.5-cm superficially infiltrating tongue cancer, T_3, may actually have a better prognosis than the 1.8-cm deeply infiltrating, endophytic T_1 tumor. Since it is almost impossible to accurately quantitate the depth of tumor infiltration, it has been wisely left out of the clinical staging schema.

Accurate assessment of the presence and extent of cervical lymph node involvement may be equally unreliable. Such assessment is based upon the size and

initial biopsy is a mandatory prerequisite to any staging system.[37]

Staging is not an exact science, nor can it be static. With increasing knowledge of tumor biology, other clinical parameters of the tumor and of the host's response may be prognostically important so that periodic revision or "upgrading" of the staging system to include this new information will be necessary.[37]

The current staging system for oral cancer uses the TNM nomenclature. T represents the primary tumor, N, regional nodal metastases, and M, distant metastases.[37]

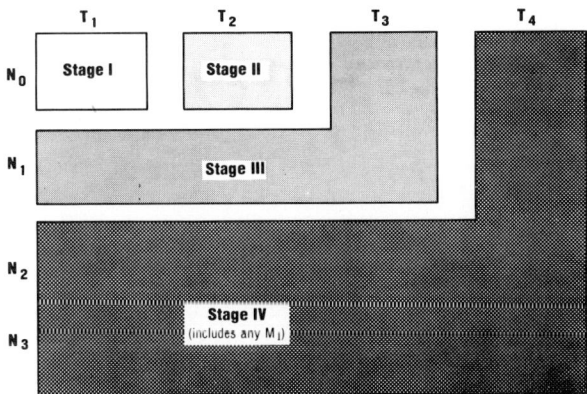

FIGURE 15-2 Block diagram summary of stage grouping of oral squamous cancer[37]

consistency of lymph nodes as evaluated by clinical palpation. The level of accuracy is less than perfect.[29,30,32-34,38] The more muscular and thick the neck, the more difficult it is to detect minimally involved lymph nodes. Some 10 to 20 percent of enlarged cervical lymph nodes will histologically show inflammatory rather than neoplastic changes. The presence of multiple enlarged lymph nodes is more reliable evidence of their involvement by metastatic tumor than is the single suspicious node. With increasing care in examination and increasing experience of the examiner, the level of clinical accuracy will improve.[38]

Histologic staging is to be preferred, but in those patients in whom there is no surgical specimen other than biopsy, this is impossible. While needle-aspiration biopsy may accurately document the presence of metastatic cancer in cervical lymph nodes (quality), it cannot document the extent of nodal involvement (quantity). The inherent inaccuracy and lack of precision in clinical staging will be common to all studies—to a greater or lesser degree.

SELECTION OF THERAPY

Surgery and Radiation Therapy

Cancer of the oral cavity may be treated by one or several different modalities. The choice of treatment will be influenced by multiple factors, including the type and extent of the primary tumor; involvement of adjacent structures, particularly bone and lymph nodes; previous treatment, if any; availability, expertise, and preference of the therapist(s); age, physical status, wishes, and needs of the patient. The small, early, superficial anterior oral cancer may be easily surgically excised, occasionally under local anesthesia via the open mouth, with good functional result and excellent prognosis. The time, expense, and morbidity of conventional fractionated external radiotherapy for the same lesion may be excessive. Since the results are similar, surgical excision is usually to be preferred.

While the more exophytic and histologically undifferentiated tumors are generally more radiosensitive, treatment results comparable to those obtained by surgical excision usually require external plus interstitial irradiation. This may require hospitalization and anesthesia in addition to the multiple treatments, all of which the elderly or debilitated patient may tolerate poorly.

Radiotherapy may be advantageous to the patient whose oral lesion is small or medium in size but with vague, indefinite margins or broad and superficial extent, or whose lesion is surgically inaccessible through the open mouth. The sequelae of therapeutic radiation on teeth, bone, salivary glands, and oral mucosa must be weighed against the functional and cosmetic sequelae of surgical resection. The patient who will not, or cannot, stop using alcohol or tobacco is a poor candidate for radiation therapy. The experience of the responsible clinician will undoubtedly influence the ultimate choice of therapy. Certainly the decision will be influenced by the histology of the primary tumor in that the infrequent nonepidermoid tumors are generally radioresistant, while the rare lymphomas are best treated by radiotherapy and/or chemotherapy.

Once the primary epidermoid carcinoma is larger and more deeply infiltrating, invading bone and regional lymph nodes, the prognosis significantly worsens.[2] Experience suggests that more effective local tumor control can be achieved by combining surgery and radiotherapy.[38,40-42] The details and sequencing of such combined treatment are beyond the scope of this chapter, but early evidence suggests that results do not significantly differ whether the radiation precedes or follows the surgical excision.[39] Most surgeons prefer to perform the surgery first with the hope of minimal complications so that radiation to full therapeutic dosage can be given soon thereafter. The surgery may be easier and the postoperative morbidity less if the radiation follows rather than precedes the surgical procedure. There is evidence to indicate that the benefits of enhanced local control by combined therapy may be lessened if the radiation is delayed for more than 8 weeks after surgery.[40] Wound healing may be slowed or impaired following 5000 rads preoperatively, but postoperative irradiation doses of 6000 to 7000 rads can be delivered with minimal additional morbidity.[41] One disconcerting factor brought out in the report of a large retrospective study of patients with head and neck epidermoid carcinoma is that distant metastases were more common in those patients who received postoperative as opposed to preoperative irradiation.[35]

The patients with stage III and IV oral cavity epidermoid carcinoma probably should receive combined surgery and radiation. The possible benefits may not be as clear as in those patients with hypopharyngeal and laryngeal cancer.[39,40,42] We currently advise postoperative radiation in those patients with large primary cancers, in those with more than minimal cervical metastatic tumor, in those whose surgical resection margins are histologically involved or very close, and in those whose specimens show extensive extracapsular lymph node and/or perineural tumor spread.[32-34,41] We prefer to start the radiotherapy no later than 4 to 6 weeks postoperatively provided wound healing is satisfactory and planned reconstruction has been completed.[40]

When bone is approached or invaded by tumor, surgery is generally preferred. Local failure occurs more often when radiation is used, and there is significant risk of bone exposure and/or osteoradionecrosis. The use of interstitial irradiation to treat large primary oral cancers further increases the risk of bone infection and necrosis, particularly when the implant approaches the mandible. The amount of bone involvement will dictate the extent of bone resection, but every attempt should be made to preserve bone continuity wherever possible without compromise of the adequacy of the tumor resection. Marginal mandibulectomy, which preserves jaw continuity by resecting only a rim of the mandible, may provide an adequate margin of resection around the tumor which approaches, but does not invade, the mandible. Portions of the maxilla may have to be resected when cancers of the hard or soft palate, upper gingiva, or buccal mucosa approach or invade the jaws. Plain x-rays often underestimate the extent of bone involvement, while bone scanning may overestimate it.[43] It is imperative that preoperative evaluation document the extent of tumor as accurately as possible in order to avoid incomplete tumor resection.

The surgical removal of involved cervical lymph nodes has generally been the treatment of choice for neck node metastases.[44] The operation may be modified to less than a classic radical neck dissection in selected patients without adversely affecting results by combining it with postoperative radiation.[45] It appears that the hallmark of success is adequate removal of bulk of disease with postoperative irradiation for control of microscopic residua.[46] While some[47,48] would advocate radiation therapy alone, our experience has been to the contrary. Whenever feasible, the neck dissection should be carried out in continuity with resection of the primary tumor, but limited experience suggests that this composite resection is not mandatory.[49] The significance of lymph node metastases upon prognosis has been amply documented[2,32,34] and the need for additional treatment beyond radical neck dissection in those patients with extensive bulky metastatic lymph node deposits has been illustrated. The propensity for such advanced tumor to be accompanied by distant metastases has also been reported.[32,35]

In the absence of clinically apparent cervical lymph node metastases (N_0) treatment of the neck may be indicated on an elective basis. When the primary lesion is sufficiently large to indicate significant risk of ultimate spread to cervical lymph nodes, appropriate elective treatment is justified. If the primary tumor is to be irradiated, the neck nodes at risk should be included within the treatment portals to destroy microscopic metastatic deposits. Dosage should be carried to at least 5000 rads with conventional fractionation.[41,46,50] Generally, both sides of the neck should be treated, particularly when the primary tumor is in an advanced stage and approaches or crosses the midline.

If the primary oral cancer is to be treated surgically and is more than T_1 or early T_2, then elective neck dissection seems justified. In general, elective neck dissection should be considered when (1) the risk of subsequent lymph node involvement is particularly high;[30] (2) when the surgical resection of the primary tumor necessitates entry into the neck for adequate exposure; (3) when the patient is unlikely or unable to return for routine follow-up examination at frequent and regular intervals; and (4) when the patient has a short, muscular neck which is difficult to clinically evaluate. Unfortunately, there are no controlled prospective studies which demonstrate enhanced local control or survival following elective neck dissection for clinically occult lymph node metastases rather than deferring such surgery until metastases become apparent.[51] Worsening of prognosis with increasing tumor burden in the cervical lymph nodes has been amply documented, however.[2,32,34,38] It clearly follows that when the decision is made to defer treatment to the neck, the patient must return frequently—at least once monthly for the first year—for reexamination so that any subsequent overt lymph node metastases will be detected as early as possible and treated promptly. Modifications of the classic dissection, which preserve the spinal accessory nerve, may be appropriate when performing the surgery for clinically uninvolved cervical lymph nodes in order to minimize the postoperative shoulder dysfunction.[45]

Studies have suggested that occult lymph node metastases can be effectively sterilized in a significant percentage of such patients after 5000- to 6000-rads radiotherapy with minimal morbidity.[50] The effectiveness of such therapy over elective neck dissection has yet to be proved by prospective randomized studies. The use of radiotherapy for the control of overt clinical metastatic disease appears to be limited to those patients with lymph nodes less than 3 cm in diameter.[47,48] The likelihood of control of large or multiple metastatic deposits by external radiotherapy alone is too small to justify its use for primary treatment of metastatic oral squamous cancer. Radiotherapy may offer some local palliation in patients with unresectable or recurrent tumor after previous surgery, but generally such palliation is temporary at best. It appears that the greatest use of radiotherapy in such patients is as an adjunct to surgical removal of bulky tumor, with the hope of eradication of any microscopic residual.[40–42,46]

Chemotherapy

Chemotherapy has been increasingly employed in the treatment of patients with advanced squamous carcinoma of the head and neck, but its value has yet to be established. Methotrexate, bleomycin, and *cis*-platinum are three currently available drugs with proven activity against squamous carcinoma. Other drugs have been used with less effectiveness. There is evidence to suggest that combination drug therapy produces a higher response rate than single agents, but the median duration of such response is short, usually limited to weeks, and none of the combinations have been proved more effective than single-agent chemotherapy in randomized trials. Both single-agent and combination chemotherapy programs have been used prior to surgery and/or radiation with significantly higher response rates than the same agents used for recurrent disease have shown, but there is no hard evidence that such adjunctive therapy has resulted in improved disease-free interval or overall survival compared with conventional treatment alone.[52] Multiple, ongoing trials are currently underway to investigate various therapeutic combinations, including the use of adjunctive chemotherapy to eradicate potential micrometastases following apparently curative local therapy. The results are not yet available, but we have expectations of beneficial results.[52] There is renewed interest in intraarterial delivery of chemotherapeutic agents, but methods of reporting response, appropriate selection of patients, and techniques for safe drug delivery need to be standardized. There is as yet no proof of greater effectiveness of the intraarterial routine over the intravenous delivery of the drug.[53]

The use of chemotherapy as first treatment modality does not appear to increase the morbidity of subsequent surgery. However, significant drug toxicity may delay definitive treatment. Only with prospective randomized clinical trials can the answers to these complex questions be obtained. At this time, it appears that adjunctive chemotherapy for head and neck epidermoid carcinoma is experimental and is not warranted as part of the routine treatment of such patients. Its role as adjunct to "standard" surgery and radiation for those patients at high risk of recurrence or metastases is currently under investigation, and answers should be forthcoming.

Other Modalities

Other modalities used for the treatment of oral cancer have included cryosurgery,[54] electrocoagulation,[55] laser,[56] chemosurgery,[57] immunotherapy,[58] and new methods of radiotherapy including neutrons, pions, and protons[59] (Table 15-2). At this time, these modalities appear to have very limited application in highly selected patients or as part of clinical research protocols. More will probably be heard in the future from researchers now investigating the immunological aspects of human cancer and the manipulation and augmentation of the human immunological mechanisms as they refer to neoplastic disease.

SPECIFIC ORGAN SITES

Cancer of the Lip

ANATOMY

The lip begins at the junction of the vermillion border with the skin and includes only that mucosa which comes into contact with the apposing lip. This red mucosal

TABLE 15-2 Treatment modalities for oral squamous cancer

Surgery

Radiation therapy
   External
   Interstitial
   Combination of both

Chemotherapy

Cryosurgery

Electrocoagulation

Laser excision

Immunotherapy

Combination of the above

surface is divided into upper and lower lips joining at the angle, or commissures, of the mouth.[37] The lymphatic drainage of the upper lip may be more rich than that of the lower. Flow is inferior and frequently bilateral to submental, submandibular, and then jugulodigastric and other deep-jugular lymph nodes.

INCIDENCE AND ETIOLOGY

Carcinoma of the lip makes up less than 1 percent of all malignant tumors, but lip cancers represent 25 to 30 percent of all cancers of the oral cavity.[37,60] There is striking variation in the geographic incidence, predominantly related to chronic exposure to solar radiation. The disease is rare in blacks and is most frequently observed in fair to ruddy complexioned individuals, particularly those with outside occupations predisposing the patient to considerable exposure to sunlight. More than 90 percent of lip cancers involve the lower lip, almost certainly related to the relative sunlight exposure and resulting actinic cheilitis.[17,18] Tobacco usage in all forms increases the risk of lip cancer.[18] The chronic thermal injury of long-standing tobacco usage, particularly pipe smoking, may be etiologically significant. Syphilis is rarely implicated in lip cancer. The role of chronic dental trauma from sharp broken teeth, ill-fitting dentures, and chronic gingival infection may be significant.[62,63] The disease most commonly affects those of middle age; less than 10 percent of reported cases are seen in patients less than 40 years of age. A reported 95 percent are seen in males, but women have a greater tendency to develop cancer of the upper lip.[37]

PATHOLOGY

Squamous cell carcinoma makes up the great bulk of malignant lip tumors. Basal-cell carcinoma from the adjacent skin may invade the lip. Melanoma of mucosal origin will rarely be seen. The few remaining tumors arise from minor salivary glands. Most of the squamous lip cancers are very slowly growing and are histologically well differentiated. The tumor may directly extend to involve adjacent structures. Cervical lymph node metastases are seen in 10 to 15 percent of patients and appear to be related to the size (stage) of the primary tumor. Distant metastases are rare but may be seen with locally advanced or recurrent cancers. As many as 10 to 15 percent of lip cancers may be multifocal, both simultaneous and metachronous.[37,60-63]

The lip chronically exposed to solar radiation will show atrophy of fat and glandular elements, loss of elastic fibers, hyperkeratosis, and chronic inflammation.

CLINICAL PRESENTATION

Lip cancer presents a varied clinical picture. It may be little more than a red granular nodule along the mucosa. Generally, the larger lesions are either exophytic, ulcerative, or verrucous (Fig. 15-3). Most of the lip cancers arise as ulcerated areas, often in areas of leukoplakia, and early may resemble an innocuous fever blister or cold sore. The verrucous type is least common and most indolent, and to the unwary it defies diagnosis by its warty, slightly exophytic, innocuous appearance. It is often treated unknowingly for months to even years as a benign dermatologic problem. Figure 15-4 illustrates such a lesion of 7 years' duration. The infiltrative lesion is often of higher histologic grade and clinically more aggressive. Spread laterally and deeply may ultimately lead to invasion of the mandible and the involvement of submental and submandibular lymph nodes and more distal internal jugular nodes and, rarely, distant sites.[37,65] In most cases this progression may require months to years, so that a high index of suspicion will enable the physician to make the diagnosis readily and to institute appropriate treatment early. Any mucosal abnormality of the lip which does not heal within 2 weeks with appropriate conservative management should be biopsied to establish the true nature of the lesion. Lesions of the size illustrated in Fig. 15-5 are rare and carry a poor prognosis, particularly with spread to cervical lymph nodes.

The tumor of minor salivary gland origin will usually

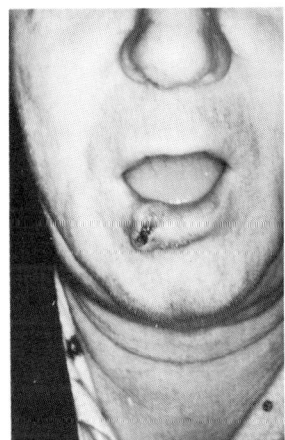

FIGURE 15-3 Moderately infiltrating T_2 squamous carcinoma of the lower lip. Excision and reconstruction with rotated upper lip flap effected cure.

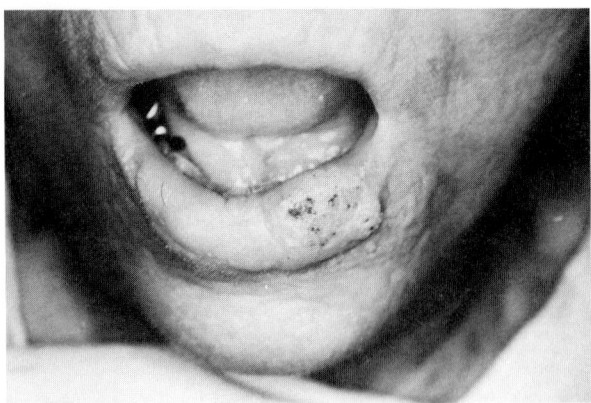

FIGURE 15-4 Typical infiltrating plaque-like verrucous carcinoma of the left lower lip treated for 7 years as a benign inflammatory process.

present as a firm, painless, nonulcerated, submucosal nodule in the lip which may appear cystic and be mistaken for a simple cyst or mucocele (Fig. 15-6). Growth, while progressive, is slow so that many months to years may be required to reach the size depicted in Fig. 15-6. Only after manipulation, usually biopsy, does mucosal ulceration appear. Lymph node metastases are uncommon, and the prognosis following adequate treatment is good.[64]

The pigmented nonulcerated lip lesion must be biopsied in order to differentiate melanoma from benign nevi, racial pigmentation, and the pigmented lesions of Peutz-Jeghers syndrome. All oral pigmented mucosal

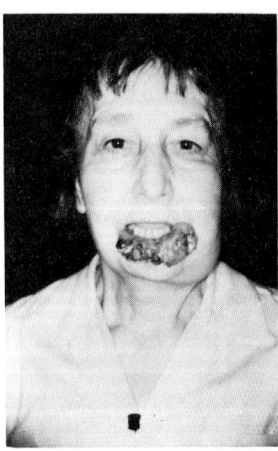

FIGURE 15-5 Massive T_4 infiltrating and destructive squamous carcinoma of the entire lower lip with left upper cervical lymph node metastases. Radical surgery and irradiation failed to locally cure this stage IV cancer.

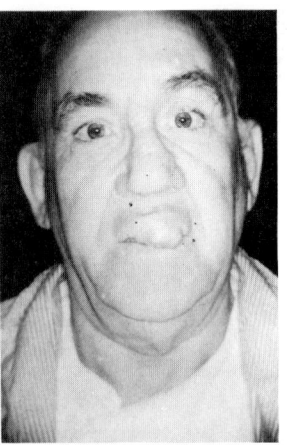

FIGURE 15-6 Large nonulcerated infiltrating adenocarcinoma of the upper lip of 5 years duration. The lesion was cured by wide surgical excision and immediate reconstruction with a pedicled flap from the lower lip.

lesions must be considered neoplastic until proven otherwise.

TREATMENT

Cancer of the lip can be effectively treated by one of several different methods. Surgery and irradiation are the most important treatment modalities, each of which has its advantages and disadvantages. Since most studies report excellent overall control rates with either modality,[60-63] the choice of treatment may be influenced by other considerations. The small lesion readily lends itself to local excision and primary closure, often under local anesthesia as an outpatient procedure, with minimal patient morbidity and expense. The obvious advantages include a surgical specimen which can be carefully studied pathologically and the savings in time and in convenience of this procedure over a prolonged course of multiple radiation exposures. One disadvantage is the shortening of the affected lip with a surgical scar. This can be minimized by appropriate choice of patient and meticulous surgical technique.

The larger lesions without extensive loss of normal lip substance may be treated by radiation with good local control and less deformity.[60,63] If extensive soft-tissue destruction by the tumor is already present, then some lip reconstruction will be necessary for maintenance of cosmesis and oral competence. In that instance, a surgical excision and immediate plastic reconstruction may be more expeditious. The large lesions with extensive soft-tissue and bone invasion will require more aggressive therapy and will usually demand a radical surgical resection and immediate restoration of oral continuity by one of several methods.[65,66] Such large lesions will often be accompanied by regional lymph node metastases, which should be resected simultaneously. Patients with advanced disease may benefit from adjunctive postoperative radiotherapy.

RESULTS

Lip cancer can and does kill.[60,65] In many patients it may prove to be little more than a nuisance which is cured by adequate local therapy. The larger the lesion, the greater the likelihood of local recurrence and of regional metastases and the more vigorous the treatment necessary for its eradication.[60-62] As many as 30 percent of these patients may have two or more malignant lesions on the skin and lip, and 10 to 15 percent may develop local recurrence after previous treatment. Most such recurrences will be detected within 2 years of initial treatment, but few may appear much later and actually represent new primary lip cancers. Some 10 to 15 percent of patients with epidermoid cancers of the lip will develop cervical lymph node metastases. The incidence is directly related to the size of the primary tumor,[63] and as many as 25 percent of recurrent lip cancers will develop cervical lymph node spread.[60] When upper neck nodes are involved, a significant risk of more distant nodal involvement is also present, so that any treatment of involved lymph nodes must include the entire neck. Since the lymph node drainage is to both sides, frequently the treatment must also be bilateral.[63,65] Bilateral supraomohyoid dissection may suffice for those patients with clinically positive but histologically negative upper cervical lymph nodes.[61]

Distant metastases from lip cancer are rare and must be treated individually. Generally such metastases are seen only in the patients with advanced or recurrent local lesions. Physical examination and periodic chest x-rays suffice for detection of recurrence and regional and distant metastases.

The treatment of lip cancer recurrent after previous treatment must be individualized. Rarely can recurrence after radiation therapy be safely and effectively reirradiated. Recurrence after surgical excision is more amenable to radiation or, in selected situations, more radical excision and appropriate reconstruction.[65,66] Once there is involvement of soft tissue, bone, and regional lymphatics, then heroic excisions and massive reconstruction efforts are frequently not curative.[65] All surgical procedures for lip cancer should combine adequate resection and immediate reconstruction to restore oral competence, thus permitting adequate speech and the resumption of a diet by mouth.[65,66] The major goals are adequate local therapy and immediate restitution of a competent oral aperture. Details of various reconstructive techniques are beyond the scope of this chapter but are adequately documented elsewhere.[65] The age and sex of the patient, the size of the mouth, the size (stage) of the primary tumor and its location of the lip(s), and the presence and extent of involvement of local and regional tissues will dictate the methods of treatment and reconstruction.

The behavior of lip cancer more closely resembles that of skin than of oral mucosal cancer. Its course is usually indolent, the tumor tending to remain localized for long periods of time, and results of treatment are good, with most series reporting 75 to 90 percent plus determinant 5-year survival.

Patients who continue their exposure to possible etiologic factors, including chronic sunlight exposure, chronic tobacco usage, and other forms of lip irritation, run a significant risk of new primary cancers of the lip. Those patients with severe actinic cheilitis are at particular risk and should be closely observed. Consideration of prophylactic lip stripping and a resurfacing of the exposed lip with mucosa advanced from the inner aspect of the lip (buccal mucosa) is appropriate. While lymph node metastases are uncommon, they will most likely appear within the first 12 to 18 months after primary treatment. Many of the patients will develop other tumors of the exposed skin and lip. Certainly patients should be strongly advised to minimize contact with the recognized etiologic factors, particularly sunlight, with appropriate use of hats and sun-screening agents when they cannot completely avoid exposure to sunlight. Any new lesions should be promptly reported and, if necessary, biopsied. With appropriate care and vigilance, new cancers can be minimized or detected early and treated appropriately with minimal morbidity and excellent results.

Cancer of the Buccal Mucosa

ANATOMY

The buccal, or cheek, mucosa includes all the mucous membrane lining the inner surface of the cheeks and lips, extending from the line of contact of the apposing lips to the line of attachment of the mucosa of the upper and lower alveolar ridges and posteriorly to the pter-

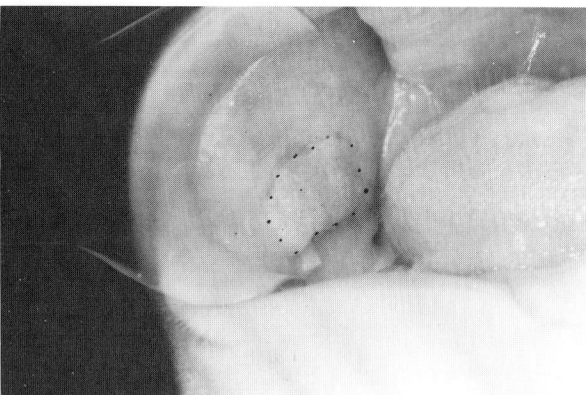

FIGURE 15-7 Granular ulcerated T$_2$ squamous carcinoma of the right buccal mucosa whose margin has been outlined by dots for emphasis.

gomandibular raphe.[37] The mucosal surface occupies some 50 to 60 cm^2 and is supported by the buccinator muscle, which interdigitates with the orbicularis oris muscle anteriorly. It is attached peripherally to the mandible, maxilla, and pterygoid plate and is perforated by Stensen's duct. It is elastic and cushioned by the buccal fat pad, which contains a network of vessels and nerves. The lymphatic drainage is to upper pre- and postvascular submandibular, upper cervical, and midjugular lymph nodes with less common spread to submental, parotid, and paraglandular parotid nodes.[67]

INCIDENCE AND ETIOLOGY

Tumors of this region of the oral cavity are uncommon, making up only 5 percent of oral cancers seen in one U.S. institution in the period reported.[68] The disease is much more common in India, where in some regions it is the most common adult cancer. This is related to the habit of chewing betel combined with tobacco and slaked lime. The quid, usually kept for hours in one buccal gingival sulcus, sets up an intense inflammatory reaction in the adjacent mucosa which may ultimately lead to neoplastic degeneration. In the southeastern United States a similar situation exists with snuff dipping. The pinch of flavored powdered, tobacco is held in the cheek during most of the patient's waking hours, stimulating similar intense mucosal irritation which may eventually lead to neoplastic change. These cancers, typically verrucous in their appearance, are usually histologically low-grade and clinically indolent. They are accompanied by a high incidence of coexisting leukoplakia, seldom metastasize to local or distant sites, but may be large, with much local destruction. Women are more likely to be afflicted, probably related to the sex difference in snuff usage.

Most buccal mucosal lesions arise opposite the plane of occlusion of the teeth. Dental trauma may be an etiologic factor. Oral hygiene and dental repair may have little significance, but there is a high correlation with smoking and leukoplakia.[67] In the United States, cancer of the buccal mucosa is rarely seen under the age of 40, and the median age at discovery is in the seventh decade. Most series report more than 60 percent of the patients to be male.[67-69]

CLINICAL PRESENTATION

The typical buccal mucosal cancer begins as a roughened or ulcerated lesion on the surface of the cheek mucosa (Fig. 15-7). Some lesions may be preceded by leukoplakia or, less commonly, erythroplakia. Occasionally, these tumors may be plaque-like and nonulcerated (Fig. 15-8). Ordinarily, lesions will develop in the mid or posterior cheek, except in the tobacco-chewing patients, whose lower sulcus is typically involved.[69,70] While the relatively rare nonsquamous lesions may present as nonulcerated mucosal or submucosal nodule(s) or induration, the

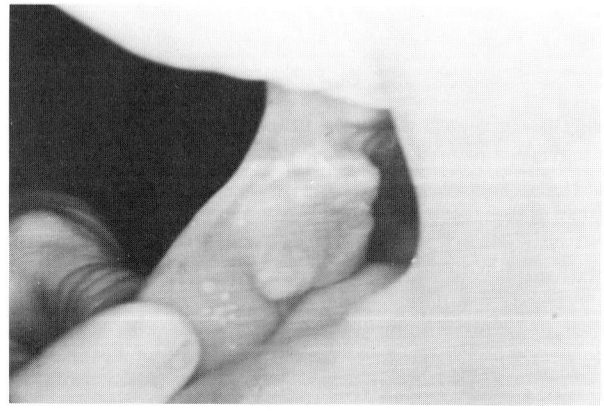

FIGURE 15-8 Atypical plaque-like essentially nonulcerated lesion of the right buccal mucosa just inside the oral commissure. While the lesion appears clinically as a minor salivary gland, tumor biopsy demonstrated it to be an infiltrating squamous carcinoma.

squamous cancer is usually a vegetative, verrucous, or infiltrating ulcerating lesion with relatively little submucosal extension. Only by definitive biopsy can the true nature of the lesion be established. With more advanced tumors of longer duration, more extensive ulceration will be seen, often accompanied by involvement of adjacent structures, including facial musculature, bone (Fig. 15-9), nerve, and even skin. Then one can see external swelling or, even more rarely, perforation, bone erosion leading to pathologic fracture, sensory and motor nerve invasion, and trismus secondary to infection and neoplastic infiltration of the muscles of mastication. Symptoms usually relate to the size of the primary tumor. In one series tumor extended beyond the cheek mucosa in 59 percent of T_2 and 83 percent of T_3 and T_4 primary cancers. Of the previously untreated patients in the same series 38 percent have clinically evident cervical lymph node metastases when first seen, and an additional 18 percent subsequently developed such nodal involvement, for a total of 56 percent. The likelihood of such metastases related directly to the T stage of the primary tumor, that is 39 percent, 56 percent, and 72 percent, for T_1, T_2, and T_3/T_4 primary cancers, respectively.[68]

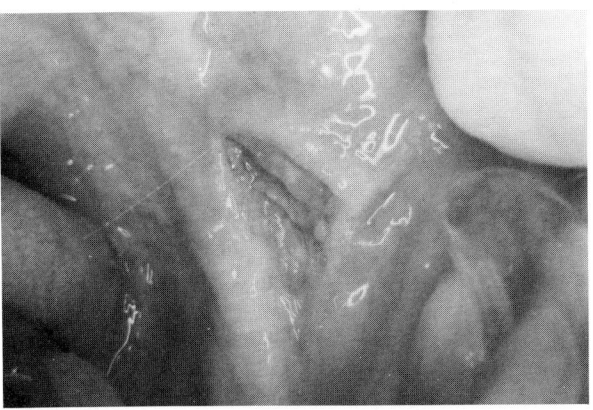

FIGURE 15-9 Infiltrating ulcerated squamous carcinoma of the left posterior buccal mucosa and adjacent retromolar trigone. For orientation, a portion of the lateral border of the oral tongue can be seen to the left of the figure.

TREATMENT

The choice of treatment will be dictated by the factors noted previously. Small T_1 lesions lend themselves well to surgical excision and primary closure or can be left open for healing by secondary intention. Excision of larger lesions will require some form of resurfacing of the cheek to prevent disabling contracture and trismus. Deeply infiltrative lesions may require through-and-through excision with immediate reconstruction using a variety of available flaps, including mucosa from the tongue, skin of the forehead or the neck, and deltopectoral or one of several myocutaneous flaps currently employed.[71,72] The use of free flaps with microvascular anastomoses to close such defects has been reported.[73] Whenever the tumor approaches bone, a portion of that bone must be removed to provide adequate clearance margins. If the bone is frankly invaded, then segmental resection is usually indicated. Radical neck dissection is usually combined with the resection, particularly when lymph nodes are clinically involved. With large lesions, particularly those extending posteriorly, elective neck dissection is justified because of the significant risk of lymph node metastases and in order to obtain more adequate exposure posteriorly for resection of the primary tumor.

Major defects should be reconstructed immediately to restore oral competence.[71] Rarely is there justification for leaving such obvious massive defects open for time-consuming secondary closure with all its attendant emotional and physical morbidity. The goal of restoration of a soft, pliable, elastic lateral wall of the mouth must be achieved if the patient is to be fully rehabilitated. Restoration of facial expression will be lost with the attendant sacrifice of the muscles of facial expression and/or the facial nerve. In a recent series[68] only 6 percent of patients required primary through-and-through excision, while primary closure of the mucosal defect was possible in only 58 percent. Skin grafting was required in 12 percent and regional or distant flaps in 28 percent. Every attempt should be made in the early postoperative period to encourage jaw-opening exercises to prevent contraction and trismus.

Other treatment modalities include radiation, either external or interstitial, and other means of local tumor excision and destruction. Careful patient selection is the key to successful treatment results. With early lesions surgical excision and radiation therapy are equally effective. When the tumor is more advanced, involves adjacent structures, or is histologically low-grade, then surgical excision is more effective than external radiation. Once the entire thickness of the cheek is involved or there is a through-and-through neoplastic fistula, then radical surgical excision with immediate reconstruction is clearly indicated.[68,70,71]

Radiation therapy may be effective in eradicating small or moderate-size lesions without significant tissue destruction or bone invasion. It is probably contraindicated in those patients whose tumors are surrounded by significant leukoplakia. External radiation may be supplemented by interstitial implantation of radioactive sources if necessary. This requires the availability of an experienced therapist, appropriate isotope, and a relatively localized accessible tumor. Since metastatic lymph nodes larger than 2 to 3 cm in diameter or multiple involved nodes are seldom controlled by external radiotherapy alone,[48] radical neck dissection is indicated. Attempts to palliate hopelessly advanced, unresectable buccal mucosal cancers by external radiotherapy alone are seldom successful, and little, if any, palliation is achieved. In many centers, clinical investigations using combinations of chemotherapy, surgery, and radiation are in progress, but long-term follow-up is not yet available, so that survival data are lacking.[52,74] Clearly these complicated, morbid, expensive trials must be carried out in controlled prospective studies by groups of interested, experienced physicians and surgeons capable of the total care of the patient with advanced head and neck cancer. Not until the benefits of such complicated multidisciplinary therapy have been confirmed should it be utilized on a more general basis.

The use of cryotherapy, electrodesiccation, or laser treatment requires small, readily accessible tumors for appropriate application. These methods have the disadvantage of providing no surgical specimen for pathologic examination and usually leave open wounds to close by secondary intention, which in the cheek usually leads to significant trismus. Most importantly, they require a skilled therapist who is sufficiently knowledgeable and experienced to recognize the limitations of the modality and therefore can be appropriately selective in the choice of patients for that treatment.

RESULTS

McComb and Fletcher[75] reported a 5-year "cure" rate of 70 percent of 115 patients, 75 of whom had T_1 or T_2 localized buccal mucosal cancers. Salvage was 92 percent, 8? percent, 65 percent, and 15 percent, respectively, in patients with stage I to IV cancer. Of the patients in the series 60 percent received radiation therapy.

Conley and Sadoyama[67] reported that 12 of 20 determinant patients who underwent surgery and 9 of 17 who were irradiated were alive and tumor-free at 5 years. Local recurrence occurred in 40 percent of their patients, and overall 5-year cure rate for all patients was 38 percent. Bloom and Spiro[68] in their series of 121 patients with squamous carcinoma of buccal (cheek) mucosa treated almost exclusively by surgery conclusively showed that survival was related to the stage of the disease at the time of treatment. Five-year determinant cure rates were 76 percent, 65 percent, 27 percent, and 18 percent, respectively, for patients with stage I through stage IV disease. Previously treated patients fared worse, with only 24 percent alive and well at 5 years. Local recurrence at the primary site occurred in 43 percent, in the neck in 37 percent, and in distant sites in 23 percent. Only 11 percent of those treated for recurrent disease after their previous treatment at Memorial Hospital were salvaged. Based upon actuarial survival data, the N stage of the neck was the most important prognostic factor. Survival was similar in patients with T_1 and T_2 tumors and was not significantly influenced by the clinical appearance or histologic grade of the primary cancer. The authors concluded that better results might follow more use of combined surgery and radiation for those patients with advanced stage III and IV buccal mucosal cancer.

Patients must be followed for life. While most local recurrences will be apparent within 2 years, the risk of a second primary cancer increases with time, particularly in those who continue their tobacco use.[2,10,11,36,76] Any mucosal abnormality, area of increasing induration, or neck nodal enlargement must be suspected as recurrence and appropriately investigated. While the treatment of recurrence is often unsuccessful, occasionally good results are seen, and the disease must be aggressively treated. To do less is to deny the patient any chance for cure.

Cancer of the Gingiva
ANATOMY

Gingivae (gums, alveolar ridges) comprise the mucosa covering the upper and lower alveolar ridges, including the alveolar processes of the mandible and maxilla, extending from the line of attachment of the mucosa in the buccal gutter to the line of free mucosa in the floor of the mouth or to the junction with the hard palate.

The posterior margin of the upper gingiva is the upper end of the pterygopalatine arch. The lower gingiva is continuous with the retromolar gingiva (trigone) at the posterior margin of the last molar tooth. The retromolar trigone is an elongated triangle of attached mucosa overlying the ascending ramus of the mandible extending superiorly to the maxillary tuberosity and bounded laterally by its junction with the buccal mucosa and medially with the anterior tonsillar pillar.[37] The fact that the gingiva surrounds the teeth and closely approximates the underlying alveolar cortical bone distinguishes cancers at this site clinically and therapeutically from other oral cancers, except those of the hard palate.

Lymphatic drainage appears to be scanty but ultimate drainage to submental, submandibular, or jugular nodes will relate to the location and size of the primary tumor. Upper gingival lesions may initially drain to buccinator or periparotid nodes in selected instances, then more distally to submandibular and jugular nodes.

INCIDENCE AND ETIOLOGY

The highest incidence of gingival cancer occurs in south India, where it constitutes roughly 9 percent of all cancers seen. In several reports from the United States, gingival cancers make up no more than 1 percent of all cancers excluding skin cancer. A study showed that 25 percent of all oral cancers in south India, 16 percent of oral cancers in Georgia, and 12 percent of oral cancers at Memorial Hospital were primary on the gingiva.[77]

History of tobacco usage in one form or another is common in most patients with squamous carcinoma of the gingiva. Nonsmokers tend to have smaller, more anterior cancers and fewer lymph node metastases. It is interesting that in the report of Cady and Catlin[77] 48 percent of the females with cancer of the gingiva were nonsmokers as compared to only 6 percent of the males. The proportion of men who were cigar or pipe smokers (34 percent) was higher than that seen in the general population. The etiologic influence of ill-fitting dentures is uncertain. Users of betel or snuff tend to have more buccal mucosal than gingival cancers.

PATHOLOGY

Most gingival cancers will be squamous (or epidermoid) tumors. Only 4 percent of the Memorial Hospital[77] series were nonsquamous neoplasms, with approximately 70 percent of these of minor salivary gland origin, 15 percent melanoma, and the remainder other, more exotic tumors. All were malignant and of varying clinical aggressiveness. The clinical behavior of the minor salivary gland tumors is similar to that of salivary gland tumors elsewhere, with a distinct tendency to bone invasion, frequent local recurrence, and cervical lymph node and occasionally distant metastases.[78] These mucosal adenocarcinomas of minor salivary gland origin should be differentiated from the rare tumors of similar histology arising from intraosseous salivary gland inclusions.[79]

CLINICAL PRESENTATION

Cancer of the gingiva is uncommon before the age of 50, and two-thirds of the patients afflicted are male. Lower gingival cancers exceed those of the upper gums by 4:1. Using the plane of the bicuspid teeth as the dividing line, more cancers of the gingiva occur posteriorly than anteriorly. Initial symptoms are generally pain, ulceration, or both. The denture wearer will frequently attribute the symptoms to the fit of the dentures and seek advice from a dentist. Not infrequently, the initial symptoms may be attributed to local infection or irritation, and inappropriate nonspecific therapy advised. The initially insignificant-appearing ulceration of early cancer of the gingiva usually arises on the apex of the alveolar ridge, and less often on the buccal or lingual surfaces. The mucoperiosteum provides 1 or 2 mm of protection over the alveolar bone, and the periosteum temporarily impedes the infiltration of the cancer. When teeth are extracted from the area of neoplastic involvement, this barrier is interrupted, and prompt bone invasion via the open socket can occur. Once the dense cortical bone is penetrated, the underlying cancellous bone and the neurovascular canal are vulnerable to invasion by the cancer, and the tumor may extend proximally or distally with ease. This adversely influences prognosis, and clearly the patient with extensive bone invasion is at a higher risk of treatment failure. In the Memorial series[77] those patients who underwent exodontia from the involved gingiva fared worse than those whose tumors were of the same stage but who had had no teeth extracted.

The precise extent of bone involvement by carcinoma of the gingiva is usually difficult to document. In the same Memorial series[77] 67 percent of those patients who underwent preoperative x-ray studies had histologic evidence of bone invasion by the cancer. The x-rays, however, were not reliable in this regard. When x-rays showed osteolysis presumably secondary to neoplastic invasion, histologic confirmation was obtained in 81 percent. On the contrary, when the x-rays were interpreted as showing no bone invasion, 33 percent of the subsequent surgical specimens had cancer invading bone. It seems clear that radiographs are not reliable in indicating either the presence or the *precise* extent of bone invasion by carcinoma of the gingiva, particularly in the early stages. Despite these inherent inadequacies, appropriate x-rays should be obtained in most patients with gingival cancer, if only to identify clinically unsuspected bone invasion or to help document radiographically the extent of gross osseous destruction in order to facilitate planning of extent of bone resection.

Rarely a cancer of paranasal sinus origin will present as a gingival lesion, and appropriate radiographs, including tomograms and computerized tomographic scanning, will confirm this fact and facilitate appropriate treatment planning. Whenever there is anesthesia of the cutaneous distribution of the inferior dental nerve or radiographic evidence of widening of the inferior alveolar canal, neoplastic invasion of bone or nerve must be suspected. Bone scanning is not yet sufficiently precise to be of great value in planning treatment. There are false positives with inflammatory changes and postextraction osteitis which cannot be differentiated from the bone reaction accompanying neoplastic invasion; however, a negative bone scan tends to rule out the possibility of bone invasion by the cancer.[43]

Most patients with gingival cancer will present with localized tumors.[77,80-82] Surprisingly, in one series[77] the size of the tumor seemed to be independent of its duration. In that same series 51 percent of the primary cancers were less than 3 cm in diameter, with only 12 percent greater than 5 cm. Pathologically only 11 percent had tumor confined to the mucoperiosteum alone, while 28 percent had spread to medial or lateral soft tissues, and 38 percent had extension to bone. Regional lymph nodes were clinically involved in 37 percent of the patients and appeared with slightly greater frequency with lower than with upper gingival cancers. If that nodal involvement was confined to the nodes in the digastric triangle, then overall prognosis was not adversely affected. When the nodal metastatic tumor involved internal jugular lymph nodes, then the prognosis was significantly worse. No patient had distant metastases at initial presentation.[77]

TREATMENT

Early superficial and anterior gingival cancers are usually excised via a peroral approach with excellent results. While radiotherapy may be employed, the risk of inducing radionecrosis in the adjacent alveolar bone is significant. The use of radiotherapy for gingival cancers with more than minimal bone erosion would appear to be contraindicated.[77,80,82] Surgical resection will almost always include removal of some alveolar bone, the extent of which will be dictated by the estimate of neoplastic bone involvement (Fig. 15-10). Since the currently available methods of such evaluation are imprecise and since intraoperative determination of the extent of bone involvement is difficult, wide bone resection is usually indicated. Extensive involvement of the upper alveolus will necessitate careful preoperative evaluation of the tumor extension beyond the alveolus, particularly into the cheek and/or antrum and the pterygomaxillary space. Partial or extended maxillectomy may be necessary. More than minimal or superficial involvement of the mandible will necessitate segmental mandibulectomy, usually accompanied by neck dissection. Whenever inferior alveolar nerve function is destroyed, the entire course of the nerve from skin to base of skull should ideally be resected with careful histologic examination of the proximal cut end of the nerve to be sure that occult cancer is not invading along the perineural sheath.

The presence of clinically involved cervical lymph nodes mandates neck dissection, but the necessity of an in-continuity monobloc procedure is uncertain. Those patients found to have large primary cancers, multiple involved cervical lymph nodes, extension beyond the lymph node capsule to adjacent tissues, or histologically involved surgical margins will probably benefit from postoperative radiotherapy to the primary site and neck.[77,79,82] The retromolar trigone cancers (Fig. 15-9) pose somewhat more complicated problems with their more posterior location and ready access to muscle, nerve, and base of skull with tumor extension. They are more inaccessible to local peroral surgery, but otherwise the principles of their treatment are the same.

Most defects created by resection of all but the largest gingival tumors can be closed by primary approximation of the wound edges. Local flaps of tongue or regional skin flaps from the neck, forehead, or chest may be required to close large defects. It is particularly important to provide adequate intraoral soft-tissue lining in those

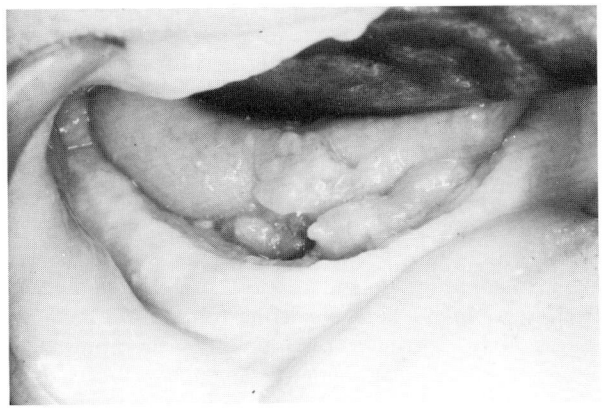

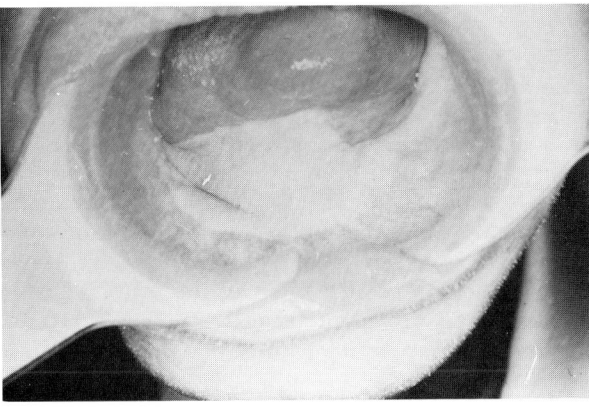

FIGURE 15-10 (a) Destructive ulcerating and infiltrative T_3 epidermoid carcinoma of the right anterior floor of mouth abutting onto the lingual gingiva. (b) Postoperative appearance after radical excision of floor of mouth, gingiva, and marginal mandibulectomy with immediate reconstruction with a rotated cervical skin flap. Excellent function is preserved with little restriction of tongue motion or disturbance of articulation while providing a thick supple base to support a lower denture.

patients in whom mandibular reconstruction is contemplated. Such bone reconstruction is usually delayed in order to avoid contamination of the wound by oral bacterial flora. The use of composite grafts containing segments of bone for reconstruction of the mandible is being explored, but long-term reliability and versatility have yet to be proved.[83,84] The advantages of myocutaneous flaps in providing soft-tissue bulk to cosmetically replace the loss of the mandible are apparent.[72] The multiplicity of methods of mandibular replacement and the complications accompanying their use suggest that the "ideal" method of reconstruction of the mandible is not yet in hand.[85] Most patients having relatively limited lateral segmental resections do not need bone replacement and can be satisfactorily rehabilitated by appropriate training aided by dental devices. Every attempt should be made to retain healthy, viable teeth in the cooperative, well-motivated patient. Upper alveolar defects can usually be very satisfactorily obturated by an appropriate dental prosthesis. The involvement of the patient from the very outset in oral and psychological rehabilitation will contribute significantly to a successful outcome.

RESULTS

There is little difference in results of treatment stage for stage between upper and lower gingival cancers.[77] Those patients with localized T_1 or T_2 lesions can expect greater than 80 percent local control, but only 20 to 30 percent of those with advanced T_3 and T_4 lesions or with multiple lymph node metastases will survive 5 years. The prognosis appears to depend on the size of the primary cancer rather than upon its location and upon the pathologic status of the regional lymph nodes.[77,80,81] Willen et al.[86] suggest that grading of cancers according to Jakobssen's classification may be helpful in suggesting therapy and pedicting prognosis. Elective dissection of the neck in those patients with cancers of the gingiva over 3 cm in diameter may be justified because of the significant risk of occult nodal metastases.

In the Memorial series[77] local failure occurred in 34 percent, regional failure in 33 percent, neck recurrence alone in 17 percent, distant metastases with regional failure in 13 percent, and distant metastases alone in only 4 percent. The failure of local therapy to control local and regional disease is the most common cause of ultimate treatment failure. Retreatment of recurrent carcinoma of the gingiva was successful in only 24 percent of those in whom it was attempted. In the past three or four decades the results of treatment of gingival cancer have significantly improved, stage for stage, in part due to more aggressive surgical resection of localized tumors.[77]

These patients should be carefully followed for the remainder of their lives. In the Memorial series[77] 19 percent developed another cancer of the oral cavity, while 8 percent developed cancers of other organs. Those patients with extensive leukoplakia would appear to be at particularly high risk of another cancer, as are those who continue their tobacco and alcohol abuse. As time passes, the risk of local recurrence lessens while the risk of another primary cancer increases.

Hard Palate

ANATOMY

The palate, comprising the hard and soft palate together with the upper alveolus, makes up the roof of the oral cavity. The hard palate is the semilunar area extending from the inner surface of the superior alveolar ridge to the posterior edge of the palatine bone at its junction with the soft palate.[37] Relatively thin mucoperiosteum overlies the palatine process of the maxillary palatine bone. It is richly supplied with minor salivary glands, distributed in an orderly manner in irregular spaces created by dense fibrous bands in the submucosa. These glands are largely placed behind the line connecting the first two molar teeth and are much less abundant in the midline or gingivae. Some 250 independent glandular aggregates are present in the hard palate compared to 100 in the soft palate. These are pure mucous glands forming a thick layer between the mucous membrane and musculature and bone of the palate.[87] Lymphatic drainage is similar to that of the upper gingiva.

INCIDENCE AND ETIOLOGY

Tumors of the hard palate are uncommon. In most large series of patients with oral cancer they make up from 0.5 to 3 percent of tumors.[88] Tumors of glandular origin constitute a higher percentage of tumors than in other oral sites, in some series up to 50 percent.[87] A recent study[89] reported a total of 392 patients with malignant tumors of the hard and soft palate. Of these, 83 had salivary gland tumor, 14 sarcoma, and 2 melanoma with the remainder squamous carcinomas. Of the previously untreated patients with single lesions, 190 were on the soft palate and 62 on the hard palate.

Chronic irritation seems an unlikely etiologic factor in carcinoma of the palate. Leukoplakia and erythroplakia may be associated factors. The habit of reverse cigarette smoking as practiced in some parts of the world is significant in producing intense mucosal irritation leading to malignant degeneration. The characteristic changes of nicotine stomatitis often seen in heavy pipe smokers are probably related to the heat to which the palatal mucosa is subjected. Of the patients in the Memorial series 94 percent smoked, 95 percent consumed alcoholic beverages, and 51 percent were heavy drinkers.[89]

PATHOLOGY

While minor salivary gland tumors represent a significant proportion of malignant palatine tumors, the bulk of the lesions are squamous carcinoma.[87,89] Their histologic appearance is similar to those squamous cancers elsewhere in the oral cavity. The vast majority of the tumors are of intermediate histologic grade, but this may not be of prognostic significance.[89]

The minor salivary gland neoplasms are more varied in their histology and clinical behavior. While a greater proportion of minor salivary gland tumors of the hard palate are benign than in othe oral sites, at least one-half are malignant. Their clinical appearance is similar, but their behavior and prognosis depend upon the stage of the lesion and its histology.[64,87] Adenoid cystic cancers are the most common, with solid duct and mucoepidermoid carcinomas less frequent. A few more rare lesions have been reported. Extension of the primary tumor into adjacent bone and soft tissues is common, but lymph node metastases are infrequent.[64]

CLINICAL PRESENTATION

Epidermoid carcinoma of the hard palate usually presents as a painful ulceration. On inspection one sees a superficial granular mucosal ulceration with rolled edges (Fig. 15-10). Growth may be exophytic or endophytic, but bone invasion tends to be late. Bleeding is occasionally reported. Some patients report difficulty with fit of dentures or change in character of speech. More than half have symptoms for at least 12 weeks, and a third for more than 6 months. The lesion may reach considerable size before the patient seeks appropriate attention. Sore throat and pain are more commonly seen with soft palate lesions.[89]

The minor salivary gland tumor presents with a usually painless, nonulcerated mass off the midline near the junction of the hard and soft palate, as illustrated in Fig. 15-11. In some patients it may reach considerable size before the abnormality is appreciated. While the two-dimensional aspect of the tumor can be readily seen,

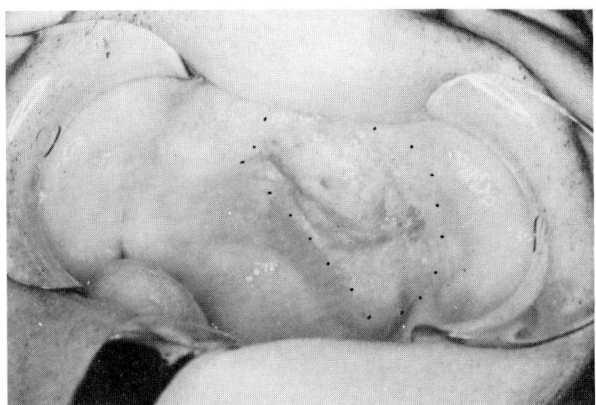

FIGURE 15-11 Granular, red, ulcerated, infiltrating T_3 squamous carcinoma of the left hard palate spreading onto the upper gingiva and bucco-gingival sulcus and lip. (*Margins of lesion are outlined by dots.*) The patient sought medical attention because of pain on wearing his denture. Radiographic studies showed no evidence of bone invasion but pathologic examination of the resected specimen documented bone involvement by cancer.

the depth of infiltration can be assessed only by appropriate radiographs. The examiner should always be wary of the possibility that the malignant lesion actually began in the nasal cavity or maxillary antrum and that its oral manifestation is secondary to invasion through the bony palate (Fig. 15-12). Certainly in advanced cases of palate cancer the nasal cavity and antrum can be readily invaded (Fig. 15-13). The squamous cancer is more prone than the adenocarcinoma to lateral extension invading upper alveolar ridge, gingivae, cheek mucosa, and lip or soft palate producing pain and difficulty in swallowing. Infiltration posteriorly and laterally will ultimately involve the pterygoid area with increased pain and trismus. In the Memorial series[89] 20 percent had T_1 lesions, 45 percent, T_2, 21 percent, T_3, and 9 percent T_4. Extension beyond the hard palate was found in 71 percent, and 29 percent had cervical lymph node metastases on admission. None had contralateral cervical lymph nodes involved without ipsilateral nodal metastases, and only 1.5 percent presented with distant metastases. Lymph nodes in the submandibular triangle are often involved initially with subsequent extension to upper jugular nodes. The larger the primary tumor, the greater the likelihood of bilateral involvement of the palate and of bilateral cervical lymph node metastases.

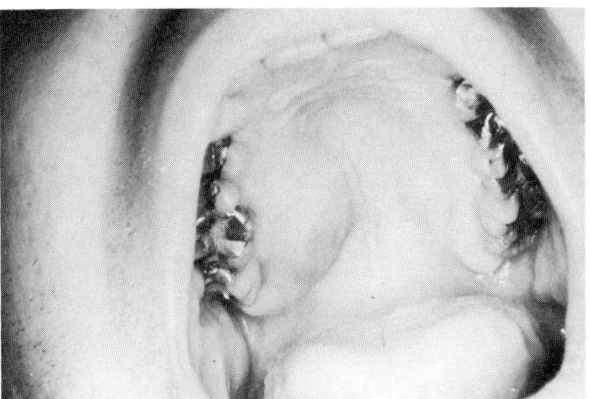

FIGURE 15-12 Adenoid cystic carcinoma of the right posterior hard palate in a 37-year-old male. The ulceration indicates the biopsy site. This is the typical location of this common tumor of the hard palate.

TREATMENT

For early epidermoid carcinoma of the hard palate without bone involvement, treatment by radiation or surgery is equally effective.[88-90] Once bone is invaded or the tumor is larger, then surgery may be more effective, but with the added morbidity of a resulting through-

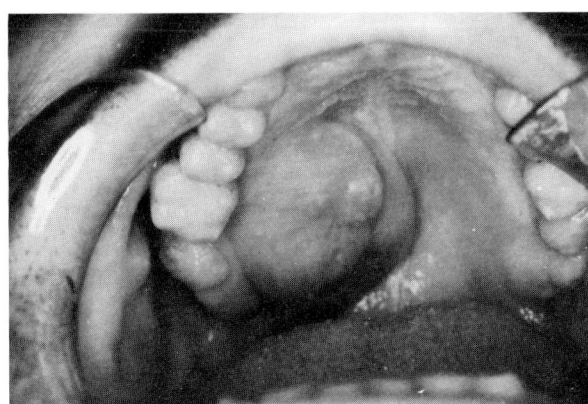

FIGURE 15-13 Very bulky, largely nonulcerated squamous carcinoma involving the palate. The tumor perforated the palatine bone and was ulcerating the floor of the nasal cavity. The exact mucosal surface from which it arose—palate or floor of nasal cavity—is uncertain. Careful clinical examination and radiographic studies are mandatory in assessing the true extent of disease.

and-through palatal defect requiring prosthetic rehabilitation. The anatomic location and extent of the primary tumor, the presence or absence of cervical metastases, and the patient's other medical problems must be considered when selecting treatment. Once bone is invaded by cancer, wide surgical excision including the entire thickness of the bony palate is indicated. The accurate assessment of the extent of the tumor is critically important in the overall treatment planning and the subsequent prognosis.

Early, superficial lesions may be excised through the open mouth. There are few instances in which the bony palate can be spared while an adequate deep margin on the malignant tumor is obtained. Benign salivary gland lesions may be excised with preservation of the palate with good results, but such is seldom the case with a malignant lesion. Small, accessible lesions may be satisfactorily excised via the open mouth, but the larger or more posterior tumors, like those in the patient with a small oral aperture, will require a lip splitting or upper cheek flap—the Weber-Ferguson—approach for adequate exposure. The contents of the antrum and lower turbinate may be excised and the defect lined with skin graft to facilitate healing and subsequent local hygiene. The advantages of insertion of an immediate palatal prosthesis in facilitating good speech and prompt resumption of a diet by mouth are apparent. The final maxillary obturator may not be constructed for 3 or more months. In the presence of cervical metastases radical neck dissection is indicated as part of the initial surgical procedure. Elective treatment of the clinically negative neck is probably not indicated. As with other sites in the oral cavity, current preference calls for postoperative irradiation within 4 to 8 weeks for those patients at high risk of local or regional recurrence.

RESULTS

The overall prognosis directly relates to the extent of the tumor at the time of the initial treatment. Of stage I cancers in the Memorial series 75 percent were alive and well at 5 years. Survival for stage II was 46 percent, for stage III, 36 percent, and for stage IV, only 11 percent. The size of the primary tumor was a slightly less satisfactory predictor of survival in the hard than in the soft palate. It was found that 50 percent of recurrences occurred at the primary site alone, 33 percent in the neck alone, 12 percent in both, 3 percent at local/regional sites with distant metastases, and in only 12 percent were distant metastases seen alone. Three-fourths of all recurrences were apparent within 8 months.[89] A significant number of patients will develop second primary cancers and for these reasons must be kept under close surveillance for the rest of their lives.

The glandular tumors represent similar problems. While the prognosis is related to the stage of the disease, it is also influenced by the histology. While the palate is the most common site of minor salivary gland tumors and the benign mixed tumor is most commonly seen there, the overwhelming proportion of the tumors in our series (77 percent) were malignant. The benign or low-grade localized malignant lesions are often successfully treated by local excision but the larger and more aggressive lesions will demand a more radical resection with a through-and-through palatal defect. Of those determinant patients with minor salivary gland tumors of the palate 45 percent survived 5 years free of disease. However, with certain histologic types the clinical course is more prolonged, and 10- and 15-year survival rates are more indicative of the true history of the disease.[64,86]

Recurrent disease of the palate may be treated by surgery or radiotherapy depending upon the site and extent of that recurrence. Recurrences involving the pterygomaxillary fossa, base of skull, extensive retropharyngeal tumor, or fixed disease in a previously treated neck are generally considered surgically unresectable. Excision of disease localized to the palate, nasal cavity, antrum, or cheek may be feasible and possibly successful, but more extensive disease is rarely cured by heroic surgery, and treatment must be even more individualized than in the primary situation. Radiotherapy with both external-beam and/or interstitial therapy may be successful in certain selected patients with appropriately located and localized disease. This is particularly true of patients with certain minor salivary gland tumors for which excellent response to irradiation can be expected for as long as 2 to 3 years but frequently recurrence will occur. In the future, fast neutron therapy may hold promise of better salvage of these patients than can be achieved with conventional proton therapy.[91] Chemotherapy for recurrent epidermoid carcinoma has been disappointing, with few patients showing objective response of limited duration.[52] Chemotherapy for salivary gland cancer is in its infancy, but some response has been reported, particularly to local and regional disease.[92] Local attempts at tumor destruction using electrocoagulation, cryotherapy, or laser may provide significant palliation, with reduction of tumor bulk, lessening of bleeding, and a cleaner defect, permitting the wearing of the palatal prosthesis, which improves speech and swallowing. The opportunity for repeated use of these modalities even after extensive, more conventional treatment is apparent, but the duration of palliation derived is usually measured in weeks to months and cure is unlikely.

Rehabilitation of the patient after excision of palate cancer essentially involves restoration of the palate. This is much more frequently accomplished with a dental obturator or prosthesis and is far less morbid, less expensive, and less time-consuming than surgical reconstruction. Perhaps most importantly, the simple removal of the obturator permits inspection and palpation of the local area which is at greatest risk of occurrence. This would be impossible after surgical palatal reconstruction. There appears to be little advantage of such surgical reconstruction over prosthetic rehabilitation.

The Floor of the Mouth

ANATOMY

The floor of the mouth is that crescent of mucosa which covers the anterior and lateral floor of the oral cavity, extending from the junction with the unattached gingiva laterally to the reflection of the mucosa of the ventral surface of the tongue, and extending posteriorly to the base of the anterior tonsillar pillars. It is divided into two halves by the frenulum of the tongue and is perforated by the two submandibular salivary gland (Wharton) ducts, which empty via their papillae on each side of the midline, and by the multiple ducts of the sublingual salivary glands.[37] Adjacent tissues include the sublingual and submandibular salivary glands, the lingual and hypoglossal nerves, and the myelohyoid muscles, the latter providing the support—the "muscular diaphragm"—of the floor of the mouth anteriorly. The mucosa is thin and relatively atrophic with shallow rete pegs and little surface keratinization, similar to the mucosa of the ventral and lateral surfaces of the tongue and of the soft palate.[93]

The lymphatic drainage is rich and continuous with that of the tongue and gingiva. There are superficial and deep systems which readily anastomose with each other and the opposite side via superficial and deep channels draining into submandibular, submental, and deep internal jugular lymph nodes. Whether or not there are lymphatic channels in man which perforate the periosteum of the mandible prior to their communication with deep cervical lymphatics is uncertain, but Ossoff et al.[94] have documented such periosteal lymphatic communication in dogs by lymphatic cannulation and injection.

INCIDENCE AND ETIOLOGY

Cancer of the floor of the mouth is the second most common oral cancer and represents 0.48 to 0.80 percent of all human cancers. The geographic incidence varies from 0.1 to 2.4 per 100,000 population for males and 0.1 to 0.8 per 100,000 for females.[95] In the past two or three decades there has been a significant change in the relative sex incidence, with a greater proportion of women afflicted.[96] The tumor is more common in older patients, most series reporting a median age at diagnosis in the seventh decade.[93,95–97] The overwhelming proportion of patients afflicted with cancer of the floor of the mouth report significant and prolonged tobacco and alcohol exposure.[95–98,100] Moore and Catlin[99] reported in their study that 75 to 80 percent of the oral cancers arose from an inferior crescent of mucosa comprising only some 20 percent of the entire oral mucosal surface. They postulated that this dependent mucosa had the most prolonged contact with carcinogens dissolved in saliva. Whether or not there are regional differences in the oral mucosa's susceptibility to malignant degeneration is uncertain. Chronic inflammation does not seem to play a major etiologic role. Local habits and customs, for example, betel and snuff exposure, are significant etiologic factors in certain geographic regions.

PATHOLOGY

Few nonepidermoid cancers are seen in the floor of the mouth.[97] These must be distinguished from such tumors primary in the sublingual or submandibular salivary glands. There is little about the squamous cancer of the floor of the mouth that is not seen in squamous cancers elsewhere in the oral cavity. Most of the tumors are histologically well differentiated,[93,96] but there is a significant propensity for multifocal neoplastic change.[36] The anatomy of the region predisposes to early involvement of adjacent structures[97] and of the rich adjacent lymphatic drainage system.[94] It is interesting to speculate upon the different frequency of floor-of-mouth and tongue cancers in the early[99] and late[101,111] oral cancers.

CLINICAL PRESENTATION

In their study of early asymptomatic oral cancers Mashberg et al.[101] found 45.5 percent of the 222 lesions involved the floor of the mouth; one-half of these were anterior, often in association with the ampulla of Wharton's duct, 15 percent arose in the mid floor of the mouth, and only 13 percent in the posterior third. Most of these early lesions had an erythroplastic component, more so than those of the gingiva, buccal mucosa, or palate.[24] Figure 15-14 illustrates a typical erythroplastic anterior floor of mouth lesion. Figure 15-15 demonstrates an infiltrating epidermoid carcinoma which is exophytic in appearance. More advanced lesions are typically ulcerated, with the characteristic rolled border and central partial necrotic ulceration. Rarely, the lesion is endophytic with little ulceration, simulating the rare nonsquamous tumors, or occasionally it is very exophytic (Fig. 15-16) or bulky[96] (Fig. 15-17). Clinical experience suggests a greater propensity to ill-defined and often multifocal lesions in the floor of the mouth. This may explain the significant incidence of second primaries in this site.[96] With tumor progression there is soon involvement of the adjacent structures, particularly the tongue and gingiva (Figs. 15-10a and 15-17). In Harrold's series[97]

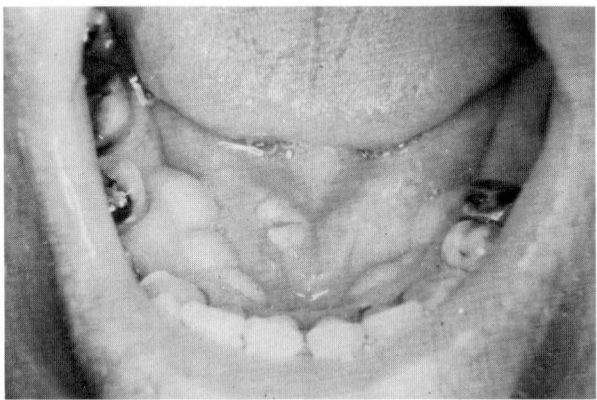

FIGURE 15-15 Small exophytic, verrucous-appearing T_1 squamous carcinoma of the right anterior floor of mouth lent itself well to wide per oral excision with closure by secondary intention. Right upper neck lymph node metastases did not appear until 7 years later.

only 23 percent had cancers confined to the floor of the mouth upon admission; 40 percent of the lesions extended beyond the midline, 11 percent were equally distributed bilaterally, and 15 percent clinically involved bone. Of the definitively treated patients 39 percent had histologically proven unilateral cervical lymph node metastases on admission (Fig. 15-18). An additional 6 percent had bilateral metastases, and 2 percent, contralateral. Another 17 percent developed such metastases

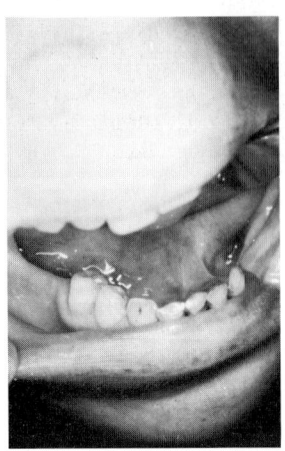 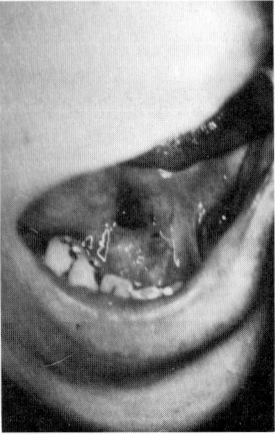

a *b*

FIGURE 15-14 (*a*) Ill-defined, erythematous, flat lesion on right anterior floor of mouth in a 50-year-old female who has had 2 previous oral squamous carcinomas. (*b*) Topical staining with toluidine blue better delineates this in situ squamous carcinoma. Note the adjacent separate foci around the margin of the dominant lesion.

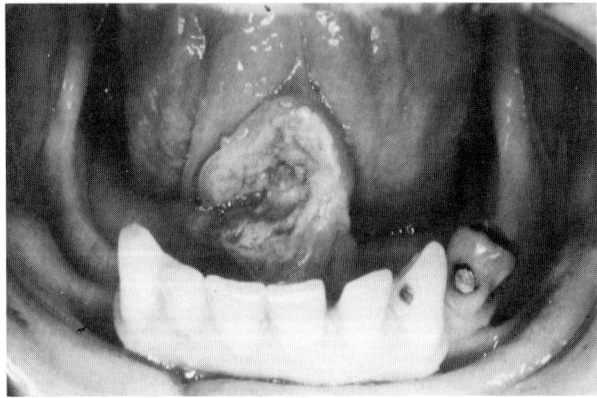

FIGURE 15-16 Large exophytic squamous carcinoma of the right anterior floor of mouth with secondary involvement of the ventral tongue.

subsequently for a total of 56 percent with cervical lymph node involvement at some time during the course of their disease. Of those who had ipsilateral nodal metastases, 24 percent developed contralateral metastases as well. Approximately half of the nodal metastases were confined to the upper third of the neck, with the rest more extensive, but 10 percent had sparing of the upper third, with their metastases confined to the lower neck.[97]

Initial symptoms do not significantly differ from those of other oral cancers except when the tumor produces obstruction of Wharton's duct. An asymptomatic, critically located anterior floor-of-mouth cancer may produce significant salivary duct obstruction, simulating benign obstructive sialadenitis. Intraoral inspection will usually reveal the true cause of the obstruction. In such circumstances it is vitally important to distinguish between the obstructed salivary gland and prevascular or intracapsular metastatic lymphadenopathy in the submandibular triangle. Pain is rarely seen, and even the larger lesion may produce only minimal pain. The pain usually results from infection, infiltration, and obstruction. Bleeding stems from trauma to the ulcerated mucosa or necrotic tumor breakdown with secondary oozing. As the disease progresses and infiltrates the tongue musculature, tongue motion is impeded, with resultant difficulties in articulation, mastication, and deglutition. Ultimately weight loss results from progressive difficulty and pain with swallowing. Disturbances of sensation and pathologic fracture of the mandible occur only with those very far advanced cancers.

In the series of Spiro et al.[64] only 17, or 3.5 percent,

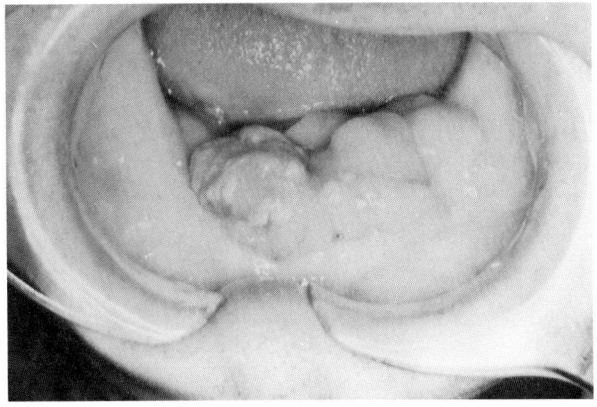

FIGURE 15-17 Massive mucoepidermoid carcinoma replacing most of the floor of the mouth and displacing the tongue posteriorly. Bilateral upper cervical lymph node metastases were also present.

of the 492 minor salivary gland tumors arose in the floor of the mouth; most of these were pathologically classified as *adenocarcinoma* (Table 15-3). Their clinical behavior was similar to that of other minor salivary gland tumors elsewhere in the oral cavity.

TREATMENT

As has been noted with the other oral sites, the early superficial T_1 and T_2 floor-of-mouth cancers can be effectively treated by either surgery or radiation with

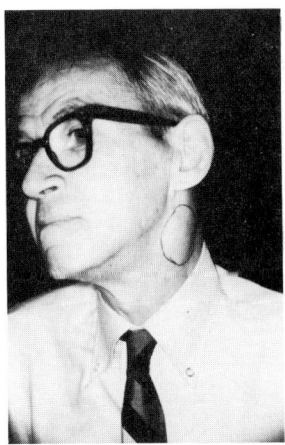
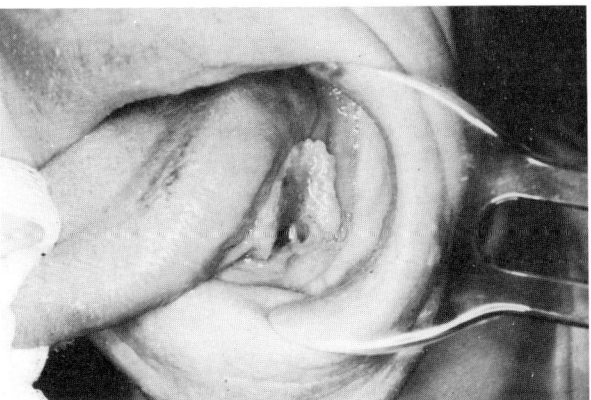

a   b

FIGURE 15-18 (*a*) This adult male presented for medical care with this painless, 4-cm firm, clinically metastatic lymph node in his left upper neck. (*b*) Appropriate clinical examination detected this 3-cm infiltrating, asymptomatic (!) ulcerated squamous cancer of the left posterior floor of mouth.

TABLE 15-3 Distribution of oral minor salivary gland tumors

Type of tumor	Palate	Tongue	Cheeks, lips	Gums	Floor of mouth	Total
Benign	41	2	9	0	0	52
Adenoid cystic	65	27	13	11	5	121
Adenocarcinoma, solid, and other	43	12	19	6	8	88
Mucoepidermoid	21	10	8	9	4	52
Malignant mixed	7	1	0	2	0	10
Oat cell	4	2	0	0	0	6
Acinic cell	0	0	0	1	0	1
Total	181	54	49	29	17	330

SOURCE: RH Spiro, LG Koss, SI Hajdu, EW Strong: Tumors of minor salivary gland origin, a clinicopathologic study of 492 cases. *Cancer* 31:117, 1973.

similar good results.[93,95–97,102] Radiation has the obvious advantage of producing no functional or cosmetic deformity but may require both external and interstitial therapy to achieve adequate dose.[98,102] Such implantation significantly adds to the risk of subsequent bone exposure and osteoradionecrosis. Anatomic site of the tumor, radiation dosage, and dental status appear to be of greatest significance in the etiology of radiation necrosis.[103] With the larger T_3 and T_4 lesions necessary radiation dosage is significantly higher, leading to unacceptable complication rates, thus favoring combined surgery and radiation therapy in these patients.[98,102]

The ease of surgical resection of any floor-of-mouth cancer relates to its size (stage), location, proximity to bone, and the presence or absence of teeth. The small, accessible lesion can be satisfactorily excised through the open mouth and the wound closed primarily or with a skin graft or left open to heal by secondary contracture and reepithelialization. The latter is remarkably well tolerated by most patients, and if the defect is not too large or abutting onto bone, the functional results are good. When the tumor approaches the mandible, marginal, or "rim," resection, including teeth, if present, is indicated (Fig. 15-10). Again every attempt should be made to conserve uninvolved mandible. The median mandibulotomy, or "mandibular swing," may allow much more adequate exposure for resection of large and posterior tumors of the floor of mouth and tongue than could be possible otherwise without bone sacrifice.[104] Whenever bone is frankly invaded, segmental mandibulectomy is usually necessary. While the relatively small lateral mandibular resection is usually well tolerated functionally and cosmetically, the necessity for arch resection often results in a cosmetic and functional disaster. One of the most obvious defects in all of head and neck surgery is that resulting from the resection of the chin. This defect is also one of the most difficult to reconstruct satisfactorily. The problems of mandibular replacement have been addressed previously, but soft-tissue deficits are equally challenging. While soft-tissue bulk can now be more readily replaced with myocutaneous[72] and free flaps,[73] adequate support and enervation of the flaps are seldom, if ever, achieved, even by multiple ingenious methods and efforts.[105–107] Whenever possible, the Wharton's duct(s) should be reimplanted more posteriorly, with the hope of reducing the incidence of postoperative submandibular salivary gland enlargement, often confused with metastatic lymphadenopathy.

We believe neck dissection to be indicated in the presence of clinically involved cervical lymph nodes. Whenever the primary cancer crosses the midline, it may be appropriate to remove the contents of the contralateral submandibular triangle to permit adequate exposure for resection of the primary tumor, and to sample the contralateral lymph nodes at risk. If these nodes are histologically involved, then further treatment of that neck is indicated, either by completion of radical neck dissection or by postoperative radiotherapy. Generally, we recommend bilateral neck dissections be done in stages and have little hesitation in the routine sacrifice of both internal jugular veins whenever necessary, but recognize the increased risk and morbidity resulting therefrom.[108]

RESULTS

Cure rates approaching 90 and 70 percent, respectively, can be achieved in patients with T_1 and T_2 tumors by surgery or radiation, including external and/or interstitial.[93,95,98,100,102] As is true elsewhere in the oral cavity, the greater the extent of the tumor, with increasing likelihood of involvement of adjacent structures, the poorer the prognosis. Treatment, often multidisciplinary, must be more aggressive and has less likelihood of success. In Harrold's series covering a 30-year span, the overall survival rates for 634 determinate patients were 69 percent, 49 percent, 24 percent and 7 percent for stages I to IV, respectively. A more recent and smaller series treated primarily by radiotherapy was reported by Fu et al. to have determinant survivals of 93 percent, 71 percent, 43 percent, and 10 percent for stages I to IV.[102] It should be pointed out that these are not entirely comparable series. Crissman et al.,[93] in their attempt to retrospectively grade cancers of the floor of the mouth by a modified Jakobsson's scheme, concluded that the extent of the primary tumor, particularly its degree of infiltration, was of value in predicting the likelihood of regional metastases. They concluded that elective treatment of cervical lymph nodes was not necessary in those patients with very superficial or microinvasive floor-of-mouth lesions but that those deeply infiltrating neoplasms with nodular or vertical growth patterns should be treated more aggressively, including elective radical neck dissection. They also confirmed the often erroneous clinical assessment of cervical lymph nodes, with 56 percent false positives and 4 percent false negatives observed. The other parameters of the histologic grading system did not seem to offer any significant predictions of prognosis. Most studies report that the state of the regional lymph nodes is the most important prognostic factor.[93,95,98,100]

The necessity for close and continuing follow-up of patients with cancer of the floor of the mouth is the same as that for other sites. Every attempt should be made to encourage the patients to stop all further exposure to possible etiologic agents and to remain under continuing observation, since they are at high risk of recurrence *and* of new primary cancers.

TONGUE

ANATOMY

The tongue is arbitrarily divided by a line connecting the circumvallate papillae into an anterior two-thirds, the mobile or oral tongue, and a posterior one-third, or base. In the 1978 revision of the *Manual for Staging of Cancer* the oral tongue is included in the oral cavity and the base in the oropharynx.[37] The oral tongue is that anterior, freely mobile portion of the organ extending from the ventral junction with the mucosa of the floor of the mouth posteriorly to the line of the circumvallate papillae. The oral tongue is divided into four areas: the tip, the lateral borders, the dorsum, and the undersurface, or ventral surface, having no papillae.[37]

The lymphatic drainage of the tongue is rich and consists of superficial and deep channels draining different portions of the tongue into four main collecting trunks, which in turn drain into submental, submandibular, jugulodigastric, and jugulocarotid lymph nodes. There is extensive bilateral drainage, especially of the central regions and the base of the tongue. In general, the more anterior neoplasms have a greater probability of draining directly to lower jugular lymph nodes. Drainage from upper to lower cervical lymph nodes is not necessarily sequential, and with these multiple lymphatic intercommunications metastasis from any part of the tongue to any level of cervical lymph nodes may occur,[109] even to contralateral nodes.

INCIDENCE AND ETIOLOGY

Cancer of the tongue is the most common oral neoplasm seen at Memorial Hospital. In Mashberg's series[101] of early asymptomatic oral cancers, tongue lesions were the second most common, numbering only 36, or 16.2 percent of the 222 lesions. Age-adjusted incidence rates for cancer of the tongue vary from 0.5 to 0.8 cases per 100,000 population for women, except in Puerto Rico, where it is 2.2 cases per 100,000, and between 1.4 and 6.6 cases per 100,000 population for men.[110] Tongue cancer may afflict patients of any sex or age, but most will be male and in the sixth or seventh decade of life.[110–113] Increasing incidence in the female and the occasional tongue cancer in the young patient are evident.

The etiology of tongue cancer is similar to that of other oral cancers. Its usual location along the lateral borders as opposed to the dorsum suggests a somewhat greater role of dental irritation than with other oral cancers, but this has not been confirmed. There appears to be an association between chronic atrophic glossitis, leukoplakia, and cancers of the dorsum of the tongue.[101] The relationship between reverse smoking and cancer of the dorsum has been previously noted.[7]

PATHOLOGY

Squamous carcinoma constitutes approximately 97 percent of all malignant tongue lesions. Glandular tumors and tumors of supporting structures make up the remainder. In the series of minor salivary gland tumors reported by Spiro et al.[64] the tongue was the third most common primary site, these tumors making up 11 percent of the total series (Table 15-3). The rare lymphoma of the tongue almost always involves the base of the organ.

The squamous cancers tend to be histologically mature, with infiltrative, ulcerative, and exophytic growth patterns. The dorsum, tip, and ventral surface are least common sites of primary tumor. While the tumors usually arise from normal epithelium, some may appear in areas of clinical leukoplakia or on preexisting chronic glossitis. Experience suggests this is frequently true with cancer of the dorsum. The tumors of the tongue base may be less well differentiated histologically than those of the oral tongue.[19]

CLINICAL PRESENTATION

Most cancers of the tongue arise in the oral, or mobile, portion of the structure. Frazell and Lucas[111] described 75 percent in the anterior tongue and 25 percent in the base, while a later study[114] from the same institution noted a two-thirds to one-third division and the frequency of base-of-tongue lesions appeared to be increasing. More oral tongue cancers will involve the posterior half of the lateral border than will be seen on the anterior half or tip, with cancer of the dorsum uncommon and midline lesions very rare.[101,111] Most of the earliest lesions will be flat, erythroplastic, and ill-defined (Fig. 15-19). With further local progression the surface will be elevated, perhaps granular, then roughened. More advanced lesions are usually ulcerated, with rolled undurated borders. An occasional verrucous lesion will be noted (Fig. 15-20). Endophytic, essentially minimally ulcerated tumors will be detected more commonly in the base than in the oral tongue. Large exophytic lesions are occasionally seen.

The most common initial symptom is the presence of a mass with local pain. Dysphasia or a lump in the neck are less frequent complaints. In the Frazell and Lucas study,[111] 80 percent of the primary lesions were estimated to exceed 2 cm, and 20 percent were in excess of 5 cm in greatest diameter. Direct extension to the floor of the mouth, alveolar ridge, soft palate, and other adjacent structures was noted in one-half of the patients, and 40 percent presented with cervical lymph node metastases,. The oral tongue lesions tend to be smaller and are detected earlier than those of the base, and only 25 percent extend to adjacent structures.[114] Regional lymph node involvement on admission in oral tongue cancer is reported to vary from 18 to 38.5 percent.[111–114,120] The likelihood of nodal metastases appears to vary directly with the size of the primary tumor and its anteroposterior location.[113,114]

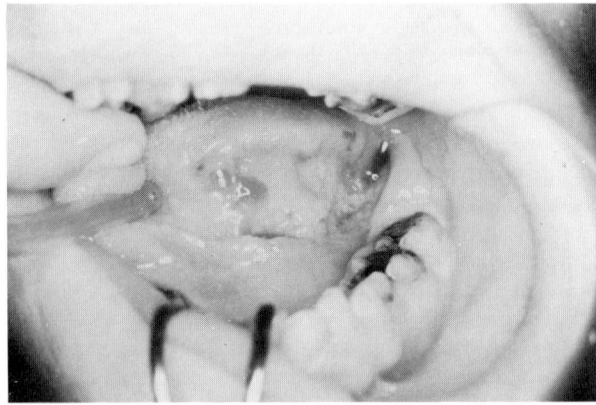

FIGURE 15-19 Diffuse, ill-defined, spreading, ulcerated squamous carcinoma of the left lateral border of the tongue.

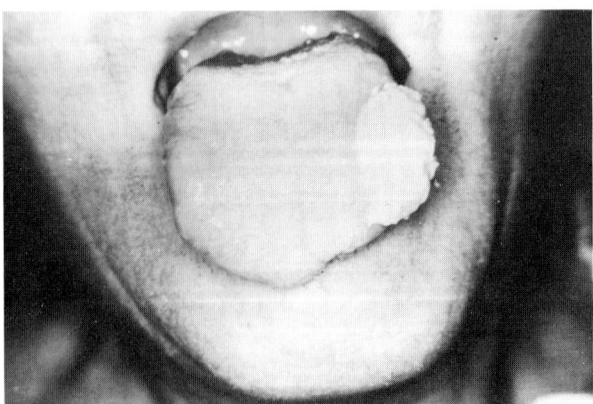

FIGURE 15-20 Two simultaneous cancers of the oral tongue, the right endophytic and ulcerated, the left exophytic and verrucous. Metastases appeared in the right neck within 6 months of partial glossectomy but no metastases ever appeared on the left.

TREATMENT

Radiation and surgery each play a major role in the treatment of oral tongue cancer, but there has been a varying preference for one modality over the other for much of this century. The ultimate decision will usually be based upon the location and stage of the primary tumor, particularly in its relationship to bone or other structures and the presence or absence of regional lymph node metastases.

In a patient with a small T_1 tumor either partial glossectomy or irradiation is highly effective treatment, with surgery offering the advantages of speed and simplicity. As the lesion increases in size or invades bone, the discrepancy between the results of surgery and radiotherapy widen, and surgery has preference. Low-voltage irradiation via peroral cones was more commonly used in the past[111] but has been largely supplanted by external and/or interstitial irradiation.[112,113] There is clear evidence of the need for increasing dose with increasing size of the primary lesion.[112–114] The primary lesion is rarely controlled by external radiation therapy alone, regardless of size, and adequate treatment requires supplementation with interstitial irradiation.[112] High doses, particularly when delivered by interstitial implant procedures, produce significant complication rates, with subsequent morbidity but minimal mortality.[112,113,115] Implantation of the tongue is an exacting technique usually requiring general anesthesia, a tracheostomy, and an experienced radiotherapist. Afterloading techniques in which plastic tubes are positioned for the subsequent insertion of the radioactive sources may be used to protect personnel from radiation exposure. This permits more precise dosimetry and the opportunity for adjustment of dosage based upon computerized calculations of dosimetry curves.[116]

Since local control rates are significantly less with large lesions, combined therapy has been used with increasing frequency. With the larger tongue lesions, surgical resection becomes more radical, necessitating more adequate exposure and consideration of various reconstructive techniques. The concerns about mandible are the same as those described for the floor of the mouth, as are the technical aspects of the procedure and subsequent reconstruction. Resection of major portions of the oral tongue will significantly interfere with mastication, deglutition, and articulation. The more extensive the necessary resection, the more likely the need for reconstruction and aggressive rehabilitative efforts. Fortunately few patients with oral tongue cancer will require total glossectomy. In no patient after total glossectomy is speech normal. Such speech is of variable intelligibility and problems of aspiration are considerable. Distant flap reconstruction will provide for lost mucosal surface but will offer little functional benefit. The effort exerted by the patient in the rehabilitation will require the cooperation of surgeon, speech pathologist, nurse, and dietitian.[117,118] Occasionally prosthetic replacement of the tongue may be of some benefit.[118] The morbidity of each radical surgery is great and only by very careful selection of patients for such procedures can their success be anticipated. The older, more debilitated, poorly motivated patient can seldom be successfully rehabilitated to swallow and to speak satisfactorily, and probably should undergo total laryngectomy as part of the procedure.

Considerations of treatment of the neck at risk are similar to those for other oral cancers. If the primary tumor is small and easily accessible and the neck clinically negative, then the neck may be observed. If the treatment of the primary tumor is by radiotherapy, the entire neck should be irradiated with good expectation of control of microscopic disease. The likelihood of regional nodal metastases increases with increasing T stage,[114,115] and with lesions greater than 2 cm in diameter, elective treatment of the neck seems justified. The larger the primary tumor, the poorer the results of its treatment by any modality, but surgery supplemented by postoperative radiotherapy may be more effective than either modality alone.[112,114,115]

RESULTS

In the report from Memorial Hospital in 1962 the 5-year cure rate in 843 patients treated for cure for carcinoma of the oral tongue was 40.7 percent.[111] By 1974 the "cure rate" in 236 patients was 49.1 percent.[114] Similar reports of comparable results from radiation therapy have appeared.[113] Cure will depend upon adequate dose being delivered to a sufficiently large volume to encompass the entire tumor. It is often impossible to compare results from different series because treatment methods have not been standardized, differing staging systems are described, and different statistical methods of reporting are used. It is clear that 90 percent of small lesions can be controlled by surgery[114] or interstitial implantation.[113,116] In the later Memorial series, 5-year determinant survival by stage for oral tongue cancer was 69.2 percent, 52.7 percent, and 36.6 percent in stages I to III, respectively. Of the three patients with stage IV disease in the series, none was salvaged.[114] In a large radiation series[113] covering a different time interval, 80 percent, 56 percent, and 25 percent of stages I to III were salvaged based upon a somewhat different staging system. With increasing T stage and increasing radiation dosage, increased complications were documented in the later study ranging from 11 percent soft-tissue and 6 percent bone complications in T_1 to 29 percent soft-tissue and 37 percent bone complications in T_3 lesions in those patients alive and free of disease at 5 years.

Attempts to predict the clinical behavior of tumor based upon histologic grading have been reported. Lund et al.[119] using Jakobsson's grading system in a careful study of a small number of tongue cancers concluded that a significant relationship existed between microscopic grading and the frequency of lymph node metastases. No correlation was found between grading score and recurrence or residual tumor, mortality, or T classification. Generally, the more anaplastic lesions have been clinically more aggressive and the results of their treatment less satisfactory. As the portion of favorable cases in any series increases, the cure rate can likewise be expected to increase. Relatively few patients with stage IV disease will be cured regardless of treatment.

Authors differ concerning the relative importance of T vs. N stage in determining prognosis. DeCroix and Ghossein[113] stated the most important prognostic factor with large cancers of the tongue was the T stage of the primary and not the degree of regional lymph node involvement. Other authors concluded that the status of the cervical lymph nodes was prognostically the most important factor.[112,120] Most have suggested[114,115,120] that more aggressive treatment of regional lymph nodes might improve prognosis.

The treatment of recurrent tongue cancer is unsatisfactory. Few of the recurrences are salvaged by any aggressive treatment. Local or regional failure is most common and will usually occur within 2 years of initial treatment.[113,120] It is suggested that higher stage lesions recur sooner than low-stage. Of the radiation failures only 10 to 15 percent are salvaged by subsequent therapy, usually surgical. Of the few who were secondarily treated, surgery salvaged one-third, but only 17 percent of radiation salvages were successful.[113] As is true with all head and neck cancers, the first treatment is that most likely to succeed.

Most series[111-113,115] report the incidence of secondary primary cancers in these patients to range between 10 and 20 percent. Most occurred in the head and neck area, with lung and esophagus also being commonly affected. Follow-up needs to be meticulous and frequent with the hope of detecting both recurrence and second primaries early and of treating them more effectively.

Cancer of the tongue is the most common oral tumor. It is subtle in its initial manifestations but is uniformly progressive. Most oral tongue cancers are clearly visible and accessible to early diagnosis and appropriate treatment. The challenge of rehabilitation of the patient following major tongue resection has not yet been met. Early detection and treatment offers the best chance of cure, with significantly less morbidity from treatment and mortality from disease.

ORAL CANCER AND THE FUTURE

There are many unanswered questions about head and neck cancer. What are its specific causes? How can it be prevented? How can it be detected earlier? What is the role of each therapeutic modality in treatment? How can these modalities be most effectively combined to produce optimum treatment results with minimal morbidity? How can we predict response to therapy? What is the best method of reconstruction? All these and many other questions require answers. The past decade has seen major accomplishments in surgical reconstruction of extensive defects after radical head and neck resections. The musculocutaneous and free flaps in all their varieties and modifications have revolutionized head and neck reconstruction.[72,73] We anticipate more of these with refinements in indications and techniques in order to achieve superior results. The recent case report of functional cheek reconstruction with microsurgical techniques and reenervation of the flap is an example of such sophistication.[121]

The concept of less radical surgical resection in combination with radiation and/or chemotherapy should be critically studied. Can unresectable tumors be rendered resectable by initial chemotherapy or radiation, permitting "adequate" subsequent removal with less cosmetic and functional defects with equally good results? Conservation surgery of the larynx is a good model of conservative surgery combined with functional preservation based upon careful patient selection and sound knowledge of patterns of disease spread and prognosis.[122]

The influence of nutrition on the response of the patient and the tumor to treatment has been recognized.[123] Future investigations will identify those important therapeutic and prognostic parameters subject to modification for the benefit of the patient. What constitutes inadequate nutrition? How can it be most adequately measured and characterized and then subsequently corrected to favorably influence treatment results? Does "adequate" nutrition favorably influence results of treatment? What will be its cost-effectiveness?

New developments in radiation therapy are on the horizon.[59,90] We anticipate identification of better combinations and sequences of treatment modalities. Under investigation are high-linear-energy transfer irradiation, hyperthermia, radiation sensitizers and protectors, and newer radioisotopes with more effective utilization of brachytherapy techniques.

New chemotherapeutic agents are appearing regularly. We need more standardized criteria in order to evaluate drug response. New drugs and new drug combinations and new methods of their delivery in both the therapeutic and adjuvant setting will be forthcoming.

In the laboratory, successful culture of squamous cancer cells has been accomplished.[124,125] This technique opens new avenues for identification of radiation and drug sensitivity, and models for studying mechanism of invasion and cell kinetics.[126,127] Serologic studies of serum proteins and of immune complexes and many in vitro assays of immune competence are being developed. Subpopulations of immune reactive cells can now be more adequately studied. We need to better characterize and to explain the profound immunodepression of the head and neck cancer patient and to investigate new means of modification and stimulation of the immune system. Cytogenic and hybridoma research may well lead to development of monoclonal antibodies for more specific treatment of squamous cancers of the head and neck.

Hand in hand with all of these is the need for better research in the prevention of head and neck cancer. Social and behavioral research may identify means of facilitating tobacco and alcohol cessation. The prevention of the disease holds greater promise than modifications of treatment of established neoplasia.

All these developments and others that will appear in the future, the combined efforts of many individuals and disciplines, may enable us to lessen the impact of head and neck cancer on our patients and their families.

REFERENCES

1. Silverberg E: Cancer statistics 1981. *CA* 31:13, 1981.
2. Farr HW et al: Epidermoid carcinoma of the mouth and pharynx at Memorial Sloan-Kettering Cancer Center, 1965–1969. *Am J Surg* 140:563, 1980.
3. Wynder EL: Etiological aspects of squamous cancers of the head and neck. *JAMA* 215:452, 1972.
4. Martin HE: The history of linqual cancer. *Am J Surg* 48:703, 1940.
5. Crile G: Excision of cancer of the head and neck with specific reference to the plan of dissection based on one hundred and thirty-two operations. *JAMA* 47:1780, 1906.
6. Blot WJ, Fraumeni JF Jr: Geographic pattern of oral cancer in the United States: Etiologic implications. *J Chronic Dis* 30:745, 1977.
7. Mahboubi E: The epidemiology of oral cavity, pharyngeal, and esophageal cancer outside of North America and Western Europe. *Cancer* 40:1879, 1977.
8. Smith EM: Epidemiology of oral and pharyngeal cancer in the United States: Review of recent literature. *J Natl Cancer Inst* 63:1189, 1979.
9. Wynder EL, Stillman SD: Comparative epidemiology of tobacco-related cancers. *Cancer Res* 37:4608, 1977.
10. Silverman S, Griffith M: Smoking characteristics of patients with oral carcinoma and the risk for second oral primary carcinoma. *J Am Dent Assoc* 85:637, 1972.
11. Moore C: Cigarette smoking and cancer of the mouth, pharynx, and larynx: A continuing study. *JAMA* 218:553, 1971.
12. Shanta V, Frishnamurthi S: A study of aetiological factors in oral squamous cell carcinoma. *Br J Cancer* 13:381, 1959.
13. Graham S et al: Dentition, diet, tobacco and alcohol in the epidemiology of oral cancer. *J Natl Cancer Inst* 59:1611, 1977.
14. McCoy GD et al: The roles of tobacco, alcohol and diet in the etiology of upper alimentary and respiratory tract cancer. *Prev Med* 9:622, 1980.
15. Rothman E, Keller AZ: The effect of joint exposure to alcohol and tobacco on risk of cancer of the mouth and pharynx. *J Chronic Dis* 25:711, 1972.
16. Mashberg A et al: Alcohol as a primary risk factor in oral squamous carcinoma. *CA* 31:146, 1981.
17. Nicolau SG, Babus L: Chronic actinic cheilitis and cancer of the lower lip. *Br J Dermatol* 76:278, 1964.
18. Keller AZ: Cellular types, survival, race, nativity, occupation, habits, and associated diseases in the pathogenesis of lip cancers. *Am J Epidemiol* 91:486, 1970.
19. Batsakis JG: *Tumors of the Head and Neck: Clinical and Pathological Considerations*, Williams & Wilkins, Baltimore, 1974.
20. World Health Organization Collaborating Centre for Oral Precancerous Lesions: Definition of leukoplakia and related lesions: An aid to studies on oral precancer. *Oral Surg* 46:518, 1978.
21. Pindborg JJ et al: Studies in oral leukoplakia, A preliminary report on the period prevalence of malignant transformation in leukoplakia based on a follow-up study of 248 patients. *J Am Dent Assoc* 76:767, 1968.

22. Einhorn J, Wersall J: Incidence of oral carcinoma in patients with leukoplakia of the oral mucosa. *Cancer* 20:2189, 1967.
23. Waldron CA, Shafer WG: Leukoplakia revisited. A clinicopathological study of 3256 oral leukoplakias. *Cancer* 36:1386, 1975.
24. Mashberg A et al: A study of the appearance of early asymptomatic oral squamous cell carcinoma. *Cancer* 32:1436, 1973.
25. Shafer WG, Waldron CA: Erythroplakia of the oral cavity. *Cancer* 36:1021, 1975.
26. Prioleau PG et al: Verrucous carcinoma. A light and electron microscopic, autoradiographic and immunofluorescence study. *Cancer* 45:2849, 1980.
27. Broders AC: Carcinoma. Grading and practical application. *Arch Pathol* 2:376, 1926.
28. Jakobsson PA: Histologic grading of malignancy and prognosis in glottic carcinoma of the larynx. *Can J Otolaryngol* 4:885, 1975.
29. Lindberg R: Distribution of cervical lymph node metastases from squamous cell carcinoma of the upper respiratory and digestive tracts. *Cancer* 29:1446, 1972.
30. Shear M et al: The prediction of lymph node metastases from oral squamous carcinoma. *Cancer* 37:1901, 1976.
31. Spiro RH, Frazell EL: Evaluation of the radical surgical treatment of advanced cancer of the mouth. *Am J Surg* 116:571, 1968.
32. Kalnins IK et al: Correlation between prognosis and degree of involvement in carcinoma of the oral cavity. *Am J Surg* 134:450, 1977.
33. Johnson JT et al: The extracapsular spread of tumors in cervical node metastases. *Arch Otolaryngol* 107:725, 1981.
34. Shah JP et al: Carcinoma of the oral cavity, factors affecting treatment failure at the primary site and neck. *Am J Surg* 132:504, 1976.
35. Merino OR et al: An analysis of distant metastases from squamous cell carcinoma of the upper respiratory and digestive tracts. *Cancer* 40:145, 1977.
36. Slaughter DP et al: "Field cancerization" in oral stratified squamous epithelium. *Cancer* 6:963, 1953.
37. American Joint Committee for Cancer Staging and End Results Reporting: *Manual for Staging of Cancer 1978*, Chicago, pp 1–10, 27–32.
38. Spiro RH et al: Cervical lymph nodes metastasis from epidermoid carcinoma of the oral cavity and oropharynx, a critical assessment of current staging. *Am J Surg* 128:562, 1974.
39. Snow JB et al: Comparison of preoperative with postoperative radiation therapy for patients with carcinoma of the head and neck. *Acta Otolaryngol* 91:611, 1981.
40. Vikram B et al: Elective postoperative radiation therapy in stages III and IV epidermoid carcinoma of the head and neck. *Am J Surg* 140:580, 1980.
41. Jesse RH, Lindberg RD: The efficacy of combining radiation therapy with a surgical procedure in patients with cervical metastases from squamous cancer of the oropharynx and hypopharynx. *Cancer* 35:1163, 1975.
42. Fletcher GH, Jesse RH: The place of irradiation in the management of primary lesion in head and neck cancer. *Cancer* 39:862, 1977.
43. Noyek AM: Bone scanning in otolaryngology. *Laryngoscope* (suppl 18): vol 89, part 2, 1979, pp 1–86.
44. Strong EW: The classical radical neck dissection, in Kagan and Miles (eds): *Head and Neck Oncology—Controversies in Cancer Management*, Hall Medical, Boston, 1981.
45. Jesse RH: Modified neck dissection with and without radiation, in Kagan and Miles (eds): *Head and Neck Oncology—Controversies in Cancer Management*, Hall Medical, Boston, 1981.
46. Suen JY et al: Evaluation of the effectiveness of postoperative radiation therapy for the control of local disease. *Am J Surg* 140:577, 1980.
47. Wizenberg MJ et al: Treatment of lymph node metastases in head and neck cancer, a radiotherapeutic approach. *Cancer* 29:1455, 1972.
48. Schneider JJ et al: Control by irradiation alone of nonfixed clinically positive lymph nodes from squamous cell carcinoma of the oral cavity, oropharynx, supraglottic larynx, and hypopharynx. *Am J Roentgenol* 123:42, 1975.
49. Spiro RH et al: Discontinuous partial glossectomy and radical neck dissection in selected patients with epidermoid carcinoma of the mobile tongue. *Am J Surg* 126:544, 1973.
50. Fletcher GH: Elective irradiation of subclinical disease in cancers of the head and neck. *Cancer* 29:1450, 1972.
51. Vandenbrouck C et al: Elective vs. therapeutic radical neck dissection in epidermoid carcinoma of the oral cavity. *Cancer* 46:386, 1980.
52. Glick JH et al: Chemotherapy for squamous cell carcinoma of the head and neck: A progress report. *Am J Otolaryngol* 1:306, 1980.
53. Muggia FM, Wolf GT: Intra-arterial chemotherapy of head and neck cancer: Worth another look? *Cancer Clin Trials* 3:375, 1980.
54. Gage AA: Five-year survival following cryosurgery for oral cancer. *Arch Surg* 111:990, 1976.
55. Patterson WB: Treatment of intraoral cancer by electrocoagulation. *Cancer* 43:821, 1979.
56. Strong MS et al: Transoral management of localized carcinoma of the oral cavity using the CO_2 laser. *Laryngoscope* 89:897, 1979.
57. Mohs FE: Chemosurgery. *Cl Plast Surg* 7:349, 1980.
58. Katz AE: Advances in the immunology of head and neck cancer. *Otolaryngol Clin North Am* 13:431, 1980.
59. Pions, ions, neutrons, protons "expanding scope of radiotherapy." *JAMA* 246:2535, 1981.
60. Petrovich Z et al: Carcinoma of the lip. *Arch Otolaryngol* 105:187, 1979.

61. Heller KS, Shah JP: Carcinoma of the lip. *Am J Surg* 138:600, 1979.
62. Baker SR, Krause CJ: Carcinoma of the lip. *Laryngoscope* 90:19, 1980.
63. Jorgensen K et al: Carcinoma of the lip. A series of 869 cases. *Acta Radiol* 12:177, 1973.
64. Spiro RH et al: Tumors of minor salivary origin. A clinicopathologic study of 492 cases. *Cancer* 31:117, 1973.
65. Brown RG et al: Advanced and recurrent squamous carcinoma of the lower lip. *Am J Surg* 132:492, 1976.
66. Wilson JSP, Walker EP: Reconstruction of the lower lip. *Head Neck Surg* 4:29, 1981.
67. Conley J, Sadoyama JA: Squamous cell cancer of the buccal mucosa. A review of 90 cases. *Arch Otolaryngol* 97:330, 1973.
68. Bloom ND, Spiro RH: Carcinoma of the cheek mucosa. A retrospective analysis. *Am J Surg* 140:556, 1980.
69. Brown RL et al: Snuff dippers' intraoral cancer: Clinical characteristics and response to therapy. *Cancer* 18:2, 1965.
70. O'Brien PH, Catlin D: Cancer of the cheek (mucosa). *Cancer* 18:1392, 1965.
71. Bakamjian VY: The surgical management of cancers of the cheek. *J Surg Oncol* 6:255, 1974.
72. Ariyan S, Cuono CB: Myocutaneous flaps for head and neck reconstruction. *Head Neck Surg* 2:321, 1980.
73. Zucker RM et al: Head and neck reconstruction following resection of carcinoma, using microvascular free flaps. *Surgery* 88:461, 1980.
74. Glick JH, Taylor SG: Integration of chemotherapy into a combined modality treatment plan for head and neck cancer: A review. *Int J Radiat Oncol Biol Phys* 7:229, 1981.
75. MacComb WS, Fletcher GH: *Cancer of the Head and Neck*, Williams & Wilkins, Baltimore, 1967, p. 122.
76. Berg JW et al: Incidence of multiple primary cancer. III. Cancers of the respiratory and upper digestive system as multiple primary cancers. *J Natl Cancer Inst* 44:263, 1970.
77. Cady B, Catlin D: Epidermoid carcinoma of the gum, A 20-year survey. *Cancer* 23:551, 1969.
78. Cady B, Hutter RVP: Nonepidermoid cancer of the gum. *Cancer* 23:1318, 1969.
79. Miller AS, Winnick M: Salivary gland inclusion in the anterior mandible. *Oral Surg* 31:790, 1961.
80. Byers RM et al: Results of treatment for squamous carcinoma of the lower gum. *Cancer* 47:2236, 1981.
81. Nathanson A et al: Prognosis of squamous cell carcinoma of the gums. *Acta Otolaryngol* 75:301, 1973.
82. Lee ES, Wilson JSP: Carcinoma involving the lower alveolus. An appraisal of results and an account of current management. *Br J Surg* 60:85, 1973.
83. Serafin I et al: Vascularized rib periosteal and osteocutaneous reconstruction of the maxilla and mandible: An assessment. *Plast Reconstr Surg* 66:718, 1980.
84. Daniel RK: Mandibular reconstruction with free tissue transfers. *Ann Plast Surg* 1:346, 1978.
85. Lawson W et al: Experience with immediate and delayed mandibular reconstruction. *Laryngoscope* 92:5, 1982.
86. Willen R et al: Squamous carcinoma of the gingiva. Histological classification and grading of malignancy. *Acta Otolaryngol* 79:146, 1975.
87. Coates HLC et al: Glandular tumors of the palate. *Surg Gynecol Obstet* 140:589, 1975.
88. Chung CK et al: Squamous cell carcinoma of the hard palate. *Int J Radiat Oncol Biol Phys* 5:191, 1979.
89. Evans JF, Shah JP: Epidermoid carcinoma of the palate. *Am J Surg* 142:451, 1981.
90. Konrad HR et al: Epidermoid carcinoma of the palate. *Arch Otolaryngol* 104:208, 1978.
91. Kaul R et al: Fast neutrons in the treatment of salivary gland tumors. *Int J Radiat Oncol Biol Phys* 7:1667, 1981.
92. Suen JY, Johns ME: Chemotherapy for salivary gland cancer. *Laryngoscope* 92:235, 1982.
93. Crissman JD et al: Squamous cell carcinoma of the floor of the mouth. *Head Neck Surg* 3:2, 1980.
94. Ossoff RH et al: Lymphatics of the floor of mouth and periosteum, Anatomic studies with possible clinical correlations. *Otolaryngol Head Neck Surg* 88:652, 1980.
95. Shedd DP et al: Cancer of the floor of the mouth in Connecticut, 1935–1959. *Cancer* 21:97, 1968.
96. Ballard BR: Squamous cell carcinoma of the floor of mouth. *Oral Surg* 45:568, 1979.
97. Harrold CC: Management of cancer of the floor of the mouth. *Am J Surg* 122:487, 1971.
98. Nakissa N et al: Carcinoma of the floor of the mouth. *Cancer* 42:2914, 1978.
99. Moore C, Catlin D: Anatomic origins and locations of oral cancer. *Am J Surg* 114:510, 1967.
100. Guillamondegui OM et al: Cancer of the anterior floor of mouth. Selective choice of treatment and analysis of failures. *Am J Surg* 140:560, 1980.
101. Mashberg A, Myers H: Anatomic site and size of 222 early asymptomatic oral squamous cell carcinomas. *Cancer* 37:2149, 1976.
102. Fu KK et al: Carcinoma of the floor of mouth: An analysis of treatment results and the sites and causes of failure. *Int J Radiat Oncol Biol Phys* 1:829, 1976.
103. Murray CG et al: Radiation necrosis of the mandible: A 10-year study. *Int J Radiat Oncol Biol Phys* 6:543, 1980.
104. Spiro RH et al: Mandibular "swing" approach for oral and oropharyngeal tumors. *Head Neck Surg* 3:371, 1981.
105. Novack AJ: Carcinoma of the anterior and lateral aspects of the floor of the mouth. *Otolaryngol Clin North Am* 2:565, 1969.
106. Barton RT, Steenerson RL: Technique for closure of the floor of the mouth in monobloc resection. *Arch Otolaryngol* 101:50, 1975.
107. Donald PJ: Surgical rehabilitation following anterior resection for oral cavity carcinoma. *Laryngoscope* 91:1941, 1981.

108. Razack MS et al: Bilateral radical neck dissection. *Cancer* 47:197, 1981.
109. Donegan JO et al: The role of suprahyoid neck dissection in the management of cancer of the tongue and floor of mouth. *Head Neck Surg* 4:209, 1982.
110. Shedd DP et al: Cancer of tongue in Connecticut, 1935–1959. *Cancer* 21:89, 1968.
111. Frazell EL, Lucas JC: Cancer of the tongue. Report of the management of 1554 patients. *Cancer* 15:1085, 1962.
112. Fu KK et al: External and interstitial radiation therapy for carcinoma of the oral tongue. A review of 25 years' experience. *Am J Roentgenol* 126:107, 1976.
113. Decroix Y, Ghossein NA: Experience of the Curie Institute in treatment of cancer of the mobile tongue. *Cancer* 47:496, 1981.
114. Spiro RH, Strong EW: Surgical treatment of cancer of the tongue. *Surg Clin North Am* 54:759, 1974.
115. Marks JE et al: Carcinoma of the oral tongue: A study of patient selection and treatment results. *Laryngoscope* 91:1548, 1981.
116. Pierquin B et al: The place of implantation in tongue and floor of mouth cancer. *JAMA* 215:961, 1971.
117. Effron MZ et al: Advanced carcinoma of the tongue. Management by total glossectomy without larygectomy. *Arch Otolaryngol* 107:694, 1981.
118. deFries HO: Reconstruction of the tongue. *Ann Otol Rhinol Laryngol* 83:471, 1974.
119. Lund C et al: Epidermoid carcinoma of the tongue. Histologic grading in the clinical evaluation. *Acta Radiol (Ther)* 14:497, 1975.
120. Whitehurst JO, Droulias CA: Surgical treatment of squamous cell carcinoma of the oral tongue. Factors influencing survival. *Arch Otolaryngol* 103:212, 1977.
121. Fujino T et al: Primary functional cheek reconstruction: A case report. *Br J Plast Surg* 34:136, 1981.
122. Russ JE et al: Conservation surgery of the larynx: A reappraisal based upon whole-organ study. *Am J Surg* 138:588, 1979.
123. Smole BF et al: The efficacy of nutritional assessment and support in cancer surgery. *Cancer* 47:2375, 1981.
124. Krause CJ et al: Human squamous cell carcinoma. Establishment and characterization of new permanent cell lines. *Arch Otolaryngol* 107:703, 1981.
125. Easty DM et al: Ten human carcinoma cell lines derived from squamous carcinomas of the head and neck. *Brit J Cancer* 43:772, 1981.
126. Salmon SE et al: Quantitation of differential sensitivity of human tumor stem cells to anticancer drugs. *N Engl J Med* 298:1321, 1978.
127. Carter SK: Predictors of response and their clinical evaluation. *Cancer Chemother Pharmacol* 7:1, 1981.

16
TUMORS OF THE NASOPHARYNX, NASAL CAVITY, AND PARANASAL SINUSES

Jose J. Terz   Walter Lawrence, Jr.

TUMORS OF THE NASOPHARYNX

Anatomical Aspects

A clear concept of the anatomical boundaries of the nasopharynx facilitates understanding of the clinical manifestations of neoplasms originating in this area (Fig. 16-1). The nasopharynx is an open chamber between the nasal cavity and oropharynx. The anterior limit is formed by the choanae, and at this point the nasopharynx communicates freely with both nasal cavities. The inferior limit is the soft palate, and the lateral boundaries are the pharyngeal walls containing the openings of the eustachian tubes. The superior and posterior wall is formed by mucosa over bony structures forming a continuous slope extending from the basisphenoid and basioccipital to the first and second cervical vertebrae. The extrapharyngeal superior boundaries are adjacent to the second and the third divisions of the trigeminal nerve; the cavernous sinuses; and second, third, and sixth cranial nerves. The lateral wall is adjacent to the pterygomaxillary space bilaterally.

Malignant Tumors

INCIDENCE AND EPIDEMIOLOGY

Nasopharyngeal carcinoma (NPC) is a rare neoplasm in many parts of the world, but it is a leading cause of cancer death in Southeast Asia. The incidence ranges from 15 to 20 per 100,000 in the population in southern China to 0.5 per 100,000 in the white populations of Europe and the United States.[1] The age curve for NPC peaks in the fifth decade and declines thereafter. It is rare in children but is seen between the ages of 10 and 15 when it does occcur.[1-3] This cancer is more frequent in males than females (2.3:1).

The high rate noted for Chinese is observed also in similar populations that have migrated to other parts of Asia and the United States.[1,4] A lower incidence has been observed in mixed populations (with Chinese), strongly suggesting genetic as well as environmental factors. The environmental role in incidence is substantiated by a higher incidence of this cancer in low-risk racial groups (non-Chinese) born and raised in a high-risk area (southern China). These geographic and ethnic variations in the incidence of NPC in adults are also seen in children and adolescents.[2,3]

An epidemiological study in the United States revealed a four- to sevenfold increase in risk among blacks under age 20 compared with the incidence in whites in the same age group. The analysis of mortality rates for NPC in the United States revealed a trimodal curve: (1) a small peak under age 10 among whites only, (2) a second peak at 15 to 24 years, predominantly in blacks, and (3) a larger peak in older adults, higher in blacks than whites but overshadowed by those of Oriental ancestry.[2]

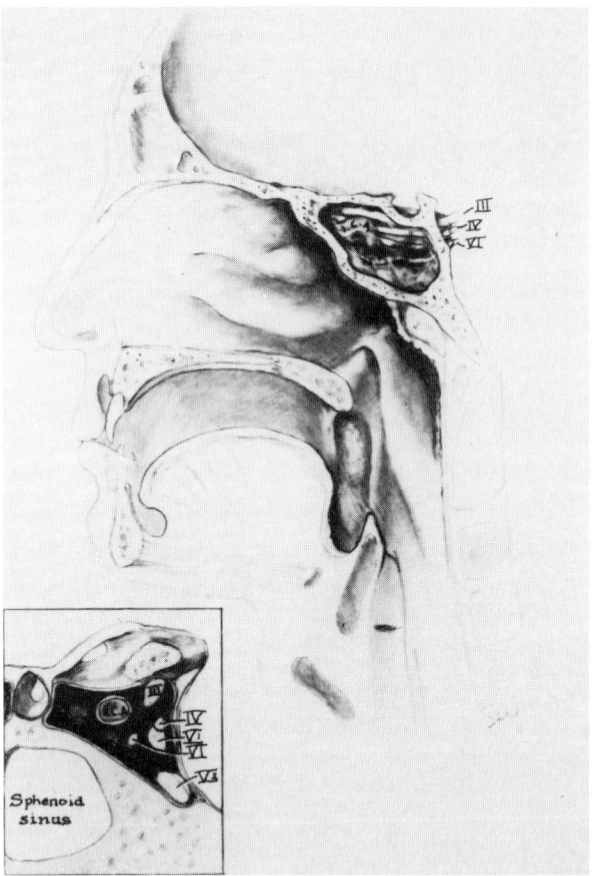

FIGURE 16-1 Anatomy of the nasopharynx showing its relationship to nasal cavity, anterior cranial fossa, sphenoid sinus, and cavernous sinus.

ETIOLOGY

The high incidence of NPC among Chinese and other Orientals, compared with that for other populations in the world, and the recent finding of an association between HLA-A2 and the presence of less than two antigens at the B locus in Chinese patients with NPC, supports the hypothesis that genetic background is a major determinant.[5-7] Now that these findings have been further confirmed, the presence of the HLA-A2 histocompatibility antigen in Chinese is considered a marker of genetic susceptibility to the development of NPC.

Well-controlled epidemiological studies carried out recently in the United States demonstrated an increased risk for NPC associated with a prior history of ear, nose, and throat disease as well as occupational exposure to various fumes and chemicals.[6]

Epstein-Barr virus (EBV), the causative agent of infectious mononucleosis, has been implicated as a factor in the genesis of both Burkitt's lymphoma and nasopharyngeal carcinoma.[8-11] These studies showed that patients with NPC have high titers of antibodies to viral capsular antigens (VCA). The high-geometric-mean titers of antibody to VCA have been shown to be directly related to the stage of disease, increasing from stage 1 to stage 4. Similar correlations were found with the titer of antibodies to the D (diffuse) antigen of the early antigen (EA) complex. The relationship of EBV to NPC was further substantiated by the detection of EBV-DNA in biopsy specimens of NPC. Also, EBV-associated nuclear antigen has been shown to be present in poorly differentiated carcinoma cells, but has not been detected in well-differentiated ones. Recently, it was reported that there are high titers of serum IgA antibodies to EBV-related antigens in 93 percent of patients with NPC, but these antibodies are practically absent in patients with head and neck carcinomas of other sites, Burkitt's lymphoma, and infectious mononucleosis.[10] Thus, the evidence that EBV plays a role in the etiology of NPC is quite impressive.

PATHOLOGY

Epidermoid carcinoma is the most common histologic type of tumor arising in the nasopharynx. This includes a well-differentiated stratified squamous carcinoma with a clear-cut histologic pattern and a poorly differentiated nonkeratinizing form. In this overall group are included the lymphoepitheliomas that are identified by the presence of a large lymphoid cell population associated with the malignant epithelial cells.[12] This lymphoid infiltrate has been the subject of wide speculation, but it has become evident lately that it is the result of a host reaction similar to that seen in other neoplasms (seminoma, pinealoma, breast and gastric cancer) or, alternatively, to the development of a carcinoma in an anatomic region that is rich in lymphoid tissue that lacks sinusoids and efferent lymphatics and, therefore, becomes incorporated in the neoplasm. In any event, these lymphoid tissues are not a histologic feature of distant metastases of this carcinoma, and this lends support to the concept that these tissues are not an integral part of the neoplasm. The other variety of poorly differentiated cancer is the so-called transitional cell cancer that resembles the epithelium of the nasal mucosa, urinary bladder, and trachea. Electron microscopic studies[13] have definitely established the epidermoid nature of both histologic patterns, failing, therefore, to demonstrate any feature to support a major separation in the histologic classification.

Metastatic spread to regional cervical nodes is a common feature of epidermoid carcinomas of the nasopharynx, and quite frequently this is the only clinical evidence of tumor. Bone, lung, and liver metastases are also common occurrences, but they are usually diagnosed late in the course of the disease and virtually always in the presence of an uncontrolled tumor at the primary site.

A less frequent form of primary nasopharyngeal cancer is non-Hodgkin's lymphoma, which must be differentiated from the poorly differentiated forms of epidermoid cancer. These lymphomas are classified into nodular or diffuse, and are well or poorly differentiated, according to the histologic pattern and the grade of maturity of the cell populations.[14] Other tumors are adenoid cystic carcinomas and mucoepidermoid carcinomas that arise from minor salivary glands in the nasopharynx, and extramedullary plasmacytoma, a localized manifestation of plasma cell myeloma.[15]

CLINICAL MANIFESTATIONS

Because of the anatomic location, tumors arising in the nasopharynx are almost never diagnosed in the asymptomatic stage. Cervical adenopathy is the most common initial symptom (44 percent). Decreased hearing due to obstruction of the eustachian tube, and nasal complaints (epistaxis, obstruction, rhinorrhea) secondary to tumor involving the choanae are initial symptoms in 29 percent of patients. Cranial nerve involvement is a rather infrequent finding at the time of the initial diagnosis (12 percent) but is a common finding in later stages of the disease.[16–18]

Compression of cranial nerves II, III, IV, V, or VI results in ophthalmoplegia and facial pain. This may be followed by palpebral ptosis and miosis (Horner's syndrome). When the local neoplasm is uncontrolled, it will eventually invade the meninges, and death then occurs as a result of sepsis, hemorrhage, and general deterioration.

DIAGNOSIS

The nasopharynx is one of the most neglected areas in a general physical examination. This is well illustrated by the fact that the mean duration of the symptoms of NPC prior to therapy is 7 months. Nasal and ear symptoms from NPC are usually mistaken for an inflammatory process, and are treated symptomatically without adequate examination. The proper diagnosis is made, finally, when significant cervical adenopathy develops or when cranial nerve involvement is clinically recognized. The nasopharynx should be suspected as the site of primary tumor in any patient with neoplastic cervical adenopathy without apparent primary tumor.

Examination of the nasopharynx does not require any unusual skill and should be performed as part of the physical examination in any patient with undiagnosed cervical adenopathy or with persistent nasal and ear symptoms that do not respond promptly to medications. With aid of a mirror and topical anesthesia, a digital exploration of the area can be easily accomplished. The retraction of the soft palate with the aid of a soft catheter introduced through the nasal cavity allows direct inspection of the nasopharynx. In the hands of the specialist the use of a nasopharyngoscope gives a clear and accurate view of the area in question.[19] Biopsy of suspicious areas will establish the diagnosis. Occasionally, the nasopharyngeal cancer is very small and not readily visible to the naked eye. For this reason, random biopsies of multiple areas in the nasopharynx should be performed in patients with metastatic cervical adenopathy if there is no clinically apparent primary cancer.

The determination of VCA, EA, and IgA antibody to EBV has proved to be of some value in the diagnosis of occult nasopharyngeal cancer, but it is particularly useful in an index of therapeutic response and prognosis.[20,21]

If the diagnosis of non-Hodgkin's lymphoma is made, the patient should have, in addition, the thorough workup appropriate for lymphomas (bone marrow and liver biopsies, liver and gallium scans) prior to initiating local therapy to the nasopharynx.

STAGING

Proper classification and staging of cancer allows the physician to determine both the appropriate treatment and the prognosis from the extent of the neoplasm. In 1976 the American Joint Committee for Cancer Staging and End Results outlined the staging of nasopharyngeal cancer as shown in Table 16-1 and Fig. 16-2.[22]

Once the diagnosis has been established, the extent of the cancer should be staged clinically according to the classification in Table 16-1. Radiographic examinations can be of great assistance in this process. The use of polytomograms of the base of the skull[23,24] as well as of the lateral soft tissues of the neck, will delineate the extrapharyngeal extensions of the tumor. The recent introduction of computerized tomography (CT)[25,26] has proved very useful also in the evaluation of tumors most commonly involving, or in close proximity to, the base of the skull (Fig. 16-3). The assessment of the extent and location of bone involvement and soft tissue extension is significantly enhanced after intravenous injection of suitable contrast material. Major anatomic landmarks, fissures, and foramina of the base of the skull, the orbit, and the nasal structures are well delineated. Transverse or axial scans for examination of the base of the skull, orbit, and nasal structures are also useful. These are usually taken with the patient in a supine position and

TABLE 16-1 Staging of Nasopharyngeal Cancer

Designation*	Description*
T_{1s}	Carcinoma in situ
T_1	Tumor confined to one side of nasopharynx or nonvisible biopsy only
T_2	Tumor involving two sites (both posterosuperior and lateral walls)
T_3	Tumor invasion of skull and/or cranial nerve involvement
N_0	No nodes
N_1	Single homolateral node less than 3 cm
N_{2a}	Single homolateral node 3 to 6 cm
N_{2b}	Multiple homolateral nodes up to 6 cm
N_{3a}	Homolateral node greater than 6 cm
N_3	Contralateral nodes
Stage 1	$T_1 N_0 M_0$
Stage 2	$T_2 N_0 M_0$
Stage 3	T_1 or T_2 or T_3, $N_1 M_0$
Stage 4	T_4, N_0 or N_1, M_0 Any T, N_2 or N_3, M_0 Any T or N, M_1

* T = tumor; N = node; M = distant metastasis.

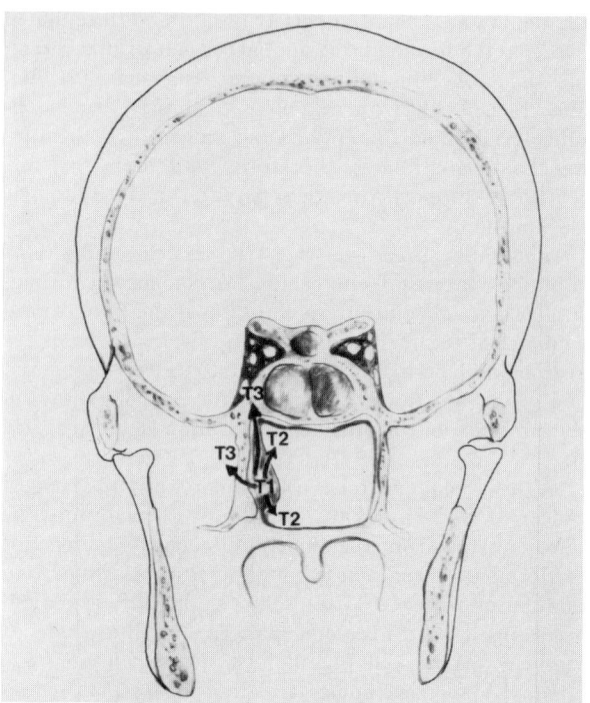

FIGURE 16-2 The stages of nasopharyngeal cancer.

the head hyperextended with cuts parallel to a line drawn between the external auditory canal and the angle of the mandible. The combination of frontal and axial planes provides a realistic assessment of the extent of the tumor, and this is of significant value in planning both treatment and follow-up evaluation.

TREATMENT

Radiation therapy is the only effective modality of primary treatment for NPC. The anatomic location of these tumors at the base of the skull precludes the use of radical surgery under any circumstance. Because of superior physical properties, the use of various forms of megavoltage therapy has changed drastically the outlook for patients with NPC, and has made radiation treatment both safer and simpler. The skin-sparing effects of megavoltage with the decreased adsorption by bone and cartilage, and diminished scatter, allow the delivery of a higher dose to the tumor with minimal damage to surrounding structures. The most common high-energy radiation sources are cobalt teletherapy

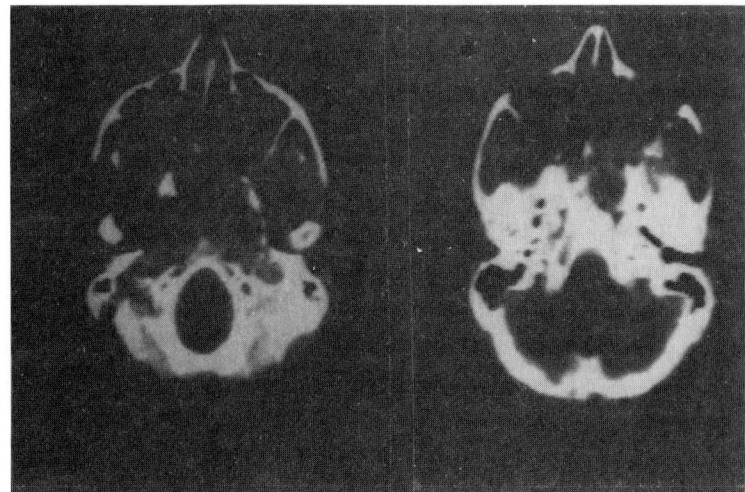

FIGURE 16-3 Computerized tomogram of the head in a patient with a carcinoma of the nasopharynx. The section is made at the level of the ear canal and shows a tumor of the nasopharynx extending into the pterygomaxillary fossa and nasal cavity.

(1.2-MeV γ radiation), the Van de Graaff generator (1- or 2-MeV x-rays), the linear accelerator (4- to 8-MeV x-rays), and the betatron (18- to 48-MeV x-rays).

The primary tumor is usually treated with opposing lateral cervicofacial fields which include the nasopharynx, base of skull, middle cranial fossa, sphenoid sinus, nasal cavity, and the upper jugular and retropharyngeal nodes (Fig. 16-4a and b). When the posterior nasal cavity is involved, anterior nasal fields are included. With the neck extended and the use of eye shields, the nasopharynx will be maintained in the radiation field. The regional lymph nodes in the lower neck and supraclavicular region are treated with opposing tangential anteroposterior fields. A midline lead bar will protect the larynx and the spinal cord, a particularly important area from the standpoint of radiation damage. After 4000 R the nasopharyngeal field is moved forward to ensure protection of the spinal cord, and the neck fields are similarly altered. The recommended size of the ports is 13.9 by 10.5 cm or 146 cm². This more extensive irradiation field has been associated with the lowest incidence of recurrence. The total dose used is 6000 to 6500 R to the nasopharynx and upper neck and 6000 R to the lower neck, delivered over a 5- to 6-week period.[18]

Complications Radionecrosis of skin and mandible are the most common serious complications of radiation therapy for NPC.[16–18] Proper dental care prior to therapy, including the removal of severely damaged teeth from periodontal, periapical, or coronal disease, with restoration when indicated, will reduce these complications significantly.[28,29] Minor complications that may accompany this therapy are xerostomia, decrease in hearing acuity, dryness of the mucous membranes, dental caries, ankylosis of the temporomandibular joint, and hypothyroidism. Ophthalmologic examinations of patients surviving 7 to 30 years after initial treatment have shown that 65 percent of treated patients have changes compatible with cataracts, with minimal chorioretinal changes, but none of the patients have shown optic nerve damage.[30] Pituitary-hypothalamic failure and hypothyroidism are seen in 50 percent of children as a result of radiation therapy. These endocrinological changes are not significant if the proper replacement is instituted early.[31]

Results The reported 5-year free-of-disease survival statistics for NPC range from 27 to 62 percent. The presence of cranial nerve involvement, bone destruction, or bilateral cervical lymph node metastasis at the time of diagnosis carries the worst prognosis.[16–18,32] Most recurrences develop within 18 months of initial treatment, but it is not unusual for recurrent disease to occur after the 5-year interval. Locally, the recurrent primary tumors are occasionally amenable to retreatment with a probability of permanent control in 20 percent of these patients.[33,34]

The histologic type of the NPC has prognostic significance also. For well-differentiated epidermoid carcinoma, the 5-year survival rate is around 30 percent, whereas that for poorly differentiated carcinoma

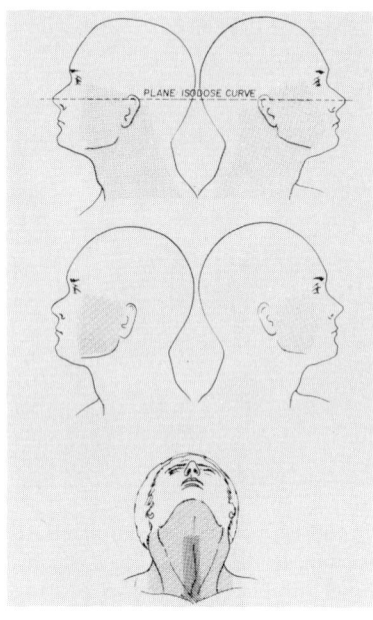
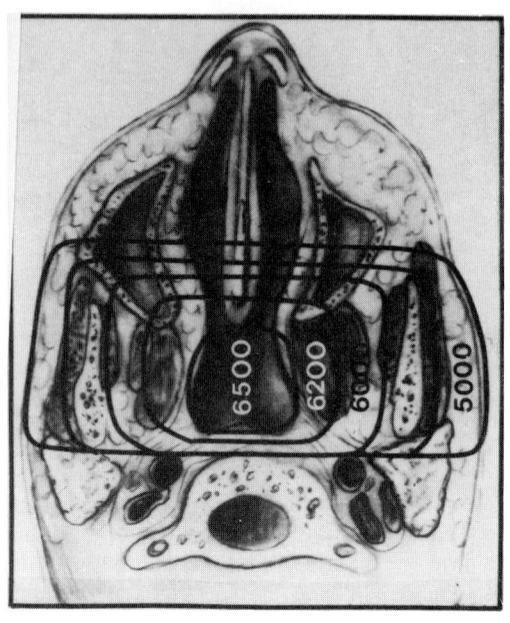

FIGURE 16-4 (*a*) The irradiation portals for the treatment of carcinoma of the nasopharynx and cervical lymph nodes. (*b*) Isodose distribution of the irradiation at the level of the TM joint.

(lymphoepithelioma) is 45 percent. The more aggressive radiotherapeutic approach adopted in the last 15 years, which includes a tumor dose no less than 6500 R, wide fields, and prophylactic irradiation of the neck nodes, is undoubtedly responsible for a significant recent improvement in treatment results.[16–18]

NASAL CAVITY AND PARANASAL SINUSES

Anatomy

NASAL CAVITY

The nasal cavities are paired spaces divided from each other by the nasal septum. They communicate externally through the nares, and posteriorly they open into the nasopharynx through the choanae. They each communicate laterally through ostia with the corresponding maxillary antrum and superiorly with the sphenoid, frontal, and ethmoid sinuses. The roof of the nasal cavity is formed by the cribriform plate that separates this cavity from the anterior cranial fossa. The most anterior part of the nasal cavity corresponding to the ala of the nose (vestibule) is lined with a squamous epithelium containing sweat and sebaceous glands and hair follicles. Posterior to the vestibule, the mucosal lining of the nasal cavity is made up of pseudostratified columnar ciliated epithelium (Schneiderian membrane or respiratory epithelium). This mucosa is highly vascular, has a large number of mucous and serous glands, and plays a role in humidification of inspired air. Above an arbitrary line passing along the superior border of the middle turbinate, the mucosa of the nasal cavity is less vascular, has a yellowish color, and contains serous glands and modified nerve cell bodies which relate to the olfactory nerve fibers (olfactory membrane). Air does not actually circulate through this upper portion of the nasal cavity.

PARANASAL SINUSES

The paranasal sinuses are a complex group of air chambers that are closely related anatomically and functionally, and are lined by stratified squamous epithelium (Fig. 16-5). The largest of these spaces is the maxillary sinus, which is also the most frequent site for neoplasms in the total sinus complex. The maxillary sinus has a pyramidal shape with its base adjacent to the lateral wall of the nasal cavity with which it communicates through an opening that is situated between the inferior and medial nasal turbinates. The anterior wall of this sinus separates it from the soft tissues of the cheeks, and the

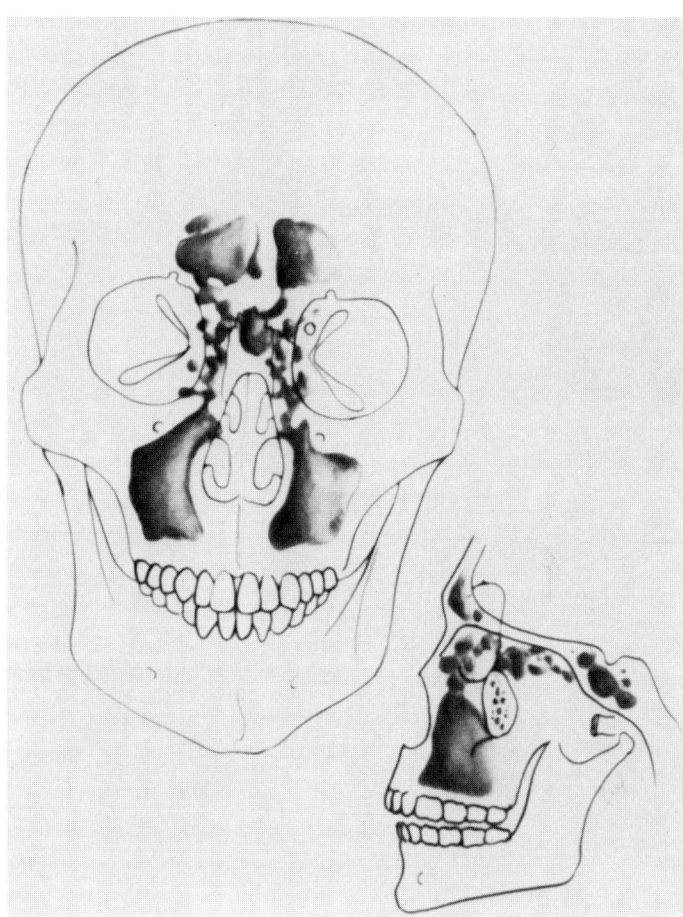

FIGURE 16-5 Anatomical distribution of the paranasal sinuses.

superior wall forms the floor of the orbit. More medially, the superior wall communicates with the complex of ethmoid sinuses. The posterior wall of this maxillary sinus is one boundary of the pterygomaxillary space (Fig. 16-6). The ethmoid sinuses, the frontal sinuses, and the sphenoid sinus form the floor of the anterior cranial fossa, and all communicate individually with the nasal cavity. These sinuses are infrequent sites for primary neoplasms, but because of their close relationship with the maxillary sinus, they are frequently involved by neoplasms originating in this sinus and must be included in the therapeutic plan.

Benign Neoplasms

Polypoid lesions are the most common benign growth observed in this area, particularly in the nasal cavity, but they also arise in the sinuses themselves. These polyps have a fibroepithelial structure, are pedunculated, often have ulcerations, and usually attain a large size before producing nasal obstruction, the common presenting symptom. Because of these well-defined characteristics, all polyps are similar, but a distinction must be made between simple polyps and papillary tumors.

Simple polyps are commonly associated with chronic inflammatory processes in the nasal cavity (allergic rhinitis, sinusitis) and are the result of mucosal hyperplasia, edema, and secondary inflammation.[35] The nasal papilloma is a true neoplastic process, less frequent than inflammatory polyps (1:25), and has no relationship to smoking, allergies, or chronic upper respiratory infections.[35-37] These lesions have been described under such various names as inverted papilloma, squamous papilloma, papillary adenoma, Schneiderian papilloma, etc.

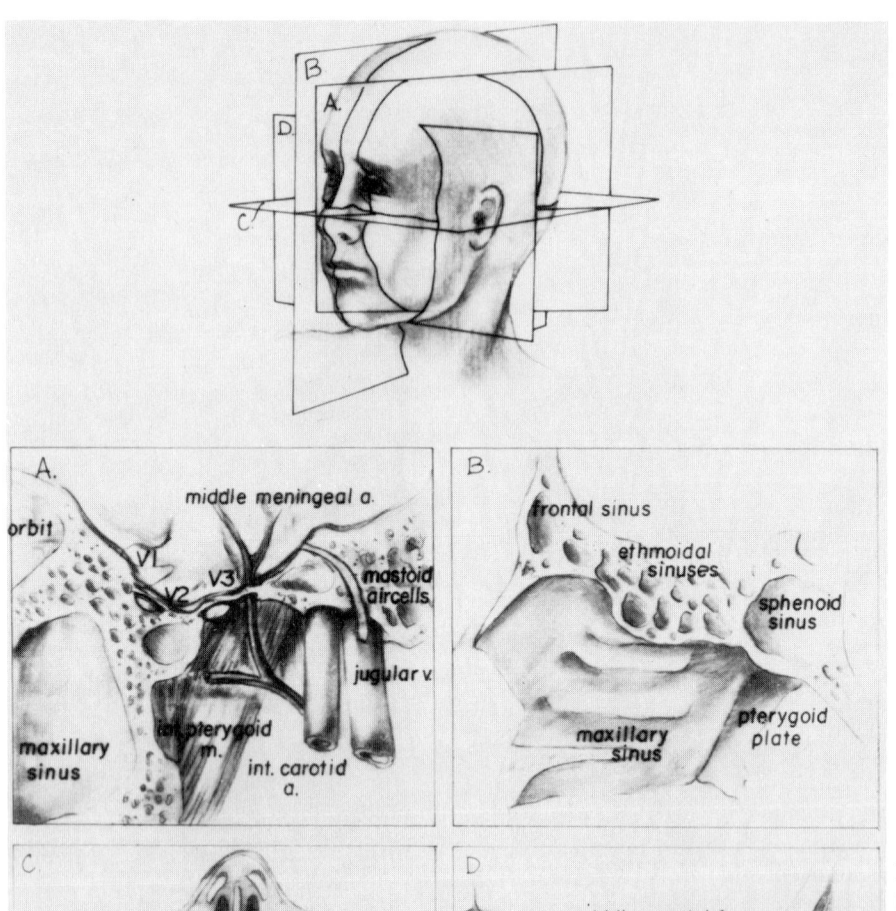
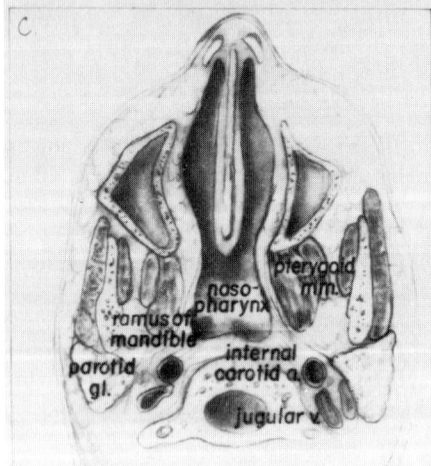
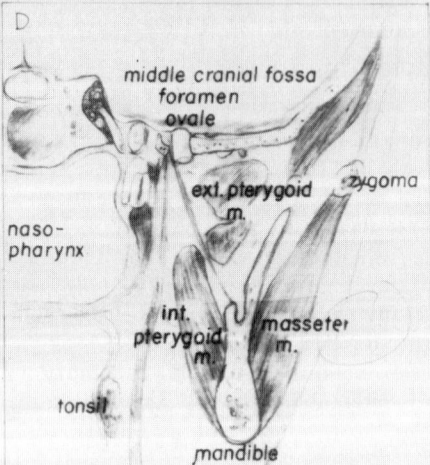

FIGURE 16-6 Anatomical relationship of the paranasal sinus in different planes. (*a*) View of the maxillary antrum and medial cranial fossa. (*b*) Paramedial sagittal view showing frontal, ethmoid, sphenoid sinuses, and anterior cranial fossa. (*c*) Horizontal section showing the boundaries of the maxillary antrum with the nasal cavity, nasopharynx, and pterygomaxillary region. (*d*) Relationship of the medial cranial fossa and pterygomaxillary region.

They commonly involve the nasal cavity, the turbinates, the nasal septum, or the paranasal sinuses. They have a cauliflower appearance and may arise from more than one site. These lesions are more common in males than females (3:1), and they occur between 40 and 70 years of age. Symptoms are usually nasal obstruction, watery discharge, and epistaxis. Nasal papilloma is considered a truly benign neoplasm, but malignant transformation has been described.[36,37]

PATHOLOGY

The histologic pattern is an important feature of the differential diagnosis of these two major entities. The ordinary nasal polyp has an edematous stroma covered by pseudostratified columnar epithelium demonstrating occasional atypia. Papillomas, on the other hand, show marked proliferation of the surface epithelium over a broad surface. This proliferation may develop in an exophytic manner, or have an inverted growth pattern with cell proliferation within the polypoid mass. Squamous metaplasia with a rare mitosis and no nuclear atypia are common findings, but all histologic sections should be screened for the presence of areas of in situ or invasive cancer.

TREATMENT

Transnasal resection is the common surgical approach, but in more extensive lesions or recurrent papillomas, lateral rhinotomy is necessary for complete eradication of the growth (Fig. 16-7). In case of cancer, a more radical procedure including maxillectomy or ethmoidectomy, or both, is indicated.[38,39]

PROGNOSIS

These tumors have a great propensity for local recurrence (50 to 70 percent).[37] Lesions arising from the nasal septum or paranasal sinuses are the most likely to recur. The presence of cellular atypia and predominance of mucin-producing epithelium in the original papilloma indicate a high likelihood of recurrence. Only on a few occasions (3 percent) has there been a well-documented development of carcinoma in a recurrent papilloma. This incidence is lower than the incidence of papillomas associated with coexisting carcinoma (10 percent).[37]

Malignant Neoplasms

Squamous cell carcinomas are the most common tumor of the nasal cavity and paranasal sinuses (80 percent).[40] They originate usually from the anterior part of the nares, the nasal septum, or the maxillary antrum. Adenocarcinomas (20 percent) arise from minor salivary or mucous glands in these same areas and are further classified as mucoepidermoid and adenoid cystic carcinomas. All of these neoplasms are more frequent in males than females (2:1) with an age peak in the fifth and the sixth decades. The maxillary antrum is the most frequent site (63 percent), followed by the nasal cavity (25 percent) and then the ethmoids (10 percent). The frontal and sphenoid sinuses are an extremely infrequent site of origin for the primary tumor, but like the ethmoid sinuses, they are frequently involved by neoplasms arising in the nasal cavity or maxillary antrum.[40,41]

CLINICAL MANIFESTATIONS AND COURSE OF THE DISEASE

An ulceration in the anterior part of the nares, or epistaxis with or without nasal obstruction, are initial manifestations of nasal cavity neoplasms that can be detected by a careful physical examination.[42,43] On the other hand, an early diagnosis of carcinoma arising from the paranasal sinuses is almost impossible because anatomic features make these lesions relatively inaccessible to routine examination. As the neoplasm increases in size, but is still limited to the antral cavity, the symptoms are quite similar to those of chronic sinusitis.[40] Throbbing pain in the face and headache are the common initial complaints. Almost invariably, these patients are treated initially with decongestants and antibiotics, since routine physical examination is usually unrevealing at this stage. Only an astute physician will obtain a radiologic study of the paranasal sinuses if specific anti-inflammatory therapy does not resolve the symptoms quickly and completely.

Radiographs of the maxillary antrum at this stage will reveal cloudiness of the antrum or the presence of a mass. These findings should lead to operative exploration of the antrum to establish both drainage and biopsy. More frequently, anti-inflammatory management will produce partial and temporary relief of the symptoms, leading to further delay in diagnosis. Dull aching facial pain, secondary to bone involvement, may then become persistent. The neoplasm can extend inferiorly, protruding into the upper gingival buccal region or the

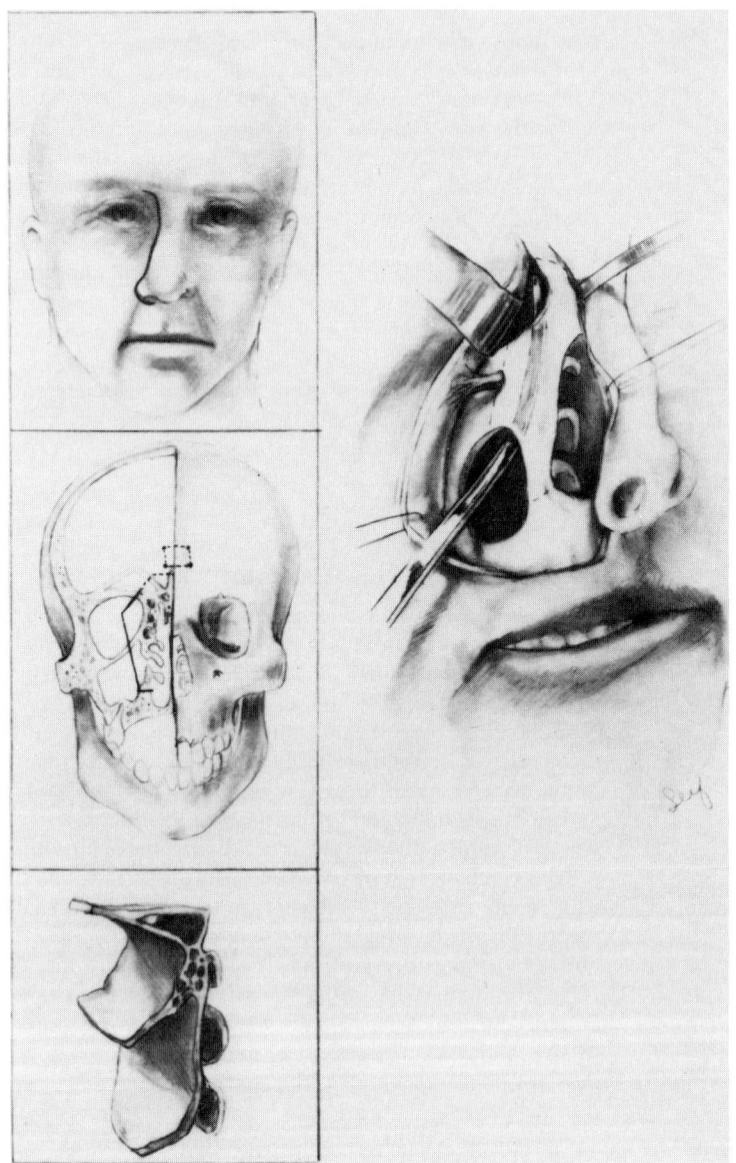

FIGURE 16-7 A lateral rhinotomy approach with partial resection of the medial wall of the maxilla for a well-localized tumor arising in the turbinates or ethmoid.

hard palate. Anteriorly, it may extend into the soft tissues of the cheek, giving the classical appearance of swelling of the face with disappearance of the nasolabial fold. Medially, the neoplasm may invade the nasal cavity, resulting in nasal obstruction, discharge, and epistaxis. Superior extension into the orbit is manifested by edema of the eyelids and proptosis. Extension through the posterior wall of the maxillary antrum into the pterygomaxillary space will lead to invasion of the pterygoid muscles and result in progressive trismus and visible swelling of the tissues in the temporal fossa. Hypesthesia of the overlying skin and severe facial pain, secondary to entrapment of the second and third trigeminal divisions, is frequently seen at this stage.

Cervical lymph node metastasis is seen in only 15 percent of these patients, regardless of the stage of the disease at the time of the initial diagnosis.[40,41] An additional 15 percent will develop neck node metastasis sometime after the initial treatment.

DIAGNOSTIC PROCEDURES

Standard radiologic examinations of the paranasal sinuses[44] (Waters' and Caldwell's projections; lateral, submental, vertical, and oblique orbital views) are an important initial diagnostic step in the management of a patient with persistent "sinus" complaints. Biopsy of suspicious nasal lesions and exploration of the sinuses, either through the nasal cavity or the gingivobuccal sulcus (Caldwell-Luc), will establish the diagnosis (Fig. 16-8). Once the presence of a malignant neoplasm has been confirmed, the use of refined radiologic techniques will properly assess all the extensions of the tumor. Polytomograms are particularly useful in confirming the suspicion of bone involvement (Fig. 16-9) as well as soft tissue extension. Computerized tomography is particularly helpful in determining the presence of pterygoid, orbital, or intracranial extension (Fig. 16-10a and b).[25,26] This information is essential for proper staging and the formulation of an appropriate therapeutic approach.

Staging The classification to be described applies to tumors arising in the maxillary antrum (Fig. 16-11).[22] The extent of tumors arising from other sources is not categorized because of the relatively low incidence of cancer in these sites. A theoretical plane (Ohngren's

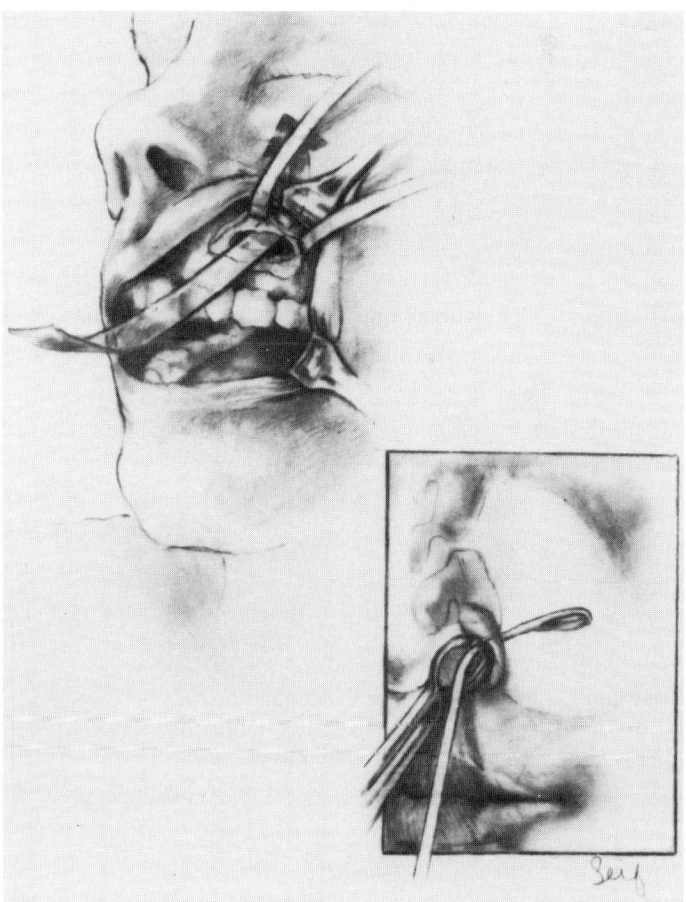

FIGURE 16-8 A nasal and gingival (Caldwell-Luc) approach to exploration of the maxillary antrum.

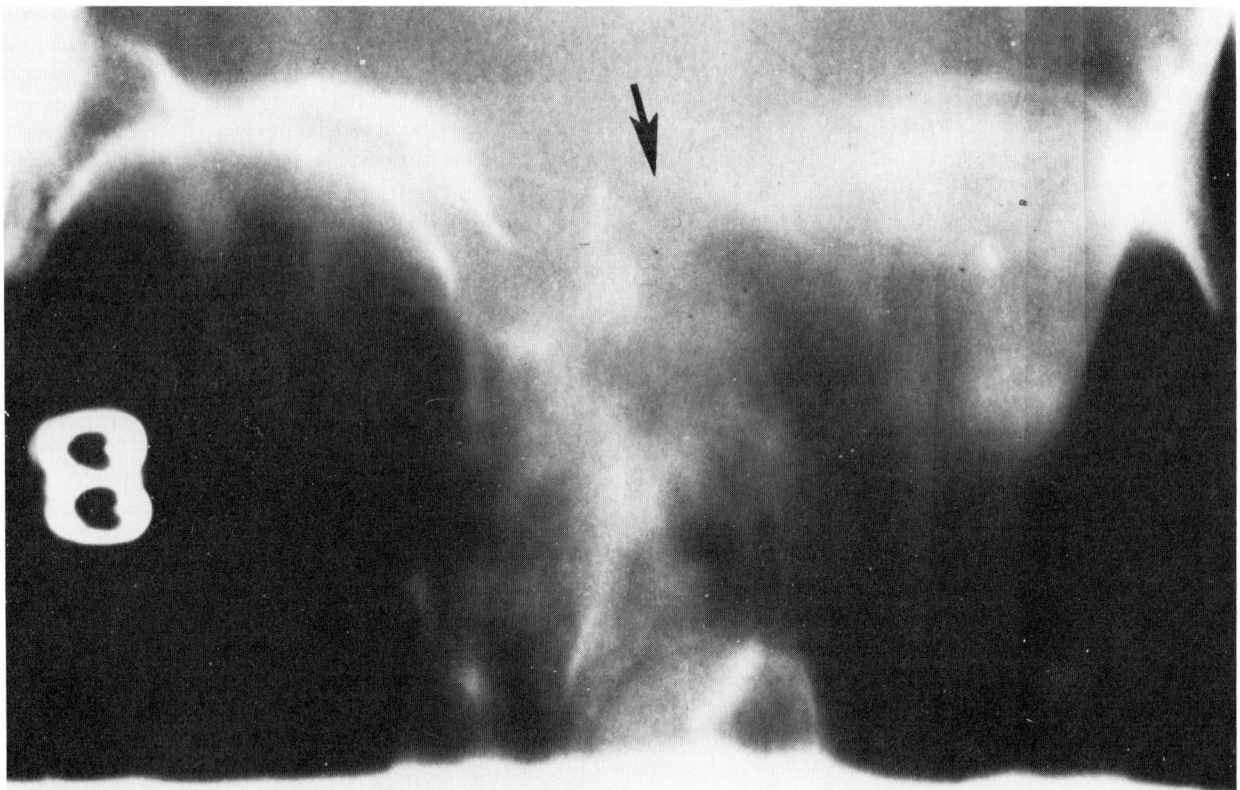

FIGURE 16-9 Polytomogram of the frontal sinuses showing a tumor involving the left orbit and anterior cranial fossa.

line), joining the medial canthus of the eye with the angle of the mandible, is often used to divide the maxillary antrum into the anterior-inferior portion (infrastructure) and superior-posterior portion (suprastructure). The original purpose of this division was to identify lesions amenable to earlier diagnosis and better therapeutic probability (infrastructure) from lesions arising posteriorly (suprastructure). The latter tend to invade the orbit, ethmoids, and pterygomaxillary space and, therefore, have a poorer prognosis. Realistically, this division is difficult to ascertain,[45] since by the time most of the maxillary antral cancers reach a diagnostic stage, the tumor actually fills most of the antrum (Table 16-2).

TREATMENT

The anatomical complexity of the paranasal sinuses, as well as the advanced stage of the disease at the time of diagnosis, has made the local control of paranasal sinus cancer a difficult accomplishment. The high incidence of involvement of more than one sinus cavity by the neoplastic process has made it mandatory to include all these cavities in any therapeutic approach to sinus cancer.

Radiation therapy has yet to be established as the primary modality of treatment, despite development of modern techniques. The close proximity of the opposite eye and brain, the presence of extensive bone involvement, tumor necrosis, or associated infection have all seriously limited radiation therapy as an aggressive and effective approach to this tumor. Nevertheless, radiation therapy still has a major role in the management of locally advanced cases, and it is favored in many centers as a preoperative adjuvant to surgical resection.

Technique Radiation therapy is administered by either a 2-MeV Van de Graaff generator or a cobalt machine.[46]

Because of the rounded contour of the cheek, maxillary antrum cancers are treated with a pair of 90°-angle wedge portals, or through an anterior field. The right-angle portals seem to give optimal coverage, but care must be taken not to treat the opposite eye. It has been suggested that a posterior angulation of the lateral field will reduce the possibility of injuring the opposite eye and will increase the exposure of the pterygopalatine region. With tumor involving the nasal cavity, ethmoids, frontal bone, and sphenoid, an anterior open portal is used with an extended L slope to include the maxilla, but this may result in inadequate irradiation of the ethmoids and middle cranial fossa. A tumor dose of 5000 R is delivered in 5 weeks, if surgery is planned afterwards. The dose is increased to 6000 to 7000 R if radiation is the only treatment.

Complications Decreased vision and blindness, central nervous system necrosis, and osteonecrosis of the maxilla represent major complications of radiation therapy

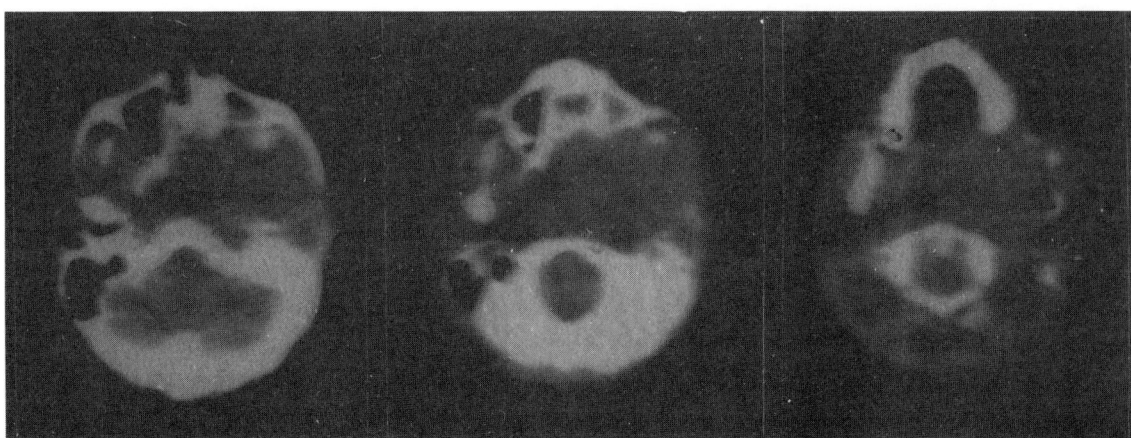

a

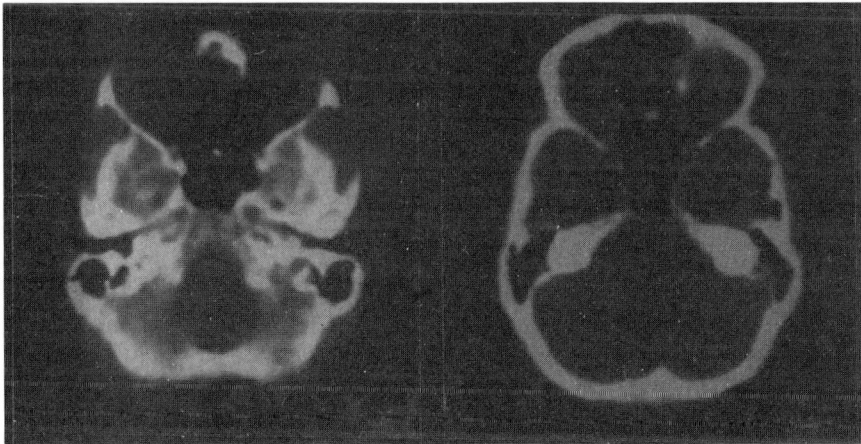

b

FIGURE 16-10 (*a*) Computerized scan of the maxillary antrum showing extension of the tumor into the nasopharynx and pterygomaxillary region. (*b*) Tumor of the ethmoids involving the nasal cavity and medial wall of the orbit.

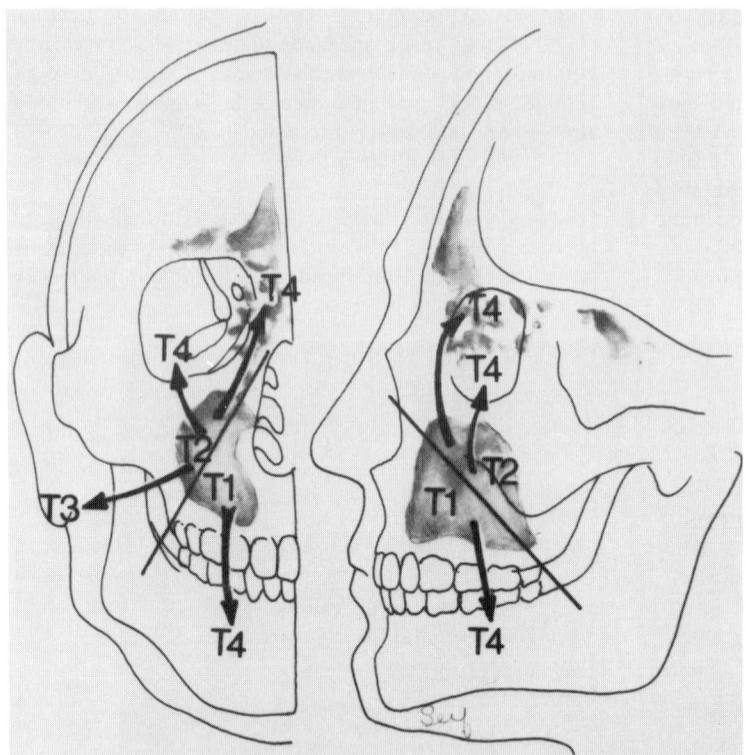

FIGURE 16-11 The staging of the tumors in maxillary antrums according to the different areas involved.

(15 percent.)[47] Less significant problems are cataract formation and epiphora (12 percent). Eye damage leading to unilateral or bilateral blindness is a significant complication (40 percent) in the management of tumors arising in the nasal cavity and ethmoids. These complications usually develop within 2 years of treatment and are due to optic nerve atrophy, retinal and macular degeneration, or central retinal artery thrombosis.

Results The 5-year survival rate for patients with paranasal sinus carcinoma treated with radiation therapy alone is between 8 and 18 percent, with some authors reporting a survival rate as high as 35 percent.[41,48–50] However, tumors of the nasal cavity and nonepithelial malignancies are included in this latter report.[48] Carcinomas of the maxillary antrum respond better than do cancers in the other sinuses, particularly if localized to the infrastructure. Tumors involving the ethmoids and the frontal sinus are seldom possible to control with radiotherapy alone.

CONVENTIONAL SURGICAL MANAGEMENT

Because of the high failure rate seen with radiation therapy, surgery has been extensively used in the management of cancers arising in the paranasal sinuses, particularly those arising in the maxillary antrum. The standard surgical procedure is designated radical maxillectomy, which entails unilateral removal of the maxillary bone. Involvement of the soft tissues of the face will sometimes require resection of the skin overlying the maxilla as well (Fig. 16-12). Orbital exenteration is required as a part of this procedure under most circumstances because of the high frequency of involvement of the orbital floor. The ethmoid sinuses are removed only partially and in piecemeal fashion. A split-thickness graft is usually employed to cover the surface defect on the interior side of the cheek flap and the exposed bony surfaces. The functional and cosmetic defects produced by these procedures are usually well corrected with properly constructed prostheses.

Complications Leakage of cerebrospinal fluid, meningitis, postoperative hemorrhage, and respiratory obstruction are the most common complications (13 percent). Leading causes of death (5 percent) are meningitis with brain abcess, and sepsis and cardiovascular complications.[40]

Results The overall 5-year disease-free survival rate after surgery alone for carcinoma of the nasal cavity is 40 percent[41,43] and for the maxillary antrum, 23 percent.[41,49,50] The presence of neck node metastases at the time of diagnosis indicates a very poor prognosis, since only 8 percent of these patients remained free of cancer at 5 years, as did only 13 percent of those patients who developed cervical metastases during the follow-up period. The survival rate for patients who never developed cervical lymph node metastases was 36 percent.[40]

TABLE 16-2 Classification of Tumors Arising in the Maxillary Antrum

Designation	Description
T_1	Tumor confined to the antral mucosa of the infrastructure with no bone erosion or destruction
T_2	Tumor confined to the mucosa of the suprastructure without bone destruction, or to the infrastructure with destruction of medial or inferior bony walls only
T_3	More extensive tumor invading skin of cheek, orbit, anterior ethmoid sinuses, or pterygoid muscle
T_4	Massive tumor with invasion of cribriform plate, posterior ethmoids, sphenoid, nasopharynx, pterygoid plates, or base of skull
SUMMARY OF STAGE GROUPINGS	
Stage 1	T_1, N_0, M_0
Stage 2	T_2, N_0, M_0
Stage 3	T_3, N_0, M_0 T_1 or T_2 or T_3, N_1, M_0
Stage 4	T_4, N_0, M_0 Any T, N_2, M_0 Any T, any N, M_1

COMBINED RADIATION AND SURGERY

Because of the limited success of radiation therapy or of surgery alone, the option of combining both treatments has been carried out in the last 10 years, but with similar results. Jesse reported a 70 percent 5-year survival rate of patients with lesions staged as T_1 and T_2 and 30 percent for T_3 and T_4.[49] These results did not differ from those obtained following either modality alone in the same institution. Similar results with the combination of preoperative radiation and surgery were also reported by Badib,[50] Cheng,[51] and Harrison.[52] The value of postoperative irradiation was also assessed by these same authors, who described a lower survival rate in this group than in those receiving preoperative irradiation.

CRANIOFACIAL RESECTION

Review of the patients who failed to be cured by the standard therapeutic modalities described demonstrates that local recurrence or persistent disease in the ethmoids and posterolateral boundaries of the resection is present 90 percent of the time.[40] Distant metastases as the sole cause of death are seen only in 10 percent of such patients. In an attempt to encompass one of the areas of local treatment failure, Ketcham et al.[53] carried out a series of combined craniofacial resections that included en bloc excision of the cribriform plate and ethmoids in addition to the standard maxillectomy. In their experience, this procedure has resulted in 65 percent of patients surviving for 3 or more years free of disease, a remarkable improvement over standard maxillectomy.[54,55]

The sound rationale and good clinical results associated with this procedure prompted the authors to adopt this technique and to extend the craniofacial resection to include the middle cranial fossa as well.[56] The purpose of this addition was to include the contents of the pterygoid fossa, a common site of involvement by cancers arising in the maxillay antrum (Fig. 16-13).

Between December 1966 and July 1977, 26 patients with T_3 and T_4N_0, or N_1 squamous cell carcinomas of the maxillary antrum, 1 patient with advanced squamous cell carcinoma of the ethmoids, and 1 patient with squamous cell carcinoma of the frontal sinus were operated upon in the Division of Surgical Oncology at the Medical College of Virginia. In 4 of the 26 patients with maxillary antrum cancer, the procedure was not com-

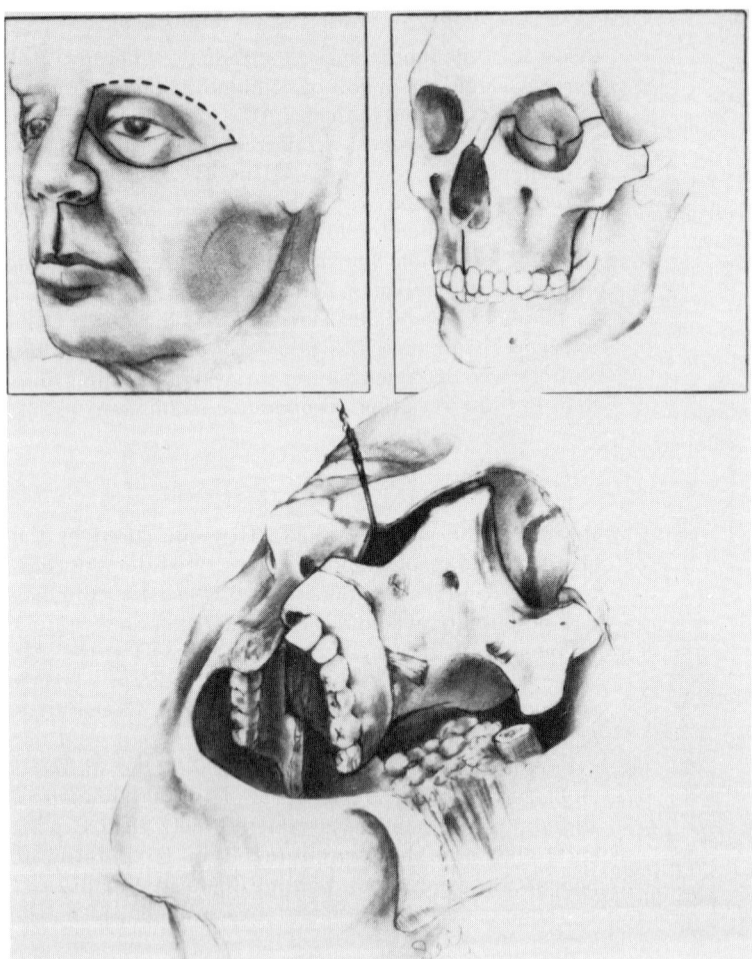

FIGURE 16-12 Radical maxillectomy outlining the skin incision and area of bony resection.

pleted when tumor was found to involve the sphenoid sinus at the time of exploration. The remaining 22 patients had combined craniofacial resections with resection of the middle and anterior cranial fossae, along with orbital exenteration and resection of soft tissue of the face. The two patients with carcinoma of the frontal and ethmoid sinuses underwent resection of the anterior cranial fossa, and of the frontal and ethmoid sinuses with orbital exenteration.

The extent of the individual lesions was determined with standard skull films, polytomograms (axial and frontal) of the paranasal sinuses, and biopsies of the nasopharyngeal mucosa in the region of the eustachian tube and cavum and of sphenoid sinus mucosa. Histologic evidence of tumor in the nasopharynx or in the sphenoid sinus mucosa is considered a definite contraindication for resection.

After the line of resection in the floor of the anterior cranial fossa is completed through an anterior craniotomy, the head is turned in preparation for exploration of the middle cranial fossa. The middle cranial fossa is approached extradurally through a subtemporal craniectomy in a fashion similar to that used for exposure of the Gasserian ganglion. The dura is elevated to expose the middle meningeal artery and the second and third divisions of the trigeminal nerve, which are transected. With an air drill, a bony incision is created connecting the foramina spinosum, ovale, and rotundum.

Attention is then directed to removal of the pharyngomaxillofacial complex. The nasal bone, maxilla, pterygoid plate, mandible, nasopharynx, oropharynx, and soft tissues of the face are resected en bloc (see Fig. 16-12). Radical neck dissection is performed in conjunction with this procedure only if the neck nodes are clinically suspected of containing metastases.

Reconstruction The forehead flap that was elevated initially is sutured to the bony edge of the anterior cranial fossa on the opposite side from the resection as well as to the margin of the floor of the middle cranial fossa. The anterior bony plate is replaced at the site of the frontal craniotomy, and this area is covered by rotation of an occipitofrontal skin flap (Fig. 16-14).

Morbidity and Mortality Rates Three of the twenty-four patients died as a result of the surgical procedure. One patient expired suddenly 48 h after operation; massive pulmonary embolism was found at autopsy. A second patient remained unresponsive following resection and expired on the tenth postoperative day. Both reexploration of the craniotomy and subsequent postmortem examination failed to show a clear-cut cause of death except for significant brain edema. The third patient developed an abscess at the tracheostomy site secondary

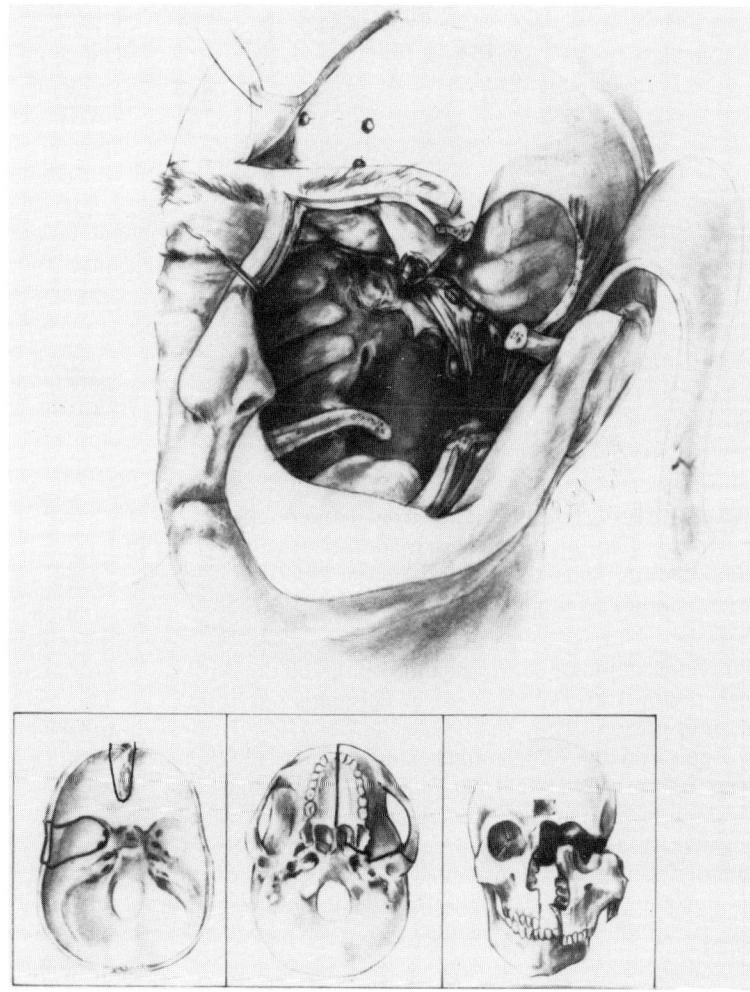

FIGURE 16-13 A combined anterior and medial cranial resection with a radical maxillectomy and orbital exenteration for carcinoma of the maxillary antrum. Top of figure shows the operation completed and the inserts outline the area of bony resections.

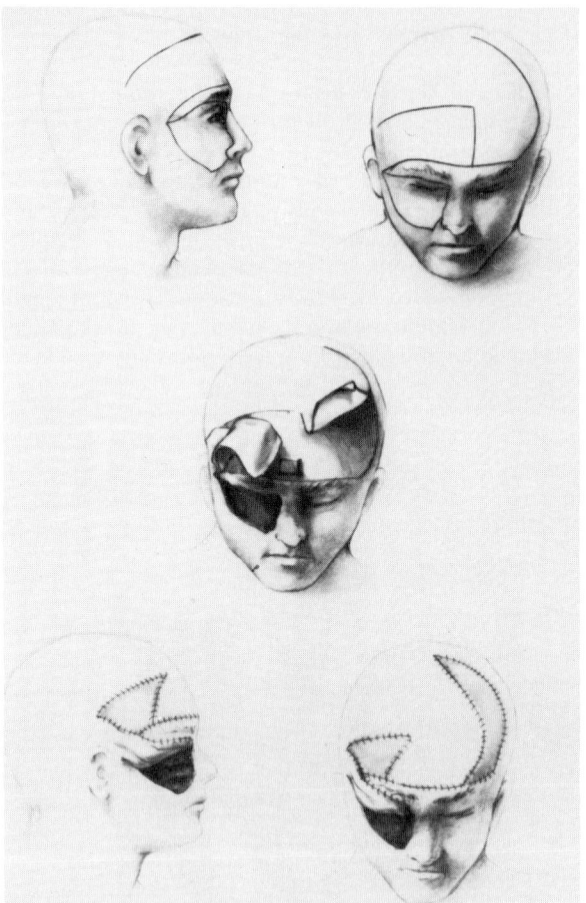

FIGURE 16-14 Outline of the frontal and occipital frontal flap for the approach and reconstruction following a combined craniofacial resection for carcinoma of the maxillary antrum.

to necrosis of the tracheal wall and expired on the thirty-fifth postoperative day. Severe mediastinitis was found at autopsy.

Eight patients had nonfatal complications (33 percent). Cerebrospinal fluid leak requiring daily spinal taps was seen in five patients. Meningitis secondary to gram-negative bacteria developed in two patients but responded to intrathecal gentamicin. Osteomyelitis of the frontal bone flap developed in two patients, and removal was required. All these patients recovered completely without sequelae.

End Results Seventy-two percent of the patients are alive and free of disease at 3 years (13:18), and four of eight patients are free of disease 5 years after operation.[57] Four patients developed neck node metastasis 4, 5, 36, and 48 months, respectively, after the primary tumor was treated without evidence of local recurrence. One of these patients died from respiratory complications following neck dissection. One died of local recurrence in the neck and lung metastasis, and the remaining two have remained free of disease 6 and 24 months, respectively, following the neck dissection.

Recurrent tumor at the original site of the primary tumor developed in 32 percent of the patients. Of the five patients who were found to have tumor in the sphenoid sinus, three developed clinical evidence of local recurrence within 9 months of operation, and all eventually died of their disease. The other two patients have remained free of disease for 36 and 48 months, respectively. All patients showing vascular invasion in the primary tumor died of recurrence. The degree of tumor differentiation did not seem to influence the end results.

It may be concluded from this experience that craniofacial resection is definitely indicated in the treatment plan for T_3T_4 carcinoma of the paranasal sinuses. It appears to be the only procedure that can control the local disease effectively in most of the patients at this stage. The problem of management of this group of patients in the past has been failure to control the local disease within the sinus complex, and the operative approach appears to have merit for selected cases.

CHEMOTHERAPY

The results of chemotherapy for cancer of the nasopharynx and paranasal sinuses have been disappointing. Multiple trials involving single or multiple agents alone or in combination with irradiation therapy resulted in only a small percentage of responses of limited duration. The introduction of new agents may well improve the prospective role of chemotherapy in the management of these cancers.[58-62]

Other Epithelial Tumors

MELANOMAS

Only 1.5 percent of human melonomas arise in the upper respiratory tract, and one-half of these arise in the nasal cavity. Most present as polypoid lesions producing epistaxis and nasal obstruction. The true diagnosis is usually unsuspected since the lesions are considered benign nasal polyps until their removal. One-third of the patients with melanoma arising in the nasal cavity present with regional cervical node metastases either at the time of diagnosis or sometime following the treatment of the primary lesion.[63,64]

Radical resection of the lesion along with the medial wall of the antrum to include all the turbinates (or radical maxillectomy when indicated) is the treatment of choice for localized lesions. Radical neck dissection is performed only when clinically positive nodes are present, since it is doubtful that elective lymph node dissection is beneficial for melanoma in this location. The prognosis is poor compared with that for cutaneous melanoma. For lesions localized to this primary site, the 5-year survival figures range from 10 to 20 percent following radical resection, but no long-term survivors have been reported among patients who developed cervical lymph node metastasis.[63]

OLFACTORY NEUROBLASTOMA (ESTHESIONEUROBLASTOMA)

Olfactory neuroblastoma is a malignant neoplasm that originates from the olfactory epithelium in the roof of the nasal cavity. These rare tumors have been described in all age groups with an equal incidence for both sexes. The tumor presents as a polypoid nasal mass or masses producing nasal obstruction, discharge, epistaxis, and anosmia. The diagnosis is usually totally unsuspected clinically, and the lesion is initially treated as a benign polyp in most instances. These tumors have a well-defined histologic pattern characterized by the presence of nerve cells (neurocytes or neuroblasts) with pseudorosettes or true rosette formation and neurofibrils. The differential diagnosis must be made from that of a neuroblastoma arising from this same site.[65,66]

Both radical maxilloethmoidectomy and radiation therapy have been used as treatment for these tumors. However, when used alone neither modality has resulted in permanent control of the disease. The overall survival rate reported at 5 years was 63 percent, but only 19 percent of patients were free of disease. The mean survival time of the patients who died because of the neoplasm was 50 months, pointing out the rather slow growth pattern of this disease.[67] A significant number of deaths occurred more than 5 and 10 years after the initial treatment. The combined use of radiation and surgery has a somewhat higher number of disease-free survivors at 5 years (33 percent), but failures have local recurrence as the common denominator. The involvement of the cribriform plate and extension of disease into the anterior cranial fossa is not adequately dealt with by standard treatment, since this is the common site of failure. A combined craniofacial resection approach should provide the best likelihood of local control.

CHORDOMA

Chordomas are rare tumors that originate from vestigial remnants of notochord. They arise in the nasopharynx where they usually present as a mass involving the basioccipital bone, but eventually extend to the basisphenoid and middle cranial fossa. The presence of calcification in the tumor mass on radiographic examination suggests the clinical diagnosis. Radiation therapy is the usual treatment, but the prognosis is very poor.[68]

Tumors of the Central Nervous System

Intranasal gliomas are very rare tumors seen soon after birth or in early childhood, but they also have been described in adults.[69] They are the result of the embryological failure of the foramen cecum to become obliterated, allowing the dura to extend into the nasal cavity. Histologically, the tumor is formed by a nest of astrocytes in a conglomeration of connective tissue stroma. Clinically, these lesions present as nasal polyps, but diagnosis of this benign condition should be seriously questioned in patients under 5 years of age. If the diagnosis of intranasal glioma is suspected clinically, neuroradiologic study will substantiate this clinical impression. When present, the tumor should be approached intracranially first, leaving removal of the nasal component for a second-stage procedure.

Meningiomas are benign intracranial tumors that usually arise from the anterior cranial fossa and involve the nasal cavity secondarily by direct extension. On rare occasions a meningioma can arise primarily in the nasal cavity from arachnoid cell nests left behind after closure of the foramen cecum. Symptoms are similar to those of other polypoid masses in the nasal cavity, and a staged cranionasal approach is used to eradicate the tumor.[69]

Tumors of Lymphoreticular Origin

Lymphomas and extramedullary plasmacytomas occasionally arise in the maxillary antrum.[14,15] Once the histologic diagnosis is clearly established by biopsy the patient should undergo a careful work-up to determine the presence or absence of a similar neoplasm in other sites. These lesions are radiosensitive, and radiation therapy uniformly will control the local disease with a dose no greater than 4500 rads. Even when tumor is present in other sites, radiation therapy is valuable for control of the local symptoms.

Midline malignant reticulosis is a descriptive name for a localized malignant neoplasm of lymphoreticular origin that classically involves the nasal cavity and hard palate.[14,68] This tumor is characterized by swelling of the soft tissues of the face, mucosal ulcerations, and nasal and maxillary bone necrosis. This clinical presentation is included in the definition of midline lethal granuloma, which also describes a series of processes of different etiology, such as syphilis, tuberculosis, bacterial and fungal infections, leprosy, and other neoplasms with similar gross findings. Histologically, this tumor is characterized by a mixed population of lymphoblasts, mature and immature lymphocytes, and extensive necrosis secondary to vascular occlusion. This tumor is quite rare and is radiosensitive. It should be differentiated from Wegener's granulomatosis, a process that may have a similar local pattern but involves not only the upper respiratory tract, but also the genitourinary and vascular systems. This latter disease is treated with both steroids and cytotoxic drugs, but without much success.

Tumors of Mesenchymal Origin

TUMORS OF VASCULAR ORIGIN

Capillary hemangiomas and cavernous hemangiomas are the most frequent vascular tumors arising in this anatomic area. They are usually located in the nasal septum or the turbinates, and epistaxis is the most common symptom. They have the gross appearance of polyps, and local excision is always curative.[70]

GLOMUS TUMORS

Glomus tumors also arise in the nasal septum and the turbinates, but pain is the cardinal clinical manifestation. Local excision is curative.

JUVENILE ANGIOFIBROMA

Juvenile angiofibromas are uncommon benign neoplasms, highly vascular and noninfiltrating, that arise in the nasopharynx and posterior naval cavity. They are seen almost exclusively in adolescent males, and seldom are found in patients over 25 years of age. However, they have been described both in females and in older patients. The marked predilection of this tumor for the adolescent male has always raised the suspicion of a possible endocrine abnormality in its etiology. Detailed endocrine studies and urinary assays for ketosteroids and other metabolites have failed to demonstrate abnormal findings in this group of patients.[70]

Pathology This tumor usually arises from the boundaries of the sphenopalatine foramen as a submucosal mass. As the tumor enlarges in the submucosa, it fills the posterior nasal cavity and flattens the turbinates posteriorly; it then extends into the nasopharynx and becomes visible behind the soft palate. The continuous growth of this neoplasm will destroy the root of the pterygoid plate by pressure, and it then extends into the pterygomaxillary space. From there, the tumor will extend into the cheek anteriorly, giving the facial deformity that is seen in some patients. The infratemporal and the middle cranial fossa become involved eventually, leading to serious problems in management.[71,74]

These tumors have a shiny, nonulcerated, rubbery appearance. Microscopically, the tumor is made up of myxomatous connective tissue with star-shaped cells and prominent vascularization. The basic histologic pattern, as described by Sternberg,[74a] is one in which endothelial-lined spaces are regularly dispersed in a stroma consisting of fibroblasts and collagen fibers. A differential diagnosis must be made between this lesion and nasal polyps, sclerosing hemangioma, hemangioendothelioma, and fibrosarcoma. The presence of mucous glands and lymphoid and eosinophilic cell infiltration is characteristic of nasal polyps. Mitotic activity and atypical vascular features are usually well identified in the other malignant neoplasms. The significant hemorrhage that is associated with management of these tumors is explained by the absence of elastic fibers and smooth muscle around the blood vessels in the lesion.[70]

Clinical Presentation and Diagnosis A young male patient with repeated episodes of epistaxis and a nasopharyngeal mass must be assumed to have a nasopharyngeal angiofibroma. Nasal obstruction, rhinorrhea, and hypoacusia may develop during the course of the disease. Facial deformity is seen in recurrent cases and in more advanced cases. Biopsy of the mass will establish the diagnosis, but due to the severity of the hemorrhage, it is recommended that this be performed in the operating room after the appropriate preliminary radiographic studies.

A coronal polytomogram will help in delineating the extent of the tumor and the degree of bone involvement. Carotid angiography with subtraction films will provide information regarding the blood supply, which comes from the internal maxillary artery on most occasions, although some feeding vessels from the ophthalmic artery have also been found. Most of the tumors receive their blood supply from one carotid artery, but larger tumors have developed a bilateral arterial supply. Of greater importance is the fact that these tumors have a classic angiographic pattern that may establish the pretreatment diagnosis without the hazard of biopsy (Fig. 16-15).[71-73]

Treatment The history of the management of these neoplasms is often characterized by repeated attempts at removal of the tumor, each associated with massive bleeding that has led to death in a few instances. This tumor often can be resected completely by a skillful surgeon or may be treated with radiation therapy as a temporizing measure. It may regress completely after the patient reaches 20 years of age. The cause of death in unsuccessfully managed cases is due to hemorrhage from attempts at removal by an inexperienced surgeon; or, on rare occasions, the tumor invades the base of the skull and leads to sepsis and/or hemorrhage.

Surgical resection can be accomplished with complete removal of the tumor in most cases, if the surgeon is familiar with the optimal surgical approach. A transpal-

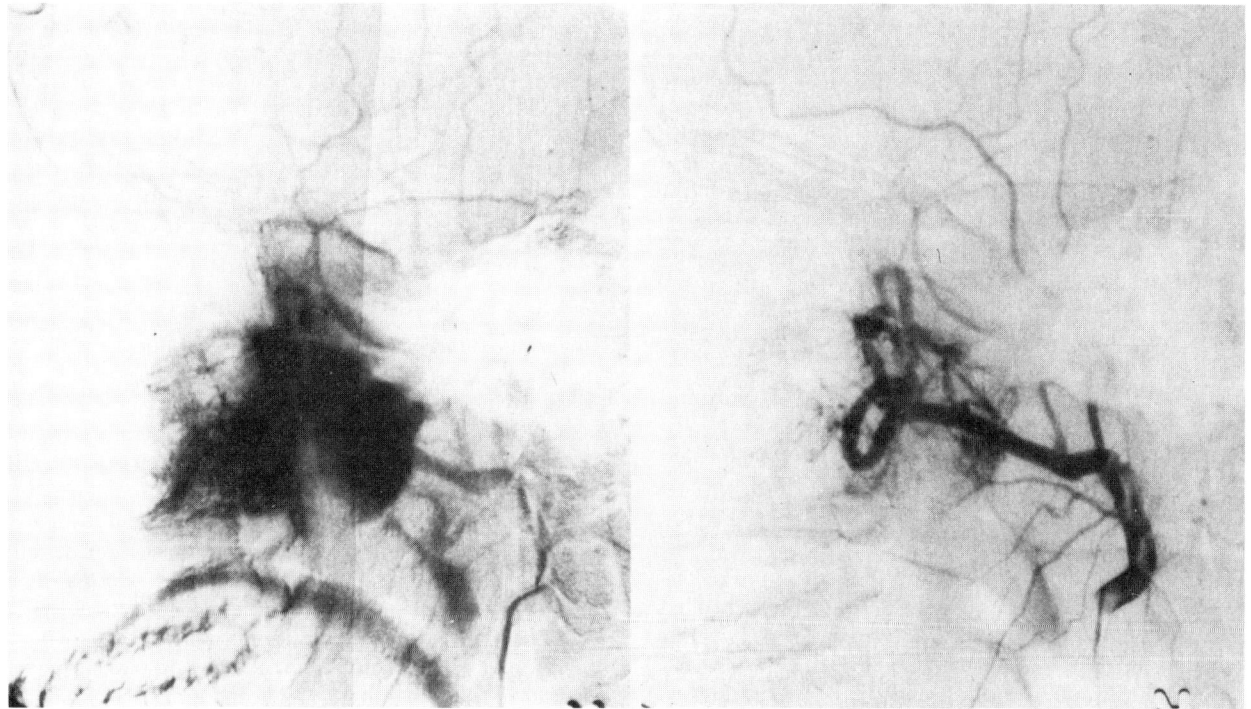

FIGURE 16-15 Carotid angiogram in a patient with juvenile angiofibroma. Notice the marked tumor blush of the pterygomaxillary region.

atine approach provides good exposure if the tumor is small or if the major component is within the nasal cavity.[74] For larger neoplasms with significant extension into the maxillary antrum or the pterygomaxillary fossa, a lateral rhinotomy combined with a Caldwell-Luc incision and transpalatine approach provides excellent exposure to all of the anatomic areas involved. Preoperative arterial embolization of the tumor through the external carotid artery has been a useful approach in some instances from the standpoint of reducing intraoperative hemorrhage.[75] Freezing the lesion prior to resection has been used with a similar purpose.

The value of radiation theapy in the control of these tumors is still undetermined. It has been used as an adjuvant to the surgical approach, either as a preoperative measure to induce regression of large tumors, or postoperatively when operative removal has been incomplete. The usual dose is 3000 to 4000 R in 3 weeks.[76] Symptomatic relief is seen almost immediately, but the bulk of the tumor will take several months to reduce in size. The use of radiation therapy in children is not favored because of the potential of additional neoplastic change.

Malignant hemangioendotheliomas and hemangiopericytomas may arise from either the nasal cavity or the maxillary antrum. They are locally aggressive and may give rise to distant metastases. Appropriate radical resection followed by postoperative radiation therapy seems to offer the best probability of prolonged local control. The incidence of both local recurrence and distant metastasis is very high.[70]

TUMORS OF FIBROUS TISSUE

Fibromas These tumors present as small polypoid masses in the nasal cavity that are usually asymptomatic and found incidentally. Histologically, they are formed by mature, well-differentiated cellular fibrous tissue. No recurrences are observed after adequate local excision.[77]

Fibromatosis This is a locally aggressive and nonmetastasizing process which can cause death by uncontrolled local invasion.[77] Histologically, it consists of well-differentiated fibrous tissue that may be difficult to differentiate from normal fibrous tissue or scar. The infiltrative behavior of the process is the best index of its neoplastic nature. Surgical resection is the only method of treatment capable of controlling this disease, but local control may be difficult in the head and neck region because of tumor extension to inaccessible anatomic areas. Recurrence is inevitable if the margins of resection are involved.

Fibrosarcoma This is a malignant tumor that shows a variable degree of collagen formation and has the ability to metastasize. It usually presents as a polypoid mass in the nasal cavity or paranasal sinuses and extends into adjacent soft tissue and bone. Histologically, a differential diagnosis must be made between this lesion and fibrous dysplasia, ossifying fibroma, and even osteogenic sarcoma. Differentiation from the latter lesion can be difficult when fibrosarcoma invades bone. Other mesenchymal malignant neoplasms may also resemble fibrosarcoma. Fibrosarcoma must be treated by a radical block excision of the neoplasm with adequate margins of normal tissue. Coley reported a 5-year "cure rate" of 79 percent for fibromatosis and 33 percent for fibrosarcoma.[77,78]

SMOOTH MUSCLE TUMORS

These tumors have been described in the nasopharynx, nasal cavity, and paranasal sinuses. Leiomyomas are benign polypoid lesions usually found in the nasal cavity and are completely eradicated by local surgical excision. Leiomyosarcoma, on the other hand, carries a poor prognosis. Surgical resections are usually followed by local recurrence and metastasis. Radiation therapy has not been successful in control of these lesions.[79]

SKELETAL MUSCLE TUMORS

Rhabdomyomas are extremely rare benign lesions of polypoid appearance that may arise in the nasopharynx, nasal cavity, or paranasal sinuses. No recurrence has been seen after adequate local excision. Rhabdomyocomas of the same site are malignant tumors that carry an extremely poor prognosis in adults. The majority of these tumors have either embryonal or botryoid features; the alveolar or pleomorphic types are rarely seen at this site. Rhabdomyosarcoma is a neoplastic process that affects children primarily; 85 percent of all patients with head and neck rhabdomyosarcoma are 15 years of age or younger. The overall survival rate of patients with rhabdomyosarcoma in this site is lower than that of patients with orbital rhabdomyosarcomas. Recent advances in combination chemotherapy, in conjunction with radiation therapy and surgery, have improved the results with these tumors in the head and neck region, but the nasal, nasopharyngeal, and other parameningeal sites are still somewhat difficult to control due to the frequency of intracranial extension.[80]

CARTILAGE TUMORS

Chondromas are benign tumors that are usually found during routine radiologic examinations. They may appear as polypoid smooth-surfaced nodules projecting into the lumen of the nasal cavity, nasopharynx, or paranasal sinuses. Chordomas also must enter into the differential diagnosis of chondroma on occasion, since a pattern showing a mixture of both has been described as "chondroid chordoma."[81]

Chondrosarcomas may arise in the nasopharynx, nasal cavity, and paranasal sinuses.[82] Clinically, they present with nasal obstruction and/or facial deformity. Pathologically, they are classified as (1) well-differentiated sarcomas (grade I), characterized by hypercellularity, hyperchromatism, nuclear atypia; (2) moderately well differentiated sarcomas (grade II), in which the cartilage is less mature and more mitoses are identified than in grade I lesions; and (3) poorly differentiated sarcomas (grade III) that show a limited amount of mature cartilage and contain numerous mitoses. Some of the chondrosarcomas are so well differentiated that the pathologist may have difficulty in differentiating these lesions from benign chondromas. Multiple sections of all surgically resected chondromas should be studied to rule out the possibility of areas of chondrosarcoma in an otherwise benign lesion. Clinical history of growth rate, the physical examination, and the radiologic findings will all aid in the differentiation between those benign and malignant cartilage tumors.

Radical en bloc resection of the tumor and adjacent structures provides local control of chondrosarcoma of these sites in 35 percent of patients. These tumors have a slow and insidious growth pattern as shown by the fact that approximately one-third of the patients live from 5 to 10 years with persistent disease. Uncontrollable local growth involving the base of the skull is the most common form of failure. Distant metastases are infrequent but, when seen, they are associated with the poorly differentiated type (grade III). The factors that seem to influence the results of treatment and subsequent prognosis are:

1. Anatomic location. Tumors involving the nasopharynx, sphenoid, or posterior nasal cavity have a poor prognosis because of the advanced size when initially diagnosed and the technical difficulties involved in accomplishing a complete resection.
2. Adequate resection. All tumors incompletely resected at initial procedure recurred, whereas those with surgical margins free of tumor remain controlled.
3. Degree of differentiation of the tumor. Only one out of six patients with grade 1 lesions died of disease, whereas most patients with grade II and III lesions died as a result of the tumor.[81]

BONE TUMORS

Osteomas and Fibrous Osteomas These tumors usually present as a painless swelling with some degree of facial asymmetry. Symptoms of nasal obstruction, headaches, and sinusitis may also be present, depending on the location of the lesion. Radiographically, they appear as a well-defined opaque, homogeneous calcified mass. Histologically, they have a well-defined bone structure. Local excision or curettage is usually successful.[83]

Fibrous Dysplasia This process also presents as facial asymmetry and painless swelling of the cheek, gum, and orbit. Radiographically, the facial bones appear replaced by a radiopaque, homogeneous mass with ill-defined margins. Pathologically, the lesion is calcified, firm, and granular, and is composed of cellular fibrous tissue with spindle-shaped fibroblastic cells and irregular trabeculae of woven bone. Nuclear atypia and mitoses are not seen. This process is definitely benign, and when localized to one bone, local excision is curative. Not infrequently this process involves several facial bones, and multiple surgical procedures may be necessary to accomplish a reasonable clinical and cosmetic result. Malignant transformation has been reported, but only when radiotherapy has been given previously.[83]

Ossifying Fibromas These lesions also present with facial deformity involving the paranasal sinuses and orbit. Histologically, this process looks like fibrous dysplasia, but there is a marked predominance of a spindle-shaped fibroblastic cell resembling those in fibrous histiocytoma, and there are occasional mitoses. Psammoma-like islands of bone are also seen. A differential diagnosis must be made between this lesion and fibromatosis, fibrosarcoma, and osteogenic sarcoma. Ossifying fibromas tend to be more locally aggressive than fibrous osteomas. Local excision and curettage are sometimes followed by local recurrence, but only if excision is incomplete.[82]

Giant Cell Tumors These benign tumors are of uncertain origin and have stromal cells which resemble reticuloendothelial cells. The multinucleated giant cells resemble osteoblasts and foreign-body giant cells. These lesions are quite similar to the giant cell tumors seen in the long bones. A differential diagnosis must be made between this tumor and the "brown tumor" of hyperparathyroidism and giant cell–reparative cell granulomas. Malignant giant cell tumor has been reported on two occasions only.[83]

Facial swelling, orbital involvement with displacement of the eyes, and nasal symptoms are the usual clinical presentations. Radical resection of the maxilla, with orbital exenteration when indicated, is the treatment of choice.

Osteogenic Sarcoma This malignant tumor also presents with facial swelling and involvement of soft tissues of the orbit, the alveolar ridge, or the hard palate. Radiologically, the lesion appears both as a mass of increased bone density and as bone destruction. These tumors have been described in association with Paget's disease, and have been seen 15 to 20 years after irradiation of the facial bones (for retinoblastoma or fibrous dysplasia), and years after the injection of thorotrast in the maxillary antrum for diagnostic purposes. Grossly, the tumor is firm, gritty, and fleshy in appearance. Microscopically, it is formed by malignant mesenchymal cells with spindle shapes and is associated with osteoid and immature bone formation.[82,83]

Radical resection has been the most frequent choice of treatment, but local recurrence as well as distant metastases are seen in most cases. The overall 5-year survival rate for osteogenic sarcoma in this site has not exceeded 10 percent, in contrast with the results seen following treatment of the mandible (30 to 50 percent). Delay in diagnosis and inadequate initial treatment may be partly responsible for the difference in results at these two sites.

TUMORS OF DENTAL ORIGIN

Ameloblastoma This benign tumor is common in the mandible but involves the maxilla in only 16 percent of cases.[83] The peak age for development is between 25 to 35 years, and patients usually present with a long history of slowly expanding mass involving the hard palate and superior gingival vestibule. They are often polycystic with the cavities lined by a smooth membrane, surrounded by a thick shell of bone, and containing brownish fluid. Differential diagnosis must include the odontogenic cyst. Complete resection of the tumor-bearing area will result in permanent control of the disease.

REFERENCES

1. Muir CS: Nasopharyngeal cancer: Epidemiology and etiology. *JAMA* 220:393–394, 1972.
2. Greene MH et al: Nasopharyngeal cancer among young people in the United States: Racial variations by cell type. *J Nat Cancer Inst* 58:1267–1070, 1977.
3. Balakrishnan V: An additional younger-age peak for cancer of the nasopharynx. *Int J Cancer* 15:651–657, 1975.
4. Henderson BE: Nasopharyngeal carcinoma: Present status of knowledge. *Cancer Res* 34:1187–1188, 1974.
5. Simons MJ et al: Immunogenetic aspects of nasopharyngeal carcinoma, I: Differences in HLA antigen profiles between patients and control groups. *Int J Cancer* 13:122–134, 1974.
6. Henderson BE et al: Risk factors associated with nasopharyngeal carcinoma. *N Engl J Med* 295:1101–1106, 1976.
7. Simons MJ et al: HLA and nasopharyngeal cancer. *Prog Clin Biol Res* 16:145–148, 1977.
8. Klein G: The Epstein-Barr Virus (EBV), in A Kaplan (ed): *The Herpes Viruses,* Academic Press, New York, 1973, pp 521–555.
9. Inuyama Y et al: Antibody to Epstein-Barr virus in patients with carcinoma of the nasopharynx. *Keio J Med,* 26:79–90, 1977.
10. Coates HL et al: Epstein-Barr virus-associated antigens in nasopharyngeal carcinoma: Relation to clinical course of American patients. *Arch Otolaryngol* 104:427–430, 1978.
11. Kottaridis SD et al: Antibodies to Epstein-Barr virus in nasopharyngeal carcinoma and other neoplastic conditions. *J Nat Cancer Inst* 59:89–91, 1977.
12. Svoboda DJ: Nasopharyngeal cancer: Pathological classification and fine structure. *JAMA* 220:394–396, 1972.
13. Michaels L, Hyams VJ: Undifferentiated carcinoma of the nasopharynx: A light and electron microscopical study. *Clin Otol* 2:105–114, 1977.
14. Fu Y, Peazin KH: Non-epithelial tumors of the nasal cavity, paranasal sinuses and nasopharynx: A clinico-pathological study, X: Malignant lymphomas. *Cancer* 43:611–621, 1979.
15. Fu Y, Peazin KH: Non-epithelial tumors of the nasal cavity, paranasal sinuses and nasopharynx: A clinico-pathological study, IX: Plasmocytomas. *Cancer* 42:2399–2406, 1978.
16. Perez CA et al: Cancer of the nasopharynx: Factors influencing prognosis. *Cancer* 24:1–17, 1969.
17. Urdaneta N et al: Cancer of the nasopharynx: Review of 43

cases treated with supervoltage radiation therapy. *Cancer* 37: 1707–1712, 1976.
18. Hoppe RT et al: Carcinoma of the nasopharynx: Eighteen years experience with megavoltage radiation therapy. *Cancer* 37:2605–2612, 1976.
19. Chiang TC, Jung PF: The nasopharyngoscope and camera examination of the primary carcinoma of the nasopharynx. *Cancer* 40:2353–2364, 1977.
20. De Schryver A et al: Virus-associated antibodies in Caucasian patients with carcinoma of the nasopharynx and in long-term survivors after treatment. *Int J Cancer* 13:319–325, 1974.
21. Lynn TC et al: Prognosis of nasopharyngeal carcinoma by Epstein-Barr virus antibody titer. *Arch Otolaryngol* 103: 128–132, 1977.
22. *Manual for Staging of Cancer*. American Joint Committee for Cancer Staging and End-Result Reporting, 1977.
23. Miller WE et al: Roentgenologic manifestations of malignant tumors of the nasopharynx. *Am J Roentgenol* 106:813–823, 1969.
24. Jing BS: Tumors of the nasopharynx. *Radiol Clin North Am* 8:323–342, 1970.
25. Dubois PJ et al: Tomography in expansile lesions of the nasal and paranasal sinuses. *Radiology* 125:149–158, 1977.
26. Nakagawa H, Wolf BS: Delineation of lesions of the base of the skull by computed tomography. *Radiology* 124:75–80, 1977.
27. Thompson RW et al: Ten-year experience with linear accelerator irradiation of cancer of the nasopharynx. *Radiology* 97:149–155, 1970.
28. Hoffmeister FS et al: Radiation in dentistry: Surgical comments. *J Am Dent Assoc* 78:511–516, 1969.
29. Hinds EC: Care of the teeth before, during and after radiotherapy of the mouth, in JC Gaisford (ed): *Symposium on Cancer of the Head and Neck*, Mosby, St. Louis, 1969.
30. DeSchryver A et al: Ophthalmologic observations on long-term survivors after radiotherapy for nasopharyngeal tumors. *Acta Radiol Ther Phys Biol* 10:193–209, 1971.
31. Fernandez CH et al: Nasopharyngeal carcinoma in children. *Cancer* 37:2787–2791, 1976.
32. McWilliams N, Hazra T: Nasopharyngeal lymphoepithelioma. *Pediatr Res* 12:469, 1978.
33. Wang CC, Schulz MD: Management of locally recurrent carcinoma of the nasopharynx. *Radiology* 86:900–903, 1966.
34. Hilaris BS et al: Therapy of recurrent cancer of the nasopharynx: Value of interstitial and intracavitary radiation. *Arch Otolaryngol* 87:500–510, 1968.
35. Alford TC, Winship T: Epithelial papillomas of the nose and paranasal sinus. *Am J Surg* 106:764–767, 1963.
36. Ridolfi RL et al: Schneiderian papillomas: A clinicopathologic study of 30 cases. *Am J Surg Pathol* 4:43–53, 1977.
37. Snyder RH, Perzin KH: Papillomatosis of nasal cavity and paranasal sinuses (inverted papilloma, squamous papilloma): A clinicopathologic study. *Cancer* 30:668–690, 1972.

38. Sessions RB, Larson DL: En bloc ethmoidectomy and medial maxillectomy. *Arch Otolaryngol* 103:195–202, 1977.
39. Harrison DFN: Lateral rhinotomy: A neglected operation. *Ann Otol* 86:756–759, 1977.
40. Frazell EL, Lewis JS: Cancer of the nasal cavity and accessory sinuses: A report of the management of 416 patients. *Cancer* 16:1293–1301, 1963.
41. Lederman M: Tumors of the upper jaw: Natural history and treatment. *J Laryngol Otol* 84:369–401, 1970.
42. Golpfert H et al: Squamous cell carcinoma of the nasal vestibule. *Arch Otolaryngol* 100:8–10, 1974.
43. Bosch A et al: Cancer of the nasal cavity. *Cancer* 37: 1458–1463, 1976.
44. Noyek AM et al: The radiologic diagnosis of malignant tumors of the paranasal sinuses and related structures. *J Otolaryngol* 6:399–406, 1977.
45. Harrison DFN: Critical look at the classification of maxillary sinus carcinomata. *Ann Otol* 87:3–9, 1978.
46. Boone MLM et al: Malignant disease of the paranasal sinuses and nasal cavity: Importance of precise localization of extent of disease. *Am J Roentgenol* 102:627–636, 1968.
47. Shukovsky LJ, Fletcher GH: Retinal and optic nerve complications in a high dose irradiation technique of ethmoid sinus and nasal cavity. *Radiology* 104:629–634, 1972.
48. Larsson LG, Martensson G: Carcinoma of the paranasal sinuses and the nasal cavities: A clinical study of 379 cases treated at Radiumhemmet and the Otolaryngologic Department of Karolinska Sjukhuset, 1940–1950. *Acta Radiol* 42:149–172, 1954.
49. Jesse RH et al: Head and neck cancer: Squamous cell carcinoma of maxillary and ethmoid sinuses. *Seventh National Cancer Conference Proceedings*, Lippincott, Philadelphia, 1972.
50. Badib AO et al: Treatment of cancer of the paranasal sinuses. *Cancer* 23:533–537, 1969.
51. Cheng VST, Wang CC: Carcinomas of the paranasal sinuses: A study of sixty-six cases. *Cancer* 40:3038–3041, 1977.
52. Harrison DFN: The management of malignant tumors affecting the maxillary and ethmoidal sinuses. *J Laryngol Otol* 87:749–772, 1973.
53. Ketcham AS et al: A combined intracranial facial approach to the paranasal sinuses. *Am J Surg* 106:698, 1963.
54. Ketcham AS et al: Complications of intracranial facial resection for tumors of the paranasal sinuses. *Am J Surg* 112:591, 1966.
55. Ketcham AS et al: The ethmoid sinuses: A re-evaluation of surgical resection. *Am J Surg* 126:469–476, 1973.
56. Terz JJ et al: Craniofacial resection for tumors invading the pterygoid fossa. *Am J Surg* 118:732–740, 1969.
57. Terz JJ et al: Combined craniofacial resection for locally advanced carcinoma of the head and neck: II. Carcinoma of the paranasal sinuses. *Am J Surg* 140:618, 1980.
58. Gorplert H et al: Arterial infusion and radiation therapy in the treatment of advanced cancer of the nasal cavity and sinuses. *Am J Surg* 126:464–468, 1973.

59. Bertino JR et al: The role of chemotherapy in the management of cancer of head and neck. *Cancer* 36:752–758, 1976.
60. Wittes RE et al: Cis-Dich-lowdia (II) in the treatment of carcinoma of head and neck. *Cancer Treatment Rep* 61:359–366, 1977.
61. Natkin GA et al: Combination chemotherapy in head and neck cancer. *Proc Am Soc Clin Oncol* 19:330, 1978.
62. Silverberg IJ et al: A phase I study of radiotherapy and multi-drug chemotherapy in advanced head and neck cancer. *Proc Am Soc Clin Oncol* 19:345, 1978.
63. Catlin D et al: Noncutaneous melanomas of the head and neck region. *Cancer J Clin* 16:75–78, 1966.
64. Harrison DFN: Malignant melanomata of the nasal cavity: Section of Laryngology. *Proc R Soc Med* 61:13–18, 1968.
65. Obert GJ et al: Olfactory neuroblastomas. *Cancer* 13:205–215, 1960.
66. Hutter RVP et al: Estesioneuroblastoma: A clinical and pathological study. *Am J Surg* 106:748–753, 1963.
67. Bailey BJ, Barton S: Olfactory neuroblastoma: Management and prognosis. *Arch Otolaryngol* 101:1–5, 1975.
68. Ackerman LV, del Regato J: Nasopharynx, in J del Regato (ed) *Cancer Diagnosis, Treatment and Prognosis.* 4th ed, Mosby, St. Louis, pp 254–276, 1970.
69. Ogura JH, Schench NL: Unusual nasal tumors: Problems in diagnosis and treatment. *Otolaryngol Clin North Am* 6:813–837, 1973.
70. Fu YS, Perzin KH: Non-epithelial tumors of the nasal cavity, paranasal sinuses and nasopharynx: A clinicopathologic study, I: General features and vascular tumors. *Cancer* 33:1275–1288, 1974.
71. Neel HB III et al: Juvenile angiofibroma: Review of 120 cases. *Am J Surg* 126:547–556, 1973.
72. Conley J et al: Nasopharyngeal angiofibroma in the juvenile. *Surg Gynecol Obstet* 126:825–837, 1968.
73. Boles R, Dedo H: Nasopharyngeal angiofibroma. *Laryngoscope* 5:364–372, 1976.
74. Biller HF et al: Angiofibroma: A treatment approach. *Laryngoscope* 84:695–706, 1974.
74a. Sternberg SS: Pathology of juvenile nasopharyngeal angiofibroma. A lesion of adolescent males. *Cancer* 7:15–28, 1954.
75. Pletcher JD et al: Preoperative embolization of juvenile angiofibromas of nasopharynx. *Ann Otol* 84:740–746, 1975.
76. Fitzpatrick PJ, Rider WD: The radiotherapy of nasopharyngeal angiofibroma. *Radiology* 109:171–178, 1973.
77. Fu YS, Perzin KH: Non-epithelial tumors of the nasal cavity, paranasal sinuses and nasopharynx: A clinicopathologic study, VI: Fibrous tissue tumors (fibroma, fibromatosis, fibrosarcoma). *Cancer,* 37:2912, 1976.
78. Conley J et al: Clinicopathological analysis of 84 patients with original diagnosis of fibrosarcomas of the head and neck. *Am J Surg,* 114:564, 1967.
79. Fu YS, Perzin KH: Non-epithelial tumors of the nasal cavity, paranasal sinuses and nasopharynx: A clinicopathologic study, IV: Smooth muscle tumors (leiomyoma, leiomyosarcoma). *Cancer* 35:1300–1308, 1975.
80. Fu YS, Perzin KH: Non-epithelial tumors of the nasal cavity, paranasal sinuses and nasopharynx: A clinicopathologic study, V: Skeletal muscle tumors(rhabdomyoma and rhabdomyosarcoma). *Cancer,* 37:364–376, 1976.
81. Fu YS, Perzin KH: Non-epithelial tumors of the nasal cavity, paranasal sinuses, and nasopharynx: A clinicopathologic study, III: Cartilaginous tumors (chondroma, chondrosarcoma). *Cancer* 34:453–463, 1974.
82. Fu YS, Perzin KH: Non-epithelial tumors of the nasal cavity, paranasal sinuses, and nasopharynx: a clinicopathologic study, II: Osseous and fibro-osseous lesions, including osteoma, fibrous dysplasia, ossifying fibroma, osteoblastoma, giant cell tumor, and osteosarcoma. *Cancer,* 33:1289–1305, 1974.
83. Ackerman LV, del Regato J: Maxillary sinuses, in J del Regato (ed) *Cancer Diagnosis, Treatment and Prognosis,* 4th ed, Mosby, St. Louis, pp 173–182.

SELECTED BIBLIOGRAPHY

Heffner DK, Hyams VJ: Low-grade adenocarcinoma of the nasal cavity and paranasal sinus. *Cancer* 50:312–322, 1982.

Kondo M, Horiuchi M: Computed tomography of malignant tumors of the nasal cavity and paranasal sinus. *Cancer* 50:226–231, 1982.

17

TUMORS OF THE OROPHARYNX, HYPOPHARYNX, AND CERVICAL ESOPHAGUS

Terence M. Davidson

A CASE HISTORY

Two years ago a 65-year-old retired Marine sergeant was admitted to the Veterans Administration Hospital in La Jolla, California, for a 30-pound weight loss. The man had been well until 2 months prior to admission when he first noted some fatigue. This did not improve with rest and he was unaware of any other problems. He stopped smoking. He had stopped in the past and had always put on 10 to 15 pounds; this time he lost 10 pounds. The weight loss continued in spite of a normal appetite. He resumed smoking and reported to the Veterans Administration Hospital for a checkup. The man was happily married, had two children, four grandchildren, and a nagging mother. His father was a coal miner and had died of lung cancer. The man smoked one pack of nonfilter cigarettes daily and had done so for 40 years. He drank one pint of whisky daily. He claimed that he was never drunk and denied any medical problems from drinking. The remainder of his history was unremarkable. His physical examination was normal. With a 30-pound weight loss he was still 10 pounds overweight. The man was admitted to the medical service, and an involved medical work-up was begun. A medical student requested a head and neck surgery consultation to evaluate left ear pain. Mirror laryngoscopy discovered a large tumor in the piriform sinus. A 2-cm mass was palpated in the left jugulodigastric lymph node chain. Barium swallow, direct laryngoscopy, esophagoscopy, and biopsy all confirmed a $T_2N_1M_0$ squamous cell carcinoma of the piriform sinus. The patient was treated with a total laryngectomy and a left radical neck dissection. Three weeks later he began postoperative radiation therapy.

All went seemingly well until 4 months later: an obvious recurrence was discovered at the base of the tongue. The patient was admitted to the hospital, and a chest x-ray revealed a new lung lesion. Fiberoptic bronchoscopy confirmed that this was a second primary tumor. The patient blossomed with cancer. It eroded through his neck. It was foul-smelling and prohibited oral alimentation. Tube feedings were necessary. Chemotherapy was ineffective. The family was distraught. The patient became depressed and soon the family avoided him. The man died slowly and horribly.

This is a common story. Carcinomas of the oropharynx, hypopharynx, and cervical esophagus grow silently. They are most commonly discovered in the advanced stages. They are often associated with second primary tumors. The cure rates are poor. The manner in which people die is not dignified.

ANATOMY

The anatomy of the oropharynx, hypopharynx, and cervical esophagus is complex. The site and the extent of the tumor are important determinants for therapy and prognosis. Thus, to diagnose, evaluate, and treat these tumors, one must know the anatomy.

The mouth and pharynx are divided into the oral cavity and the oropharynx. The oral cavity includes the lips, the cheeks, the hard palate, the mucosal covering of the maxilla and mandible, the floor of the mouth, and the anterior two-thirds of the tongue. The oropharynx includes the soft palate, the tonsils, the posterior one-third of the tongue, and the pharynx below the nasopharynx and above the hypopharynx. The division between nasopharynx and pharynx is an artificial boundary that occurs at the level of the soft palate. The base of the tongue attaches to the lateral pharyngeal wall and to the epiglottis. A midline fold joining the tongue and the epiglottis divides this area into two cuplike regions called the valleculae. Imagine an artificial line coursing circumferentially about the junction of tongue and epiglottis around the lateral and posterior pharyngeal walls. This line is the boundary between the oropharynx and the hypopharynx.

In the past, tumors of the oropharynx were staged by anatomical site, and one needed a very precise knowledge of this regional anatomy. Currently these tumors are staged by size, so that a more general knowledge of anatomy will suffice.

These tumors are classified according to the rules set up by the American Joint Committee on Cancer, which defines the anatomy of the oropharynx as follows:

The oropharynx extends from the plane of the hard palate superiorly to the plane of the hyoid bone inferiorly and is continuous with the oral cavity. The faucial arch includes both the surfaces of the entire soft palate and uvula. The anterior border and base of the anterior tonsillar pillar, and the line of the circumvallate papillae. The base of the tongue extends from the line of the circumvallate papillae to the junction with the base of the epiglottis (the vallecula) and includes the pharyngoepiglottis and glossoepiglottic folds. The lateral wall of the oropharynx is comprised largely of the tonsil and tonsillar fossae. The posterior tonsillar pillar, the narrow lateral wall, and the posterior wall comprise the pharyngeal wall.[1]

The hypopharynx is the swallowing tube beginning beneath the oropharynx. The hypopharynx ends at the upper esophageal sphincter. The upper esophageal sphincter may or may not be separate from the cricopharyngeus. The anatomists and classifiers continue to debate this issue. Topographically it is an easy separation to make, and a small error superiorly or inferiorly has no real clinical significance. The anterior wall of the hypopharynx is the back of the larynx and is called the postcricoid area. The lateral hypopharyngeal walls are the piriform fossae, and the posterior wall is the posterior hypopharynx. These regions can be difficult to visualize and tumors in these regions are easily missed. The postcricoid area and the apices or inferior tips of the piriform fossae are the most commonly missed regions.

The American Joint Committee defines the hypopharynx as follows:

The hypopharynx extends from the plane of the hyoid bone superiorly to the plane of the lower border of the cricoid cartilage inferiorly. It is made up of three distinct regions: the pyriform sinus, the posterior surface of the larynx (the postcricoid area), and the lower lateral pharyngeal wall.

The three regions of the pharynx and the sites within each region are summarized in Table 17-1.

The cervical esophagus begins where the hypopharynx stops. It is the region of the upper esophageal sphincter and/or cricopharyngeus. From this superior boundary the esophagus is a mucosa-lined conduit to the stomach. The cervical esophagus is divided from the upper thoracic esophagus at the level of the thoracic inlet. Endoscopically this can be a difficult junction to recognize. It occurs in the adult approximately 18 cm from the incisor teeth. Radiographically it occurs at the sternal notch.

The American Joint Committee on Cancer describes the anatomy of the esophagus as follows:

For purposes of classification, staging and reporting of cancer of the esophagus, the esophagus is considered as consisting of three principal regions. These regions are to be classified and reported separately. The cervical esophagus extends from the pharyngo-esophageal junction (the cricopharyngeal sphincter) down to the level of the thoracic inlet, about 18 cm from the upper incisor teeth. The upper and mid-thoracic esophagus extends from the thoracic inlet to a point 10 cm above the

TABLE 17-1 Regions and Sites of the Pharynx

Region	Site
Nasopharynx	Posterior superior wall (vault)
	Lateral wall
Oropharynx	Facial arch including soft palate, uvula, and tonsillar pillar
	Tonsillar fossa and tonsil
	Base of tongue, including glosso-epiglottic and pharyngoepiglottic folds
	Pharyngeal wall, including lateral and posterior walls and posterior tonsillar pillar
Hypopharynx	Piriform sinus
	Postcricoid area
	Posterior hypopharyngeal wall

esophagogastric junction, which is usually at the level of the eighth thoracic vertebra and about 31 cm from the upper incisor teeth. The lower thoracic esophagus extends from a point 10 cm above the esophagogastric junction to the cardiac orifice of the stomach, which is about 40 cm from the upper incisor teeth.[2]

Each of these anatomical regions has a lymphatic drainage. It is important to recognize these drainage areas for two reasons. If a tumor exists, one must know where to look for regional spread. Secondly, if a patient were to present with a suspicious neck mass, knowledge of lymphatic drainage patterns would help direct the search for the primary mucosal lesion.

The primary lymphatic drainage for oropharyngeal tumors is to the mid-high jugular region. Anterior tumors can drain to submental nodes. Tonsillar tumors often drain to retromandibular lymph nodes and to high jugular nodes. All these tumors may drain to retropharyngeal areas and to deep cervical nodes.

The primary lymphatic drainage for hypopharyngeal tumors is to midjugular and parapharyngeal nodes. The primary lymphatic drainage for the cervical esophagus is the deep cervical nodes, the low jugular nodes, the supraclavicular nodes, and the paratracheal nodes.

INCIDENCE, EPIDEMIOLOGY, AND ETIOLOGIC ASPECTS

Incidence

It is often difficult to appreciate the incidence of specific tumors in a specific anatomic site. Most authors seem determined to justify their own work and gather statistics to emphasize their own work. Similarly, different groups—regional, cultural, or socioeconomic—may also present widely varied incidences. Epidermoid carcinoma is the major tumor of the oropharynx, hypopharynx, and cervical esophagus. The following discussion focuses on this neoplasm.

In 1979 the U.S. Department of Health, Education, and Welfare published a manual entitled *Management Guidelines for Head and Neck Cancer.*[3] The numbers published in this manual are a good representation of the relative incidence of head and neck cancer. Annually, 67,000 new cases of cancer, not including superficial skin cancer, are diagnosed in the head and neck. Approximately 37,000 of these are epidermoid neoplasms of the upper aerodigestive tract. This makes the incidence about 17 in 100,000 and accounts for 5 percent of the 660,000 new cancers estimated in the United States in 1978. Table 17-2 summarizes this data.

The Third National Cancer Survey reports the following statistics:[4]

OROPHARYNX

Incidence: 1.6/100,000
3500 new cases estimated in 1978
Male-female ratio, 3.7:1

Rates for Age and Sex per 100,000

Age	Male	Female	Male/female
45–59	2.6	1.4	1.9
50–59	7.3	2.4	3.0
60–69	12.0	2.6	4.6
70–79	13.0	2.4	5.4
80 or greater	10.0	2.0	5.0

HYPOPHARYNX

Incidence: 0.8/100,000
1800 new cases estimated in 1978

Rates for Age and Sex per 100,000

Age	Male	Female	Male/female
45–49	1.3	0.7	1.9
50–59	3.7	1.2	3.0
60–69	6.0	1.3	4.6
70–79	7.0	1.2	5.8
80 or greater	5.0	1.0	5.0

Oropharynx and hypopharynx were reported together. Two-thirds of the cases were oropharyngeal and one-third hypopharyngeal. One should recognize the increasing incidence with increasing age. These tumors are more prevalent in males than females, and this disparity increases with age.

CERVICAL ESOPHAGUS

Incidence: 0.35/100,000
800 new cases estimated in 1978
Cervical esophagus contains 10 percent of all esophageal tumors
Male-female ratio for all esophageal tumors, 3:1
Black-white ratio for all esophageal tumors, 4:1

Etiology

Epidermoid carcinoma develops in response to environmental carcinogens and irritants. There is a host varia-

TABLE 17-2 Incidence of Head and Neck Cancer in the United States, 1979

	Rate per 100,000†	Percentage of			1978 U.S. incidence‡
		Oral	H&N	All	
Lip	1.9	24	12	0.6	4,200
Tongue	2.1	26	13	0.7	4,600
Other oral	2.8	35	17	0.9	6,200
Floor of mouth	(1.0)§	(13)	(7)	(0.3)	(2200)
Cheek	(0.7)	(9)	(5)	(0.2)	(1500)
Gingiva and RT	(0.7)	(9)	(5)	(0.2)	(1500)
Palate	(0.4)	(5)	(5)	(0.2)	(1500)
Salivary gland	1.1	14	7	0.4	2,400
Total oral (including salivary gland)	7.9	100	48	2.6	17,400
Nasopharynx	0.6		4	0.2	1,300
Other pharynx	2.4		15	0.8	5,300
Oropharynx			(10)	(0.5)	(3500)
Hypopharynx	(0.8)		(5)	(0.3)	(1800)
Larynx	4.2		25	1.4	9,200
Nose and paranasal sinuses	0.7§		4	0.2	1,500
Maxillary sinus	(0.5)§		(3)	(0.4)	(1100)
Other	(0.2)		(1)	(0.1)	(400)
Cervical esophagus	0.35§		2	0.1	800
Cervical trachea	0.05§		*	**	100
Ear (meatus, middle ear, mastoid)	0.15§		1	0.1	300
Unknown primary	0.35§		2	0.2	800
Total head and neck	16.7		100	5.5	36,700
Thyroid	3.6			1.2	7,900
Other H&N endocrine	0.1§			**	200
Eye and orbit	0.8			0.3	1,800
Brain and other CNS	4.7§			1.6	10,300
Soft tisse and bone (H&N)	0.5§			0.2	1,100
Melanoma, skin (H&N)	1.3§			0.4	2,900
Lymphoma (H&N primary)	2.9§			1.0	6,400
Total expanded head and neck	30.6			10.1	67,300
All invasive cancer	300.0			100.0	660,000
Nonmelanoma skin cancer					
Head and neck—90 percent¶					270,000¶
All other sites—10 percent					30,000
Total					300,000¶

SOURCE: Adapted with permission from American Joint Committee on Cancer.[3]
* Less than 1 percent.
** Less than 0.1 percent.
† Unless otherwise specified, entries are age adjusted rates from the Third National Cancer Survey.[10]
‡ Based on population estimate of 220,000,000 and 1970 age distribution.
§ From other sources and derived estimates.
¶ From American Cancer Society.[2]

bility related to genetic makeup, hormonal balance, cultural bias, psychologic stress, immunologic status, age, and sex. Other factors may also play a role. Tobacco is the major carcinogen causing epidermoid carcinoma of the upper aerodigestive tract. Alcohol is felt to enhance tobacco's carcinogenesis. In the United States alcohol alone is not a common cause of this tumor. Almost all patients with epidermoid cancer of the oropharynx and hypopharynx have a prolonged exposure to tobacco. There is a geographic variation that must be recognized. At most VA hospitals more than 95 percent of patients have a significant exposure to tobacco. Most patients smoke cigarettes. The exposure is expressed in packs per year, or simply as "pack years." Few patients with head and neck epidermoid cancer have less than a 20-pack-year history, and most have greater than a 40-pack-year history. The carcinogens in tobacco are the hydrocarbons. Whether or not low-tar cigarettes decrease the risk of head and neck cancer is not yet established.

Alcohol clearly enhances the carcinogenic effect of tobacco. This is supported by clinical experience, follow-up studies on alcoholics, and patient studies. This risk is easily seen in the work of Rothman and Keller, and is shown in Table 17-3.[5,6] The risks are expressed relative to a risk of 1.00 for persons who did not use tobacco or drink alcohol. Smoking exposure is expressed in cigarette equivalents (1 cigar = 4 cigarette equivalents and 1 pipeful = 2 cigarette equivalents).

The effect of alcohol is clearly synergistic and increases progressively. The risk for one pack of cigarettes daily increases from 1.5 to 4.13 with increasing alcohol consumption, an increase of 2.75 times. The risk of two or more packs daily increases with increasing alcohol from 2.43 to 15.5. The risk here is 6.5 times greater. The risk from alcohol is related to anatomical site and may reflect the actual contact exposure. Rothman calculated the data shown in Table 17-4 from the work of Keller and Terris.[7]

TABLE 17-3 Risk Ratio of Oral Cancer According to the Level of Exposure to Alcohol and Tobacco

Alcohol, ounces per day	Smoking, cigarette equivalents per day			
	0	1–19	20–39	40+
0	1.00	1.52	1.43	2.43
0.1–0.4	1.40	1.67	3.18	3.25
0.4–1.5	1.60	4.36	4.46	8.21
1.6+	2.33	4.13	9.59	15.50

TABLE 17-4 Risk Ratios for Heavy Drinkers vs. Nondrinkers for Head and Neck Cancer by Site

Site	Risk ratio
Floor of mouth	3.90
Tongue	3.55
Oropharynx	3.21
Uvula, soft palate	3.05
Hypopharynx	1.30
Multiple sites	3.07

It is clear that tobacco is carcinogenic and that alcohol enhances the carcinogenic effect of tobacco. If we assume that the carcinogens in tobacco are hydrocarbons, perhaps their contact with the mucosa is enhanced by the alcohol, or perhaps the alcohol destroys a protective barrier or a protective mechanism of the mucosa.

Other less prevalent risk factors are known. Syphilis is felt to be associated with carcinoma of the tongue. Whether this is an effect of the primary lesion or of the secondary or tertiary disease is not known. Woodworkers have an increased incidence of head and neck neoplasms. This is probably related to the lacquers used in finishing wood. The Plummer-Vinson syndrome is associated with carcinoma of the esophagus. This syndrome is characterized by dysphagia and hypochronic anemia. It is also associated with an upper esophageal web.

Nutritional deficiency may predispose to head and neck cancer. This probably enhances the effect of tobacco. Some authors feel the major effect of alcohol is a nutritional deficiency, specifically a vitamin B–complex deficiency. Viral etiologies and associations with head and neck cancer are being aggressively investigated. Immunosuppression, as with transplant patients, is known to increase the incidence of cancer. This increase may include head and neck cancer. Stress is recognized as playing a role in one's susceptibility to cancer. Its role in head and neck malignancies has not been studied.

In the United States and in most of the world tobacco contains the major carcinogen causing head and neck epidermoid cancer. Alcohol clearly enhances tobacco's effect. Nutritional deficiency, stress, and immunologic depression are certainly important factors, but how important is not known. Nontobacco irritants or carcinogens can cause head and neck cancer. These are rare and are probably confined to a very few specific chemicals.

SIGNS, SYMPTOMS, AND DIAGNOSIS

Tumors of the oropharynx are usually first noticed by the patient as a sore or mild discomfort. The pain may wax and wane or remain constant. Usually patients do not seek medical care until the pain progresses. Tumors of the soft palate and tonsil are more likely to cause pain as small lesions. The pharyngeal walls and the base of the tongue are not so sensitive as the palate and tonsil, and local pain will not be noticed until the tumor is more advanced. Advanced lesions will cause weight loss, which may be the first symptom. Fatigue, malaise, fever, night sweats, and other such symptoms are uncommon. If these symptoms are present, one should think of tumors other than epidermoid cancers. Initially most patients will go to a primary care physician. If the patient has not lost weight or coughed up blood, there is a low index of suspicion for malignancy. The oropharynx is not well examined by many physicians, so many tumors are not recognized. Often a course of antibiotics is prescribed and the symptoms decrease or disappear. The symptoms will return, and at some point the tumor is seen or the patient is referred to a head and neck surgeon.

These tumors metastasize to the neck, and sometimes the presenting complaint is a neck mass. The commonly recognized silent primary areas for cervical metastasis are the nasopharynx, base of tongue, and piriform fossae.

Ear pain can be the first symptom of a tumor in the nasopharynx, oropharynx, larynx, and hypopharynx. All these areas receive sensory nerve fibers from the glossopharyngeal nerve. The tympanic cavity receives its sensory fibers from the tympanic nerve, also a branch of the glossopharyngeal nerve. Auricular pain is a referred pain. Lesions in the hypopharynx and the cervical esophagus will develop symptoms even later than the oropharynx, for these are truly silent areas. Patients may complain of soreness, but more commonly they will complain of a lump in the throat, dysphagia, or odynophagia. Hemoptysis is uncommon. A lump in the neck and weight loss are more common early symptoms of hypopharyngeal and cervical esophageal tumors than of oropharyngeal tumors. Voice changes may occur if the tumor is extremely bulky and distorts the larynx or if the tumor directly invades the recurrent laryngeal nerve or the superior laryngeal nerve.

The key to diagnosis of tumors of the oropharynx, hypopharynx, and cervical esophagus is suspicion. Anyone who is a heavy drinker and smoker must be suspect. Any symptomatology must be investigated completely.

Clinically, these tumors begin as a carcinoma in situ and then become invasive. They may present initially as dyskeratosis, hyperkeratosis, or parakeratosis, and may appear as a white patch called *leukoplakia*. Alternatively the tumor may cause an erythematous response and appear simply as a reddened area. As the tumor grows, it becomes exophytic or ulcerative. Ulceration is common and is associated with pain. Tumor necrosis is found in advanced lesions and may cause a foul smell.

Diagnosis is most commonly made by the suspicious history and is confirmed by physical examination. To properly examine these areas you need a good light—either the classical head mirror or one of the more modern electric head lights. Both of the physician's hands must be free to retract and hold instruments. The two principal means of examination are inspection and palpation. Ideally two tongue blades are used to properly expose the oropharynx. The entire oropharynx can be palpated. This must be done quickly and with the patient's permission since it causes a significant gag. The base of the tongue and the hypopharynx must be examined indirectly. The classic way to do this is with a laryngeal mirror. This requires a certain expertise and practice. Recently, stiff fiberoptic endoscopes have been developed. Using these the physician can easily examine the entire nasal cavity, nasopharynx, oropharynx, larynx, and hypopharynx. One can even look inside the paranasal sinuses. Several models are available, but the most popular are those marketed under the name Hopkins rod. Different scopes are necessary for each area to be examined. If the Hopkins rods are unavailable and mirror exam has been difficult and not complete, one can pass a fiberoptic bronchoscope through the nose and visualize the nasopharynx, base of tongue, valleculae, larynx, and piriform fossae. One can also biopsy through the bronchoscope, but this is not of major benefit. The goal in detection is to suspect a tumor and then recognize a suspicious area.

At this point the patient needs a full head and neck work-up. This entails a complete history including the present illness, smoking and drinking history, exposure to other carcinogens, weight loss, dysphagia, odynophagia, hemoptysis, history of previous tumor, and history of prior irradiation. A past medical history and review of systems is necessary. One must learn the patient's psychosocial history, including personal and family support systems. A complete physical examination is necessary and must include examination of the skin, ears, eyes, nose, mouth, oropharynx, nasopharynx, larynx, hypopharynx, and neck. The patient is admitted to the hospital. Tests are ordered for a complete blood count, urinalysis, creatinine concentration, blood urea nitrogen, electrolytes, calcium, phosphorus, bilirubin total and direct, and an alkaline phosphatase. More elaborate work-ups, including a variety of scans, have been tried in the past. Their yield is so low that they are not economical or useful. Because of the high incidence of second primary tumors, a chest x-ray and a barium swallow with cervical cinefluoroscopy is also requested. The pulmonary radiologist performing the barium swallow should know you are interested primarily in the cervical esophagus. Hypopharyngeal tumors are well seen radiographically with a laryngogram. CT scanning is beginning to be useful in evaluating head and neck tumors and may become a very useful tool in the future.

The patient is brought to the operating room. Under general anesthesia inspect and palpate the entire oral cavity, oropharynx, and nasopharynx. Esophagoscopy is performed, and then a direct laryngoscopy is performed. Fiberoptic bronchoscopy is performed through the endotracheal tube. The yield on rigid bronchoscopy is low and not worth the time, effort, or risk. Any suspicious area is biopsied. Normally a biopsy is taken at the center of the lesion, but not in a necrotic area, and a second is taken at the periphery, i.e., at the junction of normal and cancerous tissue. Multiple biopsies to determine tumor borders are generally not necessary, but the extent of the tumor should be carefully noted and recorded. Standard anatomical drawings are used to indicate the location of the lesion. The neck is once again examined under general anesthesia. The biopsies are fixed in formalin and sent to pathology for permanent sectioning. A second piece is preserved in a suitable medium for electron microscopy.

If the patient is suspect not for epidermoid carcinoma but for lymphoma, a complete medical work-up is needed before biopsy. Most commonly the tonsil is involved. When a tonsil possibly contains a tumor, be it lymphoma or epidermoid carcinoma, a complete resection of the tonsil is necessary because one has a far greater chance of getting a proper diagnosis and because the risks of bleeding postoperatively are lessened. When lymphoma is suspected, bring the fresh tissue to pathology, request touch preparations, and save a piece for electron microscopy. If the tumor is submucosal, one must suspect a minor salivary gland tumor. These are most frequent in the soft palate and in the base of the tongue. Most minor salivary gland tumors are malignant. Biopsy is necessary to determine the histologic type. A significant number are pleomorphic adenomas (benign mixed tumors). These must be excised with a cuff of normal tissue. Cutting into the tumor will spill and seed it into local tissue. Thus, for all salivary gland tumors excise the entire tumor. A tumor presenting submucosally in the lateral oropharyngeal wall may be in the deep lobe of the parotid gland. Salivary gland tumors are discussed in Chap. 19 and lymphomas in Chap. 44. The reader is referred to those chapters for greater detail.

The patient is allowed to recover from anesthesia and the results of pathology are obtained. Several results are possible:

1. A diagnosis other than a neoplasm is made. This must make sense to the physician, and the slides should be reviewed by the surgeon and the case discussed with the pathologist.
2. No diagnosis can be made because the tissue is primarily necrotic. In this case a repeat biopsy is needed.
3. A positive diagnosis for tumor other than epidermoid cancer is made. The slides should be reviewed by the surgeon and then appropriate referral or treatment begun.
4. A diagnosis of epidermoid cancer is made. Generally the pathologist will comment on the degree of differentiation. Common degrees of differentiation are (1) well-differentiated, (2) moderately well differentiated, (3) poorly differentiated, (4) anaplastic. In this last case the pathologist may not be able to say it is an epidermoid cancer. A little tissue should be saved when possible for electron microscopy. Poorly differentiated and anaplastic tumors should be examined with the electron microscope to verify their cellular type. When the pathologist is unable to determine the cell type, the three most likely tumors are (1) poorly differentiated epidermoid carcinoma, (2) amelanotic melanoma, and (3) rhabdomyosarcoma. Electron microscopy should differentiate these cell types.

Additional observations by the pathologist include vascular invasion, perineural invasion, or lymphatic involvement. Some surgeons and pathologists think that microvascular invasion carries a poor prognosis. Others think microvascular invasion could be found in most cases if looked for. Major vascular invasion such as into the jugular vein or carotid artery implies a very poor prognosis. Microvascular invasion may or may not herald an unfavorable outcome. Perineural involvement is also a sign of aggressive tumor behavior. Lymphatic involvement dictates that the surgeon or radiation therapist treat the appropriate lymphatic drainage.

Many physicians feel that a well-differentiated tumor should be easier to treat than a poorly differentiated tumor. Some studies support this hypothesis, but others do not. While histologic grading may affect how aggressive the surgeon and radiation therapist will be, it has not been a definitive prognosticator.

Classification

At this juncture the patient's tumor should be classified and staged. Most surgical groups use the staging recommended by the American Joint Committee on Cancer. The classification was revised in 1977 and has not had major change since. The latest manual was published in 1980 and is called *Staging of Cancer of Head and Neck Sites and of Melanoma*. All physicians treating head and neck tumors must have a copy of this publication. It is available without charge from the executive secretary, American Joint Comittee on Cancer, 55 East Erie Street, Chicago, Illinois 60611.

The clinical diagnostic classification and staging is based on all the information learned from physical examination, radiologic studies, and endoscopic examination. The classification is made and never changed as a result of subsequent operative or pathologic findings. T classifications for oropharynx, hypopharynx, and cervical esophagus are each different.

PRIMARY TUMOR

Oropharynx TX is a tumor that cannot be assessed by rules. T_0 means no evidence of primary tumor. TIS is carcinoma in situ. T_1 is a tumor which by visual examination and by palpation is 2 cm or less in diameter. It is often difficult to make this assessment endoscopically and the surgeon is encouraged to actually measure wherever possible. T_2 is a tumor measuring more than 2 cm but not more than 4 cm in diameter. T_3 is a tumor greater than 4 cm in diameter. T_4 is a massive tumor generally greater than 4 cm across. It is invasive, with evidence of bone invasion or deep neck or muscle invasion.

Hypopharynx The hypopharynx is classified not by size but by site. T_1 is a tumor confined to the site of origin. T_2 is a tumor which extends to an adjacent site. It does not cause "fixation" of the ipsilateral hemilarynx. Vocal cord fixation can be caused by invasion of the recurrent laryngeal nerve or by direct extension into the area of the cricoarytenoid muscles and joint. Paralysis of the superior laryngeal nerve interferes with tensing of the vocal cord. It produces a slightly breathy voice, but does not affect vocal cord movement. T_3 is any tumor which fixes or paralyzes the ipsilateral hemilarynx. T_4 is a massive tumor invading bone or deep neck structures.

Cervical Esophagus T_1 is a tumor that is 5 cm or less in length, originating in the cervical esophagus, that does not extend circumferentially within the esophagus and does not grow out of the esophagus, i.e., into the trachea or other extraesophageal tissues. T_2 is a tumor that is greater than 5 cm long, but does not grow extraesophageally. T_2 is also any tumor that grows circumferentially or causes esophageal obstruction, but does not grow extraesophageally. T_3 is any tumor that grows outside the esophagus. The 1978 American Joint Committee defines obstruction as

roentgenographic evidence of significant impediment to the passage of liquid contrast material past the tumor or endoscopic evidence of esophageal obstruction.

and it defines extraesophageal spread as

extension of cancer outside the esophagus as seen by clinical, roentgenographic or endoscopic evidence of:

1. Recurrent laryngeal, phrenic, or sympathetic nerve involvement
2. Fistula formation
3. Involvement of the tracheal or bronchial tree
4. Vena cava or azygos vein obstruction
5. Malignant effusion: mediastinal widening itself is not evidence of extra-esophageal spread.

REGIONAL LYMPH NODES

Accurate assessment of regional lymph node involvement is just as important as evaluation of the primary lesion. The same node classification is now used for all epidermoid cancers of the upper aerodigestive tract. The size of the neck nodes should be measured and some allowance made for overlying soft tissues. Any midline lymph node is classified as an ipsilateral node. The nodal classification used in the 1980 manual of the American Joint Committee on Cancer is reproduced in Table 17-5. It should be referred to regularly.

TABLE 17-5 Cervical Node Classification for Head and Neck Tumors

NX	Nodes cannot be assessed
N_0	No clinically positive node
N_1	Single clinically positive homolateral node 3 cm or less in diameter
N_2	Single clinically positive homolateral node more than 3 cm but not more than 6 cm in diameter or multiple clinically positive homolateral nodes, none more than 6 cm in diameter
N_{2a}	Single clinically positive homolateral node more than 3 cm but not more than 6 cm in diameter
N_3	Massive homolateral node(s), bilateral node(s), or contralateral node(s)
N_{3a}	Clinically positive homolateral node(s), one more than 6 cm in diameter
N_{3b}	Bilateral clinically positive nodes (in this situation each side of the neck should be staged separately; that is, N_{3b}: right, N_{2a}; left N_1)
N_{3c}	Contralateral clinically positive node(s) only

SOURCE: Adapted from American Joint Committee on Cancer.[1]

DISTANT METASTASIS

Blood-borne or lymphatic spread outside the head and neck lymphatic tissue is called distant metastasis. Even with advanced tumors it is uncommon to discover distant spread clinically. The majority of patients who die of advanced head and neck tumors all have distant metastasis at autopsy, but they are all small foci. The lungs are involved 80 percent of the time and other organs only 30 percent or less. Common sites are kidney, liver, brain, bone, and heart. Techniques currently available cannot detect most distant metastasis. Extensive work-ups looking for distant metastasis are a waste of time and money.

A second mucosal lesion of the upper aerodigestive tract is called a second primary and is not considered a distant metastasis. Each tumor should be staged and treated individually. M_0 means no distant metastasis. M_1 means at least one metastasis is present.

Staging

The tumor is now classified. Staging is determined by reference to a staging table. Staging is the same for all upper aerodigestive tract tumors. Table 17-6 shows the current staging recommended by the American Joint Committee on Cancer.

The tumor is now evaluated, classified, and staged. This information should be collected and diagrammed on a summary sheet. Such a sheet is shown for pharyngeal tumors in Fig. 17-1 and Table 17-7 and for cervical esophageal tumors in Fig. 17-2 and Table 17-8.

TREATMENT

Treating head and neck epidermoid neoplasms is a controversial subject. Evaluating published treatment is difficult for several reasons.

1. Authors have used significantly different classification systems.
2. Authors report data differently.
3. Most papers report relatively successful results.
4. Numbers reported have been variable.
5. Patient follow-up is difficult and often inadequate.
6. There is a tremendous variability in attending physicians.
7. Patient desires are highly variable.

In the past, oropharyngeal tumors were classified by site, not by size as they are now. It is virtually impossible to reclassify tumors staged by alternate systems. In addition some cancer groups have modified the staging system, presumably to improve their effectiveness. Authors report their data differently. Some report only T categories. For example, T_1 tumors have a 90 percent cure rate; T_2, 60 percent; T_3, 40 percent; and T_4, 20 percent. The reader has no way of knowing whether all the T_1 tumors had N_0 necks; if so, that might be an average result. If the necks were classified as N_1 and N_2, these would be terrific results. In any case there is no means for comparison. Similarly, some authors report results primarily by stages. If one were looking for local

TABLE 17-6 Clinical Staging for Head and Neck Tumors

Stage	T	N	M
I	T_1	N_0	M_0
II	T_2	N_0	M_0
III	T_3	N_0	M_0
	$T_1, T_2,$ or T_3	N_1	M_0
IV	T_4	N_0	M_0
	T_4	N_1	M_0
	$T_1, T_2, T_3,$ or T_4	$N_2,$ or N_3	M_0
	$T_1, T_2, T_3,$ or T_4	$N_0, N_1, N_2,$ or N_3	M_1

Age _____ Sex _____ Race _____

Anatomic Site of Cancer _____________ Histologic Cell Type _____________

Grade _____________

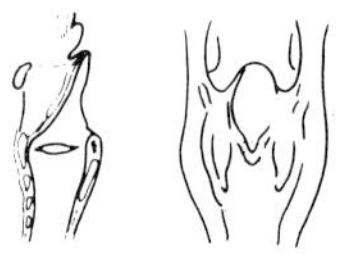

SITE-SPECIFIC INFORMATION-PHARYNX

Status Before Treatment Anywhere - Primary Tumor

Location of tumor	Site of origin (check one)	Site(s) also involved	Anatomic extent*	
Nasopharynx				
Posteriosuperior wall	______	______	T1	______
Lateral wall	______	______	T2	______
			T3	______
			T4	______

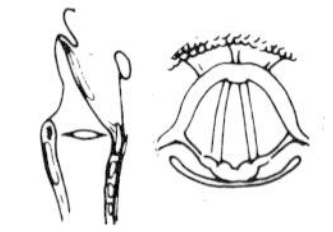

Oropharynx				
Faucial arch			T1	______
Tonsillar fossa, tonsil	______	______	T2	______
Base of tongue	______	______	T3	______
Pharyngeal wall	______	______	T4	______
Hypopharynx				
Pyriform fossa	______	______	T1	______
Postcricoid area	______	______	T2	______
Posterior wall	______	______	T3	______
			T4	______

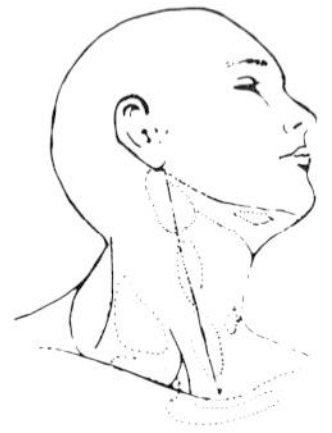

Characteristics of Tumor (check one)

Superficial ______

Exophytic ______

Moderate infiltration ______

Deep infiltration ______

Regional Lymph Nodes (check one only; diagram)

N0 ______ N3a ______

N1 ______ N3b ______

N2a ______ N3c ______

N2b ______

If bilateral nodes present, stage each side separately.

Right ______ Left ______

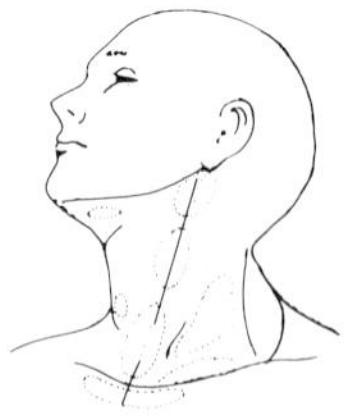

Distant Metastasis

MX ______ M0 ______ M1 ______

Sites: Lung ______ Bone ______ Liver ______

Other ______

Classification

T ______ N ______ M ______

Stage ______

FIGURE 17-1 Abbreviated data form excerpted from American Joint Committee on Cancer for Oropharyngeal and Hypopharyngeal Tumors. *See Table 17-7. (*From Staging of Cancer of Head and Neck Sites and of Melanoma, 1980.*)

control rates, it would be absurd to compare T_3N_0 lesions with T_1N_1 lesions (both are stage III). Some authors use a 2-year follow-up, others 3-year, and others 5-year. They are all adequate, but each approach is different and difficult to compare with another. For example, study 1 claims a 60 percent cure rate for T_2N_1 tumors with a 2-year follow-up. Study 2 claims a 50 percent cure rate for the same tumor with a 5-year follow-up. Such variability makes comparison of one study with another difficult if not impossible.

Most physicians do not report poor results unless they are part of a large report or unless they indicate the difficulties of a particular lesion or treatment. Therefore the data available represent noteworthy results and may not reflect average results. The numbers of cases reported are variable. Even if someone reports 100 oropharyngeal tumors, there may be only four T_2N_1 cancers of the tonsil. It is difficult to make conclusions from such data. Patient follow-up is always difficult. A patient lost to follow-up may have died of disease and yet would only be listed as lost to follow-up. Patient populations vary. One cannot compare cure rates for skid row derelicts with those of a higher socioeconomic group. It is accepted that recurrences and second primaries that can be difficult to distinguish are highly correlated to whether or not a patient continues to smoke, but patients are highly variable in their response to treatment. No known factors account for this variability, or for differences in age, sex, general health, etc.

There is also a tremendous variability among physicians. Some surgeons and radiotherapists are excellent; others are not. How do you compare a technique or an approach of a highly skilled surgery-radiotherapy team with an approach of a less highly skilled team? Or perhaps the approach of one team is superior, while the results of another team are superior; had the one team used the other team's approach, even better results might have been achieved. There is much controversy over primary treatment with radiation therapy as opposed to surgery. It is not legitimate for a weak radiation therapist to argue for radiation using figures generated by a highly skilled group. Similarly, it is not fair for a surgeon to quote results from other surgeons who are clearly superior in training and experience. Patients are also highly variable. Some will stop smoking and comply with the treatment; others will not. Patients often have to choose between treatment regimens. They are also responsible for their follow-up visits. All such factors make interpretation of published results difficult.

Certain principles do apply. The major curative treatment modalities are surgery, radiation therapy, and combinations of surgery and radiation. Chemotherapy has been useful as an adjunct to radiation therapy and as a palliative measure. Immunotherapy has not been effective even as an adjunctive modality. In choosing a treatment several factors must be considered. What are the abilities of the available surgeons and what are the abilities of the available radiation therapists? If one is excellent and the other poor, this must affect one's decision. For the most part small, nonaggressive lesions are successfully treated by either modality. Surgery is fast: the patient has the operation, heals up, and a week or so later it is finished. As long as all heals well there is no major deformity. If the surgery would destroy an important function or cause significant cosmetic deformity, this would argue against surgery. All operations carry some risks, and these risks are greater for the person with significant cardiopulmonary disease. Radiation is noninvasive and causes little cosmetic deformity. It does not interfere with major functions. It does require 5 to 7 weeks of treatment. It wreaks havoc on the teeth and destroys all salivary tissue, causing a dry mouth. High doses next to the bone, especially with radiation implants, can cause an osteoradionecrosis. All such factors must be considered. Advanced lesions require combined therapy. Surgery has a wound infection rate of around 5 percent. This increases to at least 30 percent if the surgery is performed after preoperative radiation therapy. For this reason surgery is best done prior to radiation. There are two exceptions to this rule. If the surgical reconstruction is complex and there is significant risk of wound breakdown, postoperative radiation therapy should be delayed. This jeopardizes treatment. In these cases radiation is administered first. Secondly, if the patient has a large fixed cervical lymph node, preoperative radiation may make a nonresectable mass resectable. Otherwise there are no good reasons to administer radiation prior to surgery when the two modalities are used together.

There is also great controversy about treating the lymph node drainage areas. The references by Nahum et al.[8] and Mendenhall et al.[9] should be reviewed by the interested physician.

There are several clinical situations:

1. N_0 neck with a small tumor and a small statistical chance for neck disease. In most cases these necks need no treatment.
2. N_0 neck with a higher risk of microscopic disease. These necks should be treated; it is commonly thought that 5000 rads is the best therapy available—better than a prophylactic neck dissection—assuming, of course, that the radiation therapist is skilled. To watch and plan to do a neck dissection if nodes appear seriously compromises the outcome. When there is significant risk (20 percent or more) of microscopic disease, the neck should be treated prophylactically.
3. N_1 neck. In this case the palpable disease should be removed surgically. In skilled hands limited neck dissections with postoperative radiation therapy seem to be as effective as a radical or total lymph node dissection and postoperative radiation.
4. N_2 neck. In this case, with multiple homolateral nodes a formal neck dissection should be performed. A conservative neck dissection saving the sternocleidomastoid, the jugular vein, and the spinal accessory nerve should be performed only by skilled surgeons doing this type of surgery regularly. Postoperative radiation therapy is also necessary.
5. N_3 neck. For massive homolateral nodes a neck dissection is necessary if the nodes are not fixed—most commonly to the carotid artery. If they are fixed, preoperative radiation is indicated. If they remain fixed or if there is evidence by angiography of tumor invasion of the carotid artery or jugular vein, the prognosis is poor. Therapy is palliative.

If there is a single contralateral node and one or multiple homolateral nodes, a formal homolateral neck dissection is required. If present, the node on the contralateral side is "plucked." If there are multiple nodes contralaterally, a formal neck dissection is performed on the more involved side, which is usually the ipsilateral side, and a conservative neck dissection performed on the opposite side. Postoperative radiation therapy is required. Remember that an N_3 neck makes a stage IV tumor and carries a poor prognosis.

TABLE 17-7 T Classifications for Pharyngeal Tumors

TM classification
Primary tumor (T)
  TX Tumor that cannot be assessed by rules
  T_0 No evidence of primary tumor
Nasopharynx
  TIS Carcinoma in situ
  T_1 Tumor confined to one side of nasopharynx or no tumor visible (positive biopsy only)
  T_2 Tumor involving two sites (both posterosuperior and lateral walls)
  T_3 Extension of tumor into nasal cavity or nasopharynx
  T_4 Tumor invasion of skull or cranial nerve involvement, or both
Oropharynx
  TIS Carcinoma in situ
  T_1 Tumor 2 cm or less in diameter
  T_2 Tumor more than 2 cm but not more than 4 cm in diameter
  T_3 Tumor more than 4 cm in diameter
  T_4 Massive tumor more than 4 cm in diameter with invasion of bone, soft tissues of neck, or root (deep musculature) of tongue
Hypopharynx
  TIS Carcinoma in situ
  T_1 Tumor confined to the site of origin
  T_2 Extension of tumor to adjacent region or site without fixation of hemilarynx
  T_3 Extension of tumor to adjacent region or site with fixation of hemilarynx
  T_4 Massive tumor invading bone or soft tissues of neck
Nodal involvement (N)
  NX Nodes cannot be assessed
  N_0 No clinically positive node
  N_1 Single clinically positive homolateral node 3 cm or less in diameter
  N_2 Single clinically positive homolateral node more than 3 cm but not more than 6 cm in diameter or multiple clinically positive homolateral nodes, none more than 6 cm in diameter
    N_{2a} Single clinically positive homolateral node more than 3 cm but not more than 6 cm in diameter
    N_{2b} Multiple clinically positive homolateral nodes, none more than 6 cm in diameter
  N_3 Massive homolateral node(s), bilateral nodes, or contralateral node(s)
    N_{3a} Clinically positive homolateral node(s), one more than 6 cm in diameter
    N_{3b} Bilateral clinically positive nodes (in this situation, each side of the neck should be staged separately; that is, N_{3b}: right, N_{2a}; left, N_1)
    N_{3c} Contralateral clinically positive node(s) only
Distant metastasis (M)
  MX Not assessed
  M_0 Not (known) distant metastasis
  M_1 Distant metastasis present; specify sites according to the following notations: pulmonary, PUL; osseous, OSS; hepatic, HEP; brain, BRA; lymph nodes, LYM; bone marrow, MAR; pleura, PLE; skin, SKI; eye, EYE; other, OTH

Histopathology
Predominant cancer is squamous cell carcinoma

Grade
Well-differentiated, moderately well differentiated, or poorly to very poorly differentiated.

Stage grouping
Stage I $T_1 N_0 M_0$
Stage II $T_2 T N_0 M_0$
Stage III $T_3 N_0 M_0$; T_1 or T_2 or T_3, $N_1 M_0$
Stage IV T_4, N_0 or N_1, M_0; any T, N_2 or N_3, M_0; any T, any N, M_1

Residual tumor (R)
  R_0 No residual tumor
  R_1 Microscopic residual tumor
  R_2 Macroscopic residual tumor; specify site

Host (H): Performance status of host, Karnofsky scale, %
  H_0 Normal activity, 90–100
  H_1 Symptomatic but ambulatory, 70–80
  H_2 Ambulatory more than 50 percent of time, 50–60
  H_3 Ambulatory 50 percent or less of time, 30–40
  H_4 Bedridden, 10–20

SOURCE: American Joint Committee on Cancer.[1]

One should not be heroic and operate if the chance of cure is low.

These are the basic principles of treatment. Specific situations will now be considered.

Treatment According to Site

OROPHARYNX

T_1 and T_2 tumors are common in the tonsil and soft palate and are usually discovered early. They are less commonly discovered this early in the pharyngeal walls or the base of the tongue. If the patient has an N_0 neck, radiation therapy alone is the best treatment. T_2 tumors of the tonsil or soft palate with an N_1 or an N_2 neck are best treated with combined therapy. Surgery is performed to remove the tumor and the neck disease. Tonsil tumors may require removing a portion of mandible. Radiation should include the primary site and the lymphatic drainage areas. All T_3 and T_4 tumors of the soft palate or tonsil should have combined therapy. If the neck is N_0, a suprahyoid lymph node dissection is performed simultaneously. This is done to improve the thoroughness and safety of the primary excision. Postoperative radiation is required for the primary site and the neck. Patients with N_2 and N_3 necks, if operable, should have a complete neck dissection followed by radiation therapy to the primary site and to the neck.

Tumors of the pharyngeal walls are difficult to resect. Radiation therapy is the best modality for most pharyngeal wall tumors. Palpable disease in the neck should be surgically removed. This is usually done following radiation. If the original neck node is small (less than 3 cm) and disappears with radiation therapy, additional radiation can be given to the neck for cure.

Base-of-tongue lesions are rarely discovered early. If they are, a limited resection and postoperative radiation are indicated; large lesions have the best chance for cure with combined therapy. The surgery is a total glossectomy. This destroys the ability to swallow and the patient will aspirate. Hence a total laryngectomy is also needed. This is an involved procedure and it is mutilating. It should only be performed in a patient who thoroughly understands the consequences of that procedure. For these reasons most tumors are treated with radiation therapy. Radiation implants are very useful as a means of treating base-of-tongue lesions. Neck dissection is used for palpable disease. This treatment regime is summarized in Tables 17-9 and 17-10.

The difficulty of determining cure rates from the literature has already been mentioned. Many individual papers report exceptional cure rates for small numbers of patients. A 1979 NIH publication reports 5-year survival figures which are frankly dismal. They are shown in Table 17-11.

HYPOPHARYNX

Treatment of T_1 and T_2 hypopharyngeal carcinoma is almost a hypothetical issue, for rarely are these tumors diagnosed early. For N_0 necks radiation to the primary tumor and the neck is probably sufficient. T_1 and T_2 tumors with palpable neck disease can be treated primarily with radiation for the primary tumor and combined therapy to the neck. T_3 tumors fix the vocal fold. Total laryngectomy is necessary to cure T_3 and T_4 tumors. N_0 necks should be radiated. Palpable neck disease should be excised and then the neck should be radiated. As with oropharyngeal tumors, surgery followed by radiation therapy gives the same result as reversing the order of treatment. Complications are fewer in number when surgery is performed first. If the tumor involves so much of the hypopharyngeal circumference that primary closure is not feasible, a more complex reconstruction will be needed. In these cases the risk associated with surgery without prior radiation is significant, and radiation should be performed initially. Surgery should be performed 4 to 6 weeks later. Treatment is summarized in Table 17-12. Results are poor. The results reported in *Management Guidelines for Head and Neck Cancer* are shown in Table 17-13.

CERVICAL ESOPHAGUS

As with the hypopharynx, carcinoma of the cervical esophagus is rarely diagnosed early. The treatment for all tumors is surgical excision. This may require total esophagectomy. Reconstruction is with local chest flaps, gastric pull-up, or colon interposition. Lymph node spread is often bilateral, and staged neck dissections and superior mediastinal neck dissections are often necessary. Radiation should be used in combination for all tumors. The cure rates are low. In many cases palliation may be the best therapy.

Adjuvant Therapy

Radiation and surgery are the major treatment modalities. Cryosurgery and immunotherapy have had no significant effect for curative treatment. Chemotherapy alone has not yet proved effective as a primary curative technique. It is currently being investigated as adjunctive therapy, particularly in combination with radiation.

Chemotherapy can be used in one of two ways. It can be given alone prior to surgery or radiation. The concept is to shrink the tumor mass and/or to decrease its microscopic local and regional spread. Trials have been performed, primarily with advanced tumors, using single-agent and combination programs. Ervin et al. reviewed this subject in 1981.[11] The available data are summarized in Table 17-14. Complete response means that the primary tumor disappears. In all cases radiation and/or surgery are used to complete the therapy. To date there is very little to show how this ultimately effects the

348 TUMORS OF THE HEAD AND NECK

```
                              Age _____  Sex _____  Race _____
Anatomic Site of Cancer _____  Histological Cell Type _____
                                       Grade _____

         SITE-SPECIFIC INFORMATION-ESOPHAGUS
                                              Limits
         Distance from incisors            Upper      Lower
            Cervical < 18 cm               _____      _____
            Upper thoracic 18-30 cm        _____      _____
            Lower thoracic > 30 cm         _____      _____
         Histology
            SCE _____   Other _____
         Length of tumor _____ cm
                                              Yes        No
         Encircles esophagus               _____      _____
         Evidence of obstruction           _____      _____
         Extraesophageal extension
            Nerve involvement              _____      _____
            Tracheobronchial tree          _____      _____
            Caval obstruction              _____      _____
            Pleural effusion               _____      _____
            Mediastinal widening (not necessarily
              evidence of extraesophageal spread) _____  _____
         Lymph Nodes
            Palpable                       _____      _____
            Bilateral                      _____      _____
            Fixed                          _____      _____
            Number _____
            Size of largest node _____ cm

  Location                    Clinical       Surgical       Radiologic
     Cervical                 _____        _____        _____
     Supraclavicular          _____        _____        _____
     Intrathoracic            _____        _____        _____
     Abdominal                _____        _____        _____
  Metastasis
     Distant lymph nodes      _____        _____        _____
     Lung                     _____        _____        _____
     Bone                     _____        _____        _____
     Liver                    _____        _____        _____
     Other                    _____        _____        _____
  Classification
     T _____  N _____  M _____
  Stage _____
```

FIGURE 17-2 Abbreviated data form excerpted from American Joint Committee on Cancer for Oropharyngeal and Hypopharyngeal Tumors. (*From Staging of Cancer of Head and Neck Sites and of Melanoma, 1980.*)

cure rate. For example, assume the cure rate for T_3N_2 carcinoma of the pharynx is 10 percent. One could initially treat all these patients with chemotherapy. Assuming a high complete response rate is found, one initially must document that the ultimate cure rate is significantly greater than it would have been without the chemotherapy. Studies of this nature are not yet reported. Most chemotherapy programs for cure are still experimental.

A more promising use for chemotherapy is in combination with radiation. Although the initial experiences are not favorable, there remains significant enthusiasm for this approach. Ervin et al.[11] summarize published data as shown in Table 17-15. The main goal of this regimen is to treat stage III and IV cancers, i.e. those with cure rates lower than 20 percent, and to determine if these cure rates can be improved. If so, the region can then be considered, depending on its toxicity, for stage I and II cancers.

Immunotherapy has received a lot of attention for head and neck cancer, for it is recognized that many of these patients have a marked depression of their cellular immunity even in the early stages. This subject was reviewed by Wanebo in 1979.[12] To date, most of the immunologic studies have looked at nonspecific immunity primarily as a prognosticator. Table 17-16 reproduces exemplary data from Wanebo's experience. The ultimate ability of these immunologic depressions to successfully prognosticate cure rates is not yet established. One of the major problems is that smoking, alcoholism, and malnutrition are known to depress the cellular and humoral immunity.

Immunotherapy has been tried in combination with chemotherapy for stage III and stage IV cancer patients. A variety of trials using methotrexate, BCG, INH, levamisole, and others have failed to show significant immunologic potential and have not shown significant therapeutic effects.

Follow-up

Patients are followed closely during therapy to evaluate tumor regression, patient nutrition, and possible wound infection. After treatment is completed the patient is followed at monthly intervals for the first year, and every second month for the second year. Most recurrences appear in the first 2 years. If the patient is doing well, has stopped drinking alcohol, and most importantly has stopped smoking, the chance of a second primary tumor is 10 percent and decreases over the next 5 to 10 years. If the patient continues smoking, especially if alcohol is abused also, the chance of a second primary is as high as 50 percent. Obviously a high-risk patient should be followed closely at 3- to 4-month intervals for life. Lower-risk patients can be seen at 6-month intervals for the third, fourth, and fifth posttreatment years and can then be followed as needed for new or recurrent symptoms.

Standard follow-up includes a history to see how the patient is doing, weight measurement to determine nutrition, and a good head and neck examination to look at the primary site and all other mucosal surfaces at risk. The neck is carefully palpated to evaluate regional spread. The lungs are also at risk and a yearly chest x-ray is mandatory. Any suspicious areas should be biopsied.

Recurrences can be treated. Several situations exist, as outlined below.

1. Radiation failure. In these cases additional radiation is rarely possible. Surgery is the only option. If there is only local recurrence, some surgeons will recommend concurrent neck dissection prophylactically. Others feel it is safe to observe. If the neck originally contained no palpable disease, neck dissection is not necessary for T_1 tumors, but probably is indicated for larger or more extensive tumors. The paper by Nahum et al.[8] documents the indications for prophylactic neck dissections.
2. Surgical failure. In this case reoperate if possible, removing all detectable local and regional disease. Follow this with postoperative radiotherapy to the primary site and the neck region. Two special situations are often difficult to evaluate after neck dissection. Radical neck dissection removes the homolateral submandibular gland. Inevitably the contralateral gland is not palpated until postoperatively. Without its mate for comparison it is difficult to assess if this is a normal submandibular gland or if it represents contralateral regional disease. Radiation further confuses the evaluation, for it leaves the gland scarred and firm. If in doubt it should be removed. One of the complications of radical neck surgery is fistula formation and carotid artery blowout. Most experienced head and neck surgeons cover the carotid artery with a dermal graft if the upper aerodigestive tract is entered, and a neck dissection is performed OR if a neck dissection is performed after radiation therapy. The dermal grafts seal quickly over the carotid and have been a major contribution in preventing carotid blowout. Occasionally an epidermoid inclusion cyst forms in the dermal graft. It is difficult to differentiate these cysts from recurrent regional disease. Open biopsy is usually needed to be sure of the histology.
3. Combined treatment failure. In these cases surgery is the only curative modality. If it is theoretically feasible to remove all clinical disease, then an aggressive operation should be recommended.
4. Second primary tumor
    a. No previous radiation. Treat this with the philosophies outlined for the initial tumor. Both radiation and surgery can be used.
    b. After radiation. Generally surgery is the main modality. If the second primary is out of the radiation ports of the first primary, radiation may also be used.
5. Noncurable disease and distant metastasis. If distant metastases occur they are multiple and incurable. Only palliative treatment should be given. If the patient is symptomatic and additional radiation is possible, that is the best modality.

Chemotherapy is the next best modality. This

TABLE 17-8 T Classifications for Esophageal Tumors

TNM classification
Primary tumor (T) (for all three segments of the esophagus)
T_0 No demonstrable tumor in the esophagus
TIS   Carcinoma in situ
T_1 A tumor 5 cm or less in esophageal length with no obstruction,* no circumferential involvement, and no extraesophageal spread
T_2 A tumor more than 5 cm in esophageal length with no extraesophageal spread or a tumor of any size which obstructs or has circumferential involvement and with no extraesophageal spread
T_3 Any tumor with extraesophageal spread
Nodal involvement (N)
Cervical esophagus: The regional lymph nodes in the cervical esophagus are the cervical and supraclavicular nodes
N_0 No clinically palpable nodes
N_1 Movable, unilateral, palpable nodes
N_2 Movable, bilateral, palpable nodes
N_3 Fixed nodes
Thoracic esophagus:
NX (clinical evaluation)   Regional lymph nodes for the upper, midthoracic, and lower thoracic esophagus that are not ordinarily accessible for clinical evaluation
N_0 (surgical evaluation)   No positive nodes
N_1 (surgical evaluation)   Positive nodes
Distant metastasis (M)
MX   Not assessed
M_0 No (known) distant metastasis*
M_1 Distant metastasis present

Histopathology
Squamous cell carcinoma, adenocarcinoma. Rarely do sarcomas and melanomas occur.

Grade
Well-differentiated, moderately well differentiated, or poorly to very poorly differentiated.

---

subject is reviewed by Muggia et al.[13] Low-dose methotrexate (30 to 60 mg/m²) injected IV weekly has given responses in over 50 percent of patients. Normally pain subsides, and the tumor regresses and may even disappear. Toxicity is low and remission lasts weeks to months. No better regimen has been discovered to date. Because of the success of low-dose methotrexate, high-dose methotrexate with leucovorin rescue has been widely investigated. Toxicity is greater, especially if the drugs are given correctly. Success measured in percentage of tumor remission and percentage of patients with remission or duration of remission have not been better than with low-dose methotrexate.

Bleomycin has been tried in doses of 10 to 20 mg/m² injected IM or IV once or twice weekly. Total dose should not exceed 200 mg/m². Results have not equaled those of methotrexate, and the duration of remission has been reduced to a maximum of 2 to 3 months. Toxicity has been significant.

Cis-platinum (*cis*-diamminedichloroplatinum II) is the drug being tested most recently. Dose schedules are not yet determined. In spite of an initial enthusiasm for this drug, it has failed to achieve results equaling those of low-dose methotrexate.

Combination chemotherapy has not provided results superior to single-agent chemotherapy. Toxicity, cost, and complexity are significantly greater.

Cryosurgery is also useful as a palliative treatment. When the tumor is painful, necrotic, unsightly, and foul-smelling, the patient, the family, the friends, and the medical personnel are miserable. Freezing will decrease tumor size and infection. It will also decrease the patient's pain. Optimally a large probe is used with a cold source such as liquid nitrogen. A fast deep-freeze and a slow thaw is most effective. This is done twice for each area. Treatment can be repeated weekly. This is usually done with the patient as an outpatient under local or general anesthesia. Occasional cures are reported with smaller tumors. Surgical debulking

TABLE 17-8 T Classifications for Esophageal Tumors (Continued)

Staged grouping
  Stage I
    TIS N_0M_0 Carcinoma in situ
    $T_1N_0M_0$ Tumor in any region of the esophagus that involves 5 cm or less of esophageal length, produces no obstruction, has
    $T_1NX\ M_0$ no extraesophageal spread, does not involve the entire circumference, and shows no regional lymph node metastates or remote metastases
  Stage II   A tumor of any size with no extraesophageal spread and with no distant metastases
    Cervical esophagus
    $T_1N_1M_0$
    $T_1N_2M_0$
    $T_2N_1M_0$ Any tumor with palpable, movable, regional nodes
    $T_2N_2M_0$
    $T_2N_0M_0$ A tumor more than 5 cm in length with negative nodes
    Thoracic esophagus:
    $T_2NX\ M_0$ Lymph nodes cannot be assessed (clinical-diagnostic evaluation)
    $T_2N_0M_0$ A tumor more than 5 cm in length or a tumor of any size with obstruction or circumferential involvement with no lymph node involvement (postsurgical treatment–pathologic evaluation)
  Stage III   Any esophageal cancer at any level with
    Any T_3 1. Distant metastases
    Any N_3 2. Extraesophageal spread
    (Cervical)   3. Fixed lymph node metastases
    Any N_1
    (Thoracic)   Any intrathoracic esophageal carcinoma including either upper and midthoracic region or lower thoracic region with
    Any M_1 any positive findings in regional lymph nodes

SOURCE: American Joint Committee on Cancer.[2]
* For the cervical esophagus, any lymph node involvement other than cervical or supraclavicular is considered distant metastasis. For the thoracic esophagus, any cervical, supraclavicular, scalene, or abdominal lymph node is considered distant metastasis.

of the tumor is occasionally useful and can be used in combination with cryotherapy.

CURRENT IDEAS AND PROSPECTS FOR THE FUTURE

The obvious solution to this entire problem is to ban tobacco. This would essentially eradicate head and neck and pulmonary epidermoid cancers and would seriously decrease the incidence of emphysema and would lessen the intensity of arteriosclerotic disease. The tobacco industry does not see it this way, nor do all the people who smoke. The second solution is patient education. The American Cancer Society is pursuing this approach. Education has certainly not solved the problem, for young people are still learning to smoke and older people are continuing to smoke. The third solution is the filter cigarette. Whether this will ultimately reduce the incidence of tobacco-related diseases is yet to be seen.

Local recurrence remains the major cause of treatment failure. Surgery has not significantly improved the cure rates over the last decades. Although many surgeons feel that it has, the statisticians have failed to discover the improvement. Combined therapy has been a step forward, but local recurrence remains responsible for at least 50 percent of failures. Recent work has elucidated

TABLE 17-9 Carcinoma of Soft Palate and Tonsil: Recommended Treatment

	N_0	N_1	N_2	N_3*
T_1	R†	R primary C neck†	R primary C neck	R primary C neck
T_2	R	R primary	C	C
T_3	C	C	C	C
T_4	C	C	C	C

* Palliative therapy if tumor is not curable
† R = Radiation
‡ C = Combined

TABLE 17-10 Carcinoma of Pharyngeal Walls and Base of Tongue: Recommended Treatment

	N_0	N_1	N_2	N_3*
T_1	R†	R primary C neck	R primary C neck	R primary C neck
T_2	R	R primary C neck	R primary C neck	R primary C neck
T_3	R	R primary C neck	R primary C neck	R primary C neck
T_4*				

* Palliative therapy if tumor is not curable
† R = Radiation
‡ C = Combined

TABLE 17-12 Carcinoma of Hypopharynx: Recommended Treatment

	N_0	N_1	N_2	N_3*
T_1	R†	R primary C neck‡	R primary C neck	R primary C neck
T_2	R	R primary C neck	C	C
T_3	C	C	C	C
T_4*	C	C	C	C

* Palliative treatment for noncurable tumors
† R = Radiation
‡ C = Combined

the cause for local recurrence and has suggested a solution.[14,15]

Frederick Mohs first described a new approach to difficult skin cancers in 1941. The technique was called chemosurgery and was improved over the next two decades. With this technique cure rates for recurrent and sclerosing basal cell cancers have increased from 50 percent to better than 95 percent. Its use today is a concept of frozen-section controlled surgery.

The standard frozen-section evaluation is a sampling process. Certainly a good pathologist will discover palpable disease, but in fact samples about one-thousandth of the surgical margin. Mohs's contribution was to orient the frozen sections in such a way that 100 percent of the surgical margin could be sampled. Figure 17-3 compares these two approaches.

On the right is a circular tumor removed by an elliptical excision. Frozen sections I through IV represent standard frozen-section orientation. One-thousandth of the surgical margin is examined. Obviously the chance for error is great in a tumor with significant microscopic spread. On the left is the approach recommended by Mohs. Wafers of tissue are removed, frozen, and examined microscopically; 100 percent of the surgical margin is examined.

Additional tissue is cut from areas in which tumor is identified. This process continues until all the tumor is removed.

The same process can be applied to head and neck mucosal tumors. The technical aspects of obtaining frozen sections of the entire surgical margin are more complex. Figure 17-4 shows how this might be done. Careful mapping and orientation is necessary. This technique has been used for the last 2 years at the Veterans Administration Hospital in La Jolla, California. It has been observed that over 50 percent of patients have residual microscopic tumor after conventional tumor surgery. This microscopic tumor spreads predom-

TABLE 17-11 Distribution of 2142 Patients with Carcinoma of the Oropharynx (years of diagnosis, 1950 to 1969)

Extent of disease	Distribution, %	Survival, %
Localized	29	44
Regional	50	23
Distant	15	11
Unknown	6	
All stages		28

SOURCE: Axtell et al.[10]

TABLE 17-13 Distribution of 1362 Patients with Carcinoma of the Hypopharynx (years of diagnosis, 1950 to 1969)

Extent of disease	Distribution, %	Survival, %
Localized	22	20
Regional	57	14
Distant	17	12
Unknown	4	
All stages		15

SOURCE: Axtell et al.[10]

TABLE 17-14 Chemotherapy for Advanced Head and Neck Cancer

Drug regimen	Number of trials	Number of patients evaluated	> 50 percent response, %	Complete response, %*	References
Methotrexate-leucovorin calcium	3	38	52	3	4, 17, 40
Cis-platinum	2	16	69	0	37, 38, 39
Cis-platinum methotrexate-leucovorin calcium, bleomycin sulfate	4	75	77	21	5, 7, 11, 13
Cis-platinum, bleomycin	3	71	76	23	6, 24, 44
Cis-platinum, vincristine sulfate, bleomycin	1	35	80	23	23
Cis-platinum, methotrexate-leucovorin†	1	20	60	0	46
Cyclophosphamide, vincristine, methotrexate, fluorouracil, bleomycin	1	16	56	NR‡	42
Vincristine, methotrexate, fluorouracil, bleomycin	1	30	87	NR‡	45

SOURCE: Adapted from Ervin et al,[11] tables 3,4.

* Complete responses also included in greater than 50 percent response column.
† Dose-limiting nephrotoxicity noted.
‡ Complete responses not reported.

inantly in the submucosa, but will follow other natural tissue planes as well. The tumor invades like thin fingers, and in fact these tumor strands may be as narrow as 10 cells and extend for distances of 2 to 3 cm away from clinical disease. This tumor spread is easily followed with the frozen-section approach as outlined previously. In the past 1½ years the first 20 patients on whom this technique has been used have been carefully followed. Follow-up is too short to make definite conclusions about local control, but so far all the patients are free of local

TABLE 17-15 Relation of Immune Reactivity to Stage of Disease from Wanebo*

Source, year	Number of patients	Drugs	Conclusion
Seagren et al., 1979	18	Cyclophosphamide, bleomycin sulfate	Very toxic locally; 9 in 10 patients relapsed
Glick et al., 1979	11	Vinblastine sulfate, methotrexate, bleomycin	Believed to be too toxic, 6 in 8 patients relapsed
Fu et al., 1979	15	Vinblastine, methotrexate, bleomycin	Limited to mucositis; three fatal complications; most patients relapsed
Clifford et al., 1978	102	Vinblastine, methotrexate, bleomycin	56 percent disease-free survival at 1 year; better than historical controls; $p = .001$

SOURCE: Adapted from Ervin et al.,[11] table 5.

TABLE 17-16 Percentage of Patients with Depressed Response in Each Disease State

Response	Stage I (n = 33)	Stage II (n = 32)	Stage III (n = 32)	Stage IV (n = 25)
DNCB	44	25	60	30
Lymphocyte count	21	41	49	45
PHA	32	45	45	61
Con A	24	21	32	33
PWM	9	23	33	23

SOURCE: Adapted with permission from Wanebo.[12]

disease. The technique requires active participation of a skilled pathologist. Theoretically, all microscopic disease should be traceable and local recurrence eliminated. The preliminary results are promising, but a greater and longer experience will be necessary to document success.

Another interesting treatment approach which may hold promise for the future is interstitial implant radiation therapy. This technique is not new, but is only recently being aggressively investigated for head and neck tumors. The major advantage of implant therapy is to be able to deliver a high radiation dose to the tumor but significantly lower doses to the surrounding healthy tissues. Several factors have made this possible. The radiation dose falls off as the inverse square of the distance from the implant. This rapid decline permits high radiation doses to the tumor in a controlled fashion. Computerized dosimetry can accurately predict radiation levels and is used to guide the radiation therapist to properly place the implants. A new isotope, iridium 192, is well-suited for this kind of therapy. Its half-life is 74 days, which allows it to be stored, used when needed, and even reused. Its average gamma energy is 340 keV, which is quite useful for biologic radiation. Lastly, iridium 192 decays to platinum 192. This is a stable solid. A solid decay product has the obvious advantage over a gas in that the atmosphere is not contaminated.

Normally patients are treated by conventional external beam therapy to 5000 rads. The clinical disease, including the primary tumor and regional metastases, is then implanted. The tumor dose is raised to 8000 rads. The implant radiation is delivered by threading plastic catheters into the tumor, as determined by the computerized dosimetry. This is done under general anesthesia.

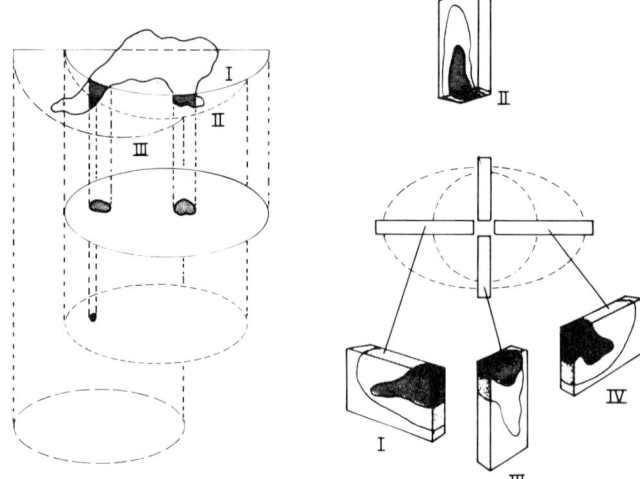

FIGURE 17-3 Comparison of orientation for Mohs chemosurgery vs. standard surgical pathology technique. (*From TM Davidson et al: Microscopic controlled excisions for epidermoid carcinoma of the head and neck, Otolaryngol Head Neck Surg 89:244–251, 1981.*)

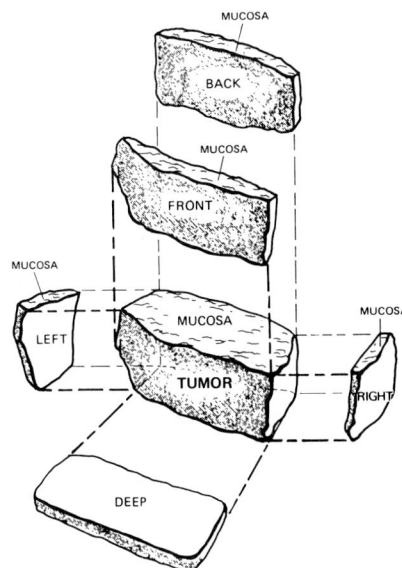

FIGURE 17-4 Orientation for frozen-section examinations of head and neck mucosal tumor. (*From TM Davidson et al: Microscopic controlled excisions for epidermoid carcinoma of the head and neck, Otolaryngol Head Neck Surg 89:244–251, 1981.*)

The catheters are then filled with iridium 192 seeds. The seeds and catheters are removed after 3 to 5 days. There is a definite skill to placing the catheters. Readily accessible sites such as the lip and anterior tongue are easier to implant than are sites such as the base of tongue. The hypopharynx and cervical esophagus are very difficult to implant.

Complications include dry mouth, increased dental disease, tumor infection, and necrosis. Osteoradionecrosis is uncommon in well-designed treatments, but can be common and very difficult to manage with less well conceived planning. Initial results reported are excellent. But, as always, follow-up is too short and cases are not randomized between implant and conventional therapy.

Occasionally a tumor biopsy is sent to pathology, and frozen section or permanent section is reported as a malignancy, cell type unknown. Special stains are immediately ordered, looking for mucin, amyloid, etc. After several days of staining, the pathologist is no closer to an answer. Ideally, a piece of tissue has been saved in a fixative suitable for electron microscopy. If not, additional tissue must be obtained. The tissue is prepared and examined in the electron microscope. This is a relatively new field and there are as of yet very few real experts in the country.[17] Conventional light microscopy can magnify up to 400 times. Electron microscopy can magnify up to 50,000 times. The microscopist looks for ultrastructural features. Small-cell tumors are the most common type of tumor requiring electron microscopy. The microscopist looks for desmosomes, tonofibrils, secretory granules, cytoplasmic processes, myofilaments, and mitochondria. The microscopist can differentiate such tumors as undifferentiated squamous cell carcinoma, rhabdomyosarcoma, melanoma (especially amelanotic melanoma), spindle-cell sarcoma, Ewing's sarcoma, enuroblastoma, and other neurogenic tumors. Electron microscopy can help in the diagnosis of adenocarcinoma and help differentiate different possible sites in the head and neck, such as thyroid or salivary gland.

Another exciting area of investigation is the use of monoclonal antibodies to examine tissue immunologically. Antibodies already exist to detect cell surface antigen of lymphomas. Surface immunoglobulins can recognize B-cell lymphoma; and different surface immunoglobulins are specific for T-cell lymphoma. A different antibody can differentiate lymphocytes and leukocytes from epidermoid cells. Antibodies will be developed in the future to recognize different carcinomas, including epidermoid carcinoma and melanoma. Immunofluorescence is fast and relatively inexpensive. Antibody can be applied to a frozen section and after 1 hour indirect immunofluorescence recognized. Similarly, peroxidase-labeled antibody can be applied and detected rapidly on permanent sections. Other antibodies are being developed for surface peptides. An antibody already exists that can detect calcitonin in medullary

TABLE 17-17 Prospective Panendoscopic Identification of Second Primary Carcinomas in 259 Patients Presenting Consecutively to the Department of Otolaryngology and Maxillofacial Surgery at the University of California Medical Center from 1977 through 1979 with Primary Squamous Cell Carcinoma of the Head and Neck

Primary tumor	Number of patients	Percentage of Registry*	Number of second primaries identified	Percentage of patients in primary tumor group	Location of second primary			
					Lung	Esophagus	Head and neck	Other†
Larynx	88	34.0	5	5.7	2	2	1	0
Oropharynx	61	23.5	11	18.0	2	1	8	0
Hypopharynx	27	10.4	2	7.4	0	1	1	0
Oral cavity	72	27.8	9	12.5	0	0	9	0
Miscellaneous	11	4.2	0	0				
Total	259	100.0	27	10.4	4	4	19	0

SOURCE: Adapted from Gluckman et al.[18]
* Department of Otolaryngology and Maxillofacial Surgery Tumor Registry.
† Sites other than lung, esophagus, and the head and neck.

carcinoma or the thyroid or in oat-cell tumors. Many of the antibody techniques are already available, and others, while still experimental, are being rapidly improved and put into regular clinical use.

The last topic to be covered in this section is not new; in fact it is quite old but is only recently becoming widely appreciated. Multicentric squamous cell carcinoma of the upper aerodigestive tract has not been widely recognized in the past—in part because second primaries were called metastases, in part because follow-up was not conducted carefully and long enough, and in part perhaps because treatment was not sufficient to allow patients time to develop second primaries. The concept of wide-field cancerization, or multicentric cancer, is known for the skin, the bladder, the breast, and the colon. It is also known for the head and neck. A very excellent paper by Gluckman et al. documents this problem:[18] 259 patients with primary squamous cell cancer of the head and neck were examined prospectively for 3 years, looking for synchronous second primary neoplasms. Table 17-17 shows the findings. Ten percent of these patients had second primaries discovered by laryngoscopy, bronchoscopy, esophagoscopy, nasopharyngoscopy, and biopsy of all suspicious areas. It must be clear to all physicians treating head and neck tumors that similar evaluations are necessary for all patients.

In this study the authors reviewed 577 cases retrospectively, looking for metachronous tumors. They defined a metachronous tumor as one that was first discovered 6 or more months after diagnosis of the initial tumor. The data is shown in Table 17-18. The authors found that 21 percent of these patients developed second primaries in the time they were followed. Not only must patients be examined carefully for synchronous tumors, they must be followed closely for the duration of their lives for metachronous tumors.

The authors identified tobacco and ionizing radiation as the primary carcinogens for head and neck mucosal epidermoid cancers. Six carcinogenic factors were also listed: alcohol, chronic sepsis predominantly associated with poor oral hygiene, poor nutrition, immunodepression, saliva as a reservoir for carcinogens, and genetic influence.

RECONSTRUCTION AND REHABILITATION

The greatest advance in reconstruction after head and neck tumor extirpative surgery is the myocutaneous flap. Prior to its advent tissue deficiencies were reconstructed by regional and axial pattern transposition flaps such as the forehead flap, flap at the nape of the neck, and the deltopectoral flap. These flaps received their blood supply from regional dermal or subdermal vessels. They often required a delay to improve their chance of survival. In spite of delay procedures, administration of vasodilators, etc., all too often the blood supply was not sufficient and the flap died. Circumferential hypopharyngeal and cervical esophageal reconstructions required multistaged chest flaps, gastric pull-up, or colon interposition. These too could fail.

Recently it has been rediscovered that the major blood supply to skin comes from musculocutaneous vessels. The different patterns of blood supply to flaps are illustrated in Fig. 17-5.

To effectively use this technique one must know the anatomy of regional muscle groups and their vascular supply. With this information, large sections of skin nourished by underlying muscle can be transferred. Several myocutaneous flaps have been recognized and tried for head and neck reconstruction.[19] By far the most safe, useful, and versatile is the pectoralis major myocutaneous flap.[20] Its dominant vascular supply arises from the thoracoacromial artery, which comes from the axillary artery. The pectoralis major muscle is large and allows one to use a paddle of skin on the chest 8 to 16 cm wide and 16 to 24 cm long. This skin can easily be used to cover oral, oropharyngeal, hypopharyngeal, transferred esophageal, and cutaneous cervical defects. It does not need delay. Its success rate approaches 100 percent, and indeed most failures are iatrogenic. The chest can be closed primarily for paddles up to 8 cm wide, and with skin grafts for wider defects. Patient disability is essentially nonexistent. The pectoralis major myocutaneous flap has become the workhorse for head and neck reconstruction.

The trapezius myocutaneous flap is technically more difficult and not so reliable.[21] It is a good flap and is useful for resurfacing cheek and scalp defects. It can be used as a backup for the pectoralis flap. Experience with this flap is limited, for the pectoralis is normally available and is used in most cases.

The latissimus dorsi is an enormous, safe, and successful flap. It is larger than is generally needed for head and neck reconstruction. Since it comes from the back it is awkward to raise. It is potentially useful and may be necessary for special circumstances.

A significant but unrecognized boon to surgery therapy is the use of hypotensive anesthesia.[22] Carefully done studies documenting its use in head and neck cancer surgery do not exist. Early experiences at the Veterans Administration Hospital in LaJolla, California, suggest that procedures which lead to a loss of more than 2000 mL of blood can be performed hypotensively with blood losses less than 400mL.

Some surgeons think that free flaps nourished by microvascular anastomosis are useful for head and neck reconstruction. This is open to question. They are technically difficult to perform and are time-consuming. They rarely offer any advantage over the myocutaneous flaps. The success rate for microvascular anastomosis is not as high as the success rate for the myocutaneous flap.

The largest problem remaining for head and neck reconstruction is reconstruction of bony defects. This is easily done in nonirradiated tissues. However, most head

TABLE 17-18 Retrospective Identification of Second Primary Carcinomas in 577 Cases of Head and Neck Cancer Entered in the Department of Otolaryngology and Maxillofacial Surgery Tumor Registry from 1974 through 1978

Primary tumor	Number of patients	Percentage of Registry*	Number of second primaries identified	Percentage of patients in primary tumor group	Location of secondary primary			
					Lung	Esophagus	Head and neck	Other†
Larynx	189	32.7	34	17.9	13	3	13	5
Oropharynx	131	22.7	27	20.6	7	3	13	4
Hypopharynx	54	9.3	21	38.8	4	4	10	3
Oral cavity	158	27.3	28	17.7	12	3	9	4
Miscellaneous	45	7.7	11	24.4	1	1	5	4
Total	577	100.0	121	20.9	37	14	50	20

SOURCE: Adapted from Gluckman et al.[18]
* Department of Otolaryngology and Maxillofacial Surgery Tumor Registry.
† Sites other than lung, esophagus, and the head and neck.

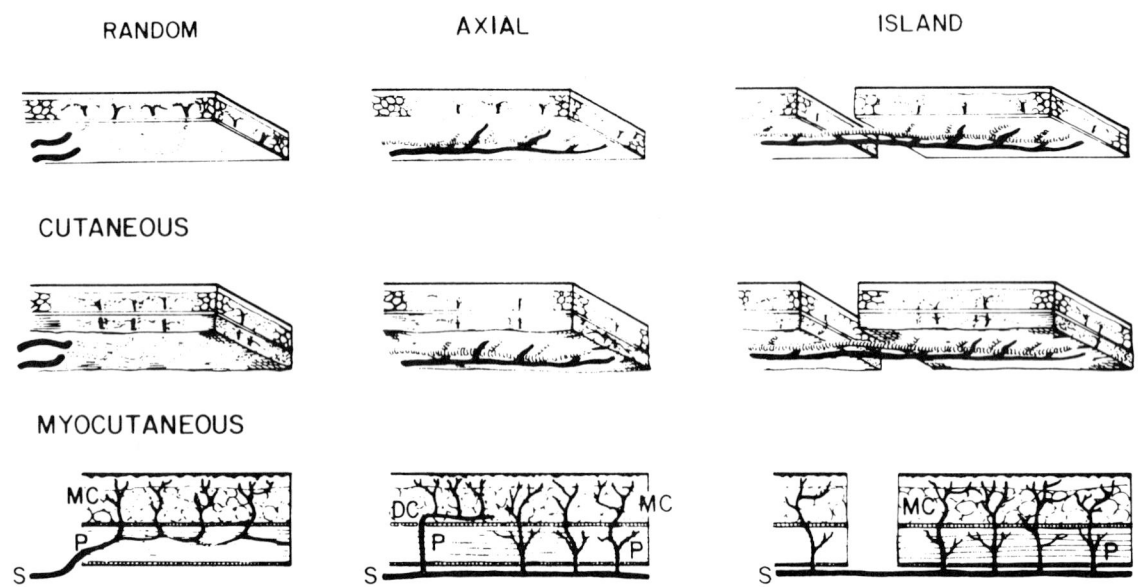

FIGURE 17-5 Artist's depiction of categories of cutaneous flaps (above) and analogous myocutaneous flaps (below). Segmental vessels (S), perforator (P), direct cutaneous (DC), and musculocutaneous (MC). (*From S Ariyan, CB Cuono: Myocutaneous flaps for head and neck reconstruction, Head Neck Surg 2(4):322, 1980.*)

and neck tumor reconstructions that require bone replacement are for advanced tumors that require radiation therapy. Techniques like rib grafts and Vitallium mesh trays filled with bone marrow do not work well in such vascular-poor areas. The ideal bone graft will bring its own blood supply with it. This may come on a myocutaneous flap, or it may ultimately require a free flap with a microvascular anastomosis. It may never come successfully.

Rehabilitation for head and neck cancer patients beyond physical reconstruction has not been well developed. For the most part the patients are reluctant to stop smoking and drinking. They are individuals who quickly put up protective defense mechanisms and do not seek or engage in psychological rehabilitation easily. Olson and Shedd studied this problem.[23] They identified the following areas of disability.

1. Physical appearance
2. Mastication
3. Salivation
4. Deglutition
5. Speech
6. Sensory deficits
7. Motor nerve deficits
8. Pain
9. Nutrition
10. Lifestyle
11. Psychosocial functioning
12. Vocalization

The various disabilities were clearly related to the tumor site and to the treatment modalities used. The majority of patients had some significant disabilities. Nine categories of rehabilitation were identified. They include

1. Surgical reconstruction
2. Dental-maxillofacial prosthetics
3. Speech therapy
4. Physical therapy
5. Rehabilitation nursing
6. Occupational therapy
7. Rehabilitation counseling
8. Vocational rehabilitation
9. Social service

Let us examine each of these areas. Surgical reconstruction has been extensively developed. Significant strides have been made and progress is being actively investigated. Dental and maxillofacial prosthetics have been available at select institutions.[24] Their availability in most major cities and institutions is increasing. External prosthetics are becoming the reconstruction of choice for total auriculectomy (excision of the ear), total rhinectomy, enucleation, and most large midface defects. Intraoral reconstruction for maxillary and palatal excision is good if there are solid remaining teeth. Mandibular reconstruction is expensive and useful only for dental restoration and for mandibular restoration. The third area of dental service is treating the oral cavity and teeth following radiation therapy. The key to treatment is prophylaxis and intensive oral hygiene for post-radiation therapy patients and for patients during chemotherapy.

Speech therapy is very useful for patients following oral and oropharyngeal surgery. Most of these patients have significant speech impediment. Their speech does not improve over time but often will improve dramatically with speech therapy.

Physical therapy is needed only for patients who have had their accessory nerve removed during neck dissection. The disability from this is manageable, but there is significant pain, which can be reduced by vigorous physical therapy. The principles of this therapy are common knowledge for physical therapists. Rehabilitation nursing can be excellent in institutions where the nursing service actively participates; it can be hopelessly inadequate when the physicians and the nurses do not commit the time and effort necessary to do a good job. Head and neck cancer patients have unique nursing requirements and require a lot of time to learn things like tracheostoma care, nutritional needs and techniques for maintaining them, oral hygiene, and physical grooming. Obtaining appropriate patient literature and giving it to the patient and family is a small step in the right direction, but it is not alone adequate. A much greater input is required by the entire medical team.

Occupational therapy is very useful for these patients, many of whom do not know what to do with themselves. Smoking and drinking too easily fills the time. An imaginative occupational therapist can find projects to involve almost all patients. Similarly, patients with a potential to work should be actively involved in vocational rehabilitation. Many can return to their former work. Others can learn new jobs. Some become hospital volunteers. Some speak to community groups about their cancer and smoking. There is a lot to do, and someone clever and skilled needs to help the patients discover and learn what they can do.

The last area to consider is psychosocial aspects of rehabilitation, an area that is all too often neglected. For example, how many patients with deforming oral resections have been counseled about oral sex? There are many difficult psychologic areas. Sex is only one example. Two modes of psychologic therapy are available. Group sessions offer these patients a great deal. Sharing their problems, experiences, and solutions and failures with people with similar problems and psychosocial backgrounds is more effective than sharing that experience with a nondiseased person of a very different psychosocial background. These sessions can be effectively led by physicians, psychiatrists, psychologists, and specially trained nurses or social workers. The leader must be skilled in facilitation and should be knowledgeable about the disease. It is wise to include husbands, wives, and loved ones in these sessions.

Individual psychotherapy is helpful for depression or other psychiatric problems. It is not so effective as the group setting for nonpsychiatric problems. A few relaxed, unhurried sessions with the treating physician can also be very useful. Physicians must remember to take the time.

The patient with terminal disease presents several special problems. Group sessions on death and dying, scheduled one day at a time, are useful for indolent disease. Most often head and neck tumor patients spend their terminal weeks in the hospital. The death from local and regional recurrent disease is miserable. Patients have problems with alimentation, respiration, speech, wound breakdown, necrotic foul-smelling tumor, and pain. No one can make that very pleasant, but much can be done to help. Most important is not to prolong the death by sustaining the patient unnecessarily with IVs, hyperalimentation, and nasogastric feedings. Many physicians worry about patient addiction to narcotics. It matters little if a patient is a drug addict for the last 2 weeks of life. Many physicians worry that they might contribute to a patient's death by generous prescription of narcotics. It is not acceptable to overdose a patient, but it is very reasonable to keep them comfortable. This may predispose them to dehydration and pneumonia. If pneumonia develops, do not treat it vigorously. There is no problem with a patient who is somnolent for most of the day if the patient is in excruciating pain when awake. A little timing will allow the patient to be awake when family members are around. Heroic surgery, chemotherapy, etc. should be discouraged for terminal head and neck cancer.

Most important for dying patients is to be honest, to be supportive, and to allow the patient control. The patient must preserve control up to the very end. If the patient wants to fight for every day, encourage this. If the patient wants to die, do not sustain life unnecessarily. If the patient wants to drink, it's okay to supply the alcohol of choice.

Dealing with the dying patient is taxing for the doctors, nurses, and other involved individuals. They too must be treated. Group sessions are useful. Occasionally individual sessions are needed. The dying patient can drain the emotional and physical energy from the involved professional staff. This must be recognized and managed. Failure to do so results in these individuals becoming insensitive or in moving to psychologically easier work.

The key to the treatment of head and neck cancer is a team. That team includes surgeon, radiation therapist, medical oncologist, nursing personnel, dentist, social worker, dietician, speech therapist, physical therapist, occupational therapist, psychiatrist, and vocational counselor. Together they can treat all aspects of this difficult disease in a fashion of which all can be proud.

REFERENCES

1. American Joint Committee on Cancer: *Staging of Cancer of Head and Neck Sites and of Melanoma*, 1980.
2. American Joint Committee for Cancer Staging and End Results Reporting: *Manual for Staging of Cancer*, 1978.
3. *Management Guideline for Head and Neck Cancer*, U.S. Dept. of Health, Education, and Welfare, National Institutes of Health Publication 80-2037, 1979.
4. National Cancer Institute, The Third National Cancer Society: *Advanced three-year report: 1969–1971 Incidence.* DHEW Publication 74-637, 1974.
5. Rothman KJ, Keller AZ: The effect of joint exposure to alcohol and tobacco on risk of cancer of the mouth and pharynx. *J Chron Dis* 25:711–716, 1972.
6. Rothman KJ: The effect of alcohol consumption on risk of cancer of the head and neck. *Laryngoscope* 88: suppl. 3(1) pt. 2: 51–55, 1978.
7. Keller AZ, Terris M: The association of alcohol and tobacco with cancer of the mouth and pharynx. *Am J Public Health* 55:1578–1585, 1965.
8. Nahum AM et al: The case for elective prophylactic neck dissection. *Trans Am Acad Ophthalmol Otolaryngol* 823:603–612, 1976.
9. Mendenhall WM et al: Elective neck irradiation in squamous-cell carcinoma of the head and neck. *Head Neck Surg* 3:15–20, 1980.
10. Axtell LM et al: *Cancer Patient Survival*, no. 5, National Cancer Institute, DHEW Publication NIA-77-992, 1976.
11. Ervin TJ et al: Chemotherapy for advanced carcinoma of the head and neck. *Arch Otolaryngol* 107:237–241, 1981.
12. Wanebo JH: Immunobiology of head and neck cancer: Basic concepts. *Head Neck Surg* 2:42–55, 1979.
13. Muggia RM et al: Role of chemotherapy in head and neck cancer: Systemic use of single agents and combinations in advanced diseases. *Head Neck Surg* 2:196–205, 1980.
14. Davidson TM et al: Microscopic controlled excisions for epidermoid carcinoma of the head and neck. *Otolaryngol Head Neck Surg* 89:244–251 (March/April), 1981.
15. Davidson TM et al: Microscopic controlled surgery for epidermoid carcinoma of the head and neck. *Trans Pac Coast Oto Ophthalmol Soc* 62:187–198, 1981.
16. Seagren SL et al: Interstitial-implant radiotherapy in upper aerodigestive tract malignancy. *Head Neck Surg* 1:409–416, 1979.
17. Battifora H, Applebaum EL: Electron microscopy in the diagnosis of head and neck tumors. *Head Neck Surg* 1:202–212, 1979.
18. Gluckman J et al: Multicentric squamous cell carcinoma of the upper aerodigestive tract. *Head Neck Surg* 3:90–96, 1980.
19. Ariyan S, Cuono CB: Myocutaneous flaps for head and neck reconstruction. *Head Neck Surg* 2:321–345, 1980.
20. Beek S et al: The pectoralis major myocutaneous flap for reconstruction of the head and neck. *Head Neck Surg* 1:293–300, 1979.
21. Panje WR: Myocutaneous trapezius flap. *Head Neck Surg* 2: 206–212, 1980.
22. Ward CF et al: Deliberate hypotension in head and neck surgery. *Head Neck Surg* 2:185–195, 1980.
23. Olson ML, Shedd DP: Disability and rehabilitation in head and neck cancer patients after treatment. *Head Neck Surg* 1: 52–58, 1978.
24. Carl W: Dental management and prosthetic rehabilitation of patients with head and neck cancer. *Head Neck Surg* 3: 27–42, 1980.
25. Shedd DP et al: Problems of terminal head and neck cancer patients. *Head Neck Surg* 2:476–482, 1980.

SELECTED BIBLIOGRAPHY

Biller H: Pectoralis myocutaneous flap. Parts I and II. Videotape distributed by The Am Acad Fac Pl & Reconst Surg, 1101 Vermont Ave NW, Suite 304, Washington, D.C., 20005.

De Santo LW, Carpenter RJ: Reconstruction of the pharynx and upper esophagus after resection for cancer. *Head & Neck Surg* 2:369–379, 1980.

Freund HR: *Principles of Head and Neck Surgery*, 2d ed. New York, Appleton-Century-Crofts, 1979.

Horwitz SD, Caldarelli DD, Hendrickson FR: Treatment of carcinoma of the hypopharynx. *Head & Neck Surg* 2: 107–111, 1979.

Mohs FE: Chemosurgery for the microscopically controlled excision of skin cancer. *Arch Surg* 42:279–295, 1941.

Mohs FE: *Chemosurgery: Microscopically Controlled Surgery for Skin Cancer.* Springfield, Ill: Charles C Thomas, 1978.

Panje WR: Myocutaneous trapezius flap. *Head & Neck Surg* 2: 206–212, 1980.

Panje W: Trapezius myocutaneous flaps. Videotape distributed by The Am Acad Fac Pl & Reconst Surg, 1101 Vermont Ave NW, Suite 304, Washington, D.C. 20005.

Silver CE: *Surgery for Cancer of the Larynx and Related Structures.* Churchill Livingstone, 1981.

18
TUMORS OF THE LARYNGEAL APPARATUS

Leslie M. Greenberg   *Donald G. Sessions*

ANATOMY

The larynx is given precise anatomical definition for the purpose of classification of laryngeal cancer. The TNM system of staging cancer and categorizing the lesions and the extent of involvement requires precise description of the primary tumor in its relation to specific anatomic landmarks, its regional nodal involvement, and its distant metastases. The following anatomic definition of the larynx allows classification of carcinoma arising in the encompassed mucous membranes, and excludes cancers arising on the lateral or posterior pharyngeal wall, piriform fossa, postcricoid area, and the vallecula or base of tongue.

The anterior limit of the larynx is composed of the anterior or lingual surface of the suprahyoid epiglottis, the thyrohyoid membrane, the anterior commissure, and the anterior wall of the subglottic region, which is composed of the inferior portion of the thyroid cartilage, the cricothyroid membrane, and the anterior arch of the cricoid cartilage.

The posterior and lateral limits include the aryepiglottic folds, the arytenoid region, the interarytenoid space, and the posterior surface of the subglottic space, represented by the mucous membrane covering the cricoid cartilage.[1]

The superolateral limits are composed of the tip and the lateral borders of the epiglottis. The inferior limit is made up of the plane passing through the inferior edge of the cricoid cartilage.

Clinically, the larynx is divided into three regions: supraglottis, glottis, and subglottis (Figs. 18-1, 18-2, 18-3). The supraglottis is composed of the epiglottis (both its lingual and laryngeal aspects), aryepiglottic folds, arytenoid cartilages, and ventricular bands (false vocal folds). The inferior boundary of the supraglottis is a horizontal plane passing through the apex of the ventricle. The glottis is composed of the true vocal folds, including the anterior and posterior commissures. The lower boundary is a horizontal plane 1 cm below the free margin of the true vocal folds. The subglottis is the region extending from the lower boundary of the glottis to the lower margin of the cricoid cartilage. The division of the larynx is summarized in Table 18-1.

Primary laryngeal tumors generally have characteristic growth patterns based on the site of origin of the tumor. Supraglottic tumors are usually slow-growing, exophytic lesions that invade locally and have a tendency toward superior, lateral, and anterior spread. These tumors spread along the mucosa of the epiglottis to the false vocal folds and aryepiglottic folds. They can invade the cartilage of the epiglottis or penetrate the natural

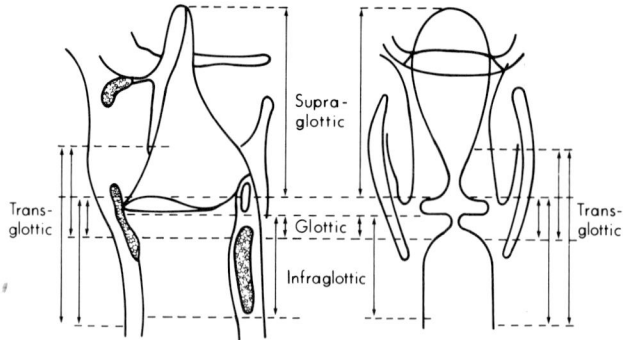

FIGURE 18-1 Classification of cancer of the larynx is determined by the anatomic regions: supraglottic, glottic, and subglottic.

fenestrations in the cartilage to reach the preepiglottic space anteriorly.

Glottic tumors are usually slow-growing, well-differentiated tumors that appear to extend locally along blood vessel planes. These tumors can extend to both anterior and posterior commissures and the contralateral true vocal fold. The anterior commissure tendon (Broyle's ligament) limits extension anteriorly. The fibrous lining of the larynx (conus elasticus laryngis) limits extension laterally. Glottic tumors infiltrate the vocalis muscle and can extend laterally to the ventricle, superiorly to the false vocal folds, and inferiorly to the subglottis.

The anterior commissure is the most common site of cartilage invasion by a glottic cancer. Ossification of the thyroid cartilage appears to predispose to cartilage invasion. When the anterior commissure and the base of the epiglottis (petiole) are invaded, 76 percent of tumors invade the thyroid cartilage or perichondrium and extend outside the larynx. The cartilaginous framework of the larynx is a natural barrier to the spread of glottic cancer, and extralaryngeal extension occurs late.

Subglottic tumors spread submucosally in all directions including circumferentially. Anterior extension through the cricothyroid membrane is common. Primary subglottic cancer is rare, whereas extension of a glottic primary tumor into the subglottic region is more common.

PATTERNS OF REGIONAL METASTASIS

The lymphatics of the larynx provide the most common route of tumor spread to the regional lymph nodes. The first-station nodes include jugulodigastric, jugulomohyoid, paratracheal, and deep cervical nodes.

The lymphatics of the larynx form two highly com-

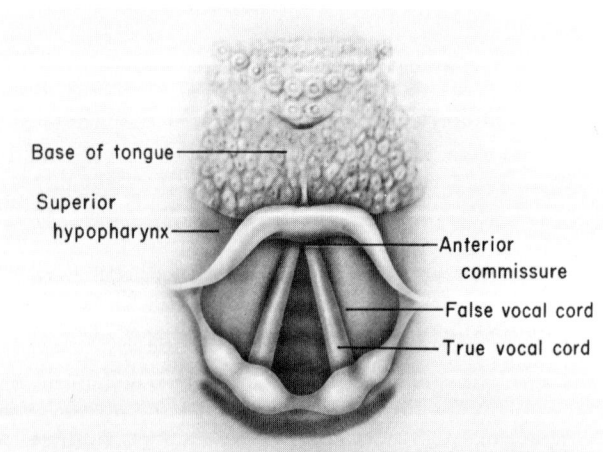

FIGURE 18-2 Endoscopic view of the larynx

partmentalized systems: superficial and deep. The superficial (intramucosal) system has free communication between the right and left sides of the larynx. The deep system of lymphatics (submucosal), which is more critical for laryngeal tumor spread, is highly specialized. It has little or no communication between the two halves of the larynx (right and left). In addition, the supraglottic and subglottic groups of lymphatics drain into different areas and are separated by an area with few lymphatics, the true vocal cords (glottis). Thus, the lymphatics of the larynx are divided into four groups: one above and one below the true vocal cords, and a right and left system.

The supraglottic lymphatics, including those of the aryepiglottic fold and false vocal cords, drain into superior channels that follow the superior thyroid artery. These pierce the thyrohyoid membrane to drain into the superior deep cervical lymph nodes situated near the bifurcation of the common carotid artery and internal jugular vein. These lymphatics drain cephalad.[2] (See Fig. 18-4).

The laryngeal ventricle lymphatics drain between the soft tissues and thyroid cartilage to pass through the cricothyroid membrane on the ipsilateral side. They pass through the ipsilateral thyroid lobe to enter the medial deep (prelaryngeal, paratracheal, prethyroidal, pretracheal) and inferior deep (supraclavicular) cervical nodes.

The free margin of the true vocal cords appears to be devoid of deep lymphatics. Dyes, radioisotopes, and lymphangiographic studies confirm localization within the vocal cord. It is a well-known clinical observation that membranous vocal cord tumors are highly curable and have low incidence of metastasis (2 percent).

The subglottic lymphatics have two inferior routes. Part of the drainage passes through the center of the cricothyroid membrane into the lymph nodes in front of the trachea (Delphian nodes) and thence to the middle deep cervical nodes. The other part of the inferior group passes to the lymph nodes accompanying the inferior thyroid artery (inferior deep lateral cervical lymph nodes) and to the paratracheal, tracheoesophageal, and subclavian lymph nodes. These have minor connections with superior lateral deep cervical nodes. The subglottic lymphatics from the cricoid area and within the cricothyroid membrane have collecting channels flowing into it from both sides of the larynx which drain to cervical nodes on both sides. This observation helps explain the fact that subglottic carcinoma has a greater tendency to early lymphatic spread. This has particular significance in limiting to the neck for long periods of time squamous

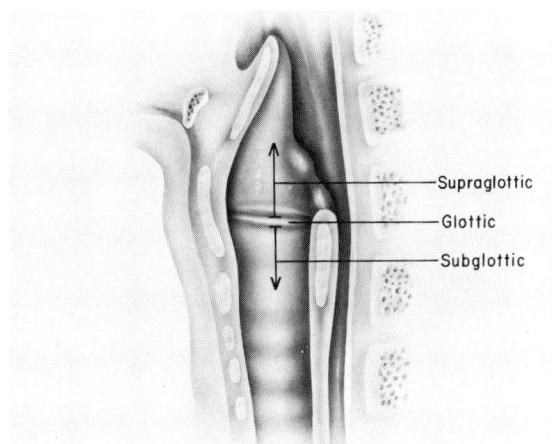

FIGURE 18-3 Anatomic regions used in classification of cancer of the larynx

cell cancer of the larynx and other epithelial organ systems in the head and neck.[3-5]

CERVICAL METASTASIS

The most important factor in determining chances for survival of patients with cancer of the larynx is the presence of tumor in cervical lymph nodes. In general, the survival rate decreases 40 percent when clinically positive nodes are present. The incidence of nodes is determined by the location, size, and cellular differentiation of the tumor. Location of the primary laryngeal

TABLE 18-1 Anatomical Division of the Larynx

Region	Site
Supraglottis	Ventricular bands (false vocal cords)
	Arytenoids
	Epiglottis (both lingual and laryngeal aspects)
	Suprahyoid epiglottis
	Infrahyoid epiglottis
	Aryepiglottic folds
Glottis	True vocal cords, including anterior and posterior commissure
Subglottis	Subglottis

SOURCE. From American Joint Committee on Cancer.[1]

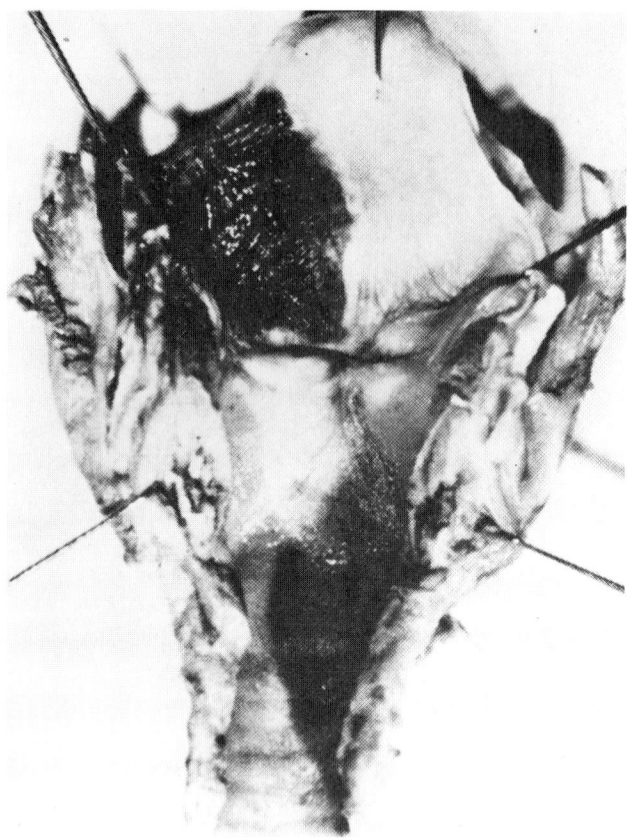

FIGURE 18-4 Dye injection of supraglottic larynx showing lymphatic supraglottic compartment

cancer results in the highest correlation with spread to the cervical lymph nodes. Location is an important guide in determining the necessity for elective radical neck dissection, especially since there is a 25 percent error in detecting lymph node metastasis by pretreatment palpation. Laryngopharyngeal and subglottic cancers metastasize more readily. Tumors larger than 2 cm are more likely to have metastasis. Less well differentiated tumors have a higher metastatic rate.

Supraglottic cancer confined to the epiglottis has a 22 to 31 percent incidence of cervical metastasis, 15 percent of which is occult. If the lesion involves the epiglottis and false vocal cord, the metastatic rate is 50 percent, of which 30 percent is occult. Supraglottic cancer extending to the true vocal cords has a 53 percent incidence of positive cervical nodes. Five percent of patients with supraglottic cancer have bilateral metastatic spread.

Glottic primary cancers have the lowest metastatic rate. Lesions confined to the middle one-third of the mobile true vocal cord have a 2 percent incidence of cervical metastasis. If the tumor invades the anterior commissure or extends more than 5 mm subglotically at the anterior commissure without vocal cord fixation, there is a 5 percent to 16 percent cervical node metastatic rate.[6,7] If there is vocal cord fixation by tumor, the incidence of positive neck nodes is 7 percent. Anterior commissure tumors have a metastatic rate of 8 percent. A positive midline deep lymph node (Delphian node) occurs in 5 percent of glottic lesions with cordal fixation and subglottic extension. In these cases the cricothyroid membrane, thyroid gland, and upper tracheoesophageal nodes are often involved and must be resected with the primary tumor.

The incidence of cervical metastasis in primary subglottic tumors or glottic tumors with more than 5 mm subglottic extension is 23 percent. In addition, a high number of these patients have paratracheal and superior mediastinal metastases.[8–11]

DISTANT METASTASES

Few patients with laryngeal cancer present with distant metastasis. It is more common for patients to develop distant metastasis more than 2 years after the onset of disease. Of the distant sites, spread to the lung is most common. Mediastinal lymph node metastases are considered distant metastases. Skeletal and liver metastases occur less often.

INCIDENCE AND ETIOLOGY

Laryngeal cancer comprises 2 to 5 percent of all malignancies diagnosed annually in the United States. The National Cancer Institute estimates that there are 9500 new cases and 3200 deaths each year. The laryngeal cancer ratio for males and females has changed in the last 20 years. A study in 1956 showed a male-female ratio for carcinoma of the larynx of 15:1. A study in 1974 showed this ratio to be 5:1. This change is thought to be due to the increase in female cigarette smokers during this period.[12,13]

Possible etiologic agents for cancer of the larynx include smoking, alcohol intake, exposure to asbestos, exposure to wood, and the herpes simplex virus. There is a correlation between cigarette smoking, alcoholism, and laryngeal carcinoma. Only 2 percent of patients with laryngeal carcinoma are nonsmokers. The risk for smokers of nonfilter cigarettes is about five times greater than for smokers of filter cigarettes. At each level of alcohol consumption there is an increase in the incidence of laryngeal cancer as smoking increases. Heavy drinkers have about three times the risk of developing laryngeal cancer as nondrinkers if they smoke, but drinking without smoking did not show an increased risk for carcinoma.

An epidemiologic study showed that laryngeal cancer patients tend to be less educated than the control group and that there was a smaller proportion of Jews and Catholics in the cancer group than the control group. The same study showed a relationship between occupations with an exposure to wood and cancer of the larynx, independent of smoking status. A number of investigations have linked asbestos exposure to cancer of the larynx. It is unclear what role nutritional status plays in the development of cancer of the larynx.[13]

Simultaneous primary malignant cancers are separate primary tumors which are diagnosed at the same time. Simultaneous tumors and laryngeal cancer occur with an incidence of 0.5 to 1 percent. Metachronous or subsequent primary malignant tumors occur with laryngeal cancer with an incidence of 5 to 10 percent. The most common areas of occurrence include the lung, upper respiratory tract, rectum, and prostate.

CLINICAL PRESENTATION

The cardinal symptom of laryngeal cancer is hoarseness. Hoarseness may be due to tumor bulk, infiltration of the muscle, or paralysis of the vocal cord. Tumor on the free margin of the true vocal cord causes hoarseness early in the course of the disease. Tumor involving adjacent structures, including the supraglottis or the subglottis, results in hoarseness only later when vocal cord motion is affected. Hoarseness persisting longer than 2 weeks is sufficient reason for examination of the larynx.

Sore throat, dysphagia, and odynophagia (pain on swallowing) are common symptoms associated with supraglottic cancer. For patients with laryngeal cancer pain in the ear may be referred via the tenth cranial nerve. Dyspnea and stridor are caused by tumor-induced airway obstruction, and present late in the course of the disease. Hemoptysis occurs in patients with large exophytic tumors. Necrotic tumor often presents with a characteristic bad breath in many patients.

DIAGNOSIS AND STAGING

Following a thorough and careful history, the initial step in diagnosis is a complete and comprehensive physical examination. Indirect laryngoscopy (mirror examination of the larynx) can yield accurate information with little discomfort or inconvenience to the patient.

The use of a head mirror or head light is essential in order to free both hands for examination. The larynx is examined with a number 4 or 6 laryngeal mirror while the tongue is held in protrusion by the examiner. Topical anesthetic is used to facilitate the examination when

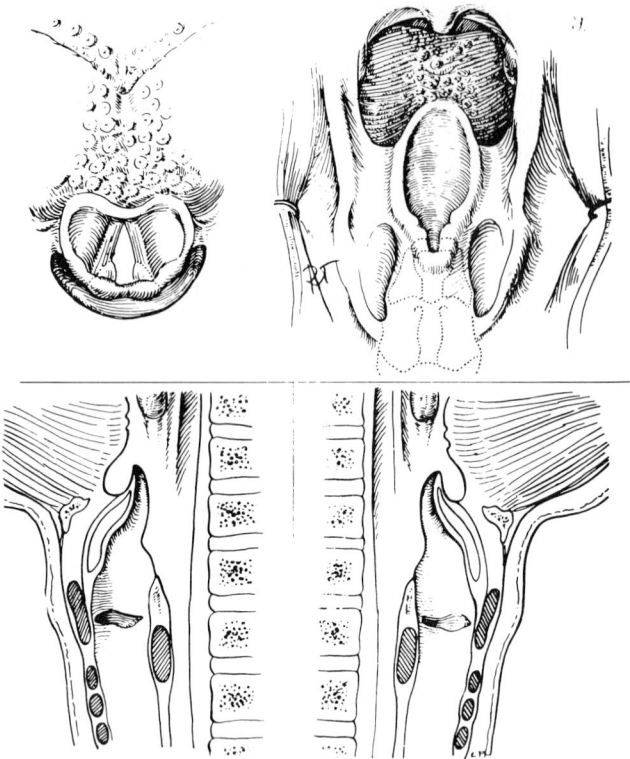

FIGURE 18-5 Diagram for pretreatment mapping of lesion

necessary. If the larynx cannot be visualized with a mirror even after the application of topical anesthetic, then examination is performed with the fiberoptic laryngoscope, which is introduced through the nose. Care is taken to examine the vallecula, base of tongue, aryepiglottic fold, epiglottis, laryngeal structures, subglottic area, piriform fossae, pharyngeal walls, and the postcricoid area. The presence or absence of vocal cord mobility is noted. Findings are recorded on a standard drawing (Fig. 18-5).

Radiologic examination of the larynx is used to help ascertain the exact extent of the lesion. These examinations are performed before tissue biopsy since biopsy of the laryngeal structures can cause edema, which produces abnormal distortion in the radiologic examination. Palin x-rays of the neck and chest reveal information about gross airway contours and possible metastases. Laminography better delineates tumor contours, size, intraluminal masses, and cartilage invasion. Xeroradiography gives 73 percent accurate information regarding thyroid cartilage destruction and 97 percent accurate information about subglottic extent of tumor (Fig. 18-6).

Laryngography is a very accurate dye study of the larynx. The laryngogram is most useful in determining the extent of tumor in the subglottic area and in outlining the anterior commissure when the epiglottis is overhanging and fixed by a bulky exophytic tumor.[18] (See Fig. 18-7.)

Computed tomography (CT) has recently been applied to the larynx. CT is most accurate in assessing the arytenoid cartilages, the superior margin of the cricoid cartilage, the anterior commissure, and the subglottic space including the conus elasticus. CT is not able to assess tumor extension into the laryngeal ventricles. It is also not useful to assess vocal cord mobility since movement results in distortion of the study[19] (see Fig. 18-8.)

After the radiologic examination is completed, the larynx is examined directly with a laryngoscope with the patient under local or general anesthesia. The operating microscope is used to detect fine mucosal abnormalities. Biopsy is performed for tissue diagnosis. This includes biopsy of the lesion itself and the various possible areas of surgical margin.

Staging

The present staging system for patients with cancer of the larynx is shown in Table 18-2. The pretreatment staging information for each of the three sites of the larynx is formed from the history, examination, radiologic evaluation, direct laryngoscopy, and biopsy results.

Problem areas in staging and classification of laryngeal cancers include tumors involving the aryepiglottic folds and those originating on the lingual surface of the epiglottis. Tumors originating on the aryepiglottic fold (marginal cancers) may invade either the larynx or the piriform fossa (inferior hypopharynx). The characteristics of growth and response to treatment of marginal cancers resemble that of cancer of the piriform fossa, and these lesions are not discussed as laryngeal lesions. Similarly, carcinoma originating in the laryngeal surface of the epiglottis is extralaryngeal in origin and takes on the growth and treatment response characteristics of base-of-tongue cancers.

PATHOLOGY

Epidermoid Carcinoma

Squamous cell or epidermoid carcinoma comprises 95 percent of all laryngeal malignancies. Table 18-3 indi-

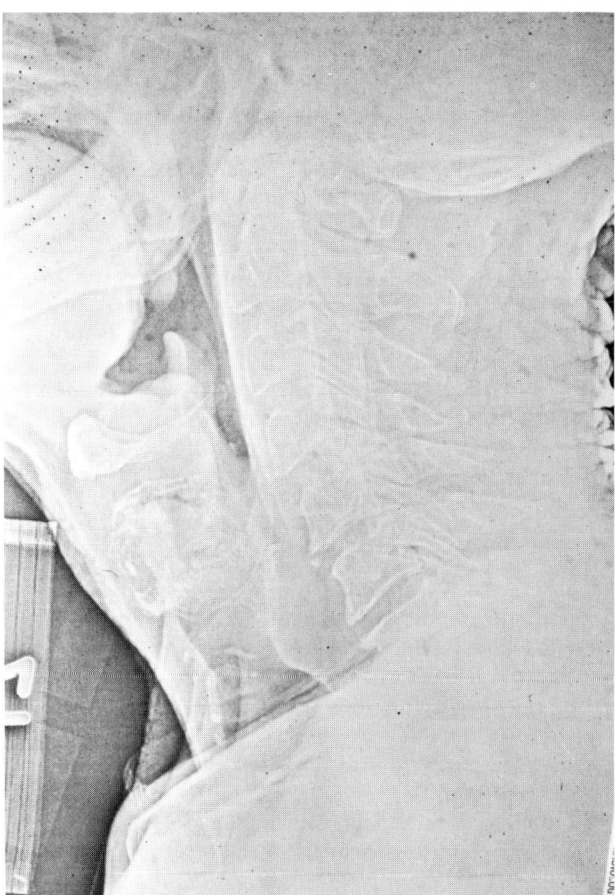

FIGURE 18-6 Xerogram of the larynx showing normal anatomy

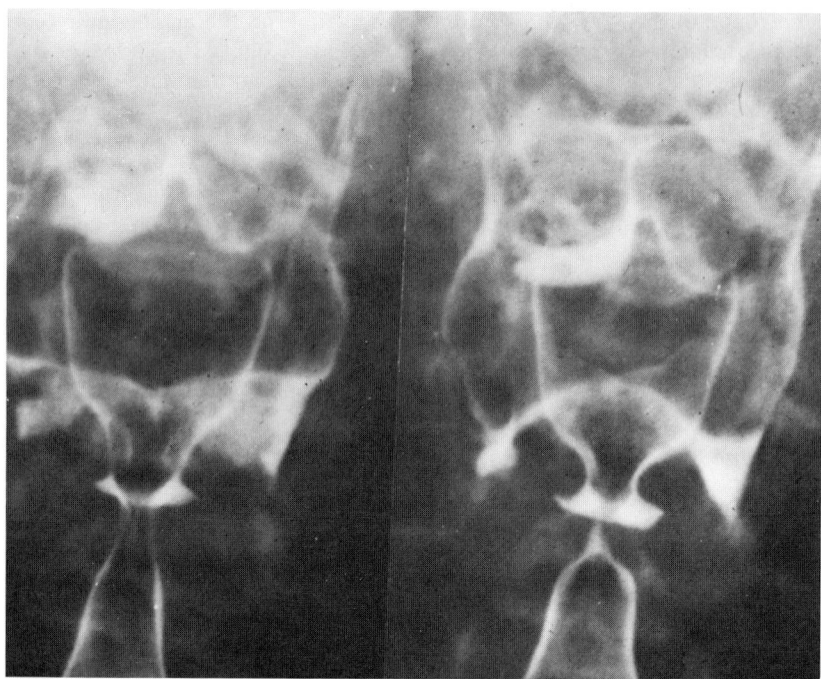

FIGURE 18-7 Laryngogram of normal larynx

cates the incidence and site of origin of a series of epidermoid cancers of the larynx. The degree of cellular differentiation varies with the region of origin. Generally, true vocal cord cancers tend to be well-differentiated and lesions involving the aryepiglottic folds are less well differentiated (Fig. 18-9).

The larynx is lined with nonkeratinizing squamous epithelium except for the laryngeal ventricle and subglottic area, which are lined with pseudostratified ciliated columnar epithelium.

Hyperkeratosis

Hyperkeratosis is a pathologic term indicating keratinization of the squamous epithelium. Hyperkeratosis is often associated with carcinoma in situ and invasive carcinoma, but the incidence of isolated hyperkeratosis becoming invasive cancer is very low (3 percent). Hyperkeratosis usually involves the true vocal cords and is related to smoking or trauma. Laryngeal examination reveals thickening of the true vocal cords. At times the lesion may appear white or gray and the term *leukoplakia* is used. Histologically, cellular atypia may be present. The treatment is conservative and consists of stripping of the true vocal cords and cessation of smoking. Frequent follow-up is mandatory.[20]

Carcinoma in Situ

Carcinoma in situ is indistinguishable grossly from hyperkeratosis or invasive carcinoma. Carcinoma in situ is intraepithelial malignancy associated with an intact basement membrane. Any area of the larynx may be involved, but characteristically it is confined to the true vocal cord. It may occur as an isolated lesion but is more commonly associated with invasive cancer. It is assumed that if left untreated, carcinoma in situ will progress to invasive carcinoma. The treatment is conservative; precise stripping of the entire lesion from the vocal cord by microlaryngoscopy is adequate. Close follow-up examinations are necessary, and repeated strippings for recurrence are indicated.[20] Irradiation is probably not indicated.

Verrucous Cancer

Verrucous cancer of the larynx is a lesion that appears to be histologically benign but is clinically malignant. It appears to be sessile and has multiple, heavy, broad, filiform projections. Histologically, hyperkeratosis with deep, swollen rete pegs is visible. Clinical invasion with destruction of cartilage may be present. Verrucous cancer is the only laryngeal lesion that should be treated as a cancer without specific histopathologic evidence of invasive malignancy. Biologically, this lesion grows slowly, and symptoms may be present for many months. Regional or distant metastasis have not been reported. The lesion is frequently amenable to conservation surgery, though total laryngectomy may be required. Irradiation is ineffective and is contraindicated. Elective neck dissection is not indicated. The prognosis is usually excellent.[21]

Malignant Tumors Other Than Epidermoid Carcinoma

Other than epidermoid cell carcinoma, most malignant tumors of the larynx are sarcomas. These are most often fibrosarcomas, but rhabdomyosarcomas, chondrosarcomas, leiomyosarcomas, hemangiosarcomas, and neurogenic sarcomas may occur also.

Laryngeal sarcomas are usually grossly indistinguishable from an epidermoid carcinoma. They present as large, fleshy, polypoid masses that are covered by mucosa. The incidence of metastasis is less than that with an epidermoid carcinoma.

The term *spindle-cell carcinoma* or *pseudosarcomatous carcinoma* refers to an epidermoid carcinoma that has a reactive stroma. The underlying stroma may appear to be sarcomatous, but the lesion should be treated like any epidermoid carcinoma.

Adenocarcinoma may occur in any area of the larynx. It is characterized by late distant metastasis in spite of adequate surgical control of the primary tumor.[20]

SURGICAL PATHOLOGY

The surgical pathology of cancer of the larynx has been studied in relation to resection margins, size, differentiation, and histopathologic characteristics of the primary tumor and position, and histopathologic characteristics of lymph node metastases.[22]

Resection Margins of the Primary Tumor

The most satisfactory survival rates occurred in patients with the report of no tumor in the specimen. Report of involved resection margins resulted in decreased survival rates in all primary sites. Treatment success for patients with positive surgical margins was reduced from 54 percent (negative margins) to 25 percent for supraglottic cancer, and from 73 percent (negative margins) to 58 percent for glottic cancer.[22,23]

Size of Primary Tumor

Twenty-five percent of patients with supraglottic cancer less than 4 cm in diameter had postive lymph nodes,

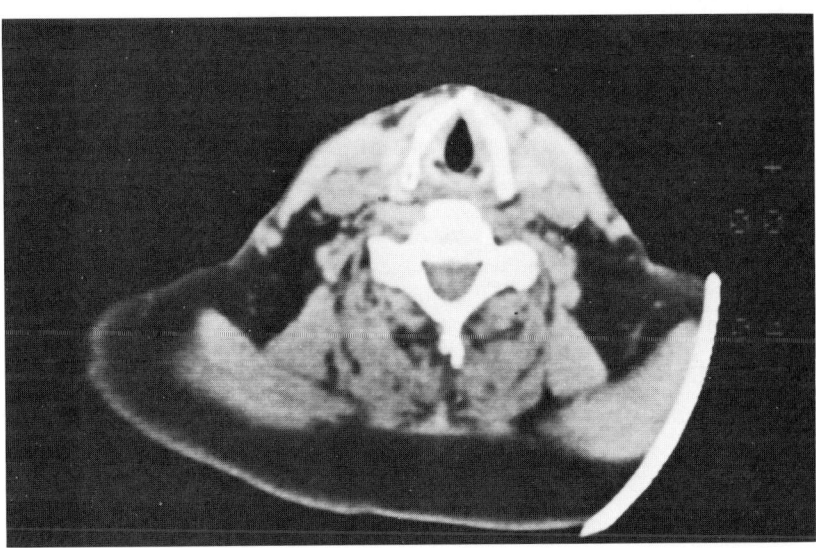

FIGURE 18-8 High-resolution computed tomogram of the normal larynx at the level of the true vocal cord. (*Courtesy Stuart S. Sagel, M.D.*)

TABLE 18-2 Staging System For Cancer of the Larynx

TNM classification
Primary tumor (T)
- TX   Tumor that cannot be assessed by rules
- T_0 No evidence of primary tumor

Supraglottis
- TIS   Carcinoma in situ
- T_1 Tumor confined to region of origin with normal mobility
- T_2 Tumor involving adjacent supraglottis site(s) or glottis without fixation
- T_3 Tumor limited to larynx with fixation and/or extension to involve postcricoid area, medial wall of piriform sinus, or preepiglottic space
- T_4 Massive tumor extending beyond the larynx to involve oropharynx, soft tissues of neck, or destruction of thyroid cartilage

Glottis
- TIS   Carcinoma in situ
- T_1 Tumor confined to vocal fold(s) with normal mobility (including involvement of anterior or posterior commissures)
- T_2 Supraglottic and/or subglottic extension of tumor with normal or impaired fold mobility
- T_3 Tumor confined to the larynx with fold fixation
- T_4 Massive tumor with thyroid cartilage destruction and/or extension beyond the confines of the larynx

Subglottis
- TIS   Carcinoma in situ
- T_1 Tumor confined to the subglottic region
- T_2 Tumor extension to vocal folds with normal or impaired fold mobility
- T_3 Tumor confined to larynx with fold fixation
- T_4 Massive tumor with cartilage destruction or extension beyond the confines of the larynx, or both

Nodal involvement (N)
- NX   Nodes cannot be assessed
- N_0 No clinically positive node
- N_1 Single clinically positive homolateral node less than 3 cm in diameter
- N_2 Single clinically positive homolateral node 3 to 6 cm in diameter or multiple clinically positive homolateral nodes, none over 6 cm in diameter
- N_{2a} Single clinically positive homolateral node, 3 to 6 cm in diameter
- N_{2b} Multiple clinically positive homolateral nodes, none over 6 cm in diameter
- N_3 Massive homolateral node(s), bilateral nodes, or contralateral node(s)
- N_{3a} Clinically positive homolateral node(s), none over 6 cm in diameter

---

while those patients with supraglottic cancer greater than 4 cm had positive lymph nodes 85 percent of the time. There was no statistical correlation between the size of the primary tumor and survival rate.

Cellular Differentiation of the Primary Tumor

Glottic tumors showed a significant increase in cervical metastasis with increasing tumor dedifferentiation.[22] The metastatic rate of 26 percent for poorly differentiated glottic cancers might suggest elective radical neck dissection in these patients.

Histopathologic Characteristics of the Primary Tumor

Increased lymph node metastasis was noted in supraglottic lesions with invasion of epiglottis, vessel, extralaryngeal soft tissue, and infiltrating borders; and in glottic lesions with invasion of thyroid cartilage, muscle, nerve, and extralaryngeal soft tissue. Decreased survival

TABLE 18-2 Staging System For Cancer of the Larynx (*Continued*)

N_{3b}	Bilateral clinically positive nodes (in this situation, each side of the neck should be staged separately; that is, N_{3b}: right, N_{2a}; left, N_1)	
N_{3c}	Contralateral clinically positive node(s) only	
Distant metastasis	(M)	
MX	Not assessed	
M_0	No (known) distant metastasis	
M_1	Distant metastasis present	
	Specify sites according to the following notations: pulmonary, PUL; osseous, OSS; hepatic, HEP; brain, BRA; lymph nodes, LYM; bone marrow, MAR; pleura, PLE; skin, SKI; eye, EYE; other, OTH	

Histopathology
Predominant cancer is squamous cell carcinoma of undifferentiated carcinoma—also adenocarcinoma and others

Grade
Well-differentiated, moderately well differentiated, poorly to very poorly differentiated, or numbers 1, 2, 3–4

Stage grouping
Stage I $T_1N_0M_0$
Stage II $T_2N_0M_0$
Stage III $T_3N_0M_0$
          T_1 or T_2 or T_3, N_1, M_0
Stage IV T_4, N_0 or N_1, M_0
          Any T, N_2 or N_3, M_0
          Any T, any N, M_1

Residual tumor (R)
  R_0 No residual tumor
  R_1 Microscopic residual tumor
  R_2 Macroscopic residual tumor Specify site

	ECOG/ Zubrod scale	Karnofsky scale, %
Host (H)—Performance status of host	0	90–100
H_0 Normal activity	1	70–80
H_1 Symptomatic but ambulatory—cares for self	2	50–60
H_2 Ambulatory more than 50 percent of time—Occasionally needs assistance	3	30–40
H_3 Ambulatory less than 50 percent of time—Nursing care needed	4	10–20
H_4 Bedridden—may need hospitalization		

SOURCE: American Joint Committee for Cancer Staging.[1]

rates were noted in patients with supraglottic lesions whose pathology report showed tumor invasion of nerve, vessel, or epiglottic cartilage.

Lymph Node Metastasis

The presence of lymph node metastasis results in decreased survival rates in patients with either supraglottic or glottic cancer. Supraglottic and glottic cancer spreads most commonly to the ipsilateral upper jugular lymph nodes. The next most common site is the lower jugular lymph nodes. The position of the positive lymph nodes significantly correlated with survival rates only if the nodes were found in the posterior inferior triangle or inferior cervical node areas. All patients with positive nodes in these areas were treatment failures. The presence of ipsilateral lymph node metastasis causes a significant decrease in treatment success with both supraglottic and glottic primaries.

Tumor regularly involved structures in the neck other

TABLE 18-3 Squamous Cell Carcinoma of the Larynx

	Number	Percent
Supraglottis	183	30.7
Glottis	410	68.8
Subglottis	3	0.5
Total	596	100.0

SOURCE: Sessions.[22]

than lymph nodes. Invasion of neck muscle, vessels, or into extranodal soft tissue decreased treatment success by a factor of 5:1, independent of primary site. Invasion of laryngeal cancer into the submandibular gland or the thyroid gland, though rare, carries a poor prognosis.

TREATMENT

The major treatment modalities in the management of cancer of the larynx are surgery and radiation therapy. These may be used individually or in planned combination. Treatment must be individualized for each patient. The choice of therapy is based on the expected cure rate, the probable functional capacity after treatment, and the possible complications that may occur.

Radiation Therapy

Radiation therapy as a curative modality is used for early cancer of the true vocal cords, small lesions of the epiglottis, lesions in patients who are poor operative risks, and lesions on patients with either distant metastases or an unresectable second primary tumor.[24-26]

Combined Radiation Therapy and Surgery

Preoperative radiation therapy combined with surgery has been shown to increase cure rates in certain cancers of the larynx. The optimal dose of preoperative irradiation is not known at the present time. There is evidence that high-dose preoperative irradiation (4500 to 5500 rads) decreases the local recurrence rate for lesions of the lingual epiglottis. In patients receiving preoperative radiation therapy of the larynx, the ipsilateral neck nodes are treated in those patients with an expected high

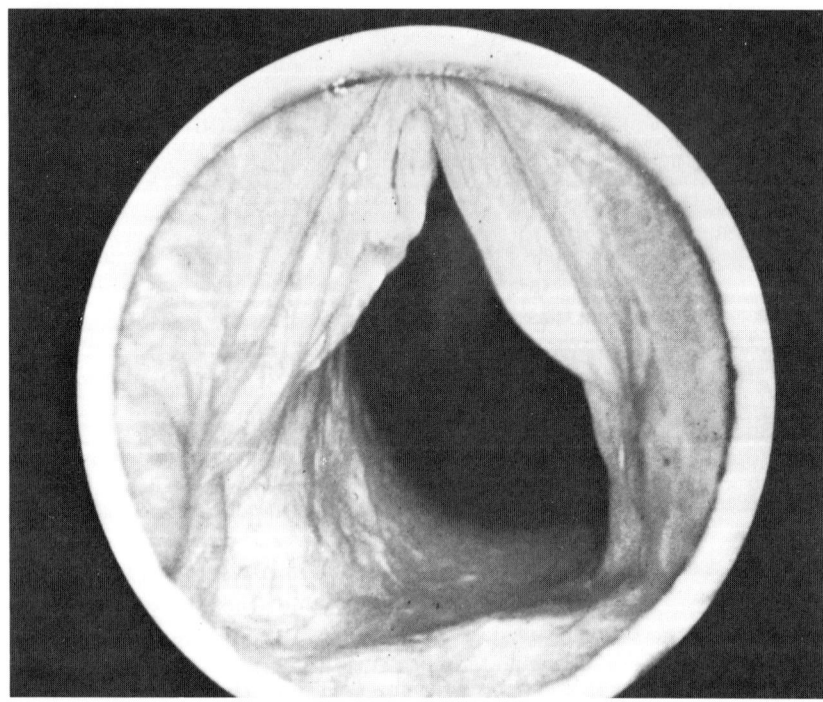

FIGURE 18-9 Epidermoid carcinoma of the left true vocal cord (direct laryngoscopy)

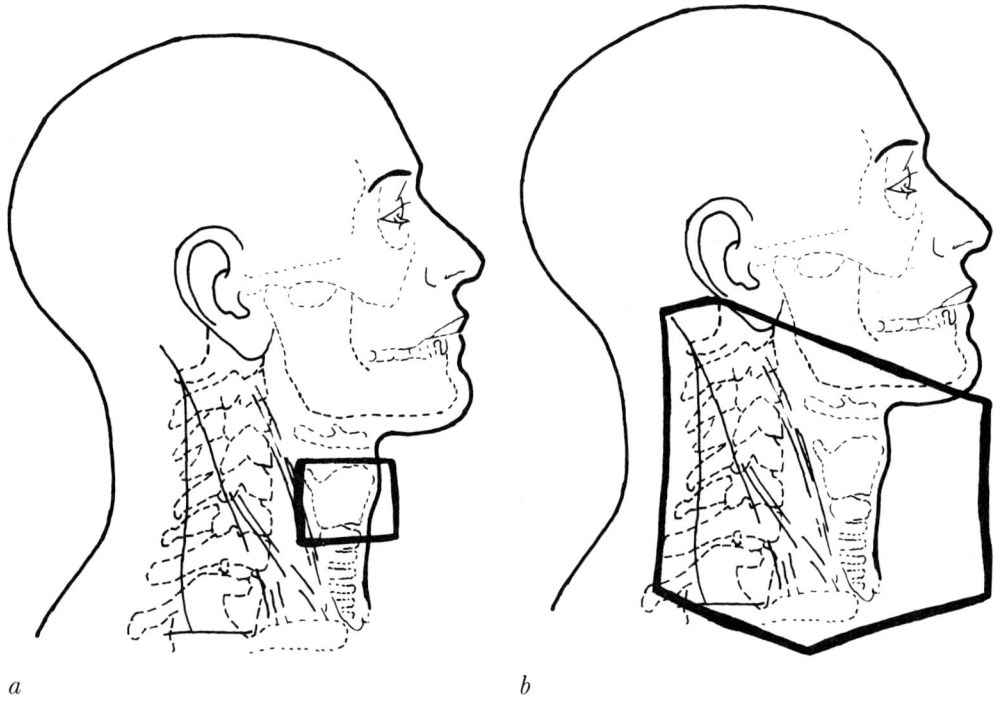

FIGURE 18-10 (*a*) Standard ports for radiation therapy of glottic carcinoma. (*b*) Standard ports for radiation therapy of cervical nodes.

incidence of metastases. This includes patients with lesions originating in the supraglottis, subglottis, and aryepiglottic fold.

More recently, combined therapy has included resection followed by a planned, full-course, postoperative radiation therapy. An attempt is made to begin the postoperative radiation within 3 weeks of the surgical excision. The neck nodes are included in the ports of the planned treatment (Fig. 18-10).[27-30]

Surgery

MICROLARYNGOSCOPY AND VOCAL CORD STRIPPING

Carcinoma in situ and superficially invasive cancer of the true vocal fold can be effectively treated with stripping of the vocal cord, using the operating microscope. Patient cooperation and close follow-up are mandatory. In properly selected patients cure rates resulting from vocal cord stripping for superficially invasive glottic cancer are as good as more extensive procedures.[31,32]

LASER TREATMENT

The CO_2 laser has recently been introduced in the transoral treatment of cancer of the larynx (Fig. 18-11). The laser has been particularly valuable in establishing an airway in patients with large, bulky tumors. This eliminates the need for preoperative tracheostomy and its attendant problem of stomal recurrence. The laser has also been used for decreasing the size of tumors prior to the use of radiation therapy. The use of the laser in the treatment of carcinoma in situ and superficially invasive cancer of the vocal cord is controversial.[33-35]

CONSERVATION SURGERY OF THE LARYNX

Conservation surgery for carcinoma of the larynx refers to adequate surgical excision of laryngeal malignancies with preservation of deglutition, respiration, and phonation. The principles of conservation surgery demand that it be precision surgery. The diagnostic appraisal and

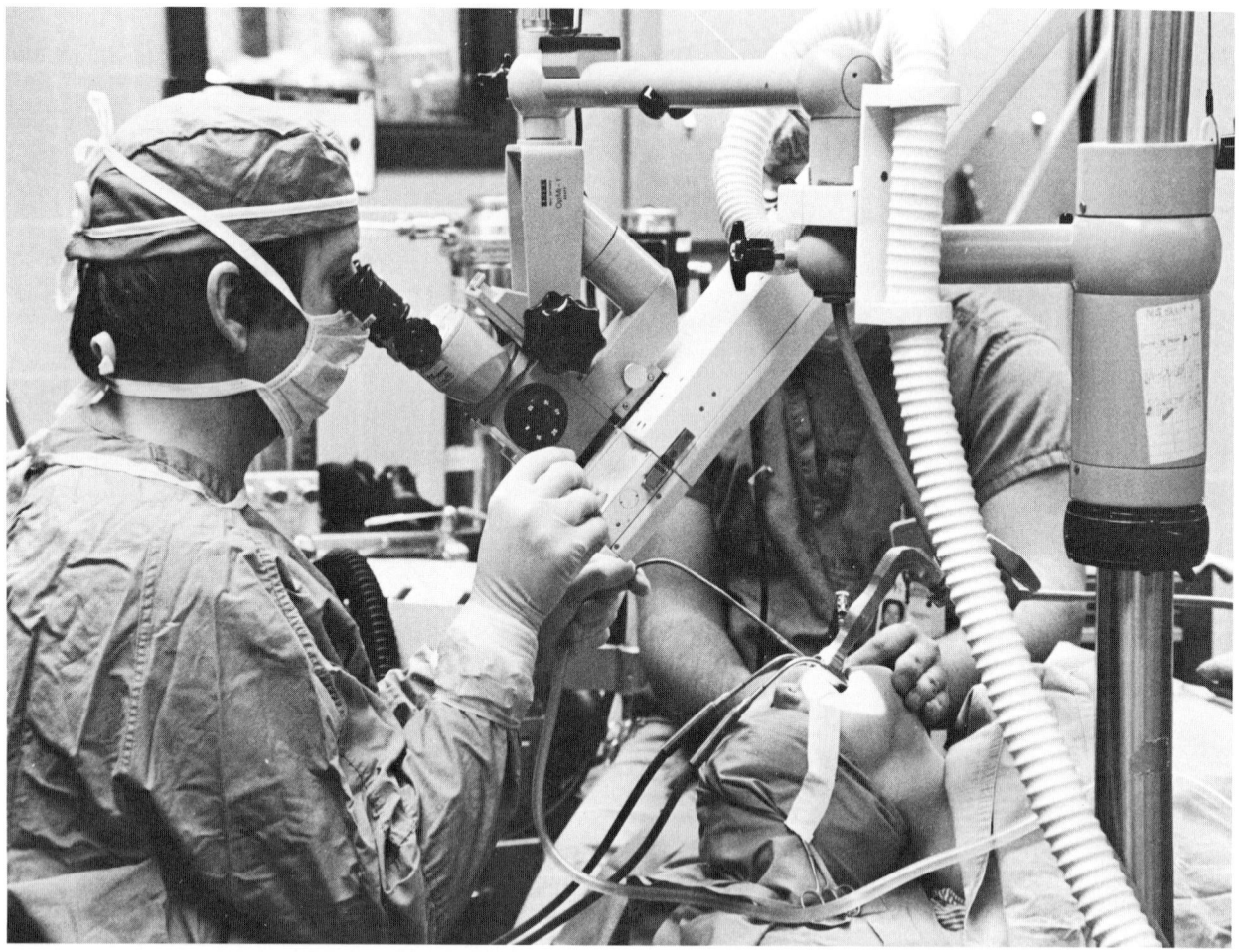

FIGURE 18-11 Carbon dioxide laser attached to operating microscope for use in direct laryngoscopy

subsequent exact mapping of the lesion permits an exact resection, which is consistent with complete removal of the tumor and restoration of function. The technique can be combined with en bloc radical neck dissection. Conservation surgery of the larynx can be used in combination with planned preoperative or postoperative irradiation.

Conservation surgery in selected patients with lesions of the glottis, supraglottis, piriform fossa, hypopharynx, or base of tongue can be performed without compromising survival chances. Approximately 60 percent of all cancers in these areas can be treated in this fashion.

Table 18-4 indicates the surgical management presently used in patients with cancer of the larynx.

TREATMENT OF GLOTTIC CANCER

Early glottic cancer (T_1 or T_2) can be treated with radiation therapy or surgery. Radiation is frequently reserved for lesions involving the membranous true vocal cord. Glottic cancer is treated with 6000 to 7000 rads administered via 4×5 to 5×5 cm ports.

Resection of early glottic cancer can be accomplished by hemilaryngectomy or resection of the anterior commissure. Indications for partial vertical hemilaryngectomy include (1) lesions of the true vocal cord, involving the anterior commissure or vocal process; (2) lesions which extend less than 1 cm below the free margin of the vocal cord; (3) lesions producing limited but not total loss of vocal cord mobility; (4) lesions involving the arytenoid cartilage; (5) selected glottic radiation failure or recurrence.[36-38] (See Fig. 18-12.) Partial vertical hemilaryngectomy is a frontolateral vertical resection and is followed by immediate reconstruction (Fig. 18-13). Lesions involving both the vocal cords and the anterior commissure are treated by frontoanterior resection of the anterior commissure.[39,40]

Larger lesions with fixation of the vocal cord (T_3 and T_4) are treated with resection or a combination of radiation therapy and resection by total laryngectomy. Total laryngectomy in the treatment of glottic cancer is indicated for (1) lesions involving one or both vocal cords with fixation of the cord; (2) cancer of the vocal cords with fixation which invades across the ventricle superiorly (transglottic); (3) cancer of the vocal cord with subglottic extension of more than 1 cm; (4) cancer extending beyond the endolarynx; (5) interarytenoid cancer; (6) cancer extending to the cricopharyngeous, preepiglottic space, or postcricoid area; and (7) cancer causing laryngeal cartilage destruction (Fig. 18-14). The technique of total laryngectomy is shown in Fig. 18-15.

TREATMENT OF SUPRAGLOTTIC CANCER

Small (T_1) epiglottic cancers can be treated with radiation therapy as a curative modality. Because of the high incidence of bilateral metastases to the cervical lymph nodes, radiation ports are used to include the neck in the treatment area. Treatment includes 6000 to 6500 rads to the primary site and 4500 rads to the neck.

Most supraglottic cancer is treated by resection or combined resection and postoperative radiation therapy to the primary and the neck. A majority of these lesions are amenable to conservation surgery. Subtotal supraglottic laryngectomy is indicated in patients with cancer of the epiglottis, false vocal cords, and aryepiglottic folds. This procedure may be extended to include the ipsilateral arytenoid and true vocal cords. It is then called a three-quarter laryngectomy. Selected cancers of the lingual epiglottis and vallecula can be treated by extended supraglottic subtotal laryngectomy. Extralaryngeal tumor spread, cartilage destruction, subglottic tumor extension, or involvement of the piriform apex are contraindications to the use of this technique. At least one normally functioning arytenoid and vocal cord must be present for adequate postoperative function.[41-43] (See Fig. 18-16.)

Cancer of the supraglottic area is managed by a horizontal supraglottic subtotal laryngectomy along with an en bloc radical neck dissection (Fig. 18-17). Radical neck dissection is indicated for patients with N_1 to N_3 necks. Patients with no palpable, involved, pretreatment lymph nodes may have either radical neck dissection or postoperative radiation therapy to the neck.

Total laryngectomy is indicated for supraglottic cancer involving the glottis with greater than 1-cm subglottic extension, lesions with thyroid cartilage destruction, and lesions involving the postcricoid area or piriform apex.

TREATMENT OF SUBGLOTTIC CANCER

Subglottic cancer is rare and symptoms occur late in the disease process.[43] (See Fig. 18-18.) Curative treatment of subglottic cancer usually requires total laryngectomy and ipsilateral radical neck dissection, followed by postop-

TABLE 18-4 Surgical Treatment of Cancer of the Larynx[22]

Primary site	T_1	T_2	T_3	T_4
Larynx				
Supraglottis	SSL* ± ND†	SSL ± ND	Extended SSL ± ND or TL‡ + ND	TL + ND
Glottis	Hemi§	Hemi	Hemi or TL ± ND	TL + ND
Subglottis	Local resection or TL + ND	TL + ND	TL + ND	TL + ND

SOURCE: Sessions.[22]
* Subtotal supraglottic laryngectomy
† Neck dissection
‡ Total laryngectomy
§ Hemilaryngectomy

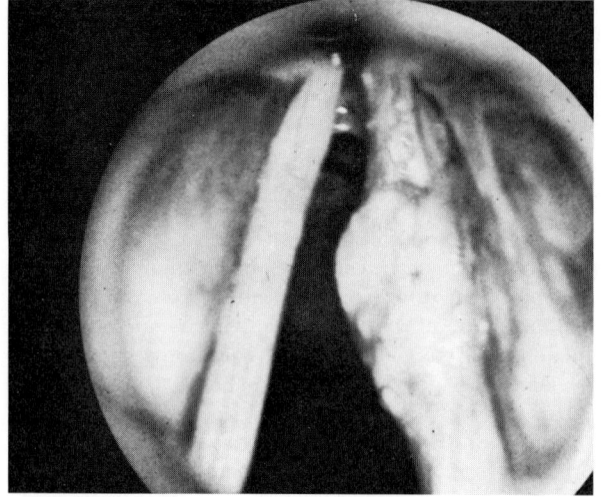
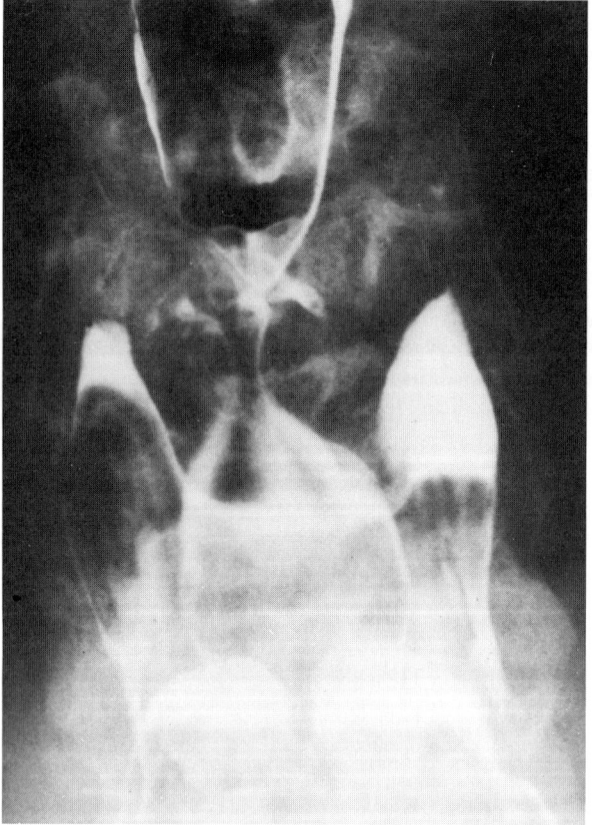
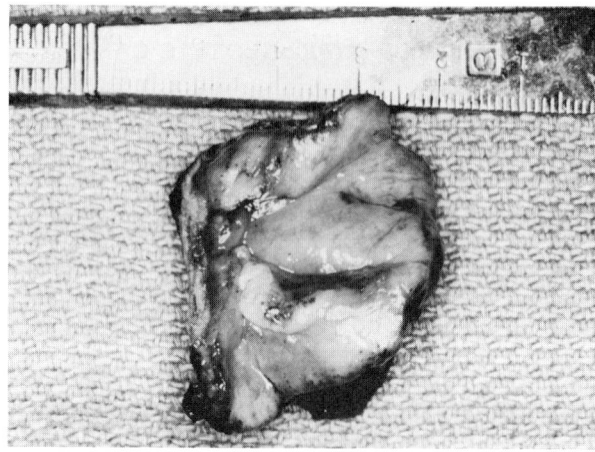

FIGURE 18-12 (*a*) Epidermoid carcinoma (T_1) of the right true vocal cord (direct laryngoscopy). (*b*) Laryngogram of early glottic cancer (*Courtesy Stuart S. Sagel, M.D.*). (*c*) Pretreatment diagram showing mapped T_1 glottic cancer. (*d*) Hemilaryngectomy specimen showing resected T_1 glottic cancer.

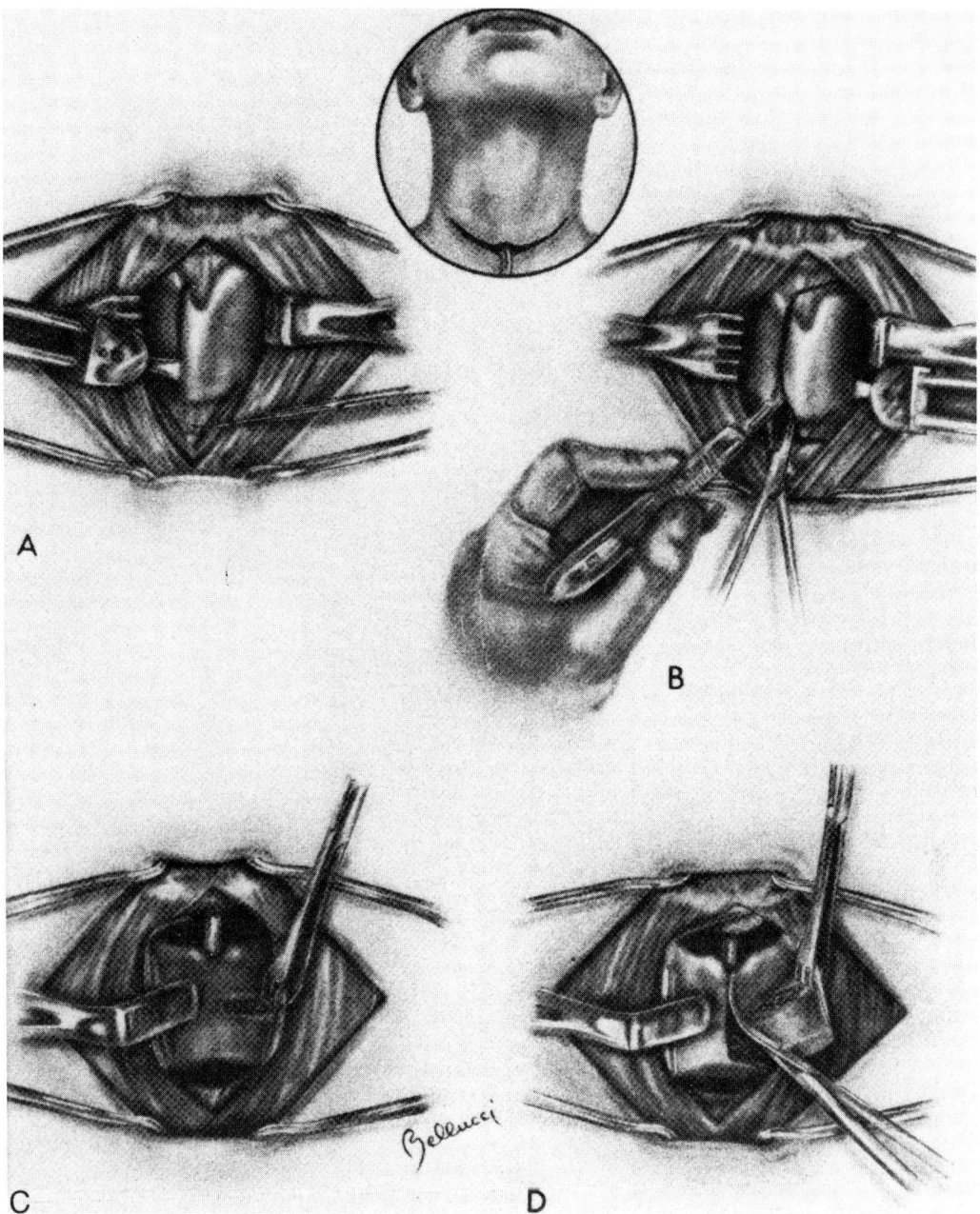

FIGURE 18-13 Hemilaryngectomy for glottic cancer. (*a*) Cartilage cut for a left cord lesion with anterior commissure involvement. Cricothyroid membrane incised at inferior margin. (*b*) Thyrotomy completed under direct vision. (*c*) Retraction of involved side exposes posterior extent of lesion. (*d*) Posterior soft tissue cut. (*From JH Ogura, HF Biller: Conservation surgery in cancer of the head and neck, Otolaryngol Clin North Am, October 1969.*)

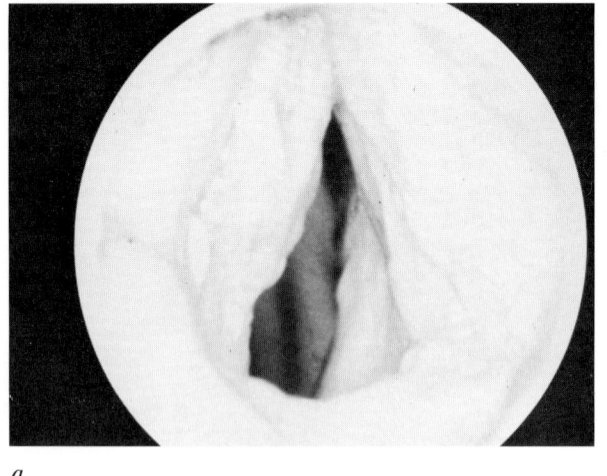
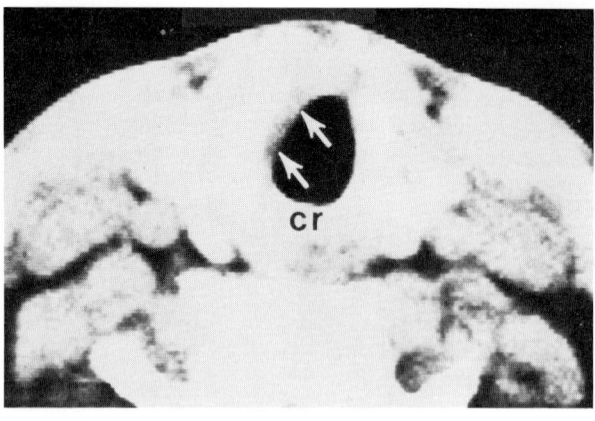
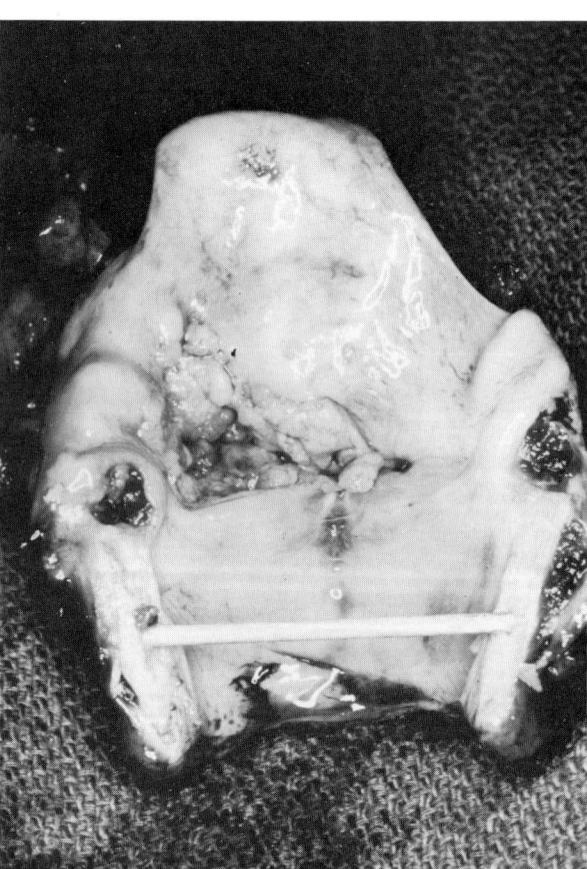

FIGURE 18-14 (*a*) Transglottic epidermoid cancer of the larynx (direct laryngoscopy). (*b*) High-resolution computed tomogram of a transglottic cancer showing thyroid cartilage destruction (at the level of cricoid cartilage—CV). (*Courtesy Stuart S. Sagel, M.D.*) (*c*) Pretreatment diagram of mapped transglottic cancer. (*d*) Total laryngectomy specimen showing transglottic cancer of the vocal fold (T_3).

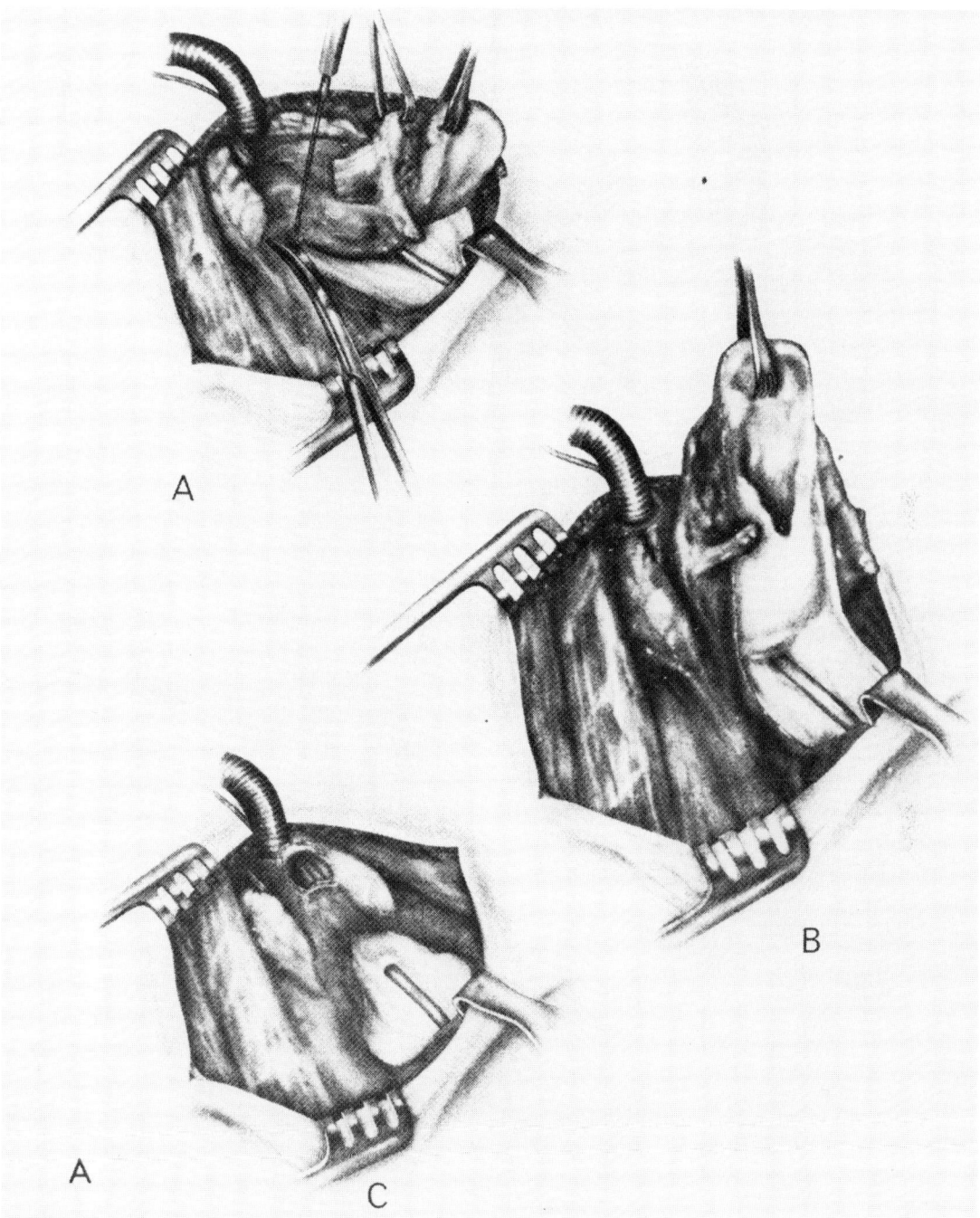

FIGURE 18-15 Total laryngectomy. (*a*) Entrance into hypopharynx through the vallecula. (*b*) The larynx delivered except for inferior mucosal cut at inferior border of the cricoid. (*c*) Specimen removed with open pharynx.

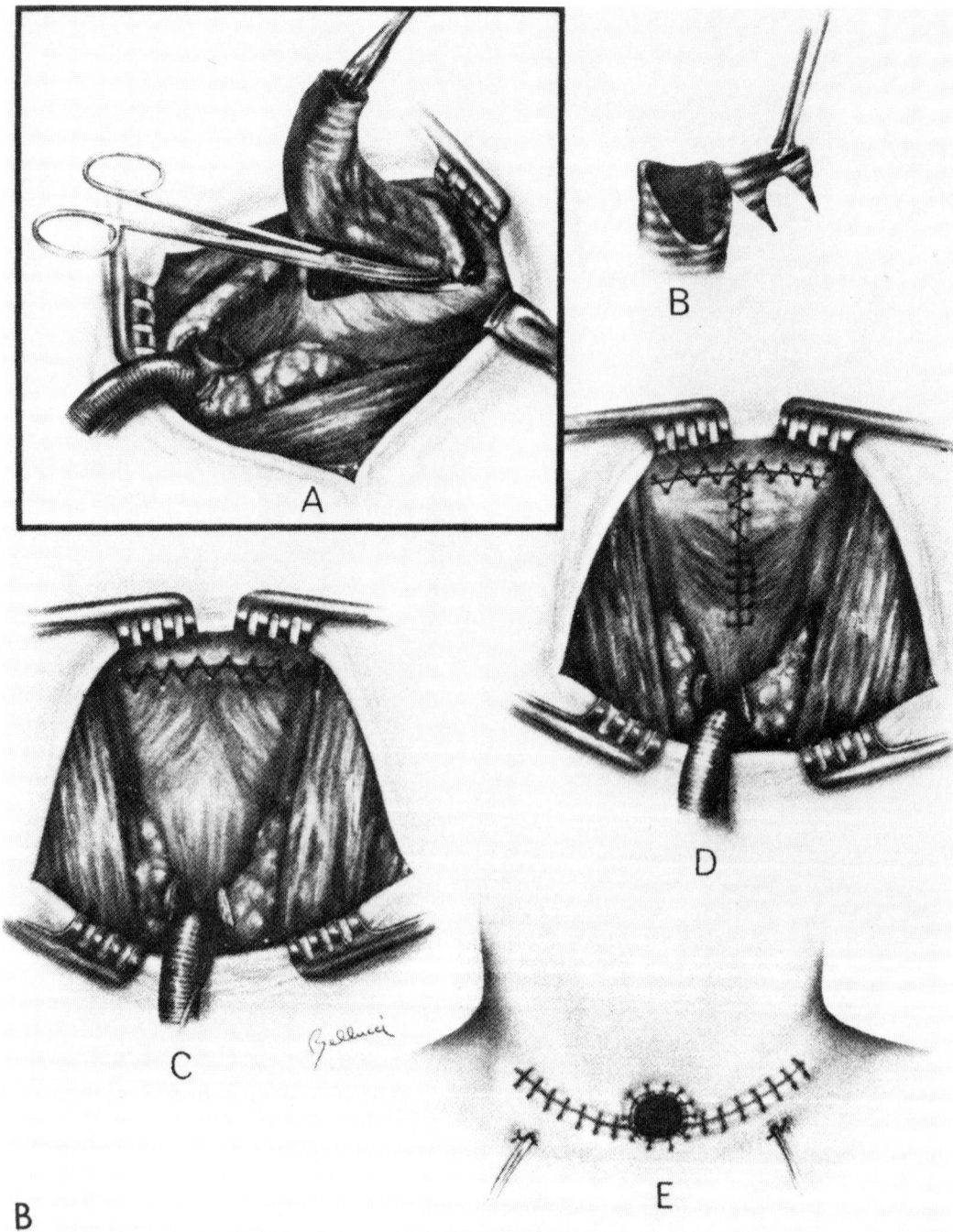

FIGURE 18-15 (Continued) (a) Entrance to hypopharynx through piriform sinus. (b) Beveling trachea for stomal reconstruction. (c) Transverse pharyngeal closure. (d) T pharyngeal closure. (e) Skin closure. (*From JH Ogura, HF Biller: Partial and total laryngectomy and radical neck dissection, in Otolaryngology, vol 4, Harper & Row, Hagerstown, Md, 1971.*)

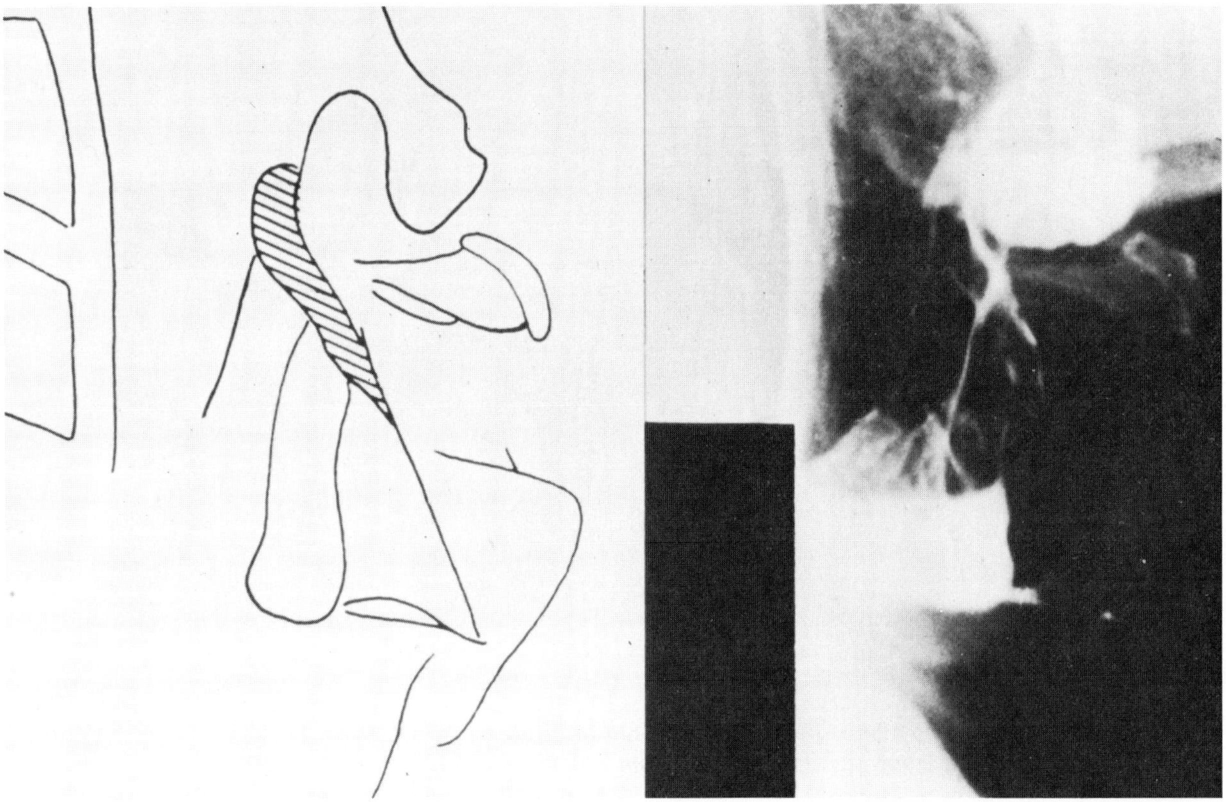

TUMORS OF THE LARYNGEAL APPARATUS **381**

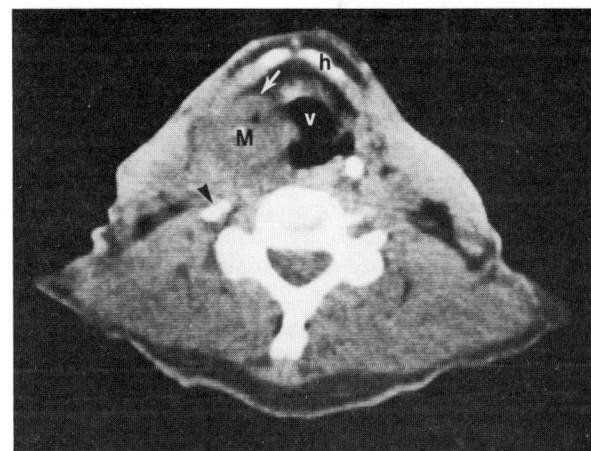

FIGURE 18-16 (a) Supraglottic cancer: Laryngogram of an exophytic epidermoid cancer of the supraglottic larynx (lateral). (b) High resolution computed tomogram of a bulky epidermoid cancer (M) of the supraglottic larynx at the level of the hyoid (H) and the vestibule (V). (*Courtesy of Stuart S. Sagel, M.D.*)

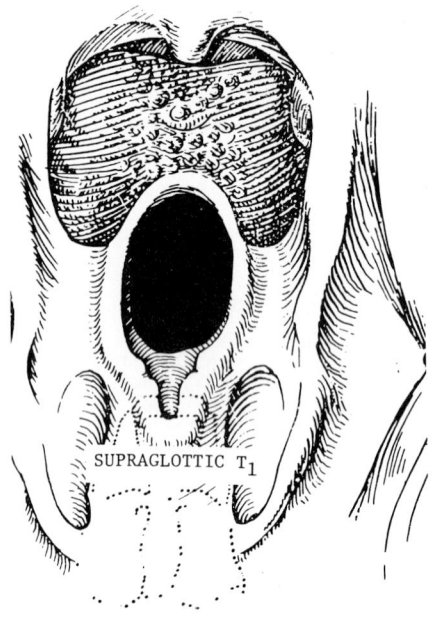
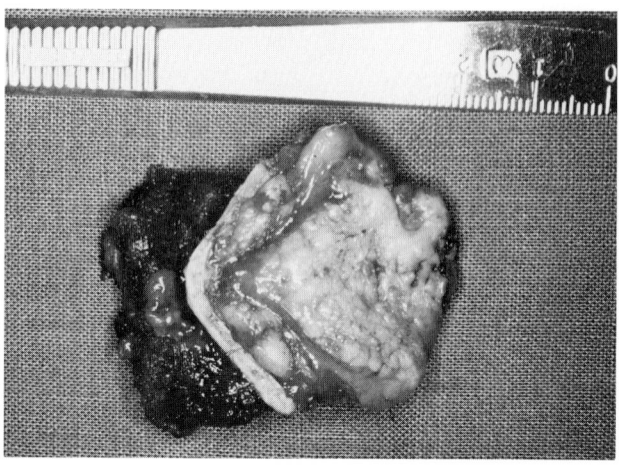

FIGURE 18-16 (*Continued*) (*c*) Pretreatment diagram showing mapped T_1 supraglottic cancer. (*d*) Subtotal supraglottic laryngectomy specimen showing exophytic tumor with adequate margin.

erative radiation therapy with particular attention to the paratracheal and upper mediastinal node-bearing areas.

CHEMOTHERAPY

The role of chemotherapy in the treatment of head and neck and laryngeal cancer in particular is not established. Methotrexate, *cis*-platinum, and bleomycin have shown significant, reproducible activity as single agents in locally advanced laryngeal carcinomas. Although recent studies with the combination of *cis*-platinum and bleomycin in previously untreated, locally advanced head and neck cancer show increased complete and partial tumor response rates, no agents or methods appear to have a higher response rate than methotrexate used alone on a weekly schedule.[44–54]

RESULTS

The treatment of laryngeal cancer results in very satisfactory survival rates. The length of survival is related to the extent of the primary tumor and the degree of spread to the regional lymph nodes. Early distant metastasis is rare. Table 18-5 shows survival rates by stage for a series of laryngeal cancers. Small glottic tumors result in the best survival rates. Treatment of these tumors results in 5-year cure rates approaching 90 percent.[55]

REFERENCES

1. American Joint Committee for Cancer Staging and End Result Reporting: *Manual for Staging Cancer,* 1977.
2. Pressman JA et al: Lymphatics of the larynx. *Ann Otol Rhinol Laryngol* 65:963, 1965.
3. Johner CH: The lymphatics of the larynx. *Otolaryngol Clin North Am* 3:439, 1970.
4. Ruviere H: *Anatomy of the Human Lymphatic System,* Edward Bros., Ann Arbor, Mich, 1938.
5. Pressman JA et al: Anatomical studies related to the dissection of cancer of the larynx. *Trans Am Acad Ophthalmol Otolaryngol* 64:628, 1960.

6. Kirchner JA: Cancer of the anterior commissure of the larynx results with radiotherapy. *Arch Otolaryngol* 91:524, 1970.
7. Kirchner JA, Fischer JJ: Anterior commissure cancer—A clinical and laboratory study of 39 cases. *Can J Otolaryngol* 4:637, 1975.
8. O'Keefe JJ: Evaluation of laryngectomy with radical neck dissection. *Laryngoscope* 69:914, 1959.
9. McGavran MH et al: The incidence of cervical node metastasis from epidermoid carcinoma of the larynx and their relationship to certain characteristics of the primary tumor. *Cancer* 14:55, 1961.
10. Reed GF, Rabuzzi DD: Neck dissection. *Otolaryngol Clin North Am* 2:547, 1969.
11. Staley CJ, Herzon FS: Elective neck dissection in carcinoma of the larynx. *Otolaryngol Clin North Am* 3(3)543, 1970.

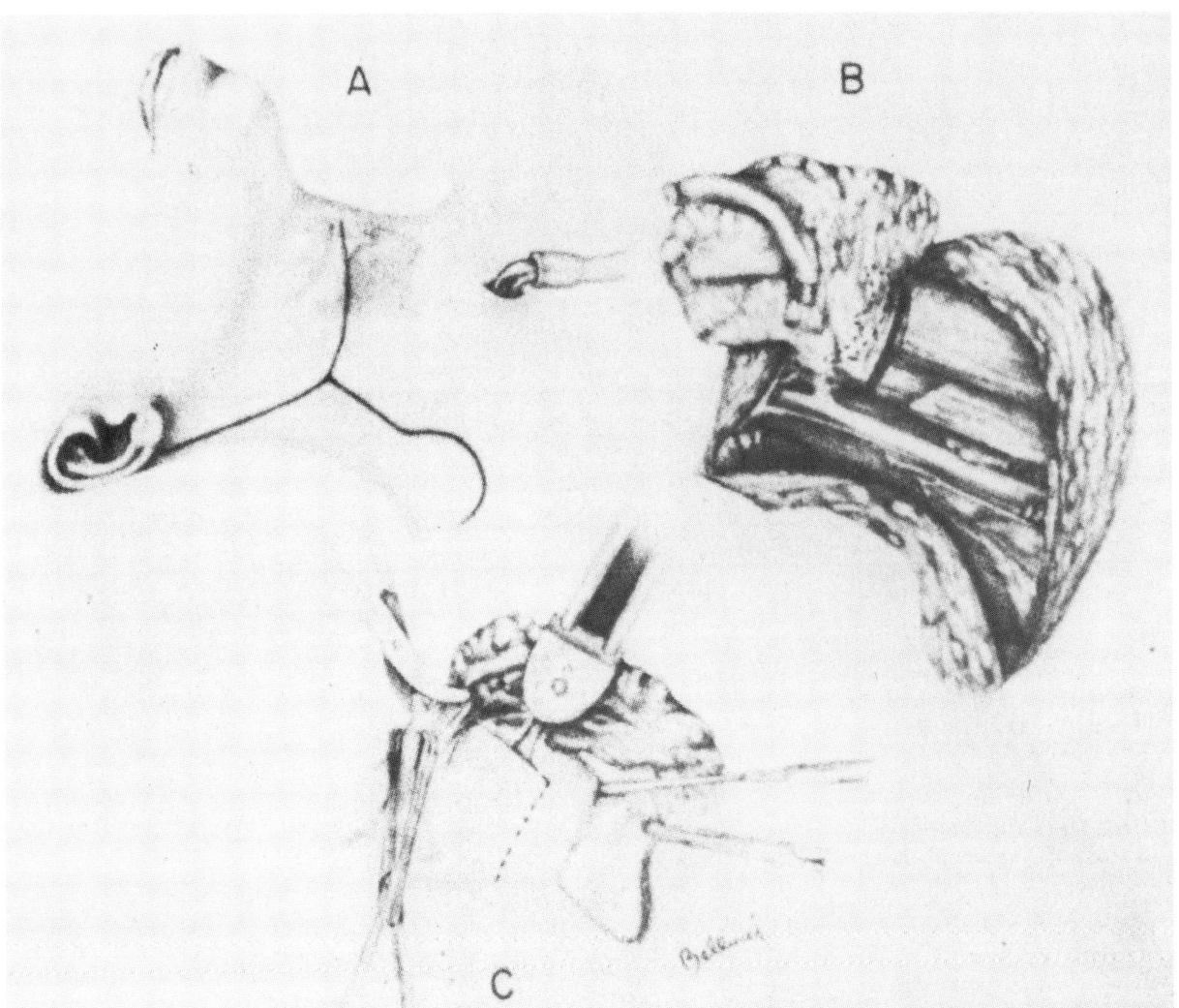

FIGURE 18-17 Subtotal supraglottic laryngectomy with radical neck dissection. (*a*) Skin incision for partial laryngectomy. (*b*) Neck dissection attached to thyrohyoid area; strap muscles incised at superior border of thyroid cartilage. (*c*) Thyroid perichondrium reflected; thyroid and hyoid cartilage cuts.

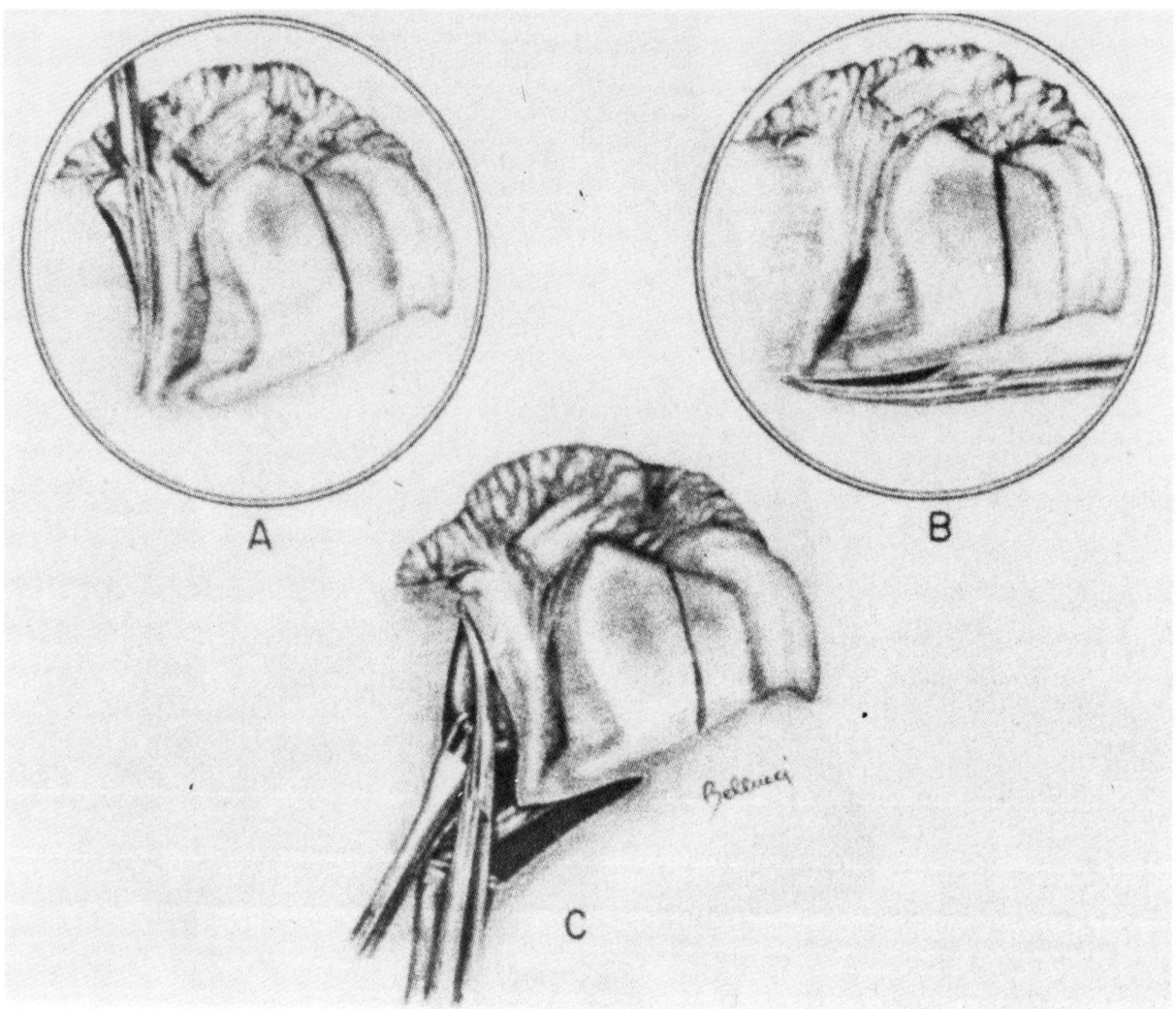

FIGURE 18-17 (Continued) (*a*) Pharyngectomy performed at vallecula. (*b*) Pharyngotomy performed at piriform sinus. (*c*) Enlarging the pharyngostoma by incising opposite vallecula.

12. Wynder E et al: Study of environmental factors in cancer of the larynx. *Cancer* 9:86, 1956.
13. Wynder E et al: Environmental factors in cancer of the larynx—A second look. *Cancer* 38:1591, 1976.
14. Lawry WS: Alcoholism and cancer of the head and neck. *Laryngoscope* 85:1277, 1975.
15. Auerback O et al: Histologic changes in the larynx in relation to smoking habits. *Cancer* 25:92, 1975.
16. Hollinshead AC et al: Antibodies to herpesvirus nonvirion antigens in squamous carcinomas. *Science* 182:713, 1973.
17. Leborgne R: Tomographic study of cancer of the larynx. *Am J Roentgenol* 43:493, 1940.
18. Bao-Shan J: Malignant tumors of the larynx. *Radiol Clin North Am 16:247, 1978.*
19. Marcus AA et al: Computed tomography of the larynx. *Radiol Clin North Am* 16:195, 1978.

20. Batsakis JG: *Tumors of the Head and Neck,* Williams & Wilkins, Baltimore, 1974, pp. 68–75.
21. Biller HB et al: Verrucous cancer of the larynx. *Laryngoscope* 81:1323, 1971.
22. Sessions DG: Surgical pathology of cancer of the larynx and hypopharynx. *Laryngoscope* 86:814, 1976.
23. Bauer WC et al: The significance of positive margins in hemilaryngectomy specimens. *Laryngoscope* 85:1, 1975.
24. Perez CA et al: Radiation therapy of early carcinoma of the true vocal cords. *Cancer* 21:764, 1972.
25. Hibbs GG et al: Radiotherapy for early stages of vocal cord cancer. *Ann Otol Rhinol Laryngol* 78:319, 1969.
26. Wang CC: Treatment of squamous cell carcinoma of the larynx by radiation. *Radiat Clin North Am* 16:209, 1978.
27. Powers WE, Ogura JH: Preoperative irradiation in head and neck cancer surgery. *Arch Otolaryngol* 81:153, 1965.
28. Powers WE, Ogura JH: Low dose preoperative radiation in head and neck cancer. *Otolaryngol Clin North Am* 2:533, 1969.
29. Biller HF, Ogura JH: Planned preoperative radiation for laryngeal and laryngopharyngeal carcinoma. *Front Radiat Ther Oncol* 5:100, 1970.
30. Constable WC et al: High dose preoperative radiotherapy and surgery for cancer of the larynx. *Laryngoscope* 82:1861, 1972.
31. Lilla JC, DeSanto LW: Transoral surgery of early cordal carcinoma. *Trans Am Acad Ophthalmol Otolaryngol* 77:92, 1973.
32. Stutsman AC, McGavran MH: Ultraconservative management of superficially invasive epidermoid carcinoma of the true vocal cord. *Ann Otol Rhinol Laryngol* 80:507, 1978.
33. Lyons DG et al: CO_2 laser laryngoscopy in a variety of lesions. *Laryngoscope* 86:1658, 1976.

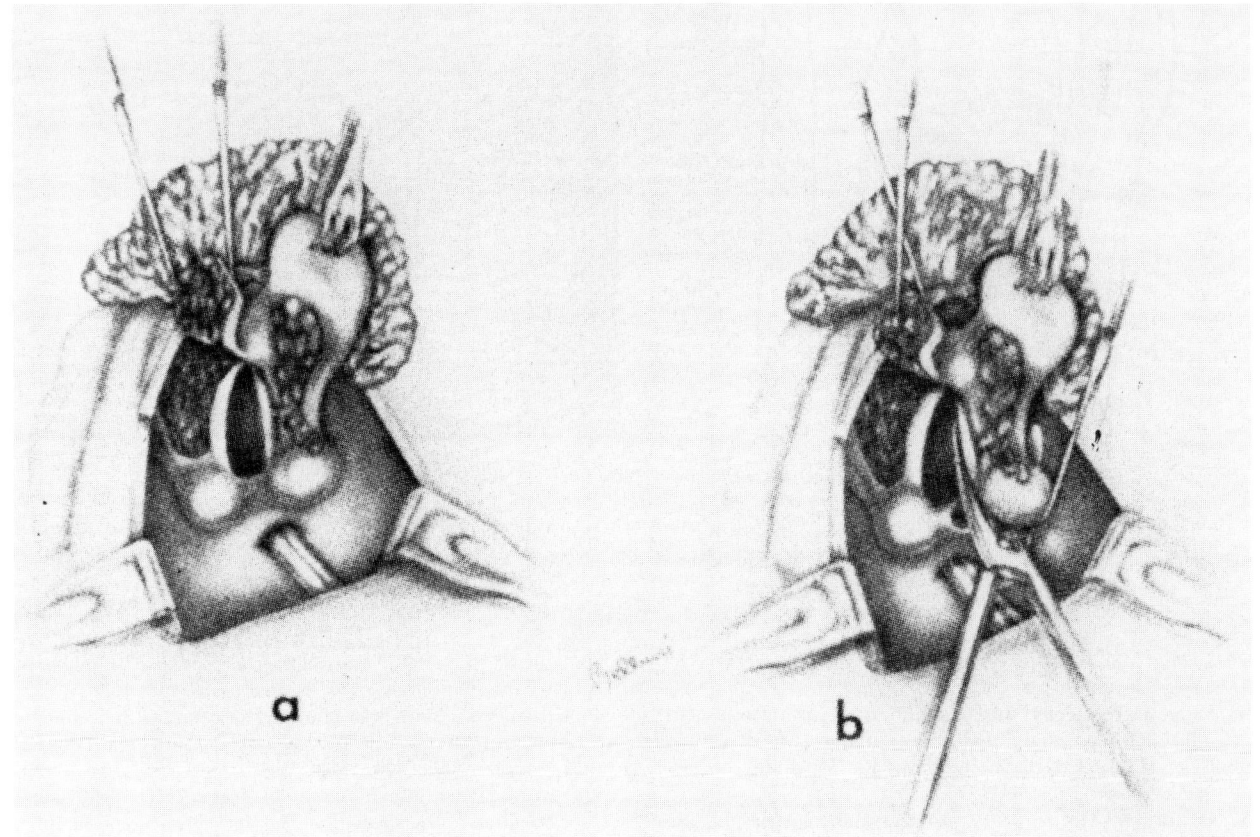

FIGURE 18-17 (*Continued*) Separating uninvolved side initially, thereby obtaining improved visibility of involved side when arytenoid is to be resected. (*From DG Sessions et al: Head and Neck, in J Horton, GH Hill (eds): Clinical Oncology, Saunders, Philadelphia, 1977.*)

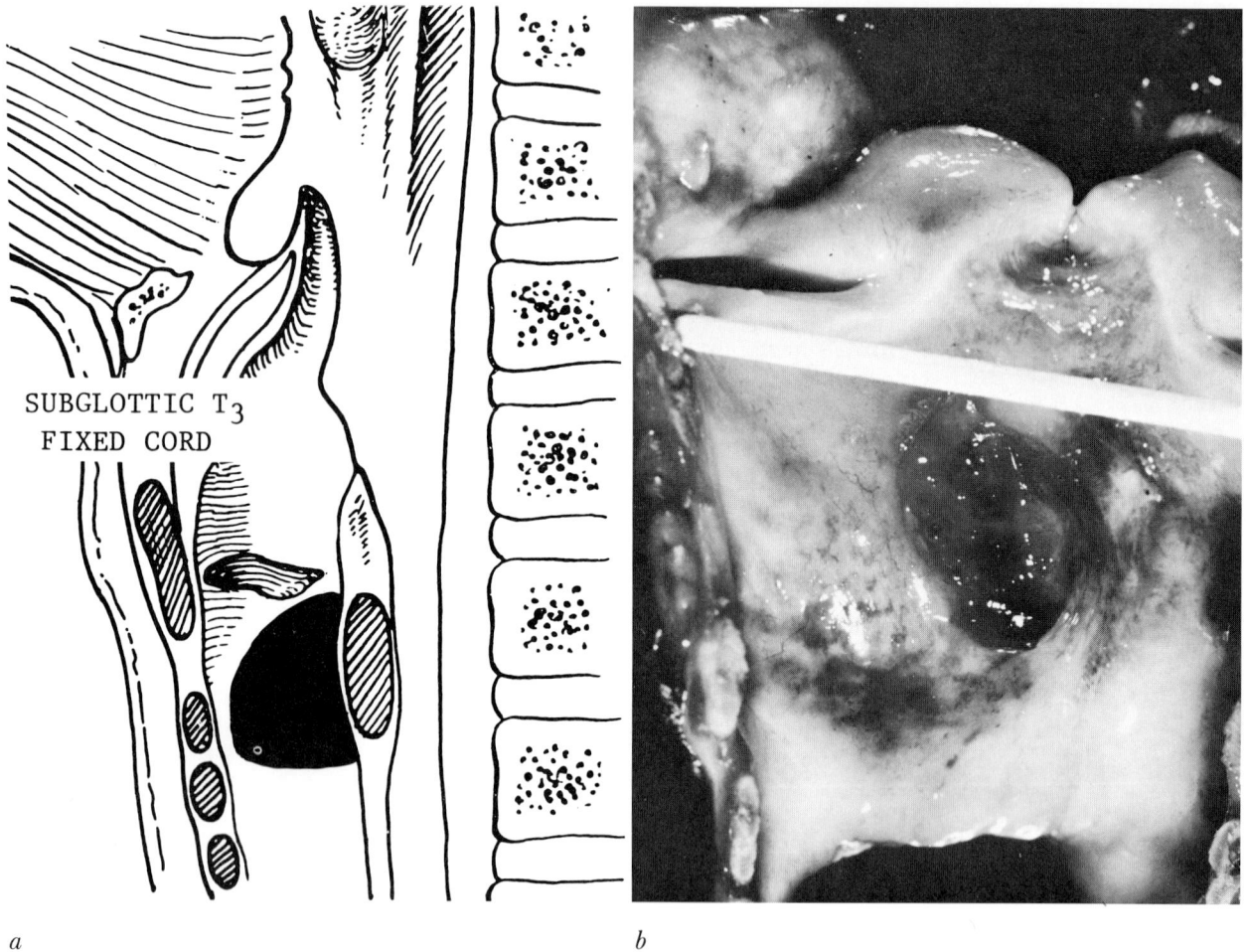

FIGURE 18-18 (a) Pretreatment diagram showing mapped T_3 subglottic cancer. (b) Total laryngectomy specimen of resected T_3 subglottic chondrosarcoma of the larynx.

34. Strong MS: Laser excision of carcinoma of the larynx. *Laryngoscope* 85:1286, 1978.
35. Vaughn CW et al: Laryngeal carcinoma: Transoral treatment utilizing the CO_2 laser. *Am J Surg* 136:490, 1978.
36. Biller HF et al: Hemilaryngectomy for T2 glottic cancers. *Arch Otolaryngol* 93:238, 1971.
37. Ogura JH, Heeneman H: Conservation surgery of the larynx and hypopharynx—Selection of patients and results. *Canad J Otol* 2:11, 1973.
38. Ogura JH: Selection of patients for conservation surgery of the larynx and pharynx. *Trans Am Acad Ophthalmol Otolaryngol* 76:741, 1972.
39. Som ML, Silver CE: The anterior commissure technique of partial laryngectomy. *Arch Otolaryngol* 87:138, 1968.
40. Kirchner JA, Soun ML: The anterior commissure technique of partial laryngectomy clinical and laboratory observations. *Laryngoscope* 85:1308, 1975.
41. Ogura JH et al: Conservation surgery for epidermoid carcinoma of the supraglottic larynx. *Laryngoscope* 85:1808, 1975.
42. Ogura JH et al: Supraglottic carcinoma with extension to the arytenoid. *Laryngoscope* 85:1329, 1975.
43. Sessions DG et al: Carcinoma of the subglottic area. *Laryngoscope* 85:1417, 1975.

TABLE 18-5 Laryngopharyngeal Cancer: 3-Year Survival by Stage

Primary site	Tumor-free (T_1)		Death from (T_1)		Tumor-free (T_2)		Death from (T_2)	
	Number	%	Number	%	Number	%	Number	%
N_0								
Supraglottis	62	71	22	25	6	60	3	30
Glottis	190	80	37	16	43	77	12	21
Subglottis	0	0	0	0	0	0	0	0
N_1								
Supraglottis	6	38	9	56	2	22	7	78
Glottis	4	67	2	33	3	43	3	43
N_2								
Supraglottis	3	43	4	57	1	50	1	50
Glottis	0	0	1	100	1	100	0	0
Subglottis								

SOURCE: Sessions.[22]

44. Constanzi JJ et al: Intravenous bleomycin infusion as a potential synchronizing agent in human disseminated malignancies. *Cancer* 38:1503, 1976.
45. Blum RH et al: A clinical review of bleomycin—A new antitumor agent. *Cancer* 31:903, 1973.
46. Tarpley JL et al: High dose methotrexate as a preoperative adjuvant in treatment of epidermoid carcinoma of the head and neck. *Am J Surg* 130:481, 1975.
47. Pitman SW et al: Initial adjuvant therapy in advanced squamous cell carcinoma of the head and neck employing weekly high-dose methotrexate with leukovorin rescue. *Laryngoscope* 88:632, 1978.
48. Wittes RE et al: Cis-diaminedichloroplatinum (II) in the treatment of epidermoid carcinoma of the head and neck. *Cancer Treat Rep* 61:359, 1977.
49. Wittes RE et al: DPP in epidermoid carcinoma of the head and neck. *J Hematol Oncol* 6:85, 1976.
50. Wittes RE et al: Combination chemotherapy with cis-diaminedichloroplatinum (II) and bleomycin in tumors of the head and neck. *Oncology* 32:202, 1975.
51. Randolph VL et al: Combination therapy of advanced head and neck cancer. *Cancer* 41:460, 1978.
52. Goldberg NH et al: Preoperative high-dose methotrexate—A well tolerated regimen in head and neck cancer. *Proc AACR-ASCO* 18:292, 1977.
53. Rozencweig M et al: Cis-diaminedichloroplatinum: A new anti-cancer drug. *Ann Intern Med* 86:803, 1977.
54. Rozencweig M et al: Investigational chemotherapeutic agents in head and neck cancer. *Semin Oncol* 4:425, 1977.
55. Ogura JH et al: Analysis of surgical therapy for epidermoid carcinoma of the laryngeal glottis. *Laryngoscope* 85:1522, 1975.
56. Sessions DG et al: Head and neck, in J Horton, GJ Hill (eds): *Clinical Oncology,* Saunders, Philadelphia, 1977.

SELECTED BIBLIOGRAPHY

Harwood AR et al: T_3 glottic cancer: An analysis of dose time-volume factors. *Int J Radiat Oncol Biol Phys* 6:675, 1980.

Lee F et al: Laryngeal radiation after hemilaryngectomy. *Laryngoscope* 90:1534, 1980.

Neel HB III et al: Laryngofissure and cordectomy for early cordal carcinoma: Outcome in 182 patients. *Otolaryngol Head Neck Surg* 88:79, 1980.

Pennacchio JL et al: Combination of *cis*-platinum and bleomycin prior to surgery and/or radiotherapy compared with radiotherapy alone for the treatment of advanced squamous cell carcinoma of the head and neck. *Cancer* 50:2795, 1982.

Vogl SE et al: Mitomycin-C, methotrexate, bleomycin and *cis*-diaminedichloroplatinum II in the chemotherapy of advanced squamous cancer of the head and neck. *Cancer* 50:6, 1982.

Woodhouse RJ et al: Treatment of carcinoma of the vocal cord: A review of twenty years' experience. *Laryngoscope* 91:1155, 1981.

19

TUMORS OF THE MAJOR AND MINOR SALIVARY GLANDS

Harvey W. Baker

A variety of tumors and tumorlike lesions arise in salivary tissue. Surgeons who are called upon to manage these conditions must be aware of far more than the standard operative approaches. They must be familiar with diagnostic measures, and with the pathology of a complex group of neoplasms and their clinical behavior and prognosis.

ANATOMICAL CONSIDERATIONS

The salivary glands consist of the paired major salivary glands—the parotid, the submaxillary, and the sublingual—as well as minor salivary glands which occur in scattered locations about the upper airways and digestive tracts.

Parotid Gland

The parotid is the largest of the salivary glands and probably for this reason gives rise to the large majority of salivary tissue tumors. While the parotid is anatomically a unilobar structure it is useful for clinical purposes to employ the terms "superficial lobe" and "deep lobe" in designating portions of the gland which lie on either side of the plane of the facial nerve. The superficial lobe is molded over the masseter muscle and angle of the mandible, extending superiorly to the zygoma and inferiorly into the upper cervical region. Posteriorly it is applied closely to the cartilage of the external auditory canal. The facial nerve, after exiting from the stylomastoid foramen, enters the posterior aspect of the parotid and in traversing the gland gives off its major divisions and branches. The smaller deep lobe of the parotid curves around the posterior border of the ramus of the mandible and extends into the lateral pharyngeal space where it is close to the pharynx. It is traversed by the posterior facial vein and the terminal portion of the external carotid artery. Stensen's duct emerges from the anterior edge of the parotid and extends forward and medially to enter the mouth. Ectopic bits of parotid tissue occasionally lie along the course of the duct and may give rise to salivary tumors which are separate from the parotid.

A number of lymph nodes lie directly upon the superficial aspect of the parotid (preauricular nodes) and drain the face and upper scalp. They communicate with a number of lymph nodes lying within both the superficial and deep lobes of the gland. Nodes about the lower pole of the parotid occasionally contain heterotopic salivary tissue which may give rise to neoplasms, usually Warthin's tumors. Lymphatic drainage from the parotid is principally to the superior nodes in the jugular chain.

Submaxillary Gland

The submaxillary gland lies deep to the body of the mandible extending downward to fill most of the digastric triangle of the neck. The bulk of the gland lies upon the hyoglossus muscle; anteriorly it extends to the mylohyoid and is folded about both the superficial and deep aspects of the free posterior edge of this muscle. Wharton's duct leaves the gland anteriorly to course beneath the mucosa of the floor of the mouth to enter the oral cavity near the frenulum of the tongue.

The anterior facial vein crosses the external aspect of the gland in a vertical direction, and the vein itself is crossed horizontally by the mandibular branch of the facial nerve, which courses about 1 cm below the midportion of the body of the mandible. The facial artery is closely applied to the deep aspect of the gland. A number of lymph nodes lie superiorly adjacent to the facial vessels; others are located along the anterior and posterior surfaces of the gland. The submaxillary gland lies immediately upon the hypoglossal nerve as it traverses the floor of the digastric triangle. The superior surface of the gland is also in close relationship to the lingual nerve and is connected to it by several nerve filaments (submaxillary ganglion).

Sublingual Gland

The sublingual, smallest of the salivary glands, lies immediately beneath the mucosa of the floor of the mouth. Laterally the gland is close to the body of the mandible and medially it lies upon the hyoglossus and styloglossus muscles. The lingual nerve curves from laterally to medially beneath the gland to reach the tongue. The two sublingual glands almost meet anteriorly in the midline. Each gland has numerous tiny ducts extending superiorly into the sublingual fold of the floor of the mouth.

Minor Salivary Glands

The minor salivary glands include many small collections of salivary tissue composed largely of mucus-secreting cells and short ducts. They are found in numerous locations in the mucous membrane lining the upper air and food passages, most often the palate, but also the lip, tongue, pharynx, nasal cavity, paranasal sinuses, larynx, and trachea.

PATHOLOGY AND NATURAL HISTORY

A complex group of benign and malignant neoplasms arise in salivary tissue. The site of origin is of importance; over 75 percent of parotid tumors are benign, while over 50 percent of tumors arising in the submaxillary gland are malignant. The great majority of tumors in minor salivary glands are also malignant. While some salivary tumors may be difficult to classify, it is important to obtain an exact diagnosis whenever possible since the behavior of each neoplasm is closely related to its histologic appearance.

It is probable that most epithelial salivary tumors arise from stem cells in the excretory and intercalated ducts.[1,2] Myoepithelial cells closely related to acinar and ductal epithelium also play a part in the histogenesis of some neoplasms, particularly mixed tumors and adenoid cystic carcinomas. While the etiology of most salivary tumors is unknown there is increasing evidence of the role played by radiation in the development of some neoplasms, both benign and malignant. As in the case of radiation-induced thyroid cancer, the radiation, usually given for a benign condition, precedes the appearance of a salivary tumor by an interval of 12 to 25 years.[3] The majority of salivary tissue tumors related to prior radiation have appeared in the parotid, but some have been reported in the other salivary glands as well. In the author's experience most of these tumors have been adenoid cystic carcinomas; others have noted a predominance of mixed tumors. The author has noted one acinic cell carcinoma of the sublingual gland arising 21 years after irradiation of the face for acne. It is probable that if patients are questioned more closely about prior radiation many more instances of this association will be noted.

A number of varying classifications for salivary tumors have been published.[1,4,5] Table 19-1 lists the major lesions which may be encountered. Some authorities have proposed dividing malignant neoplasms into two groups, those of low-grade and high-grade malignancy. The author no longer feels this is useful since some tumors considered low-grade, such as adenoid cystic carcinoma, while often having a sluggish growth rate eventually have a poor prognosis. Both clinically aggressive and

TABLE 19-1 Classification of Salivary Gland Tumors

1. Epithelial tumors
   a. Benign
      (1) Mixed tumor (pleomorphic adenoma)
      (2) Papillary cystadenoma lymphomatosum (Warthin's tumor)
      (3) Oncocytoma (oxyphil cell adenoma)
      (4) Other adenomas
   b. Malignant
      (1) Malignant mixed tumor
      (2) Mucoepidermoid carcinoma
      (3) Adenoid cystic carcinoma
      (4) Acinic cell carcinoma
      (5) Miscellaneous adenocarcinomas
      (6) Squamous cell carcinoma
2. Nonepithelial tumors
   a. Benign
      (1) Hemangioma, hemangioendothelioma
      (2) Lymphangioma
      (3) Lipoma
      (4) Neurilemmoma, neurofibroma
   b. Malignant
      (1) Malignant lymphoma
      (2) Malignant mesenchymal tumors
3. Metastatic tumors
4. Tumorlike conditions
   a. Benign lymphoepithelial lesion
   b. Cysts
   c. Lymphoid hyperplasia

relatively benign forms of a number of tumors can also be identified.

Benign Mixed Tumor

Benign mixed tumors (pleomorphic adenomas) are the most common salivary neoplasms, comprising over half of all parotid tumors, benign and malignant, as well as the predominant benign tumors of the submaxillary and minor salivary glands.

PATHOLOGY

A benign mixed tumor typically presents as a rounded, well-circumscribed, often encapsulated mass in a salivary gland. Its cut surface bulges and is homogenous, glistening white or gray in appearance; larger tumors may have areas of cyst formation or hemorrhage. Histologically benign mixed tumors contain a variety of cell types, some distinctly epithelial and others probably originating from myothelial cells. In some instances epithelial cells predominate with a dense collection of sheets of cells and irregular attempts at gland formation. In others the cellular elements are scanty and the tumor is composed largely of a loose myxomatous type of connective tissue, at times with actual cartilage formation. A single tumor may contain both the cellular and the chondromucoid components.[6] The fibrous capsule or pseudocapsule may be incomplete and may contain nests of tumor cells, some extending beyond the capsule.

NATURAL HISTORY

Benign mixed tumors are encountered at all ages; they have been reported in newborns as well as the very old. They are seen most often in the third and fourth decades and are somewhat more common in females than males. Typically a benign mixed tumor presents in a major salivary gland as a rounded, well-circumscribed mass which has been present for months or years with almost imperceptible growth. The tumors are generally painless and in the parotid are never accompanied by facial weakness. While the usual mixed tumor encountered measures 1 to 2 cm in diameter, an occasional early lesion may be only a few millimeters in size, and long-neglected tumors may form huge, grotesque masses. As a rule, the tumors arise in one salivary gland; involvement of more than one gland is extremely rare. The tumors are noted both for their slow growth and for their propensity to recur after enucleation or inadequate excision. The recurrence may be prompt or long delayed; the average time for clinical recurrence is 4 years following surgery. In contrast to the unicentric appearance of origin of a primary benign mixed tumor, the recurrences frequently present as multiple nodules in the operative field and even involve the skin in the area of the surgical scar. There is no constant relation between the histologic appearance of the tumor and its recurrence. The recurrence rate is more related to the size and location of the primary tumor and technical factors involved in its removal. In minor salivary glands benign mixed tumors are also slow-growing, painless, rounded masses almost always covered with intact mucosa.

Papillary Cystadenoma Lymphomatosum

These tumors are entirely benign neoplasms which contain both epithelial and lymphoid elements. They are commonly called Warthin's tumors, named after one of the first to describe them. They are the second most common benign salivary tumor and are encountered only within or adjacent to the parotid.

PATHOLOGY

Warthin's tumors are rounded, soft, encapsulated masses; the cut surface discloses cystic spaces of varying size with a fine papillary lining and containing a brownish mucoid fluid. Microscopically the tumors are readily recognized by pale eosinophilic epithelial cells forming cystic spaces and papillary projections. There is an underlying lymphoid matrix, often with germinal centers.

NATURAL HISTORY

The majority of Warthin's tumors occur in males, usually in the fifth or sixth decades. They most commonly appear as a mass with a cystic consistency in the lower pole of the parotid gland. It is not unusual to obtain a history of fluctuation in the size of the mass, occasionally with intermittent pain and local tenderness suggesting inflammation. A preoperative diagnosis of Warthin's tumor is likely when an elderly male presents with a cystic mass in the lower pole of the parotid and a history of increasing and decreasing size. The tumors are generally slow-growing and up to 10 percent may be bilateral, an incidence of bilateralism unique among salivary tissue neoplasms. Recurrences may appear after inadequate surgery but are far less common than recurrences of mixed tumors. While there have been a few reports of malignant transformation of Warthin's tumors, the evidence for malignant potential has not been convincing.

Oncocytoma

The oncocytoma or oxyphil cell adenoma is an uncommon epithelial neoplasm which has most often been reported as arising in the parotid.

PATHOLOGY

The tumor presents grossly as a rounded, well-circumscribed mass with a firm pink or brownish cut surface. Histologically, dense sheets and cords of oncocytes, large uniform acidophilic cells with a scanty connective tissue stroma, are seen.

NATURAL HISTORY

The majority of oncocytomas appear as slow-growing, firm parotid masses in elderly patients. The usual clinical diagnosis is benign mixed tumor. Recurrences after complete excision have not been reported. While the majority of oncocytomas are entirely benign, rare malignant variants have been reported.

A variety of other adenomas have been infrequently noted arising in salivary tissue. These include clear cell tumors, basal cell adenomas, and other benign neoplasms composed of a single cell type.

Malignant Mixed Tumor

In most reported series malignant mixed tumors are said to comprise 5 percent or less of salivary neoplasms, but these tumors are being recognized with increased frequency.

PATHOLOGY

These are bulky salivary tissue tumors which often have a grossly malignant appearance. While a capsule may be present, it is often incomplete with extension of the tumor beyond it. Foci of hemorrhage are often seen as well as areas of softening and cyst formation. Histologically these are noted to be malignant epithelial neoplasms, usually adenocarcinomas, but occasionally with an undifferentiated or even epidermoid appearance. The diagnosis of malignant mixed tumor depends on the presence of areas of myxomatous or chondroid tissue resembling a benign mixed tumor.[7]

NATURAL HISTORY

The average age of patients with malignant mixed tumors is about 10 years older than those with benign mixed tumors. As is true of the benign lesions this neoplasm is more common in females. The typical history is that of a sudden change in a long-standing, slow-growing salivary mass with rapid growth and frequently pain. A similar change may occur in a known benign mixed tumor with several recurrences over a period of years. Less often the tumor may appear de novo as a rapidly growing painful mass. The tumors are bulky, irregular rather than rounded, and often fixed to adjacent structures. Ulceration of overlying skin or mucosa may occur, and there is often facial nerve weakness when the parotid is involved. These tumors are among the more aggressive of the salivary neoplasms with early recurrence and a high incidence of distant metastasis. While cervical node metastases may occur, vascular spread to the lungs and bone is far more common.

Mucoepidermoid Carcinoma

Mucoepidermoid carcinoma is a distinct type of salivary neoplasm which may involve the major or minor salivary glands. It comprises about 10 percent of all salivary tumors. Mucoepidermoid carcinomas are divided into several groups on the basis of their histologic appearance and clinical behavior. Some separate them into "low-grade" and "high-grade" tumors while others add an "intermediate" group.[8,9]

PATHOLOGY

Low-grade mucoepidermoid tumors are generally small, encapsulated masses arising in a salivary gland. The cut surface is soft and often cystic. The higher-grade tumors are bulky, unencapsulated infiltrative tumors which appear clearly malignant. The tumors are characteristically composed of several cell types: mucus-secreting cells, epidermoid cells, and intermediate cell types. In the low-grade lesions the mucus-secreting cells predominate with pools of mucus, areas of fibrosis, and a histologic appearance often more of inflammation than neoplasia. In the higher-grade tumors the epidermoid and intermediate cells predominate, with a poorly differentiated and highly malignant appearance, and mucus-secreting cells may be rare.

NATURAL HISTORY

The low-grade mucoepidermoid carcinomas have a clinical presentation similar to benign mixed tumors. They are among the most common epithelial salivary neoplasms in children. The tumors are slow-growing and generally encapsulated. While they are capable of recurrence and metastasis, these events are rare and the prognosis is generally excellent. In contrast, there is seldom clinical doubt as to the malignant nature of the high-grade tumors. These are rapidly growing, often painful neoplasms which invade adjacent structures and metastasize early to cervical lymph nodes as well as to distant sites.

Adenoid Cystic Carcinoma

Adenoid cystic carcinoma or cylindroma arises in both major and minor salivary glands. While it comprises only about 10 percent of all salivary tissue neoplasms, it is one of the more common malignant lesions of minor salivary glands. This tumor has generally been considered to have a slow growth rate. A clinicopathological review of our material, however, has indicated a group of these tumors with an aggressive behavior which might be considered "high-grade," contrasted with others which fall into a "low-grade" group.[10] Eneroth[5] and others have confirmed this, and Conley has even suggested a third group of tumors of "intermediate-grade" malignancy.

PATHOLOGY

These tumors present as firm, rounded masses. On cut section the hard, yellow-white tissue appears unencapsulated and infiltrative. The most typical histologic appearance is of masses of small dark-staining cells surrounding cystic spaces, forming a cribriform pattern. The pattern is rather uniform and monotonous in the low-grade lesions, and the tumor margins appear blunt and "pushing" rather than infiltrative. In the more aggressive high-grade tumors, in addition to the cribriform pattern there are prominent sheets of malignant cells, often with central areas of necrosis and with irregular infiltrating tumor margins. Extension of tumor cells along perineural spaces is prominent in all these tumors.

NATURAL HISTORY

An asymptomatic lump or swelling is the presenting symptom in most cases, and the mass is often believed to be a benign salivary tumor. In the high-grade tumors, which comprise about one-fourth of all cases, local recurrence after aggressive surgical treatment is usually prompt and distant blood-borne metastases appear early. Death occurs within 2½ years in the majority of high-grade lesions. The low-grade tumors, on the other hand, have a protracted clinical course, and while recurrences and metastases may eventually appear, patients survive for many years with their tumors.

Acinic Cell Carcinomas

These are rare salivary tissue neoplasms which arise most commonly in the parotid. They are generally small, rounded tumors with a predominance of one cell type, usually resembling acinar cells of salivary tissue. Histologic criteria of malignancy may be difficult to find, but since recurrences and regional or distant metastases occur in over 10 percent of these tumors, they must all be classified as low-grade carcinomas.

Squamous Cell Carcinomas

These are uncommon tumors which arise in the parotid and submaxillary gland. They are highly malignant with rapid growth and early metastasis, most often to regional lymph nodes. The diagnosis of squamous cell carcinoma of salivary tissue, in the author's opinion, must be accepted with reservation. It is probable that some tumors previously placed in this category were in reality high-grade mucoepidermoid carcinomas with a predominant epidermoid pattern or carcinomas metastatic to salivary tissue from some other site.

Miscellaneous Adenocarcinomas

A small miscellaneous group of adenocarcinomas of salivary tissue are encountered which defy further classification. These vary from extremely anaplastic tumors to somewhat better differentiated forms with attempts at gland formation. They are generally rapidly growing aggressive lesions with predominantly vascular metastases and recurrences in spite of aggressive treatment.

Malignant Lymphomas

While malignant lymphomas are often omitted from lists of salivary neoplasms, the author's material includes 17 instances in which the first evidence of a malignant lymphoma was a mass presenting in the parotid or occasionally the submaxillary gland. While at times it can be demonstrated that the malignant process originated in a node lying within or upon the parotid, on other occasions there is only a diffuse infiltration of the gland by malignant lymphocytic tissue. Others have noted this origin of malignant lymphomas in the parotid and also emphasized that lymphomas may supervene on benign lymphoepithelial lesions of the parotid or Sjögren's syndrome. All varieties of the malignant lymphomas, including Hodgkin's disease, have been reported.[11]

Metastatic Carcinoma

Lymph nodes lying within and upon the parotid or adjacent to the submaxillary gland may be the site of metastatic carcinoma, and the clinical presentation may resemble a primary salivary gland tumor. The primary tumors metastasizing to the parotid region are most often squamous cell carcinomas or malignant melanomas of the face or scalp.[12,13] Tumors spreading to nodes lying upon the submaxillary gland usually arise from the lower part of the face, the lips, and anterior oral cavity.

Mesenchymal Tumors

Lymphangiomas, hemangiomas, and hemangioendotheliomas are among the most common parotid lesions of infants and children. Lipomas within the parotid are occasionally encountered; they are usually mistaken for a benign salivary tissue tumor or cyst. The author has treated one neurofibroma diffusely involving the parotid as well as two neurilemmomas arising from the facial nerve. Malignant mesenchymal tumors of the parotid are rare, but malignant fibrous tissue tumors have been noted, and one primary liposarcoma has been encountered.

Benign Lymphoepithelial Lesion

Benign lymphoepithelial lesion is a term proposed by Godwin[14] to designate an uncommon salivary lesion which in the past has been called Mikulicz's disease. The latter term has been confused with Mikulicz's syndrome, an enlargement of salivary and lacrimal glands which may occur in the course of leukemia, lymphomas, Boeck's sarcoid, and tuberculosis. It seems most likely that a benign lymphoepithelial lesion should be classified as an autoimmune process rather than a neoplasm.

PATHOLOGY

Benign lymphoepithelial lesions may present as a poorly circumscribed salivary gland mass or more often as diffuse swelling of one or more salivary glands. Histologically there is diffuse infiltration of lymphocytes, occasionally arranged in follicles, with disappearance of normal salivary tissue except for small islands containing epithelial and myoepithelial cells arranged in a ductlike pattern.

NATURAL HISTORY

Benign lymphoepithelial lesions are generally encountered most often in middle-aged women. The parotid is most often involved but rarely the submaxillary gland is involved as well. Clinical findings are generally a diffuse firm swelling of one or more salivary glands; less often there is a discrete mass. There is usually a history of swelling of several years' duration with slow increase in size. Benign lymphoepithelial lesion is similar to, and probably identical to, Sjögren's syndrome, an antoimmune condition associated with rheumatoid arthritis, dry mouth and eyes, and other systemic manifestations. A number of reports of malignant lymphomas appearing in Sjögren's syndrome have been published.[15] The lymphomas may first appear in the parotid or in multiple sites.

DIAGNOSIS

The diagnosis of a salivary gland tumor can usually be made on the basis of the history and physical findings and the surgeon can often suspect a benign or a malignant tumor on clinical grounds. Radiologic aids to diagnosis are occasionally helpful. Exact histologic diagnosis, of course, must await biopsy or excision of the lesion.

Parotid Tumors

The typical benign parotid tumor presents as a painless mass usually located just anterior to or below the lobe of the ear. There is generally a history of several months or years prior to medical consultation with slow or imperceptible increase in size. On examination the mass is nontender and usually freely movable, with no attachment to the overlying skin or deeper structures. The mass may be firm, rubbery, or occasionally cystic in consistency. There is never evidence of facial nerve dysfunction. At times a small mass may seem to lie immediately beneath the skin and its parotid origin is not suspected by the inexperienced examiner.

Many of the malignant tumors of the parotid have a presentation similar to the above and are clinically indistinguishable from a benign mixed tumor. There are a number of findings, however, which suggest the presence of a malignant tumor.[16] Rapid growth of the mass is highly suspicious as is a change in the growth rate of a previous indolent mass. Pain is an ominous symptom suggesting nerve invasion, and weakness of muscle groups innervated by the facial nerve is almost conclusive of malignancy.[17] Invasion of branches of the greater auricular nerve may result in anesthesia of the lobe of the ear and areas of skin overlying the parotid. Impaired mobility or fixation of the tumor to the overlying skin, the mastoid process, or the mandible are also suspicious, as are palpably enlarged regional lymph nodes. The author has encountered two instances in which local pain and facial paralysis preceded a palpable mass; both were diagnosed as Bell's palsy and both proved later to be high-grade mucoepidermoid cancers.

DEEP-LOBE PAROTID TUMORS

By far the greatest number of parotid tumors arise in the superficial lobe of the gland. However, the small number which arise deep to the plane of the facial nerve are of particular interest. They may present clinically in one of three ways: (1) the tumor may bulge outward in the upper neck and over the angle of the mandible; (2) the tumor may present itself only in the pharynx; (3) the tumor may be visible and palpable both in the pharynx and externally in the neck.[18] Those neoplasms which present externally cannot be distinguished clinically from tumors of the superficial lobe of the gland, and the unusual location is discovered only at operation. While the facial nerve may be stretched far out of its usual course into a superficial position, no facial weakness has been noted in benign tumors of the deep lobe.

The retromandibular tumors are encountered as firm rounded masses in the lateral pharyngeal wall covered by intact mucosa. They usually lie superior to the tonsil and extend outward and upward into the soft palate and may reach as far as the midline before discovery. In one patient the tumor presented mainly in the lateral wall of the nasopharynx, where it caused unilateral deafness and only slight distortion of the soft palate. The usual complaint of a patient with a retromandibular parotid tumor is of a sense of fullness and discomfort in the throat. There may be slight dysphagia and change in the voice. The diagnosis may be quite obscure to one who is not familiar with this form of presentation of parotid neoplasm, particularly when no external component is palpable in the neck. In one patient the pharyngeal mass was thought to represent a peritonsillar abscess and was incised twice in a fruitless search for pus. Bimanual palpation through the pharyngeal wall and upper neck has been an aid to diagnosis. By this maneuver the continuity of the mass with the more superficial portion of the parotid can be demonstrated.

DIFFERENTIAL DIAGNOSIS OF PAROTID SWELLINGS

A number of conditions other than a primary tumor may result in diffuse enlargement of the parotid or even a localized mass. While these can usually be differentiated from a parotid tumor, surgical exposure is occasionally required for diagnosis.

Chronic parotitis with or without calculi, can generally be recognized by the recurrent nature of the attacks, by diffuse involvement of the gland, and signs of an inflammatory lesion. A calculus may be palpable in Stensen's duct. A sialogram points to the correct diagnosis.

Mikulicz's syndrome is a condition characterized by diffuse enlargement of one or more of the salivary glands and often the lacrimal glands. It occurs rarely during the course of leukemia, malignant lymphomas, sarcoidosis, tuberculosis, and syphilis.

Benign lymphoepithelial lesion (Mikulicz's disease) also most often presents as a diffuse swelling of one or more salivary glands. It is closely related or perhaps identical to Sjögren's syndrome.

Nonspecific and unexplained parotid enlargement may occur during the course of pellagra, beriberi, diabetes mellitus, and cirrhosis.[19] This swelling is usually bilateral and symmetrical; it is believed to be associated with endocrine abnormalities and disturbed carbohydrate metabolism.

Benign hypertrophy of the masseter muscle (phantom parotid) is occasionally mistaken for a parotid tumor and has even resulted in unnecessary surgery.[20] The swelling in the parotid region may be quite marked; its true nature is detected by having the patient clench the jaws while the area is palpated. It will be noted that the mass is in the muscle and little or no overlying parotid tissue can be felt. The masseteric hypertrophy is often due to a faulty bite on one side of the mouth with missing or poorly aligned teeth. It has also been noted in psychiatric patients and those who have the habit of clenching their jaws; in such patients the swelling may be bilateral.

A hyperplastic lymph node lying within or upon the surface of the parotid often cannot be differentiated from a small parotid tumor. Surgical exposure and even parotidectomy may be required for diagnosis. This condition is particularly common in children. A few weeks' observation of a questionable small parotid nodule in a child or young adult will often resolve the problem.

Metastatic carcinoma must always be considered in the evaluation of a parotid mass. Scars on the face or local atrophic skin changes from prior radiation may be a diagnostic clue. Complete head and neck examination and search for a primary tumor must be part of the evaluation of any parotid mass. Bulky tumors arising in the lower pole of the parotid and filling the upper neck are particularly difficult diagnostic problems. They must be differentiated from branchial cleft cysts and from metastatic carcinoma in the superior deep cervical nodes.

Submaxillary Gland Tumors

A benign tumor of the submaxillary gland presents as a firm rounded mass below the body of the mandible extending downward in the neck. The tumor is painless and extremely slow in its growth. Bimanual palpation with one finger in the floor of the mouth and the other hand on the external surface is most useful in determining the extent of the tumor as well as confirming its origin in the submaxillary gland. As in parotid tumors, malignancy is suggested by pain, rapid growth, and extension to surrounding structures.[21] While the submaxillary gland is in close relation to the lingual and hypoglossal nerves as well as the mandibular branch of the facial nerve, impairment of nerve function is seldom seen in untreated malignant tumors.

Sialadenitis is the most common cause of swelling of the submaxillary gland and must be differentiated from a tumor. It presents as a diffuse enlargement of the entire gland usually with signs of inflammation. Submaxillary calculi are often the cause of the process and may be palpable along the course of Wharton's duct or visible on roentgen studies. Metastatic carcinoma in nodes lying immediately adjacent to the submaxillary gland must also be considered in differential diagnosis. The history of prior removal of a lesion of the lip, skin of the face, or oral cavity should always arouse suspicion, and examination of these sites in search of a primary tumor must always be carried out.

Sublingual Gland Tumors

Neoplasms of the sublingual gland are quite rare. When benign they appear as painless, slow-growing masses in the floor of the mouth covered by intact mucosa. Malignant tumors, in addition to their more rapid evolution, tend to invade and ulcerate the mucosa with resulting pain and infection. Involvement of the adjacent tongue and mandible occurs with local progression. Benign tumors must be differentiated from ranulas, which are cystic swellings associated with obstruction of one of the sublingual ducts. Malignant lesions may be confused with the far more common squamous cell carcinomas arising in the mucosa of the floor of the mouth.

Minor Salivary Gland Tumors

The most characteristic location of a minor salivary gland tumor is in the palate, usually near the junction of the soft and hard palate.[22] Here a benign tumor presents as a painless rounded mass covered by intact mucosa. Malignant tumors are usually larger and frequently ulcerated. They may involve the adjacent bone and invade the maxillary sinus. Other relatively common sites of appearance of minor salivary gland tumors include the mucosa of the lips, the tongue (particularly its base), the pharyngeal wall, nasal cavity, and paranasal sinuses. Malignant tumors in all of these locations must be differentiated from squamous cell carinomas arising from the lining mucosa.

Biopsy

In many if not most cancers preliminary biopsy is essential before definitive therapy is undertaken. This step is certainly warranted for tumors of minor salivary glands and probably also the sublingual gland. Exceptions to this rule are frequently made, however, in dealing with neoplasms of the parotid and submaxillary glands. The main objection to biopsy is the danger of spreading tumor cells in the operative field. Salivary gland tumors are among the most easily implanted of neoplasms, and the author feels that the risk of recurrence following open biopsy is significant. It might be argued that the risk would be minimized by a needle aspiration biopsy, but even here there is a proven risk of tumor implantation in the needle tract unless it is encompassed by a later operation. The main disadvantage of needle biopsy, however, is that the specimen obtained is seldom large enough or representative enough for the pathologist to make an accurate histologic diagnosis.

The majority of benign and malignant neoplasms of the parotid are contained within one lobe of the gland and in the case of the submaxillary gland contained within its substance. When the tumor can be encompassed by the standard operative procedure, parotid lobectomy or total excision of the submaxillary gland, no preliminary biopsy seems necessary. In the author's opinion biopsy is indicated only when the clinical or operative findings suggest that a significant extension of the standard operative approach will become necessary. For example, if there is ulceration of the skin overlying a tumor or obvious tumor invasion of the skin, preliminary biopsy of this area is certainly justified. If a regional lymph node is palpably enlarged, it is wise to excise this at the time of surgery and to obtain a frozen-section diagnosis before proceeding. If a high suspicion of malignancy exists it is advisable during preliminary surgical exposure to look for nodes about the parotid and to perform excision biopsies and frozen sections on any nodes which appear enlarged. When there is clinical evidence of involvement of the facial, lingual, or hypoglossal nerves it is the author's practice to perform an open biopsy of the tumor with an immediate frozen section at the time of surgery. Even though nerve paralysis is not known to be caused by benign tumors, it seems wise to obtain histologic proof of malignancy before a nerve is irrevocably sacrificed. Likewise, during a standard operative approach if it becomes evident that a tumor extends to the nerve or surrounds it, the general rule must be broken and an open biopsy performed. On such occasions every precaution must be taken to avoid contaminating the wound with tumor cells. Precautions should include taking a small biopsy with a scalpel and discarding all instruments used, coagulation of the biopsy site with the electrocautery, and copious irrigation of the wound with saline or half-strength Dakin's solution at the conclusion of the operation.

Radiologic Aids to Diagnosis

In the usual clearly evident localized tumor of a major salivary gland no roentgen studies are indicated other than a routine chest x-ray. On other occasions specific radiologic techniques play an important part in pretreatment evaluation. They are particularly useful in the study of more advanced or recurrent tumors, of many lesions of the minor salivary glands, and of certain diagnostic problems which arise.

Suspected bone invasion can often be confirmed by plain films or tomograms. Invasion of the hard palate by minor salivary gland tumors is of particular importance and may be noted on studies of the palate and views of the paranasal sinuses. Soft-tissue films including xeroradiographs are useful in determining the extent of certain tumors, particularly minor salivary gland tumors of the soft palate, base of tongue, or pharyngeal wall. Computerized tomography is also proving to be an important aid in determining tumor extent, particularly in the evaluation of bulky or recurrent malignant tumors in less accessible locations. CT scans have proved useful in studying tumor involvement of the pterygoid space or the base of the skull.

The place of sialography in the evaluation of tumors of the parotid and submaxillary glands remains somewhat controversial. Displacement of ducts by tumors within the gland can certainly be demonstrated by a sialogram, but this technique seems unnecessary for most obvious tumors. The sialogram may disclose displacement of the entire gland by an adjacent mass, and this is of occasional value in differentiating a submandibular mass from a submaxillary tumor.[23] The main use for sialography is in the differentiation of chronic sialadenitis from other cases of diffuse salivary gland enlargement. The cystic dilatation of ducts noted with inflammatory lesions is usually diagnostic. Calculi frequently associated with sialadenitis can be demonstrated on conventional radiographs or by the use of dental films.

Warthin's tumors, alone among primary salivary gland neoplasms, have an affinity for the radioisotope technetium pertechnate, and an isotope scan will confirm the presence of this tumor. This study is occasionally valuable in the evaluation of a mass which appears to be located either in the lower pole of the parotid or the upper cervical region.

CLINICAL STAGING

The Task Force on Salivary Glands of the American Joint Committee for Cancer Staging and End-Results Reporting has recently completed an extensive retrospective survey of over 800 malignant tumors of the major salivary glands.[24] Numerous demographic variables and clinical findings as well as histologic diagnoses were analyzed in the light of survival rates after tumor-directed therapy. A simplified TNM staging system has been recommended which appears to be statistically valid.

A number of characteristics of the primary tumor were found to be of significance including its histologic diagnosis, cellular differentiation, size, degree of fixation or local extension, and nerve involvement.

It was found that the prognosis was principally related to the size of the tumor and any significant local extension to the overlying skin, soft tissues, bone, or the facial or lingual nerves. The following T categories relating to the primary tumor were recommended:

T_0 No evidence of primary tumor
T_1 Tumor 2.0 cm or less in diameter without significant local extension
T_2 Tumor more than 2.0 cm but not more than 4.0 cm in diameter without significant local extension
T_3 Tumor more than 4.0 cm but not more than 6.0 cm in diameter without significant local extension
T_{4a} Tumor over 6.0 cm in diameter without significant local extension
T_{4b} Tumor of any size with significant local extension

On a similar analysis of regional nodes palpable and suspicious of containing metastases a number of factors were of significance, including degree of fixation, number of nodes involved, and laterality. It was found, however, that node palpability alone was the major factor in prognosis and could be utilized without considering the other variables:

N_0 No evidence of regional node involvement
N_1 Evidence of regional node involvement

The definitions of the M factor are as follows:

M_0 No distant metastases
M_1 Distant metastases present

The stage grouping for salivary gland cancer based on the above clinical variables is listed in Table 19-2. The 5-year survival rate for each stage indicates the validity of this simple system in which only tumor size, lymph node palpability, and distant metastases are considered.

An important recommendation of this and other task forces of the American Joint Committee was that uniform data collection forms be utilized in the clinical records of patients with salivary gland cancer. This will be of inestimable value in future collection of end results and avoid the difficulties encountered in this and other retrospective surveys. The suggested data collection form or checklist is illustrated in Fig. 19-1.

TREATMENT

The treatment of salivary gland tumors is primarily surgical. Radiation therapy, however, is playing an increasingly important role as an adjuvant to surgery and for palliation of advancing disease. The most commonly

TABLE 19-2 Stage Grouping in Salivary Cancer*

Stage	TNM set	No. of patients	5-Year survival probability, %	SE, %
Stage I	$T_1N_0M_0$	136	90.1	2.6
	$T_2N_0M_0$	151	85.9	2.9
	Overall	287	87.9	2.0
Stage II	$T_3N_0M_0$	51	56.9	6.9
Stage III	$T_1N_1M_0$	4		
	$T_2N_1M_0$	16	0	0
	$T_{4a}N_0M_0$	30	40.2	9.3
	$T_{4b}N_0M_0$	106	45.2	4.9
	Overall	156	39.4	4.0
Stage IV	$T_3N_1M_0$	8		
	$T_{4a}N_1M_0$	12	17.7	10.8
	$T_{4b}N_1M_0$	38	7.9	4.4
	Any T, any N, M_1	8		
	Overall	66	9.1	3.5

* Staging system proposed by the Task Force on Salivary Glands, American Joint Committee for Cancer Staging and End-Results Reporting, 1980.

seen well-localized primary tumors are managed by standard operative techniques which have been widely described. Advanced and recurrent tumors require more extensive and often unorthodox approaches which may tax the ingenuity of the most experienced surgeon.

Parotid Tumors

The most frequently observed parotid tumor which appears to be confined to the superficial lobe of the gland is managed by resection of this lobe of the gland (Fig. 19-2). It is the author's conviction that this operation is entirely adequate if the tumor can be removed intact with a surrounding rim of uninvolved salivary tissue. The essential element in this procedure is, of course, identification and protection of the facial nerve and its branches.[25] Most commonly the main trunk of the nerve is identified close to its exit from the stylomastoid foramen; it is followed distally, preserving its two major divisions and their branches as the overlying superficial parotid lobe is removed. Some surgeons prefer first to isolate a peripheral branch of the nerve, usually the marginal mandibular, and follow it proximally to accomplish the same result. Various technical aids to dissection have been reported and advocated. These include the use of an electrical nerve stimulator, the preliminary injection of Stensen's duct with methylene blue dye, and the local infiltration of vasoconstrictors. It is the author's opinion that these measures are superfluous for the experienced surgeon, who is an expert in locating and protecting the nerve.

TOTAL PAROTIDECTOMY

When a tumor arises deep to the plane of the facial nerve or involves both lobes of the gland, a total parotidectomy is performed. The superficial lobe is mobilized in the usual manner, isolating and preserving the facial nerve and its branches. If the tumor is confined to the deep lobe it is simpler to completely remove the superficial lobe as a preliminary step. The nerve and its branches are then gently elevated from the underlying parotid tissue and retracted superiorly or inferiorly. The termination of the external carotid artery is divided and ligated below the inferior pole of the gland. Dissection is then carried behind the ramus of the mandible to mobilize the deep portion of the parotid, delivering it above or below the main trunk of the nerve. If the tumor involves both lobes of the gland without compromising the facial nerve, a total parotidectomy is carried out as a monobloc procedure, retracting the nerve or its branches to allow removal of the intact tumor mass. Various techniques have been described for removal of the bulky tumor of the deep parotid lobe filling the parapharyngeal space. These include an oral or a submandibular approach and even division of the mandible just anterior to its angle. The author prefers the standard parotid approach, first performing a superficial lobectomy and then delivering the deep-lobe tumor downward in the neck beneath the retracted facial nerve (Fig. 19-3).

RADICAL PAROTIDECTOMY

Malignant tumors of the parotid, with the exception of those which can be removed by superficial lobectomy, require a more extensive procedure. Any tissues which are grossly involved by contiguity or extension of the neoplasm must be sacrificed. At times this involves wide excision of the overlying skin or the underlying masseter and digastric muscles and even portions of the mandible and cartilaginous auditory canal. With many bulky malignant tumors, no attempt is made to preserve the facial nerve; it is severed at the stylomastoid foramen. Less extensive tumors may occasionally justify the attempt to preserve one or more uninvolved nerve branches. If

SITE-SPECIFIC INFORMATION — SALIVARY GLANDS

Location of Tumor
    Parotid   _____
    Submaxillary   _____
    Sublingual   _____
    Side
        Right   _____
        Left   _____
        Bilateral   _____

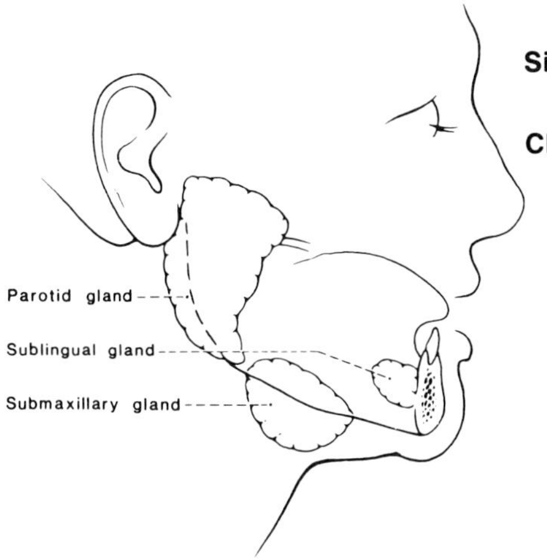

Size of Tumor
    Largest diameter   _____ cm

Characteristics of Tumor
    Mobile   _____
    Limited mobility   _____
    Fixed   _____
    Hard   _____
    Soft   _____
    Cystic   _____
    Adjacent tissues involved   No _____   Yes _____
    Nerve involvement
        None   _____
        Facial   _____
        Hypoglossal   _____
        Lingual   _____
        Vagus   _____
        Other _____
        Partial paralysis   _____
        Complete paralysis   _____

Regional Lymph Nodes (check one only)
    NX _____
    N0 _____
    N1 _____

Distant Metastasis
    MX _____ M0 _____ M1 _____ Specify _____
    Sites: Lung _____ Bone _____ Liver _____ Other _____

Classification
    T _____   N _____   M _____

Residual Tumor
    R _____

Host — Performance Status (H)
    H _____ Scale used: AJC _____ Zubrod _____ Karnofsky _____

*cTNM, clinical-diagnostic; sTNM, surgical-evaluative; pTNM, postsurgical treatment-pathologic; rTNM, retreatment; aTNM, autopsy.

FIGURE 19-1 Data collection sheet for salivary gland neoplasms. (*From Manual for Staging of Cancer, American Joint Committee for Cancer Staging and End-Results Reporting, 1978.*)

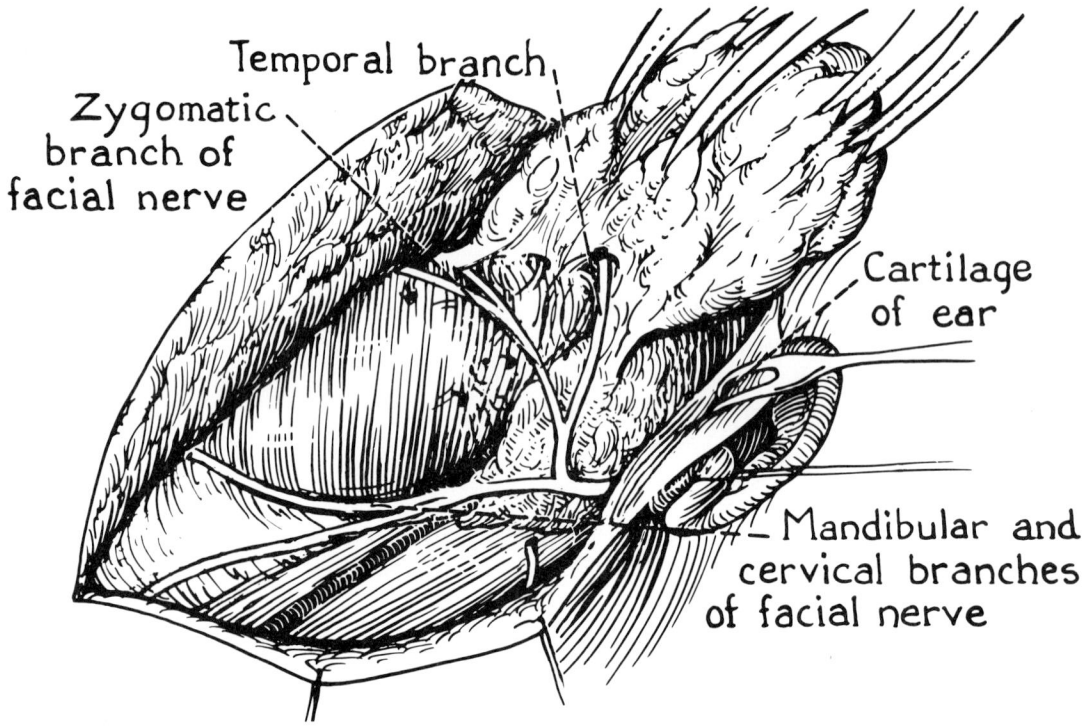

FIGURE 19-2 Superficial parotid lobectomy being completed for tumor confined to superficial lobe of the gland. (*From RA Wise, HW Baker: Surgery of the Head and Neck, ed 3, Chicago, Year Book Medical, 1968.*)

there is clinical evidence of cervical lymph node metastasis, a radical neck dissection is performed at the time of parotidectomy. An elective neck dissection is not performed for most parotid neoplasms. It may well be justified, however, for squamous cell carcinomas and high-grade mucoepidermoid carcinomas because of their propensity for lymphatic spread.

METASTATIC CARCINOMA

An elective parotidectomy is performed as part of a regional lymph node dissection for deeply invasive malignant melanomas of the face, temporal region, ear, or scalp (see section on melanomas for indications for node dissection). A similar elective procedure is indicated for a deeply invasive squamous cell carcinoma arising in the skin of the parotid region. The author believes that a superficial parotid lobectomy is adequate for these elective or prophylactic operations. However, when there is clinical evidence of metastasis to the parotid a total parotidectomy must be performed. The lymph nodes overlying or contained within the superficial lobe act as a primary drainage site for skin neoplasms in this region. With clinical metastasis to these superficial nodes one cannot neglect the nodes in the deep lobe and these too must be removed, usually in conjunction with a radical neck dissection.

RECURRENT PAROTID TUMORS

Recurrences of both benign and malignant parotid tumors are managed surgically although adjuvant radiation therapy may play an important role (see below). In the case of recurrent cancer all possible measures must be taken prior to surgery to determine the local extent of the tumor as well as the presence of distant metastases.

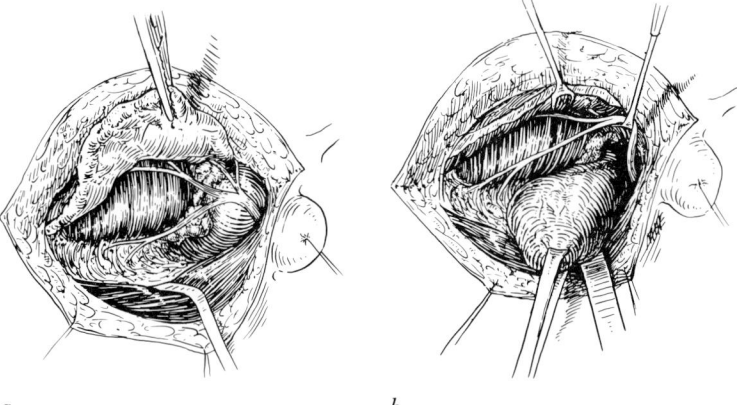

FIGURE 19-3 (*a*) Superficial lobectomy being completed prior to removal of deep lobe parotid tumor. (*b*) Elevation of facial nerve and delivery of deep lobe. (*From RA Wise, HW Baker: Surgery of the Head and Neck, ed 3, Chicago, Year Book Medical, 1968.*)

Recurrent benign mixed tumors present as a single nodule or, more often, as multiple nodules in the previous operative field, with frequent involvement of the overlying skin. In surgical removal the facial nerve and its branches must be identified in the dense scar tissue and preserved if not grossly involved by tumor. It is occasionally necessary to excise segments of nerve to adequately encompass tumor nodules.

Recurrent malignant tumors when localized require radical surgical procedures for their adequate removal. Wide areas of skin must be excised as well as portions of the mandible and the mastoid process. Part or all of the external ear may be sacrificed in addition to the external auditory canal. On some occasions temporal bone resection will allow a complete bloc excision of the recurrent carcinoma. After many of the procedures necessary for recurrent cancer, repair must be accomplished with pedicle flaps of skin from the scalp, the forehead, or the deltopectoral region. Free skin flaps with microvascular anastomoses have also been found useful.

Facial Nerve Injury and Repair   The implications of the facial nerve traversing the operative field must always be discussed with the patient in obtaining informed consent for parotid gland surgery. In experienced hands there should be no permanent facial paralysis after parotidectomy for a primary benign tumor. In approximately 10 percent of superficial parotid lobectomies and 40 percent of total parotidectomies some transient paralysis of muscle groups innervated by the facial nerve is noted in the postoperative period. This is most often manifested by weakness of the corner of the lower lip. If it has been ascertained that the nerve and its branches are intact at the conclusion of the operation, the surgeon can predict with confidence that functional recovery will occur within a 3-month period.

Approximately 10 percent of patients with malignant tumors of the parotid will present with some impairment of facial function, and in another 10 percent the nerve will be found to be grossly involved by tumor or uncomfortably close to it at operation. In these circumstances the facial nerve or its major divisions and branches must be resected. In view of the propensity for extension of salivary tumors proximally and distally along perineural spaces it is generally advisable to remove a long segment of nerve. Frequently the main trunk of the nerve is divided at the stylomastoid foramen or even within its bony canal. Less often a segment of the nerve or a major branch is removed.

Great strides are presently being made in facial rehabilitation by improved microsurgical techniques and increased understanding of muscle reinnervation. When a segment of nerve has been removed immediate repair should be carried out with a free graft of the greater auricular nerve using magnification and fine perineural sutures.[26,27] The extent of resection of the main trunk of the nerve often precludes a free graft. The older procedures of anastomosing the hypoglossal or spinal accessory nerve to the facial have been abandoned by the author since the results have been unsatisfactory. A tarsorrhaphy is performed to prevent the lower eyelid from sagging, and the patient's face is later supported with suspensory strips of fascia to achieve at least resting symmetry. A small number of patients will undergo spontaneous recovery of facial function. It is unsettled whether this is due to regrowth of filaments from the stump of the facial nerve or to innervation from the trigeminal. It is probable that both mechanisms may occur as well as some cross-innervation from the contralateral facial nerve. Reinnervation by small pedicles of innervated muscle is an exciting development.[28] The masseter muscle is ideal for this, and some have even suggested suturing the posterior borders of facial muscles to the bared masseter.

Submaxillary Gland Tumors

Masses in the submaxillary gland are managed surgically by dissection of the digastric triangle of the neck with total excision of the gland. This operation is accomplished through a submandibular incision; as skin flaps are elevated the mandibular branch of the facial nerve is identified and preserved. As the submaxillary gland with adjacent lymph nodes is removed it is freed from the lingual nerve coarsing superiorly and elevated away from the hypoglossal nerve on the hyoglossus muscle. Wharton's duct is divided far anteriorly beneath the mylohyoid (Fig. 19-4).

The above procedure is adequate for benign submaxillary tumors as well as malignant lesions confined to the gland. More aggressive carcinomas which have broken through the capsule of the gland and recurrent cancers require a more radical approach. Skin, soft tissues, and nerves must be resected widely, and removal of part or all of the body of the mandible may be required as well. A radical neck dissection should accompany the local procedure when there is clinical evidence of cervical node metastasis or when frozen sections of nodes adjacent to the gland reveal metastatic tumor. In all reported series of salivary gland carcinomas, the prognosis for tumors arising in the submaxillary gland is distinctly worse than for similar tumors of the parotid. Knowledge of this should encourage the surgeon to be more aggressive in managing submaxillary gland tumors

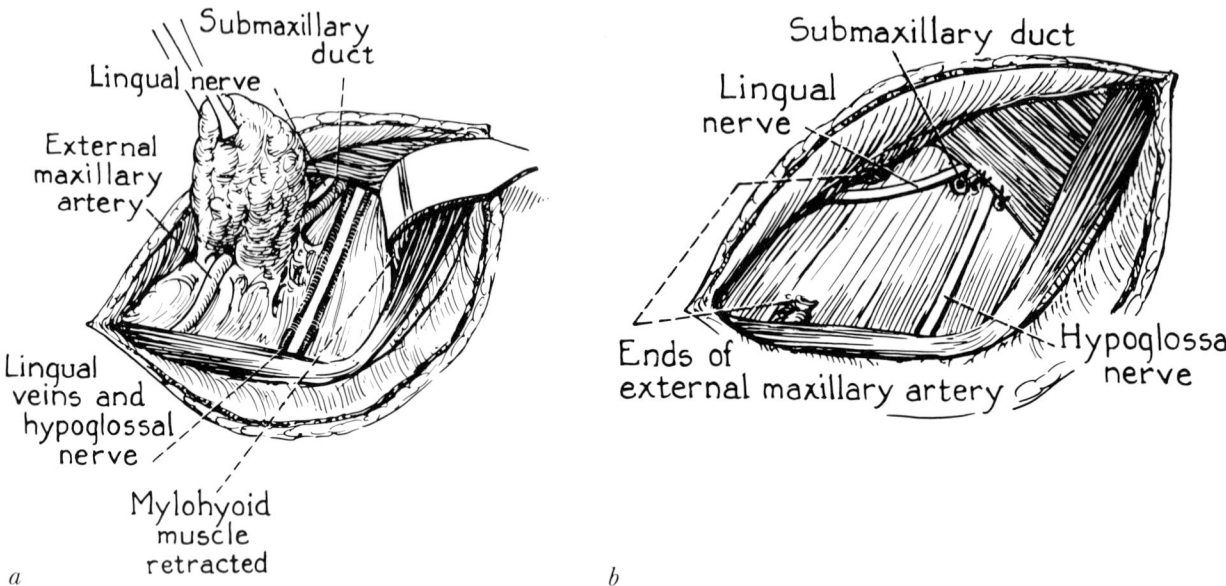

FIGURE 19-4 (*a*) Dissection of right digastric triangle for tumor of the submaxillary gland. (*b*) Dissection completed. (*From RA Wise, HW Baker: Surgery of the Head and Neck, ed 3, Chicago, Year Book Medical, 1968.*)

and to sacrifice suspiciously involved adjacent structures without hesitation.

Sublingual Gland Tumors

Benign tumors of the sublingual gland are managed by transoral excision of the gland. Malignant tumors which have ulcerated through the overlying mucosa require more extensive operative procedures similar in scope to those for the more common cancers of the floor of the mouth or tongue.

Minor Salivary Gland Tumors

When biopsy discloses a salivary tissue of the upper air or food passages the lesion must be surgically removed. The approach varies with the location and extent of the tumor as well as its histologic appearance. Benign mixed tumors, other adenomas, and low-grade mucoepidermoid carcinomas are locally excised with a small rim of surrounding tissue. In the common location in the hard palate, local removal with curettage of the underlying bone is generally adequate. Malignant tumors of the palate require a wide excision of bone; if the tumor has invaded the maxillary sinus a maxillary resection is indicated. Malignant minor salivary gland tumors in other locations are managed according to the same surgical principles governing the resection of the more common squamous cell carcinomas in such sites.

Radiation Therapy

Radiotherapy has its more definitive place in the management of malignant lymphomas which arise in lymph nodes within or adjacent to the parotid or submaxillary glands. When the diagnosis of lymphoma has been made by surgical excision or biopsy, a search for other foci of tumor should be made by appropriate staging measures, including bone marrow biopsies and abdominal lymphangiograms. If the tumor appears localized, irradiation is given to the primary site and usually the entire ipsilateral neck, with the administration of a dose of 3500 to 4000 rads in approximately 4 weeks.

While epithelial lesions of salivary tissue were at one time thought to be quite radioresistant, this is no longer considered valid and certain tumors have been found to be quite responsive. Radiation plays its most important role as an adjuvant to surgery when the bulk of a tumor has been removed but the risk of recurrence is significant. Even benign mixed tumors show a response to radiation, and postoperative therapy is indicated following surgical treatment of a recurrent mixed tumor in which numerous nodules are found scattered widely in the previous scar. Postoperative radiation therapy is similarly indicated following surgical removal of any high-grade malignant salivary gland tumor. There is increasing evidence that this is useful in preventing local recurrence and is far more effective than deferring radiation until gross recurrence appears. Therapy is usually given with megavoltage equipment in a full cancericidal dose of 5500 to 6000 rads in $5\frac{1}{2}$ to 6 weeks.

The most radiosensitive of the malignant salivary tumors are adenoid cystic carcinomas and mucoepidermoid carcinomas. While other neoplasms are more resistant their response is not entirely predictable, and a trial of radiation is indicated for palliation of any nonresectable recurrent malignant tumor.

Chemotherapy

At present no clinically useful regimen of chemotherapy exists for the management of malignant epithelial tumors of salivary tissue. Trials with several combinations of drugs have produced temporary partial responses in some advanced lesions, but the effects have been quite transient and of limited value. Further clinical trials with newer agents are needed. If useful drug combinations for advanced or disseminated salivary cancer can be developed, their use as an adjuvant to surgery to destroy distant undetected micrometastases will be justified.

PROGNOSIS

The prognosis for permanent cure of benign parotid tumors following adequate surgery is excellent. The recurrence rate of benign mixed tumors was formerly reported to be as high as 40 percent following enucleation. Most present-day series report a recurrence rate of less than 5 percent following parotidectomy. In the author's personal series there have been three recurrences in a group of over 150 primary benign mixed tumors followed for up to 25 years. There have been five recurrences in a group of 21 recurrent mixed tumors operated on one or more times previously.

The prognosis for malignant salivary gland tumors varies considerably with the histologic type and the site of origin. Survival rates for malignant parotid neoplasms are significantly better than for those arising in the submaxillary salivary gland. Patients with malignant tumors of minor salivary glands in the oral cavity also have a more favorable prognosis than those with submaxillary tumors. Minor salivary gland neoplasms in less accessible locations (nasal cavity, paranasal sinuses, hypopharynx) have the poorest prognosis.

The prognosis is also affected by a number of other important factors, regardless of the histologic type. The following ominous findings are generally associated with a poor outcome: (1) gross nerve invasion or the presence of perineural extension of tumor cells on microscopy; (2) invasion of periglandular soft tissues; (3) an aggressive histologic grade of any given tumor type; (4) regional lymph node metastases.

Five-year survival figures do not give an accurate portrayal of the ultimate prognosis of many salivary gland neoplasms, particularly those classified as low-grade. There is a continued drop-off for years after the traditional 5-year milestone. For example, while 40 percent or more of patients with adenoid cystic carcinoma may appear free of disease in 5 years, less than 30 percent will be controlled at 10 years, and there is a continued loss even beyond the 15-year period.

Following adequate surgical therapy the recurrence rate for acinic cell carcinomas and low-grade mucoepidermoid carcinomas is less than 15 percent. The more aggressive tumors have a distinctly less favorable prognosis. Malignant mixed tumors have an overall control rate of less than 50 percent, and fewer than 30 percent of the high-grade mucoepidermoid carcinomas are controlled by therapy. Success in management of the unclassified adenocarcinomas and squamous cell carcinomas is also poor with survival rates of 20 percent or less cited in most reports. Early results from the combined use of surgical excision with postoperative radiation of these aggressive neoplasms are encouraging and suggest that some improvement in their prognosis can be expected.

REFERENCES

1. Batsakis JG, Regezi JA: The pathology of head and neck tumors: Salivary glands, part 1. *Head Neck Surg* 1:59, 1978.
2. Batsakis, JG, Regezi JA: The pathology of head and neck tumors: Salivary glands, part 2. *Head Neck Surg* 1:167, 1978.
3. Svelstad JA et al: Irradiation induced polyglandular neoplasms of the head and neck. *Am J Surg* 135:820, 1978.
4. Foote FW Jr, Frazell EL: Tumors of the major salivary glands. *Atlas of Tumor Pathology*, sec IV, fasc II, Armed Forces Institute of Pathology, Washington, DC, 1954.
5. Eneroth CM: Incidence and prognosis of salivary gland tumors at different sites. *Acta Otolaryngol* 263:174, 1970.
6. Ryan RE et al: Cellular mixed tumors of the salivary glands. *Arch Otolaryngol* 104:451, 1978.
7. Batsakis JG, Regezi JA: The pathology of head and neck tumors: Salivary glands, part 3. *Head & Neck Surg* 1:260, 1979.
8. Connell HC, Evans JC: Mucoepidermoid carcinoma of the salivary gland. *Am J Surg* 124:519, 1972.
9. Spiro RH et al: Mucoepidermoid carcinoma of salivary gland origin. *Cancer* 132:461, 1978.
10. Eby LS et al: Adenoid cystic carcinoma of the head and neck. *Cancer* 29:1160, 1972.
11. Morgan WS, Castleman B: A clinicopathologic study of "Mikulicz's disease." *Am J Pathol* 29:471, 1953.
12. Conley JJ, Arena S: Parotid gland as a focus of metastasis. *Arch Otolaryngol* 87:69, 1963.
13. Cassisi NJ et al: Squamous cell carcinoma of the skin metastatic to parotid nodes. *Arch Otolaryngol* 104:336, 1978.
14. Godwin JT: Benign lymphoepithelial lesion of the parotid gland. *Cancer* 5:10089, 1952.
15. Lichtenfeld JL et al: Familial Sjögren's syndrome with associated primary salivary gland lymphoma. *Am J Med* 60:286, 1976.
16. Spiro RH et al: Cancer of the parotid gland: A clinicopathologic study of 288 primary cases. *Am J Surg* 130:452, 1975.
17. Eneroth CM: Facial nerve paralysis: A criterion of malignancy in parotid tumors. *Arch Octolaryngol* 95:300, 1972.
18. Wise RA, Baker HW: Tumors of the deep lobe of the parotid gland. *Am J Surg* 100:323, 1960.
19. Borsanyi S, Blanchard CL: Asymptomatic enlargement of the parotid glands. *JAMA* 174:102, 1960.
20. Barton RT: Benign masseteric hypertrophy. *JAMA* 164:1646, 1957.
21. Byers RM et al: Malignant tumors of the submaxillary gland. *Am J Surg* 126:458, 1973.
22. Chung CK et al: Malignant salivary gland tumors of the palate. *Arch Otolaryngol* 104:501, 1978.
23. White IL: Submandibular gland sialography in the differential diagnosis of lesions in the submandibular triangle. *Am J Surg* 126:539, 1974.
24. Levitt SH et al: Clinical staging system for cancer of the salivary gland. 1980.
25. Beahrs OH, Chong GC: Management of the facial nerve in parotid surgery. *Am J Surg* 124:473, 1972.
26. Conley, JJ: Facial nerve grafting. *Arch Otolaryngol* 73:322, 1961.
27. Kitamura T, et al: Extratemporal facial nerve surgery. *Arch Otolaryngol* 95:369, 1972.
28. Adour KK et al: Trigeminal neurotization of paralyzed facial musculature. *Arch Otolaryngol* 105:13, 1979.

20

TUMORS OF THE THYROID AND PARATHYROID

Arthur G. James   *William B. Farrar*   *Marc Cooperman*

Cancer of the thyroid gland is a comparatively rare disease. In the 1981 issue of *Facts and Figures,* The American Cancer Society estimated that a total of 9900 new cases of thyroid cancer would occur in the United States in 1981, 2800 in men and 7100 in women. It was also estimated that 1050 Americans would die of thyroid cancer in the same year.

Even though the incidence of thyroid cancer is low, in many instances the patient is a young woman and treatment is associated with much controversy and emotion. For example, papillary adenocarcinoma of the thyroid often occurs in young persons. The prognosis of this disease was known to be good, but because neck metastases were found in a majority of these patients,[1] the advocated treatment was radical operation, and the resulting deformity contributed to an emotional reaction in patients and their families. In 1970, Hutter et al.[2] established that the prognosis of patients with papillary cancer and clinically negative nodes was not altered by excision of the nodes, and therefore surgical procedures have become much more conservative.

BENIGN THYROID ENLARGEMENTS

Although any enlargement of the thyroid must be considered a possible indication of thyroid cancer, most enlargements are benign and are due to adenomas, goiters, or thyroiditis. These should be reviewed to provide a differential diagnosis with the malignant lesion.

Adenomas may be follicular (Fig. 20-1), papillary, Hürthle cell (Fig. 20-2), or fetal (Fig. 20-3). These may have been present for many years when they are first detected. There is some agreement that most thyroid cancers originate in a previously existing adenoma.[3,4]

Goiters may be toxic or nontoxic. The incidence of cancer in the toxic goiter is low, and this type will not be discussed further. Nontoxic goiter may be diffuse or nodular, and the nontoxic nodular goiter often must be considered in the differential diagnosis of thyroid cancer.

Patients with nodular goiter are still frequently seen by a surgeon, but very large goiters are not as common as they were 30 or 40 years ago. The incidence of cancer in patients with nontoxic multinodular adenomas has been reported to be 4 to 17 percent;[5] the incidence of solitary nodules is higher.[6] An autopsy study showed the incidence of cancer in patients with normal glands to be 2.1 percent.[7] Most surgeons agree that a patient with a cold, nontoxic thyroid nodule on scan, or a nodule which is increasing in size despite suppressive medication, should be investigated for cancer.

Thyroiditis may be acute, subacute (Fig. 20-4), or chronic. Suppuration occurs rarely, and only in the acute form is operation indicated. The chronic form with

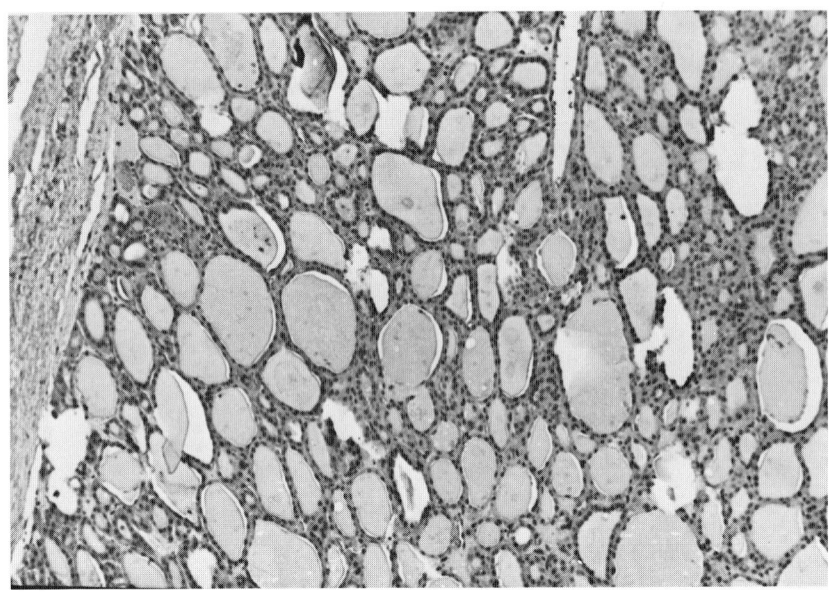

FIGURE 20-1 Follicular adenoma. The adenoma is composed of well-formed follicles and has a thick fibrous capsule. (H&E stain; 120×.)

dense fibrosis (Riedel's struma) is very rare, but occasionally operation to relieve compression symptoms is indicated. The severe subacute form usually responds to steroid therapy.

Hashimoto's disease is another form of chronic thyroiditis; it is also known as *struma lymphomatosa* because of the diffuse infiltration of lymphocytes noted on microscopic sections (Fig. 20-5). This disease most often occurs in women, usually involves both lobes, and is often accompanied by hypothyroidism. Most patients can be treated by medical management. Aspiration biopsy has been suggested by some surgeons as a method

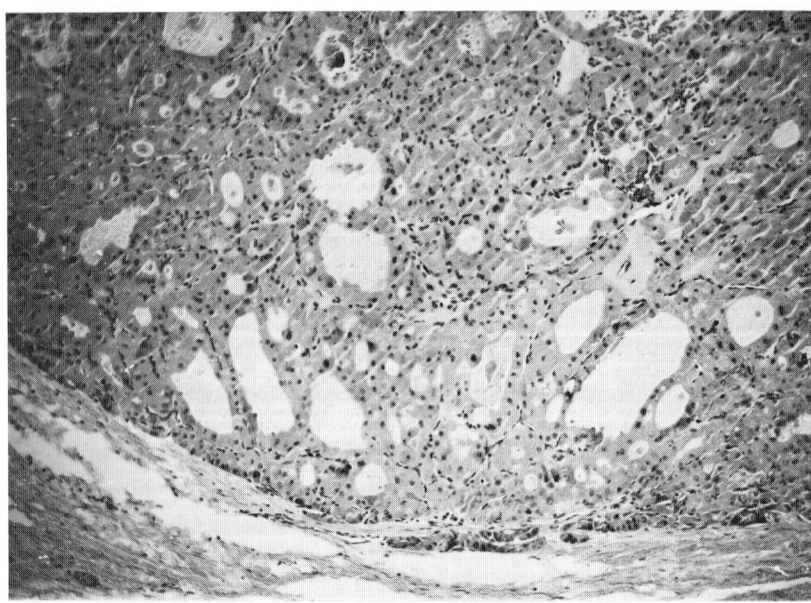

FIGURE 20-2 Hurthle cell adenoma. The adenoma is well demarcated. The cells show abundant eosinophilic cytoplasm and are arranged in solid nests and cords as well as follicles. (H&E stain; 120×.)

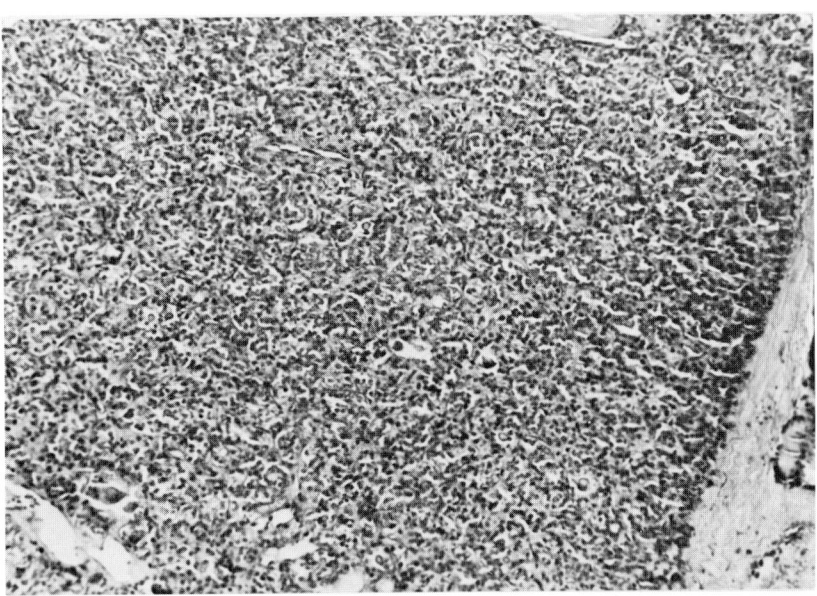

FIGURE 20-3 Fetal adenoma. The adenoma is composed of small cells arranged in nests. There is minimal colloid formation. (H&E stain; 120×.)

of diagnosis. Occasionally, this disease is associated with nodular goiter that does not regress on treatment or forms a mass that is clinically suggestive of cancer. Surgical resection is indicated in these circumstances.

CLASSIFICATION OF MALIGNANT TUMORS

Carcinoma of the thyroid gland may fall into one of the following categories:

1. Papillary
2. Follicular
3. Anaplastic
4. Medullary
5. Hürthle cell

The most commonly occurring thyroid cancer is papillary; the next most common type is follicular. Anaplastic cancers are rare. Medullary and Hürthle cell cancer occur even more rarely. However, if one or two families with medullary cancer are being treated at one institution, many cases of the disease may be reported from that institution.

Papillary Carcinoma

Papillary carcinoma may occur in either sex but has a higher incidence in the female. It is the most frequently occurring thyroid cancer in the young, but may occur at any age. As age increases, risk of death from thyroid cancer also increases in both sexes.

Physical findings that suggest a serious prognosis are recurrent laryngeal nerve paralysis, primary tumors greater than 5 cm in diameter, and the presence of pulmonary metastases. Microscopically, this type of cancer is characterized by a papillary structure lined by malignant cells of uniform size (Fig. 20-6). In many, a small amount of follicular structure is also present. The stroma is composed of thin, vascularized fibrous connective tissue. Papillary carcinoma is usually an unencapsulated tumor, sharply demarcated from thyroid parenchyma, which is usually grossly and histologically normal. It may be multicentric and may involve both lobes.[8]

Hazard and Hawk classified the histologic types of papillary carcinomas as principally follicular, mixed papillary and follicular, those with solid areas, and those composed of "tall" cells.[9] Commonest are the mixed forms composed of nearly equal portions of papillary and follicular areas.

According to Thompson et al., the histologic subtype of papillary carcinoma has no effect on the life expectancy of patients, even when seemingly ominous solid or squamous areas are present. The prognosis for the "tall" cell subtype is worse.

The size of the papillary carcinoma influences the

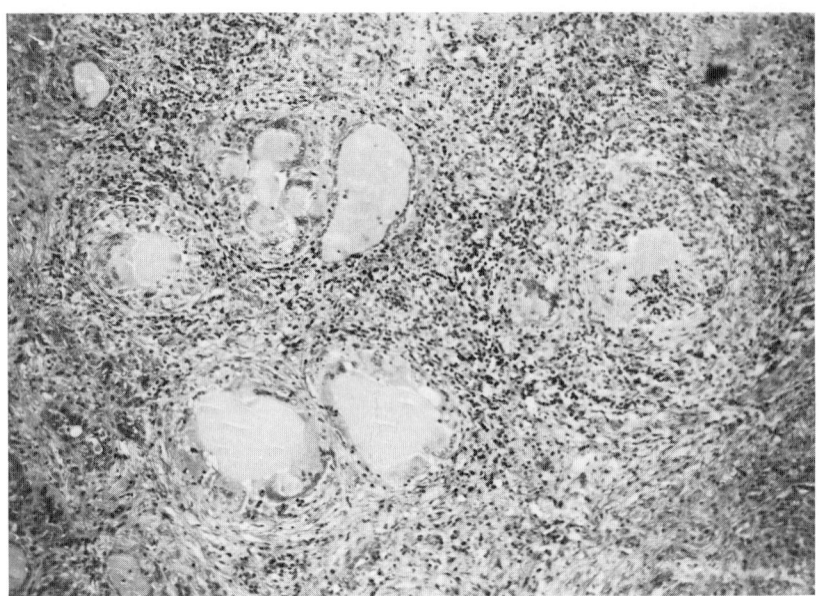

FIGURE 20-4 Subacute thyroiditis. There is active destruction of follicles. Giant cells are seen surrounding colloid. There is early granuloma formation. The stroma shows a lymphocytic infiltration. (H&E stain; 120×.)

prognosis. Woolner and others divided papillary carcinomas into occult, intrathyroidal, and extrathyroidal types, according to the size and invasiveness of the lesion.[10] Occult carcinomas are less than 1.5 cm in diameter, and are usually incidental findings in thyroid glands removed for other conditions. Intrathyroidal carcinomas are larger but are still confined within the gland. Extrathyroidal carcinomas extend beyond the thyroid gland and invade the tracheal or esophageal areas.

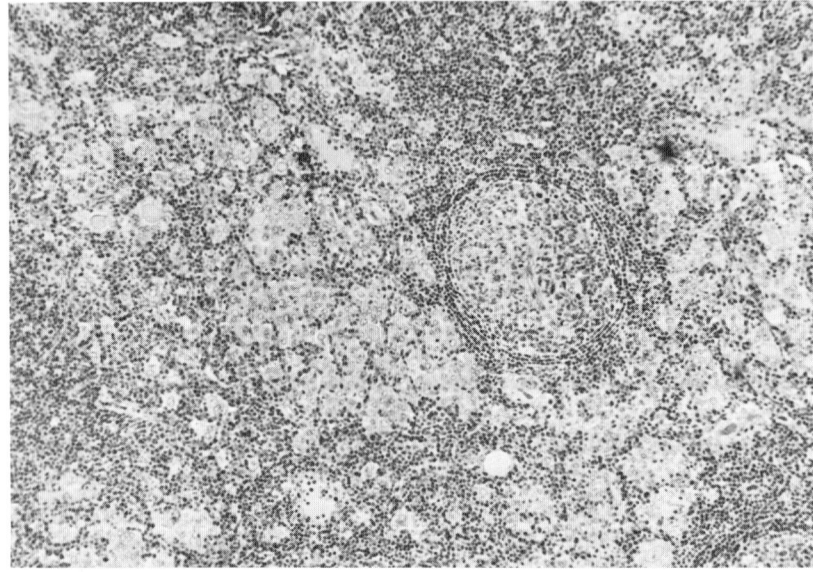

FIGURE 20-5 Hashimoto's thyroiditis. There is a marked lymphocytic infiltration with lymphoid follicle formation. There is prominent metaplasia of the follicular cells, showing abundant eosinophilic cytoplasm (Askanazy cells). (H&E stain; 120×.)

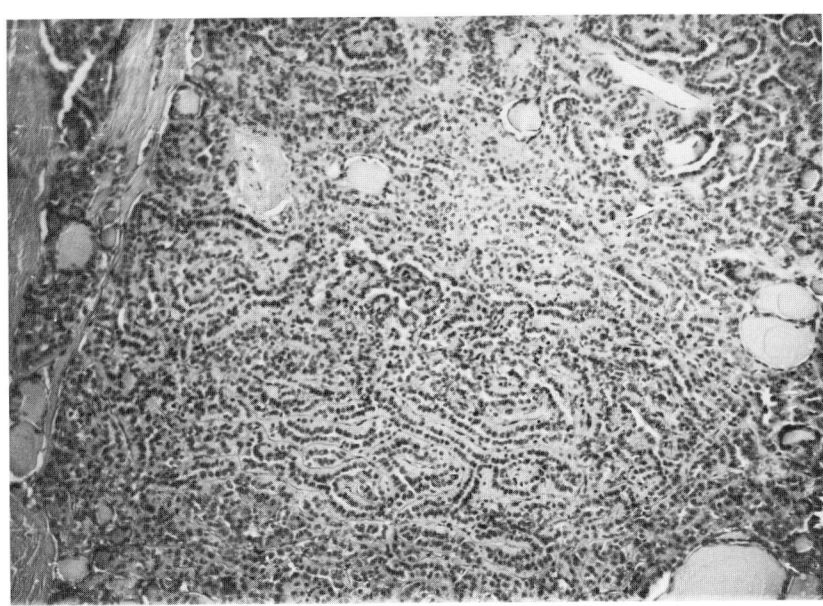

FIGURE 20-6 Papillary thyroid carcinoma. The papillary pattern is quite apparent, even in this relatively solid area of the tumor. (H&E stain; 120×.)

At an international workshop conference on thyroid cancer in Chicago in 1976, the designation *minimal thyroid cancer* was given to those cancers 1 cm or less in diameter. The high incidence of minimal cancers recently documented is related to the thoroughness of microscopic studies of thyroid specimens. Sampson reported a high incidence of minimal cancer in the Japanese.[11] By cutting thyroid tissue at 2- to 3-mm intervals, minimal cancer was detected in 28 percent of Japanese patients. In contrast, a similar study in Minnesota found the incidence to be 5.7 percent. The 5-year survival rate for papillary carcinoma was reported as 90 percent at the Memorial Cancer Center in New York City.

Follicular Carcinoma

Follicular carcinoma has many of the characteristics of the papillary form. The primary difference is that although it also may metastasize through the lymphatics, dissemination takes place chiefly through the bloodstream. Microscopically (Fig. 20-7), the pure follicular type reproduces the structural unit of the gland.[12] The follicles vary from the immature to mature and demonstrate colloid formation. Follicular carcinoma occurs often as a mixed type, with elements of both papillary and follicular forms.

These tumors are usually well encapsulated; they do not often spread to the lymph nodes but spread easily to the bones and lungs. They are more common in the middle-aged and elderly.

Classification is based on the invasiveness of the neoplasm. Woolner classifies follicular carcinoma as noninvasive, with slight capsular invasion and with moderate to extensive invasion. The noninvasive form is well encapsulated, with obvious malignant changes but no evidence of invasion. The slightly invasive forms demonstrate minimal invasion of blood vessels and the capsule. The moderate to severely invasive forms demonstrate extensive invasion of blood vessels and surrounding thyroid tissue.

Beaugie divided follicular carcinomas into two types: *microinvasive*, with invasion restricted to the capsular venous sinuses, and *angioinvasive*, with invasion into extracapsular veins, rarely involving the deep jugular vein.[13]

Some data indicate that follicular carcinomas are more prevalent in areas of endemic goiters, while papillary carcinoma occurs commonly in uninvolved thyroid gland. Follicular carcinomas are rarely found in children and young adults.

Thompson et al. indicated that the incidence of follicular carcinoma decreased from 19 percent, observed 20 years ago to 10 percent during the past 10 years. They do not believe that geographic differences

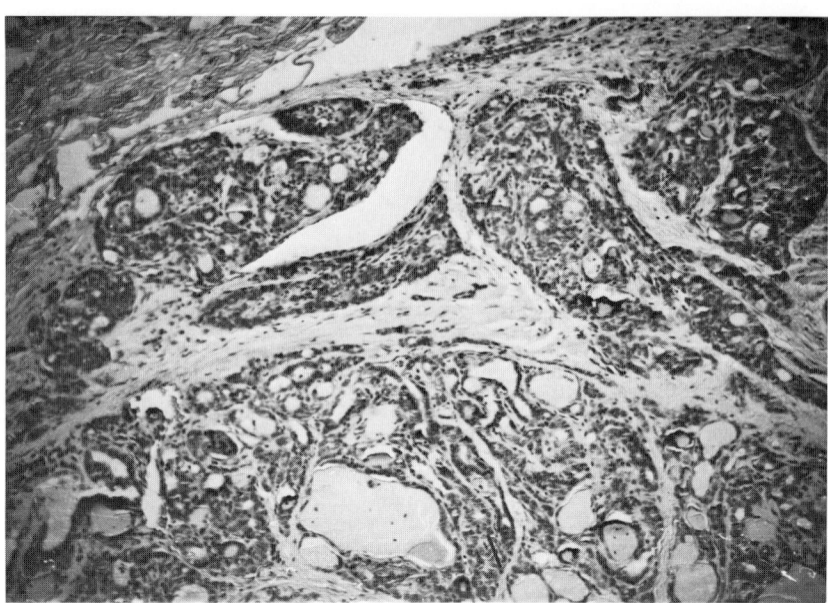

FIGURE 20-7 Follicular carcinoma of the thyroid. The stromal and vascular invasion is quite evident. (H&E stain; 120×.)

account for these changes but do believe that the high dietary intake of iodine may be a factor in the United States. Another factor which helps to account for the apparent decrease is the use of different classifications. The follicular variant of papillary cancer may be classified by some as papillary and by others as follicular carcinoma. Other distinctive characteristics of pure follicular carcinomas are the lack of association with previous radiation and the almost complete absence of an occult form. Huvos reported that 5-year survival rate of this disease to be 70 percent.[14]

Anaplastic Carcinoma

Anaplastic carcinoma is also called *undifferentiated carcinoma;* it includes such variants as small cell, spindle cell, and giant cell carcinoma. This type of cancer may be confused with thyroiditis. When first detected, this process has usually involved both lobes, which feel firm and fixed. About 10 to 15 percent of thyroid cancers are of the anaplastic type.[15] They usually occur in older persons, grow rapidly, and spread both by lymphatics and by the bloodstream.

Microscopically, the tumor is often composed of irregular cords and masses of poorly differentiated epithelial cells (Fig. 20-8a and b) which vary in size and shape and exhibit no definite tendency toward glandular or papillary formation. In some, spindle and giant cells predominate. Aldinger reported a 5-year survival rate of 7.1 percent in a group of anaplastic carcinomas treated at the M. D. Anderson Hospital in Houston.[16]

Medullary Carcinoma

Medullary carcinoma, which has been recognized for 20 years, constitutes only about 5 to 10 percent of all thyroid carcinomas; it is slightly more common in women. It may occur sporadically or, more rarely, as a familial disease with an autosomal dominant pattern of inheritance. This tumor may be part of a multiple endocrine neoplasia syndrome, and the most commonly associated lesion is pheochromocytoma. Block cited reports of 37 patients with medullary thyroid carcinoma, most of whom had associated pheochromocytoma.[17] He indicated that either the thyroid cancer or the pheochromocytoma may dominate the clinical manifestations, and either lesion may precede the other. Of 9 patients for whom data were available, both lobes were involved in 8; 6 had metastases to the cervical lymph nodes; and 6 had distant metastases. Five had died of their thyroid malignancy. Of 29 patients for whom the distribution of pheochromocytoma was recorded, 21 had bilateral tumors; 2 had died; and 3 had associated parathyroid tumors. Two patients demonstrated clinical hyperparathyroidism, and in both pa-

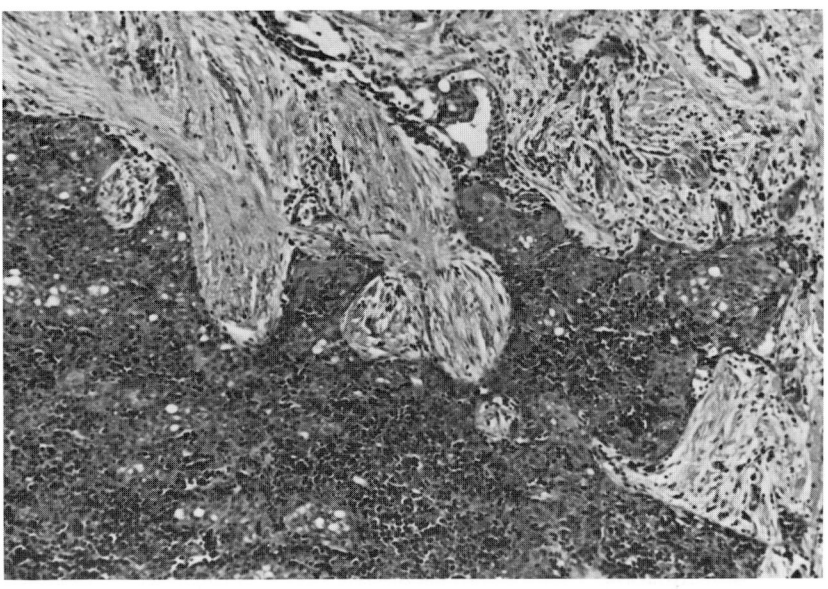

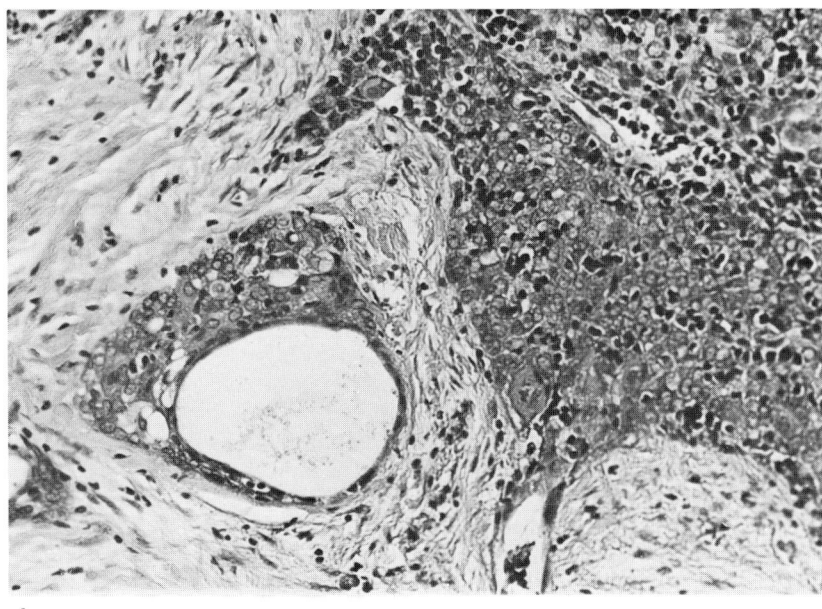

FIGURE 20-8 (*a*) Undifferentiated thyroid carcinoma. The tumor is composed of anaplastic cells showing fingerlike projections into the stroma. No follicular or papillary pattern is evident. (H&E stain; 120×.) (*b*) Undifferentiated thyroid carcinoma. Higher magnification of the same tumor. (H&E stain; 300×.)

tients multiple parathyroid glands were enlarged. Nonfamilial coexistence of these lesions also occurs.

Symptoms vary, depending on whether the medullary carcinoma is part of an endocrine syndrome. The first manifestation may be a firm, nodular mass in the thyroid with or without enlarged cervical nodes. If a pheochromocytoma is present, symptoms may be referable to this tumor.

The diagnosis is confirmed by an assay of calcitonin. Determination of peak thyroid calcitonin response to

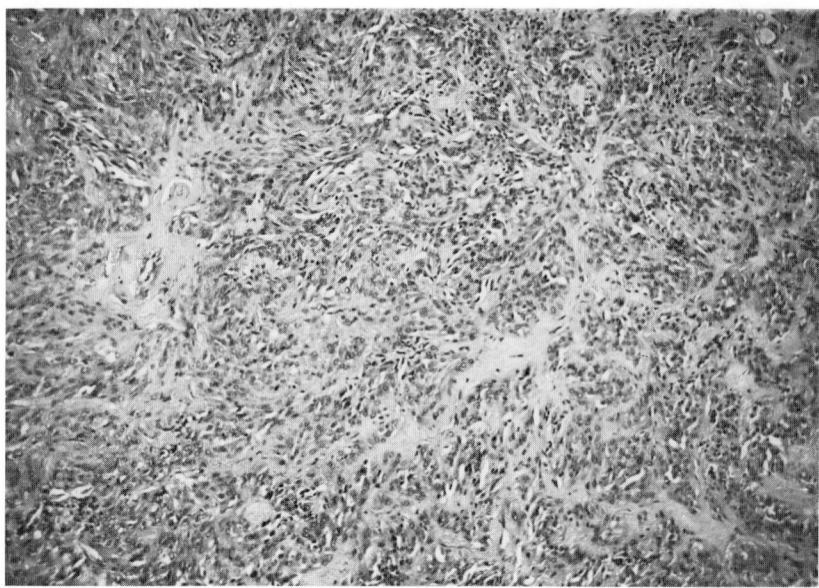

FIGURE 20-9 Medullary carcinoma of the thyroid. There is a moderate amount of intercellular eosinophilic hyaline material (amyloid) present in this tumor. This area of the tumor is composed principally of spindle cells. (H&E stain; 120×.)

pentagastrin[18,19] provides a method for diagnosing medullary carcinoma in asymptomatic members of the family of a patient with MEN II syndrome.[20] Pheochromocytoma diagnostic studies should be performed in all patients with medullary carcinoma of the thyroid. Microscopically (Fig. 20-9), the cell type varies from small and round to large and ovoid or polyhedral. The stroma contains differing amounts of amyloid. Black et al. reported a 10-year survival rate of 61 percent in 49 patients with medullary carcinoma.[21]

Hürthle Cell Carcinoma

Hürthle cell carcinoma is a tumor composed entirely of Hürthle cells, large eosinophilic cells whose function is unknown. Pathologists differ in the diagnosis of this lesion. Since these cells can occur in nodules in Hashimoto's thyroiditis, in Graves' disease, and in nodular goiter, many malignant lesions are called benign. The more obvious malignant lesions demonstrate invasiveness or the presence of metastases.

Some classifications consider Hürthle cell carcinomas to be variants of follicular or papillary carcinomas. Thompson et al. indicate that this disease should be considered a separate entity, but agree that the presence of Hürthle cells makes the evaluation of such lesions difficult. In contrast to follicular carcinomas, Hürthle cell carcinomas rarely, if ever, concentrate radioactive iodine, and they most commonly metastasize to lymph nodes (Fig. 20-10). Tollefsen et al. reviewed 35 patients with Hürthle cell carcinomas initially treated at Memorial Hospital from 1930 to 1966.[22] Patients with the diagnosis of Hürthle cell adenoma were excluded. The peak incidence occurred in the sixth decade, and none of the patients were under 20 years of age. At the time of the first clinical evaluation, the tumor was confined to the thyroid gland in 26 patients and to the thyroid gland and cervical nodes in 4 patients; distant metastases were already evident in 5 of the patients. During the follow-up period, 6 patients had distant metastases, 3 had pulmonary metastases, 2 had osseous metastases, and 1 had metastases to multiple organs. The rates of survival were 76 percent at 5 years and 40 percent at 25 years.

STAGING

Comparison between series of patients with thyroid cancer should be made only if each series has the same number of cases of equal involvement. An alternative is to compare total experience. The method of comparison differs among institutions.

Staging according to the TNM method facilitates comparison of different modes of treatment or experience. The American Joint Committee for Cancer Staging and End-Results Reporting has evaluated over 1000 protocols with the goal of establishing a staging system for cancer of the thyroid, but currently there is no satisfactory system. The temporary classification, using TNM symbols recommended by this committee, is outlined in Table 20-1.

Stage Grouping

No stage grouping for thyroid cancer is recommended at this time.

DIAGNOSIS

Many factors must be considered in the detection and diagnosis of thyroid cancer. Age and sex of the patient are important. A solitary mass that has recently developed in the thyroid is more likely to be cancer in a child or a man than in a woman. A patient who lives by the seashore and develops a thyroid mass is more likely to have thyroid cancer than a person living in a goiter belt who develops such a mass. Patients who have had previous radiation to the head and neck have a higher incidence of thyroid cancer.

Physical examination may disclose a firm, fixed mass, although many thyroid cancers are neither fixed nor hard. The presence of enlarged cervical lymph nodes in addition to a thyroid mass should increase suspicion of a malignant process. A fixed vocal cord along with a thyroid mass is an ominous finding. The senior author has never seen cord paralysis resulting from pressure from benign thyroid disease, but has seen cord paralysis resulting from localized central nervous system lesions.

Thyroid function tests should be performed on all patients with thyroid masses. If hyperthyroidism exists, the chances are less that the mass is malignant. Before subjecting a patient with a thyroid mass to an operation, the patient's thyroid function should be determined.

Thyroid scans are helpful, although not diagnostic. A scan showing a functioning nodule could represent a well-differentiated carcinoma in a small percent of patients. A nonfunctioning nodule, or "cold" nodule on scan, is a more significant finding; it could represent a colloid nodule, a benign cyst, or hemorrhage into a preexisting nodule, but thyroid cancer must be considered.

Iodine is a basic metabolite used by the thyroid gland in the biosynthesis of its major hormones T_3 and T_4. Because the thyroid is the only organ in the body which accumulates and stores iodine for appreciable periods of time, measurement of thyroid iodine uptake reflects

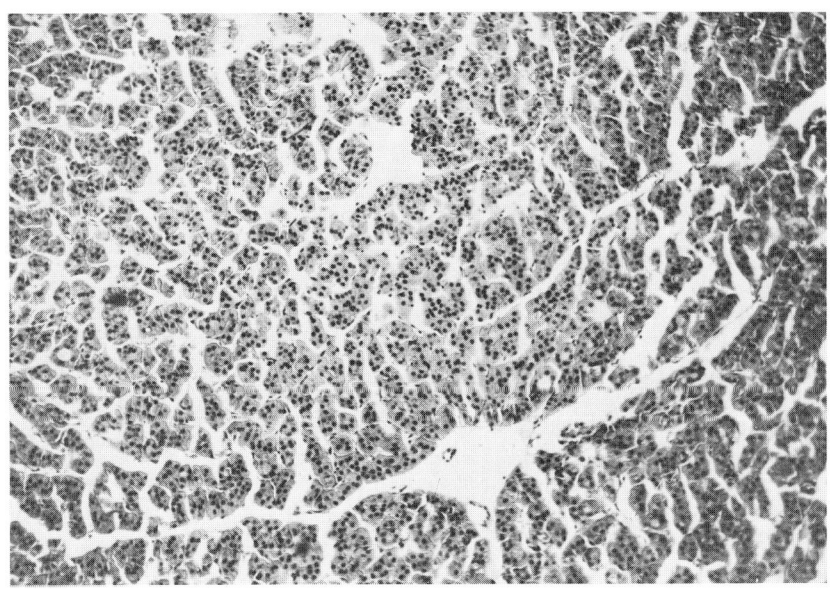

FIGURE 20-10 Metastatic Hurthle cell carcinoma. Tumor found in cervical lymph node 13 years post resection of thyroid with Hurthle cell carcinoma. The tumor is composed of well-differentiated cells with abundant eosinophilic cytoplasm. The cells are arranged in nests and cords with little follicle formation. (H&E stain; 120×.)

TABLE 20-1 TNM Classification

PRIMARY TUMOR (T)

T_X	Tumor that cannot be assessed by rules
T_0	No available information on primary tumor
T_1	Mobile tumor
$\quad T_{1a}$	Mobile tumor 4 cm or less in greatest diameter
$\quad T_{1b}$	Mobile tumor more than 4 cm in greatest diameter
T_2	Partial fixation of tumor, any size, with or without neurologic involvement
$\quad T_{2a}$	Lateral position
$\quad T_{2b}$	Midline position
T_3	Complete fixation of tumor, any size, with or without neurologic involvement; fistula

NODAL INVOLVEMENT (N)

N_X	Nodes cannot be assessed
N_0	No palpable nodes
N_1	Palpable mobile node or nodes
$\quad N_{1a}$	Homolateral only
$\quad N_{1b}$	Contralateral only
$\quad N_{1c}$	Bilateral and/or midline
N_2	Any palpable fixed node

DISTANT METASTASES (M)

M_X	Not assessed
M_0	No (known) distant metastasis
M_1	Distant metastasis present
	Specify _____

the physiologic state of the thyroid gland. A thyroid scan may be performed at the same time that the iodine uptake is determined, using only a small dose of radioactive iodine.

Commonly used are iodine 131 and technetium 99m; the former has a half-life of 8.05 days and the latter, 6 h. Iodine 125, with a half-life of 60 days, and iodine 123, with a half-life of 13 h, are also available for scanning. Although each of these agents has specific advantages, in general the one with the lesser half-life results in less radiation to the thyroid gland. One advantage of ^{131}I is its relatively high energy, making it a better agent for identifying substernal or mediastinal thyroid tissue. ^{123}I is expensive, as commercially prepared, but it is the radionucleotide of choice for thyroid imaging, and as methods are developed to produce it more economically it will probably be used more widely.

The pertechnetate ion is a chemical analogue of iodine, and is trapped by the thyroid gland in a similar manner. Localization of pertechnetate in the thyroid gland occurs early and reaches a maximum about 20 min following intravenous injection. The amount of pertechnetate decreases slowly in proportion to its clearance from the blood by the kidneys and other organs. ^{99m}Tc has almost ideal physical properties for x-ray imaging. Its short half-life results in less radiation to the thyroid gland and other body organs. It is readily available and inexpensive. The fact that a scan can be carried out in 20 min after injection rather than the 24 h required for ^{131}I makes its use much more practical. Numerous case reports in the literature, however, document the fact that both benign and malignant tumors of the thyroid gland may take up pertechnetate but not iodine.[23]

In most cases, the result of scintiscan should not be the decisive factor in choosing treatment for a thyroid nodule. Thyroid scintiscans only supplement the findings of a physical examination, which is usually more definitive in outlining a thyroid nodule. In a small percentage of cases, the scan may demonstrate a nodule that is "hyperfunctioning"; such a nodule may even be autonomous in its function, forming a so-called hot nodule. Hot nodules are not likely to be malignant.

Thallium 201 has recently been reported to be of value in the diagnosis of thyroid cancer.[24] Nodules which appear cold with ^{131}I or ^{99m}Tc have been shown to be hot when ^{201}Tl is administered. If additional clinical use substantiates early reports, use of ^{201}Tl will aid in the diagnosis of cancer of the thyroid.

Thyroid Suppression

The anterior pituitary secretes TSH, which stimulates the thyroid gland. Exogenous thyroid blocks TSH secretion, the thyroxin level is lowered, and functioning thyroid tissue decreases in size. If the scan shows the nodule to be functioning, it may be worthwhile to attempt suppression with thyroid. If it is a cold, nonfunctioning nodule, the odds are that there will be no change, although an occasional malignant nodule has shown temporary regression. Cole treated 111 patients with nontoxic nodules with 2 to 8 g of desiccated thyroid per day for varying periods and concluded that, in general, thyroid suppression is ineffective in treating thyroid nodules.[25] If the mass is diffuse and functional, it is more likely to regress when treated with adequate thyroid medication. Some advocate routine attempt of thyroid gland suppression for any thyroid nodule, reasoning that even if the nodule proves to be papillary carcinoma, treatment for 3 to 6 months probably does not alter the ultimate prognosis.

Echography may be helpful in differentiating a cystic from a solid mass, and is of value mainly when dealing with a cold nodule. Aspiration may be performed on lesions suspected of being cystic. A fine-needle aspiration may determine that a cold nodule is a colloid cyst and thus obviate the need for operation. Echography, used during the last 5 years, appears to be accurate in about 95 percent of cases, but, unfortunately, its usefulness is limited because cystic lesions comprise less than 10 to 20 percent of solitary thyroid nodules.

Aspiration biopsies may be performed on solid thyroid masses as safely as elsewhere in the neck, but we do not employ this procedure often. A nodule that should be removed is better removed by lobectomy with histologic examination by frozen section. In a patient with a medical contraindication to operation, aspiration biopsy is an ideal method of determining whether a thyroid nodule is benign or malignant. We usually use a 16-gauge needle fitted with a stylet for the procedure. After the skin has been cleansed with an antiseptic solution, a small nick is made in the skin with a pointed blade, the needle is introduced into the mass, and the stylet is removed. A 30-mL syringe is attached, and suction is produced by partially withdrawing the plunger. With a rotary, to-and-fro motion, it is usually possible to obtain an adequate amount of tissue for a paraffin block and sectioning. This technique is also of value in a patient suspected of having thyroiditis, although tissue may be a little more difficult to obtain. A negative aspiration biopsy does not mean the patient does not have cancer, and other measures should be taken to make sure.

SURGICAL MANAGEMENT

Papillary Carcinoma

The treatment of this disease has varied widely during the past 30 years. Because papillary carcinoma metastasizes to the neck nodes so often, treatment in the forties and fifties was radical. In the sixties it was demonstrated that in patients lacking clinical evidence of nodes, the prognosis was the same whether or not radical neck dissections were performed. Since then, the surgical management of cervical lymph nodes has become more conservative. The extent of operations performed both for the primary lesion and for nodal involvement varies widely.

MANAGEMENT OF THE PRIMARY LESION

Total Thyroidectomy Advocates of this procedure perform a total thyroidectomy even though a mass can be felt grossly in only one lobe of the gland.[26] Some advocate total thyroidectomy because they believe that lesions are all multicentric and that the opposite lobe is involved in a high percentage of cases. Others believe that the entire thyroid gland should be removed so that when radioactive iodine uptake studies are performed postoperatively, or if it becomes necessary to administer radioactive iodine later, no remaining thyroid tissue will actively compete with the possible metastatic deposits for the iodine. The morbidity of both hoarseness due to laryngeal nerve damage and hypoparathyroidism is greater following total thyroidectomy than that which follows lesser procedures.

Total Lobectomy, Isthmusectomy, and Subtotal Lobectomy on the Contralateral Side This "near-total" thyroidectomy is widely performed in the United States for the treatment of papillary carcinoma.[27] A small rim of thyroid tissue and the posterior capsule are left to protect the recurrent nerve and parathyroid glands on the opposite side. Preservation of the recurrent laryngeal nerve is not difficult with the proper surgical technique. Prevention of hypoparathyroidism is difficult after total thyroidectomy because of the common blood supply of the thyroid and parathyroid glands. Hypoparathyroidism has been reported in as many as 30 percent of patients after total thyroidectomy, which is the main reason some surgeons perform the near-total procedure. Excellent results have been reported with this method. Again, those who advocate the total removal of the thyroid gland object to leaving a small portion of the opposite lobe for fear of leaving behind areas of carcinoma, and because if thyroid tissue is left behind, the competition for ^{131}I interferes with the detection of metastases. If a remnant of tissue is left and it later becomes necessary to administer radioactive iodine, the remnant could be ablated by an initial dose of radioactive iodine.

Unilateral Total Lobectomy and Isthmusectomy Total extracapsular lobectomy is performed on the side of the palpable nodule, and the isthmus is excised in continuity. The recurrent nerve is identified and dissected free up to its point of entrance into the larynx. Both parathyroid glands are identified. If no mass is felt in the opposite lobe, it is not resected. Advocates of this procedure emphasize that recurrence of cancer in the opposite lobe is low, roughly 5 percent, despite the fact that whole-organ sectioning of the opposite lobe has shown that over 80 percent contain malignant thyroid cells. Nevertheless, if only a low percentage of patients exhibit recurrent masses, unnecessary lobectomies have been performed, not without serious morbidity. Insofar as the remaining thyroid gland interferes with radioactive iodine pickup, only a small percentage of patients with thyroid cancer develop metastases, and in those few cases the opposite lobe can be removed if necessary before administering iodine.

Subtotal Lobectomy A subtotal lobectomy is done when carcinoma is not suspected or when the report of frozen section examination is false negative. This is an undesirable situation because it means that the patient must undergo a second operative procedure if the permanent section examination indicates that the lesion was malignant. If a total lobectomy is performed for any solitary lesion within a lobe, such situations are avoided.

MANAGEMENT OF CERVICAL NODES

Since the Hutter et al. paper on elective radical neck dissection, practically everyone agrees that neck dissection for papillary carcinomas is not indicated if the nodes are not clinically positive for cancer. If the nodes are involved, several different methods of management have been employed.

Radical Neck Dissection Complete dissection of the neck is still performed by some if (1) there are many nodes in the neck of an older person; (2) the nodes are bulky and technically very difficult to remove without taking the deep jugular vein and sternocleidomastoid muscle (this occurs most frequently in an adult); (3) the primary lesion is large and multiple nodes are present in an older person. Papillary carcinoma is a more virulent process in the older person, and complete resection offers a better chance of local control of disease.

Modified Neck Dissection Some surgeons believe that a complete radical neck dissection is seldom necessary for cervical carcinoma. They alter the procedure either by performing the node dissection primarily through an extended collar incision, or by leaving such structures as the spinal accessory nerve, deep jugular vein, or the sternocleidomastoid muscle.

Local Excision of Nodes Some surgeons believe that nodes may be managed by individually shelling them out ("berry picking"). Others advocate a block excision of the locally involved nodes. The nodes in the recurrent nerve area and in the lower neck region may easily be removed by block excision.

Follicular Carcinoma

One of the most difficult diagnoses to establish is well-differentiated follicular carcinoma with no invasion of the capsule or blood vessels. The surgical treatment is similar to that for papillary adenocarcinoma of the thyroid.

MANAGEMENT OF THE PRIMARY LESION

The patient may have a solitary nodule, which should be removed by total lobectomy. Depending upon the degree of differentiation, the pathologist may not be able to make the diagnosis on frozen section examination. If the nodule is well differentiated, it is difficult for even the most experienced pathologist to make the diagnosis until permanent sections are examined. Options for the local management of this disease are the same as for papillary carcinoma. Some advocate removal of all thyroid tissue, especially since this type picks up radioactive iodine very readily and they prefer not to have any thyroid tissue competing with metastases for iodine uptake. Other surgeons perform less than a total thyroidectomy unless metastases are present; the opposite lobe can be removed if metastases occur.

MANAGEMENT OF CERVICAL LYMPH NODES

If the neck is clinically negative, prophylactic neck dissections are not advocated for this lesion. Nodes are not involved nearly as often as they are in the presence of papillary carcinoma, but if they are involved, options for treatment are the same as those for papillary carcinoma.

Anaplastic Carcinoma

Local structures, including the trachea, are often invaded and death may be due to an impaired airway. Only rarely can such carcinomas be removed surgically. They often regress with radiation therapy but usually recur rapidly, and the prognosis is very poor. Since a low percentage of nontoxic nodular goiters eventually degenerate into this type of carcinoma, the removal of large nodular goiters in patients in their fifties and sixties may prevent some of these from developing.

Medullary Carcinoma

Medullary carcinoma is characterized biologically by a greater virulence and lethal potential than the more common papillary and follicular varieties. Pheochromocytoma, if present, should be removed first. The parathyroid glands should be explored. In the presence of hypercalcemia, a large single gland should be removed if the remaining three are normal, and 3½ glands should be removed if hyperplasia of the gland exists.

This tumor does not respond to radioactive iodine treatment, external radiation, or thyroid hormone. The prognosis is worse than that for either papillary or follicular carcinoma of the thyroid.[28]

MANAGEMENT OF THE PRIMARY LESION

The familial type is uniformly bilateral. The lesion is usually well demarcated and is located in the upper midportion of each lobe. Both lobes of the thyroid gland should be removed. If the familial type of carcinoma has been detected by screening tests, the lesions in each lobe may be small. In these situations, some have advocated near-total thyroidectomy, leaving a small rim of thyroid tissue on one side or bilaterally to preserve the parathyroid glands. However, even in the sporadic type, which may be unilateral, it is safer to perform a total lobectomy on the involved lobe and a subtotal of the opposite lobe with immediate pathologic examination of tissue.

MANAGEMENT OF NECK NODES

Clinically negative nodes need not be resected. The extent of node dissection depends upon the extent of involvement. If the central paratracheal nodes are involved and extend inferiorly into the mediastinum, recommended procedure is to split the sternum if necessary and perform resection of the upper mediastinal nodes in continuity with the paratracheal nodes. In the familial type, lateral neck nodes can be removed by block dissection of the involved area or by modified neck dissection. The sporadic unilateral type is usually a more virulent form of the disease, and if lateral neck nodes are present, they should be adequately removed by a formal radical neck dissection.

The patients should be followed at regular intervals postoperatively. A serum calcitonin determination should be made immediately after surgery. Some advocate performing a pentagastrin test at 6-month intervals to detect elevated levels of thyrocalcitonin. If a patient has had negative responses and then develops an elevated calcitonin after pentagastrin stimulation, it becomes necessary to look for recurrent medullary carcinoma. Wells advocated selective venous catheterization in an attempt to localize disease in one side of the thyroid gland or the other.[19] If disease is found in the thyroid, the patient should be subjected to neck reexploration. If the patient has not had the lateral cervical nodes removed, the question of neck dissection comes up for consideration. Some believe that unless the disease can be localized in some way, it is better to continue observation without surgical intervention. Wells reported two patients with minimally elevated thyrocalcitonin levels after pentagastrin stimulation which did not change much over a 3-year period in spite of known metastatic disease outside the neck.

Not enough data are available to make it possible to outline a definite routine to follow. It would seem at least practical at this time simply to continue following a patient who suddenly develops increased calcitonin levels until the recurrent disease can be definitely localized.

At the Memorial Hospital Cancer Center, the overall survival rate for medullary thyroid carcinoma was 71.4 percent for 5 years and 57.6 percent for 10 years.

Hürthle Cell Carcinoma

PRIMARY

When a lobectomy is performed and the frozen section examination indicates Hürthle cell carcinoma, the treatment is the same as for any other thyroid carcinoma. If changes can be felt in the opposite lobe, that lobe should be removed also. This diagnosis is difficult to establish on examination of frozen section, and some pathologists advocate that the disease be considered malignant if a nodule measuring over 2 cm containing Hürthle cells is present.

CERVICAL LYMPH NODES

These nodes should be removed by block excision of the central compartment and upper mediastinum if they are located along the trachea and by the standard radical neck dissection if they are located laterally. The lesions are radioresistant, so cure depends on adequate excision.

RADIATION THERAPY

External

Thyroid cancers, whether well-differentiated or undifferentiated, are usually resistant to radiotherapy. However, their radiosensitivity is sufficiently unpredictable to warrant a "curative" attempt with radiotherapy when the disease is still localized in the thyroid area.

Postoperative radiation therapy may be directed toward areas of residual disease after meticulous efforts to remove all possible tumor have been made.

In general, radiotherapy for cancer of the thyroid is reserved as a palliative measure to alleviate symptoms associated with distant metastases. External radiation may also be a valuable adjunct to surgery in the definitive treatment of advanced or recurrent papillary and follicular carcinomas which do not concentrate radioactive iodine.

Radioactive Iodine

The rationale for the use of radioactive iodine, ^{131}I, is that some tumor tissue will concentrate enough of the radioactive isotope to cause self-destruction. Radioactive iodine is effective in treating papillary and follicular carcinomatous tissue, but it is ineffective in treating undifferentiated, Hürthle cell, or medullary carcinomas.

If postoperative treatment with ^{131}I is planned, it is advisable to remove all the thyroid gland. If all thyroid tissue has not been removed, an initial dose of 50 to 100 millicuries (mCi) of ^{131}I will usually ablate the residual tissue.

At M. D. Anderson Hospital, when metastases are to be treated with radioactive iodine, thyroid tissue remaining after thyroidectomy is first treated with ^{131}I. No thyroid replacement is given for a 6-week period. This permits intense stimulation of the thyroid tissue by TSH. A tracer dose of ^{131}I is then given. If concentration is demonstrated, an ablative dose of ^{131}I is given. Replacement thyroid therapy is given for 3 months and then discontinued. When the patient becomes myxedematous again, the tracer procedure is repeated. If there is evidence of ^{131}I concentration, a second treatment dose of ^{131}I is given. No single treatment dose of more than 200 mCi is ever administered, and dosages are not repeated oftener than every 3 months.

The alternative is to begin thyroid replacement immediately after operation and employ ^{131}I only when metastases becomes clinically evident. If metastases become evident, replacement therapy is stopped for 6 weeks. A tracer dose of ^{131}I is given, and if it is positive, a treatment dose is administered.

Thompson et al. reported that only a small percentage of patients with papillary or follicular carcinoma have distant metastases at the time of their initial treatment. Distant metastases will occur in 5 to 20 percent of patients with papillary carcinoma, 3 to 5 percent with microinvasive follicular carcinoma, and approximately 50 percent of those with extensive (angioinvasive) follicular carcinoma. Nearly all patients under 42 years of age with distant metastases of differentiated thyroid carcinoma concentrate ^{131}I. It is not uncommon for patients 60 years of age with metastatic papillary carcinoma to fail to concentrate ^{131}I. Inability of older patients with follicular carcinoma to concentrate ^{131}I is uncommon, although all the metastatic areas may not respond. Pochin found that 50 percent of patients with differentiated thyroid carcinoma treated with ^{131}I had excellent responses and that an additional 25 percent had good palliation.[29]

The possible complications following the use of ^{131}I include leukemia, pulmonary fibrosis, sterility, and genetic abnormalities. It is estimated that 75 percent of patients with distant metastases from differentiated thyroid carcinoma will die of their disease within 5 years of diagnosis.

In a study by Harness et al. 28 patients with distant metastases from papillary thyroid carcinoma were treated with ^{131}I at the University of Michigan. The average follow-up period was 15 years, and 20 patients were followed 10 years or more. Seventy percent were under 40 years of age. Each received an average total dose of 383 mCi of ^{131}I. Eight additional patients had metastases from follicular carcinoma. Of the 36 patients who received ^{131}I, 10 died. The average survival time was 8 years. Of the patients who died, 6 had papillary carcinoma and 4 had follicular carcinoma. The survival rate of those with pulmonary metastases treated with ^{131}I was 87 percent at 10 years and 67 percent at 20 years.

Of 10 patients with osseous metastases, 8 had died at the end of 10 years. The conclusion was that ^{131}I is nearly always successful in patients under 40 years of age with metastatic papillary carcinoma and in some patients, regardless of age, with follicular carcinoma. Pulmonary metastases appear to be more radiosensitive than osseous metastases. Patients over 60 years of age with metastatic papillary carcinoma are less likely to respond.

Radiation-Associated Thyroid Cancer

Beginning in the 1920s, x-ray therapy was used in the treatment of patients with respiratory diseases, many children who were presumed to have enlarged thymus glands, and in the treatment of patients with chronic tonsillitis, adenoiditis, cervical adenitis, eczema, and severe acne. In 1950, Duffy and Fitzgerald reported 28 patients under 18 years of age with thyroid cancer, 10 of whom had received x-ray therapy to the thymus during infancy.[31] In 1966, Winship and Rosvoll reviewed 704 cases of thyroid cancer and noted that 80 percent of the patients had received radiation therapy during infancy.[32] Even as small a dose as 6.5 rads to the thyroid given for tinea capitis resulted in an increased incidence of thyroid cancer. In dose ranges of 400 to 1500 rads, the incidence of nodular goiter was about 27 to 40 percent and the incidence of thyroid cancer varied from 5 to 9 percent.

Greenspan reviewed 94 patients with a history of radiation exposure with or without known thyroid enlargement and found 46 patients with thyroid cancer.[33] Of these, 34 had cancer alone, 7 had adenomas, 3 had Hashimoto's thyroiditis, and 2 had both adenomas and thyroiditis. In the 48 patients without thyroid cancer, no thyroid disease was present in 18; multiple adenomas were found in 12, Hashimoto's thyroiditis in 8, and hot nodules in 3. The other 7 exhibited a variety of other lesions.

The incidence of thyroid cancer in irradiated persons is not known. It is estimated that the risk of developing palpable benign abnormalities as the result of irradiation is about four times the risk of developing cancer.

The length of the latent period between administration of radiation and the appearance of carcinoma cannot be predicted; it varies from 3.5 to 35 years. There is no way of knowing what percentage of persons exposed to radiation will later develop cancer, although a clinical estimate is that as many as 7 to 9 percent may. In a series of 100 patients who had received radiation therapy, Refetoff found that 7 percent had carcinoma. In another series of 1056 patients who had previously received radiation to the head and neck, mainly to the thymus and tonsils, Favus found that 9 percent had carcinoma, 16 percent had palpable nodular thyroid glands, and an additional 10.7 percent had thyroid lesions on scintiscans. These figures suggest an incidence of about 8000 cases of thyroid disease per 100,000 persons who receive radiation, whereas the incidence for persons who have not received radiation is 4 thyroid cancers per 100,000.

The commonest type of thyroid cancer occurring after radiation is papillary carcinoma. There is no definite evidence that radiation-induced carcinomas are more lethal than any other.

Management of Patients after Radiation Therapy to Thyroid Glands

The connection between the exposure of infants and children to radiation and the later appearance of thyroid cancer has been widely publicized, so it is not uncommon for a patient to seek medical advice even though no symptoms are present. What should be advised? Varying types of management have been suggested. Greenspan recommends that if there is thyroid enlargement without nodularity, hypothyroidism, or a strongly positive antibody test, the patient should receive thyroxine therapy for life. If the scan shows a cold nodule, he recommends thyroidectomy and indicates that incidence of malignant disease in this group is approximately 50 percent. If multinodular goiter is present, he recommends a trial of thyroxine medication, but if discrete, firm nodules remain, he advocates thyroidectomy. Thompson et al. recommend a meticulous physical examination. If the gland feels normal to palpation and no cervical nodes are palpable, annual physical examination is advocated. They believe that a scintiscan is not necessary in a person who previously received radiation to the head and neck but whose thyroid gland is normal to palpation. If a scan is to be done, they recommend the use of [99mTc]pertechnetate since it delivers a lower dose of radiation to the thyroid, while utilizing ^{131}I for scans at intervals adds additional radiation to the thyroid gland. If a scan shows a defect that cannot be confirmed by physical examination, they do not believe that operation is necessary, since they doubt that occasional small papillary carcinomas undetected until they become palpable jeopardize the life expectancies of patients.

The recommended procedure for dealing with this

problem is first to perform a careful clinical examination. A scan is not advised unless there is some doubt about physical findings. If the thyroid gland is diffusely enlarged, thyroid function studies should be obtained. If the patient is euthyroid or shows lowered function, suppressive thyroid medication is advised. If one or more nodules are present, thyroidectomy is advised, with total lobectomy on one side and a subtotal on the other to remove most of the thyroid gland.

CHEMOTHERAPY

Chemotherapy has proved to be relatively ineffective in patients with disseminated or recurrent thyroid carcinoma. Of the chemotherapeutic agents currently in use, Adriamycin is the most widely employed and the most useful in the treatment of metastatic thyroid malignancies refractory to ^{131}I or external radiation therapy. Gottlieb and Hill reported that of 30 patients with refractory distant or local metastases, 11 (37 percent) achieved a partial remission.[34] Survival was signficantly greater in responding than in nonresponding patients. The highest response rates occurred in medullary carcinoma, and the lowest in spindle or giant cell types. Pulmonary metastases responded most frequently, followed by bone and cervical metastases.

In a subsequent report, Gottlieb and Hill reported 3 objective responses in 6 patients with medullary carcinoma treated with Adriamycin.[35] In responding patients, the median duration of the remission was 21 months, and median survival was 26 months.

In view of the lack of effectiveness of current chemotherapeutic agents in the treatment of thyroid carcinoma, chemotherapy should be reserved for patients with metastatic disease refractory to ^{131}I or external radiation therapy. Adriamycin appears to be the drug of choice at this time and is most effective against medullary carcinomas. Currently the use of chemotherapy to treat thyroid carcinoma must be viewed as experimental, awaiting the development of an effective new drug or combination of drugs.

EXPERIENCE IN THYROID CANCER, THE OHIO STATE UNIVERSITY HOSPITALS

From 1952 to 1977, 174 patients at the Ohio State University Hospitals underwent surgery as the initial treatment for thyroid carcinoma: 124 (71 percent) had papillary carcinoma, and 31 (18 percent) had follicular carcinoma. There were 7 cases of medullary carcinoma (4 percent), 7 cases of undifferentiated carcinoma (4 percent), and 5 cases (3 percent) of either adenocarcinoma or Hürthle cell tumors. In cases of mixed papillary and follicular histologic types, the tumors were classified as papillary. Only patients with papillary or follicular carcinomas were included in the study.

Of the 155 patients with papillary or follicular carcinoma, 29 were treated with total thyroidectomy, and the remaining 126 had less than total thyroidectomy. The types of operation that were less than total thyroidectomy are shown in Table 20-2. In all but 7 patients, a total lobectomy was performed on the side of the tumor, either alone or in combination with removal of the isthmus. Enlarged cervical lymph nodes were removed either by formal radical neck dissection or by simple excision in all patients regardless of whether the primary tumor was treated by total or less than total thyroidectomy. None of the patients had distant metastases at the time of operation. At the time of operation, 62 patients had lymph node involvement and 93 patients had no lymph node involvement.

Pathologic examination demonstrated multicentric foci of tumor in 41 patients. A solitary tumor was present in the remaining 114 patients. Of the 41 patients with multicentric tumors, 29 were treated by less than total thyroidectomy and 12 by total thyroidectomy.

These 155 patients have now been followed from 1

TABLE 20-2 Operative Procedures for Carcinoma of the Thyroid

Type of operation	Number
Total thyroidectomy	29
Less than total thyroidectomy:	
Lobectomy	15
Lobectomy and isthmus removal	20
Lobectomy and removal of nodes	2
Lobectomy, isthmus removal, and radical neck dissection (RND)	55
Lobectomy and isthmus removal subtotal	17
Lobectomy, isthmus removal and RND subtotal	10
Bilateral subtotal	7

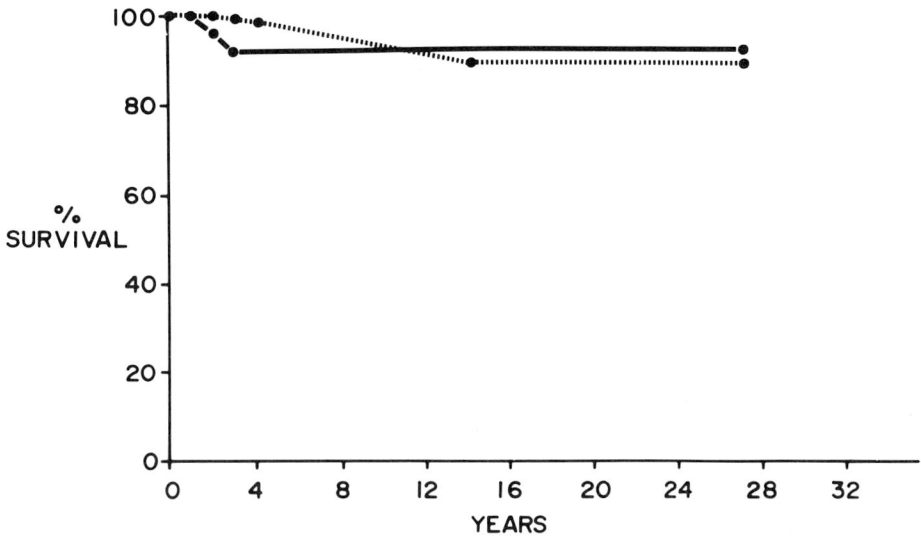

FIGURE 20-11 Survival curves comparing total and less than total thyroidectomy for papillary or follicular carcinoma of the thyroid.

to 25 years, with a mean follow-up period of 10 years. There has been regular follow-up on 70 percent of the patients for over 5 years, and on 43 percent for over 10 years. Follow-up data were obtained from the Ohio State University Tumor Registry, by direct contact with the patient, or from the patient's regular physician.

Factors influencing survival and incidence of recurrent disease were analyzed for statistical significance by means of either chi-square or Fisher's exact test, as were differences in incidence of complications between patients undergoing total and those undergoing less than total thyroidectomy.

Survival

Cumulative survival rate was 92.6 percent in patients treated by total thyroidectomy and 90.4 percent in those treated by less than total thyroidectomy (Fig. 20-11). Statistical analysis showed no significant difference in cumulative survival between the two groups of patients.

In patients with multicentric foci of thyroid carcinoma, total thyroidectomy also failed to improve chances for survival. Of 12 patients with multicentric disease treated by total thyroidectomy, 1 patient died of thyroid carcinoma; of 29 patients with multicentric disease treated by less than total thyroidectomy, 1 died.

The presence of lymph node metastases at the time of operation did not significantly affect survival (Fig. 20-12). Cumulative survival rate for patients with positive nodes was 87.7 percent; for patients without lymph node involvement, it was 93.6 percent.

Surprisingly, no significant difference in survival rate could be demonstrated between patients with papillary carcinoma and those with follicular carcinoma (Fig. 20-13). Cumulative survival rate was 92.3 percent in the 31 patients with follicular cancer, and 90.8 percent in the 124 patients with papillary tumors.

Recurrent Disease

No difference in the incidence of recurrence of thyroid carcinoma could be demonstrated between patients treated by total thyroidectomy and those treated by less than total thyroidectomy (Table 20-3). Recurrent tumor developed in 5 of the 29 patients (17 percent) treated by total thyroidectomy, and 16 of the 126 patients (13 percent) treated by less than total thyroidectomy.

Tumor recurrence was more frequent in patients with lymph node metastases at the time of the initial operation. Recurrent tumor developed in 17.7 percent of those with lymph node involvement, and in 10.7 percent of those without lymph node involvement. This difference was not statistically significant ($p > .2$).

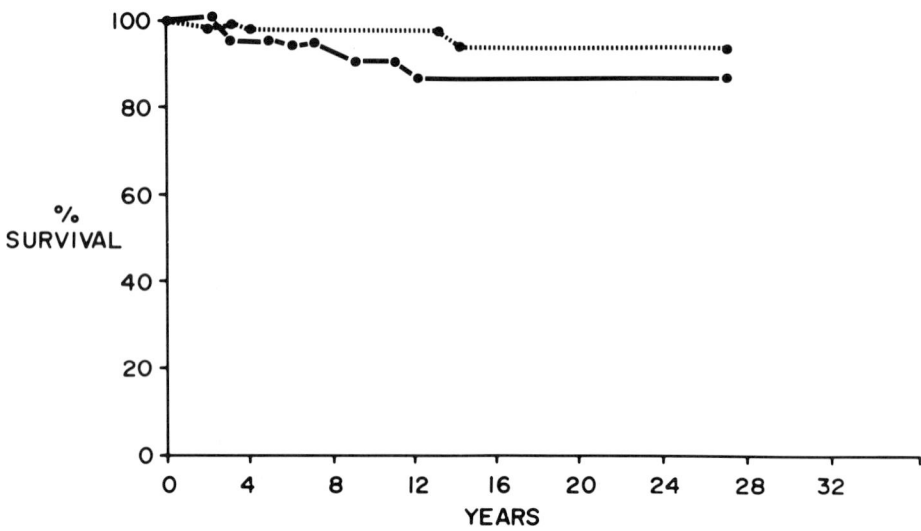

FIGURE 20-12 Survival curves comparing patients with papillary or follicular carcinoma of the thyroid with or without positive lymph nodes.

Postoperative Complications

Serious postoperative complications occurred significantly more often following total thyroidectomy than after less than total thyroidectomy (Table 20-4). Of the 29 patients undergoing total thyroidectomy, 6 developed hypoparathyroidism (20.7 percent) and 1 developed permanent unilateral recurrent laryngeal nerve damage (3.4 percent); the overall complication rate was 24.1 percent. In contrast, only 2 of 126 patients undergoing less than total thyroidectomy became hypoparathyroid (1.6 percent), and there was only 1 case of recurrent laryngeal nerve damage (0.8 percent). The overall complication rate after less than total thyroidectomy was 2.4 percent, which statistically is significantly less than the complication rate after total thyroidectomy ($p < .001$).

TABLE 20-3 Comparison of Tumor Recurrence in Patients with Papillary or Follicular Carcinoma Treated by Total or Less Than Total Thyroidectomy

Total thyroidectomy	5:29	17.2%
Less than total thyroidectomy	16:126	12.7%

Discussion

The data clearly support the concept that total thyroidectomy is not required for the treatment of papillary and follicular thyroid carcinomas. Survival in patients treated by less than total thyroidectomy (90.4 percent) was virtually identical to that in patients treated by total thyroidectomy (92.6 percent). Total thyroidectomy did not result in a reduction in the incidence of recurrent disease. Recurrent thyroid cancer developed in 17 percent of patients treated by total thyroidectomy, and in 13 percent of patients treated by less than total thyroidectomy.

While offering no benefit in terms of either increased chance for survival or lowered incidence of disease recurrence, total thyroidectomy has been associated with a significantly higher incidence of postoperative complications. Our data also fail to support the concept that total thyroidectomy is necessary because of the high incidence of multicentric disease in thyroid carcinoma. Of the 29 patients treated by less than total thyroidectomy who were subsequently shown to have multiple foci of tumor within the gland, only 1 subsequently died of thyroid carcinoma. Of the 12 patients with multicentric disease who were treated with total thyroidectomy 1 also eventually died of thyroid cancer. Clearly, although multicentric disease is often present in papillary and follicular tumors, these small foci of cancer are usually of no clinical significance.

On the basis of the results of this study, the following recommendations can be made. The lobe on the side of

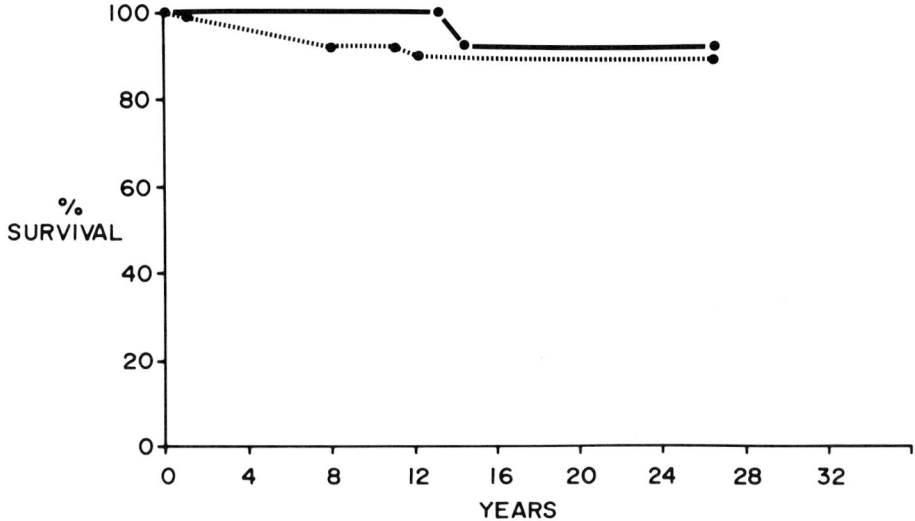

FIGURE 20-13 Survival curves comparing patients with papillary or follicular carcinoma of the thyroid.

the tumor should be removed, and the thyroid isthmus should be resected. If enlarged cervical lymph nodes are present, they should be excised. Lymph node involvement does not appear to alter the favorable prognosis of this disease and does not always justify a formal radical neck dissection. Equally good results can be obtained in papillary and follicular tumors by resection of the involved nodes.

Unilateral lobectomy and removal of the thyroid isthmus provide long-term results equally as good as those obtained by total thyroidectomy and result in considerably less postoperative morbidity. In the rare patient in whom a recurrence occurs in the contralateral lobe, removal of the remaining thyroid tissue is indicated.

In the past, radical neck dissections were often performed for papillary carcinoma of the thyroid in patients with clinically negative necks. Over 60 percent of these patients were found to have positive nodes. However, now that it is known that the prognosis is not altered by failure to resect the nodes, most surgeons do not perform radical neck dissections when the nodes are clinically negative. There is no question but that thyroid cancer cells are being left in the nodes of many of these patients and apparently they do not alter the prognosis. For this group of patients, some practitioners are advocating what could be termed "radical medical measures," involving a thyroidectomy plus scans with ^{131}I to determine if residual tumor persists. If the findings are positive, it is then recommended that therapeutic doses of ^{131}I be given, even in the very young.

If leaving the positive nodes at operation does not make a difference in prognosis, the question could be raised why treatment with ^{131}I should be employed. The morbidity of radical surgery was the resulting deformity, but it could be argued that no one really knows what the morbidity of therapeutic doses of ^{131}I are or will be. Other forms of radiation, especially in the young, have all been carcinogenic in a low percentage of patients and after a varying number of years. There is no definite proof that radiation from ^{131}I will not also prove to be carcinogenic.

ANATOMY OF THE PARATHYROID

Precise knowledge of the anatomy of the anterior cervical compartment is mandatory. The parathyroid glands are located in the anterior half of the neck, arising from the IIId and IVth branchial pouches, the superior glands from the IVth and the inferior glands from the IIId. They descend into the anterior neck along with the other branchial structures (thyroid and thymus). Although there are usually four glands, the presence of two to nine has been reported.

TABLE 20-4 Complications Following Total and Less Than Total Thyroidectomy for Papillary or Follicular Carcinoma of the Thyroid

Total thyroidectomy:		
Hypoparathyroidism	6:29	20.7%
Recurrent nerve damage	1:29	3.4%
		24.1%
Less than total thyroidectomy:		
Hypoparathyroidism	2:126	1.6%
Recurrent nerve damage	1:126	0.8%
		2.4%

The average size of a parathyroid gland is 6 × 4 × 2 mm, and the average weight is 30 to 35 mg per gland. The glands are located in a variety of positions. The superior glands are relatively consistent in position; in nearly 75 percent of cases, they lie on the posterior capsule of the middle third of the thyroid gland directly about the inferior thyroid artery.[36] The inferior glands, in 50 percent of cases, are located on the posterior surface of the lower pole of the thyroid directly inferior to the junction of the inferior thyroid artery and the recurrent laryngeal nerve (Fig. 20-14). Other inferior glands may lie anywhere along the embryonic line of descent, including the anterior mediastinum.

Blood is supplied to all four glands by the inferior thyroid arteries, although the superior glands may be partly supplied by the superior arteries. The venous drainage parallels the arterial supply.

TUMORS OF THE PARATHYROID

The most commonly occurring tumor of the parathyroid glands is an adenoma. Parathyroid hyperplasia constitutes the second most commonly occurring enlargement. Carcinoma of the parathyroid glands is rare.

Tumors of the parathyroid glands have an interesting historical background. In 1891, von Recklinghausen first described a group of patients with multiple cystic tumors of bone associated with pathologic fractures. This entity was named *osteitis fibrosa cystica generalisata*. Twelve years later, in 1903, Askanazy noted the relationship between this bone disease and parathyroid tumors on autopsy specimens. Erdheim, in 1907, proposed that the parathyroid tumors were secondary to the bone disease; and in 1915, Schlagenhaufer suggested that the bone disease was actually secondary to the parathyroid tumors. Ten years later, in 1925, Mandl performed the first successful removal of a parathyroid adenoma. The first parathyroid exploration in the United States was performed in 1927 at the Massachusetts General Hospital. No tumors were disclosed, but the patient underwent six additional operations over the next 5 years, with demonstration of a mediastinal parathyroid adenoma in the last operation in 1932. The patient subsequently died from electrolyte imbalance. The first successful operation in America was reported by Barr and Bulger in 1930, and the first carcinoma was reported in 1934 by Hall and Chaffin. In 1934 Albright described water-clear cell hyperplasia. Primary chief cell hyperplasia was described by Cope in 1958.[37]

Hyperparathyroidism

Functioning tumors of the parathyroid glands result in hyperparathyroidism: primary, secondary, or tertiary. *Primary hyperparathyroidism* is defined as persistent elevation in the secretion of parathyroid hormone associated with hypercalcemia. This may be due to a parathyroid adenoma, hyperplasia of the parathyroid glands, carcinoma, or a nonparathyroid tumor producing parathyroid hormone. *Secondary hyperparathyroidism* is characterized by hypophosphaturia, hyperphosphatemia, hypocalcemia, and parathyroid hyperplasia usually caused by chronic renal failure.[38] The parathyroid glands secrete more hormone in an effort to maintain the calcium-phosphate ratio, and this results in hyperplasia of the glands. The increased circulatory hormone causes increased calcium release from bone, producing in advanced disease the condition called renal rickets.

Tertiary hyperparathyroidism occurs when a hyperplastic gland of a patient with secondary hyperparathyroidism becomes autonomous and hypercalcemia develops.

Primary hyperparathyroidism affects 1 to 3 per 100,000 persons and is often asymptomatic. It is discovered most frequently between the ages of 35 and 65 and is more common in women. Because of the increasing use of laboratory screening tests, this disease has been detected more often during the past several years.

Primary hyperparathyroidism may be caused by a single enlarged gland, referred to as a parathyroid adenoma, by multiple adenomas, by chief cell or Wasserhalle hyperplasia, or by carcinoma. The most frequent pathologic finding is the enlarged single adenoma (83

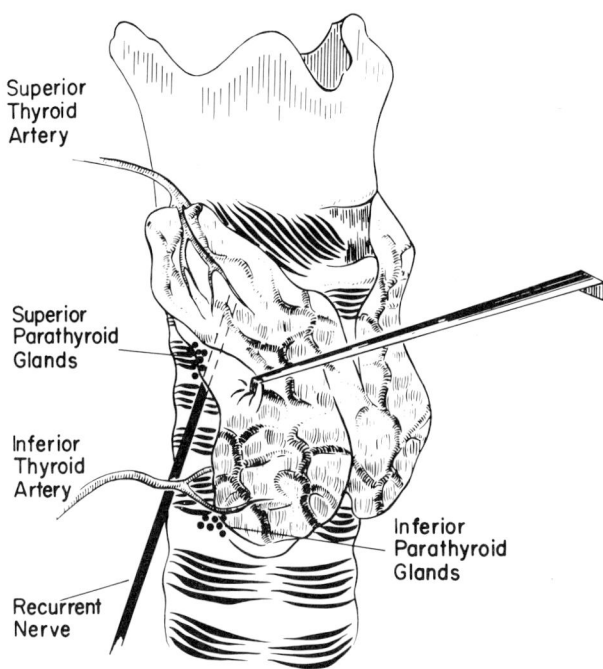

FIGURE 20-14 Anatomic relationship of recurrent nerve and parathyroid glands.

percent).[39] Most adenomas are composed predominantly of chief cells, although careful search usually demonstrates all cell types. A single adenoma is found in the inferior glands in 75 percent of cases.

Primary hyperplasia occurs in two forms: water-clear cell hyperplasia and primary chief cell hyperplasia. Since 1958, when Cope first described chief cell hyperplasia, it has been identified more often than water-clear cell hyperplasia. Most pathologists consider a single hyperplastic gland to be grossly and histologically indistinguishable from an adenomatous gland, making specific pathologic identification difficult for the surgeon. In most cases, however, the presence of a single normal parathyroid gland indicates that the enlarged gland represents an adenoma rather than hyperplasia.

Carcinoma

Malignancy of the parathyroid glands is rare, representing 1 to 4 percent of all parathyroid neoplasms.[40] They are found equally in both sexes, usually in the fourth to sixth decade of life. Compared to adenoma or hyperplasia, carcinoma produces more severe symptoms, higher calcium levels (15.9 mg per 100 mL), higher evidence of bone lesions (62 percent), urolithiasis (30 percent), palpable neck mass (30 to 50 percent), and pancreatitis.[41] Parathyroid carcinomas are usually biochemically functional, although parathyroid malignancies without hypercalcemia have been reported. Owing to the histologic similarities between adenoma and carcinoma, the diagnosis is often difficult. Mitosis, bizarre nuclei, and giant cells can be seen in both carcinoma and functioning adenomas. Therefore, clinical evidence of invasion of contiguous structures, presence of involved lymph nodes, and distal metastases are the best means of diagnosing carcinoma.[42]

Clinical Manifestations

Hyperparathyroidism may not cause clinical symptoms but often is detected by hypercalcemia demonstrated by routine laboratory examinations. Most patients found to have primary hyperparathyroidism are being evaluated for recurrent renal calculi (65 percent). Conversely, 5 to 10 percent of patients presenting with nephrolithiasis have hyperparathyroidism.

Many other associated symptoms are related to the affects of hypercalcemia. Musculoskeletal symptoms are usually vague and include weakness, hypotonia, and bone and joint pain. Pathologic fractures and shortening of stature may occur in severe cases. The earliest roentgenographic skeletal change is subperiosteal absorption, classically noted in the distal phalanges of the hand but also noted in the distal third of the clavicle and the distal ulna.

Anorexia, constipation, nausea, vomiting, peptic ulcer disease, and pancreatitis may be present; peptic ulcer disease is present in about 10 percent of cases and pancreatitis in a lower percent.

Symptoms referable to the central nervous system range from depression to coma and may be life-threatening.

Primary hyperparathyroidism may also present as one of a class of endocrine disorders, the multiple endocrine adenopathies. These are divided into two groups: MEA I, consisting of hyperparathyroidism, Zollinger-Ellison syndrome, and chromophobe adenomas; and MEA II, consisting of hyperparathyroidism, medullary carcinoma of the thyroid, pheochromocytoma, and adrenal cortical tumors. A recognized subgroup, MEA IIb, consists of medullary carcinoma of the thyroid; pheochromocytomas; mucosal neuromas of the lips, tongue, and/or conjunctiva; and ganglioneuroma of the bowel. Primary hyperparathyroidism in these syndromes is usually due to chief cell hyperplasia. A surgeon should always be aware of these syndromes and related diseases before neck exploration is undertaken.

Clinical Evaluation

Hypercalcemia is the predominant finding in primary hyperparathyroidism. Serum calcium levels should be obtained at intervals of several weeks before undertaking extensive laboratory and x-ray studies. Once hypercalcemia has been substantiated, other disease processes that may cause hypercalcemia must be ruled out. Routine laboratory studies should include plasma phosphate and chloride, BUN, creatinine, serum alkaline phosphatase, and serum parathyroid hormone level. Serum plasma phosphate is a less reliable index, although values consistently below 2.5 mg per 100 mL are significant. BUN and creatinine help to evaluate renal function. It has been reported that 80 to 90 percent of patients with primary hyperparathyroidism have some degree of renal impairment. Serum chloride levels below 102 meq/L are seldom seen in primary hyperparathyroidism. Will and McGowan reported that of 61 patients, 33 had serum chloride levels greater than 102 meq/L and all but one of these had hyperparathyroidism; the 28 with values below 102 meq/L had hypercalcemia due to other causes.[43] Serum alkaline phosphatase gives some clue to the amount of bone destruction.

The recent development of serum parathyroid hormone assay has been exciting, giving a direct measure of the amount of hormone circulating in the bloodstream. Levels are elevated in 80 to 90 percent of patients with either primary or tertiary hyperparathyroidism. Chest x-ray, bone scan, and contrast studies, including upper gastrointestinal series, barium enema, and intravenous pyelogram, should be obtained to help rule out an unrecognized malignancy which might produce ectopic parathyroid hormone. The chest x-ray and upper gastrointestinal series may also demonstrate a mass lesion, possibly representing a parathyroid tumor. Other x-ray studies which may aid in the diagnosis include skull and hand films. X-rays of the skull may demonstrate the "moth-eaten," ground-glass appearance of hyperparathyroidism, while the hand films may show the classic subperiosteal bone resorption of the middle and distal phalanges.

An accurate, safe, economical noninvasive method for localizing parathyroid tumors is not presently available. Therefore, any effort toward localizing the tumor should be reserved for only those patients to be reoperated upon. Most experienced surgeons can identify and remove the abnormal parathyroid gland in more than 90 percent of patients at initial exploration.

Preoperative attempts to localize the parathyroid glands are warranted if a second neck exploration is required. Arteriograms of the superior and inferior thyroid arteries may demonstrate a parathyroid tumor "blush." At certain centers, results of this procedure have been good, with little morbidity or mortality. Selective venous sampling from the inferior thyroid veins to measure serum levels of PTH has helped to define on which side the abnormal gland is located. Unilateral elevation (twice that of the peripheral plasma sample) usually suggests a single parathyroid adenoma, while bilateral high concentration usually indicates hyperplasia.

A new test described by Reiss, called the *parathyroid squeeze test,* is performed by massaging both sides of the neck at different intervals and testing PTH levels after each side is massaged.[44] A rise in serum PTH after one side is massaged indicates that an adenoma is likely on that side. If both sides are elevated, disease is bilateral and hyperplasia is usually present. The time delay in obtaining PTH levels makes this test impractical.

Localization of parathyroid glands by selenium methionine scan has been attempted recently. Although some excellent visualization of parathyroid adenomas has been reported, false positives and false negatives are common.

Differential Diagnosis

If unnecessary neck exploration is to be avoided, several other diseases which can cause hypercalcemia must be differentiated from primary hyperparathyroidism (Table 20-5). Malignant tumor with or without osseous metastases is the most common cause of hypercalcemia. It may be very difficult clinically to distinguish between a parathyroid adenoma and a PTH-producing tumor. Tumors producing similar symptoms include bronchogenic tumors, hypernephromas, hepatomas, epidermoid cancer, tumors of the bladder, ovary, uterus, vulva, pancreas, liver, and lymphatic malignant tumors. Although both

TABLE 20-5 Differential Diagnosis of Hypercalcemia

Metastatic carcinoma

Primary hyperparathyroidism

Osteoporosis

Sarcoidosis

Hypervitaminosis D

Paget's disease of bone

Milk-alkali syndrome

Renal tubular acidosis

Immobilization

Dysproteinemias

entities have high serum PTH levels, it has recently been demonstrated that serum immunoreactive parathyroid hormone levels are lower in ectopically produced PTH than in primary hyperparathyroidism.

A good history will identify milk-alkali syndrome, vitamin D intoxication, use of thiazide, or immobilization if any of these is the cause of hypercalcemia. The remaining possible diagnoses can be tested by the appropriate use of laboratory and x-ray examinations.

The primary concern is to be sure that all possible causes of hypercalcemia have been explored before the patient is subjected to a neck exploration.

Treatment

Treatment of primary hyperparathyroidism is surgical extirpation of the hyperactive tissue. It is definitely advantageous to prevent the severe renal and bone changes which will eventually occur if the patient is not operated upon. Since specific medical therapy for hypercalcemia is generally adequate, it is seldom necessary to perform emergency parathyroid surgery. Calcium levels can usually be controlled temporarily with a variety of agents.

Most patients respond to isotonic saline infusions (1 L every 3 to 4 h), which can be supplemented with intermittent use of furosemide (100 mg/h). This combination places drastic stress on the vascular compartment. Complications include pulmonary edema, hypernatremia, hypokalemia, and volume depletion, and all patients should be carefully monitored. Steroid medication quickly lowers the calcium in multiple myeloma and some malignant processes, but has little effect on elevated serum calcium secondary to primary hyperparathyroidism. Other agents used include oral phosphate, calcitonin, and mithramycin. Mithramycin given intravenously (25 μg per kilogram of body weight) has been shown to be very effective when other agents have failed, but complications include hemorrhage and thrombocytopenia.

Parathyroid surgery is performed through a standard transverse low collar incision. After mobilizing the thyroid, the inferior thyroid artery and recurrent laryngeal nerve should be identified. Exploration should begin at the junction of these two structures. The inferior gland is usually found anterior to the recurrent laryngeal nerve, while the superior gland is usually located posterior to the nerve (Fig. 20-14).

A single parathyroid adenoma is found in 83 percent of the cases, but the other parathyroid glands should be identified to be sure multiple adenomas are not present. If all glands are enlarged (hyperplasia), a subtotal parathyroidectomy should be performed, removing $3\frac{1}{2}$ glands. If possible, the specimens should be preserved by freezing; they may be transplanted at a later date if permanent hypocalcemia occurs postoperatively.

If the surgeon has difficulty identifying the parathyroid glands, it is sometimes helpful to divide the superior pole vessels to further mobilize the thyroid. The carotid sheath and superior mediastinum should also be thoroughly explored. Staining the glands by injecting the inferior thyroid artery with toluidine blue has been helpful in isolated cases.

Postoperative complications include hemorrhage, hypoparathyroidism, recurrent nerve damage, and recurrent disease. Hypocalcemia is possible after the excision of a large parathyroid adenoma. The remaining glands are hypoplastic and usually require 1 to 2 weeks to regain normal function.

Recurrent disease is most commonly seen if primary chief cell hyperplasia is not recognized. A second exploration is usually required.

Treatment of carcinoma of the parathyroid gland consists of en bloc excision of the ipsilateral thyroid lobe and isthmus, skeletonization of the trachea, excision of adherent strap muscles, and ipsilateral radical neck dissection. For recurrent disease, surgical exploration for removal of metastases is used as a palliative measure to aid in controlling hypercalcemia. Radiation and chemotherapy have proved to be ineffective. The 5-year survival rate is reported to be 50 percent.[45]

ACKNOWLEDGMENT

We wish to thank John T. Brandt, M.D., Clinical Instructor, Department of Pathology, Ohio State University, College of Medicine, for preparing the thyroid and parathyroid microphotography and legends.

REFERENCES

1. Frazell EL, Foote FW Jr: Papillary thyroid carcinoma. *Cancer* 8:1164, 1955.
2. Hutter RVP, Frazell EL, Foote FW: Elective radical neck dissection: An assessment of its use in the management of papillary thyroid cancer. *CA* 20:87, 1970.
3. Ackerman, Regato: *Cancer,* Mosby, St. Louis, 1947.
4. Ward GE, Hendrick JW: *Tumors of the Head and Neck,* Williams & Wilkins, Baltimore, 1950.
5. Welch CE: Therapy for multinodular goiter, *JAMA* 195:95, 1966.
6. Cole WH, Majarkis JD, Slaughter DP: Incidence of carcinoma of the thyroid in nodular goiter. *J Clin Endocrinol Metab* 9:1007, 1949.
7. Mortensen JD, Bennett WA, Woolner LB: Gross and microscopic findings in clinically normal thyroid glands. *J Clin Endocrinol* 15:1270, 1955.
8. Thompson NW, Nishiyama RH, Harness JK: Thyroid carcinoma. *Curr Prob Surg* 15:5, 1978.
9. Hawk WA, Hazard JB: The many appearances of papillary carcinoma of the thyroid. *Cleveland Clin Q* 43:207, 1976.
10. Woolner LB: Thyroid carcinoma: Pathologic classification with data on prognosis. *Semin Nucl Med* 1:481, 1971.
11. Sampson RJ, Woolner LB, Bahn RC, Kurland LT: Occult thyroid carcinoma in Olmstead County, Minn. *Cancer* 34:2072, 1974.
12. MacComb WS, Fletcher GH: *Cancer of the Head and Neck,* Williams & Wilkins, Baltimore, 1967.
13. Beaugie JM: *Principles of Thyroid Surgery,* Grune & Stratton, New York, 1975, p. 144.
14. Tollefsen HR, Shah JP, Huvos AG: Follicular carcinoma of the thyroid. *Am J Surg* 126, 1973.
15. Edis AJ: Surgical treatment for thyroid cancer. *Surg Clin North Am* 57:533, 1977.
16. Aldinger KA, Naguib AS, Ibanez M, Hill CS: Anaplastic carcinoma of the thyroid. *Cancer* 41:2267, 1978.
17. Block MA, Horn RC, Miller JM, Barrett JL, Brush, BE: Familial medullary carcinoma of the thyroid. *Ann Surg* 166:403, 1967.
18. Block MA, Jackson CE, Tashjian AH Jr: Medullary thyroid carcinoma detected by serum calcitonin assay. *Arch Surg* 104:579, 1972.
19. Wells SA Jr, Ontjes DA, Cooper CW, Hennessy JF, Ellis GJ, McPherson HT, Sabiston DC: The early diagnosis of medullary carcinoma of the thyroid gland in patients with multiple endocrine neoplasia, type II, *Ann Surg* 182:362, 1975.
20. Schwartz SI: *Principles of Surgery,* McGraw-Hill, New York, 1979.
21. Black BM, YaDeau RE, Woolner LB: Surgical treatment of thyroidal carcinomas. *Arch Surg* 88:610, 1964.
22. Tollefsen HR, Shah JP, Huvos AG: Hurthle cell of the thyroid. *Am J Surg* 130, 1975.
23. Hoffer PB, Gottschalk A, Quinn J: *Thyroid in Vivo Studies, Diagnostic Nuclear Medicine,* Williams & Wilkins, Philadelphia, 1975, pp. 255–277.
24. Kyoichi U, Hariki K, Tatsumura T: The value of thallium-201 imaging in the diagnosis of thyroid cancer in a patient with negative ^{99m}Tc and ^{131}I scans. *Clin Nucl Med* 3:447, 1978.
25. Glassford GH, Fowler EF, Cole WH: The treatment of nontoxic nodular goiter with desiccated thyroid. *Surgery* 58:621, 1965.
26. Mazzaferri EL, Young RL, Oertel JE, Kemmerer WT, Page CP: Papillary thyroid carcinoma: The impact of therapy in 576 patients. *Medicine* 56:171, 1977.
27. Remine WH, McConahey WM: Management of thyroid nodules. *Surg Clin North Am* 57:523, 1977.
28. Gordon PR, Huvos AG, Strong EW: Medullary carcinoma of the thyroid gland. *Cancer* 31, 1973.
29. Pochin EE: Prospects from the treatment of thyroid carcinoma with radioiodine. *Clin Radiol* 18:113, 1967.
30. Harness JK, Thompson NW, Sisson JC, Beierwaltes WH: Differentiated thyroid carcinomas: Treatment of distant metastases. *Arch Surg* 108:410, 1974.
31. Duffy BJ Jr, Fitzgerald PJ: Thyroid cancer in childhood and adolescence: Report on 28 cases. *J Clin Endocrinol* 101:1296, 1950.
32. Winship T, Rosvoll R: Childhood thyroid carcinoma. *Cancer* 14:734, 1961.
33. Greenspan FS: Radiation exposure and thyroid cancer. *JAMA* 237:2089, 1977.
34. Gottlieb JA, Hill CS Jr: Chemotherapy of thyroid cancer with adriamycin: Experience with 30 patients. *N Engl J Med* 290:193, 1974.
35. Gottlieb JA, Hill CS Jr: Adriamycin therapy in thyroid carcinoma. *Cancer Chemother Rep Part 3* 6:283, 1975.
36. Schwartz SI: *Principles of Surgery,* McGraw-Hill, New York, 1979.
37. Beahrs OH, Hoehn JG: Surgery of the parathyroid glands, *Head and Neck Surgery Textbook,* Harper & Row, New York, 1974.
38. Robbins SL, Angell M: *Basic Pathology,* Saunders, Philadelphia, 1976, pp. 614–617.
39. Sabiston DC: *Textbook of Surgery.* Saunders, Philadelphia, 1977.
40. Hardy JD: *Textbook of Surgery,* Lippincott, Philadelphia, 1977.

41. Schantz A, Castleman B: Parathyroid carcinoma, *Cancer,* 31: 600, 1973.
42. Kay S, Hume DM: Carcinoma of the parathyroid gland. *Arch Pathol* 96:316, 1973.
43. Wills MR, McGowan GK: Plasma-chloride levels in hyperparathyroidism and other hypercalcemia states. *Brit Med J* 1:1153, 1964.
44. Reiss E, Canterbury JM: Application of radioimmunoassay to differentiation of adenoma and hyperplasia and to preoperative localization of hyperfunctioning parathyroid glands. *N Engl J Med* 280:1381, 1969.
45. McGarity WC, Boehm G: Carcinoma of the parathyroid. *South Med J* 68:2, 1975.

SELECTED BIBLIOGRAPHY

Brennan MF, Bloomer WD: Cancer of the endocrine system: The thyroid gland, in DeVita VT Jr et al (eds): *Cancer: Principles and Practice of Oncology,* Lippincott, Philadelphia, 1982, pp 971–985.

Goldman JM et al: Anaplastic thyroid carcinoma: Long-term survival after radical surgery. *J Surg Oncol* 14:389, 1980.

Norton JA et al: Localization and resection of clinically inapparent medullary carcinoma of the thyroid. *Surgery* 87:616, 1980.

Russell CF et al: The surgical management of medullary thyroid carcinoma. *Ann Surg* 197:42, 1983.

Saxe AW, Brennan MF: Technique of reoperative parathyroidectomy. *Surgery* 89:497, 1981.

Simpson WJ et al: Management of medullary thyroid cancer. *Am J Surg* 144:420, 1982.

PART THREE

INTRATHORACIC NEOPLASMS

21
PULMONARY NEOPLASMS

E. Carmack Holmes

Lung cancer is the leading cause of death from cancer in men and is rapidly increasing in the female population. In 1978, lung cancer accounted for 15 percent of cancers and 23 percent of cancer mortality. Lung cancer is now the second most frequent cause of cancer deaths in the female population, and it is anticipated that it will become the most common cause of cancer death among females in the near future. While the death rates from cancer at other organ sites have remained essentially constant during the past decade, there is every indication that the incidence of lung cancer will continue to increase at an alarming rate. While much is known regarding the cause of lung cancer, it has been difficult to implement measures to prevent the development of the disease. At the present time, surgery provides the only reliable cure. Radiation therapy is an excellent palliative treatment. While chemotherapy remains essentially experimental, there are several new combination chemotherapeutic regimens which appear to be effective. Clinical investigators are now exploring the possibility of combining two or more of these modalities in an effort to improve results. New developments in early detection and improved staging techniques are leading to a better knowledge of the natural history of the disease and to an increased ability to effect cures.

RISK FACTORS

In the past, lung cancer was a problem primarily in the male population. However, the disease is now increasing very rapidly in women.[1,2] It is clear that oat-cell and squamous cell carcinoma are closely related to smoking; however, the relationship between adenocarcinoma and smoking is less clear. Adenocarcinoma of the lung is the most common carcinoma in nonsmokers.[3] Asbestos, arsenic, chromates, and nickel have been strongly indicated as causative agents.[4] (See Table 21-1.) Recently, a strong association between uranium dust and the development of bronchogenic carcinoma has been described.[5-7] Mesotheliomas are associated with exposure to asbestos, and family members of workers exposed to asbestos also have an increased incidence of mesothelioma. Since it appears that the majority of lung cancers are associated with certain carcinogenic agents, the majority of lung cancers should be preventable. Of interest is the recent discovery that retinoids may be effective in preventing the development of cancer in experimental animals. Although it has not yet been demonstrated that retinoids are preventive agents in humans, they may, in the future prove effective in helping prevent lung cancer.[84]

Environmental factors are probably superimposed on

TABLE 21-1 Agents Associated with Lung Cancer In Man

Asbestos
Nickel
Chromium
Uranium
Polycyclic aromatic hydrocarbons

genetic patterns that predispose individuals to the development of lung cancer. Studies have indicated that genetic factors may exert an influence on the development of lung cancer equal to that of cigarette smoking.[8] One such genetic factor may be the presence of the inducible enzyme arylhydrocarbon hydroxlyase (AHH), which converts the polycyclic hydrocarbon of cigarette smoke into highly carcinogenic hypoxides. The inducibility of AHH by these hydrocarbons appears to be controlled by a single gene. Individuals who smoke and who have a high inducibility of this enzyme have a significantly greater risk of developing lung cancer.[9] It is clear, therefore, that the etiology of lung cancer involves more than a simple association with smoking. Undoubtedly, other environmental carcinogens have an additive effect, and certain genetic characteristics probably increase susceptibility to these environmental carcinogens.

CLASSIFICATION

The World Health Organization has developed a classification system that has been accepted by most pathologists and oncologists (Table 21-2). Epidermoid carcinomas tend to be centrally located and are less likely to have metastases at the time of presentation than are the other histologic types. Epidermoid carcinoma is most likely to be resectable and is associated with the best prognosis. In addition, epidermoid tumors may cavitate and, therefore, suggest a lung abscess.

Small-cell carcinomas arise from the Kultschitzsky cells of neuroectodermal origin. They tend to be more centrally located and are likely to have distant metastases at the time of presentation. Sites of metastases include brain, bone, bone marrow, liver, adrenal glands, and abdominal lymph nodes. These patients are not usually considered candidates for surgery in view of the high incidence of metastatic disease. However, a few patients with localized small-cell carcinoma have survived for a prolonged period of time following surgery.[10]

Adenocarcinomas of the lung arise from the bronchoalveolar epithelium or from the mucous glands and they tend to be peripheral. Adenocarcinomas obviously represent a spectrum of tumors, each with a different histiogenesis. An adenocarcinoma can arise from a bronchial mucous gland cell, a Kultschitzsky cell, ciliated columnar cells, nonciliated columnar cells, or alveolar pneumocytes (type I or type II). These tumors may all have different growth patterns and different responses to therapy. Chronic interstitial pulmonary disease, pulmonary scars, and fibrosis may predispose to adenocarcinoma. Adenocarcinomas frequently involve the pleura and often metastasize to the extrathoracic lymph nodes. These tumors have a tendency for hematogenous dissemination, and chances for survival following surgery are considerably worse than with epidermoid carcinomas. Bronchoalveolar carcinoma is a form of adenocarcinoma, but it has a much better prognosis.[11] This tumor has a tendency to involve multiple areas of the lung, and when it reaches this stage it is rarely curable. Early detection and surgical resection are, therefore, very important. This tumor is interesting, since infectious agents have been implicated as causative agents.[12] Large-cell carcinoma of the lungs is similar to adenocarcinoma and may represent a more undifferentiated form of adenocarcinoma.

TABLE 21-2 Histologic Types of Lung Cancer

1. Epidermoid carcinomas
2. Small-cell anaplastic carcinomas
3. Adenocarcinomas
4. Large-cell carcinomas
5. Combined epidermoid and adenocarcinomas
6. Carcinoid tumors
7. Bronchial gland tumors
8. Papillary tumors of the surface epithelium
9. "Mixed" tumors and carcinosarcomas
10. Sarcomas
11. Unclassified
12. Mesotheliomas
13. Melanomas

Bronchial carcinoid tumors, like small-cell carcinomas, are related to Kultschitzsky-type cells. Although only 10 to 12 percent of bronchial carcinomas metastasize to the regional nodes, they are frequently locally invasive. These tumors tend to be centrally located, and produce symptoms such as cough, wheeze, dyspnea, and hemoptysis. Because of their central location, they are easily visualized with the bronchoscope. However, caution should be exerted when biopsying these tumors since they are very vascular. Bronchial carcinoids rarely produce the carcinoid syndrome. Great care should be taken to adequately resect these tumors, since they will recur locally if inadequately resected. However, more conservative resection for these tumors is indicated when the anatomy is appropriate.[13]

DIAGNOSIS

Screening programs for the early detection of lung cancer have been instituted in a variety of institutions, including the Mayo Clinic, Johns Hopkins Medical Institutions, and the Memorial Hospital for Cancer and Allied Diseases.[14–18] At 4-month intervals, these programs screen men of 45 years of age or older who smoke one or more packs of cigarettes per day, using chest x-rays, 3-day pooled sputum cytologies, and health lung questionnaires. The early data from these studies suggest that these screening techniques may detect a prevalence rate of approximately 5 per 100,000 and that patients who are detected early are more curable than those who present with symptoms. These studies indicate that early detection of radiologically occult lung cancer may lead to improved survival following surgery, and such screening programs will likely be indicated in all high-risk patients in the future.[18]

It is becoming apparent that patients with small localized early carcinomas of the lung have a decided tendency to develop second primaries. For this reason, surgical procedures that conserve lung tissue are indicated for these early lesions,[19,20] and patients can be treated with less than a complete lobectomy. Very often, segmental resection or generous wedge excision of the small primary tumor will be appropriate. However, in all cases, the regional lymph nodes should be adequately and thoroughly examined.

Chest x-rays are the most common means of detecting pulmonary tumors. Comparison with previous x-rays whenever possible is essential. It should be remembered that segmental or lobar pneumonia often accompanies carcinoma of the lung because of bronchial obstruction. Any segmental or labor pneumonia that does not respond to the usual medical management should be considered a possible indication of carcinoma of the lung. Continued technological improvement in the examination of sputum cytology has made sputum cytology the primary diagnostic tool in patients with lung cancer, and at least 75 percent of all lung cancers can be diagnosed by this means. Patients who have radiologically apparent tumors on the chest x-ray should have bronchoscopy and sputum cytology examination, as well as full lung tomograms, to evaluate the characteristics of the nodule as well as to evaluate the mediastinum. Conventional tomography has been recommended to delineate mediastinal lymphadenopathy and has been shown to be more effective than plain radiography for detecting mediastinal nodes.[21,22] Computed tomography is particularly useful in detecting mediastinal lymphadenopathy and holds great promise as a staging and diagnostic tool.[23] Cytology may be obtained at the time of bronchoscopy, but the highest yields occur on the morning following bronchoscopy. A positive finding on cytologic examination is very reliable for the diagnosis of lung cancer (98 percent) and quite good (75 percent) in identifying the cell type.[24,25] It should be remembered that rarely a positive finding on sputum cytology examination may be due to aspirated tumor cells shed from a head and neck malignancy. More recently, the technique of percutaneous needle aspiration biopsy for the purpose of diagnosing peripherally located tumors has become popular. The complication rate is low, and the risk of tumor dissemination is negligible.[26] The aspirated cytology from these procedures is also highly accurate, and needle aspiration is a very useful diagnostic tool.

STAGING

Since there is a significant morbidity rate associated with the surgical treatment of lung cancer, it is important to identify and to exclude from surgery those patients who are likely to have disseminated disease. The staging of patients with lung cancer can be divided into two general categories: evaluation of the extent of extrathoracic disease and evaluation of the extent of intrathoracic disease. Hepatic metastases are frequently suspected from physical examination or routine screening of liver chemistries. These metastatic lesions are almost always associated with an elevated alkaline phosphatase, and routine liver scanning should only be done in those patients who have evidence of hepatic metastases on physical examination or elevated alkaline phosphatase. Several studies have indicated that routine multiorgan scanning for the purpose of staging patients with lung cancer is not useful.[27–29] The use of computed tomography instead of the usual radioisotopic brain scan might increase diagnostic accuracy; however, this technique is still under investigation.[30] Obviously, any patient whose physical examination or history suggests bone, liver, or brain metastases should be further evaluated. However, in the asymptomatic patient with a normal physical examination and liver profile, routine use of these scans is an expensive, time-consuming, and low-yield diagnostic maneuver. It has been suggested that whole-body gallium scans may be useful as a staging procedure and may obviate the need for other scans. However, further study is needed in order to precisely define the role of this technique.[31,32] All patients with the diagnosis of small-cell carcinoma (oat-cell carcinoma) should be evaluated with multiorgan scanning techniques, and an evaluation of the bone marrow for metastatic disease should be made. Since small-cell carcinoma of the lung is frequently a disseminated and systemic disease, these staging procedures should be practiced routinely.

Recently, considerable interest has centered on intrathoracic staging by mediastinoscopy. However, the indications for mediastinal exploration in patients with bronchogenic carcinoma are controversial. The yield varies between 10 and 75 percent, depending on the histology of the tumor, the size of the tumor, and the extent of the disease at the time of mediastinoscopy. Therefore, the percentage of positive findings depends entirely on patient selection. Although some surgeons recommend routine cervical mediastinal exploration prior to thoracotomy,[33] while others use it infrequently, it is clear that the development of mediastinoscopy has increased the incidence of resectability at the time of thoracotomy. While the advantages of mediastinal exploration are generally recognized, many surgeons feel that not all patients with bronchogenic carcinoma require the procedure.[34–36] Most surgeons now feel that mediastinal exploration should be employed in all patients in whom x-rays suggest mediastinal involvement and in those patients who have a high risk of surgery due to medical problems. Indirect tests such as mediastinal tomography and barium swallow may erroneously suggest metastases, and mediastinoscopy should be performed in all these instances to prove the presence of mediastinal metastatic disease. Indeed, one study indicated that there was no correlation between the diagnosis at mediastinoscopy and that made using various indirect diagnostic tests.[37]

Mediastinal exploration can be performed either by the cervical or parasternal route.[38] Cervical mediastinal exploration is especially useful for right or left paratracheal lymph node sampling. The carina, as well as the right main stem bronchus, can be easily reached by the cervical approach. Since the aortic arch is on the left side, cervical mediastinoscopy is not useful in evaluating left hilar lesions. Therefore, parasternal mediastinoscopy is used more frequently for these lesions.

The American Joint Commission for Cancer Staging and End Results Reporting has developed a classification for the staging of lung cancer.[39] This classification is outlined in Table 21-3. In this TNM system, T designates the characteristics of the primary tumor, N the regional lymph nodes, and M the distant metastases. The staging may, therefore, be determined by clinical classification (presurgical evaluation) or by surgical classification based on the actual pathologic findings. As indicated in the table, the TNM classification is used to characterize the stage of the disease. Patients with T_1N_0, T_1N_1, or T_2N_0 are considered stage I. Patients with T_2N_1 are stage II and patients with stage III disease are those with a T_3 lesion or any N_2 or M_1. This staging system correlates very well with survival rate following surgery.[40] Patients with T_1N_0 lesions can anticipate an 80 to 90 percent 3-year survival rate following surgical resection.[41,42] Patients with T_2N_0 and T_1N_1 lesions have a 30 to 40 percent recurrence rate at 2 years. Patients with squamous carcinoma who have positive hilar nodes but with negative mediastinal involvement can expect a 50 percent 5-year survival rate following surgery. However, the prognosis for patients with adenocarcinoma of the lung with positive hilar lymph node involvement is much worse.[43] Generally, the presence of mediastinal lymph node involvement is associated with a very poor 5-year survival rate. However, recent studies have indicated that patients with squamous cell carcinoma of the lung and undifferentiated large-cell carcinoma with limited mediastinal lymph node involvement may have a 30 to 40 percent 5-year survival rate following adequate resection. Therefore, mediastinal lymph node involvement is no longer considered an absolute contraindication to surgical resection if the mediastinal lymph node involvement is limited.[85] However, patients with adenocarcinoma and mediastinal lymph node involvement have a survival rate of only 5 to 15 percent following pulmonary resection and mediastinal lymph node resection. Every patient undergoing thoracotomy for carcinoma of the lung should be staged according to the TNM classification (Fig. 21-1). Even if the regional lymph nodes do not appear to be involved, representative samples of mediastinal and hilar lymph nodes should be taken and submitted for pathologic examination, since there is at least a 10 percent error in the assessment of mediastinal lymph node involvement at thoracotomy if the nodes are not removed and studied histologically. It is likely that in previous reports on survival rate many patients who were classified as having stage I lung cancer may have had occult stage II and stage III disease. Therefore, careful intraoperative staging is important in that it provides useful prognostic information and permits a better understanding of the natural history of the disease.

TREATMENT

Surgery

All cell types of lung cancer with the exception of small-cell carcinoma are amenable to surgical resection in the appropriate stage. It is generally believed that small-cell carcinoma should not be resected, although, rarely, patients with this form of cancer who present with a small peripheral nodule may benefit from pulmonary resection.[10]

Surgery remains the most effective therapy for lung cancer. While pneumonectomy was once considered the treatment of choice for all lung cancers, it has become clear that pneumonectomy provides no advantage over lobectomy if the tumor can be properly encompassed with the lesser procedure.[44,45] Radical pneumonectomy has been evaluated; however, this procedure is not now routinely applied.[46] Indeed, segmental resections for very small lung cancers can produce good 5-year survival rates. These operations are particularly indicated in patients with small primary tumors who are at high risk for developing second primaries in the future.[13] The involvement of the chest wall, phrenic nerve, or diaphragm does not contraindicate resection. The diaphragm can be resected and reconstituted with prosthetic material, as can the chest wall. Chest wall resection can be performed with excellent survival rates provided that the mediastinal nodes are negative.[47,48]

TABLE 21-3 Staging of Carcinoma of the Lung

T, N, M

T: Primary tumor
  T_0: No evidence of primary tumor
  T_X: Tumor occult of primary tumor
  T_1: Tumor 3 cm or less in diameter, surrounded by lung pleura or parenchyma, and without evidence of invasion of lobar bronchus.
  T_2: Tumor more than 3 cm in diameter or tumor extending to the hilar region; must be 2 cm or more distal to the carina and not have T_3 characteristics
  T_3: Tumor of any size with direct extension into adjacent structures (e.g., chest wall, diaphragm, mediastinum) or tumor less than 2 cm distal to carina or tumor associated with atelectasis or obstructive pneumonitis of an entire lung or with pleural effusion

N: Regional lymph nodes
  N_0: No demonstrable metastasis to regional lymph nodes
  N_1: Metastasis to lymph nodes in the ipsilateral hilar region (including direct extension)
  N_2: Metastasis to lymph nodes in the mediastinum

M: Distant metastasis
  M_0: No distant metastasis
  M_1: Distant metastasis, such as scalene, cervical or contralateral hilar lymph nodes, brain, bones, lung, liver, and so forth

Stage grouping
  Occult carcinoma: $T_X N_0 M_0$
  Stage I: $T_1 N_0 M_0$, $T_1 N_1 M_0$, or $T_2 N_0 M_0$
  Stage II: $T_2 N_1 M_0$
Stage III: Any T_3; any N_2; any M_1

SOURCE: Adapted from DT Carr, CF Mountain: *Semin Oncol* 1:229, 1974.

Carcinoma of the lung involving the superior sulcus may give rise to the Pancoast syndrome.[49] While these tumors were originally considered incurable, it has become apparent that a substantial percentage of these patients will benefit from resection of the tumor and the involved chest wall. This procedure may require the resecting of the spinal roots of T8 and C1, resulting in a significant ulnar nerve palsy. It has been reported that with the use of preoperative radiation therapy, 35 percent of patients with superior sulcus tumors will survive 5 years after this operation.[50]

There are certain absolute contraindications to pulmonary resection in patients with lung cancer. Obviously, the presence of clinically apparent metastases beyond

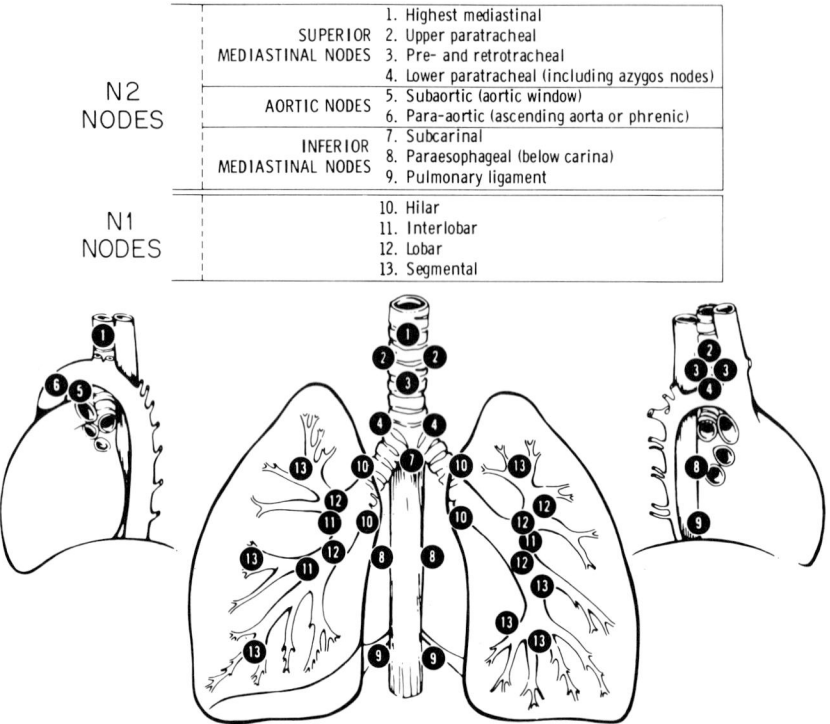

FIGURE 21-1 Anatomical distribution of bronchopulmonary, hilar, and mediastinal lymph nodes.

the thorax contraindicates pulmonary resection. In addition, pleural effusion containing malignant cells is a contraindication to pulmonary resection. As indicated above, the presence of chest wall involvement is not a contraindication to surgery. However, recurrent laryngeal nerve paralysis on the side of the tumor is considered an absolute contraindication, as is superior vena caval obstruction. Involvement of the main stem bronchus within 2 cm of the carina indicates that an adequate surgical resection may not be feasible.

With the development of more effective adjuvant therapy such as chemotherapy for both small-cell and non-small-cell carcinoma of the lung, the role of surgery and the indications for surgical resection may change in the not too distant future. The development of combination chemotherapeutic regimens which are capable of controlling systemic disseminated tumor will likely increase the role of the surgeon in the treatment of lung cancer. The development of effective adjuvant therapy which could control disseminated visceral metastatic disease would justify using more radical procedures in an attempt to totally extirpate the local disease.

Radiation Therapy

Radiation therapy in the management of lung cancer may be used as a curative measure or a palliative measure. The 5-year survival rate after radical radiation therapy is 3 to 9 percent.[51] Potentially curative radiation therapy requires doses of 5500 to 6500 rads delivered over a 6- or 7-week period.[52] Dosages in this range cause radiation pneumonitis and progressive pulmonary fibrosis. In addition, esophagitis may occur, and radiation myelitis is a risk. Generally, patients do not receive potentially curative doses of radiation therapy unless they are found to be surgically unresectable or are in good general condition and have no evidence of disseminated disease.

Radiation therapy can be a very effective palliative treatment for complications of lung cancer in 75 to 80 percent of patients. Hemoptysis, bronchial obstruction, superior venal caval obstruction, bone pain, and chronic cough can frequently be relieved with relatively moderate doses of radiation therapy.

Preoperative radiation therapy is valuable in the treatment of superior sulcus tumors. The usual dose is

3000 to 3500 rads given in 10 treatments, followed by surgical resection in 3 weeks. The results of preoperative radiation therapy for other forms of bronchogenic carcinoma have been disappointing, and indeed some studies have indicated that preoperative radiation therapy results in a lower survival rate than surgery alone.[53,54] No prospective randomized studies comparing postoperative radiation therapy with surgery alone have been reported. A retrospective study has indicated that patients with squamous carcinoma with mediastinal lymph node metastases benefit from postoperative therapy.[43] However, the role of radiation therapy following surgery at the present time is unclear. There are several ongoing prospective randomized trials evaluating postoperative radiation therapy with surgery alone.

Therefore, while relatively high doses of radiation therapy may result in the cure of a small percentage of patients with lung cancer, this treatment is usually reserved for palliation. Radiation therapy is a very effective palliative tool for patients with lung cancer and should be used primarily on this basis. Radiation therapy is indicated on a preoperative basis for patients with superior sulcus tumors; however, the role of postoperative radiation therapy at this time remains obscure.

Immunotherapy

Patients with lung cancer are among the most profoundly immunosuppressed of all patients with solid neoplasms. Both delayed cutaneous hypersensitivity reactions and in vitro lymphocyte function are suppressed in patients with lung cancer.[55] The mechanism of this immunosuppression is not clear, but it has been shown that serum from patients with lung cancer is capable of suppressing normal lymphocyte function and that patients with lung cancer have suppressor cells which may play a role in the immunosuppression of lung cancer.[56,57] In view of these findings, it seems reasonable to assume that manipulation of immune response might have beneficial therapeutic effects.

Bacillus Calmette-Guérin (BCG) was one of the first agents evaluated as an immunotherapeutic agent in lung cancer. Several studies have evaluated the use of BCG given intradermally following surgery. Two studies using intradermal BCG have indicated a therapeutic effect.[55,59] A third study, in which patients received one dose of BCG postoperatively, showed a difference in favor of the BCG treatment but the final results did not reach statistical significance.[60] BCG has also been evaluated by the intrapleural route by several investigators. The most notable of these studies is that of McNeally, who treated patients postoperatively with intrapleural BCG or no further treatment. Intrapleural BCG appeared to have no effect on patients with stage II and stage III resected lung cancer; however, intrapleural BCG significantly prolonged survival of patients with stage I disease.[61] Another study indicates a definite trend toward a better survival rate in the group receiving intrapleural BCG; however, the differences have not yet reached significance.[62] There is evidence in these studies that only those patients that convert their PPD (purified protein derivative) skin tests from negative to positive have a beneficial effect from the intrapleural BCG. Patients who do not convert their PPD or who are PPD-positive at the time of treatment do not appear to benefit from BCG immunotherapy. Recently, a third study has been published in which there was no apparent benefit from postoperative intrapleural BCG.[63] BCG administered by direct injection into the tumor is also being evaluated. Intratumoral BCG has been effective in treating animal tumors and in various cutaneous human malignancies. For these reasons, it is now being evaluated in patients with lung cancer. Patients are injected with BCG prior to surgery, and the tumors are completely resected 2 weeks following BCG injection.[64]

A review of the completed trials evaluating BCG as a surgical adjunct in lung cancer indicates that there have been few entirely negative studies. Most of these studies do show a definite trend in favor of BCG treatment, although not all the results are statistically significant. Unfortunately, it is very difficult to compare studies. Different strains of BCG have been used, and there has not been proper definition of prognostic factors, such as careful surgical and pathologic staging. There are several ongoing clinical trials in which the prognostic factors are being carefully documented and the patients are being properly stratified. Although the studies to date suggest that BCG has a biological effect, it is clear that BCG immunotherapy in the treatment of lung cancer remains experimental. Its role, if any, in treatment is not clear at this time.

Levamisole (L-tetramisole) has been widely used as an antihelminthic agent in animals and in humans. Levamisole, in contrast to BCG, is a chemical that can be taken orally. It is felt that this agent is an immunopotentiator or an antianergic agent. Some studies indicate that levamisole may be able to reverse the suppression of lymphocyte function.[65] Levamisole has been evaluated in at least two prospective randomized trials in resected lung cancer patients. In these double-blind, randomized studies, patients who were candidates for theracotomy received levamisole or placebo preoperatively and postoperatively. In the original studies there was a trend in favor of the levamisole-treated group. However, when the patients were evaluated on the basis of body weight, there was a striking difference in favor of levamisole in patients who weighed less than 70 kg. The investigators felt that patients who weighed over 70 kg were underdosed and they now recommend a dose of 2.5 mg per kilogram of body weight.[66] A second study evaluating levamisole did not corroborate the original findings.[67] Therefore, while theoretically levamisole is an attractive immunotherapeutic agent, its true value in the treatment of lung cancer is yet to be determined.

Specific immunotherapy requires the use of tumor cells containing tumor antigens or the use of fractions of the tumor cells in various degrees of purification, hopefully containing tumor antigen. Specific immunotherapy using whole tumor cells or tumor antigens has been applied to patients with resectable lung cancer. Unfortunately, these studies have not been performed in a manner which allows careful interpretation. There are now, however, a number of ongoing trials testing the efficacy of specific immunotherapy in patients with lung cancer.[68,69]

At the present time, our understanding of the immunologic relationship between the tumor and the patient is incomplete. Mechanisms of immunosuppression in lung cancer are poorly understood, and the mechanism of action of the various therapeutic agents is even more poorly understood. There is evidence to suggest that BCG immunotherapy may be effective in the early stages of lung cancer. However, it is clear that if immunotherapeutic techniques as currently applied have an effect, it is minor. With the current agents available, if immunotherapy is to be applied at all, it should be applied in combination with the standard therapeutic modalities such as surgery, radiation therapy, and chemotherapy.

Chemotherapy

Patients with advanced lung cancer have been treated with chemotherapy in attempts to palliate symptoms and to prolong survival. Earlier trials involving single-agent chemotherapy were not very successful in the treatment of non-small-cell carcinoma. However, for small-cell carcinoma of the lung, positive response rates with single-agent chemotherapy using nitrogen mustard, vincristine, or Cytoxan were in the range of 30 to 40 percent. In addition, Adriamycin, hexamethylmelamine, procarbazine, BCNU, and methyl CCNU have showed activity in small-cell carcinoma of the lung. Regimens using combinations of these agents and radiation therapy have resulted in response rates of 70 to 100 percent, with a median survival rate of from 8 to 12 months and a few long-term disease-free survivors.[71]

Histologic types other than non-small-cell carcinoma have not responded nearly as well to chemotherapy. Combination chemotherapeutic regimens including various combinations of Adriamycin, Cytoxan, vincristine, *cis*-platinum, and CCNU have resulted in response rates up to 40 percent. In these studies, responders generally had a significantly improved survival rate.[32,72,73] Chemotherapy is less effective in those patients with a low response rate and most effective in patients with the highest response rates. In general, it appears worthwhile to treat non-small-cell carcinoma patients with combination chemotherapy, choosing a regimen with manageable toxicity in an attempt to identify the responders. Prolongation of survival is most likely to occur in patients who are responders.[74] While adjuvant single-agent chemotherapy has been extensively studied in patients with non-oat-cell carcinoma of the lung following surgical resection, none of the agents tested have been of any value.[75] However, new, more effective combination chemotherapy is now being evaluated in the surgical adjuvant setting, and the preliminary results are encouraging.

It is quite clear that regardless of the stage of the disease at the time of pulmonary resection, the site of the first recurrence in the majority of patients is outside the chest. Local recurrence has not been the major problem in resected lung cancer. The distant metastases observed as the first sites of failure were most commonly the brain, the contralateral lung, and the skeletal system. The majority of the failures occur within 2 years following operation. Therefore, it is clear that adjuvant therapy should be primarily directed toward systemic disease. Immunotherapy has some promising aspects as a systemic agent in lung cancer, but the early trials indicate only a marginal effect at best. Also, previous studies have indicated that single-agent chemotherapy given postoperatively has not been effective. However, with the development of newer and more effective combination chemotherapy regimens, it is anticipated that postoperative adjuvant chemotherapy will have a greater effect on the systemic disease. There is also some evidence that preoperative chemotherapy will be useful in converting unresectable patients to a resectable status. Unfortunately, however, the brain is a very common site for the first site of recurrence following pulmonary resection. Since many chemotherapeutic agents do not cross the blood-brain barrier, the control of systemic disease in the brain remains a difficult problem. Experience with oat-cell carcinoma has indicated that prophylactic whole-brain irradiation helps to prevent cerebral metastases. Perhaps similar prophylaxis in non-small-cell carcinoma would also be useful.

Surgical Management of Pulmonary Metastatic Disease

In the past, the indications for resection of pulmonary metastases were poorly defined. Survival rate following resection of pulmonary metastases was variable and unpredictable.[76,77] However, in recent years the criteria for selection of patients for resection of pulmonary metastases have become more standardized. Consideration is given to such factors as the tumor growth rate, the histologic type of primary, the disease-free interval from resection of the primary to the onset of pulmonary metastases, and, finally, the availability of effective adjuvant therapy. When these factors are considered and the patients are carefully selected, 5-year survival rates of from 30 to 60 percent can be obtained even in patients with multiple bilateral pulmonary metastases.[78-80] The histologic type of the tumor is also an important consideration in the management of patients with metastatic disease. Since melanoma, breast cancer, and gastrointestinal tumors frequently metastasize to other viscera, these tumors do not lend themselves as well to resection as do the genitourinary tumors and the sarcomas. In general, the longer the disease-free interval between the control of the primary and the onset of pulmonary metastases, the more favorable the prognosis. In patients in whom

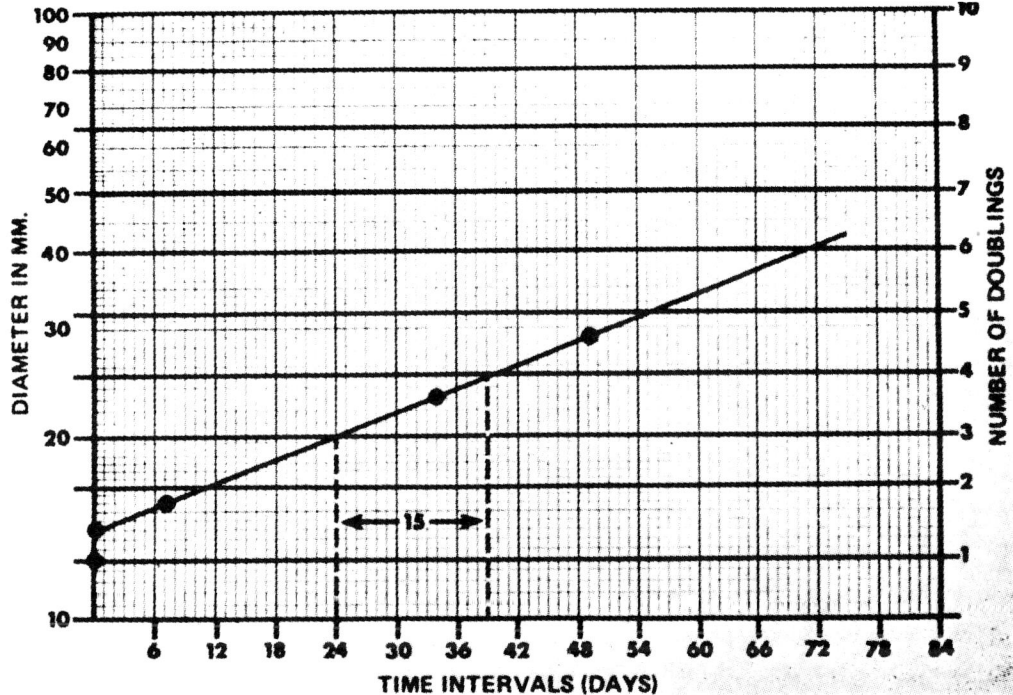

FIGURE 21-2 Technique of calculating tumor doubling time. Diameter plotted at 2 time intervals at least 14 days apart. The point at which the line bisecting these two crosses one tumor doubling represents the tumor doubling time.

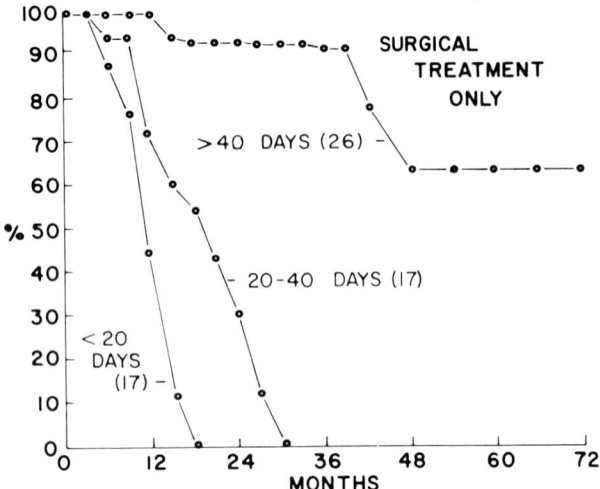

FIGURE 21-3 Survival following surgery based on tumor doubling time.

sarcoma and metastatic nonseminomatous testicular tumors are excellent examples of tumors for which effective adjuvant therapy is available; these tumors respond very well to aggressive resection of metastases.

The concept of *tumor doubling time* has made an important contribution to the management of patients with pulmonary metastatic disease.[81] Tumor doubling time has been used to predict the response following resection of pulmonary metastases (Fig. 21-2). These studies indicate that the tumor doubling time correlates closely with the biological aggressiveness of the neoplasm. Sixty percent of patients with tumor doubling times greater than 40 days can anticipate a prolonged survival following pulmonary resection. However, patients with tumor doubling times less than 20 days do not benefit from surgery (Fig. 21-3).[82,83] Therefore, a determination of the tumor doubling time is an excellent aid in the selection of patients for pulmonary resection.

The availability of effective adjuvant therapy is becoming an important consideration in the selection of patients for resection. In patients with osteosarcoma, 5-year survival rates as high as 70 percent have been reported in patients undergoing pulmonary resection and receiving adjuvant chemotherapy. A study at UCLA involving 38 consecutive pulmonary resections for metastatic sarcoma is diagramed in Figure 21-4. As with other studies, a 5-year survival rate in excess of 35 percent is

the disease-free interval is 12 months or more, a median survival time of greater than 2½ years can be obtained. However, when effective adjuvant chemotherapy is available, the resection of pulmonary metastases that present simultaneously with the primary tumor can frequently result in prolonged survival and cure. Metastatic osteo-

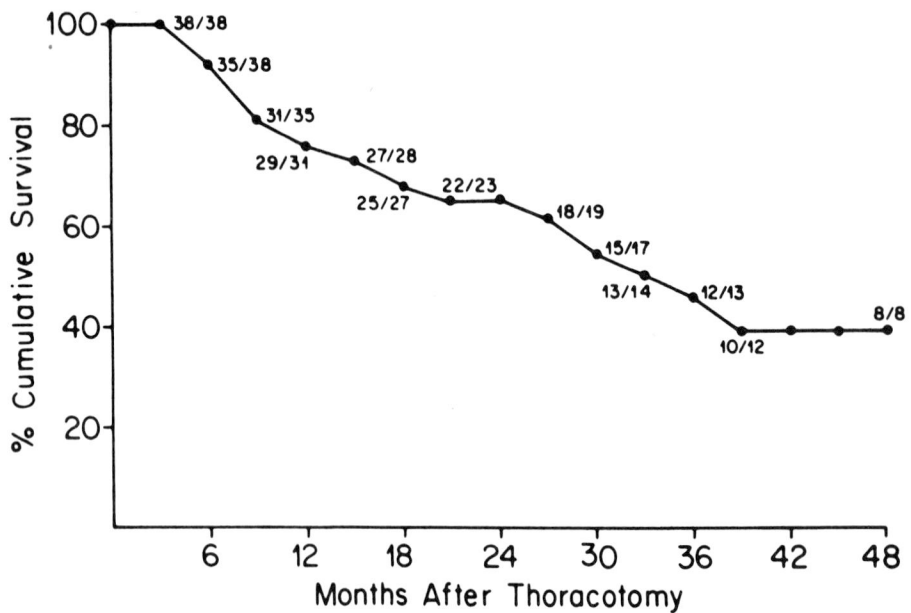

FIGURE 21-4 Survival of patients with metastatic sarcoma to the lungs following pulmomary resection.

anticipated. The effect of tumor doubling time is indicated in Fig. 21-5. Patients with metastatic sarcomas with tumor doubling times of greater than 40 days have a higher survival rate than those patients with doubling time less than 40 days. Figure 21-6 indicates that patients with a disease-free interval of greater than 12 months have a better survival following resection of pulmonary metastases than those with a disease-free interval of less than 12 months. The most common site of recurrence following pulmonary resection of sarcoma is the lung. This local recurrence is not due to inadequate resection, since the recurrence rates in patients with operated lungs are similar to those in patients with unoperated lungs. The greatest cause of failure is micrometastatic disease within the lung. More effective systemic therapy needs to be developed in order to control this microscopic residual disease. However, recurrent pulmonary disease following surgical resection should be resected if technically feasible. Frequently, three or even five thoracotomies are necessary before recurrent disease is controlled and a prolonged disease-free interval results. More recently, patients who have pulmonary metastases with tumor doubling times less than 40 days are evaluated with preoperative chemotherapy. If the chemotherapy is effective in reducing the tumor doubling time, the patients are operated upon and treated with adjuvant systemic chemotherapy (Figs. 21-7 and 21-8). The early results indicate that this in vivo evaluation of the sensitivity of the chemotherapy is a good predictor of the postoperative survival.

Nonseminomatous testicular tumors also lend themselves well to pulmonary resection. The availability of potent systemic chemotherapeutic agents in this disease allows for a very aggressive surgical attack on these pulmonary metastases. Experience at UCLA has indicated that with surgical resection and adjuvant chemotherapy, 60 percent of patients with nonseminomatous tumors metastatic to the lung can be cured with surgery and chemotherapy. It should be emphasized that the presence of multiple bilateral metastases are not contraindications to surgery. The biological features such as tumor doubling time, length of disease-free interval, and susceptibility to chemotherapy are the major criteria.

Resection of pulmonary metastases may be accomplished by wedge excision, lobectomy, or pneumonectomy. Patients with bilateral metastatic disease should

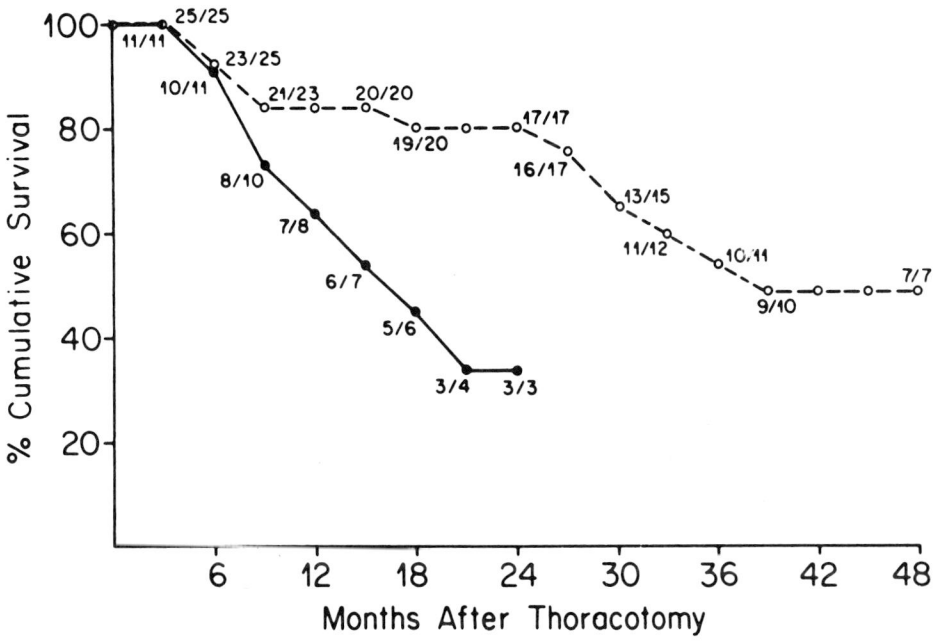

FIGURE 21-5 Survival following pulmonary resection in patients with tumor doubling times of greater than 40 days and less than 40 days.

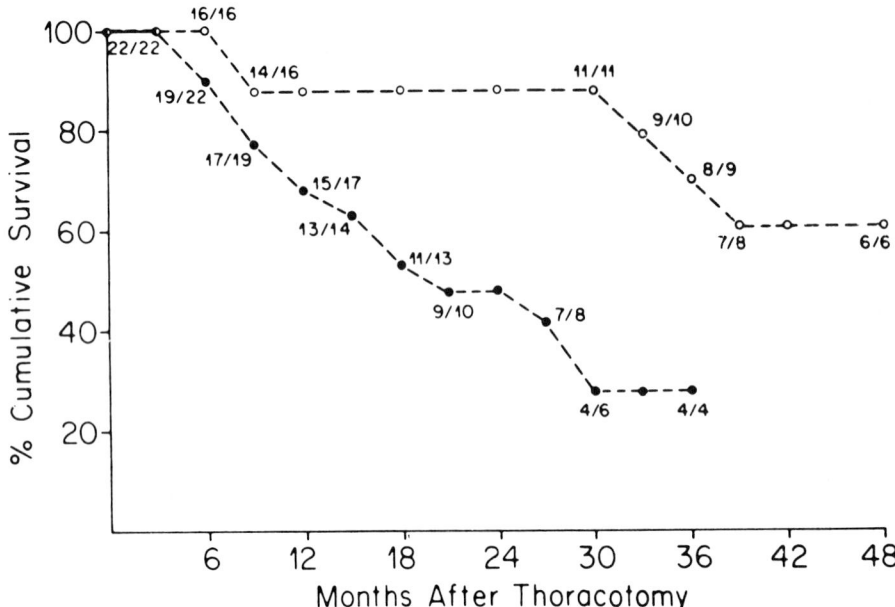

FIGURE 21-6 Survival of patients with surgically resected pulmonary metastasis from sarcoma according to the disease-free interval of less than 12 months or greater than 12 months.

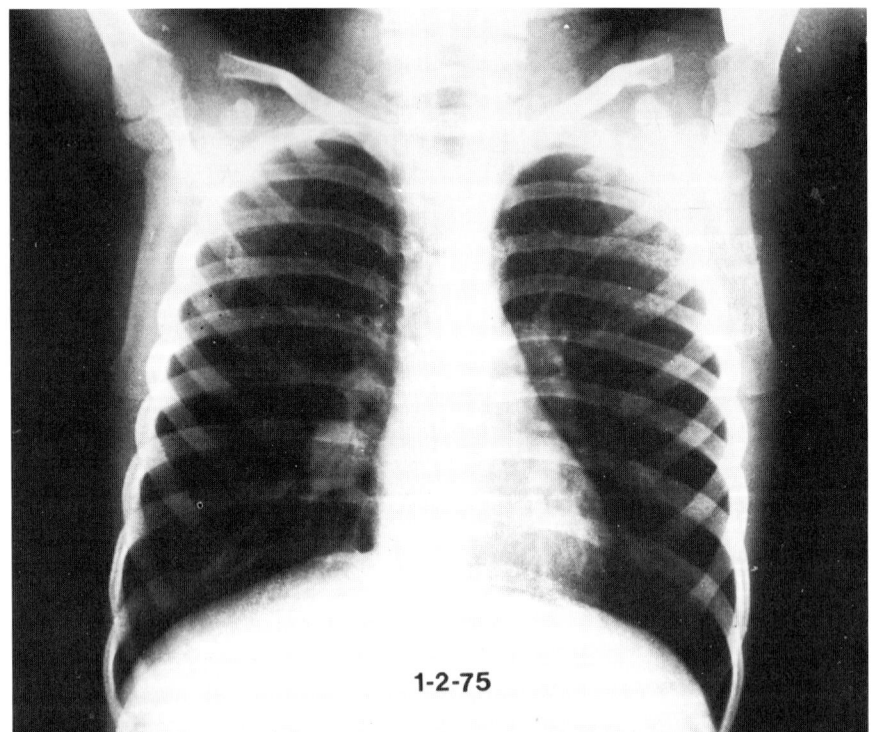

FIGURE 21-7 This young patient had a metastatic osteosarcoma in the right midlung field. Following chemotherapy, there was significant regression of the tumor (see Fig. 21-8).

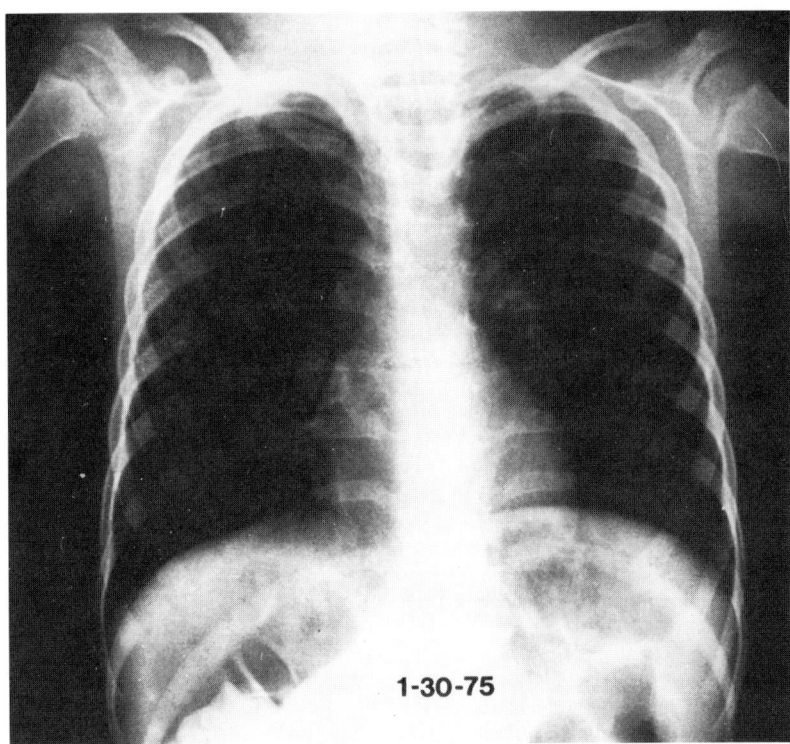

FIGURE 21-8 Same patient as in Fig. 21-7. The response to chemotherapy is evident. This kind of preoperative response to chemotherapy indicates that a good result will be obtained with surgical resection followed by adjuvant chemotherapy.

have staged bilateral thoracotomy; in some instances, a median sternotomy can be performed with simultaneous bilateral resections. Adequate exposure of the posterior portion of the left lower lobe, however, is difficult through this approach. Most pulmonary metastases are subpleural in location and can be removed by wedge excision. At the time of surgery, the lungs are examined in both the inflated and deflated positions. All lesions are carefully marked by sutures before excision. Needless to say, all disease should be removed and there is no place for subtotal resection or "debulking" procedures.

The results following resection of metastatic carcinoma have not been as good as those obtained in cases of sarcoma and nonseminomatous testicular tumor. However, in those patients who do satisfy the strict criteria outlined, the 5-year survival following resection of metastatic carcinomas is 25 percent. It is clear that the results of pulmonary resection for metastatic disease in general are quite encouraging. This is particularly true in patients with sarcomas, nonseminomatous testicular tumors, and hypernephromas. Properly selected patients with carcinomas also will occasionally benefit from pulmonary resection. The development of more effective adjuvant chemotherapy will obviously increase the indications for the resection of pulmonary metastases.

REFERENCES

1. Jensen OM: Lung cancer and smoking in Danish women. *Int J Cancer* 15:954, 1975.
2. Beamis JF, Stein A, Andrew JL: Changing epidemiology of lung cancer: Increasing incidence in women. *Med Clin North Am* 59:315, 1975.
3. Auerback O, Garfinkel L, Parks VR: Histologic type of lung cancer in relation to smoking habits, year of diagnosis, and sites of metastases. *Chest* 67:382, 1975.
4. Hueper WC: *Occupational Tumors and Related Diseases*. Springfield, Ill., Charles C Thomas, 1942.
5. Saccomanno G et al: Development of carcinoma of the lung as reflected in exfoliated cells. *Cancer* 33:364, 1974.
6. Wright ES, Couves CM: Radiation induced carcinoma of the lung—The St. Lawrence tragedy. *J Thorac Cardiovasc Surg* 74:495, 1977.

7. Saccomanno G et al: Cancer of the lung: Cytology of sputum prior to the development of carcinoma. *Acta Cytol (Balt)* 9:413, 1975.
8. Kazazian HH: A geneticist's view of lung disease. *Am Rev Respir Dis* 113:261, 1976.
9. Kellerman G, Shaw CR, Luyten-Kellerman M: Arylhydrocarbon-hydroxylase inducibility in bronchogenic carcinoma. *N Engl J Med* 289:934, 1973.
10. Higgins GA, Shields TW, Keehan RJ: The solitary pulmonary nodule (10-year followup Veterans Administration–Armed Forces Cooperative Study). *Arch Surg* 110:570, 1975.
11. Munnell ER et al: Reappraisal of solitary bronchiolar (alveolar cell) carcinoma of the lung. *Am Thorac Surg* 25:289, 1978.
12. Coolson RE et al: Alveolar cell carcinoma: An in vitro study. *Lab Inves* 28:38, 1973.
13. Jensik RJ et al: Bronchoplastic and conservative resectional procedures for bronchial adenoma. *J Thorac Cardiovasc Surg* 68:556, 1974.
14. Sanderson VR, Fontana RE: Early lung cancer detection and localization. *Am Octol Rhinol Laryngeal* 84:583, 1975.
15. Fontana RS et al: The Mayo Lung Project for early detection and localization for bronchogenic carcinoma: A status report. *Chest* 65:511, 1975.
16. Marsh BR et al: New horizons in lung cancer diagnosis. *Cancer* 37:437, 1976.
17. Melamed M et al: Preliminary report of the lung cancer detection program in New York. *Cancer* 39:369, 1977.
18. Fontana RS: Early diagnosis of lung cancer. *Am Rev Respir Dis* 116:399, 1977.
19. Martini N, Melamed MR: Multiple primary lung cancers. *J Thorac Cardiovasc Surg* 70:606, 1975.
20. Abbey-Smith R, Nigam BK, Thompson JM: Second primary lung carcinoma. *Thorax* 31:507, 1976.
21. Fennessy JJ: The radiology of lung cancer. *Med Clin North Am* 59:95, 1975.
22. Shevland JE et al: The role of conventional tomography and computed tomography in assessing the resectability of primary lung cancer. CT: *J Comput Tomgr* 2:1, 1978.
23. Crowe JK, Brown LR, Muhn JR: Computed tomography of the mediastinum. *Radiology* 128:75, 1978.
24. Lukeman JM: Reliability of cytologic diagnosis in cancer of the lung. *Cancer Chemother Rep* 4:79, 1973.
25. Gagneten CB, Geller CE, del Carmen Saenz M: Diagnosis of bronchogenic carcinoma through the cytologic examination of sputum, with special reference to tumor typing. *Acta Cytol (Balt)* 20:530, 1976.
26. Pavy RD, Antic R, Begley M: Percutaneous aspiration biopsy of discrete lung lesions. *Cancer* 34:2109, 1974.
27. Ramsdell JW et al: Multiorgan scans for staging lung cancer. *J Thorac Cardiovasc Surg* 73:653, 1977.
28. Delaney JF, Gertz D, Shreiner DP: Usefulness of brain scans in metastatic carcinoma of the lung. *J Nucl Med* 17:406, 1976.
29. Muggia FM, Shervu L: Lung cancer: Diagnosis and metastatic sites. *Semin Oncol* 1:217, 1974.
30. Paxton R, Ambrose J: The EMI scanner. A brief review of the first 650 patients. *Brit J Radiol* 47:530, 1974.
31. Mintz U et al: Sequential staging in bronchogenic carcinoma. *Chest* 76:653, 1979.
32. Eagan RT et al: Platinum-based polychemotherapy versus dianhydrogalactitol in advanced non-small cell lung cancer. *Cancer Treat Rep* 61:1339, 1977.
33. Baker RR, Stitik FP, March BR: The clinical assessment of selected patients with bronchogenic carcinoma. *Am Thorac Surg* 20:520, 1975.
34. Hutchinson CM, Mills NL: The selection of patients with bronchogenic carcinoma from mediastinoscopy. *J Thorac Cardiovasc Surg* 71:768, 1976.
35. Whitcomb ME et al: Indications for mediastinoscopy in bronchogenic carcinoma. *Am Rev Respir Dis* 113:189, 1976.
36. Stanford W et al: Mediastinoscopy. *Am Thorac Surg* 19:121, 1975.
37. Fishman NH, Bronstein MH: Is mediastinoscopy necessary in the evaluation of lung? *Am Thorac Surg* 20:678, 1975.
38. Jolly PC et al: Parasternal mediastinotomy, and mediastinoscopy. *J Thorac Cardiovasc Surg* 66:549, 1973.
39. Anderson WAD et al: *Clinical Staging System for Carcinoma of the Lung*, The American Joint Committee for Cancer Staging and End Results Reporting, Chicago, American College of Surgeons, 1973.
40. Mountain CF: Assessment of the role of surgery for control of lung cancer. *Am Thorac Surg* 24:365, 1977.
41. Martini N, Beattie E: Results of surgical treatment in stage I lung cancer. *J Thorac Cardiovasc Surg* 74:499, 1977.
42. The Lung Cancer Study Group: Surgical adjuvant immunotherapy in non-oat cell carcinoma, in WD Terry and WD Rosenberg (eds): *Immunotherapy Trials in Man* (in press).
43. Kirsch MM et al: Carcinoma of the lung: Results of treatment over 10 years. *Am Thorac Surg* 21:271, 1976.
44. Shields TW: *Bronchial Carcinoma*, Springfield, Ill., Charles C Thomas, 1974.
45. Overholt RH, Neptune WB, Ashraf MM: Primary Cancer of the lung. *Am Thorac Surg* 20:511, 1975.
46. Ramsey HE et al: The importance of radical lobectomy in lung cancer. *J Thorac Cardiovasc Surg* 58:225, 1969.
47. Burnard RJ, Martini N, Beattie EJ, Jr: The value of resection in tumors involving the chest wall. *J Thorac Cardiovasc Surg* 68:530, 1978.
48. Ramsey HE, Clifton EE: Chest wall resection for primary carcinoma of the lung. *Am Surg* 167: 342, 1968.
49. Pancoast HK: Superior pulmonary sulcus tumor. *JAMA* 99:1391, 1932.
50. Paulsen DL: Carcinoma in the superior pulmonary sulcus. *J Thorac Cardiovasc Surg* 70:1095, 1975.
51. Lee RE: Radiation therapy in the management of carcinoma of the lung. *Semin Oncol* 1:245, 1974.

52. Perez CA: Radiation therapy in the management of carcinoma of the lung. *Cancer* 39:901, 1977.
53. Collaborative Study: Preoperative irradiation of cancer of the lung: Preliminary report of a therapeutic trial. *Cancer* 23:419, 1969.
54. Shields TW: Preoperative radiation therapy in the treatment of bronchiolar carcinoma. *Cancer* 30:1388, 1972.
55. Holmes EC, Golub SH: Immunologic defects in lung cancer patients. *J Thorac Cardiovasc Surg* 71:161, 1976.
56. Giuliano A et al: Serum-mediated immunosuppression in lung cancer. *Cancer* 43:917, 1979.
57. Jerrells TR et al: Suppressor activity in immunosuppressed lung and breast cancer patients (abstracts). *Proc Am Assoc Cancer Res* 19:73, 1978.
58. Perlin E et al: Immunotherapy of carcinoma of the lung with BCG and allogeneic tumor cells, in RH Crispen (ed): *Neoplasm Immunity: Solid Tumor Therapy,* Philadelphia, The Franklin Institute Press, 1977.
59. Pouillart P et al: Trial of BCG immunotherapy in the treatment of resectable squamous cell carcinoma of the bronchus (stage I and stage II). *Cancer Immunol Immunother* 1:271, 1976.
60. Edwards FR, Whitwill F: Use of BCG as an immunostimulant in surgical treatment in carcinoma of the lung: A five year follow-up report. *Thorax* 33:250, 1978.
61. McKneally MF, Maver CM, Kausel HW: Regional immunotherapy of lung cancer using intrapleural BCG, in WD Terry and D Windhorst (eds): *Immunotherapy of Cancer: Present Status of Trials in Man,* New York, Raven, 1978.
62. Wright PW et al: Adjuvant immunotherapy with intrapleural BCG and levamisole in patients with resected non-small cell lung cancer (abstract). *Proc Second Intern Conf Immunother Cancer,* 1980.
63. Lowe J et al: Intrapleural BCG in inoperable lung cancer. *Lancet* 11:13, 1980.
64. Holmes EC et al: Intralesional BCG immunotherapy of pulmonary tumors. *J Thorac Cardiovasc Surg* 77:362, 1979.
65. Golub SH, Holmes EC: In vitro assays of immunocompetence in patients with lung cancer treated with levamisole. *Cancer Immunol Immunother* 7:143, 1979.
66. Amery WK: A placebo-controlled levamisole study in resected lung cancer, in WD Terry and D Windhorst (eds): *Immunotherapeutics of Cancer: Present Status of Trials in Man,* New York, Raven, 1978.
67. Anthony HM et al: Levamisole and surgery in bronchial carcinoma patients: Increase in death from cardiorespiratory failure. *Thorax* 34:4, 1979.
68. Stewart THM et al: A survival study of specific active immunochemotherapy in lung cancer, in RG Crispen (ed): *Neoplasms Immunity: Solid Tumor Therapy,* Philadelphia, The Franklin Institute, 1977.
69. Takita H et al: Adjuvant immunotherapy of stage III lung carcinoma, in WD Terry and D Windhorst (eds): *Immunotherapy of Cancer: Present Status of Trials in Man,* New York, Raven, 1978.
70. Greco FA, Einhorn LH, Richardson RL et al: Small cell lung cancer: Progress and perspective. *Semin Oncol* 5:323, 1978.
71. Cohen MH: Small cell bronchogenic carcinoma: A prolonged remission following chemotherapy. *JAMA* 237:2528, 1977.
72. Sarna GT: Chemoimmunotherapy for unresectable bronchogenic carcinoma. *Cancer Treatment Rep* 62:181, 1978.
73. Livingston RB: Combination chemotherapy of bronchogenic carcinoma. I. Non-oat cell. *Cancer Treatment Rev* 4:153, 1977.
74. Sarna GP, Holmes EC, Petrovich Z: Lung Cancer, in CM Haskell (ed): *Cancer Treatment,* Philadelphia, Saunders, 1980.
75. Shields TW et al: Adjuvant cancer chemotherapy after resection of Carcinoma of the lung. *Cancer* 40:2057, 1977.
76. Ochsner A Sr et al: Treatment of metastatic pulmonary malignant lesions. *Lancet* 83:16, 1963.
77. Alexander J, Haight C: Pulmonary resection for solitary metastatic sarcomas and carcinomas. *Surg Gynecol Obstet* 85:129, 1947.
78. Morton DL et al: Surgical resection and adjunctive immunotherapy for selected patients with multiple pulmonary metastases. *Am Surg* 178:360, 1973.
79. Telander RL et al: Resection of pulmonary metastatic osteogenic sarcoma in children. *Surg* 84:335, 1978.
80. Takita H et al: Surgical management of multiple lung metastases. *Am Thorac Surg* 24:359, 1977.
81. Collin SD, Leofflar RK, Tivey H: Observation on growth rates of human tumors. *Am J Roentgenol* 76:988, 1956.
82. Holmes EL, Morton DL: Pulmonary resection for sarcoma metastases. *Orthop Clin North Am* 8:805, 1977.
83. Joseph WL, Morton DL, Adkins PC: Variation in tumor doubling time in patients with pulmonary metastatic disease. *J Surg Oncol* 3:143, 1971.
84. Sporn MD, Newton DL, Smith JM: Retinoids and cancer prevention: The importance of the terminal group of the retinoid molecule and modifying activity and toxicity, in AC Griffin and CR Shaw (eds): *Carcinogenesis: Identification and Mechanism of Action,* New York, Raven, 1979.
85. Martini N et al: Prospective study of 445 lung carcinomas with mediastinal lymph node metastases. *J Thorac Cardiovasc Surg* 80:390–399, 1980.

SELECTED BIBLIOGRAPHY

Chahinian AR: Lung cancer, in Burchenal JH, Oettgen HF (eds): *Cancer: Achievements, Challenges and Prospects for the 1980's,* vol II, Grune & Stratton, New York, 1981, pp 539–550.

Golomb HM (ed): Non-small cell carcinoma of the lung. *Sem Oncol* 10:1–126, 1983.

22
MALIGNANT TUMORS OF THE ESOPHAGUS

Samuel E. Wilson   *John R. Benfield*

Malignant, derived from the Latin verb *malignare,* means "to act maliciously." There is no better application of this word than for carcinoma of the esophagus. This least common of the visceral malignancies is the most difficult to treat surgically and has among the worst prognoses. Diagnosis is late because the esophageal smooth muscle initially dilates easily and painlessly to accommodate an obstruction. Thus, the usual first symptom, dysphagia, implies an advanced lesion. The absence of serosa probably facilitates rapid invasion of contiguous vital mediastinal structures. Cure by resection is frequently impossible, and the primary goal most often becomes palliation of dysphagia.

During the past decade, a brighter outlook has evolved in several areas. First, there has been a steady lowering of operative mortality so that resection can be performed with a mortality of 10 percent or less in some centers. Secondly, modern radiotherapy has resulted in better quality of survival. Finally, these poorly nourished patients have been helped by the use of perioperative total parenteral nutrition.

Commonly, the esophagus may suffer from *squamous cell carcinoma* arising in the mucosal epithelial lining, or *adenocarcinoma* as an invader from the glandular epithelium of the esophagogastric junction. The latter, however, may also begin primarily in the esophagus in an area of Barrett's epithelium. *Primary adenocarcinoma* of the esophagus is so uncommon that until the last decade some pathologists doubted its existence. The diagnosis may be safely made only if there is unquestioned glandular carcinoma in the esophagus and the absence of tumor in the stomach. The incidence of this tumor is only 0.76 percent of all cancers of the esophagus and consequently only limited experience in treatment has been accumulated.[1]

Rarely, leiomyosarcoma or other mesenchymal neoplasms develop in the muscularis layer of the esophagus.

HISTORICAL ASPECTS

After cervical esophagotomies for removal of foreign bodies and palliative esophagostomies early in the nineteenth century, the first resection of a carcinoma of the esophagus in the neck was accomplished by Czerny in 1877.[2] The first successful resection of the thoracic esophagus for carcinoma was performed by Torek in 1913.[3] His patients lived for 11 years, nourished through a rubber tube which passed externally from the cervical esophagus to the stomach. Advances in anesthesia paved the way for successful one-stage transpleural esophageal resection and reconstruction. This was reported in Japan by Oshaswa[4] in 1933, and in the United States by Marshall[5] and by Adams and Phemister[6] in 1938.

INCIDENCE AND EPIDEMIOLOGY

The characteristics of epidermoid carcinomas vary in different geographic locations. Even within the United States there is regional variation in the occurrence of the disease with a four to five times greater incidence in South Carolina as compared to Connecticut. In our country the annual incidence is approximately 4 per 100,000 population, accounting for some 7500 new cases per year, while in other areas, the incidence is much higher.[7] Cancer of the esophagus in the Transkei province of South Africa has approximately a 25 times greater incidence than in the United States.[8,9] In northwest France, the incidence is 56 per 100,000, and in the northeastern part of Iran, bordering the Caspian Sea, known as the Caspian littoral, the incidence is 62 new cases per 100,000 population annually.[10,11] Perhaps the highest incidence is in Hunan province in northern China where there are 108 cases per 100,000[11] (Fig. 22-1).

Incidence varies according to sex and race. The peak incidence occurs during the sixth decade of life. Black men are at highest risk. In the United States the ratio of men to women with esophagus cancers in blacks is 4:1, and in whites, it is 2:1. In South Africa this ratio in blacks is 9:1, and in whites it is 4:1.[7,8]

Certain *predisposing conditions* may be associated with squamous cell cancer of the esophagus. These include the presence of primary squamous cell carcinoma of the head and neck or of the oral cavity.[12] All these malig-

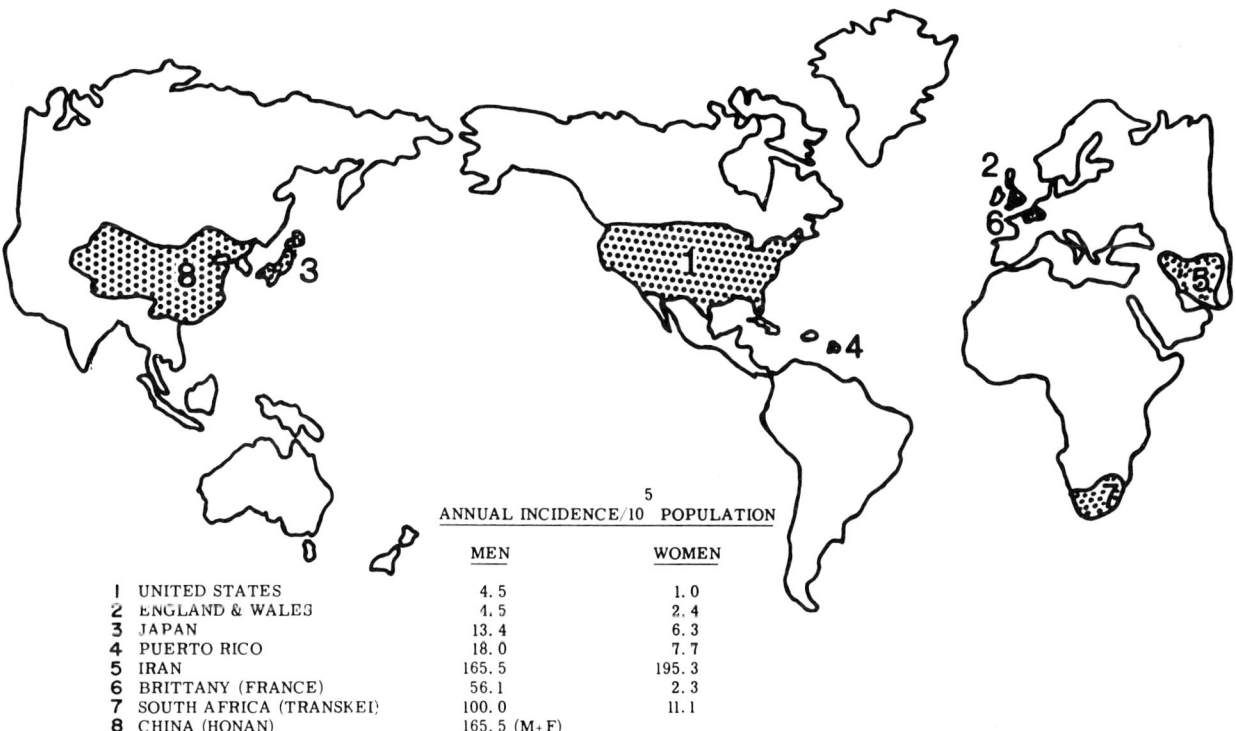

FIGURE 22-1 Epidemiologic studies indicate widespread geographic variation in the incidence of epidermoid cancer of the esophagus.

nancies are related to excess consumption of alcohol and tobacco; thus, suggesting similar oncogenic factors. Lye burns of the esophagus with stricture predispose to squamous cell carcinoma. The incidence of esophageal cancer in such patients is estimated as 1000 times that of the general population.[13] The belief that carcinomas arising after caustic injury may have a better prognosis due to limitation of tumor invasion by scar tissue is not fully substantiated.

The Plummer-Vinson syndrome, consisting of esophageal webs and anemia, is related to a higher risk of cancer of the upper third of the esophagus among women.[14] This type of tumor usually presents at a younger age than other esophageal cancers.

Tylosis is generally considered a benign disorder; however, it was recognized to occur with carcinoma of the esophagus in 1958.[15] The name was derived from the Greek word for *woody*, an appropriate description of an ectodermal anomaly characterized by thickening of the skin of the palms and feet. This hereditary abnormality is caused by the expression of a single, autosomal gene in heterozygous state, showing high penetrance.

Etiologic factors in epidermoid esophageal cancer occurring in the United States include excessive use of alcohol and tobacco. These factors, however, are not prerequisites. For example, in northern Iran where cigarette smoking or abuse of alcohol are uncommon due to religious prohibition, esophageal cancer is a relatively frequent tumor. Nitrosamines, which readily induce experimental esophageal cancer, have been incriminated in the etiology of human esophageal cancer.[16,17] A connection between these carcinogens and alcoholic beverages has been sought. So far, no volatile nitrosamines have been detected in the various alcoholic spirits which have been examined.[17] Nitrosamines may also be formed in vivo by the interaction of nitrites and nitrosatable amines. Nitrites are either ingested or formed from nitrates by the action of oral microorganisms. No difference has been found in the salivary secretions of esophageal cancer patients and normal subjects in the capacity to form nitrites. Interesting observations have been made relevant to tobacco and alcohol among the highly susceptible population south of the Taihang Mountains in northern China where esophageal cancer has been prevalent for centuries.[9] There the incidence is stable and apparently not connected with smoking and drinking. Instead, the ingestion of pickled cabbage mixed with the fungus *Geotrichum candidum* has been incriminated. Although speculation about the role of potential environmental carcinogens continues, to date no definite or single causative factor has been discovered.

Adenocarcinoma of the lower esophagus may arise in the columnar epithelium lining of Barrett's esophagus. In his original description, Barrett believed that this columnar epithelium belonged to a thoracic stomach situated below a congenitally short esophagus. Others contended that the anomaly was simply congenital rests of gastric epithelium in the distal esophagus. It appears clear now that this is usually an acquired lesion in patients with reflux esophagitis. For many years the development of adenocarcinoma of the esophagus in a hiatal hernia had been noted anecdotally. Recently it has been demonstrated conclusively in 1225 patients with reflux esophagitis that 140 patients (8.7 percent) had deposition of glandular mucosa in response to continued gastroesophageal reflux. This reparative epithelium undergoes continued replacement and exhibits varying degrees of dysplastic changes. Barrett's epithelium should be considered a premalignant lesion which gives rise to multifocal hyperplasia, dysplasia, and eventually, in a small number of patients, adenocarcinoma. For example, among 140 patients with esophageal reflux with Barrett's epithelium, 12 were discovered to have esophageal adenocarcinoma.[18]

SIGNS, SYMPTOMS, AND DIAGNOSTIC CONSIDERATIONS

Pathology

The esophagus is traditionally divided into three anatomical zones: in adults, the cervical segment is about 18 cm long above the clavicles; the middle third of the esophagus is approximately 18 to 31 cm long; and the distal third and cardia span about 32 to 45 cm from the incisors. The distribution of tumors (Fig. 22-2) is similar in most large series with about 8 percent of cancers occurring in the cervical esophagus, 25 percent in the middle third, and 17 percent in the lower third.[19] Of the lower-third cancers, 50 percent occur within 5 cm of the cardia. Thus, about one-half of all esophageal tumors involve the gastroesophageal junction, and most neoplasms in this location are adenocarcinomas arising in the proximal stomach infiltrating the distal esophagus.

Early squamous cell carcinomas appear either as small, gray-white plaquelike thickenings and elevations of mucosa or as granular, friable, erythematous, or

MALIGNANT TUMORS OF THE ESOPHAGUS **451**

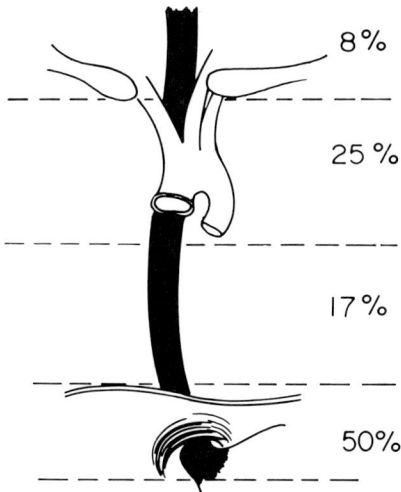

FIGURE 22-2 Distribution of 170 cases of carcinoma of the esophagus.

eroded mucosa. Extension occurs primarily in the long axis of the esophagus, but encirclement of the lumen occurs. Although the time required for the formation of circumferential cancers is uncertain, it is thought to be within a year. Larger carcinomas develop central ulceration. The malignant ulcer has elevated margins and a necrotic, shaggy center. Progressive invasion occurs through the wall of the esophagus into the mediastinum and adjacent structures as well as under adjacent normal mucosa. Epidermoid esophageal cancers spread for remarkable distances within the submucosa, and skip areas are known to occur.

Upper-third esophageal tumors disseminate through the lymphatics to the cervical nodes, especially the supraclavicular nodes. Midesophageal tumors spread to the peritracheal and esophageal nodes, as well as to the supraclavicular and subdiaphragmatic area. Tumors of the lower third and cardia involve primarily lymphatics in the celiac axis and local mediastinal nodes. In the midthoracic esophagus, tumor fixation to the aorta and the trachea is common. Deepening of the ulcerative lesion leads to tracheoesophageal and aortoesophageal fistulas. Autopsy studies show metastases to the liver in 72 percent of patients, to the lungs 56 percent, and to bones in 23 percent. Other frequent sites of metastatic involvement include the adrenal and kidney.[20]

The natural history of esophageal cancer can be reasonably predicted by staging the anatomical extent of the tumor at the time of diagnosis. In the contrast to many other cancers, remote metastases from cancers of the esophagus are less ominous than tumors which extend outside the esophagus into the tracheobronchial tree or aorta.

We recommend adhering to TMN terminology using the clinical staging system of the American Joint Committee for Cancer Staging and Results Reporting,[21] summarized in Table 22-1. *Stage I* tumors ($T_1M_0N_0$) involves 5 cm or less of the esophageal lumen. They produce no obstruction and have no extraesophageal spread. The entire circumference of the esophagus is not involved, and there are no regional lymph node or remote metastases. In *stage II* ($T_2N_0M_0$), the cancer involves more than 5 cm of the esophageal lumen without evidence of local extension outside the esophagus, without regional lymph node metastases, and without distant metastases. These neoplasms often produce obstruction or involve the entire circumference of esophagus. *Stage III* ($T_2N_1M_0$ or $T_2N_1M_1$) is any esophageal cancer with distant metastases, extraesophageal extension, or regional lymphatic metastases.

Clinical Manifestations

The typical patient with esophageal cancer presents with a 3-month history of progressive difficulty swallowing and a weight loss of approximately 20 lb. Thoracic or

TABLE 22-1 Clinical Staging for Carcinoma of the Esophagus

Stage	
Stage I	Less than 5 cm of length; no obstruction; not circumferential; no extraesophageal spread; no regional node metastasis; no distant metastasis; ($T_1N_0M_0$).
Stage II	More than 5 cm of length; no evidence of extension outside the esophagus; no regional node or distant metastasis; obstructs or involves the entire circumference of the esophagus; no evidence of extraesophageal spread or node metastasis; ($T_2N_0M_0$). Cervical tumors limited to the esophagus with regional node metastasis which are not fixed are included in stage II.
Stage III	Any esophageal tumor with distant metastasis, extraesophageal extension, or regional node metastasis; (T_1 or T_2N_1 or M_1).

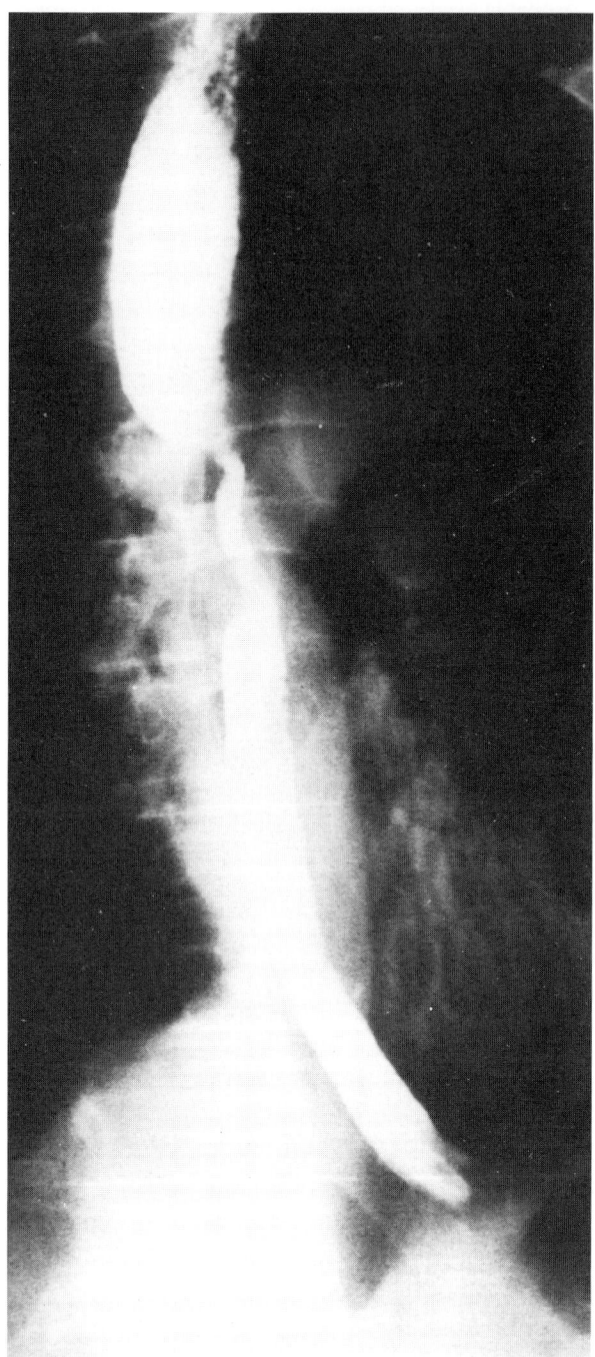

FIGURE 22-3 Typical radiographic appearance of a middle esophageal carcinoma.

abdominal pain is an uncommon symptom. It occurs in only 25 percent of esophageal tumors, and hence dysphagia rather than pain usually triggers the search for medical care. Dysphagia in any American man over the age of 40 should be assumed due to esophageal cancer until proven otherwise. Dysphagia rarely becomes prominent until there is about 50 percent narrowing of the diameter of the esophagus. Initially, difficulty is experienced with swallowing solid foods, particularly meat. Complaints may include regurgitation, substernal distress, or a constant sense of pressure or pain in the lower esophageal area. Voluntarily restriction of diet ensues and at presentation to the physician, patients' meals are usually limited to soft foods or liquids. The results are weakness, malnutrition, and extreme weight loss. As the disease progresses, obstruction becomes more severe, and bouts of aspiration develop. In far-advanced cases paralysis of the recurrent laryngeal or phrenic nerves may be seen, but these concomitants have been rare in our experience.

The diagnosis is usually apparent on the barium esophagram. Multiple projections, rotating the patient in a vertical axis, will outline a tumor mass which extends into the lumen and is often bulky. Mucosal disruption and irregular ulcerations are common (Fig. 22-3). Undermining of the normal mucosa by the tumor may result in an irregular stricture extending over several centimeters of the esophageal lumen (Fig. 22-4).

Differential diagnosis includes peptic stricture and achalasia. The degree of esophageal dilatation above an obstruction due to cancer is not usually as marked as that due to achalasia, and the narrowing of inflammatory strictures is typically conical and relatively smooth. However, radiographic differentiation is occasionally very difficult.

In stage I esophageal carcinomas, the initial accuracy of radiologic examination is limited.[22] These tumors are most frequently misdiagnosed as varices, or occasionally as a leiomyoma or esophageal stricture. Air-contrast esophagography is a useful additional technique since it shows excellent mucosal detail and allows detection of small ulcerations, mass lesions, or submucosal invasion. The double contrast is achieved by insufflating air following the barium swallow. Another helpful radiographic sign is thickening of the posterior tracheal stripe to wider than 4.5 mm on the lateral chest x-ray.[23] This retrotracheal thickening is due to periesophageal lymphatic involvement. In the nonobstructed esophagus, this early diagnostic clue has become apparent on the lateral chest x-ray as early as 6 months prior to the development of dysphagia. Anterior bowing of the posterior wall of the trachea is also a frequent finding on the lateral chest x-ray in patients with retrotracheal lymphatic spread. These radiographic findings have prognostic significance in that 22 percent of patients with retrotracheal abnormality due to esophageal cancer will ultimately develop esophagobronchial fistulas.[24]

Endoscopy should be performed in all patients who have dysphagia even if the esophagogram is normal. At the time of biopsy specimens should be obtained from the base and edge of the lesion. A brush rotated on the lesion for a Papanicolaou preparation provides good specimens for cytologic study. Multiple biopsies are essential, and it is helpful to obtain biopsies at various levels of apparently normal esophagus in order to delineate the proximal extent of the lesion.

Difficulty arises in diagnosis with stricture of the distal esophagus in the patient who has a hiatal hernia and reflux esophagitis (Fig. 22-5). When it is impossible to differentiate between cancer and narrowing due to benign reflux esophagitis, the conservative approach is to bypass repeat barium studies and proceed promptly to endoscopy. The finding of the inflammatory changes in the mucosa of a biopsy specimen from the lumen proximal to a stricture taken through the flexible endoscope does not rule out malignancy. The brush cytology technique is particularly useful for establishing accurate etiology of a stricture, since the specimen may be collected from the lumen and represents field rather

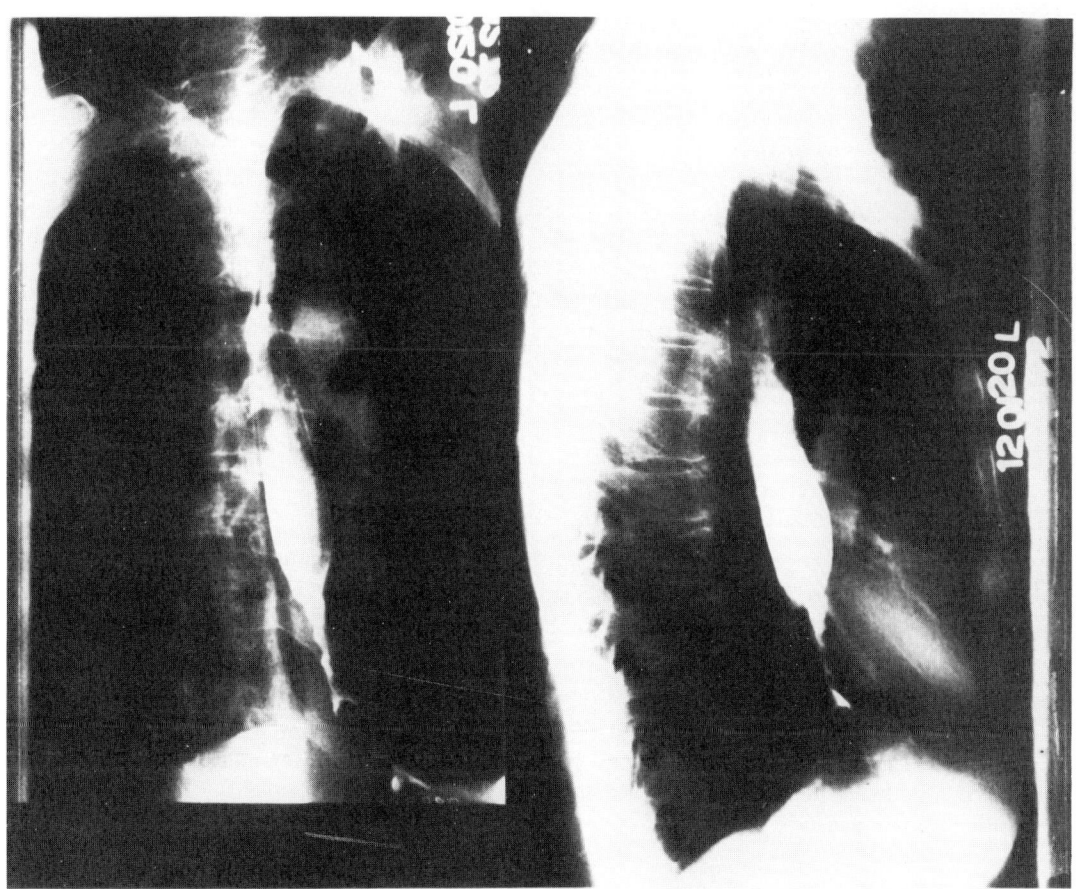

FIGURE 22-4 The entire thoracic esophagus is involved by longitudinal extension of this carcinoma.

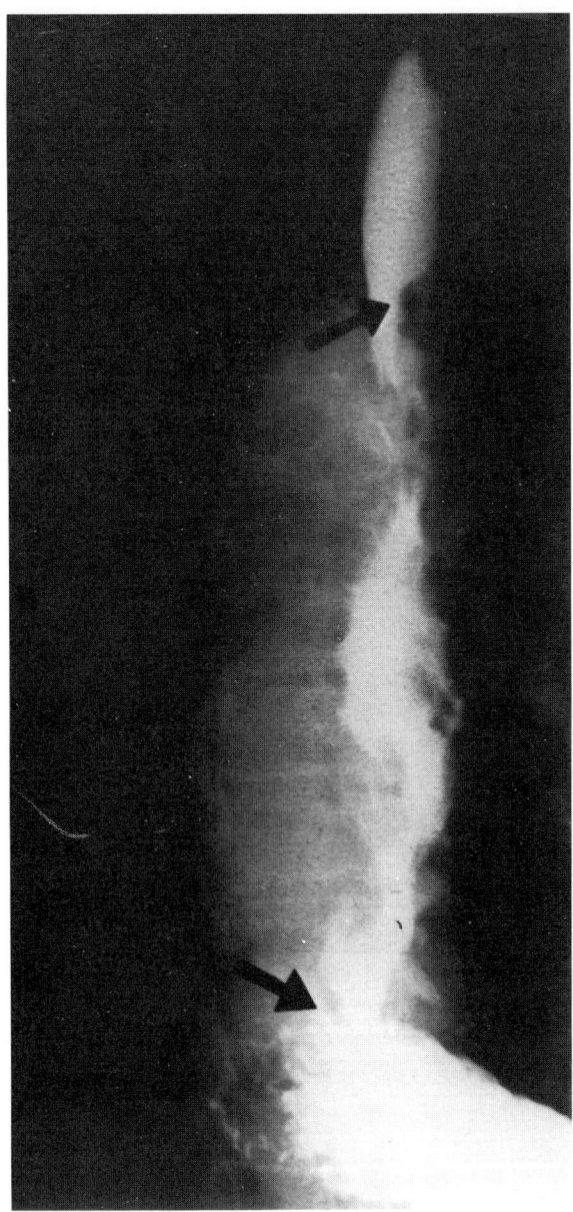

FIGURE 22-5 This distal esophageal stricture associated with a large hiatal hernia on biopsy was found to be an adenocarcinoma.

than focal sampling.[25] Patients with a worrisome distal esophageal stricture should have dilatation and subsequent rigid esophagoscopy in order to obtain deep biopsies from the stenotic area (Fig. 22-6). On rare occasions all attempts at biopsy of a suspicious stricture will be negative, and exploratory laparotomy is necessary to establish the diagnosis.

Bronchoscopy is recommended routinely for lesions involving the middle third of the esophagus to rule out extension to the tracheobronchial tree. Routine biopsy of the carina is obtained even when it appears grossly normal. In some cases even though the bronchoscopy is negative, tracheal washings will yield a positive cytology. In such cases both the possibility of primary bronchogenic carcinoma and tracheal invasion from esophageal cancer should be considered. We consider tracheobronchial involvement with cancer of the esophagus a contraindication to resection.

Operations for staging include mediastinoscopy, and cervical or scalene lymph node biopsies. We employ mediastinoscopy and scalene biopsies only in circumstances where the information to be derived would modify treatment. For example, excision of enlarged scalene nodes containing metastatic cancer may be the least trying and most direct way to prove the presence of stage III carcinoma, thus effectively eliminating the patient from an opportunity for cure by resection of the primary tumor. Mediastinoscopy can be helpful for staging cancers of the middle third of the esophagus. Despite the fact that we advocate mediastinoscopy to evaluate lung cancer patients, we rarely use it for staging esophageal lesions. In general the findings at esophagoscopy and bronchoscopy combined with angiographic evaluation of the mediastinum can provide the necessary information regarding the extent of local invasion in the midmediastinum. Mediastinal lymph node involvement alone does not eliminate consideration of resection for palliation.

Laparoscopy may be useful in staging lower-third carcinomas where intraabdominal metastasis is expected. General anesthesia and a formal exploratory laparotomy can be avoided in patients with peritoneal carcinomatosis or extensive liver metastasis by laparoscopy and biopsy of the tumor implants.

Angiography to outline the azygous vein can be helpful. In 1964 we postulated that azygous venography could reflect the extent of mediastinal spread.[26] This hypothesis proved correct. Obstruction or occlusion of the azygous vein (Fig. 22-7) was reliably associated with

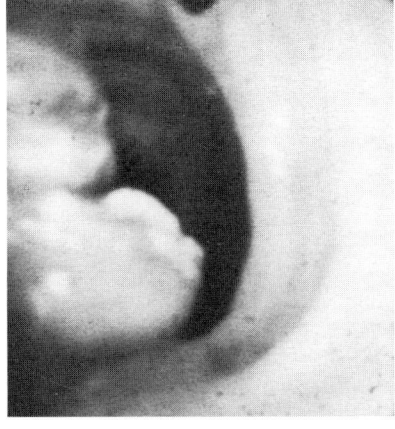 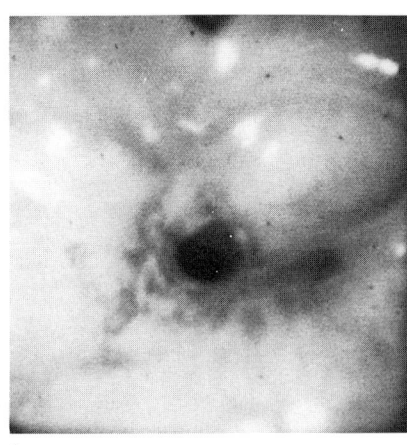

FIGURE 22-6 Venography shows occlusion of the azygous vein, a sign of unresectable tumor. (*a*) extensive cancer. (*b*) occluded azygous vein.

unresectability despite the fact that the azygous vein itself is not a vital structure. For the past decade we have used azygous venography to stage cancers of the middle third of the esophagus and to evaluate the effects of preoperative radiotherapy. Our current practice is to reserve transthoracic operation for middle-third carcinomas for patients who have patent azygous veins and to rely on other forms of palliation when there is mediastinal extension signalled by a blocked vein. Occasionally azygous vein obstruction can be relieved by radiotherapy, and then further consideration is given to esophagectomy.

THERAPEUTIC CONSIDERATIONS FOR PRIMARY TREATMENT

Patients who have carcinoma of the esophagus are usually incurable. For example, of 461 patients treated at Memorial Hospital in New York, only 2.4 percent survived more than 5 years, and of 713 patients treated at the Lahey Clinic, only 2.1 percent were alive after 5 years.[27,29] Resection and irradiation can be used to achieve the best available results for patients who can be cured and effective palliation for those who are incurable. The therapy selected depends on the histology, the clinical stage of the lesion, its anatomical site, and the patient's nutrition and general medical status. Preoperative decisions regarding the advisability of parenteral nutrition and the role of radiotherapy are as important as the choice of operation.

Cervical Carcinomas

Tumors of the cervical esophagus are particularly difficult problems since involvement of the larynx is frequent, and may involve pharyngolaryngoesophagectomy. Resection of such tumors deprives the patient of speech. This operation usually is excessively radical treatment when palliation is the goal. For local control of cervical cancers megavoltage radiation therapy with the linear accelerator or radiocobalt has been a significant contribution. Reports of radiotherapy results before 1960 such as Jacobson's review of eight centers and 1160 cases cited cure rates of 3 to 14 percent.[29] Advances in irradiation techniques have improved survival in some centers. To our knowledge, the best results by far have been achieved by Pearson at Edinburgh.[25] This Radiation Therapy Center serves the entire population of southeastern Scotland. In 46 patients with upper-third lesions, the 5-year survival was 30 percent. Other radiotherapists have not been as successful as Pearson. In Toronto, patients at the Princess Margaret Hospital treated for upper-third lesions with megavoltage irradiation had a 5-year survival of 10 percent.[31] At the V.A. Wadsworth Campus of UCLA we have had no 5-year survivors in 18 patients treated with irradiation alone. Thus, results vary widely, but radiation therapy is now generally accepted as the

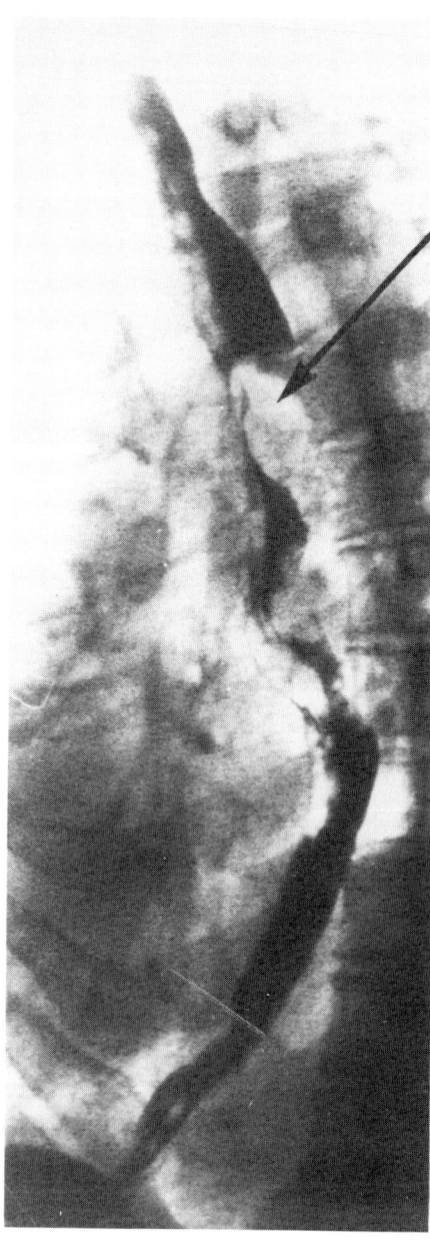
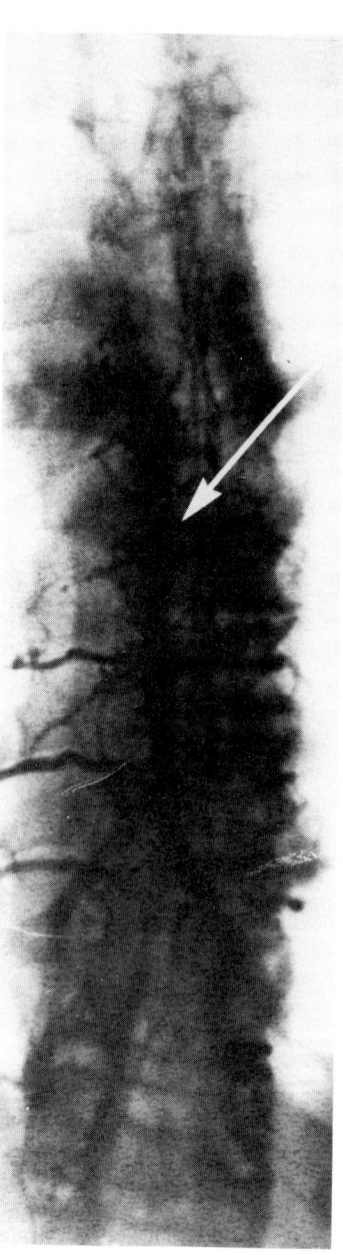

FIGURE 22-7 (a) Endoscopic view of a typical bulky esophageal carcinoma readily proven by biopsy. (b) An esophageal stricture. Proof of cancer may require brush biopsy, dilatation, and repeated biopsies.

most effective primary treatment for cancers of the upper esophagus.

Excision of cervical esophageal cancers can be accomplished. It is probably best confined to cancer centers with multidiscipline expertise and facilities necessary for the complex reconstruction procedures required after extirpation.[32,33] Adequate surgery for carcinoma of the cervical esophagus may require contiguous resection of larynx and pharynx. Even though this may remove the lesion, most patients still will not be cured. To achieve true palliation, it is essential to be able to provide reliable reconstruction of the pharyngoesophageal segment.

Transposition of the stomach and its attached blood supply either through the posterior mediastinum or subcutaneously with pharyngogastric anastomosis accomplishes these goals with a single-stage operation. Resection and reconstruction can be performed without thoracotomy. For detailed discussion of this technique, and other methods of reconstruction including esophagocoloplasty and reversed gastric tube esophagoplasty, the reader is referred to Silver's excellent monograph.[33]

Middle- and Lower-Third Carcinomas

Primary treatment of middle-third carcinomas is the subject of much controversy. Cure is so unusual that many surgeons view all resections of these lesions as palliative. For example, in over 50 patients treated by one of us (John Benfield) only 1 patient survived 5 years free of cancer. Three alternate methods of potentially curative therapy are currently practiced: (1) resection with one stage or multiple-stage reconstruction; (2) radiotherapy; and (3) combination of radiotherapy with resection.

One-stage resection and reconstruction of middle-third lesions is accomplished by esophagogastrectomy or esophagocoloplasty. We have found the combined abdominal and right thoracic approach for esophagogastrectomy first described by Ivor Lewis in 1946 to be excellent one-stage procedure for resection of midesophageal lesions.[34] The patient is placed on the operating table in the left lateral position with the right side elevated and the pelvis rotated almost flat on the operating table (Fig. 22-8).[35] The operation is begun through an abdominal incision, and the greater curvature of the stomach mobilized. Care is taken to divide the omental vessels without injuring the gastroepiploic artery, which will provide blood supply to the stomach after it is advanced into the thorax. The short gastric vessels are divided gently, leaving the spleen intact. The lesser curvature is then detached from the gastrohepatic ligament, but the right gastric artery is preserved. The left gastric artery is divided near its origin in order to preserve communication with the right gastric for collateral supply to the fundus. The esophagogastric junction is completely freed from its attachments to the diaphragm, and the lower esophagus is mobilized for about 5 cm. We do a pyloromyotomy or pyloroplasty, although we are not certain that this is necessary for gastric drainage. The operating table is now rotated to the left, and a right posterolateral thoracotomy is done through the fifth intercostal space. Recently we have successfully been using median sternotomy extension of the abdominal incision with right anterior thoracotomy extension. The lung is retracted anteriorly after division of the inferior pulmonary ligament, and the azygous vein is divided. The esophagus is dissected from the mediastinum. In most cases resection can be accomplished even though the lesion may be invading the adventitia of the aorta. After dilatation of the esophageal hiatus, the stomach is drawn into the right thorax (care is taken to avoid twisting). We use a stapler device to transect and close the esophagogastric junction. A vascular clamp is placed on the esophagus, approximately 5 cm above the lesion, and the esophagus divided. One of us (John Benfield) prefers not to clamp the esophagus. A full thickness of the proximal margin is always sent for frozen section to assure clearance of tumor. An anastomosis is performed, using an outer layer of silk sutures which incorporate the parietal pleura. The mucosal layer is constructed using synthetic absorbable suture. The anterior sutures are used to "serosalize" the anastomosis by plicating the stomach around the anastomosis. A nasogastric tube is placed in the stomach. Alternatively a circumferential stapling device may be used to construct satisfactory anastomosis, but our experience with this device to date has been limited. A gastrotomy is needed to introduce the stapler, and the

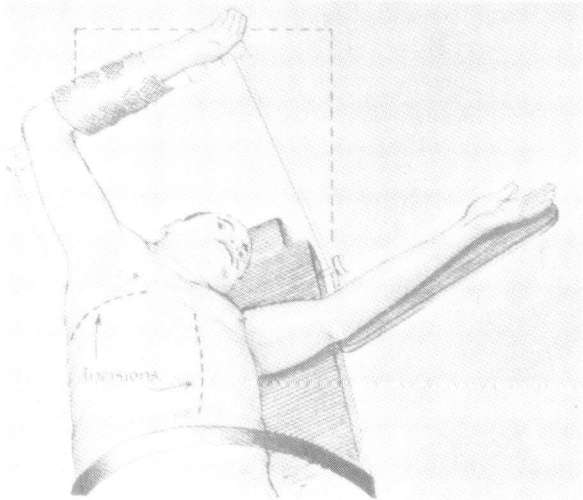

FIGURE 22-8 Positioning of the patient for the Lewis operation. The tube may be rotated to the left or right to improve exposure. (*From J S Carey et al: Ann Thorac Surg 1459–1468, 1972.*)

rather bulky instrument has been difficult to position at use. However, the principle is sound, and with more experience and better-sized instruments staple anastomotic methods may technically simplify construction of the anastomosis. The right thoracic and upper midline approach may be performed by two teams simultaneously with one operating in the chest and the other in the abdomen. We have found it simpler to begin in the abdomen and proceed to the thorax; however, both incisions may be closed at the same time.

Few surgeons have mastered Belsey's technique for middle-third carcinomas, in which a right thoracotomy is used for both resection of the esophagus and mobilization of the stomach through an enlarged hiatus.[36] The abdomen is not opened unless the patient is obese or there has been previous upper-abdominal surgery.[37]

For lower-third squamous cell tumors or adenocarcinomas of the cardia where infiltration of the esophagus is minimal, many surgeons use a thoracoabdominal incision, which permits wide resection of the distal esophagus and proximal stomach along with the spleen, omentum, and regional lymphatics. We prefer a left thoracotomy. The diaphragm is divided in circumferential rather than in radial fashion. Transthoracic pyloromyotomy can usually be done safely, but we do not hesitate to make a separate small transverse upper abdominal incision over the pylorus for pyloroplasty or pyloromyotomy if necessary. The left thoracotomy has several advantages over the thoracoabdominal incision. The latter permits wide resection of the distal esophagus and proximal portion of the stomach, but we have found healing to be better and postoperative pain to be less if transection of the coastal margin is avoided. There is evidence to support our clinical observations and prejudice. Pulmonary function studies were done by Black et al. in patients after esophageal resection via a left thoracolaparotomy and after laparotomy followed by separate thoracotomy.[38] The pronounced hypoxemia which occurred in the first few days after esophageal resection with thoracolaparotomy in most patients was reversed more rapidly after separate thoracic incisions. Whenever reasonable, we favor thoracotomy with or without laparotomy as needed in preference to transection of the costal margin by a thoracoabdominal incision.

Lower-third squamous cell carcinomas may extend further in the esophageal submucosa than anticipated, forcing the surgeon who is approaching the tumor from the left side to perform an unexpected and potentially dangerous anastomosis high in the left chest near the aortic arch. In our experience some adenocarcinomas of the gastroesophageal junction, like squamous cell cancers, will have extensive submucosal extension in the esophagus undetected on preoperative barium esophagram. (Fig. 22-9a and b). Therefore, except for smaller cancers in the distal esophagus, abdominal incision and right thoracotomy is used.

Alternative in primary treatment of thoracic esophageal cancer is resection with colon interposition.[39,40] To decide the suitability of the colon substitution, barium enema is done to rule out colonic abnormalities. Arteriography is advisable in the older patient to ascertain that an adequate mesenteric blood supply for the colonic segment is present. The operation can be done in one or two stages. The single-stage approach begins with abdominal exploration and mobilization of the right colon for transplantation into the thorax. The esophageal tumor is excised through a right thoracotomy. The anastomosis between the esophagus and colon is made through a neck incision. Some surgeons prefer to use the left colon for interposition. The length, blood supply, and smaller left colonic diameter are given as significant advantages. Depending on individual anatomic features, our experience has been that the right or left colon may be used equally well. The colon is usually placed in the anterior mediastinum, but it can be placed subcutaneously. We have reserved colon interposition for palliation in highly selected cases.

Nakayama has advocated a staged approach.[41] In his well-renowned experience, esophageal resection is done as the first stage, and about 6 months later, colon interposition is done as the second stage. When adjunctive radiotherapy has been used before excision of the tumor, a gastrostomy is placed, and cervical esophagostomy is done during the first-stage exploration. Esophagectomy follows radiation, and 6 to 12 months later reconstruction by colon bypass is done. This staged approach allows an important degree of natural selection to occur from the behavior of the cancers during the therapeutic intervals. We are reluctant to use staged operations routinely, wishing to avoid repeated hospitalizations when life expectancy is short. The use of colon interposition in the treatment of esophageal cancer must be weighed against the risks of the procedure. Although in 685 patients the operation carried an acceptable mortality of 7.5 percent, the death rate among patients operated because of esophageal malignancy was 25 percent.[36] With the exception of Gregory's report of 29 patients undergoing one-stage colon interposition for

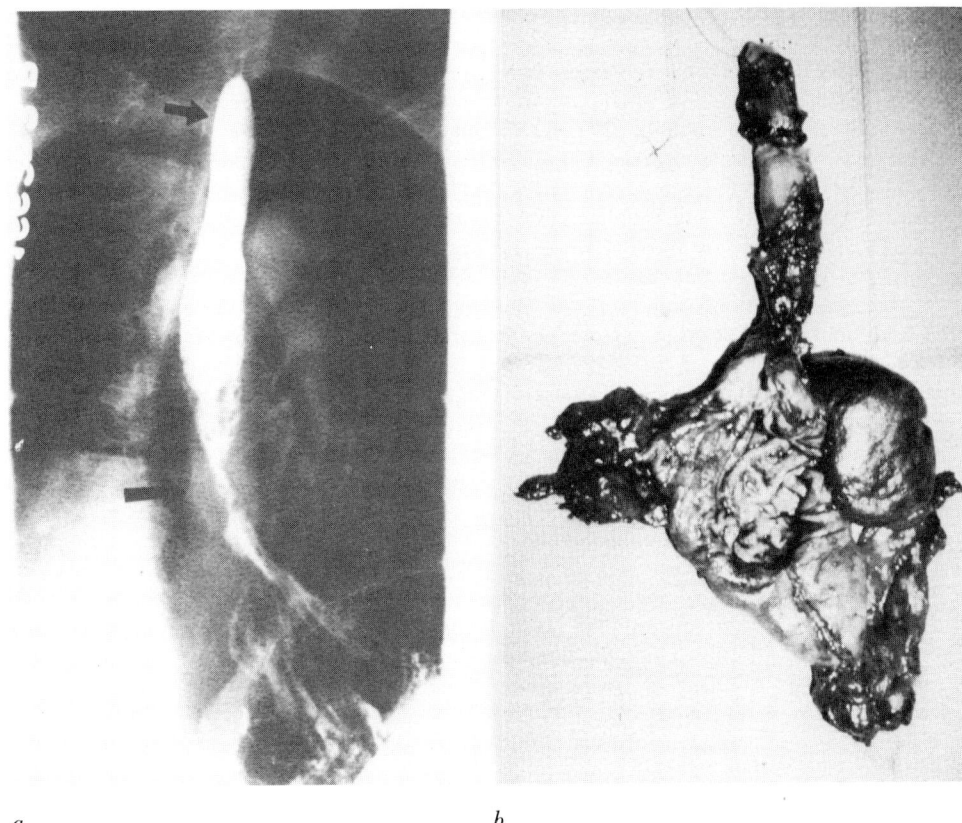

FIGURE 22-9 (*a*) Adenocarcinoma of the gastroesophageal junction associated with a hiatal hernia. The lower arrow indicates site of biopsy; the upper arrow shows extent of submucosal invasion present at operation. (*b*) Operative specimen showing transection of esophagus at three levels before frozen section was negative for carcinoma.

esophageal cancer where the mortality was 10.3 percent, the results of esophagogastrectomy have generally been better than those for colon interposition.[39]

POSTOPERATIVE COMPLICATIONS

Most patients with esophageal cancer have been heavy smokers, and atelectasis, pneumonia, and respiratory insufficiency after operation are significant risks. There are few situations where preoperative and postoperative prophylactic measures are more rewarding. If at all possible, we insist that our patients stop smoking for a full week before operation. Sputum cultures are obtained preoperatively and again before endotracheal extubation. After operation we maintain endotracheal intubation with assisted respiration until satisfactory blood gases and spontaneous tidal volumes, vital capacities, and inspiratory and expiratory forces have been achieved. Usually this requires 12 to 24 h of postoperative respiratory assistance, and occasionally 30 to 72 h of assistance is necessary. The endotracheal tube is well tolerated when patients are advised of this plan before operation. It is well established that several days of indicated and well-managed nasal or orotracheal intubation is quite safe in well-monitored intensive care setting. Troublesome postintubation laryngeal edema is rare; tracheostomy is rarely needed. Before and after extubation tracheal aspiration and bronchoscopy are used liberally when indicated.

Anastomotic leak is the dreaded complication of esophageal surgery. After colonic interposition, temporary leakage in the neck occurs in about 20 percent of patients. Cervical anastomotic leak is rarely a significant contributor to death if effectively and promptly drained. In contrast, the mortality from esophagogastric leaks still exceeds 50 percent in the most modern and aggressive centers.[42,43] In 56 of our patients (Samuel Wilson's) with lower-third cardia lesions undergoing esophagogastrectomy, four anastomotic leaks (7 percent) resulted in three deaths.

Before feeding any patient after an esophagogastrectomy, it is good practice to obtain a barium esophagogram on the fifth to seventh day. Not infrequently a small sinus tract may be seen leading from the anastomosis. If feeding is withheld in these patients for another week and hyperalimentation is maintained, the leak will heal in almost all cases.

Esophagogastric leaks of major proportion become evident on the fifth to seventh day, with fever and accumulation of fluid in the chest. If chest tubes are still in place, increased drainage of gastric content may be noted. On occasion the pleural fluid signifying a leak may present in the contralateral hemithorax. The risk of leaks is enhanced by extensive proximal gastric resection for lesions of the cardia, since antrum to esophagus anastomosis may be technically difficult. Anastomotic leak is due either to insufficient blood supply, tension, or technical error. The blood supply of the stomach after mobilization into the chest is critical.[43] Likewise, the blood supply of the midthoracic esophagus derives from small branches of the aorta and intercostals, and it may be comprised by mobilization of an excessive length. The blood supply for high anastomoses arises largely from the inferior thyroid vessels, and previous thyroidectomy may jeopardize vascularity.

When a leak is recognized, optimum chest drainage must be assured. Chest tubes should be reinserted if they have already been removed (Fig. 22-10). Serial chest x-rays are obtained daily to check for undrained accumulations of fluid or unsuspected empyema. These should be anticipated. Upon discovery careful placement of a new tube will ensure drainage (Fig. 22-11). If the nasogastric tube has been removed, it may be cautiously replaced by the surgeon, and suction reinstituted. For major uncontrolled leaks, or complete anastomotic disruption, it will be necessary to take down the anastomosis, close the proximal stomach, return it to the abdomen, and fashion a gastrostomy. The esophagus is mobilized until healthy, uninfected tissue is obtained, and it is stapled closed. A cervical esophagostomy is performed. Radical as this treatment may appear, most patients will die unless it is carried out; therefore, aggressive, early management is justified in serious leaks or anastomotic disruption. To ensure healing and maintenance of the host-defense mechanisms, good nutrition, i.e., a positive nitrogen balance, must be maintained by total parenteral and enteric tube feedings.

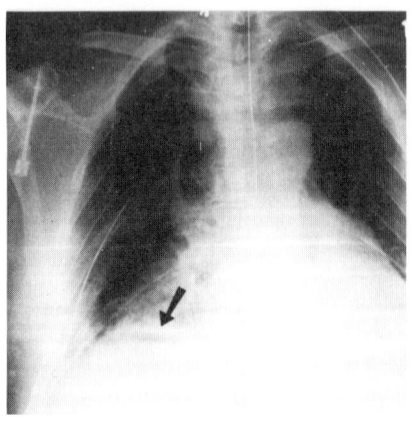
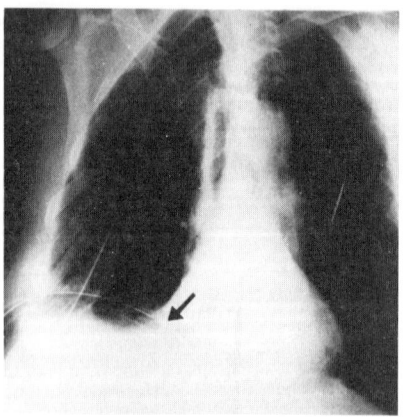

a *b*

FIGURE 22-10 (*a*) Accumulation of an air fluid level signified an anastomotic leak on the sixth postoperative day. (*b*) Accurate placement of an additional chest tube drains the collection satisfactorily. This patient survived the small leak.

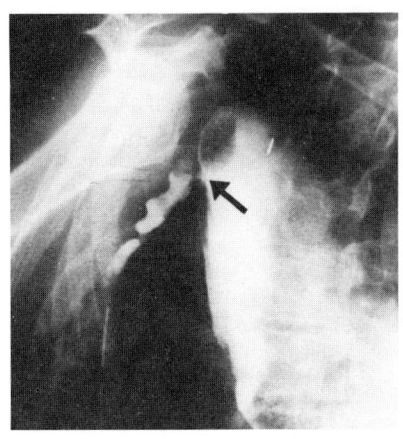 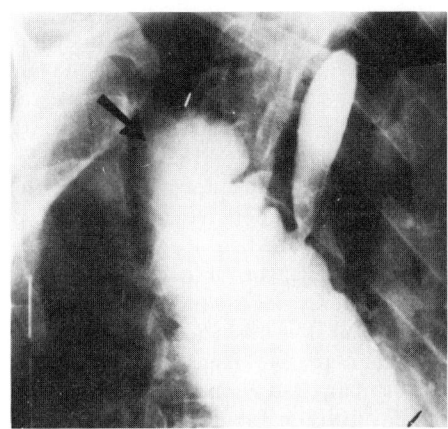

FIGURE 22-11 (*a*) A leak from the gastric closure, probably due to ischemic necrosis, has formed a well-delineated fistula. (*b*) After 1 month of parenteral nutrition the leak has closed. This was confirmed not only by barium x-ray but also by the more sensitive test of methylene blue ingestion prior to removing the chest tubes.

Radiation therapy is an alternate method seeking curative treatment of squamous-cell carcinoma of the midesophagus.[30] The field length is usually 13 to 15 cm to encompass submucosal spread, and 5000 to 6000 rads (cobalt 60 unit or 6 to 18 linear MeV accelerators) are divided into 20 fractions over 4 to 6 weeks.[31] These are frequently employed doses, but radiotherapy technique varies with the patient's medical status and development of toxicity. We concur that radiotherapy should be the treatment of choice in patients where general medical condition does not justify operation. Discouragement with poor survival rates as the cost of a high-risk operation has led physicians to employ irradiation frequently as primary treatment. We do not seriously quarrel with this approach, but the choice should be made after multidisciplinary consultation, preferably in the form of a tumor board. Irradiation has several disadvantages and, therefore, only limited applicability to lower esophageal carcinomas. The main route of metastasis is to nodes of the celiac axis, lesser curvature of the stomach, hilum of the spleen, and the mediastinum. To encompass this spread, the radiation field must be enlarged to the extent that it is difficult to give an adequate dose safely. Our treatment for such lesions, therefore, is resection when at all possible.

Combination preoperative radiotherapy and resection as a primary therapeutic modality has several theoretical advantages. Nonresectable lesions may be decreased enough in size to permit resection. The risk of implantation or dissemination of viable tumor cells during operation may be decreased. At least three regimens of preoperative radiation therapy are under investigation in several centers. A total dose of 2000 to 2500 rads fractionated over 4 to 5 days followed by a short interval has been given prior to esophagectomy by Nakayama.[41] Akakura employs 5000 to 6000 rads over 4 to 6 weeks and delays operation for 3 weeks after completion of the irradiation.[44] In the United States most surgeons have given 4000 to 4500 rads preoperatively over 30 to 40 days followed by surgery in 3 to 4 weeks. The following regimen has been developed at Harbor-UCLA Medical Center and City of Hope National Medical Center for middle-third esophageal cancers: (1) staging to include bronchoscopy and angiography (azygous vein); (2) preoperative radiation to approximately 3000 rads; (3) operation with one-stage resection for patients with patent azygous veins and reasonable nutrition; or (4) completion of radiotherapy as definitive treatment for patients who are prohibited operative risks, or whose azygous veins remain occluded.

THERAPEUTIC OPTIONS: PALLIATION

Palliation of esophageal cancer consists largely of restoring the ability to swallow and of providing nutrition and relief of pain. We believe treatment should be selected which has demonstrated benefit and is least expensive of the patient's time and money. If at all possible palliative therapy should permit the patient to remain at home with his or her family until the terminal stages.

Normally a saliva volume of 1 to 1½ L each 24 h is swallowed without any awareness of this important function. With complete esophageal obstruction and inability to swallow, the patient has constantly to spit into a basin. When the patient falls asleep, oral secretions are aspirated into the tracheobronchial tree. The available therapeutic modalities should be considered competitive, and care must be taken not to allow hope and enthusiasm to outstrip reason. The selection of palliative measures will be tempered by bearing in mind that survival of patients with incurable esophageal carcinoma is approximately 6 months.

For cancers of the upper esophagus irradiation is currently the most widely used palliative dose. A dose of 2000 to 3000 rads over two weeks may relieve symptoms of pain or hemorrhage and improve swallowing enough to permit the patient to sleep.[45]

For midesophageal lesions, operation, radiation, or intubation may be appropriate for primary use. Carey and associates at the V.A. Wadsworth Center of UCLA hold the view that resection with an acceptable mortality and morbidity affords superior palliation and extends life better than radiation therapy.[35] In their patients, palliative resection for middle-third lesions gave a mean survival of 11 months, as compared with 5 months for patients who had radiation therapy.[46] Of 20 patients undergoing resection and esophagogastrostomy, all experienced permanent relief of dysphagia, whereas swallowing was restored to normal in only 4 of 20 irradiated patients. They found that 16 of 20 patients who had resection and 6 of 20 irradiated patients survived beyond 6 months. The authors attempted to match both sets of patients according to stage, but only cautious conclusions are warranted. Patients offered palliative operations are generally in better condition than patients selected for radiotherapy, thus weighing results in favor of operative palliation. To date no randomized, prospective study has tested these two methods for palliation of midthoracic cancers, and the choice of operation or radiation is somewhat subjective. We are certain, however, that resection when it can be done safely is an excellent palliative approach in selected patients with middle-third cancer.

Studies to compare resection and radiotherapy are not available for lower-esophageal squamous cell carcinoma. The difficulty in giving adequate radiation therapy to this region and the potential for cure suggests that these lesions should be resected if possible. The mean survival after palliative resection for patients with lower-third and cardia lesions is 11 months, compared with a 3-months survival for patients without resection.[20] In patients with liver metastases, survival after resection averages only 6 months; therefore, resection is probably not indicated for most patients with hepatic spread. However, in patients undergoing resection of the primary cancers, despite the presence of gross tumor remaining in the mediastinum, survival of over 1 year has been achieved. Resection may be worthwhile under these less than ideal circumstances. Symptomatic local recurrence has not been noted in our patients after palliative resection; death from hepatic metastasis usually precedes recurrent dysphagia.

Palliation may be accomplished with *bypass of the lesion without resection*. In addition, radiation therapy can be given to the primary tumor after the patient's recovery from surgery. The operation may be the previously described colon interposition, which passes the colon to the neck in the substernal or subcutaneous position. Others have used the reversed gastric tube, fashioned from the greater curve of the stomach, and supplied by the gastroepiploic arteries.[47] In patients with a relatively large stomach, it is possible to bring the gastric tube up to the pharynx through a subcutaneous tunnel. Through an abdominal incision, a tube from the greater curvature of the stomach is constructed with a suitable stapler. An incision is made in the neck for anastomosis to the cervical esophagus. Advocates of this procedure point out that the reversed gastric tube is invariably of adequate length, and has sufficient blood supply to heal per primum or to close anastomotic leaks spontaneously when they occur. We have not used the reversed gastric tube, and we therefore refer the reader to its advocates.

Intubation of the obstructed esophagus has been utilized for palliation of advanced disease since the 1840s when a decalcified animal tusk was inserted through an esophageal tumor. Tubes in current use are either pulled or pushed through the cancer.[48,49] The Celestin tube is an example of the traction type. Introduction requires that the tapered leading edge be guided through the tumor by a previously passed string. The tube is grasped in the stomach through a gastrotomy and fixed to the stomach wall after the tube is well positioned through the tumor. Endoscopic visualization of the proximal end of the tube may be made to ensure a snug fit. These pull-through tubes are most useful for lesions of the lower-third esophagus and gastroesophageal junction.

Pulsion intubation of the esophagus by oral insertion of a tube has the advantages of not requiring a laparotomy or gastrotomy. A suitable tube is the Procter-Livingstone prosthesis.[50] Other types in general use include the Souttar and Makler tubes. After identifying the tumor with a rigid esophagoscope, a bougie is passed and left in situ as the esophagoscope is removed. A well-lubricated Procter-Livingstone tube of soft latex rubber with an internal diameter of 12 mm and external diameter of 18 mm is inserted over the bougie and passed through the stricture, using the esophagoscope as a pulsion device until the expanded proximal end of the tube reaches the upper extent of the tumor. The bougie and the esophagoscope are then removed. The push-through tube is best used for short-segment tumors (8 cm) of the upper and middle thirds of the esophagus.

The main advantage of the pulsion type of tube is that it can be inserted without an abdominal operation. Our preference has been the traction approach, because the likelihood of esophageal perforation is lessened after a guide for traction has been passed into the stomach. Blind insertion of a pulsion tube can perforate the esophagus, resulting in fatal mediastinitis. Complications of the tube prostheses include pressure necrosis and erosion of the esophagus by the flanged upper end of the tube; in some patients this has led to aortoesophageal fistula. Migration of the tube proximally or distally can occur, especially after radiation therapy. If the patient is extremely malnourished, healing of the abdominal incision may be delayed, and wound dehiscence is not uncommon. The overall in-hospital mortality for pull-through intubation is 23.5 percent with a direct technical mortality of 6.6 percent.[51] Any esophageal intubation prosthesis may become obstructed by food, tumor growth, or pills.

Intubation has been used in some patients for treatment of tracheoesophageal fistula or perforation with the hope that the tube will serve as a stent. In our practice we do not usually recommend esophageal tubes once a tracheoesophageal fistula has formed. Most of these patients are near death from pneumonia, and we believe maintaining their comfort is perhaps the best form of palliation at this late stage.

Cervical esophagostomy is not a satisfactory palliative technique for relief of dysphagia. Management of the cervical stoma may require continual changing of gauze dressings, or at best collection of saliva in disposable plastic colostomy bags.

ADJUVANT THERAPIES

Nutrition is a most important adjuvant therapy in both curative and palliative approaches to esophageal cancer. The alternatives in order of preference are to restore the patient's ability to eat by surgery or radiation therapy, to use *temporary* parenteral hyperalimentation, or to place gastrostomy. We decline to use either hyperalimentation or gastrostomy except as an adjunct to other forms of palliation. It is highly appropriate to enhance preoperative nutrition with total parenteral nutrition when palliative or curative resection is planned. In addition a jejunostomy, e.g., Intracath, or a tube placed at operation can be useful for enteric alimentation should oral feedings be delayed by anastomotic complications. It is often worthwhile to place a small silastic nasogastric tube before a course of radiotherapy in anticipation of temporary worsening of the obstruction due to inflammation and edema from tumor necrosis. An elemental diet given through the tube may sustain nutrition until the obstruction is relieved. We consider it inappropriate to use either hyperalimentation or to place a new gastrostomy until all other palliative means have failed. The nutritional deficit in most patients suffering from unresectable cancer of the esophagus have been reversed following intubation by oral alimentation, using an elemental dietary supplement.

Limited experience with adjuvant chemotherapy or palliative chemotherapy in esophageal epidermoid carcinoma has been obtained almost entirely with bleomycin. In 64 Japanese patients treated preoperatively with bleomycin, histological examination of the regional lymph nodes showed degenerative changes in the metastatic tumor cells to a greater degree than in nodes of untreated patients.[52] Seventeen East African patients with advanced esophageal squamous cell cancer were treated with intramuscular bleomycin. Improvement in swallowing after 2 to 6 months was noted in 12 patients.[53] Another report from the West Indies detailed the use of cyclophosphamide and 5-fluorouracil given both intravenously and by injection into the tumor.[54] An average survival period of 9 months was achieved with this technique, but meaningful controls were lacking. At present, chemotherapy for esophageal squamous cell carcinoma is not of proven efficacy and agents such as *cis*-platinum are best administered within the confines of a study rather than an ad hoc treatment in desperation.

The experience obtained with chemotherapy for gastric adenocarcinomas may be applied to proximal gastric tumors involving the esophagus. The Gastrointestinal Tumor Study Group has found a combination of 5-fluorouracil (5-FU) and methyl-chloroethylcyclohexyl-nitrosurea (MeCCNU) to be superior to radiation and chemotherapy (5000 rads plus 5-FU plus MeCCNU) in treatment of locally advanced gastric adenocarcinoma.[55] Improved survival for advanced gastric carcinoma has also been obtained with a combination chemotherapy program consisting of 5-FU, mitomycin C, and Adriamycin. This regimen gave a partial response to 16 to 29 treated patients (55 percent) for a median duration of 9.5 months.[56] This should be reserved for locally unresected carcinoma or metastasis. Again, despite promising reports with these chemotherapeutic agents, we recommend that they best be employed as part of an ongoing study.

THERAPEUTIC OPTIONS: OVERALL RESULTS

Operations

The 5-year survival rates for esophageal cancer are dependent on the stage of disease at diagnosis and on the anatomical site in the esophagus. Of all patients entering the hospital with esophageal cancer, just under one-half will have tumors initially judged to be resectable potentially, and only 30 percent of the initial group selected for operation will have apparently curable tumors. The resectability rate for patients undergoing exploration varies from 60 to 75 percent depending on the surgeon's attitude towards palliative resection. In general a higher resectability rate is accompanied by an increase in operative mortality. At the V.A. Wadsworth Campus of UCLA, 60 percent of patients undergo exploration, and resectability is 77 percent of all patients with lower-third and cardia lesions and 90 percent for middle-third lesions. A compilation of reports prepared for a Veterans Administration Cooperative Study showed that of 4000 patients only 1105 patients had lesions judged to be resectable.[57] The postoperative mortality ranged from 11 to 50 percent. The 5-year survival of all patients has been 0.9 to 6.3 percent; of those having resections, 6.2 to 13.8 percent have survived 5 years (Table 22-2).

The tendency for early invasion of vital mediastinal structures gives carcinoma in the midthoracic section the worst prognosis. The 5-year survival is approximately one-half of that for the same tumor stage in the lower thoracic esophagus or at the gastroesophageal junction. For example, a stage 1 carcinoma of the thoracic esophagus has an 11 percent 5-year survival rate following resection, as compared to 21 percent for a stage 1 cancer in the lower third of the esophagus.

As many as 75 percent of patients with lower esophageal and cardia tumors have exploratory operations, and the resectability rate is about 60 percent. The overall 5-year survival for lesions in this area ranges between 6 and 14 percent, with selected reports indicating 5-year survival as high as 40 percent for stage 1 lesions in this area (Table 22-2).

Radiotherapy

The best overall results are from Scotland, where Pearson obtained a 16 percent 5-year survival for midesophageal lesions, and 12 percent 5-year survival for lower esophageal lesions, in carefully selected patients (Table 22-3). To our knowledge, these results have not been reproduced by radiotherapists in North America. Complications of radiation therapy include radiation peumonitis, constrictive pericarditis, and spinal cord injury. Radionecrosis of tumor involving the full thickness of the esophageal wall may accelerate formation of a bronchoesophageal fistula or result in perforation. Thus irradiation cannot be viewed as without risk. The advantages of preoperative radiation therapy include reduction in size of the primary lesion permitting greater resectability, and perhaps minimizing dissemination during surgery by decreasing the viability of surviving or implanted tumor cells.

Results with the combination of radiotherapy and surgical resection as primary therapy are promising (Table 22-4). Nakayama, employing a 2000 to 2500 rads total dose, fractionated in 500 rads daily dose, allows a 4- to 5-day interval prior to surgery. His reported 5-year survival rate of 37.5 percent is based on a small number of patients (three of eight patients at risk after 5 years).[58] Akakura, employing a total dose of 5000 to 6000 rads over a period of a month, to 6 weeks, with a 2- to 4-week

TABLE 22-2 Results of Resection of Carcinoma of Esophagus and Gastroesophageal Junction, Selected Reports 1970–1977

Cancer	Number of patients			Operative mortality, %	Five-year survival after resection, %
	Total	Operated	Resected		
CARCINOMA OF MIDESOPHAGUS					
Younghusband[63]	191	108	87	14	13.8
Spath[64]	—	388	107	11	13.7
Goodner[65]	1859	—	260	23	6.2
Akakura[44]	—	346	187	17	10.7
CARCINOMA OF DISTAL ESOPHAGUS AND GASTROESOPHAGEAL JUNCTION					
Gunnlaugsson et al.[49]	458	—	169	15	12.0
	366	—	198	10	—
Boyd and Kim[66]	286	244	160	—	6.0
Teitler et al.[67]	157	130	89	16	8.0
Skinner[37]	59	—	40	25	8.0
Stone et al.[20]	86	68	52	11	14.0

delay in surgery, has achieved a 5-year survival of 25 percent.[44] Unfortunately, results with trials of preoperative radiation therapy in the United States have not been as good as in Japan. Parker reported a 12 percent 2-year survival in 138 patients treated with combination surgery-radiation therapy.[59] Marks, employing a total dose of 4500 rads over a period of 3 weeks, then delaying operation for 6 weeks, achieved a 5-year survival of 13.9 percent.[60] In summary, reports, primarily from Japan, indicate increased survival with preoperative radiation therapy. Similar results have not yet been demonstrated by randomized study in the United States.

FOLLOW-UP CONSIDERATIONS

Postoperative radiation is recommended when the surgeon has performed a palliative resection leaving tumor in the mediastinum. Marking the residual tumor with hemostatic clips is a valuable aid to the radiotherapist. We do not routinely employ postoperative radiation for patients with positive nodes in the specimen, and do not recommend radiotherapy if nodes are negative.

Recurrence at the anastomosis is suspected with new onset of dysphagia. Endoscopy should be carried out, and if biopsy indicates recurrent tumor instead of fibrotic stricture, we begin radiation therapy. Metastases are usually evident first in the liver, but it is not our practice to treat them unless significant right upper quadrant pain develops. Radiation to the liver has proved a satisfactory method for relief of pain from metastases.

On follow-up examination patients who have had esophagogastrectomy may have distressing symptoms of reflux esophagitis, caused by reflux alkaline duodenal contents through the anastomosis. A high esophagogastrostomy is less likely than a low anastomosis to produce endoscopic changes of esophagitis. Symptoms are not usually severe and are well controlled by avoiding late evening meals, maintaining an upright position after eating, and prescribing antacids for heartburn. In truth, the morbidity and mortality of esophageal carcinoma so far outstrip the problems of reflux esophagitis that it is rarely an important problem.

In recent years there has been increasing enthusiasm for the use of intrathoracic fundoplication techniques in an attempt to prevent reflux. While this procedure serves to reinforce suture lines, it may be equally important in the prevention of reflux esophagitis in those fortunate enough to be long-term survivors. We have usually not found this technique possible after the proximal stomach is removed.

TABLE 22-3 Results of Radiation Therapy of Carcinoma of Midesophagus

Author, year	Total number of patients	Number treated with irradiation	5-year survival
Pearson,[30] 1971	575	144	$\frac{31}{144}$ (22%)
Watson,[68] 1967	178	37	$\frac{4}{37}$ (10%)
Nakayama,[69] 1967	261	142	$\frac{6}{77}$ (8%)
Marcial,[70] 1966	413	151	$\frac{22}{151}$ (15%)
Leborgne,[71] 1963	541	431	$\frac{13}{431}$ (3%)
	1968	905	3–22% (11.6%)

In a few patients, particularly if there has been an anastomotic leak, postoperative stricture may occur. We recommend that the first dilatation be done by the surgeon through a rigid esophagoscope so as to exclude the possibility of recurrent carcinoma. Our preference is the Maloney dilators since they have a weighted tapered tip. If desirable, for subsequent per oral dilatations, we teach patients to pass bougies themselves. Only rarely is long-term bouginage necessary.

CURRENT AREAS OF RESEARCH AND PROSPECTS FOR THE FUTURE

Carcinoma of the esophagus may be the ideal neoplasm for epidemiologic research. Studies of highly susceptible populations, within narrow geographic boundaries, hold great promise for discovery of environmental oncogenic factors. Epidemiologic data to date clearly point to environmental causes rather than genetic factors, and although no single carcinogen has been identified, we look forward to continued investigation of the role of alcohol, tobacco, nitrosamines, trace element deficiencies, and other possible causes. The observation that immigrants traveling from Mozambique to Rhodesia acquired the higher cancer rate of the latter area raises the possibility of an "elusive virus" as in Burkitt's lymphoma.[8] Definition of these environmental factors in esophageal carcinogenesis will ultimately lead to preventive measures.

Early diagnosis will be facilitated by implementation of screening techniques for high-risk populations. Such a group in the United States might constitute males over the age of 45 who are both heavy smokers and drinkers.

TABLE 22-4 Results of Preoperative Radiation and Surgery for Carcinoma of Esophagus

Author, year	Radiation dose	Total number of patients	Five-year survival
Akakura et al.,[44] 1970	5000–6000 rads over 4–6 wks	117	25.0%
Nakayama and Kinoshita,[41] 1974	200–2500 rads over 4–5 days	191	37.5% ($\frac{3}{8}$)
Parker,[59] 1978	4500 rads over 3–4 wks	138	12% (17)*
Marks,[60] 1976	4500 rads over 3–4 wks	137	13.9% (20)

* Two-year survival.

Already diagnosis of superficial cancers has been achieved by obtaining specimens with a brush introduced via a nasogastric tube or by a net-covered balloon catheter.[11]

Clinical experience with carcinoma in situ of the esophagus is still extremely limited.[61] In a few patients carcinoma in situ has been found by exfoliative cytology, or on endoscopic examination and biopsy. Multifocal carcinoma in situ with areas of superficial invasion have also been reported.

Surgeons in Japan and China are recognizing superficial esophageal cancer, defined in 1969 by the Japanese Society for Esophageal Diseases as tumor invasion limited strictly to the submucosa.[62] When detected in this early stage, approximately 75 percent of patients are free from lymph node metastases. About 100 cases of superficial esophageal cancer have been reported in Japan as of 1975. The Chinese Research Group from Linhseen, Hunan, detected 136 cases among 11,564 persons.[11] They report a 5-year survival rate of almost 90 percent for those patients. The awareness that early detection of upper gastrointestinal cancer is possible has not yet influenced our diagnostic approaches, but again, we anticipate progress in this direction in the next decade.

Mortality from resection in these nutritionally depleted patients will probably continue to decrease primarily due to greater use of preoperative parenteral nutrition. In addition, esophageal anastomotic leaks will be managed more safely with combined parenteral and enteral feeding.

The promise of increased resectability and greater survival rates obtained with preoperative radiation therapy in Japan merits additional testing by selection of patients for randomized alternate treatment. Well-controlled, nationwide, cooperative studies are essential in the United States.

While no chemotherapeutic agents show promise at present, we are confident that continued trials will eventually make significant inroads. The histological finding of minimal lymphocytic and histocytic infiltration in tumors with exceedingly poor prognoses warrants investigation of immune mechanisms,[63] In our most optimistic view, we would project earlier diagnosis by screening susceptible populations, increased recognition of superficial lesions by cytologic techniques, further reduction in operative mortality, confirmation of the benefits of preoperative radiation, and development of adjuvant chemotherapy.

REFERENCES

1. Hankins JR et al: Adenocarcinoma involving the esophagus. *J Thorac Cardiovasc Surg* 68:148–158, 1974.
2. Czerny J: Neu Operationen: Resection des Oesophagus. *Zentralbl Chir* 4:433, 1877.
3. Torek F: The first successful case of resection of the thoracic esophagus. *Surg Gynecol Obstet* 16:614, 1913.
4. Oshawa T: The surgery of the esophagus. *Arch Jpn Chir (Nippon Geka Hokan)* 10:605, 1933.
5. Marshall SF: Carcinoma of the esophagus: successful resection of lower end of esophagus with re-establishment of esophageal gastric continuity. *Surg Clin North Am* 18: 643–648, 1938.
6. Adams WE, Phemister DB: Carcinoma of lower thoracic espohagus: Report of successful resection and esophagogastrectomy. *J Thorac Cardiovasc Surg* 7:621–632, 1938.
7. Seidman H et al: Cancer statistics, 1976: A comparison of black and white populations. *CA* 26:2–29, 1976.
8. Gilder SSB: Carcinoma of the esophagus. *Ann Intern Med* 87:494, 1977.
9. Cancer of the esophagus, editorial. *Br Med J* 2(6028):1356, 1976.
10. Turyns AJ, Masse G: Cancer of the esophagus in Brittany: An incidence study in Ille-et-Vilaine. *Int J Epidemiol* 4:55–59, 1975.
11. Dowlatshahi K et al: Early detection of cancer of the esophagus along Caspian littoral. *Lancet* 1:125–126, 1978.
12. Cahan WG et al: Separate primary carcinomas of the esophagus and head and neck region in the same patient. *Cancer* 37:85–89, 1976.
13. Lansing PB et al: Carcinoma of the esophagus at the site of lye stricture. *Am J Surg* 118:198–111, 1969.
14. Wynder EL, Bross IJ: A study of etiological factors in cancer of the esophagus. *Cancer* 14:389–398, 1961.
15. Shine I, Allison PR: Carcinoma of the esophagus with tylosis. *Lancet* 1:951–953, 1966.
16. Gough TA: A search for volatile nitrosamines in East Africa spirit. *Gut* 18:301–302, 1977.
17. Lowenfels AB et al: Nitrite studies in oesophageal cancer. *Gut* 19:199–201, 1978.
18. Naef AP et al: Columnar-lined lower esophagus, an acquired lesion with malignant predisposition. *J Thorac Cardiovasc Surg* 70:826–835, 1975.
19. Gunnlaugssan GH et al: Analysis of the records of 1,657 patients with carcinoma of the esophagus and cardia of the stomach. *Surg Gynecol Obstet* 130:997, 1970.
20. Stone R et al: Carcinoma of the gastroesophageal junction: A ten-year experience with esophagogastrectomy. *Am J Surg*, 134:70–76, 1977.
21. Clinical staging system for carcinoma of the esophagus. *CA* 25:50–57, 1975.

22. Moss AA et al: Initial accuracy of esophagogram in detection of small esophageal carcinomas. *Am J Roentgenol* 127:909–913, 1976.
23. Putnam CE et al: Thickening of the posterior tracheal stripe: A sign of squamous cell carcinoma of the esophagus. *Radiology* 121:533, 1976.
24. Daffner RH et al: Retrotracheal abnormalities in esophageal carcinoma: Prognostic implications. *Am J Roentgenol* 130:719–723, 1978.
25. Eastman MC et al: An assessment of the accuracy of modern endoscopic diagnosis of oesophageal stricture. *Br J Surg* 65:182–185, 1978.
26. Crummy AB et al: Azygous venography: An aid in the evaluation of esophageal carcinoma. *Ann Thorac Surg* 6:522–527, 1968.
27. Beatti EJ Jr, Goodner JT: Treatment of carcinoma of the esophagus. *Am Surg* 33:100, 1967.
28. Boyd DP, Kim MCC: Survival in cancer of the esophagus. *Surg Clin North Am* 47:613, 1967.
29. Jacobson F: Carcinoma of the hypopharynx. *Acta Radiol* 35:1–21, 1951.
30. Pearson JG: The value of radiotherapy in the management of squamous esophageal cancer. *Br J Surg* 58:794–798, 1971.
31. Rider WD, Mendoza RD: Some opinions on treatment of cancer of the esophagus. *Am J Roentgenol* 105:514–517, 1969.
32. Postlethwait RW: Carcinoma of the esophagus, in *Current Problems in Cancer*, Year Book, Chicago, vol 12, 8, 1978.
33. Silver CE: Surgical management of neoplasms of the larynx, hypopharynx, and cervical esophagus, in *Current Problems in Surgery*, Year Book, Chicago, vol 14, 1977
34. Lewis I: The surgical treatment of carcinoma of the oesophagus with special reference to new operation for growths of the middle third. *Br J Surg* 34:18–31, 1946.
35. Carey JS et al: Esophagogastrectomy: Superiority of the combined abdominal–right thoracic approach (Lewis operation). *Ann Thorac Surg* 14:59–68, 1972
36. Belsey R, Hiebert CA: An exclusive right thoracic approach for cancer of middle-third of the esophagus. *Ann Thorac Surg* 18:1–15, 1974.
37. Skinner DB: Esophageal malignancies: Experience with 110 cases. *Surg Clin North Am* 56:137–147, 1976.
38. Black J et al: The effect of the surgical approach on respiratory function after oesophageal resection. *Br J Surg* 64:624–627, 1977.
39. Postlethwait RW et al: Colon interposition for esophageal substitution. *Ann Thorac Surg* 12:89–109, 1971.
40. Gregorie HB Jr: Esophagocoloplasty. *Ann Surg* 175:740–751, 1972.
41. Nakayama K, Kenoshita Y: Surgical treatment combined with preoperative concentrated irradiation. *JAMA* 227:171–181, 1974.
42. Pearlstein L et al: An experimental assessment of esophageal anastomotic integrity. *Surg Gynecol Obstet* 146:545–550, 1978.
43. Cole WR et al: Factors affecting incidence of anastomotic leak following esophagogastrectomy: An analysis. *Ann Thorac Surg* 6:396–400, 1968.
44. Akakura I et al: Surgery of carcinoma of the esophagus with preoperative radiation. *Chest* 57:47–57, 1970.
45. Ellis FH, Salzman FA: Carcinoma of the esophagus. Surgery versus radiotherapy. *Postgrad Med* 61:167–174, 1977.
46. Wilson SE et al: Esophagogastrectomy versus radiation therapy for midesophageal carcinoma. *Ann Thorac Surg* 10:195–202, 1970.
47. Griffen WO et al: Unified approach to carcinoma of the esophagus. *Ann Surg* 183:511–516, 1976.
48. Celestin LR: Permanent intubation in inoperable cancer of the esophagus and cardia. *Ann R Coll Surg Engl* 25:165, 1959.
49. Duvoisin GE et al: The value of palliative prosthesis in malignant lesions of the esophagus. *Surg Clin North Am* 47:827–831, 1967.
50. Hegarty MM et al: Pulsion intubation for palliation of carcinoma of the esophagus. *Br J Surg* 64:160–165, 1977.
51. Girardet RE et al: Palliative intubation in the management of esophageal carcinoma. *Ann Thorac Surg* 4:417–430, 1974.
52. Fujmaki M et al: A new chemotherapy as a preoperative treatment for esophageal cancer surgery. *Acta Med Bio* 19:181–191, 1972.
53. Edsyr F et al: Clinical efficiency of bleomycin in oesophageal and skin carcinoma in East Africa. *East Afr Med J* 50:449–453, 1973.
54. Nelson CS: Chemotherapy as the definitive form of therapy in esophageal carcinoma. *J Thorac Cardiovasc Surg* 63:827–837, 1972.
55. Gastrointestinal Tumor Study Group. A randomized trial of combined modality therapy (5,000 R + 5-FU + MECCNU) vs. combination chemotherapy (5-FU + MECCNU) in the treatment of locally advanced gastric cancer. *Gastroenterology* 74:1057, 1978.
56. McDonald J et al: Improved survival in patients responding to 5-fluorouracil, mitomycin C, and Adriamycin: A new combination chemotherapy program for advanced gastric carcinoma. *Digestion* 16:257, 1977.
57. Veterans Administration, Surgical Adjuvant Group, Protocol 32: Esophagus-trial of radiation therapy and surgery, alone or in combination, August, 1975.
58. Nakayama K: Preoperative irradiation in the treatment of patients with carcinoma of the oesophagus and of some other sites. *Clin Radiol* 15:232–241, 1964.
59. Parker EF, Gregorie HB: Carcinoma of the esophagus: Long-term results. *JAMA* 235:1018–1020, 1976.
60. Marks RD Jr et al: Preoperative radiation therapy for carcinoma of the esophagus. *Cancer* 38:84–89, 1976.
61. Sotus PC et al: Carcinoma in situ of the esophagus. *JAMA* 239:335–336, 1978.
62. Itai Y et al: Superficial esophageal carcinoma. *Radiology* 126:597–601, 1978.

63. Younghusband JD, Aluiwihare APR: Carcinoma of the esophagus: Factors influencing survival. *Br J Surg* 57:422, 1970.
64. Spath F: Heutige Operative Moglichkeiten beim Thorakelen Oesophaguskarzinom und Prognose. *Bruns Beitr Klin Chir* 218:289, 1970.
65. Goodner JT: Combined (irradiation and surgery) therapy for cancer of the thoracic esophagus. *Prog Clin Cancer* 4: 375, 1970.
66. Boyd DP, Kim MC: Survival in carcinoma of the esophagus. *Surg Clin North Am* 47:613, 1967.
67. Teitler RF et al: Cancer of the cardia. *Am J Surg* 129:89, 1975.
68. Watson FA: Radiotherapy in the treatment of cancer of the esophagus. *Radiol Clin* 36:1–14, 1967.
69. Nakayama K et al: Surgical treatment combined with pre-operative concentrated irradiation for esophageal cancer. *Cancer* 20:778–788, 1967.
70. Marcial VA: Role of radiotherapy in esophageal carcinoma. *Radiology* 87:231, 1966.
71. Leborgne R: Carcinoma of esophagus: Results of radiotherapy. *Br J Radiol* 36: 806–811, 1963.

SELECTED BIBLIOGRAPHY

Bains MS: Cancer of the esophagus, in Alfonso AE, Gardner B (eds): *The Practice of Cancer Surgery*, Appleton-Century-Crofts, New York, 1982, pp 171–183.

Bains MS et al: Management of esophageal cancer, in Carter SK et al (eds): *Principles of Cancer Treatment*, McGraw-Hill, New York, 1982, pp 444–455.

Beatty JD et al: Carcinoma of the esophagus. *Cancer* 43:2254, 1979.

Earle J et al: A controlled evaluation of combined radiation and bleomycin therapy for squamous cell carcinoma of the esophagus. *Int J Rad Onc Biol Phys* 6:821, 1980.

Ellis FH, Gibb SP: Esophagectomy for carcinoma: Current hospital mortality and morbidity rates. *Ann Surg* 190:699, 1979.

Giuli R, Gignoux M: Treatment of carcinoma of the esophagus—retrospective review of 1400 patients. *Ann Surg* (7):44, 1980.

Kolaric K et al: Combination of bleomycin and Adriamycin (doxorubicin) with and without radiation in the treatment of inoperable esophageal cancer. *Cancer* 45:2265, 1980.

Mori S et al: Pre-operative assessment of resectability for carcinoma of the thoracic esophagus. Part I: Esophagogram and azygogram. *Ann Surg* 190:100, 1979.

Payne WS: Palliation of esophageal carcinoma. *Ann Thor Surg* 28:208, 1979.

Piccone VA et al: Reappraisal of esophagogastrectomy for esophageal malignancy. *Am J Surg* 137:32, 1979.

Postlethwait RW: Esophagectomy without thoracotomy. *Ann Thor Surg* 27:395, 1979.

Postlethwait RW: Technique for isoperistaltic gastric tube for esophageal bypass. *Ann Surg* 198:673, 1979.

Rosenberg JC et al: Cancer of the esophagus, in Devita VT Jr et al (eds): *Cancer: Principles and Practice of Oncology*, Lippincott, Philadelphia, 1982, pp 499–533.

Rosenberg JC et al: Squamous cell carcinoma of the thoracic esophagus: An interdisciplinary approach. *Curr Probl Cancer*, vol 5, no 5, 1981.

Schuchmann GF et al: Treatment of esophageal carcinoma: A retrospective review. *J Thorac Cardiovasc Surg* 79:67, 1980.

Steichen FM, Ravitch MM: Mechanical sutures in esophageal surgery. *Ann Surg* 191:373, 1980.

vanAndel JG et al: Carcinoma of the esophagus: Results of treatment. *Ann Surg* 190:684, 1979.

23

TUMORS OF THE MEDIASTINUM

John R. Benfield   *Robert M. Bearman*   *John L. Werner*

Mediastinal masses defy diagnosis until they have been sampled or excised. Primary tumors are uncommon, constituting approximately 1 of 3400 admissions at a university center whose faculty has a particular interest in these lesions.[1] In the practice of oncologic surgery, mediastinal tumors necessitate differential diagnosis between primary and metastatic neoplasms. This chapter concerns itself solely with primary lesions.

HISTORICAL ASPECTS

Safe access to the mediastinum was the prerequisite for the modern management of mediastinal masses. With reference to the posterior and middle mediastinum, this required development of the principles of thoracic surgery, including progression from the negative pressure chamber of Sauerbruch to the routine use of endotracheal anesthesia.[2] For the anterior mediastinum, the problem of access related to sternotomy. At the turn of the century, Milton extensively studied the feasibility of sternotomy,[3] and thereafter Heuer and Andrus laid the foundation for current principles of management.[4] Until perhaps 10 years ago, entering the pleural space during anterior mediastinotomy via the sternal splitting approach was considered undesirable. There has now been extensive experience with median sternotomy in part as a by-product of cardiac surgery, and it is clear that mediastinotomy with unilateral, and even bilateral, simultaneous thoracotomy can be done safely. The reluctance to achieve wide exposure of the anterior mediastinum and contiguous pleural spaces via median sternotomy has disappeared.

Tumors of the mediastinum are of great historical interest because they were among the first examples in human beings of a relationship between neoplasia and function. One of the first links in a fascinating and still incomplete chain of observations was the recognition of the beneficial effects of resecting a thymic tumor in a patient with myasthenia gravis by Blalock.[5] Subsequently, clear evidence of the major role of the thymus in immunity has emerged.[6] This is exemplified by the better acceptance of allografts following thymectomy in certain animal systems.[7] From this follows the logical supposition that thymectomy may alter the immune competence of adults. Although of potential relevance to tumors, this hypothesis has not as yet been substantiated in human beings. This theme of functional neoplasms in the mediastinum is continued by certain endocrine and neurogenic tumors. Thyroid tumors, parathyroid neoplasms, and pheochromocytomas may be found in the mediastinum as well as in their more usual locations. Thus, the mediastinum is an area replete with examples of actual or potential functional tumors. This implies that important chapters in tumor biology will be forthcoming from further study of mediastinal neoplasms.

INCIDENCE AND ETIOLOGIC ASPECTS

A comprehensive account of the relative incidence of mediastinal neoplasms and cysts was recently compiled by Silverman and Sabiston.[8] In records of 1687 patients compiled from six reports, neurogenic tumors, thymomas, and cysts together accounted for 61 percent of the lesions. Neurogenic tumors made up 21 percent while each of the other two represented 20 percent. Lymphomas and teratoma tumors accounted for 12 percent and 10 percent, respectively; and neoplasms of mesenchymal or endocrine origin constituted 7 and 6 percent, respectively. Primary tumors of pure germ-cell origin were rare, e.g., only 1 percent. The series included 55 cases of primary carcinoma of the mediastinum; these should be viewed with considerable caution since the possibility of an occult extramediastinal primary always exists. In a patient with an undiagnosed mediastinal mass, the likelihood of malignancy is about 30 percent.[8,9] We believe, however, that provided with a complete history and thorough diagnostic evaluation, the histological diagnosis can be approximated preoperatively with reasonable certainty in most instances.

DIAGNOSTIC ASPECTS

Table 23-1 lists the classification of the most common primary tumors of the mediastinum according to the broad categories suggested by Ackerman and Rosai.[10] The aggregate of neurogenic tumors, thymomas, cysts, lymphomas, teratomas, and endocrine tumors accounts for almost 90 percent of lesions. When metastatic lesions are excluded, there is a high probability that a new mediastinal mass will be in one of the six mentioned categories. The thyroid and parathyroid tumors and certain neurogenic masses have functional hallmarks, hormonal markers, or the ability to concentrate radionuclides, thus making specific preoperative diagnosis quite probable within this group.

TABLE 23-1 Primary Tumors of the Mediastinum

Thymoma
Neurogenic tumors
Malignant lymphoma:
   Hodgkin's disease
   Non-Hodgkin's lymphoma
Germinal tumors
Thyroid tumors
Parathyroid tumors

SOURCE: Ackerman and Rosai.[10]

Further refinement of preoperative diagnostic accuracy rests on anatomic considerations. We concur with Burkell et al.[11] in their suggestion that the mediastinum be divided into three regions rather than the traditional four. Figure 23-1 shows the division of the mediastinum into anterosuperior, middle, and posterior compartments; it also includes the common neoplasms and cysts found in each region. In effect, unless there are endocrine considerations to the contrary, a mass in the anterosuperior mediastinum is likely to be a thymoma, a teratoma, or a lymphoma. In the middle mediastinum, pericardial or bronchogenic cysts tend to be characterized by their location and smooth outline while lymphomas tend to be multifocal. The predominant neoplasms of the posterior mediastinum are neurogenic.

SIGNS, SYMPTOMS, AND DETECTION

Chest roentgenograms are the single most effective way to detect mediastinal masses because about one-third of patients with these lesions are asymptomatic. Even in symptomatic patients, chest x-ray is the essential first step in recognizing the presence of a mediastinal mass.

The spectrum of symptoms ranges from ill-defined chest discomfort (with or without cough) to overt systemic manifestations. More than 90 percent of carcinomas are symptomatic, while most benign neoplasms are asymptomatic.[9]

In general, pain is a manifestation of an expanding or degenerating lesion, and its distribution reflects the location of the tumor. For example, Figure 23-2 shows a mass high in the posterior mediastinum. It did not arise from the brachial plexus, but the proximity of the neoplasm to the plexus was sufficient to cause pain that originated in the chest and radiated to the arm. Removal of the tumor resulted in relief of the symptoms. However,

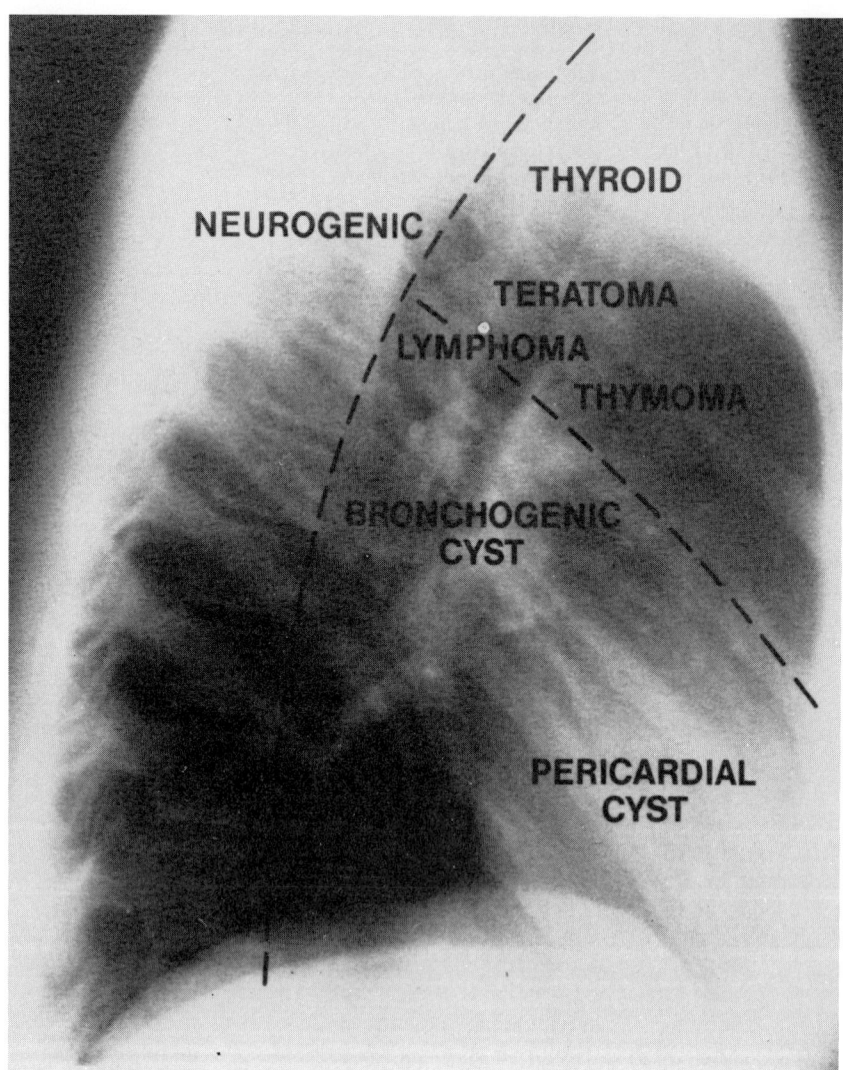

FIGURE 23-1 Divisions of the mediastinum and common cystic neoplasms in various locations.

clear anatomical correlations are the exception rather than the rule.

Superior vena caval compression, Horner's syndrome, recurrent laryngeal nerve palsy, and dysphagia from esophageal displacement are examples of mechanical compression of specific structures by mediastinal masses. However, the significance of these signs when due to compression is not the same as when they are caused by invasion from lung or esophageal carcinomas. For example, recurrent laryngeal nerve palsy, generally accepted as a sign of incurability when it results from lung cancer, does not necessarily mean that a mediastinal neoplasm is incurable.

The common systemic manifestations of mediastinal neoplasms are summarized in Table 23-2. The endocrine syndromes are reasonably straightforward, because the symptoms can be attributed to hormones. For example, hyperparathyroidism from a mediastinal adenoma or thyrotoxicosis due to substernal goiter differ from their cervical counterparts in location and perhaps by surgical access route, but not by function. Our experience has been that parathyroid adenoma is rarely recognized as

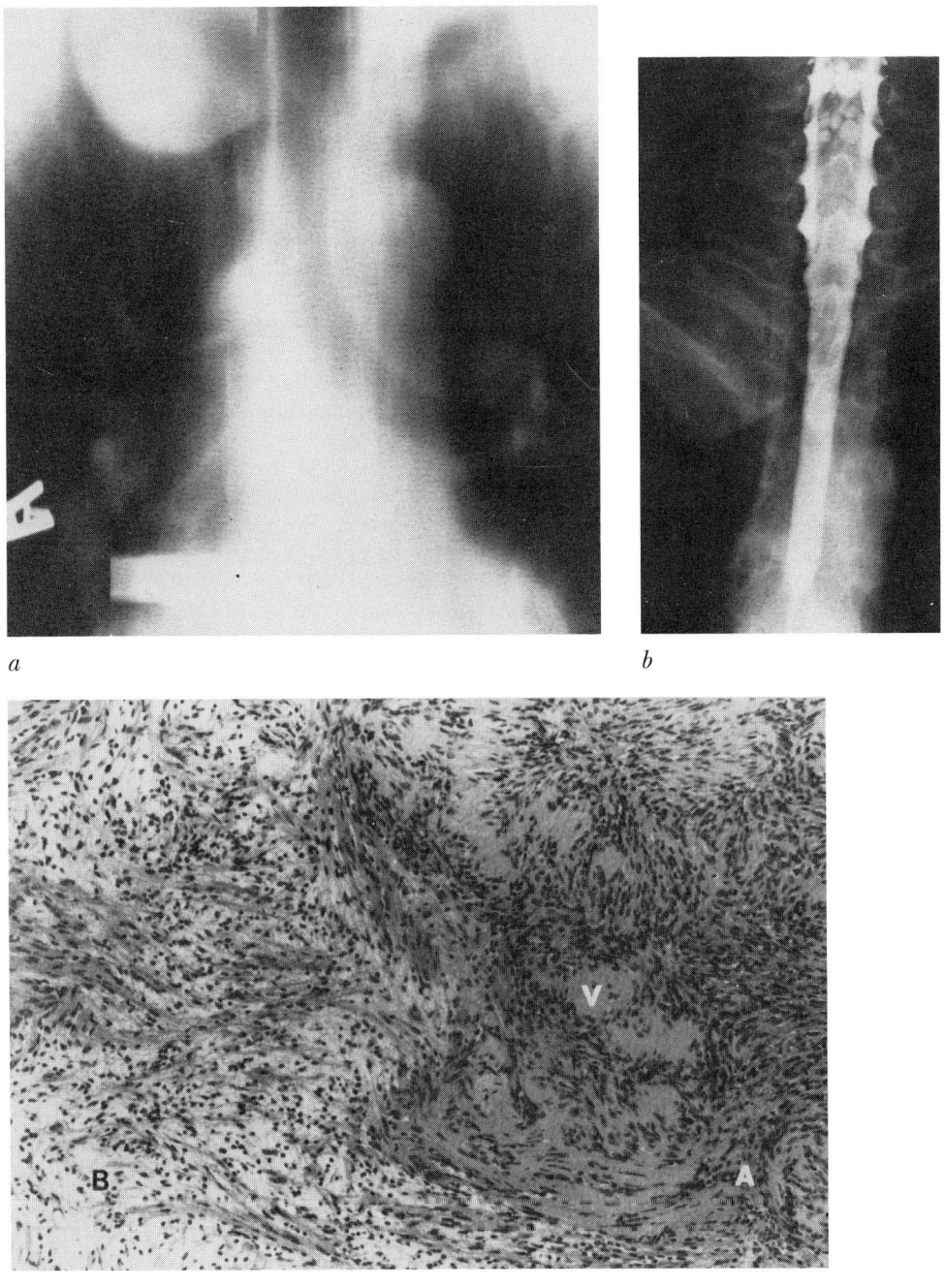

FIGURE 23-2 Cystic neurilemmoma. (*a*) Coronal plane tomogram at 9.5 cm—sharply defined mass in posterior mediastinum. (*b*) Myelogram performed to exclude neural canal component. (*c*) Photomicrograph shows neural elements in wall of cyst.

TABLE 23-2 Systemic Manifestations of Mediastinal Tumors

ENDOCRINE SYNDROMES	
Thyrotoxicosis	Intrathoracic goiter
Hypercalcemia	Parathyroid tumors—hyperplasia
Hypertension	Pheochromocytoma, neurogenic tumors
Hypoglycemia	Mesothelioma, teratoma

OTHER SYNDROMES	
Myasthenia	Thymoma
Red-cell aplasia	Thymoma
Collagen disease	Neurogenic tumors
Fever	Hodgkin's lymphoma
Osteoarthritis	Neurogenic tumors

a mass on chest x-ray, but rather is detected only after extensive search. Hypoglycemia rarely may be associated with mesotheliomas or teratomas of the mediastinum. Although teratomas may include ectopic pancreatic islets, the hypoglycemia is most likely a manifestation of insulin antagonist production rather than overproduction of insulin.

The most common systemic syndromes associated with mediastinal neoplasms are those which accompany thymomas, Hodgkin's disease, or neurogenic tumors. Although patients with thymomas are usually asymptomatic, they may have systemic signs and symptoms. The best known of these is myasthenia gravis, occurring in 10 to 15 percent of patients with a thymoma.[8] The pathogenesis is not completely understood, but there is evidence for the concept of an autoimmune disorder.[12] However, myasthenia gravis frequently occurs unassociated with a thymoma, and the systemic symptoms are not regularly relieved when the thymus (or thymoma) is removed. In fact, after thymectomy, only about 25 percent of patients with thymomas have relief of their myasthenic signs and symptoms, while 75 percent of patients without a thymoma become asymptomatic. Other systemic manifestations of thymomas include hypogammaglobulinemia, erythroid hypoplasia, myositis, and an increased incidence of carcinoma. It is of interest that, on rare occasions, patients develop myasthenia gravis years after the removal of a thymoma.

Hodgkin's disease is well known for the repetitive fevers which it may cause. Neurogenic neoplasms may be the cause of osteoarthritis.

DIAGNOSTIC TECHNIQUES, EVALUATION, AND STAGING

Despite ever-increasing sophistication in means of assessment, which now include computerized axial tomography (CT) and immunologic evaluations related to the possibility of autoimmune disease, chest roentgenography (including tomography) and mediastinotomy are the primary methods of diagnosis. Although this is both preliminary and concluding, other diagnostic techniques nonetheless warrant comment.

Contrast radiography, e.g., esophagograms, angiograms, bronchograms, and myelograms, may be used for the purpose of assessing extent, and sometimes origin, of the neoplasm. For example, we have operated on two patients with esophageal leiomyomas initially detected as mediastinal mass lesions on plain radiography of the chest. Esophagograms were helpful in establishing a preoperative diagnosis.

Angiograms are not regularly used, but may be particularly helpful in determining whether or not the mass is a vascular abnormality. This pertains particularly to the thoracic inlet, where the vena cava may be unusually prominent without pathologic significance, and to the middle mediastinum, where pulmonary artery aneurysm may mimic either lung carcinoma or bronchogenic cyst. An additional aim of the procedure is to seek evidence for involvement of major blood vessels. Our experience in this regard has shown that angiography is reliable as an indicator of blood vessel invasion or occlusion. However, the finding of vessel compression is often quite compatible with resectability.[13] We reserve angiography for those special circumstances in which the location and radiographic chracteristics of the mediastinal mass warrant such studies, since in some instances, ordinary fluoroscopy by an experienced radiologist can exclude vascular lesions.

Bronchograms are rarely indicated for the evaluation of mediastinal masses. Bronchogenic cysts usually do not communicate with the tracheobronchial tree, while demonstration of airway compression can usually be well accomplished by tomography.

Myelograms are occasionally needed for complete evaluation of posterior mediastinal masses suspected of extension into the vertebral canal (Fig. 23-2). Our practice is to limit myelography to patients with neurologic abnormalities on physical examination. Since CT can provide much of the information which a myelogram might yield, at present we use myelography, and most often at the instigation of our neurosurgical consultant in those instances wherein his or her intraoperative participation is anticipated.

Endoscopy of the tracheobronchial tree or esophagus is employed in evaluating mediastinal masses only when there are strong indications that the tumor either is primary in these structures or is invading them. Mediastinoscopy, the procedure most frequently requested by the referring internist, adds little to the evaluation of primary mediastinal neoplasms, with the exception of lymphomas. The usual cervical mediastinoscopy visualizes the paratracheal and parahilar middle mediastinum without providing adequate exposure for resection of neoplasms or cysts. Its main advantage is the possibility of establishing a histological diagnosis of lymphoma with a minimally invasive procedure.

Because of its frequent inadequacy as a therapeutic exposure, we do not use anterior mediastinotomy via the cervical approach as a diagnostic or staging method, preferring instead to proceed directly to full sternal splitting mediastinotomy.

CT may be very useful, but it is not often imperative. Examples are shown in Figs. 23-3, 23-6, and 23-7. The value of the study is to determine if a mass is cystic or solid and to assess whether or not it involves or originates from structures in such a way as to materially effect therapeutic approaches. For example, CT can be helpful in differentiating bronchogenic or pericardial cysts from solid tumors; it is particularly useful in evaluating the relationship of neurogenic tumors to the neural foramina.

Ultrasonography has little application in the mediastinum because of interference by the bony thorax and the lungs.

With improvements in imaging technology and newer isotopes, nuclear medicine may play an increasingly important role in the diagnostic evaluation of mediastinal masses. Radioiodine imaging of suspected thyroid lesion is the classic application. While less specific, gallium uptake within numerous mediastinal neoplasms including thymoma and lymphoma is a promising technique that is receiving increased attention. Technetium flow studies have been useful in documenting superior vena caval obstruction, and may aid in differentiating vascular lesions from solid neoplasms.

Endocrine neoplasms are discussed in depth elsewhere in this volume. However, it is important to remember that appropriate hormonal evaluation should be done in certain patients with mediastinal masses. For example, venous catheterization in search of occult parathyroid tumors may be very useful. Primary choriocarcinomas of the mediastinum may also be identified in that way, as these secrete chorionic gonadotropins.

The most direct and definitive diagnostic and staging procedure is mediastinotomy. We recommend median sternotomy for anterosuperior mediastinal masses and posterolateral thoracotomy as the approach to masses in the middle and posterior mediastinum. The side chosen for the thoracotomy depends on which hemithorax contains the major portion of the tumor.

THERAPEUTIC ASPECTS

Treatment of masses in the mediastinum depends upon the location and extent of the lesion as well as on the natural history of the specific disease.

Neurogenic Tumors

Neurogenic tumors typically occur in the posterior mediastinum. Although rarely such tumors may be found in the anterior mediastinum associated with the phrenic or the vagus nerve, the usual origin is from the nerve trunks or sheaths of the autonomic or intercostal nerves. Of these neoplasms, 10 to 20 percent are histologically malignant.[14] The incidence of malignancy in published series is variable and depends on the number of children included in the review, since neurogenic tumors in pediatric practice are more often malignant.

Although many neurogenic tumors are asymptomatic, both the large and the malignant varieties tend to be associated with signs and symptoms which include chest wall pain and evidence of compression of the sympathetic ganglia, of brachial plexus involvement, or of encroachment on nerve roots or the spinal cord. The latter possibility is of particular importance because it is usually preferable to treat the intraspinal component of the neoplasm first and then subsequently to excise the intrathoracic portion. The management of such "dumbbell"-shaped lesions requires both preoperative and intraoperative collaboration between neurosurgeons and thoracic surgeons.

Systemic findings may reflect the secretion of cate-

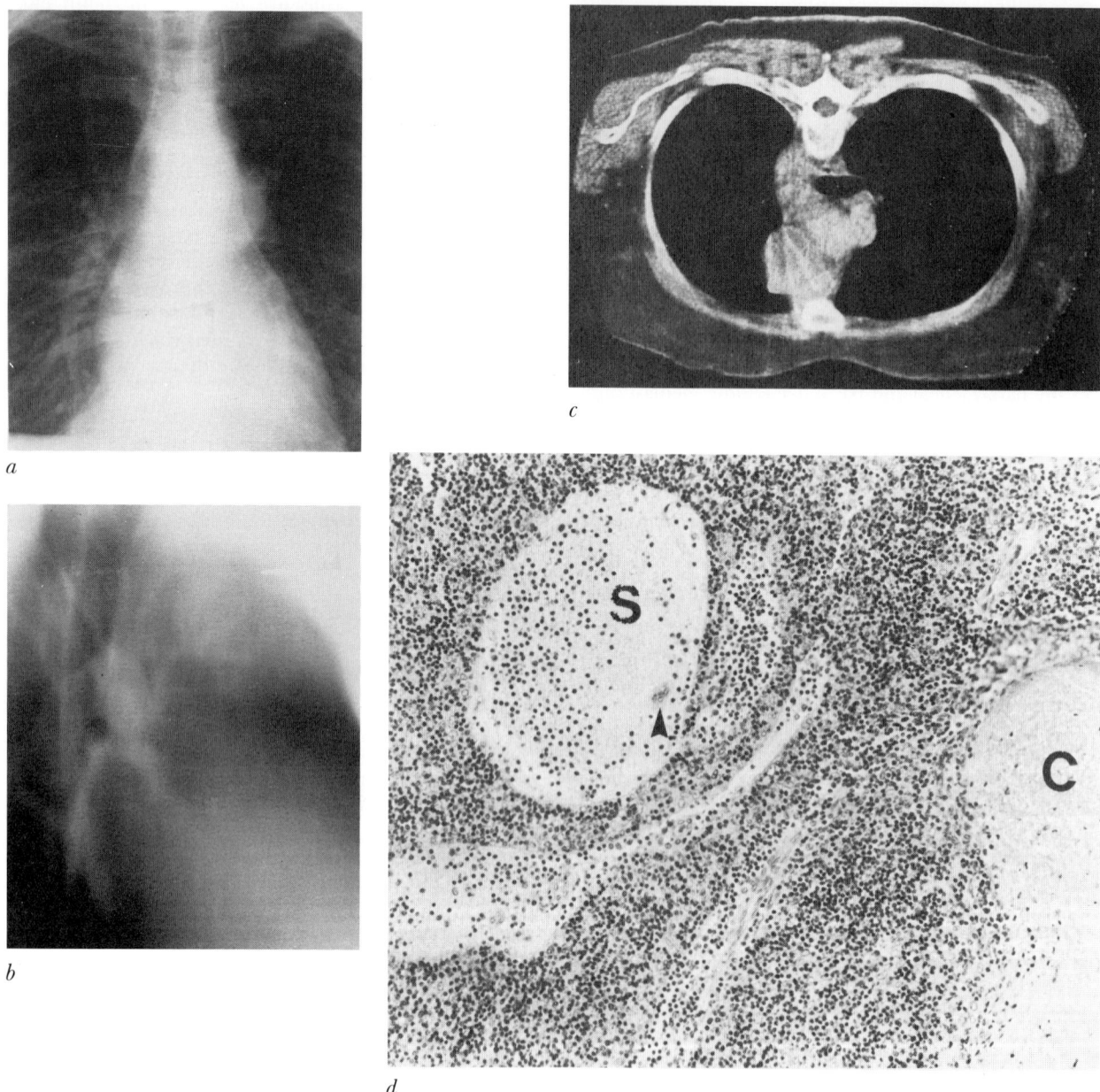

FIGURE 23-3 Thymoma. (*a* and *b*) PA and lateral views—lobulated mass in mediastinum. Gallium imaging showed uptake in mass consistent with thymoma. (*c*) CT imaging—defines solid nature of lesion, as well as relation of margins to adjacent structures. (*d*) Characteristic collagen bands (C) and the dilated perivascular spaces (S) containing vessels (arrowhead); lymph and white blood cells are evident. The cellular population consists of lymphocytes and larger cells having vesicular nuclei; the latter are epithelial cells (H&E stain; 120×).

cholamines or vasoactive amines by a pheochromocytoma, a neuroblastoma, a ganglioneuroma, or a chemodectoma. Pheochromocytoma, the more common catecholamine-producing tumor, is neurogenic. Its occurrence outside the adrenal gland in the mediastinum is uncommon, and its management when in the mediastinum is not significantly different than when it arises elsewhere. Preoperative preparation with adrenergic blocking agents, intra- and postoperative availability of α-adrenergic blocking agents, and proper fluid replacement are vital to the management of patients with these neoplasms. These issues are discussed in detail elsewhere in this volume but are mentioned here merely to reinforce that these considerations pertain equally to adrenal and to mediastinal pheochromocytomas. In addition, when mediastinal pheochromocytoma is encountered, we consider it important to measure serum calcitonin levels in search of associated medullary carcinoma of the thyroid to exclude the presence of multiple endocrine adenomatosis and to consider the possibility of metastasis to the chest from an adrenal primary.

In patients without hypertension or symptoms of a vasoactive tumor, vanillylmandelic acid (VMA) screening of the serum probably suffices, but direct measurement of serum and urine catecholamine levels is recommended to evaluate even subtle findings discovered by history or physical examination. Carcinoidlike symptoms, osteoarthritis, or elevated insulin levels may also occur with neurogenic tumors. In general, the systemic signs and symptoms due to abnormal secretory products can be expected to disappear if complete tumor excision can be accomplished. The issue of whether or not to undertake partial excision when total tumor removal is not feasible is complex and unresolved. In our view, the likelihood of significant regression of symptoms after subtotal resection warrants this therapeutic approach.

Neurilemmomas (schwannomas) arise from nerve sheaths and tend to be cystic. Complete excision is frequently possible, and the subsequent prognosis is good. However, the biologic behavior of the tumor does not correlate well with its histologic appearance. A patient with a cystic neurilemmoma of the posterior mediastinum is shown in Fig. 23-2.

Neurofibromas arise from nerves and are usually solid. They may be part of generalized neurofibromatosis (von Recklinghausen's disease), a syndrome associated with meningocele in the posterior mediastinum.[8] Some neurofibromas appear histologically benign with slow growth rates, but at operation there is local invasion of blood vessels. When we have encountered this situation, we have proceeded with resection and have omitted postoperative radiotherapy. Even in cases of incomplete excision we have achieved long-term (greater than 10-year) control of the disease without evidence of continuing growth.

Neurofibrosarcomas have a poor prognosis, causing death by local invasion and extension into vital structures. It has been said that "when a neurofibroma or a neurilemmoma undergoes malignant degeneration, it becomes a neurofibrosarcoma," and the incidence of this transformation has been quoted as 25 to 29 percent.[8] We are not aware of proof based on serial observations that tumors which were originally benign later become malignant; hence, we consider that the differentiation between neurofibrosarcomas and similar benign tumors rests not only on histology, but also on gross findings at operation and on factors of natural history which we have not yet learned to measure or anticipate.

Thymomas

These are one of the two most common solid tumors of the mediastinum. Classically they lie in the anterosuperior mediastinum as illustrated in Fig. 23-3, but we have operated on three patients whose thymomas presented as mass lesions which appeared as if they were in the pulmonary hilum. In most instances plain chest radiographs and mediastinal tomograms suffice to localize the lesion. CT is an optional diagnostic adjunct which can help to detect thymic cysts, and occasionally angiography is needed to exclude the possibility of vascular origin of a mass or to establish angiographic evidence of vascular invasion.

Thymoma is perhaps the best example of a solid neoplasm which does not reveal its natural history or biology by histological morphology; rather, the judgment as to malignancy depends on the operative findings. Malignant tumors invade contiguous structures such as the pericardium and the great vessels, while benign thymomas are localized and easily dissected free of their surroundings.

The thymus has its embryologic origin in the third and fourth branchial cleft, and developmentally descends into the mediastinum from the neck. In adults this origin continues to be expressed by the normal configuration of the gland, with its bilateral cervical extensions giving it a shape not unlike a bicornuate uterus. The thymic isthmus is regularly encountered during routine mediastinoscopy when it must be reflected from the trachea to gain access to the mediastinum. The cervical extensions lie sufficiently within the neck to preclude complete thymectomy via posterolateral thoracotomy from either side.

There are three operative approaches to thymomas. The safest and most widely used is median sternotomy. Its advantage is excellent exposure of the mediastinum as well as the neck; dissection of the thymus away from the innominate vessels is readily accomplished, and the short veins which drain the gland can be easily ligated in continuity. The second approach is via unilateral thoracotomy, which may be used when the mass projects predominantly into one thorax. However, there is no real access to cervical extensions of the gland, and resection of thymoma via unilateral thoracotomy cannot include total thymectomy.

The third, and most controversial, access to thymectomy is via the neck. We have found this a technically satisfying challenge, readily mastered by an experienced mediastinoscopist also experienced in excision of substernal goiters. The controversy is quite clearly reflected in the report of Jaretzki et al.[15] Proponents favor cervical thymectomy because of a low morbidity and results believed comparable to those of thymectomy via sternotomy. Antagonists deplore suboptimal exposure during operation and inability to accomplish a truly total extirpation of the thymus through the neck. They stress that thymomas may be multicentric, and that myasthenia gravis may be inadequately treated if thymic tissue is left behind.

Our approach is to use median sternotomy for resection of thymomas and the cervical approach for thymectomy in the treatment of myasthenia gravis in patients without apparent tumors. Should the cervical approach not prove optimal, we are prepared to proceed with sternotomy. We have removed thymomas via posterolateral thoracotomy, but only in cases in which the thymic origin of the neoplasm was not appreciated before operation. In one such instance, we proceeded with a second-stage thymectomy via median sternotomy in an unrewarding search for additional foci of tumor. Currently we do not believe that a second-stage thymectomy is required if the initial resection of the neoplasm via posterolateral thoracotomy was apparently complete.

Lymphomas

Lymphomas are a fascinating family of diseases, sufficiently multifaceted that a Lymphoma Task Force was established in 1968. The Pathology Panel and Repository Center for Lymphoma Studies, an outgrowth of the task force, now exists at our institution, the City of Hope National Medical Center.[16] Hodgkin's and non-Hodgkin's lymphomas have been carefully classified,[17,18] and there is an ongoing review of clinicopathologic correlations. While the broad topic of lymphomas is covered elsewhere in this volume, a review of mediastinal tumors would be incomplete without reference to these diseases. For example, it has recently been observed that 36 percent of patients with the most aggressive form of Hodgkin's disease present with mediastinal involvement, and also that the presence of disease within the mediastinum is in fact a favorable prognostic feature.[19]

The surgeon's role in the management of lymphomas is largely diagnostic. A lymphoma limited to the mediastinum is shown in Fig. 23-4. In the absence of peripheral lymph node enlargement, histologic diagnosis is best established by mediastinoscopy. Radionuclide scanning with ^{66}Ga or technetium pertechnetate is useful as a staging adjunct, but neither scanning nor lymphangiography can replace a biopsy. Our practice is to work closely with the pathologist during mediastinoscopy to determine whether or not sufficient tissue for a definitive diagnosis has been submitted. We prepare our patients for the possibility of limited thoracotomy so that this can be accomplished during the same anesthesia if diagnostically necessary. In general, cervical mediastinoscopy yields sufficient lymphoid tissue for diagnostic purposes.

Cysts

The importance of these lesions is twofold: they may rupture or become infected, and they may be manifestations of malignant tumors, although rarely. Most mediastinal cysts are not malignant. The signs and symptoms they cause are usually manifestations of pressure exerted on contiguous structures.

Bronchogenic cysts are illustrated in Fig. 23-5. They are lined by bronchial epithelium, and their wall commonly contains cartilage. There is usually no connection with the tracheobronchial tree, and thus neither bronchography nor bronchoscopy is useful in their evaluation except perhaps for assessment of compression effects. Since these cysts are usually in the middle mediastinum near major bronchi, they may be associated with recurrent pneumonias. Resection is indicated, and can often be accomplished without sacrificing any lung tissue.

Pericardial cysts characteristically occur in the middle

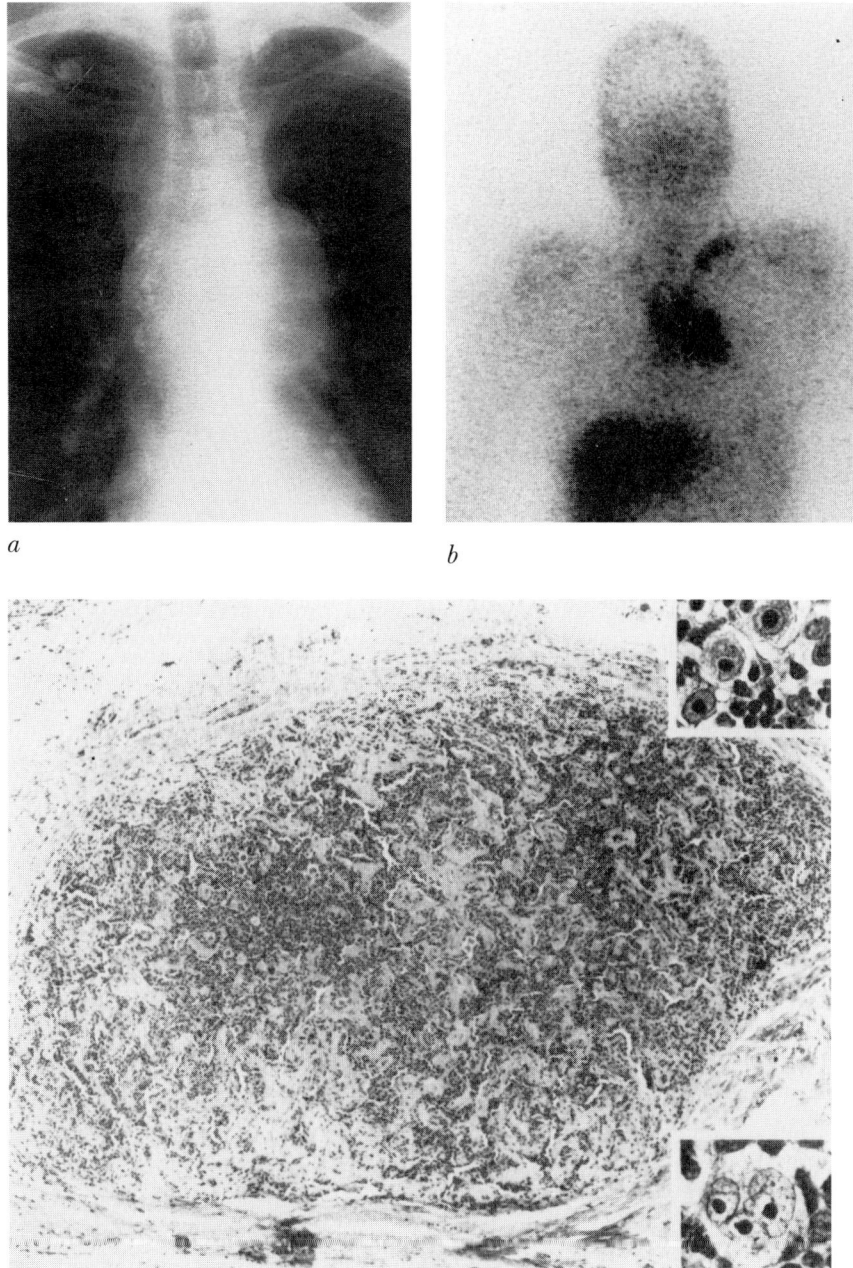

FIGURE 23-4 Hodgkin's disease. (*a*) PA projection—enlarged lymph nodes in middle mediastinum, opacified following lymphangiogram. (*b*) Gallium imaging—increased uptake in mediastinum and left subclavian area consistent with lymphoma. (*c*) Hodgkin's disease, nodular sclerosing type. A nodule of lymphoid tissue is surrounded by collagen bands (H&E stain; 48×). (*Inset, upper right*) Mononuclear Hodgkin's cells (H&E stain; 480×). (*Inset, lower right*) A Reed-Sternberg cell (H&E stain; 480×).

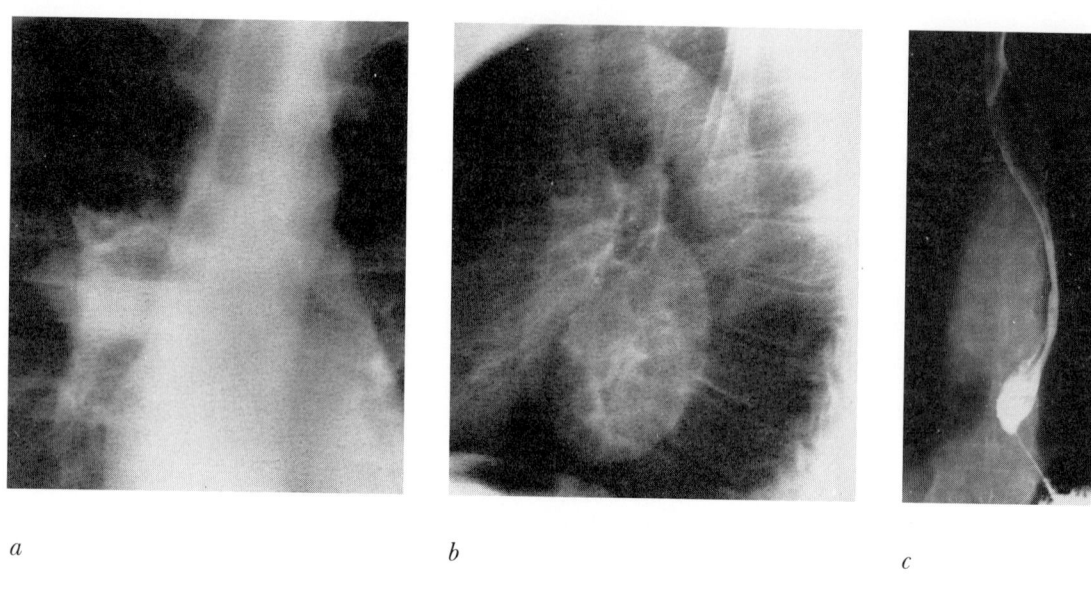
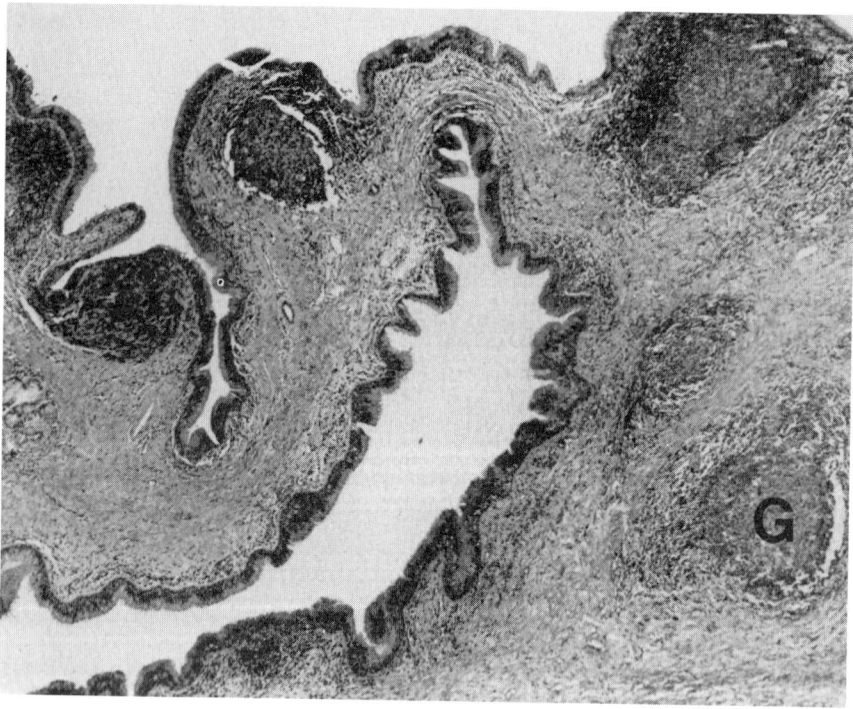

FIGURE 23-5 Bronchogenic cyst. (*a*) PA view demonstrates unusual but diagnostically useful air-fluid level. (*b* and *c*) Lateral view and barium swallow show very clear margins of tumor and extrinsic esophageal displacement. (*d*) The cyst lining (top) is respiratory epithelium. Germinal centers (G) are prominent. Also present are mucus glands and a portion of a bronchiole (H&E stain; 30×).

mediastinum. We are not aware of their becoming infected, and significant compression effects from them are rare. However, their excision is safe, and it is indicated to exclude neoplasia and obviate potential pressure phenomena.

Thymic and other cysts occurring in the mediastinum include those of dermoid origin, which shall be discussed later.

At times the origin of a cyst cannot be determined, presumably because of atrophy or degeneration of the connection between the cyst and its parent structure. In such instances the cyst often contains a clear aqueous fluid, hence the older, colorful but nondiagnostic term, "spring-water" cyst.

Teratomas

Teratomas occur predominantly in the anterosuperior or middle mediastinum. They are not common, accounting for 10 percent of a collected series of over 1600 mediastinal neoplasms.[8] The incidence of malignancy is about 20 percent, but neither malignancy nor resectability can be determined with certainty prior to operation. Choice of operative approach depends on the location and extent of the mass. Our policy is to use posterolateral thoracotomy when the tumor is predominantly in one hemithorax and median sternotomy when the mass is largely in the anterior mediastinum.

A dermoid cyst is illustrated in Fig. 23-6. These lesions often enlarge if left untreated, and without excision it is not possible to differentiate benign from malignant enlarging tumors. Ultrasound and CT are useful in preoperative evaluation since they may identify structures such as teeth and bone in the cyst wall. At operation, it is highly desirable to avoid rupture of the cyst, since the material within it is often quite irritating to the pleural space.

Germ-Cell Tumors

Germ-cell neoplasms account for only about 3 percent of mediastinal masses, but they are of proportionally greater interest because of the potential for cure in otherwise ominous diseases. The availability of endocrine markers for both diagnosis and assessment of disease status after treatment is an important factor in management. Adjuvant chemotherapy has become a mainstay of treatment.

Choriocarcinomas elaborate gonadotropins which can be detected in the serum. It is not common for these tumors to present with a mediastinal mass as the solitary focus, but even in cases where this occurs, aggressive adjuvant chemotherapy is required because of the high likelihood of occult metastases. Dramatic results can sometimes be obtained (Fig. 23-7).

Seminomas occurring in the mediastinum alone are rare. Adjuvant irradiation and chemotherapy are indicated.

Endocrine Tumors

In addition to pheochromocytoma, discussed above as a neurogenic tumor, thyroid and parathyroid neoplasms occur within the mediastinum. Both of these entities are discussed in depth elsewhere in this volume, and our remarks here concern only management of the mediastinal aspects of these tumors.

An intrathoracic goiter, as illustrated in Fig. 23-8, is shown to emphasize that neck masses can appear to be lower in the mediastinum by radiography than they are at operation. In our experience, it is hardly ever necessary to remove the intrathoracic portion of thyroid tumors via sternotomy.

Parathyroid tumors are traditionally included in reviews of mediastinal neoplasms,[8] and with this we have no quarrel. However, in our experience with parathyroid tumors, no benign neoplasm has been initially discovered because a mediastinal mass was noted on a chest radiogram. Indeed, even with the use of esophagograms and mediastinal tomograms in the evaluation of biochemical hyperparathyroidism, mediastinal tumors are rarely found before operation. Perhaps our experience is inexplicably skewed, but in nearly 100 personal operations for the treatment of hyperparathyroidism, only once have we needed to use median sternotomy for excision of a parathyroid adenoma which otherwise eluded detection.

ADDITIONAL THERAPIES

The distinction should be made between classic surgical adjuvant therapy and ancillary treatment. The former is treatment provided following operation for patients without overt metastasis in whom complete removal of tumor was apparently accomplished, but in whom historical information regarding the disease indicates a high probability of existing micrometastasis, either regional

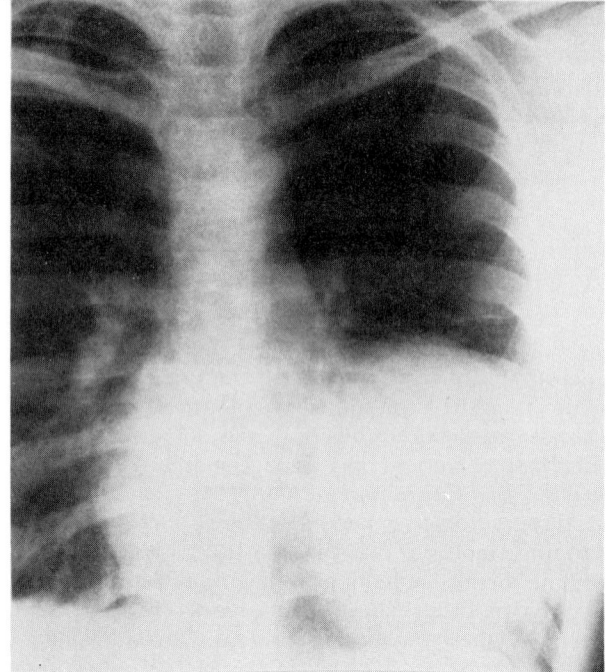

a

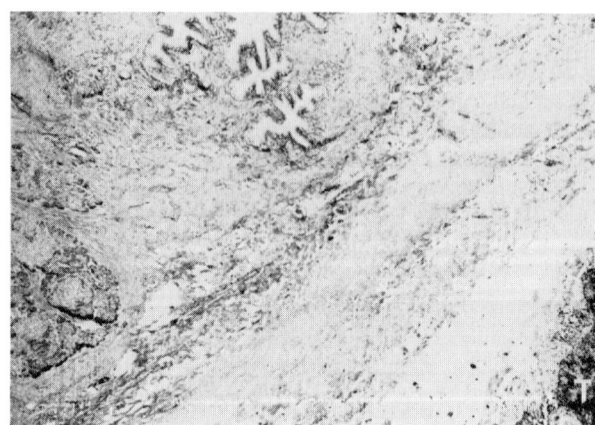

d

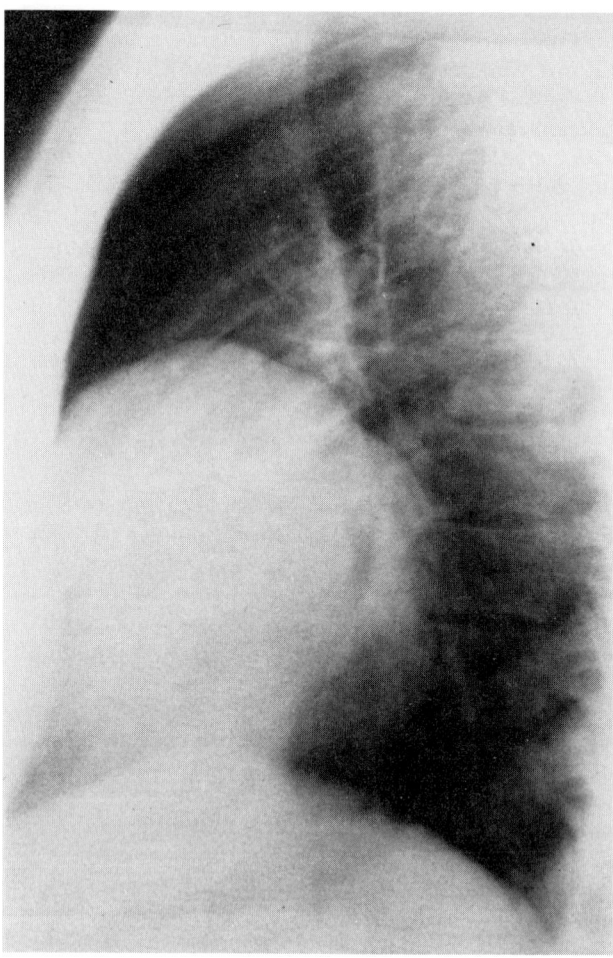

b

FIGURE 23-6 Teratoid (dermoid) cyst. (*a* and *b*) PA and lateral views—well-defined mass contiguous with middle and anterosuperior divisions of mediastinum. (*c*) CT imaging—fluid level indicates multicomponent cystic nature consistent with dermoid. (*d*) A portion of thymus (T) with a Hassall's corpuscle is at lower right. Pancreatic tissue, a not infrequent component of mediastinal teratomas that may result in hypoglycemia, is at lower left. Also present is bronchial epithelium (H&E stain; 30×).

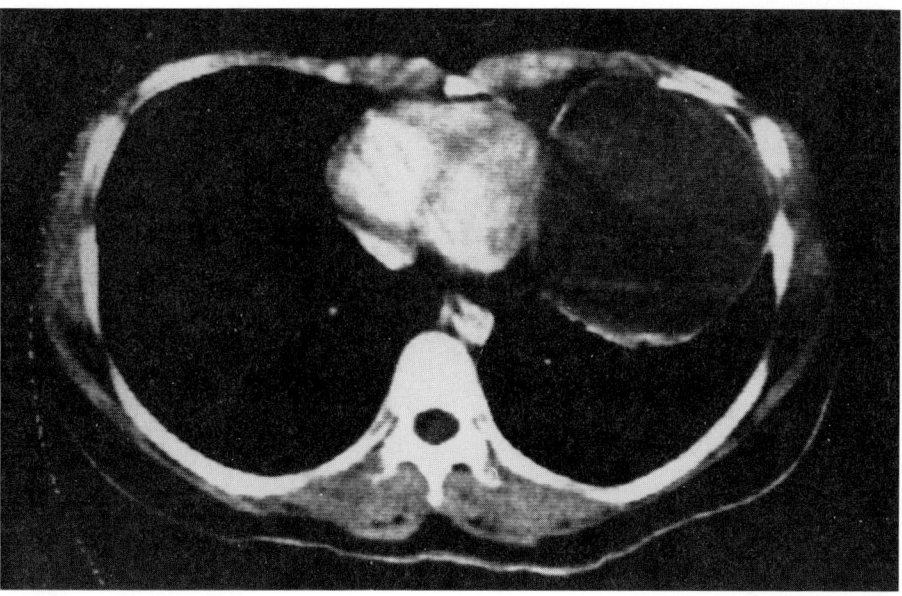

c

or systemic. Ancillary therapy is treatment rendered following operation when known residual disease remains at the site of excision of the primary tumor (usually due to tumor invasion of vital structures) or when there are regional metastases in instances wherein regional node dissection is not feasible as part of the operation for removal of the primary tumor.

Since operations are utilized predominantly for diagnosis and staging in the treatment of mediastinal lymphoma, radiation therapy and systemic chemotherapy are, in this context, considered as primary treatment modalities.

Adjuvant Therapy

Neuroblastoma primary in the mediastinum which can be completely excised is rare, but in such cases, adjuvant therapy with the current Adriamycin-Cytoxan regimen is warranted in all instances except in very young children. Neonates and children up to 4 to 6 months old have a significantly different natural history of their disease, and in them vigorous chemotherapy should be withheld until such time as recrudescent overt disease occurs.

A full course of thoracic radiation therapy following excision of a seminoma is most important. The use of adjuvant chemotherapy in this neoplasm is still undergoing evaluation. It is our present view that systemic chemotherapy for seminoma is inappropriate as a surgical adjuvant and should be reserved for recrudescent disease.

Following resection of mediastinal choriocarcinoma, a course or courses of methotrexate similar to that used for choriocarcinoma elsewhere is indicated. Further details regarding the chemotherapy of choriocarcinoma will be found elsewhere in the volume.

The use of both radiation and systemic chemotherapy as adjuvants in the treatment of neurosarcomas, malignant dermoids, and malignant thymomas has not been critically evaluated, largely because of the infrequency of these disorders. Available experience precludes clear recommendations at present. Although there are anecdotal instances of real benefit, many varied regimens have been utilized, and none have consistently met with significant success.

Ancillary Therapy

In malignant thymomas, neuroblastomas, and malignant teratomas, thoracic radiation therapy following known incomplete excision should be used for local control. (It is helpful to the radiotherapist if the extent of known

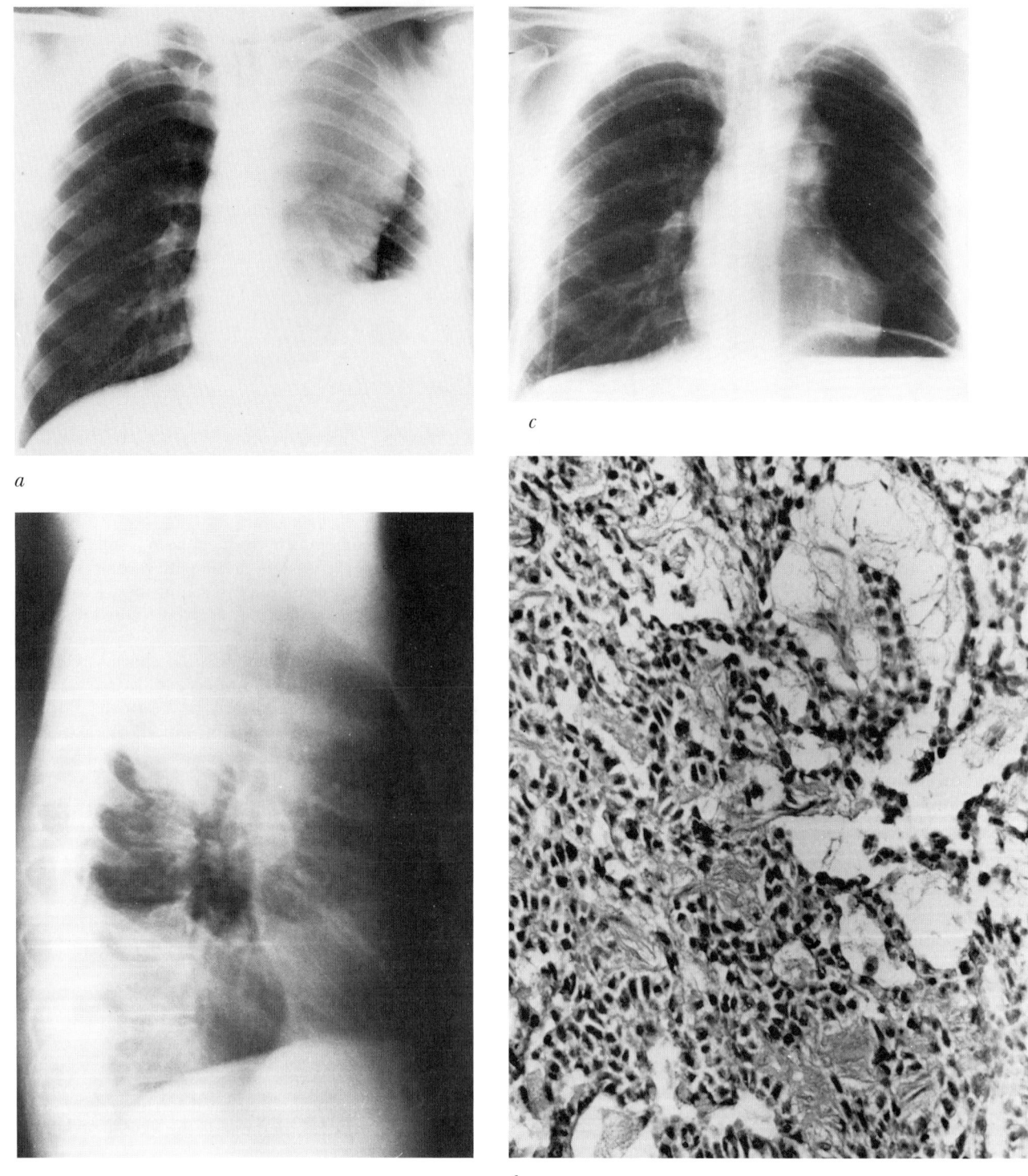

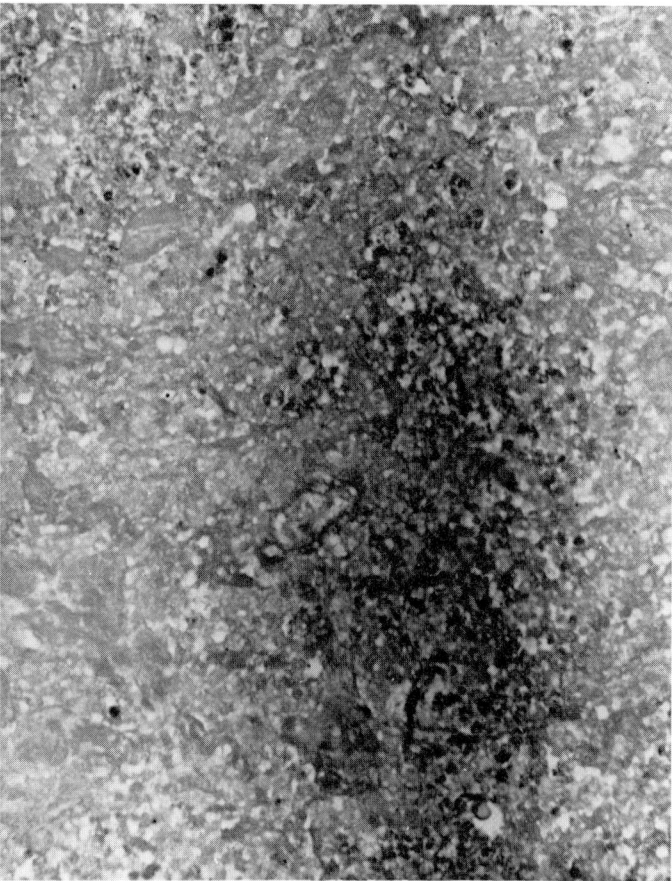

FIGURE 23-7 Germ-cell tumor of the mediastinum. (*a* and *b*) Radiographs demonstrating large mass originating in the mediastinum and occupying much of the left chest prior to diagnosis by limited left anterior thoracotomy or incisional biopsy. (*c*) Radiographs after completion of chemotherapy with *cis*-platinum, bleomycin, and Velban. (*d*) Germ-cell tumor with groups and clusters of polygonal cells with areas of gland formation. Foci of teratocarcinomatous differentiation were also found in other areas (H&E stain; 120×). (*e*) The residual tumor, resected by median sternotomy 4 months after initial biopsy via anterior thoracotomy, showing complete necrosis without viable cells. Chemotherapy had consisted of *cis*-platinum, bleomycin, and Velban.

e

residual tumor is outlined at operation by radiopaque markers.) Prognosis for success of such treatment is guarded because these are not highly radiosensitive neoplasms.

FOLLOW-UP TECHNIQUES

The basic technique for follow-up of mediastinal neoplasms is radiography of the chest. After complete excision of benign lesions, chest x-rays at 6- to 12-month intervals for several years is sufficient. Following apparently complete excision of malignant neoplasms, follow-up radiographs should be obtained at 3- to 4-month intervals for 2 years and thereafter at 6- to 12-month intervals. The usual assessments for the presence of distant metastases should be carried out at 6- to 12-month intervals. In the case of incomplete excision of malignant neoplasms, frequency of follow-up roentgenography will be guided by the needs of the ancillary therapy being provided and by the clinical course of the patient.

In those patients for whom circulating tumor markers (predominantly endocrine) are available, such tests should be performed at the same intervals as roentgenography.

More complex thoracic imaging studies, such as CT or radioisotope studies, are reserved for specific indications from history or chest radiographs. In situations where these tests are likely to be needed, we recommend baseline studies 3 to 6 months after operation.

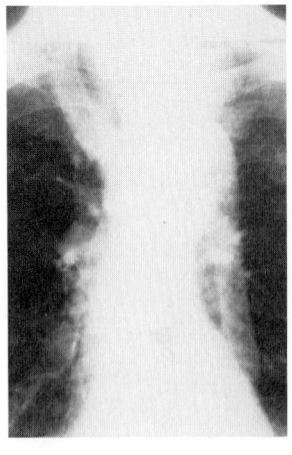
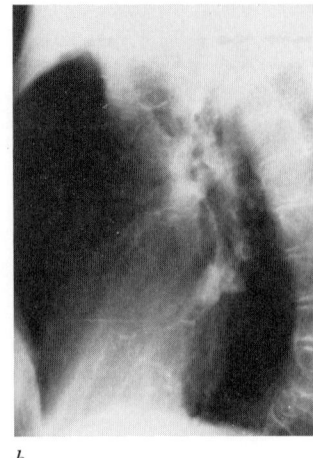
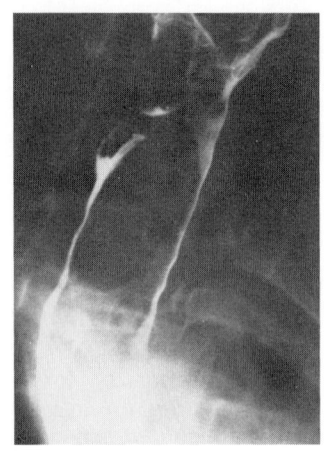

a *b* *c*

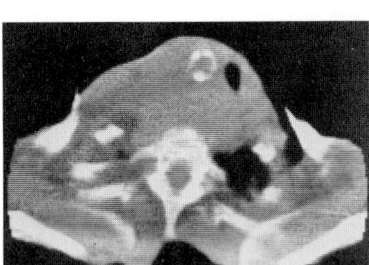

FIGURE 23-8 Thyroid carcinoma. (*a* and *b*) PA and lateral films—widening of mediastinum. (*c*) Oblique esophagram—mild esophageal displacement and anterior curvilinear calcification usually associated with benign disease. (*d*) CT imaging of thoracic inlet—curvilinear calcification and tracheal displacement.

d

TREATMENT OF RECURRENCES

Clinical recurrences of malignant mediastinal neoplasms occur from two sources—continued growth of residual tumor following incomplete excision, and growth of regional metastases not overt at the time of excision of the primary tumor. Since growth of residual tumors usually occurs in patients who have had a full course of radiation therapy to the mediastinum, the only operation potentially useful in such instances would be a debulking procedure in preparation for a course of systemic chemotherapy. Patients with malignant thymoma are the ones most likely to benefit from repeated incomplete reexcisions of gross disease. Other neoplasms in which regional metastases become apparent following presumed complete excision of the primary have a natural history such that the presence of these regional metastases is almost certainly accompanied by the development of systemic disease; thus systemic chemotherapy is the treatment of choice. On rare occasions, removal of recurrent masses of hyperfunctioning endocrine tumors may be useful for palliation of the systemic effects of this endocrine hyperfunction. Also rarely, debulking secondary procedures may be of some benefit prior to efforts at vigorous systemic chemotherapy in the presence of distant metastatic disease. These instances are rare and still largely experimental.

CURRENT AREAS OF RESEARCH AND PROSPECTS FOR THE FUTURE

Further advances in the operative management of mediastinal neoplasms appear unlikely, since the present impediment to complete resection is tumor invasion of great vessels and major tracheobronchial structures. Prosthetic replacement, even with the use of cardiopulmonary bypass, is unlikely to assume a major role in mediastinal cancer therapy. Future hopes for improved treatment of malignant neoplasms of the mediastinum rest on the development of improved chemotherapy regimens and radiotherapeutic modalities, and possibly effective systemic immunotherapy.

REFERENCES

1. Oldham HN, Sabiston DC: Primary tumors and cysts of the mediastinum. *Monogr Surg Sci* 4:243, 1967.
2. Meade, RH: *A History of Thoracic Surgery,* Charles C Thomas, Springfield, Ill, 1961.
3. Milton, H: Mediastinal surgery. *Lancet* 1:872–975, 1897.
4. Heuer GJ, Andrus WO: The surgery of mediastinal tumors. *Arch Surg* 50:146, 1940.
5. Blalock A et al: Myasthenia gravis and tumors of the thymic region: Report of a case in which tumor was removed. *Ann Surg* 110:544, 1939.
6. Bach JF, Carnand C: Thymic factors. *Prog Allergy* 21:342–408, 1976.
7. Osoba D: The effects of thymus and other lymphoid organs enclosed in Millipore diffusion chambers on neonatally thymectomized mice. *J Exp Med* 122:633, 1965.
8. Silverman NA, Sabiston DC Jr: Primary tumors and cysts of the mediastinum, in RC Hickey (ed): *Current Problems in Cancer,* Year Book, Chicago, vol II, no 5, 1977.
9. Fontenelle LJ et al: The asymptomatic mediastinal mass. *Arch Surg* 102:98–102, 1971.
10. Ackerman LV, Rosai J: *Surgical Pathology,* 5th ed, Mosby, St. Louis, 1974.
11. Burkell CC et al: Mass lesions of the mediastinum, in RM Ravitch (ed): *Current Problems in Surgery,* Year Book, Chicago, 1969.
12. Goust JM et al: Delayed hypersensitivity to muscle and thymus in myasthenia gravis and polymyositis. *Clin Exp Immunol* 18:39–47, 1974.
13. Benfield JR et al: Azygograms and pulmonary arteriograms in bronchogenic carcinoma. *Arch Surg* 99:4;6–409, 1969.
14. Oberman HA, Abell MR: Neurogenous neoplasms of the mediastinum. *Cancer* 13:882–898, 1960.
15. Jaretzki A III et al: A rational approach to total thymectomy in the treatment of myasthenia gravis. *Ann Thorac Surg* 24:120–130, 1977.
16. DeVita VT et al: Announcement of formation of the lymphoma task force and pathology reference center. *Cancer* 22:1087–1088, 1968.
17. Nathwani BN et al: Non-Hodgkin's lymphomas—A clinicopathologic study comparing two classifications. *Cancer* 41:303–325, 1978.
18. Lukes RJ, Collins RD: Lukes-Collins classification and its significance. *Cancer Treat Rep* 61:971–979, 1977.
19. Bearman RM et al: Hodgkin's disease, lymphocyte depletion type—A clinicopathologic study of 39 patients. *Cancer* 41:293–302, 1978.

SELECTED BIBLIOGRAPHY

Ariaratnam LS et al: The management of malignant thymoma with radiation therapy. *Int J Radiat Oncol Biol Phys* 5:77, 1979.
Beattie EJ Jr: Mediastinal germ cell tumors (surgery). *Semin Oncol* 6:109, 1979.
Gray GF, Gutowski WT: Thymoma: A clinicopathologic study of 54 cases. *Am J Surg Pathol* 3:235, 1979.
Hurt RD et al: Primary anterior mediastinal seminoma. *Cancer* 49:1658, 1982.
Levitt LJ et al: Primary non-Hodgkin's lymphoma of the mediastinum. *Cancer* 50:2486, 1982.
Livesay JJ et al: The use of computed tomography to evaluate suspected mediastinal tumors. *Ann Thorac Surg* 27:305, 1979.
Marti JR: Considerations in the management of mediastinal tumors, in AE Alfonso, B Gardiner (eds): *The Practice of Cancer Surgery,* Appleton-Century-Crofts, New York, 1982, pp 341–350.
Polansky SM et al: Primary mediastinal seminoma. *Am J Roentgenol* 132:17, 1979.
Reynolds TF et al: Chemotherapy of mediastinal germ cell tumors. *Semin Oncol* 6:113, 1979.
Rosenberg JC: Neoplasms of the mediastinum, in VT DeVita Jr et al (eds): *Cancer: Principles and Practice of Oncology,* Lippincott, Philadelphia, 1982, pp 475–498.
Rostock RA et al: CT Scan modification in the treatment of mediastinal Hodgkin's disease. *Cancer* 49:2267, 1982.
Wilkins EW, Castleman B: Thymoma: A continuing survey at the Massachusetts General Hospital. *Ann Thorac Surg* 28:252, 1979.

PART FOUR

TUMORS OF THE BREAST

24
BREAST CANCER

Yosef H. Pilch

This chapter will deal primarily with carcinoma of the female breast, since breast cancer is very uncommon in the male and the vast majority of breast cancers in the female are adenocarcinomas. At the end of the chapter, we will review male breast cancer and sarcomas of the breast briefly.

Carcinoma of the female breast is by far the most common cancer in the American female, accounting for 26 percent of all neoplasms (excluding nonmelanoma skin cancers and carcinoma in situ).[1] Breast cancer is also the leading cause of death from cancer in American women, accounting for 19 percent of all cancer-related deaths. The American Cancer Society estimates that approximately 112,000 new cases of breast cancer will arise in 1982 in the United States and over 37,000 American women will die of this disease in the same year.[1] Since 80 to 90 percent of breast biopsies are performed for benign disease, usually in order to rule out the diagnosis of breast cancer, and since by no means every woman with a breast lump seeks medical attention because of the fear of breast cancer, the 112,000 cases of actual breast cancer represent only the "tip of the iceberg" of the huge population of women receiving medical attention in the United States because of actual breast cancer or the possibility thereof. Certainly, this represents a public health problem of the first magnitude.

Moreover, most women treated for primary breast cancer in the United States today undergo a total mastectomy as part of their therapy. The problems resulting from breast loss frequently include serious aberrations of self-image, feelings of loss of femininity, sexual, social, and marital problems, alterations in style and manner of dress, occupational and career disruptions, and serious alterations in lifestyle. These factors result in a morbidity from breast cancer far in excess of that directly attributable to the disease process itself. These problems will be dealt with in greater detail later.

ESTABLISHING THE DIAGNOSIS OF BREAST CANCER

Screening of Asymptomatic Women

Screening may be defined as the presumptive identification of unrecognized disease or defect by the application of tests, examinations, or other procedures which can be performed rapidly and simply. Screening tests sort out asymptomatic, apparently well individuals who probably have a disease from those who probably do not. The goal of screening for breast cancer is early detection. The hope is that women who are discovered to have breast cancer by screening, prior to the onset of symptoms, will have a higher proportion of small tumors and a lower incidence of nodal and/or distant metastases than women with breast cancer who present themselves in the usual way, i.e., after the onset of symptoms. Furthermore, it is hoped that treatment of such women with conventional therapy will result in increased disease-free survival and overall survival. In the case of screening for breast cancer, it appears likely that these hopes may be warranted, although final conclusions are probably premature.

Beginning in 1960, preliminary reports from periodic examination programs for the detection of breast cancer among asymptomatic patients indicated that a higher proportion of breast cancer cases were detected at a localized stage than was experienced in the general population, and some reports suggested an increase in the survival rate among such patients.[2-7] Despite these findings, considerable doubt remained about the contribution such routine examinations might make in reducing breast cancer mortality in the population at large. These early screening programs suffered from a central flaw in study design which made definitive conclusions impossible. The programs involved persons who volunteered for the examinations or patients who appeared for other forms of medical care at a clinic. Therefore, it was difficult to determine the selectivity factors associated with these groups, and suitable comparison groups could not be established for the women studied.

At the same time, mammography emerged as a significant new radiographic technique which had obvious applications to breast cancer screening. In 1961, Gershon-Cohen et al., in the report of their periodic examination survey using this new technique, established that occult, nonpalpable breast cancers could be detected by means of mammography.[4] Egan, in 1962, demonstrated the value of mammography in the differential diagnosis of breast masses and in detecting occult lesions.[8]

THE HIP STUDY

These developments were sufficiently impressive for the National Cancer Institute (NCI) to contemplate a long-term study of the effectiveness of periodic screening with mammography and clinical examinations of the breast in reducing breast cancer mortality. Under the leadership of Dr. Michael Shimkin, who was, at the time, head of NCI's biometry branch, suitable performance sites were sought for the conduction of the trial. Concurrently, Dr. Philip Strax, a radiologist in the Health Insurance Plan of Greater New York (HIP), was exploring the applications of mammography. Other favorable circumstances that led to the selection of HIP to conduct the study were the size of the population covered by the plan (about three-quarters of a million individuals) and the presence of an experienced research department. A pilot study was initiated in 1963, followed by a full-scale prospective screening program.

Two random samples of women 40 to 64 years of age with membership of at least 1 year in HIP were selected. The total number of women in each sample was about 30,000, and each study individual was "paired" with a control woman. The pairs of study and control group women were randomized, and study women were drawn in sequence from a list in scheduling screening examinations.

Study group women were offered screening examinations at their medical group centers. Each examination consisted of a clinical examination of the breast and mammography. Pregnant women were excluded. If a woman with a prior mastectomy appeared, she was examined, but the findings were not included in the study. Every woman who had an initial examination was asked to return for three annual follow-up examinations, even if she was no longer a member of HIP. The only exceptions were women who, in their screening examination, were found to have conditions that required earlier follow-up. Women in the control group followed their usual practices in receiving medical care. No special effort was made to encourage them to have general physical examinations. On the other hand, they were not discouraged from having such examinations. Mammography was not routinely included in the general physical examinations offered to all members, but it was being used increasingly within HIP for differential diagnostic purposes.

About 20,000 women, or 65 percent of the study group, appeared for their initial screening examinations, and of those, 80 percent participated in the first annual repeat examination, 75 percent in the second annual follow-up examination, and 69 percent in the third annual examination. Information obtained through surveys of subsamples of the total study population and control population demonstrated the comparability of these two groups.[9] However, study women who refused screening differed from those examined in several respects, e.g., they were slightly older; had a lower level of educational attainment; and were less likely to be Jewish, to have been married, to be multiparous or premenopausal, or to have ever reported having a lump in the breast. Also, they differed markedly from the others in basic attitudes toward preventive health examinations and were more apt to avoid physical examinations in general.[10] There were 302 breast cancers detected among the 30,000 study women and 929 breast cancers in the control group. Of the 302 breast cancers found in the study group, 55 were detected due to the initial screening examination among the 20,188 women who appeared for their initial examination, 77 were detected due to annual follow-up examinations, and 93 were detected as a result of routine medical care and not as a result of screening examinations. The prevalence rate of breast cancer among screened women, as determined from the results of the initial examinations, was 2.72 per 1000 women screened. The detection rate among women who returned for subsequent annual screening examinations was 1.49 per 1000 person-years. Breast cancers diagnosed among screened women whose biopsies did not result from findings at the screening examinations occurred at a rate of 0.93 per 1000 person-years. Of the 93 cases in this group, 45 were detected within 12 months after screening, while the other 48 were detected after 12 months and up to 5 years after their last screening examination. Incidence rates among study group women who refused screening and among control group women were 1.56 per 1000 and 1.92 per 1000, respectively. (The relatively low rate in the group not accepting screening examinations suggests that study women with a higher risk for breast cancer tended to self-select themselves for screening.)

It is of considerable importance that mammography alone was responsible for the biopsy recommendation in 33.3 percent of the cancers detected by screening. Of the 132 breast cancers diagnosed as a result of screening 44 would have been missed if mammography had not been utilized. Among women aged 50 to 59, 41.5 percent of cancers were detected by mammography only, whereas among women between the ages of 40 and 49 only 19.4 percent of cancers were detected by mammography only. Among women aged 60 or older, 31.4 percent of cancers were detected by mammography only.[11] These results clearly established the value of mammography as a screening technique but pointed out that its importance probably varied among different age groups. It is also important to note that 59 cases of breast cancer (47 percent) were detected by physical examination alone and would have been missed had mammography been relied upon alone.

But were cancers detected by screening diagnosed at an earlier stage, and did such patients, when treated with conventional therapy, experience a lower mortality? The answer appeared to be yes to both questions. Among the women whose breast cancers were detected by screening, the proportion with no evidence of axillary nodal involvement was high (71 percent). In the group of cancers diagnosed among screened women for whom screening was not responsible for case detection, the proportion of patients with no nodal involvement was only 51 percent. The figure was 40 percent for study women who refused screening and 46 percent for control group women, a difference that could readily be due to chance. For the total group of study women, the proportion with no nodal involvement was 57 percent.

As of December 31, 1978, through the tenth year after entry into the study, the differential in breast cancer mortality between the study group (including both women who were screened and women who refused screening) was 30 percent—94 deaths in the study group and 133 deaths in the control group ($p = .01$). The impact of the screening program was greatest in women 50 years of age or older. Women aged 50 to 59 who underwent screening had a highly significant improvement in survival. There was no significant benefit from screening observed in women 40 to 49 years of age. This may have been due to the relatively small number of cancers arising in women in this age group. The survival differences between the study group and control group for women over 60 years of age was also relatively large, but the small numbers involved resulted in differences which were not statistically significant.

The major conclusions drawn from the HIP study were as follows: Periodic screening with mammography and palpation by physicians among women aged 40 to 64 years resulted in a reduction in mortality due to breast cancer. The decrease measured over a 10-year interval was close to 30 percent. Women 50 years of age and older clearly benefited. Benefit was not clearly established for women of ages 40 to 49. (This may be due to the small numbers in the study or to the degree of development of mammographic techniques at the time of the study.) Mammography appeared to be critically important in achieving the benefits which were observed in the screened population of women.

THE BREAST CANCER DETECTION DEMONSTRATION PROJECT

In 1973, soon after the early results of the HIP study became available, the Breast Cancer Demonstration Project (BCDDP) was implemented. This ambitious program, which was funded jointly by the National Cancer Institute and the American Cancer Society (ACS), was designed to answer operational questions related to the introduction of breast cancer screening into a wide variety of communities and to disseminate the techniques of early breast cancer detection to both the general public and the medical profession. By 1975, there were 29 BCDDP centers at 27 locations throughout the United States, and more than 280,000 women had enrolled for a 5-year screening program. Participants were screened annually using a combination of history, physical exam, mammography, and thermography. Thermography was discontinued in 1977 on the recommendation of the special working group that was asked by the NCI to review the BCDDP (see below). Breast self-examination (BSE) was taught at the screening sessions, and all participants were encouraged to practice BSE on a monthly basis. The screening was completed in March, 1981. Although the BCDDP was not designed as a scientific investigation of the efficacy of breast cancer screening, the data derived from the program offered a unique opportunity to obtain new information on the benefits of periodic screening, especially in women under 50 years of age, and on the contribution of mammography to the benefits of screening.

Although most centers accepted all women who wished to participate in the breast cancer screening program, 99.4 percent of the participants were between the ages of 35 and 74 when they entered the program. The median age was 49.5 years, so that the population was almost evenly divided between women under 50 years of age and women over 50. Remarkably, regardless of age, over half the women (51.7 percent) who entered the program attended all of the five annual screening sessions.[12] In 1977, two policy changes occurred that affected women during the third to fifth annual screenings. Thermography was dropped as a screening modality, and restrictions were placed on the utilization of mammography for women under 50 years of age.

A total of 4440 breast cancers was recorded as of September, 1981. Of these, 3557 cancers (over 80 percent) were detected at BCDDP centers, and 886 were detected outside the project. Of the 3557 "project-detected" cancers, 3293 were detected as a result of annual screening examinations or early recall exams, and 264 were detected when women who had been scheduled for an early recall exam chose to consult a surgeon prior to the scheduled examination. Of the 886 cancers detected outside the program, 744 were classified as "interval cancers" because they were detected within the one-year interval between screening examinations, and 142 were classified as "postscreening cancers" because they were detected more than 1 year after the women's last annual exam. Significantly, minimal breast cancers, which have been defined as noninfiltrating cancers and infiltrating cancers less than 1 cm in diameter, constituted 32.4 percent of all cancers detected in the BCDDP.[12] Of the infiltrating breast cancers detected in the BCDDP, 16.5 percent were less than 1.0 cm in size. Minimal breast cancers are associated with an excellent prognosis. In addition, more than 80 percent of all breast cancer patients in the BCDDP program had negative axillary nodes. (This figure is considerably higher than the corresponding proportion of minimal cancers in the HIP study, which was 12 percent.) Again, such patients, with localized disease, should have a very good prognosis.

The HIP study was designed to determine whether periodic screening played a significant role in reducing mortality from breast cancer. The results of that study (see above) suggested that it did—at least for women over 50 years of age. Unfortunately, the BCDDP was not designed to address research issues on the efficacy of breast cancer screening in reducing mortality from breast cancer. Unlike the HIP study, which included a matched control group of women, there is no control group within the BCDDP population, and, therefore, no conclusions can be drawn from the results of the BCDDP program as to whether or not the screening program resulted in a reduction in breast cancer mortality. However, the program did provide very valuable data on the contribution of mammography to the detection of early breast cancer.

Whereas the HIP study maintained strict independence of observations between mammography and physical examination, in the BCDDP the degree of independence of such examinations varied among the 29 centers and tended to be decreased in women under 50. As a result of this greater dependence between modalities in the BCDDP, the percentage of cancers detected by either modality alone tends to be reduced. Despite this fact, 41.6 percent of the cancers detected in the BCDDP were detected by mammography alone as compared to 33.3 percent in the HIP study. In the HIP study, mammography appeared to be a less effective screening modality for women 40 to 49 years of age than for women 50 to 59 years old. Only 19.4 percent of the cancers detected in the HIP study in women 40 to 49 years of age were detected by mammography alone, whereas in women 50 to 59 years of age, 41.5 percent of cancers in the HIP study were detected by mammography only. In the results of the BCDDP, this striking difference was not apparent. Larger numbers of cancers were detected in the 40 to 49 age group, and mammography alone was responsible for the biopsy recommendation in 35.4 percent of cancers detected. In the 50 to 59 age group 42.1 percent of BCDDP cancers were detected by mammography alone. It is clear that mammography alone was a more important contributor to the detection of breast cancer in the BCDDP than in the HIP study for women in the 40 to 49 age group. This may be due to the larger number of breast cancers detected in this age group by the BCDDP but is most probably due to technical changes in the quality of mammography.

As mentioned above, less than 20 percent of all cancers detected within the BCDDP had positive nodes at the time of surgery. This is considerably less than would be expected in the general population of breast cancer patients, in which approximately half (53 percent) of patients have positive nodes at the time of initial treatment.[12] As expected, noninfiltrating breast cancers either did not have findings warranting node dissection or had negative nodes. Only 14.3 percent of infiltrating cancers less than 1.0 cm in diameter had positive nodes, and, more importantly, only 29.2 percent of infiltrating cancers greater than 1.0 cm in diameter had positive nodes.

Although there was no preselected comparison group, these patients should have an extremely good prognosis.

In March of 1978, the special working group appointed by the NCI in March of 1977 published its findings and recommendations.[13] They reached the following conclusions:

The BCDDP's experience is unusual in the extent to which minimal breast cancer has been reported in screened women at all ages and the degree to which mammography was an important factor. This experience raises the important possibility that screening may be beneficial for women under the age of 50 years and that mammography may be a significant factor for women at all ages.

However, the observations from the BCDDP cannot be used to measure the overall benefit of the screening program or the effect of mammography in reducing mortality due to breast cancers. The principal reason is that no suitable comparison group is available. The use of patient survival rates to measure benefit poses an additional difficulty; i.e., at this state of knowledge, it is not known how large an error results when such rates for cases detected in clinical practice at different stages of disease are applied to the experience in screening programs.

The encouraging observations in the BCDDP make it imperative that randomized controlled trials be designed and conducted to provide information required for national recommendations regarding screening. These trials would have, in the background, the fact that the HIP study has demonstrated efficacy of annual screening with physical examination and mammography for women above the age of 50 years. For women under 50 years of age, there are still no data that demonstrate an effect on mortality through screening, but the BCDDP's experience is consistent with a possible reduction.

The working group's recommendations relative to screening with the two principal modalities, palpation, and mammography follow:

Physical examinations should be continued in the BCDDP as a routine screening modality for women of all ages.

Mammography (or xeroradiography) should be continued in the BCDDP as a routine screening modality for

1. all women 50 years of age and older,
2. women 40 to 49 years of age only when they have a personal history of breast cancer or a history of breast cancer in first-degree relatives (mother or sisters),
3. women 35 to 39 years of age only when they have a personal history of breast cancer.

CURRENT STATUS OF BREAST CANCER SCREENING

In June of 1978, the NCI published a statement on the recommendations of the Consensus Development Panel on Breast Cancer Screening[14] which promulgated the same guidelines for breast cancer screening as those recommended by the NCI Working Group, which appear above. Since the appearance of the 5-year summary report of the BCDDP, the American Cancer Society (ACS) has, more recently, issued its own guidelines for the detection of breast cancer in asymptomatic women.[15] They are as follows:

1. Women 20 years of age and older should perform breast self-examination every month.
2. Women 20 to 40 should have a physical examination of the breast every 3 years, and women over 40 should have a physical examination of the breast every year.

3. Women between the ages of 35 and 40 should have a baseline mammogram.
4. Women under 50 should consult their personal physicians about the need for mammography.
5. Women over 50 should have a mammogram every year when feasible.
6. Women with personal or family histories of breast cancer should consult their physicians about the need for more frequent examinations, or about beginning periodic mammography before age 50.

Guidelines numbers 1, 2, 3, and 5 are quite straightforward. However, guidelines 4 and 6 are vague. The adoption here of the NCI consensus panel's recommendations with respect to periodic mammography prior to age 50 in women with personal or family histories of breast cancer seems appropriate. The guidelines presented below are an attempt to synthesize and amalgamate both sets of recommendations and to expand slightly upon them:

1. Women 20 years of age and older should perform breast self-examination every month.
2. Women 20 to 40 should have a physical examination of the breast every 3 years, and women over 40 should have a physical examination of the breast every year.
3. Women between the ages of 35 and 40 should have a baseline mammogram.
4. Women with a personal history of breast cancer should have a physical examination of the breast at least once a year and a mammogram every year when feasible, regardless of age.
5. Women over 40 with a history of breast cancer in a first-degree relative (mother or sister) should have a mammogram every year, when feasible.
6. Women over 50 should have a mammogram every year, when feasible.
7. Women under 40 with a history of breast cancer in a first-degree relative with onset prior to age 40 or with a history of multiple first-degree relatives with breast cancer should consult an oncologist concerning the need for more frequent examinations, or about beginning periodic mammography before age 40.

Establishing the Diagnosis of Occult Breast Cancers

Breast cancers may be palpable or they may be occult, i.e., nonpalpable. Occult breast cancers may only be detected as a result of mammography performed as part of the breast cancer screening program or obtained in order to evaluate a different, palpable breast lesion.

An occult carcinoma may appear mammographically as a soft-tissue density or mass without calcifications, (see Figs. 24-1a and b), a cluster or tiny calcifications without a mass (see Figs. 24-2a and b), or a mass with calcifications (see Figs. 24-3a and b). A cluster of tiny, finely stippled calcifications is characteristic, although not pathognomonic of carcinoma. Unfortunately, only approximately half the cases of cancer exhibit mammographic evidence of calcification. All suspicious clusters of calcifications merit excisional biopsy, with the expectation that in some cases they will be found to result not from malignancy, but from benign disease—usually sclerosing adenosis. Similarly, alterations of breast architecture that could signify a malignant desmoplastic reaction require biopsy, although benign disorders such as sclerosing adenosis and fat necrosis may both manifest an identical fibrous connective tissue response. Until recently, resection of a quadrant of the breast was often necessary to be certain that the mammographically suspicious area was encompassed within the margins of the excision. To reduce the size of the biopsy specimen and to improve the accuracy of localization of the suspicious findings, percutaneous transfixion of the lesion with a 22-gauge needle may be performed just prior to operation (see Figs. 24-4a and b and 24-5a and b.

First, the relationship of the lesion to the nipple and skin edge is determined from the cephalocaudal radiograph. From the mediolateral radiograph, the relative height of the lesion in relation to the nipple is ascertained. From these factors, the most advantageous position for needle introduction is ascertained. This site is then cleansed with antiseptic and locally anesthetized. Since the breast tissue beneath the skin is insensitive to pain, anesthesia is easily obtained. The localizing needle is then inserted through the lesion, and taped in position. Cephalocaudal and mediolateral mammograms are then obtained to confirm that the needle is close to or within the lesion. If the needle placement is adequate, a soft dressing is placed over the hub of the needle, and the patient is sent to the operating room. As an alternative to leaving the needle in place, or in addition to needle placement, a drop of methylene blue or other dye may be injected. The needle is then withdrawn or left in place, the dye acting as a surgical landmark. Preoperative needle localization does not alter the need for specimen radiography to confirm that the lesion is actually in the biopsy specimen.

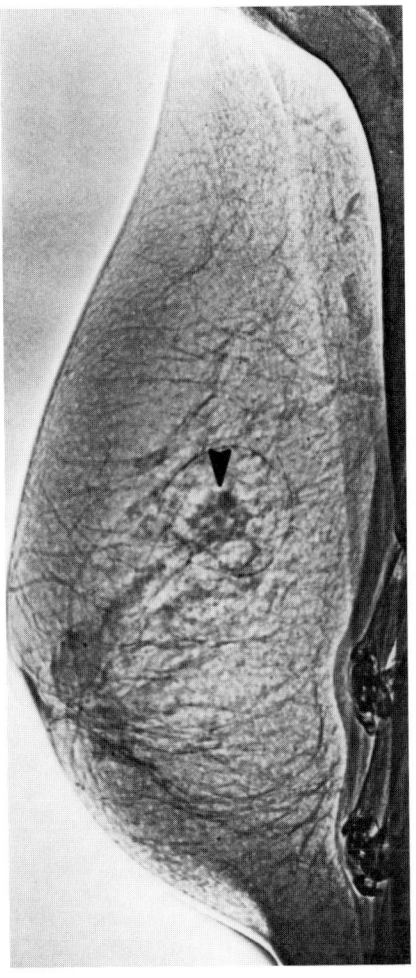 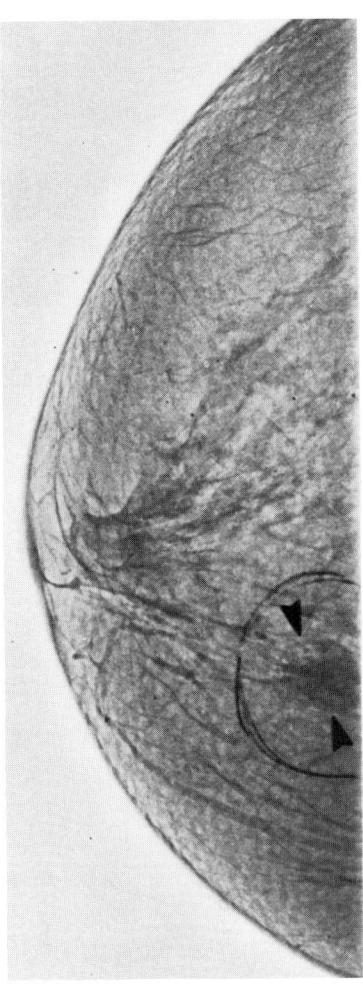

FIGURE 24-1 Lateral (*a*) and cephalocaudal (*b*) xeromammograms demonstrating a dominant mass which could not be palpated clinically. It proved to be an infiltrating ductal carcinoma.

Biopsy of nonpalpable mammographic lesions should be followed immediately by specimen radiography (see Figs. 24-6 and 24-7), since it is necessary for a radiograph to be made of the surgical specimen in order to confirm that the lesion has indeed been excised. If radiographs of the specimen fail to reproduce the suspicious findings, excision of additional tissue followed by specimen radiography is required until the lesion is finally identified within the specimen. The patient therefore must remain on the operating table until this process is complete. The surgeon is notified by the mammographer or pathologist as to the presence or absence of the previously identified findings within the specimen.

Another important reason for specimen radiography is to localize the lesion for the pathologist, who will perform a frozen section examination of the lesion and submit a specimen for estrogen and progesterone receptor analysis if a carcinoma is found. This may be accomplished in several ways. One is to place the specimen on a wire grid and obtain another radiograph (see Figs. 24-6 to 24-8). Alternatively, the specimen may be cut into slices, the slices laid out and numbered with radiopaque markers, and a radiograph obtained. The mammographer may then identify for the pathologist the radiographically suspicious region within each slice that is likely to provide the most fruitful area for

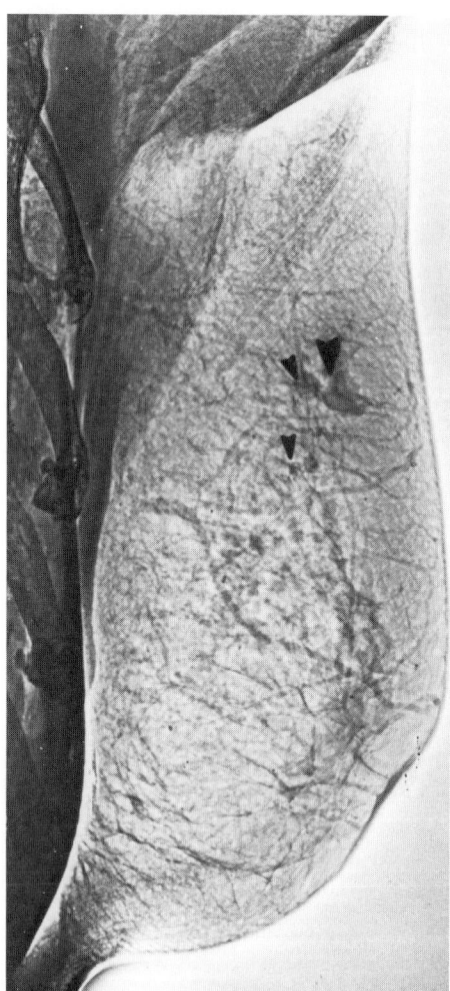 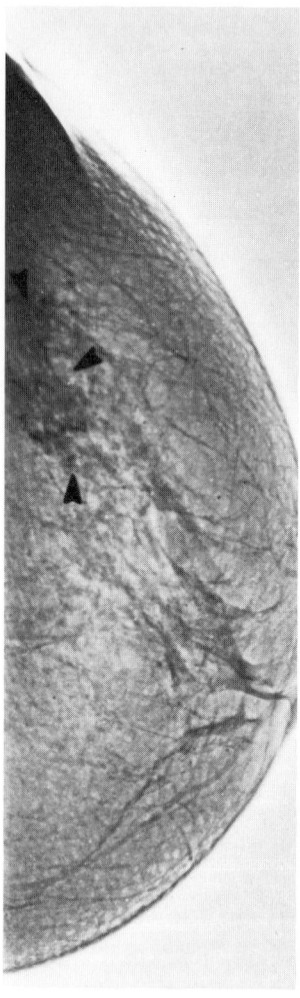

a *b*

FIGURE 24-2 Lateral (*a*) and cephalocaudal (*b*) xeromammograms demonstrating two occult lesions, both of which proved to be invasive ductal carcinomas. The more central lesion is characterized by clustered microcalcifications without an associated mass.

histologic examination. It is important to perform a frozen section examination in all cases since if a malignancy is identified, this may be the only opportunity to obtain fresh frozen tissue for hormone receptor determination.

Establishing the Diagnosis of Carcinoma when a Mass is Palpable

Palpable breast masses which merit biopsy include those that are suggestive of carcinoma on mammography, those which are suspicious on clinical grounds, and those that suggest cancer both clinically and radiographically. A breast mass is clinically suggestive of malignancy if it fulfills five characteristics beginning with the letter *D*: dominant, different, discrete, definite, and dense. It should be possible in most instances to distinguish a carcinoma from a cyst or fibroadenoma, since the latter are very smooth, round, and regular. Moreover, cysts may be fluctuant, and fibroadenomas tend to be very freely movable. In addition, the presence of associated signs of malignancy, i.e., skin thickening or edema, nipple retraction or pointing, skin retraction, or the presence of enlarged, firm axillary and/or supraclavicular

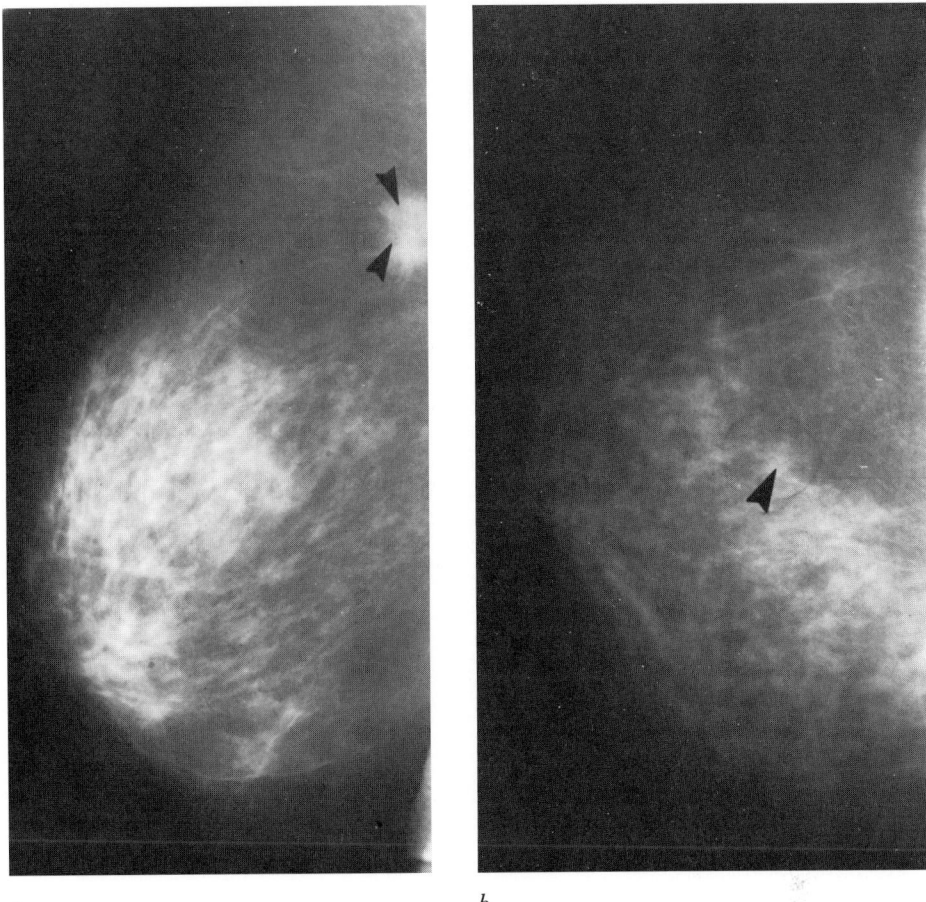

FIGURE 24-3 Lateral (*a*) and cephalocaudal (*b*) mammograms demonstrating a dominant mass containing clustered microcalcifications which was not palpable clinically. It proved to be an invasive ductal carcinoma.

nodes, will help to confirm the clinical diagnosis of breast cancer when and if such signs are present.

Clinical diagnosis of palpable breast masses based on mammography and physical examination is quite accurate. Diagnostic accuracy rates of 85 to 95 percent are usual.[16-18] Despite this fact, approximately 80 percent of all women coming to biopsy prove to have benign lesions.[17] This is, no doubt, due in part to the fact that some breast biopsies are performed in order to excise lesions which are thought preoperatively to be benign, e.g., fibroadenomas. However, in large measure it is due to a justifiable desire on the part of surgeons not to miss cancers in vue of a false-negative rate of approximately 10 percent in the clinical assessment of breast masses.[17]

The traditional method for biopsy prior to the early 1970s involved admitting the patient to the hospital, obtaining an operative consent for excisional biopsy and "possible" mastectomy, and submitting the patient to a general anesthetic. The biopsy specimen was examined by frozen section, and if a carcinoma was found, an immediate mastectomy was performed. Since that time, several changes have occurred. First, it has become evident that breast biopsy for cancer may safely be performed as a separate procedure days to a few weeks prior to definitive treatment. Moreover, most workers in the field now feel that this procedure *should* be followed routinely. Second, it has been shown that breast biopsy may safely be performed on an outpatient basis and may

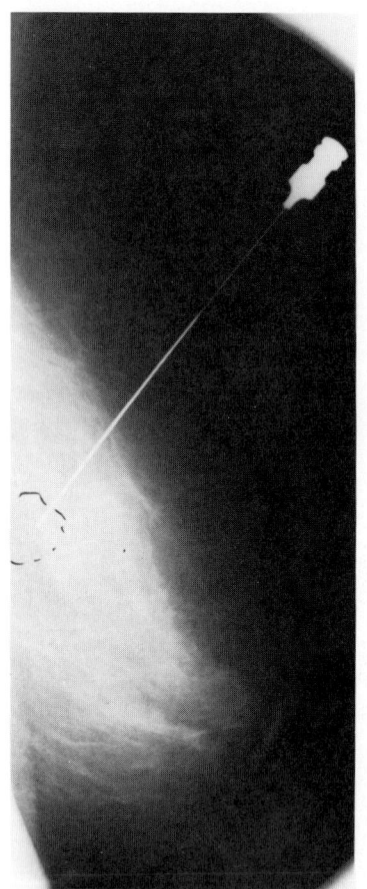 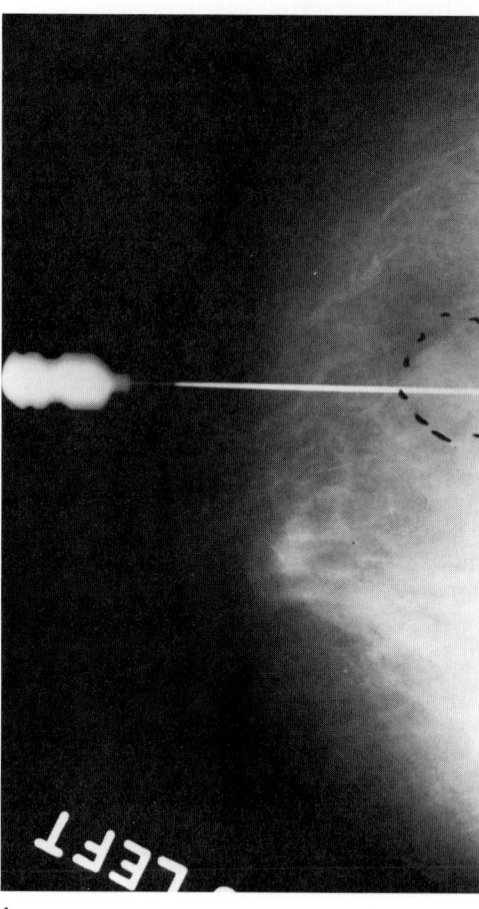

FIGURE 24-4 Lateral (*a*) and cephalocaudal (*b*) mammograms obtained prior to biopsy demonstrating the technique of localizing an occult lesion with a needle under radiographic control. The patient is the same as that in Fig. 24-1.

routinely be performed under local anesthesia (with a few exceptions where general anesthesia is required.[17,18] This approach is sensible, human, and cost-effective. Women with benign breast masses need not be subjected to the risk and cost of biopsy under general anesthesia and can usually be spared the fear of awakening without a breast. In addition, the cost of hospitalization is avoided. Women with cancer may receive the benefit of a full preoperative diagnostic work-up for metastatic disease. Moreover, a firm preoperative diagnosis means that the patient can be informed with certainty of the nature of the definitive operative procedure which is proposed, and she and her family have time to prepare themselves emotionally for the recommended treatment.

Since 1975, increasing emphasis has been placed on the use of percutaneous needle biopsy and thin-needle aspiration cytology to establish a definitive pathologic diagnosis of breast cancer. Needle biopsy provides a tissue specimen for histologic evaluation and has been reported to be 67 to 88 percent accurate.[17,19,20] Thin-needle aspiration cytology provides a cytologic specimen and is highly accurate (usually greater than 90 percent).[18,21] The advantages of these techniques are obvious. They are inexpensive, simple, painless, and rapid. When a definitive diagnosis of cancer is made, open surgical biopsy may be obviated. It is important to remember, however, that because of sampling error a negative needle biopsy and/or aspiration cytology can never exclude the diagnosis of cancer. A negative needle biopsy or aspiration cytology report has no clinical significance in the face of a clinically suspicious breast mass, and further investigation, namely open surgical biopsy, usu-

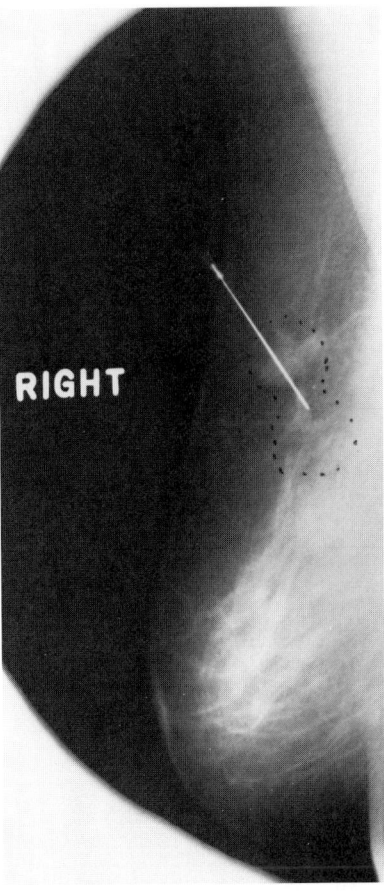 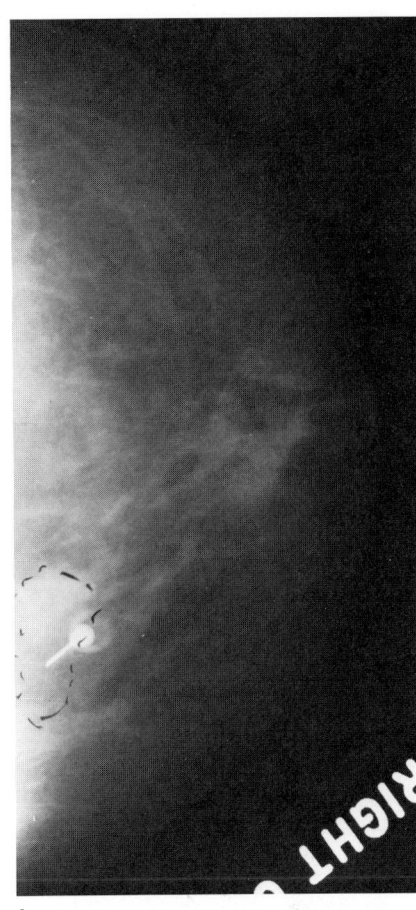

FIGURE 24-5 Lateral (*a*) and cephalocaudal (*b*) mammograms obtained prior to surgery on the patient whose preoperative xeromammograms are depicted in Fig. 24-2. The technique of needle localization under radiographic control is again demonstrated.

ally under local anesthesia as an outpatient, is mandatory. Because of this, we have chosen to perform these procedures only in women with breast masses which we believe to be cancer on clinical grounds. For breast masses which we consider benign, we advocate excisional biopsy, preferably under local anesthesia, on an outpatient basis.

Needle biopsy is objected to by some surgeons, who allege that edema and inflammation tend to obscure physical findings in subsequent examinations. In our experience, the inflammatory response is short-lived, and we have encountered little difficulty in evaluating or excising a mass previously biopsied percutaneously. Others object on grounds that disturbing the cancer by needle biopsy may contribute to an increased risk of dissemination. To our knowledge, there is no evidence to support this view. On the contrary, available evidence indicates that no increased risk of dissemination can be demonstrated in patients treated by needle biopsy.[22,23]

A salient advantage of needle biopsy is that sufficient tumor tissue remains to measure estrogen receptors at the time of definitive operation. This critically important determination can easily be lost either when a malignant mass is excised in its entirety for diagnosis or when cancer is unexpectedly found on permanent section.

Other advantages of needle biopsy include the facility with which segmental mastectomy can subsequently be performed. This procedure is often made technically difficult by previous excisional biopsy with its attendant edema, hemorrhage, and inflammation. The financial advantages are also significant.

Apprehension has been expressed that some breast

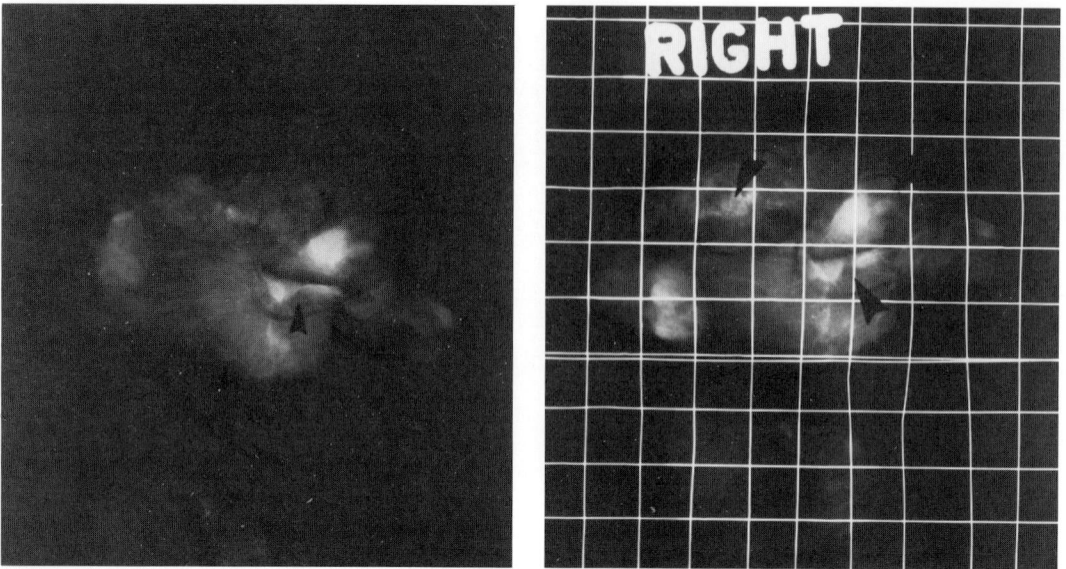

FIGURE 24-6 Specimen radiographs of the biopsy specimen obtained from the patient whose mammograms appear in Figs. 24-2 and 24-5. The two lesions are both in the specimen. The technique of specimen radiography on a wire grid is illustrated.

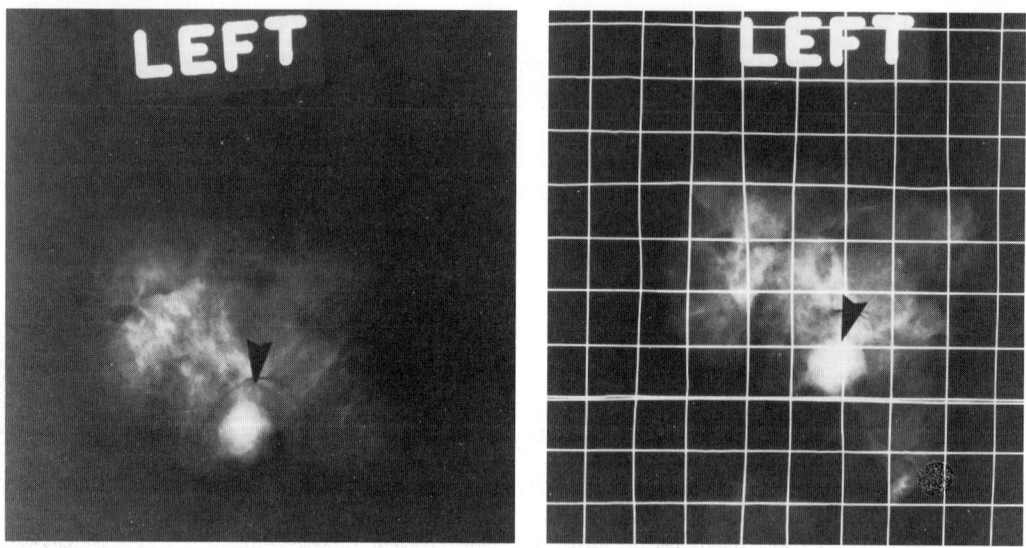

FIGURE 24-7 Specimen radiographs of the biopsy specimen obtained from the patient whose mammograms are depicted in Figs. 24-1 and 24-4. Again the lesion can be seen within the specimen and the technique of specimen radiography on a wire grid is illustrated.

cancer patients subjected to needle biopsy or excisional biopsy under local anesthesia might subsequently refuse mastectomy. In our experience, very few patients refused mastectomy after biopsy under local anesthesia. We believe that these patients would also likely have refused to permit mastectomy after biopsy under general anesthesia with frozen section diagnosis.

Our policy has been to carry out excisional biopsy when an equivocal or benign diagnosis is obtained by needle biopsy. In our view, a negative needle biopsy has no clinical significance and necessitates further investigation, namely, excisional biopsy. All masses considered benign are excised under local anesthesia. A frozen section is always performed to allow for an estrogen and progesterone receptor determination if the lesion should prove to be malignant.

TYPES OF BREAST CARCINOMA

Breast carcinoma may be ductal or lobular (approximately 80 percent are ductal). Both types exist in invasive or infiltrating and noninvasive forms. Thus, there is invasive or infiltrating lobular carcinoma and lobular carcinoma in situ, and there is invasive or infiltrating ductal carcinoma and intraductal carcinoma, its noninvasive form. The bulk of this chapter will deal with invasive breast cancer, but first we shall consider, briefly, the two types of noninvasive breast cancer and certain differences between invasive lobular and ductal carcinoma.

Noninvasive or In Situ Breast Carcinoma

INTRADUCTAL CARCINOMA

There are three histologic patterns discerned in noninfiltrating ductal cancer: comedo, cribriform, and micropapillary. The comedocarcinoma form of intraductal carcinoma is more easily detected by mammography due to its tendency to produce microcalcifications.[13] It has also been reported to differ from the other types in having a higher incidence of bilaterality, approaching that of lobular carcinoma in situ.[24]

Foci of intraductal carcinoma are not an uncommon component of invasive breast cancer. In its pure form it is generally regarded as a preinvasive form of the latter, although this concept has been challenged. Gillis and his associates found no less than 14 of 50 tumors originally believed to be preinvasive to exhibit invasion

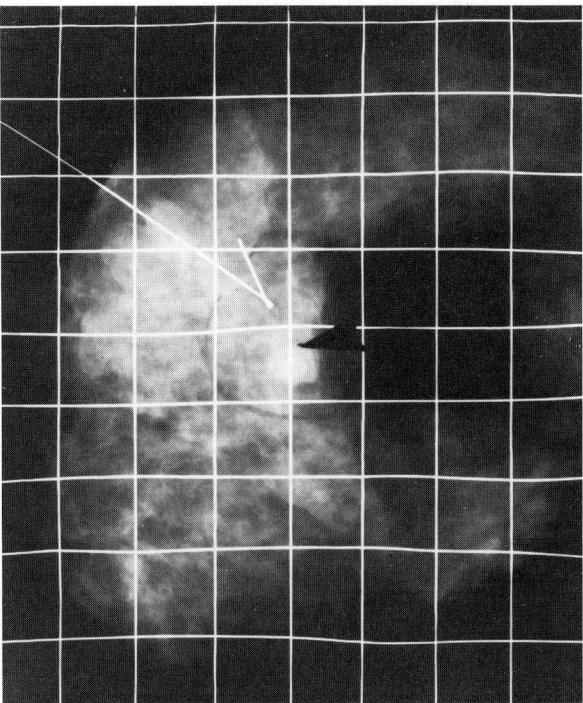

FIGURE 24-8 Specimen radiograph of the biopsy specimen obtained from the patient whose preoperative mammograms appear in Fig. 24-3. A different type of needle has been used for needle localization. This needle has a barb at its end similar to a fish hook which prevents it from being dislodged from the specimen during surgery.

after more careful and thorough examination.[25] This often required more than the six sections recommended by McDivitt et al. for this purpose.[26] Ozello and Sanpitak found electron microscopic evidence of disruption and loss of continuity of the lamina basalis (the ultrastructural basement membrane) in examples of cancers regarded histologically as purely intraductal.[27] Fisher has reported a similar experience in intraductal foci of invasive cancers examined by this technique.[20] In this regard the dichotomy between light and electron microscopic findings is comparable to that observed with lobular carcinoma in situ. Further, there have been reports of metastases in regional lymph nodes in cases of so-called pure intraductal cancer where no actual stromal invasion could be detected microscopically.

The risk of developing subsequent invasive ipsilateral breast cancer or new foci of intraductal carcinoma following excisional biopsy of intraductal carcinoma is incompletely understood, and no prospective study has ever addressed this issue. The true risk of axillary nodal involvement is also not known precisely, and the incidence of positive axillary nodes has never been correlated with the *size* of the primary intraductal cancer. (It would seem logical that the risk of missing an area of microscopic invasion due to sampling error should increase with increasing size of the primary tumor.) Clearly, the prognosis for patients with "pure" intraductal cancer is excellent, and a number of studies suggest that such patients have a normal life expectancy. Furthermore, although many reports have noted that intraductal carcinoma tends to be multicentric within the ipsilateral breast, the proclivity of intraductal cancer for bilaterality is not well known. In 1968, McDivitt et al. reported a retrospective series of 10 patients who had cribriform or micropapillary intraductal carcinoma treated by excisional biopsy and then subsequently developed invasive or recurrent intraductal carcinoma.[29] The average interval between biopsy and mastectomy was only 1.6 years. At mastectomy eight patients had infiltrating duct carcinoma, and two had recurrent intraductal carcinoma. All carcinomas were in the same breast quadrant as the prior biopsy, and most developed subjacent to the biopsy scar. Four of 8 patients developed invasive carcinoma and lymph node metastases at mastectomy, and 3 of these 4 subsequently died of disease 8, 9, and 12 years post mastectomy. Haagensen subsequently described 11 patients who had papillary intraductal carcinoma treated initially by biopsy or partial mastectomy.[30] During a follow-up period that varied from 1 to 10 years eight patients developed recurrent invasive carcinoma, and seven of these subsequently died of disease. Farrow, in reviewing the records from 200 intraductal carcinomas treated at Memorial Sloan-Kettering Cancer Center, found 25 cases that had been treated initially by biopsy only. Five (25 percent) subsequently developed recurrent carcinoma during follow-up periods that varied from 1 to 8 years.[31] More recently, Betsill et al. reported follow-up on 25 papillary intraductal carcinomas from the same institution that were initially treated by biopsy only.[32] The follow-up periods varied from 10 months to 24 years, averaging just under 10 years. Overall 7 of 25 patients (28 percent) developed recurrent ipsilateral carcinoma. However, among ten patients for whom complete follow-up information was available, seven were known to have developed subsequent invasive carcinoma. Four of these patients either died of disease or were alive with metastatic disease.

These various small retrospective series suggest that intraductal carcinoma treated by excisional biopsy presents a significant threat of subsequent recurrent invasive carcinoma, and that these invasive carcinomas carry with them a significant threat of mortality from the disease. However, because of variations in the quality and time of follow-up, they do not permit a precise calculation of risk or how it relates to time-at-risk subsequent to excisional biopsy. Furthermore, it would appear that the risk is more unilateral, i.e., confined to the ipsilateral breast, than is the case for lobular carcinoma in situ.

The treatment for intraductal carcinoma is somewhat controversial. Essentially all workers in the field would agree that radical mastectomy is unwarranted for intraductal cancer. Most recommend total mastectomy as the treatment of choice for the breast based on the risks of recurrent cancer reported after local excision which have just been cited for treatment by excisional biopsy alone. Recently, however, some investigators, on the basis of their interpretation of what is known concerning the natural history of this disease as well as the uncertainty concerning the biologic significance of multicentric cancer, have advocated segmental mastectomy followed by periodic mammographic and physical examinations. Nonetheless, at the present time, total mastectomy remains the "standard" treatment for this disease. However, if results of the segmental mastectomy trial of the National Surgical Adjuvant Breast Project (NSABP) indicate that segmental mastectomy, with or without breast irradiation, is appropriate treatment for *invasive* ductal cancer (see below), a trial of segmental mastectomy as treatment for intraductal carcinoma will clearly be warranted.

Whether or not complete or partial axillary dissection is indicated is a more debatable point. The reason usually given for including this dissection is that a small (0 to 2 percent) percentage of patients with intraductal cancer will be found to have occult axillary metastases even though no infiltration was identified in the biopsy specimen.[27,33-35]

The presumption appears to be that were this metastatic disease not removed, it would continue to spread and be responsible for a certain number of patient deaths. However, it is not known whether there would be any difference in mortality were one to delay axillary dissection until axillary metastases became clinically palpable in this small group of patients. If this were the case (and the results of NSABP protocol B-04 discussed later suggest that it is), then axillary dissection could be avoided in patients with intraductal carcinoma. One might consider reserving axillary dissection for those patients with larger primary tumors in which the sampling errors in histopathologic evaluation would be higher. Alternatively, as some authors have suggested, "axillary sampling", i.e., removal of a few low-lying axillary nodes, might suffice to identify the occasional patient with axillary nodal involvement.

Treatment of the contralateral breast in patients with intraductal carcinoma has attracted less attention than it has for patients with lobular carcinoma in situ, presumably because the risk of bilaterality is less. Although most of the previously quoted carcinomas have been discovered in the contralateral breast, Farrow in his review of 200 intraductal carcinomas treated at Memorial Hospital between 1949 and 1967 projected a 15 percent risk of bilaterality for intraductal carcinoma as compared to a 44 percent risk for in situ lobular carcinoma.[31] Although Farrow did not stratify this risk of bilaterality according to histological type of intraductal carcinoma, Berg and Robbins' data suggest that perhaps it might be highest for the comedo type.[36] In this 20-year follow-up study of 1458 women whose first breast cancer was treated by radical mastectomy, they found the highest rate of subsequent bilaterality (13.6 percent) among women whose first breast cancer was of the comedo type. Therefore, it would seem adequate to monitor the contralateral breast of patients with intraductal carcinoma by means of repeated physical examinations and mammography. The known risk to the contralateral breast does not seem sufficient to warrant empirical contralateral biopsy or empirical contralateral mastectomy.

LOBULAR CARCINOMA IN SITU

In 1941, Robert Muir[37] and Foote and Stuart[38] independently published papers describing an in situ form of carcinoma of the female breast apparently arising within the terminal portions of the lobule which they designated as *lobular carcinoma in situ*. These authors observed that this lesion was associated frequently with a linear type of invasive cancer which they postulated to be of lobular origin. This relatively distinct histologic type of invasive breast cancer was designated as *infiltrating lobular* or *invasive lobular carcinoma*. The incidence of lobular carcinoma in situ has been reported to vary from 2.8 to 6 percent of all breast cancers, including invasive as well as noninvasive forms of the disease. Lobular carcinoma in situ was found by Farrow to represent almost one-half of all noninvasibe breast cancers seen at Memorial Hospital between 1949 and 1965.[31]

The frequency with which lobular carcinoma in situ progresses to invasive lobular cancer is not known. Furthermore, the risk of invasive cancer that subsequently accrues when and if lobular carcinoma in situ is treated by excisional biopsy only is also not known precisely, although it has been defined more accurately than that of intraductal carcinoma. In 1966, Newman reported finding evidence of lobular carcinoma in situ in 72 of 73 examples of the invasive variety and concluded that the in situ and invasive forms represented a continuum.[39] A similar view was expressed a year later by McDivitt et al., who followed 50 patients with lobular carcinoma in situ who were treated by local excision and estimated that the risk of developing the invasive form was 8 percent after 5 years, 15 percent at 10 years, 27 percent at 15 years, and 35 percent after 20 years.[40] A slightly higher incidence of the development of invasive cancer has been reported by Toker in a similar type of study.[41] Anderson, in 1974, reported on 44 lobular carcinomas in situ which had been treated by excisional biopsy only.[42] During a follow-up period that averaged almost 16 years, 11 patients developed 13 invasive breast cancers. The incidence appeared to be bilateral, since four cancers developed in the contralateral breast. More recently, Rosen et al. have published a review of lobular carcinoma in situ treated by excision only with an average follow-up of 24 years. They estimated the frequency of subsequent invasive cancer of the breast (including the contralateral breast) to be 9 times greater than the expected frequency and death from breast cancer to be 11 times greater.[43] Moreover, the incidence of development of invasive breast cancer appeared to be equal bilaterally, with 19 patients developing cancer in the ipsilateral breast and 16 patients developing cancer in the contralateral breast. In addition, 10 in situ carcinomas were detected in ipsilateral breasts, and 5 in situ carcinomas developed in contralateral breasts. They also noted, as had McDivitt et al., that the risk of subsequently developing invasive breast cancer increased with increasing time-at-risk, in that 38 percent of the women who developed invasive breast cancer did so 20 years or more after their initial treatment for lobular carcinoma in situ by excisional biopsy.

Haagensen et al. have also reported recently a study of 211 patients with a lesion they call "lobular neoplasia" who were treated by excisional biopsy only.[44] (McDivitt notes that "it seems fair to assume that 'lobular neoplasia' is roughly equivalent to lobular carcinoma in situ, but the authors' illustrations suggest that the category may include some lesions others would designate lobular hyperplasia."[45] During an average follow-up period of 14 years, 19 invasive cancers were noted in 205 contralateral breasts, an essentially equal incidence. They concluded that the subsequent cumulative risk of developing invasive breast cancer, when lobular neoplasia was treated by excisional biopsy only, was 7 percent at 10 years, 10 percent at 15 years, 18 percent at 20 years, and 22 percent at 25 years for the ipsilateral breast, and 7 percent at 10 years, 9 percent at 15 years, and 15 percent at 20 years for the contralateral breast.

It is important to note that in all the studies discussed above the invasive cancers which subsequently developed in women initially treated for lobular carcinoma in situ were of both the ductal as well as the lobular variety. It would appear that, in such patients, the risk of subsequently developing invasive breast cancer is by no means confined to the development of lobular carcinoma. Of the 10 patients in the series of McDivitt et al.[40] who had unilateral lobular carcinoma in situ treated by excisional biopsy only and who subsequently developed invasive cancers, 8 of the latter were infiltrating duct carcinomas and only 2 of the infiltrating lobular type. The association of invasive cancers of either histologic type with intraductal and in situ lobular carcinomas provokes the conjecture that factors resulting in the development of in situ cancers may also affect the development of invasive cancer but that there is not necessarily a direct causal relationship between the two.

In summary, it would seem that patients with intraductal cancer have a risk of developing subsequent invasive breast cancer which is primarily ipsilateral and expresses itself within 1 to 10 years following excision of the intraductal carcinoma. In patients with lobular carcinoma in situ, the risk of subsequently developing invasive breast cancer is bilateral but requires much longer to express itself.

In their paper describing the disease,[37] Foote and Stewart recommended that lobular carcinoma in situ be treated by total mastectomy without axillary node dissection (simple mastectomy). This became the generally accepted form of treatment and proved to be extremely effective. However, occasionally in dissecting mastectomy specimens of this type, pathologists found a small focus of occult infiltrating carcinoma. For this reason, surgeons gradually began to include proximal axillary dissection in their treatment, a prophylaxis that seemed reasonable since it did not increase morbidity significantly. It seems certain that this method of treatment will eliminate risk derived from the ipsilateral breast.[31]

Recently, a number of investigators, notably Haagensen,[44] have suggested that lesser therapy may be equally effective. Haagensen recommends that patients with lobular carcinoma in situ (lobular neoplasia) be treated by excisional biopsy and repeat physical examination each 4 months for the remainder of their lives. He does not use mammography in these follow-up examinations because of his concern for its expense and possible radiation hazards. Although 8 of the 210 patients in Haagensen's series are either dead of disease or living with metastatic disease, Haagensen stresses that none of these patients participated in the follow-up program that he recommends.

In considering the risks associated with treating lobular carcinoma in situ by excisional biopsy, it is important to know the morbidity and mortality that may result from infiltrating carcinomas that subsequently develop. Anderson summarized the available literature on the subject in 1977, and reported that, among 288 patients who subsequently developed invasive breast cancer, 13 (5.7 percent) had lymph node metastases at the time the invasive cancer was detected, and 9 (4 percent) subsequently died of the disease.[42] Among the 28 patients reported by Rosen et al. in whom lymph node status could be determined at the time of mastectomy, 54 percent of patients with ipsilateral invasive cancers and 47 percent of patients with contralateral invasive cancers were found to have axillary metastases.[43] Of their patients who developed invasive cancer 59 percent eventually died of their disease. The differences in mortality reported by Anderson and that reported by Rosen et al. may be, in part, explained by the latter's significantly longer period of follow-up. Finally, Haagensen et al. reported that of their 36 patients who subsequently developed invasive cancer, 6 (17 percent) are dead of disease and 2 others are living with distant metastases.[44]

Treatment of the contralateral breast in patients with lobular carcinoma in situ also poses special problems in view of the data suggesting that both the ipsilateral and contralateral breast have approximately the same subsequent risk. It should follow that they would be treated similarly. However, many surgeons who perform total mastectomy and partial axillary dissection as treatment for the ipsilateral breast have been reluctant to perform a contralateral mastectomy. Urban has recommended that an empirical contralateral biopsy be done at the time of the ipsilateral mastectomy. If there is any palpable or mammographic abnormality in the contralateral breast,[46] this area is selected for biopsy. Otherwise a liberal biopsy of the upper outer quadrant as well as a mirror image biopsy of the proven cancer is suggested. Detection rates reported for occult carcinomas discovered by empirical biopsy of contralateral breasts vary between 25 and 40 percent.[47-50] When occult carcinomas are detected in the contralateral breast, these authors perform a contralateral mastectomy. If the biopsies are negative, the contralateral breast is observed. However, the benefit from this approach in terms of reducing mortality from contralateral breast cancer has never been documented or quantified.

Since the subsequent risk derived from each breast is the same, it should follow that the treatment for both breasts should be the same and that the reduction in risk should be proportional to the total volume of breast tissue removed regardless of whether it is removed from the ipsilateral breast or the contralateral breast. Yet the therapy advocated in the past by Urban and others[46-50] utilizes different treatments for each breast. However, not even the most aggressive surgeons have advocated bilateral total mastectomies with low axillary dissections.[51] Bilateral subcutaneous mastectomy with implantation has been suggested by McDivitt.[45] He points out that this procedure would remove a greater total volume of breast tissue than unilateral total mastectomy and contralateral breast biopsy and should produce a superior cosmetic result. He does not indicate *when* these procedures should be performed with relation to the excisional biopsy which is found to contain lobular carcinoma in situ. Since the risk of developing invasive breast cancer in such patients manifests itself many years following excision of lobular carcinoma in situ, would it not be appropriate to delay mastectomy, at least for a few years?

RECOMMENDATIONS FOR TREATMENT

At the risk of joining the ranks of those who advocate therapies without the benefit (or encumbrance) of data, I am prepared to offer some suggestions of my own for the treatment of patients with in situ breast cancers. At least the lack of data makes it difficult, but by no means impossible, to argue against my recommendations.

In patients with intraductal carcinoma, the risk of developing a new occurrence of invasive breast cancer following excisional biopsy is primarily unilateral, and this risk manifests itself within a relatively few years. Therefore, total mastectomy of the ipsilateral breast appears appropriate. This procedure should probably be performed shortly after the biopsy which revealed the intraductal cancer, i.e., within a year or so. Subcutaneous mastectomy and implant insertion (with or without nipple preservation) seems an equally appropriate alternative. Since the incidence of axillary node involvement is only 0 to 2 percent, axillary dissection, even for staging purposes, does not seem to be indicated. At the very least, axillary sampling should be reserved for those patients presenting with very large primary tumors, in whom foci of invasive cancer are more likely to be missed by the pathologist. The contralateral breast should be followed with periodic physical and mammographic examinations, especially in cases of comedocarcinoma, but not otherwise treated.

In patients with lobular carcinoma in situ, the risk of developing a new occurrence of invasive breast cancer following excisional biopsy is bilateral, but this risk manifests itself many years (usually 10 or more) following detection of the in situ carcinoma. Therefore, it would seem possible to delay all treatment other than the excisional biopsy for several years (up to 5 years, at least). Treatment is prophylactic and should be bilateral. Bilateral total mastectomies or bilateral subcutaneous mastectomy and implant insertion, with or without nipple preservation, seems appropriate. No treatment to either axilla is required. I will quote from McDivitt,[45] whose recommendations were similar, only changing his use of the singular to the pleural: "Although I am certain that (these) suggestion(s) will encounter resistance from traditionalists, I, nevertheless, believe (they) deserve a serious trial."

Histologic Types of Invasive Breast Cancer

As mentioned above, cancer of the female breast may arise from the epithelium of the mammary ducts or the mammary lobules, and both types exhibit noninvasive and invasive forms. Although there is only a single histologic subtype of infiltrating lobular carcinoma, a number of morphologic variants of infiltrating ductal carcinoma have been described. These histologic subtypes will be considered briefly.

INVASIVE LOBULAR CARCINOMA

Invasive lobular carcinomas make up approximately 6 percent of invasive breast cancers. The prognosis of invasive lobular carcinoma is not significantly different from that of invasive ductal carcinoma. The main significance of this histologic type of breast cancer is its association with lobular carcinoma in situ and its tendency to multicentricity and bilaterality, which has raised questions concerning the appropriate approach to the contralateral breast.

Invasive lobular carcinoma has been reported to be associated with a higher incidence of subsequent cancer development in the contralateral breast than is the case with invasive ductal cancer. A 20 percent incidence of bilaterality is usually cited.[52] As is the case with lobular carcinoma in situ, the cancers arising in the contralateral breast are not regularly lobular in type. Since foci of lobular carcinoma in situ are frequently found in association with invasive lobular carcinoma, it is unclear whether the risk to the contralateral breast can be directly attributable to the invasive lobular cancer or the in situ component of the disease.

Urban and others[46-50] have advocated routine biopsies of the contralateral breast in patients with invasive lobular carcinoma. However, there is no good evidence to indicate that this procedure significantly reduces the mortality risk from contralateral breast cancer.

INVASIVE DUCTAL CARCINOMA

In addition to infiltrating ductal carcinoma without special features, a number of subtypes have been described which display certain characteristic histopathologic features. These subtypes include scirrhous carcinoma, mucinous, or comedo, carcinoma, medulary carcinoma, tubular carcinoma, and papillary carcinoma. Not all pathologists employ all these terms, and many prefer not to use them at all.

The term *sirrhous carcinoma* refers to ductal cancers in which a dense desmoplastic reaction results in a very dense fibrous stroma in which a relative paucity of neoplastic cells are found. Although it has been alleged that this histologic variant is associated with a poor prognosis, there is little reliable data to support this contention.

Mucinous carcinomas are sometimes referred to as *colloid carcinoma* or *comedocarcinoma*. They are characterized by aggregates of tumor cells within pools of mucin.

Mucinous and tubular carcinomas have been alleged to be the most favorable histologic types of breast cancer, when found in "pure" forms.[53] Medulary carcinoma has also been regarded as a prognostically favorable form of breast cancer on the basis of retrospective studies. However, recent data has failed to confirm such a favorable prognosis.[53]

Papillary carcinoma is a rare type, representing 1 percent or less of all mammary cancers, and very little data exists regarding its clinical behavior. This pattern is occasionally found in combination with other types.

STEROID HORMONE RECEPTOR ASSAYS

Steroid hormone receptor assays have become critically important in the management of patients with breast cancer. They not only are of vital importance in selecting appropriate therapy for patients with recurrent and or metastatic disease but may be useful in selecting appropriate adjuvant therapy for patients following initial therapy for primary breast cancer. In addition, they may provide information of prognostic significance. Because the opportunity to obtain specimens of tumor tissue for receptor analysis presents itself either at the time of biopsy or at the time of initial therapy, this topic will be discussed at this time.

The two steroid hormone receptors of proven importance in breast cancer are the estrogen receptor (ER) and the progesterone receptor (PR). Their place in the mechanism of steroid hormone action within the cell is presented in Table 24-1. Both are proteins. They are related to each other in that the progesterone receptor itself is a protein whose synthesis is induced by estrogen and, therefore, is dependent upon the presence and intact function of estrogen receptor. The absence or low concentration of PR in ER-positive tumors may indicate a defect in the mechanism of action of estrogen distal to

TABLE 24-1 Steps in Steroid Hormone Action

1. Hormone enters cell.
2. Binding to specific receptor protein.
3. Receptor activation.
4. Translocation of hormone-receptor complex to nucleus.
5. Binding to chromatin.
6. Altered gene transcription.
7. mRNA translocation to ribosome.
8. Changes in protein synthesis.
9. Net biochemical consequences of hormone action.

receptor binding. The measurement of PR, therefore, provides the basis for the estimation of an end product of estrogen activity within the cell and may be a better marker of hormone dependence than the measurement of ER alone. Several techniques exist for the measurement of ER and PR in human breast cancer tissue. These methods have recently been reviewed in detail.[54] There is now conclusive evidence that these assays predict response to endocrine therapy in patients with recurrent and/or metastatic disease.

The concentration of ER and PR in human breast cancer specimens varies over a wide range from 0 (i.e., below the sensitivity of the assay) to over 100 femtomol (fmol) per milligram of cytoplasmic protein. Variations in receptor content may be due to a variety of factors related to the tumor cells themselves, the nature of the biopsy specimen, the manner of obtaining and handling the specimen, the source of the specimen, and the internal hormonal milieu of the patient from whom the specimen is obtained. It is important for the clinician to know these factors in order to maximize the opportunity of obtaining accurate and clinically relevant assays and minimize the possibility of obtaining spuriously low results. In addition, absolute values for ER and PR may be expressed differently from laboratory to laboratory, and the cut-off values for receptor-positive and -negative are not uniform among laboratories, but are based on the assay sensitivity of a particular laboratory or on results of correlations with clinical information. This may confuse some physicians, since an absolute value for ER or PR in one laboratory may not be equivalent to that obtained in another. Finally, the assays themselves require considerable experience from a technical and interpretive point of view. Valid results depend on proper handling of the specimen by the surgeon and pathologist, proper transport and storage in the laboratory, and precise methodology. The 5 to 10 percent response rate to endocrine therapy in receptor-negative tumors may partially reflect "false-negative" assays due to undetected procedural errors. Specimens should be sent to laboratories providing evidence for quality control of their assay.

Sources of Variability in Results of Receptor Assays

OBTAINING AND HANDLING THE SPECIMEN

The initial tumor tissue specimen for receptor assay may be obtained either at the time of biopsy or at the time of primary therapy. Additional specimens should be obtained, whenever possible, if and when recurrence or metastasis occurs and at the time of each and every clinical relapse, since receptor content may change during the course of the disease and its treatment. If an excisional or incisional biopsy is performed, part of that specimen should be sent for receptor determination. If the diagnosis is established by needle biopsy or aspiration cytology, a specimen of the tumor should be obtained at the time of primary surgical therapy. If, at the time of primary therapy, one or more grossly involved axillary nodes are apparent, a tumor specimen should be obtained from the involved node(s) as well, since there may be discordance between the receptor content of specimens from primary tumors and metastatic nodal deposits. The specimen should be (1) representative, (2) composed entirely of tumor, i.e., free of fat and normal breast tissue, (3) free of necrosis and/or hemorrhage, (4) of adequate size, and (5) fresh. The specimen should be at least 500 mg in size, and 1 g or more is preferable. It should be obtained within 30 min of the time of excision or devascularization and promptly frozen in liquid nitrogen or dry ice–acetone. A frozen section from the specimen itself or from adjacent tissue should always be obtained in order to confirm the suitability of the specimen. The specimen should be stored in liquid nitrogen, dry ice, or an ultra-low-temperature (65°C or lower) freezer and transported to the laboratory in dry ice. A household freezer is inadequate for specimen storage. Failure to follow these procedures will result in spuriously low receptor values, since the receptor proteins are subject to degradation.

THE SPECIMEN ITSELF

Some variability in receptor content may be due to factors pertaining to the tumor tissue itself. There may be heterogeneity within the tumor cell population wherein receptor content varies with the proportion of cells in the biopsy specimen which contain receptor. There may be differences in the amount of receptor content among different receptor-containing cells. The degree of epithelial cellularity of the tumor biopsy has also been correlated with results of receptor analysis. One might expect that tumors with a prominent fibrotic reaction and a relative paucity of tumor cells might have a negative receptor assay even if the tumor cells contained receptor, since these cells would be contributing only a minority of the total protein assayed. Surprisingly, data addressing this question are controversial. Several small studies suggest that the tumor cell content of the biopsy specimen may influence ER determinations and should be considered in the interpretation of the assay.[55–57] However, in a larger study, Rosen et al. found no relationship between tumor cell density and the qualitative results of the ER assay.[58] This result may be due to the fact that this study grouped tumors according to a relatively broad range of tumor cellularity. The "low-density" group included tumors with up to 30 percent epithelial cellularity. Perhaps a correlation between tumor cellularity and ER would have been observed if tumors with an even lower cell density were examined as a subject. The observation that on occasion tumor tissue from axillary lymph nodes may be higher in receptor content than tissue obtained at the same time from the primary tumor of the same patient may be due to increased cellularity and diminished stomal content of tumor deposits within lymph nodes.

Tumor receptor content may also depend partially on the source of the tissue obtained for assay. For instance, a greater proportion of primary tumor samples are ER-positive than are specimens from metastatic sites.[59] Perhaps this reflects a gradual depletion of receptor-positive cells and a selective increase in receptor-negative cells from a heterogeneous primary tumor over the course of the disease, or it may be due to contamination of the biopsy specimen from metastatic sites with normal receptor-negative cells, resulting in a falsely low ER value. No major correlation has been found between ER status and the organ from which the biopsy is taken.

There is only sparse information regarding receptor content in multiple simultaneous or sequential tumor samples from the same patient. However, a surprising variation in ER content (15 to 38 percent) has been reported from the limited number of patients studied.[60,61] These qualitative discrepancies in ER in multiple simultaneous biopsies may partially explain the prognostic inaccuracy of a qualitative ER assay, since the ER level in the tissue site chosen for biopsy may not be representative of the residual neoplastic tissue. Another report suggests that the tumor ER level in a given patient tends to decrease as the duration of the disease increases, perhaps indicating further dedifferentiation of the tumor during the metastatic process or selective growth of ER-negative cells. These observations suggest that ER determined on tumor tissue obtained early in the course of the disease may not always be useful in predicting response to endocrine therapy at a later date. The effect of systemic therapy or radiotherapy on tumor receptor content has not been well defined. Interestingly, one study does report a tendency for tumor ER to decline after endocrine therapy and to increase after chemotherapy, suggesting that endocrine therapy depletes the tumor of ER-positive cells, whereas chemotherapy primarily reduces the number of ER-negative cells.[62] This conclusion remains unconfirmed. In any event, because of the potential for change in receptor status (and presumably in hormone dependence) of breast cancer with time, it seems advisable, if possible, to repeat the receptor determinations on accessible tumor tissue just prior to instituting or changing therapy.

THE HORMONAL MILIEU OF THE PATIENT

Estrogen receptors are present in about one-third to two-thirds of human breast cancer specimens. About one-third of breast cancers contain both ER and PR. Another one-third contain neither ER nor PR, and one-third contain ER but no PR. Finally, tumor specimens rarely are found to contain PR in the absence of ER. This finding conforms to the observation that PR synthesis is induced by estrogen and requires a functionally intact estrogen response mechanism.

Most studies agree that postmenopausal women have a greater proportion of ER-positive tumors and/or higher tumor ER concentrations than premenopausal women. The explanation for this observation is not totally clear. One possibility is that this phenomenon does not really represent biological differences between tumors as a function of age or menopausal status, but simply reflects the fact that younger women have higher circulating estrogen levels that bind to and mask receptors, resulting in falsely lower ER content. Several studies suggest that alternative explanations deserve consideration. First, it is doubtful that physiological estradiol concentrations ever reach levels sufficient to saturate all of the available receptor sites, which would result in a negative ER assay.[63] Second, tumors from pre- and postmenopausal women have been found to have similar levels on endogenously bound ER.[63] Third, an inverse relationship between the concentration of estrogen and progesterone in plasma or in tumor tissue itself and ER and PR has not been observed consistently.[64] Finally, perimenopausal patients have been reported to have a lower incidence of ER-positive tumors than premenopausal patients.[55] These data collectively suggest that mechanisms for the differences in ER levels between pre- and postmenopausal women are complex and are not due simply to differences in endogenous estrogen concentration.

However, it may be appropriate to determine plasma estrogen and progesterone levels in premenopausal and perimenopausal women on a blood sample drawn the same day on which a tissue specimen for ER and PR content is obtained.

Other Steriod Hormone Receptors in Breast Cancer

Recently the presence of androgen receptors (AR) and glucocorticoid (GR) receptors in human breast cancer tissue has been established. AR and GR have now been identified in up to 50 percent of tumors studied. The presence of each of the receptors studied (ER, PR, AR, and GR) correlates with the presence of all of the other receptors. In addition, preliminary evidence suggests that the presence of AR or GR may have some value in predicting response to endocrine therapy. Thus, one might expect that the presence of multiple receptors in a biopsy specimen might improve the selection of hormone-dependent tumors, as was observed with ER and PR. Preliminary evidence from a small number of patients supports this notion. Additional studies will be required to determine whether measurements of these steroid hormone receptors have any clinical significance in the management of breast cancer patients.

Uses for Steroid Receptor Assays

CORRELATION WITH RESPONSE TO ENDOCRINE THERAPY

The value of ER and PR determinations in selecting appropriate therapy for patients with recurrent and/or metastatic disease is well established and will be discussed later. In addition, these assays may be of value in selecting appropriate adjuvant therapy following primary treatment for breast cancer. This, too, will be discussed in a later section.

PROGNOSTIC FACTORS IN PRIMARY BREAST CANCER

Several recent studies have shown that the ER content of a primary breast cancer appears to be an important prognostic marker. Moreover, the relationship between ER and prognosis tends to be independent of other variables such as axillary nodal status, age or menopausal status, size or location of the tumor, and the degree of histologic differentiation of the tumor. The most often cited study is that of Osborne and McGuire, who found that the number of axillary node–negative patients with recurrent disease 20 months after mastectomy was three times higher if the tumor was ER-negative (22 percent) than if the tumor was ER-positive (7 percent).[65] Similarly, 50 percent of ER-negative, node-positive patients had recurrences at 20 months compared to 25 percent of the ER-positive group. A few recent studies have reported that progesterone receptor content may also be an important prognostic variable. These observations have obvious implications for clinical trials, in that it may be important to include receptor status in the stratification of patients.

AN AID IN THE DIFFERENTIAL DIAGNOSIS OF METASTATIC ADENOCARCINOMAS OF INAPPARENT PRIMARY

Since breast cancer is the most prevalent cancer in the American female, it must be considered a serious diagnostic possibility in any women presenting with metastatic adenocarcinoma without a readily apparent primary site of origin. This is particularly true if axillary and/or supraclavicular nodes are involved. In approximately two-thirds of women with metastatic adenocarcinoma in axillary lymph nodes and no apparent site of origin, a primary breast cancer may be found in the ipsilateral breast (usually in the upper outer quadrant) if the ipsilateral breast is removed. This is true even if mammography and physical examination of the ipsilateral breast are entirely negative. The presence of ER and/or PR in metastatic tumor tissue strongly suggests a breast primary although absence of ER and PR by no means excludes breast carcinoma, since many breast cancers lack receptors. Because of this, it is extremely important to obtain a freshly frozen sample of unfixed tumor tissue for receptor analysis in such patients whenever a biopsy is performed on a metastatic tumor mass, especially if the disease involves axillary and/or supraclavicular lymph nodes.

PREDICTING RESPONSE TO CHEMOTHERAPY

Recently, several studies have suggested that ER-negative tumors tend to respond better to chemotherapy than ER-positive tumors.[66] In support of their results, these investigators postulate that ER-negative tumors proliferate more rapidly, and that chemotherapy generally is more effective in rapidly dividing cells. On the other

TABLE 24-2 The Manchester Classification

Stage I	The growth is confined to the breast. Involvement of the skin directly over and in continuity with the tumor may be present, provided the area is small in relation to the size of the breast.
Stage II	The growth is confined to the breast, but palpable mobile lymph nodes are present in the axilla.
Stage III	The growth extends beyond the mammary parenchyma as shown by 1. Skin invasion or fixation over an area large in relation to the size of the breast or skin ulceration. 2. Tumor fixation to the underlying muscle of fascia; axillary nodes, if present, are mobile.
Stage IV	The growth extends beyond the breast area as shown by fixation or matting of the axillary nodes, complete fixation of tumor to chest wall, deposits in supraclavicular nodes or in the opposite breast, satellite nodules, or distant metastases.

hand, several other studies report opposite results, and other studies find no association between these two parameters. All of these studies are retrospective analyses, chemotherapy was not uniform even within individual studies, and the chronological sequence of the ER assay and the chemotherapy was variable. Some investigators studied patients with an ER assay performed on metastatic tissue immediately prior to the initiation of chemotherapy, others used ER data obtained earlier from the primary tumor, and still others accepted patients for study who had their ER status determined after completion of chemotherapy. Perhaps these or other methodologic variables account for the disparate results. Prospective clinical trials are required to answer this question, which has important ramifications in treatment planning.

STAGING OF INVASIVE BREAST CANCER

A clinical staging system, which records accurate information with regard to the extent of the disease prior to the onset of definitive treatment, is absolutely necessary for planning therapeutic strategy, estimating prognosis, and providing a mechanism for comparing the results of different therapeutic procedures performed in different centers. In addition, histopathologic staging may be performed following surgical intervention and is based on histologic findings. It is, therefore, often more precise than clinical staging and may be used as a guide for planning subsequent adjuvant therapy.

The practice of grouping and classifying breast cancer patients according to the extent of their disease has been in existence for almost a century. In 1905, only a decade after Halsted's first report of the radical mastectomy, Steinthal observed that patient survival was directly related to the extent of disease at the time of diagnosis.[67] He made the first known attempt to clinically stage breast cancer by proposing to divide patients into three groups: group I—small primary tumor without skin involvement and without clinically positive axillary nodes, group II—larger primary tumors with skin involvement and positive axillary nodes, and group III—large primary tumors and involved supraclavicular nodes. Because of the dismal results of surgery in group III patients, he recommended conservative management for patients with advanced disease. In 1940, Paterson developed a much more sophisticated staging system which was widely accepted in England and became known as the Manchester Classification.[68] This staging system, which is presented in Table 24-2, was based exclusively on clinical findings and served as an objective basis for comparing treatment results.

In 1943, Haagensen and Stout designed a new clinical staging system known as the Columbia Clinical Classification.[69] It is presented in Table 24-3. This classification evolved from a study of criteria for inoperability and was based on data derived from a careful analysis of 27 years of experience with breast cancer patients at the Columbia-Presbyterian Hospital in New York. In this staging system, not only the presence or absence of clinically positive axillary nodes but the size and character of the involved nodes were considered as important prognostic factors. In addition, "grave signs" of locally advanced primary tumors were taken into consideration. However, this system ignores the size of the primary tumor. Despite its shortcomings, this staging system gained wide acceptance both in the United States and abroad.

In 1944, Pierre DeNoix,[70] of the Institute Gustave Roussay in France, conceived of the TNM system of classification, which was based on Raven's[71] suggestion that letters be used as symbols to describe the extent of the disease, emphasizing three components: tumor size (T), regional lymph nodes (N), and distant metastases

(M). The staging system proposed by Denoix was accepted by the International Union against Cancer (UICC) in 1961,[72] and the TNM method of staging rapidly gained general acceptance. The TNM system was also adopted by the American Joint Committee for Cancer Staging and End Results Reporting (AJC), which published their staging system, differing in some respects from that of the UICC, in 1962, 1 year after the UICC version appeared. Numerous efforts to evaluate the two systems and to reconcile the differences between them resulted in several revisions. The current version, endorsed by both organizations, appeared in 1977.[73] In addition to clinical-diagnostic staging it provides for the separate categorization of histopathologic information obtained from surgical biopsies (surgical-evaluative staging) and therapeutic resections (postsurgical treatment–pathologic staging).

For clinical-diagnostic staging, the following are required: physical examination including careful inspection of skin and palpation of mammary glands and regional nodes, determination of the degree of fixation with and without flexing pectoral muscles, routine laboratory studies and hemograms, and chest films. Mammography and thermography are optional staging procedures.

For surgical-evaluative staging, needle biopsy or excisional biopsy of nodes with a sampling of axillary internal mammary or supraclavicular nodes must be noted separately and is not considered part of the clinical staging system. Suspected skin involvement should be confirmed by biopsy.

For postsurgical treatment–pathologic staging, evaluation of the breast in its entirety and/or the axillary contents with careful pathologic evaluation of all nodes is commonly done. This should never be substituted for clinical evaluation.

The AJC-UICC clinical-diagnostic classification system is presented in Table 24-4. It takes most of the clinical features of breast cancer into consideration and is certainly the most elaborate and complex system to date. Unfortunately, its complexity makes it cumbersome to use and difficult to remember. Its stage grouping scheme probably assigns too great an importance simply to the size of the primary tumor. It will probably be revised again as results from current clinical trials become available.

Finally, there is an operational "shorthand" form of clinical staging which, although unofficial, is part of the general parlance of most workers in the field. *Stage I*,

TABLE 24-3 The Columbia Clinical Classification

Stage	
Stage A	No skin edema, ulceration, or solid fixation of tumor to chest wall; axillary nodes not clinically involved
Stage B	No skin edema, ulceration, or solid fixation of tumor to chest wall; clinically involved axillary nodes, but less than 2.5 cm in transverse diameter and not fixed to overlying skin or deeper structure of axilla
Stage C	Any one of five grave signs of comparatively advanced carcinoma: 1. Edema of skin of limited extent (less than one-third of the skin over the breast) 2. Skin ulceration 3. Solid fixation of tumor to chest wall 4. Massive involvement of axillary lymph nodes (2.5 cm or more in transverse diameter) 5. Fixation of the axillary nodes to overlying skin or deeper structures of the axilla
Stage D	All other patients with more advanced breast carcinoma, including 1. A combination of any two or more of the five grave signs listed in stage C 2. Extensive edema of skin (involving more than one-third of the skin over the breast) 3. Satellite skin nodules 4. The inflammatory type of carcinoma 5. Supraclavicular metastases, clinically 6. Parasternal metastases, clinically 7. Edema of the ipsilateral arm 8. Distant metastases

without further definition, refers to a tumor confined to the breast without "grave signs," involvement of adjacent tissues, or signs of metastases to axillary nodes. *Stage II* denotes a similar tumor associated with clinically involved axillary lymph nodes. *Stage III* indicates advanced loco-regional disease without clear evidence of incurability, and *stage IV* implies obvious incurability either due to the presence of distant metastases or because of unusually extensive loco-regional disease.

Clinical staging, however precise, has certain inherent limitations and inaccuracies, both with regard to estimates of tumor size and to the assessment of axillary nodal involvement. Irving and his associates studied the correlation between preoperative estimates of tumor size and the actual tumor size. They found on pathologic examination[74] marked discrepancies between the two.

TABLE 24-4 Clinical-Diagnostic Classification (AJC-UICC, 1977)

PRIMARY TUMOR (T)

T_X Tumor cannot be assessed.

T_0 No evidence of primary tumor.

T_{IS} Paget's disease of the nipple with no demonstrable tumor. Note: Paget's disease with a demonstrable tumor is classified according to size of the tumor.

T_1*   Tumor 2 cm or less in greatest dimension.
    T_{1a} No fixation to underlying pectoral fascia or muscle.
    T_{1b} Fixation to underlying pectoral fascia and/or muscle.

T_2*   Tumor more than 2 cm but not more than 5 cm in its greatest dimension.
    T_{2a} No fixation to underlying pectoral fascia and/or muscle.
    T_{2b} Fixation to underlying pectoral fascia and/or muscle.

T_3*   Tumor more than 5 cm in its greatest dimension.
    T_{3a} No fixation to underlying pectoral fascia and/or muscle.
    T_{3b} Fixation to underlying pectoral fascia and/or muscle.

T_4 Tumor of any size with direct extension to chest wall or skin.
Note: Chest wall includes ribs, intercostal muscles, and serratus anterior muscle, but not pectoral muscle.
    T_{4a} Fixation to chest wall.
    T_{4b} Edema (including peau d'orange), ulceration of the skin, or satellite skin nodules confined to the same breast.
    T_{4c} Both of above.
    T_{4d} Inflammatory carcinoma.†

NODAL INVOLVEMENT (N)

N_X Regional lymph nodes cannot be assessed clinically.

N_0 No palpable homolateral axillary nodes.

N_1 Movable homolateral axillary nodes.
    N_{1a} Nodes not considered to contain growth.
    N_{1b} Nodes considered to contain growth.

N_2 Homolateral axillary nodes containing growth and fixed to one another or to other structures.

N_3 Homolateral supraclavicular or infraclavicular nodes containing growth or edema of the arm.‡

Note: Edema of the arm may be caused by lymphatic obstruction, and lymph nodes may not then be palpable.

DISTANT METASTASIS (M)

M_X Not assessed.

M_0 No (known) distant metastasis.

M_1 Distant metastasis present.
Specify _____.
Specify sites according to the following notations:
Pulmonary PUL	Bone marrow MAR
Osseous OSS	Pleura PLE
Hepatic HEP	Skin SKI
Brain BRA	Eye EYE
Lymph nodes LYM	Other OTH

STAGE GROUPING

Stage	T	N	M
Stage I	T_{1a}	N_0 or N_{1a}	
	T_{1b}	N_0 or N_{1a}	M_0
Stage II	T_0	N_{1b}	
	T_{1a}	N_{1b}	
	T_{1b}	N_{1B}	M_0
	T_{2a} or T_{2b}	N_0, N_{1a}, or N_{1b}	
Stage III	T_{1a} or T_{1b}	N_2	M_0
	T_{2a} or T_{2b}	N_2	M_0
	T_{3a} or T_{3b}	N_0, N_1, or N_2	M_0
Stage IV	T_4	Any N	Any M
	Any T	N_3	Any M
	Any T	Any N	M_1

* Dimpling of the skin, nipple retraction, or any other skin changes except those in T_{4b} may occur in T_1, T_2, or T_3 without changing the classification.

† Inflammatory carcinoma is a clinicopathologic entity characterized by diffuse brawny induration of the skin of the breast with an erysipeloid edge, usually without an underlying palpable mass. Histologically infiltrating mammary carcinoma diffusely permeates dermal lymphatics. (Inflamed cancers that are clinically similar to the above and are due to inflammation, infection, or necrosis but lack microscopic dermal lymphatic permeation are not classified as inflammatory carcinoma.)

‡ Homolateral internal mammary nodes considered to contain growth are included in N_3 for surgical-evaluative classification and postsurgical treatment–pathologic classification.

Furthermore, clinical evaluation of axillary nodal status is notoriously difficult and unreliable. The incidence of falsely assessing axillary nodes as negative is between 30 and 45 percent, and the incidence of false-positive clinical staging is approximately 15 percent. Therefore, even in experienced hands, clinical staging of the axilla is inaccurate approximately half the time.

The presence or absence of axillary nodal involvement has been shown to be the single most important prognostic factor in predicting eventual outcome. Moreover, it has been shown that not only the presence or absence of axillary node involvement influences prognosis but the extent of nodal disease closely correlates with survival.[75] The number of positive axillary nodes has been demonstrated to have a profound influence on prognosis,[76-79] with involvement of one to three axillary nodes having a significantly better prognosis than involvement of four or more nodes.[80] In addition, the size of nodal metastases is of prognostic importance. Those patients with occult or microscopic nodal involvement (i.e., < 2 mm in size) fare better than those with larger metastatic deposits. Finally, evidence of gross nodal disease (i.e., >2 mm) or evidence of extracapsular spread are particularly poor prognostic signs.[81] Because of the considerations discussed above, a histopathologic staging system is extremely valuable. The AJC-UICC postsurgical treatment–pathologic classification system is depicted in Table 24-5. Its value is as a supplement to the clinical-diagnostic staging system, not as a replacement for it. Both the clinical-diagnostic and postsurgical treatment–pathologic staging systems represent parts of a dynamic process and are subject to modification periodically as new data and information on the biology and natural history become available. The current staging systems do not consider the presence or absence of estrogen and progesterone receptors within the tumor, which has been shown to be of considerable prognostic importance. Receptor status will probably be included in future revisions, as may other prognostic discriminants which are not well understood at the present time.

SURGICAL TREATMENT OF INVASIVE BREAST CANCER STAGES I AND II

Radical Mastectomy

The operation which came to be known as the "radical mastectomy" was first reported by William Stewart Halsted in 1894.[82] Although Halsted has been given exclusive credit for developing this operation, Willy Meyer developed a similar operation independently at about the same time and reported his experience the same year, i.e., 1894.[83] The radical mastectomy was adopted enthusiastically throughout the United States and abroad, and resulted in an immediate and dramatic reduction in chest wall recurrences which were, at this time, occurring at rates as high as 82 percent following lesser operations. This operation was based on the theory that breast cancer spread circumfugally with time to

TABLE 24-5 Postsurgical Treatment–Pathologic Classification (AJC-UICC, 1977)

PRIMARY TUMOR (T)

T_X Tumor cannot be assessed.

T_0 No evidence of primary tumor.

T_{IS} Preinvasive carcinoma (carcinoma in situ), noninfiltrating intraductal carcinoma, or Paget's disease of nipple.

T_{1a} and T_{1b} are the same as clinical-diagnostic classification.

T_{1a}

T_{1b}
  1. Tumor < 0.5 cm
  2. Tumor 0.5–0.9 cm
  3. Tumor 1.0–1.9 cm

T_{2a} and T_{2b} are the same as clinical-diagnostic classification.

T_{3a} and T_{3b} are the same as clinical-diagnostic classification.

T_{4a} and T_{4b} are the same as clinical-diagnostic classification.

T_{4d} Inflammatory carcinoma.

NODAL INVOLVEMENT (N)

N_X Regional lymph nodes cannot be assessed clinically.

N_0 No metastatic homolateral axillary nodes.

N_1 Movable homolateral axillary metastatic nodes not fixed to one another or to other structures.
  N_{1a} Lymph nodes with only histologic metastatic growth.
  N_{1b} Gross metastatic carcinoma in lymph nodes.
    1. Micrometastasis smaller than 0.2 cm.
    2. Metastasis (larger than 0.2 cm) to 1 to 3 lymph nodes.
    3. Metastasis to 4 or more lymph nodes.
    4. Extension of metastasis beyond the lymph node capsule.
    5. Any positive node greater than 2 cm in diameter.

N_2 Homolateral axillary nodes containing metastasis tumor and fixed to one another or to other structures.

N_3 Homolateral supraclavicular or infraclavicular nodes containing tumor or edema of the arm.*

* Edema of the arm may be caused by lymphatic obstruction and lymph nodes may not then be palpable.
NOTE: The postsurgical treatment–pathologic classification of the 1977 TNM system is based upon histologic demonstration of cancer. It grades the sizes of primaries smaller than 2 cm in diameter and gives well-deserved importance to the number of involved axillary lymph nodes as well as to their size and to the presence of extracapsular extension of cancer.

contiguous structures and could, therefore, be encompassed by a wide en bloc resection. The "permeation theory" of breast cancer spread promulgated by W. S. Handley, in 1906, supported this concept.[84] Although the radical mastectomy certainly reduced the incidence of local recurrence profoundly, little evidence can be found that this resulted in an increased number of cures or, indeed, significantly prolonged survival.

After the early 1900s, the radical mastectomy was often supplemented with postoperative irradiation, particularly if the axillary lymph nodes were found to contain metastases and/or if the primary tumor was located in the medial half of the breast, where spread to internal mammary nodes was more likely. Although the operation tended to be employed as the sole treatment only for particularly favorable cases, i.e., small tumors arising in the lateral half of the breast with negative axillary nodes, it remained the standard initial therapy for "primary operable breast cancer" for eight decades. It resulted in 5-year relative survival rates of approximately 75 percent in stage I patients and 50 percent in stage II patients, and 10-year relative survival rates of approximately 70 percent for stage I and 40 percent for stage II patients.

For those who subscribed to the permeation theory of breast cancer spread, it soon became obvious that the radical mastectomy ignored the fact that the internal mammary nodes constitute one of the primary routes of lymphatic drainage of the breast. This fact led many surgeons to extend the conventional radical mastectomy to include resection of the ipsilateral internal mammary nodes. In addition, Halsted, Meyer, and others extended the operation to include dissection of the supraclavicular lymph nodes. Some surgeons even dissected mediastinal nodal groups.

Extended Radical Mastectomy

Of all the "supraradical," or extended radical, mastectomies which were devised, only that operation utilized by Urban, Sugarbaker, and others,[85,86] which removes the internal mammary nodal chain and an overlying portion of the chest wall en bloc with the radical mastectomy specimen, has ever been widely practiced. Enthusiasm for this procedure was engendered by reports of high incidences of unsuspected metastases to internal mammary nodes when such nodes were biopsied at the time of radical mastectomy. Handley and Thackray reported, in 1949, that when internal mammary node biopsies were performed in 50 unselected cases of breast cancer, metastases were found in 38 percent, ostensibly making them incurable by radical mastectomy.[87] In 1954, they reported on the results of internal mammary node biopsies in 250 patients.[88] They found a 44 percent incidence of positive internal mammary nodes in patients with inner hemisphere and central tumors and a 22 percent incidence of positivity in patients with outer hemisphere tumors. When the axillary nodes were negative, internal mammary nodes were rarely positive with outer half primary tumors, but some 10 percent of patients with inner hemisphere tumors were found to have involved internal mammary nodes. When the axillary nodes were positive, approximately one-third of patients with outer half primary lesions and almost two-thirds of patients with inner half lesions were shown to have involved internal mammary nodes.

Based on these findings it appeared logical to treat the internal mammary nodes either by surgical excision or by postoperative irradiation in patients who had inner hemisphere or central primary tumors and/or involved axillary nodes. Since only a few surgeons practiced the extended radical mastectomy, most such patients received postoperative radiation therapy.

At this point, it seems appropriate to discuss the following question before going on to discuss alternatives to the radical mastectomy based on lesser surgical procedures: Is either extended radical mastectomy (i.e., radical mastectomy plus internal mammary node dissection) or the addition of postoperative irradiation to the radical mastectomy superior to the radical mastectomy alone in terms of local control, disease-free survival, or overall survival for any subset or subsets of patients with clinical stage I or II breast cancer? In other words, are there subsets of patients for whom routine treatment of the internal mammary nodes, either by surgery or by radiation therapy, is beneficial? Several lines of evidence suggest that the answer to this question is no.

First it would appear that in spite of the relatively high frequency of occult microscopic involvement of internal mammary nodes noted when they are removed, a much smaller percentage of patients go on to develop clinical parasternal recurrences when the internal mammary nodes are left untreated. Donegan, in 1977, reported the latter incidence to be only 10 percent despite a 22 percent incidence of positive internal mammary node biopsies.[89] Moreover, it could not be demonstrated that positive internal mammary nodes increased chest wall recurrence or decreased survival independently of axillary nodal involvement, and the survival of five patients with internal mammary node involvement who were treated with postoperative irradiation or castration was not superior to that of 20 patients with untreated mammary nodal metastases. Veronesi and Valagussa have reported that only 49 percent of their patients treated by radical mastectomy developed clinically relevant internal mammary metastases despite a 20.5 percent incidence of occult microscopic involvement in a comparable group of patients treated by extended radical mastectomy.[90]

Second, the results of both prospective and retrospective studies indicate that the extended radical mastectomy has no survival advantage over the radical mastectomy even for patients with medial hemisphere primary tumors and/or positive axillary nodes. Although Urban and Morjani,[91] in 1971, reported a reduction in parasternal chest wall recurrences and Donegan,[92] in 1972, reported slightly fewer local recurrences when patients undergoing extended radical mastectomies were compared with "matched" patients undergoing radical mastectomy, overall survival was not improved. Moreover, a number of carefully performed retrospective analyses have failed to demonstrate a survival advantage in patients treated by the extended operation.[93]

Third, it appears doubtful that treatment of the internal mammary nodes by irradiation or surgery influences outcome. It has been well shown in a prospectively randomized clinical trial from Denmark that irradiating internal mammary and supraclavicular nodes is as efficacious as removing them.[94] Results from at least two large prospectively randomized clinical trials have indicated that irradiation of internal mammary (and supraclavicular) lymph nodes provides no advantage in disease-free survival or overall survival regardless of the location of the primary tumor and axillary nodal status.[95,96]

Finally, extended radical mastectomy has been compared directly to radical mastectomy in a prospectively randomized multinational clinical trial in which 1580 patients were randomized to receive either radical mastectomy or radical mastectomy plus internal mammary node dissection. No irradiation was given. The results of this study after 5 years of follow-up were reported by Lacour et al. in 1976.[97] In 1981, Veronesi and Valagussa reported on the 737 patients from this trial who were randomized at the Cancer Institute in Milan and for whom 10-year follow-up data was available.[90] Lacour et al. reported that after 5 years of observation, the survival rates of the two groups were statistically indistinguishable (69 percent vs. 72 percent). Of dubious significance was the observation that in one small subset of patients, those with T_1 and T_2 medial hemisphere tumors *and* positive axillary nodes, survival seemed to favor extended radical mastectomy (71 percent vs. 52 percent). However, a small advantage in survival was observed for radical mastectomy in patients with tumors of similar size arising in the lateral hemisphere and with negative axillary nodes (87 percent vs. 78 pecent). The results of the Milan experience, based on 10 years of observation, were much more clear-cut. No significant difference in either disease-free survival or overall survival was noted between the two groups. This was true for the groups as a whole and for all subsets of patients regardless of location of the primary tumor, tumor size, and/or axillary nodal status.[90]

In summary, it may be concluded that surgical removal of internal mammary (or supraclavicular) lymph nodes as part of primary therapy for breast cancer does not contribute appreciably to cure. Internal mammary node dissection may possibly reduce the incidence of parasternal chest wall recurrences, but this occurs very infrequently in any case and survival is not affected. An argument might be made for performing internal mammary node biopsies for staging in order to identify patients who are at high risk for recurrence and, therefore, candidates for adjuvant therapy. However, there is no evidence that this procedure would provide improved staging information over that obtained from pathologic examination of axillary lymph nodes. Finally, there appears to be no indication for routine treatment of internal mammary lymph nodes by surgery or irradiation even in patients with medial hemisphere primary tumors and/or positive axillary nodes.

Modified Radical Mastectomy

Modified radical mastectomies are operations which remove the entire breast and axillary contents en bloc while preserving the pectoralis major muscle. (The term *total mastectomy plus axillary dissection* is equally appropriate.) Two general types of modified radical mastectomy exist. They differ with respect to whether or not the pectoralis minor muscle is resected (the Patey procedure) or preserved (the Auchincloss-Madden procedure). The benefits to the patient from preservation of the pectoralis major are entirely cosmetic but significant. A normal contour and softness of the shoulder and anterolateral chest wall is preserved. The patient is left with a stronger arm. Serious lymphedema of the arm is less frequent, and breast reconstruction is greatly facilitated. In addition, placement of incisions are horizontal, resulting in scars which do not extend to the shoulder. These factors permit patients to wear a wider variety of clothing styles, including "low-cut" and "sleeveless" styles, without exposing the disfiguring sequelae of their operation.

It has been alleged, or rather assumed, by several prominent surgeons that preservation of the pectoralis minor muscle ipso facto results in a partial or incomplete axillary dissection, equating not removing the pectoralis minor muscle with not removing apical lymph nodes to the degree that would normally be accomplished if the pectoralis minor were removed.[93,98,99] Although this contention seems logical, I have been unable to find any data to support it. What few data exist are either inconclusive or tend to refute this contention. In 1975, Nemoto and Dao reported that the mean and median numbers of axillary nodes removed in the course of 121 consecutive radical mastectomies was the same as the mean and median numbers of axillary nodes removed during 111 consecutive modified radical mastectomies.[100] Unfortunately, the pectoralis minor muscle was neither removed nor preserved during the course of the modified radical mastectomies. It was divided. Therefore, this report fails to resolve the issue. In unpublished data from the National Surgical Adjuvant Breast Project (NSABP), the average number of axillary nodes removed during radical mastectomy (from protocol B-04) was the same as the average number of nodes removed during "total mastectomy plus axillary dissection" (from protocol B-06).[101] In the vast majority of these modified radical mastectomies, the pectoralis major muscles had been preserved.

Results obtained with the modified radical mastectomy reported in the late 1960s and early 1970s appeared comparable to those achieved with the radical mastectomy.[102-105] Gradually, and without the benefit of substantial scientific data, the modified radical mastectomy replaced the radical mastectomy as the "standard" treatment for clinical stage I and II breast cancer (and for some cases of stage III breast cancer) in the United States and in many foreign countries. This occurred despite the fact that *no prospectively randomized clinical trial had ever been reported comparing the two operations*. During the same period, several clinical trials were undertaken in order to study alternatives to the radical mastectomy, the then standard operation. By the time the results of most of these trials were published, indicating no difference in results of treatment, the modified radical mastectomy had become the new standard operation.

This dilemma is graphically illustrated in the rather complex figure of W. L. Donegan which is reproduced as Fig. 24-9. In it Dr. Donegan illustrates the various "clinical trials of different techniques of irradiation and surgery for carcinoma of the breast . . . all of which resulted in no significant difference in survival." Some trials studied extended operative procedures, more extensive in scope than the radical mastectomy; some studied lesser procedures; and some studied the addition

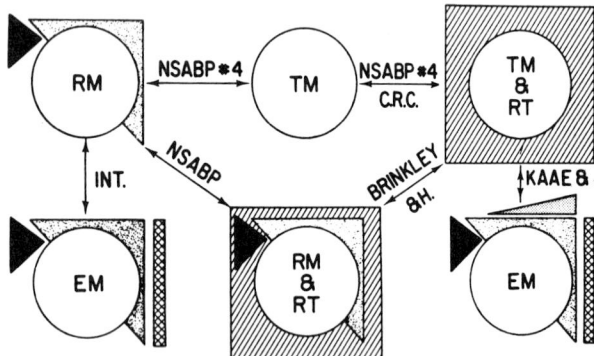

FIGURE 24-9 Illustrated are clinical trials of different techniques of irradiation and surgery for carcinoma of the breast, all of which included removal of the entire breast and all of which resulted in no significant differences in survival. The geometric figures represent anatomic structures that were treated. Diagonal crosshatches indicate irradiation of the chest wall and regional nodes; circles represent the breast; lightly shaded triangles indicate the pectoralis major and minor muscles; dark triangles represent removal of internal mammary lymph nodes; stippled triangles superior to the pectoralis muscles indicate removal of supraclavicular lymph nodes; NSABP = National Surgical Adjuvant Breast Project; CRC = Cancer Research Campaign; INT = the International Cooperative Study of Radical and Extended Mastectomy[90,97]; Kaae & J. = Kaae and Johansen;[94] Brinkley & H = Brinkley and Haybrittle[105]; RM = radical mastectomy; TM = total mastectomy; RT = radiation therapy; and EM = extended mastectomy. (*From WL Donegan: Staging methods, primary treatment options, and end results, in WL Donegan, JS Spratt (eds): Cancer of the Breast, (Saunders, Philadelphia, 1979.)*

of postoperative radiation therapy to mastectomy. *Note that the modified radical mastectomy does not appear* among the six forms of treatment which were studied. Therefore, while most workers in the field accept the modified radical mastectomy as providing results which are equivalent to those achieved with any of the other therapies depicted in the figure, this assumption has never been definitively proved. In fact, only a single randomized clinical trial has ever directly compared the modified radical mastectomy with the radical mastectomy, and the results of this trial conducted in the United Kingdom did not appear until 1981.[106] The results, as might be expected, showed no difference between the two treatments.

Total (Simple) Mastectomy with and without Radiation Therapy

As early as 1936, Grace and Moitrier reported that total (simple) mastectomy plus radiation therapy was an effective treatment for early stages of breast cancer.[106a] However, it remained for McWhirter, in the early 1960s, to champion combining total mastectomy plus postoperative irradiation as an alternative to the radical mastectomy.[107] Total mastectomy combined with irradiation of the regional lymph nodes is, in fact, no different from the radical mastectomy conceptually. It simply raises the question of whether nodal irradiation is as efficacious as surgical extirpation. The bulk of the evidence suggests that it certainly is.[105]

The question of whether or not total mastectomy *alone* is appropriate initial treatment for clinical stage I breast cancer (i.e., with clinically negative axillary nodes) is more interesting and fundamental. When applied to patients with clinically negative axillary lymph nodes, both the radical mastectomy and the modified radical mastectomy include prophylactic axillary lymphadenectomies. One might, and indeed should, question whether this approach is superior to performing delayed *therapeutic* axillary dissection only in that subset of patients who go on to develop clinically relevant axillary nodal involvement following no initial treatment to the axillary nodes. This addresses two basic questions of tumor biology: Will all patients in whom occult nodal metastases can be demonstrated on prophylactic lymphadenectomy proceed inevitably to develop clinically relevant nodal disease, and will their opportunity for cure be impaired if treatment to these nodes is delayed until nodal involvement is clinically evident?

In 1971, after almost a decade of planning, investigators from 34 institutions in the United States and Canada began participation in protocol B-04 of the National Surgical Adjuvant Breast Project (NSABP). This protocol, whose schema is presented in Fig. 24-10, compared alternative treatments for primary operable breast cancer with the radical mastectomy. The specific aims of the study were to determine, in patients with clinically negative axillary nodes, if total (simple) mastectomy is as effective as radical mastectomy (provided that patients undergoing total mastectomy who subsequently develop axillary nodal involvement have axillary dissection at that time), and whether total mastectomy plus postoperative regional irradiation is as effective as radical mastectomy or total mastectomy with delayed therapeutic axillary node dissection in patients who develop nodal involvement. In patients with clinically involved axillary nodes the primary aim was to ascertain whether total mastectomy with regional irradiation and radical mastectomy are equivalent treatments. As Fisher has pointed out, "This protocol does not compare total mastectomy alone with radical mastectomy," since patients having total mastectomy without regional irradiation who subsequently develop clinically apparent axillary node involvement have the nodes treated by axillary dissection at that time. The finding of such nodes does "not represent a treatment failure unless they cannot be removed." However, the occurrence of such nodes in patients receiving total mastectomy and radiation does represent a treatment failure."[108] No significant difference in disease-free survival (treatment failure) or survival has been noted between patients with clinically negative nodes treated by radical mastectomy and those treated by total mastectomy followed by postoperative regional irradiation; nor has a significant difference been observed between patients treated by radical mastectomy and patients treated by total mastectomy and delayed axillary dissection only if and when positive axillary nodes subsequently occurred. Similarly, no significant difference in disease-free survival or overall survival has been observed between patients with clinically positive nodes treated by radical mastectomy and those treated by total mastectomy followed by regional irradiation.[96,108]

The clinical course of those patients with clinically negative nodes who were treated initially with total mastectomy without regional irradiation is of special interest. Among those patients with clinically negative nodes who underwent radical mastectomy (and in whom, therefore, *histopathologic* staging of axillary nodes was

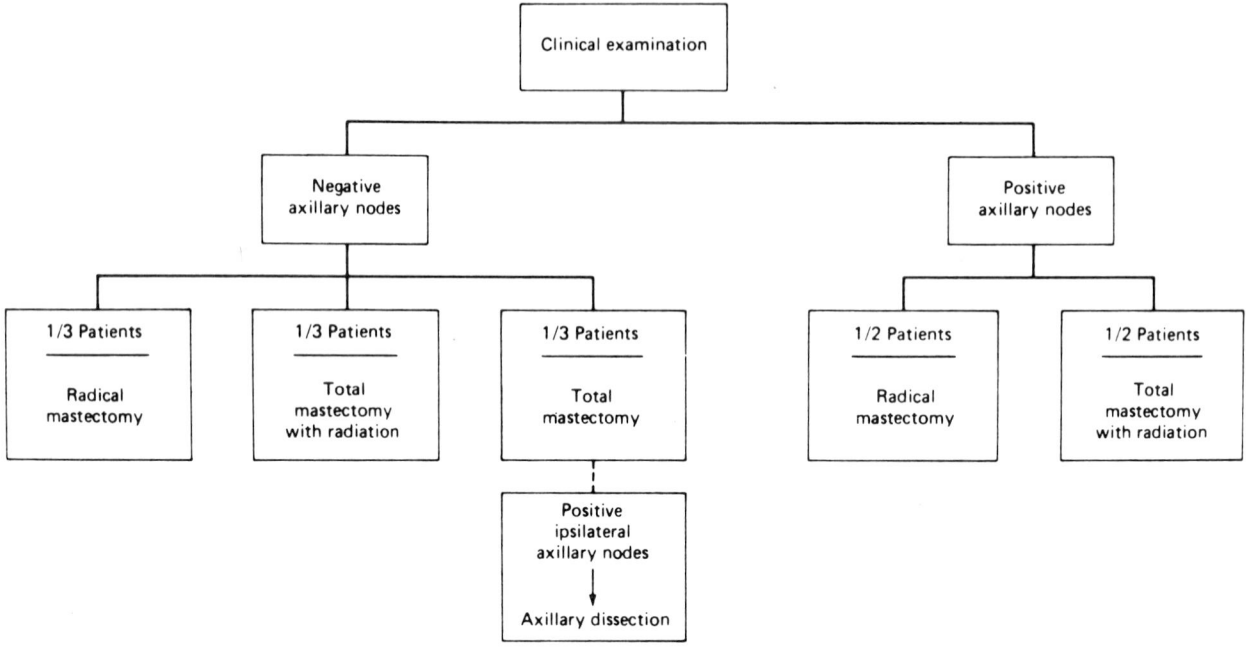

FIGURE 24-10 The schema of NSABP protocol B-04.

possible), 40 percent were found to have histologically positive nodes. Consequently, approximately 40 percent of those patients treated by total mastectomy alone could be expected to harbor occult metastases in axillary nodes which were neither removed nor irradiated. Yet, with a mean of 5 years of follow-up, only 15 percent of such patients developed clinically evident positive axillary nodes requiring axillary dissection. This finding reinforces the view that small tumor deposits in lymph nodes do not invariably assume clinical significance, and supports the concept that occult axillary nodal metastases need not be removed prophylactically, but may be removed therapeutically, at a later date, without loss of benefit. Moreover, it is apparent that failure to remove occult nodal metastases initially did not increase the incidence of distant metastases or the overall proportion of treatment failures. "Tertiary metastasis" from retained tumor deposits in nodes seems to be minimal and/or is inconsequential to the overall course of the disease.

One should also make note of the fact that the data from NSABP protocol B-04 indicate that preservation of clinically uninvolved lymph nodes did not *benefit* the patient, since some have suggested that immunologic host resistance might be impaired by removal of functioning regional lymph nodes, thereby accelerating the progress of the disease.[109] Patients in whom axillary nodes were preserved did not manifest a decreased incidence of treatment failure, as one might expect if the regional nodes made a clinically relevant contribution to host defense mechanisms.

Results from another recent clinical trial confirm that prophylactic treatment of regional lymph nodes (by irradiation in this case) does not affect survival or tumor dissemination, although it does prevent subsequent progressive tumor growth in those nodes. This multicenter, international trial was conducted under the auspices of the Cancer Research Campaign between 1970 and 1975, and was coordinated at King's College Hospital in London. Patients with clinical stages I and II breast cancer were randomized between two treatment arms: total (simple) mastectomy alone or simple mastectomy followed by regional irradiation.[110] After 5 years of follow-up, there were no differences in survival or in the incidence of dissemination between the two treatment arms. This was true for both stage I patients and stage II patients. Loco-regional recurrences occurred more frequently in both stage I and stage II patients when postoperative irradiation was withheld. However, 70 percent of recurrences were successfully controlled by additional treatment.

In summary, it is apparent that surgical removal and radiation therapy are equally effective in controlling the growth of breast cancer in axillary lymph nodes. Prophylactic treatment, by either modality, of clinically uninvolved axillary nodes does not improve disease-free survival or overall survival, but does prevent subsequent development of clinically apparent nodal disease in a subset of patients. Whether or not one should treat all clinical stage I patients prophylactically in order to spare some patients a "second bout of treatment" seems to be a moot question. Delayed treatment of axillary nodal metastases by either method seems neither to enhance nor to jeopardize chances for cure. The fact that a disproportionate number of treatment failures in the total mastectomy group of NSABP protocol B-04 occurred in those patients who subsequently required axillary dissection supports the position that involved axillary lymph nodes are not the predecessor or cause of distant spread of tumor but are rather an indicator or manifestation of diseminated disease.[108] However, in recent years, the need to remove axillary lymph nodes, whether clinically positive or negative, in order to obtain material for accurate histopathologic staging of breast cancer so that appropriate adjuvant therapy may be instituted (see below) where indicated has superseded all of the above considerations. Axillary dissections, even in clinically negative node patients, are now routinely performed for staging purposes rather than because of any therapeutic imperatives, and irradiation of axillary nodes (as opposed to their removal) has been abandoned, since this precludes histopathologic staging.

Segmental Mastectomy

All of the surgical procedures for the treatment of primary operable breast cancer discussed heretofore have one facet in common—total mastectomy, i.e., removal of the entire breast including the nipple-areola complex. Therefore, despite variations in the total extent of the overall operative procedure, the impact on the patient and her self-image is not radically dissimilar—total breast loss has invariably resulted. Since "prophylactic" treatment of clinically uninvolved axillary lymph nodes appears to be unnecessary and since treatment of lymph nodes by irradiation appears to be equivalent to surgical excision, it seems appropriate to ask the following two questions: (1) Is "prophylactic" treatment of clinically uninvolved breast tissue necessary or advantageous in the initial management of early primary breast cancer? (2) Is irradiation of clinically uninvolved breast tissue equivalent to surgical removal, i.e., mastectomy? In other words, is total mastectomy the essential sine qua non of all treatment schemes for invasive breast cancer, or is excision without sacrifice of the entire breast, with or without irradiation to the retained breast, an acceptable alternative, at least for women with relatively small primary tumors? Is it feasible to treat women for breast cancer and, at the same time, preserve a cosmetically acceptable breast?

In the nineteenth century, local excision of breast cancers usually failed to cure and was associated with a very high incidence of local treatment failure. However, at that time most patients presented with large tumors, and irradiation was not yet available. It seemed entirely reasonable to a number of investigators to reevaluate conservative surgery in the twentieth century. Local excision of primary breast cancers has been referred to as *lumpectomy, tumorectomy,* or *tylectomy* (from the Greek word *tylow,* which means lump). Operations which remove the primary tumor together with some surrounding normal breast parenchyma and, usually, a small amount of overlying skin have been termed *partial mastectomy, sector mastectomy, extended tylectomy,* or *segmental mastectomy.* We prefer the latter term and shall employ it whenever possible. (These operations are *not* similar to *quadrantectomy,* "the aim of which is the radical removal of the entire quadrant of the breast containing the primary carcinoma (together with) the overlying skin and fascia of the major pectoral muscle."[111]

Initially, segmental mastectomy was performed primarily in older patients, in patients with serious coexisting systemic diseases, or, occasionally, in women who refused mastectomy. Adair et al. reporting on the results of treating 1419 patients with breast cancer reviewed 63 cases of "local removal" and found results so good that they took pains to try to explain them away.[112] In 1964, Porritt reported retrospectively on a 12-year experience comparing 107 patients treated by segmental mastectomy plus radiation therapy when axillary nodes were involved with 156 patients treated by radical mastectomy.[113] At both 5 and 10 years, survival after segmental mastectomy was *greater* than survival following radical mastectomy, (65 percent vs. 50 percent at 5 years and 45 percent vs. 34 percent at 10 years). However, these differences were not statistically significant. In 1971, Taylor et al. reported a series of 77 patients treated by "sector mastectomy" plus postoperative radiation therapy to the breast and axilla with favorable 5- and 10-year survival statistics.[114] In the United States, the champion of segmental mastectomy was George Crile, Jr., who, in 1955 began performing partial mastectomies on carefully selected patients at the Cleveland Clinic.[115] Between 1957 and 1972, 160 patients with invasive breast cancer underwent partial mastectomy at the Cleveland Clinic.[116] Of these, 115 patients underwent segmental mastectomy without axillary dissection or axillary irradiation. Of the total group, 75 percent survived 5 years and 45 percent survived 10 years. Among the 115 patients who had no treatment to the axilla, lymph node metastases developed in only 8 patients (7.9 percent). These patients were then treated with axillary dissection or nodal irradiation. Eight patients (7.9 percent) developed cancer in the ipsilateral breast and underwent total mastectomy.[117]

The first randomized clinical trial of partial mastectomy was initiated in 1961 at Guy's Hospital in London.[118] Between 1961 and 1971, 370 women aged 50 years or over with clinical stage I and II breast cancer were randomized so as to receive either wide local excision (partial mastectomy) or radical mastectomy. All patients received postoperative radiation therapy to regional lymphatics at a relatively small dose (2500 to 2700 rads) which would not be considered adequate by today's standards. In addition, patients treated by partial mastectomy received 3500 to 3800 rads of postoperative radiation therapy to the breast. Prior to 1969, all patients also received three doses of thiotepa. While wide local excision plus 3800 rads was associated with a higher incidence of locoregional recurrences, primarily in axillary nodes, there were no statistically significant differences between the two treatment groups in 5-year or 10-year survival rates.[119] However, in clinical stage II patients, limited surgery plus limited radiation therapy was associated with inferior survival as well as increased local recurrences, presumably due to inadequately treated axillary nodal metastases.

In 1976, the NSABP initiated a prospectively randomized clinical trial of segmental mastectomy (with and without breast irradiation). The schema for this trial NSABP protocol B-06 is presented in Fig. 24-11. Before discussing the protocol in some detail, a few comments relating to the study design are in order.

The results of both NSABP protocol B-04 and the Cancer Research Campaign of Great Britain trial,[110,120]

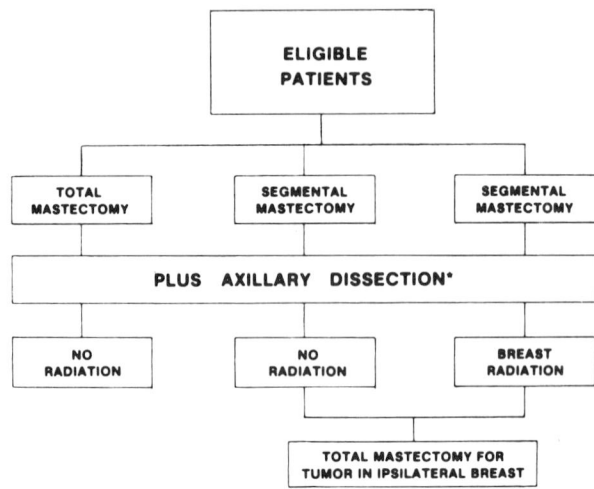

FIGURE 24-11 Schema for NSABP protocol B-06. *Patients with one or more histologically positive axillary nodes receive adjuvant chemotherapy consisting of L-PAM plus 5-FU.

discussed in the last section, had indicated that prophylactic treatment of the axilla was not necessary in clinically negative node patients. However, in the mid 1970s it became apparent that adjuvant chemotherapy was beneficial in at least some, if not all, patients with histologically positive axillary lymph nodes. Therefore, it became appropriate to include an axillary dissection for all patients *as a staging procedure* and to administer adjuvant chemotherapy to those patients found to have one or more histologically positive axillary nodes. This feature of the study design also made it possible to include clinical stage II patients in the trial. Furthermore, in the intervening years between the design of protocol B-04 and protocol B-06, the modified radical mastectomy (total mastectomy plus axillary dissection) had replaced the radical mastectomy as the "standard" treatment for stage I and II breast cancer. It is the former operation that constitutes the "control" or "standard therapy" arm of protocol B-06.

It is important to note that the only difference between the three treatment arms is the treatment of the breast itself. All patients undergo axillary dissection, and all patients with histologically positive nodes receive the same chemotherapy. Eligible patients must have a primary tumor no more than 4 cm in its greatest transverse diameter and must have a favorable tumor size-to-breast size ratio. In addition, the primary tumor must be so located as to permit sparing of the nipple-areola complex. Fixation to the underlying muscle fascia or skin involvement must be absent, as must other "grave signs." Eligible patients are then randomly assigned to receive total mastectomy, segmental mastectomy without postoperative irradiation to the breast, or segmental mastectomy followed, within 6 weeks, by external-beam radiation therapy, using high-energy equipment, consisting of 5000 rads to the entire breast over 5 weeks. All patients found to have one or more positive axillary nodes receive L-phenylalanine mustard (L-PAM) and 5-fluorouracil (5-FU) for 2 years. Patients in the two segmental mastectomy arms who subsequently develop a new occurrence of cancer (either a recurrence or a new primary) within the ipsilateral breast, proven by biopsy, undergo total mastectomy at that time.

One of the important aspects of the design of this trial is that it will answer certain fundamental questions concerning the multicentricity of breast cancer. One of the arguments for total mastectomy as the primary treatment for invasive breast cancer has been the risk of subsequently developing new primary breast cancers. Yet there is substantial evidence that this risk is to a large extent *bilateral*, and few advocates of total mastectomy have advised bilateral total mastectomy as treatment for cancer of one breast. Crile, who followed 132 patients treated by segmental mastectomy for an average period of 5 years, found 4 new primary cancers arising in the ipsilateral breast and 6 in the contralateral breast.[121]

At the time of this writing, almost 1500 patients have entered the trial since June, 1976. Although, no data is available at the present time, "findings to date provide no evidence for not continuing the trial, since ... no undesirable consequences have been noted:[122] Cosmetic results in patients undergoing segmental mastectomy have been, by and large, good to excellent (see Figs. 24-12 to 24-15).

Another important trial of partial mastectomy is that of the National Cancer Institute of Milan.[111,123] It differs from the NSABP trial in a number of important ways. From 1973 to 1980, patients with clinical stage I breast cancers less than 2 cm in diameter and with no palpable axillary lymph nodes (T_1, N_0, M_0) were randomized to receive either radical mastectomy or quadrantectomy (described above) with axillary dissection and postoperative radiotherapy consisting of 5000 rads to the ipsilateral residual breast tissue and a "boost" of 1000 rads to the skin surrounding the scar. The axillary dissection was performed en bloc with the quadrantectomy for tumors in the upper quadrants and through a separate incision for tumors in the lower quadrants. (In the NSABP trial axillary dissection is always performed in discontinuity, through a separate incision, except for primary tumors in the axillary tail of the breast.) Patients with positive axillary lymph nodes in the quadrantectomy group were further randomized to receive either additional radiotherapy (4000 to 4500 rads) to the supraclavicular and internal mammary node areas or no additional radiotherapy. In January, 1976, the protocol was changed so that all patients with positive nodes received adjuvant chemotherapy with cytoxan, methotrexate, and 5-fluorouracil (CMF) for 1 year. From 1976 to 1980, nodal radiotherapy was no longer utilized. A total of 701 patients were entered between 1973 and 1980. No differences in disease-free survival or overall survival were noted between the two groups.[111]

It is important to remember that this trial was limited to a small subset of breast cancer patients with very small primary tumors and clinically negative axillary nodes. Such patients constitute no more than 10 to 15 percent of all patients who present with primary breast cancer. Moreover, quadrantectomy involves removal of substantially more breast tissue and skin than does segmental mastectomy, and is, therefore, a less attractive procedure from a cosmetic point of view. Furthermore, all patients received postoperative radiation therapy. Nonetheless, this is an important study with far-reaching implications.

PRIMARY RADIATION THERAPY FOR INVASIVE BREAST CANCER

Coincident with and in parallel with attempts to reduce the scope of primary surgical therapy, increasing attention has been paid to replacing surgical excision with irradiation. Enthusiasm for primary radiation therapy is based on the laudable goal of preserving structure and function which surgery ablates; specifically, in the case of breast cancer, the preservation of a cosmetically acceptable breast. This is the same goal which is being pursued in NSABP protocol B-06. Just as many schemes for "primary surgical therapy" include some radiation therapy, so all schemes for "primary radiation therapy" involve varying amounts of surgery. The difference is one of emphasis, or the degree to which irradiation is used to replace surgical removal.

The pioneering work of McWhirter, from Edinburgh, which began in 1941, had suggested that, at least with

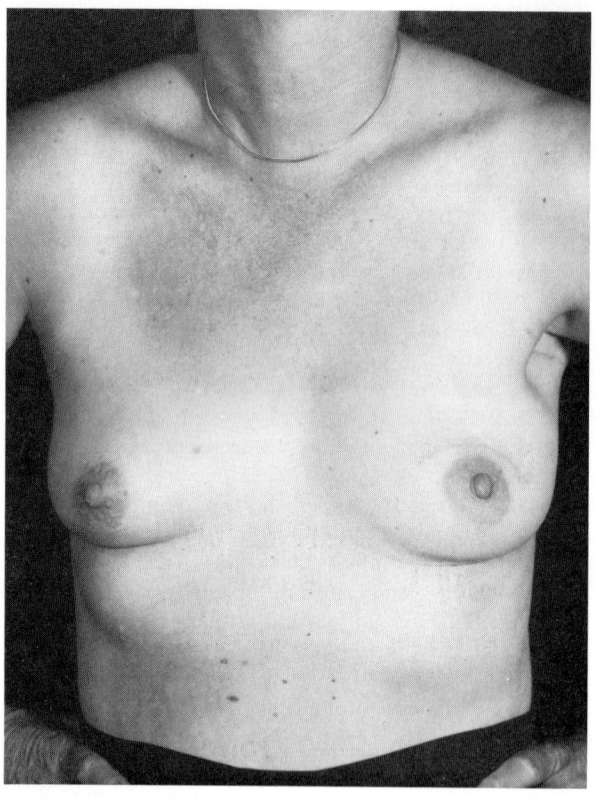 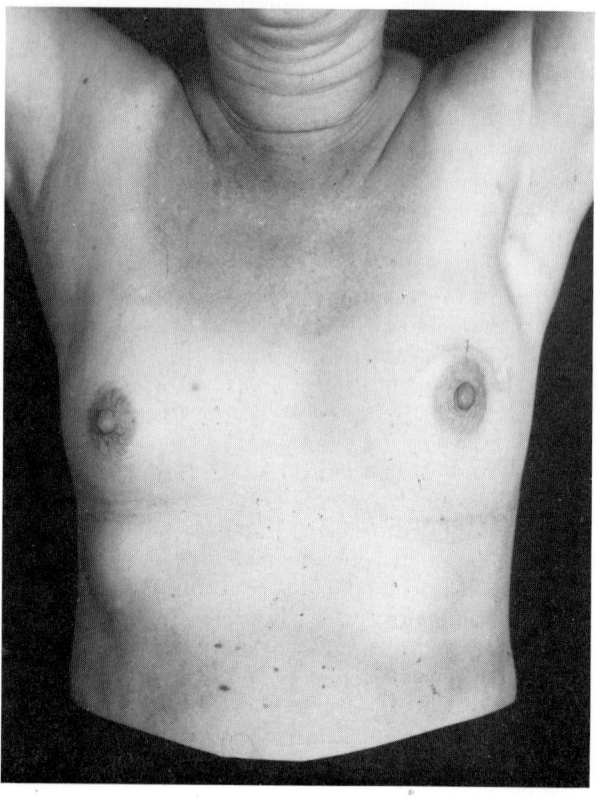

FIGURE 24-12(a) and (b) Two frontal views of a patient who underwent segmental mastectomy and axillary dissection without breast irradiation on NSABP protocol B-06 3 months before these photographs were obtained.

respect to treatment of regional lymph nodes, the therapeutic efficacy of surgical excision and irradiation appeared equivalent.[124] Beginning around the same time, Mustakillo, from Helsinki, employed simple excision of primary tumors followed by irradiation as primary therapy for patients with clinical stage I breast cancer.[125] The radiation therapy he employed, using 180- to 250-kilovolt equipment, would be considered inadequate by today's standards, i.e., 2100 rads in six fractions. Although 20 percent of his patients developed locoregional recurrences within 10 years, he reported a 5-year survival rate of 79 percent and a 10-year survival rate of 61 percent. At around the same time, Peters, from Toronto, began treating patients with T_1 or T_2, N_0, M_0 breast cancer with simple excision plus radiation therapy.[126] Between 1939 and 1969, she treated 217 patients in this manner. When these patients were "matched" with similar patients treated at the same hospital by radical mastectomy, overall survival was found to be similar for both groups with follow-up periods of up to 30 years.

With the development of megavoltage radiotherapy equipment, efforts at primary radiation therapy intensified. Pierquin and his colleagues, in France, began treating clinical stage I and II breast cancer patients with external-beam radiotherapy in 1960, and, in 1976, reported excellent results in 310 patients followed for periods of 3 and 5 years.[127] Results of the Guy's Hospital trial (discussed earlier) further stimulated interest in treatment methods based on primary radiation therapy with breast preservation, and other reports of the results of primary radiation therapy, both from the United States and abroad, followed in the mid 1960s.[128–131]

However, it was Hellman and his group at the Joint Center for Radiation Therapy at Harvard Medical School, who most profoundly influenced the acceptance of primary radiation therapy by radiation oncologists in the United States.[132–134] (Why he and his particular technique for primary radiation therapy achieved such unique approbation, I cannot state with assurance.)

In July, 1968, Hellman and his group began treating patients with T_{1-3}, N_{0-1}, M_0 breast cancer with primary radiation therapy. Local control in patients with T_3 tumors was found to be poor, and later in their study such patients were usually excluded. In some instances, excisional biopsy was performed; in others, incisional or needle biopsy was utilized to establish the diagnosis. Axillary dissection was not performed. The technique of radiation therapy "gradually evolved" over the course of their series. During the later years of their experience, "a small low axillary incision to sample axillary nodes in premenopausal women to aid in determining the need for adjuvant chemotherapy" was employed.[135]

Between July, 1968, and December, 1976, Hellman and his group treated 135 clinical stage I and II breast cancers in 129 patients (6 women had bilateral breast cancers). Of the 135 breasts treated, 118 tumors had been removed by excisional biopsy, while 17 had incisional or needle biopsies. In those patients undergoing excisional biopsy, no attempt was made to achieve wide excision, and the volume of tissue removed was "kept to the minimum necessary for gross excision of the mass." External-beam radiotherapy was then administered to the breast and regional lymph nodes. The dose was usually 5000 rads, but ranged from 4000 to 6300 rads.

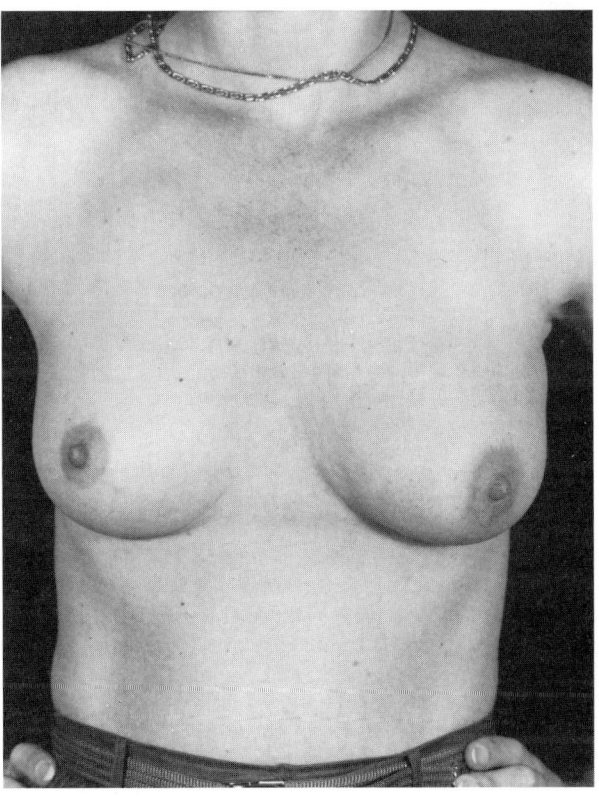
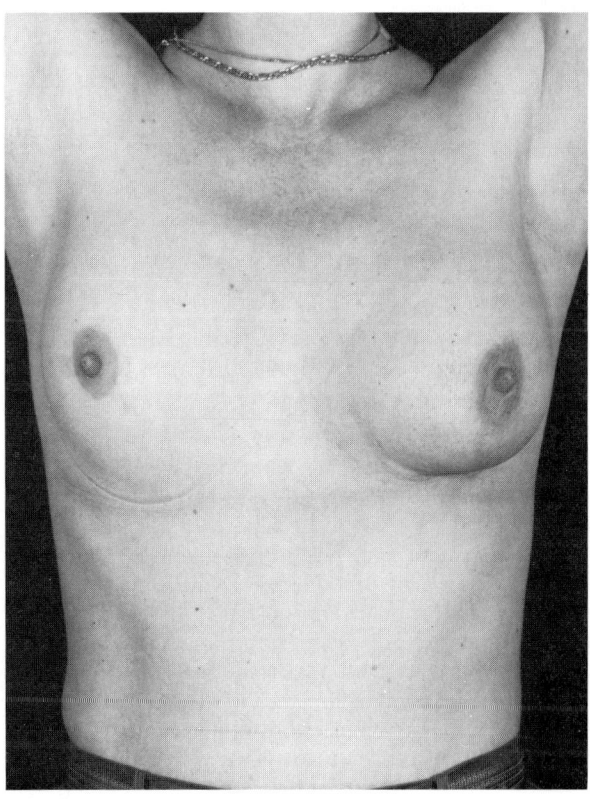

a *b*

FIGURE 24-13(a) and (b) Two frontal views of a patient who underwent segmental mastectomy, axillary dissection, and breast irradiation on NSABP protocol B-06 3 months before these photographs were obtained.

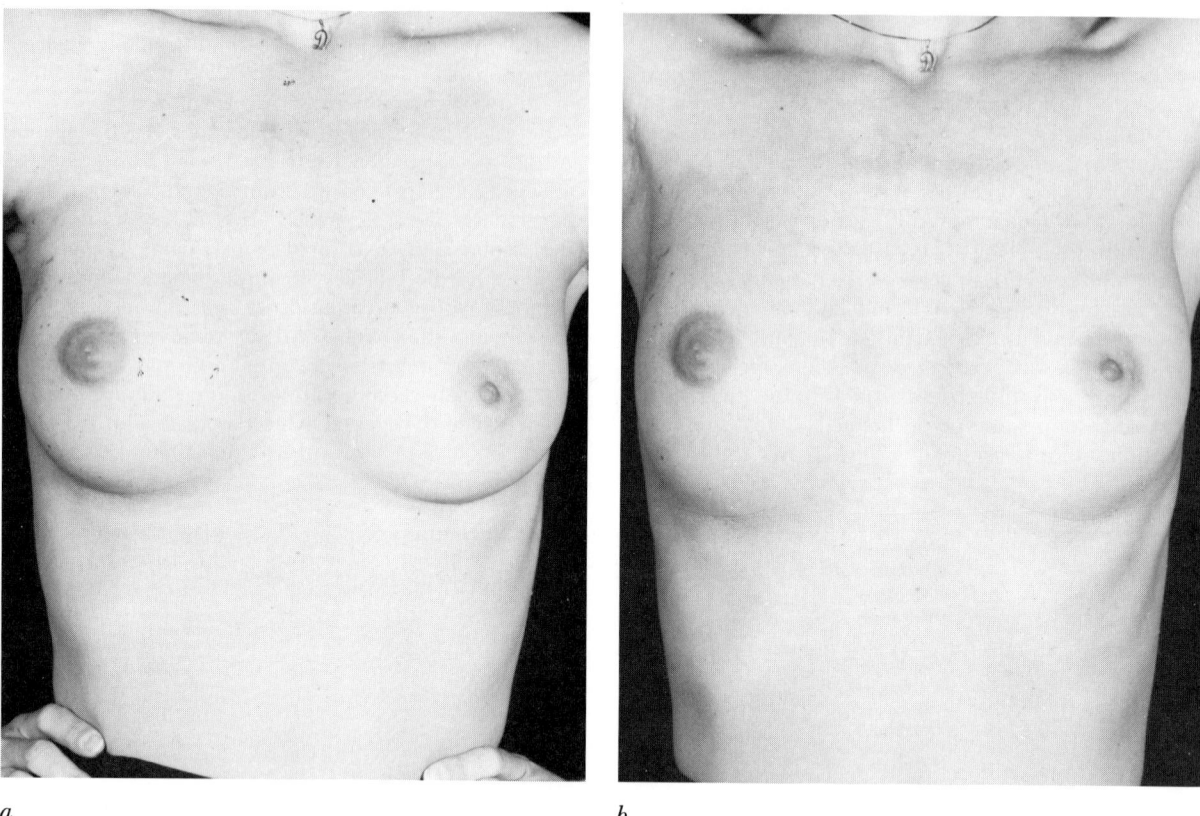

FIGURE 24-14(a) and (b)   Two frontal views of a patient who underwent segmental mastectomy, axillary dissection, and breast irradiation on NSABP protocol B-06 3 months before these photographs were obtained.

In 32 of the patients, an interstitial implant of the primary tumor or "tumor bed" was also performed using iridium.[192] At the time of the reports of 1977 and 1978, only seven patients had local recurrences (1 of 47 tumors in stage I and 6 of 88 tumors in stage II), and results reported as "cumulative probability of local control" were impressive, i.e., 94 percent for stage I and 86 percent for stage II. All recurrences were in the breast. "Actuarial likelihood of survival" was equally impressive, i.e., 91 percent for stage I and 66 percent for stage II. When local recurrence was analyzed in relation to biopsy procedure and interstitial implantation, it was noted that 4 percent of patients undergoing incisional biopsy recurred locally, as opposed to 18 percent of patients in whom incisional or needle biopsy had been performed ($p < .05$). None of the 32 patients treated with interstitial implants recurred locally, whereas 7 percent of patients who were not implanted recurred. As of 1978, "this difference (had) not reached statistical significance, but since patients with greater likelihood of local recurrence were implanted, this difference (was) felt to be of importance."[134] Based on these data and data from 49 additional patients treated after 1976, Hellman, in 1980, recommended the treatment regimen outlined in Table 24-6.

Unfortunately, none of the studies of primary radiation therapy methods include controls treated by "standard" surgical techniques. Therefore, claims of comparable efficacy are difficult to substantiate. Criteria for patient selection are not uniform and, even within a single series, patients have not been treated in an identical manner. The absence of good staging information on

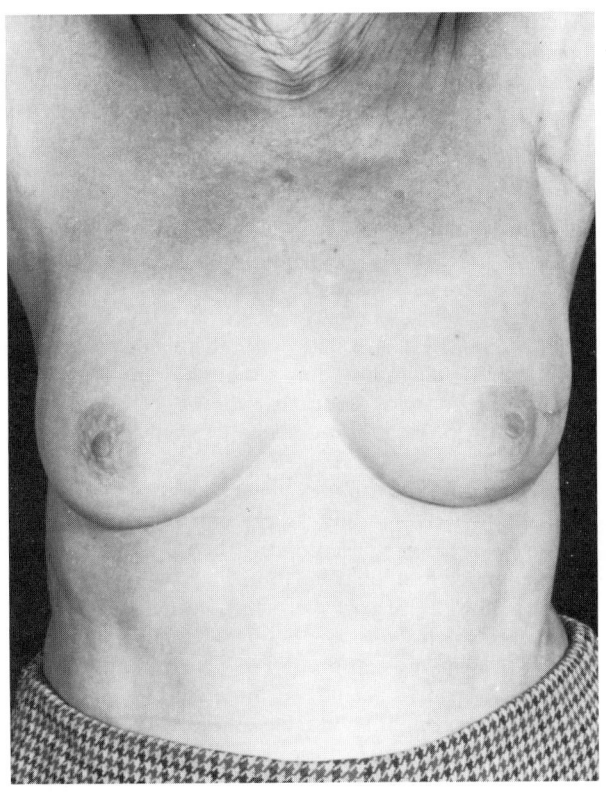 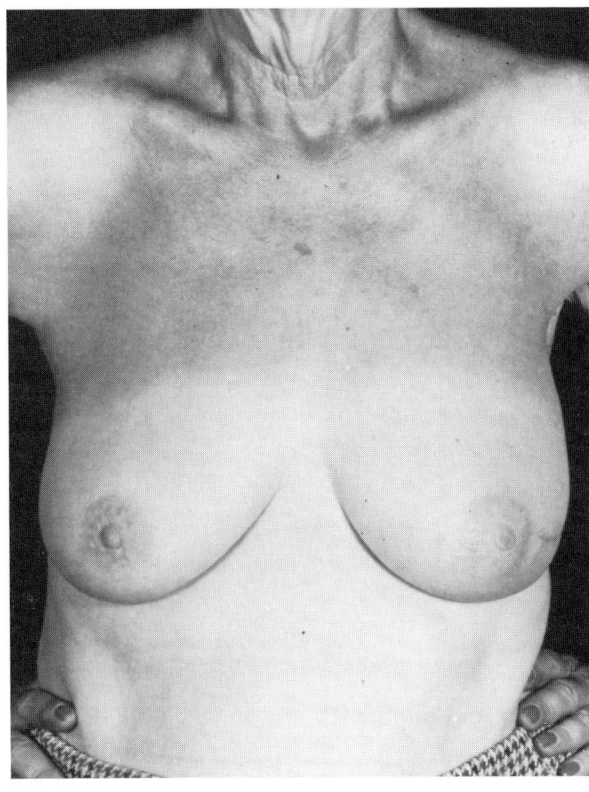

FIGURE 24-15(a) and (b) Two frontal views of a patient who underwent segmental mastectomy and axillary dissection without breast irradiation on NSABP protocol B-06 3 months before these photographs were obtained.

axillary nodal status prevents careful analysis of the recurrence risk factors of patients in these studies. Unless complete axillary dissections are performed routinely, such data will not become available in the future. The need for an interstitial implant in all patients has not yet been definitely established. Several series in which implants have not been employed, report results comparable to Hellman's. Clearly, a rigidly controlled randomized clinical trial comparing the therapeutic regimen outlined in Table 24-6 with "standard" surgical therapy, i.e., modified radical mastectomy, is vital before this form of treatment can be recommended routinely. Such a trial is presently underway at the surgery branch of the National Cancer Institute, and, hopefully, will yield much valuable information. Clearly, cosmetic results are very good (see Figs. 24-16a and b). However, cosmetic results

TABLE 24-6 Current Cancer of the Breast Treatment Program at the Joint Center for Radiation Therapy

Surgery	Tumor excision; determination of estrogen receptor status; axillary sampling
External radiation	4600 rads over 4.5–5 3 wks to breast, axilla, and internal mammary lymph nodes; 4-MeV linear accelerator; no bolus; compensating filters; no field overlap; fraction size, 200 rads or less
Interstitial radiation	Afterloading ^{192}Ir implant; 2200 rads to target volume at 35–40 rads/h

SOURCE: S Helman: Improving the therapeutic index in breast cancer treatment. *Cancer Res* 40:4335, 1980.

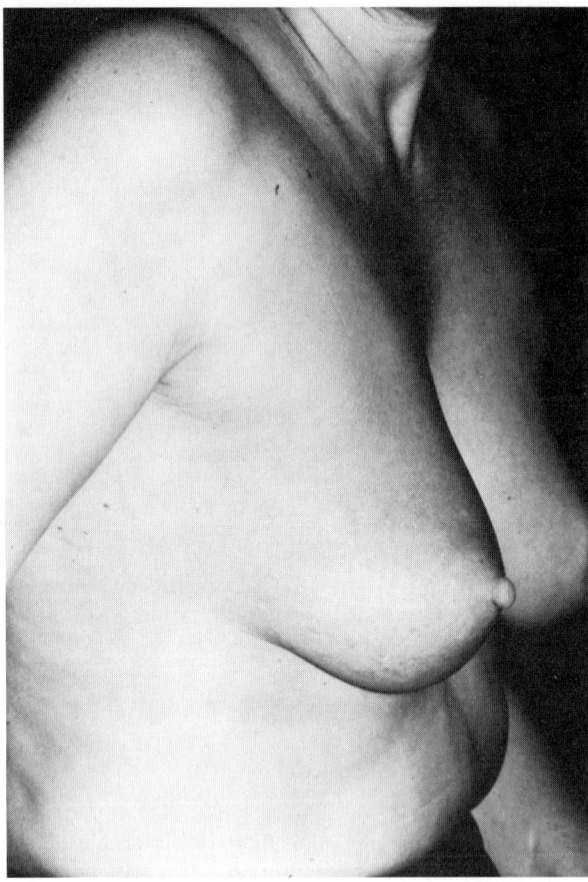

FIGURE 24-16(a) Patient treated according to the method of Hellman at the University of California San Diego Medical Center. (*Courtesy of J. Utley.*)

obtained with segmental mastectomy with or without breast irradiation are comparable (see Figs. 24-12 to 24-15). If either of these approaches to the treatment of breast cancer with breast preservation is proved to be equivalently efficacious to "standard" surgical therapy, the days of the modified radical mastectomy may be numbered.

ADJUVANT THERAPY

Strictly speaking, adjuvant therapy refers to adjunctive therapy, usually employing a different treatment modality, given to a patient in addition to the main or primary treatment regimen in the hopes of improving disease-free survival and overall survival over and above that obtainable with primary treatment alone. However, primary treatment remains the sine qua non of the therapeutic regimen. Adjuvant therapy is desirable in patients in whom the risk of recurrence after primary treatment alone is high. Although adjunctive radiotherapy and endocrine ablation (usually following radical mastectomy) were studied in the adjuvant setting in the 1950s, these trials failed to improve results and will not be reviewed here. We shall concentrate on modern trials of adjuvant chemotherapy, although some of the programs also employ endocrine therapy or even immunotherapy in the adjuvant setting. Usually, the latter two types of agents are combined with chemotherapy rather than being used as single agents.

Early trials of adjuvant chemotherapy in operable breast cancer were based on the theory that tumor cells, disseminated into the circulation from the primary tumor at the time of surgery, were responsible for the subsequent development of distant metastases. Therefore, chemotherapy was administered only for a few doses in the perioperative period. In these studies single agents rather than combination chemotherapy were employed. The most notable of these early trials was that of the NSABP, in which thiotepa was administered at the time of operation and for 2 days postoperatively to one group of patients undergoing radical mastectomy, while a second group of patients was treated with surgery only. Although disease-free survival and overall survival was not different between the two groups as a whole, analysis of subsets of patients revealed that the administration of thiotepa led to a reduction in recurrences and improved survival in premenopausal patients with four or more positive axillary nodes.[136] Another trial from Scandinavia demonstrated improved survival following a few doses of cyclophosphamide given postoperatively.[137]

In more recent trials, the circulating tumor cell concept has been abandoned in favor of the assumption that occult metastases already exist in many patients at the time of diagnosis and require prolonged and intensive treatment. Furthermore, therapy has been planned recognizing that cytotoxic drugs act by first-order kinetics, i.e., a certain proportion of cells are killed by a single dose of chemotherapy, following which regrowth may occur. Therefore, chemotherapy should be given intermittently, in full doses, for prolonged periods, allowing for bone marrow recovery between courses.

In 1972, a clinical trial was initiated by the NSABP

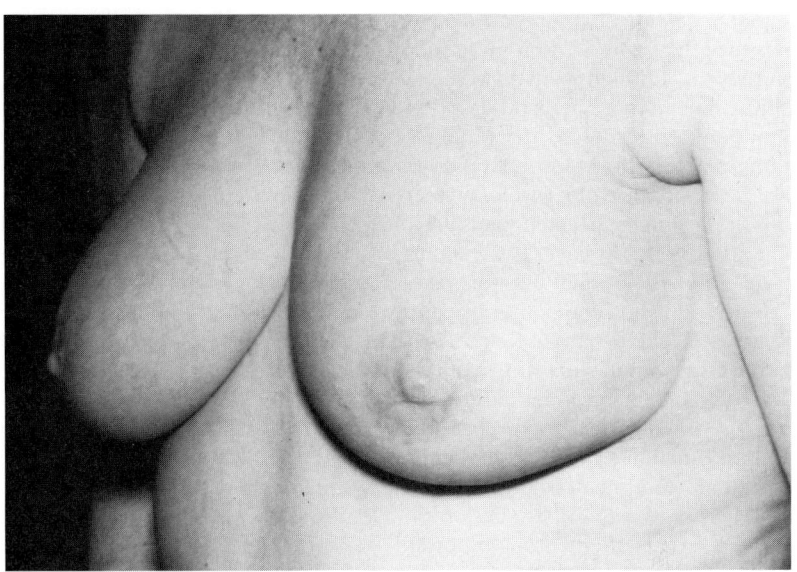

FIGURE 24-16(b) Patient treated according to the method of Hellman at the University of California San Diego Medical Center. (*Courtesy of J. Utley.*)

(protocol B-05) in cooperation with the Eastern Cooperative Group. Women treated by radical mastectomy or modified radical mastectomy and found to have one or more histologically positive axillary nodes were randomized to receive either a placebo or L-phenylalanine mustard (L-PAM) orally for 5 days every 6 weeks for 2 years. Preliminary results of this trial showed a significant improvement in disease-free survival in the group receiving L-PAM ($p = .01$).[138] This benefit was largely confined to premenopausal women (age less than 50 years), in whom treatment failures were markedly reduced by L-PAM ($p = .008$). A similar trend was noted in postmenopausal women, but the difference was not statistically significant. Later analyses indicated that only premenopausal patients with one to three involved axillary nodes experienced a diminished rate of recurrence on L-PAM. No significant benefit occurred in postmenopausal women (age 50 or older) or in premenopausal women with 4 or more positive axillary nodes.[139,140]

In 1973, Bonadonna and his group at the Instituto Nationale Tumori of Milan initiated an adjuvant therapy trial employing combination chemotherapy with cytoxan, methotrexate, and 5-fluorouracil (CMF). The criteria for entry into the study were the same as those for NSABP protocol B-05, i.e., one or more histologically positive nodes at the time of surgery. (In the Milan study, all patients were treated with radical mastectomy.) The rationale for electing to employ CMF in a trial of adjuvant therapy was based on its success in the therapy of advanced disease, and the dosage schedule was the same as that employed for the treatment of advanced disease, except that after the first year of the trial, a reduced dosage schedule was instituted in patients over 65 years of age in order to reduce toxicity. Chemotherapy was continued for 12 cycles lasting 1 year.[141] A striking reduction in recurrence rate was noted in patients receiving CMF. Like the NSABP trial, this benefit appeared to be confined to premenopausal women ($p < .0001$), and no significant benefit was observed in postmenopausal patients. However, unlike the NSABP L-PAM trial, this benefit was observed in premenopausal patients with four or more positive nodes as well as in those with one to three positive nodes.[141,142] In a subsequent study restricted to premenopausal women, 6 cycles of CMF (6 months) was compared to the previous 12 cycles (12 months). Although the relapse rate using 12 cycles of CMF was slightly less than that observed using 6 cycles, this difference was not significant ($p = .25$), suggesting that 6 cycles of CMF was probably as effective as 12 cycles.[143]

Recently, Bonadonna and his group have performed a retrospective analysis of the importance of administering the full dose of CMF.[144] This analysis revealed a clear dose-response relationship indicating that the CMF regimen was effective only at near-full doses, i.e., ≥85 percent of full dose. When these full doses were administered to postmenopausal women, the results were comparable to those observed in premenopausal women. Bonadonna interpreted the failure of CMF to achieve significant benefit in postmenopausal women to the fact that fewer of these older women received full doses than did the younger premenopausal women. (Remember that after the first year of the trial, his protocol specified lower doses for women over 65 years of age.)

Since adjuvant chemotherapy appeared to be more effective in premenopausal women than in postmenopausal women and since approximately half of premenopausal patients receiving adjuvant chemotherapy developed amenorrhea, it was presumed that decreased ovarian function as a result of chemotherapy ("chemical castration") might be responsible for the finding. In both the Milan and NSABP studies, review of the data has suggested that "there is an important trend but not a significant correlation between incidence of relapse and drug-induced amenorrhea."[143] It is likely that while ovarian suppression may account for some of the adjuvant chemotherapeutic effect in premenopausal women, other factors could well be responsible for some or much of the effect.[140]

After completion of the L-PAM trial (protocol B-05) evaluating the effectiveness of a single agent, the NSABP proceeded to implement two additional sequential protocols to evaluate the efficacy of chemotherapeutic regimens involving combinations of two or three drugs.[145] The first, protocol B-07, compared L-PAM with L-PAM plus 5-FU (PF), and the second, protocol B-08, compared PF with L-PAM, 5-FU, and methotrexate (PMF). As in protocol B-05, chemotherapy was administered for 2 years. Results from protocol B-05 suggest that PF is superior to L-PAM alone and benefits both premenopausal and postmenopausal women. In premenopausal patients, both those with four or more as well as those with one to three positive nodes achieved significant benefit. Among postmenopausal patients, those with four or more positive nodes benefited significantly from PF. However, the difference in disease-free survival between women receiving L-PAM and those receiving PF was not significant for postmenopausal women with one to three positive nodes. Early results from protocol B-08 suggest that, at least for most patients, the addition of a third drug (PMF) did not significantly improve results over those obtainable with the two-drug, PF, combination.

Protocol B-09 of the NSABP studied the possibility that the addition of tamoxifen to L-PAM plus 5-FU (PF) would enhance the benefit observed with those two drugs and compared PF with PF plus tamoxifen. Results of this trial at 2 years of follow-up have recently been published.[146] Recurrences were reduced at 2 years in patients receiving PF plus tamoxifen whose tumor estrogen and progesterone receptor levels were ≥10 fmol/mg cytosol protein. Among patients 50 years of age or older, treatment failure was significantly reduced ($p < .001$): by 51 percent in those with 1 to 3 positive nodes and by 64 percent in those with 4 or more positive nodes. Higher receptor levels were associated with a greater probability of benefit. Patients less than 50 years old were less responsive. Those with one to three positive nodes received no benefit from tamoxifen regardless of receptor level, whereas those with four or more positive nodes appeared to exhibit reduced recurrence rates with higher receptor levels. Interestingly, patients over 50 appeared to benefit even when receptor levels were low. It is important to note that PF plus tamoxifen is contraindicated in patients under age 50 whose tumor estrogen or progesterone levels are below 10 fmol, since it appeared that, in this subset of patients, recurrence rates were *higher* among patients receiving PF plus tamoxifen than in those receiving PF alone. However, recurrence rates in the former group of patients (i.e., 50 years of age with receptor levels under 10 fmol receiving PF plus tamoxifen) were not greater than those associated with surgery alone in previous protocols. Therefore, it seems that in this particular subset of patients the addition of tamoxifen to PF abrogates some or all of the benefit of adjuvant therapy.

Yet another recent NSABP protocol (protocol B-10) has compared adjuvant chemotherapy with PF to chemoimmunotherapy using PF plus intravenous *Corynebacterium parvum* and hydrocortisone. Early, unpublished results suggest that no additional benefit is achieved by adding *C. parvum* to the basic PF regimen.

Recently, the NSABP has initiated two new protocols for patients treated by modified radical mastectomy and found to have one or more positive nodes. Protocol B-11 compares PF to PF plus Adriamycin, while protocol B-12 compares PF plus tamoxifen (PFT) to PFT plus Adriamycin. Allocation of patients to these protocols depends on age and tumor levels of estrogen receptor (ER) and progesterone receptor (PR) and is based on the results of protocol B-09. Patients under 50 whose ER and PR levels are both over 10 fmol are allocated to protocol B-12 while all other patients under 50 enter B-11. Between ages 50 and 59, all patients with PR levels above 10 fmol enter B-12 regardless of ER level, while those whose PR is under 10 fmol enter B-11. All patients over age 59 enter protocol B-12 regardless of ER and PR levels.

Many other groups have mounted adjuvant chemotherapy trials in node-positive patients. It is beyond the scope of this chapter to list them all or discuss them in detail. Two trials are of special interest, however. The Cancer and Leukemia Group B (CALGB) has recently completed a trial suggesting that CMF plus vincristine and prednisone (CMFVP) is superior to CMF as an adjuvant therapy combination for patients with four or more positive nodes, regardless of menopausal status.[147] (The addition of MER did not increase efficacy.) In addition, a recent trial from the Southwest Oncology Group (SWOG) has indicated that CMFVP is significantly superior to treatment with L-PAM as a single agent.[148]

It is important to remember that all of these trials included only patients whose primary therapy consisted of radical or modified radical mastectomy and who were found to have one or more histologically involved axillary lymph nodes. To date, no trials of adjuvant therapy in negative-node patients have been completed although two have recently been initiated by the NSABP—protocols B-13 and B-14. Protocol B-13 randomizes patients between surgery alone and surgery plus a chemotherapy regimen consisting of sequential high-dose methotrexate with citrovorum rescue and 5-fluorouracil (M → F). Protocol B-14 is a double-blind trial between tamoxifen and placebo. Allocation of patients is on the basis of tumor ER level alone. PR level and age are not allocation factors. Patients whose tumor ER levels are below 10 fmol enter protocol B-13, while patients whose ER levels are 10 fmol or greater enter B-14.

In summary, it is appropriate to provide some guidelines concerning the present state of adjuvant therapy.

1. It is of proven value only in node-positive, i.e., histopathologic stage II, patients. Negative-node patients probably should not be treated outside of a study setting.
2. It is probably indicated in both premenopausal and postmenopausal patients, although its value in postmenopausal patients, especially with one to three positive nodes, has not been demonstrated as convincingly as has been the case in premenopausal patients.
3. There are no clear differences in efficacy between any of the regimens of combination chemotherapy, although combinations are certainly superior to L-PAM as a single agent.[149] CMF for 6 months or 1 year, PF for 2 years, or CMFVP for a year are all good regimens although the CALGB trial has suggested that CMFVP may be superior to CMF in patients with four or more positive nodes. PMF does not appear to offer any therapeutic advantage over PF. The regimen to be used for a given patient, therefore, should probably depend primarily on which is most familiar to the oncologist who is administering the therapy.
4. The addition of tamoxifen to any of the chemotherapy regimens should be approached with caution. Although there is some evidence that CMF plus tamoxifen may be superior to CMF, in receptor-positive patients, this issue requires further study. The results of NSABP protocol B-09 strongly suggest that PF plus tamoxifen is superior to PF alone for older patients, especially those whose tumors are receptor-positive, but should be used in younger women only if both ER and PR are over 10 fmol, and even in this subset of patients the increased benefit achieved by adding tamoxifen may not be substantial. Further data is needed before the routine use of tamoxifen in adjuvant therapy regimens can be recommended unequivocally.
5. There is no data to suggest that it is necessary or desirable to add postoperative radiotherapy to any of these regimens.

THE TREATMENT OF LOCO-REGIONALLY ADVANCED AND INFLAMMATORY CARCINOMA

Loco-regionally advanced and inflammatory carcinoma cases include patients with certain T_3 tumors and T_4 tumors and patients with N_2 disease in the axilla. They are considered together because their treatment is similar in many respects. The implication is that these patients are rarely, if ever, cured by surgery alone. Many patients in this category have disease which is technically irresectable by virtue of fixation to the chest wall. Until recently, radiation therapy was the cornerstone of therapy for these patients, and irradiation continues to be a useful modality in many instances. Recently, however, chemotherapy has assumed a prominent role in the treatment of these patients.

Initial surgical therapy is not feasible when the primary tumor, the axillary nodes, or both are fixed to the chest wall. Even if chest wall fixation is absent, skin grafts are often necessary to close defects remaining following resection of large tumors. Skin grafts do not tolerate radiotherapy well if and when this modality is employed. Primary radiation therapy also presents problems when large tumors are treated. Large doese are required (up to 7000 rads) with correspondingly increased toxicity. In addition, local control is achieved in only some 50 percent of such patients.

Since some 80 percent or more of previously untreated breast cancer patients will respond significantly to combination chemotherapy, initial treatment with combination chemotherapy in order to reduce local tumor bulk has seemed an attractive approach to several investigators. Many initially irresectable tumors are converted to potentially operable status by this "induction chemotherapy."[150] Moreover, less extensive operative procedures may often be employed and skin grafts avoided. The CALGB has been conducting a trial of such induction chemotherapy in patients with stage III breast cancer.[150] Three courses of CMFVP* chemotherapy have led to significant reduction of tumor size in most patients. Patients, whose tumors are considered to be technically resectable after the chemotherapy, are then randomized to receive mastectomy or radiotherapy.

Several other studies are currently in progress to evaluate the use of chemotherapy in combination with surgery and/or radiation therapy in these types of patients. In one such study 70 percent of patients achieved either a complete or partial response after 4 cycles of Adriamycin and vincristine, and were then treated with radiotherapy. After completion of radiation therapy, 83 percent were free of detectable disease. Moreover, 89 percent of all patients in the study were alive at 36 months.[151] A second study, utilizing a combination of 5-fluorouracil, Adriamycin, and cyclophosphamide (FAC) plus bacillus calinethe-guirin (BCG) by scarification, has also yielded promising results. Only 3 percent of patients with stage III disease entered on this trial have relapsed within 24 months.[152]

A similar approach to inflammatory carcinoma has been pioneered by Montague and her group at the M. D. Anderson Hospital in Houston except that radiotherapy rather than surgery is used in all patients.[153] Her group has also employed the combination of FAC-BCG. Three or four courses of FAC-BCG are given prior to irradiation. Chemotherapy is resumed 3 weeks after the completion of radiotherapy and is continued until a total

* Cytoxan, methotrexate, 5-fluorouracil, vincristine, prednisone.

dose of Adriamycin of 450 mg/m^2 is reached. Methotrexate is then substituted for Adriamycin, and CMF-BCG is continued for a total of 2 years. Chu et al. have also published encouraging results recently using a similar regimen (CMFVP or CMF without BCG).[154] Although it appears that such approaches have facilitated local control, their impact on disease-free survival and overall survival are not yet known. The data from the M. D. Anderson Hospital experience suggests that this approach does not improve cure rates but does delay the appearance of distant metastases.[153]

At the University of California, San Diego Medical Center, we now prefer to treat locally advanced breast cancer initially with induction chemotherapy, using three to six cycles of CMVP or CMF. Surgical excision is then undertaken whenever feasible, and the chemotherapy is resumed postoperatively. Primary skin closure is always attempted and almost always accomplished. If surgery is not feasible, radiation therapy is administered and the chemotherapy resumed 4 to 6 weeks after the cessation of radiotherapy. We treat inflammatory carcinoma of the breast in a similar manner, except that radiotherapy rather than surgery is employed as the preferred regional treatment modality.

TREATMENT OF RECURRENT AND METASTATIC BREAST CANCER

Local or Regional Recurrence with No Evidence of Distant Metastases

Regional recurrences may be treated with regional modalities. Solitary chest wall recurrences may be treated by simple surgical excision alone, provided negative margins can be obtained. More extensive local recurrence requires radiation therapy. The same is true of axillary recurrences. Recurrence in supraclavicular nodes or parasternal areas also demands radiotherapy. It is appropriate to withhold systemic therapy until systemic disease is noted. This is especially important if no untreated disease remains with which to evaluate response to systemic therapy. Although these patients have a very high probability of developing disseminated disease, there is no evidence that survival is adversely affected by withholding systemic therapy until systemic disease is detected.

Skeletal Metastases

Regardless of other manifestations of metastatic disease and of the type of systemic therapy utilized, radiotherapy is often indicated in the treatment of bony metastases. Irradiation at doses of 2500 to 4000 rads often results in effective pain relief. Lesions of the long bones should also be irradiated if there is danger of pathologic fracture. This is particularly important for lesions in the weight-bearing bones of the lower extremities. Finally, irradiation is indicated for large metastases to the spine where compression fracture may produce neurologic sequelae.

Systemic Metastases in Receptor-Positive Patients

Tumor levels of estrogen and progesterone receptor are the most important guides to the selection of appropriate therapy for disseminated disease. Endocrine manipulation is usually the initial treatment of choice in patients with receptor-positive tumors unless extensive liver involvement is present. In such patients, and in patients with life-threatening disease, combination chemotherapy should be utilized.

In premenopausal or perimenopausal patients oophorectomy has been the usual procedure. However, in recent years, tamoxifen (usually given at a dose of 40 mg/day) has emerged as an acceptable alternative. In the postmenopausal patient tamoxifen, estrogens, or even androgens are appropriate, tamoxifen probably being the preferable agent due to its few and mild side effects.

If the receptor-positive patient responds to the initial hormonal therapy and then relapses, additional endocrine manipulation is appropriate. Adrenalectomy or hypophysectomy remain useful procedures in such patients. For patients who fail to respond to the initial hormonal therapy, combination chemotherapy should be instituted. Eventually, all patients with endocrine-sensitive tumors become refractory to hormonal therapy and become candidates for combination chemotherapy.

Although there is some data to support the use of chemotherapy immediately following oophorectomy, the value of concomitant hormonal therapy and chemotherapy is unproven and remains investigational, especially in the postmenopausal patient.

Systemic Metastases in Receptor-Negative Patients

In the receptor-negative patient, whether premenopausal or postmenopausal, response to endocrine manipulation is extremely unlikely, and combination chemotherapy is the treatment of choice. Historically, the five-drug combination of CMFVP was the first to gain widespread acceptance. Attempts were then made to eliminate one drug or another. In general, the elimination of either vincristine or prednisone did not appear to change overall response rates, and the CMF regimen emerged. However, the Eastern Cooperative Oncology Group has recently shown that the four-drug combination CMFP is more effective than CMF.[155] Adriamycin-containing combinations has also been shown to be extremely active. These include Adriamycin and vincristine, Adriamycin and cyclophosphamide, and cyclophosphamide, Adriamycin, and 5-fluorouracil (CAF or FAC). The last combination is considered by many to be the most active combination available for the treatment of metastatic breast cancer.[156] Often patients who respond initially to a CMF-based regimen and then relapse may respond again to treatment with an Adriamycin-containing regimen.

SARCOMAS OF THE BREAST

Nonepithelial malignant neoplasms of the female breast are rare, accounting for less than 1 percent of all cases of breast cancer.[157,158] Of these, the overwhelming majority are sarcomas of mammary stromal origin. The origin of these neoplasms is poorly understood. Many may arise de novo, but others, especially malignant cytosarcoma phylloides, may arise from preexisting fibroadenomas.[159] In 1962, Berg et al. classified only malignant cystosarcoma phylloides, lymphomas, and angiosarcomas as specific, well-defined entities and grouped all other pleomorphic tumors as "stromal sarcomas."[160] We shall adhere to his classification, although other authors have continued to identify a large variety of different histologic types of sarcomas.

Sarcomas of the breast often present as large masses. Metastases to regional lymph nodes are quite uncommon, and enlarged axillary lymph nodes are therefore seldom present. Attachment to skin and chest wall is also infrequent. Hematogenous dissemination occurs primarily to the lungs. The risk of pulmonary metastases varies with histologic type and, perhaps, with the degree of differentiation. Lymphogenous dissemination is rare. Therefore, treatment of regional nodes is not indicated in most cases.

Cystosarcoma Phylloides

Cystosarcoma phylloides is a neoplasm of mammary stroma containing both mesenchymal and epithelial elements arranged in a distinctive pattern. It is peculiar to the breast and is associated with a much better prognosis than that of pure sarcomas. It is by far the most common sarcoma of the breast and accounts for 50 percent or more of the nonepithelial neoplasms of the breast.[157,158] Although some cystosarcomas probably arise within preexisting fibroadenomas, the possibility of independent de novo origin cannot be excluded. There are benign and malignant variants, but the histologic features and clinical behavior are often discordant. Tumors which lack the histologic criteria of malignancy may exhibit malignant behavior, and not all histologically "malignant" cystosarcomas metastasize. However, histologic grade, i.e., degree of anaplasia, is of prognostic value in the histologically malignant group and may be used as a guide to therapy. Benign cystosarcomas have been termed *giant fibroadenomas* because of their histologic similarity to certain types of fibroadenomas. This term is misleading and has been largely abandoned.

The overall incidence of malignancy in cystosarcoma phylloides is unknown and is difficult to determine with certainty because of the lack of good correlation between histologic appearance and clinical behavior. When cystosarcomas metastasize, the more common sites are lung, bone, and subcutaneous tissue. Although metastases to lymph nodes are uncommon, they have been reported. The metastatic deposits themselves invariably consist only of stroma and never include epithelial elements. The degree of anaplasia in metastatic deposits may be greater than that of the primary tumor. Local recurrences occur more frequently than metastases. Recurrences tend to occur earlier with more anaplastic tumors, often within a year, while well-differentiated cystosarcomas may recur many years after resection of the primary tumor. It appears that risk of recurrence may be a function of the degree of differentiation of the tumor.

Therapy is surgical, since there is no evidence to suggest that either radiation therapy or chemotherapy is of significant value as primary treatment. The extent of surgical therapy is problematic, since cystosarcomas exhibit such widely varying clinical behavior. Segmental mastectomy is probably suitable for small tumors (under 4 cm in diameter) which are relatively well differentiated and have low mitotic indices. In all other cases, total mastectomy appears to be the treatment of choice. There is no reason to perform an axillary dissection, since metastases to axillary lymph nodes rarely occur. When recurrence or metastases develop, endocrine therapy is not effective. Chemotherapy has been similarly ineffective, although experience is scant. Local recurrences tend to respond poorly to radiotherapy.

Lymphosarcoma

Lymphosarcomas occasionally occur as localized tumors within the breast, with or without involvement of regional lymph nodes. A variety of therapeutic measures have been reported ranging from local excision to radical mastectomy with and without radiation therapy. The frequency of dissemination supports the view that frequently these tumors may represent a mammary manifestation of a more generalized lymphomatous process. These tumors are radiosensitive, and irradiation of locally "bulky" disease often provides satisfactory local control.

Angiosarcoma (Hemangiosarcoma)

Angiosarcoma of the breast is a rare but well-recognized entity. It is a highly lethal neoplasm which tends to occur primarily in relatively young women. Seventy-five percent of reported cases have occurred in women under 40 years of age. Angiosarcoma usually presents as a rapidly enlarging, painless mass of brief duration, although a few small tumors have been reported. It rarely, if ever, metastasizes to regional lymph nodes.

Angiosarcoma of the breast is almost invariably fatal. Only three probable cures and one additional long-term survival have been reported. Of the probable cures, two had small lesions, less than 3 cm in diameter. Dissemination is hematogenous and tends to be rapid and widespread. Local recurrence is also common. Most patients succumb to disseminated disease rapidly. The average survival is in the range of 2.5 years from the time of diagnosis.

There have been so few therapeutic successes that appropriate treatment is essentially unknown. Since axillary nodal metastases essentially never occur, total mastectomy, without axillary dissection, would seem to be a logical form of initial therapy. Radiation therapy has been reported to produce prompt, albeit temporary, regression of recurrent and metastatic lesions. However, its efficacy as an adjunct to surgery in primary treatment remains unproven. Chemotherapy has been reported to produce responses in a few sporadic cases, but remains of uncertain value.

Stromal Sarcomas

Sarcomas other than angiosarcoma that appear to arise within the breast and that lack an epithelial component (thereby excluding cystosarcoma phylloides) are usually grouped together under the designation *mammary stromal sarcoma*, following the suggestion of Berg et al.[160] This group of tumors is histologically diverse, but since their clinical features tend to be similar, this classification is useful. Stromal sarcomas occur primarily in women but have occasionally been reported in men. These tumors are highly variable in histologic appearance, and many histologic types have been reported, including liposarcoma, osteosarcoma, chondrosarcoma, rhabdomyosarcoma, leiomyosarcoma, and fibrosarcoma. Their clinical behavior is also highly variable, but generally is intermediate between angiosarcoma and cystosarcoma phylloides. As is the case with other sarcomas of the breast, nodal metastases rarely occur. The lungs and bones are frequent sites of metastatic spread. Local recurrence is also common. The 5-year survival in collected reports is approximately 60 to 70 percent.[158]

Total mastectomy seems to be the most appropriate form of initial therapy. Axillary dissection is not indicated. The value of radiation therapy and chemotherapy is uncertain.

CARCINOMA OF THE MALE BREAST

Carcinoma of the breast has been reported to represent between 0.38 to 1.5 percent of all cancers in the male and less than 1 percent of all breast cancers.[161] A subareolar mass is the presenting symptom in approximately 90 percent of patients. Nipple discharge is more common in men with breast cancer than in women. A striking feature of male breast cancer is the high incidence of fixation to and/or retraction of the nipple. Crichlow reported frank ulceration of the nipple in 28 percent of his collected cases, and some other nipple abnormality, including fixation, edema, retraction, and encrustation, in an additional 37 percent.[161] Therefore, no signs of nipple abnormality were present in only 35 percent of his cases.

The primary treatment of male breast cancer has tended to be much the same as for cancer of the female breast. While most authors have advocated radical mastectomy, others have suggested total mastectomy alone, if axillary nodes are uninvolved, particularly in elderly patients.[162] Many breast cancers in the male are irresectable at the time of presentation. In a review published in 1941, the primary tumor was considered irresectable in 26 percent of 264 cases.[163] Over the next 30 years, improvement in initial operability was noted. By the time of Crichlow's report, in 1972, only 19 percent were classified as inoperable. Among the remaining patients, 68 percent underwent radical mastectomy and 13 percent were treated by total mastectomy.[161] Skin grafts are more frequently required in the male than in the female because of the smaller pectoral skin area in the male.

The relative prognosis of breast cancer in the male as opposed to breast cancer in the female remains uncertain. The issue is confused by the lack of comparable populations of men and women treated coincidentally, the very small data base available for male breast cancer, the absence of uniform criteria for reporting results, and the failure to accurately record vital clinical and pathologic parameters. In 1964, Moss reported 5-year survival rates of 59 percent for clinical stage I patients, 39 percent for clinical stage II patients, and 16 percent for patients with distant metastases.[164] In 1974, Schieke, employing the 1968 version of the TNM classification, reported 5-year survival rates of 58 percent for clinical stage I patients, 38 percent for stage II patients, 29 percent for stage III patients (the most frequent stage of presentation for male breast cancer in his series), and 4 percent for stage IV patients.[165] Ten-year survival rates in his series were 38 percent, 10 percent, 9 percent, and 0 percent.

According to Crichlow,[162] two trends seem to be apparent: The first is a gradual improvement in survival during this century (probably due to less delay in diagnosis), and the second is the "persisting survival advantage for the female." There are several factors which might lead to a poor prognosis for men. Males with breast cancer tend to be older and to present for treatment after relatively long delays. The sparseness of breast tissue in the male results in a very high frequency of early skin and nipple involvement as well as a relatively high incidence of fixation to underlying pectoral fascia. Skin ulceration is much more common in the male than in the female. Therefore, a much greater percentage of males present with clinical stage III or stage IV disease. Finally, the obligatory central location of breast cancer in the male may be an unfavorable factor of significance.

No trials of adjuvant chemotherapy in males have as yet been performed; however, there is some evidence that advanced cancer of the male breast may respond to the same chemotherapeutic agents which have proven useful in female breast cancer. Meyskens et al. have recently reported responses to chemotherapy in three of four males with advanced breast cancer.[166]

Endocrine ablation has proved effective in males with advanced breast cancer, although the hormonal mechanisms involved are uncertain and good data on tumor hormone receptor content is lacking. Orchiectomy produces tumor regression in between 45 and 88 percent of cases, with response durations averaging 16 to 29 months.[167] In the collected review of Meyskens et al.,[166] 67 percent of evaluable patients responded to orchiectomy. Responses to adrenalectomy and hypophysectomy have also been reported. In the same review by Meyskens et al., 19 of 25 patients responded to adrenalectomy, including 4 who had not responded to prior orchiectomy. Of 17 patients treated with hypophysectomy, 10 (60 percent) responded. Although estrogen receptor protein has been found frequently in male breast cancers, data on clinical correlation between estrogen receptor content and response to endocrine therapy is lacking.[168,169]

Additive hormone therapy has been considered to be much less effective in male breast cancer than in female breast cancer. Occasional responses to estrogen therapy have been reported.[170] Androgens have been considered to be contraindicated, largely on the basis of a few early reports of cases in which it appeared to accelerate the progress of the disease. A few remissions of brief duration have been reported following the administration of adrenocorticosteroids.[170]

REFERENCES

1. Cancer statistics, 1982. *CA* 32:15, 1982.
2. Holleb AI et al: Breast cancer detected by routine physical examinations. *NY State J Med* 60:823, 1960.
3. Day E, Venet L: Periodic cancer detection examinations as a cancer control measure, in *Proc Fourth Natl Cancer Conf*, Lippincott, Philadelphia, 1961.
4. Gershon-Cohen J et al: Detection of breast cancer by periodic x-ray examination. *JAMA* 176:1114, 1961.
5. Wolfe JN: Mammography as a screening examination in breast cancer. *Radiology* 84:703, 1965.
6. Stevens GM, Weiger JF: Mammography survey for breast cancer detection. *Cancer* 19:51, 1966.
7. Gilbertsen VA: Survival of asymptomatic breast cancer patients. *Surg Gynecol Obstet* 122:81, 1966.
8. Egan RL: Mammography, an aid to diagnosis of breast carcinoma. *JAMA* 182:839, 1962.
9. Fink R et al: The reluctant participant in a breast cancer screening program. *Public Health Rep* 83:479, 1968.
10. Fink R et al: Impact of efforts to increase participation in repetitive screenings for early breast cancer detection. *Am J Public Health* 62:328, 1972.
11. Shapiro S: Evidence on screening for breast cancer from a randomized trial. *Cancer (Suppl)* 39:2772, 1977.
12. Baker LH: Breast cancer detection demonstration project: Five-year summary report. *CA* 32:194, 1982.
13. Beahrs OH et al: Report of the working group to review NCI/ACS breast cancer detection demonstration projects. *J Natl Cancer Inst* 62:708, 1979.
14. Statement on recommendations of the concensus development panel on breast cancer screening. *J Natl Cancer Inst* 60:1523, 1978.
15. Mammography 1982: A statement of the American Cancer Society. *CA* 32:226, 1982.
16. Caffee HH, Benfield JR: Data favoring biopsy of the breast under local anesthesia. *Surg Gynecol Obstet* 104:88, 1975.
17. Coates MR et al: Changing concepts in establishing the diagnosis of breast masses. *Am J Surg* 134:77, 1977.
18. Shabot MM et al: Aspiration cytology is superior to Tru-Cut needle biopsy in establishing the diagnosis of clinically suspicious breast masses. *Ann Surg* 196:122, 1982.
19. Salzstein SL: Histologic diagnosis of breast carcinoma with the Silverman needle biopsy. *Surgery* 48:366, 1960.
20. Roberts JG et al: The "Tru-Cut" biopsy in breast cancer. *Clin Oncol* 1:297, 1975.
21. Kline T, Neal H: Role of needle aspiration biopsy in diagnosis of carcinoma of the breast. *Surg Gynecol Obstet* 46:89, 1975.
22. Kaae S: The risk involved by biopsy in breast cancer. *Acta Radiol* 37:469, 1952.
23. Robbins GF et al: Is aspiration biopsy of breast cancer dangerous to the patient? *Cancer* 7:774, 1954.
24. Adair F et al: Long-term follow-up of breast cancer patients: The 30-year follow-up. *Cancer* 33:1145, 1974.
25. Gillis DA et al: Pre-invasive intraductal cancer. *Surg Gynecol Obstet* 110:555, 1960.
26. McDivitt RW et al: *Tumors of the Breast. Atlas of Tumor Pathology*. Armed Forces Institute of Pathology, Washington, DC, 1968.
27. Ozello L, Sanpitak P: Epithelial-stromal junction of intraductal carcinoma of the breast. *Cancer* 26:1186, 1970.
28. Fisher ER: Ultrastructure of the human breast and its disorders. *Am J Clin Pathol* 66:291, 1976.
29. McDivitt RW, Holleb AI: Prior breast disease in patients treated for papillary carcinoma. *Arch Pathol* 85:117, 1968.
30. McDivitt RW: Breast carcinoma. *Hum Pathol* 9:3, 1978.
31. Farrow JH: Current concepts in the detection and treatment of the earliest of breast cancers. *Cancer* 25:458, 1970.
32. Betsill WL et al: Intraductal carcinoma, long-term follow-up after treatment of biopsy alone. *JAMA* 239:1863, 1978.

33. Westbrook KC, Gallager HS: Intraductal carcinoma of the breast. *Am J Surg* 130:667, 1975.
34. Ashikari R et al: Intraductal carcinoma of the breast. *Cancer* 28:1182, 1971.
35. Silverberg SG, Chitale AR: Assessment of the significance of proportions of intraductal and infiltrating tumor growth in ductal carcinoma of the breast. *Cancer* 32:830, 1975.
36. Berg J, Robbins GF: Twenty year follow-up on breast cancer. *Acta Unio Int Contra Cancrum* 19:1575, 1963.
37. Muir R: The evolution of carcinoma of the mamma. *J Pathol Bacteriol* 52:155, 1941.
38. Foote FW Jr, Stewart FW: Lobular carcinoma in situ, A rare form of mammary cancer. *Am J Pathol* 17:491, 1941.
39. Newman W: Lobular carcinoma of the female breast: A report of 73 cases. *Ann Surg* 164:305, 1966.
40. McDivitt RW et al: In situ lobular carcinoma. A prospective follow-up study indicating cumulative patient risks. *JAMA* 201:82, 1967.
41. Toker C: Small cell dysplasia and in situ carcinoma of the mammary ducts and lobules. *J Pathol* 114:47, 1974.
42. Anderson JA: Lobular carcinoma in situ. A long-term follow up of 52 cases. *Acta Pathol Microbiol Scand [A]*, 82:519, 1974.
43. Rosen PP et al: Lobular carcinoma in situ of the breast. Detailed analysis of 99 patients with average follow-up of 24 years. *Am J Surg Pathol* 2:225, 1978.
44. Haagensen CD et al: Lobular neoplasia (so-called lobular carcinoma in situ) of the breast. *Cancer* 42:737, 1978.
45. McDivitt RW: In situ carcinoma, in B Hoogstraten, RW McDivitt (eds): *Breast Cancer*, CRC Press, Boca Raton, Florida, 1981, pp 137–153.
46. Urban JA: Bilaterality of cancer of the breast—biopsy of the opposite breast. *Cancer* 20:1867, 1967.
47. Donegan WL, Perez-Mesa CM: Lobular carcinoma: An indication for elective biopsy of the second breast. *Ann Surg* 176:178, 1972.
48. Newton W: Lobular carcinoma of the female breast. *Ann Surg* 164:305, 1966.
49. Urban JA: Biopsy of the "normal" breast in treating breast cancer. *Surg Clin North Am* 49:291, 1969.
50. Urban JA: Bilateral breast cancer. *Cancer* 24:1310, 1969.
51. Leis HP Jr: Selective, elective, prophylactic contralateral mastectomy. *Cancer* 28:956, 1971.
52. Donegan WL, Spratt JS: Cancer of the second breast, in WL Donegan, JS Spratt (eds): *Cancer of the Breast*, Saunders, Philadelphia, 1979, pp 464–483.
53. Fisher ER: The pathologist's role in the diagnosis and treatment of invasive breast cancer. *Surg Clin North Am* 58:705, 1978.
54. Chamness GC, McGuire WL: Methods for analyzing steroid receptors in human breast cancer, in WL McGuire (ed): *Breast Cancer, Advances in Research and Treatment*, vol 3, Plenum, New York, 1979, pp 149–197.
55. Kiang DT, Kennedy BJ: Factors affecting estrogen receptors in breast cancer. *Cancer* 40:1571, 1977.
56. Antoniades K, Spector H: Estrogen receptor levels in human mammary carcinoma, histologic correlation (abstract). *Am J Clin Pathol* 69:212, 1978.
57. Hawkins RA et al: Reproducibility of measurements of estrogen-receptor concentration in breast cancer. *Br J Cancer* 36:355, 1977.
58. Rosen PP et al: Estrogen receptor protein (ERP) and the histopathology of human mammary carcinoma, in WL McGuire (ed): *Hormones, Receptors and Breast Cancer*, Raven, New York, 1978, pp 59–70.
59. McGuire WL et al: Predicting hormone responsiveness in human breast cancer, in WL McGuire et al (eds): *Estrogen Receptors in Human Breast Cancer*, Raven, New York, 1975, pp 17–30.
60. Rosen PP et al: Estrogen receptor protein (ERP) in multiple specimens from individual patients with breast cancer. *Cancer* 39:2194, 1977.
61. Webster DJT et al: Estrogen receptor levels in multiple biopsies from patients with breast cancer. *Am J Surg* 136:337, 1978.
62. Allegra JC et al: Changes in multiple or sequential estrogen receptor determinations in breast cancer. *Cancer* 45:792, 1980.
63. Sakai F, Saez S: Existence of receptors bound to endogenous estradiol in breast cancers of premenopausal and postmenopausal women. *Steroids* 27:99, 1976.
64. Saez S et al: Estradiol and progesterone receptor levels in human breast adenocarcinoma in relation to plasma estrogen and progesterone levels. *Cancer Res* 38:3468, 1978.
65. Osborne CK, McGuire WL: Current use of steroid hormone receptors in the treatment of breast cancer. *Surg Clin North Am* 58:777, 1978.
66. Osborne CK, McGuire WL: The use of steroid hormone receptors in the management of patients with breast cancer, in B Hoogstraten, RW McDivitt (eds): *Breast Cancer*, CRC Press, Boca Raton, 1981, pp 155–169.
67. Steinhal CF: Zue Dauerheilung des Brustkrebses. *Beitr of Klin Chir* 47:226, 1905.
68. Paterson R: *The Treatment of Malignant Disease by Radium and X-rays.* Arnold, London, 1948, p 309.
69. Haagenson CD, Stout AP: Carcinoma of the breast, II, Criteria of operability. *Ann Surg* 118:859, 1943.
70. DeNoix PF: Projet d'une organization bibliographique pour faciliter les études. *Acta Unio Int Contra Cancrum* 9:270–271, 1953.
71. Raven RW: Clinical-pathological classification of cancer of the breast. *Br Medical J* 1:611–613, 1939.
72. Committee on Clinical Stage Classification and Applied Statistics: Malignant tumours of the breast, clinical stage classification and presentation of results. *Acta Unio Int Contra Cancrum* 17:544, 1961.

73. *Manual for Staging of Cancer,* American Joint Committee for Cancer Staging and End Result Reporting, Chicago, 1977.
74. Irving AD et al: Pathological staging of breast cancer. *Clin Oncol* 5:193, 1979.
75. Johnston FR: Results of treatment of carcinoma of the breast based on pathological staging. *Surg Gynecol Obstet* 134:211, 1972.
76. Wallace IWJ, Champion HR: Axillary nodes in breast cancer. *Lancet* 1:217, 1972.
77. Berg JW, Robbins GF: Factors influencing short and long term survival of breast cancer patients. *Surg Gynecol Obstet* 122:1311, 1966.
78. Fisher ER et al: Pathologic findings from the National Surgical Breast Project (Protocol No. 4). V. Significance of axillary micro and macro metastases. *Cancer* 42:1382, 1978.
79. Fisher ER et al: The pathology of invasive breast cancer, syllabus derived from findings of the National Surgical Adjuvant Breast Project (Protocol No. 4). *Cancer* 46:1, 1975.
80. Fisher ER et al: Pathologic findings from the National Surgical Adjuvant Breast Project (Protocol No. 4), VI: Discriminants for five-year treatment failures. *Cancer* 46: 908, 1980.
81. Huvos AG et al: Significance of axillary macrometastases and micrometastases in mammary cancer. *Ann Surg* 173: 44, 1971.
82. Halsted WS: The results of operations for the cure of cancer of the breast performed at the Johns Hopkins Hospital from June 1889 to January 1894. *Johns Hopkins Hosp Rep* 4:297, 1894.
83. Meyer W: An improved method of radical operation for carcinoma of the breast. *NY Med Rec* 46:746, 1894.
84. Handley WS: *Cancer of the Breast and Its Operative Treatment.* John Murray, London, 1906.
85. Urban JA, Baker HW: Radical mastectomy with en bloc resection of the internal mammary lymph node chain. *Cancer* 5:992, 1952.
86. Sugarbaker ED: Radical mastectomy combined with resection of the internal mammary node chain. *Cancer* 6:969, 1953.
87. Handley RS, Thackray AC: The internal mammary lymph chain in carcinoma of the breast. *Lancet* 2:276, 1949.
88. Handley RS, Thackray AC: Invasion of internal mammary lymph nodes in carcinoma of the breast. *Br Med J* 1:61, 1954.
89. Donegan WL: The influence of untreated internal mammary metastases upon the course of mammary cancer. *Cancer* 39:533, 1977.
90. Veronesi V, Valagussa P: Inefficacy of internal mammary nodes dissection in breast cancer surgery. *Cancer* 47:170, 1981.
91. Urban JA, Marjani MA: Significance of internal mammary lymph node metastases in breast cancer. *Am J. Roentgenol Radium Ther Nucl Med* 111:130, 1971.
92. Donegan WL: Mastectomy in the primary management of invasive mammary carcinoma, in DH Hardy (ed): *Advances in Surgery,* vol. 6, Year Book Medical, Chicago, 1972, pp 1–101.
93. Donegan WL: Staging methods, primary treatment options and end results, in WL Donegan, JS Spratt (eds): *Cancer of the Breast,* Saunders, Philadelphia, 1979, pp 221–301.
94. Kaae S, Johansen H: Simple versus radical mastectomy in primary breast cancer, in APM Forrest, PB Kunkler (eds): *Prognostic Factors in Breast Cancer,* William & Wilkins, Baltimore, 1968, pp 93–102.
95. Fisher B et al: Postoperative radiotherapy in the treatment of breast cancer: Results of the NSABP trial. *Ann Surg* 172:711, 1970.
96. Fisher B et al: Comparison of radical mastectomy with alternative treatments for primary breast cancer: A first report of results from a prospective clinical trial. *Cancer* 39:2827, 1977.
97. Lacour J et al: Radical mastectomy versus radical mastectomy plus internal mammary node dissection: Five-year results of an international cooperative study. *Cancer* 37: 206, 1976.
98. Leis HP Jr: Selective moderate surgical approach for potentially curable breast cancer, in HS Gallager et al (eds): *The Breast,* Mosby, St Louis, 1978, pp 232–247.
99. Herman RE, Steiger RE: Modified radical mastectomy. *Surg Clin North Am* 58:743, 1978.
100. Nemoto T, Dao TL: Is modified radical mastectomy adequate for axillary lymph node dissection? *Ann Surg* 182: 722, 1975.
101. Fisher B: Personal communication.
102. Patey DH: A review of 146 cases of carcinoma of the breast operated on between 1930 and 1943. *Br J Cancer* 21:260, 1967.
103. Handley RS: A surgeon's view of the spread of breast cancer. *Cancer* 24:1231, 1969.
104. Haagensen CD: The choice of treatment for operable carcinoma of the breast. *Surgery* 76:685, 1974.
105. Brinkley D, Haybittle JL: Treatment of stage II carcinoma of the female breast. *Lancet* 2:291, 1966.
106. Turner L et al: Radical versus modified radical mastectomy for breast cancer. *Ann Royal Coll Surg Eng* 63:239, 1981.
106a. Grace EG, Moitrier W Jr: Simple mastectomy with x-ray in the treatment of cancer of the breast. *NY State J Med* 26:1, 1936.
107. McWhirter R: Should more radical treatment be attempted in breast cancer? *Am J Roentgenol* 92:3, 1964.
108. Fisher B et al: Clinical trials and the surgical treatment of breast cancer. *Surg Clin North Am* 58:723, 1978.
109. Bond WH: The influence of various treatments on survival rates in cancer of the breast, in AA Jarett (ed): *The Treatment of Carcinoma of the Breast,* Excerpta Medica, New York, 1967, pp 24–39.
110. Murray JC et al: Management of early cancer of the breast.

110. Report on an international multicenter trial supported by the Cancer Research Campaign. *Br Med J* 1:1035, 1976.
111. Veronesi U et al: Comparing radical mastectomy with quadrantectomy, axillary dissection and radiotherapy in patients with small cancers of the breast. *N Engl J Med* 305:6, 1981.
112. Adair F et al: Long-term follow-up of breast cancer patients: The 30-year report. *Cancer* 33:1145, 1974.
113. Porritt A: Early carcinoma of the breast. *Br J Surg* 51:214, 1964.
114. Taylor H et al: Sector mastectomy in selected cases of breast cancer. *Br J Surg* 58:161, 1971.
115. Crile G Jr: Results of simplified treatment of breast cancer. *Surg Gynecol Obstet* 118:517, 1964.
116. Crile G Jr: Results of conservative treatment of breast cancer at 10 and 15 years. *Ann Surg* 181:26, 1975.
117. Cooperman MA et al: Partial mastectomy. *Surg Clin North Am* 58:737, 1978.
118. Atkins H et al: Treatment of early breast cancer, Ten years of clinical trial. *Br Med J* 20:423, 1972.
119. Hayward JL: The Guy's trial of treatments of early breast cancer. *World J Surg* 1:314, 1977.
120. Murray JC et al: Cancer research campaign study of the management of "early" breast cancer. *World J Surg* 1:317, 1977.
121. Crile G Jr: Management of breast cancer. Limited mastectomy. *JAMA* 230:95, 1974.
122. Fisher B, Gebhardt MC: The evolution of breast cancer surgery: Past, present and future. *Semin Oncol* 5:385, 1978.
123. Veronesi U: Conservative treatment of breast cancer, A trial in progress at the Cancer Institute of Milan. *World J Surg* 1:317, 1977.
124. McWhirter R: Simple mastectomy and radiotherapy in the treatment of breast cancer. *Br J Radiol* 28:128, 1955.
125. Mustakillo S: Conservative treatment of breast cancer, Review of 25 years of follow-up. *Clin Radiol* 23:110, 1972.
126. Peters MV: Cutting the "Gordian Knot" in early breast cancer. *Am R Col Physicians Surg Canada* 8:186, 1975.
127. Pierquin B et al: Radiation therapy in the management of primary breast cancer. *Am J Roentgenol* 127:645, 1976.
128. Fletcher GH et al: Combination of conservative surgery and irradiation for cancer of the breast. *Am J Roentgenol* 126:216, 1975.
129. Spitalier J et al: Cesium therapy of breast cancer, A five-year report of 400 consecutive patients. *Int J Radiat Oncol Biol Phys* 2:231, 1977.
130. Prosnitz LR et al: Radiation therapy as initial treatment for early stage cancer of the breast without mastectomy. *Cancer* 39:917, 1977.
131. Ghossein NA et al: Local control of breast cancer with tumorectomy plus radiotherapy or radiotherapy alone. *Radiology* 121:455, 1976.
132. Levene MB et al: Treatment of carcinoma of the breast by radiation therapy. *Cancer* 39:2840, 1977.
133. Hellman S: Improving the therapeutic index in breast cancer treatment. *Cancer Res* 40:4335, 1980.
134. Harris JR et al: The role of primary radiation therapy in the primary treatment of carcinoma of the breast. *Semin Oncol* 5:403, 1978.
135. Levene MB et al: Primary radiation therapy for operable carcinoma of the breast. *Surg Clin North Am* 58:767, 1978.
136. Fisher B et al: Ten-year follow-up results of patients with carcinoma of the breast in a cooperative clinical trial evaluating surgical adjuvant chemotherapy. *Surg Gynecol Obstet* 140:528, 1975.
137. Nissen-Meyer R et al: Preliminary report from the Scandinavian Adjuvant Chemotherapy Study Group. *Cancer Chemother Rep* 55:561, 1971.
138. Fisher B et al: L-Phenylalanine mustard (L-PAM) in the management of primary breast cancer. A report of early findings. *N Engl J Med* 292:117, 1975.
139. Fisher B et al: L-Phenylalanine mustard (L-PAM) in the management of primary breast cancer. An update of earlier findings and a comparison with those utilizing L-PAM plus 5-fluorouracil (5-FU). *Cancer* 29:2883, 1977.
140. Fisher B et al: L-Phenylalanine mustard (L-PAM) in the management of premenopausal patients with primary breast cancer. Lack of association of disease-free survival with depression of ovarian function. *Cancer* 44:847, 1977.
141. Bonadonna G et al: Combination chemotherapy as an adjuvant treatment in operable breast cancer. *N Engl J Med* 294:405, 1976.
142. Bonadonna G et al: The CMF program for operable breast cancer with positive axillary nodes. Updated analysis on the disease-free interval, site of relapse and drug tolerance. *Cancer* 39:2904, 1977.
143. Bonadonna G et al: Are surgical adjuvant trials altering the course of breast cancer? *Semin Oncol* 5:450, 1978.
144. Bonadonna G, Valagussa P: Dose-responses effect of adjuvant chemotherapy in breast cancer. *N Engl J Med* 304:10, 1981.
145. Fisher B et al: Disease-free survival at intervals during and following completion of adjuvant chemotherapy. The NSABP experience from three breast cancer protocols. *Cancer* 48:1273, 1981.
146. Fisher B et al: Treatment of primary breast cancer with chemotherapy and tamoxifen. *N Engl J Med* 305:1, 1981.
147. Tormey DC et al: Five drug versus three drug IMER postoperative chemotherapy for mammary carcinoma, in SE Salmon, SE Jones (eds): *Adjuvant Therapy of Cancer III*, Grune & Stratton, New York, 1981, pp 377–384.
148. Glucksberg H et al: Combination chemotherapy (CMFVP) versus L-phenylalanine mustard (L-PAM) for operable breast cancer with positive axillary nodes. *Cancer* 50:423, 1982.
149. Fisher B, Wolmark N: The current status of systemic adjuvant therapy in the management of primary breast cancer. *Surg Clin North Am* 61:1347, 1981.

150. Holland JF: Adjuvant chemotherapy for breast cancer. *Surg Clin North Am* 61:1361, 1981.
151. De Lena M et al: Combined chemotherapy (CT)–radiotherapy (RT) in primary inoperable (T3b-T4) breast cancer. *Proc AACR-ASCO* 18:356, 1977.
152. Buzdar AV et al: Intensive postoperative chemoimmunotherapy for patients with stage II and stage III breast cancer. *Cancer* 41:1064, 1978.
153. Barker JL et al: Clinical experience with irradiation of inflammatory carcinoma of the breast with and without chemotherapy. *Cancer* 45:625, 1980.
154. Chu AM et al: Inflammatory breast carcinoma treated by radical radiotherapy. *Cancer* 45:2730, 1980.
155. Canellos GP et al: Combination chemotherapy for metastatic breast carcinoma: Prospective comparison of multiple drug therapy with L-phenylalanine mustard. *Cancer* 38:1882, 1976.
156. Carbone PP, Davis TE: Medical treatment for advanced breast cancer. *Semin Oncol* 5:417, 1978.
157. Dennegan WL: Sarcomas of the breast, in WL Donnegan, JS Spratt (eds): *Cancer of the Breast,* Saunders, Philadelphia, 1979, pp 504–542.
158. Martin RG, Gallager HS: Sarcomas of the breast, in HS Gallager et al (eds): *The Breast,* Mosby, St Louis, 1978, pp 539–554.
159. Curran RC, Dodge OC: Sarcoma of the breast, with particular reference to its origin from fibroadenoma. *J Clin Pathol* 15:1, 1962.
160. Berg JW et al: Stromal sarcomas of the breast. A unified approach to connective tissue sarcomas other than cystosarcoma phylloides. *Cancer* 15:418, 1962.
161. Crichlow RW: Carcinoma of the male breast. *Surg Gynecol Obstet* 134:1011, 1972.
162. Crichlow RW: Breast cancer in men. *Semin Oncol* 1:145, 1974.
163. Sachs MD: Carcinoma of the male breast. *Radiology* 37:458, 1941.
164. Moss NH: Cancer of the male breast. *Ann NY Acad Sci* 114:1937, 1964.
165. Scheike O: Male breast cancer. 6: Factors influencing prognosis. *Br J Cancer* 30:261, 1974.
166. Meyskens FL Jr et al: Male breast cancer. A review. *Cancer Treat Rev* 3:83, 1976.
167. Neifield JP et al: The role of orchiectomy in the management of advanced male breast cancer. *Cancer* 37:992, 1976.
168. Le Clercq G et al: Oestrogen receptors in male breast cancer. *Biomed* 25:327, 1976.
169. Rosen PP et al: Estrogen receptor protein in lesions of the male breast. A preliminary report. *Cancer* 37:1866, 1976.
170. Treves N: The treatment of cancer, especially inoperable cancer, of the male breast by ablative surgery (orchiectomy, adrenalectomy, and hypophysectomy) and hormone therapy (estrogens and corticosteroids): An analysis of 43 patients. *Cancer* 12:820, 1959.

SELECTED BIBLIOGRAPHY

Bedwinek JM et al: Concurrent chemotherapy and radiotherapy for nonmetastatic, stage IV breast cancer: A pilot study by the Southeastern Cancer Study Group. *Am J Clin Oncol (CCT)* 6:159, 1983.

Bland KI et al: A clinicopathologic correlation of mammographic parenchymal patterns and associated risk factors for human mammary carcinoma. *Ann Surg* 195:582, 1982.

Harris JR et al: Clinical-pathologic study of early breast cancer treated by primary radiation therapy. *J Clin Oncol* 1:184, 1983.

Mann BD et al: Delayed diagnosis of breast cancer as a result of normal mammograms. *Arch Surg* 118:23, 1983.

Rosen PP et al: Discontinuous or "skip" metastases in breast carcinoma: Analysis of 1228 axillary dissections. *Ann Surg* 197:276, 1983.

Shapiro S et al: Ten- to fourteen-year effect of screening on breast cancer mortality. *JNCI* 69:349, 1982.

PART FIVE

INTRAABDOMINAL NEOPLASMS

25
CARCINOMA OF THE STOMACH

E. Douglas Holyoke Harold O. Douglass, Jr.

HISTORICAL ASPECTS

Gastric cancer has shown a decline in incidence in a number of the developed, industrialized nations over the last 40 years. This trend has been particularly noticeable in the United States, where rates have fallen from perhaps 29 per 100,000 in 1947 to a level of 9 per 100,000 in 1969, as reported by Haenszel.[1,2]

Surgery for gastric cancer was first successfully performed by Billroth and was developed by McNeer, among many others.[3-5] The overall result of surgery in the United States and many parts of the world allows salvage of some 10 percent of individuals, with a better success rate with patients who present with early disease.[6,7] Attempts have been made to extend surgery toward total gastrectomy and toward meticulous systematic node removal with selective splenectomy.[8,9] The usefulness of pushing surgery to this extent remains debatable. Many clinicians feel that the extent of surgery has already reached its limit; as more disease involves more distant lymph nodes, extension of the surgical procedure will not be of much value.[10,11] On the other hand, many eminent Japanese surgeons endorse meticulous extensive node dissection and believe their results are improved by this approach.

There is a startling contrast in the outlook toward the success of the treatment of gastric cancer across the Pacific. Most reviewers of the management of gastric cancer in the Americas feel that the rate of frequency of cure by surgery alone has been nearly static for 20 years.[12,13] In contrast, our Japanese colleagues have demonstrated quite consistently and convincingly that they could improve 5-year survival rates over this time.[14,15] In Japan, these results stem largely from earlier diagnosis and surgical therapy at an earlier stage. The earlier diagnosis appears to be mainly the result of mass screening techniques in a high-risk population. Double-contrast radiography and endoscopy are widely used. The percentage of early gastric cancer (using the now widely accepted Japanese definition as tumor penetration not beyond the muscularis mucosa) encountered at surgery has risen from 7 to 11 percent to 36 percent and more over 25 years. The result is that survival among the Japanese has risen to more than 50 percent.[16,17] Of course, the question remains as to how rapidly these early gastric cancers will become advanced. However, it appears to most thoughtful scholars that survival rates exceed the artifact of earlier diagnosis.[18,19]

In contrast to the situation in Japan, the net effect of endoscopy in the United States has been to establish

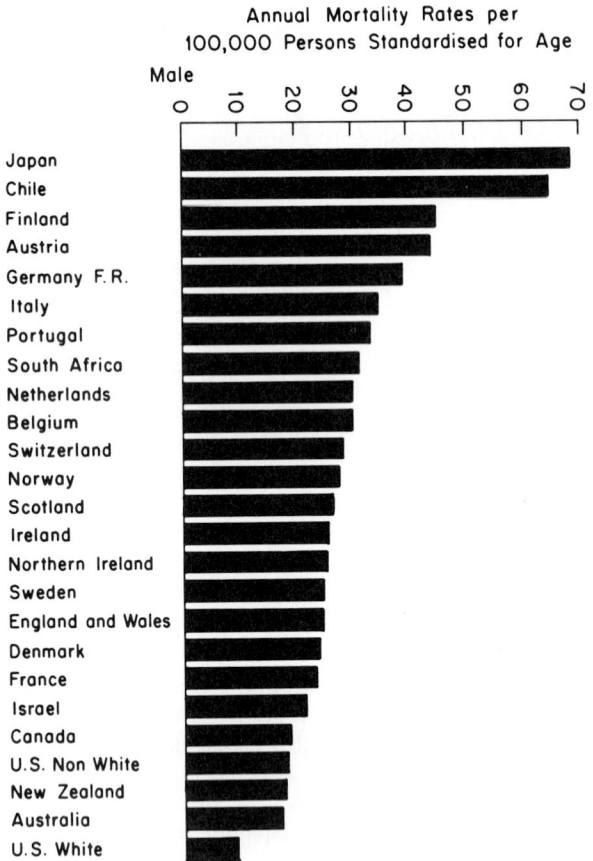

FIGURE 25-1 The fact that gastric cancer seems to occur almost seven times as frequently in the Japanese populations as in the U.S. population and that migration of Japanese to the United States results in a decreased incidence in nisei and sansei populations, approaching that of the European citizens, indicates clearly the considerable importance of exogenous factors. (*Adapted from J Higginson.*[56])

preoperatively a definitive histologic diagnosis, which is technically helpful to reduce morbidity and mortality. However, only 1 to 3 percent of patients are encountered with early disease, a lower figure than was seen in Japan 25 years ago.[20,21] The question remains as to whether within the bounds of a reasonable diagnostic program this percentage will increase in the next decade in the United States.[22] There is a general exhortation for the first-line practitioners to be sensitive to any persisting gastric symptoms, even when quite vague.[23,24]

INCIDENCE, EPIDEMIOLOGY, AND ETIOLOGIC ASPECTS

At the present time, emphasis has been placed on the role of environmental factors in the development of a variety of cancers.[25] In the increasingly industrialized world in which we live, with the continuing alterations in preparation and techniques of preservation of our foods, one might expect the incidence of gastric cancer to increase.[26] The increased incidence of lung cancer and apparent increased incidence in pancreatic cancer (both probably related to smoking) represent such an event.[27] However, the incidence of gastric cancer around the world is declining. As Ochsner and Blalock noted, cancer of the stomach was the leading cause of cancer death in the United States in the early years of this century.[28] But over the last 40 years, mortality from gastric cancer in the United States has dropped in absolute numbers from 26,000 to 14,000 annually, and incidence, as we have stated, has fallen from 29 to 9 per 100,000 persons per year. The National Cancer Institute's *Third National Cancer Survey* showed a 63 percent decrease in the incidence of gastric cancer from 1950 to 1970.[29] As an example of the meaning of this in the care setting, at UCLA a comparison of the decades 1956 to 1965 and 1965 to 1975 shows a 14 percent drop in admissions for gastric cancer at a time when total admissions rose by 70 percent.[30] Recent studies from Chile and even Japan show a leveling off or decline in incidence. These changes are pronounced enough and have been noted over a long enough period to establish them as true phenomena.

A great difference in incidence between various populations around the world persists. As a matter of fact, *Cancer Facts and Figures* for 1980 reports the United States as ranking forty-second in incidence, gastric cancer remaining eight times more frequent in Japan.[31] The maximum range varies from a low value of 7.9 per 100,000 in El Paso, Texas, to 95.3 per 100,000 in the Miyami Prefecture of Japan.[32] Higginson reviewed the epidemiology of gastric cancer in a 1977 WHO monograph. Figure 25-1 presents the mortality for males in 25 countries around the world showing a range from the United States to Japan.[56]

Still another factor to arise from population incidence studies is that migrant workers and their children often demonstrate, after a period of time, the incidence of cancer endemic to their new environment. Haenszel and Kurihara have demonstrated this clearly with their studies of Japanese migrants in the United States. Of course, as Kriebel and Jowett have noted, the influx of a foreign population may be associated with a local ripple effect, or change of incidence, in local nationals. These studies all point strongly to a role for exogenous factors as a major cause of gastric cancer.

Pfeiffer listed a number of exogenous factors which have been related at least tentatively to gastric cancer.[34] Table 25-1 is modified from his presentation. Some recent studies have shown a high risk for farmers.[34] Others continue to show a high risk for fishermen.[35] A relationship between gastric cancer and smoking is also becoming apparent.[36] In addition, a study of rubber workers indicates some risk.[37] All of these findings concur as to the importance of exogenous factors in the induction of gastric cancer.

There are reported instances in which cancer of the stomach is concentrated in families.[38] In a study of 300 patients with adenocarcinoma of the stomach Cruze et al. found 13 in whose immediate family a similar type of cancer was identified, a 3 percent incidence suggesting some type of familial grouping.[39] Graham and Lilienfeld have pointed out that there are difficulties with family studies since family groups often experience similar environmental stimuli for many years. Mosbeck and Videbaek also reported a high familial incidence of this disease in their studies.[40]

Osborne and Degorge and Maddock inferred from available epidemiologic and host-defense-mechanism studies that the data support the concept of a genetic susceptibility exposed to an environmental sequence leading to gastric cancer, with exogenous factors overshadowing heredity as a cause of gastric cancer.

Creagan and Fraumini[41] studied a seven-generation family with two first-cousin marriages and 12 members with gastric cancer. A high frequency of living kindred demonstrated immunologic impairment as determined by lymphoblastogenesis assay, skin test response, and lymphopenia. The approach was imaginative, but the immune assays used have severe limitations, and it is difficult to more than speculate.

The occurrence of gastric cancer simultaneously in twins certainly suggests that there is a hereditary factor.[42] Although data suggest a tendency for persons with blood group A to develop gastric cancer,[43] the evidence is contradictory, and the trend not strong.[44]

Various models for the induction of gastric cancer have been proposed. Among these, the model developed by Lilienfeld predicts the crucial event to be a deficiency in the mucopolysaccharides protecting the underlying mucosa.[45] Other consequences of such an event could be mucosal injury and resultant reduced acidity, followed by overgrowth of bacteria in the stomach leading to the formation of carcinogenic nitrosamines. This hypothesis could provide an explanation for the increased incidence of gastric cancer patients with blood group A and also could explain the protective effect of fresh vegetables and vitamin C.

The conclusions from the available evidence are that exogenous factors are of major importance in this disease. It is probable that changes in the diet in the United States have either resulted in less carcinogenesis or have been protective for the stomach. It is highly desirable to continue to observe selected populations to identify with as much certainty as possible both carcinogenic and protective materials, and to watch for any reversal of the trend of the last 50 years which would warn that this fortuitous state of affairs might be changing.

SIGNS, SYMPTOMS, AND ATTEMPTS AT EARLY DETECTION

Unfortunately, most symptoms usually don't occur until the disease is at least moderately advanced, large enough to cause rigidity and dysfunction of a significant portion

TABLE 25-1 Exogenous Factors Associated with an Increased Risk for Gastric Cancer

Environmental: Acidic soil, urban residency, nitrate fertilizers, soft water, lead or zinc in the water supply, volcanic rock, talc

Dietary: Highly salted or smoked foods, high fat or oil intake (nitrite preservatives)

Smoking and drinking: Cigarette smoking and whiskey

Economic: Lower social class, miners and quarry workers, metal workers, fisherman, printers and bookbinders, construction workers, painters, transport repair and maintenance workers, textile workers, ceramic workers, and clerical workers

In contrast, milk, fresh vegetables, vitamin A or C and other antioxidants may decrease the incidence of cancer.

SOURCE: Pfeiffer.[34]

of the stomach wall, or large enough to impede ingress or outflow of gastric content. Symptoms are initially vague and are related to indigestion, fullness after meals, heartburn, or loss of appetite.

Weed reviewed 265 patients with gastric cancer seen at the Ochsner Clinic from 1958 to 1978.[46] This report is typical of other American series in that only about 1 percent of patients presented with disease limited to the submucosa. The two symptoms most often encountered in this series were pain and a weight loss of more than 10 percent. Pain was a symptom in two-thirds of the patients and weight loss in nearly one-half. Pain may occur in up to 85 percent of patients with more advanced disease at the time of diagnosis. In the series reported from UCLA by Adashek, pain and weight loss were also the two most common symptoms.[30] The striking physical findings have been the presence of a mass in a third or more of these patients, and abdominal tenderness in many others.

Other symptoms include nausea, vomiting, weakness, dysphagia, gastrointestinal bleeding, anorexia, and dyspepsia. These symptoms occur in 10 to 25 percent of patients presenting for diagnosis in most series. Interestingly, a history of peptic ulcer is present in about one quarter of these patients and probably delays diagnosis.[47] Other physical findings include signs of metastatic spread, such as a Virchow's node or Blumer's shelf.

Symptoms can be related to the location of the tumor within the stomach.[48] About 50 percent of gastric malignancies are located in the antrum and pyloric area and cause symptoms related to gastric outflow. Tumors in the body of the stomach are often asymptomatic until ulceration or extension through the serosa takes place. Dysphagia is usually associated with proximal or cardial tumors.

All writers stress that in order to improve our results in treating this disease, we have to make our diagnosis earlier. The question first to be asked is whether or not we can develop a mass screening program similar to that found in Japan. In 1975, about 3 million individuals were screened in a mass gastrography and endoscopy program for gastric cancer as a part of a national screening effort.[19] Approximately 3000 gastric cancer patients, 45 percent of them "early," were identified by this program. Hirayama comments that following treatment, the 5- and 10-year survivals for these patients are too high to be due to "lead time" bias or artifact. His data indicate that over the decade before 1976, the detectable rate for gastric cancer from this screening program fell from 1.45 to 0.95 per 1000 persons screened. This translates to an expected detection rate for early gastric cancer of 40 per 100,000 people. The cost of screening in 1979 in Japan was $15 for the gastrography with six exposures. This comes out to $1,500,000 per 40 persons identified with early cancer or about $30,000 per patient identified. To visualize the problem as applied to the United States, we simply can state that on a similar basis, excluding a possible higher x-ray cost, the cost per patient for an early diagnosis of gastric cancer could be expected to be 5 times as high. This does not include problems of compliance. It is clear that we cannot develop mass screening on the same basis for our population.

Hakkinen published an interesting screening study based on use of a biologic marker in 1980.[49] Fifteen early gastric cancers were identified after screening 39,000 persons in southern Finland by obtaining a sample of gastric juice for analysis for fetal sulfaglycoprotein antigen (FSA) and then endoscoping some 3000 secretion-positive individuals. Again, this would not appear economically feasible in the United States, but if the false-positive (for malignancy) rate for FSA, or some other antigen was 2 percent instead of 6.5 to 8.5 percent, a screening program might be possible. Thus, Hakkinen's report deserves study.

Tataryn et al. reported on the identification of gastric cancer with the LAI assay.[50] This is an interesting approach, especially for earlier, stage I disease, but consistency and antigen stability have been problems.[51]

At the present time, it is clear that mass screening is not practical in the United States. We should continue to look for epidemiologic studies to identify high-risk populations, and we should constantly warn the public and physicians that even though vague, persistent dyspeptic symptoms should be evaluated and studied vigorously.

DIAGNOSTIC TECHNIQUES, WORK-UP, AND STAGING

With a strong emphasis on the vigorous investigation of persistent symptoms of dyspepsia, even if quite vague, we should first consider the classic diagnostic means through radiologic study. Allan and Coates examined their accuracy of x-ray diagnosis and determined that on first barium meal, approximately 72 percent of tumors were found.[52] Figures in the literature run from 65 to 85 percent, depending on the number of views obtained and meticulousness of technique. Several studies from Japan and elsewhere have stressed the superiority of the double-contrast series in the detection of small or early lesions.[53,54] Cineradiography and image amplification may augment this approach.[55,56] Many reports review the characteristics seen in gastric ulcer, and the surgical oncologist should be familiar with them.[57,58] The classic sign of a cancer as an ulcer in a raised mass may help, particularly when the ulcer is located in the distal or prepyloric portion of the stomach. The study of Schulman and Simpkins reviews the gastric ulcer–cancer problem and attempts to develop helpful criteria to assist the clinician in an assessment.[59] The point which is universally stressed is that gastric ulcers should be followed until they are healed, and it should be ascertained that they remain healed. It is necessary to keep in mind that in about 10 percent or more of patients, a definitive diagnosis of malignant ulcer is not possible by x-ray.

Weed's series reported results for diagnosis of gastric cancer by barium, by endoscopy, and by endoscopy and biopsy. Table 25-2 reproduces this data.[46] In this unrandomized comparison, 66 percent of upper gastrointestinal series in patients with cancer were read as consistent with malignancy, 17 percent with benign gastric ulcer disease, and 8 and 9 percent as obstruction of the gastroesophageal junction or normal. Endoscopy was not performed in exactly the same patients, but in this series, 75 percent were correctly diagnosed as having cancer with the older Horowitz endoscopy and 87 percent were so identified with the newer fiberoptic equipment. Endoscopy carried out with meticulous biopsy technique led to an accurate diagnosis of gastric cancer in over 90 percent of instances.[60] Attention to rim biopsy of visible craters was important.[61]

Winawer and others have reported that brush cytology is superior to endoscopic lavage cytology, particularly in the case of infiltrative lesions and lesions in the cardia.[62] Brushings should precede biopsy. Nomura et al. indicated that in vivo methylene blue staining of the lesion improves biopsy accuracy.[63]

An immunodiagnostic tool would be of great value in helping us identify early gastric cancer; but as pointed out by Hakkinen, most tumor-associated antigens can only be identified in circulation after mucosal invasion, which usually implies at least a moderate-sized lesion.[49]

As we discussed, the antigen FSA first identified by Hakkinen in 1967 may turn out to be useful as a criterion of possible risk of malignancy in evaluation of peptic ulcer.[64] An elevated secretory IgA level in gastric aspirate

TABLE 25-2 Diagnosis of Gastric Cancer (Tumor Present In All Patients)

	Tumor, % diagnosed	Peptic ulcer, % diagnosed	Other, % diagnosed	Normal, % diagnosed
Barium	66	17	8	9
Endoscopy	71	15	7	6
Endoscopy and biopsy	79	21	—	—

SOURCE: Weed.[46]

in patients with malignant neoplasms has been reported, but further information concerning the possible usefulness of this assay is not available.

There are several histologic classifications of gastric cancer to consider in staging. These include the World Health Organization's classification, which is useful for communication, the Lauren classification, and those of Mulligan, of Rember, and of Ming.[65–67] There has always been debate about how useful these classifications, as well as earlier, similar attempts at description of histologic appearance of gastric cancer, are from a staging point of view.[68] Lauren reports some improvement in survival in his patients with "intestinal" type of tumor over that in patients with diffuse tumors, and in general it appears that more diffuse tumors or more poorly differentiated tumors are at high risk in all classifications.[66] Several reports indicate that a pushing edge has a better prognosis than an infiltrating one.[69,70] As for some other tumor types, the claim has been made that lymphocyte or plasma-cell infiltration may be associated with an improved survival.[71]

We know without question that both depth of tumor penetration and lymph node involvement are predictive of outcome and should be carefully assayed by the surgical oncologist.[72–74] Resection of early gastric cancer, not extending deeper than the muscularis mucosa, led to an average 95 percent 5-year survival in a collective series for Japan.[75] Paile reported only a 5 percent survival with submucosal tumors, but when the muscles were involved, this value fell to 20 percent.[76]

Several studies indicate that lymph node involvement is critical and that not only the presence or absence of nodes but also their number and location can be equated to chances for survival.[77]

Figure 25-2 presents the classification of early cancer developed in Japan based on endoscopic appearance of these tumors. This is useful in developing a precise way

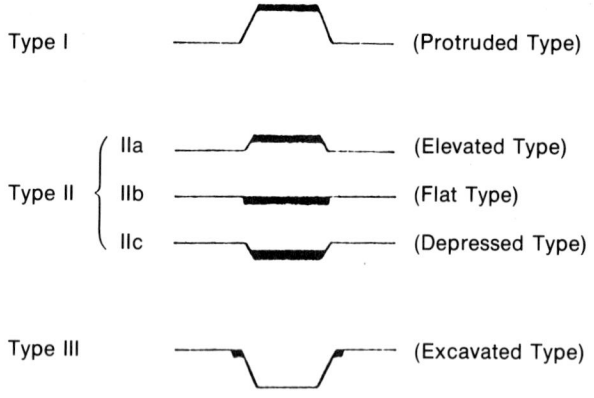

FIGURE 25-2 The Japanese classification of early gastric cancer based on endoscopic appearance. Types IIa and IIc are the predominant forms.

of viewing these lesions endoscopically, but the recurrence rate for early gastric cancer is so low that it is not difficult to assign a prognostic meaning of one versus the other to these various early macroscopic tumor types unless ulceration has occurred.

Table 25-3 presents the TNM histopathological staging system for gastric cancer of the American Joint Committee for Cancer Staging and End Result Reporting (AJC). Figs. 25-3 and 25-4 portray this system graphically. This staging system is published as an alternate to the system of the International Union against Cancer. Figure 25-5 indicates the usefulness of the original AJC staging as it relates to prognosis, and it appears to be a quite sensitive staging system. The AJC and Japanese staging differ in that the Japanese emphasize the importance of seroal invasion more and adjacent lymph nodes less and have data to support it. This would seem to offer the most precise method of staging that can be carried out at a majority of treatment centers. This, together with the WHO and the Lauren or Ming histopathologic staging systems, should be considered in evaluating a patient with gastric cancer or in trying to ascertain the effects of a therapy applied.

THERAPEUTIC OPTIONS FOR PRIMARY TREATMENT

Surgery is still, despite its acknowledged limitations, the primary treatment of this disease. Surgery dates back to 1881, when Billroth performed his first successful gastrectomy. Subsequent events proved apocryphal, as this

TABLE 25-3 The American Joint Committee Staging System (TNM)

Stage	Description	Code
Stage I	No metastasis in regional lymph nodes	
	No distant metastasis	
	A Carcinoma confined to the mucosa	T_1
	No metastasis in regional lymph nodes	N_0
	No distant metastasis	M_0
	T_1, N_0, M_0	
	B Carcinoma involving the submucosa or serosa but not penetrating through the serosa	
	No metastasis in regional lymph nodes	T_2
	No distant metastasis	N_0
	T_2, N_0, M_0	M_0
	C Carcinoma with penetration through the serosa with or without invasion of contiguous structures	
	No metastasis in regional lymph nodes	T_3
	No distant metastasis	N_0
	T_3, N_0, M_0	M_0
Stage II	Diffuse involvement of the stomach wall	T_4
	No lymph nodes involved	N_0
	No distant metastasis	M_0
	or	
	Any involvement of the stomach wall as defined by T_1 to T_4, and including involvement of the perigastric lymph nodes in the immediate vicinity of the primary tumor	
	No distant metastasis	
	T_1, N_1, M_0	
	T_2, N_1, M_0	
	T_3, N_1, M_0	
	T_4, N_1, M_0	
Stage III	Tumor involving the stomach wall in any classification of T_1 to T_4, but including involvement of the perigastric regional nodes at a distance from the primary tumor or on both curvatures of the stomach	
	No distant metastasis	
	T_1, N_2, M_0	
	T_2, N_2, M_0	
	T_3, N_2, M_0	
	T_4, N_2, M_0	
Stage IV	Any carcinoma of the stomach with distant metastasis (M_1), including those with T_X or N_X	

SOURCE: American Joint Committee for Cancer Staging and End Result Reporting: *Manual for Staging of Cancer,* Chicago, 1977.

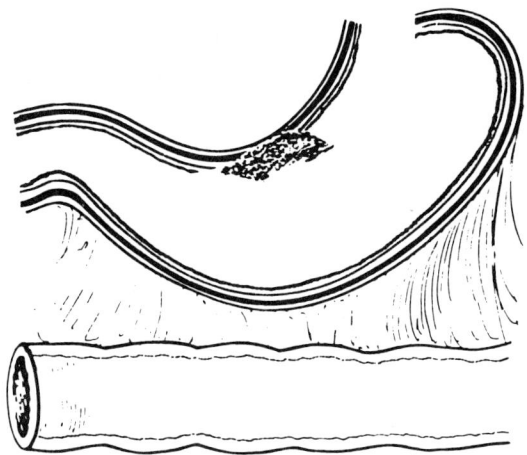

FIGURE 25-3 Schematic presentation of a T_2 primary tumor involving the mucosa, the submucosa, including the muscularis propria, and extending to or into the serosa but not penetrating through the serosa.

first patient died after 14 months with advanced gastric cancer. In 1891, Schaller performed a successful total gastrectomy, but reports of successful gastric resection were scattered and very limited until well into the 1930s.

A number of technical modifications to the surgery have been made over the years, but the basic operations are still modeled on the Billroth II procedure, the proximal gastric resection, or, in selected patients, on total gastrectomy. We do have some evidence that an effort to extend the role of total gastrectomy to include the majority of patients with gastric cancer resulted in higher mortality and less survival than was achieved basing most surgery on partial gastrectomy.[78,79]

As pointed out by Lawrence, there is general consensus today that all patients with gastric cancer (except those with ascites positive for tumor cells or with rectal shelf or documented liver or distant metastasis) deserve an exploration and, if possible, resection of the primary tumor and possible involved nodal areas.[80]

Current standard surgical treatment for gastric adenocarcinoma is a "radical" subtotal gastric resection with en bloc omentectomy, removing 80 to 85 percent of the stomach, the first portion of the duodenum, a portion of the hepatoduodenal pedicle, and the gastrohepatic and gastrocolic omentum. Splenectomy and omentectomy may be done, but this does not enhance survival. Pathologic studies have shown proximal extension of tumor cells among the submucosal lymphocytes of the gastric wall 6 cm or more from any visible tumor, particularly when the primary lesions are located in the proximal stomach or distal esophagus. For this reason, care must be taken, using frozen section, to ensure that the line of resection is proximal to the tumor.

The reason that a portion of duodenum is usually included in a radical subtotal gastrectomy is that serosal extension of tumor may occur up to 3 cm beyond the pylorus via the serosal lymphatics. Supra- and intrapyloric lymph nodes may also be removed with this resection.

Total gastric resection including splenectomy with or without distal pancreatectomy may be performed for more advanced lesions. Hoerr has documented the long-term survival of vigorous elderly patients with quite advanced tumors following surgery.[81] He points out that, overall, about one-third of his patients have been able to live out a normal life span, but in a small group of patients late recurrence of the cancer, appearing after 5 years, had been well-documented.

Overall, it is now reasonable to expect 75 to 80 percent operability in our patient populations presenting for treatment of gastric cancer, but fewer people than this

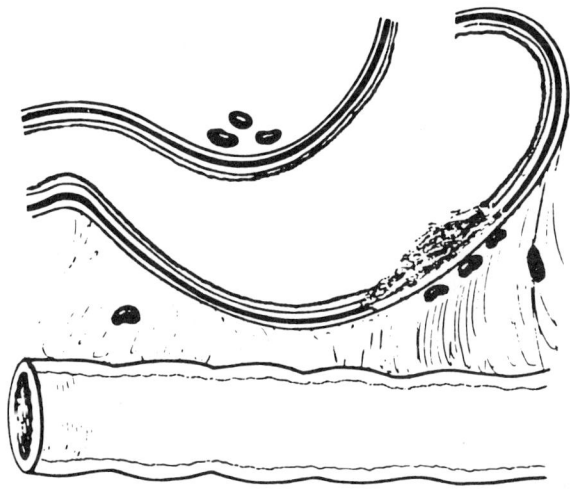

FIGURE 25-4 Schematic presentation of an N_2 lesion. Perigastric lymph nodes are involved some distance from the primary tumor or on both curvatures of the stomach.

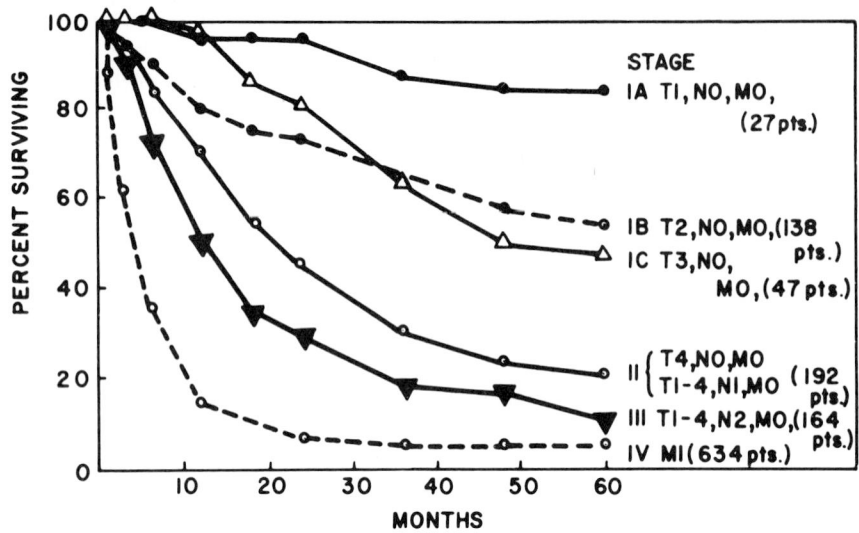

FIGURE 25-5 The TNM classification is predictive and offers meaningful staging as is seen in the spread in survival between stages IA and IV. (*American Joint Committee for Cancer Staging and End Result Reporting: Manual for Staging of Cancer, Chicago, 1977.*)

percentage warrants are actually explored. A resectability rate in 12 studies ranging from 31 to 66 percent and averaging 45 to 50 percent was reported by Dupont et al.[12] In this series LSU from "radical subtotal gastrectomy" was associated with the best rate of 5-year survival, with the gain becoming more apparent after 2 years, as compared to subtotal gastrectomy, total gastrectomy, esophagogastrectomy, or no resection. Survival was 22 percent. In this series, *radical* was defined as at least a 75 percent distal gastrectomy with omentectomy and excision of those groups of lymph nodes accompanying the right and left gastric arteries plus, in selected patients, splenectomy, examination of lymph nodes at the celiac axis and along the porta hepatitis, and, more rarely, excision of the tail of the pancreas or a portion of the transverse colon.

One point that needs to be stressed is that the surgical oncologist should be aware of the difficulty of defining whether or not adjacent organ involvement is malignant or inflammatory. Because of this difficulty many resections may be designated at operation as palliative which are in fact curative, and vice versa. Failure to appreciate the error involved in gross inspection by the surgeon is also apparent in the evaluation of grossly enlarged lymph nodes without a histologic diagnosis. The failure to biopsy can result in surgery that is less than curative and to misinterpretation of results from immune therapy or other adjuvant treatment.

Addressing the problem of the gastric cardia, Lawrence suggests that resection of proximal tumor usually requires that the proximal line of resection be through the esophagus.[80] Thus, the major hazard of total gastrectomy has already been encountered, and there appears to be little gain in retaining the distal portion of the stomach. However, the persisting practice of proximal gastrectomy would indicate that not all surgeons agree.

Papachristou and Fortner reviewed a series of 100 patients and examined their results for extended total gastrectomy versus proximal subtotal gastrectomy in a retrospective nonrandomized study.[82] In this series, smaller groups of patients underwent total gastrectomy and extended proximal subtotal gastrectomy, but not enough to give any idea of their relative efficacy. In TNM stage I and II patients, these investigators felt that extended total gastrectomy was superior to the subtotal procedure. There is pathoanatomic data which shows for these proximal cancer patients a high incidence of tumor-involved pyloric, greater curvature, splenic, and pancreatic lymph nodes. It may be that in stage I and II tumors these nodes are involved with microscopic tumor, which explains the efficacy of the more extensive procedure.

Whether peforming proximal or total gastrectomy for adenocarcinomas of the cardioesophageal junction and those arising in gastric mucosa in the lower esophagus, the risk of submucosal tumor spread proximally in the esophagus almost always mandates a line of resection high enough to require thoracotomy. Because of restrictions on extent of excision caused by the arch of the aorta, we routinely employ an approach through the abdomen and right chest approach utilizing two separate incisions, rather than a thoracoabdominal or left chest approach. In this way, not only does the dissection tend to be more complete, but the anastomosis is technically easier to perform.

For patients with impaired pulmonary function, we have utilized the abdominal and cervical approach with proximal gastrectomy, anastomosing the distal stomach to the cervical esophagus. Although the mediastinal dissection is less complete, the palliation achieved is superior to nonresection with or without colon bypass.

As we have already discussed, surgery may mandate colon resection on occasion because of direct tumor extension. Indeed, no gastric resection of any sizable tumor should be planned without preparation of the gastrointestinal tract, as the flora of the tumor-containing stomach is much like that of the colon.

Excision may extend to the mesocolon or liver. The possibility of adding a pancreatoduodenectomy to this procedure is raised from time to time.[83] Pathologic study of lymphatic spread by Berry and Rottschafer gave no indication that this would be helpful.[83] It is generally felt that there is too little gain for the added morbidity with this procedure.

Palliative surgery may be undertaken in the face of distant metastases, and resection probably represents the best palliation if it is possible without extensive node dissection.[84,85] We perform resection for palliation up to total gastrectomy except in the face of peritoneal studding or ascites, and we hope to obtain perhaps 10 to 12 months for these patients.[86] We do gastrojejunostomies on occasion but are not advocates of feeding jejunostomy or gastrostomy. We find a Celestin or other tube useful occasionally in relieving obstruction to allow swallowing of saliva and ingestion of a specially designed diet. The procedure is not without morbidity and mortality.[87,88]

ADJUVANT THERAPY

Less information concerning the effects of chemotherapeutic agents in gastric cancer is available than we would like. In part, this is related to the difficulty of identifying measurable parameters in patients other than those with rather advanced cancer. Furthermore, early U.S. trials used meager stratification and only short duration of treatment with moderate doses of chemotherapy. As could have been anticipated, a poor result was attained.[89,90] All current programs emphasize the extreme importance of careful staging and stratification in designing clinical trials in this disease.

5-Fluorouracil (5-FU) has activity in gastric cancer. This agent is widely used, and an anticipated response rate approaches 20 percent with a median duration of 4 to 5 months.[91] Most evidence indicates that mitomycin C has a somewhat higher, but shorter response rate. Kovach and Moertel studied 5-FU together with 1,3-bis-(2 chloroethyl)1-nitrosuria (BCNU) at the Mayo Clinic.[92] Forty-one percent of their gastric and pancreatic cancer patients (or 14 of 34 patients) who were evaluable responded, compared to a 29 percent response rate seen in the same study of patients treated with 5-FU alone. The Eastern Cooperative Oncology Group also indicated a better than 40 percent response rate for advanced gastric cancer patients with 5-FU and methyl-chloro-ethylcyclohexynitrosurea (MeCCNU). With the possibility of response rates that approach those seen in breast cancer, the way seemed open for adjuvant studies. Three studies have developed as a result of these preliminary reports: the above-mentioned Eastern Cooperative Oncology Group Study, the Veterans Administration Group Study, and the Gastrointestinal Tumor Study Group Protocol (GITSG). All groups compared patients treated with the chemotherapeutic regimes MeCCNU and 5-FU to a group of patients who were to have been followed with equal intensity but received no treatment beyond surgery. To date, analysis of these group studies is inconclusive, although the GITSG study does show an advantage for treatment. Other studies are not yet confirmatory. Details of stratification and eligibility are being verified for all these protocols.

Koyama, in 1978, summarized a major portion of the Japanese work completed by the National Hospitals Group.[93] Seven controlled studies were carried out. The first study reported on the use of thiotepa and mitomycin C in moderate dosage. This was followed by a low-dose study. In the third study, mitomycin C was administered together with Cytoxan and Chromomycin A3. In the fourth protocol, more mitomycin C was administered at surgery. This was a push protocol for mitomycin C.

In the fifth study, mitomycin C in large dose, Cytoxan, and 5-FU were given together. The fifth study alternated mitomycin C with 5-FU. The next study combined these agents with the mitomycin C given at the time of surgery. The seventh study combined mitomycin C 5-FU and carbazilquin-one. In most studies drugs were not ad-

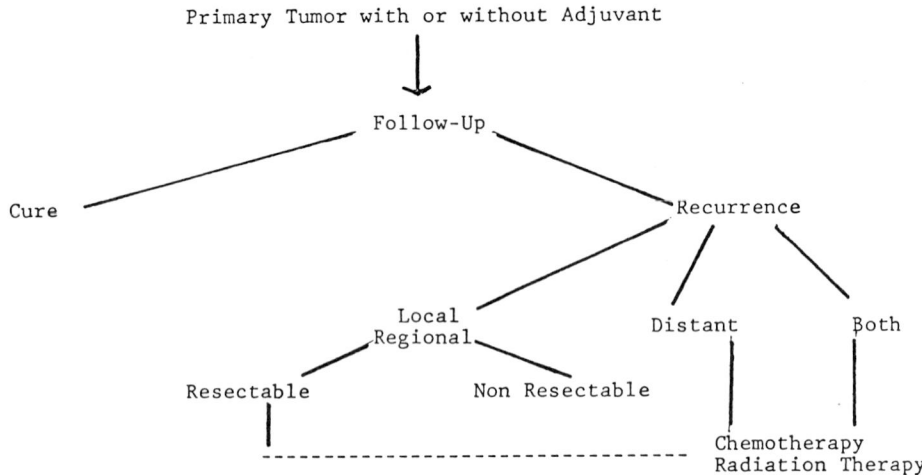

FIGURE 25-6 An orderly plan of follow-up and treatment of recurrent disease must be kept in mind. Recurrence is the more common outcome of primary surgery. Where feasible, surgery is superior palliation but cannot be used alone for systemic disease. (*Adapted from R Pichlmayr, HJ Meyer.*[101])

ministered beyond 6 weeks. No effect was seen in patients with adenocarcinoma, but a possible effect was seen in the relatively small number of patients stratified as having carcinoma simplex.

Other Japanese groups studies also showed improved survival in more recent series, but in most instances survival increments appear to be due to improvement in staging and surgical result when dealing with earlier stage disease. Most Japanese studies of adjuvant therapy for gastric cancer still retain control arms.[94]

A number of other studies are completed or underway which combine radiation therapy and chemotherapy, including intraoperative radiotherapy.[95,96] A European Organization on Research and Treatment of Cancer (EORTC) study tested 2000 rads of radiation together with short-term, long-term, and combined chemotherapy dosage of 5-FU. No beneficial effects were seen. This approach is based on studies by Moertel and others which suggest some potentiation for 5-FU on radiotherapy.[97,98]

Schein et al. commented on the United States' experience with mitomycin C and gastric cancer and indicated that it would be a useful drug.[99] MacDonald et al. continued this work and reported on the combination 5-FU, Adriamycin, and mitomycin C (FAM) in advanced gastric cancer. They felt that they obtained in measurable patients a 42 percent response rate. Further developments from the use of combined radiation and systemic chemotherapy with intraoperative radiation with FAM and possible newer combinations are awaited. It is necessary to be aware of the difficulties in staging in reviewing these studies.[100]

FOLLOW-UP AND TECHNIQUES FOR EARLY IDENTIFICATION OF RECURRENCE AND METASTASIS

Except for those patients who are fortunate enough to be diagnosed with early gastric cancer, the results of treatment of primary gastric cancer are really quite poor. For most patients, recurrence is the order of the day. The anticipated failure rate with subsequent clinical progression is over 80 percent following resection with curative intent. Figure 25-6 posed our problem.[101]

Gastric cancer spreads by direct organ invasion, by transcoelomic passage, via lymphatics, and by hematogenous routes. Often more than one type of recurrence or spread occurs simultaneously. Koga et al. reported on recurrence rates in a series of over 1000 patients with gastric cancer.[102] In this series, two-thirds had recurrence in less than 2 years, but a little more than 15 percent of recurrences (or 2 percent of all operated patients) occurred after 5 years. Poorly differentiated cancer with serosal involvement tended to recur earlier. Earlier recurrence was located more frequently in the peritoneum and regional nodes, with later recurrence relatively more common in the liver.

Lymphatic spread may be submucosal or subserosal, and, as we have stressed, does not necessarily stop at the cardia or pylorus. Extragastric lymphatic spread is important, and over 20 percent of patients will have involvement of nodes in the splenic-pancreatic region regardless of the location of the primary tumor within the stomach. A particularly disturbing spread may extend to the parenchyma of the liver along the omentum. Peritoneal spread is via lymphatics and transserosal seeding with peritoneal implant. It is important to note that perhaps 10 to 15 percent of recurrences will be localized in the gastric remnant, and not more than 25 to 30 percent of recurrences will be regional.[103] The rest will either be distant or mixed.

In spite of the above data, we advocate a frequent revisit program following curative surgery for gastric cancer. We are especially concerned with following patients whose cancers were found to be poorly differentiated, penetrating, or metastatic to lymph nodes at the time of definitive surgery. The options for follow-up available to us include the diagnosis of metastasis or clinical recurrence by symptomatology, physical findings, routine laboratory evaluation, aspiration cytology, barium swallow, endoscopy, and the use of tumor markers. We believe that our patients should be seen at least every 3 months during the first 2 to 2½ years following surgery and at 6-month intervals thereafter. If they are on adjuvant therapy, of course, they may be seen more often, but they should have a careful symptom review and physical examination done at least as often as described above. A posttreatment barium swallow should be carried out 3 months following surgery and repeated yearly over 5 years.

The role of endoscopy versus radiologic diagnosis is not clear in this disease. In a series of 176 patients Groitl et al. reported 34 recurrences detected using endoscopy in follow-up, none of which was seen on barium swallow. For patients who, based on the stage of their disease at initial surgery, appear to be at risk of recurrence, we recommend endoscopy at 1, 2, and 3 years. Otherwise, we recommend pursuing diagnosis with endoscopy in the face of symptoms, questionable x-ray findings, or other evidence of possible recurrence. In this instance, endoscopy should be accompanied by brush cytology and biopsy.

At present, we do not believe that such tumor markers as carcinoembryonic antigen (CEA), α-fetoprotein, or other serum or plasma markers are useful for follow-up on this disease because of low sensitivity.[104,105] With the presence of an expert laboratory, aspiration cytology may be incorporated into a follow-up schema to increase diagnostic accuracy.

Hirose et al. reported 77 patients with recurrent gastric cancer following initial gastrectomy.[106] Seven of these had localized disease and were re-resected. Of the other 70 patients, 32 had local invasion through the serosa, 33 demonstrated peritoneal seeding, 2 had liver metastasis, and 3 showed positive paraaortic nodes. In the judgment of the authors, some 14 of 18 patients operated on with nonresectable local recurrence could have been diagnosed earlier with a more rigorous paraaortic follow-up, which might have allowed re-resection. These authors advocate a barium swallow every 6 months, particularly for patients with primary disease in the middle portion of the stomach with serosal invasion.

THERAPEUTIC OPTIONS FOR THE TREATMENT OF RECURRENCE AND/OR METASTASIS

When feasible, re-resection of recurrences should be considered.[106] Most series indicate that a percentage of gastric stump recurrences can be re-resected with success.[108] Such reoperation may entail splenectomy and resection of the body or tail of the pancreas as well as of the gastric remnant.[109] The question of the usefulness of gastrojejunostomy as a bypass procedure for obstruction or threatened obstruction remains a moot point. Most surgeons feel there is a benefit to palliative resection, although many would not ordinarily support total gastrectomy as a palliative procedure.[110,111] Most feel there is a better relief of outlet obstruction from resection than from a bypass procedure.

For obstructing lesions of the cardia which are not amenable to resection, a Celestine tube or other endoprosthesis may be employed.[112,113] We prefer to seat the tube using an endoscopist and surgical team in order to properly secure the tube and obtain good drainage.[114]

Perhaps half of the patients so treated are able to go home for a few weeks or months at least, without a nasogastric tube, but morbidity and mortality remain a problem.[115]

When we considered adjuvant therapy, we discussed 5-FU and mitomycin C, as well as 5-FU combined with BCNU or MeCCNU. Adriamycin has also been shown to produce a response in a significant proportion of patients with gastric cancer. As we discussed, initial reports of a benefit from combining 5-FU with nitrosourea have not stood up under repeated study.[92,116]

Newer combinations include the regimen of mitomycin C, 5-FU, and cytosine arabinoside, which has been reported as giving a response rate of 17 percent, and the regimen of 5-FU, Adriamycin, and MeCCNU (FAME), reported as producing a 47 percent partial response rate.

As reported by MacDonald et al., the use of 5-FU, Adriamycin, and mitomycin C (FAM) showed a 42 percent partial response rate lasting 9 months, with one patient converting from inoperable to operable on this treatment program.[100] This FAM response rate of 40 to 50 percent has been confirmed in two other studies which suggest that it currently represents the state of the art.

When disease is localized, the use of radiation therapy may be considered. Radiation alone, when applied at a dose of 3000 to 4000 rads to localized residual disease, does not seem to accomplish significant palliation.[117] The Mayo Clinic as well as Falkson and coworkers indicated some benefit from radiation therapy combined with 5-FU.[97,118] The Mayo Clinic series, in particular, contained a few long-term survivors.

The Gastrointestinal Tumor Study Group studied patients with localized unresectable or residual gastric cancer treated with 5-FU + MeCCNU combined with radiation versus chemotherapy alone.[119] Their result is interesting in that it illustrates among other phenomena the need for prolonged follow-up in these treatment studies. Initially, the combined treatment appeared to do much more poorly than the chemotherapy alone. It appears that this was due in part to toxicity and in part to a delay in beginning the chemotherapy portion of treatment. However, after 4 years, eight patients who received the combined therapy remained clinically free of disease although several later relapsed. It is possible that a regimen which allowed for earlier administration of the chemotherapy and provided more nutritional support might be of use for this somewhat regionalized disease. We do know, thanks to the studies of Dent et al., that more than 2000 rads must be given, as he found no benefit from a combined 2000-rads cobalt therapy with 5-FU over no treatment for gastric cancer.[120]

CURRENT AREAS OF RESEARCH AND PROSPECTS FOR THE FUTURE

Although the incidence of gastric cancer has fallen quite precipitously over the last 50 years in this country, this is a fortuitous result, and the evidence is inescapable that exogenous factors, and probably multiple factors, affect the incidence of gastric cancer. Among those areas which need study are the causes and effects of achlorhydria, the role of bacteria in the stomach, and the frequency with which we encounter *N*-nitroso compounds. Other studies of chronic atrophic gastritis, gastric polyps, and reflux gastritis may help. In addition, possible mechanisms of action of foods which seem in particular to be protective, such as fruits, milk, and greens, must be understood for long-term protection.

Diagnosis needs to be improved. There is at present no economic way for us to screen for gastric cancer in the United States. More sensitive glycoprotein markers, perhaps in gastric secretion, will have to be identified, and some basic simplifications of the sampling technique for gastric juice will have to come about to gain wider acceptance. As a part of this effort, the collection and characterization of gastric tumor antigens needs further study. In this area, improved awareness of the danger of prolonged use of antacids without careful study may be of help. Technical advances in x-ray technique may also help.[121] As to screening, with the incidence of tumor seen in the United States at present, new means will have to be found except for high-risk groups.

Testing of new means of combined modality therapy must be carried on in study settings, since current evidence for an adjuvant effect of radiation or chemotherapy is less than conclusive. Newer drugs will have to be tried, as will new forms of radiation, although neutron radiation, for example, is proving to have some delayed scarring effects.[122] In special instances, the use of tissue sensitization with hematoporphyrin derivatives and light may help with obstruction, as may direct (intratumor) administration of chemotherapeutic agents injected via the endoscope.[123] At present, palliation from drugs for gastric cancer is modest.[124,125] For gastric cancer it would appear that the significant advances lie ahead once increased cellular, metabolic, and immunologic knowledge are available.

RECONSTRUCTION AND REHABILITATION

Two aspects of reconstruction and rehabilitation stand out. The first is the correction to some degree of the inanition due to gastric cancer. Parenteral alimentation and elemental nutrition make this possible to an extent not possible previously. It is desirable preoperatively, for good postoperative healing, to reverse the weight loss usually present with at least some weight gain.[126] In addition, there is evidence that radiation is better tolerated in the presence of an active effort to maintain alimentation.

Postsurgically, mechanical rearrangements of the gastrointestinal continuity result in decreased absorption and rapid transit of ingested materials. Both can be quite troublesome. The construction of a reservoir or Hunt-Lawrence pouch will reduce these effects to some degree.

REFERENCES

1. Haenzel W: Report of the working group on studies of cancer and related diseases in migrant populations. *Int J Cancer* 4:364–371, 1969.
2. Haenzel W et al: Stomach cancer in Japan. *J Natl Cancer Inst* 56:265–174, 1976.
3. Billroth T: Open letter to Dr. L. Wittelshofer, in A Hurwitz, GA Degenshein (eds): *Milestones in Modern Surgery,* Hoeber-Harper, New York, 1958, pp 276–280.
4. McNeer G et al: End results in the treatment of gastric cancer. *Surgery* 43:879–896, 1958.
5. Lumpkin WM et al: Carcinoma of the stomach: Review of 1,035 cases. *Ann Surg* 159:919–932, 1964.
6. Kidokoro T: Frequency of resection of metastasis and five-year survival rate of early gastric carcinoma in a surgical clinic, in T Murakami (ed): *Early Gastric Cancer,* Jpn Cancer Assoc, Gann Monograph on Cancer Research, no 11, University Park, Baltimore, 1972.
7. Lahey FH, Marshall SF: Should total gastrectomy be employed in early carcinoma of the stomach? Experience with 139 total gastrectomies. *Ann Surg* 132:540–565, 1950.
8. Marshall SF: Total versus radical partial resection for cancer of the stomach. *SGO* 104:497–498, 1957.
9. Rush BF Jr et al: Total gastrectomy: An evaluation of its use in the treatment of gastric cancer. *Cancer* 13:643–648, 1960.
10. Paulino F, Roselli A: Carcinoma of the stomach with special reference to total gastrectomy. *Curr Prob Surg* 10:3–72, 1973.
11. Longmire WP: The place of radical surgery in gastric cancer, in JW Fielding et al (eds): *Gastric Cancer,* Pergamon, Oxford, 1981; *Adv Biosci* 32:203–217, 1981.
12. Dupont JB Jr et al: Adenocarcinoma of the stomach: Review of 1,497 cases. *Cancer* 41:941–947, 1978.
13. Walters WH et al: Prognosis and end results in the treatment of cancer of the stomach. *Arch Surg* 46:939–943, 1943.
14. Kajitani T, Takagi K: Cancer of the stomach at Cancer Institute Hospital, Tokyo, in Kajitani et al (eds): *Gann Monograph on Cancer Research,* no 22, Tokyo Japan Sci, Tokyo, 1979, pp 77–87.
15. Muto S: Factors influencing surgical results for gastric cancer. *Nichiishi Kaishi (Jpn)* 47:135, 1962.
16. Mine M et al: End results of gastrectomy for gastric cancer. *Surgery* 68:753–758, 1970.
17. Muto S et al: Improvement in the end results of surgical treatment of gastric cancer. *Surgery* 63:229–235, 1968.
18. Sakamoto K et al: Surgical concept and long-term prognosis of early gastric cancer surgery, diagnosis, and treatment. *Geka Shinryo* 13:37, 1971.
19. Hirayama T: Methods and results (cost effectiveness) of gastric cancer screening, in JW Fielding et al (eds): *Gastric Cancer,* Pergamon, Oxford, 1981; *Adv Biosci* 32:77–84, 1981.
20. Friesen G et al: Superficial carcinoma of the stomach. *Surgery* 51:300–312, 1962.
21. Gilbertson VA, Hollenberg M: The results of surgery for cancer of the stomach. *SGO* 115:543–546, 1962.
22. Hirayama T: Changing patterns in the incidence of gastric cancer, in JW Fielding et al (eds): *Gastric Cancer,* Pergamon, Oxford, 1981; *Adv Biosci* 32:1–15, 1981.
23. Gear MWL et al: Gastric cancer simulating benign gastric ulcer. *Br J Surg* 56:739–742, 1969.
24. Holyoke ED: Cancer of the stomach, in JM Seigel, PD Chadoff (eds): *The Aged and High Risk Surgical Patient,* Grune & Stratton, New York, 1976.
25. Hill M: Nitrates and bacteriology: Are these important etiological factors in gastric carcinogenesis? in JW Fielding et al (eds): *Gastric Cancer,* Pergamon, Oxford, 1981; *Adv Biosci* 32:35–45, 1981.
26. Hoffman D, Wynder EI: A study of tobacco carcinogenesis. XI. Tumor initiators, tumor accelerators and tumor-promoting activity of condensate fractions. *Cancer* 27:848–864, 1974.
27. Tayler R, Piper DW: The carcinogenic effect of cigarette smoke on human gastric mucosal cells in organ culture. *Cancer* 39:2520–2523, 1977.
28. Ochsner A, Blalock J: Carcinoma of the stomach. *JAMA* 151:1377–1384, 1953.
29. Nealson TF: *Management of the Patient with Cancer.* Saunders, Philadelphia, 1976.
30. Adashek et al: Cancer of the stomach: Review of consecutive ten-year intervals. *Ann Surg* 189(1):6–10, 1979.

31. American Cancer Society: *Cancer Facts and Figures,* American Cancer Society, New York, 1980.
32. MacDonald EJ: Cancer of the gastrointestinal tract: Epidemiological aspects. *JAMA* 228:884–886, 1974.
33. Higginson J: *Worldwide Review of Epidemiology of Gastric Cancer,* WHO-CC Monograph, no. 1, 1977, pp 81–92.
34. Pfeiffer CJ: Exogenous factors in the epidemiology of gastric carcinoma, in C Herfarth, P Schlag (eds): *Gastric Cancer,* Springer-Verlag, Berlin, 1979, pp 2–8.
35. Pfeiffer CJ et al: An epidemiologic analysis of mortality and gastric cancer in Newfoundland. *J Can Med Assoc* 108:1374–1388, 1973.
36. Wolff G, Lauter J: On the epidemiology of gastric cancer. *Arch Geschwulstforsch* 46:1–14, 1976.
37. McMichael AJ et al: Cancer mortality among rubber workers: An epidemiologic study. *Ann NY Acad Sci* 271:125–137, 1976.
38. Maimon SN, Zinninger MM: Familial gastric cancer. *Gastroenterology* 25:139–152, 1953.
39. Cruzek et al: Familial aspects of gastric adenocarcinoma. *Am J Dig Dis* 6:7–10, 1961.
40. Mosbeck J, Videbaek A: Mortality from and risk of gastric carcinoma among patients with pernicious anemia. *Br Med J* 2:390–394, 1950.
41. Creagan ET, Fraumeni JF Jr: Familial gastric cancer and immunological abnormalities. *Cancer* 32:1325–1331, 1973.
42. Cworn M et al: Simultaneous occurrence of gastric carcinoma in identical twins. *Am J Gastroenterol* 75:41–47, 1981.
43. Roberts JAF: Associations between blood groups and disease. *Acta Genet Statist Med* (Basel) 6:549–560, 1957.
44. McConnell RB: *The Genetics of Gastrointestinal Disorders,* Oxford, London, 1966.
45. Lilienfeld DE et al: Model for gastric cancer epidemiology. *Lancet* 1(7949):45, 1976.
46. Weed TE et al: Carcinoma of the stomach: Why are we failing to improve survival? *Ann Surg* 193:407–413, 1981.
47. LaDue JS et al: Symptomatology and diagnosis of gastric cancer. *Arch Surg* 60:305–335, 1950.
48. Longmire WP: Carcinoma of the stomach, in D Sabiston (ed): *Davis-Christopher Textbook of Surgery,* Saunders, Philadelphia, 1977, pp 983–993.
49. Hakkinen IP et al: The use of oncofetal antigen FSA in discrimination between benign and malignant gastric ulceration. *Acta Chir Scand* 146:507–510, 1980.
50. Tataryn DN et al: Tube leukocyte adherence inhibition (LAI) assay in gastrointestinal (GIT) cancer. *Cancer* 43:898–912, 1979.
51. Goldrosen M: Personal communication.
52. Allen S, Coates RH: The accuracy of the barium meal in the diagnosis of carcinoma of the stomach. *Australas Radiol* 20:236–238, 1976.
53. Suzuki H: Barium spray method to improve radiographic and endoscopic diagnosis. *Gastrointest Endosc* 19:125–128, 1973.
54. Denny M et al: The double contrast barium meal in relation to the diagnosis of early mucosal lesions in the stomach and duodenum. *Front Gastrointest Res* 5:1–13, 1979.
55. Keto P et al: Double contrast examination of the stomach compared with endoscopy. *Acta Radiol (Diagn) Stockh* 20:762–768, 1979.
56. Burhenne HJ: The radiologic diagnosis of carcinoma of the digestive tract, in RJ Cohen et al (eds): *Current Concepts in the Diagnosis and Treatment of the Intra-abdominal Cancer,* Proc San Francisco Cancer Symp 1974, San Francisco, 1975.
57. Koga M et al: Roentgen features of the superficial depressed type of early gastric cancer. *Radiology* 115:289–292, 1975.
58. Bernadino ME et al: Differentiating gastric tumors from benign ulcers. *VA Med* 105:140–141, 1978.
59. Schulman A, Simpkins KC: The accuracy of radiological diagnosis of benign primary and secondary malignant gastric ulcers and their correlation with three simplified radiological types. *Clin Radiol* 26:317–325, 1975.
60. Moshakis V, Hooper AA: The accuracy of endoscopic diagnosis of gastric carcinoma and the conventional barium meal. *Clin Oncol* 4:359–368, 1978.
61. Prolla JC et al: Gastric cancer: Some recent improvements in diagnosis based upon the Japanese experience. *Arch Intern Med* 124:238–246, 1969.
62. Winawer SJ et al: Endoscopic diagnosis of advanced gastric cancer: Factors influencing yield. *Gastroenterology* 69:1183–1187, 1975.
63. Nomura H et al: A study of intestinal metaplasia of gastric mucosa by in vivo dye staining, *Meeting Abstract, Proc. 39th Ann Meet Jpn Cancer Assoc, Tokyo,* November, 1980.
64. Hakkinen IP: Differentiation of antigenic gastric cancer sulphopolysaccharides from metaplastic "intestinal" type sulphosaccharides. *Scand J Gastroenterol* 2:37–43, 1967.
65. Oota K: *Historical Types of Gastric and Esophageal Tumors,* WHO International Histological Classification of Tumors, no 18, Geneva, 1977.
66. Lauren, P: The two histological main types of gastric carcinoma diffuse and so-called intestinal type carcinoma: An attempt at a histo-clinical classification. *Acta Pathol Microbiol Scand* 64:31–49, 1965.
67. Mulligan RM, Rember RR: Histogenesis and biologic behavior of gastric carcinoma. *Arch Pathol* 58:1–25, 1954.
68. Day DW: Histopathology of gastric cancer, in JWL Fielding et al (eds): *Gastric Cancer,* Oxford, 1981; *Adv Biosci* 32:95–109, 1981.
69. Steiner PD et al: Gastric cancer morphologic factors in five-year survival after gastrectomy. *Am J Pathol* 24:947–969, 1948.
70. Martin C, Kay S: The prognosis of gastric carcinoma as related to its morphologic characteristics. *SGO* 119:319–322, 1964.
71. Larmi TK, Saxen L: "Host Reactions" in gastric cancer: A preliminary study of 119 cases of gastrectomy. *Acta Chirugica Scand* 125:144–146, 1963.

72. American Joint Committee for Cancer Staging and End Result Reporting: *Manual for Staging of Cancer,* Chicago, 1977.
73. Hawley PR et al: Pathology and prognosis of carcinoma of the stomach. *Br J Surg* 57:877–883, 1970.
74. Cantrell EG: The importance of lymph nodes in the assessment of gastric carcinoma at operation. *Br J Surg* 58:384–386, 1971.
75. Kidokoro T: Frequency of resection, metastasis and five-year survival of early gastric carcinoma in a surgical clinic, in T Murakami (ed): *Early Gastric Cancer,* Gann Monograph on Cancer Research, no 11, Univ. Tokyo, Tokyo, 1971, pp 45–49.
76. Paile A: Morphology and prognosis of carcinoma of the stomach. *Ann Chir Gynaecol (Fenniae)* 60 (Suppl 175):1–56, 1971.
77. ReMine WH et al: Long-term survival 10–56 years after surgery for carcinoma of the stomach. *Am J Surg* 117:177–184, 1969.
78. Rush BF, Ravitch MM: The evaluation of total gastrectomy *SGO* 114:411–423, 1962.
79. Scott HW Jr, Longmire WP Jr: Total gastrectomy: Report of 63 cases. *Surgery* 26:488–498, 1949.
80. Lawrence WL: Carcinoma of the stomach. *CA* 23(5):286–304, 1973.
81. Hoerr SO: Long-term results in patients who survived five or more years after gastric resection for primary carcinoma. *SGO* 153:820–822, 1981.
82. Papachristou DN, Fortner JG: Adenocarcinoma of the gastric cardia. *Ann Surg* 192:58–64, 1980.
83. Berry RE, Rottschafer W: The lymphatic spread of cancer of the stomach observed in operative specimens removed by radical surgery including total pancreatectomy. *SGO* 104:269–279, 1957.
84. Lawrence W Jr, McNeer G: The effectiveness of surgery for palliation of incurable gastric cancer. *Cancer* 11:28–31, 1958.
85. ReMine WH: Preoperative assessment and palliative surgery, in JWL Fielding et al (eds): *Gastric Cancer,* Pergamon, Oxford,1981; *Adv Biosci* 32, 1981.
86. Stern J et al:Evaluation of palliative resection in advanced carcinoma of the stomach. *Surgery* 77:291–298, 1975.
87. Celestin LR: Permanent intubation in inoperable cancer of the oesophagus and cardia: A new tube. *Ann R Coll Surg Engl* 25:165–170, 1959.
88. Fry DD: Technique for introducing celestine tube. *SGO* 139:252–253, 1974.
89. Rochlin D et al: A chemotherapy of malignancies of the gastrointestinal tract. *Am J Surg* 109:43–46, 1965.
90. Hurley JD et al: Treatment of advanced cancer of the gastrointestinal tract with antitumor agents. *Gastroenterology* 41:557–562, 1961.
91. Kennedy BJ, Theoligides A: The place of 5-fluorouracil in malignant disease. *Ann Intern Med* 55:719–730, 1961.
92. Kovach JS et al: A controlled study of 1-3-bis-(2-chloroethyl)-1-nitrosourea and 5-fluorouracil therapy for advanced gastric and pancreatic cancer. *Cancer* 33:563–567, 1974.
93. Koyama Y: The current status of chemotherapy for gastric cancer in Japan with special emphasis on mitomycin C. *Recent Results Cancer Res* 63:135–147, 1978.
94. Nakajima T et al: Adjuvant chemotherapy with mitomycin-C and with a multidrug combination of mitomycin-C, 5-fluorouracil and cytosine arabinoside after curative resection for gastric cancer. *Jap J Clin Oncol* 10:187–194, 1980.
95. Goffin JC, Machin D: Treatment of patients with gastric cancer by surgery, radiotherapy and chemotherapy: Preliminary results of an EORTC radomized study. *Recent Results Cancer Res* 68:208–211, 1978.
96. Tobe T: Treatment of gastric cancer with combined surgery and intra-operative radiotherapy. *World J Surg* 3:715–719, 1979.
97. Childs DS et al: Treatment of unresectable adenocarcinomas of the stomach with a combination of 5-fluorouracil and radiation. *Am J Roentgenol* 102:541–544, 1968.
98. Moertel CG, Reitemier RT: Advances in gastrointestinal cancer, in *Clinical Management and Chemotherapy,* Harper & Row, New York, 1969, p 164.
99. Schein PS et al: Mitomycin C, Experience in the United States with emphasis on gastric cancer. *Recent Results Cancer Res.* 63:148–151, 1978.
100. MacDonald JS et al: 5-Fluorouracil, doxorubicin and mitomycin (FAM) combination chemotherapy for advanced cancer. *Ann Intern Med* 93:533–536, 1980.
101. Pichlmayr R, Meyer HJ: Patterns of recurrence in relation to therapeutic strategy, in JWL Fielding et al (eds): *Gastric Cancer,* Pergamon, Oxford, 1981; *Adv Biosci* 32:171–184, 1981.
102. Koga et al: Clinical and pathological evaluation of patients with recurrence of gastric cancer more than five years postoperatively. *Am J Surg* 136:317–321, 1970.
103. Iwanaga T: Mechanisms of late recurrence after radical surgery for gastric carcinoma. *Am J Surg* 135:637–640, 1978.
104. Holyoke ED, Cooper EH: CEA and tumor markers. *Semin Oncol* 3:377–385, 1976.
105. Ravry M et al: Carcinoembryonic antigen and alpha-fetoprotein in diagnosis of gastric and colonic cancer: A comparative clinical evaluation. *J Natl Cancer Inst* 52:1019–1021, 1974.
106. Hirose S et al: Recurrent carcinoma after gastrectomy and primary carcinoma of the residual stomach. *J Jpn Soc Cancer Ther* 12:59–60, 1975.
107. Ekbom GA et al: Gastric malignancy: Resection for palliation. *Surgery* 88:476–481, 1980.
108. Klasfeld J, Resnick G: Gastric remnant carcinoma. *Cancer* 44:1129–1133, 1979.
109. Papachristou DN et al: Anastomotic recurrence in the esophagus complicating gastrectomy for adenocarcinoma of the stomach. *Br J Surg* 66:609–612, 1979.

110. Lawrence W, NcNeer G: The effectiveness of surgery for palliation of incurable gastric cancer. *Cancer* 11:28, 1958.
111. Leinster SJ et al: The role of resection in advanced gastric carcinoma. *Clin Oncol* 6:55–61, 1980.
112. Sander WR: The celestin tube in the palliation of carcinoma of the oesophagus and cardia. *Br J Surg* 66:419–421, 1979.
113. Turnbull A et al: Palliative prosthetic intubation in gastric cancer. *J Surg Oncol* 15:37–42, 1980.
114. Nava H: Personal communication.
115. Hartog-Jager FC et al: Palliative treatment of obstructing esophagogastric malignancy by endoscopic positioning of a plastic prosthesis. *Gastroenterology* 77:1008–1014, 1979.
116. Moertel CG et al: Chemotherapy of gastric carcinoma. *Proc Am Assoc Cancer Res Am Soc Clin Oncol* 20:288, 1979.
117. Gundersson LL: Radiation therapy, Research and value possibilities. *Clin Gastroenterol* 5:743–776, 1976.
118. Falkson et al: Combined telecobalt and 5-fluorouracil therapy in cancer of the stomach. *S Afr Med J* 36:712–717, 1963.
119. Schein PS, Novak JW for the Gastrointestinal Tumor Study Group: A comparative assessment of combination chemotherapy in advanced cancer. *Proc AACR & ASCO* 21:420 (c403), 1980.
120. Dent DM et al: Prospective randomized trial of combined oncological therapy for gastric carcinoma. *Cancer* 44:385–391, 1979.
121. Treichel J: Double contrast radiography of the stomach, Technique and results in early gastric cancer. *J Radiol* 60:299–305, 1979.
122. Kingsley D et al: Adenocarcinoma of the stomach: Radiological and pathological correlation of effects of treatment with fast neutrons. *Gut* 17:624–632, 1976.
123. Yamada et al: Comparison of intramural 5-fluorouracil and more conventional routes of drug administration on concentration in gastric regional lymph nodes: A potential for transendoscopic adjuvant chemotherapy. *J Surg Oncol* 11:341–349, 1979.
124. Moertel CG: Chemotherapy of gastrointestinal cancer. *Clin Gastroenterol* 5:777–793, 1976.
125. Lavin PJ et al: Phase II–III chemotherapy studies in advanced gastric cancer. *CT Rep* 63:1863–1869, 1979.
126. Jorgensen ST: Conservative treatment with total parenteral nutrition in patients with gastroesophageal anastomotic leaks (anastomotic leaks conservatively treated). *Acta Chir Scand* 145(3):173–175, 1979.

26
HEPATOBILIARY AND PERIAMPULLARY NEOPLASMS

Joseph G. Fortner

Primary liver cancer is one of the most common cancers afflicting human beings, for it is the most common cancer in certain areas of Asia and Africa.[1,2] (Table 26-1.) Although this tumor is less commonly seen in Western countries, it is estimated that in the United States, 13,000 new cases of cancer of the liver and biliary tract will have been diagnosed in 1981.[3] Major developments seem very likely in this field since so many promising clues to the etiology of these cancers are being actively pursued.

ETIOLOGY

Primary Liver Cancer

There is abundant evidence that primary liver cancer is the cumulative result of several etiological agents.[4]

HEPATITIS B VIRUS

One of the most important suspects is hepatitis B virus (HBV). This infection and virus-induced postnecrotic cirrhosis are associated with the majority of hepatomas in Asian and African populations.[5,6] This association has been less evident in Western populations, but radioimmunoassay and other new techniques are permitting reevaluation of incidence.[7] Some degree of caution in accepting the causal relationship between HBV and liver cancer is necessary, however. HBV is hyperendemic in Greenland (serological evidence of infection is found in over half the adult population), but the incidence of hepatoma is low.[8] HBV infection is at least 10 times more prevalent in Greenland than in Europe, but neither cirrhosis nor primary liver cancer is more common. Eskimos of Greenland show no evidence that HBV per se contributes to their developing cirrhosis or primary liver cancer. Any causal relationship hopefully will be clarified upon completion of the mass vaccination program against HBV infection currently underway.[9]

Genetic factors appear to play a role in the development of hepatoma. The lack of hepatoma formation in the Greenland population in spite of their high rate of hepatitis B infection has been explained on this basis. Further evidence that genetic factors are important is shown in the history of a Peruvian family in which the mother and three sons were all hepatitis B antigen–positive. The oldest son developed hepatoma and died. The second son developed hepatoma and had a left hepatic lobectomy (Fig. 26-1), and was alive and well 2

560 INTRAABDOMINAL NEOPLASMS

TABLE 26-1 Geographic distribution of primary cancers of the liver and intrahepatic bile ducts. Incidence figures are given as new cases per 100,000 population per year.

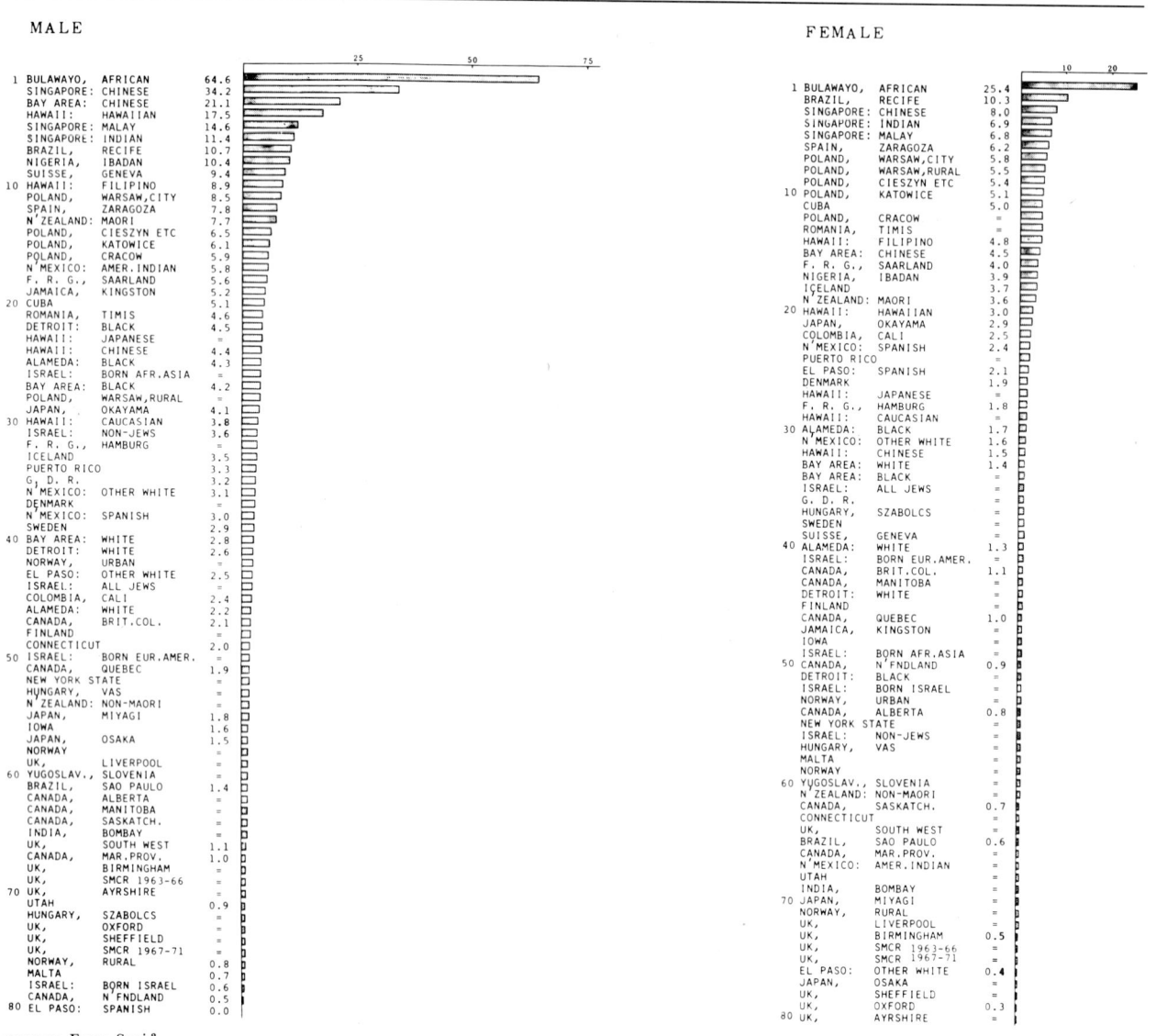

SOURCE: From Segi.[2]

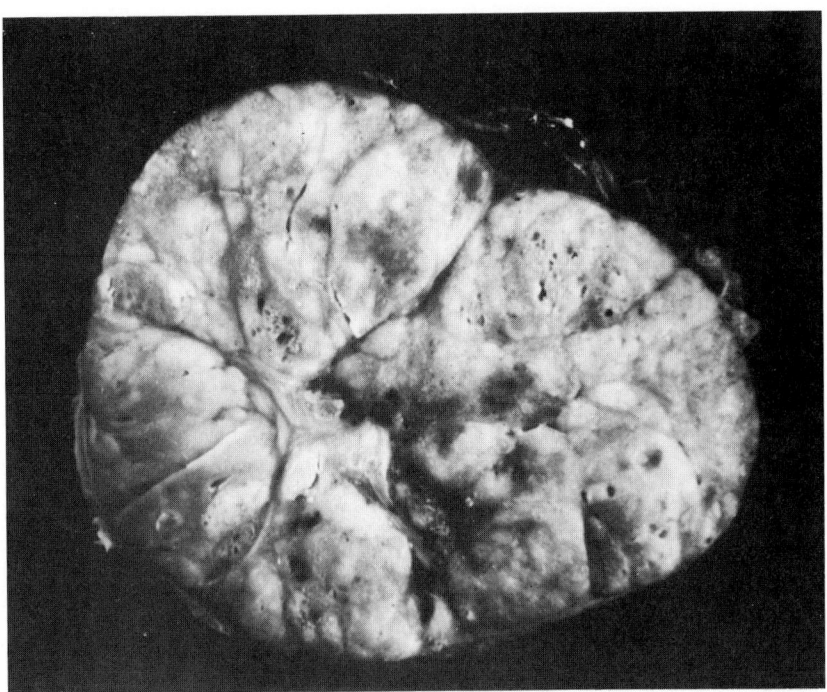

FIGURE 26-1 Hemisection of left lobe of liver showing severe cirrhosis and hepatoma formation.

years later. The third and youngest son is being observed closely for signs of malignant degeneration of his liver.

HEREDITARY TYROSINEMIA

A fascinating phenomenon is the development of hepatoma in children who are afflicted with tyrosinemia.[10–12] In this rare and tragic disease, an inborn error of metabolism results in increased levels of tyrosine in plasma and urine. In the more indolent form, patients may survive into childhood, manifesting continued hepatic and renal dysfunction and early development of macronodular cirrhosis. This form is called *chronic tyrosinemia* with hepatorenal involvement and is associated with abnormal *p*-hydroxyphenylpyruvate hydroxylase activity. Weinberg et al.[12] reported on 29 patients with chronic tyrosinemia and hepatorenal disease surviving through 2 years of age and found that 35 percent developed hepatoma. Another 14 patients with a presumptive diagnosis of chronic tyrosinemia and hepatorenal disease who survived to 2 years of age had a 43 percent incidence of hepatoma. The overall prevalence of hepatoma was 37 percent in the combined group of 43 patients. Death from hepatocellular carcinoma occurred in 66 percent of the females and 57 percent of the males. The median age at time of death from cancer in the known tyrosinemia group was 5 years with a range of 4 to 25 years. The peak incidence of tumor is between 4 and 5 years. Many patients were alive with cirrhosis with no clinical evidence of malignancy at the time of the report. All of the tumors were hepatocellular carcinoma and were often extensive, multicentric, and associated with cirrhosis. Figure 26-2 shows the appearance of such a liver in a 2-year-old patient. It has been proposed that the cirrhosis and hepatoma are results of the toxic effects of tyrosine or some metabolite of tyrosine. The disease is inherited as an autosomal recessive trait. There is an area in Quebec Province where the prevalence is high.[13,14] Hereditary tyrosinemia has also been reported from Scandinavia.

AFLATOXIN

Aflatoxin ingestion appears also to be important in the etiology of hepatoma.[15] The Inhambane district of Mo-

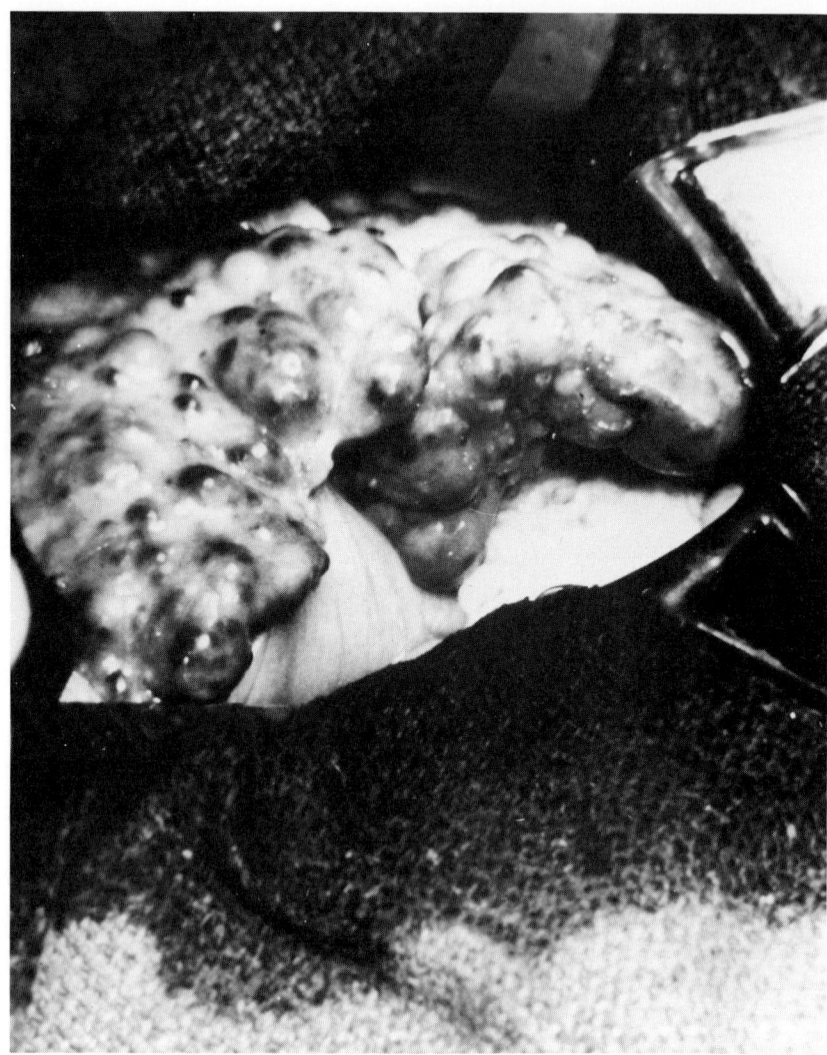

FIGURE 26-2 Appearance of liver at laparotomy of 2-year-old girl with hereditary tyrosinemia. Liver shows severe micro- and macronodular cirrhosis and hepatoma.

zambique, for example, has the highest aflatoxin intake and the highest crude liver cancer rate of any of the four countries studied (Table 26-2). A similar relationship exists for other areas of Africa and Thailand where there is a high degree of positive correlation between the calculated levels of ingestion of aflatoxin and adult incidence of hepatocellular carcinoma.

DIETARY FACTORS

The problem becomes even more complex when the modifying influences of dietary factors are considered.[16]

The ratio of metabolic activation to detoxification appears to be a most important determinant of the net effect of various food substances. Flavonoids, for example, affect the in vitro metabolism of foreign chemicals by human liver. Flavone, tangeretin, and nobiletin activate the hydroxylation of benzo[a]pyrene and the metabolism of aflatoxin B_1 to mutagens. Other flavonoids such as quercetin and kaempferol inhibit in vitro hydroxylation of benzo[a]pyrene by human liver microsomes. Benzo[a]pyrene and other polycyclic aromatic hydrocarbons such as benzanthracene and dibenzanthracene are widespread. Investigations in this complex field appear to have unusual potential for significant contributions toward the prevention of cancer.

ALCOHOLIC CIRRHOSIS

A variety of other agents influence the development of liver tumors. Alcoholic liver cirrhosis is considered the main cause of primary liver cancer according to one study from West Germany.[17] In that study, the risk of hepatoma developing was apparently greatly enhanced by the presence of more than one risk factor. This included HBsAg antigenemia and/or acute hepatitis, as well as alcoholic liver cirrhosis.

VARIOUS AGENTS

Hepatic angiosarcoma has been related to exposure to vinyl chloride, thorium dioxide (Thorotrast), or arsenic.[18-21] Pesticides are of concern as hepatic carcinogens. They are biologically active and are significant environmental contaminants.[22] Only a few have been subjected to short- or long-term evaluation, and some are hepatic carcinogens for experimental animals, usually mice.

CONTRACEPTIVES

Three liver tumors appear possibly to be affected by use of oral contraceptives. These are focal nodular hyperplasia, liver cell adenoma, and hepatocellular carcinoma. Focal nodular hyperplasia is not causally related but develops a hemorrhagic tendency on use of oral contraceptives. The annual incidence of hepatocellular adenoma in long-term users of oral contraceptives is estimated as 3 to 4 per 100,000 persons; a causal relationship is unproven but possible.[23] Christopherson and Mays[24] have reported on 19 women with hepatoma who have used steroids, but the causal relationship here is also nebulous. Experimentally, diethylstilbestrol promotes the growth of hepatomas that are initiated by carcinogens.[25]

Extrahepatic Biliary Tract

The overall risk of developing cancer of the biliary tract increases with age. There is an excess risk, however, after age 55 for whites compared with blacks.[26] A high rate has been reported in Mexicans[27] and American Indians.[28] Cancer of the gallbladder predominates in females, while other biliary tract cancer is more common in males.[26,29] The ratio of gallbladder to bile duct cancer is 3:1;[30] age-adjusted incidence rates are shown in Table 26-3.[26,29]

Certain diseases are associated with these neoplasms. Gallstones are found in 70 to 90 percent of patients with cancer of the gallbladder.[31-33] Ulcerative colitis[34] may be associated with cancer of the extrahepatic biliary tract, while Clonorchis sinensis (Asia)[35] has been associated with intrahepatic biliary tract cancer (Fig. 26-3). Periampullary cancer and Gardner's syndrome[36] are associated in a greater-than-expected frequency. Second primary cancers are found in 27 percent of patients with periampullary cancer.[37] This is significantly higher than the expected overall incidence of multiple primary cancer in the population.

TABLE 26-2 Summary of the Available Data on Aflatoxin Ingestion Levels and Liver Cancer Incidence

Study area	Subarea	Aflatoxin intake, ng/kg·D	Crude liver cancer rate, ×10⁵ per year
Kenya	High altitude	3.5	1.2
Thailand	Songkhla	5.0	2.0
Swaziland	High veld	5.1	2.2
Kenya	Midaltitude	5.9	2.5
Swaziland	Midveld	8.9	3.8
Kenya	Low altitude	10.0	4.0
Swaziland	Lubombo	15.4	4.3
Thailand	Rat Buri	45.0	6.0
Swaziland	Low veld	43.1	9.2
Mozambique	Inhambane	222.4	13.0

SOURCE: Linsell CA: Environmental chemical carcinogens and liver cancer, in K Lapis, JV Johannessen (eds): Liver Carcinogenesis, Hemisphere Publishing Corporation, Washington, D.C., 1979.

TABLE 26-3 Age-Adjusted Incidence Rates in the United States for Biliary Tract Cancer, 1969–1971

	WHITE		BLACK	
	M	F	M	F
Gallbladder	1.1*	2.2	0.7	1.6
Other biliary passages	1.6	1.0	1.2	0.8

*Annual rate per 100,000 population.
SOURCE: Fraumeni.[26]

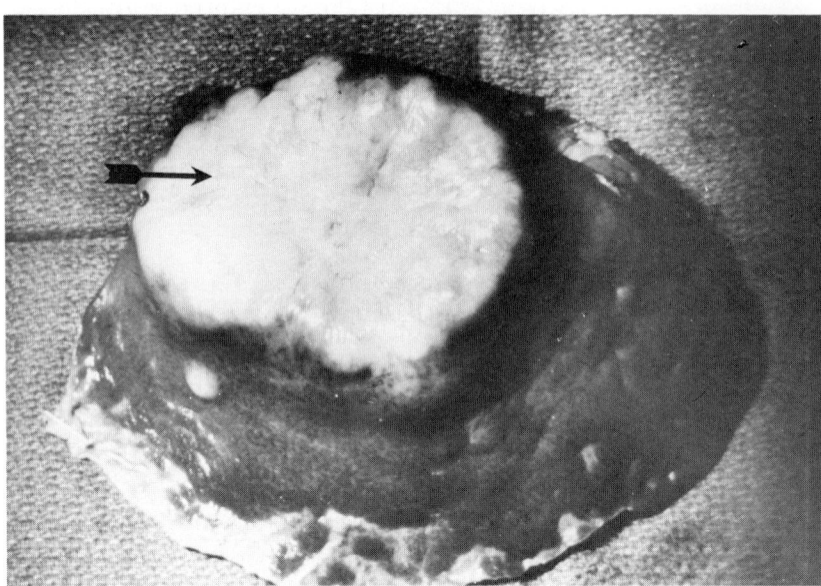

FIGURE 26-3 Cholangiocarcinoma in left lobe of liver. Myriads of Clonorchis sinensis were evident in the bile ducts.

Any causal relationship which may exist between gallstones and gallbladder cancer has been attributed to chronic irritation,[38,39] to a low level of radioactive material in the gallstones,[39-41] or to a carcinogen incorporated within the stone.[42-44] These various possibilities[45] were investigated in a study in which the radioactivity of stones from patients with cancer of the gallbladder was measured and found to be inconsequential.[46] In a series of experiments, the domestic cat was found to be a suitable experimental model for the study of gallbladder carcinogenesis,[47] because of the ability to induce gallbladder cancer with methylcholanthrene pellets implanted in the cat's gallbladder. Using this experimental model, gallstones from patients with and without cancer of the gallbladder were tested.[48] Unfortunately, the mortality rate of the cats was high. Of the surviving animals, however, two cats developed adenocarcinoma of the gallbladder, and one also developed a primary adenocarcinoma of the ampulla of Vater. These stones came from a patient with gallbladder cancer and had been in situ in the cats for about 5½ years. Precancerous changes of papillary hyperplasia with atypical foci developed in the gallbladder of a third cat with stones from a patient with breast cancer and benign biliary tract disease. These stones had been in situ for 6 years and 4 months. A presumably spontaneous islet-cell carcinoma arose in a fourth cat in whose gallbladder stones from a patient with benign biliary tract disease and an adenomatous polyp of the colon had been placed 4 years previously. This massive islet-cell tumor invaded the gallbladder and bile ducts. These data suggest that gallstones might act as promoters for carcinogens excreted in the biliary tract. Another possibility is that the implanted stones might contain either a carcinogen which is a metabolic derivative of ingested chemicals or an endogenous carcinogen which had been excreted in the bile of the patient from which the gallstones had come.

DIAGNOSIS

Liver Cancer

SIGNS AND SYMPTOMS

The possibility of primary or metastatic cancer in the liver should be considered in all patients who have hepatomegaly.[49,50] The upper abdominal mass may be asymptomatic, an incidental finding of the patient or of an examining physician. In other instances, mild discomfort or pain in the epigastrium or right upper quadrant may develop along with weight loss. At times, particularly in Asian and African patients, the presence of a primary hepatoma is heralded by a sudden severe pain and shock from spontaneous rupture of the tumor and hemoperitoneum.[51] This is a rare presentation for patients with hepatoma in Western countries. Jaundice is seldom present at first; fever is rare, occurring in only about 10 percent of patients. Symptoms increase with progression of the disease; at the time of hospital admission of 67 patients studied by Ihde et al.,[52] 71.6 percent of the series presented with right upper quadrant or epigastric pain of a chronic nature accompanied by a right upper quadrant mass or a hard enlarging liver in a setting of weight loss or increasing abdominal girth. Curutchet et al.[53] found pain was present in 88 percent of 65 patients and weight loss in 77 percent of patients with hepatoma at time of admission. Intermittent fever developed in 47 percent. Gastrointestinal bleeding developed in 30 percent, the majority of whom had cirrhosis associated with the hepatoma. Hepatomegaly, ascites, and jaundice were the most frequent physical findings in this series of patients, many with advanced disease.

The clinical history is important in ruling out previous cancers that may have metastasized to the liver. The incidence of cirrhosis in hepatoma patients in Western countries is difficult to obtain. Surgical experiences are weighted heavily toward patients who do not have cirrhosis, while nonsurgical experience is weighted heavily toward those with cirrhosis.

Metastatic cancer of the liver, particularly colorectal cancer, may manifest itself as an asymptomatic mass occurring some months or years after the colon resection.[49] It may, of course, be found at the time of detection of the primary colon tumor. The disease progresses in much the same fashion as described for primary liver tumors.

The physical examination is particularly important in evaluating patients with primary and secondary liver cancer. The findings can be misleading, for tumors in the right lobe commonly cause marked distortion leading to the erroneous conclusion that both right and left lobes of the liver are involved. In addition, a left-lobe tumor may cause rotation of the liver to the right so that the right lobe is no longer palpable and the left lobe gives the appearance of being an enlarged right lobe of the liver.

Serum biochemical tests of importance include the serum bilirubin, total and conjugated, SGOT, alkaline phosphatase, 5'-nucleotidase, serum protein electrophoresis, uric acid, CEA levels and serum α-fetoprotein concentration, HBV antigen and antibody, and a coagulogram.

TUMOR MARKERS

The prevalence with which α-fetoprotein is detected in patients with primary liver cancer varies significantly in different countries. While the average frequency is 63 percent, it is only 53 percent in Europe and in the Africa-Asia group it is 71 percent.[54] The prevalence is even less in the United States, where Caucasians have been reported to have 31 percent[55-57] and 51 percent[58] positivity, and the Negro and non-Caucasian populations 71 percent[55-57] and 76 percent.[58] Mass screening programs have been carried out in mainland China utilizing the α-fetoprotein marker to detect hepatomas.[59] The high incidence there of hepatoma makes this effort feasible.

Carcinoembryonic antigen (CEA) is elevated in about two-thirds of one series of patients with metastatic colorectal cancer in the liver.[50,60] These elevations range from 5.9 to 20,000 ng/mL. Sequential CEA estimations following treatment for metastatic colorectal cancer in the liver are particularly valuable. Table 26-4 indicates that recurrent metastatic colorectal cancer after major hepatic resection can be detected by CEA elevations if the recurrence is intraabdominal. Extraabdominal disease was not found to be associated with an elevation in the CEA titer. Particularly interesting is the rate with which elevated CEA levels fall after major hepatic resection. Figure 26-4 indicates that it can take as long as 3 months for a greatly elevated CEA level to return to normal.

Human chorionic gonadotropin (HCG) has been reported elevated in patients who have primary liver cancer.[61] 5-Hydroxyindoleacetic acid will be excreted in the urine of patients with a carcinoid.

RADIOLOGICAL INVESTIGATIONS

CAT scanning and/or sonography and selective celiac and superior mesenteric angiography are the two most important radiological investigations. CAT scanning and sonography are noninvasive. For patients with hepatomegaly the presence of a tumor and its location can be detected. Invaluable clues as to the type of tumor can be

TABLE 26-4 Recurrence Subsequent to Hepatic Resection for Metastatic Colorectal Cancer

Site of recurrence	CEA > 5 ng/mL
Liver	6/6
Lungs	0/5
Colorectum	2/2
Ovaries, peritoneum	1/1
Bone	0/1
Total	9/15 (60%)

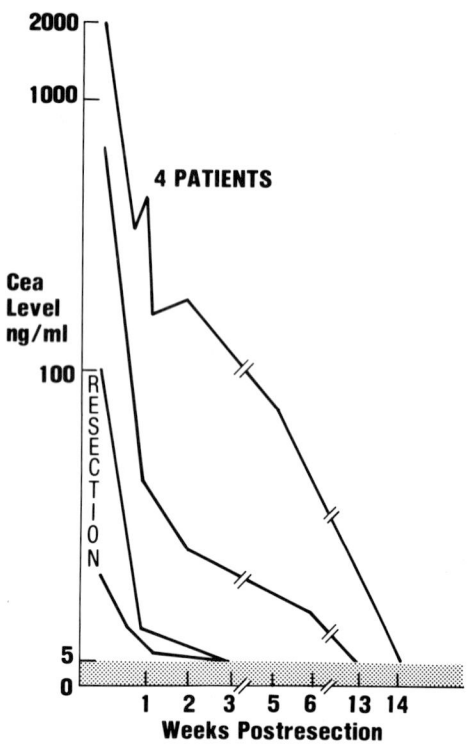

FIGURE 26-4 CEA levels after hepatic resection for metastatic colorectal cancer.

gained (Fig. 26-5). Angiography provides a "road map" for hepatic vasculature; it can disclose the presence of a tumor, its degree of vascularity, and important information as to the type of tumor (Fig. 26-6). It is essential for the proper placement of catheters in the hepatic artery and portal vein for infusional chemotherapy. Within a given type of cancer, vascular lesions tend to be more sensitive to chemotherapy than nonvascular lesions; hepatomas tend to be more vascular than metastatic colorectal cancers.[62]

The evaluation should include posteroanterior (PA) and lateral views of the chest, as well as selected use of such studies as an upper GI series, small-bowel series, barium enema, and bone scan. Gastroscopy or colonoscopy may be useful in evaluation of patients with gastric cancer which is invading the liver or who have metastatic colon cancer in the liver. A technetium-99 liver scan can be useful in detecting the presence of a tumor in the liver but can be quite erroneous in localizing the areas of the liver which are invaded by tumor.[63]

BIOPSY

Preoperative biopsy of the liver by needle, minilaparotomy, or otherwise is contraindicated except for advanced incurable lesions. There is great danger of spreading cancer. Tissue reaction even to needle biopsy causes adherence of the diaphragm or other structures, requiring en bloc removal of the adherent areas, thus needlessly complicating the operation. A diagnosis based on the small amount of tissue obtained is often tentative. Furthermore, the information is not needed in managing such patients at this stage of treatment. If the tumor can be removed, with a potential for cure, it will be regardless of its histological classification. Incurable metastases from a pancreatic or lung cancer will be evident. In contrast, it is essential to obtain a formal biopsy of tumors which are not resected.

Cancer of the Extrahepatic Biliary Tract

Cancer of the gallbladder is often first detected as an incidental finding in patients who are having a routine cholecystectomy. Otherwise, about 50 percent of patients present with jaundice and about 70 percent with pain.[31,64] Fifty percent have a palpable gallbladder; blood in the stool is practically never found, and the gallbladder is, of course, not visualized on cholecystectomy.

Signs and symptoms of cancer of the extrahepatic biliary tract and periampullary region are similar to those of cancer of the pancreas.[65] Jaundice is present in about 95 percent of patients.[66,67] Abdominal pain, weight loss, and anorexia are present in more than three-fourths of patients. The gallbladder is palpable in about 50 percent, and an enlarged liver is a common finding, being seen in about 85 percent of patients. Occult blood can be detected in the stool in over 80 percent.

In the evaluation of the jaundiced patient, four diagnostic techniques are particularly valuable: CAT scanning and sonography, endoscopic retrograde cholangiopancreatography (ERCP), selective celiac and superior mesenteric angiography, and percutaneous transhepatic cholangiography. CAT scanning or sonography is noninvasive and gives valuable information as to whether the head of the pancreas contains a tumor (Fig. 26-7). Assumptions regarding the presence of liver metastases may be hazardous in the jaundiced patient

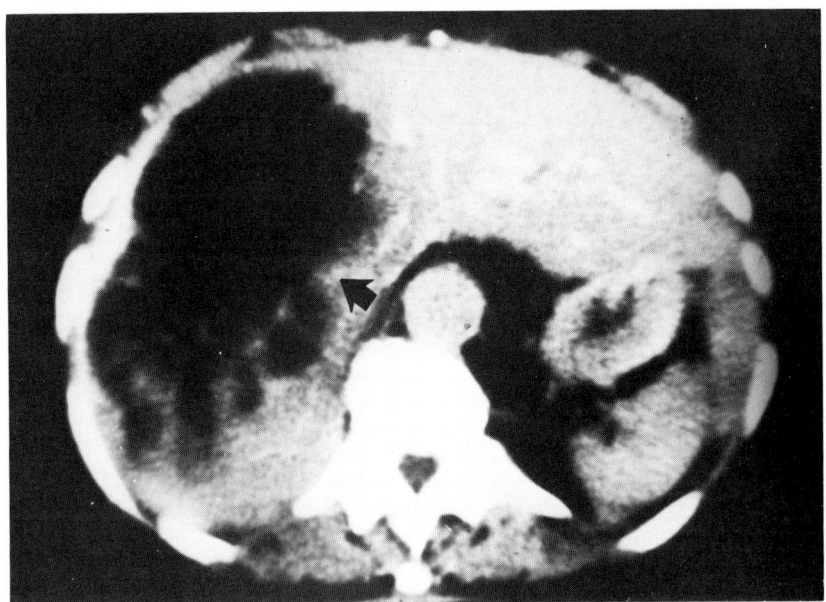

FIGURE 26-5 CAT scan of metastatic colon cancer in right lobe of liver.

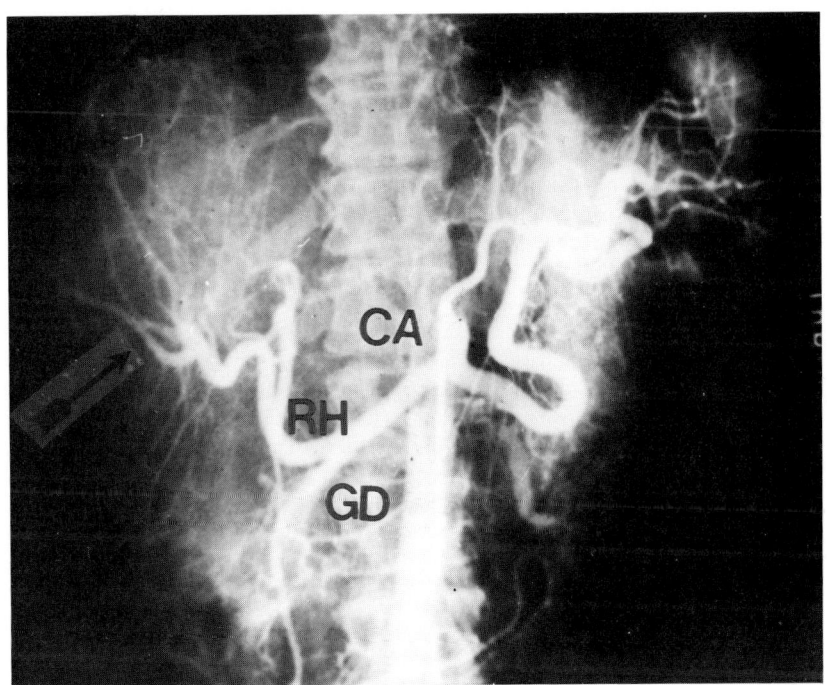

FIGURE 26-6 Celiac arteriogram in patient with metastatic colon cancer in liver. The lesion is avascular. Intrahepatic vessels are stretched over the tumor (arrow). CA = celiac axis; RH = right hepatic artery; GD = gastroduodenal artery.

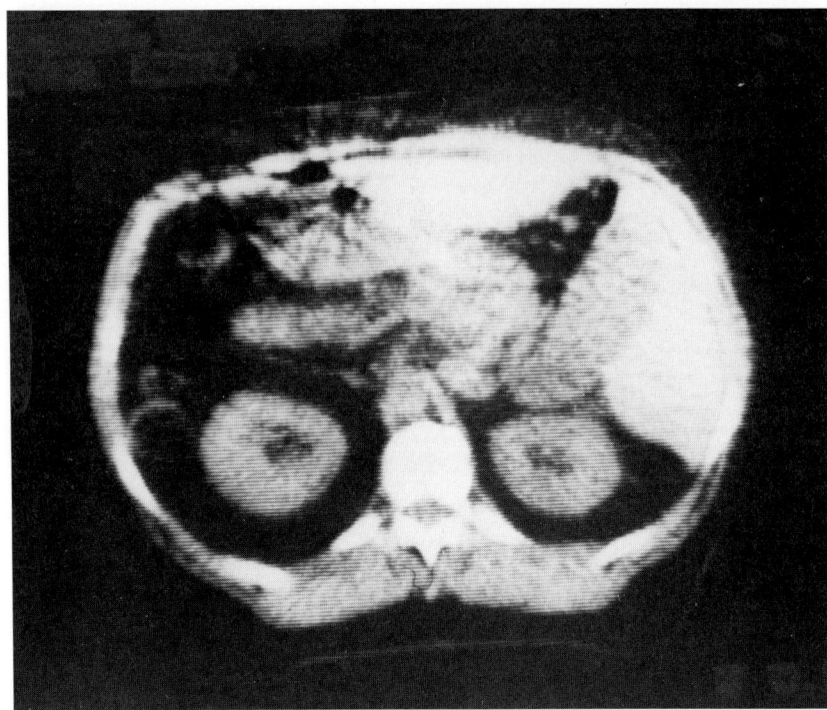

FIGURE 26-7 CAT scan of mass in head of pancreas.

because dilated intrahepatic bile ducts can give the appearance of metastatic disease.

The next order of invasiveness is the ERCP. It is particularly important in detecting ampullary or periampullary lesions. Cannulation of the pancreatic duct or common bile duct may be possible so that the nature of the obstructive lesion can be more fully defined. Retrograde cannulation of the obstructed common bile duct is possible in some instances, providing temporary relief from the jaundice in preparation for later surgical intervention.

Percutaneous transhepatic cholangiography (Fig. 26-8) enables the level of obstruction to be determined for patients with obstructive jaundice. The clinical picture is essentially the same for the jaundiced patient whose tumor involves the major hepatic ducts, common hepatic or common bile ducts, the periampullary region, or head of the pancreas. The test also gives valuable information as to the type of obstruction, and the catheter can be left in place for temporary decompression of the biliary tract.

Angiography is essential so that the course of major vessels, the presence of vascular anomalies, and vascular involvement by the tumor can be shown. The most commonly encountered anomaly is the origin of the right hepatic artery from the superior mesenteric artery. The right hepatic artery will then usually course immediately posterior to the head of the pancreas or through it, going to the right, abutting the posterior surface of the common bile duct. Other vascular anomalies, such as arcuate ligament compression of the celiac axis, must be recognized prior to any surgical approaches.[68]

Preoperative evaluation of the patient's physiological state must be individualized. This may include pulmonary function studies, blood volume estimations, and evaluation of renal function.

MANAGEMENT

The liver has been a source of mystery and wonderment from the beginnings of recorded history. The ancients inspected the liver of sacrificed animals in an effort to obtain guidance for many of their activities and to prophesy future events. The regenerative capacity of the liver was well known as illustrated in the legend of Prometheus, who was chained to the rock as punishment by Zeus for returning fire to the earth. During the day a vulture ate his liver, which then regenerated during the night. The portrait by Rubens[69] (Fig. 26-9) indicates that the vulture's approach was through a small right subcostal incision.

Hepatic Resection

The modern era of major hepatic resection began in 1949 when Honjo and Araki[70] performed a right hepatic lobectomy using preliminary hilar ligation.[71-73] Their report was delayed. In 1952 Lortat-Jacob and Robert[74] in France, and in 1953 Quattlebaum[75] in the United

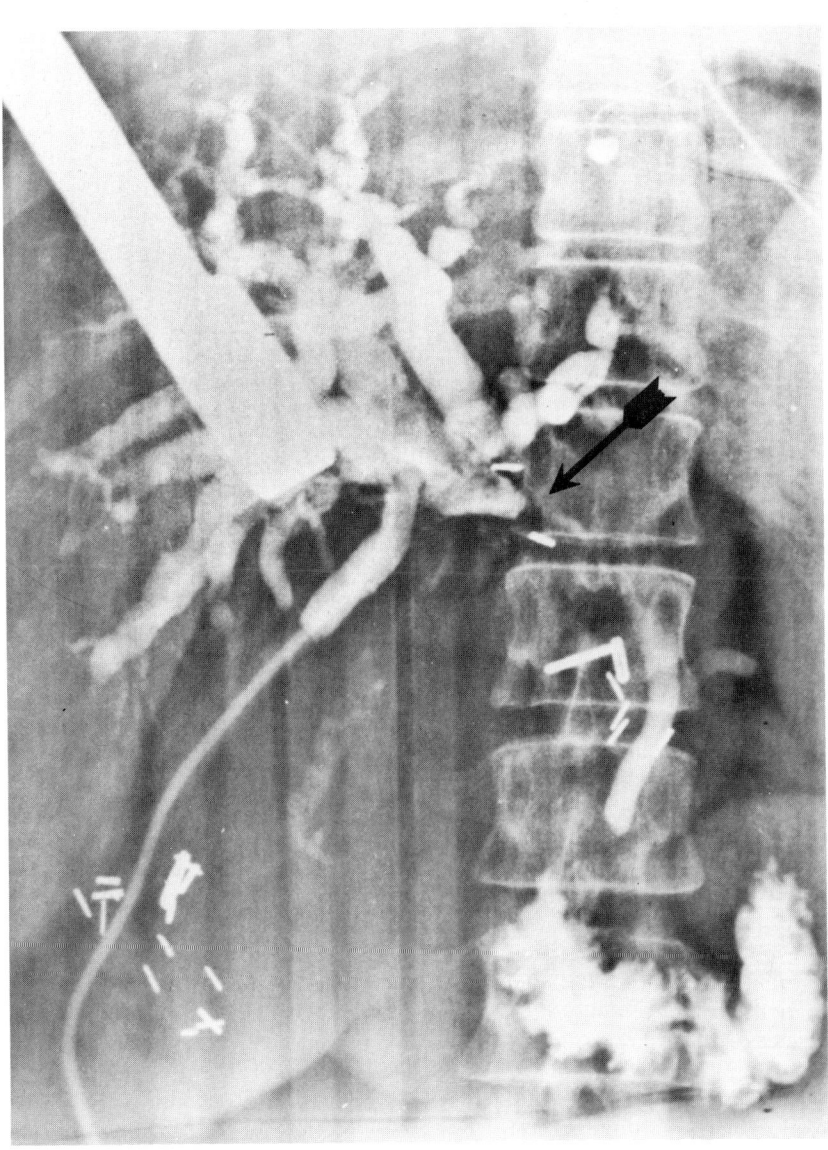

FIGURE 26-8 Percutaneous transhepatic cholangiogram showing obstruction (arrow) of common hepatic duct secondary to primary carcinoma.

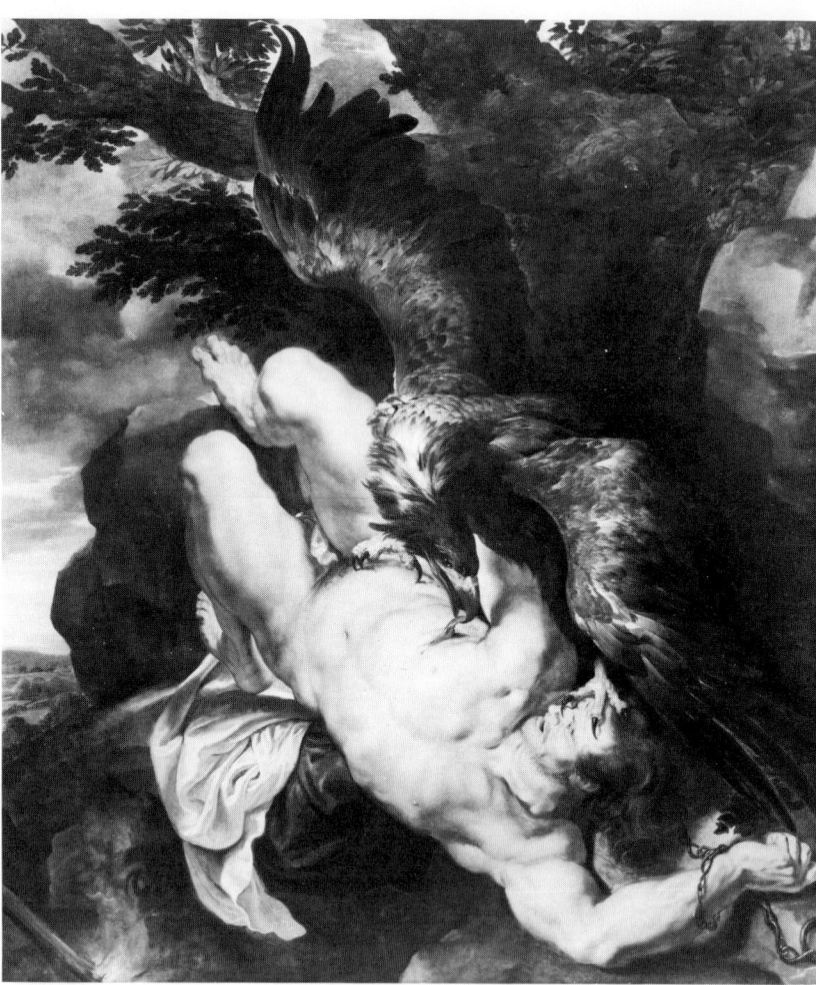

FIGURE 26-9 *Prometheus Bound* by Pieter Paul Rubens. Philadelphia Museum of Art. Purchased: The W. P. Wilstach Collection. Photographed by Philadelphia Museum of Art.

States, independently reported on clinical hepatic lobectomy utilizing preliminary hilar ligation with anatomic removal of the lobe. In 1953 Healey[76,77] described lobar segments. In 1954 Lin et al.[78] reported on their experience with finger-fracture technique. In 1957 Goldsmith and Woodburne[79] made their very important contribution on the blood supply to the medial segment of the left lobe of the liver. Various authors have contributed to knowledge about liver surgery since that time.[80-90]

It has been the policy of the author for the past 11 years to explore most patients with primary or metastatic liver tumors who do not have evidence of extrahepatic metastases and who are satisfactory surgical risks. At exploratory laparotomy, careful evaluation of the abdominal contents is carried out. Where the disease is confined to one surgically resectable area of the liver, it is removed either by wedge excision or by major hepatic resection.[50,60] The natural history of the particular cancer is taken into consideration. This approach would not be rational for patients with pancreatic cancer or lung cancer, for example. It would apply where there is direct invasion of the liver by gastric cancer, but not where there are metastases from gastric cancer. Hepatoma and metastatic colon cancer are tumors especially suited to this approach. Patients are placed on systemic adjuvant chemotherapy when it is feasible. Otherwise, catheters are placed in the hepatic artery and/or portal vein and a course of infusional chemotherapy is given. If extensive extrahepatic cancer is found, the patient is only biopsied and closed.

From 1970 to 1981, 485 patients were treated in this fashion. The operations carried out are listed in Table 26-5. The resectability rate is 32 percent. Table 26-6 shows the types of tumors removed in the 151 major hepatic resections of this series. The 30-day operative mortality rate since 1975 was only 5 percent (5 of 96). The deaths were as follows. One patient died of uncontrollable hemorrhage when resection of a massive tumor of the caudate lobe was attempted. A second death occurred in a 72-year-old man 3 days after an uneventful hepatic lobectomy. Myocardial infarction and completely occluded coronary vessels were found at autopsy. Two patients died of liver failure of undetermined cause after an extended right hepatic lobectomy. The fifth patient died of thrombosis of the portal vein after a catheter had been placed for infusional chemotherapy.

Complications which have been encountered since 1978 are shown in Table 26-7.[50] Particularly important is the low incidence of subphrenic abscess, in striking contrast to experience prior to 1978. A sharp decrease in this complication was associated with substitution of closed drainage of the subphrenic space for placement of multiple Penrose drains into this area. Early removal of the drains also appears to be important. Patients undergoing major hepatic resection are now usually discharged from the hospital about 10 days after resection; they are on a regular diet and fully ambulatory. Abnormalities in serum chemistries after major hepatic resection are minimal with the less traumatic techniques employed today.

Table 26-8 shows the staging by which patients undergoing liver resection are classified. Estimates of 3-year survival rates (product limit method)[91] for 30 patients with hepatocellular carcinoma are shown in Table 26-9. It will be noted that 78 percent with stage I disease were alive and 36 percent with stages II & III disease were alive, an overall survival rate of 65 percent.[92]

Two new developments make total hepatectomy and orthotopic liver transplantation therapeutic options to be considered in the management of patients with primary liver cancer. This possibility would apply where the cancer is confined to the liver but involves all segments or where associated cirrhosis was so severe as to preclude a safe resection. One development is the use of cyclosporin A with steroids for immunosuppression. Starzl[92a,92b] and Calne[92c,92d] both report major improvement in survival rates over those previously expressed.

TABLE 26-5 Surgical Experience, 1970–1981: 485 Patients

Operation	Number
Extended lobectomy	40
Lobectomy	80
Segmentectomy	31
Wedge resection	22
Ligation/cannulation	205
Unroofing giant cyst	10
Chemoperfusion	4
Exploratory laparotomy and liver biopsy	93
Total	485

Starzl estimates his 1-year survival rate to be 75 to 80 percent.

The second new development is improved liver storage so that the liver can be maintained ex vivo for at least 24 hours with 48 hours a real possibility. Monden and Fortner[92e] using the dog model preserved the liver at refrigerator temperature using modified Sacks' solution and prostacyclin. Orthotopic liver transplantation then was performed.

Five of 6 livers preserved 24 hours and 3 of 5 livers preserved 48 hours were able to sustain life for more than 5 days. This increased preservation capability may allow for better liver exchanges with fewer transportation problems. The limited function which has previously been seen in grafted livers due to poor preservation may no longer be a factor.

Table 26-10 indicates figures for metastatic colorectal cancer where resection has been possible. The data do not indicate a benefit from adjuvant chemotherapy with resection of primary or metastatic cancer, owing to relatively small number of cases and the elapsed time. Certain aspects of the problem of metastatic colorectal cancer to the liver deserve special comment. Wedge

TABLE 26-6 Major Hepatic Resection: 151 Patients

Primary tumor	Number
Liver	43
Colorectal	49
Miscellaneous	21
Hepatoblastoma	6
Gallbladder	5
Bile duct	3
Benign	24

TABLE 26-7 Complications of Major Hepatic Resection, 1978–1980: 27 Patients*

Pleural effusion	7
Intraabdominal bleeding	3
Subphrenic abscess	2
Pneumonia	2
Hepatorenal failure	1
GI bleeding	1
Pneumothorax	1
Wound infection	1
Phlebitis	1
Postoperative psychosis	1

SOURCE: Fortner.[50]
*Excludes two 30-day postoperative deaths.

resection of metastatic disease, or of primary hepatoma for that matter, can be curative provided an adequate margin is obtained around the primary or metastatic focus and there is no other disease. Our policy is to obtain a finger-breadth's margin of normal tissue around the gross limits of the tumor in all three dimensions. Wedge excision has the same prognosis as major hepatic resection (Fig. 26-10).[93] Multiple metastases to the liver from colorectal cancer have the same prognosis after resection as a solitary metastasis.[50,60] A 5-year survival rate of 37 percent was reported after wedge excision of hepatic metastases from colorectal cancer,[98] compared with a 30-percent survival estimate after major hepatic resection.[98a]

Infusional Chemotherapy

Patients whose primary or metastatic cancer cannot be removed surgically are treated with infusional chemo-

TABLE 26-8 Extent of Disease Staging in Hepatic Resection Patients

Stage	Description
I	Tumor confined to the resected portion of the liver without involvement of the hepatic vascular or biliary structures or the margins of resection.
II	Regional spread such as vascular involvement, residual disease, direct extension into adjacent structures, bile duct involvement, or tumor rupture.
III	Any metastasis such as to lymph nodes, neighboring organs, or distant sites.

TABLE 26-9 Hepatocellular Carcinoma

		Survival estimate, %		
Resection	Number	1 year	2 year	3 year
Stage I	11	100	100	78 (8)*
Stages II and III	19	80	51	36 (4)
Total	30	94	80	65 (12)

*Numbers in parentheses represent number of patients alive beyond that period.

therapy, unless extensive intraabdominal disease is present.[94,95] The hepatic artery is cannulated through the gastroduodenal artery. The portal vein is cannulated via the inferior mesenteric vein or the middle colic vein. Raimondi catheters are inserted and the patient given chemotherapy after recovering from the surgical procedure.

As indicated in Table 26-11,[95] 184 patients have been treated from 1971 to 1980. In recent years the hepatic artery has not been ligated since patients rarely feel well after this procedure. It also may decrease the efficiency with which drugs are delivered. Hepatic artery ligation is effective in killing a large portion of vascularized tumors, but significant numbers of cells still remain which must be treated chemotherapeutically. Since 1975 there have been only four postoperative fatalities; two of these were in patients who had more than 70 percent of their liver involved by tumor. The third death was in a patient in whom macronodular postnecrotic cirrhosis precluded resection of a lesion involving approximately 25 percent of the liver. The fourth patient died of unknown causes on the twenty-fifth postoperative day, after having been discharged and then readmitted to the hospital.

It is important to stage the extent of disease at the time of laparotomy. Each segment of the liver is inspected, and the percent of tumor involvement is estimated. Almersjö et al.[96] devised a staging method in which the disease was designated as stage I if less than 20 percent of the liver was involved; stage II if 20 to 70 percent was involved; and stage III if more than 70 percent of the liver was involved. Response to chemotherapy and survival figures seem to correlate with this staging system in initial studies of patients with hepatic metastases from colorectal cancer. Responses were seen in two of three patients with stage I disease, in 55 percent of those with stage II disease, and in 14 percent of those with stage III disease. Median survival times were 14 months for those with stage II disease and 9 months for those with stage III disease.[97] In a more recent evaluation by Fortner et al., it was found that patients with more than 80 percent liver involvement did not appear to benefit from intrahepatic chemotherapy. In patients with hepatocellular carcinoma, there appears to be little difference in response rates and survival times for up to 70 percent of liver involvement. Median survival times were 21 months if less than 70 percent of the liver was involved, compared with 6 months if there was more extensive hepatic involvement. Twenty-four individuals had less than 70 percent liver involvement and disease so extensive as to preclude surgical resection; 2 of these patients are living more than 5 years and 6 are living more than $2\frac{1}{2}$ years.[92]

Surgical Treatment of Cancer of the Gallbladder

There appears to be a consensus that major hepatic resection for gallbladder cancer is ineffective. This is rather surprising since only 24 patients have been reported in the English literature during the past two decades to have had an extensive hepatic resection.[98] Experience at Memorial Sloan-Kettering Cancer Center is also limited, for most patients had extensive disease when first explored. Since 1941 there have been six long-term survivors of gallbladder cancer who were

TABLE 26-10 Metastatic Colorectal Cancer

Resection	Number	Survival estimate, %		
		1 year	2 year	3 year
Stage I	35	93	75	66 (10)*
Stages II and III	22	79	55 (2)	
Total	57	89	69	

*Numbers in parentheses represent number of patients alive beyond that period.

treated at Memorial Sloan-Kettering Cancer Center (Table 26-12).[31,99–100a] Two of the patients had extensive infiltrating cancer requiring resection of adjacent viscera. Two of the long-term survivors had lymph node metastases. Other authors have reported long-term survivals of patients with locally invasive gallbladder cancer.[101–105] These results and a limited experience with major hepatic resection for this cancer would appear sufficient basis for further evaluation of the procedure. It should be combined with hilar and celiac axis lymph node dissection in order to encompass the regional lymph node drainage basin.

A major consideration is the management of the incidental cancer of the gallbladder found on routine cholecystectomy for presumed inflammatory disease. It is of paramount importance to avoid contamination of

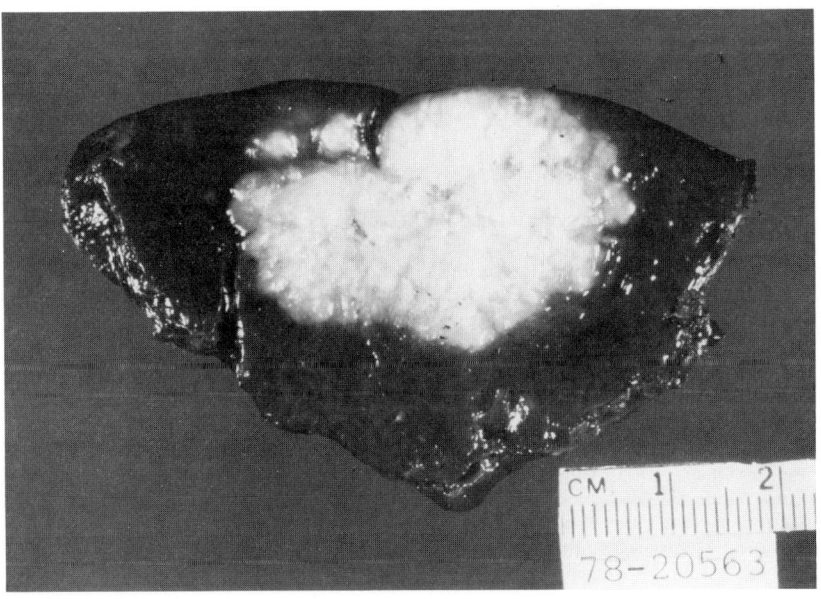

FIGURE 26-10 Wedge resection for metastatic colon cancer in liver. Fingerbreadth margin around gross limit of the tumor is desirable.

TABLE 26-11 Ligation/Cannulation, 1971–1980

	PRIMARY CANCER		
	Liver	*Colorectal*	*Other*
HALC*	29	26	26
HALC, PVC†	5	15	2
HAC, PVC	2	22	5
HAL	1	3	3
HAC	3	3	11
PVC	3	9	7
HAL, PVC	3	4	2
Total	46	82	56

SOURCE: Fortner.[95]
*HALC = hepatic artery ligation and cannulation. Includes individuals in whom the infusional catheter was never functional and who were evaluated as undergoing HAL only, in earlier publications.
†PVC = portal vein cannulation.

the area by cutting into the cancer. In situ, intraepithelial cancer can be treated satisfactorily by cholecystectomy alone. Any invasion of the gallbladder wall necessitates further surgery. A second-stage hepatic resection with hilar and celiac axis node dissection would appear to provide the best chance for cure. However, if the tumor has been cut into during the dissection, any further surgical treatment appears doomed to failure. Judicious use of needle biopsy or cytological examination of aspirated fluid from the gallbladder lumen may be helpful in resolving a surgical dilemma as to whether cancer of the gallbladder or severe cholecystitis is present. The anatomic relationship of the gallbladder to the liver segments and hilar structures will determine whether a right or extended right hepatic lobectomy is required.

Extrahepatic Biliary Tract

Several excellent reviews of this subject have been published recently.[106–110] These studies and experience at Memorial Sloan-Kettering suggest that the initial treatment of jaundiced patients with extrahepatic bile duct obstruction as demonstrated by sonography or CAT scan should be by preliminary decompression using percutaneous transhepatic intubation. Passage of the decompressing catheter into the duodenum for internal drainage is desirable but carries the risk of perforation and cannot always be done. If either external or internal catheter drainage is successful, then laparotomy can wait

TABLE 26-12 Cancer of the Gallbladder: Long-Term Survivors

Age	Sex	Operation	Adenocarcinoma of gallbladder	Survival
68	M	Extended R hepatic lobectomy, R and partial transverse colectomy	Infiltrating and extending into liver, omentum, colon	55 months NED
51	F	Wedge resection liver; segmental resection common bile duct; resection omentum, duodenal wall; LN* dissection	Infiltrating, with common bile duct LN metastases	60 months NED
71	F†	Cholecystectomy, segmental resection colon	Infiltrating	8 years NED
64	F‡	Cholecystectomy, LN excision	Grade III with two LN metastases	11 years died cancer(?) of gallbladder or gastric primary
53	F§	R hepatic lobectomy	Infiltrating with focal invasion liver	15 years died cancer distal bile duct
40	F¶	Cholecystectomy	Multiple adenomatous polyps; in situ cancer in one	30 years NED Resection ampullary cancer 8 years ago

*LN-lymph node
†Patient of Dr. W. Knapper.
‡Patient of the late Dr. G. Pack.[103]
§Patient of the late Dr. R. Brasfield.[104]
¶See JG Fortner, GT Pack[31] and EJ Tabah, G McNeer.[100a]
NOTE: NED = no evidence of disease.

TABLE 26-13 Extrahepatic Bile Duct Cancer, 1962–1981

	Number	30-day postoperative mortality rate	Survival, months
Proximal bile duct	36	6/36 (17%)	Median: 17 (2–61)
Complete tumor resection	7	1/7 (14%)	Median: 44.5 (23–61)
Major hepatic and bile duct resection	5	1/5	23, 30, 44,* 57
Bile duct resection	2	0/2	45,* 61
Other procedures	29	5/29 (17%)	Median: 11 (2–37)
Incomplete tumor resection	3	1/3	13, 17
T-tube insertion	12†	2/12	2, 5, 7, 11,* 13, 19, 22,* 29
with HAL, PVC	1	0/1	35
Biliary enteric bypass	5	1/5	2,* 2, 7, 21
Intrahepatic catheter	6‡	1/5	2, 3, 31, 37*
Orthotopic liver transplant	2	0/2	37 days, 95 days
Middle one-third	6	0/6	Median: 12 (8–22)
Complete tumor resection	3		
Excision liver; bile duct resection	1		19
Bile duct resection	1		10
Pancreaticoduodenectomy	1		9
Other procedures	3		
Incomplete tumor resection	2		8, 22*
T-tube insertion	1		14
Distal one-third	9	2/9 (22%)	Median: 13 (3–85)
Complete tumor resection	7	1/7	
Regional pancreatectomy type 1	3	0/3	6, 27,* 34*
Regional subtotal pancreatectomy	2	1/2	3
Pancreaticoduodenectomy	1	0/1	85*
Bile duct resection	1	0/1	13
Other procedures	2	1/2	
Biliary enteric bypass	2	1/2	7
Diffuse	3	1/3	
Other procedures	3	1/3	
Incomplete tumor resection	1	0/1	11
Intrahepatic catheter	2	1/2	2

*Alive.
†Indicates two patients without follow-up information.
‡Indicates one patient without follow-up information.

until normal or near-normal bilirubin levels are recorded and the patient has been prepared for surgery.

Some authors advise a nonoperative approach, particularly for hilar lesions.[111] In somewhat idealized circumstances, biopsy is obtained by percutaneous skinny-needle biopsy; decompression is obtained by percutaneous cannulation and the lesion is treated by external radiation therapy. The risk in this approach is that nonoperative or indirect evaluation of upper abdominal cancer is frequently misleading, and not all hilar or Klatskin[112] tumors are radiosensitive. For these reasons the author explores such patients to assess the tumor as accurately as possible.[113] A localized tumor which is resectable may be found, or internal decompression may be possible by dilation of the obstructed bile ducts with Bakes' dilators. This permits U-tube[114] or T-tube drainage of the biliary tract. Localized but nonresectable lesions can be marked by metal clips to direct external radiation, and interstitial implantation into the tumor can be carried out. Hepaticojejunostomy may be done utilizing dilated bile ducts peripheral to the tumor mass. A convenient approach in this regard is a Roux en Y hepaticojejunostomy utilizing the bile duct to the anterior segment of the left lobe (segment III). This duct is readily found by cutting the bridge of liver tissue between the medial and lateral segments of the left lobe, progressing to the left of the round ligament at its base. External radiation therapy is given postoperatively.

Localized tumors in the midportion or lower end of the common bile duct lend themselves more commonly to resection than upper-third lesions.[115] A pancreaticoduodenectomy with resection of the bile duct to just above the bifurcation, combined with removal of lymphatics and soft tissue in the porta hepatis and celiac node dissection, appears optimal. Some tumors arising from the lower end of the common bile duct cannot be differentiated from pancreatic or ampullary lesions until the resected specimen is examined by the pathologist. Their treatment will be that of pancreatic cancer.[116]

Relatively few bile duct cancers are curable, but many lend themselves to long-term palliation. Tompkins et al.[110] reported a resectability rate of 47 percent for upper-third lesions, with a mortality rate of 23 percent. All 47 patients in their series were dead by 60 months postoperatively. There was not a statistically significant difference in survival time between resected and bypassed patients in this group. Lesions in the middle third of the bile ducts had a resectability rate of 67 percent with no operative deaths. The 5-year survival rate was 12 percent. Lower-third lesions had the best prognosis; overall 5-year survival rate was 28 percent.

Tompkins et al.[110] advise use of the operative choledochogram in all cases of choledochotomy for stones. They reported three cases of small distal duct carcinomas found in such patients.

The author has treated 54 patients at Memorial Sloan-Kettering Cancer Center with extrahepatic bile duct cancer from 1962 to 1981. Most frequently, the tumors were located in the proximal bile duct—67 percent (36 of 54); 11 percent (6 of 54) were in the middle one-third; 17 percent (9 of 54) in the distal one-third; and 5 percent (3 of 54) were too diffuse in nature to identify the site of origin. The 30-day operative mortality rate was 17 percent (9 of 54) (Table 26-13). Excluding the postoperative deaths, the median survival time for patients with tumors at each of the three bile duct segments was approximately 1 year: 17 months, 12 months, and 13 months for proximal, middle, and distal one-third, respectively. For patients with proximal bile duct cancer, the median survival time was 44.5 months in those in whom all clinically evident tumor could be resected. Those who had more extensive tumor and hence underwent a palliative procedure had a median survival time of 11 months. Survival times for all patients are shown in Table 26-13, although the small number of cases does not allow comparison of treatment results.

Periampullary Cancer

The favorable reputation which this tumor has is applicable only to small tumors without lymph node metastases.[117] In the Memorial Sloan-Kettering Cancer Center experience no patient with lymph node metastases lived free of disease 5 years after resection.[37] Six of nine patients (67 percent) with no evident lymph node metastases were alive at 5 years. Patients whose tumors were 2 cm or larger in diameter succumbed prior to the 5-year mark. These results are the basis for the recommendation that periampullary cancers which are not superficial and less than 2 cm in diameter be considered comparable to pancreatic cancer. Regional pancreatectomy with its relatively wide soft-tissue margin and regional lymph node dissection would appear to be a realistic approach. The number of cancers treated by this approach is still too small for evaluation.

REFERENCES

1. Maltz C, et al: Hepatocellular carcinoma. *Am J Gastroenterol* 74:361, 1980.
2. Segi M: *Graphic Presentation of Cancer Incidence by Site and by Area and Population.* Compiled from data published in *Cancer Incidence in Five Continents,* vol III, Segi Institute of Cancer Epidemiology, Nagoya, Japan, 1977.
3. *American Cancer Society: 1981 Cancer Facts and Figures,* American Cancer Society, New York, 1980.
4. Fortner JG: The liver and cancer, in G Gitnick (ed): *Current Hepatology,* vol I, Houghton Mifflin, Boston, 1980.
5. Kew MC et al: Hepatitis B virus infection in southern African blacks with hepatocellular cancer. *J Natl Cancer Inst* 62:517, 1979.
6. Reys LL et al: The relationship between hepatitis B virus infection and hepatic cell carcinoma in Mozambique. *Trop Geogr Med* 29:251, 1977.
7. Omata M et al: Hepatocellular carcinoma in the U.S.A.: Etiologic considerations. *Gastroenterology* 76:279, 1979.
8. Skinhof P et al: Occurrence of cirrhosis and primary liver

cancer in an Eskimo population hyperendemically infected with hepatitis B virus. *Am J Epidemiol* 108:121, 1978.
9. Blumberg B: Hepatitis B virus and the prevention of primary liver cancer, in JG Fortner, JE Rhoads (eds): *Accomplishments in Cancer Research 1981*, vol. III, Lippincott, Philadelphia, 1982 (in press).
10. Fisch RO et al: Homotransplantation of the liver in a patient with hepatoma and hereditary tyrosinemia. *J Pediatr* 93:592, 1978.
11. LaDu BN, Gjessing LR: Tyrosinosis and tyrosinemia, in JB Stanbury et al (eds): *The Metabolic Basis of Inherited Disease*, McGraw-Hill, New York, 1978.
12. Weinberg AG et al: The occurrence of hepatoma in the chronic form of hereditary tyrosinemia. *J Pediatr* 88:434, 1976.
13. Laberge C: Hereditary tyrosinemia in a French Canadian isolate. *Am J Human Genet* 21:36, 1969.
14. Scriver CR et al: Hereditary tyrosinemia and tyrosyluria in a French Canadian geographic isolate. *Am J Dis Child* 113:41, 1967.
15. Linsell CA: Environmental chemical carcinogens and liver cancer, in K Lapis, JV Johannessen (eds): *Liver Carcinogenesis*, Hemisphere Publishing Corporation, Washington, D.C., 1979.
16. Conney AH et al: Regulation of human drug metabolism by dietary factors, in D Evered, G Lawrenson (eds): *Environmental Chemicals, Enzyme Function and Human Disease*, Exerpta Medica, The Netherlands, 1980.
17. Lehmann FG, Wegener T: Etiology of human liver cancer: Controlled prospective study in liver cirrhosis. *J Toxicol Environ Health* 5:281, 1979.
18. Delorme F, Theriault G: Ten cases of angiosarcoma of the liver in Shawinigan, Quebec. *J Occup Med* 20:338, 1978.
19. Popper H et al: Development of hepatic angiosarcoma in man induced by vinyl chloride, Thorotrast, and arsenic: Comparison with cases of unknown etiology. *Am J Pathol* 92:349, 1978.
20. Tamburro CH, Wyatt S: Vinyl chloride: Present findings concerning health effects. *Tex Rep Biol Med* 37:126, 1978.
21. Underwood JC, Huck P: Thorotrast-associated hepatic angiosarcoma with 36 years' latency. *Cancer* 42:2610, 1978.
22. Sugar J et al: Role of pesticides in hepatocarcinogenesis. *J Toxicol Environ Health* 5:183, 1979.
23. Rooks JB et al: Epidemiology of hepatocellular adenoma: The role of oral contraceptive use. *JAMA* 242:644, 1979.
24. Christopherson WM, Mays ET: Relation of steroids to liver oncogenesis. *J Toxicol Environ Health* 5:207, 1979.
25. Gindhart TD: Liver tumors and oral contraceptives: Pathology and pathogenesis. *Ann Clin Lab Sci* 8:443, 1978.
26. Fraumeni JF Jr: Cancers of the pancreas and biliary tract: Epidemiological considerations. *Cancer Res* 35:3437, 1975.
27. Bornstein FP: Gallbladder carcinoma in the Mexican population of the southwestern United States. *Pathol Microbiol* 35:189, 1970.
28. Creagan ET, Fraumeni JF Jr: Cancer mortality among American Indians: 1950–1967. *J Natl Cancer Inst* 49:959, 1972.
29. Biometry Branch, National Cancer Institute: *The Third National Cancer Survey Advanced Three-Year Report 1969–1971 Incidence*, Department of Health, Education, and Welfare Publication 75:637, 1975.
30. Shani M et al: Cancer of the biliary system: A study of 445 cases. *Br J Surg* 61:98, 1974.
31. Fortner JG, Pack GT: Clinical aspects of primary carcinoma of the gallbladder. *Arch Surg* 77:742, 1958.
32. Parkash O: On the relationship of cholelithiasis to carcinoma of the gallbladder and on the sex dependency of the carcinoma of the bile ducts. *Digestion* 12:129, 1975.
33. Ramandanis G, Fortner JG: Carcinoma of the gallbladder: A twenty-five year study (unpublished data).
34. Ritchie JK et al: Biliary tract carcinoma associated with ulcerative colitis. *Q J Med* 43:263, 1974.
35. Belamaric J: Intrahepatic bile duct carcinoma and *C. sinensis* infection in Hong Kong. *Cancer* 31:468, 1973.
36. Mir-Madjlessi SH et al: Adenocarcinoma of the ampulla of Vater associated with familial polyposis coli: Report of a case. *Dis Colon Rectum* 16:542, 1973.
37. Williams JA et al: Twenty-two year experience with periampullary carcinoma at Memorial Sloan-Kettering Cancer Center. *Am J Surg* 138:662, 1979.
38. Burrows H: An experimental inquiry into the association between gallstones and primary cancer of the gallbladder. *Br J Surg* 20:607, 1933.
39. Petrov NN, Krotkina NA: Experimental carcinoma of the gallbladder: Supplementary data. *Ann Surg* 125:241, 1947.
40. Lazarus-Barlow WS: A lecture on the cause and cure of cancer viewed in the light of recent radio-biological research. *Br Med J* 1:1001, 1914.
41. Lazarus-Barlow WS: An attempt at the experimental production of carcinoma by means of radium. *Proc R Soc Med (Pathol)* 2:1, 1918.
42. Burrows H: Gall-stones and cancer: A problem of aetiology, with special reference to the role of irritation. *Br J Surg* 27:166, 1939.
43. Desforges G et al: Carcinoma of the gallbladder: An attempt at experimental production. *Cancer* 3:1088, 1950.
44. Nelson AA, Woodward G: Tumors of the urinary bladder, gall bladder and liver in dogs fed *o*-aminoazotoluene or *p*-dimethylaminoazobenzene. *J Natl Cancer Inst* 13:1497, 1953.
45. Fortner JG: An appraisal of the pathogenesis of primary carcinoma of the extrahepatic biliary tract. *Surgery* 43:563, 1958.
46. Fortner JG, Norris WP: Determination of the radioactivity of gallstones obtained from cases of gallbladder cancer. *Cancer* 8:687, 1955.
47. Fortner JG: The experimental induction of primary carcinoma of the gallbladder. *Cancer* 8:689, 1955.

48. Fortner JG, Randall HT: Endogenous carcinogens for the extrahepatic biliary tract, in *Proceedings of the VIII International Cancer Congress 1962,* Moscow, 1963.
49. Fortner JG et al: Surgery in liver tumors, in MM Ravitch (ed): *Current Problems in Surgery,* Year Book, Chicago, 1972.
50. Fortner JG et al: The seventies evolution in liver surgery for cancer. *Cancer* 47:2162, 1981.
51. Ong GB: Techniques and therapies for primary and metastatic liver cancer. *Curr Prob Cancer* 2:1, 1977.
52. Ihde DC et al: Clinical manifestations of hepatoma: A review of 6 years' experience at a cancer hospital. *Am J Med* 56:83, 1974.
53. Curutchet HP et al: Primary liver cancer. *Surgery* 70:467, 1971.
54. Masseyeff RF: Factors influencing α-fetoprotein biosynthesis in patients with primary liver cancer and other diseases, in H Hirai, T Miyaji (eds): *Alpha Fetoprotein and Hepatoma,* Gann Monograph on Cancer Research, no 14, University of Tokyo Press, Tokyo, 1973.
55. Hull EW et al: Serum α-fetoprotein in U.S.A. *Lancet* 1:779, 1970.
56. Hull EW et al: Serum α-fetoprotein (AFP) in cancer patients. *Clin Res* 17:403, 1969.
57. Hull EW et al: Synthesis of α-fetoprotein by monkey hepatoma cells *in vitro. Proc Am Assoc Cancer Res* 10:41, 1969.
58. Alpert E et al: α-Fetoprotein in human hepatoma: Improved detection in serum and quantitative studies using a new sensitive technique. *Gastroenterology* 61:137, 1971.
59. Tang Z et al: Evaluation of population screening for hepatocellular carcinoma. *Chin Med J* 93:795, 1980.
60. Fortner JG et al: Major hepatic resection for neoplasia: Personal experience in 108 patients. *Ann Surg* 188:363, 1978.
61. Vaitukaitis J et al: Gonadotrophins and their subunits: Basic and clinical studies. *Rec Progr Hormone Res* 32:289, 1976.
62. Kim DK et al: Tumor vascularity as a prognostic factor for hepatic tumors. *Ann Surg* 185:31, 1977.
63. Kim DK et al: Tumors of the liver as demonstrated by angiography, scan and laparotomy. *Surg Gynecol Obstet* 141:409, 1975.
64. Del Regato JA, Spjut HJ: *Ackerman and del Regato's Cancer Diagnosis, Treatment and Prognosis,* Mosby, St. Louis, 1977.
65. Bowden L, Pack GT: Cancer of the head of the pancreas: A collective review of the experiences of the Gastric Service of the Memorial Cancer Center 1926–1958. *Separata de GEN* 23:339, 1969.
66. Cooper WA: Carcinoma of the ampulla of Vater. *Ann Surg* 106:1009, 1937.
67. Lieber MM et al: Carcinoma of the peripapillary portion of the duodenum. *Ann Surg* 109:219, 1939.
68. Fortner JG, Watson RC: Median arcuate ligament obstruction of celiac axis and pancreatic cancer. *Ann Surg* (in press).
69. Wedgwood CV et al (eds): *The World of Rubens 1577–1640,* Time-Life Books, New York, 1967.
70. Honjo I, Araki C: Total resection of the right lobe of the liver. *J Int Coll Surg* 23:23, 1955.
71. Adson MA, Beart RW Jr: Elective hepatic resections. *Surg Clin North Am* 57:339, 1977.
72. Fineburg C et al: Right hepatic lobectomy for primary carcinoma of the liver. *Ann Surg* 144:881, 1956.
73. Foster JH, Berman MM: *Solid Liver Tumors,* Saunders, Philadelphia, 1977.
74. Lortat-Jacob JL, Robert HG: Hepatectomie droite réglée. *Presse Med* 60:549, 1952.
75. Quattlebaum JK: Massive resection of the liver. *Ann Surg* 137:787, 1953.
76. Healey JE Jr, Schroy PC: Anatomy of biliary ducts within human liver, analysis of prevailing patterns of branching and major variations of biliary ducts. *Arch Surg* 66:599, 1953.
77. Healey JE Jr et al: The intrahepatic distribution of the hepatic artery in man. *J Int Coll Surg* 20:133, 1953.
78. Lin TY et al: Study on lobectomy of the liver: A new technical suggestion on hemihepatectomy and reports of 3 cases of primary hepatoma treated with left lobectomy of the liver. *J Formosan Med Assoc* 57:742, 1958.
79. Goldsmith NA, Woodburne RT: The surgical anatomy pertaining to liver resection. *Surg Gynecol Obstet* 105:310, 1957.
80. Adson MA, Van Heerden JA: Major hepatic resections for metastatic colorectal cancer. *Ann Surg* 191:576, 1980.
81. Almersjö O et al: Liver resection for cancer. *Acta Chir Scand* 142:139, 1976.
82. Brasfield RD et al: Major hepatic resection for malignant neoplasms of the liver. *Ann Surg* 176:171, 1972.
83. Cady B et al: Elective hepatic resection. *Am J Surg* 137:514, 1979.
84. Calne RY: Transplantation of the liver. *Ann Surg* 188:129, 1978.
85. Hasegawa H et al: Major hepatic resection for metastatic neoplasia. *Rinsho Hoshasen* 24:1067, 1979.
86. Joishy SK, Balasegaram M: Hepatic resection for malignant tumors of the liver: Essentials for a unified surgical approach. *Am J Surg* 139:360, 1980.
87. Longmire WP et al: Elective hepatic surgery. *Ann Surg* 179:712, 1974.
88. Pack GT, Baker HW: Total right hepatic lobectomy. *Ann Surg* 138:253, 1953.
89. Starzl TE et al: Right trisegmentectomy for hepatic neoplasms. *Surg Gynecol Obstet* 150:208, 1980.
90. Yu Y et al: Experience in resection of small hepatocellular carcinoma. *Chin Med J* 93:491, 1980.
91. Kaplan EL, Meier P: Nonparametric estimation from incomplete observations. *J Am Stat Assoc* 53:457, 1958.

92. Fortner JG, Silva J, Maclean BJ: Hepatocellular carcinoma. (Unpublished data.)
92a. Starzl TE et al: Liver transplantation with use of cyclosporin A and prednisone. *N Engl J Med* 305:266, 1981.
92b. Starzl TE: Personal communication.
92c. Calne RY: Transplant surgery: Current status. *Br J Surg* 67:765, 1980.
92d. Calne RY: Personal communication.
92e. Monden M, Fortner JG: Twenty-four and forty-eight hour canine liver preservation by single hypothermia with prostacyclin. Submitted for publication.
93. Attiyeh FF et al: Hepatic resection for metastasis from colorectal cancer. *Dis Colon Rectum* 21:160, 1978.
94. Fortner JG, Pahnke LD: A new method for long-term intrahepatic chemotherapy. *Surg Gynecol Obstet* 143:979, 1976.
95. Fortner JG: What's new in surgical oncology: Infusion chemotherapy, in J Shah (ed): *Current Concepts in Surgical Oncology 1980,* Memorial Sloan-Kettering Cancer Center, New York, 1980.
96. Almersjö O et al: Evaluation of hepatic dearterialization in primary and secondary cancer of the liver. *Am J Surg* 124:5, 1972.
97. Fortner JG, Hoffman JP: (Unpublished data.)
98. Piehler JM, Crichlow RW: Primary carcinoma of the gallbladder. *Surg Gynecol Obstet* 147:929, 1978.
98a. Fortner JG et al: Metastatic colorectal cancer to the liver (unpublished data.)
99. Booher RJ, Pack GT: Cancer of the gallbladder: Report of a five-year cure of anaplastic carcinoma with metastases. *Am J Surg* 78:175, 1949.
100. Brasfield RD: Right hepatic lobectomy for carcinoma of the gallbladder, a five year cure. *Ann Surg* 153:563, 1961.
100a. Tabah EJ, McNeer G: Papilloma of the gall bladder with in situ carcinoma. *Surgery* 34:55, 1953.
101. Fahim RB et al: Carcinoma of the gallbladder: A study of its modes of spread. *Ann Surg* 156:114, 1962.
102. Finsterer H: *Med Klin* 28:432, 1932.
103. Marcial-Rojas RA, Medina R: Unsuspected carcinoma of the gallbladder in acute and chronic cholecystitis. *Ann Surg* 153:289, 1961.
104. Nagakawa T: Radical operation for carcinoma of the gallbladder. *Gastroenterol Surg (Japan)* 4:1117, 1981.
105. Sheinfeld W: Cholecystectomy and partial hepatectomy for carcinoma of the gallbladder with local liver extension. *Surgery* 22:48, 1947.
106. Bismuth H, Malt RA: Current concepts in cancer: Carcinoma of the biliary tree. *N Engl J Med* 301:704, 1979.
107. Corlette MB, Bookwalter JR: Individualization of treatment for hilar bile duct cancers. *Cancer* 46:415, 1980.
108. Evander A et al: Evaluation of aggressive surgery for carcinoma of the extrahepatic bile ducts. *Ann Surg* 191:23, 1980.
109. McDermott WV, Peinert RA: Carcinoma in the supra-ampullary portion of the bile ducts. *Surg Gynecol Obstet* 149:681, 1979.
110. Tompkins RK et al: Prognostic factors in bile duct carcinoma: Analysis of 96 cases. *Ann Surg* 194:447, 1981.
111. Lawrence RW: Discussion. *Ann Surg* 194:456, 1981.
112. Klatskin G: Adenocarcinoma of the hepatic duct at its bifurcation within the porta hepatis: An unusual tumor with distinctive clinical and pathological features. *Am J Med* 38:24, 1965.
113. Fortner JG et al: Surgical management of carcinoma of the junction of the main hepatic duct. *Ann Surg* 184:68, 1976.
114. Terblanche J: Carcinoma of the proximal extrahepatic biliary tree—Definitive and palliative treatment. *Surg Annu* 11:249, 1979.
115. El-Domeiri AA et al: Carcinoma of the extrahepatic bile ducts. *Ann Surg* 169:525, 1969.
116. Fortner JG: Surgical principles for pancreatic cancer: Regional total and subtotal pancreatectomy. *Cancer* 47:1712, 1981.
117. Cooperman AM: Cancer of the ampulla of Vater, bile duct and duodenum. *Surg Clin North Am* 61:99, 1981.

SELECTED BIBLIOGRAPHY

Blumberg BS, London WT: Primary hepatocellular carcinoma and hepatitis B virus. *Curr Prob Cancer* vol 6, no 12, 1982.

27
TUMORS OF THE PANCREAS
Bimal C. Ghosh

HISTORICAL ASPECTS

The pancreas has challenged the interest of anatomists and surgeons for centuries. The word itself is of Greek origin (*pan,* "all," "every"; *kreas,* "flesh," "meat"). John Conrad Brunner (1653–1727) was the first surgeon to excise portions of the pancreas from a dog that survived the operation. Morgagni (1771–1862) is credited with being the first to record observing a cancer of the pancreas; his diagnosis was made on the basis of necropsy findings in a patient whom he described as having hard, enlarged pancreatic nodules and a dilated gallbladder with a thickened wall.

In 1858, Dacosta reviewed 35 cases, the first large contribution on the subject to American literature. In 1869, Langerhans published the first description of the pancreatic islets that bear his name. In 1980, Mehring and Minkowski produced fatal diabetes mellitus in a dog by performing a total pancreatectomy.

The contributions of Whipple and Brunschwig laid the foundation for present-day treatment of carcinoma of the pancreas. In 1935, Whipple[1] performed the first two-stage radical excision of an ampullary carcinoma, which led to a resurgence of interest in operative treatment of ampullary pancreatic neoplasms. In 1937, Brunschwig[2] reported the first successful combined resection of the pancreas and duodenum. Present-day knowledge of the secretions of the pancreas in digestion, its endocrine function, and its action in different stages of metabolism have had great impact on the development of surgery of pancreatic tumors. Table 27-1 gives a classification of tumors of the pancreas.

INCIDENCE, EPIDEMIOLOGY, AND ETIOLOGIC ASPECTS

In 1979, there were 765,000 new cancers in the United States, 377,000 in males and 388,000 in females; approximately 23,000 of these were pancreatic cancers. The number of deaths from cancer of the pancreas in 1979 was 20,200, of which 10,900 were males and 9300 were females.[3]

The underlying etiologic factors in carcinoma of the pancreas are not yet known, although chemical carcinogens and environmental, endocrinologic, and dietary factors have been implicated. Many environmental and chemical carcinogens are biologically inert until they are enzymatically activated. Polynuclear aromatic hydrocarbon and dimethylbenzanthracene (DMBA) are examples of such chemical carcinogens. Benzpyrine is one of several chemical carcinogens found in tobacco smoke and in the atmosphere. Harris et al.[4] found that metabolism of benzpyrine in cultured human bronchus and pancreas is mediated by polar nuclear aromatic hydrohormones, which are the intermediaries converting benzpyrine into ultimate pancreatic carcinogen.

One of the most attractive hypotheses concerning the cause of cancer of the pancreas implicates the bile duct reflux mechanism. The majority of pancreatic cancers are found in the head of the pancreas, where the alleged carcinogens in the human bile constantly irritate the pancreatic parenchyma at the junction of the common bile duct and the pancreatic duct at the ampulla of Vater.

The distribution and the histogenesis of pancreatic cancers also seem to point to a carcinogen present in systemic circulation. This mechanism would readily explain the development of tumors in the hamster pancreas following subcutaneous injection of N-nitrosomethyl urea (NMU). An association between diabetes and pancreatic cancer has been reported; however, diabetes seems in general to increase a predisposition to all cancers.[5] Chronic pancreatitis, chronic alcoholism, and exposure to certain industrial carcinogens such as coal tar, betanaphthalamine, and benzidine have also been associated with an increased incidence of cancer of the pancreas.

CLINICAL FEATURES

Carcinoma of the head of the pancreas is predominantly a disease of middle age or later, especially the sixth and seventh decades. The youngest patient on record, however, was only 7 months old.[6] Pancreatic cancer is more common in males than in females, the ratio being approximately 2 to 1.

TABLE 27-1 Classification of Tumors of the Pancreas

I. Adenocarcinoma
   A. Small-duct
      Scirrhous
      Poorly differentiated
      Colloid (mucoid)
   B. Large-duct
      Papillary adenocarcinoma
      Mucoepidermoid carcinoma
      Squamous-cell carcinoma
      Cystadenocarcinoma
   C. Acinar-cell carcinoma

II. Pleomorphic
   Spindle-cell carcinoma
   Giant-cell carcinoma
   Carcinosarcoma

III. Benign tumors of the pancreas and extrahepatic bile duct
   Papilloma
   Adenoma
   Granular-cell myoblastoma
   Fribroma
   Schwannoma
   Leiomyoma
   Hamartoma

IV. Endocrine pancreatic tumors
   Insulinoma
   Gastrinoma (Zollinger-Ellison syndrome)
   Vernier-Morrison
   Glucagonoma
   Somatostatinoma
   Carcinoid

Jaundice

The classic symptom of carcinoma of the head of the pancreas is progressive painless jaundice, or icterus. In a series of cases reported by Bowden,[7] jaundice was the initial symptom in more than 90 percent. In resectable cases, the median duration of the jaundice was 4 weeks. In nonresectable cases, the duration of the jaundice was from 1 to 11 months, the median being 6 weeks.

Weight Loss

Weight loss is also a common symptom in patients with carcinoma of the pancreas. The average weight loss in patients with operable pancreatic carcinoma is about 20 pounds.

Pain

Occasionally a patient with pancreatic carcinoma may initially complain of either a colicky pain in the abdomen or a deep posterior abdominal aching or gnawing sensation. Colicky pain with jaundice is also a classic symptom in patients with common duct obstruction due to a stone, and it is therefore necessary to differentiate between the two conditions.

Anorexia, Diarrhea, and Steatorrhea

Diarrhea and anorexia sometimes are the first symptoms of pancreatic carcinoma, particularly in advanced cases. The tumor may obstruct the second or third portion of the duodenum and may be responsible for nausea and vomiting. These symptoms may be due to obstruction of the pancreatic duct resulting from a lack of pancreatic secretion in the intestine, producing steatorrhea (excessive loss of fat in the intestine).

Physical Signs

An abdominal mass is usually not present in the early stages. A palpable, nontender gallbladder, known as Courvoisier's sign, is present in about one-third or one-half of patients. Other abdominal masses or an enlarged nodular liver are usually a sign of advanced disease. Ascites may be present, particularly in advanced disease. It may also be present as a result of portal vein occlusion, which causes portal hypertension. Tenderness of the abdomen is not common but may be present in a small degree, particularly in patients with advanced and unresectable pancreatic carcinoma.

Laboratory Findings

In the vast majority of patients, there is elevated bilirubin with altered liver enzymes of alkaline phosphatase. Although the liver enzymes are intermediate, in many patients the increased lactic dehydrogenase level signifies liver involvement. Hyperglycemia may also be present. It has been reported that serum enzymes such as ribonuclease and glutamyl transpeptidase differentiate pancreatic cancers from other cancers in 90 and 76 percent of all cases, respectively.

Thrombophlebitis

Thrombophlebitis has been described as a significant physical finding on initial examination of patients with carcinoma of the pancreas. Due to the apparent increase of phlebitis and thrombosis in patients with carcinoma of the pancreas, emphasis has been placed on this finding as an important factor in clinical evaluation of patients suspected of having deep abdominal cancer. However, it is important to recognize that thrombophlebitis is also associated with other types of intraabdominal visceral cancer, for example, ovarian cancer.

Thrombophlebitis is a common finding in cancer of the body and tail of the pancreas. It is difficult to ascertain the exact incidence and significance of this disorder, since most of the studies have been done at autopsy. In one report,[8] 30 percent (5 out of 16) of the patients with cancer of the body and tail of the pancreas had thromboemboli at autopsy, compared to 10 percent (3 out of 31) of patients with cancer of the head of the pancreas. Although there is no denying that with cancers of the pancreas there is an increased possibility of peripheral venous thrombosis and occasional microemboli, a definite serum coagulating factor has not yet been isolated.

DIAGNOSTIC TECHNIQUES

Laboratory Tests

The standard biochemical and immunologic tests that are reliable for detecting carcinoma of the pancreas in the early stages are alkaline phosphatase, bilirubin, lactic dehydrogenase and glutamic oxaloacetic transaminase, 5-nucleotidase, alpha fetoprotein carcinoembryonic antigen amylase, and, recently, serum pancreas ribonuclease.

Radiography, Sonography, and Endoscopic Retrograde Cholangiopancreaticography

A standard radiologic examination is essential. Hypotonic duodenography (Fig. 27-1) can reveal a tumor of the head of the pancreas at an early stage with the impression over the duodenal wall. Inversion of the C loop of the duodenum is usually a sign of advanced carcinoma of the pancreas. A percutaneous transhepatic cholangiogram is also helpful (Fig. 27-2). A scan of the pancreas with an injection of 75 mL of selanomethanine and the use of gamma cameras is useful in selected patients. Ultrasonography is another noninvasive test that is sometimes useful in differentiating a solid from a cystic lesion of the pancreas (Fig. 27-3).[9,10] Endoscopic retrograde cholangiopancreaticography has been found helpful in detecting early carcinoma of the pancreas (Figs. 27-4 and 27-5). This technique is performed by introducing a flexible fiberoptic endoscope into the duodenum and following with an injection of 60% dye (Renographin) into the pancreatic and the biliary ductal system. The progression of the dye through the ductal system is observed on a fluoroscopic screen, and representative radiographs are taken. If an abnormal area suggests a neoplasm, a biopsy and cytologic examination of the pancreatic fluid should be done. If a specimen of fluid cannot be obtained from inside the pancreatic duct, a specimen from the duodenum will sometimes provide the diagnosis.

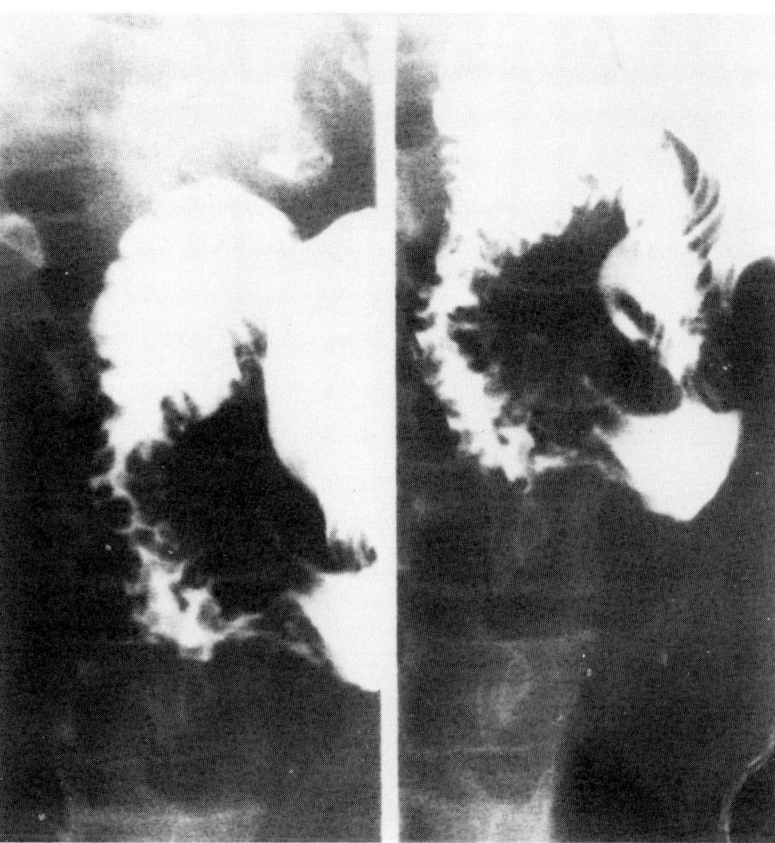

FIGURE 27-1 Hypotonic duodenography showing deformity of the second and third portions of duodenum from extrinsic pressure of a carcinoma of the pancreas.

Celiacangiography

Celiacangiography and selective pancreaticoduodenal angiography are of value in the diagnosis and staging of pancreatic neoplasms (Figs. 27-6 to 27-9).[11,12] Percutaneous transfemoral selective injections of a radiopaque dye in the celiac axia and the superior mesenteric artery can give a broad idea of lesions in these locations.[13,14] Selective pancreatic angiography is a promising method in pancreatic investigation. Since the pancreas is richly vascular, ample information can be obtained by injecting contrast media into the superior and inferior pancreaticoduodenal arteries.[15–20] This technique is useful in preoperative staging of the disease and in determining resectability. Angiographic findings of pancreatic carcinoma reflect poorly vascularized infiltrative lesions with invasion of the blood vessels and the serpiginous encasement. In advanced pancreatic carcinoma, the arterial branches become prominent and irregular and show an increased parenchymal accumulation of contrast media in the capillary phase. In adenoma, the findings are well circumscribed around the areas of contrasted accumulation in the capillary and venous phases. No true malignant vessels can be seen. This technique has been investigated in depth for the isolation of functioning islet-cell tumors. Since Olsson[12] published his findings in 1963, nonfunctioning islet-cell tumors have received little attention. A typical angiographic appearance of insulinoma is that of gradual tumor opacification via an inconspicuous supplying artery.[21–24] The opacification persists through the parenchymal and capillary phases. Within the tumor, the contrast medium slowly diffuses from small arterial channels into blood spaces, where it is only gradually replaced by nonopacified blood. Venous drainage channels are not seen in these circumstances. Undue abdominal compression during angiography may

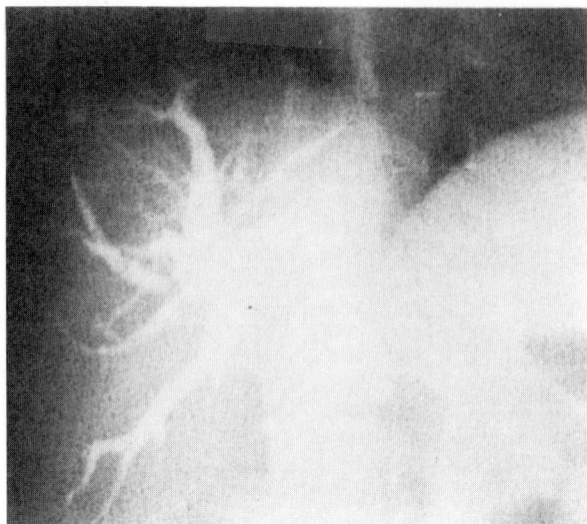

FIGURE 27-2 Percutaneous transhepatic cholangiography showing dilated common bile duct, common hepatic duct, and dilated intrahepatic ducts.

interfere with the diffusion of the contrast medium into the tumor and should be avoided. In certain instances, malignant insulinomas have been reported which showed poor opacification because of encasement and occlusion of arteries within the tumors. Second lesions in the liver show abundant neovascularity. Angiography is helpful in many instances for differentiating pancreatic tumors

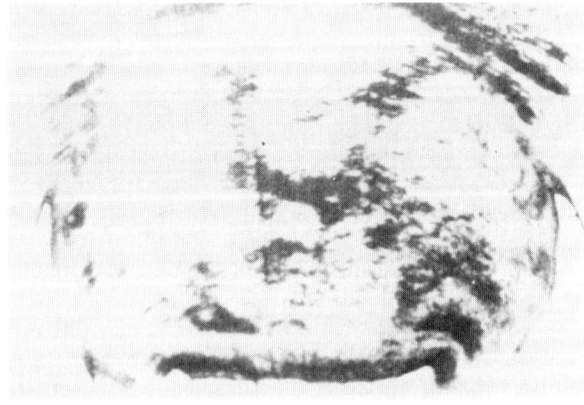

FIGURE 27-3 Ultrasound of the pancreas showing a mass over the pancreas.

from cysts and pancreatitis. In pancreatitis, the pancreas is swollen, and there is increased vascularity, with an occasional stretched vessel. There may be increased parenchymal accumulation of the contrast medium in the capillary phase in more advanced pancreatitis. In pseudocysts, stretching of the vessels without invasion by the tumor is diagnostic. In advanced carcinoma, the tumor vessels are found outside the pancreas, signifying unresectability.

Computerized Axial Tomography (CAT)

The technique of CAT scanning has been recently introduced for detecting lesions in deep-seated organs (Fig. 27-10). A lesion of the pancreas which is not accessible through clinical and laboratory testing is now detectable by this method. A CAT scan is a noninvasive and reasonably accurate method of diagnosis of pancreatic cancers in the early stage of the disease. Although there are still some artifacts in this method, with increasing use sufficient data will be generated to make diagnosis and assessment of operative feasibility more accurate in the future.

Percutaneous Transhepatic Cholangiography

Percutaneous transhepatic cholangiography is commonly used in evaluating pancreatic carcinoma or carcinoma of the common bile duct. In obstructive jaundice, this examination may show the site of obstruction.

With the invention of the Chibba needle, transhepatic percutaneous cholangiography has become a safe procedure. In cases of bile duct obstruction with dilatation of the common duct or the intrahepatic duct, a success rate of 98 percent has been reported by Ariyama et al.[25] Percutaneous transhepatic cholangiography is useful not only for diagnosis but also for the treatment of pancreatic carcinoma with jaundice. Percutaneous biliary drainage by introducing a cannula in the obstructed bile duct hastens reduction of the jaundice and improves the general status of the patient. In a patient with progressive obstructive jaundice, operation for pancreatic carcinoma results in a high incidence of mortality, and in selected cases preoperative drainage can be of help in reducing mortality and morbidity.

Percutaneous Aspiration Biopsy of the Pancreas

Making a preoperative diagnosis of carcinoma of the pancreas is difficult.[26-29] A curative operation for pan-

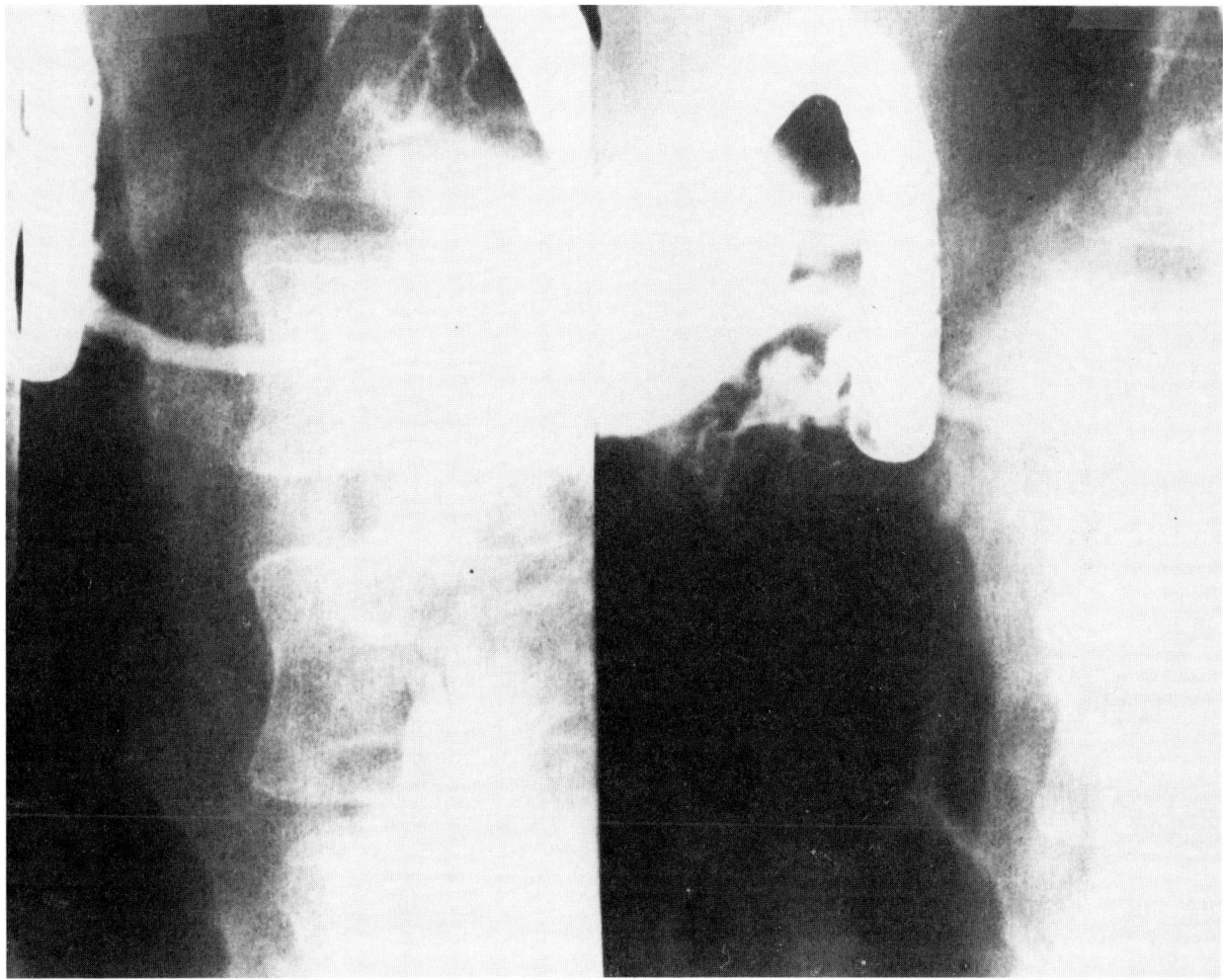

FIGURE 27-4 Endoscopic retrograde cholangiopancreaticography (ERCP).

creatic carcinoma is a major procedure, requiring radical resection of the pancreas, the duodenum, and the surrounding organs; an accurate preoperative histologic diagnosis is therefore desirable. Macroscopic examination of the diseased pancreas on the operating table is of little use, since it is impossible to distinguish between chronic pancreatitis and carcinoma by appearance alone. The technique proposed by Goldman et al.,[30] a preoperative percutaneous biopsy of the pancreatic tissue, has great potential. It provides histologic material not usually available conventionally. By this means, an accurate diagnosis of malignancy can be made without undue rush. Also, a needless laparotomy can sometimes be avoided. An aspiration biopsy of the pancreas can be done under sonographic control.[30,31] The skin directly over the portion of the pancreas is punctured with the Chibba needle, and under fluoroscopic guidance the needle is directly advanced to the region of the abnormal vessel seen earlier by angiography. The needle may pass through the stomach loops of the small intestine or through the liver prior to its entry into the pancreatic mass. Pancreatic tissue aspirate is then spread on a slide and sent for cytologic examination. Kline and coworkers[27] reported a 90 percent accuracy rate in their series

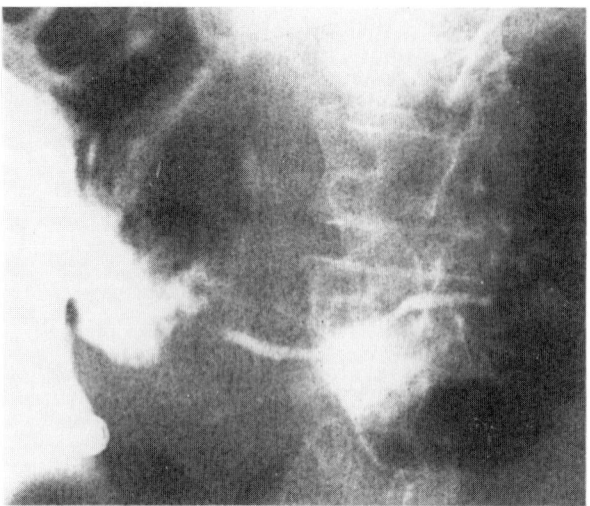

FIGURE 27-5 Endoscopic retrograde cholangiopancreaticography showing obstruction of pancreatic duct, "sharp cut of" suggestive of carcinoma of the pancreas.

of intraoperative needle aspiration biopsies of pancreatic neoplasms (Figs. 27-11 and 27-12).

TREATMENT OF PANCREATIC NEOPLASMS

Surgery

In Whipple's 1935 paper on the treatment of carcinoma of the pancreas,[1] he remarked that in the preceding five or six years while doing surgery of the pancreas he had noted brilliant cures of hyperinsulinism effected by the removal of adenomas and by excision of a large part of the pancreatic tumor. In the series of cures reported to date by American surgeons there has been no mortality. The overall results of surgical treatment of pancreatic tumor, however, have been unsatisfactory. The mortality and morbidity rates after surgery of the pancreas are significantly high.

After an initial wave of interest in radical resection in cases of carcinoma of the pancreas, there was a period of disenchantment, and the technique was nearly abandoned. Recently, however, improvements have been reported in a few series.[32-38] This renewed interest in the procedure has produced an increased survival rate in cases of pancreatic neoplasms, particularly ampullary tumors.

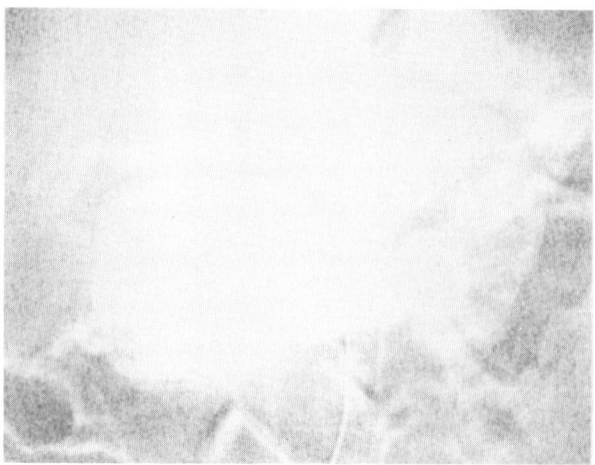

FIGURE 27-6 Angiogram of the pancreas showing large mass at the head of the pancreas (Zollinger-Ellison syndrome).

Whipple[1] initially described the technique of pancreaticoduodenectomy in 1935 for periampullary carcinoma (Fig. 27-13). He performed the surgery in two stages. This technique has subsequently been modified by several authors. The results of Whipple's procedure are excellent for periampullary lesions but not encour-

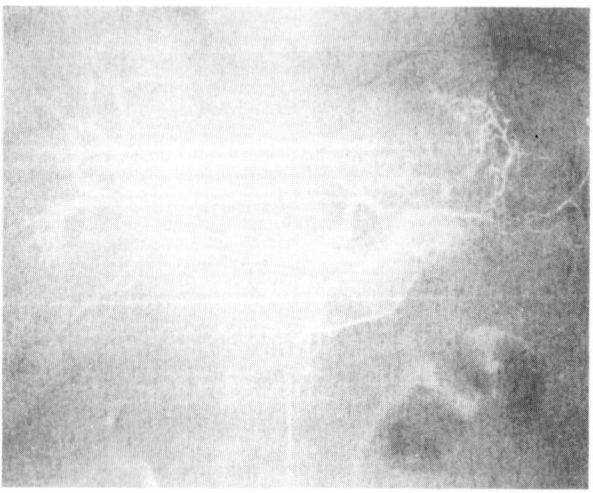

FIGURE 27-7 Angiogram of the pancreas showing carcinoma of the head and body of the pancreas and encasement of the splenic artery.

aging for carcinoma of the head of the pancreas. Brunschwig[2] performed the first one-stage resection of cancer of the head of the pancreas. He also popularized the method of ligation of the pancreatic duct as a preferred alternative to the pancreatic jejunostomy originally described by Whipple. Although ligation of the pancreatic duct theoretically could involve impairment of the exocrine function of the pancreas, we have never encountered any such problems. In fact, in our experience the incidence of postoperative complications such as pancreatic fistula has been reduced. The endocrine function of the pancreas has also been found to be unimpaired after ligation of the pancreatic duct. Although treatment of carcinoma of the pancreas has continued to present a dismal outlook, there has been some improvement reported in the operative results. In 1959, Ross[39] made a plea for treating carcinoma of the pancreas by total pancreatectomy. However, objections to this procedure were made both because of the high mortality rate and because the operation often resulted in metabolic deficiency. These problems led to a loss of popularity for the procedure. In 1971, Hicks and Brooks[40] found total pancreatectomy superior to partial pancreatectomy. The mortality rate for total pancreatectomy was 9 percent, compared to 36 percent for partial pancreatectomy. None of their patients who underwent total pancreatectomy had intestinal-tract complications. Interestingly enough, 4 of the 11 patients that had total pancreatectomy showed the presence of a distal tumor at the usual resection line. Also, 6 of the 36 patients with partial pancreatectomy showed lesions beyond the line of the resection, with residual tumor in the remaining pancreas. This finding clearly demonstrates the need for total pancreatectomy for cure of pancreatic carcinoma. With present-day knowledge, replacement of the pancreatic enzymes and the insulin is not a great technical problem.

Recently, a technique of en bloc resection of the pancreas, duodenum, surrounding nodal area, superior mesenteric artery and vein and celiac axis, with immediate prosthetic reconstruction of the blood vessels, has been described.[41] This is termed a regional pancreatectomy. So far, this method of treatment has not provided any improvement in the cure rate. Furthermore, the morbidity and mortality rates are extremely high, and we think it is a procedure without any redeeming feature. In our present judgment, total pancreatectomy is probably the ideal way to treat cancers of the head of the pancreas (Fig. 27-14).

In terms of cure, carcinoma of the body of the pancreas probably requires an approach similar to that for carcinoma of the head of the pancreas. Carcinoma of the tail of the pancreas is sometimes present as a small lesion, and in selective instances it may be justifiable to perform a distal pancreatectomy and splenectomy (Fig. 27-15).

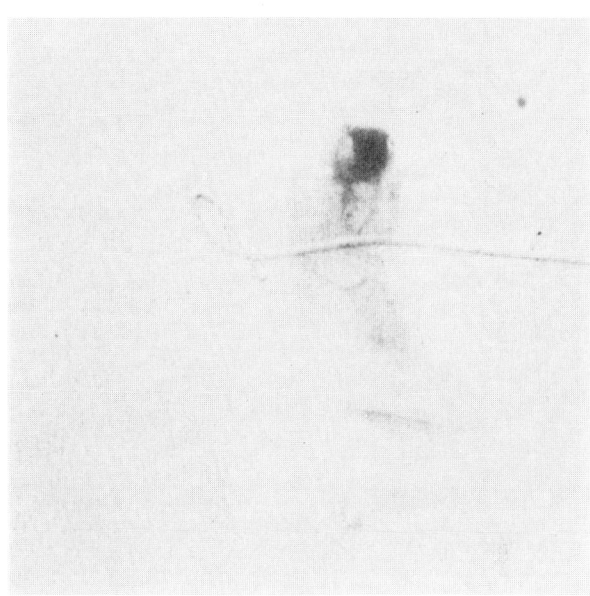

FIGURE 27-8 Capillary phase of angiogram of the pancreas. The small tumor at the tail is an insulinoma.

ENZYME REPLACEMENT FOLLOWING PANCREATECTOMY

The pancreas is vital to normal bowel function. Normally, the pancreas secretes biocarbonates, lipase, trypsin, amylase, and about 2000 mL of fluid per day. These activities may be curtailed following pancreatectomy. One of the striking symptoms of pancreatic insufficiency is severe steatorrhea. This means that there is more than 25 g of fat in the stool per day, which leads to malnutrition, weight loss, and difficulty in controlling coexistent diabetes if it is present. Patients who undergo a partial or total pancreatectomy may suffer from pancreatic enzyme insufficiency, which is treated by oral use of pancreatic enzymes extracted from hog pancreas[48,49] and will require this enzyme replacement. A patient who undergoes partial pancreatectomy without reimplantation of the pancreatic duct to the intestinal tract, or one who has had total pancreatectomy, will need replacement therapy

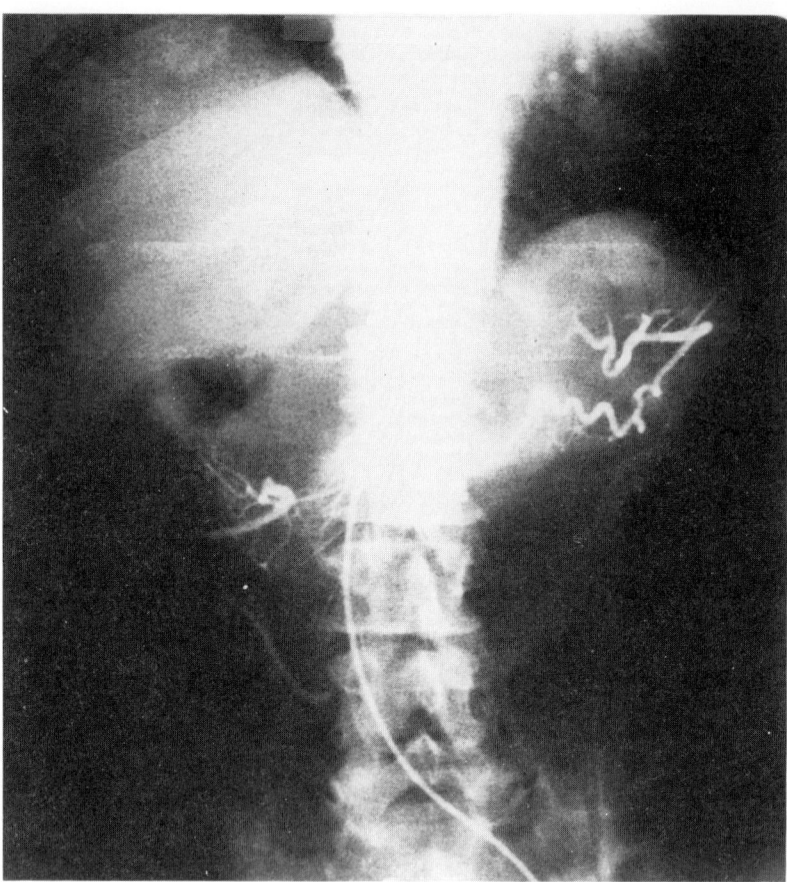

FIGURE 27-9 Angiogram of the pancreas showing carcinoma at tail of the pancreas and encasement of the blood vessels.

more often than one who had partial pancreatectomy with anastomosis of the pancreas distal to the intestines. After pancreatectomy, most patients may be given pancreatic enzyme replacement. Once the pancreatic insufficiency has been documented as the cause of steatorrhea, replacement therapy is mandatory. There are several enzymes available on the market, some of which are pH-sensitive and protected by an enteric coating.[50] Microspores have been found on short- and long-term follow-up to be effective for replacement therapy following pancreaticoduodenectomy or pancreatectomy.

INSULIN REPLACEMENT FOLLOWING PANCREATECTOMY

Insulin, secreted solely by the pancreas, is of utmost importance for the maintenance of life. It is essential for the metabolism of carbohydrates. Diabetes mellitus will develop in the patient who undergoes total pancreatectomy, as well as in many patients who undergo distal pancreatectomy. These patients usually develop very fragile diabetes, since carbohydrate metabolism is solely controlled by the outside replacement of insulin. Most will require a small amount of insulin, and careful adjustment is mandatory. Usually, patients are controlled well with 15 to 40 units of insulin daily; the average dose is 27 units.[40]

Radiation Therapy

Radiation therapy has not proved to be highly successful as a primary treatment for carcinoma of the pancreas,[42,43] although implantation of radioactive iodine or radon seeds into the pancreas may be a good choice in selected cases in which the tumor is technically unresectable but not disseminated. In this technique, a high dose of

TUMORS OF THE PANCREAS **589**

radiation is used. The implantation of radioactive seeds into pancreatic cancers was first performed by Handley in 1925, and then by Pack in 1926, mostly for tumors that were locally unresectable. However, there has not been much improvement in the long-term survival rate with this treatment. Reports have appeared in which betatron therapy was used for unresectable pancreatic cancers.[44,45] Borgelt et al.[44] recently recommended this technique for treatment of small, unresectable pancreatic tumors. Historically, the role of radiation therapy has been largely one of palliation. Irradiation in high dosages could not be given because of the deep location of the pancreas and its close proximity to the spinal cord, kidneys, intestines, and liver. Now, with the advent of high-energy protons and electron beams, it is possible to deliver a minimum tumor dose of 6700 rads to the target region of the pancreas while sparing the adjacent critical structures. This new technique will probably be useful in selected cases of unresectable pancreatic cancer.

Intraarterial Chemotherapy Infusion

A few selected cases of locally unresectable pancreatic carcinoma can be palliated with intraarterial infusion of chemotherapeutic agents.[46,47] This technique could be used in conjunction with radon or radioactive iodine

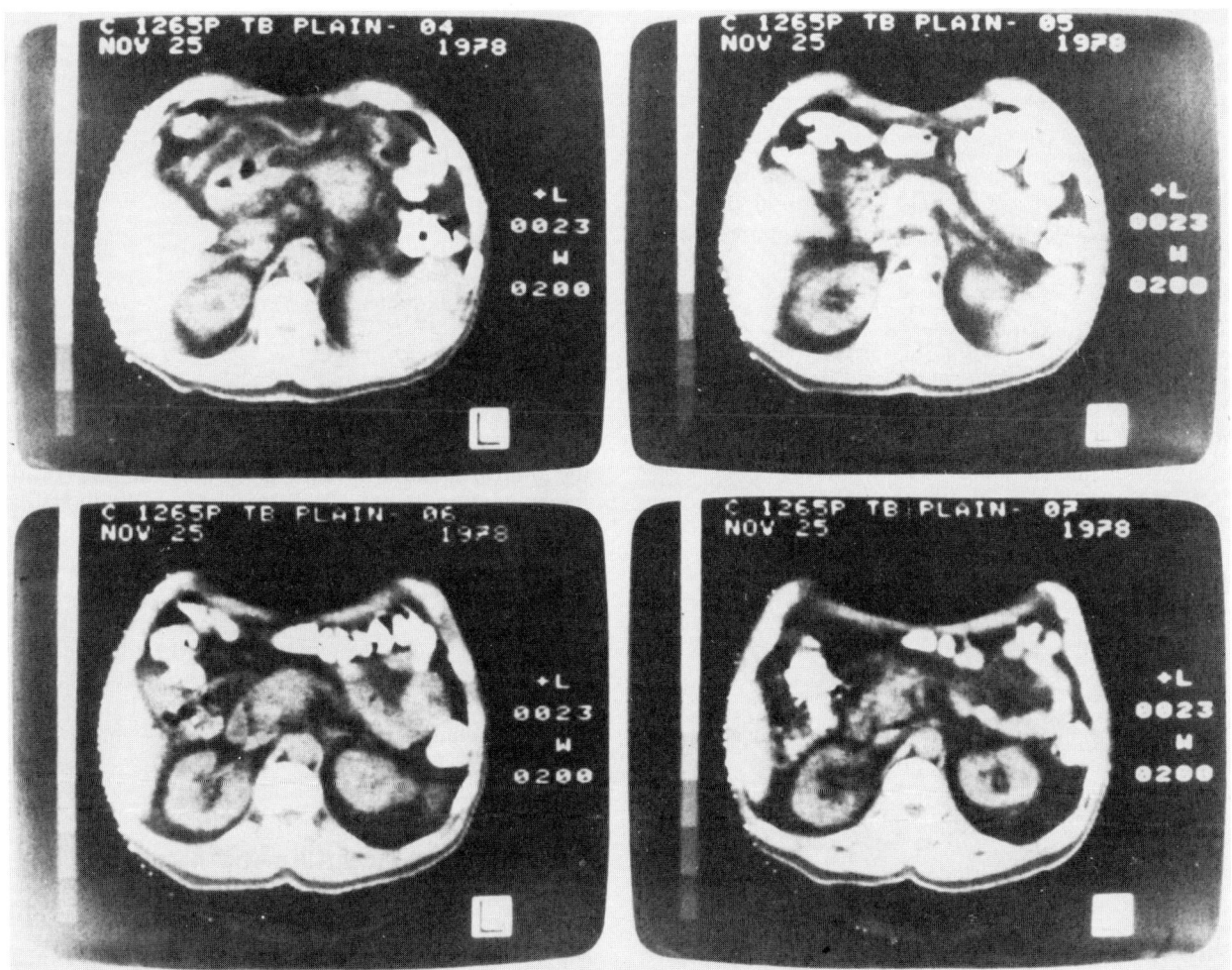

FIGURE 27-10 Computerized axial tomogram suggestive of pancreatic neoplasm.

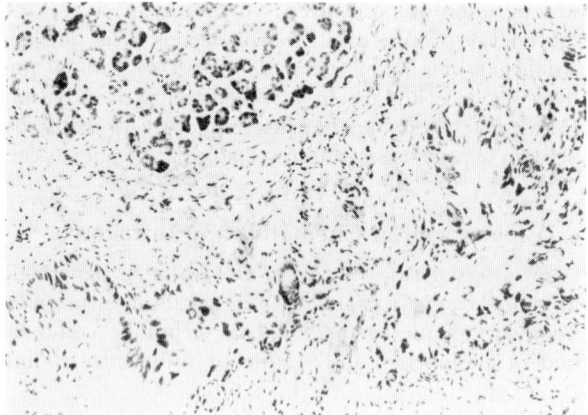

FIGURE 27-11 Histologic findings in chronic pancreatitis—extensive fibrosis, no carcinomatous cells, areas of some pancreatic lobules and islets (H&E, ×280).

implants. The combination of radiation and chemotherapy has been reported to yield better results than any other conventional treatment of locally unresectable pancreatic carcinomas.

Adjuvant Therapies

The role of adjuvant chemotherapy is presently being investigated by several national cooperative study groups, but success has been limited.

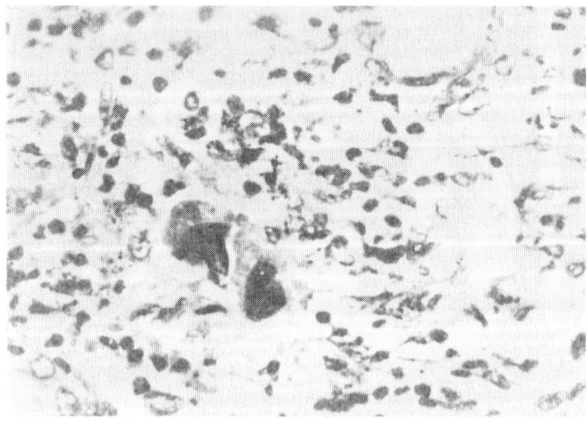

FIGURE 27-12 Anaplastic adenocarcinoma of the pancreas—hyperchromatic nucleus with mitosis (H&E, ×280).

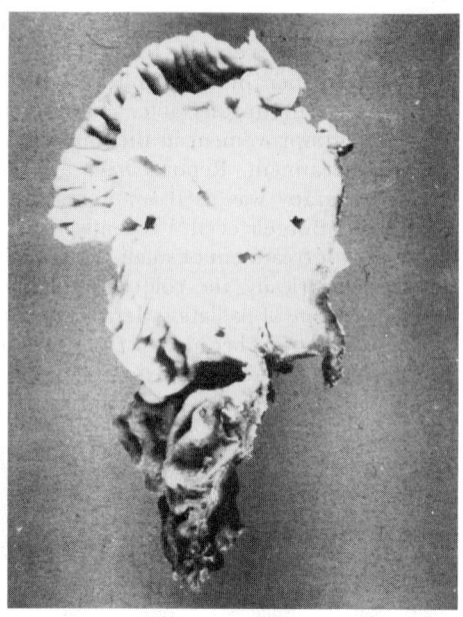

FIGURE 27-13 Specimen of standard Whipple procedure showing duodenum and head of the pancreas. (*Courtesy of A. G. Lawrence.*)

The Gastrointestinal Tumor Study Group studied the locally unresectable pancreatic carcinoma. In a prospective randomized and controlled clinical trial, high-dose (6000-rad) radiation therapy alone was compared with radiation therapy at two dose levels (6000 and 4000 rad) administered in conjunction with fluorouracil. The two regimens using fluorouracil resulted in a higher survival rate, with no differences in toxicity.

Postoperative radiation therapy has also been used in several centers. If the tumors are resected and if they are properly marked with radioptic clips, postoperative radiation therapy alone might be tried. Yet the combination of irradiation and chemotherapy seems to be a more logical choice.

CANCER OF THE BODY AND TAIL OF THE PANCREAS

The body and tail of the pancreas, along with the superior portion of the head, derive from the dorsal pancreatic duct embryologically. The ratio of cancer of the body and tail of the pancreas to that of the head of

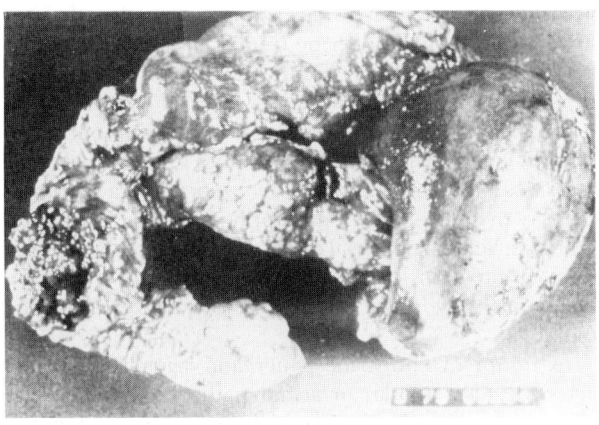

FIGURE 27-14 Specimen of total pancreatectomy showing duodenum, pancreas, and spleen.

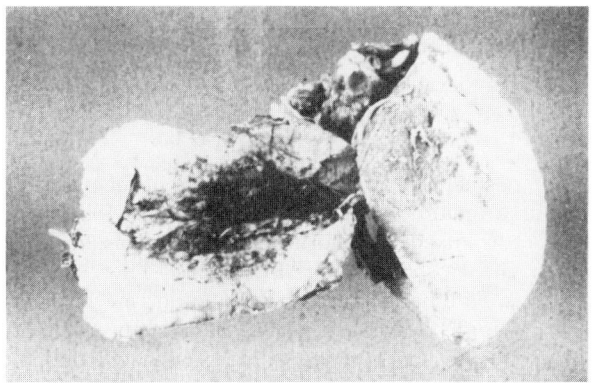

FIGURE 27-15 Specimen of distal pancreatectomy. (*Courtesy of A. G. Lawrence.*)

the pancreas is about 1:2. These tumors are usually found at laparotomy or at autopsy. Although adenocarcinoma is the commonest variety of cancer of the body and tail of the pancreas, large numbers of endocrine tumors, such as insulinomas, also occur in these locations. The clinical symptoms are quite different from those of carcinoma of the head of the pancreas. Notably, the jaundice that occurs early in carcinoma of the head of the pancreas is seen much later in carcinomas of the tail or body. Certain cases present with gripping upper abdominal pain, constipation, splenomegaly, upper gastrointestinal bleeding, skin lesions, phlebitis, arterial embolisms, and local bursitis. Functional endocrine abnormality might provide a clue to the diagnosis of carcinoma of the body of the pancreas.

CYSTOADENOCARCINOMA

Without exploration and biopsy, a cystoadenocarcinoma of the pancreas, if very large, can be difficult to distinguish from a pancreatic cyst (Fig. 27-16).[51] The absence of pancreatitis, trauma, alcoholism, or drug addiction should arouse suspicion of a pancreatic cystoadenocarcinoma. The presence of a large tumor involving any segment of the pancreas without extension or metastasis is highly suggestive of cystocarcinoma of the pancreas.[52] The majority occur in women and are situated in the body or tail of the pancreas. Because of the possibility of neoplasmic change, an operation should be performed for cystoadenoma of the pancreas.[53] Aspiration, intra-abdominal biopsy, and internal or external drainage are not recommended for cystoadenomas of the pancreas, since there might be an associated carcinoma or subsequent change to the existing carcinoma. However, internal or external drainage may occasionally be required for palliation of a large, metastatic cystoadenocarcinoma.

BENIGN NEOPLASMS OF THE PANCREAS AND EXTRAHEPATIC BILIARY TRACTS

Benign neoplasms of the pancreas are extremely rare. Burhans and Myers[54] in 1971 reported a series of 85 cases. The benign neoplasms that have been recorded constitute clinical varieties rather than any significant

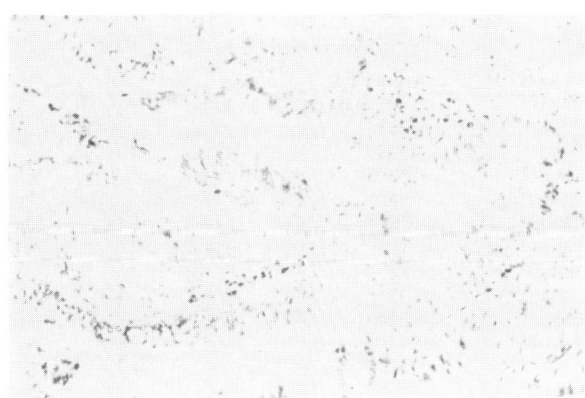

FIGURE 27-16 Papillary cyst adenocarcinoma (H&E, ×280).

problem. Operative cholangiography is an important tool for diagnosing these rare entities.

ENDOCRINE TUMORS OF THE PANCREAS

In the normal human pancreas the islets of the pancreas contain a multitude of endocrine cells. Only four types have been linked with hormones, namely, insulin, glucagon, somatostatin, and APUD cells. There might, however, be other cell types whose endocrine function remains to be established. Recently, it has been found that pancreatic polypeptide cells secrete a polypeptide that exerts an effect on the gastrointestinal tract as an antagonist to cholecystokinin. It has also been observed that the pancreas has cells capable of producing carcinoid-type tumors. Recently a type of cell, known as a P cell, has been found in the fetal pancreas and in the lungs, the exact function of which is not known.

Most endocrine pancreatic tumors produce one or several hormones. Hyperplasia of the islet tissue indicates a nonductal origin of the hyperplastic cells. It has been suggested that several peptide hormone–producing cells are closely related embryonically. Polypeptide hormone–producing cells are called APUD cells; APUD tumors are composed of APUD cells. These cells have certain enzymes which can be shown by both light and electron microscopy to be a definite characteristic of cytoplasmic granules.

Pancreatic endocrine tumors are usually classified according to the particular symptom produced. It is known that many endocrine tumors are multihormonal and contain different peptide hormones. The clinical symptoms are due to excess secretion of one particular hormone, which produces a specific symptom. The present consensus is that diagnosis and follow-up of these cases should be monitored by a specific radioimmunoassay or several different peptide hormones or tumor markers. Selective arterial catheterization, combined with duct cannulation for radioimmunoassay of polypeptide hormones, may be the best of all the available diagnostic tools.

A tumor of endocrine pancreatic origin has a characteristic solid tubular or acinar pattern and sometimes resembles a carcinoid. The cells have lightly staining, pale nuclei, with granular cytoplasm (Fig. 27-17). The metastasis shows a well-developed pattern. The size of the tumor varies considerably and has no relation to the severity of symptoms. Several special stains are available for electron microscope histochemical studies and light microscopy examination. Endocrine tumors of the pancreas are not difficult to diagnose. Several methods of studying the different polypeptide hormones by immunohistochemistry are technically feasible.

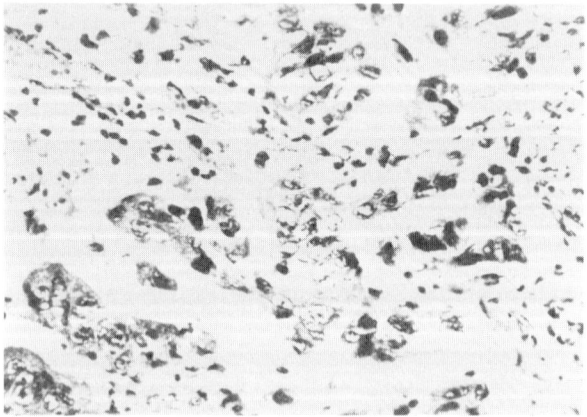

FIGURE 27-17 Endocrine tumor of the pancreas (H& E, ×280).

Insulinomas

Hypoglycemia is usually present, and frequently the patient has neuropsychiatric disturbances. The hypoglycemia can be relieved by administration of glucose. Laboratory findings show a high insulin-to-glucose ratio and often an increased proportion of proinsulin-like material. Proinsulin is converted into insulin in the pancreas with C peptides, which may explain the high ratio of proinsulin secretion in the blood. Localized beta-cell hyperplasia may produce the same symptoms that occur in insulinomas.

Gastrinomas

A gastrinoma is a distinct endocrine tumor of the pancreas that is frequently malignant.[55,56] These tumors often multiply, and on initial examination many patients show signs of metastasis. Gastrinomas occur also in the duodenum and, rarely, in the antrum of the stomach. Gastrinomas are part of the Zollinger-Ellison syndrome, which consists of gastric hyperacidity, intractable peptic ulcer, and the pancreatic tumor. There may also be abdominal pain, diarrhea, and gastrointestinal bleeding.

The type of peptic ulcer found in this syndrome usually occurs in the duodenum, but occasionally is found in the jejunum. Hypertrophic gastric mucosa, with high basal and histamine stimulations, and gastrin-stimulated gastrin acid secretion, as well as high overnight gastric secretion, are definitely diagnosed by gastrin radioimmunoassay. Gastrin may also be produced in islet-cell hyperplasia, and it is important to differentiate between gastrinomas and islet-cell hyperplasia.

Verner-Morrison Tumors

These tumors are also known as WHDA tumors.[57] Usually the symptoms are watery diarrhea and hypokalemia. There are several hypotheses concerning the particular type of hormone that produces these symptoms: gastrin plus glucagon, secretin, vasoactive polypeptide, or intestinal pancreatic polypeptides. Extrapancreatic tumors, such as neuroblastomas, produce similar symptoms.

Glucagonomas

Glucagon-producing tumors and diabetes are usually associated. Glucagonomas produce occasional enterocolitis, migratory erythema, diabetes, stomatitis, weight loss, a high rate of venous thrombosis, and, sometimes, diarrhea. Psychiatric disturbances may also be present.

Somatostatinomas

Pure somatostatin-producing tumors are uncommon. They produce a diabetic-type glucose tolerance curve, and in some cases steatorrhea and diarrhea are present. It has been reported that with this type of tumor glucagon concentration is significantly below normal and insulin concentration is in the low to normal range. Usually, angiography will show a high capillary gradient, which indicates active secretion from these tumors.

Other Types

The carcinoid tumor which produces hydrotryptaphen or tumorlike ACTH or MSH, although uncommon, has been reported in the pancreas. Rarely, Cushing's syndrome is associated with this type of tumor. Several other peptide hormone–producing tumors originating in the pancreas have recently been reported.

Treatment

The treatment of endocrine pancreatic tumor is surgical removal if diagnosis is made sufficiently early to make this possible. Gastrinomas are in most instances malignant. Widespread metastases to the nodes and liver are usually found. The ulcer symptoms can be relieved by removal of the target organs. Gastrinomas produce the symptoms that arise from hypersecretion of gastric acid, and total gastrectomy will relieve these symptoms, even in the presence of metastatic disease. If the tumor is small and localized in the pancreas, surgical removal will relieve the symptoms and the patient should have a long, symptom-free life.

CURRENT AREAS OF RESEARCH AND PROSPECTS FOR THE FUTURE

Most research on pancreatic tumors is directed toward finding methods of early detection, discovering the etiologic factors involved, and studying the behavior of the tumors. In recent studies, pancreatic carcinomas have been induced in Syrian hamsters by injection of chemical carcinogens.[58,59] These tumors are transplantable to inbred hamsters and can be produced within a period of 4 to 5 months. They mimic most of the features of human pancreatic adenocarcinoma, including its behavior in relation to invasion and metastasis, and therefore are an excellent model. Several earlier models are also very promising. The pancreatic disposition of chemical carcinogens has also been studied recently.[60] Carcinogenesis in pancreatic ductal tissue and continuation of pancreatic carcinoma is being studied using tissue cultures.[61,62] Turner[63] studied antigens associated with pancreatic tumors. Similar analysis in experimental pancreatic carcinoma has opened a new line of experimental carcinogenesis. Pancreatic secretion has also been studied to establish the presence of carcinogens.[64,65] One theory about the origin of pancreatic carcinoma involves the bioreflex mechanism. Although this hypothesis has not yet been proved in experimental models, the bile reflex mechanism is a factor in blood-mediated carcinogens, and could be a factor in the development of human pancreatic carcinoma. The exciting development of secretory proteins from the pancreas could be a significant indication of pancreatic disease long before the appearance of clinical symptoms. This encouraging study may find the parameter which singly or in combination would permit the detection of early pancreatic malignancies. Scheele[66] compared exocrine pancreatic protein from hospital patients with cancer of the pancreas with that from patients with pancreatitis. Using radiolabeled soluble elastin, Scheele performed a sensitive assay for elastosis, and was able to identify two forms of protelastose.

The most important objective of research studies of pancreatic carcinoma is to develop a technique for detecting such tumors at an early stage. Coordinated clinical research across the country would result in improved communication between research scientists and clinicians. Fiberoptic endoscopy, biochemical markers, antigens, enzymes, angiography, and pancreatic scan should be evaluated for their possible use in early diagnosis. The development of new drugs and the study of the effect of existing drugs on pancreatic carcinomas should be undertaken. Immunotherapy, either alone or in combination, should be explored in depth. Current studies are leading to promising lines of research for the future. Research scientists and clinicians together will arrive at a better understanding of tumors of pancreatic origin and develop improved methods of treatment for patients with pancreatic carcinoma.

REFERENCES

1. Whipple AO et al.: Treatment of carcinoma of the ampulla of Vater. *Ann Surg* 102:1935.
2. Brunschwig A: Pancreatoduodenectomy: A "curative" operation for malignant neoplasms in the pancreatoduodenal region. *Ann Surg* 136:610, 1952.
3. Cancer Statistics. *CA* 27:26, 1977.
4. Harris CC, Autrup H, Stoner G et al: Metabolism of benz(a)pyrene and 7-12-dimethylbenz(a)anthracine in cultured human bronchus and pancreatic duct. *Cancer Res* 37: 3349, 1977.
5. Cecil RL: A study of the pathological anatomy of the pancreas in ninety cases of diabetes mellitus. *J Exp Med* 11: 266.
6. Goldsmith HS et al.: Ligation versus implantation of the pancreatic duct after pancreaticoduodenectomy. *Surg Gynecol Obstet* 132:87, 1971.
7. Bowden L, Pack GT: Cancer of the head of pancreas: A collective review of the experiences of the Gastric Service of the Memorial Cancer Center 1926–1958. *Separata de G.E.N. Organo de la Sociedad Venezolara de Gastroenterologia* 23:339, 1969.
8. Arlen M, Brockunier A Jr: Clinical manifestations of carcinoma of the tail of the pancreas. *Cancer* 20:1920, 1967.
9. Gosink BB, Leopold GR: The dilated pancreatic duct: Ultrasonic evaluation. *Radiology* 163:475, 1978.
10. Nordshus T et al.: Cystademona of the pancreas: Report of a case studied by ultrasound and endoscopic retrograde pancreaticography. *Ann Chir Gynaecol* 67:33, 1978.
11. Ghosh BC et al.: The role of angiogram in pancreatic neoplasm. *Am J Surg* (in press).
12. Gray RK et al.: Anteriography in the diagnosis of islet cell tumors. *Radiology* 97:39, 1970.
13. Orlov VA: Significance of angiography of the pancreas in the diagnosis of chronic pancreatitis. *Am J Gastroenterol* 68: 461, 1977.
14. Olsson O: Angiographic diagnosis of an islet cell tumor of the pancreas. *Acta Chir Scand* 126:346, 1963.
15. Alfidi RJ, Skillern PG Jr: Arteriographic manifestations of the Zollinger-Ellison Syndrome: Report of a case. *Cleveland Clin Quart* 36:41, 1968.
16. Baghery S et al.: Angiography of nonfunctioning islet cell tumors of the pancreas. *Radiology* 120:57, 1976.
17. Baum J et al.: Clinical application of selective celiac and superior mesenteric anteriography. *Radiology* 84:279, 1965.
18. Berger A et al.: Zur Diagnostik des Inselzellademons mittles viazeraler Angiographic. *Zbl Chir* 92:2184, 1967.
19. Buranasiri S, Baur S: The significance of the intravenous phase of celiac and superior mesenteric anteriography in evaluating pancreatic carcinoma. *Radiology* 102:11, 1972.
20. Nebesar RA, Pollard JJ: A critical evaluation of selective celiac and superior mesenteric angiography in the diagnosis of pancreatic diseases, particularly malignant tumor: Facts and "artefacts." *Radiology* 89:1017, 1967.
21. Deutch V et al.: Angiographic diagnosis and differential diagnosis of islet-cell tumors. *Radiother Nucl Med* 119:121, 1973.
22. Fujii K et al.: Arteriography in insulinoma. *Radiother Nucl Med* 120:634, 1974.
23. Fulton RE et al.: Preoperative angiographic localization of insulin producing tumors of the pancreas. *Radiother Nucl Med* 123:367, 1975.
24. Herlinger H: The angiographic diagnosis of insulinoma. *Proc R Soc Med* 69: 1976.
25. Ariyama J et al.: The diagnosis of the small resectable pancreatic carcinoma. *Clin Radiol* 28:437, 1977.
26. Carlson RI: The problems of diagnosis at the time of operation in tumors of the head of the pancreas. *Surgery* 28:672, 1950.
27. Kline TS, Hunter SN: Needle aspiration biopsy: A safe diagnostic procedure for lesions of the pancreas. *Am J Clin Path* 73: 1975.
28. Kline TS, Hunter SN: Needle biopsy: a pilot study. *JAMA* 224:1143, 1973.
29. Kline TS et al.: Needle aspiration biopsy of the pancreas at laparotomy. *Am J Gastroenterol* 68:30, 1977.
30. Goldman HM et al.: Preoperative diagnosis of pancreatic carcinoma by percutaneous aspiration biopsy. *Dig Dis* 22: 1977.
31. Forsgren L, Orell S: Aspiration cytology in carcinoma of the pancreas. *Surg* 73:38, 1973.

32. Aston SJ, Longmire WP Jr: Pancreaticoduodenal resection: Twenty years' experience. *Arch Surg* 106:813, 1973.
33. Braasch JW, Gray BN: Technique of radical pancreatoduodenectomy, with consideration of hepatic arterial relationships. *Surg Clin North Am* 65:631, 1978.
34. Brooks JR, Culebras JM: Cancer of the pancreas: Palliative operation, Whipple procedure, or total pancreatectomy. *Am J Surg* 131:516, 1976.
35. Cattell RB, Pytek LJ: An appraisal of pancreatoduodenal resection: A followup study of 61 cases. *Ann Surg* 129:840, 1949.
36. Cattell RB, Warren KW: *Surgery of the Pancreas*, Saunders, Philadelphia, 1953.
37. Cattell RB: Polypoid epithelial tumors of the bile ducts. *N Engl J Med* 266:57, 1962.
38. Howard JM: Pancreatico-duodenectomy: Forty-one consecutive Whipple resections without an operative mortality. *Ann Surg* 168:629, 1968.
39. Ross DE: Cancer of the pancreas: A plea for total pancreatectomy. *Am J Surg* 87:20, 1956.
40. Hicks RE, Brooks JR: Total pancreatectomy for ductal carcinoma. *Surg Gynecol Obstet* 133:16, 1971.
41. Fortner JG: Regional resection of cancer of the pancreas: A new surgical approach. *Surg* 73:307, 1973.
42. Dobelbower RR et al.: Pancreatic carcinoma treatment with high-dose, small volume irradiation. *Cancer* 41:1087, 1978.
43. Miller TR, Fuller L: Radiation therapy of carcinomas of the pancreas: Report on 91 cases. *Am J Roentgenol* 80:787, 1958.
44. Borgelt BB et al.: Betatron therapy for unresectable pancreatic cancer. *Am J Surg* 135:76, 1976.
45. Green N et al.: Carcinoma of pancreas palliative radiotherapy. *Am J Roentgenol* 117:620, 1973.
46. Barone RM: Treatment of carcinoma of the pancreas with radon seed implantation and intra-arterial infusion of 5-FUDR. *Surg Clin North Am* 55:117, 1975.
47. Itkin AB: Regional intra-arterial chemotherapy of cancer of the pancreas. *Khirurgiia* (Moscow) 48:22, 1972.
48. Graham DY: Enzyme replacement therapy of exocrine pancreatic insufficiency in man. *N Engl J Med* 296:1314, 1977.
49. Meyer JH: The ins and outs of oral pancreatic enzymes. *N Engl J Med* 196:1347, 1977.
50. Blythe RH et al.: The formulation and evaluation of enteric coated aspirin tablets. *Am J Pharm* 131:206, 1959.
51. Lichenstein L: Papillary cystadenocarcinoma of the pancreas: Case report, with notes on classification of malignant cystic tumors of the pancreas. *Am J Cancer* 21:524, 1934.
52. Warren KW et al.: Carcinoma of the pancreas. *Surg Clin N Am* 48:601, 1968.
53. Hodgkinson DJ et al.: A clinicopathological study of 21 cases of pancreatic cystadenocarcinoma. *Ann Surg* 188:679, 1978.
54. Burhans R, Myers RT: Benign neoplasms of the extrahepatic biliary ducts. *Am Surg* 37:161, 1971.
55. Mihas AA et al.: Zollinger-Ellison syndrome associated with ductal adenocarcinoma of the pancreas. *N Engl J Med* 198:144, 1978.
56. Zboralski FF, Amberg JR: Detection of the Zollinger-Ellison syndrome: The radiologist's responsibility. *Am J Roentgenol* 104:529, 1968.
57. Thomas ML et al.: Angiographic demonstration of a pancreatic "Vipoma" in the WDHA syndrome. *Am J Roentgenol* 127:1037, 1976.
58. Bockman DE: Experimentally-induced pancreatic carcinoma. *National Pancreatic Cancer Society Newsletter* 3:22, 1978.
59. Gingell R, Pour P: Metabolism of the pancreatic carcinogen N-nitroso bisamine (2-oxopropyl) after oral and interiperitoneal administration to Syrian golden hamsters: Brief communication. *J Nat Cancer Inst* 60:911, 1978.
60. Epstein SS: Chemical carcinogens in the pancreas. *National Pancreatic Cancer Society Newsletter* 3:19, 1978.
61. Githens S: Carcinogenesis of pancreatic ductal tissue in vitro. *National Pancreatic Cancer Society Newsletter* 3: 1978.
62. Yunis AA: Pancreatic carcinoma in continuous culture. *National Pancreatic Cancer Society Newsletter* 3:7, 1978.
63. Turner MD: Pancreatic tumor associated antigens. *National Pancreatic Cancer Society Newsletter* 3:10, 1978.
64. Reber HA: Pancreatic secretion in pancreatic cancer. *National Pancreatic Cancer Society Newsletter* 3:13, 1978.
65. Rinderknechu H: Pancreatic secretory proteins in cancer of the pancreas. *National Pancreatic Cancer Society Newsletter* 3:18, 1978.
66. Scheele, GA: Exocrine pancreatic protein in cancer of the pancreas. *National Pancreatic Cancer Society Newsletter* 3:23, 1978.

SELECTED BIBLIOGRAPHY

Beazley RM: Needle biopsy diagnosis of pancreatic cancer. *Cancer* 47:1685, 1981.
Chu MY et al: Growth and innovative chemotherapeutic approaches to human pancreatic carcinoma. *Proc Amer Assoc Cancer Res* 22:231, 1981.
Dobelbower RR Jr: Current radiotherapeutic approaches to pancreatic cancer. *Cancer* 47:1729, 1981.
Fortner JG: Surgical principles for pancreatic cancer: Regional total and subtotal pancreatectomy. *Cancer* 47:1712, 1981.
Freeny PC, Ball TJ: Endoscopic retrograde cholangiopancreatography (ERCP) and percutaneous transhepatic cholangiography (PTC) in the evaluation of suspected pancreatic carcinoma: Diagnostic limitations and contemporary roles. *Cancer* 47:1666, 1981.
Holyoke DE: New surgical approaches to pancreatic cancer. *Cancer* 47:1719, 1981.
Longmire WP Jr, Traverso WL: The Wipple procedure and other standard operative approaches to pancreatic cancer. *Cancer* 47:1706, 1981.

28
CANCER OF THE COLON AND RECTUM

E. Douglas Holyoke   Arnold Mittleman

Background and Historical Aspects

Cancer of the colon and rectum is treatable. For patients with this disease in whom the primary curative modality is surgery, the outlook should be better than for patients with breast cancer who have undergone radical mastectomy.[1,2] Treatment and evaluation of cancer of the colon and rectum have been changing over the last decade, and today a high rate of cure must be the goal for those patients who are technically operable for removal of all grossly visible tumor. In addition to reviewing the general characteristics, diagnosis, and treatment of this disease, this discussion will present the authors' view that vigorous, active surgical intervention, combined-modality treatment, and close follow-up in an organized treatment program results in a higher survival rate than a more traditional, possibly less organized program.

Table 28-1 lists chronologically the major developments in the care of patients with colorectal cancer. It is evident that our understanding of colorectal cancer is still changing and that there are relatively recent developments with therapeutic implications. The results of surveys for colon and rectal cancer by the American College of Surgeons also indicate, in the authors' opinion, the need for increased effort to use the tools already at hand to obtain the best possible outcome for these patients.[9]

Incidence, Epidemiology, and Etiologic Aspects

Colorectal cancer is about as common as lung cancer among the solid tumors, although chances for survival are better for colorectal cancer patients.[10,11] Overall survival rate for these patients is about 45 percent.[12] At the present time, 1 in 25 Americans will develop this disease during a lifetime, and each year over 100,000 individuals in this country will be diagnosed as new patients with this disease.[13] In addition, with an estimated 50 percent recurrence rate, approximately 25,000 patients a year will be candidates for palliative reductive surgery for recurrent regional or metastatic colorectal cancer.

Colorectal cancer does have an environmental cause. The disease is found in high incidence in the West as opposed to many third world nations.[14] It is believed that this higher incidence is related to diet. Increased protein and animal fat intake, increased refined carbohydrate intake, and/or reduced fiber intake have been implicated. Incidence ranges for both males and females from 5 per 100,000 population in Japan or Chile to 15 per 100,000 in Canada or Scotland. This difference in incidence by a factor of 3 is surveyed for some 24 countries. Figure 28-1 shows the apparent relationship between dietary fat intake and the incidence of colorectal cancer. The data for males and females are similar.

TABLE 28-1 Progression in the Care of Patients with Colorectal Cancer

Abdominal perineal resection (Miles[3])	1908
Classification of colorectal cancer (Dukes[4])	1958
Identification of colon tumor–associated antigens (Gold[5])	1965
Development of the stapler for colonic anastomosis (Androsov[6])	1970
Use of the flexible colonoscope (Overholt[7])	1975
Publication of results for treatment of colorectal cancer following accurate staging (Enker[1])	1980
Demonstration of an advantage in disease-free survival for combined-modality therapy of the rectum (Mittleman[8])	1981

Figure 28-2 reports the most convincing studies relating environmental factors to colorectal cancer.[15] Immigrants from Japan to the United States show a steady generation-by-generation change in incidence rate for both colorectal and gastric cancer, a rate which finally approaches that of the entire U.S. population. These figures are striking and their significance cannot be ignored, even though the specific environmental factors (probably dietary) and their mechanism of action have not been precisely established.

Genetic factors also play a role. Families show a high incidence of colon cancer. Both members of families in which familial polyposis occurs, and individuals with moderate to numerous adenomatous polyps have been found to be at risk.[16] Familial polyposis is an autosomal dominant disease characterized by the development of multiple polyps usually after the age of 10 and before the age of 40.[17,18] Series have been reported in which up to 50 percent of patients have presented with carcinomatous changes at the time of original diagnosis of familial polyposis. Over a 10-year period, virtually 100 percent of these individuals will develop cancer in the colon or rectum. Figure 28-3 is a colon specimen from an individual with familial polyposis.

The role of the development of other "benign" polyps in the development of colon cancer is uncertain. Ackerman and Del Regato discuss a series of lesions which demonstrates that colon cancer can indeed arise in polyps. Occasional discrete polyps of the colon may be classified as adenomatous, or as villoglandular or villous adenomas. Adenomatous polyps may develop in 10 to 15 percent of an adult population and make up 80 percent of the benign polyps of the large bowel. Perhaps 75 percent are located distal to the sigmoid colon, but a significant number, more than was appreciated prior to modern endoscopy, occur proximally. Symptoms depend on the size and location of the lesion. Malignant change is usually reported as unlikely in lesions less than 1.0 cm in diameter, as occurring in about 5 percent of lesions greater than 1.0 and less than 2.0 cm in diameter, and as occurring in 10 percent or greater of lesions more than 2.0 cm across. Villoglandular adenomas comprise approximately 10 percent of colonic polyps. They demonstrate histologic changes found in both adenomatous polyps and villous adenomas. About 20 percent of those reported are found to be malignant.[19] Villous adenoma also makes up about 10 percent of polyps of the colon and rectum. Most of these are located in the rectosigmoid and rectum. Malignant change occurs in at least 15 percent, and in lesions greater than 5 cm in diameter, the rate of malignancy approaches 50 percent. The malignant potential of villous adenoma is 5 to 10 times greater than that of simple adenomatous polyps.[20] The oncologist should be aware that other "genetic" syndromes occur that are associated with polyposis. These include Gardner's syndrome, in which multiple osteomas and bony exostosis as well as varied soft-tissue tumors may be associated with polyposis.[21] Peutz-Jeghers syndrome, Turcot syndrome, and associated multiple endocrine abnormalities and colonic polyposis may rarely be encountered. One problem which may arise is the tendency of some family members to form desmoid tumors following colectomy in the resulting healed abdominal wound. In any event, treatment is complete excision, endoscopically or surgically, depending on size, gross configuration, and histology.

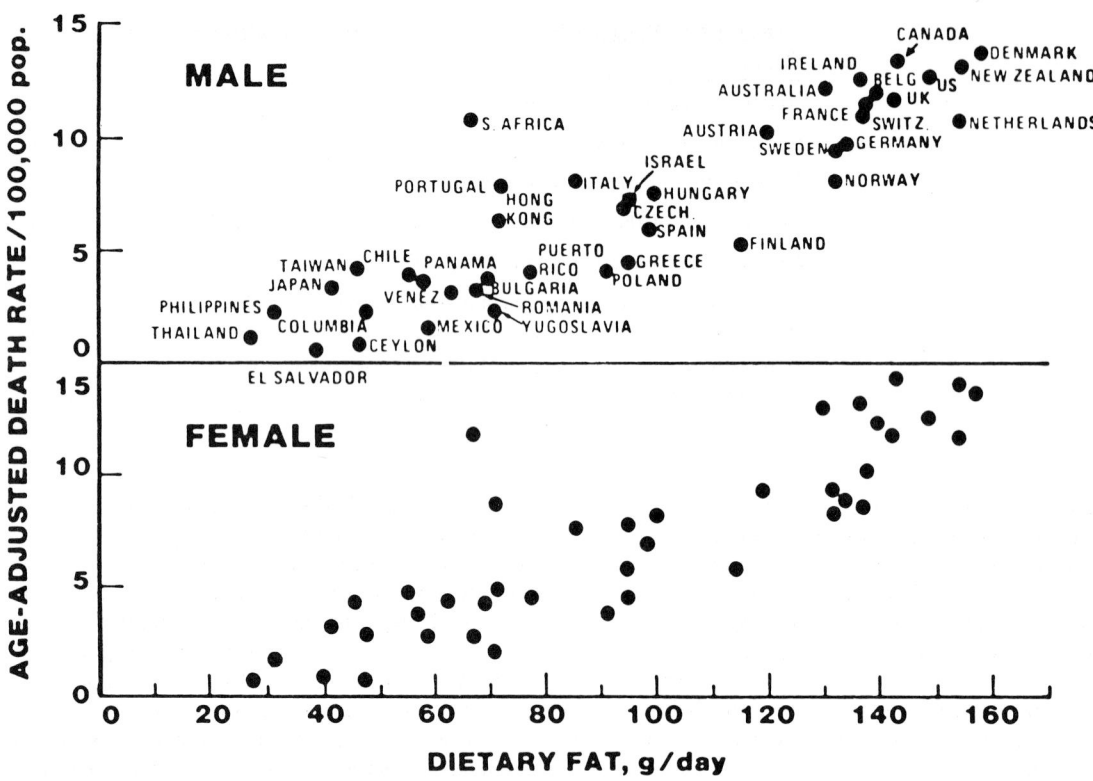

FIGURE 28-1 The age-adjusted death rate for males and females in different countries as related to daily intake of dietary fat. A threefold change in tumor incidence relates remarkably well to dietary fat.

For the initial excision of polyps the development of endoscopy has altered the surgical approach, and even quite large polyps, 3 to 4 cm in diameter with a stalk, as well as smaller sessile polyps, can be removed. Complications are few, with no severe bleeding and only one perforation in some 600 polypectomies via endoscopy.[22] An area of difficult decision are those polyps removed endoscopically, usually of moderate size, with microscopic invasive malignancy. The question arises as to whether to perform subsequent segmental colon resection. This procedure is recommended if the submucosal tissue can be seen to be invaded in the polyp itself, and it should certainly be carried out if the stalk is invaded.

For multiple polyposis proctocolectomy has in the past been performed as a standard procedure. A consideration always has been retention of the rectum with ileorectosigmoidostomy. Moertel et al. in 1970 published figures which suggest that the rate of occurrence of cancer in the retained rectum in those patients may approach 50 to 60 percent 20 to 25 years following initial colon resection.[23] A new recommended approach is the removal of the rectal mucosa with ileal anal anastomosis and pull-through, preserving the lower rectal musculature and rectal sphincter.[24] The long-term feasibility of this approach is satisfactory to date.[25]

Ulcerative colitis is associated with a somewhat lower, but still significant, incidence of colorectal cancer.[26,27] In these individuals, over time, cancer occurs 5 to 10 times more frequently than in the general population. When chronic ulcerative colitis is present for over 10 years, the incidence of cancer approaches 15 to 30. When ulcerative colitis begins before the age of 25, the risk is still higher.[28] Carcinoma developing in patients with ulcerative colitis is often multifocal and may be more malignant, although this is difficult to establish stage by stage.

encountered between 40 and 60 years of age and improves a little for older patients. However, it should not be forgotten that this disease can occur before 50 years of age.[29,30]

Successful diagnosis of asymptomatic patients is followed by improved survival rates,[31] but screening is difficult. The preponderance of evidence does not indicate in the authors' opinion an established screen for use in the general population. Many physicians believe hemoccult testing is useful as a screen for colorectal cancer.[32,33] The test involves the collection of two small samples of stool on a specially prepared sealable paper slide for 3 consecutive days.[34] It has been established that a meat-free diet and avoidance of vitamins and drugs which irritate the GI tract while the test is in progress, as well as prompt testing of the slides, improves efficiency.

Greegor in 1971 reported favorably on the use of this type of assay as a screen.[35] In his test population 95 percent of individuals tested as negative. Of the 5 percent who were positive, one in five, or 1 percent, of the overall population were diagnosed as having cancer of the colon and rectum. About 3 percent were found either to have no pathology or reported as having diverticulosis. This is fine in a population where 1 percent of those tested eventually are found to have colorectal cancer, but, as well described by Henderson,

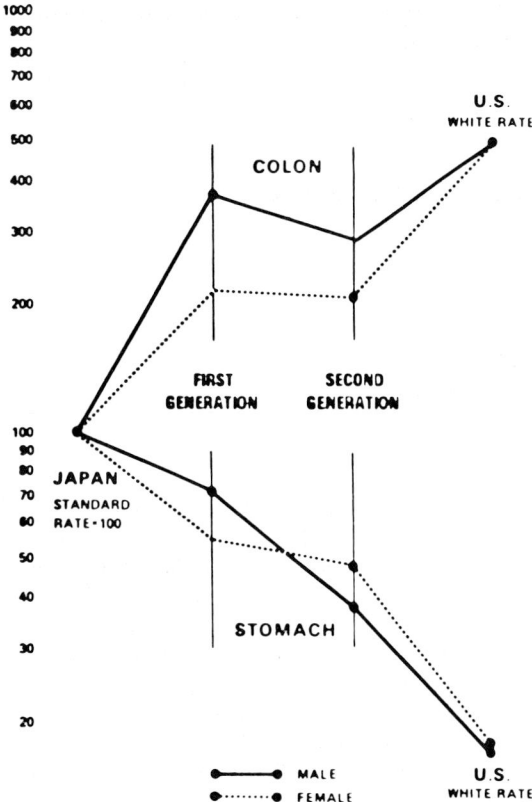

FIGURE 28-2 Mortality rates for colon cancer among Japanese families after immigration to the United States. Clearly with time the incidence of both colon and gastric cancer in this population adjusts to that of indigenous rates in the new country. (*From WM Haenszel et al: J Natl Cancer Inst 40:43, 1968.*)

Signs, Symptoms, and Attempts at Early Diagnosis

Early diagnosis is productive. Survival rates for patients designated as having localized tumors are about twice that of patients having regional spread of both colon and rectal cancer, as described by Burdette in 1973. In 1976, Cutler pointed out that patient age is a factor in any diagnosis of colorectal cancer. Approximately 30 percent of younger patients first staged for colon or rectal cancer have localized tumor at diagnosis. This figure improves to more than 50 percent for patients

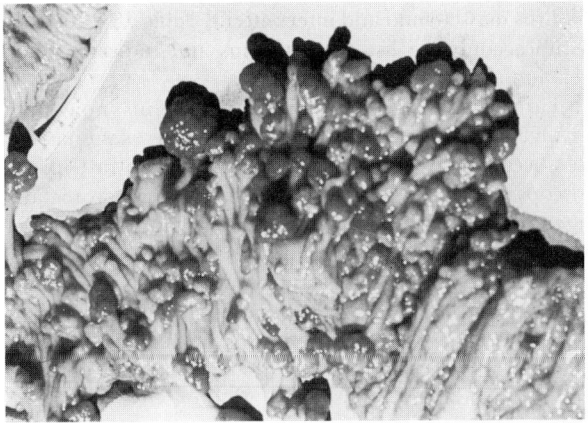

FIGURE 28-3 This colon indicates the profusion of polyps which develop in familial polyposis victims. Left for 10 years, close to 100 percent of these individuals will develop cancer.

low prevalance makes screening of the population at large difficult even with a very low incidence of false positivity.[36] If 100,000 individuals are screened with a false-positive rate of 2 percent, 2000 will have a positive hemocult test. Somewhat less than 20 or 30 individuals will have cancer even in a somewhat restricted population, and this means approximately 99 of 100 individuals would undergo further study to detect possible malignancy where none was to be found. This is the limitation to this approach. The usual solution suggested is to screen only high-risk groups. This is, in fact, not so significant as it may sound, since high-risk groups often consist of very small, specialized subgroups among the total population at risk.

As has been indicated, high-risk groups include those with familial polyposis or ulcerative colitis. Most screening efforts have been confined to patients over the age of 40 years because the incidence of disease increases with age.[37] The largest significant group of patients at risk are those who have previously undergone resection, since for them it has been found that the risk of metachronous cancer is 0.5 to 1.0 percent per annum.

Symptoms of colorectal cancer unfortunately may be very insidious early in the disease. Vague lower abdominal crampy pain, mild diarrhea, weakness, evidence of obstruction, eventually more advanced evidence of obstruction with more severe pain, constipation, and perhaps vomiting may occur.[38] Rectal pain may occur with defecation. One important point is that the crampy abdominal pain need not be progressive and for some months may be mild and intermittent. Table 28-2 records a more complete list of symptoms and indicates their relation to tumor location.[39]

Early diagnosis of symptomatic patients now may involve physical examination with rectal examination, hemocult assay, barium enema with air contrast, proctoscopy or flexible sigmoidoscopy, carcinoembryonic antigen (CEA) assay, and possibly colonoscopy. It is important that the investigation of these patients follow an orderly format that has been found useful in the particular practitioners' milieu. Figure 28-4 suggests such a schema. Properly employed means of diagnosis should enable the detection of better than 95 percent of colorectal cancers.

Diagnostic Techniques, Work-Up, and Staging

For complete work-up prior to surgery colonoscopy is recommended. This will allow precise definition of the size and extent of a tumor when the bowel is not obstructed and will also allow a careful search of the entire colon for other lesions. One should also obtain a chest x-ray and intravenous pyelogram (IVP) prior to surgery, looking for metastatic disease and, with the latter, particularly for low-lying lesions, to anticipate any possible ureteral involvement.

Today, prognosis and staging are becoming increasingly important as combined modalities of therapy, with their attendant risks and complications, are considered in order to improve chances for survival. Several general statements can be made. In most reports, tumors of the rectum and splenic flexure have a poorer prognosis than other colon tumors, with tumors of the left colon in turn having a poorer prognosis than those of the right colon.[40,41] This applies in the absence of obstruction or perforation.[42] It is interesting that, although there is some correlation, size is not necessarily related to the presence of lymph nodes. Also, invasion of adjacent organs by colorectal cancer or of soft tissue does not necessarily imply a poor prognosis. In spite of many efforts to determine prognosis through estimate of clinical size, circumference, etc. for clinical staging, the most important method of estimating prognosis is the histologic examination of the resected specimen.

According to Dukes's staging system, as shown in Fig. 28-5, staging is based on depth of penetration of the resected specimen. By 1954, Astler and Coller refined Dukes's classification (see Table 28-3).[43] This allowed the identification of five subgroups of patients with colorectal cancer with a variation in prognosis for survival from 22 to 100 percent. Other parameters to be considered are

TABLE 28-2 Symptoms of Colorectal Cancer: Right and Left Malignant Lesions

	Right	Left
Occult blood in stools	+	−
Anemia	+	−
Gallbladder disease–like symptoms	+	−
"Sentinel polyps"	+	−
Bright blood on stools	−	+
Obstructive signs	−	+
"Sentinel hemorrhoids"	−	+
Small caliber of stools	−	+

SOURCE: Sabistan.[39]

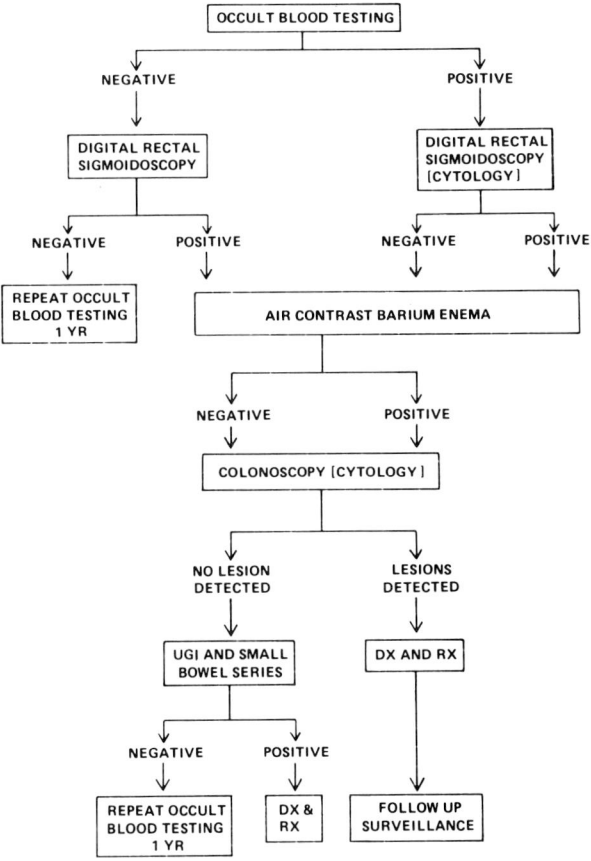

FIGURE 28-4 It is important that the practitioner develop an orderly method of screening and diagnosis. It will vary depending on changing evaluation of, for example, colonoscopy versus air contrast barium enema, but it should be rational and orderly.

lymph node location (for example, whether the node lies near to the lesion or to the root of the mesentery), venous invasion, tumor grade, exophytic or invasive growth, so-called pushing margin or invasive margin, and inflammatory infiltrate.[44,45] Table 28-4 presents the TNM system suggested by the American Joint Committee on Cancer, which illustrates another approach to staging. At present in the United States most clinicians use the Astler-Coller system, but it is probably desirable when reporting results to use the TNM system as well for comparison.

Therapeutic Options for Primary Therapy

Accurate bowel resection for carcinoma of the colon or rectum mandates complete excision of the tumor with adequate free margins of normal tissue and en bloc resection of the vascular and lymphatic structures that supply and drain the involved bowel. The anatomic limits of bowel, lymph node, and soft-tissue removal are well diagramed in Enker's text on colon cancer.[46] For

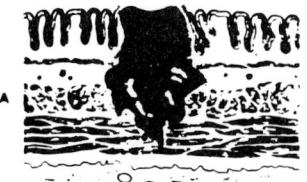

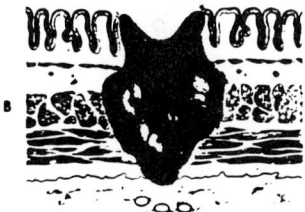

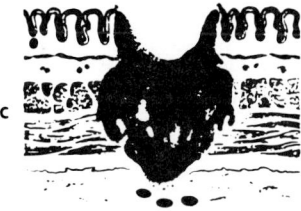

FIGURE 28-5 Dukes related this classification to depth of tumor penetration, whether partly or completely through the bowel wall. He also noted the presence of nodes. (*a*) Invasion of muscularis propria; (*b*) invasion to serosa; (*c*) invasion through serosa with involvement of regional lymph nodes. (*From JA del Regato, HJ Spjut, Cancer, Mosby, St Louis, 1977, p 540.*)

TABLE 28-3 Classification of Colorectal Cancer

Class	Extent	5-year survival rate, %
A	Lesions limited to mucosa	100.0
B_1	To muscularis propria Negative nodes	66.4
B_2	Penetrating muscularis Proptid with negative nodes	53.9
C_1	Limited to wall with positive nodes	42.8
C_2	Through the wall with positive nodes	22.4

SOURCE: Astler and Coller.[43]

resection of the rectum a knowledge of the vessels serving the rectum and the anatomy of the levator muscles is necessary. For low-lying rectal lesions the authors recommend removal of the ovaries for staging, as well as removal of uterus,[47] vaginal fornix, and posterior wall. At present we have no 5-year survivors who have demonstrated ovarian involvement. However, the recurrence rate in a series of over 100 patients with well-advanced tumors locally who have undergone abdominal perineal resection, as the procedure is performed at Roswell Park Memorial Institute, is less than 5 percent.[48]

For preoperative preparations the patient is put on

TABLE 28-4 American Joint Committee Trial Staging*

T
- T_0 No tumor
- T_1 Mucosa or submucosa
- T_2 Muscular wall or serosa
- T_3 All layers and extension
- T_4 With fistula
- T_5 Other organs
- T_x Unknown

N
- N_0 Negative nodes
- N_1 Positive nodes
- N_x Unknown

M
- M_0 No metastases
- M_1 Metastases

* This is a clinical assessment: A pTNM pathological assessment is made after surgery.

a 3-day regimen of a low-residue to liquid diet, magnesium sulfate cathartics, enemas, intravenous supplement, and a short-term neomycin and erythromycin preparation of the bowel. Betadine shower is given the evening of surgery.[49]

In determining the precise extent of surgery to be performed intramural spread is considered, aiming for at least 5 cm of bowel proximal and distal to the lesion free of tumor. Also considered are lymphatic spread, venous spread, direct extension, transperineal spread, and the possibility of implantation during surgery.

In the last few years the use of the EEA stapler has allowed a gradual increase in the number of patients spared abdominal-perineal resection, and there is a nationwide trend in this direction. In the authors' opinion a resection can be performed satisfactorily for tumors whose lower edges reach to 6 to 7 cm above the anal verge. The incidence of complications is probably less than previously encountered.[50] The deciding factor, however, is still meticulous anatomic surgery.

There are reported instances of cure of inoperable lesions by radiation therapy, but these are so few as to make this an unexpected event.[51] Papillon has described an intrarectal radiation technique which has now been widely applied and has proved useful for smaller lesions that are movable and of favorable configuration in the rectum.[52,52]

Adjuvant Therapies

The rationale for chemotherapy and radiation therapy as adjuvant therapy to surgery lies in the fact that both are more effective against small amounts of tumor. Chemotherapy kills a constant percentage of cells present; radiation therapy is effective possibly because privileged hypoxic areas and sheltered nests of cells are removed with bulk excision.[54,55] Adjuvant therapy for colon cancer is not, however, a substitute for good surgical resection; it is not a treatment regimen without risk; it is not yet the proven standard practice for colorectal cancer; and it is not a substitute for careful follow-up of patients operated on for colon cancer. Chemotherapy or radiation therapy may result in toxicity that causes severe vomiting or bone marrow suppression that may be life-threatening, and there are delayed effects of radiation on the small bowel which may be of a serious nature.[56,57] It is also theoretically possible that such treatment may result in selection of a resistant tumor cell population through a premature exposure to a low dose of selected chemotherapeutic agents or a significant impairment of host resistance which in some instances might have an adverse effect.

A number of studies have tested 5-fluorouracil (5-FU) and FUdR as adjuvants following potentially curative colorectal surgery.[58,59] Higgins and the Veterans Hospital Study Group reported several studies, not one of which indicated a marked effect of 5-FU.[60] However, in reviewing all of the cumulative veterans studies Higgins et al. have proposed that they indicate a trend. Although no study was statistically significant alone, when considered as a total they indicated that 5-FU has an effect on survival rates.[61] This suggestion is open to criticism, however. Since not all patients in these groups were clearly resected for cure, they constitute a somewhat different group from those ordinarily designated for adjuvant therapy. Other studies by Lawrence and Grage et al. for the Central Oncology Group have failed to show a clear-cut effect. Studies such as that reported by Kim et al. suggest that 5-FU is effective, but this type of nonrandomized review probably should not be definitive since the sample population is too small.[62]

Following reports from the Eastern Cooperative Oncology Group concerning an enhanced effect of methyl-CCNU and 5-FU over 5-FU alone in the treatment of gastric cancer, the Gastrointestinal Tumor Study Group (GITSG) prepared two protocols which were begun in 1975. The first was adjuvant treatment of colon carcinoma.[63] There were four treatment groups. One group received surgery alone. The second group received methanol-extracted tubercle bacilli residue (MER) following surgery, the third group 5-FU in 5-day cycles at 5-week intervals with MeCCNU in 10-week cycles, and the fourth group chemotherapy and immunotherapy.

As of August 1981, no clear-cut effect of any of the adjuvant treatments in this protocol was apparent; however, patients in this study are still being followed.

The work of Taylor and Brooman in Liverpool kindled a considerable interest in local hepatic treatment as a means of developing an adjuvant approach based on the prophylactic treatment of the liver as a prime organ for the appearance of metastases in patients with colon cancer.[64] The last published reports indicate that 7 days of portal vein infusion with 500 mg/m^2 per day of 5-FU has resulted in a reduction in the later appearance of metastases.[65] The GITSG has a current study of radiation therapy to the liver in patients with class B_2 and C colon cancer. Two thousand rads as well as two cycles of chemotherapy against a surgery-alone group is being tested. The study is ongoing and no results are available as yet.

For rectal cancer the treatment picture may be changing. In 1975 the GITSG began its study of the adjuvant treatment of rectal cancer with chemotherapy and radiation therapy. A number of studies have suggested a possible effect of preoperative radiotherapy for rectal cancer.[66,67] The GITSG felt that a study with four treatment arms was in order. The study began with a surgery-only treatment arm, a chemotherapy group, a radiotherapy group, and finally a combined chemotherapy and radiation therapy arm. The chemotherapy was 5-FU and MeCCNU, and because, in part, of the previous difficulties of gaining acceptance of a presurgical radiation therapy program, the radiation therapy was given following definitive surgery. Figure 28-6 shows the basic schema for this study. Radiation therapy was 4000 or 4800 rads in about 5 weeks with 5 days a week of therapy. Chemotherapy consisted of 130 mg/m^2 MeCCNU PO on day 1 of a 5-day course, with 325 mg/m^2 5-FU IV on days 1 to 5; alternating with 375 mg/m^2 5-FU alone IV on days 1 to 5 every other cycle.

All three treatment groups are somewhat better than the surgery-only group, with the combination group possibly better than the other two adjuvant programs. The relationship has continued to the present (August 1981). There is a definite effect on disease-free survival rates, but final data must await the passage of more time.

The GITSG has begun a new study attempting to determine whether chemotherapy can be reduced to 6 months' duration and still be effective. This would be of great benefit in reducing the toxicity which occurs from 18 months of the MeCCNU–5-FU treatment and should be much better tolerated than the previous regimen. At

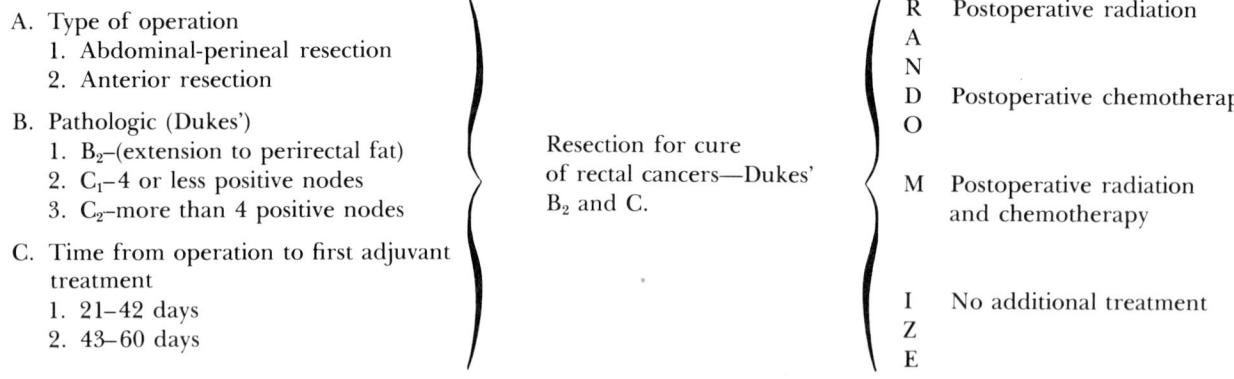

FIGURE 28-6 The basic schema for the four-arm Gastrointestinal Tumor Study Group rectal adjuvant treatment program with surgery, surgery and chemotherapy, surgery and postsurgical radiation therapy, and surgery followed by both chemotherapy and radiation treatment.

present, however, there is considerable indication from prospective randomized studies that adjuvant therapy improves results in the treatment of rectal cancer.

Follow-Up and Techniques for Early Identification of Recurrence and Metastases

A vigorous follow-up program can result in survivors. In the case of early detection of recurrence 10 to 40 percent of instances may provide an opportunity for "curative" retreatment. The schedule of follow-up should be based on anticipated progression according to site, stage, and therapy of the primary tumor.

The basic instrument for follow-up remains the periodic careful history and physical examination. A complaint of weight loss and aching perineal pain or discomfort aggravated by sitting, low abdominal, pelvic, or back pain may represent recurrence and needs careful evaluation. The physical examination includes the original area of tumor occurrence, any incisions, anastomotic suture lines, and the liver, which is a very likely site for recurrence. Any abdominal masses or fullness should be sought. In addition to the periodic history and physical examination, follow-up at Roswell Park Memorial Institute is based on annual colonoscopy. This examination should be repeated yearly for several years, although it may be possible to reduce the frequency to every 2 years after some time. This recommendation is based on a study of 304 colonoscopies in 240 patients performed between 1975 and 1979. Of these colonoscopies per-

formed for postoperative surveillance, 236, or 78 percent, were negative, while in 68 (22 percent) there was some significant finding. The lesions in this group of patients included 11 metachronous cancers, 17 recurrent malignancies, 43 tubular adenomas, and 9 villous adenomas. It is interesting that the median time to recurrence of cancer was 20 months, and the median time to occurrence of metachronous cancer was 40 months. Table 28-5 indicates the relative number of patients with each condition diagnosed using the colonoscope who were symptomatic vs. those who remained asymptomatic. In this series of over 300 colonoscopies only four complications of note were encountered: three instances of mild bleeding not requiring transfusion and one coagulation syndrome.[68] Subsequently, one perforation in 600 procedures has been encountered.

Although the numbers in these series are small, barium enema never identified a lesion not seen on colonoscopy if the latter was carried to completion. Furthermore, about half of the metachronous tumors, 20 percent of the recurrent tumors, and half of the adenomatous polyps were not seen on barium enema even when the films were rereviewed.

Of the 17 recurrent tumors identified, 6 were able to be resected, but it is too early to ascertain what can be accomplished with this approach. At any rate if colonoscopy is economically feasible, it is recommended that follow-up be based on this examination; if it is not feasible, an air-contrast barium enema should be performed yearly for at least 5 years.

TABLE 28-5 Postoperative Surveillance of Colorectal Neoplasms

Pathology	Symptoms	Asymptomatic
Metachronous cancer	4	7
Recurrent cancer	11	6
Tubular adenomas	5	37
Villous adenomas	3	6

In addition to the use of annual colonoscopy, assay for serum carcinoembryonic antigen (CEA) is recommended. This should be performed preoperatively, at 1 month to 6 weeks following surgery, and preferably monthly, or bimonthly if it is necessary to limit cost, between 5 and 24 months in patients in whom there is a reasonably high expectation of recurrence. A quarterly assay for 2 additional years may be of benefit. There is a period of CEA elevation postoperatively caused by the trauma of surgery per se and also by slow clearance of the CEAs which were more highly elevated prior to surgery. For this reason patients who show an elevated value of more than 4 to 5 ng/mL should have their postoperative base line done later rather than earlier.

There is a lag time following CEA elevation before other clinically detectable manifestations of tumor become apparent. This is significant in about a third of the patients being monitored and may be 5 months or more. This is the group that hopefully will be helped by repetitive CEA assay. Table 28-6 summarizes a number of studies of CEA in follow-up, and the predominance of evidence is that CEA is useful in this setting.[69-78] In addition, the preoperative CEA may assist in determining which patients should be followed using the CEA assay, at least for B lesions, since B lesions with an elevated CEA are at a significant risk of recurrence, while those whose initial CEA is normal have such a low expectation of recurrence that the cost of such an elaborate follow-up is probably not justified.

The next section examines the evidence which suggests that recurrent and metastatic colorectal cancer can be successfully treated by the recommended approach in a significant percentage of patients.

Therapeutic Options for the Treatment of Recurrence and/or Metastases

Can recurrent colorectal cancer be successfully treated? Will earlier detection of recurrence by careful follow-up make even more successful treatment possible? These questions need answering. The authors recently reviewed 91 patients who developed recurrence between January 1968 and December 1978. During the last few years of the study colonoscopy and CEA surveillance of postsurgical patients have been maintained. It has been known for some years that single hepatic metastases can be successfully treated in patients with colorectal cancer. But the surgical approach now has been extended, and definitive surgery with removal of all gross tumor wherever reasonably possible is being attempted, for example, in the face of two, three, or four smaller hepatic metastases. The only exception to this today is based on the finding that a surgical approach to cerebral metastases undertaken even for single cerebral metastases has not improved patients' survival chances enough to justify such surgery.[48] Table 28-7 shows the results following surgery for a series of patients with anastomotic, intra-abdominal, and hepatic recurrence and metastases. These patients are divided into three groups: those with

TABLE 28-6 Recent Studies of CEA and Recurrence

Tumor site	Follow-up	Author	Date	Result
Colorectal	Follow-up	Sugarbaker et al.[69]	1976	+
Gastrointestinal	Follow-up	Martin et al.[70]	1977	+
Gastrointestinal	Follow-up	Koch et al.[71]	1977	+
Lung	Follow-up	Gropp et al.[72]	1977	+
Colorectal	At recurrence	Moertel et al.[73]	1978	−
Colon	Follow-up	Minton et al.[74]	1978	+
Breast	Follow-up	Wahren et al.[75]	1978	+
Gastrointestinal	Follow-up	Cooper et al.[76]	1979	+
Colon	Follow-up	Martin et al.[77]	1979	+
Colorectal	Follow-up	Cohen et al.[78]	1979	+

TABLE 28-7 Median Survival Time and Estimated 5-year Survival Rate

	Anastomotic recurrence			Intraabdominal recurrence			Distant metastasis		
	Number of patients	Median survival, months	5-Year survival rate, %	Number of patients	Median survival, months	5-Year survival rate, %	Number of patients	Median survival, months	5-Year survival rate, %
Complete resection	15	59.3	49	12	41.64	34	14	46.25	Not reached yet
Minimal residual tumor	10	17.5	12	20	21.26				
Gross residual tumor	5	8.0		15	13				

complete resection, those with only minimal disease remaining at the time of surgery or disease at the margins of resection, and those in whom gross tumor is apparent after surgery.

Recurrence is divided by location into anastomotic, intraabdominal, or hepatic metastases. All patients in the last several years of this period received chemotherapy with a variety of agents following the surgery. It is apparent even with the low numbers of patients in these studies that there is very little surgical benefit when grossly apparent disease is left behind. There is no long-term survival with minimal-residue disease either, but median survival time approaches 1½ to 2 years, a fact which must be considered in deciding whether or not to attempt a surgical approach as part of a combined-modality treatment program. In contrast, where disease is amenable to technical removal—even with one, two, or three small liver metastases, for example—a 50 percent survival rate at 5 years is possible. It is because of these findings that surgery is recommended as part of a combined-modality approach to recurrent or metastatic colorectal cancer whenever a complete resection seems feasible. A great deal more work needs to be done in this area to determine parameters which delineate who should be operated upon and what results can be anticipated, but the possibility of success is present for some patients subjected to reoperation for recurrence and "second adjuvant" therapy.

Current Areas for Research and Proposals for the Future

Rather than any remarkable breakthrough in the next several years progress will probably come from the thoughtful application and organization of the technology already available. In the area of diagnosis public concern and the use of the hemoccult test and the techniques of colonoscopy in selected patients should help to detect the disease earlier, when surgery allows a high rate of cure, reducing the present 20- to 30-week delay encountered following initial symptoms.

With the use of the stapler a shift in surgery is anticipated, which means that fewer abdominal perineal resections, with attendant emotional trauma, will be required. With improved knowledge of the natural history and precise staging, it should be easier to identify more precisely those patients who are at risk and who are proper candidates for adjuvant therapy and close postsurgical monitoring. While the use of chemotherapy as an adjuvant remains to be established as effective for colon cancer, radiation therapy and chemotherapy appear to improve survival rates for rectal cancer. Hoped for are improvements that will allow physicians to minimize the side effects of this therapy and determine optimal schedules of therapy.

Following patients at risk with CEA assay and colonoscopy may allow identification of recurrent disease earlier than previously. The use of aggressive surgery in recurrent disease where resection is feasible combined with chemotherapy may allow additional survival time. Hopefully the proper application of all these methodologies will improve the cure rate. The key seems to be combined-modality treatment and careful organization of the care of these patients.

Reconstruction and Rehabilitation

Rehabilitation for colorectal cancer patients should include education of those at risk to participate in follow-up care. Otherwise, rehabilitation lies in the care of patients who have had an abdominal perineal resection. Bladder problems may require teaching the patient how to empty urine fully, and these problems may need attention postsurgically. Modern colostomy apparatus is much improved and expert instruction is now widely available from professional enterostomy therapists, who can help with dietary and housekeeping tips, skin care, irrigation, etc. Sexual counseling and psychiatric support may also be helpful. This disability is consistent with a full, productive life when appropriate support is given.

REFERENCES

1. Enker WE et al: Enhanced survival of patients with colon and rectal cancer is based on wide anatomic resection. *Ann Surg* 190:350–360, 1979.
2. Corman ML et al: Colorectal carcinoma: A decade of experience at the Lahey Clinic. *Dis Colon Rectum* 22:477–479, 1979.
3. Miles WE: A method of performing abdominal-perineal excision for carcinoma of the rectum and of the terminal portion of the pelvic colon. *Lancet* 2:1812, 1908.
4. Dukes CE, Bussey HJR: The spread of rectal cancer and its effect on prognosis. *Br J Cancer* 12:309–320, 1958.
5. Gold P, Freedman SO: Demonstration of tumor specific antigens in human colonic carcinomas by immunological tolerance and absorption techniques. *J Exp Med* 121:139–162, 1965.
6. Androsor PL: Experience in the application of the instrumental mechanical suture in surgery of the stomach and rectum. *ACTA Chir Scand* 136:57–63, 1970.
7. Overholt BF: Colonoscopy—A review. *Gastroenterology* 68:1308–1320, 1975.
8. Mittelman A, Gastrointestinal Tumor Study Group: Adjuvant chemotherapy and radiotherapy following rectal surgery: An interim report from the Gastrointestinal Tumor Study Group (GITSG), in SE Salmon, SE Jones (eds): *Adjuvant Therapy of Cancer*, vol. 3, Grune & Stratton, New York, 1981.
9. Evans JT et al: Management and survival of carcinoma of the colon: Results of a national survey by the American College of Surgeons. *Ann Surg* 188:716–720, 1978.
10. Phil E et al: Carcinoma of the rectum and rectosigmoid: Cancer special long-term survival: A series of 1061 cases treated by one surgeon. *Ann Surg* 192:114–117, 1980.
11. Miller DR, Albbitten FF Jr: Carcinoma of the colon and rectum: A review of results of surgical treatment in 164 patients. *Arch Surg* 111:692–696, 1976.
12. Alarcon J, Greenwood GR: Adenocarcinoma of the colon and rectum: A review of surgical treatment in 302 patients. *Dis Colon Rectum* 22:35–39, 1979.
13. American Cancer Society: *1981 Facts and Figures*.
14. Segi M, Kurlhara M: *Cancer Mortality for Selected Sites in 24 Countries*, no 6 (1966–1967), Japan Cancer Society, Tokyo, 1972, p 137.
15. Haenzel WM, Kurihara M: Studies of Japanese migrants, I: Mortality from cancer and other diseases among Japanese in the United States. *J Nat Cancer Inst* 40:43–68, 1968.
16. Smith WG: The cancer family syndrome and heritable solitary colonic polyps. *Dis Colon Rectum* 13:362–367, 1970.
17. Bussey, HJR: *Familial Polyposis Coli*, Johns Hopkins Press, Baltimore, 1975.
18. McKusick VA: Genetics and large bowel cancer. *Dig Dis* 19:954–958, 1974.
19. Muto T et al: The evolution of cancer of the colon and rectum. *Cancer* 36:2251–2270, 1975.
20. Morson BC, Abell MR: Polyps and cancer of the large bowel, in JH Yardley (ed): *The Gastrointestinal Tract*, Int Acad Path Mon, Williams & Wilkins, Baltimore, 1900, pp 101–108.
21. Gardner E, Richards R: Multiple cutaneous and subcutaneous lesions occurring simultaneously with hereditary polyps and osteomatosis. *Am J Hum Genet* 5:139–148, 1953.
22. Nava HR: Roswell Park data (unpublished).
23. Moertel CG et al: Surgical management of multiple polyposis: The problem of cancer in the retained bowel segment. *Arch Surg* 100:521–526, 1970.
24. Katz J: An operation for multiple polyposis with preservation of rectal function. *Intern Surg* 51:202–209, 1969.
25. Heimann T, Greenstein AJ: Familial polyposis coli: Management by total colectomy with preservation of continence. *Arch Surg* 113:1104–1105, 1978.
26. Bargen JA: Chronic ulcerative colitis associated with malignant disease. *Arch Surg* 17:561–576, 1928.
27. Brooke BN: Ulcerative colitis and carcinoma of the colon. *J R Coll Surg Edin* 14:274, 1969.
28. Hughes RG et al: The prognosis of carcinoma of the colon and rectum complicating ulcerative colitis. *Surg Gynecol Obstet* 146:46–48, 1978.
29. Recalde M et al: Carcinoma of the colon and rectum and anal canal in young patients. *Surg Gynecol Obstet* 179:902–913, 1974.
30. Simstein NL et al: Colorectal carcinoma in patients less than 40-years-old. *Dis Colon Rectum* 21:169–171, 1978.
31. Hertz BE et al: Value of periodic examinations in detecting cancer of the rectum and colon. *Postgrad Med J* 27:290–294, 1960.
32. Gilbertsen VA et al: The earlier detection of colorectal cancers: A preliminary report of the results of the occult blood study. *Cancer* 45:2899–2901, 1980.
33. Winawer SJ et al: Progress report on controlled trial of fecal occult blood testing for the detection of colorectal neoplasia. *Cancer* 45:2954–2964, 1980.
34. Bralow SP, Kopel J: Hemoccult screening for colorectal cancer: Impact study on Sarasota, FL. *T Fl Med Assoc* 66:915–919, 1979.

35. Greegor DH: Diagnosis of large bowel cancer in the asymptomatic patient. *JAMA* 201:943–945, 1967.
36. Henderson, M: Validity of screening. *Cancer* 37:573–581, 1976.
37. Falterman KW et al: Cancer of the colon, rectum and anus: A Review of 2313 Cases. *Cancer* 34:951–959, 1974.
38. Holliday HW, Hardcastle JD: Delay in diagnosis and treatment of symptomatic colorectal cancer. *Lancet* 1(8111)309–311, 1979.
39. Cohn I Jr, Nance FC: Intermediate or precancerous lesions and malignant lesions, in D Sabiston (ed): *Davis-Christopher Textbook of Surgery,* 11th ed, Saunders, Philadelphia, 1977, pp 1100–1109.
40. Buckwalter JA, Kent TH: Prognosis and surgical pathology of carcinoma of the colon. *Surg Gynecol Obstet* 136:465–472, 1973.
41. Silverberg G, Holleb AI: Major trends in cancer: 25-year survey. *CA* 25:2–7, 1975.
42. Gennaro AR: Obstructive colonic cancer. *Dis Colon Rectum* 21:346–351, 1978.
43. Astler VA, Coller FA: The prognostic significance of direct extension of carcinoma of the colon and rectum. *Ann Surg* 136:846–852, 1954.
44. Dukes CE, Bussey HJR: The spread of rectal cancer and its effect on prognosis. *Br J Cancer* 12:309–320, 1958.
45. DeMascarel A et al: The prognostic significance of specific histologic features of carcinoma of the colon and rectum. *Surg Gynecol Obstet* 153:511–514, 1981.
46. Enker WE: *Carcinoma of the Colon and Rectum,* Year Book, Chicago, 1979.
47. Knopp LF et al: Ovarian metastasis from colorectal cancer. *Dis Colon Rectum* 16:305–311, 1973.
48. Mittelman A: Roswell Park data (unpublished).
49. Herter FP: Preparation of the bowel for surgery: Symposium on diseases of the colon and rectum. *Surg Clin North Am* 52:859–870, 1972.
50. Laitnen S et al: Experience with the EEA stapling instrument for colorectal anastomosis. *Ann Chir Gynecol* 69:102–105, 1980.
51. Williams IG, Horwitz H: The primary treatment of adenocarcinoma of the rectum by high voltage roentgen rays (1,000 KV). *Am J Roentgenol Radium Ther Nucl Med* 76:919–928, 1956.
52. Papillon J: Endocavity irradiation of early rectal cancers for cure: A series of 123 cases. *Proc R Soc Med* 66:1179–1181, 1973.
53. Papillon J: Intracavity irradiation of early rectal cancer for cure. *Cancer* 36:696–701, 1975.
54. Griswold DP, Corbett TH: A colon tumor model for anticancer agent evaluation. *Cancer* 36:2441–2444, 1975.
55. Steel GG, Peckham MJ: Exploitable mechanisms in combined radiotherapy-chemotherapy: The concept of additivity. *Int J Rad Oncol Biol Phys* 5:85–91, 1979.
56. Davis S, Park YK: Chemotherapy for colorectal cancer with a combination of 5-fluorouracil, mitomycin C, Adriamycin, and cytosine arabinoside: A pilot study. *Cancer Treat Rep* 62:1557–1559, 1978.
57. Knowlton AH: The role of radiation therapy in large bowel cancer. *Curr Concepts Oncol* 3:8–16, 1981.
58. Grage T et al: Adjuvant therapy with 5-FU after resection of colo-rectal cancer. *Proc Am Assoc Clin Oncol* 16:258, 1975.
59. Dwight RW et al: FUdR as an adjuvant to surgery in cancer of the large bowel. *J Surg Oncol* 5:243–249, 1973.
60. Higgins GA et al: Adjuvant chemotherapy in the surgical treatment of large bowel cancer. *Cancer* 38:1461–1467, 1976.
61. Higgins GA et al: The case for adjuvant 5-fluorouracil in colorectal cancer. *Cancer Clin Trials* 1:35–41, 1978.
62. Kim RH et al: Chemoprophylaxis for patients with five year follow-up. *Proc Am Soc Clin Oncol* 16:231, 1975.
63. Holyoke ED et al: Adjuvant therapy and immune therapy following colon surgery: An interim report from the Gastrointestinal Tumor Study Group (GITSG), in SE Salmon, SE Jones (eds): *Adjuvant Therapy of Cancer,* vol 3, Grune & Stratton, New York, 1981.
64. Taylor I, Brooman P: Adjuvant liver perfusion of 5-fluorouracil in the treatment of the colorectal cancer: Initial results of a controlled clinical trial. *Br J Surg* 64:838, 1977.
65. Taylor I et al: Adjuvant cytotoxic liver perfusion for colorectal cancer. *Br J Surg* 66:833–837, 1979.
66. Arnott SJ: The MRC Trial of low dose preoperative radiotherapy in operable rectal cancer, in *Controversies in Cancer: Design of Trials and Treatment,* Proceedings of an EORTC Symposium, April 26–29, 1978, EORTC, Brussels, Belgium, 1978, pp 139–143.
67. Stearns M: Preoperative radiotherapy in rectal cancer, in *Controversies in Cancer: Design of Trials and Treatment,* Proceedings of EORTC Symposium, April 26–29, 1978, EORTC, Brussels, Belgium, 1978, pp 244.
68. Nava HR, Pagana TJ: Postoperative surveillence of colorectal cancer. (in press).
69. Sugarbaker PH et al: Assessment of serial carcinoembryonic antigen (CEA) assays in postoperative detection of recurrent colorectal cancer. *Cancer* 38:2310–2315, 1976.
70. Martin EW et al: A retrospective and prospective study of serial CEA determinations in the early detection of recurrent colon cancer. *Am J Surg* 137:167–171, 1979.
71. Koch MM et al: Carcinoembryonic antigen: 3 Years' experience in a cancer clinic. *Can Med Assoc* 116:769–771, 1977.
72. Gropp C et al: Carcinoembryonic antigen, alpha 1-fetoprotein, ferritin, and alpha 2-pregnancy associated glycoprotein in the serum of lung cancer patients and its demonstration in lung tumor tissues. *Oncology* 34:267–272, 1977.
73. Moertel CG et al: Carcinoembryonic antigen test for recurrent colorectal carcinoma inadequacy for early detection. *JAMA* 239:1065–1066, 1978.
74. Minton JP et al: The use of serial carcinoembryonic antigen

determinations to predict recurrence of carcinoma of the colon and the time for a second look operation. *Surg Gynecol Obstet* 146:208–211, 1978.
75. Waaren B et al: Carcinoembryonic antigen and other tumor markers in tissue and serum or plasma of patients with primary mammary carcinomas. *Cancer* 42:1870–1878, 1978.
76. Cooper MJ et al: A reappraisal of the value of carcinoembryonic antigen in the management of patients with various neoplasms. *Br J Surg* 66:120–123, 1979.
77. Martin EW Jr et al: The use of CEA as an early indicator in gastrointestinal tumor recurrence and second-look procedures. *Cancer* 39:440–446, 1977.
78. Cohen AM, Wood WC: Carcinoembryonic antigen levels as an indicator for reoperation in patients with carcinoma of the colon and rectum. *Surg Gynecol Obstet* 149:22–26, 1979.

SELECTED BIBLIOGRAPHY

Ledesma EJ et al: Surgical treatment of isolated abdominal wall metastasis in colorectal cancer. *Cancer* 50(9):1884–1887, 1982.

Shinya H et al: Colonoscopic diagnosis and management of rectal bleeding. *Surg Clin North Am* 62(5):897–903, 1982.

Sugarbaker PH: Partial sacrectomy for en bloc excision of rectal cancer with posterior fixation. *Dis Colon Rectum* 25(7): 708–711, 1982.

Watne AL: Syndromes of polyposis coli and cancer. *Curr Prob Cancer* vol 7, no 1, 1982.

Yanamoto RH: Techniques of resection in lesions of the colon-rectum. *Curr Prob Cancer* vol 6, no 1, 1982.

29

ADRENAL TUMORS

Glenn W. Geelhoed

THE ADRENAL GLANDS

There are two adrenal glands—not in the simple sense of left and right—but two totally different endocrine glands that coexist in the same space, the adrenal cortex and the adrenal medulla. The difference between these glands is embryologic (each being derived of different germ layers), biochemical (each has different enzyme systems and produces different species of hormones), and genetic (the adrenal medulla is chromaffin tissue with APUD* properties and may be linked to other APUD neoplasms in the same patient and in families, whereas the adrenal cortex and its neoplasms exhibit neither of these features). The reason for considering these very different tissues and their tumors together as "a gland" is their anatomic propinquity.

Common Structure and Different Functions

The shared anatomic location, and particularly one structure both glands have in common—the adrenal vein—is significant because it confers a common structural fate on these near neighbors despite their complete functional independence. Adrenalectomy removes both glands. Although independent in function, the two adrenal glands are interdependent in ablation.

For surgical purposes, the two halves of the adrenal gland are considered an *organ;* and ablation by operation or disease (e.g., Waterhouse-Friderichsen syndrome) requires treatment of the patient for the loss of the essential half—the adrenal cortex.

Tumors—that is, "mass lesions"—of the adrenal gland may arise in either the cortex or the medulla. A tumor in one site does not seem to affect the function in the other until the whole gland is ablated. As seen in Fig. 29-1, the adrenal cortex appears normal in size, and no abnormal adrenal cortical function could be inferred despite its displacement by a very large adrenal medullary tumor.

Ablation of both adrenals does not result in catecholamine deficiency, since these hormones are still produced from nerve endings and other ganglia in the sympathetic nervous system. But the adrenal cortex is the only source of adrenocortical steroids of the mineralocorticoid and glucocorticoid varieties (except under unusual circumstances in which they may be generated by the gonads—the only other mesodermally derived endocrine glands that synthesize steroid hormone), and both gluco- and mineralocorticoids are necessary for life. This means that "adrenal replacement" following total

---

* Amine precursor uptake and decarboxylation.

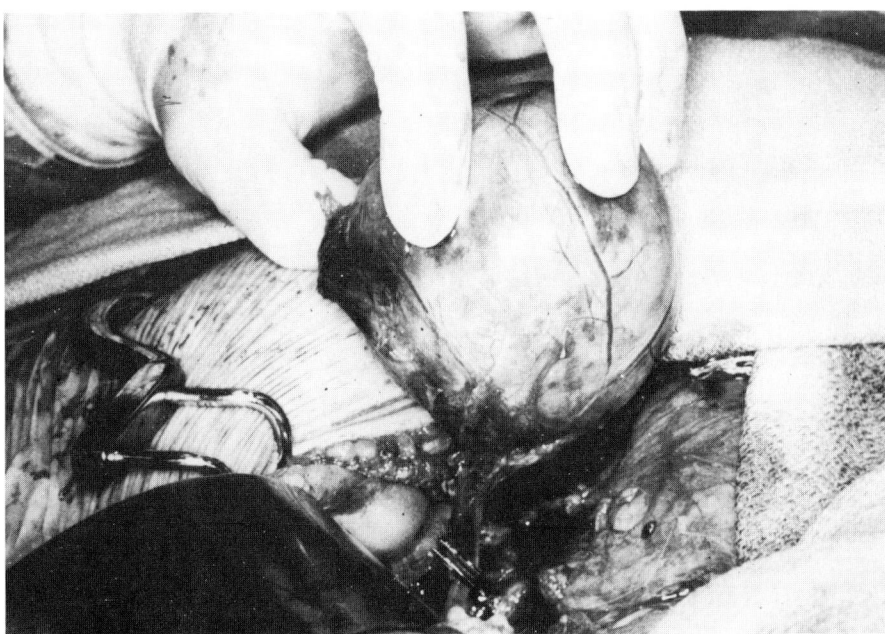

FIGURE 29-1 A large pheochromocytoma shows the special relationship of this adrenal medullary tumor to the minimally distorted adrenal cortex and the enlarged adrenal vein, the common venous drainage for both the normal adrenal cortex and the medullary neoplasm.

adrenalectomy is the replacement of these two types of essential steroids, the products of the cortical zona glomerulosa and zona fasciculata.

ADRENAL TUMORS

Morphology

Adrenal tumors of this common organ may be classified by a morphologic description of the mass lesion: hemorrhage, cyst, hyperplasia, adenoma, carcinoma, or nonadrenal tumor metastases.

Adrenal hemorrhage can occur as a result of trauma or inflammation, injuring cortex and medulla together because of their common arterial supply and single venous drainage. Blunt or penetrating trauma may cause adrenal hemorrhage. An invasive diagnostic maneuver—especially extravasation from adrenal venography (Fig. 29-2)—may be an iatrogenic trauma that ablates the adrenal glands. Meningiococcemia may cause hemorrhagic destruction of both adrenal glands in the Waterhouse-Friderichsen syndrome.

An adrenal cyst may constitute a congenital adrenal mass that can present as an adrenal tumor (Fig. 29-3).

Besides the diagnostic problem of confusion with other adrenal tumors, an adrenal cyst may rarely be a source of renovascular hypertension[1] or rupture in blunt trauma.[2]

The ratio of cortical to medullary tissue is 4:1 in a normal adrenal gland that weighs from 3 g (for the right gland) to 6 g for the left. Hyperplasia is a well-known finding in the adrenal cortex, and may in some instances precede or accompany benign neoplasia in "nodular hyperplasia," but there is no evidence that cortical hyperplasia is premalignant. It is a matter of debate whether adrenal medullary hyperplasia exists at all,[3] but if it does, it is probably limited to the remaining chromaffin tissue of patients who have had resection of familial pheochromocytoma.

Both adenomas and carcinomas can occur in the adrenal medulla or cortex. As in any endocrine neoplasm, microscopic examination may fail to distinguish benign from malignant tumors by histologic or cytologic criteria, and determination of malignancy may rely in some instances simply on the size of the primary tumor or gross or histologic evidence of invasion. A common malignant tumor of the adrenal glands may be metastasis from nonadrenal cancers, particularly carcinoma of the lung or breast, or bowel primary tumors.

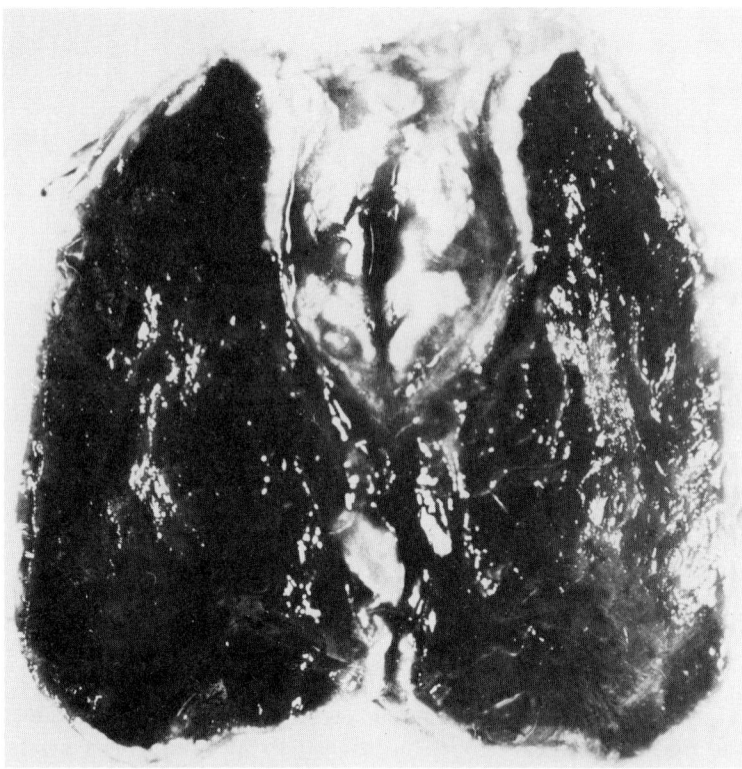

FIGURE 29-2 This adrenal mass is an adrenal hemorrhage that occurred following extravasation during adrenal venography.

Mass Effects

The suprarenal fossa is a very "silent" area of the body in which mass lesions may become very large in asymptomatic patients. Some nonfunctioning adrenal tumors may exceed "volleyball size" without causing symptoms in the patient who bears such a lesion (see Fig. 29-4). Most mass lesions in the body that simply occupy space depend on impingement on, erosion into, or obstruction of vital contiguous structures that may be impaired (such as the biliary tract, gastrointestinal tract, ureter, etc.) or superficial tumefaction that is palpable.

There are few vital, and no unpaired, structures for the expanding adrenal mass to interfere with in the suprarenal fossa. In its retroperitoneal location, the adrenal tumor gives little intraabdominal evidence of its presence, and its nearest neighbor, the kidney, is very mobile, showing no early disturbance in function when displaced. A mass in one-half of the adrenal gland does not even disturb the function in the other half of the same gland. Since a similar anatomic position is nearly the only relationship shared by cortex and medulla, function of one continues oblivious to the presence of the tumor in the other (as seen in Fig. 29-1), whereas great changes in form and function more closely follow changes in some remote area of the body such as the anterior pituitary.

Nonfunctioning mass lesions are more frequent and of greater variety in the adrenal cortex than the medulla.

Functional Effects

Adrenal tumors that are functional betray their presence early by the secretion of endocrine "markers"—mature hormones, their precursors, or their breakdown products. Without these hormones and their biologic effects—classified clinically as "syndromes" (Table 29-1)—small tumors, such as a 0.5-cm-diameter aldosterone-secreting adenoma as seen in Fig. 29-5, could never be clinically detectable by mass alone. Even when the presence of a tumor is suspected by the effects produced by its hormones, identification and localization of the primary lesion is difficult, even with exacting techniques. The endocrine excess leads the clinician from findings in distant target organs to infer a primary problem in an adrenal source.

Structure-Function Relationship

Tumors of the adrenal gland may or may not be functional; they may also gain or lose function. The size of the tumor does not always correlate with the severity of symptoms of endocrine hyperfunction. Some tumors dedifferentiate as they grow, losing the enzymatic capability of producing finished hormones, and sometimes they lose the ability to synthesize the precursors or any hormone at all.

Some adrenal tumors, particularly chromaffin neoplasms in children, mature from rapidly expanding malignant tumors to stable benign neoplasms with or without treatment. An example of such a fortunate transformation is seen in the occasional neuroblastoma that becomes sympathicogonioma to finally mature as a ganglioneuroma. This maturation may be reflected in endocrine secretions and the breakdown products to which they are degraded. At present, the presence of these markers gives a means of following these tumors at various stages of enzymatic activity which may reflect the neoplastic status of the tumor. For the future, this repression and maturation process suggests that the tumor cells still follow regulatory systems that might possibly be induced to modify the tumor's behavior.

For some adrenal tumors an inverse size-function correlation exists, simply because the smaller functional lesions are less likely to escape earlier detection on the basis of the endocrine evidence they produce. Nonfunctioning neoplasms must often await symptoms based on mass lesion effects for their earliest signs. Some large tumors that are nonfunctional, meaning they do not make finished-product hormones, may still produce humoral products of incomplete hormone synthesis or breakdown which may be detectable on screening for urinary metabolite excretions.

Diagnostic Techniques for Study

Diagnostic tests for adrenal tumors depend on the function and mass characteristics of the tumor. The work-up for adrenal tumors follows the classic pattern of screening symptomatic patients for quantifying hor-

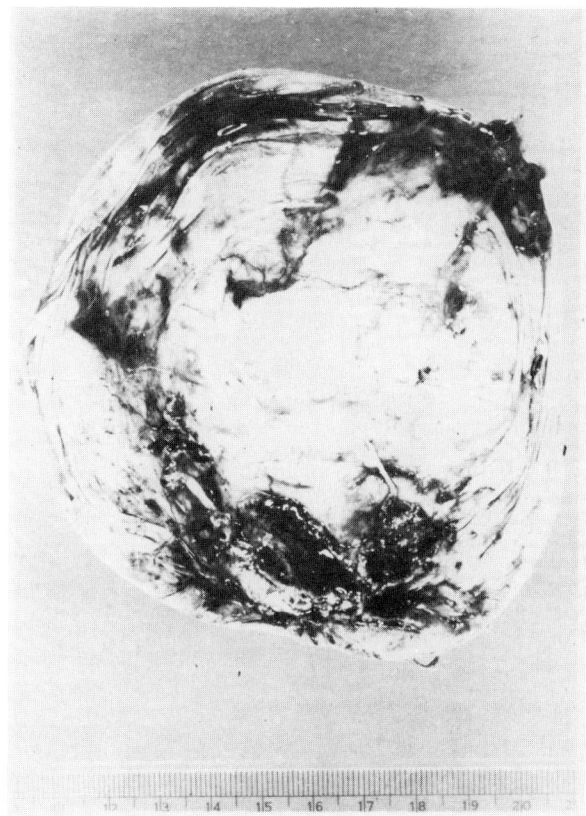

FIGURE 29-3 A very large adrenal cyst that was confused with an adrenal tumor.

mone elevations as a method of case finding, then diagnostic confirmation usually by suppression testing and then finally tumor localization (see Table 29-2). To rule out false-negative tests, cautious administration of provocative testing may stimulate endocrine output from adrenal tumors that are nonfunctional or function only intermittently. Provocative studies and invasive localization tests which may themselves stimulate activity from adrenal tumors are not performed for chromaffin neoplasms unless careful endocrine blockade has been initiated to protect the host from excessive hormone release.

The tumor localization studies progress through anatomic distinctions using techniques that are noninvasive or progressively more invasive. The retroperitoneal pneumography listed in Table 29-2 has been rendered

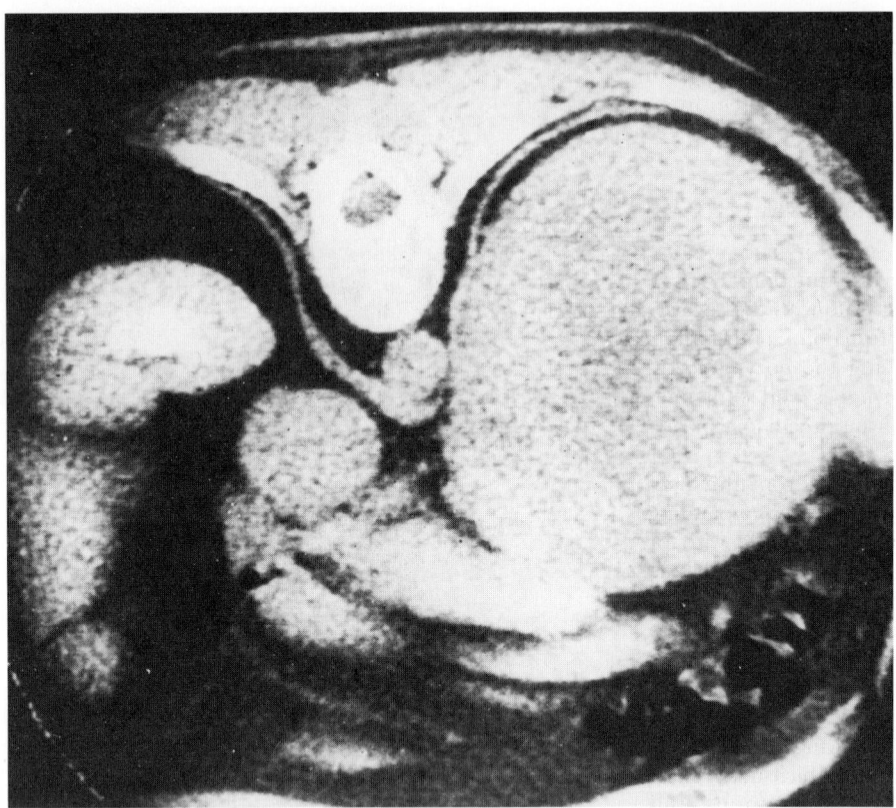

FIGURE 29-4 A large adrenocortical carcinoma as it appeared on a CAT scan of the upper abdomen.

nearly obsolete by the better resolution of less invasive imaging studies such as sonography and contrast-enhanced CAT scanning.

Therapy

The simple curative treatment for adrenal tumors is adrenalectomy—removing the gland involved with the tumor. The retroperitoneal adrenal gland can be approached from either anterior or posterior directions. Different surgical approaches are indicated for adrenalectomy depending on the type of disease being treated (see Table 29-3). Ablation of the adrenal gland may be primary treatment for adrenal tumors, but is only one step in controlling the symptoms of endocrine hyperfunction. These symptoms may also be treated by antineoplastic drugs, by synthesis blockade preventing the production of functional hormone, or by blockade of the effects of the tumor's endocrine products at the target tissues.

ADRENOCORTICAL TUMORS

History

The earliest anatomic descriptions of the adrenal glands are found in the 1563 plates of the text of Bartholomaeus Eustachius of Rome. The function of these glands was not appreciated for several centuries until Thomas Addison of Guy's Hospital in London suggested that they were necessary for life. He described in 1855 a fatal syndrome in 11 patients, noting that the adrenal glands were destroyed in each patient who died because of this wasting syndrome.[4]

Another century slipped by before the several steroid hormones were correlated with production in general anatomic layers of the adrenal cortex. (Table 29-1). The

TABLE 29-1 Hyperfunction of Anatomic Layers of Adrenal Gland Gives Rise to Distinctive Hormone Excess Syndromes

1. Mineralocorticoid ("salt")—Aldosteronism—Zona glomerulosa
   a. Primary
   b. Secondary
2. Glucocorticoid ("sugar")—Hypercortisolism—Zona fasciculata
   a. Cushing's disease
   b. Cushing's syndrome
3. Ketosteroid ("sex")—Androgens or estrogens—Zona reticularis
   a. Virilizing
   b. Feminizing
4. Catecholamine ("panic")—Pheochromocytoma—Medulla

different species of corticosteroids were found to have different physiologic effects: the outermost zona glomerulosa producing mineralocorticoids ("salt") regulated electrolyte metabolism; the middle fasciculata layer producing glucocorticoids ("sugar") regulated carbohydrate metabolism; and the inner reticular layer producing ketogenic steroids ("sex") regulated secondary sexual differentiation by virilizing or feminizing effects of androgens or estrogens. Syndromes of corticosteroid excess were described as listed in Table 29-4. The first syndrome to be described well was that of hypercortisolism; aldosteronism was known immediately following discovery of aldosterone. Occasional adrenal tumors were found to give rise to feminization or virilization, but a review of the adrenogenital syndromes was the latest of these corticosteroid-excess syndromes to be published.

Each of the syndromes in Table 29-4, listed according to each anatomic and biochemical division of the adrenal cortex, was found to result from hyperplasia as well as neoplasia. The differentiation between primary hypercorticosteroid syndromes (usually due to neoplasia) and secondary hypercorticosteroid syndromes (often due to adrenal hyperplasia) remains a chief diagnostic distinction upon which treatment is predicated.

Incidence, Epidemiology, and Etiology

Syndromes of adrenocortical hyperfunction are not common, but case finding is significant, because each syndrome represents a potentially treatable lesion. The number of the syndromes based on adrenocortical tumors is less than half the incidence of the proven syndromes because the majority of hypercorticism is based in hyperplasia rather than autonomous neoplasia.

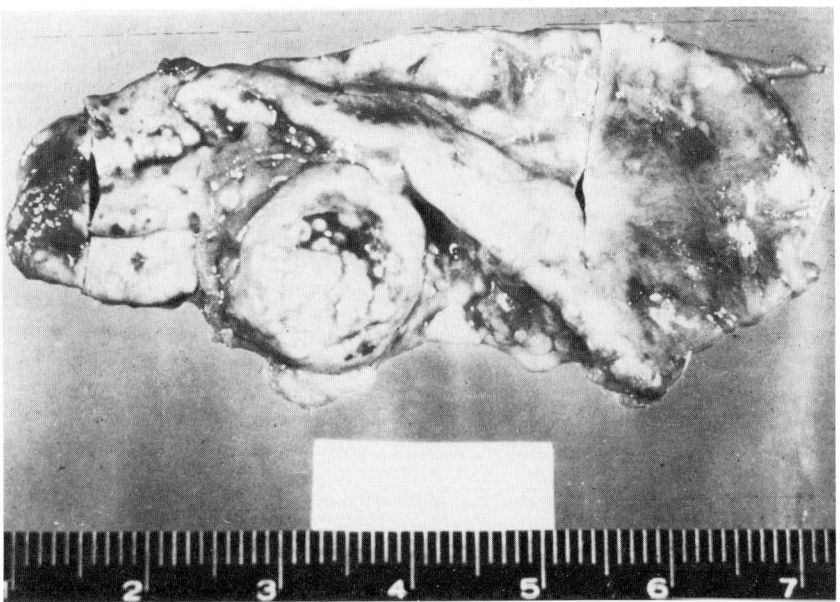

FIGURE 29-5 A small benign adrenocortical adenoma that secreted aldosterone; following unilateral adrenalectomy, the patient's symptoms of primary aldosteronism and hypertension cleared.

TABLE 29-2 Diagnostic Techniques for Screening, Confirming, and Localizing Adrenal Tumors

1. Function tests
   a. Metabolite excretion studies—Screening tests
   b. Suppression tests—Confirming diagnosis
   c. Provocative tests—Rule out false negatives
2. Localization of space-occupying adrenal masses
   a. Noninvasive
      (1) Abdominal x-ray and fluoroscopy
      (2) Sonography
      (3) CAT scan
   b. Minimally invasive
      (1) Urography and nephrotomography
      (2) Iodocholesterol adrenal scanning
   c. Invasive
      (1) Arteriography
      (2) Venography
      (3) Venous sampling
      (4) (Retroperitoneal pneumography)

The prevalence of primary aldosteronism has been revised downward from initial estimates that a substantial proportion of the hypertensive population might trace their hypertension to this etiology. Approximately 1 percent of patients with primary hypertension may have primary aldosteronism,[5] which would mean a very large number of the 25 million people with hypertension in the United States alone. The majority of this population goes undiagnosed because the symptoms are not severe enough to bring them to detection. Cushing's syndrome is diagnosed about once per 1000 autopsies, with a somewhat lower incidence detected by clinical presentation of the syndrome. The adrenogenital syndromes are fortunately very rare, occurring usually as congenital salt-losing grave illness or as an acquired paraneoplastic syndrome in the adult.

Each of the syndromes is more common in females than in males. No specific external etiologic agents are suspected in the development of the syndromes.

Signs and Symptoms

Signs and symptoms, even if incomplete, that suggest a clinical syndrome are the earliest indications of adrenocortical disease, as is the case with most other endocrine abnormalities. Almost no patients with adrenocortical tumors present with mass symptoms of the primary lesion. Hypertension is a finding common to many of the adrenocortical excesses, and abnormalities in blood sugar and electrolytes give rise to such symptoms as muscle weakness. Changes in some urine constituents may lead to polydipsia and polyuria. Classic stigmata of Cushing's syndrome are the features of exaggerated cortisol activity. Most of the features can be seen in patients subjected to prolonged treatment with high doses of exogenous corticosteroids: truncal obesity, hypertension, hirsutism, striae, psychiatric disturbance, osteoporosis, and fragile skin with poor wound healing.

The clinical features of the ketogenic steroid excesses are either feminizing or masculinizing across gender, or the showing of signs of precocious development of secondary sex characteristics within gender.

Diagnosis, Work-Up, and Staging

PRIMARY ALDOSTERONISM

The diagnosis of aldosteronism is made by proving excessive aldosterone secretion or excretion of aldosterone metabolites. Plasma aldosterone can be measured by radioimmunoassay, and aldosterone secretion rate can be calculated. Measurement of serum potassium in a known state of sodium balance can suggest the need for aldosterone measurements.

The chief distinction to be made in aldosteronism is to distinguish primary from secondary aldosteronism. Underlying confirmation of aldosteronism comes by way of plasma and urine electrolytes and steroids; but *differentiation* between primary and secondary aldosteronism

TABLE 29-3 Adrenalectomy

1. Operative approaches for adrenal tumors
   a. Anterior, transabdominal
   b. Posterior, retroperitoneal
2. Selection of operative approach
   a. Anterior
      (1) Benign lesions with potentially dangerous secretion, e.g., catecholamines from active pheochromocytoma
      (2) Malignant lesions for staging and en bloc resection, e.g., mass suspected of being adrenocortical carcinoma
      (3) Ectopic or multicentric lesions, e.g., exploring chromaffin chain
   b. Posterior
      (1) Benign cortical adenoma, e.g., aldosterone-secreting adenoma
      (2) Ablation as therapy for other malignant disease, e.g., adrenalectomy for breast cancer

TABLE 29-4 Historical Development of Adrenocortical Hyperfunction Syndromes from Neoplasia or Hyperplasia

Anatomic division	Steroid biochemistry	Syndrome	Date	Investigator
Zona fasciculata	Glucocorticoid	Cushing's syndrome (hypercortisolism)	1932	H. Cushing
Zona glomerulosa	Mineralocorticoid	Primary aldosteronism	1955	J. Conn
Zona reticularis	Sex steroid	Adrenogenital syndrome	1962	A. Bongiovanni, et al.

comes by determination of plasma *renin*. In primary aldosteronism plasma renin activity is suppressed, and in secondary aldosteronism the renin (angiotensin) activity is the drive to the elevated secretion of aldosterone. High renin activity may result from low effective blood volume states such as congestive heart failure, nephrotic syndrome, or cirrhosis. High renin activity may also result from a primary renal hypersecretion as in Bartter's syndrome. But renin activity is low or absent in primary aldosteronism, reflecting the normal feedback inhibition in the renin-regulated aldosterone physiology.

Spironolactone response tests and DOCA suppression tests also are designed to differentiate primary from secondary aldosteronism, but these tests are less useful since they are judged against the main standard for primary aldosteronism, low-renin excess aldosterone.

The differential diagnosis of the adrenal lesion in primary aldosteronism is made by noninvasive and invasive studies in patients to distinguish those with adrenocortical adenomas secreting aldosterone from the nearly equal number who may have idiopathic hyperaldosteronism due to hyperplasia of one or both glands. The noninvasive studies that have been particularly helpful in distinguishing adenoma from idiopathic hyperplasia have been the tilt test and iodocholesterol adrenal imaging. Of the invasive studies, adrenal venous sampling is particularly useful. To detect a true elevation in an adrenal steroid and not simply a sampling error that may be occasioned by technical differences in adrenal venous sampling, assays of one species of steroid are controlled with steroid determinations from another adrenal cortical layer. For example, if one finds an elevated aldosterone in the samples of blood obtained from one adrenal gland that is three times the concentration seen in a sampling of the opposite adrenal effluent, these data are valid if the cortisol determinations are approximately the same, and one could infer a true difference in adrenal aldosterone output. Similarly, adrenal venous sampling strongly suggests an adrenal cortical adenoma as the source of Cushing's syndrome if the cortisol determinations are several times higher on one side than on the other in the presence of similar aldosterone concentrations.

Aldosterone-secreting adenomas are small benign cortical lesions (see Fig. 29-5). These small tumors are best treated by unilateral adrenalectomy. As benign lesions, excision is curative with nearly all patients so treated reverting to normal blood pressure if nephrosclerosis has not already taken place secondary to the hypertension.

Since adenomas that give rise to primary aldosteronism are small benign lesions, no further discussion will be considered for staging or follow-up as will be done for the other adrenal tumors considered in this chapter. Spironolactone medical therapy can be used for those patients who are not operative candidates, and for the majority of patients with idiopathic hyperaldosteronism on the basis of adrenal hyperplasia. This drug is not appropriate therapy on a long-term basis for most operative candidates, since adverse side effects have been reported. Some adrenal tumors that give rise to symptoms of primary aldosteronism have been reported to be malignant, but this possibility is remote in the classic patient with primary aldosteronism.

CUSHING'S CORTICAL TUMOR

The majority of patients with Cushing's syndrome from endogenous hypercortisolism have bilateral hyperplasia due to excess adrenocorticotropic hormone (ACTH). This ACTH-driven cortisol excess is classical Cushing's *disease*. Some paraneoplastic syndromes elaborate ACTH-like hormones that can similarly stimulate hyperplasia in the adrenal cortex. About one-fourth of all patients who have Cushing's syndrome have adrenal tumors as the source of the excess cortisol. The majority

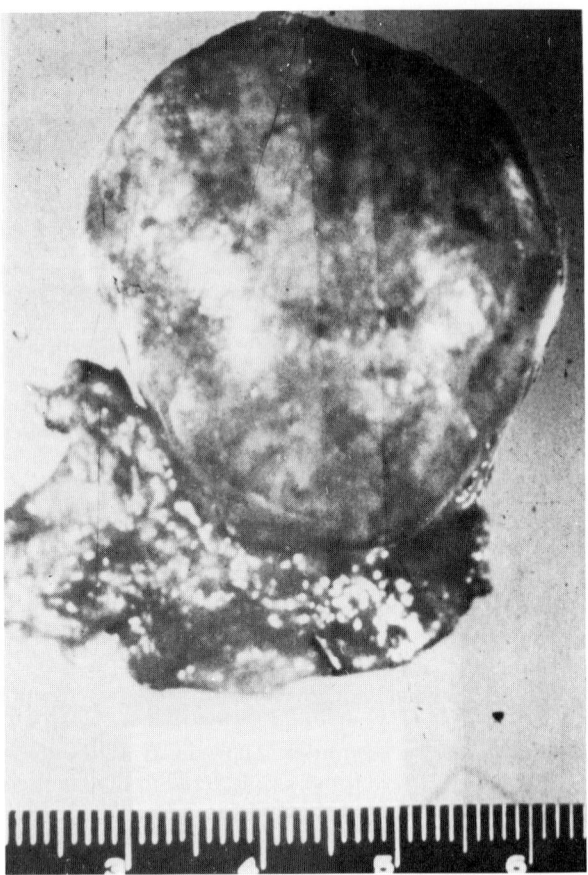

FIGURE 29-6 Appearance of a benign adrenocortical adenoma that gave symptoms of Cushing's syndrome before curative resection.

of these tumors are benign cortical adenomas in the adult, whereas the tumors are usually carcinomas in children.

The single most important biochemical feature of this disease is loss of circadian rhythm in the normal ACTH ebb and peak in an average daily cycle, lagged by cortisol variation. The definition of Cushing's syndrome does not rest upon an elevated cortisol determination as much as the demonstration of an absence in diurnal rhythm. For this reason, urinary excretions of cortisol metabolites are of less significance than plasma cortisol determinations at ebb and peak in the circadian cycle.

Differentiation of primary versus secondary hypercortisolism depends largely on dexamethasone suppression tests. Low doses of this cortisol congener suppress the pituitary to inhibit cortisol secretion in the normal individual but not in the patient with Cushing's syndrome. A high-dose suppression test should suppress the plasma cortisol secretion in patients with adrenal hyperplasia that are ACTH-responsive, but would fail to decrease cortisol secretion from autonomous tumors. The stimulation test for hypercortisolism uses ACTH administration or metyrapone inhibition of cortisol feedback, again depending on the autonomy of the adrenal neoplasia for the distinction of adrenal tumors versus hyperplasia secondary to ACTH from pituitary or other tumor sources.

After the work-up in confirmation of Cushing's syndrome and differentiating it by suppression or stimulation tests, if adrenal tumor is suspected, the noninvasive and invasive localization tests listed in Table 29-2 are followed. Much of the information obtained in localization is useful in staging the tumor. If the preoperative data suggest a benign cortical adenoma of the type seen in Fig. 29-6, further staging information would not usually be indicated before curative resection.

Some very large adrenal cortical tumors exhibit a characteristic feature that is crucial in preoperative staging. Some adrenocortical carcinomas send intravenous extensions from the tumor through the adrenal vein into the cava.[6] These intravascular extensions must be recognized preoperatively for modification of the surgical approach and successful and safe extirpation of the entire tumor with its intravascular component. An example of preoperative staging that implies a significant difference in operative management is seen in Fig. 29-7, in which the preoperative cavagram demonstrates the large intravenous tumor extension from an adrenocortical carcinoma. Further information from scans, x-rays, and biochemical surveys for evidence of metastatic disease are also carried out in staging a tumor diagnosed preoperatively as probably an adrenal cortical adenocarcinoma.

ADRENOCORTICAL MASCULINIZING-FEMINIZING SYNDROMES

Virilization in adrenogenital syndrome occurring in infants is due to a defect in steroidogenesis. This inherited inborn error of metabolism is due to an enzyme deficiency at one of three points in the synthesis of mineralocorticoids: a 21-hydroxylase, 11-hydroxylase, or 3-β-hydroxysteroid dehydrogenase. Deficiencies in one

pressive or destructive pituitary radiation. An option in the treatment of Cushing's disease is the performance of bilateral total adrenalectomy. A subtotal adrenalectomy is generally not successful since the high ACTH drive will cause hyperplasia of the adrenocortical remnant. An advantage of total adrenalectomy is that it rapidly gets rid of the excess cortisol by ablating the tissue of the hormone's origin. A late sequel that can complicate adrenalectomy for Cushing's disease is the evolution of pituitary hypersecretion in the absence of cortisol feedback. Patients who have this syndrome can eventually develop adenomas in the pituitary as well as darkening of the skin in Nelson's syndrome.

For adrenal tumors, however, primary treatment usually consists in unilateral adrenalectomy. In the case of benign cortical adenomas, simple adrenalectomy is curative. For the patient with adrenocortical carcinoma, radical adrenalectomy may be considered including the contents of Gerota's fascia in an en bloc resection of the retroperitoneal contents on the side affected (Fig. 29-8). A radical adrenalectomy is an operation performed for cure of an invasive malignant disease. Debulking of the primary tumor also will accomplish the reduction in the

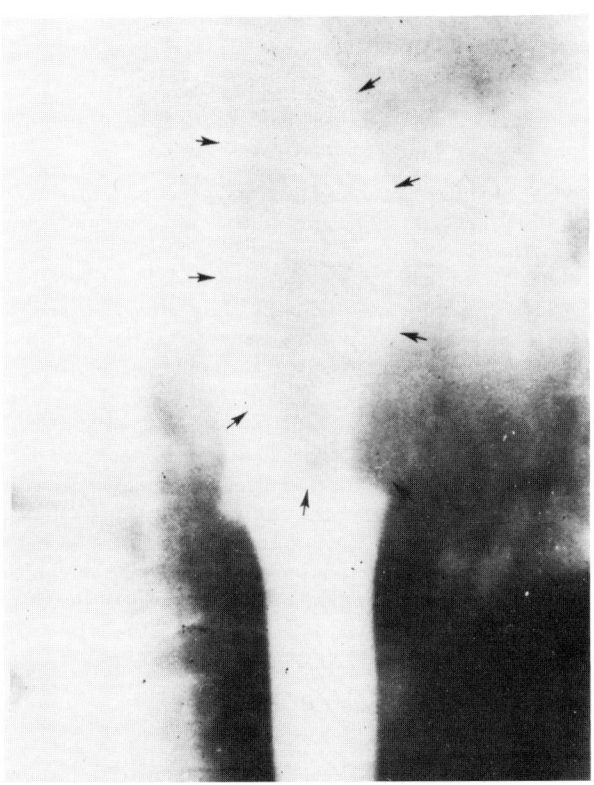

FIGURE 29-7 Venography can be crucial in preoperative staging of adrenocortical carcinoma in demonstrating intravenous extensions of the tumor as seen in this cavogram.

of these enzymes can be inherited as an autosomal recessive trait. Acquired defects in steroid synthesis usually result from neoplasia and usually give rise to feminizing characteristics. Presentation is usually in the male beginning with gynecomastia. High urinary estrogens and other 17-ketosteroids can be detected on urinary screening. Feminizing tumors are almost always carcinomas and carry a poor prognosis.

Options for Primary Treatment

For adrenocortical hyperfunction secondary to adrenal hyperplasia, treatment may be directed at the driving stimulus. In Cushing's disease, this may take the form of an hypophyseal attack by hypophysectomy or sup-

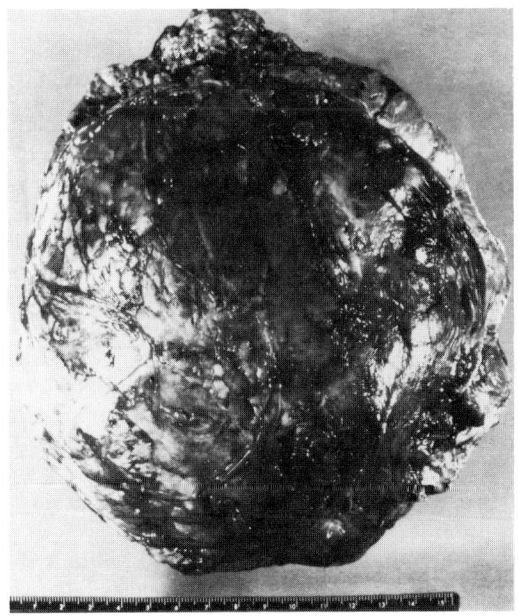

FIGURE 29-8 Large adrenocortical carcinoma resected in radical adrenalectomy.

mass of the cells that are producing the hormone that gives rise to the clinical symptoms.

Another form of primary surgical therapy is any operation directed at paraendocrine tumors that are giving rise to ACTH-like hormones that are driving the adrenals to production of excess cortisol through hyperplasia. Most paraendocrine tumors that produce ACTH or similar paraneoplastic hormones have a poor prognosis for response to surgical therapy. Radiotherapy has shown poor results in primary control of adrenal tumors.

Adjunctive Therapies

Adrenocorticolytic drugs may have some limited role in adjunctive management of adrenal cortical tumors. A DDT derivative, o,p'-DDD, is useful as an adrenocorticolytic drug, but its usefulness is in palliation, which may be limited by the patient's tolerance of the side effects of this toxic agent. The drug is a useful adjunct after bulk disease is removed in reducing to a minimum the amount of functional tissue present.

An experimental agent used to inhibit the synthesis of cortisol is aminoglutethimide. This drug can give significant endocrine palliation even though it may not impair further spread of the metastatic adrenocortical adenocarcinoma.

A significant problem in adjunctive treatment of patients with adrenocortical tumors is steroid therapy. The patient who has undergone bilateral adrenalectomy has an obvious need for complete replacement of the daily secretion of mineralocorticoid and glucocorticoid. Furthermore, this minimum daily secretion rate must be supplemented under circumstances of stress, such as fever, infection, or high metabolic demand. In patients who have a secreting adrenocortical tumor, the high level of circulating cortisol suppresses ACTH so that the opposite adrenal gland is often involuted and atrophic. Following resection, the suppressed adrenal gland may not be capable of corticosteroid secretion at normal or stress levels of demand. A postoperative patient who has had Cushing's syndrome generally requires excess cortisol over daily maintenance for some weeks, but eventually will arrive at a glucocorticoid equivalent of 37.5 mg/day of cortisone and 0.1 mg of the mineralocorticoid 9-fluorocortisol. A patient who has had an adrenalectomy or who has been maintained on replacement corticosteroids for some period of time should have adequate instructions and also some form of medical alert indicating that proper doses of parenteral corticosteroids should be administered in any stressful situation.

Follow-Up and Detection of Recurrence or Metastases

After an adrenal tumor resection, the patient should be followed by regular clinical examinations and urinary corticosteroid metabolite determinations made at intervals or for clinical indications. A disheartening experience for the surgeon caring for patients for several years following the report of a successful resection of a large benign cortical adenoma is the discovery of recurrent Cushing's syndrome, later to be found based in metastatic adrenocortical carcinoma. The usual studies in postoperative patients such as chest x-ray and biochemical and radioisotope screening may raise suspicion before the patient is found to have recurrent Cushing's syndrome. The close check on urinary cortisol metabolites also allows the physician to monitor the adequacy of steroid replacement in the patient who has had an adrenalectomy.

Treatment of Recurrence and Metastases

The recurrent adrenocortical carcinoma may be responsive to surgical resection of evident bulk disease. When bulk disease has been reduced, an adrenocorticolytic drug such as o,p'-DDD may sometimes control minimal residual disease within the tolerance of the patient for the target cells. Aminoglutethimide administration can give successful palliation for the excess hormone without inhibiting the advance of the metastatic tumor.

Future Prospects

Objectives in therapy for adrenocortical tumors would include better screening techniques to determine the diagnosis of adrenocortical cancer earlier than the late stages in which most present. Better medical control of the illness resulting from corticosteroid excess would be achieved if the drugs for corticosteroid synthesis inhibition or antimetabolite chemotherapy were less toxic. A controllable medical adrenalectomy has been a long-sought goal that might enable the physician to reduce hyperfunction to normal levels without ablating the normal adrenal gland.

At present, with safe surgical techniques and steroid

replacement therapy available, the removal of any functional tumor responsible for the illness of hypercortisolism is practical. However, this is not often done with the reduction of hypercortisolism toward normal, including the preservation of normal pituitary and adrenal function and their ability to respond to stress. The ideal treatment of adrenocortical tumor and the syndrome of its excess hormone would be the extirpation of mass lesions and reduction of hormone excess with the return to the normal physiologic autoregulation of pituitary-adrenal control.

CHROMAFFIN TUMORS

The adrenal medulla may give rise to tumors that may seem oncologically benign but are physiologically malignant. The adrenal medulla consists of chromaffin tissue which is not limited to the adrenals but is found in a predictable distribution from the base of the skull to the pelvis along the sympathetic chain. Chromaffin tissue, wherever it is distributed in its migration from its origins in the primitive neural crest, carries with it the staining properties that lead to its name, and the enzymatic properties that make synthesis of its amine hormones possible. These APUD features allow chromaffin tissue to take up amine precursors and decarboxylate them in the synthesis of catecholamines. Pheochromocytomas are classic "apudomas," or APUD tumors.

History

The history of the recognition of this form of adrenal tumor is summarized in Table 29-5. The pioneering studies made by von Euler of catecholamine neurotransmitters were awarded the Nobel Prize in 1970, a prize von Euler's father had received 40 years earlier.

Incidence, Epidemiology, and Etiology

Pheochromocytoma is not so much a rare tumor as a rarely detected tumor. In large autopsy series, performed on patients dying of all causes, pheochromocytoma is found in about 0.1 percent of patients. Of the patients known to have diastolic hypertension, 0.1 percent have hypertension on the basis of pheochromocytoma; a larger number may be found in the large groups of the population who do not know they are hypertensive. The most unfortunate presentation of the tumor is in the sudden death of the patient not suspected of having the tumor. It is estimated that approximately 1000 deaths per year in the United States are due to pheochromocytoma, and perhaps 30 times that number of patients in the United States alone harbor this tumor.[8] No external etiologic inciting causes are known for pheochromocytoma, but a genetic predisposition to the tumor is known in some instances. Pheochromocytoma usually occurs as a sporadic finding in individuals, but may also be associated within families. Pheochromocytoma alone is familial in some cases, and in others there is a familial inheritance of pheochromocytoma along with other APUD neoplasms (see "Multiple Endocrine Adenopathy," below). Patients with neurofibromatosis and patients with one of the phacomatoses have a much higher incidence of pheochromocytoma which may be associated with the neuroectodermal lesions.

TABLE 29-5 History of the Recognition of Pheochromocytoma

Author	Date	Description
Frankel	1886	Bilateral adrenal tumors in girl who died in "attack"
Manasse	1896	"Chromaffin" stain reaction of adrenal tumor
Alezais	1908	"Paraganglioma"—Extraadrenal chromaffin tumors
Pick	1910	Coined term "pheochromocytoma"
Suzuki	1910	Neurofibromas and adrenal tumors
Vaquez	1926	Paroxysmal hypertension syndrome
Mayo	1927	Successful resection of pheochromocytoma
Blashko	1939	Suggested biosynthesis pattern of "adrenaline"
Roth	1945	Histamine stimulation test
von Euler	1946	Norepinephrine is sympathetic transmitter
Iseri	1951	Phentolamine blocking test
Manger	1954	Plasma catecholamines elevated in pheochromocytoma
Armstrong	1957	VMA urinary metabolite excretion
Axelrod	1959	*o*-Methyl transferase activity in blood and tissue

Signs, Symptoms, and Early Detection

Pheochromocytoma has been called the "great mimic," and many of its signs are insidious. Nearly all patients with pheochromocytoma have characteristic sustained diastolic hypertension. Better known, but less frequently observed, are paroxysms of hypertensive attacks. Although these paroxysms may be more typical of pheochromocytoma than they are of other causes of hypertension, only about one-third of adults and less than 10 percent of children with pheochromocytoma experience these attacks. A paroxysmal attack can be precipitated by stress. One such stressful state is pregnancy and labor. A patient may have hypertension in pregnancy that is usually ascribed to some form of toxemia and may enter labor with an undetected pheochromocytoma carrying a very high risk of both maternal and fetal mortality. If the pheochromocytoma is unrecognized, and the patient delivers successfully, the symptoms may subside only to return at a later time, sometimes at the time of a subsequent pregnancy. The first indication of some pheochromocytomas comes during elective or emergency operation. The pheochromocytoma that is unknown and not prepared for is a devastating surprise with a very high mortality rate.

Although hypertension and headache with sweating and nausea and palpitations with paroxysmal attacks under stimulation may be thought of as the "classic" presenting symptoms, the manifestations of pheochromocytoma are protean and a wide variety of atypical patterns are observed. Patients may exhibit such unusual features as psychiatric imbalance, nervousness, and depersonalization—reflecting functional and behavioral changes. The central nervous system employs catecholamine neurotransmitters, and other signs such as restlessness, diplopia, muscle spasms, seizures, and even coma may be other central nervous system signs of pheochromocytoma.

Another nervous system uses the same humoral neurotransmitters—the autonomic (sympathetic) system. Autonomic symptoms may include sweating, flushing, nausea, chill, weakness, tachycardia, hunger, and visceral pain.

The best method for early detection of pheochromocytoma is a very high awareness and willingness on the part of the physician to elicit unusual symptoms and explore them for the possibility of this diagnosis. It is probably not feasible to screen all patients with hypertension for pheochromocytoma. But any index that raises clinical suspicions that a patient could have a pheochromocytoma as an etiology for any of the symptoms listed might be an occasion for screening. This is especially true for any patients who may be undergoing an elective surgical procedure with the remote possibility of an uncontrolled pheochromocytoma as the source for some symptoms. This is particularly true for patients who have a known history of problems with their blood pressure or blood sugar.

Diagnosis, Work-Up, and Staging

Screening studies for initial diagnosis consist of determination of urinary catecholamines and their metabolites, metanephrine, normetanephrine, and vanillylmandelic acid (VMA). If the urinary catecholamine determinations suggest hypercatecholaminemia, this can be confirmed by measurements of plasma catecholamines. If these values are equivocal, gentle suppression tests (such as the phentolamine test) or very cautious provocative tests such as the tilt test, or glucagon or histamine stimulation, may be used under strict physician's supervision. If biochemical confirmation is achieved, the next step is localization of the tumor.

As reviewed in Table 29-2, localization studies may be noninvasive or invasive. The noninvasive studies for pheochromocytoma are acceptable without preparation of the patient by synthesis blockade or receptor blockade. However, the invasive studies require adequate protection of the patient prior to their performance in order to guard against an uncontrolled injection of large quantities of the catecholamine into the patient's circulation during the diagnostic studies. Some suggestion as to the localization of the tumor may be achieved with the biochemical tests, since the predominant species of catecholamine secreted by the tumor may give evidence for an inference as to its location. Catechol-o-methyl transferase (COMT) is an enzyme that is found in greater abundance in the adrenal medulla than it is in peripheral nerve endings or other areas of the extraadrenal chromaffin system. Therefore, a tumor that secretes predominantly epinephrine has a higher probability of being within the adrenal medulla than one which secretes predominantly norepinephrine, which might be presumed to have an extraadrenal location with a higher probability.

A very promising and new technique for noninvasive localization may be forthcoming in the form of adrenal medullary imaging with radiolabeled adrenergic neu-

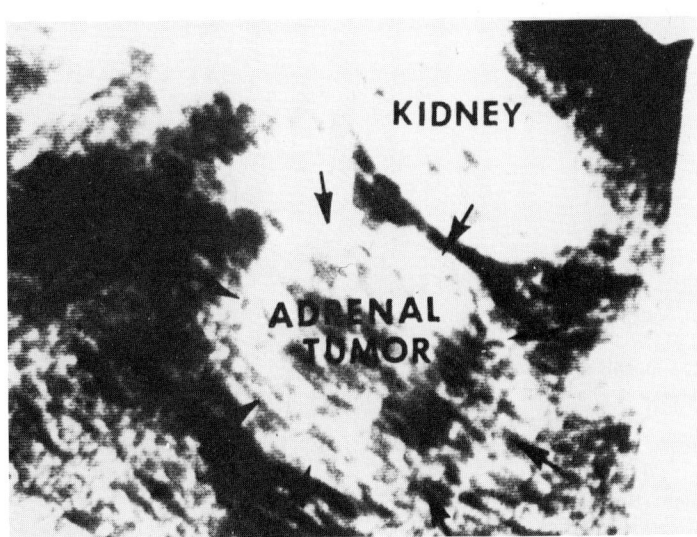

FIGURE 29-9 Sonography is a noninvasive study that safely established the location of this pheochromocytoma.

ron-blocking agents.[9] Imaging of adrenal medullae has been achieved with radiolabeled iodobenzylguanidine in animal experiments and is currently under investigation for human adrenal medullary and extraadrenal chromaffin tissues. The radiolabeled adrenergic blocking agents make possible an autoradiograph when taken up in the chromaffin tissues with high affinity for such adrenergic blocking agents. This technique shows promise in being noninvasive and nonprovocative, but does carry the disadvantage of ionizing radiation release, a feature of several of the radiologic techniques with the exception of ultrasonography.

An example of a noninvasive study that localizes the adrenal tumor is seen in Fig. 29-9. In this case, retroperitoneal sonography established the presence of a left adrenal tumor in a patient who was safely studied by this technique without activation of paroxysmal attack.

Venous sampling by selective placement of a caval catheter and the gravity drainage of a venous sample at sites in the superior and inferior vena cava and adjacent to the adrenal vein may "map" the location of secreting chromaffin tissue. This technique is especially helpful in locating ectopic small lesions and multiple or recurrent pheochromocytoma. An example obtained from such venous sampling data is seen in Fig. 29-10. These data from caval sampling might suggest further localization efforts by selective study of the left perirenal region. It is important that the technique be performed carefully, since the catecholamine concentrations might differ if blood were drawn directly from a catheter-occluded left adrenal vein, or from a mixed pool adjacent to the right adrenal vein. Such a bias would yield a higher catecholamine activity on the basis of sampling technique. The technique to be performed is the "laminar flow" technique in which the caval catheter is placed adjacent to the wall of the vena cava and the blood flows by gravity into the chilled collecting tube.

An invasive test requiring adequate patient protection by receptor blockade (see below) is adrenal venography. As seen in Fig. 29-11, adrenal venography can give a precise localization of the adrenal tumor, but the technique can also stimulate activation of the tumor to secrete dangerous quantities of catecholamine into the patient's circulation. This is particularly true if the venography technique yields extravasation or adrenal infarction or hemorrhage as seen in Fig. 29-2.

Selective arteriography has remained the "gold standard" against which all localization studies are judged, but it is rapidly being made obsolete by the increasing application of CAT scanning. Arteriography is particularly helpful for its high degree of resolution and applicability for ectopic lesions. However, it shares the disadvantages of the invasive studies, and requires adequate patient preparation by adrenergic blockade prior to its use. CAT scanning is a noninvasive study that may circumvent some of the disadvantages of arteriography, but it remains to be seen whether it has the same capability of resolution that arteriography has for pheo-

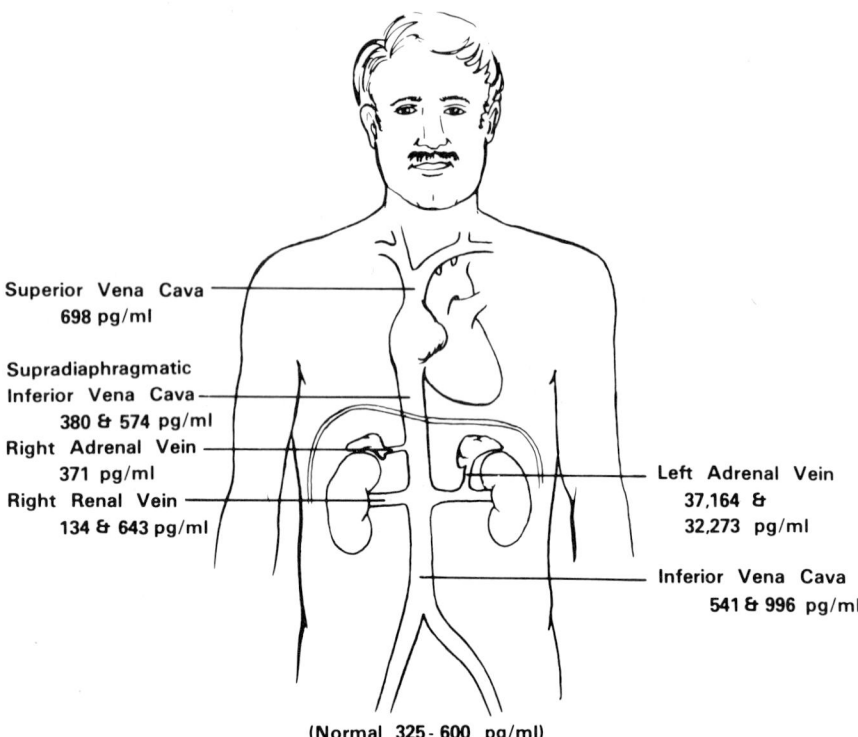

FIGURE 29-10 Caval sampling for catecholamine analysis is useful for "mapping" small, recurrent, or multiple ectopic pheochromocytomas.

chromocytoma. A note of caution must be employed with the use of CAT scanning for the purpose of localization of pheochromocytoma, since many radiologists use an injection of glucagon to change the appearance of the gastrointestinal tract when employing contrast-enhanced CAT scanning. As noted, glucagon is a potent stimulus to the release of catecholamines from pheochromocytoma, and should be avoided in the patient who is not prepared for such a provocative stimulus.

Primary Treatment of Pheochromocytoma

The primary treatment for pheochromocytoma is surgical extirpation of the tumor that has been localized preoperatively. This mode of treatment is also treatment for recurrence or a new primary lesion.

The operative excision of a pheochromocytoma requires careful preparation of the patient and a close collaboration between anesthesiologist and surgeon. The patient with a pheochromocytoma that is secreting considerable quantities of catecholamine vasoconstrictors is frequently contracted in blood volume; the blood volume should be measured and expanded preoperatively as the patient undergoes vasodilatation with adrenergic blockade. The patient may also experience "catecholamine myocarditis," and these changes should be looked for by cardiography and cardiotonic support employed as indicated. Preparation of pressor drugs and antihypertensive agents in the form of readily available intravenous "drips" must be carried out before the patient is brought into the operating room for induction. The induction of anesthesia is a very dangerous time for a patient with pheochromocytoma, and extreme care must be exercised during induction, intubation, and maintenance of the patient with an anesthetic agent that does not potentiate myocardial problems in the presence of large quantities of circulating catecholamines. Frequently, after the tumor is removed, the patient may experience hypotension under anesthesia, as a reflection of the still-contracted blood volume as vasomotor tone is relaxed. Volume therapy is important in supporting such patients. If the patient experiences hypotension prior to the removal of the tumor, epinephrine shock is suggested, and large doses of corticosteroids may be used. Sometimes, patients

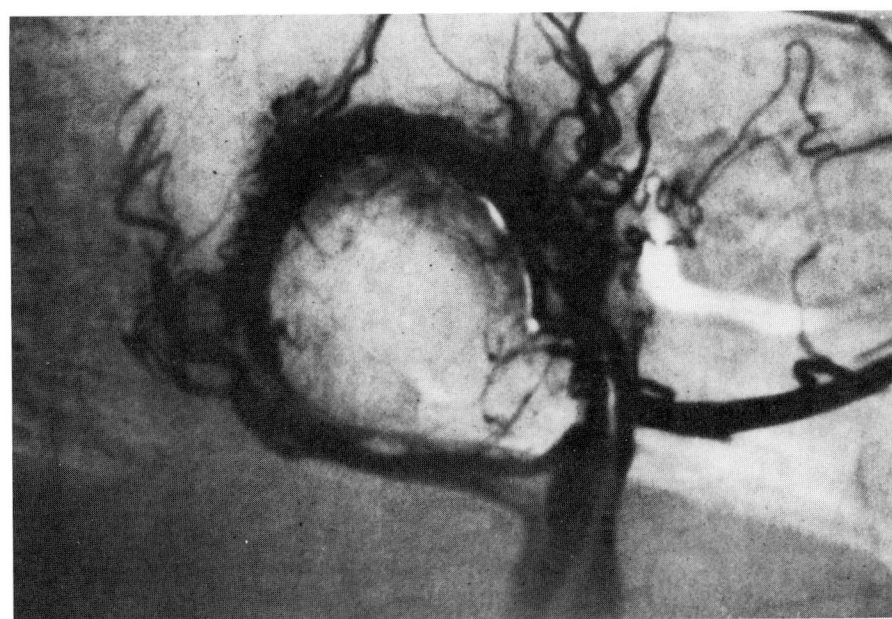

FIGURE 29-11 Adrenal venography is an invasive test that requires patient preparation through catecholamine blockade and careful technique to avoid extravasation or adrenal hemorrhage.

may require administration of pressor agents in addition to fluid volume therapy immediately following the removal of a secreting pheochromocytoma (see Fig. 29-12).

Antiseptic preparation of the abdomen must be carried out very gently to avoid massaging the tumor in these patients, and incision must be carried out with the plan to approach the tumor without manipulation. Preoperative localization of the tumor obviates the need for exploratory palpation, and the first objective of surgical extirpation is rapid and deliberate control of the venous effluent from the tumor. As seen in the case of the patient whose anesthesia record is illustrated in Fig. 29-12, the immediate securing of the adrenal vein (Fig. 29-1) resulted immediately in falling blood pressure, and a turnaround in anesthetic management from antihypertensive agents to volume and pressor therapy. After the excision of the left adrenal tumor, careful exploration of the entire chromaffin chain that is accessible from the abdominal approach is done to rule out bilateral, multiple, or ectopic chromaffin tumors. Special attention is paid to the opposite adrenal gland and the area of the organ of Zuckerkandl.

Simple adrenalectomy that removes a solitary benign pheochromocytoma as seen in Fig. 29-13 is the only therapy that 90 percent of patients will need for primary surgical treatment. However, 10 percent of patients will have bilateral adrenal involvement, 10 percent will have multiple pheochromocytomas in extraadrenal locations, and 10 percent of the total number of patients with pheochromocytoma will have a metastasizing malignant disease. It is in location of these extraadrenal and multiple tumors that the preoperative localization studies are especially helpful.

Adjunctive Treatment

Any patient who is undergoing invasive localizing diagnostic studies for a suspected pheochromocytoma, or who is taken to the operating room for treatment of a confirmed pheochromocytoma, must have readily available drugs to combat a hypertensive crisis, arrhythmia, or hypotension. These drugs must be prepared in a form that can be delivered to the circulation quickly in the management of such complications. If the patient has had severe hypertension or evidence of arrhythmias regularly, β-adrenergic blockade may be indicated (see Table 29-6). Some surgeons prefer to manage a patient without chronic receptor blockade, but a majority will agree that patients with pheochromocytoma are safer with the protection of the adrenergic blockade if employed according to the indications listed in Table 29-6.

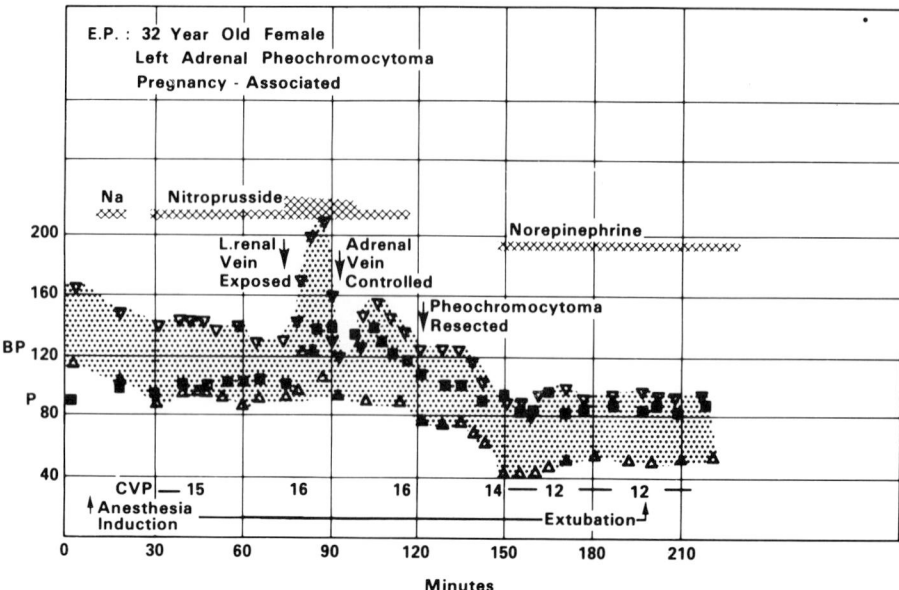

FIGURE 29-12 Anesthetic management for a patient undergoing excision of a pheochromocytoma is of critical importance and may require supplementary adrenergic blockade and antihypertensive drugs following induction and intubation, and volume and pressor therapy after control of the adrenal vein and excision of the tumor.

The α-adrenergic blockade helps overcome the high vasoconstrictor tone of the patient preoperatively and allows adequate volume restitution. It is important to recognize that the use of β-adrenergic blockade obligates α-adrenergic blockade, since many patients who are known to be hypertensive are now being placed on propranolol therapy for management of their hypertension. One such patient was seen by this observer; severe pulmonary edema in this patient was brought under control only with the addition of α-adrenergic blockade.

Another adjunctive agent that can be used successfully in the management of these patients is sodium nitroprusside.[10] Such an agent can be titrated over a short term to protect the patient's circulation during periods of stress (see Fig. 29-12) and overcome some of the disadvantages of adrenergic blockade. Inhibitors of catecholamine synthesis have recently become more generally available for blockade of the production of catecholamines. Such agents are useful in the management of patients, particularly those with metastatic residual pheochromocytoma, but they carry with them disadvantages of their own.

Follow-Up and Detection of Recurrence or Metastases

The patient who has had a pheochromocytoma diagnosed should have regular medical surveillance for life. The author has recently seen a patient who experienced a severe crisis during an operation to fix a fractured hip. After vigorous resuscitation efforts, a pheochromocytoma was confirmed and localized to the right adrenal gland. Only after this intraoperative crisis could the patient recall that she had undergone a previous operation 14 years earlier for the removal of a pheochromocytoma of the left adrenal gland!

In addition to the possibility of multiple primary tumors, either in the adrenal glands or in other chromaffin tissue sites, the patient may experience recurrence

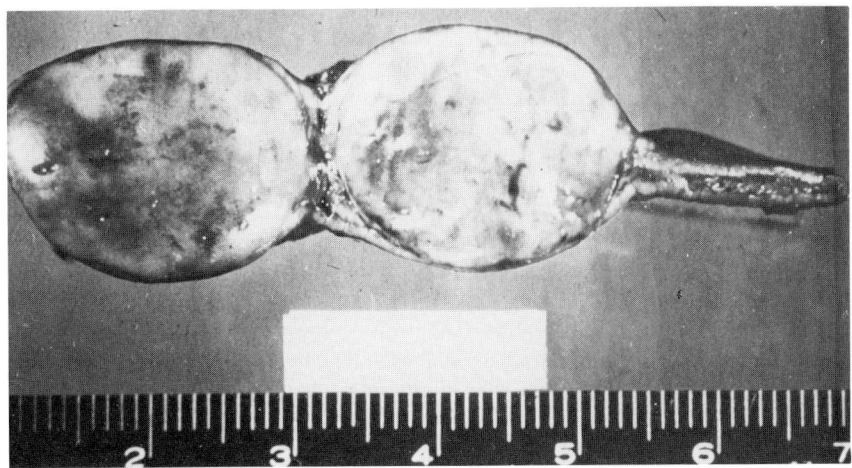

FIGURE 29-13 Adrenalectomy is curative for 90 percent of patients with adrenal pheochromocytoma with the typical appearance seen in this specimen.

or metastasis after initial successful treatment of an apparently benign tumor. Histologic criteria, as previously pointed out, are not uniformly successful in predicting the behavior of endocrine neoplasms. Furthermore, the patient should be followed closely for any evidence of abnormality in related endocrine systems, such as the parathyroid glands or thyroid (see "Multiple Endocrine Adenopathy," below). The patient should also be made aware that he or she might represent an index case in a familial syndrome, and the other members of the first-order kindred should be alerted to the symptoms of pheochromocytoma for the possibility of earlier detection among relatives.

The means for detection of recurrent disease are the same screening techniques for detection and confirmation of hypercatecholaminemia. In addition, the means for detection of mass lesion recurrence are as for other neoplasms, such as chest x-ray, excretory urography, and biliary enzyme studies.

Treatment of Recurrence or Metastases

Surgical removal of functioning pheochromocytoma tissue is the only curative therapy. Moreover, surgical extirpation is also more successful palliative treatment than other options available. Radiotherapy and antimetabolite chemotherapy are of little benefit in metastatic pheochromocytoma. Some medical management has been designed to palliate the endocrine manifestations of the metastatic disease, although the tumors are resistant to most cytotoxic agents.

α-Methyl-p-tyrosine is an agent that has been used to decrease synthesis of catecholamines.[11] A remarkable reduction in catecholamine excretion and metabolite

TABLE 29-6 Indications for Adrenergic Blockade in Patients with Pheochromocytoma.

α-Adrenergic receptor blockade (phentolamine, phenoxybenzamine):
Severe diastolic or systolic hypertension (>200/120)
Frequent, severe paroxysmal attacks
Contracted plasma volume (hematocrit >50%)
Use of β-receptor blockade
β-Adrenergic receptor blockade (propranolol):
Tachycardia (pulse >120/min)
Arrhythmia
Ventricular extrasystole
Pure epinephrine-secreting tumor

SOURCE: Courtesy of Dr. Timothy S. Harrison[4] with modifications from the original.

recovered from the urine is seen, but adequate reduction in blood pressure is not always correlated with this catecholamine reduction. The drug itself has considerable side effects including a Parkinsonian appearance to the patient taking the agent and a significant renal impairment.

α-Methyldopa reduces urinary excretion of catecholamine metabolites and controls blood pressure, but leads to orthostatic hypotension. Phenoxybenzamine given over prolonged periods of time appears to be the most successful method of management of the endocrine illness of patients with unresectable pheochromocytoma. Since the metastatic pheochromocytoma itself is often slow-growing, the use of phenoxybenzamine may make the patient more comfortable during the course of the progressive disease.

Prospects for the Future

Over the past two decades, a better understanding of the physiology of pheochromocytoma and its clinical management has been gained. The genetics and interrelationship of this APUD neoplasm and other endocrine abnormalities have recently opened up and will be an area of further exploration in the future. At present, the clinician might wish for adequate cytotoxic therapy for the control of metastatic neoplasm, or even less ambitiously, might wish development of adequate catecholamine synthesis–blockade agents that would have less toxicity than those that have been tested. But each of these treatments directed at the tumor or its mediators would be "halfway technologies." The more exciting area that is opening at this time is in the control and prevention of APUD neoplasia by better understanding of the mechanisms of derepression in apudomas.

MULTIPLE ENDOCRINE ADENOPATHY

A major advance in our understanding of endocrine neoplasia has evolved in the last two decades with the discovery of heritable clinical syndromes of multiple endocrine adenopathy. Coupled with these descriptions of kindreds with multiple endocrine abnormalities was the development of the APUD concept by Pearse, Weichert, Zollinger, and others linking the dispersed argentaffin cells and their secretions into a unified concept of pathophysiology by way of the understanding of neural crest cell dysplasia. Clinical features of both the adrenal cortex and the adrenal medulla and their hormones are found in these unified concepts of endocrine abnormalities—in the form of *tumors* of the adrenal medulla but *hyperplasia* of the adrenal cortex. The adrenal cortex has no fellow within the APUD system, since the adrenal cortex is mesodermally derived and secretes steroid hormones. But, except for those autonomous adrenal tumors discussed earlier in this chapter, the adrenal cortex is under the direct control of the anterior pituitary, which, in turn, is controlled by hypothalamic neurotransmitters. Thus, the connection between the adrenal cortex and medulla is not in their common location near the kidney, but is seated in the APUD neurohumoral control system.

The first of the multiple endocrine adenomatoses was discovered in an association of gastrointestinally linked glands—the pancreatic islets, pituitary, and parathyroid

TABLE 29-7 History of the Typing of Multiple Endocrine Adenopathy (MEA)

Author	Date	Description
MEA-I (WERMER'S SYNDROME)		
Wermer	1954	Familial adenomatosis of parathyroid, pancreatic islets, pituitary
Zollinger-Ellison	1955	Ulcerogenic syndrome
Vernor-Morrison	1958	Diarrheogenic syndromes
MEA-II (SIPPLE'S SYNDROME)		
Hazard	1959	Medullary carcinoma thyroid (MCT)
Sipple	1961	Autopsy case of bilateral pheochromocytoma and thyroid cancer
Copp	1962	Calcitonin (TCT)
Manning	1963	Hyperparathyroidism added to Sipple's syndrome
Williams, Schimke	1965	MCT is thyroid cancer in familial pheochromocytoma
Steiner	1968	MEN-II large kindred described
Tashjian	1970	TCT immunoassay for subclinical MCT
Chong	1975	Subclass MEA-IIb: normal parathyroids, but distinctive phenotype and mucosal neuromas

(see Table 29-7). Tumors that develop in these glandular sites are discussed in other chapters.

The second major association of multiple endocrine abnormalities is also reviewed in Table 29-7, in the historical development of type II multiple endocrine adenopathy (MEA). In this syndrome, pheochromocytoma is the most urgent diagnosis because of its physiologic malignancy. But, the medullary carcinoma of the thyroid (discussed in Chap. 20) is a metastasizing cancer that deserves attention immediately after the threat of pheochromocytoma is removed. The significance of these MEA syndromes is that a predictable combination of glands is involved, either synchronously or evolving over time. This feature has considerable significance for the follow-up of a patient who has been treated for one of the endocrine tumors in an MEA syndrome. Involvement within a glandular system is most often multiple in the hereditary syndromes, such as the bilaterality of pheochromocytoma in MEA II, and hyperplasia is a frequent histologic finding as well as neoplasia giving rise to the hormone excess.

The genetic significance of these endocrine adenopathies is that they generally occur in younger patients and are typically autosomal dominant characteristics with a high degree of penetrance. Since symptoms may vary in severity from absence of symptoms to latent subclinical disease to severe crises, screening of family members is a productive case-finding method when one relative has obvious clinical disease.

Unlike most autonomous tumors, suppressibility is an occasional feature with hyperplasia or microadenomatosis a histologic correlate. Operation within these MEA syndromes usually requires total or nearly total organ ablation for control because of the involvement of all the affected endocrine tissue; it is a "genetic field change" rather than focal neoplasia as is seen with sporadic endocrine tumors. The intriguing observation made about treatment of these syndromes has major implications for understanding of carcinogenesis: that is, treatment that disrupts hormonal feedback may lead to regression—for example, hyperplasia may progress to neoplasia or revert back with repression.

Endocrine tumors are fascinating instructors in physiology. Their clinical management is often very gratifying. These tumors, particularly those that are linked in heritable syndromes, may yet teach us much about oncogenesis.

REFERENCES

1. Geelhoed GW, Spiegel CT: "Incidental" adrenal cyst: A correctible lesion possibly associated with hypertension. *Southern Medical Journal* 74:626, 1981.
2. Aronsohn RS et al: Blunt trauma to an adrenal cyst producing abdominal pain and anemia. *Am Surg*, 44: 605, 1978.
3. Harrison TS, Gann DS: Adrenal medullary hyperplasia: An opinion. *Surgery*, 85:353, 1979.
4. Harrison TS et al: *Surgical Disorders of the Adrenal Gland*, Grune and Stratton, New York, 1975.
5. Conn JW et al: Preoperative diagnosis of primary aldosteronism. *Arch Intern Med* 123:113, 1969.
6. Geelhoed GW et al: Management of intravenous extensions of endocrine tumors and prognosis after surgical treatment. *Am J Surg* 139:844, 1980.
7. Scott HW et al: Surgical experience with Cushing's disease. *Ann Surg*, May 1977.
8. Manger WM, Gifford RW: *Pheochromocytoma*, Springer-Verlag, New York, 1977.
9. Wieland DM et al: Radiolabeled adrenergic neuron-blocking agents: Adrenomedullary imaging with (^{131}I) iodobenzylguanidine. *J Nucl Med* 21:349, 1980.
10. Lipson A et al: Nitroprusside in the management of a patient with a pheochromocytoma. *JAMA* 239: 427, 1978.
11. Sjoerdsma A et al: Pheochromocytoma—Current concepts of diagnosis and treatment. *Ann Intern Med* 65:1302, 1966.

SELECTED BIBLIOGRAPHY

Vieto RJ et al: Type I multiple endocrine neoplasias. *Curr Prob Cancer*, vol 7, no 5, 1982.

30

THE CARCINOID CELL, TUMORS, AND SYNDROMES

Glenn W. Geelhoed

HISTORY

Carcinoid Tumor

Carcinoid tumors have been described as the "missing link" between benign and malignant tumors. The name *karzinoide* was coined by Oberndorfer in 1909 to suggest that carcinoid was a benign tumor with a morphologic appearance of carcinoma. Several nineteenth-century authors described tumors of the appendix, which probably were carcinoids, since it is now known that the most common neoplasm of the appendix is carcinoid. The clinical behavior of these appendiceal carcinoids was definitely more like a benign neoplasm than the carcinoma they resembled under the microscope. Similar carcinoid tumors outside the appendix were described in 1888, by Lubarsch, who found at autopsy that two patients had multiple small ileal tumors he called "little carcinomata" in the crypts of Lieberkühn.

Carcinoid Cell

The cell of origin of the carcinoid tumor was recognized by Kultschitzky in 1897, when he pointed out the granularity of these cells in the crypts of the intestinal lining, cells which were later called *enterochromaffin cells* by Ciaccio in 1906. Carcinoid tumor was first suggested to arise from Kultschitzky's cells by Hubschmann in 1910, and the Oberndorfer name transliterated into "carcinoid" designated the tumor from this point in history to the present.

There were some suggestions earlier that this carcinoma-like tumor did not always behave like a benign neoplasm. Ransom reported in 1890 a tumor of the ileum with hepatic metastases that were much larger and more extensive than the primary tumor. Most pathologists continued to regard the carcinoid as a benign tumor, describing it at locations throughout the alimentary canal, overlooking the obscure reports of carcinoids with malignant characteristics.

As seen in the history of the carcinoid concept (Table 30-1), there was a gap between the accumulation of understanding about structural and functional characteristics of this neoplasm. Further morphologic refinements took place in the early twentieth century when the carcinoid cells were noted to have affinity for silver stains, and tumors of these "argentaffin" cells were considered "argentaffinomas." But nearly a half-century elapsed before the functioning features of the carcinoid tumor were suggested. After serotonin had been discovered, it was identified in a carcinoid tumor by Lembeck

TABLE 30-1 History of Carcinoid Concept

Date	Author	Observation
1867	Langhans	"Drusenpolyp" of ileum
1882	Berger	"Adenocarcinoma" in appendix
1888	Lubarsch	Autopsies of multiple small ileal tumors
1890	Ransom	Malignant ileal tumor with massive liver metastases
1897	Kultschitzsky	Granular cells in crypts of Lieberkühn
1906	Ciaccio	"Enterochromaffin" cells
1909	Oberndorfer	"Karzinoide," benign tumor with appearance of carcinoma
1910	Hubschmann	Carcinoid tumors arise from Kultschitzsky cells
1914	Gossett, Masson	Silver-stain affinity in "argentaffin" cells and tumors
1948	Rapport	Serum vasoconstrictor = "serotonin"
1952	Biorck	Carcinoid and cardiopulmonary changes linked
1953	Lembeck	Serotonin in carcinoid tumors
1954	Pernow, Waldenstrom	Serotonin in blood and urine of two carcinoid patients
1954	Thorson	"Carcinoid syndrome" in 16 patients
1964	Sjoerdsma	Role of kinins, other hormones, in carcinoid syndrome
1971	Pearse	Carcinoid shares APUD characteristics

and from the circulation of patients with carcinoid tumors by Pernow and Waldenstrom. The *carcinoid syndrome* was clearly described in a report of 16 patients by Thorson in 1954, bringing a third entity into being: first the carcinoid tumor, then the carcinoid cell, and finally the carcinoid syndrome.

Carcinoid Syndrome

The clear association of carcinoid and serotonin and its metabolites facilitated the understanding of the syndrome, but several inexplicable features of the syndrome could not be accounted for by serotonin's actions. A dozen other active substances have now been isolated from carcinoids, and many of the features of the syndrome are more characteristic of mediators such as kinins than of serotonin alone.

The current understanding of carcinoids that rests on this historical base (Table 30-1) regards the carcinoid tumor as a part of the "apudoma" spectrum. In 1971 Pearse synthesized the concept that APUD cells share a common heritage embryologically as well as several biochemical properties, among them the capacity for amine precursor uptake and decarboxylation (APUD). These multipotential argentaffin cells share in the APUD properties and may secrete multiple amine and polypeptide hormones. The tumor itself may also have a widely variable range of malignant behavior, and the carcinoid syndrome is a functional feature of malignant carcinoid, whereas the majority of these carcinoid tumors in their gut-derived primary sites exhibit benign behavior.

INCIDENCE, EPIDEMIOLOGY, AND ETIOLOGY OF CARCINOID TUMOR

A distinction to be made throughout this chapter is the difference between the cell, the tumor, and the syndrome when the term *carcinoid* is used. The carcinoid cell is nearly ubiquitous, but predictably found in tissues derived from entoderm—therefore associated with the gut and the bronchial and genitourinary tracts. The carcinoid cell is neuroectodermal in origin, derived from neural crest. It masquerades under several synonyms: the enterochromaffin cell, argentaffin cell, Kultschitzsky cell, argyrophil cell, and APUD cell. But, wherever this neuroectodermal derivative is found in its dispersion throughout the body in coexistence with gut derivatives, it carries its APUD birthright, manifested by (1) common cytochemistry, (2) similar cytoarchitecture and ultrastructure, and (3) amine and polypeptide hormone synthesis and secretion. These features are shared with other APUD cells in anatomically distant sites with which the carcinoid cells have more in common than with their near neighbors of entodermal origin.

The carcinoid tumor may arise wherever the carcinoid cell is found, that is, from derivatives of the primitive entoderm or from teratomas containing entodermal elements. The majority of carcinoid tumors arise in midgut derivatives—carcinoids are the most common neoplasms of the small intestine and of the appendix. Nearly half of the known carcinoid tumors are present in the appendix; over a quarter of the total are found in the ileum. The third most common site is the rectum—between 10 and 15 percent of the reported abdominal cases—and bronchial carcinoids constitute 10 percent of the total number of carcinoid tumors. In a review of over 2000 neoplasms of the gastrointestinal tract, Ariel once calculated a 1.3 percent incidence of carcinoid tumors. The incidence of carcinoid tumors in the population is probably less than the product of this figure and the incidence of gastrointestinal cancer shown by clinical findings; but there is probably a higher proportion of "silent" carcinoids that are never diagnosed than there are carcinomas.

Table 30-2 summarizes the data from the George Washington University Hospital on carcinoid tumors obtained by review of surgical pathology specimens over a 20-year period in which the diagnosis of carcinoid tumor was made in 119 patients. The distribution as to the primary site is not congruent with figures from the literature in that a higher percentage of bronchial and rectal tumors is noted, perhaps on the basis of atypical referral patterns. With these exceptions, the pattern is otherwise compatible with the figures of the incidence of tumor from the collected series of nearly 4000 abdominal carcinoid tumors reviewed by Wilson.

There are no specific environmental carcinogens linked with the development of carcinoid. One important feature in the epidemiology of this neoplasm is in the personal and family history of the patients at risk. If the patient has had a previous carcinoid tumor—or an apudoma of another type—that patient is at higher risk for development of another. Further, if multiple endocrine neoplasms are found within a patient, the family should be checked for similar heritable endocrine disorders. Moreover, carcinoid tumors are found frequently associated with nonendocrine malignancy as well as with other endocrinopathy. The finding of a carcinoid tumor in a patient is indication for a thorough search for another tumor of endocrine or nonendocrine origin.

CARCINOID SYNDROME

An unusual manifestation of carcinoid tumor that has metastasized so that the endocrine products of the tumor have access to the systemic circulation (usually by liver metastases) is the carcinoid syndrome. This syndrome consists of cutaneous flushing, diarrhea, and asthma experienced by the patient in episodes triggered by known or unknown stimuli.

Although the syndrome is classic for endocrine-active neoplasm, the minority of patients with carcinoid tumor—even those that metastasize—experience the discomforts of the carcinoid syndrome. Approximately 15 percent of patients with carcinoid tumors will have systemic metastases, and only 6 percent of the patients with metastases show some form of carcinoid syndrome. Table 30-2 shows a series of carcinoid tumors with infrequent metastases and rare presentation of the carcinoid syndrome.

Clinical features of the syndrome may be considered typical if experienced by 50 percent or more patients with carcinoid syndrome, or nontypical if the majority of carcinoid patients exhibit these features.[1]

Typical Features

Cutaneous flush, a characteristic sign of the carcinoid syndrome, may be the harbinger of the tumor's presence. The flush resembles the florid rubor of alcoholism, but is episodic. Hypotension may accompany the vasomotor flushing.

TABLE 30-2 Incidence of Carcinoid Tumor

Site	Number of cases	Metastases, %	Carcinoid syndrome, %
Bronchus	32	*	*
Stomach	3	33	33
Small intestine	10	60	20
Appendix	25	0	0
Colon	4	75	50
Rectum	37	75	*
Pancreas (two with islet cell carcinoma)	6	33	*
Ovary (metastatic from bowel primary)	2	100	100
Liver biopsies	5	100	30

* Incomplete information.
SOURCE: From George Washington University Hospital Surgical Pathology Records (see text).

Hepatomegaly is another common feature. The liver is often very much enlarged by, and sometimes nearly replaced by, bulk metastatic carcinoid tumor in patients who show the carcinoid syndrome. Many carcinoid tumors arise in the distribution of the portal vein, i.e., the gut, and any endocrine secretion into the portal vein carries these mediators to the liver where they are detoxified. Liver metastases of the carcinoid tumor may pass the hormones (e.g., serotonin, kinins) from the metastases directly into the systemic circulation.

Gastrointestinal symptoms are present in the majority of patients with carcinoid syndrome.

Diarrhea is the most common disability in the syndrome. Diarrhea and borborygmi are correlated with hyperserotoninemia. Crampy abdominal pain may also result from the changes in transit time and flux across the bowel mucosa.

In addition to episodic cutaneous flushing, a persistent skin change may be found in half the patients with carcinoid syndrome. *Venous telangiectasis,* which resembles acne rosacea of alcoholism with which it may be confused, occurs in a "butterfly" pattern over the nose and the malar eminences.

Edema is a feature in many patients, with at least two reasons for its appearance. Right-sided heart failure can be an explanation for the edema; most of these patients have carcinoid tumor replacing much of the hepatic parenchyma, and hypoproteinemia results from this failure of protein synthesis. The right-sided heart failure results from endocardial fibrosis occurring in the right-sided chambers and valves; it may be found on both the right and left sides of the heart if a bronchial carcinoid is responsible for the syndrome, or if intracardiac shunting is present.

Occasional Findings

Wheezing may occur in some patients with the syndrome; although most of the mediators known to come from carcinoid tumors are bronchoconstrictors, only the minority of patients show asthmalike wheezing.

A few patients may have *pellagra* signs. This is a genuine vitamin deficiency, since tryptophan is diverted to serotonin synthesis, leaving a relative deficiency in niacin production.

Arthralgias and myopathies have been associated with excess serotonin in the circulation. *Fibrosis* may occur elsewhere than in the right-sided heart chambers, including the retroperitoneum and in Peyronie's disease.

CARCINOID HORMONES

Secretions isolated from carcinoid tumors and from the circulation of patients with carcinoid syndrome have included over a dozen amine hormones.[2] Among these are serotonin, 5-hydroxytryptophan, kallikrein, histamine, ACTH, prostaglandins, growth hormone, prolactin, calcitonin, gastrin, and glucagon. These several mediators reflect the multiple-potential endocrine properties of these APUD-derived carcinoid cells. Furthermore, the carcinoid syndrome can originate not only from noncarcinoid tumors, but from other APUD-derived neoplasms as well. Carcinoid syndrome has been reported from medullary carcinoma of the thyroid, oat-cell carcinoma of the lung, pancreatic islet cell tumors, and chromaffin tumors.

SIGNS, SYMPTOMS, AND ATTEMPTS AT EARLY DETECTION OF CARCINOID TUMOR

Carcinoid is an endocrine tumor, and like most other endocrine neoplasms, it elaborates a marker of its presence—the "hormone handle." This tumor marker may be useful in diagnostic screening, detecting recurrence, or monitoring the effect of therapy in many endocrine tumors; but this is less true in carcinoid. By definition, the carcinoid syndrome is a sign of the carcinoid tumor's presence, but only after functioning metastases are present. Carcinoid syndrome is in no way useful for "early detection," but is more like an occasional feature of end-stage disease. Presence of an abdominal mass, occasionally intestinal intussusception with a carcinoid lead point, and, rarely, intestinal obstruction may signal an abdominal carcinoid. Wheezing, atelectasis, or hemoptysis may be signs of a bronchial carcinoid. The usual sign of a carcinoid tumor is no sign at all, and its discovery is not often based on accountable symptoms.

Several characteristics of the carcinoid tumor carry important clinical implications. First is its tendency to multicentricity. As noted, it is frequently associated with other concurrent malignancies. Carcinoids are usually slow-growing, but all carcinoids are potentially malignant, that is, invasive and metastasizing. Metastases from carcinoid may exponentially outgrow the size of the primary tumor. Carcinoid tumor that presents as a space-occupying mass lesion is often a function of the metastasis rather than primary tumor.

The malignant potential of the carcinoid tumor depends on the site of origin of the primary tumor and the size of the primary tumor (Table 30-3). These two features of the primary tumor are related; for example, appendiceal carcinomas are alleged to be benign compared to ileal carcinomas, but this benignancy is less apparent when corresponding tumors of the same size are considered.

Early detection, then, means discovery of the primary tumor when it is small; this eliminates the usefulness of the endocrine tumor marker, and the space-occupying mass of the primary lesion must be the feature upon which early detection is based. This resolves to the observation that nearly all early detection of primary carcinoid tumors is incidental.

DIAGNOSTIC TECHNIQUES, WORK-UP, AND STAGING

Primary Tumor

Positive diagnosis of carcinoid tumor is by biopsy and histologic verification of the presence of argentaffin cells (Fig. 30-1). As with most endocrine neoplasms, a judgment as to malignant potential cannot be made by a review of the microscopic features of the tumor at the primary site. Because of the submucosal location of most primary carcinoid tumors, exfoliative cytology is not often helpful.

BRONCHUS

In some instances in which a small intraluminal mass lesion occurs in a position that would cause obstructive symptoms, such as in the bronchus, diagnosis by endoscopy and biopsy occurs early. Obstruction is not a major presenting feature of carcinoids—including appendiceal

TABLE 30-3 Malignant Potential of Carcinoid Tumor

Site of origin	Percent metastasized at operation
Appendix	2
Jejunoileum	34
Colorectal	60

Size of primary tumor, cm	Percent metastasized at operation
<1.0	2
>2.0	100

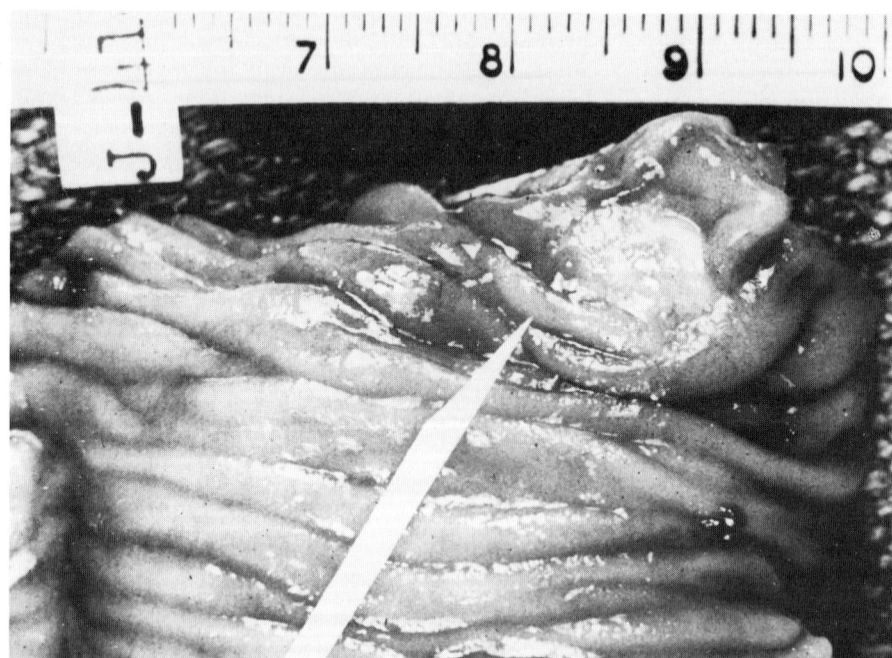

FIGURE 30-1 Carcinoid cells are distinctive, here present in an appendiceal "argentaffinoma."

carcinoids—in the gastrointestinal tract. Another indication favoring early diagnosis by bronchial carcinoids is the relative density differential between the solid tumor and the air-filled lung around it that makes the tumor density apparent on routine chest roentgenogram (Fig. 30-2).

GASTROINTESTINAL TRACT

In the gastrointestinal tract, submucosal mass lesions are read by reversing this density difference by filling the lumen with radiodense contrast; some gastrointestinal primary carcinoid tumors have been seen as "filling defects" on barium gastrointestinal series (Fig. 30-3). Endocrine tumors have generally been visualized by arteriography because of their rich blood supply; this is less true with carcinoids than with several of the other endocrine adenomas. Isotopic scans and ultrasonography have been directed largely at localizing liver metastases of carcinoid tumors and have not been useful in early detection of primary tumors.

TESTS FOR ASSOCIATED DISORDERS

Since carcinoid tumors are found in frequent association with other tumors, a careful search should be carried out for (1) other nonendocrine malignancies, (2) other endocrinopathy of the apudoma type, and (3) multiple carcinoids. Routine screening techniques are employed to search for the first-mentioned neoplasms, and specific assays can help uncover the related endocrine disorders mentioned second. These include serum gastrin, glucagon, insulin (and fasting blood sugar), parathyroid hormone (PTH), ACTH, and calcitonin assays.

The Carcinoid Syndrome and Staging

The presence of the carcinoid syndrome is an important piece of information in staging a carcinoid tumor. The carcinoid syndrome signifies that considerable metastatic disease from a gastrointestinal primary tumor is present beyond regional lymph nodes. This is true because patients do not become symptomatic unless serotonin and other mediators have access to the systemic circulation, for example, when secreted by liver metastases. Serotonin secreted in the portal vein distribution would be metabolized in the liver and inactivated as it is passed into the systemic circulation, so that symptoms of carcinoid syndrome mean that metastatic tumor is secreting into the transhepatic circulation.

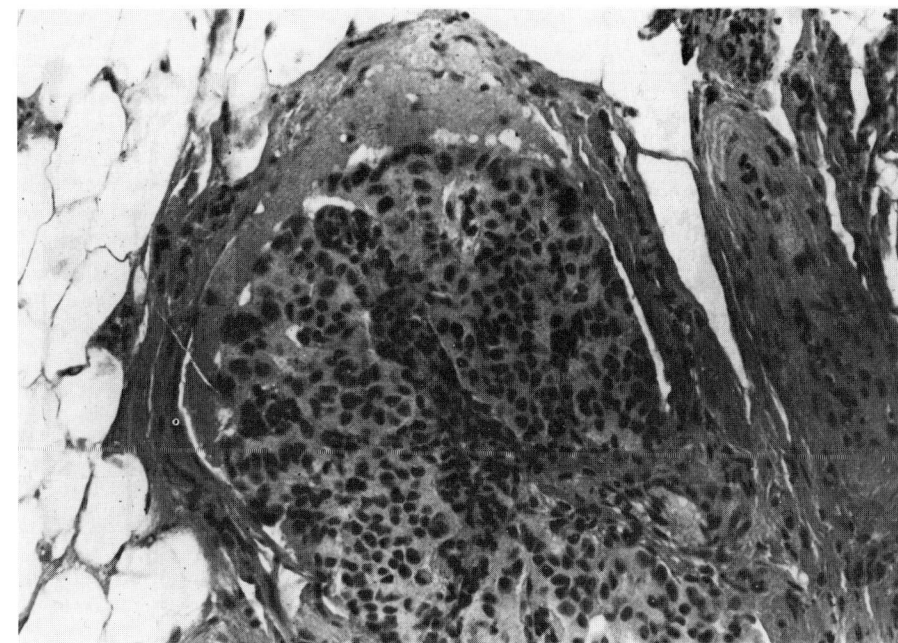

FIGURE 30-2 Bronchial carcinoid tumor, the most common adenoma in peripheral major bronchi, may present early because of mass effect obstructing the bronchus and because of the contrast in density with the surrounding air-filled lung when seen on chest x-ray.

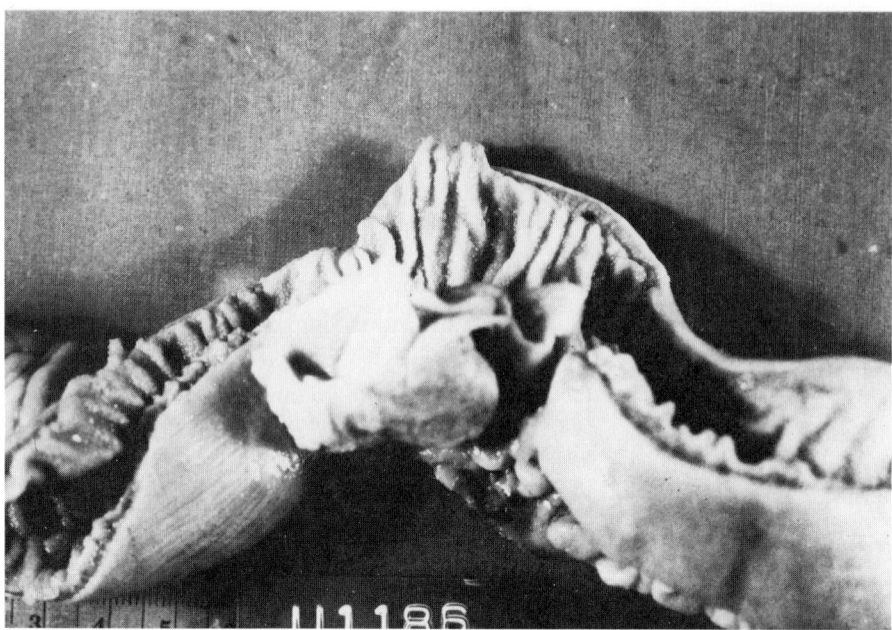

FIGURE 30-3 Intestinal carcinoid may be seen as a "filling defect" in the contrast-filled gut.

Absence of carcinoid syndrome, however, cannot be taken as evidence that carcinoid tumor has not metastasized. Only 6 percent of carcinoid tumors *with* metastases result in the carcinoid syndrome. Most of the metastatic carcinoid tumors are nonfunctional, including some tumors which can be shown to have produced elevated quantities of serotonin metabolites in patients who have never experienced the syndrome.

Most of the carcinoid staging information comes at the time of operation, and staging is as good as the surgeon's measurement of the size and description of the site of the primary tumor and any evident regional nodal or distant disease.

Tests for Diagnosing Carcinoid Syndrome

SERUM TESTS

Some blood tests may be used to confirm a diagnosis of carcinoid syndrome, usually after the diagnosis is suggested by clinical criteria and elevated urinary metabolites. Blood serotonin and histamine levels can be measured, and prostaglandin and bradykinin blood levels may be assayed in special research facilities. A positive test for elevations in these mediators would confirm the diagnosis, but false-negative results would be obtained if the carcinoid tumor and its metastases were not functionally active, or were not secreting as actively at the time of blood sampling as they would be during the carcinoid syndrome episode.

PROVOCATIVE TESTS

Such an episode can be induced by one of a number of provocative tests. Alcohol ingestion seems to trigger the carcinoid secretion. An epinephrine test has been designed to achieve a positive test endpoint—the carcinoid cutaneous flushing and hypotension. (The preponderance of serotonin and other depressor mediators overcomes the epinephrine pressor response to give a positive depressor test.) A calcium-provocative test has also been used to induce flushing and to provoke the cardiopulmonary and gastrointestinal features of a carcinoid attack.

METABOLITE SCREENING TESTS

The urinary 5-hydroxyindoleacetic acid (5-HIAA) excretion is the most useful single test of the presence of the carcinoid syndrome. A urine sample from a carcinoid syndrome patient during an attack is shown in Fig. 30-4 both before and after the addition of the reagent to show the presence of 5-HIAA in the darker urine sample. A 24-h urine collection is sampled for this breakdown product of serotonin (5-hydroxytryptamine) while the patient is on a diet free of serotonin-containing foods (such as fruits or nuts) or drugs which may interfere in the assay of 5-HIAA. Quantities of 2 to 9 mg of 5-HIAA are excreted normally in 24 h, and values above 15 mg per 24 h are strongly suggestive of an abnormal endogenous source of excess serotonin.

PRIMARY TREATMENT OF CARCINOID TUMOR

The primary treatment of carcinoid tumor is operation, and to this date at the present state of the art, there is no other option. Radiation therapy of carcinoid tumors has proved ineffective.

Surgical excision of the primary tumor itself is of great importance, giving the best chance of management of carcinoid for cure. The carcinoid tumor is amenable to surgical management because it is slow-growing, and local control is often curative. "Second-look" operations are often recommended because of the gratifying patient response to an operation that removes bulk tumor.

Regardless of the site of origin, isolated solitary carcinoid tumors are treated on the basis of the size of the primary lesion. Carcinoids smaller than 1.0 cm are locally excised, but carcinoids greater than 1.0 cm in diameter are treated as any other frank carcinoma by a "cancer operation," that is, en bloc resection of the tumor with wide margins that include the intervening regional nodes.

Anesthesiologic considerations are especially critical in the operative management of the patient with carcinoid. The anesthesiologist should maintain a careful awareness of the effects of carcinoid humors in the circulations, and should particularly exercise care to ensure a stable cardiovascular response to the potential infusion of multiple unknown mediators.

If the circulation is being supported with pharmacologic stimulation, a paradoxic response to injection of β-adrenergic agonists called "bradykinin shock" is seen. In response to catecholamine infusion, the carcinoid might release its mediators which may overwhelm the pharmacologic pressor response with their depressor actions. Compare this response to the anesthesiologist's pressor drug support with the provocative epinephrine test (see above) which seeks to induce flushing and hypotension.

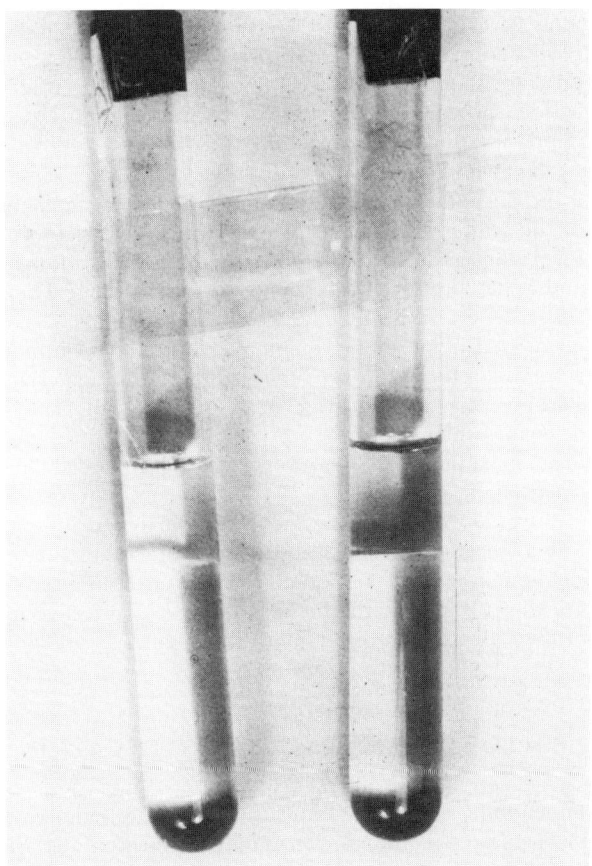

FIGURE 30-4 A positive urine test for 5-HIAA, a principal serotonin metabolite, for a patient with carcinoid syndrome during an attack of cramping abdominal pain and diarrhea.

ADJUNCTIVE THERAPY

Primary Carcinoid Tumor

Adjunctive therapy may be called in to help control the physiologic derangements of functionally active residual carcinoid tumor. No adjunctive treatment is needed if primary surgical excision has been successful and no neoplasm persists. Carcinoid syndrome is a special indication for adjunctive therapy. Special consideration will also be given to atypical carcinoid variants arising from carcinoid tumors at different primary sites.

Treatment of Carcinoid Syndrome

The pharmacology of carcinoid syndrome palliation is aimed at intervention in the serotonin pathway and in kinin mechanisms, at nutritional replacement and symptomatic drugs to reduce response at the target organ, and at antimetabolite chemotherapy.

Antiserotonin drugs are given chiefly to help in management of diarrhea, which is largely serotonin-dependent. Antiserotonin therapy does not do so much for flushing attacks, which seem to be dependent on other mechanisms (see below concerning antikinin therapy). Methysergide is a known serotonin antagonist, which—interestingly—has fibrosing complications in heart valves and retroperitoneum like those of the agonist serotonin it is given to counteract. But methysergide is helpful in controlling diarrhea, if given by a properly graded loading dose, with a period of interruption in therapy every few months to avoid the fibrosing complications of continuous treatment.

Another drug that is commercially available is cyproheptadine, which has both antiserotonin and antihistamine actions. It can be given continuously for management of carcinoid diarrhea. Two drugs that are investigational at this time are 5-fluorotryptophan, an analog of 5-hydroxytryptophan, and parachlorophenylalanine, an enzyme inhibitor that acts on tryptophan hydroxylase. Each of these experimental drugs interferes in serotonin synthesis, whereas available drugs have antiserotonin properties, blocking serotonin action at the target organ.

Antikinin treatment is designed to control the cutaneous flushing episodes experienced by many patients with carcinoid syndrome. The antiserotonin drugs are not effective in controlling flushing, which suggests that other humoral mechanisms may be more important than the serotonin that may come from the tumor. Several types of flushing are recognized in variants of the syndrome (see below), and there is poor correlation of the serum serotonin and urine 5-HIAA levels with flushing episodes. Direct infusion of serotonin does not often produce the characteristic carcinoid flush, although administration of catecholamines, kinins, ethanol, and calcium can provoke a flushing attack. Pentagastrin may provoke and somatostatin inhibit the carcinoid flush as recently described by Frolich.[3]

Blocking some of the agents that provoke flushing may prevent or ameliorate the flushing attack. Phenoxybenzamine is effective in those patients whose attacks are correlated with catecholamine provocation. Corticosteroids, though they have mild antiserotonin activity, are not uniformly beneficial in carcinoid syndromes, although they may be useful in the atypical prolonged flushing of bronchial carcinoid syndrome (see below). Another agent that can help patients with a specific variant of the carcinoid syndrome is methyldopa, which may prevent the atypical flush of the patients whose tumors lack the enzyme decarboxylase (see "Gastric Carcinoid" below). Somatostatin may be used in instances of life-threatening bronchoconstrictions.

Symptomatic management with an empiric agent to treat diarrhea includes the use of opiates, codeine, and Lomotil-type agents to slow transit times. Phenothiazines and antihistamines are sometimes useful in the management of flushing or asthmatic wheezing.

Nutritional support for the patient with carcinoid syndrome involves replacing the niacin that is not synthesized, since the carcinoid diverts most of the tryptophan substrate to serotonin production. To maintain protein synthesis and to prevent pellagra-like deficiency symptoms, every patient with carcinoid syndrome should receive supplementary niacin in the daily diet. Decreasing the transit time with the other antiserotonin drugs listed, besides preventing diarrhea, is an important step in improving nutrient absorption.

Antimetabolite chemotherapy of the carcinoid tumor itself is usually palliative as is the pharmacologic management of the symptoms of the carcinoid syndrome. Streptozotocin is an agent used somewhat specifically in apudomas, and it has produced a response in tumor size. 5-Fluorouracil, cyclophosphamide, and methotrexate have been used alone or in combination, with some tumor response reported. The carcinoid tumor is generally slow-growing, and the rate of response is not usually dramatic when chemotherapy is given. Carcinoid syndrome symptoms may be worse during antimetabolite chemotherapy.

Surgical therapy can be used as adjunctive treatment, with a "second look" or "debulking" of metastatic tumor yielding a positive response in the functioning slow-growing tumors. Radiotherapy has been ineffective as primary or adjunctive carcinoid treatment.

FOLLOW-UP AND EARLY IDENTIFICATION OF METASTASES

Functioning carcinoid tumor usually secretes endocrine markers, so screening for recurrent or persistent disease in follow-up can take the form of clinical examination for evidence of new primary tumors, or for development of carcinoid syndrome, checking for urinary metabolites (5-HIAA) and for evidence of dysfunction in liver or other organs that are commonly affected by metastatic disease.

The patient who has had a carcinoid tumor or tumors is at high risk for developing (1) other carcinoid tumors, (2) a nonendocrine malignancy, (3) endocrinopathy in another APUD-derived system.

Prognosis for the patient with treated carcinoid tumor is very favorable if the operative staging shows that the tumor was localized at the primary site. With regional and distant metastases, the survival rate falls progressively, as seen in Table 30-4, but the overall 5-year survival rate of patients with carcinoid tumor of all stages at all sites is an encouraging 82 percent.

CONSIDERATIONS FOR CHARACTERISTICS OF SPECIAL CARCINOID TUMORS

Bronchial Carcinoid

Bronchial carcinoid tumor is the most common bronchial adenoma, representing 85 percent of adenomas occurring in the bronchi. They occur in the periphery of major bronchi, and may cause few early symptoms, entering the differential diagnosis of "coin lesions" seen on chest x-ray of asymptomatic individuals (see Fig. 30-2).

Bronchial carcinoids may present earlier than carcinoid tumors elsewhere because they may give rise to obstructive symptoms such as intermittent wheezing. Hemoptysis is a major sign in clinical presentation, and was the means by which the bronchial carcinoid seen in Fig. 30-5 was first diagnosed.

Although composed of the same APUD-derived cells as other carcinoid tumors, the argentaffin reaction is *negative* for bronchial carcinoids. The tumor itself is more malignant in behavior than carcinoids elsewhere of similar size, and it metastasizes more frequently than corresponding midgut carcinoids. Bronchial carcinoids are also associated in familial multiple endocrine adenomatoses much more often than are other carcinoids.

Bronchial carcinoid syndrome can result from bronchial carcinoid, but it has a unique characteristic flushing, distinctive from that seen in gut carcinoids with metastases.[3] The flushing, rather than occurring in frequent brief spells, may be severe and protracted for days. Cholinergic-type effects are seen in tearing, drooling, vomiting, and diarrhea with a hot puffiness of the face that may persist through the length of the attack.

TABLE 30-4 Prognosis: 5-Year Relative Survival Rates by Site and Stage

Site	Stage			All stages, %
	Local, %	Regional, %	Distant, %	
Stomach	93	23	0	52
Small intestine and ileocecum	75	59	19	54
Appendix	99	100	27	99
Colon except rectosigmoid	77	65	17	52
Rectum and rectosigmoid	92	44	7	83
Lung and bronchi	96	71	11	87
All sites	94	64	18	82

SOURCE: Modified from the collected series reported by Godwin,[4] used with permission.

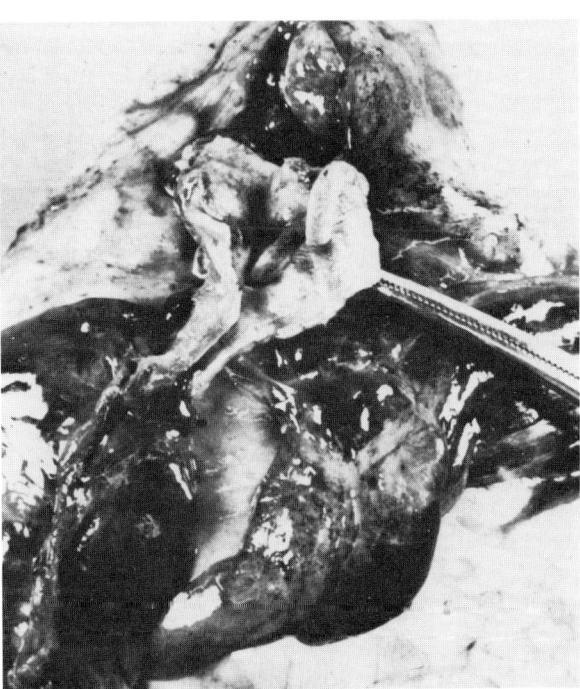

FIGURE 30-5 Gross appearance of a bronchial carcinoid that presented with hemoptysis and obstructive symptoms.

Asthmatic wheezing may occur from bronchoconstriction in the attack, and left-sided heart valvular disease of the fibrosing type may occur. Unlike gut carcinoids, liver metastases are not necessary for the syndrome to be present, and the endocardial lesions in the bronchial carcinoid syndrome are not predominantly right-sided. Patients with the bronchial carcinoid syndrome may be treated by corticosteroid drugs during the attack. Since corticosteroids are known to have an antikinin action, and because of a lack of evidence for a predominance of other carcinoid syndrome mediators, kinin release has been thought to be the major reason for the distinctiveness of the bronchial carcinoid syndrome.

Gastric Carcinoid

Gastric carcinoid tumors have the silver-staining characteristic of all other gut carcinoid tumors, but have a therapeutically important histochemical deficiency. These tumors lack the decarboxylase enzyme. Although they show an elevated 5-HIAA urinary excretion, the secretion that makes up most of the urinary catabolite is 5-hydroxytryptophan. This difference in hormone output makes for a clinically distinctive appearance, and for at least one significant pharmacologic management method.

Patients with gastric carcinoid tumors have attacks provoked by meals—particularly beef meals. Two mediators are implicated in further findings of the clinical features of these patients—the release of histamine and of gastrin. Peptic ulceration is higher in incidence in gastric carcinoid patients. The rash is a flare of coalescing patches. Pentagastrin administration can provoke such a flush in gastric carcinoid patients, and somatostatin can inhibit it as described by Frolich and coworkers.

The lack of the decarboxylase enzyme means that gastric carcinoid syndrome patients can be treated with methyldopa. This drug inhibits the functioning of the carcinoid tumors without decarboxylase, but does nothing to slow the growth rate. The drug slows neither the growth nor functioning of the majority of carcinoid tumors that have the decarboxylase.

Small-Bowel Carcinoid

Carcinoid tumor is the most common primary tumor of the small bowel. It has been described at every point from the pylorus to the ileocecal valve, especially including Meckel's diverticuli.[5,6] The closer the site is toward the appendix, the higher the reported incidence of carcinoid.

The usual clinical presentation of a small-bowel carcinoid tumor is an asymptomatic patient. Rarely does it give evidence of its presence by focal mass lesion effects, such as intestinal obstruction. When it does so, it may be because of its presence as a lead point for an intussusception. In retrospect, patients may report crampy abdominal pain of years' duration. A large number of the small-bowel carcinoids are encountered as incidental findings.

One-fourth of small-bowel carcinoids are multiple, and one-third of these tumors show metastases when first encountered at operation. Ten percent of all patients with small-bowel carcinoid show the carcinoid syndrome—a late presentation after liver metastases. Small-bowel carcinoids are frequently (up to 50 percent of cases) associated with another cancer, and often exploration for that other tumor uncovers the asymptomatic carcinoid.

Therapy for small-bowel carcinoid is surgical in both primary and secondary stages. An en bloc "cancer resection" is performed for the primary tumor and regional nodes. Residual metastatic disease, such as liver metastases, may also be subject to surgical attack, reducing the bulk of this slow-growing and possibly functional tumor. At the time of operation, a careful search is carried out for multiple carcinoids and also for another cancer.

Primary bowel carcinoids often have a fibrosing reaction around them if they penetrate serosa, possibly provoked by endocrine activity, which may cause adhesions in the peritoneal cavity. A further peculiarity is that metastases may exponentially outgrow the size of the primary tumor, growth of which may be much more indolent than presumably later tumor growth in lymph nodes and liver.

Appendiceal Carcinoids

The appendix is the most common site of carcinoid, and carcinoid is the most common neoplasm of the appendix.[7] The first encounter of many surgeons with this distinctive site of carcinoid comes through the medium of a pathology report 3 days after appendectomy showing carcinoid tumor in an appendix removed incidentally or because of classic indications of appendicitis.

In fact, about 0.5 percent of all surgically removed appendices are reported to show carcinoid tumor, usually not appreciated at the time of the operation. The rather benign behavior of these appendiceal carcinoids when not further treated after their incidental discovery in the appendectomy has led to their consideration as a different species of carcinoid tumor. The carcinoid cells and the tumor look the same (see Fig. 30-1) in microscopically examined appendiceal carcinoids, but rarely do these tumors metastasize, and almost never give rise to the carcinoid syndrome.

The case has been made that appendiceal carcinoids behave as all other carcinoids do when correlated as to size; Moertel has noted that only 2 percent of ileal carcinoids less than 1 cm in diameter metastasize. Even though it is said that appendiceal carcinoids present earlier at smaller size because they are more likely to obstruct the appendiceal lumen, this is not reconciled with the fact that for the majority of appendixes with carcinoid removed for appendicitis the carcinoid could not be implicated as an obstruction of the appendiceal lumen. Despite lymphatic invasion, serosal extension, invasion of the mesoappendix, or location at the appendiceal base—all formerly thought to be indications for reoperation and hemicolectomy—such indications have been discredited by Moertel's review of over 1000 appendiceal carcinoids treated only by appendectomy with only two recurrences. Appendiceal carcinoid seems to behave as a more benign disease, therefore, and reoperation for carcinoid at this site should *not* take place unless the tumor is over 2 cm in diameter, and has positive specimen margins, residual tumor, or node disease recognized at operation.

Rectal Carcinoid

Rectal carcinoid tumors behave as two diseases. As in the case of ileal compared with appendiceal carcinoids, there is no histologic difference between the two kinds of rectal carcinoids: the carcinoid cells look the same in each type and there is no histochemical difference as in bronchial or gastric carcinoids. But rectal carcinoids behave as benign (compare with appendiceal carcinoid) or very malignant tumors. The only suggested correlation with behavior is the size of the primary tumor; those patients with rectal carcinoids smaller than 2 cm in diameter had a good prognosis after limited local excision.

The term *metastasizing carcinoid of the rectum* is applied to those larger lesions which exhibit aggressive malignant behavior.[8] These tumors are treated as any rectal carcinoma with en bloc resection. Although the aggressive rectal carcinoid may invade and metastasize widely, it almost *never* gives rise to the carcinoid syndrome. Follow-up of such lesions relies on mass lesion findings discovered by rectal examination and proctosigmoidoscopy rather than checking for functional signs or hormone markers in urine or serum.

FUTURE PROSPECTS FOR CARCINOID TUMORS

The carcinoid tumor is a fascinating neoplasm balanced halfway between malignancy and benignancy. It is a good model to study for malignant transformation from tumor coexisting with the host to a cancer taking over and destroying its host. At each point along the way it gives off a dozen tumor markers by which its maturation, degeneration, or involvement with other organs can be assessed. Subtle biochemical shifts in its natural history can be reflected in its predominant hormone production, conditioned, to some extent, by the sophistication and differentiation of its enzymatic capabilities. It may revert to "wild" primitive metabolism, but still carries its APUD heritage.

As such, carcinoid may be a good model of tumor predeterminism versus how much behavior modification can be manipulated over its usually slow-growing history. The primary tumor often seems constrained by some inhibitions to which its daughter metastases are not sensitive in their more rapid growth. As with other APUD neoplasms, there are suggestions of regression with host or target manipulation, and successful surgical palliation may result by tipping the balance in favor of the host through removal of bulk disease.

The several variant subtypes of carcinoid syndromes are reflections of different pathophysiology of endocrine functions, but also of oncologic potential. That these tumors and their markers are found in association with multiple carcinoids, other endocrine neoplasms, and other cancers within the same patient and within MEA families is a fascinating "window" into genetic potential for cancer development within at least one system—the chromaffin system. This family of tumors broadens our concept of "field changes" and predisposition to malignant transformation.

The multipotential endocrine tumor cannot usually be judged under a microscope by usual cytologic criteria to be oncologically benign or malignant. Most of its injury to the host comes from overproduction of hormone or hormones, or—in the case of carcinoid—stealing nutrient from the host for its own overproduction. Some of these cells carry their innocent appearance with them to distant metastatic sites where they keep on producing their DNA-determined endocrine products. Two vital questions with respect to the function of endocrine tumors that represent different sides of the same coin are: What turns them "on"? How can they be turned "off" from their hormone production?

Several other questions remain that could be answered in the context of the mediator or the host: What host receptor modification can be accomplished to change the response at the target organ? What determines that bronchial carcinoids produce kinins predominantly, whereas carcinoids identical in appearance found lower down the enterochromaffin path produce predominantly serotonin? Can production be changed from one hormone type to another type for which there is better pharmacologic control—e.g., gastric carcinoid—by specific enzyme inhibitors?

In carcinoid tumor, as the archetype of endocrine neoplasm, the surgical investigator is less concerned with mass lesions than with function, modifying either hormone secretion or its receptor response. New understanding of the biochemical mechanisms have brought forth new pharmacologic agents in blocking or diverting synthesis or masking response. The next bright step in the future is in genetic understanding of repression or derepression of the faulty hormone-synthesis machinery, in which case multiple endocrinopathy such as represented in patients with carcinoid tumor can be prevented not only in the afflicted patient, but in the patient's family.

REFERENCES

1. Kaplan EL: The carcinoid syndromes, in SR Friesen (ed): *Surgical Endocrinology*, JB Lippincott, Philadelphia, 1978, p 120.
2. Pearse AGE et al: Polypeptide hormone production by "carcinoid" apudomas and their relevant cytochemistry. *Virchows Arch* 16:95, 1974.
3. Frolich JC et al: The carcinoid flush. *New Engl J Med* 299: 1055, 1978.
4. Godwin JC II: Carcinoid tumors: An analysis of 2837 cases. *Cancer* 36:560, 1975.
5. Ariel IM: Argentaffin (carcinoid) tumors of the small intestine. *Arch Pathol* 27:25, 1939.
6. Moertel CG et al: Life history of the carcinoid tumor of the small intestine. *Cancer* 14:901, 1961.
7. Moertel CG et al: Carcinoid tumors of the vermiform appendix. *Cancer* 21:270, 1968.
8. Wilson H et al: Carcinoid tumors. *Curr Probl Surg* 7:1, 1970.

SELECTED BIBLIOGRAPHY

Frolich JC et al: The carcinoid flush: Provocation by pentagastrin and inhibition by somatostatin. *New Engl J Med* 299: 1055, 1979.

Herbsman H et al: Tumors of the small intestine. *Curr Prob Surg* 17:121, 1980.

Marks C: *Carcinoid Tumors: A Clinico-Pathologic Study*. GK Hall, Boston, 1979.

Moertel CG, Hanley JA: Combination chemotherapy trials for metastatic carcinoid tumor and the malignant carcinoid syndrome. *Cancer Clin Trials* 2:327, 1979.

PART SIX

UROLOGIC NEOPLASMS

31
MALIGNANT TUMORS OF THE KIDNEY
Jean B. deKernion

RENAL-CELL CARCINOMA

History

The first recognition of carcinoma of the human kidney occurred sometime prior to 1883, the year in which Grawitz[1] described nephrectomy for a malignancy in the adult kidney. Several years later the name *hypernephroma* was attached to the Grawitz tumor in support of the misconception of Grawitz, that the tumor arose from adrenal tissue.[2] It is unclear from the literature how often total nephrectomy was attempted for renal carcinoma prior to the description of intravenous pyelography by Swick in 1929.[3] Contrast imaging of the renal parenchyma made possible the diagnosis of renal tumors and facilitated their early excision. Further progress in the managing of renal carcinoma awaited the development of diagnostic studies which more accurately segregated malignant from benign lesions of the kidney. Refinements in radiographic contrast studies, including improvements in nephrotomography, added significant accuracy to the diagnosis of renal carcinoma. Subsequently, the introduction of ultrasound further enabled the clinician to segregate cystic from solid renal masses, and thereby significantly influenced the treatment and decision-making process. Improvement in angiographic techniques, especially the development of aortic catheterization techniques, provided a high degree of accuracy in the study of renal parenchymal lesions.

The acknowledged therapy for renal carcinoma has been nephrectomy, since the original description by Grawitz. Recognition by Robson[4] of the importance of the excision of Gerota's fascia with the kidney was a major contribution to the surgical management of the tumor. Since this work, few important advances have been made in the therapy for renal carcinoma, and the major emphasis has been on early detection and treatment of metastatic tumor.

Epidemiology and Etiology

Renal carcinoma is a tumor of adults, occurring primarily in the fifth through the seventh decades of life, but it may occasionally occur in younger age groups.[5,6] Most studies have identified the origin of the tumor as the proximal convoluted tubule,[7] from the same cell of origin as renal adenomas. Numerous etiologic agents have been identified in various animals,[5] but no specific etiologic agent has been identified for human renal carcinoma. Several epidemiologic studies have incriminated tobacco as an etiologic agent although the specific carcinogen has not been described.[8,9] Bennington and Laubscher found a high incidence of renal carcinoma in British males who smoked pipes or cigars.[10] Although diethylstilbestrol causes typical renal-cell carcinomas in adult Syrian hamsters,[11] the hormone has not been shown to be associated with an increased risk of cancer in humans.

Occupational and industrial carcinogens have not yet been firmly linked to renal carcinoma. A recent study suggested an increased risk in male cigarette smokers who were exposed to industrial contaminants of cadmium.[12] No other relationship has been established, although research in this area has been limited. The radiographic agent thoratrast has been associated with a high incidence of renal carcinoma in one study.[13]

Adult renal carcinoma is a relatively rare tumor, accounting for approximately 3 percent of adult malignancies.[5] The tumor is more common among urban dwellers, and is most commonly found in males with a male-to-female ratio of approximately 2:1. Familial renal carcinoma has been reported, with as many as five family members being affected. Patients with von Hippel-Lindau disease[14] are known to have a higher incidence of carcinoma, and patients with polycystic kidney disease appear to have a predisposition to the development of renal carcinoma.

Signs and Symptoms

The classic triad of pain, hematuria, and presence of a flank mass is actually found in relatively few patients and usually indicates the presence of far-advanced disease. Patients more frequently present with one of these symptoms or with stigmata of local extension and tumor metastases, and complaints such as diffuse pain, weight loss, or anemia. Not infrequently, the tumor is an incidental finding on physical examination, or the presence of metastases is detected during examination for nonspecific symptoms. Fever, loss of appetite, malaise, or sudden onset of a varicocele in the male may be the only presenting complaint. We have seen numerous patients who were found to have multiple pulmonary metastases when a chest x-ray was performed for a vague, dry cough. Patients may occasionally present with symptoms secondary to paraneoplastic syndromes.

Renal carcinoma is associated with a variety of paraneoplastic syndromes. Erythrocytosis has long been recognized as a sign of renal carcinoma, and approximately 3 percent of patients with elevated red blood count have been found to have occult renal cancer. This is presumably due to a secretion of an erythropoetinlike substance. Hypercalcemia may occur but usually is due to extensive skeletal metastases. However, parathyroidlike hormone production by primary renal tumors has been reported.[15] The most common paraneoplastic syndrome is that of hepatic dysfunction in the absence of liver metastases. This has been reported to occur in approximately 40 percent of patients with renal carcinoma. Liver function may return to normal, and the hepatomegaly may resolve after nephrectomy, but the presence of the hepatopathy is a dire prognostic sign, and few such patients survive 5 years.[16] The syndrome, the etiology of which is unclear, is characterized by hepatosplenomegaly, elevated phosphatase levels, prolonged prothrombin time, and sometimes elevated serum haptoglobin level. Recently, Sufrin et al.[17] reported elevated peripheral renin blood levels in patients with high-stage and anaplastic lesions. Nephrectomy caused a fall in the plasma renin level, and the authors suggest that this may be a useful determinant of occult disease. Increase in the erythrocyte sedimentation rate has also been reported in renal carcinoma, and a marked elevation correlates with poor prognosis.[18,19]

Diagnostic Methods

Since the advent of pyelography, numerous advances have been made in the study of renal mass lesions. Numerous invasive and noninvasive methods have been devised primarily to segregate benign cysts from solid tumors. The degree to which each of the multitude of diagnostic methods contributes to the decision-making process, and the cost-effectiveness ratio of each, are still subjects of controversy among radiologists and urologists. In addition to contrast imaging methods of pyelography and arteriography, ultrasound, radionuclide scan, computerized axial tomography, venacavography, and percutaneous needle aspiration and biopsy have all been added to the diagnostic armamentarium. Disagreement exists as to the sequence in which these should be used and as to the point at which diagnostic studies have given sufficient information to yield to exploration and treatment. A schematic approach used by this author is depicted in Fig. 31-1.

The scheme is initiated on the basis of the presence or absence of symptoms, and relies upon the accuracy of infusion nephrotomography and ultrasound to determine the sequence of renal angiography and puncture of the renal mass. Nephrotomography has been shown to be highly accurate in diagnosing renal cysts, and when cyst puncture is added, the accuracy approaches 100 percent.[20] Ultrasonography should be used only as an adjunct in the diagnosis of renal mass lesions. In view of the small but definite misinterpretation of ultrasonography, even in the most skilled hands, it should never be the final step in the diagnostic evaluation of renal masses. It should assist in deciding when the presence

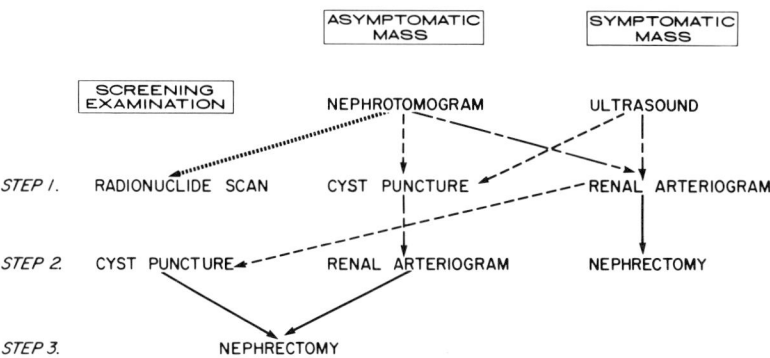

FIGURE 31-1 Schematic approach to the diagnosis of renal masses. The evaluation is based on whether or not the mass is symptomatic. Cyst puncture is not utilized unless the mass is cystic and avascular by ultrasound or nephrotomography, or renal arteriogram. *Solid line* = inconclusive, or diagnostic of renal cancer; *dotted line* = column of Bertin; *evenly dashed line* = avascular, cystic; *unevenly dashed line* = not proven cyst by all criteria.

of a benign cyst is likely, making aspiration a rational next step.

The imposition of needle aspiration and biopsy of suspected cysts has been promulgated by interested radiologists, who view this procedure as an extension of their diagnostic acumen. The procedure is not without complications such as hemorrhage and perforation of adjacent viscera. However, in skilled hands, with proper radiologic monitoring, major complications rarely occur.[21] The major concern has been the prospect of seeding tumor in the needle tract, and this has been reported.[22] We have also observed tumor growth in needle tracts in two patients after percutaneous aspiration of renal carcinoma metastases. However, with the use of the thin-walled 20-gauge needle, this has never been reported. Nonetheless, blind percutaneous puncture of a mass which has a high possibility of containing tumor is not warranted, and will add little to accuracy or decision making. Percutaneous puncture needle aspiration should be limited to patients in whom the diagnosis, by nephrotomography and/or ultrasound, is benign cyst, or in whom mitigating circumstances make angiography or surgery unduly hazardous.

This approach to the evaluation of renal mass is controversial, especially with respect to the use of percutaneous needle aspiration and the role of ultrasound. Many of these issues may become moot if computerized axial tomography proves to be reliable in the detection and differential diagnosis of renal mass lesions.

Staging

As with any malignant tumor, staging must be based on factors which influence survival. Renal vein involvement has long been thought to be associated with a poor prognosis,[23] but recent studies fail to show such a correlation.[24] This is perhaps due to the emphasis in recent years on complete excision of the renal veins, and identifying renal vein involvement preoperatively. Properly managed, extension of tumor into the renal veins and inferior vena cava does not significantly compromise survival.[24,25] The size of the primary tumor is only loosely correlated with survival, and is not a major factor in staging.[18]

The factors which have been shown to influence prognosis are regional lymph node involvement, invasion through the renal capsule, extension to contiguous organs, and distant dissemination. The presence of tumor in the lymph nodes draining the renal parenchyma is a dire prognostic sign, and the 5-year survival is approximately 33 percent. Invasion through Gerota's fascia into the perinephric fat was a greater detriment to survival prior to the widespread adoption of radical nephrectomy, because the renal capsule was not excised. Even after radical excision of Gerota's fascia with the kidney, the extension of tumor into the perinephric fat decreases 5-year survival to about 45 percent.[24] When tumor extends to contiguous organs, rarely does a patient survive 5 years, even after surgical excision. The significance of local tumor recurrence or persistence is reflected in our study of patients with metastatic renal carcinoma.[26] Those who had the tumor incompletely excised (usually due to contiguous extension) had a much poorer prognosis than those who developed distant metastases without local recurrence of tumor.

The staging system commonly in use is Robson's[4] modification of the system of Flocks and Kadesky, graphically depicted in Fig. 31-2. The shortcomings of the system become obvious when it is noted that the survival of patients with stage 2 (or B) tumor is less than that of patients with stage 3 (or C) disease, indicating an inappropriate assignment of prognostic factors. The group-

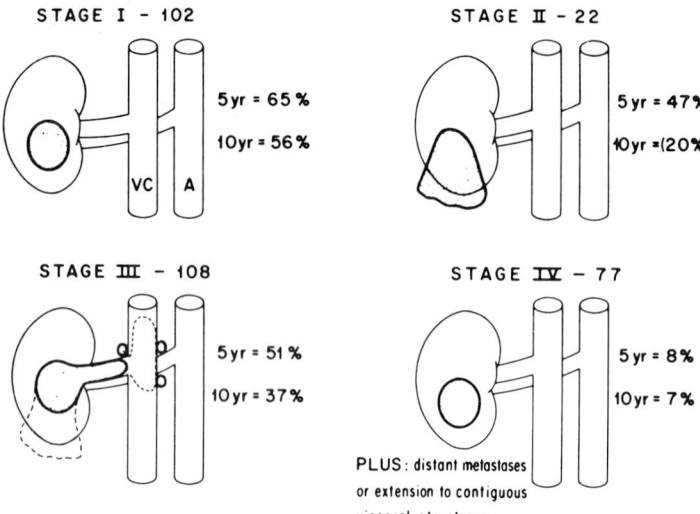

FIGURE 31-2 The commonly used staging classification after Robson's modification of the system proposed by Flocks and Kadesky. Renal vein involvement is placed on an equal prognostic scale as lymph node involvement. Vena caval extension is not segregated as to whether the tumor involves the infradiaphragmatic or supradiaphragmatic vena cava. The extent of the lymph node involvement is not quantitated. (*From Skinner DG et al: Surgical management of renal cell carcinoma. J Urol 107:705, 1972.*)

ing of renal vein, vena caval, and lymph node involvement into stage 3 causes survival to be higher since simple renal vein extension is not a dire prognostic factor. The TNM system proposed by the American Joint Committee for Cancer Staging and End-Results Reporting (Table 31-1) separates venous involvement from nodal invasion and quantitates each, and as such is an improvement over the system in common use. Tumors extending into the capsule are grouped with those extending into the vein in the T_3 category, but are separated by subclasses (T_{3a}, T_{3b}, T_{3c}). The shortcoming of the proposed TNM system is the number of subgroups, which are cumbersome and deter enthusiastic acceptance by clinicians.

Critical to any staging system is an accurate assessment of the degree of local spread, and the presence of distant dissemination. The assessment of the primary lesion should include determination of invasion of adjacent organs or abdominal wall invasion, the presence of extension into the renal vein or vena cava, and the presence of metastases to regional organs and lymph nodes. The angiogram is the single most important test in the assessment of the primary lesion. In addition to establishing the size and malignant nature of the tumor with great accuracy, selective renal arteriography may detect adrenal metastases and invasion of abdominal wall or adjacent viscera. A selective arteriogram of the contralateral kidney is also important to rule out the presence of bilateral tumors, which occur in a small percentage of patients. Considerable information is also obtained from the aortic injection. Knowing the size and number of arteries to the involved kidney is helpful in the planning of surgery. Extension of tumor to the paraspinous muscle or to the paraaortic lymph nodes can often be detected by the presence of neovascularity arising from the small lumbar arteries. Whenever feasible, hepatic angiography should be performed at the same time as the selective renal visualization, especially for right-sided lesions. Invasion of the liver by direct extension or through metastases can often be detected with considerable accuracy in this manner.

Extension of tumor into the renal veins and vena cava can influence surgical approach and prognosis. Although the angiogram often gives valuable information about the presence of renal vein invasion, an inferior venacavogram is vital to the determination of extension of tumor thrombus into the vena cava.

The use of lymphangiography to assess extension into the regional lymph node has not proven to be beneficial. While massive extension of tumor may be detected in the high paraaortic nodes, the reliability of the test does not warrant its routine use as a staging method. The advent of computerized axial tomography has provided a new method of assessing the primary tumor. The axial tomography not only assists in the diagnosis of the renal mass lesion but can provide valuable insight into extension of adjacent structures. Extension of tumor into regional nodes can also be detected by the tomography,

TABLE 31-1 Stage Classification of Renal-Cell Carcinoma

Tumor status	Robson	TNM
No primary	—	T_0
Small primary, minimal distortion	A	T_1
Large tumor, renal distortion	A	T_2
Involving perinephric tissues	B	T_{3a}
Involving renal vein	C	T_{3b}
Involving renal vein and inferior vena cava	C	T_{3c}
Invading adjacent structures	D	T_{4a}
Involving superior vena cava	C	T_{4b}
No nodes involved	A, B	N_0
Single, ipsilateral node involved	C	N_1
Involvement of multiple regional nodes	C	N_2
Fixed regional nodes	C	N_3
Involving juxtaregional nodes	C	N_4
Distant metastases	D	M_1

but the reliability of detection of nodal metastases has not yet been determined. The role of axial tomography in the diagnosis and staging of renal tumors may well become more important in the future.

In addition to lymphogenous dissemination, the most common sites of distant metastases from renal carcinoma are lungs, skeletal system, and liver. Chest x-ray is therefore important, but full-lung tomography is usually restricted to patients who have poorly defined or suspicious pulmonary lesions on the plain films. Computerized axial tomography may prove to give greater resolution than routine radiographic studies, but the interpretation of the many small lesions detected by axial tomography has not been satisfactorily studied. Chest radiographs will also demonstrate the presence of extensive mediastinal involvement, which, although unusual, can occur as the only detectable site of metastasis.

Radioisotope scanning of the skeletal system has supplanted the skeletal survey in the routine evaluation of renal carcinoma patients. Subclinical metastases can occasionally be detected. The value of the isotope bone scan is markedly enhanced by simultaneous radiographs of suspected regions, especially in the joint areas. In this way, localized increased isotopic uptake in areas of inflammation or arthritis can be detected and properly interpreted. Occasionally, lesions cannot be interpreted with assurance, and biopsy of suspected lesions is important if the presence of metastases will change the treatment decision. Liver scan was previously a routine part of the evaluation of patients with renal carcinoma. Recent studies have, however, shown that in the patient with a normal liver function test, liver scan will rarely detect hepatic metastases. We therefore reserve liver scan for the patient who has abnormal liver function tests and/or enlarged liver on physical examination. Similarly, although cerebral metastases are not common, radioisotope brain scan or computerized axial tomography of the skull are worthwhile when the patient has central nervous system symptoms.

Prognosis

The natural history of renal-cell carcinoma is more unpredictable than that of most tumors, and has been a subject of interest to urologists for many decades. The tumor is the second most common tumor to undergo spontaneous regression, many times after removal of the primary lesion. Thus far, over 70 cases of spontaneous regression of renal-cell carcinoma have been reported in the literature, although biopsy confirmation of metastases was documented in only 52 cases.[27] A further unusual manifestation of renal-cell carcinoma is the variability in growth of the primary tumors, which occasionally have remained localized for many years. Occasionally metastatic foci appear to have a propensity for long periods of growth arrest, and metastatic lesions have been identified many years after complete removal of the primary tumor. Finally, the behavior of metastatic foci is unusual in the frequently observed varying growth and tumor doubling time of metastases, particularly pulmonary lesions. Pulmonary parenchymal metastases may temporarily regress or undergo growth arrest for varying periods, followed by sudden decrease in tumor doubling time. The unusual behavior in some patients, however, does not detract from the lethality of this neoplasm.

The largest series of patients with untreated renal-cell carcinoma was reported by Riches in 1964.[28] The 3-year survival rate was 4.4 percent and the 5-year survival was 1.7 percent for 443 untreated patients. Only occasionally have patients with disease limited to the kidney

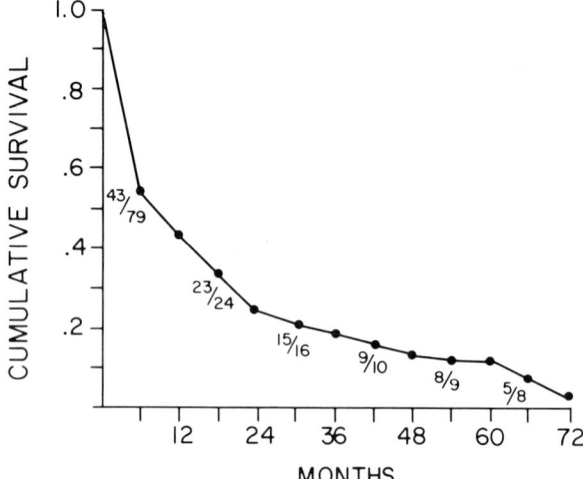

FIGURE 31-3 The cumulative survival of patients with metastatic renal cell carcinoma depicts the poor prognosis. The 1-year survival rate was 42 percent and the 5-year survival rate was 12 percent. All patients eventually died of metastatic renal carcinoma.

not been operated upon, and most develop local progression and metastatic spread within 5 years.

Survival appears to be dependent mainly upon the extent to which thumor has invaded and spread locally, and upon the presence of absence of distant metastases. The influence of local invasion and spread will be discussed below. Once metastases develop, survival depends primarily on the extent of the disease and the interval between nephrectomy and appearance of metastases.[26] Figure 31-3 demonstrates the cumulative survival for 86 patients with metastatic renal-cell carcinoma who were followed at UCLA and affiliated hospitals between 1972 and 1976. The 1-year survival rate of 42 percent and the 5-year survival rate of 12 percent are higher than those previously reported.[4,29] However, when the patients are segregated into groups according to the time of appearance of metastases, the dire prognosis of those with metastases when first diagnosed is apparent. Figure 31-4 demonstrates that patients who had metastases at the time of diagnosis, or developed them within 6 months, had a 1-year survival of only 10 percent, and all were dead by 2½ years. Those who developed metastases more than 2 years after nephrectomy had a 1-year survival of 55 percent and a 5-year survival of 22 percent. Katz and Davis[29] reported an 18 percent 1-year survival in such patients, and Middleton[30] reported no survival after 2 years. These statistics emphasize that most patients who develop metastases have an unrelenting progression of tumor within a short time. The incidence of regression is less than 1 percent, showing the rarity with which this occurs. Furthermore, some of these may not have been permanent spontaneous cures, but simply transient regressions of lesions which were never biopsied.

TREATMENT OF RENAL-CELL CARCINOMA

Localized Renal Carcinoma (Stages A, B, and C)

The mainstay of treatment of primary renal carcinoma is surgical excision. The role of adjuvant preoperative or postoperative radiotherapy is discussed in a subsequent section of this chapter. The object must be to completely excise the local tumor. In the past, simple nephrectomy was advocated, but the current practice of radical nephrectomy appears to have significantly increased patient survival.[31,32] Radical nephrectomy includes excision of Gerota's fascia and its contents, including the kidney and adrenal gland. In all previous reports, invasion of perinephric fat has been shown to be an important determinant of survival, and survival can be expected to be seriously compromised by the leaving of microscopic or gross tumor in Gerota's fascia after a simple nephrectomy.[24,25,31] Similarly, although the importance of renal vein invasion has been debated, failure to remove gross tumor from the renal vein results in decreased survival. The importance of the radical nephrectomy is, therefore, obvious.

Those who have reported improved survival in renal carcinoma following radical nephrectomy have also attributed this improvement to excision of the regional lymph nodes.[4,24] Regional nodal involvement is unquestionably an important prognostic factor, since it indicates dissemination. In most series, it is not possible to segregate and analyze the survival of patients with lymph node metastasis and assess its influence on survival. Skinner[24] reported a 17 percent 10-year survival in patients with regional lymph node involvement. The extent and location of the involvement of regional nodes, as well as the number of patients who received postoperative radiotherapy, is not known. It seems reasonable that the improved survival rate since the advent of radical nephrectomy with lymphadenectomy is more likely to be due to more complete excision of the tumor rather than excision of involved regional lymph nodes. Although an occasional patient might be cured when only one or two nodes contain tumor, the true contribution of lymphadenectomy to survival has not been demonstrated. It is, however, a valuable method of staging and will become more important as adjuvant clinical treatment trials are instituted.

The surgical technique of radical nephrectomy has been graphically described by several authors,[33,34] and the approach is guided more by individual preference than by necessity. Stewart[35] prefers a transperitoneal approach since this allows early ligation of the renal artery and vein before tumor manipulation. This is an essential factor in surgery for renal carcinoma, and any approach used must incorporate this prerequisite. Others have employed extraperitoneal and extrapleural flank incisions.

The thoracoabdominal incision described by Chute et al.[36] is especially suitable for large and upper pole lesions. The surgical technique of this intrapleural approach, along with the modification of reflecting the peritoneum medially and approaching the kidney extraperitoneally, has been thoroughly described.[33] Considerable dissection is performed prior to ligating the vessels, but this can be done safely without manipulation. The dorsolumbar osteoplastic flap, as described by Nagamatsu[37] also provides excellent exposure. The main limitation of transperitoneal anterior approaches is difficulty in dissecting the paraaortic and paracaval lymph nodes above the renal pedicle, especially on the left side. Advocates of this approach, however, feel comfortable with the thoroughness of the procedure, and have little difficulty removing the large upper pole tumors after early ligation of the vessels. Occasionally, a flank approach utilizing the eleventh interspace allows excellent exposure without producing the added morbidity caused by entering the chest or peritoneum. We have used this approach for lower pole as well as upper pole renal tumors, and had excellent exposure as long as the eleventh rib costovertebral ligaments were divided, allowing the rib to be deflected downward.[38]

The outcome of surgical therapy for renal carcinoma is affected by tumor stage, by the grade of the tumor, and by the histological type. The type of surgical therapy also influences survival, and statistics prior to the widespread practice of radical nephrectomy cannot be compared to more recent survival figures. In addition, the use of various staging systems makes comparison of data impossible. Broad statements can be made, however, with respect to survival after surgical therapy.

After radical nephrectomy for stage A renal carcinoma, 5-year survival is from 65 to 75 percent, while survival for patients with stage 2 lesions varies from approximately 47 to 65 percent.[4,18,24,39] In Robson's series,[4] in which all patients underwent radical nephrectomy, the survival of patients with stage B tumors (extension through capsule) was identical to that for patients with stage A disease, presumably due to more thorough excision of tumor and a decreased local tumor recurrence. The survival of patients with stage C disease varied from 35 to 51 percent, again depending upon the number of patients included who had renal vein involvement without lymph node involvement or extracapsular extension. It is also important to note that interpretation of renal vein invasion varies among pathologists.

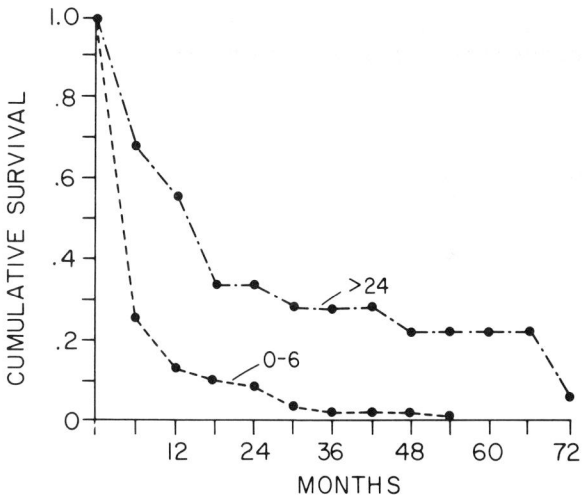

FIGURE 31-4 Prognosis of patients with metastatic renal cell carcinoma is dependent upon the interval between the diagnosis of the primary tumor and the clinical appearance of metastases. Patients who either had metastases at the time of diagnosis (0) or develop them within 6 months (6) had a more favorable prognosis than those who developed metastases more than 24 months after removal of the primary lesion.

RENAL ARTERY OCCLUSION

With the advent of more sophisticated angiographic methods, preoperative percutaneous transaortic occlusion of the renal artery has been advocated as a routine procedure. This makes radical nephrectomy technically easier since the renal vein can then be divided without first having to dissect the renal artery, which has already been occluded. The maneuver also decreases hemorrhage, especially in patients with large locally extensive tumors. Another reason given for routine preoperative renal arterial occlusion is that the destruction of tumor is associated with a stimulation of host immune response. This, however, has not been conclusively demonstrated. Furthermore, the procedure is sometimes associated with complications even in the best of hands, and the patients suffer considerable pain, fever, and nausea which may occasionally compromise their ability to tolerate extensive surgery. Urologic surgeons have safely and effectively performed radical nephrectomy, including early ligation of the renal artery and vein, for years without the benefit and the cost of catheter occlusion. Thus far, little evidence has been produced to suggest that this is appropriate as a routine measure. However, in patients with very vascular tumors or very large bulky tumors, this procedure can facilitate radical nephrectomy.

RADIATION THERAPY

Radiation therapy has been applied in the treatment of renal-cell carcinoma in two major areas: the treatment of metastatic foci, and as an adjuvant to surgical therapy. The role of preoperative radiotherapy is still controversial. Several reports have shown an increased survival with the preoperative use of radiotherapy.[40,41] The Genitourinary Oncology Group has completed a prospective cooperative study to evaluate preoperative radiation therapy (4500 rads) followed by radical nephrectomy versus nephrectomy alone. Preliminary data* suggest that the radiotherapy has a slight impact on survival, but further long-term follow-up will be necessary to determine the significance of the findings. The randomized study conducted by Werf-Messing[42] compared 3000 rads of preoperative therapy to no preoperative radiotherapy. Five-year survival was not improved, although the incidence of recurrence in the renal fossa was significantly diminished.

---

* Personal communication, Claire Cox, M.D., 1979.

Postoperative radiotherapy has not been shown to affect survival.[43,44] Indeed, survival after postoperative radiotherapy was diminished in several studies.[44,46]

Treatment of Stage D Renal Carcinoma

The only definitive treatment for the patient with invasion of adjacent structures by primary renal carcinoma is extensive surgery. Renal tumors usually are encapsulated and do not directly invade adjacent organs. However, liver invasion is not uncommon, and invasion of the psoas muscle occurs with aggressive, anaplastic lesions. Whenever possible, attempts should be made to excise the tumor completely even if excision of adjacent organs such as bowel, spleen, and muscle are required. En bloc partial hepatectomy is rarely curative, and I know of no patient cured of renal carcinoma once tumor involved the liver. Although extensive regional lymph node metastases usually indicate that the patient is not curable, excision of the regional node in patients with limited nodal involvement may occasionally be curative and certainly is warranted when there is no evidence of distant metastasis. The importance of extended radical surgery to remove completely the primary tumor is obvious when one realizes that no effective systemic therapy for recurrent or persistent tumor now exists, and when the prognosis of patients with incomplete resection is understood. Figure 31-5 shows the cumulative survival of patients who had incomplete excision of renal carcinoma. Although many patients had only very minimal or even microscopic tumor remaining, no patients survived longer than 12 months.

Approximately one-third of patients with renal carcinoma have distant metastases when the diagnosis is first made. For many decades, the treatment of such patients has been palliative or adjunctive nephrectomy in spite of the distant metastases.

The practice of excision of the primary renal carcinoma in the presence of metastases has been advocated both for relief of symptoms secondary to the primary lesion, and in the hope of inducing spontaneous remission of the metastatic foci. Palliative nephrectomy for severe symptoms, such as local pain, hemorrhage, and endocrinopathy, appears to be justified in the patient who has a reasonable expectation of survival for at least 6 months. Several factors, however, influence the palliation produced by such surgery. First, although pain is a common symptom, few patients have pain which cannot be controlled by narcotic analgesics. The presence of

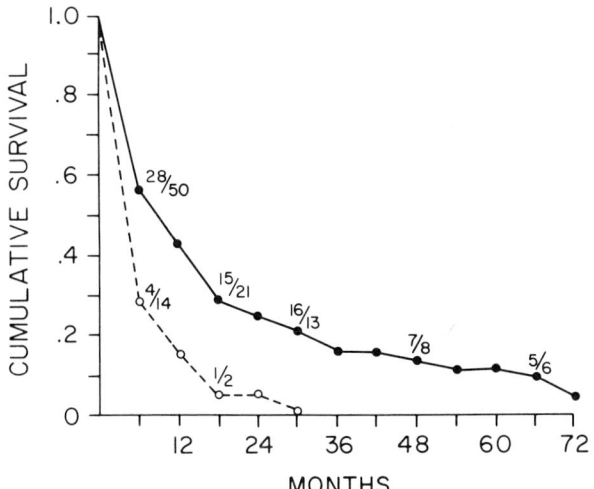

FIGURE 31-5 Patients who had incomplete excision of the primary tumor had a poorer prognosis than patients who did not develop local recurrence but rather developed distant metastases. *Solid line* = no; *dashed line* = yes.

severe pain usually indicates invasion of the abdominal wall, precluding complete surgical excision. As noted above, patients in whom tumor is incompletely excised rarely survive for 6 months after surgery.[26] Secondly, life-threatening hemorrhage from the primary tumor is not a common occurrence. Thirdly, when performing surgery for palliation, it is important to understand the prospects for survival. The mean survival of patients with metastases at the time of diagnosis is approximately 4 months, and only 10 percent of such patients survive 1 year.[26] In spite of these qualifiers, however, nephrectomy can produce relief of troublesome symptoms and improve quality of life in a selected group of patients.

The practice of nephrectomy in patients who present with metastases at the time of diagnosis, in whom the primary tumor is not producing severe symptoms, was based upon the hope of inducing spontaneous regression of metastases or prolonging survival.[47] No clinical trials have affirmed the benefit of this practice, which stems from several observations about the natural history of renal carcinoma rather than from established fact. No therapy for disseminated renal carcinoma is currently effective, and the surgeon is compelled to pursue any method of therapy which has even the most remote potential for benefit. The natural history of renal carcinoma suggests that intrinsic host factors play a role in growth and dissemination of the tumor. From these observations was extrapolated the concept that an association existed between the behavior of the distant foci and the presence of the primary lesion. Finally, spontaneous regression of metastases has been reported, in some instances, after removal of the primary tumor.[27,48]

Since the phenomenon of spontaneous regression is most often inculcated to justify the practice of palliative or adjunctive nephrectomy, it is important to scrutinize the literature to ascertain the validity of the observations and the incidence with which regression occurs. In 1973, Bloom[48] reported approximately 40 cases of spontaneous regression of renal carcinoma, and many more have been anecdotally described in recent years. In all but two instances, regression occurred in patients with pulmonary metastases, and in 80 percent of cases, the patients were males. It is important to note that most of the patients did not have histologic documentation of the metastatic foci, and regression as reported cannot be equated with long-term cure. The incidence in which the spontaneous regression of metastases occurs is more important than the absolute number of reported anecdotal cases. The incidence of regression is only 0.4 percent or 1 in 250.[49] In many series, spontaneous regression was never noted. No instance of regression was noted in 533 patients reviewed at the Mayo Clinic,[23] and Mostifi[52] reported only two survivors 2 years after diagnosis among patients with metastases at the time of diagnosis.

The incidence of regression of distant metastases after palliative adjunctive nephrectomy is, perhaps, more germane to the discussion. A summary of a recent series of patients undergoing palliative nephrectomy indicated that the incidence of regression was only 0.8 percent.[50] It is important to reiterate that many of the metastatic lesions were not documented by biopsy, and that regression was often only for a brief period of time. Furthermore, the mortality rate varies from 2 to 15 percent, depending upon patient selection. Based on these statistics, it is difficult to support the routine practice of palliative nephrectomy for the purpose of inducing regression of metastatic lesions.

The impact of palliative or adjunctive nephrectomy on survival of patients with metastatic disease rather than on the induction of spontaneous regression may be important. Johnson et al.[51] did not find a significant difference in survival between patients who underwent palliative nephrectomy and those who did not, except in the case of patients with metastases confined to the skeletal system. In our series, we noted a significant greater survival of patients who underwent palliative nephrectomy.[26] However, this was obviously on the basis of selection, since only patients in good clinical condition were considered to be candidates for surgery. In order to assess the influence of palliative nephrectomy on survival, we compared the cumulative survival of all patients who underwent palliative nephrectomy to the cumulative survival of the entire series of patients with metastatic renal carcinoma, regardless of therapy (Fig. 31-6). It is obvious that the survivals of the two groups are identical, suggesting that factors other than the nephrectomy determined the clinical course. In certain situations, however, palliative nephrectomy can be supportable.

Patients occasionally present with a limited number of metastases which are treatable by surgery or by definitive radiotherapy. Following excision of pulmonary metastases, 5-year survival rate is between 25 and 35 percent.[39] Excision of other solitary foci or tumors can sometimes produce significant palliation. In the series of patients studies by this author,[26] aggressive therapy of solitary skeletal, central nervous system, and skin or subcutaneous lesions produced a significant palliation interval. It seems reasonable, therefore, to recommend nephrectomy in such patients along with definitive therapy of the limited metastatic foci. A second potential indication for palliative nephrectomy is in the patient who has been shown to respond to some form of systemic therapy. Our current management of the patient with an asymptomatic primary lesion and widely disseminated metastases is to recommend a 3- to 4-month trial of systemic therapy, either chemotherapy or immunotherapy or a combination of both modalities (see below). If at the end of the trial period the metastatic lesions have either decreased in size or remained stable, no new lesions have developed, and the patient's general clinical status has not deteriorated, we then offer palliative nephrectomy to the patient. It is difficult to determine whether the therapy or simply the growth characteristics of the tumor are operative. Regardless, such patients can be expected to have a reasonable survival period and might be well served by excision of the large primary lesion.

Johnson et al.[52] have recently advocated a combination of percutaneous renal artery occlusion followed by nephrectomy and hormonal therapy. Several patients in their series have undergone regression of metastases following the combination of infarction and nephrectomy, suggesting an immunologic effect. However, long-term survival occurs rarely, and the data do not yet support this approach in routine practice.

Tumor in the Solitary Kidney and Bilateral Simultaneous Tumors

Renal-cell carcinoma in the solitary kidney has been reported in over 90 cases in the literature and has recently been the subject of an extensive review by Wickham.[53] Only in recent years have aggressive attempts been made and techniques devised to excise the tumors yet leave sufficient renal parenchyma to maintain the patient's life without renal dialysis. In addition to standard partial nephrectomy, more elaborate methods have been devised for larger tumors and tumors which are centrally located in the renal parenchyma: in vivo partial nephrectomy with regional hypothermia, ex vivo ("work-

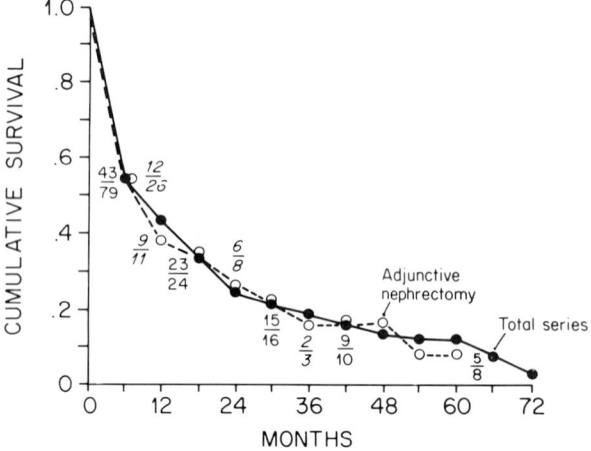

FIGURE 31-6 The cumulative survival of patients who underwent adjunctive nephrectomy is demonstrated on the same graph as the cumulative survival of the entire series of patients with metastatic renal carcinoma. The total series included patients who either presented with metastases or developed metastases at various times in their follow-up and included patients who did or did not undergo adjunctive nephrectomy. The survival is almost identical, suggesting that it is more dependent on factors of natural history than on the surgical intervention.

bench") excision, and autotransplantation. The choice of the surgical procedure depends upon the location of the tumor and the projected degree of difficulty and time required for complete excision with a rim of normal renal parenchyma. Small tumors or tumors peripherally located or situated in the upper or lower pole can often be excised very simply by partial nephrectomy. The Kaufman partial nephrectomy clamp is extremely useful in this situation. The clamp can be applied above or below the involved renal pole without the need to occlude the main renal artery, thereby obviating the need for regional hypothermia. After excising the tissue adjacent to the clamp, the collecting system can be repaired and large vessels ligated in a relatively bloodless field. Troublesome bleeding can be partially controlled by the judicious use of synthetic collagen preparations.

When the tumor is large or is centrally located in the solitary kidney, simple partial nephrectomy is not practical. The major renal artery must be isolated and occluded. This can be most simply accomplished by using either regional hypothermia in vivo or by employing the newer techniques of workbench surgery. In vivo partial nephrectomy with hypothermia has the obvious advantage of not requiring autotransplantation with its potential complications. Most tumors can be adequately treated in this manner unless extensive microsurgical reconstruction or multiple vascular anastomoses are required. Also, a large tumor in a large patient can sometimes best be managed in this way. After exposing the kidney through either a thoracoabdominal extraperitoneal excision or a modified flank incision, the renal artery is isolated. The patient is given a diuretic, usually 25 g of mannitol, and the renal artery is gently occluded with a Rummel tourniquet. The kidney, in Gerota's fascia, is then mobilized and surrounded with a plastic sheet. The sheet is then filled with iced saline slush and the surrounding tissue is insulated by multiple gauze packs surrounding the plastic sheet. The tumor along with the attached Gerota's fascia is then excised with a small margin of normal renal parenchyma. Next the collecting system is carefully and meticulously closed with nonabsorbable suture material. The transected vessels are ligated with suture ligatures prior to releasing the arterial clamp. The remaining blood vessels are then transfixed after the arterial flow is reconstituted. The use of fat or fascia over the denuded kidney often assists hemostasis and healing. The actual safe ischemia time has not been definitely determined, but occlusion with hypothermia for up to 60 min is well tolerated.

Ex vivo surgery has certain advantages over the simpler in vivo methods. First, the tumor is better visualized and the collecting system and vascular systems are more rapidly identified and repaired. Second, ex vivo angiography is possible, although this is seldom necessary or practical. Thirdly, a standard radical nephrectomy with regional lymphadenectomy is possible by this method. This last advantage is of minimal value, since regional lymphadenectomy probably seldom improves survival and is more important as a staging procedure. Furthermore, excision of the Gerota's fascia adjacent to the tumor is all that is necessary, and this is possible by in vivo surgery. Distinct disadvantages of ex vivo surgery are the complexity of the technique, the need for vascular and sometimes ureteral anastomosis, increased operating time and morbidity, and prolonged hospitalization. In selected cases, however, the procedure may be the only way to excise the tumor and preserve functioning renal parenchyma.

After isolating the vessels, the renal artery is clamped close to the aorta, and the renal artery is infused either with a cold electrolyte solution or with continuous mechanical perfusion. The standard radical nephrectomy is performed, except that the ureter may sometimes be left attached to the bladder. When possible, this is preferable, but the ureter should be temporarily and gently occluded during the procedure so that the ureteral blood supply does not continuously warm the kidney. After excision of the tumor and meticulous reconstruction of the vessels and collecting systems, an autotransplantation is carried out in the ipsilateral pelvic fossa. When the ureter has not been divided, the upside down position of the kidney and the uphill ureteral drainage appear to present no problems in the postoperative period.

Using the various methods of excision of tumor in the solitary kidney has brought very satisfactory results. Most recent series relate the 5-year survival to whether the contralateral kidney had been either agenetic or removed for benign disease, or had been removed for the presence of a renal carcinoma. In patients who had not previously had a renal carcinoma in the contralateral kidney, the 5 year survival rate is approximately 65 to 70 percent. However, when the patient previously underwent nephrectomy for a renal carcinoma, the 5-year survival has been only approximately 40 percent. This is approximately equal to the 5-year survival obtained by excision of a solitary metastasis. Furthermore, the results of excision are directly related to the interval between the nephrectomy on the contralateral side and the appearance of the tumor in the remaining solitary kidney. Both facts suggests that the tumor in the remaining kidney is often actually a metastatic focus rather than a second tumor, although this is purely circumstantial evidence. It is important to note that a recent report showed that survival is not related to the presence or absence of tumor in the contralateral kidney, suggesting that the difference in survival may be due to more conservative, less definitive surgery in the patient previously known to have a renal carcinoma.[54] Regardless, the resectable tumor in the solitary kidney should be aggressively treated and definitively excised whenever the patient's general condition permits.

Prognosis of patients with simultaneously appearing bilateral renal carcinomas is uniformly poorer. When radical nephrectomy on one side and partial nephrectomy on the other side is practiced in such patients, less than 20 percent of patients survive 2 years. Although the follow-up on such patients is not detailed, it appears that most actually die from other distant metastases rather than from local regrowth or recurrence. This suggests that most patients have other metastases when first diagnosed, and supports the contention that simultaneous renal tumors actually represent metastasis from one kidney to the other. Indeed, in most cases one kidney harbors a large tumor, and the other kidney harbors a much smaller lesion. Regardless of the poor prognosis, if the presence of distant metastases has been ruled out, the patient should undergo a radical nephrectomy on the side with the largest tumor, and partial nephrectomy on the side of the smaller lesion. The surgical technique depends on the surgeon's choice. We usually prefer to excise both lesions simultaneously through a Chevron incision or a midline incision which can be carried transthoracically and intrapleurally on the most involved side. In a very obese patient, separate oblique flank incisions are preferable. When extensive intrarenal dissection or ex vivo surgery is required, the operations should be performed several weeks apart. Also, when serious doubts exist about the ability to preserve sufficient parenchyma to maintain the patient without dialysis, the kidney with the less extensive tumor which will be expected to maintain renal function should be operated first. In this way, if renal parenchyma cannot be preserved or if a nephrectomy is necessitated by technical considerations, the patient may prefer to simply live as long as possible with the tumor in the remaining kidney off of dialysis. Some such tumors often are fairly slow growing, and the patient may live a satisfactory life for several years.

A final option for the patient with simultaneous renal tumors or with tumor in the solitary kidney is radical and complete nephrectomy followed by chronic hemodialysis. This is seldom a chosen method of treatment for obvious reasons but should be mentioned to the patient as a potential method of completely excising the renal carcinoma. Renal transplantation in such patients has not been practiced often, but immunosuppression following transplantation may potentially activate microscopic slow-growing occult foci of tumor.

FOLLOW-UP CARE

The most likely areas of renal-cell carcinoma recurrence or metastasis following the nephrectomy are in the wound, in the renal fossa, the lung, liver, bone, and mediastinal lymph nodes. Patient follow-up after nephrectomy must be designed to detect recurrence in these areas. The patient should have a careful physical examination every 3 months during the first year and every 6 months thereafter. Chest x-ray, CBC, and liver function tests are also important every 3 months for the first year and every 6 months thereafter. Liver chemistries are especially important in patients who had the renal carcinoma–induced hepatopathy prior to nephrectomy since subsequent return of abnormal enzyme assays may indicate early tumor recurrence. Similarly, serum calcium determination should be performed in order to detect early hypercalcemia due to skeletal metastases. We routinely obtain a radioisotope bone scan at 6 and 12 months following nephrectomy and then yearly thereafter. Bone scan is also performed whenever the patient complains of skeletal or joint discomfort. Routine use of bone scan is a debatable issue since its expense mitigates against its frequent use, and thus far, there is little systemic therapy that can be offered the patient when diffuse skeletal metastases are found. As treatment for widespread metastases improves, bone scan may occupy a more significant role in the follow-up. Detection of renal fossa recurrence is difficult and often is not suspected until the patient has significant weight loss and chronic discomfort. We have treated many patients who complained of vague pain deep in the region of the previous surgery, in whom physical examination failed to reveal evidence of tumor mass. In such patients, ultrasound examination occasionally reveals a solid mass. However, ultrasound in this situation often fails to identify small masses and the "sheetlike" spread or recurrence of tumor in the retroperitoneum. The distorted anatomy following radical nephrectomy and lymphadenectomy also can make interpretation of the computerized axial tomography difficult, unless the mass is large. The modality, however, may play an increasingly important part in the detection of retroperitoneal and paraspinal recurrence. Aortography will often identify tumor recurrence with a high degree of accuracy. The flush aortogram and selective catheterization of enlarged lumbar vessels or hepatic arteries can often unveil metastatic foci not detectable by physical examination. Once the presence of the metastasis is confirmed by any of the above modalities, it is often important to perform a confirmative percutaneous needle biopsy before initiating radical systemic therapy. This is best performed by the skilled radiologist using the thin-walled needle, directed either by fluoroscopic or ultrasonic control.

A second major reason for follow-up of patients following nephrectomy is for detection of tumor in the remaining contralateral kidney. Although this is not a usual occurrence, approximately 3 percent of patients will present with tumors in the opposite kidney after nephrectomy. As mentioned above, surgical therapy can often be curative in such circumstances, and the early detection of the lesion is therefore important. The patient should have a urinalysis every 6 months thereafter. We recommend intravenous pyelogram at 6 and 12 months following nephrectomy, and once a year thereafter. Any patient who develops gross or microscopic hematuria or discomfort in the region of the remaining kidney also undergoes pyelography at that time.

TREATMENT OF TUMOR RECURRENCE

The primary factors influencing the treatment of recurrent renal carcinoma are the number of metastases (single or multiple), the location, the interval from nephrectomy to identification of recurrent tumor, and the general age and condition of the patient. The patient who presents with a single metastasis or several metastases adjacent to each other is best treated by surgical excision, with an expected survival as high as 30 percent for 5 years. This is especially applicable to patients with isolated pulmonary recurrence, small wound recurrence, or skin and subcutaneous metastases. We have treated several patients who underwent repeated excision of isolated metastases over an 8- to 12-year period. Although the 5-year survival is reasonable, few such patients are cured of their tumor, and almost all succumb to advanced metastatic disease at sometime during their follow-up. Figure 31-7 illustrates the cumulative survival of patients who underwent excision of isolated metastases, and indicates that a significant palliation interval can be achieved by such surgery. The patients who profit most by excision of metastases are those whose metastases occur at more than 2 years after their nephrectomy, probably because such tumors have a less aggressive malignant potential.

Occasionally, a single metastasis to the skeletal system presents as first evidence of tumor recurrence, and such patients may be cured by amputation of a finger or part of a limb. This, however, seems to be rather drastic therapy in view of the fact that solitary skeletal metastases are a rarity, and most patients manifest diffuse skeletal involvement within a few months. External beam radiotherapy is very effective in the management of skeletal metastases, and the patient with an apparently solitary metastasis should undergo definitive therapy to that

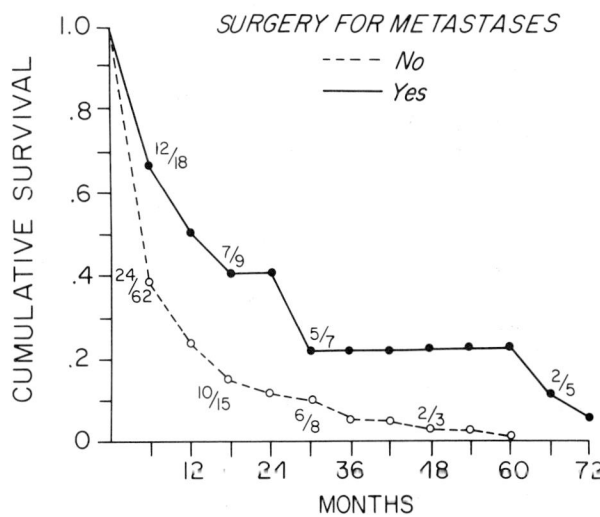

FIGURE 31-7 Patients who underwent excision of isolated lesions had a period palliation which was greater than for patients who could have excision of tumor, and was greater than that of the population of patients as a whole (see Fig. 31-2).

lesion. Also, patients with painful skeletal lesions often have dramatic pain relief following radiation therapy.

Since renal carcinoma metastases are lytic lesions, extensive bony destruction is common. When this occurs in the upper extremities or weight-bearing areas of the pelvis or lower extremities, consideration should be given to prophylactic orthopedic intervention. Prophylactic nailing with stabilization by use of methylmethacrylate may decrease the morbidity which follows pathologic fracture.[55] Definitive orthopedic treatment of such lesions is practical in patients who have a 3-month or greater life expectancy, since it will enable them to remain ambulatory, and it will decrease the pain of an unstable fracture.

The presence of multiple and diffuse metastases demands systemic therapy, in the form of chemotherapy or hormonal therapy.

The observation that the progestational agents inhibit the growth of the stilbestrol-induced tumor of the golden Syrian hamster provided the stimulus for clinical trials in humans.[56] The initial report was encouraging, and isolated reports of regression of tumor after progestational therapy continued to appear. In 1973, Bloom[48] reviewed the literature and reported an objective response rate of approximately 15 percent in patients with metastatic renal carcinoma. These statistics were derived from nonrandomized studies, and it is possible that the "responses" were simply manifestations of the natural history of the tumor. In recent years, no report has substantiated the role of progresterones in the treatment of this disease. In 65 patients we reviewed who were treated with either progestational agents and/or androgens at UCLA between 1971 and 1974, no evidence of a single objective response was noted. Although the toxicity of progestational therapy (nausea, vomiting, edema, and breast tenderness and uterine bleeding in the female) is usually not severe, little evidence exists in support of its benefit in this disease.

Chemotherapeutic agents had no significant effect on metastatic renal-cell carcinoma. Numerous review articles have documented trials of many single agents with dismal results.[44,57,58] Hrushesky[59] recently reviewed retrospectively the activity of 35 chemotherapeutic agents. He found a 25 percent objective response rate following therapy with vinblastine sulfate. This surpassed the activity of any other single agent, or any combination of agents. We have treated 14 patients with vinblastine sulfate and noted stabilization of growth of metastatic lesions in three patients and partial regression in one patient. No patient had complete regression of tumor. No response to any other chemotherapeutic agent or combination of agents was observed in 71 patients reviewed. It therefore appears that vinblastine sulfate is the most effective agent currently available, although its true effect in inducing regression must be established by future randomized trials.

WILMS'S TUMOR

History

In 1899, Wilms[60] described the renal tumor of childhood and reviewed the current literature to that time. The tumor was almost uniformly fatal in this era, prior to the advances in antisepsis and anesthesia. In the early part of the twentieth century, surgical management improved, but the surgical cure rate was less than 25 percent; death was usually due to distant metastasis or inability to completely resect the lesion. The introduction of cancer chemotherapy provided the impetus for evaluation of cytotoxic agents in the pediatric age group, and in 1963 Sutow[61] reported significant results with vincristine and the treatment of Wilms's tumor patients. Since 1969, the National Wilms's Tumor Study has been responsible for further strides in therapy through controlled clinical trials in a cooperative fashion.

Wilms's tumor is an uncommon malignancy, occurring in 1 live birth per 150,000 in the United States.[62] Most lesions occur in the first 7 years of life, although adult Wilms's tumor has been reported in patients in the second or third decade of life. There is no sex predominance, and bilaterality occurs in approximately 6 percent of patients.

Signs and Symptoms

Most childern have few symptoms unless the disease is allowed to progress extensively prior to medical attention. The most common method of presentation is palpation of an abdominal mass, and this occurs in over 90 percent of the patients. Abdominal discomfort, weight loss, and fever also may occur. Hematuria is not a common complaint, although microscopic hematuria occurs in up to 30 percent of patients. Renin levels are increased, and the instance of hypertension has been reported in as high as 60 percent.[63]

An unusual characteristic of this tumor is the high incidence of associated congenital anomaly. Aniridia and hemihypertrophy occur in a small but significant percent (3 percent) of patients, and the finding of either anomaly strongly suggests the presence of Wilms's tumor. Genitourinary malformations, umbilical hernias, and microcephaly have been associated with Wilms's tumor, although the relationship is not well founded as with aniridia and hemihypertrophy.

Diagnostic Methods and Staging

The intravenous urogram is the single most important test in the diagnosis of Wilms's tumor. Total nonfunction of the kidney is rare, and differentiation from neuroblastoma is usually possible on the basis of the pyelogram. Wilms's tumor tends to distort and displace the calyceal system whereas neuroblastoma tends to displace the entire kidney and collecting system. Calcification occurs in approximately 10 percent of Wilms's tumors and is much more common (50 percent) in neuroblastoma. A venacavogram can be obtained at the time of the pyelogram by injecting the contrast through a leg vein or by retrograde injection of the inferior vena cava. The degree of displacement of the vena cava or of involvement by tumor is of some value in surgical planning.

Arteriography is seldom indicated in the young child, and the diagnosis of Wilms's tumor seldom depends on the selective angiographic study. However, the angiogram is invaluable in the assessment of the extent of bilateral or recurrent tumor. In the patient with very poor function and severe distortion of the collecting system, ultrasound is a help in discerning cystic from solid mass. Similarly, the computerized axial tomography will have an increasingly important role in both the diagnosis and staging of this tumor.

Laboratory studies should include complete blood count, liver function studies, serum electrolyte levels, and renal function analysis, either by serum analysis or by quantitative differential renal scan. If liver function tests are abnormal, liver scan is necessary. Skeletal scan or survey and pulmonary tomograms are important staging tests.

Although the urgency to complete the diagnosis and staging evaluation of patients with suspected Wilms's tumor is not emphasized as it was in the past, the entire work-up should be expiditious and can usually be completed within 48 to 72 h.

The staging system most commonly in use is that proposed by the National Wilms's Tumor Study, outlined in Table 31-1. This staging system emphasizes the factors which influence prognosis. In addition to the presence of metastases, invasion of the renal capsule and extension to the regional lymph nodes are associated with a decreased survival.[64] The degree of anaplasia[65] and the size of the tumor also influence prognosis. The age of the patient appears to be an important factor, since patients under the age of 2 at the time of diagnosis have a better prognosis. After age 2, the tumor is diagnosed in a higher stage, accounting for the decreased survival.

Therapy

The treatment of Wilms's tumor is a multimodality effort. No single method of therapy has been proved as effective as a critical intermingling of surgery, radiation therapy, and chemotherapy.

The surgical procedure must accomplish several goals. First, the exact extent of the tumor must be ascertained by careful exploration and excision of the regional lymph nodes, exploration of the liver, and thorough visual examination of the exposed opposite kidney. Secondly, the entire tumor must be excised if possible. A transabdominal approach affords the needed exposure and allows exploration of the contralateral kidney. A true radical nephrectomy should be performed with minimal manipulation of the tumor prior to occlusion of the artery and vein. Tumor spillage changes the prognosis, and every effort should be made to avoid entering the tumor mass. The regional lymph nodes along the aorta and vena cava should be excised to facilitate accurate staging. Tumors extending into the spleen, muscle, or tail of the pancreas may be removed along with the involved organs. However, a "super-radical" approach with excision of major organs seems to be unwarranted and does not improve survival.[66] It is better in such instances to biopsy the lesion and demur in favor of radiation therapy and subsequent reexploration.

Radiation therapy is usually administered according to the program outlined by the National Wilms's Tumor Study. The amount of therapy is adjusted according to the age of the patient, and is begun within 48 hours after surgery. The remaining kidney is shielded, and the entire operative field is radiated. All patients receive radiotherapy, including those in groups I and II. Preoperative irradiation does not appear to be beneficial unless the tumor is initially unresectable.[67] In children under the age of 2 with group I tumors which are completely resected, postoperative radiotherapy appears to be of no benefit and is reserved for older children with group I disease or patients with higher stage tumors. Metastatic lesions to lung, bone, liver, and brain appear to respond to aggressive radiotherapy

Chemotherapy is probably the single most important factor accounting for the improvement in survival of Wilms's tumor patients, both as adjuvants to surgical therapy, and in the treatment of metastatic disease. Vincristine and actinomycin D are the current mainstays of cytotoxic therapy, and are used either as single agents or in combination. Therapy is begun as soon as a diagnosis is secure and is continued on a carefully prescribed program for up to 15 months. The details of the current program have been formulated by the National Wilms's Tumor Study.[68]

Follow-Up Care

Follow-up is facilitated by the program of postoperative adjuvant chemotherapy which the patient undergoes. Careful physical examination and chest x-ray should be performed every 3 months during the first 2 years. Recurrence after 2 years is unusual. Periodic blood counts and liver function tests are important to detect early hepatic or skeletal malignancies. Since approximately 3 percent of patients without evidence of tumor in the contralateral kidney will later develop lesions in the opposite kidney, intravenous pyelography should be performed every 6 months for the 2 years, or whenever either hematuria or change in renal function suggests the occurrence of tumor.

Treatment Results

Survival seems to be directly related to the stage of the disease and the other prognostic factors stated in the previous section. Nonetheless, with optimal combination of surgery, radiation therapy, and chemotherapy, the difference in survival between patients with group 1 disease and those with group 4 disease is not as striking as expected with other tumors. The best survivals obtained in the National Wilms's Tumor Study I were as follows: group 1, 97 percent; group 2, 89 percent; group 3, 86 percent; and group 4, 77 percent. Current and future clinical trials with other cytotoxic agents may further improve this already impressive cure rate.

Treatment of Bilateral Wilms's Tumor

Bilaterality at the time of diagnosis occurs in approximately 5 percent of patients with Wilms's tumor. It is important to note that approximately 30 to 40 percent of such patients are not suspected of having bilateral disease until the time of exploration. In the review by Bishop[69] 87 percent of patients survived 2 years or more, and survival was common even in patients with residual disease. In view of these promising results, overly aggressive surgery is not indicated, and excessive doses of radiotherapy are probably not warranted.

Treatment of Tumor Recurrence

Since the use of postoperative radiotherapy to the tumor bed, tumor recurrence in the renal fossa is unusual. Most metastases occur in the lung, liver, bone, brain, and superficial lymph nodes. Multiple pulmonary metastases or nonresectable metastases in brain or liver often respond to radiotherapy. Solitary or several metastases in the lung and even the liver are best treated, when possible, by surgical resection. Recurrences in the abdomen should be excised when feasible, and all patients with recurrence or metastatic disease should have the benefit of aggressive multidrug chemotherapy.

NEUROBLASTOMA

Etiology

Neuroblastoma is the most common solid tumor of childhood and infancy, and occurs most in children under the age of 5 years. The tumors arise from primordial neural crest cells derived from the fetal spinal cord. The stimulus for neoplastic transformation is unknown, and no significant evidence incriminating maternal exposure to viral or chemical agents has been presented.

Neuroblastomas may arise in any area where neuroblasts are found, usually adjacent to the spinal column. Seventy-five percent arise in the abdomen, most of them in the adrenal. The next most common site is the thorax (15 percent), but tumors have also been identified from the cervical area to the pelvis.

Signs and Symptoms

Most patients with neuroblastoma present with evidence of an abdominal mass which is usually large and frequently fixed and which frequently crosses the midline. Abdominal pain is a common presenting complaint along with abdominal distention and gastrointestinal complaints. Frequently, the child is noticed to be constitutionally ill with failure to thrive, pallor, and irritability. Since a significant number of children, approximately 80 percent, have skeletal metastases at the time of diagnosis, bone pain and fever are common presenting complaints.

Retroorbital metastases are common, causing proptosis and occasionally hemorrhage. This is sometimes the initial presenting complaint in the patient with neuroblastoma.

Diagnosis and Staging

The diagnosis of neuroblastoma is suspected in the infant with an abdominal mass, or with presenting complaints as just discussed. The major differential diagnosis is between neuroblastoma and Wilms's tumor. Flocculent calcifications occur in approximately 50 percent of patients with neuroblastoma, and this is a helpful differentiating sign. Neuroblastomas seldom cause hydronephrosis, and calyceal distortion is usually produced by extrinsic compression and displacement rather than the intrinsic distortion of the Wilms's tumor. The laboratory determination most likely to confirm the diagnosis is urine assay for vanillymandelic acid, which is elevated in approximately 75 percent of patients.[70]

Once the diagnosis is established, metastatic work-up is critical. Bone survey will be the most helpful test in detecting metastatic disease, especially in the spine, femur, and humerus. Radioisotope bone scans will sometimes detect lesions not found on plain radiographs.

The prognostic factor determines the basis for the staging system depicted in Table 31-2. The size of the primary lesion, involvement of adjacent structures, and the presence of distant metastases are primary prognostic factors. The distribution of metastases also appears to be important. Patients who do not have radiographically evident skeletal metastases appear to have a better prognosis than patients in either stages III or IV. The site of origin of the tumor is also important since tumors of the thorax and pelvis have a more favorable prognosis than tumors elsewhere. The age at diagnosis also markedly influences prognosis. Patients under 1 year of age have approximately a 70 percent chance of long-term survival, whereas patients over age 2 survive for 2 years in less than 10 percent of cases.[71]

Treatment

In contrast to Wilms's tumor, the cure rate for neuroblastoma has not materially changed in recent decades.

TABLE 31-2 Staging of Neuroblastoma

Stage 1	Confined to organ of origin
Stage 2	Extends beyond organ but does not cross midline (ipsilateral nodes possibly involved)
Stage 3	Extends beyond midline (nodes possibly involved bilaterally)
Stage 4	Remote metastases
Stage 4-S	Stage 1 or 2 patients whose remote disease is confined to one or more of the following sites: liver, skin, bone marrow

Surgical excision is still the major and most effective method of cure. When possible (stages I and II), complete surgical removal of the tumor with the kidney or adrenal gland, if indicated, is usually possible. When the tumor is not completely resectable, some controversy exists as to the advisability of removal of as much tumor as possible. If such a procedure appears to be feasible without undue risks to the patient, excision of the major part of the tumor may be salutary. Massive operations with resection of vital structures do not seem to be indicated and do not appear to improve survival. Excision of the primary lesion in the face of widespread metastasis does not appear to be beneficial unless the patient is in stage IV-S, without demonstrable skeletal metastases.

An alternative approach to the patient with nonresectable neuroblastoma is simple exploration, staging, and biopsy, followed by chemotherapy and radiation therapy with a subsequent "second look" procedure. In the patient who demonstrates a good response to radiation and chemotherapy, the second look procedure with excision of residual tumor appears to be rational.

Chemotherapy has not had a major impact on the outcome of neuroblastoma. Cytoxan, vincristine, and dimethyltriazeno-imidazole-carboxamide are the mainstays of therapy.[72] Other agents such as doxorubicin and immunotherapeutic agents such as methanol-extractable residue of bacillus Calmette-Guérin have also shown some antitumor action, but their role in the treatment of the tumor is as yet poorly defined.

The results of treatment reflect our current inability to cure the majority of patients with neuroblastoma. The 2-year survival of patients with abdominal neuroblastoma in all stages reported by the Children's Hospital of Philadelphia was 23 percent, and was 65 percent for those with tumor in the thorax.[71] When all patients were considered, the total survival was 32 percent at 2 years.

Survival by stage was as follows: stage I, 82 percent; stage II, 50 percent; stage III, 38 percent; stage IV, 14 percent; stage IV-S, 57 percent. It is important to note that 5-year survival, especially for patients with stage III and IV disease, would be considerably less. It is hoped that future development of new chemotherapeutic and immunotherapeutic agents will improve the cure rate of this common malignancy of childhood.

REFERENCES

1. Grawitz P: Die sogennanten lipome de Niere. *Virchows Arch [Pathol Anat]* 93:39, 1883.
2. Birch-Hirshfeld FV Doederlein A: *Zentralbl Krankh Horn Sex Org* vol. 3, 1894.
3. Marshall V: Methods in urographic diagnosis, In, J Emmett, S Witten (eds): *Clinical Urography,* Saunders, Philadelphia, p 1, 1971.
4. Robson CJ et al: The results of radical nephrectomy for renal cell carcinoma. *Trans Am Assoc Genitourin Surg* 60:122, 1968.
5. Bennington JL, Beckwith JB: Tumors of the kidney, renal pelvis, and ureter, in *Atlas of Tumor Pathology,* fasc 12, Armed Forces Institute of Pathology, Washington, DC, 1975.
6. Ward JS, Middleton RG: Renal-cell carcinoma in children. *Urology* 2:50, 1973.
7. Tannenbaum M: Ultrastructural pathology of human renal cell tumors. *Pathol Annu* 6:249, 1971.
8. Weir JM, Dunn JE Jr: Smoking and mortality: A prospective study. *Cancer* 25:105, 1970.
9. Kantor AF et al: Epidemiology of renal cell carcinoma in Connecticut. *J Natl Cancer Inst* 57:495, 1976.
10. Bennington JL, Laubscher FA: Epidemiologic studies on carcinoma of the kidney: I. Association of renal adenocarcinoma with smoking. *Cancer* 21:1069, 1968.
11. Kirkman H: *Natl Cancer Inst Monogr* 1:1, 1959.
12. Kolonel LN: Association of cadmium with renal cancer. *Cancer* 37:1782, 1976.
13. Wenz W: Tumors of the kidney following retrograde pyelography with colloidal thorium dioxide. *Ann NY Acad Sci* 145:806, 1967.
14. Lauritsen JG: Lindau's disease: A study of one family through six generations. *Acta Chir Scand* 139:482, 1973.
15. Goldberg MF et al: Renal adenocarcinoma containing a parathyroid hormone–like substance and associated with marked hypercalcemia. *Am J Med* 36:805, 1964.
16. Boxer RJ et al: "Non-metastatic" hepatic dysfunction associated with renal cell carcinoma. *J Urol* 119:468, 1978.
17. Sufrin G et al: Hormones in renal cancer. *J Urol* 117:433, 1977.
18. Bottiger LE: Prognosis in renal cell carcinoma. *Cancer* 26:780, 1970.
19. Kaufman JJ, Mims MM: Tumors of the kidney, in MM Ravitch et al (eds): *Current Problems in Surgery,* Year Book, Chicago, p 1, 1966.
20. Lang EK: Asymptomatic space-occupying lesions of the kidney: A programmed sequential approach and its impact on quality and cost of health care. *South Med J* 70:277, 1977.
21. Zelch J et al: Complications of renal cyst exploration versus renal mass aspiration. *J Urol* 7:244, 1976.
22. Gibbons RP et al: Needle tract seeding following aspiration of renal cell carcinoma. *J Urol* 118:865, 1977.
23. Myers GH et al: Prognostic significance of renal vein invasions by hypernephroma. *J Urol* 100:420, 1968.
24. Skinner DG et al: Extension of renal cell carcinoma into the vena cava: The rationale for aggressive surgical management. *J Urol* 107:711, 1972.
25. McCullough DL, Gittes RF: Ligation of the renal vein in the solitary kidney: Effects on renal function. *J Urol* 113:295, 1975.
26. deKernion JB et al: Natural history of metastatic renal cell carcinoma: Computer analysis. *J Urol* 120:148, 1978.
27. Freed SZ et al: Idiopathic regression of metastases from renal cell carcinoma. *J Urol* 118:538, 1977.
28. Riches E: The natural history of renal tumors, in *Tumors of the Kidney and Ureter,* Livingston, Edinburgh, p 124, 1964.
29. Katz SA, Davis JE: Renal adenocarcinoma: Prognosis and treatment reflected by survival. *Urology* 10:10, 1977.
30. Middleton RG: Surgery for metastatic renal cell carcinoma. *J Urol* 97:973, 1967.
31. Robson CJ: Radical nephrectomy for renal cell carcinoma. *J Urol* 89:37, 1963.
32. Patel NP, Lavengood RW: Renal cell carcinoma: Natural history and results of treatment. *J Urol* 119:722, 1978.
33. Skinner DG, deKernion JB: in DG Skinner, JB deKernion (eds): *Genitourinary Cancer* Saunders, Philadelphia, p 107, 1978.
34. Graham JB: Renal malignancies, in J Glenn (ed): *Urologic Surgery,* Harper & Row, Hagerstown, p 73, 1975.
35. Stewart BH: Radical nephrectomy, in Stewart BH (ed): *Operative Urology: The Kidney, Adrenal Gland, and Retroperitoneum,* Williams & Wilkins, Baltimore, 1975.
36. Chute R et al: The value of the thoraco-abdominal incision in the removal of kidney tumors. *N Engl J Med* 241:951, 1949.
37. Nagamatsu G et al: Dorsolumbar approach to the kidney and adrenal with osteoplastic flap. *J Urol* 63:569, 1950.
38. deKernion JB: Radical nephrectomy, in RE Ehrlich (ed): *Modern Techniques in Surgery.* Futura, New York, pp 1–14, 1980.
39. Skinner DG et al: Diagnosis and management of renal cell carcinoma. *Cancer* 28:1165, 1971.
40. Cox CE et al: Renal adenocarcinoma: Twenty-eight year review with emphasis on rationale and feasibility of preoperative radiotherapy. *J Urol* 104:53, 1970.
41. Riches EW: The place of radiotherapy in the management of parenchymal carcinoma. *J Urol* 95:313, 1966.

42. Van der Werf-Messing B: Carcinoma of the kidney. *Cancer* 32:1056, 1973.
43. Middleton RG, Presto AJ III: Radical thoracoabdominal nephrectomy for renal cell carcinoma. *J Urol* 110:36, 1973.
44. Lokich JJ, Harrison JH: Renal cell carcinoma: Natural history and chemotherapeutic experience. *J Urol* 114:371, 1975.
45. Finney R: An evaluation of post-operative radiotherapy in hypernephroma treatment: A clinical trial. *Cancer* 32:1974.
46. Peeling WB et al: Postoperative irradiation in the treatment of renal cell carcinoma. *Br J Urol* 41:23, 1969.
47. Goodwin WE et al: Under what circumstances does "regression" of hypernephroma occur? in JS King Jr (ed): *Renal Neoplasia*, Little, Brown, Boston, 1967.
48. Bloom HJG: Hormone-induced and spontaneous regression of metastatic renal cancer. *Cancer* 32:1066, 1973.
49. Monti J et al: The role of adjunctive nephrectomy in patients with metastatic renal cell carcinoma. *J Urol* 117:272, 1977.
50. deKernion JB, Berry D: The diagnosis and treatment of renal cell carcinoma. *Cancer* 45:1947, 1980.
51. Johnson DE et al: Is nephrectomy justified in patients with metastatic renal carcinoma? *J Urol* 114:27, 1975.
52. Johnson DE, Swanson DA: The management of renal carcinoma. *Weekly Urology Update Series*, 1:2, lesson 36, 1978.
53. Wickman JEA: Conservative renal surgery for adenocarcinoma: Natural history and results of treatment. *J Urol* 119: 722, 1978.
54. Novick AC et al: Partial nephrectomy in the treatment of adenocarcinoma. *J Urol* 118:932, 1977.
55. deKernion JB, Grant T: Treatment of skeletal metastases from urological malignancies. *Urology* 11:563, 1978.
56. Bloom HJB: Medroxyprogesterone acetate (provera) in the treatment of metastatic renal carcinoma. *Br J Cancer* 25:250, 1971.
57. Hahn RG: Megace, VP-16, Cytoxan, and Galactitol Phase II treatment trials in advanced renal cell cancer. *Proc Am Soc Clin Oncol* 18:332, 1977.
58. Tally R: Chemotherapy of adenocarcinoma of the kidney. *Cancer* 32:1062, 1973.
59. Hrushesky EJ: What's old and new in advanced renal cell carcinoma? *Proc Am Soc Clin Oncol* 18:318, 1977.
60. Wilms M: *Die Misgeschwulste der Nieren*, Arthur Geogi, Leipzig, 1899.
61. Sutow W et al: Vincristine (leurocristine) sulfate in the treatment of children with metastatic Wilms's tumor. *Pediatrics*, 32:880, 1963.
62. Young JL, Miller R: Incidence of malignant tumors in United States children. *J Pediatr* 86:254, 1975.
63. Ganguly A et al: Renin-secreting Wilms's tumor with severe hypertension: Report of a case and brief review of renin-secreting tumors. *Ann Intern Med* 79:835, 1973.
64. Lemerle J et al: Wilms's tumor: Natural history and prognostic factors. *Cancer* 37:2557, 1976.
65. Beckwith JB, Palmer NG: Information bulletin #5 for contributing pathologists. National Wilms's Tumor Study, June 15, 1977.
66. Leape L: Diagnosis and management of Wilms's tumors and neuroblastomas, in DG Skinner, JB deKernion (eds): *Genitourinary Cancer*, Saunders, Philadelphia, p 179, 1979.
67. LeMerle J et al: Preoperative versus postoperative radiotherapy: Single versus multiple courses of actinomycin D in the treatment of Wilms's tumor. *Cancer* 38:647, 1976b.
68. Cromie WJ, Duckett JW: Wilms' tumor. *Weekly Urology Update Series*, 1, lesson 21, 1979.
69. Bishop HC et al: Survival of bilateral Wilms' tumor: Review of 30 national Wilms' tumor study cases. *J Pediatr Surg* 12: 631, 1977.
70. BaBrosse EH et al: Catecholamine metabolism in neuroblastoma. *J Natl Cancer Inst* 57:633, 1976.
71. Duckett JW: Neuroblastoma. *Weekly Urology Update Series*, 1, lesson 5, 1979.
72. Evans AE et al: Diagnosis and treatment of neuroblastoma. *Pediatr Clin North Am* 23:161, 1976a.

SELECTED BIBLIOGRAPHY

Cherrie R, Goldman D, Lindner A, deKernion JB: Prognostic implications of vena caval extension of renal cell carcinoma. *J Urol* 128:910, 1982.

deKernion JB, Berry D: Diagnosis and treatment of renal cell carcinoma. *Cancer* 45:1947, 1980.

deKernion JB: Lymphadenectomy for renal cell carcinoma: Therapeutic implications. *Urol Clin North Am* 7:697, 1980.

deKernion JB: Surgical management of high stage renal cell carcinoma, in D Paulson (ed), *Genitourinary Cancer*, Martinus Nijhoff, Boston, 1982.

32

TUMORS OF THE RENAL PELVIS AND URETER

Jerome P. Richie

Although tumors of the upper urinary tract are relatively uncommon, the implications of etiologic association with various carcinogens are far-reaching. The overwhelming majority of these tumors of the upper urothelial system are transitional-cell carcinomas and are similar to transitional-cell tumors located elsewhere in the urinary tract. However, certain features of these neoplasms are unique and, thus, dictate a different plan of management.

Because of their common transitional epithelial surface, urothelial tumors of the upper urinary tract, both of the renal pelvis and ureter, will be considered together and discussed in detail. Other intrinsic tumors of the ureter and pelvis will be described briefly.

HISTORICAL ASPECTS

Tumors of the upper urinary tract were rarely recognized prior to the development of adequate uroradiography, except by incidental finding at exploration. Rayer,[1] in 1841, observed at autopsy tumors in the right renal pelvis, ureter, and bladder of a patient with a history of hematuria. The first authentic case report of a carcinoma of the lower ureter in the ureteral stump after nephrectomy was reported in 1884. On rare occasions, the tumor of the ureter was seen protruding from the ureteric orifice at cystoscopy.

Aschner,[2] in 1922, reviewed the literature and compiled a series of 47 patients with primary tumors of the ureter. With improvements in radiological techniques, diagnosis of renal pelvic and ureteral tumors increased in frequency. Abeshouse,[3] in 1956, reviewed 592 cases from the literature.

Removal of the entire kidney and ureter en bloc, first performed by Albarran[4] in 1898, was regarded for many years as the treatment of choice. Vest,[5] in 1945, suggested that conservative measures, with sparing of the kidney or portion of the ureter, were preferable. These two proponents have touched off a controversy of operative management that exists to this date.

INCIDENCE AND ETIOLOGY

Primary carcinoma of the upper urinary tract is relatively rare, accounting for only 5 percent of all tumors of the kidney. During a 20-year study conducted by the Bristol Bladder Tumor Registry,[6] 43 cases of transitional-cell carcinoma of the renal pelvis, 54 cases of carcinoma of the ureter, and 2770 cases of carcinoma of the bladder were admitted, a ratio of 51 to 1 to 1 (bladder–renal pelvis–ureter). A similar 16-year study[7] in Oakland described 238 patients with bladder tumors, 14 with renal pelvic tumors and only 5 with ureteral tumors, a ratio of 50 to 3 to 1. In autopsy studies, the incidence has been no higher than 1 in 1000.[3]

The peak occurrence is in the sixth or seventh decade of life, and tumors are rare in persons less than 30 years of age. Males predominate by a ratio of 2 or 3 to 1. The majority of ureteral tumors occur in the lower third of the ureter. There is no predilection for unilaterality for either renal pelvic or ureteral tumors, and bilateral occurrences are distinctly uncommon.

Petkovic[8] has suggested that the incidence of carcinoma of the ureter and renal pelvis is increasing. However, Bennington and Beckwith attribute this apparent increase to improved recognition by better diagnostic techniques, education of physicians, and health reporting data.

Carcinogens

Mucosal surfaces of the collecting tubules, calyces, renal pelvis, ureter, bladder, and urethra share a common embryologic origin. The term *urothelium* has been utilized by Melicow[9] to describe this entire mucosal system. Carcinogens that are excreted in the urine would theoretically effect malignant transformation of exposed urothelial cells in proportion to their surface area. Thus, one would predict that transitional-cell tumors would occur more frequently in the bladder than in the upper urothelial tract. The rapid transit time of urine down the upper urinary tract, as well as activation of carcinogens by hydrolyzing enzymes, results in an even lower ratio of upper urothelial tumors to lower (bladder) urothelial tumors than would be predicted.

Cancer of the renal pelvis or ureter rarely occurs naturally in animals; therefore, most basic research has been directed by clinical observations. The epidemiologic observation that urothelial cancer was more common in urban as opposed to rural populations led to the eventual specific association of certain chemicals with transitional-cell carcinoma of the urinary tract. Long-term workers in a variety of industries, including those involving aniline dye, certain chemicals in the rubber textiles and plastics industries, and a variety of other chemicals, have a higher reported incidence of transitional-cell carcinoma. Excellent reviews on the chemical induction of cancer of the urinary tract have been prepared by Kerr and Barkin,[10] and Oyasu and Hopp.[11]

Various agents have been shown to incite neoplasm in the renal pelvis, ureter, or bladder. Makar[12] documented the development of bladder and ureteral neoplasms in patients with schistosomiasis. Scott and Boyd[13] administered β-naphthylamine to dogs and produced neoplastic lesions in the ureter and renal pelvis. Other potent carcinogens for the urothelium are benzadine, 4-amino-biphenyl, and β-naphthylamine. Renal pelvic carcinoma has also been produced by chronic consumption of aflatoxin B[14] or chronic consumption of lead compounds.[15]

Smoking has been implicated as an etiological factor in the increased incidence of transitional carcinoma of the urinary tract, especially the bladder. Kerr and Barkin[10] postulated that abnormal metabolites of tryptophan may be the intermediary agent. Bennington and Beckwith[7] have suggested that the incidence of renal pelvic cancer is increased in patients with a long history of cigarette consumption. An intriguing association of renal pelvic carcinoma with viral particles has been described by Elliott et al.[16] This concept is especially appealing because of the multifocal and widespread nature of transitional carcinomas of the urinary tract. The DNA simian virus 40 (SV40) has been shown to produce neoplastic transformation of urothelium in vitro. Experimentally, bovine papilloma virus produces papillomas when injected into bladder mucosa in cows.[17] Furthermore, Elliott et al.[16] isolated an RNA virus from cultured human transitional-cell carcinomas. Although this association is intriguing, Fraley et al.[18] suggest that there is a lack of evidence to support the RNA virus as a consistent mechanism in induction of transitional cell carcinoma. Nevertheless, viruses can transform normal uroepithelial cells in vitro and may be causally related to tumor induction.

Associated Nephropathy

Two clinical situations occur in which known chemical carcinogens may be directly involved in carcinoma of the renal pelvis: analgesic nephropathy and Balkan nephropathy. In both instances, the usual male predominance is reversed, with females predominating by a ratio of 2 to 1. The term *analgesic nephropathy* is applied to patients with chronic phenacetin ingestion in whom a form of interstitial nephritis is associated with the destruction of the renal papillae and papillary necrosis. In those patients who develop papillary necrosis, two-thirds will also develop cancer of the renal pelvis. However, rarely do chronic analgesic abusers develop renal pelvic tumors without papillary necrosis as an antecedent event. Therefore, the chronic inflammation may be a causative factor together with phenacetin metabolites. Experimentally, it has been shown that increased ingestion of phenacetin results in increased N-hydroxylated metabolites, especially acetoamenophenol in the urine, a compound structurally resembling known urothelial carcinogens.[19]

An intriguing geographic localization is that there is a high rate of renal pelvic, ureteral, and bladder tumors in parts of Bulgaria, Rumania, and Yugoslavia. Patients in these areas are also afflicted with an endemic chronic renal disease known as *Balkan nephropathy*. Petkovic[8] has made an extensive study of patients in this geographic area and has attempted to identify epidemiological etiologies without success. The cancers of the renal pelvis and ureter that arise in association with Balkan nephropathy are multifocal and relatively slow growing. Many of the patients have some degree of renal failure secondary to the nephropathy, and this factor, in conjunction with an increased incidence of bilaterality, mandates conservative management. The etiology of these tumors, as well as that of the Balkan nephropathy itself, remains unclear.

SIGNS AND SYMPTOMS

At least 75 percent of patients with renal pelvic and ureteral tumors will have hematuria during the course of the disease. Although usually painless, severe hematuria may be associated with the passage of vermiform blood clots and with ureteral colic. Rarely, obstruction of the renal pelvis or upper ureter may present a syndrome similar to that of congenital ureteropelvic junction obstruction. Scott and McDonald[20] have reported terminal hematuria as the initial symptom when a lower ureteral tumor protruded through the ureteral orifice.

In addition to symptoms of hematuria and/or pain, these patients commonly have complaints of frequency, malaise, weight loss, or fever of unexplained etiology. Positive physical findings are unusual. The ureteral tumor rarely may produce sufficient hydronephrosis to result in a palpable renal mass in a thin patient.

Urinary cytology may be an important screening adjunct for the diagnosis of upper urinary tract or bladder tumors. Indeed, at the Mayo Clinic, routine cytologies performed on every patient in the Urology Clinic revealed a population of patients with only carcinoma in situ in the bladder or upper urinary tracts. At the present time, however, the yield of routine urinary cytology is not sufficient to warrant this as a routine screening procedure.

Urinary irritative symptoms, such as frequency or dysuria, are seen in 50 percent of patients with ureteral tumors,[21] as compared with 10 percent of patients with renal pelvic tumors.[22] It is worthwhile to recall that patients with upper tract urothelial tumors may have bladder tumors as well, accounting for some of the hematuria and irritative urinary symptoms, especially in patients with carcinoma in situ.[23]

The average duration of symptoms prior to treatment has ranged from 2 years in earlier series to 2 months in a recent study.[24] The inconclusive nature of the symptoms, as well as patient procrastination, contribute to this inordinate delay and may account in part for a relatively dismal overall prognosis.

PATHOLOGIC GRADING AND STAGING

Classification of tumors of the renal pelvis or ureter is similar to Broder's classification for bladder tumors. The various types of urothelial tumors are shown in Table 32-1. The histologic criteria for transitional-cell carcinoma, grades 1 to 4, are based on the thickness of the papillary wall, nuclear characteristics, loss of differentiation and progression from basal layers to surface, and prominence of mitotic figures.

Transitional-Cell Tumors

The true papilloma of the renal pelvis is a relatively benign lesion and may be connected to the urothelium by a narrow base or stalk. Although these lesions are benign, they may portend development of additional tumors in the remainder of the urinary tract. Bennington and Beckwith[7] reported that patients with a solitary papilloma have a 25 percent chance of developing carcinoma somewhere else in their urinary tract. For patients with multiple papillomas, 50 percent will eventually develop an invasive tumor.

Pathologic staging of renal pelvic or ureteral tumors is similar to the Jewett and Strong[25] staging classification for bladder tumors. Because the calyces, infundibuli, and renal pelvis are surrounded by renal parenchyma,

TABLE 32-1 Malignant Tumors of Renal Pelvis and Ureter

PRIMARY

Epithelial:

    Transitional-cell carcinoma (71%)

    Transitional-cell carcinoma with differentiation (20%)
        Squamous differentiation
        Glandular differentiation
        Mixed

    Squamous-cell carcinoma (8%)

    Adenocarcinoma (1%)

    Undifferentiated carcinoma (1%)

Mesodermal:

    Leiomyosarcoma

SECONDARY

Metastases via blood or lymph

Direct extension

Drop metastases

SOURCE: Modified from JL Bennington and JB Beckwith.[7]

the staging is necessarily different. Staging of pelvic and ureteral tumors proposed by Grabstald[22] is illustrated in Fig. 32-1. A parallel staging system for ureteral tumors has been described by Bloom et al[21] and Batata et al.[24] Stage 0 disease is limited strictly to the mucosa. In stage A tumors, the lamina propria has been invaded, but no progression of tumor into the muscularis is evident. Stage B tumors are confined by the muscularis, whereas stage C tumors have invaded through the adventitia to involve adjacent structures. Stage D tumors involve distant metastases. Since prognosis seems to be more related to stage than grade, a uniform staging system is desirable. Because of the surrounding renal parenchyma in renal pelvic tumors, a tumor that has extended through the wall of the calyx or renal pelvis into surrounding renal parenchyma but is still contained by the parenchyma should be analogous to a stage C ureteral tumor. Stage D with regard to renal pelvic tumors should designate direct invasion of adjacent structures or distant metastases.

Transitional-cell carcinomas may spread by direct extension or may metastasize via bloodstream or lymphatics. The regional lymph nodes, both for renal pelvic and ureteral tumors, are commonly involved before other sites of metastases are evident. For this reason, surgical treatment should include regional lymphadenectomy, as described in the section on surgical treatment.

Distant metastases may be found in the lungs, liver, lymph nodes, and bones. However, almost any organ may receive metastases from a transitional-cell tumor of the upper urinary tract.

Squamous-Cell Carcinoma of the Renal Pelvis and Ureter

Pure squamous-cell carcinoma of the upper urinary collecting system accounts for only 8 percent of all renal tumors. The age range is similar to that for transitional-cell tumors, and there is no predilection for either sex. Over 50 percent of the cases are associated with a renal pelvic calculus.[26] Chronic inflammation is believed to be an etiologic factor, as the majority of cases of squamous-cell carcinoma of the upper tract are associated with chronic infection and preexisting squamous metaplasia or leukoplakia. Only rarely have cases been reported without preexisting inflammation or irritation.[27]

Squamous-cell carcinomas of the renal pelvis frequently extend into the ureter or deeply into the renal parenchyma. They tend to follow a rapid course and are often not discovered until metastases are already present. Hematuria occurs late in the disease. Squamous-cell carcinoma in the renal pelvis tends to be flat, extensive, and ulcerated, spreading in a scirrhous fashion. Cytology is of limited value.

Radical surgical intervention is the treatment of choice; however, 5-year survivals are only rarely reported.[28] It is unlikely that radiation therapy or chemotherapy will substantially alter the natural history of this aggressive tumor.

Adenocarcinoma of the Renal Pelvis

Adenocarcinoma of the renal pelvis is exceedingly rare; less than 60 cases have been reported to date. The tumor is often associated with chronic infections and tends to metastasize early. The etiology of adenocarcinoma of the renal pelvis is unclear, and radical nephroureterectomy is the procedure of choice.

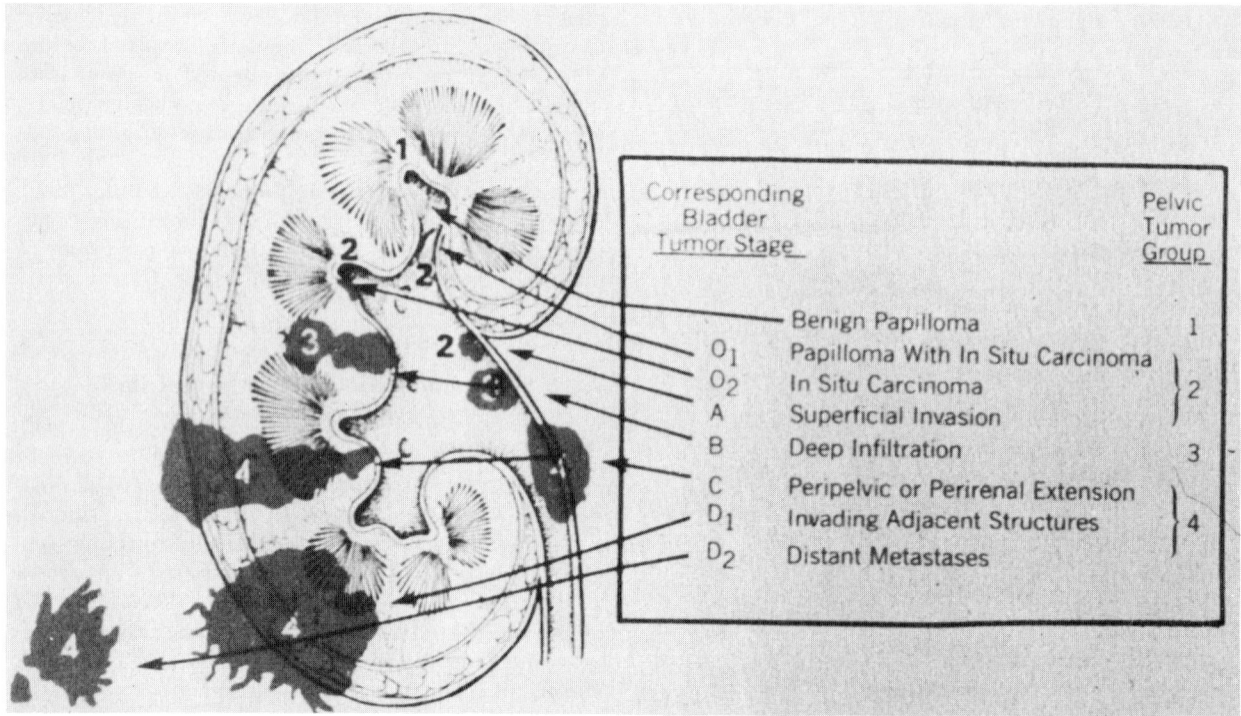

FIGURE 32-1 Proposed staging system for renal pelvic tumors with corresponding bladder tumor stage. (*From H Grabstald et al.*[22])

DIAGNOSTIC TECHNIQUES

Excretory Urography

In any patient with hematuria, an intravenous pyelogram should be the first major step in diagnostic evaluation. Commonly, tumors of the renal pelvis or ureter may be outlined as a radiolucent defect. The differential diagnosis of radiolucent defect is detailed in Table 32-2. A typical renal pelvic tumor with papillary growths, as confirmed by the gross pathologic specimen, is illustrated in Fig. 32-2.

In ureteral tumors, intravenous pyelography has previously been thought to be of little diagnostic value. However, recent advances in technique, including tomography, abdominal compression, and improved contrast agents, have altered the diagnostic accuracy of this study. Williams and Mitchell[29] found intravenous pyelograms to be of value in 28 of 30 patients examined. Almgard et al.[30] reported abnormal intravenous pyelogram findings in all 41 patients with ureteric tumor in whom nephrectomy had not been previously performed.

Although excretory urography may suggest a ureteral tumor, the obstruction must usually be defined further by retrograde or antegrade pyelography. Retrograde urography is much more likely to demonstrate the presence of a lesion and accurately define its lower margin (Figs. 32-3 and 32-4). In addition, multiple ureteral tumors may occur and have important therapeutic and prognostic significance.

Because of the chronic nature of obstruction, excretory urography may reveal absence of function of the kidney. This was reported in as many as one-third of the cases reviewed by Scott and McDonald.[20] Batata et al.[24] reported findings of unilateral nonvisualization in 46 percent of their patients with ureteral tumors, hydronephrosis in 34 percent, and filling defect in 19 percent.

Retrograde Pyelography

Cystoscopy and retrograde pyelography have a definite place in the diagnosis of renal pelvic or ureteral tumors,

TUMORS OF THE RENAL PELVIS AND URETER **669**

TABLE 32-2 Differential Diagnosis of Radiolucent Filling Defect (Presumed Renal Pelvic Cancer)

INTRINSIC
Uric acid calculus
Blood clot
Submucosal hemorrhage
Pyelitis cystica
Malacoplakia
Cholesteatoma

EXTRINSIC
Renal artery aneurysm
Parapelvic cyst

SOURCE: Modified from EE Fraley: Cancer of the renal pelvis, in DG Skinner, J deKernion (eds): *Genitourinary Cancer,* Saunders, Philadelphia, 1978.

even with an obvious tumor of the renal pelvis noted with excretory urography. Retrograde study permits collection of washings for histology and cytology and, in some cases, passage of a ureteral brush for histologic confirmation. Furthermore, retrograde pyelography may clarify the differential diagnosis of an intraluminal filling defect. If the defect moves about with injection of contrast material, a radiolucent calculus or a blood clot may be diagnosed. Occasionally, the fine stalk of a polypoid tumor may be demonstrated on retrograde pyelogram. In cases of extrinsic compression of the renal pelvis, gentle pressure may completely eradicate the defect, excluding the likelihood of a malignant process.

In ureteral tumors, retrograde pyelography and ureterography may be the only way to define the lesion accurately. A ureteral lesion may appear radiographically as either an intraluminal lesion or as a diffuse stricturelike obstruction of the ureter. Prior to the retrograde pyelogram, endoscopic examination can yield valuable information. Efflux of bloody material may be noted from the affected side, or, rarely a ureteral tumor may prolapse through the ureteral orifice. In addition, with a tumor in the intramural portion of the ureter, a bulge may be noticed in the ureteral ridge similar to the presentation of a ureteral calculus.

An intraluminal lesion will often produce a filling defect accompanied by local dilatation of the ureter distal to the growth. Contour of the lower margin of the

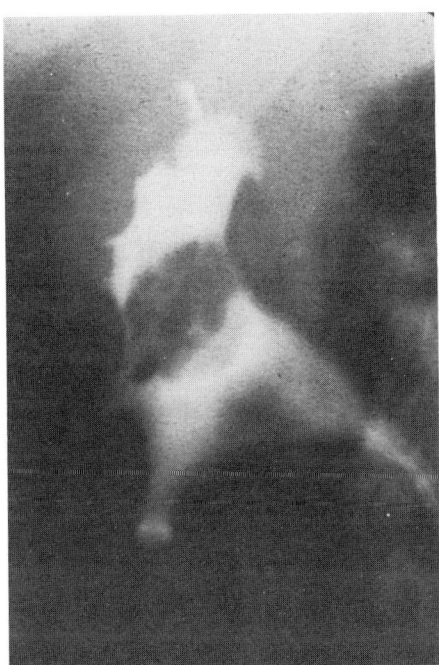
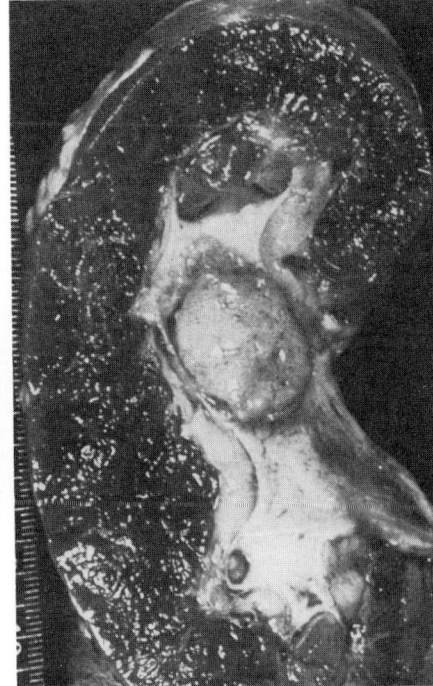

FIGURE 32-2 (*a*) Radiolucent filling defect occupies majority of right renal pelvis. (*b*) Gross pathologic specimen confirms transitional cell carcinoma.

a *b*

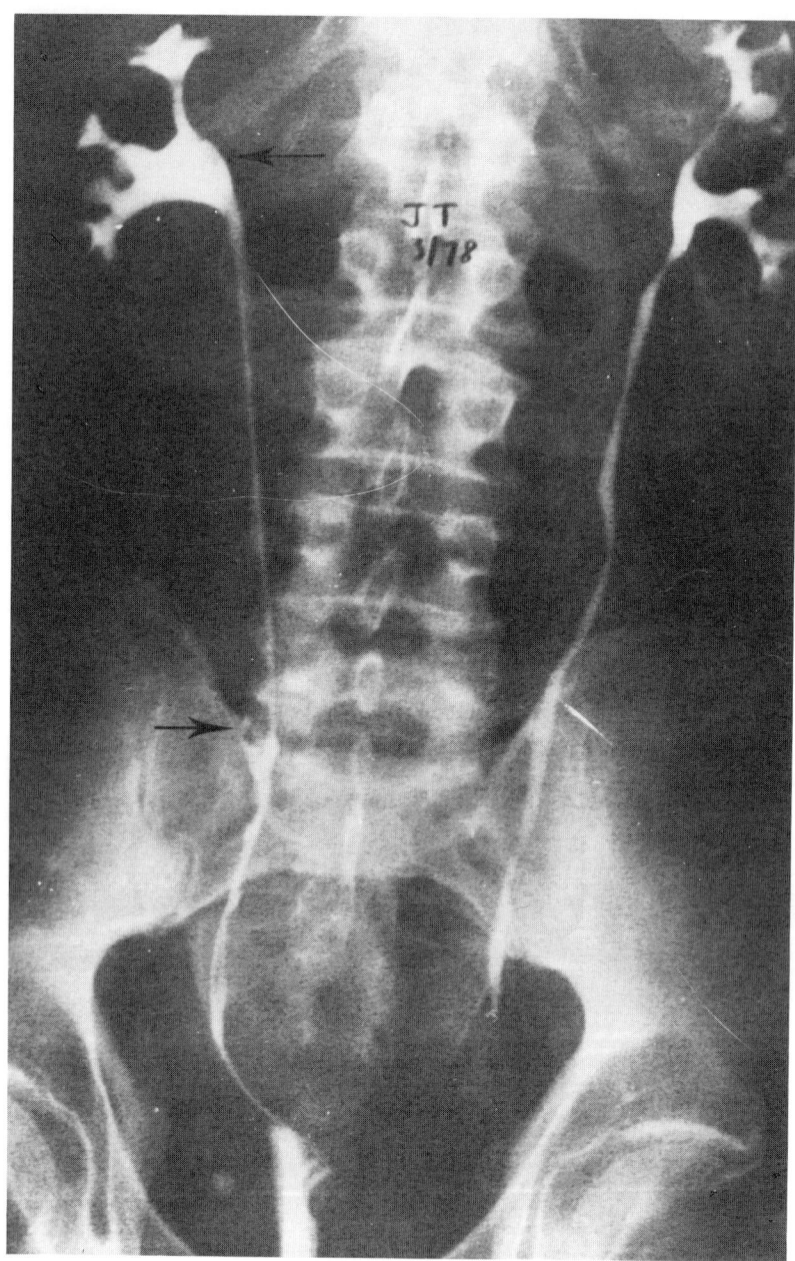

FIGURE 32-3 Retrograde pyelogram demonstrates filling defects in right renal pelvis and right mid-ureter (*arrows*). The ureteral defect was not appreciated on excretory urogram.

tumor may cause dilatation of the ureter distal to the tumor. When contrast material is injected by occlusive bulb ureterogram, the tumor may be lifted proximally toward the kidney. The dilated segment of ureter has been described as wine goblet– or meniscus-shaped (Fig. 32-4). Bergman and associates,[31] in 1961, described this shape as an important diagnostic sign distinguishing ureteral tumor from radiolucent calculus. The ureteral catheter has a tendency to coil in the dilated space below a ureteral tumor, producing *Bergman's sign*, which is

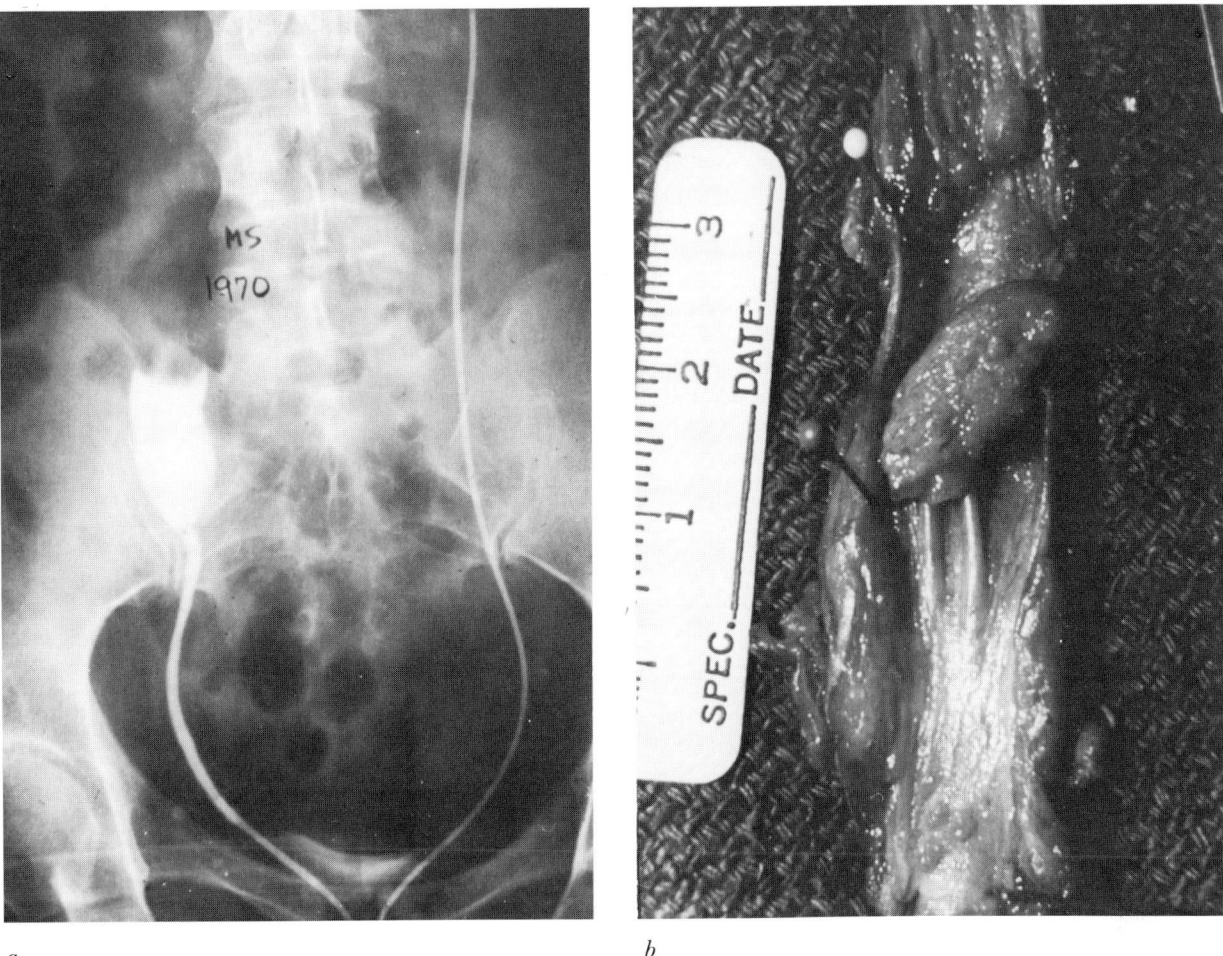

FIGURE 32-4 (*a*) Retrograde ureterogram demonstrates "chalice" sign of ureteral tumor with distal dilatation. (*b*) Gross pathologic specimen. Note additional tumors proximal to large tumor that were not seen on retrograde pyelogram.

almost pathognomonic for ureteral tumor. The differential diagnosis of a ureteral filling defect, however, includes nonopaque calculi, blood clots, ureteritis cystica, and seedling metastases from a renal pelvic or bladder tumor. The presence of a calculus in the ureter should not prevent visualization of the entire ureter by retrograde pyelogram, as calculus and tumor may occur in conjunction.[32] The presence of a defect in the renal pelvis does not exclude additional defects in the ureter, as shown in Fig. 32-3. Although in this patient the right ureter had been described as "normal" on the intravenous pyelogram, retrograde ureterogram clearly demonstrated an additional defect in the ureter at the pelvic brim.

Additional Techniques

ANTEGRADE PYELOGRAPHY

The diffuse, stricturelike obstructive lesion of the ureter causes considerable consternation in diagnosis. In addition to infiltrate of primary carcinoma of the ureter, other entities, such as varicosities, ureteritis, extension of an extraureteral carcinoma, ureteritis cystica, retroperitoneal fibrosis, and endometriosis must be considered. In some patients, delineation of the upper ureter and collecting system would be impossible, especially if a ureteral filling defect occludes the lumen. This problem has led to the development of additional techniques to improve the accuracy of preoperative diagnosis. Antegrade pyelography, described by Casey and Goodwin,[33] will delineate the upper urinary tracts and ureter as well as provide material for cytologic examination. This study, however, should be used only after failure of retrograde studies. Blind puncture of the upper collecting system may lead to spillage of carcinomatous cells and preclude a potentially curative cancer procedure. In patients with complete obstruction of the lower urinary tract, however, no other technique may be applicable, and thus the risk is warranted. The technique consists of percutaneous puncture with a long spinal needle guided by fluoroscopy or ultrasound into the hydronephrotic collecting system. Computer tomography–guided needle aspiration is a recent development that may further enhance the safety of this procedure. Once the needle has entered the collecting system, fluid is aspirated for cytology, and contrast material is injected to visualize the collecting system.

ANGIOGRAPHY

Renal pelvic and ureteral tumors lack a characteristic appearance on angiography. In advanced tumors of the renal pelvis, arteriographic findings of encasement of arterial branches on the arteriogram or an increase in the blood supply to the renal pelvis may suggest a neoplasm of the upper urinary tract.

Arteriography is most useful in order to delineate a renal-cell carcinoma or a radiolucent defect in the collecting system secondary to congenital vascular malformation.

In patients with carcinoma of the ureter, elective ureteral arteriography has been suggested as a diagnostic tool to differentiate diffuse stricturelike lesions of the ureter.[34] Ureteral carcinoma lacks a characteristic, reproducible angiographic pattern, but angiography will allow differentiation of primary carcinoma from endometriosis, hemangioma, or metastatic tumors.[35]

Angiography may become particularly important in patients with tumor of the renal pelvis or calyx in a solitary kidney in whom segmental surgical resection is contemplated.

Cytology

Cullen et al.[36] have documented the value of cytologic examination of freshly voided urine in the diagnosis of transitional-cell tumors of the upper urinary tract. With the use of a filter preparation, they reported positive cytologies in 80 percent of their patients with tumors of the pelvis or ureter. Numerous investigators, however, have questioned the value of voided urinary cytology because of its low yield in low-grade tumors and because of the possibility of concomitant bladder tumors.[22,37] The addition of furosemide diuresis to retrograde collections yields much better results than voided specimens alone; Zincke et al.[38] found that 61 percent of patients had positive cytology on retrograde collections as opposed to 33 percent on voided cytology. A pathologist with a genuine interest in cytology is essential to the accurate evaluation of urinary cytologic specimens.

Nuclear cytologic characteristics can provide a strong clue to the histological grade of a tumor, but correlation with invasiveness is usually lacking. In a study of 43 patients with upper tract urothelial tumors, Eriksson and Johansson[39] found 35 percent of patients with a negative or atypical cytology to have invasive tumors. Batata and Grabstald[24] found positive cytology in only 29 percent of patients with proven invasive ureteral tumors. Therefore, although cytology may be useful as a screening test in patients with hematuria, its value in accurate staging is markedly limited.

Brush Biopsy

A technique adapted from bronchoscopic brushing by Gill et al.[40] has permitted increased diagnostic accuracy of radiolucent filling defects in the ureter and renal pelvis. In patients with cytology suggestive of a high-grade lesion, brush biospy is contraindicated because of the additional risk to the patient. In patients with a radiolucent filling defect in the renal pelvis or ureter and a negative cytology, however, brush biopsy may be useful to substantiate the diagnosis as well as to direct the appropriate form of therapy.

The technique of brush biopsy consists of the passage of a special number 5 or 6 French ureteral catheter transurethrally into the affected ureter. A small nylon- or steel-bristled brush is encased within the lumen of the ureteral catheter until properly positioned (Fig. 32-5). By means of a manipulating handle, the tip of the ureteral brush can be maneuvered to reach a defect in any infundibulum or calyx (Fig. 32-6). Under fluoro-

cell carcinoma of the renal pelvis or ureter. This technique evolved after the finding of numerous failures by local recurrence of lesions in the ureteral stump after nephrectomy alone. Colston and Arcadi[41] reported recurrences in the ipsilateral ureteral stump to be as high as 84 percent. Scott and McDonald[20] reported that 20 percent of ureteral tumors were treated with a kidney-conserving operation. The major controversy over preferred treatment of renal pelvic and ureteral tumors centers on the difficulty of diagnostic accuracy of staging. Proponents of radical nephroureterectomy with removal of a cuff of bladder emphasize the difficulty in distinguishing the histological grade of the tumor as well as in making an accurate estimation of the stage. McIntyre

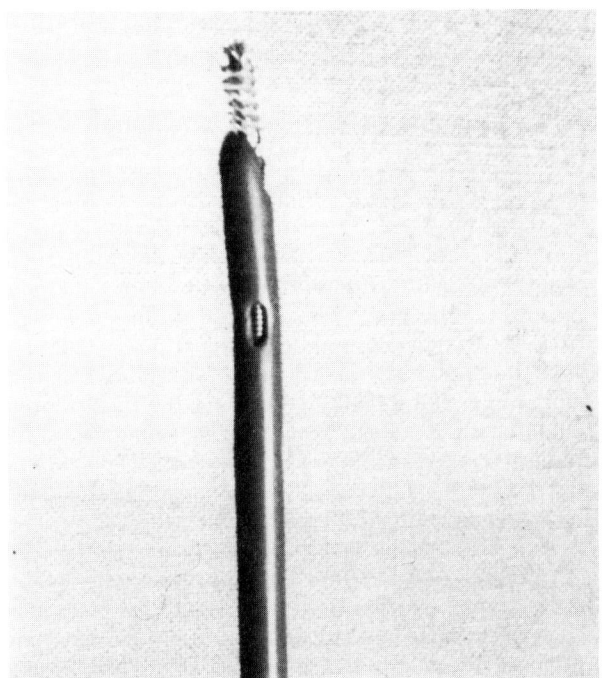

FIGURE 32-5 Retrograde brush biopsy catheter with bristle tip extended from sheath.

scopic control, the bristle brush is extended and rubbed against the lesion to gather material for histologic examination. Once the brush catheter is removed, the barbitage with normal saline will allow collection of small fragments of tissue for histological examination in addition to the material trapped by the bristle brush. Collection of urine for 24 h after brushing provides additional material (Fig. 32-7). Gill et al.[40] have reported this technique to be accurate in diagnosis of moderately differentiated transitional-cell carcinoma in two of six patients. A recent report* has found brush biopsy to be at least 80 percent accurate and important in the planning of therapy.

TREATMENT

Radical Operative Therapy

Nephroureterectomy that includes a cuff of bladder has been considered the classic treatment for transitional-

* RF Gittes, personal communication.

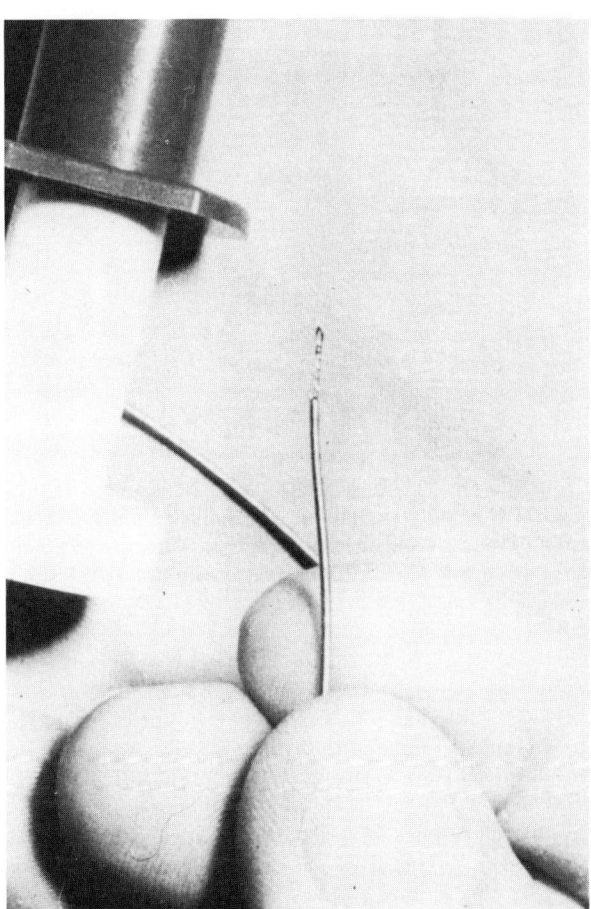

FIGURE 32-6 Handle to manipulate brush into various positions, enabling brush to be negotiated into any calyx.

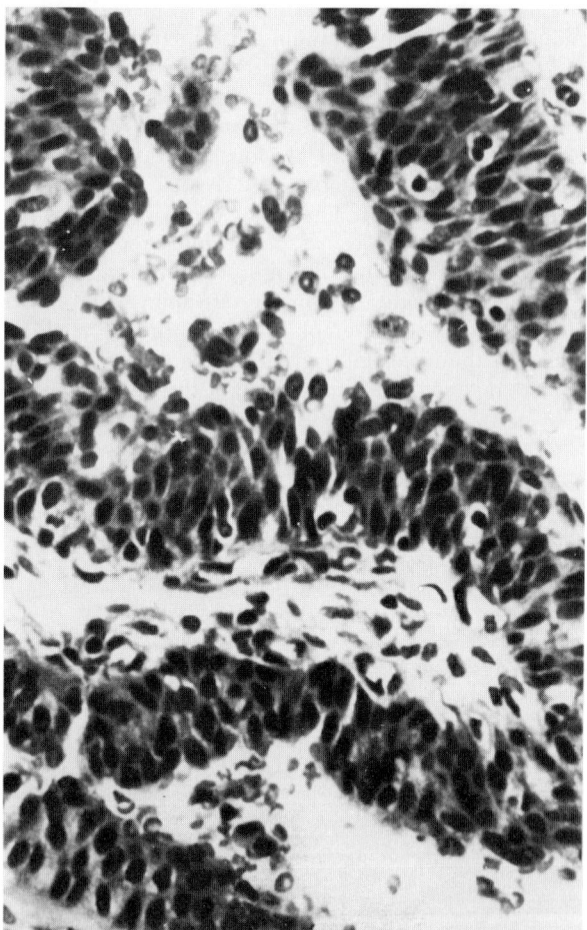

FIGURE 32-7 Histologic specimen obtained from brush biopsy. Papillary and nuclear characteristics confirmed a grade II transitional cell carcinoma. (H&E stain; reduced from 425×.)

et al.[42] decried ureterotomy in assessment of the tumor because of the danger of spillage of tumor cells and the likelihood of implantation in the surgical wound. Half of all cases of ureteral tumor invade the muscular layer and have lymphatic involvement. When one considers the high incidence of ipsilateral recurrence as well as in situ lesions, removal of the entire ureteral segment as well as the kidney would seem preferable to partial ureterectomy as a cancer operation. Furthermore, the well-known phenomenon of recurrence in the remaining ureteral stump has been reported in more than 30 percent of patients treated by nephrectomy and partial ureterectomy alone.[43]

Conservative Operative Therapy

The concept of less radical procedures has been championed by such noted authorities as Vest,[5] Colston and Arcadi,[41] and Carroll.[44] Advocates of less radical procedures have been steadily gaining converts. These opponents of radical surgical intervention indict the poor prognosis associated with advanced lesions that have invaded through the ureteral or renal pelvic wall, and the higher operative mortality rate with more extensive procedures. These authors attribute the dismal prognosis, regardless of the form of surgical therapy, to the thin ureteral wall, difficulty in accurately diagnosing ureteral tumors, lack of early presenting symptoms, and the rich lymphatic plexus surrounding the ureter.

Most large series have reported survival data for patients treated by radical nephroureterectomy (Table 32-3). Unfortunately, there are no good comparative data to determine how efficacious conservative treatment would be in similarly staged lesions.

In certain instances, renal sparing or less radical procedures must be considered. These procedures may consist of local excision of the tumor, ureteral anastomosis, ureteral reimplantation, ureterocutaneous diversion, replacement of the ureter with a segment of ileum, and renal autotransplantation. In the patient with a

TABLE 32-3 Correlation of 5-Year Survival with Stage of Tumor

Stage	Renal Pelvic Tumors		
	Blute and Richie[45]	Grabstald[22]	Total
0–A	$\frac{10}{10}$	$\frac{17}{24}$	$\frac{27}{34}$ (79%)
B	$\frac{4}{5}$	$\frac{4}{9}$	$\frac{8}{14}$ (57%)
C	$\frac{0}{1}$	$\frac{1}{12}$	$\frac{1}{13}$ (7%)
D	$\frac{0}{3}$	$\frac{0}{8}$	$\frac{0}{11}$ (0%)

Stage	Ureteral tumors		
	Blute and Richie[45]	Batata et al[24]	Total
0–A	$\frac{5}{6}$	$\frac{8}{8}$	$\frac{13}{14}$ (93%)
B	$\frac{1}{1}$	$\frac{3}{7}$	$\frac{4}{8}$ (50%)
C	$\frac{0}{3}$	$\frac{2}{12}$	$\frac{2}{15}$ (13%)
D	$\frac{0}{5}$	$\frac{0}{9}$	$\frac{0}{14}$ (0%)

solitary kidney, embarrassed renal function, bilateral lesions, or endemic Balkan nephropathy, conservatism is essential. The preferred treatment should be removal of the ureter with replacement by a segment of ileum. Local excision and reanastomosis should be limited to patients with a localized polypoid filling defect that is presumably grade 1 and stage A after retrograde brush biopsy.

If a solitary kidney or simultaneous bilateral tumors necessitate conservative procedures, several caveats must be remembered. Partial nephrectomy can be performed for a tumor located in a calyx, but it is important to isolate the calyx early in the procedure to prevent spread or implantation of tumor cells. The Gil Vernet approach has proved useful in isolating the major infundibulum prior to partial nephrectomy. Operative nephroscopy should be utilized to define the position and configuration of the tumor prior to the decision for a partial nephrectomy. The remaining intrarenal collecting system should be carefully inspected before it is considered to be free of tumor. In any patient in whom the collecting system will be opened for treatment of a tumor, careful packing of the wound to prevent wound implantation is mandatory.

Technique

The surgical technique of nephroureterectomy with removal of a cuff of bladder should consist of en bloc removal of the kidney and the entire ureter with surrounding segment of bladder and surrounding lymphatics. Various techniques have been described, some utilizing two incisions and others using a single flank incision with extension as a paramedian incision.

The two-incision technique necessitates repositioning the patient and repreparing the operative field midway through the procedure. For an en bloc dissection, the dissected kidney and ureter must remain in situ while the primary incision is closed. Untoward anesthetic events that might occur during the repositioning of the patient would create a difficult problem. Furthermore, exposure for a regional lymphadenectomy in conjunction with the radical procedure is compromised by the two-incision technique.

This author prefers a single incision with the patient positioned in a torque position, with the pelvis nearly supine and the shoulders angled approximately 50°. With flexion of the table, this creates a position similar to that utilized for thoracoabdominal retroperitoneal lymphadenectomy for patients with testis tumor. The peritoneal envelope is mobilized completely across the midline, allowing exposure of the entire retroperitoneum. This approach facilitates the performance of regional lymphadenectomy.

Regional lymphadenectomy clearly provides a more accurate staging of renal pelvic or ureteral tumors and may have therapeutic implications as well. The regional lymph nodes appear to be the earliest and most common site of metastatic spread. In the series by Batata et al.[46] 17 of their 22 patients had metastases involving the regional lymph nodes. Lymphatic metastases were ipsilateral in 90 percent of lower ureteral tumors and 60 percent of upper ureteral or renal pelvic tumors. This high incidence of predominantly ipsilateral regional lymphatic involvement lends credence to the addition of extensive regional lymphadenectomy as an integral part of the radical surgical approach.

The removal of the kidney should be by technique of radical nephrectomy, including all of Gerota's fascia as well as the regional lymph nodes. Early ligation of the renal artery and renal vein, prior to manipulation of the tumor, is recommended.

In removal of the distal ureter and cuff or bladder, the bladder should be open and the ureter approached intravesically as well as extravesically. Removal of the distal ureter by an extravesical approach only by tenting up the distal ureter represents an inadequate cancer procedure. Strong and Pearse[43] reported nine cases in which this maneuver was utilized; on subsequent cystoscopy, all nine patients were noted to have a remaining ureteral orifice and intramural ureter on the ipsilateral side. Recurrence of tumor was subsequently noted in the ureteral stump in two of the nine patients. This method, therefore, is mentioned only to be condemned. Once the bladder is open, the mucosa surrounding the ureteral orifice should be sutured over the end of the ureter to prevent any malignant cancer cells from being manipulated into the normal bladder mucosa. This is especially important in view of the reports by Soloway[47] of implantation of tumor cells in damaged urothelial mucosa. The cuff of bladder should include a 1-cm circumferential margin around the ureteral orifice.

ADJUVANT THERAPIES

Radiation Therapy

Radiation therapy is an unproven adjunct for control of residual tumor, unresectable disease, and lower recurrence. Brady et al.[48] reported three of five patients with advanced disease to have survived 5 years after operation and adjunctive radiation therapy. Holtz[49] suggested the use of postoperative radiotherapy. Batata et al.[46] recommended postoperative irradiation, 6000 rads, for ureteral tumors that involved the muscular layer or deeper. Preoperative radiotherapy has not been shown to be of efficacy in the treatment of ureteral or renal pelvic carcinoma, largely because of the difficulty in establishing a preoperative diagnosis and accurate staging of the tumor. Postoperative radiation therapy in invasive disease would seem to be a logical extension of the combination of radiation therapy and surgery for bladder tumors.

Chemotherapy

Unfortunately, adjuvant chemotherapy for advanced renal pelvic or ureteral tumors has been notoriously ineffective. Only sporadic reports of the use of adjuvant chemotherapy have appeared. Batata et al.[46] reported on two patients who received postoperative therapy with actinomycin D and thiophosphamides; both patients continued to have advanced disease. *cis*-Platinum, which has been shown to have objective response rates in advanced carcinoma of the bladder, is currently being evaluated in patients with advanced carcinoma of the upper urothelial system.

Topical thiotepa and mitomycin C have been used in patients with recurrent superficial bladder lesions. Although absorption of thiotepa is enhanced in the upper urinary tracts, this local chemotherapy should be considered as a method of preventing recurrences, especially in patients with positive cytology from the upper tract but without demonstrable lesions.

FOLLOW-UP AND EARLY IDENTIFICATION OF RECURRENCE

Several authors have reported that 40 percent of patients with tumors of the renal pelvis or ureter will have associated bladder tumors at some time during their evaluation. Additionally, patients who have undergone conservative treatment with the ipsilateral ureter in situ are at high risk of recurrence in that ureter. Consequently, cystoscopic evaluation is indicated at 3 to 6-month intervals for a minimum of 2 years and for probably 5 years after the occurrence of a documented tumor in the upper urinary tract.

In addition to cystoscopic follow-up, urinary cytology should be performed on an annual or a semiannual basis indefinitely. Because the likelihood of diagnosis by cytology improves with higher-grade lesions, this test should continue to be important in the overall management of patients with upper tract or bladder urothelial lesions.

Should an ipsilateral ureteral stump be left in place, special attention must be paid to this. The likelihood of recurrence approaches 30 percent, and strong consideration should be given for removal of the stump. If this is not feasible for medical reasons, careful follow-up with retrograde studies and/or fulguration of the mucosa inside the ureteral stump should be utilized.

Of increasing import with the advent of cytologic examination is the patient without demonstrable upper tract lesions but with positive cytology localized to one upper urothelial system. This patient may have carcinoma in situ in the renal pelvis and/or ureter, but the decision to perform nephroureterectomy should require demonstration of an actual lesion. Those patients deserve random biopsies of the bladder, careful retrograde pyelograms to be certain there are no filling defects, and periodic x-ray studies every 3 to 6 months in order to define a lesion early in its course. The instillation of topical thiotepa or mitomycin C with reduction of dosage and careful attention to the pressure of instillation should be considered in these patients.

THERAPEUTIC OPTIONS FOR RECURRENCES

In patients who have been treated by a conservative operation, ipsilateral ureteral recurrences are not uncommon. In such an individual, strong consideration should be given for nephroureterectomy with removal of a cuff of bladder. Should the contralateral kidney be compromised or surgically absent, resection of the entire ureter with replacement by a segment of ileum would be the procedure of choice. In patients with numerous or high-grade recurrences in the bladder, radical cystectomy should be strongly considered. In patients with compromised renal function and ureteral tumors in a remaining solitary kidney, resection of the ureter and replacement with a short segment of ileum as a cutaneous diversion may be the only available procedure short of radical nephrectomy and transplantation. That latter procedure should be reserved for the exceptional patient.

CURRENT AREAS OF RESEARCH

As indicated earlier in "Incidence and Etiology," breakthroughs in the understanding of carcinoma of the renal pelvis and ureter, as well as bladder, will require further knowledge of carcinogens and their effect on the urothelium. In terms of diagnosis, automated cytologic screening may provide a method of earlier diagnosis of urothelial tumors, especially those of high grade. The operative approach has been well described and utilized over the years, but the addition of regional lymphadenectomy and our understanding of the role of the host immune system may hold important clues for the future. The development of new and more powerful chemotherapeutic agents in order to provide an adjuvant setting would be most desirable but will depend upon the development of agents that can produce an objective response in advanced disease. As in many fields of urological oncology, further advances in diagnosis and therapy will depend upon enhanced understanding of the basic disease process of neoplasia, of the immune system, and of methods of manipulation of host immunocompetence. Earlier diagnosis, as well as more judicious use of radiotherapy, chemotherapy, and possibly immunotherapy as adjuncts to the operative removal of urothelial tumors, should result in improved overall survival rates in patients with all stages of upper tract urothelial tumors.

REFERENCES

1. Rayer PFO: *Traité des Maladies des Reins,* Ballière, Paris, 1841.
2. Aschner PW: Primary tumors of the ureter. *Surg Gynecol Obstet* 35:749, 1922.
3. Abeshouse BS: Primary benign and malignant tumors of the ureter. *Am J Surg* 91:237, 1956.
4. Albarran J: In JFA Le Dentu, P Delbet (eds): *Traité de Chirugie,* Paris, vol 8, 1889.
5. Vest SA: Conservative surgery in certain benign tumors of the ureter. *J Urol* 53:97, 1945.
6. Williams CB, Mitchell JP: Carcinoma of the ureter: A review of 54 cases. *Br J Urol* 45:377, 1973.
7. Bennington JL, Beckwith JB: Tumors of the kidney, renal pelvis, and ureter, in *Atlas of Tumor Pathology,* Armed Forces Institute of Pathology, Washington, DC, fasc 12, 1975.
8. Petkovic SD: A plea for conservative operation for ureteral tumors. *J Urol* 17:220, 1972.
9. Melicow MM: Tumors of the urinary drainage tract: Urothelial tumors. *J Urol* 54:186, 1945.
10. Kerr WK, Barkin M: Aetiology and biochemistry of cancer of the bladder, in E Riches (ed): *Modern Trends in Urology,* 3d ed, Appleton-Century-Crofts, New York, p 163, 1970.
11. Oyasu R, Hopp ML: The etiology of cancer of the bladder. *Surg Gynecol Obstet* 138:97, 1974.
12. Makar N: Bilharzial ureter: Some observations on surgical pathology and surgical treatment. *Br J Surg* 36:148, 1948.
13. Scott WW, Boyd HL: A study of the carcinogenic effect of betanaphthylamine on the normal and substituted sigmoid loop bladder of dogs. *J Urol* 70:914, 1953.
14. Butler WH, Barnes JM: Carcinogenic action of ground nut meal containing aflatoxin in rats. *Food Cosmet Toxicol* 6:135, 1968.
15. Boyland E et al: The induction of renal tumours by feeding lead acetate to rats. *Br J Cancer* 16:283, 1962.
16. Elliott AY et al: Isolation of RNA virus from a papillary tumor of the human renal pelvis. *Science* 179:393, 1973.
17. Olson C et al: Oncogenicity of bovine papilloma virus. *Arch Environ Health* 19:827, 1969.
18. Fraley EE et al: Recent studies on the immunobiology and virology of human urothelial tumors. *Urol Clin North Am* 3:31, 1976.
19. Johansson S et al: Uroepithelial tumors of the renal pelvis associated with abuse of phenacetin-containing analgesics. *Cancer* 33:743, 1974.
20. Scott WW, McDonald DF: Tumors of the ureter, in MF Campbell, JH Harrison (eds): *Urology,* 3d ed, Saunders, Philadelphia, 1970.
21. Bloom NA et al: Primary carcinoma of the ureter: A report of 102 new cases. *J Urol* 103:590, 1970.
22. Grabstald H et al: Renal pelvic tumors. *JAMA* 218:845, 1971.
23. Skinner DG et al: The clinical significance of carcinoma-in-situ of the urinary bladder and its association with overt carcinoma. *J Urol* 112:68, 1974.
24. Batata M, Grabstald H: Upper urinary tract urothelial tumors. *Urol Clin North Am* 3:79, 1976.
25. Jewett HJ, Strong GH: Infiltrating carcinoma of the bladder: Relation of depth of penetration of the bladder wall to incidence of local extension and metastases. *J Urol* 55:366, 1946.
26. Deming EL, Harvard BM: Tumors of the kidney, in MF Campbell, JH Harrison (eds): *Urology,* 3d ed, Saunders, Philadelphia, 1970.
27. Higgins CC: Tumors of the renal pelvis: Review of 47 cases. *Ann Surg* 137:95, 1953.
28. Carlson HE: Squamous cell carcinoma of the renal pelvis: A five year cure. *J Urol* 83:812, 1960.
29. Williams CB, Mitchell JP: Carcinoma of the ureter: A review of 54 cases. *Br J Urol* 45:377, 1973.
30. Almgard LE et al: Carcinoma of the ureter, with special reference to malignancy grading and prognosis. *Scand J Urol Nephrol* 7:165, 1973.
31. Bergman H et al: New roentgenologic signs of carcinoma of the ureter. *Am J Roentgen* 86:707, 1961.

32. Devlin HB: Carcinoma of the ureter associated with a ureteric calculus invading the sigmoid colon. *Br J Surg* 52:553, 1965.
33. Casey WC, Goodwin WE: Percutaneous antegrade pyelography and hydronephrosis. *J Urol* 74:64, 1955.
34. Boijsen E, Folin J: Angiography in carcinoma of the renal pelvis. *Acta Radiol* 56:81, 1961.
35. Lang EK, Nourse M: The roentgenographic diagnosis of obstructive lesions of the ureter. *J Urol* 101:812, 1969.
36. Cullen TH et al: Urine cytology and primary carcinoma of the renal pelvis and ureter. *Aust NZ J Surg* 41:230, 1972.
37. Grace DA et al: Carcinoma of the renal pelvis: A 15-year review. *J Urol* 98:566, 1967.
38. Zincke H et al: Significance of urinary cytology in the early detection of transitional cell cancer of the upper urinary tract. *J Urol* 116:781, 1976.
39. Eriksson O, Johansson S: Urothelial neoplasms of the upper urinary tract: A correlation between cytologic and histologic findings in 43 patients with urothelial neoplasms of the renal pelvis or ureter. *Acta Cytol* 20:20, 1976.
40. Gill WB et al: Retrograde brushing: A new technique for obtaining histologic and cytologic material from ureteral, renal pelvic, and renal caliceal lesions. *J Urol* 109:573, 1973.
41. Colston JAC, Arcadi JA: Bilateral renal papillomas: Transpelvic electro-resection with preservation of kidney. *J Urol* 73:460, 1955.
42. McIntyre D et al: Primary ureteric neoplasms, with a report of forty cases. *Br J Urol* 37:160, 1965.
43. Strong DW, Pearse HD: Recurrent urothelial tumors following surgery for transitional cell carcinoma of the upper urinary tract. *Cancer* 38:2178, 1976.
44. Carroll G: Bilateral transitional cell carcinoma of the renal pelvis. *J Urol* 93:132, 1965.
45. Blute RD Jr, Richie JP: Tumors of the renal pelvis and ureter. *J Urol* (in press).
46. Batata MA et al: Primary carcinoma of the ureter: A prognostic study. *Cancer* 35:1626, 1975.
47. Soloway MS: Intravesical and systemic chemotherapy of murine bladder cancer. *Cancer Res* 37:2918, 1977.
48. Brady LW et al: Radiation therapy, a valuable adjunct in the management of carcinoma of the ureter. *JAMA* 206:2871, 1968.
49. Holtz F: Papillomas and primary carcinoma of the ureter: Report of 20 cases. *J Urol* 88:380, 1962.

SELECTED BIBLIOGRAPHY

Johnson DE, Samuels ML (eds): *Cancer of the Genitourinary Tract.* Raven Press, New York, 1979.

Skinner DG, deKernion JB (eds): *Genitourinary Cancer.* Saunders, Philadelphia, 1978.

Yagoda A: Chemotherapy of genitourinary tumors, in Burchenal JH, Oettgen HF (eds): *Cancer Achievements, Challenges and Prospects for the 1980's,* vol. 2, Grune & Stratton, New York, 1981.

33

BLADDER CARCINOMA

George R. Prout, Jr.

Bladder cancer has been known since ancient times, but, like the weather, no one could do anything about it until Thomas Alva Edison invented the incandescent bulb in 1880. Cytoscopes had already been imagined and developed, but Nitze immediately recognized the applicability of the bulb to the scope. Diagnoses hitherto guessed at were made, and some improvement in treatment was realized. However, urology remained in its infancy until intravenous contrast material was developed in Germany, in 1929, and introduced in this country by Moses Swick of the Mount Sinai Hospital (think of the bureaucratic trials he'd now face!). The compound "Uroselectan" had side effects, and lethal reactions occurred, but modern urology was born. The next major event was the development of the resectoscope. This reached useful proportions by the late 1930s and with its development it became inevitable that urologists, long a separate body within the surgical community, would be for the foreseeable future a discrete group of specialists, destined to study and learn in great depth about the disorders which they treated.

By 1925, urologists could diagnose preoperatively renal cell carcinoma, hydronephrosis, calculi, renal tuberculosis, and a host of upper tract diseases. Appropriate therapeutic strategies could be planned and carried out. Ureteral calculi could be visualized, located, and extracted (sometimes too often). Benign prostatic hyperplasia could be resected transurethrally instead of enucleated from above, and both large and small bladder tumors could be seen and treated. At last, patients no longer needed to die of hemorrhage or clot retention.

Advances in other specialties and other scientific disciplines have been adopted by urologists to benefit their patients. Eugene Bricker made radical pelvic urological surgery with its associated urinary diversion a medically and socially acceptable form of treatment.[1] Prior to the repopularization of the ileal conduit, urinary diversion was accomplished via the colon or skin in a variety of ways. This, plus suitable skin appliances, made radical cystectomy acceptable. Interestingly, it brought about a new body of nursing specialists through patient organization and demand. A huge void in patient care was filled when patients organized themselves into "ostomy societies," whence arose the indispensable enterostomal therapists of today.

The incidence of bladder carcinoma can only be estimated. About 30,000 individuals will develop their first bladder tumor in 1982.[2] There will be a sex distri bution of male to female of 4:1. About 10,000 patients will die of bladder carcinoma in 1982. These figures are important, but they scarcely reflect the real incidence of the disease. Bladder carcinoma is prone to recur, not because the tumor(s) was(were) incompletely treated, but because new tumors arise. Heney et al.,[3] reporting for the National Bladder Cancer Project Collaborative Group A (CGA), found that recurrence of superficial carcinoma (T_a, T_1) depends on several variables. However, over a median of 39 months of observation of 238 patients who had never before had a tumor, half experienced at least one recurrence in 12 to 18 months. Since these were superficial tumors initially and most of the recurrences were superficial, it follows that repetitive tumor expression and multiplicity of tumors in the same patient at the same time makes the incidence figure given a nearly meaningless estimate. Probably bladder carcinoma is the most commonly diagnosed neoplasm in the United States, leaving skin cancer aside.

Workers in certain industries seem to suffer a higher initial incidence that the population at large. In fact, human bladder carcinoma is said to be the first neoplasm produced by an industrial compound. In 1895, Rehn reported on "aniline cancers" which occurred in workers who were in contact with dyestuffs.[4] Forty years went by before it was appreciated that the causative agent was probably an aromatic amine. This untimely discovery was reported by Ferguson et al.,[5] who obtained the information from 23 patients who had worked in a plant that opened in the United States in 1917. These workers had been exposed to 2-naphthylamine. Feeding this compound to dogs produced bladder carcinomas;[6] urinary diversion in dogs produced ureteral and pelvic tumors, but no bladder cancers were found.[7] The metabolite, 2-amino-1-naphthol sulphuric acid, could be found in the urine,[8] and this metabolite was carcinogenic for the mouse bladder.[9] Subsequently, the causal relationship between human and animal bladder carcinoma and 4-aminobiphenyl, 4-4'-diaminophyl (benzidene), and 4-nitrobiphenyl has been established.[10-12]

It is difficult to identify many carcinogens, particularly those that are "weak." Even more difficult is to identify the proximate carcinogen. In human beings, 2-naphthylamine is hydroxylated to 2-amino-1-naphthol (see Fig. 33-1). This compound may be the proximate carcinogen responsible for human bladder carcinoma. N-hydroxylation may be important,[13] and Troll and Belman have produced evidence suggesting that an N-hydroxy-ortho-OH metabolite is the proximate carcinogen.[14]

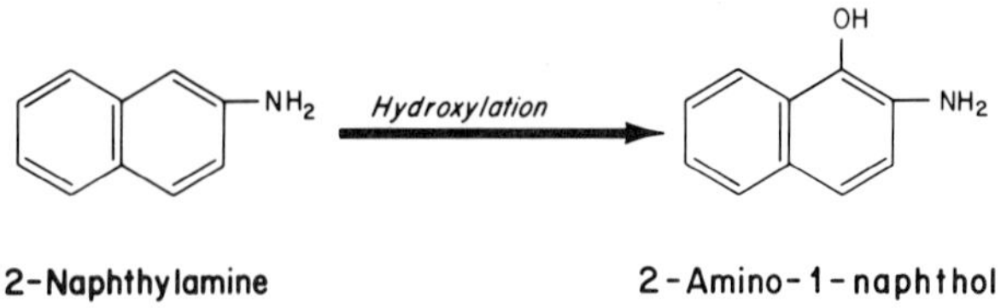

FIGURE 33-1 The probable proximate carcinogen of 2-naphthylamine.

Characterization of carcinogens plays an important role in identifying compounds that may be otherwise unsuspected. For instance, it is known that at least one tryptophan metabolite will alter the heat stability and RNA-priming ability of treated DNA,[15] that tryptophan metabolites are carcinogenic in mice,[16] that the addition of tryptophan to the diets of animals fed acetylaminofluorene makes the diet carcinogenic,[17] and that 50 percent of patients with bladder carcinoma excrete excessive amounts of hydroxy-kyurenine, acetylkynurenine, and kuyrenic acid when given a loading dose of tryptophan.[18]

Epidemiological studies suggest that as many as 40 percent of the patients with bladder carcinoma would never have developed the disease if they had not smoked cigarettes.[19] No one has even suggested what the nature of the proximate carcinogen might be that results from smoking cigarettes. Initially, women were spared bladder carcinoma, but today, even though the sex ratio is three or four times more prevalent in males, the incidence of bladder carcinoma, like that of lung cancer, is increasing in females.

Much has been written about saccharin and cyclamates as causes of human bladder cancer. Hicks and Chowaniec[20] conducted a series of studies which demonstrated that these compounds were strong promoters but were, overall, weak carcinogens. Animals fed the sweeteners alone had a very low incidence of bladder carcinoma, but those whose bladders had been insulted with subcarcinogenic doses of methyl-nitrosourea (MNU) had a very high incidence of bladder carcinoma. The lay press produced much copy when these data were released and even more when some preliminary results of studies in humans were made public. Cyclamates had previously been banned for consumption, but careful epidemiological studies in humans revealed that prodigious amounts of saccharin in food and drink would be required to increase the risk of bladder cancer to a detectable level.

Coffee drinking has been suspect for years. Again, epidemiological studies have ruled this out as a cause. Parenthetically, these types of studies are very difficult to perform since the variables, e.g., cigarette smoking, industrial exposure, sweeteners, are so many in the population at large.[21,22]

Regarding bilharziasis and bladder carcinoma, an exhaustive review of the subject demonstrates a very close relationship between the two disorders.[23] A recent publication[24] indicates that nitrite was present in the urine of patients with bilharzial cystitis (25 percent) and when carcinoma was present, two-thirds of the patients had urinary nitrite present. Controls had no nitrite present. Urinary tract infection was associated with urinary nitrite and commonly found with urinary dysplasia. Nitrosourea may be one of the products of infection, thus producing a proximate carcinogen. The figures are persuasive, but much more investigation is clearly necessary.

SIGNS, SYMPTOMS, AND EARLY DETECTION

Painless hematuria is the most common symptom of which patients with bladder carcinoma complain. It is usually total but may be at the end of the stream or, less likely, at the beginning. Terminal hematuria may be associated with suprapubic pain or discomfort, since the bladder mucosa, which slides so readily over the detrusor under normal circumstances, is fixed by the tumor. The mucosa splits at the end of voiding; hence, the terminal hematuria. Lack of vesical compliance produces the discomfort.

It is important not to neglect evaluation of patients microscopic hematuria, even those on anticoagulant therapy. In men, a two-glass test may be very helpful to locate the site of bleeding. Many red blood cells in the first 30 mL would suggest the cause for bleeding is below the bladder neck. Equal numbers of red blood cells would suggest the cause of the bleeding is above the bladder neck.

Frequency and nocturia may also occur as bladder compliance is limited or as infection involves necrotic tumors. Clots may be present, of course. Vermiform clots are often casts of the ureter, and careful inquiry should be made, since there may be laterlizing signs to suggest unilateral renal or ureteral bleeding.

The most important thing about hematuria is to recognize it as evidence of serious urological disease until proven otherwise.

Cystitislike symptoms may occur with gross or microscopic hematuria. When this occurs, the patient may have carcinoma in situ. Sometimes the irritative symptoms precede the hematuria by several months.

Always be alert for the 45- to 60-year-old man with frequency, urgency, nocturia, and dysuria, who has no residual urine and a smooth or mildly trabeculated bladder. Carcinoma in situ may be responsible for this constellation of symptoms, and every physician should be aware of their implications.

Rarely, flank pain due to pyelonephritis with obstruction of a ureteral orifice may be the presenting symptom. This is quite uncommon, as are metastases evident in some other organ without urinary symptoms. This almost never happens. In fact, incidentally found bladder carcinoma is very rare. Urinary symptoms of some sort are nearly always present when bladder carcinoma is found.

While intravenous urography is an important diagnostic study, it is folly to depend on this alone to detect carcinoma of the bladder. Cystoscopy is the definitive step. If one's index of suspicion is high, urinary and saline bladder washings should be obtained for cytological examination.

"Early" detection is a fruitless effort. About 65 percent of the patients with invasive bladder carcinoma have never had a previous bladder tumor, and their delay in seeking help averaged about 2 weeks.[25] The frequency of bladder carcinoma in the population at large makes screening programs ineffectual and/or impractical. Therefore, if physicians would proceed with appropriate diagnostic studies instead of treating the hematuria with pills and/or watchful waiting, the source of bleeding and the cause could be determined and correct therapy instituted.

DIAGNOSTIC TECHNIQUES

Given the patient with hematuria, a complete history and physical examination are essential and should not be left to the internist. If the patient has a bladder tumor, in one way or another, the urologist and the patient are going to be together for a long time, and so the urologist must be familar with all the patient's problems, current medications, and past operations. An aortoiliac graft is a very major matter with which to deal if a cystectomy is planned, and special strategies must be considered if the urinary diversion is not to be a very eventful occasion. Yet, matters of this magnitude have escaped careful consideration by the vascular surgeon, internist, and urologist, with disastrous results.

Intravenous urography has a high yield in this age group. The tumor(s) may be visible, ureterectasis or hydronephrosis may be present, synchronous ureteral or pelvic tumors may be visualized, diverticula which may harbor tumors may be seen, and, above all else, the physician will discover if the patient has two kidneys and where they are.

Cystendoscopy under anesthesia is the next step. If the patient is bleeding when first seen, then a quick examination with a small cytoscope is indicated. It is often a missed chance not to cytoscope a bleeding patient since examination may be very revealing. This will often indicate whence the patient is bleeding, if not from what. Blood may be seen issuing from one ureteral orifice, a bladder tumor may be seen; a host of conditions may be identified because the bleeding localizes the source. Leaving the currently bleeding patient aside, urinary and saline bladder washings should be obtained at cystoscopy. These studies are very important because they may reflect the existence of hidden or invisible tumor in the bladder or in one or both upper tracts. Further, the differential of urinary cytology and saline cytology may help to isolate the neoplastic process. Patients should be well-hydrated before a sample is submitted for cytology. Never submit the first voided urine in the morning for cytology because hypertonic urine is very destructive to exfoliated cells. Cytology may be positive in a urinary specimen and negative in saline washings, suggesting that the source of the tumor cells lies in one upper tract or the other. Positive urinary cytology alone strongly suggests that a urothelial tumor is present but gives no hint as to site unless washings are also done. Visible tumors and suspicious areas should be biopsied with a cold cup. Today's instruments allow for biopsies into muscle, if one wishes. This is advantageous when the visible tumor(s) is small, the bladder wall thin, or the tumor placed so that tangential bites with a resectoscope may cut deeper than one wishes.

Bimanual examination under anesthesia is an important and often omitted step. There is no hope of palpating the majority of bladder carcinomas, but this information, even though negative, is important. Further, extraurinary pathological processes may be discovered. Palpable tumors are commonly high-stage. This determination should be made in conjunction with microscopic examination of deep parts of the tumor. The International Union against Cancer classification of bladder tumor allows for a sample biopsy of tumor and a record of bimanual palpability or lack of same to stage of a tumor.[26] This is unsuitable for staging, in the view of the American Joint Committee's Task Force on the Staging of GU Neoplasms.[27]

Transurethral resection of tumors over 2 or 3 cm is appropriate after cold cup biopsies have been taken. Often it is simpler, quicker, and, in women, safer to fulgurate after biopsies have been obtained. Jewett has advocated transurethral resection of larger tumors in two or three separate collections.[28] The superficial part of the tumor is resected and the bladder evacuated. Those resected chips constitute the first specimen. The muscularis is resected next, and these chips represent the second specimen. Deep bites represent the third. This practice is a good one providing the bladder wall is suitably thick and the tumor large. However, the deep bites are often charily obtained and charred so badly that the pathologist has difficulty in identifying tumor cells even though they may be present. Practice today usually follows the more direct lines of simple resection with the request that each chip be sectioned. The World Health Organization (WHO) has proposed that a deeply invasive tumor is one that provides a bite of resected tissue in which the tumor has invaded the entire piece, from one edge to the other. Superficially invasive tumors are those that have invaded only parts of chips. While there are objections to these stipulations, e.g., orientation of the resected bite, an oblique cut, and so on, it seems to be a worthwhile proposal. The data base for this system is lacking, and so it would be a useful project to evaluate its accuracy. Certainly, our current means of clinical staging are grossly inadequate (see later).[29]

Invasive bladder carcinoma is a potentially lethal disease. It often metastasizes before urinary symptoms have brought the patient to the physician. It is very rare, however, for metastatic disease to be clinically evident before urinary symptoms, i.e., hematuria, frequency, dysuria, have occurred. Upon diagnosis, a chest roentgenogram, a radionuclide bone scan, and liver and renal function studies should be performed. A study of the first site of failure in patients who had undergone cystectomy revealed that bones and lungs were most commonly involved.[30] Therefore, these areas, along with the liver, should be evaluated.

Modern day staging had its beginnings with the observations of Jewett and Strong,[31] Jewett,[28] and Marshall.[32] Intravenous urography, bimanual examination, and transurethral resection (TUR) formed the basis of the system (see Fig. 33-2). It provided a good basis for communication, creating order out of chaos. However, as time has passed, it is evident that the system has several shortcomings and should be changed.

Some of the problems are as follows:

1. It does not automatically indicate whether the stage is clinical or pathological.
2. It fails to indicate grade.
3. It does not provide for indicating multiplicity.
4. It does not provide for carcinoma in situ to be separated from papillary tumors confined to the mucosa.
5. It does not provide any description of the primary tumor if the stage is D_1 or D_2.
6. There is no provision for indicating evidence of lymphatic invasion in the primary tumor.
7. There is no provision for indicating metastatic sites, aside from lymph nodes in D_1.

While any system which remedies these deficiencies will be more cumbersome, it seems appropriate that we think of neoplastic processes in these ways. The American Joint Committee has provided those involved in the care of patients with urological carcinoma with a logical system that is based on a shorthand system of describing a tumor, its domains, and the means by which the information was obtained. It is as follows:

1.0 ANATOMY OF THE BLADDER

1.1 Primary site: The urinary bladder is a hollow viscus consisting of three layers: the mucosa and submucosa (lamina propria), the muscularis, and the serosa (peritoneum covering the superior surface and upper part of the base). In the male, it is in relationship to the rectum and seminal vesicles posteriorly, the prostate inferiorly, and the pubis and peritoneum anteriorly. In the female, the vagina is located posteriorly and the uterus superiorly. The bladder is extraperitoneal in location.

1.2 Nodal stations: The regional lymph nodes are the nodes of the true pelvis, whose anatomical boundaries are subtended by the arcuate line and planes involved. Its fixed points are the pubic crest, the pectineal line, medial border of ilium, ala of sacrum, and sacral promontory. Distant nodes are all others.

1.3 Metastatic sites: Distant spread to lung, bone, and liver is most common.

2.0 RULES FOR CLASSIFICATIONS

2.1 Clinical-diagnostic staging: Primary tumor assessment includes bimanual examination under anesthesia before and after endoscopic surgery (biopsy or transurethral resection) and/or histologic verification of the presence or absence of tumor. Add "m" for multiple tumors. Lymphography is neces-

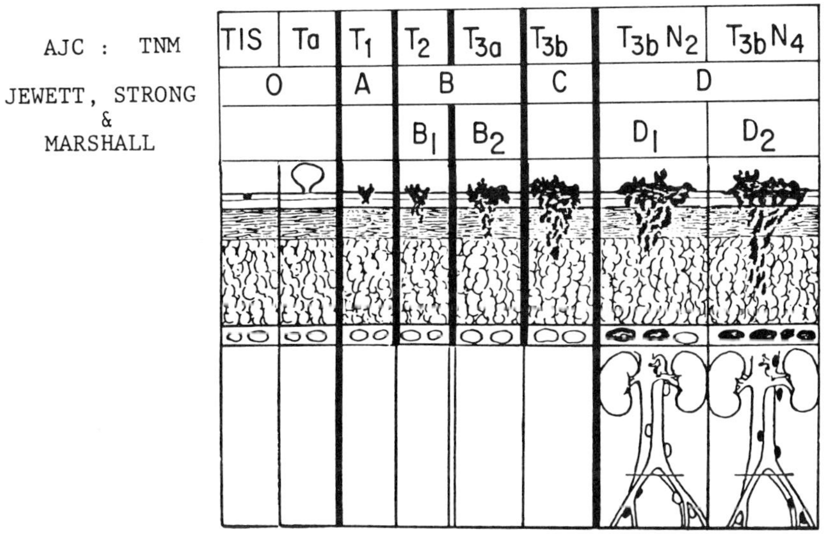

FIGURE 33-2 The Jewett-Strong-Marshall system of staging compared with the American Joint Committee system.

sary for nodal evaluation. Evaluation for distant metastases requires chest films, biochemical and blood profiles, and isotopic studies as indicated.*

2.2 Surgical-evaluative staging: Laparotomy or extraperitoneal surgical evaluation of primary tumor and lymph nodes with biopsy material other than endoscopic are required for this staging. Histologic confirmation of tumor involvement or lack of same is required for use of this stage.

2.3 Postsurgical treatment–pathologic staging: Histologic examination and confirmation of extent is required. Total cystectomy and lymph node dissection are required to utilize this staging.

2.4 Retreatment staging: Biopsy confirmation when feasible is desirable to determine persistence after irradiation or surgery. Other procedures as noted above may be utilized, particularly in distant visceral sites.

NB: See Appendix A for the use of subscripts ("c," "s," "p," and "r") to indicate source of material used for determining T, N, and M.

3.0 TNM CLASSIFICATION

3.1 Primary tumor (T)
The suffix "m" should be added to the appropriate T category to indicate multiple lesions. Papilloma is classified as "G0."
 T_X Minimum requirements cannot be met.
 T_0 No evidence of primary tumor.
 T_{IS} Carcinoma in situ (if used without subscript, T_{IS} indicates bladder alone).
  b   bladder
  u   ureter
  pr u prostatic urethra
  p d prostatic ducts
 T_a Papillary noninvasive carcinoma.
 T_1 There is carcinoma without microscopic invasion beyond the lamina propria. On bimanual examination a freely mobile mass may be felt; this should not be felt after complete transurethral resection of the lesion.
 T_2 There is microscopic invasion of superficial muscle of the bladder. On bimanual examination there may be induration of the bladder wall, which is mobile. There is usually no residual induration after complete transurethral resection of the lesion.
 T_3 On bimanual examination there may be induration or a nodular mobile mass palpable in the bladder wall which persists after transurethral resection (T_3 may not be used alone).
  T_{3a} Microscopic invasion of deep muscle which is defined as histological evidence of tumor clearly extending through muscle bundles to both edges of a resected specimen.
  T_{3b} Invasion into perivesical fat.
 T_4 There is microscopic evidence of muscle invasion and tumor is fixed or invading neighboring structures. The following subclassifications should be used when conditions are met:
  T_{4a} Tumor invading substance of prostate (microscopically proven), uterus, or vagina.
  T_{4b} Tumor fixed to the pelvic wall and/or infiltrating the abdominal wall.

3.2 Nodal Involvement (N)
The regional lymph nodes are those within the true pelvis. All others are distant nodes. Histological examination is required for stages N_0 through N_3, except for subscript "c."
 N_X Minimum requirements cannot be met.
 N_0 No involvement of regional lymph nodes.
 N_1 Involvement of a single homolateral regional lymph node.
 N_2 Involvement of contralateral, bilateral, or multiple regional lymph nodes.
 N_3 There is a fixed mass on the pelvic wall with a free space between this and the tumor.

3.3 DISTANT METASTASES (M)
 M_X Not assessed.
 M_0 No (known) distant metastases.
 M_1 Distant metastases present.
  Specify _____.
  Specify sites according to the following notations:

Distant lymph nodes	LYM
Pulmonary	PUL
Osseous	OSS
Hepatic	HEP
Brain	BRA
Bone marrow	MAR
Pleura	PLE
Skin	SKI
Eye	EYE
Other	OTH

---

* Computerized body scan and/or other modalities may subsequently be used to supply information concerning minimal requirements for staging.

4.0 POSTSURGICAL TREATMENT RESIDUAL TUMOR (R)

R_0 No residual tumor.
R_1 Microscopic residual tumor.
R_2 Macroscopic residual tumors.
    Specify _____.

5.0 STAGE GROUPING

Follow 2.0 rules for classification:
Stage   I: cT_a, T_{IS} restricted to bladder, T_1, N_0, M_0
Stage II: cT_2, N_0, M_0
Stage III: cT_{IS} in prostatic urethra and/or ducts, $cT_{3a}, T_{3b}, N_0, M_0$
Stage IV: cT_4, pT_{IS} in prostatic substance, Any pN+, any M+

6.0 HISTOPATHOLOGY

The predominant cancer is a transitional-cell cancer. Grading of the tumor is as follows:

6.1 Tumor grade (G)

G_1 Well-differentiated.
G_2 Moderately well-differentiated.
G_{3-4} Poorly to very poorly differentiated.
Use whichever indicator is most appropriate (either term or G + number).

7.0 PERFORMANCE STATUS OF HOST (H)

		ECOG/ Zubrod scale	Karnofsky, %
H_0	Normal activity.	0	90–100
H_1	Symptomatic but ambulatory—cares for self.	1	70–80
H_2	Ambulatory more than 50% of the time—occasionally needs help.	2	50–60
H_3	Ambulatory 50% or less of time—nursing care needed.	3	30–40
H_4	Bedridden—may need hospitalization.	4	10–20

APPENDIX A Subscripts and Their Use to Indicate the Manner in Which Extent of Tumor was Determined

Under most circumstances a clinical estimate of tumor extent will be made according to the TNM classification. This may vary according to the rules of classification for a given site, but this initial classification will not be altered, regardless of subsequent events. Further information obtained by surgical-evaluative procedures (s), post-surgical-treatment pathologic staging (p), or other techniques that relate to a determination of extent of disease should be used as appropriate subscripts to the relevant part of T, N, or M (see below). In some circumstances, as the neoplastic process progresses either locally (T), in regional nodes (N), or in distant sites (M), further clinical evidence of extent of disease may be obtained. In such instances, cT or some element of TNM may be altered. By such additions, one might subsequently characterize a patient as being stage $cT_3 \, sN_2 \, pM$ (PUL) indicating clinical extent of the local tumor, regional nodal involvement as proven by a surgical-evaluative procedure, and actual pathological proof of a metastatic pulmonary lesion. Again, it should be emphasized that the first clinical staging classification which determined the initial therapeutic plan should not be changed. This remains with the patient for the duration of the disease. Further subsets of TNM classification are introduced to provide a means of communicating the changes in disease status and in reporting the results of therapeutic strategies employed at given stages in the progression of the disease.

Some examples of how the foregoing classifications might be used are as follows:

AJC Stage

Patient undergoes TURB, and pathology report reveals tumor invading into perivesical fat. Because of severe urinary symptoms an ileal loop is done. During surgery several lymph nodes are removed from the pelvis and histologically confirmed as metastatic. Following surgery a bone scan is done which reveals bony metastases. $cT_{3b}sN_2cM_{10SS}$

A patient comes in following preoperative radiotherapy. Chest x-ray, bone scan, and liver scan are negative. A radical cystectomy is performed. The pathology report reveals no residual bladder cancer, but one lymph node is positive from the obturator group. $pT_0pN_1cM_0$

A patient has negative bladder biopsies, but a biopsy of a suspicious area in the prostatic urethra reveals TCC. Chest x-ray is negative. $cT_{ISpr.u.}N_xM_x$

Computerized axial tomography has been evaluated for the staging of bladder carcinoma. It seems to be most useful in staging large tumors and those that are invading the perivesical tissues. In one's personal experience, a CAT scan was reported positive for an extensive invasive tumor when the patient actually had several low-grade tumors contiguous to an area where a previous cystostomy had been performed. Enlarged nodes lying low in the mesentery have been reported as positive in another patient. Some of these were calcified, as well.

Subsequent generations of CAT scanners will surely have improved resolution and result in better, more accurate estimates of tumor size, bladder wall, and extravesical involvement.

Pedal lymphangiogram (LAG) has had its supporters[34,35] and will have its detractors. Johnson and his associates perform the study routinely in patients who may be candidates for cystectomy. They have observed positive nodes, obtained biopsies using small-bore needles, and avoided unnecessary operations. The procedure has been criticized on several grounds. Pelvic nodes in this group of aged individuals often appear abnormal, and, further, there has been the complaint that pedal LAGs do not fill the obturator nodes. Merrin has demonstrated that these nodes are visualized. More importantly, a search of authoritative anatomical texts fails to describe nodes in the obturator space. We have studied the nodes of 12 patients who had bilateral pedal LAGs.[36] Pelvic roentgenograms preoperatively revealed the customary distribution of iliac nodes, and postoperative roentgenograms revealed all the visualized nodes to be removed. The dissections were done with great care, labeling nodes anterior, lateral, medial and posterior external iliacs, and, where possible, hypogastric and inferior common iliac nodes. We also removed the tissue from the obturator space on each site. This was separately labeled as obturator. All nodes removed had oil droplets in them, and the tissues of the obturator space rarely contained any nodes. These uncommonly encountered nodes also had oil droplets present (Fig. 33-3). While one may complain that the source of nodes is simply that which one wishes to designate them, our dissections were meticulous with regard to anatomical structures, and when we finished dissecting the external iliac vessels we still had a mass of tissue in and around the obturator nerve and vessels. As indicated, these tissues rarely harbored a node. Regardless of the question about anatomical dissection, we did remove all the visualized nodes, and none were free of oil droplets. Therefore, we agree with Merrin.[35] Pedal lymphangiography will visualize all the nodes customarily dissected in a lymphadenectomy. It will not fill presacral and other posteriorly

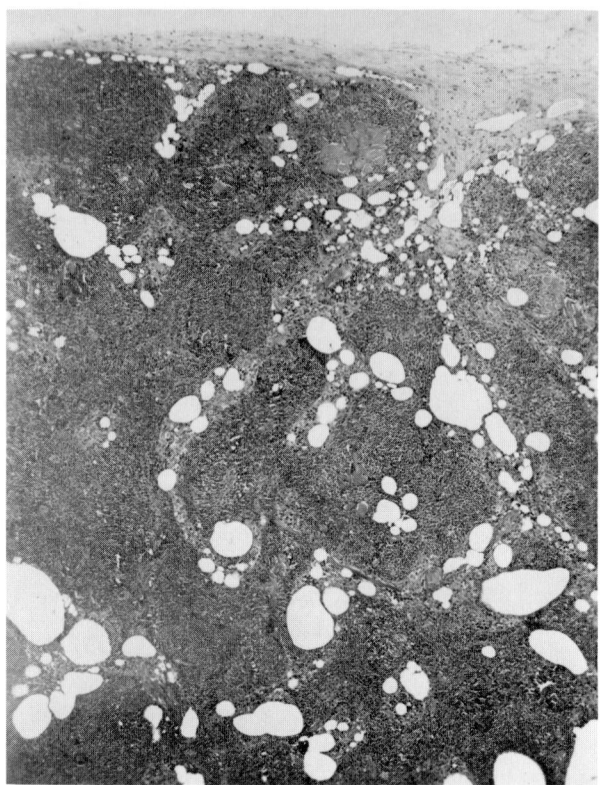

FIGURE 33-3 Obturator lymph nodes with oil droplets present.

placed lymph nodes, but these are not customarily removed during radical cystectomy, in any event. Thus, we must conclude that pedal LAG will reveal grossly involved pelvic nodes. Given a patient with a nodular invasive tumor, LAG may help identify nodes that may be aspirated by slender-needle biopsy, thus obviating an unnecessary surgical procedure when the aspirate of the suspicious node is positive for tumor cells.

Vesical sonography is in a preliminary stage regarding the staging of bladder carcinoma. Abdominal, transrectal, and intravesical routes have all been attempted. The most effective and accurate method thus far developed has been via the intravesical route when two angle sources, 90° and 120°, have been used. Lower-stage tumors have been most accurately staged, but the procedure requires great skill and experience.[37,38]

THERAPY

Superficial Tumors: Stages O, A (T_{IS}, T_a, and T_1)

The conventional means of treating superficial papillary tumors have been by cystoscopy, biopsy, TUR, and/or fulguration (F). Satisfactory 5-year survival rates have been reported which taken at face value would suggest that little further need be done to improve the status of these patients (Table 33-1). Evaluation of the course of these patients indicates that survival rates are an inaccurate means of judging the results of this type of therapy, however.

There are now many reports which indicate that there is an almost unacceptable recurrence rate of tumors in many patients.[3,39] Karyotypic data, animal models,[40,41] and site of recurrence in humans all strongly support the concept that most of these tumors arise from implantation of viable cells that originated from a single cell. Althausen et al.[42] have reported that of 129 patients with initially superficial tumors, after 5 years only 20 failed to have another tumor. Seventy-nine patients had gratuitously selected mucosa which was taken with the tumor. Of these 79, 12 patients had T_{IS} in the mucosa surrounding papillary tumors and 26 had atypia. Of the 12 patients with T_{IS} 10 and 9 of the 26 patients with atypia 9 developed invasion of the bladder muscle.

Heney et al.[39] have demonstrated that after conventional TUR and fulguration, grade II and, particularly, grade III tumors will progress (45 percent of 31 tumors) to a higher stage, even though the histological sections demonstrated complete removal of the tumor. Progression was also closely related to T_1 tumors (30 percent of 63 tumors) and to the presence of moderate to severe dysplasia in biopsies of preselected sites. National Bladder Cancer Collaborative Group A (CGA) has shown that triethylene thiophosphoramide (TTPA) will prevent recurrences for periods of time far in excess of a control group, providing the original tumor was sensitive to the agent. CGA is currently testing the hypothesis that immediate instillations of TTPA (60 mg/60 mL) after TUR, followed by either observation only or three more instillations at weekly intervals, will significantly diminish recurrences.[43]

One is faced, then, with two issues regarding superficial tumors. Each has its subsets. The ideal antitumor agent would be completely effective in ablating superficial tumors. To be effective, only a single instillation would be required (the ultimate would be a single oral dose of the agent); it would have no systemic or local toxic effects, and the patient would remain tumor-free. We may never reach such a perfect state. A host of agents have been used and the results reported. They are fairly consistent, but one should keep in mind that many variables influence outcome. For instance, in the decade after TTPA was introduced by Jones and Swinney[44] and Veenema et al.[45] this agent was used only when the quantitative aspects of tumor growth were overwhelming or had overwhelmed the urologist who had been doggedly resecting tumors from such a patient for months or, more likely, years. If the TTPA failed, cystectomy was the next step, providing the patient was a suitable physical candidate. In contrast, the characteristics of tumor diathesis listed by Koontz et al.[43] indicate that the success rate (CR) drops markedly when multiple tumors are present and/or when the tumors are >4 cm.

This seems to be true for other drugs, as well, though these types of data are often lacking. To judge the ablative effectiveness of an agent, reports should include data concerning the patients—what proportion were experiencing their first tumor event, what proportion had had prior tumors treated by TUR, what proportion had been treated with other cytotoxic agents (failure to respond to TTPA usually means that a significant decrease in the proportion of responders to mitomycin C will result)?[46] Tumor size, multiplicity, grade, and stage should also be included, along with the results of cytology and biopsies of preselected sites of urothelium. These matters all bear on the ultimate result of intravesical therapy as an ablative agent.

Equally, how might one best select patients for prophylactic TTPA and, probably, other agents, as well? Since the tumors in question are low stage, and few, if any, aside from T_{IS}, represent an immediate threat to the host, the writer reasoned that an index lesion might

TABLE 33-1 Five-Year Survival for Patients with Bladder Tumors in Low Stage Treated by Transurethral Resection and Fulguration

	Stage O	Stage A
Flocks[104]		77 percent
Milner[105]		70 percent
Nichols and Marshall[106]		82 percent
Barnes et al.[107]		63 percent
Althausen et al.[42]		81 percent

provide a good in vivo test of that tumor's sensitivity to a given agent, in this case, TTPA. Obviously, if eight instillations of TTPA did not eradicate the index lesion, then there would be no purpose in continuing with prophylactic therapy on a monthly basis.

Different therapeutic regimens for TTPA have varied from 15 to 60 mg instilled weekly[45,47-49] or more frequently for several weeks. The toxicity reported by Abbassian and Wallace[47] resulted in a silent consensus that weekly doses of 60 mg in 60 mL of distilled water would be adequate. The CGA experience[43] demonstrated that concentration, not total dose, would yield the same result; 30 mg/30 mL distilled water was associated with a CR equivalent to 60 mg/60 mL distilled water, nearly 50 percent for each. A matter of considerable importance intrudes here. The patients to be treated need a white blood cell and platelet count before each treatment, and they also should have fasted overnight. One has seen patients who failed to respond to TTPA when it was administered after lunch, but who did respond after fasting. This prevented the dilution of the drug by a coffee- or beer-induced diuresis over the 2-h period of retention.

There are now numerous reports of other agents which, when instilled intravesically, are effective in destroying tumors. They seem to have the same or a slightly higher rate of response than TTPA. Mitomycin C (MMC) is possibly the most widely used of these other agents.[50] A phase I and II study has shown that the most effective dosage regimen was 40 mg weekly for 8 weeks.[51] There are no systemic effects, though it has been reported that some patients develop a rash on the hands and feet within days of instillation.[52-54] One has also observed edema and redness of the prepuce in a patient. This was correct by having the patient retract his foreskin completely before voiding and washing carefully afterwards. The evidence suggests that the rash is due to local contact with the drug. There have also been irritative vesical symptoms. These may be severe enough to cease treatment.[52] MMC may have a very high CR rate in patients not previously treated with TTPA, but patients who fail TTPA therapy may not respond nearly so well.[52,55] This may be because both are alkylators or because of some inherent biological characteristics of certain tumors.

Doxorubicin has been used with varying degrees of success in the treatment of superficial tumors.[56,57] It may be a very effective agent, but dosage and schedules have not been worked out. The response rates have varied from nil (CR) to 80 percent.[58] The agent has been used in amounts as high as 60 mg 3 times a week for 2 weeks.[56] The higher the dose, the more likely irritative symptoms are to occur. Systemic toxicity has not occurred in the patients reported.

Immunotherapy has been reported to reduce the size and number of tumors present when bacillus Calmette-Guérin had been administered intravesically (120 mg) and intradermally (5 mg) weekly for 6 weeks.[59,60] This form of therapy is experimental and should be used only after further data have been obtained and more extensive trials conducted.

Doxorubicin has been used as an adjuvant to TUR of T_a and T_1 tumors by a group of Belgian urologists.[61] The drug was instilled within 24 h after TUR (50 mg/50 mL normal saline) and retained for 1 h. This was repeated twice in the next week, then weekly for a month, and then monthly for a year. Of the 110 patients accessioned 82 were evaluable at 1 year. Of the "primary" patients (23), 19 were tumor-free; 4 had T_1 recurrence. Of the 59 recurrent patients, 31 were tumor-free while 28 (47 percent) had had a recurrence. Of the 82 patients 5 developed $>T_1$ recurrent tumors. Supporting the proposition that we still lack adequate data to determine the most effective and least toxic adjuvant regimen for doxorubicin is the fact that 22 percent of the patients accessioned developed severe local irritative symptoms and withdrew from the study.

Koshiba has used 2000-mL solutions over 24 h containing either 40 mg of MMC, 100 mg Adriamycin (ADM), or 120 mg of bleomycin (BLM).[62] Starting after surgery, one of these solutions was administered for 3 days through a three-way catheter. MMC (13 patients), ADM (17 patients), and BLM (14 patients) resulted in 2-year recurrence rates of 25 percent, 24 percent, and 20 percent, respectively. The control group had a 2-year recurrence rate of 48 percent. These are very interesting results, because no further treatment was given during follow-up, and the three agents were given in very dilute concentrations. The study should be repeated and the observations confirmed, since it is based on the concept that total drug exposure is equally important to drug concentration in an adjuvant setting.

Prophylactic chemotherapy might better be kept separate from adjuvant chemotherapy, since they are conceptually different. As indicated above, therapeutic regimens are empiric, and prophylactic and adjuvant programs are no different. They all provide some advantage for the patients who receive TTPA.[43,49,63–66] To achieve maximum advantage, selection by in vivo testing (see above) would seem the proper tactic.

Adjuvant intravesical treatment is gradually being accepted as an appropriate addition to TUR. There are several reports concerning the effectiveness of immediate post-TUR treatment with TTPA.[55] Burnand et al.[64] instilled 90 mg for 30 min immediately after resection and Gavrell et al.[64a] used either 30 mg twice a day for 3 days or weekly for 6 weeks. Side effects were scant in each study, and both were very effective in reducing incidence of recurrences. As mentioned above, CGA is testing single versus multiple instillations of TTPA in an adjuvant role.

Carcinoma in Situ

This type of urothelial carcinoma deserves special consideration. Melicow and Hollowell first described it in 1952,[67] and since it was associated with invasive carcinomas, little attention was directed to it. Franks and Chesteman then described an apparent variant of the disease with predominant involvement of the prostatic urethra.[68] In 1960, Eisenberg et al.[69] described carcinoma in situ (C_{IS}/T_{IS}) with other mucosal lesions, i.e., all of which were associated with superficial papillary carcinoma. One-third of these patients did well, another one-third had multiple operations, and one-third had disastrous outcomes, regardless of the therapy involved. Many reports then followed in quick succession.[42,70–72] It became evident that T_{IS} was a very serious disorder in many patients and that invasive carcinoma of the nodular type may well have its origin as T_{IS}. For instance, Soto et al.[73] prepared giant sections of bladders containing invasive carcinomas. They found that T_{IS} merged with the invasive carcinoma in 33 cases. The neoplasia in these cases was largely multifocal. In 10 patients there was no T_{IS} in contact with the invasive carcinoma, and there was none elsewhere in those bladders.

Therapy has consisted of TUR, fulguration, cytotoxic agents, segmental resection (usually with very poor results), and radical cystectomy. The disease has a great propensity for moving laterally in all directions, or, as indicated above, it may be multifocal. It has an equally great propensity for appearing in the bladder, prostatic urethra, and prostatic ducts, and for invading the prostatic substance. Most treatment has been in reaction to the type of symptoms and/or dissemination that the disease exhibits. Farrow et al. have described the various forms of the disease, the treatments given, and the results obtained with respect to survival.[74]

It is clear that no single therapeutic plan is universally applicable. The patient crippled with dysuria, urgency, and frequency represents no massive intellectual challenge. Cystectomy is the only choice, but if the patient can retain TTPA or MMC for even an hour, initially, it is worth the effort, because an occasional bladder may be saved. Patients with disease in the prostatic urethra should have a cystectomy promptly. Preoperative radiotherapy (350 rads × 3) should be given to reduce the likelihood of local implants.[75]

The real problem lies with the patient who may have mild dysuria and/or hematuria, positive cytology, may or may not have a papillary tumor(s) T_1 or less, and for whom, when selected mucosal biopsies or biopsies of a suspicious area are taken and T_{IS} is reported, treatment might consist of refulguration and a course of TTPA. The response rate with respect to ablation is about 50 percent (Koontz).[43] The duration of response is not yet known.

Recently, we have evaluated the results of conservative therapy (TUR, TTPA) in 59 consecutive patients with T_{IS}.[76] These patients were followed and evaluated according to protocols 1, 2, and 3 of CGA. Thirty patients (51 percent) did not develop muscle invasion or metastatic disease. Twenty-one had associated T_a lesions, five had associated T_1 lesions, and only four had T_{IS} alone. Only six patients never had a disease-free period (negative cytologies and biopsies). The remaining 24 patients had an average disease-free period of 17.5 months (3 to 60 months' range). The average follow-up period from the date of diagnosis of T_{IS} was 25 months (12 to 78 months' range).

In contrast, 29 patients (49 percent) progressed with muscle invasion (10), metastatic disease (6), extension to the prostatic urethra (3), to the prostatic ducts (4), or invasion of the prostatic substance (6). Of these patients 7 had associated T_a papillary tumors, while 14 had associated T_1 papillary tumors. Eight patients had T_{IS} not associated with other tumors. Fifteen patients never had a disease-free period; six were disease-free at one contact only, while the remaining five had a disease-free interval ranging from 6 to 60 months. The average follow-up period from the first diagnosis of T_{IS} to the first evidence of progression or extension was 26 months (3 to 54 months' range).

In summary, of the 59 patients who were treated conservatively, progression or extension occurred in half, particularly in patients who developed T_1 lesions at some time during the course of their neoplastic diathesis. At high risk were those patients who never achieved a complete remission—negative biopsies and negative cytology. In this group of patients, another agent may be tried. Should it, too, fail, then cystectomy should be considered.

SEGMENTAL RESECTION

Segmental resection is being considered separately because of the frequency with which this operation is employed.

The operation is ideal in many ways. It is simple to perform, has scant morbidity and mortality, and preserves sexual function. The 5-year survival rates are shown in Table 33-2, for all stages. These are surely the best results that one might expect. Careful selection of patients is imperative. The lesion must be single, situated away from the bladder neck and ureteral orifices (one is not convinced that more than a very small proportion of the patients who have a segmental resection which requires ureteroneocystostomy are cured by such an operation), and surrounded by at least 2 cm of normal mucosa. Further, selected biopsies about the periphery of this area should be negative for dysplasia and/or tumor. Other biopsies from preselected sites should be histologically normal, as well.

From this writer's viewpoint, the operation is used far too frequently because of its positive attributes, while the stringent requirements for selection of patients are not so frequently met.

Invasive Carcinoma

This section will deal with the treatment of transitional cell carcinoma (TCC) squamous cell carcinoma, and adenocarcinoma. They account for over 90 percent of all carcinomas arising in the bladder. All cell types may be found in the same tumor, though adenocarcinomas are believed to arise from cloacal rests in the trigone and/or in the dome at the site of the urachus. The remainder consist of a variety of sarcomas, hemangiomas pheochromocytomas, and other unusual neoplasms that do not fall within the scope of this chapter.

The successful treatment of any neoplasm depends upon the ability of the physician to destroy the lesion completely and to do so before metastases have occurred. As noted above, T_a, G_1 tumors are very, very unlikely to metastasize, and so destruction of these will result in a cure, for the time being at least.

While Geraghty was probably among the first to relate depth of invasion to metastases and depth of invasion into the bladder wall,[77] Jewett and Strong were the first to dissect more precisely this relationship.[31] In brief, the deeper tumors infiltrate, the more likely they are to metastasize. While great emphasis has been placed on lymph node involvement as being a primary site for metastasis to occur, careful evaluation of patients who have undergone cystectomy suggests that there is a relationship between lymphatic invasion and metastases[78] and that failure to survive in the absence of positive pelvic nodes is due to metastatic disease found in the lungs, bones, and liver.[30] One other analysis[88] concerning lymphatic metastases, nodal metastases, and distant metastases revealed that the majority of tumors in the patients studied had a "solid" configuration and a poorer prognosis than those with papillary tumors (27 percent of patients surviving 5 years compared to 50 percent, 19 of 70 and 6 of 12 patients, respectively), and that the presence of small vessel invasion was an ominous portent even in the negative node group of patients studied (the absence of small vessel invasion conferred a 52 percent survival rate compared to 30 percent for the L+ group). Further studies are needed in this area and should encompass other contributing factors, as well, such as the possibility of tumor cell dissemination during cystectomy and the radiosensitivity of various tumor types.

Proponents of transurethral resection must depend

TABLE 33-2 Five-Year Survival for Patients with Bladder Carcinoma Treated by Segmental Resection by Stage

	Stage, %					
	0	A	B_1	B_2	C	D
Flocks[104]		38				
Marshall et al.[108]		62	22			
Jewett[109]		70		8		
Riches[110]	58		36			0
Resnick and O'Conor[111]	75	70.7	77	18	12.5	20
Utz et al.[112]		68	47	40	29	0

TABLE 33-3 Five-Year Survival of Patients According to Their Clinical Stage [Separated into Those Who Received Adjuvant Therapy or Did Not and Did or Did Not Have Tumor(P) in Their Specimens]

	Number	% 5-Year survival
CLINICAL STAGE B_1		
No XRT – P_0	7	57
XRT – P_0	18	44
XRT – P_+	30	37
No XRT – P_+	44	27
CLINICAL STAGE B_2		
XRT – P_0	14	57
XRT – P_+	33	33
No XRT – P_+	61	31
CLINICAL STAGE C		
XRT – P_0	7	16
XRT – P_+	13	31
No XRT – P_+	24	21

SOURCE: Prout.[83]

on at least fairly well localized tumors if cure is to be expected. The survival rate decreases as stage increases (see Table 33-3). There is some validity to the claim that invasive neoplasms not cured by TUR may not be curable. This opinion is contrary to that held by more aggressive surgeons, but the difference in survival is not so great that this opinion should be totally disregarded. Confronted with a single tumor which invades the muscle superficially in an 80-year-old patient, TUR may be vastly more desirable than radical surgery.

Cystectomy, whether simple or radical, has been used to eradicate invasive carcinoma. The survival of patients thus treated by the best urological surgeons is shown in Table 33-4. Because of the subsequent development of persistent pelvic disease, whether due to microscopic tumor left after cystectomy or to inadequate dissection, these poor results caused urologists to turn to adjuvant radiotherapy as a means of improving survival.[79–85] The initial hypothesis was that two agents would be better than one, even though each left much to be desired when used separately. There was also the likelihood that radiotherapy (XRT) would reduce wound implants and the viability of neoplastic cells that might be exfoliated during cystectomy. Further, adjuvant XRT might destroy extravesical tumor cells left behind after cystectomy.

Combinations of adjuvant radiotherapy and cystectomy have been employed for 20 years, and there are certain things that have emerged. They are as follows:

1. There is no certain evidence that XRT improves the 5-year survival rate for these patients, because it has been impossible to do an impeccable phase 3 study on this aged population. Valid questions have been raised in this regard.[86]
2. Many uncontrolled studies have been reported. The authors declare varying degrees of enthusiasm for the combination of XRT and radical surgery, but they are universally convinced that XRT improves the 5-year survival rate. The amounts of XRT have varied from 5000 to 2000 rads or less, and in these uncontrolled studies (some depend on historical controls to demonstrate improved results) there have been continued claims that the combination yields superior results.
3. When 4000 to 5000 rads are given, a small proportion, about 25 percent, of patients will have no tumor in their surgical specimens (P_0). These patients seem to be those who derive the greatest advantage in survival.[78,87]
4. Operative mortality for radical cystectomy, when ini-

TABLE 33-4 Five-Year Survival for Patients with Bladder Carcinoma Treated by Cystectomy by Stage

	Stage, %					
	0	A	B_1	B_2	C	D
Brice et al.[113]		37		9		
Bowles and Cordonnier[114]		52	50		20	0
Jewett[109]		50		9		
Wajsman et al.[115]		50		31		0

tially introduced, was 12 to 15 percent. This has now reached almost irreducible lows of 2 to 4 percent. This reduction, as well as better selection of patients for surgery, may play a role in the apparent improvement in survival.

Surrounding these facts are matters of interest. Van der Werf-Messing reported that downstaging from T_3 to P_0 or P_1 (the pathological stages of the surgical specimen) was essential if improved survival were to occur.[87] In her series, 80 percent of these patients survived more than 5 years. If the surgical specimen was P_3, the survival rate was 20 percent. This suggests that either clinical staging is immensely inaccurate or there are different types of invasive tumors which exhibit great differences in radiosensitivity. Since clinical staging at extreme ends of the spectrum is quite accurate, one must opt, reasonably, for the latter explanation. The Surgical Adjuvant Bladder Group, the only investigators to attempt a randomized study (see Table 33-5), found that XRT P_0 patients had a statistically significant difference in 5-year survival (44 percent) when compared to non-irradiated controls who were P+ (see Fig. 33-4). There seemed no way to approximate the Rotterdam group's experience, however. The very best survivorship (66 percent) was that of the small number of patients who had not received XRT, but whose TUR was both diagnostic and therapeutic. This might be best explained because the tumors had invaded only the superficial muscle, and most had not had an opportunity to metastasize. This did add support to the hypothesis that we were dealing with a group of tumors that were not

TABLE 33-5 Participants in the Surgical Adjuvant Bladder Study[78]

Urologist	Radiotherapist	Institution
Marvin W. Woodruff	Donald H. Baster	Albany Medical College
William H. Boyce Clair E. Cox	Damond D. Blake	Bowman Gray School of Medicine
Joseph Kaufman	Justin J. Stein	University of California at Los Angeles
Lester Persky	John Soraasli	Case Western Reserve University
James Glenn Joseph Malin	Patrick J. Cavanaugh	Duke University
Rubin H. Flocks David Culp Mark Immergut	H. B. Latourette	University of Iowa
William Valk	Galem N. Tice	University of Kansas
George R. Prout, Jr.	Milford Schultz	Massachusetts General Hospital
Ian M. Thompson Gilbert Ross	Gus R. Ridings	University of Missouri
Chester Winter	Frank Batley	Ohio State University
Clarence V. Hodges Gerry D. Giesy	Clifford V. Allen	University of Oregon
Harry C. Miller	Philip Rubin	University of Rochester
Gerald P. Murphy Gerald Hardner	John H. Webster	Roswell Park Memorial Institute
M. V. Vernon Smith Warren W. Koontz, Jr.	Seymour H. Levitt	Medical College of Virginia

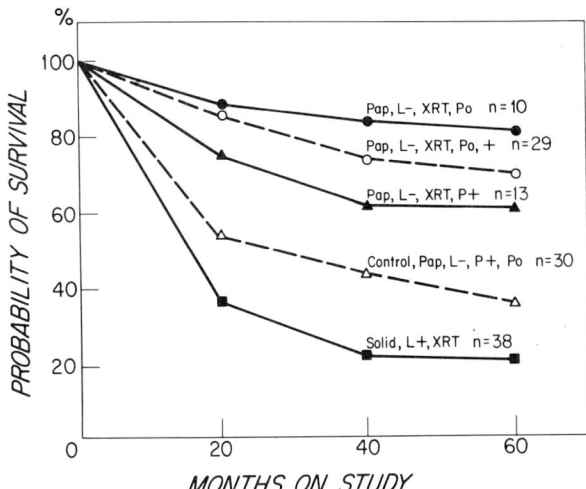

FIGURE 33-4 Five-year survival of P_0 patients who received adjuvant XRT compared to nonirradiated controls who were P+.

Prout but also emphasizes the need for further studies on the relationship between lymphatic invasion and survival.[88]

Both Whitmore[89] and Swanson et al.[90] have reviewed their data concerning these factors and have reached different conclusions. The Memorial group have found that smaller tumors respond favorably to XRT and are most likely to yield P_0 cystectomy specimens. Swanson et al. were unable to find any correlation between tumor type, lymphatic invasion, and tumor-free specimens. They have noted the importance of P_0 surgical specimens and their relationship to a higher proportion of 5-year survivors. Unhappily, Swanson et al. have little data on pelvic lymph node involvement, and neither group has a control population for comparison.

Clearly, much work needs to be done in this area. Opinion favors T_{IS} as the (pre?)malignant lesion which subsequently invades the detrusor and establishes a potentially lethal circumstance for the host.[30,71–74,91] The superficial cells of T_{IS} have the appearance of very malignant cells, yet they do not demonstrate the characteristic cathodic shift of lactic dehydrogenase. Only

homogeneous, but it was already known that superficial tumors might be well resected and thus destroyed locally. Success, as already indicated, depended on this factor. Slack and I then decided to retrieve all the prospectively collected data available from the Surgical Adjuvant Bladder Group on tumor types and whether lymphatic invasion was evident in the resected tissues and to establish whether there might be a relationship between these variables and downstaging.[78] One point should be made clear: the results of our review represent an hypothesis, because the data are not complete. Our observations suggest that invasive bladder carcinomas are heterogeneous. We could identify two tumor types, papillary and solid, or nodular. The latter were more commonly encountered, and they were twice as likely to exhibit lymphatic invasion and much less likely to be downstaged to P_0 by adjuvant XRT. When separated into different groups depending on tumor type, L+, L−, P+, and P_0, the data suggest that adjuvant XRT is most effective in patients with papillary, invasive tumors and least effective in solid tumors (see Fig. 33-5). While adjuvant XRT did not influence solid tumors, survival for patients with papillary tumors was doubled by adjuvant XRT (71 percent versus 35 percent, $p < .05$).

A recent blinded analysis of 86 Massachusetts General Hospital patients tends to support the data of Slack and

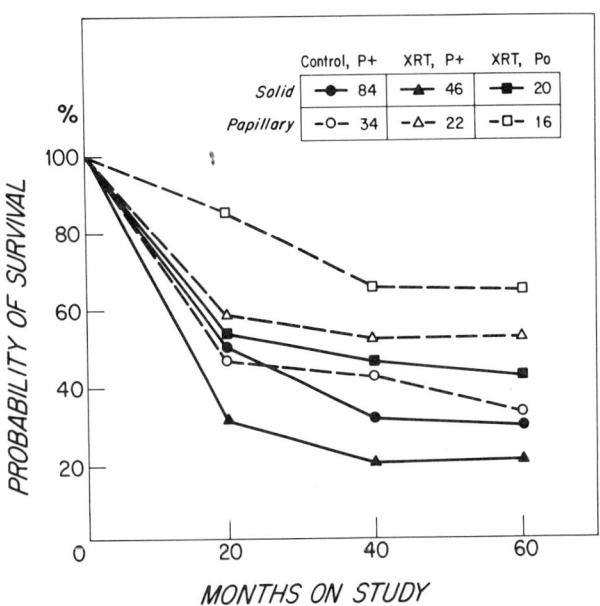

FIGURE 33-5 Survival of patients with papillary, invasive tumors and adjuvant XRT versus those with solid tumors.

high-grade invasive tumors demonstrate this shift.[92] Perhaps other studies, prospective in nature, on the biochemical, cytogenetic, and morphological characteristics of the cells that make up different tumor types might assist us in selecting patients for adjuvant XRT and selecting other patients for different treatments. What is needed most is to help change the perception of clinicians who treat invasive bladder carcinoma. Each tumor may be capable of destroying the host, but tumors may differ appreciably in their capability to do so. This may depend on the routes the cells will travel to do so, the speed with which they metastasize, and the organs they select as metastatic sites. Invasive carcinomas are heterogeneous, and this heterogeneity should be the subject of careful characterization so that differences may be exploited in treatment programs.

Definitive radiotherapy as an alternative to cystectomy with or without adjuvant irradiation is used in many parts of the world, including this country. Shipley has recently reviewed the subject thoroughly.[93] In brief, dosage techniques are extremely important to avoid unnecessary irradiation of normal tissues. Conventional doses of irradiation range between 6000 and 7000 rads given over 6 to 8 weeks. Five-year survival figures range between 12 and 33 percent,[94,95] at least 10 percent less than that obtained by adjuvant XRT and cystectomy. However, other considerations bear on the decision to accept or reject definitive radiotherapy. Two randomized trials comparing definitive XRT with XRT and cystectomy have shown that XRT alone produces inferior results, though in one of these the difference in survival never reached statistical significance.[94,96] Further, the complications of definitive XRT are appreciably less than XRT and cystectomy. Sexual activity may be retained after definitive XRT, something that rarely occurs after cystectomy. Another problem intrudes, though. Radiotherapy may destroy one invasive carcinoma only to have another appear within a few months or years of the treatment. From what is known about T_{IS}, definitive XRT for an invasive TCC would be a second choice for a patient who had an invasive lesion and multifocal T_{IS}, in addition. On the other hand, a patient with a single, 2- to 3-cm invasive papillary lesion without T_{IS} and without lymphatic invasion might be the perfect patient for definitive irradiation. Granted, the data are imperfect, but we are learning more and more about the biology of this disease, and multifocal T_{IS} is probably a powerfully negative indicator.[97]

The patient who fails definitive XRT is not necessarily lost. Much depends on the original stage and other characteristics of the treated tumor, because this is the patient's primary risk. If XRT does not destroy the tumor to a biopsy-negative status by 3 months, or if there is any recurrence other than a single <1 cm T_a tumor, salvage cystectomy is the only viable choice. These operations are not simple. Planes have been obliterated; the bowel is fragile, and the ureteral blood supply feeble. The surgeon must make every effort to obtain the radiotherapy records and have good consultative radiotherapeutic advice as to where one might expect trouble. It is usually safe to use bowel from the lower or mid jejunum. The conduit should be as short as possible and the ureters severed at the umbilicus or just below it. This leaves little room for maneuvering, but published results demonstrated the value of such operations.[98–101]

Chemotherapy for Metastatic TCC

The interested reader is referred to a comprehensive review by Stump and Corder.[102] The CGA has conducted an extensive trial using CDDP versus CDDP and Cytoxan. They treated 109 patients. There were 10 responders (20 percent) among the 50 evaluable patients who received CDDP alone, with 5 CR and 5 PR. Of the 59 evaluable patients who received CDDP and Cytoxan there were seven responders (11.9 percent). Three achieved complete response, and four had a partial response. There was no statistical significance between the response rates in the two arms. These rates fall far below the reported phase II study from the Memorial group.[103]

Currently, CGA is testing methotrexate against CDDP and MTX in patients with advanced metastatic disease.

There is no drug with a level of activity that makes it suitable for use as an adjuvant.

REFERENCES

1. Bricker M: Substitution for the urinary bladder by the use of isolated ileal segments. *Surg Clin N Am* 36:1117, 1956.
2. American Cancer Society: Cancer statistics, 1979. *Ca* 29:15, 1979.
3. Heney NM et al: Ta and Tl bladder cancer: Location, recurrence and progression. *Br J Urol* 54:152, 1982.
4. Rehn L: Blasengaschwultste Bei Anilinarbeitern. *Arch Klin Chir* 50:588, 1895.
5. Ferguson ES et al: Symposium on aniline tumors of the bladder. *J Urol* 31:121, 1934.
6. Hueper WC et al: Experimental production of bladder

tumors in dogs by administration of beta-naphthylamine. *J Indust Hyg Toxicol* 20:46, 1938.
7. Scott WW, Boyd HL: A study of the carcinogenic effect of betanaphthylamine on the normal and substituted isolated sigmoid loop bladder of dogs. *J Urol* 70:914, 1953.
8. Wiley FH, Blood F: Metabolism of betanaphthylamine. *J Biol Chem* 124:627, 1938.
9. Hueper WC: Environmental and industrial cancers of the urinary bladder in the U.S.A. *Acta Unio Int Contra Cancerum* 18:585, 1962.
10. Melick WF et al: The first reported cases of human bladder tumors due to a new carcinogen—Xenylamine. *J Urol* 74:760, 1955.
11. Vigliani EC, Barsotti M: Environmental tumors of the bladder in some Italian dye-stuff factories, in *Symposium on Cancer of the Urinary Bladder*, Hafner, New York, 1963, p 151.
12. Deichmann WB (ed): *Bladder Cancer: A Symposium*, Aesculapius, Birmingham, Ala, 1967, p 10.
13. Miller JA, Miller EC: A survey of molecular aspects of chemical carcinogenesis. *Lab Invest* 15:217, 1966.
14. Troll W, Belman S: Studies on the nature of the proximal bladder carcinogens, in *Bladder Cancer: A symposium*, Aesculapius, Birmingham, Ala, 1967, p 35.
15. Belman S, Troll W: The reaction of bladder carcinogens and mutagens with deoxyribonucleic acid, in *Bladder Cancer: A Symposium*, Aesculapius, Birmingham, Ala, 1967, p 58.
16. Allen MJ et al: Cancer of the urinary bladder induced in mice with metabolites of aromatic amines and tryptophan. *Br J Cancer* 11:212, 1957.
17. Dunning WF et al: The effect of added dietary tryptophan on the occurrence of 2-acetylaminofluorene–induced liver and bladder cancer in rats. *Cancer Res* 10:454, 1950.
18. Price JM, Brown RR: Studies on the etiology of carcinoma of the urinary bladder, in *Symposium on Cancer of the Urinary Bladder*, Hafner, New York, 1963, p 166.
19. Cole P et al: Smoking and cancer of the lower urinary tract. *N Engl J Med* 284:129, 1971.
20. Hicks RM, Chowaniec J: Experimental induction, histology and ultrastructure of hyperplasia and neoplasia in the urinary bladder epithelium. *Int Rev Exp Pathol* 18:199, 1978.
21. Cole P et al: Occupation and cancer of the lower urinary tract. *Cancer* 20:1250, 1972.
22. Wynder EL et al: An epidemiological investigation of cancer of the bladder. *Cancer* 16:1388, 1963.
23. Symposium on the geographical pathology of neoplasms of the urinary bladder, in *Symposium on Cancer of the Urinary Bladder*, Hafner, New York, 1963, p 4.
24. El-Asar AA et al: A study on the etiological factor of bilharzial bladder cancer in Egypt: 5-Urinary nitrite in a rural population. *Tumori* 66:409, 1980.
25. Cutler SJ et al: Factors associated with disease recurrence and progression, in WW Bonney, GR Prout Jr (eds): *Bladder Cancer*, AUA Monographs, vol I, Williams & Wilkins, Baltimore, 1982, p 35.
26. International Union against Cancer: TNM Classification of Malignant Tumors, 2d ed. International Union against Cancer, Geneva, 1974, p. 79.
27. American Joint Committee for Cancer Staging and End-Results Reporting: *Manual for Staging of Cancer*, 2nd ed, Lippincott, Philadelphia, 1982.
28. Jewett HJ: Carcinoma of the bladder: Influence of the depth of infiltration on the five-year results following complete extirpation of the primary growth. *J Urol* 67:672, 1952.
29. Prout GR Jr: The surgical management of bladder carcinoma in GR Prout Jr (ed): *Symposium on Ureoepithelial Tumors, Urol Clin North Am* 3:149, 1976.
30. Prout GR Jr et al: Bladder carcinoma as a systemic disease. *Cancer* 43:2532, 1979.
31. Jewett HJ, Strong GH: Infiltrating carcinoma of the bladder: Relation of depth of penetration of the bladder wall to incidence of local extension and metastases. *J Urol* 55:366, 1946.
32. Marshall VF: The relation of the preoperative estimate to the pathologic demonstration of the extent of vesical neoplasms. *J Urol* 68:714, 1952.
33. Koss JC et al: CT staging of bladder carcinoma. *Am J Radiol* 137:359, 1981.
34. Johnson DE et al: Lymphangiography as an aid in staging bladder carcinoma. *South Med J* 69:28, 1976.
35. Merrin C et al: The clinical value of lymphangiography: Are the nodes surrounding the obturator nerve visualized? *J Urol* 117:762, 1977.
36. Prout GR Jr, Griffin PP: Unpublished data, 1981.
37. Denis, L.: Accuracy in staging by ultrasound, in *Proc Int Bladder Cancer Conf 1981, Mt Fugi, Japan* (in press).
38. Niijima T, Nakamura S: Transurethral ultrasonography—bladder cancer, in LJ Dennis et al (eds): *Clinical Bladder Cancer*, Plenum, New York, 1982, p 47.
39. Heney NM et al for National Bladder Cancer Collaborative Group A: Superficial bladder cancer: Progression and recurrence (in press).
40. Sandberg AA: Chromosome markers and progression in bladder cancer. *Cancer Res* 37:2950, 1977.
41. Falor WH, Ward RM: Prognosis in well differentiated and non-invasive carcinoma of the bladder based on chromosomal analysis. *Surg Gynecol Obstet* 144:515, 1977.
42. Althausen AF et al: Non-invasive papillary carcinoma of the bladder associated with carcinoma in situ. *J Urol* 116:575, 1976.
43. Koontz WW Jr et al: The use of intravesical thio-tepa in the management of non-invasive carcinoma of the bladder. *J Urol* 125:307, 1981.
44. Jones HC, Swinney J: Thio-TEPA in the treatment of tumors of the bladder. *Lancet* 2:615, 1961.

45. Veenema RJ et al: Bladder carcinoma treated by direct instillation of thio-tepa. *J Urol* 88:60, 1962.
46. Prout GR Jr et al: Carcinoma in situ of the urinary bladder with and without associated vesical neoplasms. *Cancer* (in press).
47. Abbassian A, Wallace DM: Intracavitary chemotherapy of diffuse non-infiltrating papillary carcinoma of the bladder. *J Urol* 96:461, 1966.
48. Edsmyr F, Bowman J: Instillation of thio-tepa (Tifosyl) in vesical papillomatosis. *Acta Radiol (Ther) (Stockh)* 9:395, 1970.
49. Pavone-Macaluso M: Chemotherapy of vesical and prostatic tumors. *Br J Urol* 43:701, 1971.
50. Mishina T et al: Mitomycin C bladder instillation therapy for bladder tumors. *J Urol* 114:217, 1975.
51. Crooke ST et al: A phase I–II study of mitomycin C (MMC) topical therapy in early transitional cell carcinoma of the bladder—a preliminary report. *Proc Am Assoc Cancer Res* 19:321, 1978.
52. Prout GR Jr et al: Intravesical therapy of low stage bladder carcinoma with mitomycin C: Comparison of results in untreated and previously treated patients. *J Urol* 127:1096, 1982.
53. Defuria MD et al: Phase I–II study of mitomycin C topical therapy for low-grade, low-stage transitional cell carcinoma of the bladder: An interim report. *Cancer Treat Rep* 64:225, 1980.
54. Defuria MD: Personal communication, 1979.
55. Soloway MS: Rationale for intensive intravesical chemotherapy for superficial bladder cancer. *J Urol* 234:461, 1980.
56. Niijima T: Intravesical therapy with adriamycin and new trends, in *Diagnostics and Treatment of Superficial Urinary Bladder Tumors*, Montedison Lakemedel, A.B., Stockholm, 1979, p 37.
57. Edsmyr F et al: Intravesical therapy with adriamycin in patients with superficial bladder cancer, in *Diagnostics and Treatment of Superficial Urinary Bladder Tumors*, Montedison Lakemedel, A.B., Stockholm, 1979, p 45.
58. Jacobi GH et al: On the biological behavior of T1-transitional cell tumors of the urinary bladder and initial results of the prophylactic use of topical adriamycin under controlled and randomized conditions, in *Diagnostics and Treatment of Superficial Urinary Bladder Tumors*, Montedison Lademedel, A.B., Stockholm, 1979, p 83.
59. Morales A et al: Intracavitary bacillus Calmette-Guérin in the treatment of superficial bladder tumors. *J Urol* 116:180, 1976.
60. Lamm DL et al: BCG immunotherapy of superficial bladder cancer. *J Urol* 124:38, 1980.
61. Schulman CC et al: Early adjuvant Adriamycin in Ta T1 bladder cancer, in *Proc Int Bladder Cancer Conf 1981, Mt Fuji, Japan* (in press).
62. Koshiba K: TUR and implantation, in *Proc Int Bladder Cancer Conf 1981, Mt Fuji, Japan* (in press).
63. Wescott JW: The prophylactic use of thio-tepa in transitional cell carcinoma of the bladder. *J Urol* 92:913, 1966.
64. Burnand KG et al: Single dose intravesical thiotepa as an adjuvant to cystodiathermy in the treatment of transitional cell bladder carcinoma. *Br J Urol* 48:55, 1976.
64a. Gavrell GJ et al: Intravesical thiotepa in the immediate postoperative period in patients with recurrent transitional cell carcinoma of the bladder. *J Urol* 120:410, 1978.
65. Byar D, Blackard C: Comparisons of placebo, pyridoxine and topical thiotepa in preventing recurrence of stage I bladder cancer. *Urology* 10:556, 1977.
66. Schulman C et al: Adjuvant therapy of T1 bladder carcinoma: Preliminary results of an EORTC randomized study *Urol Res* (in press).
67. Melicow MN, Hollowell JW: Intraurothelial cancer, Carcinoma in situ, Bowen's disease of the urinary system: Discussion of thirty cases. *J Urol* 68:763, 1952.
68. Franks LM, Chesteman FC: Intraepithelial carcinoma of the prostatic urethra, peri-urethral glands and prostatic ducts (Bowen's disease of urinary epithelium). *Br J Cancer* 10:223, 1956.
69. Eisenberg RB et al: Bladder tumors and associated proliferative mucosal lesions. *J Urol* 84:544, 1960.
70. Schade RO, Swinney J: Pre-cancerous changes in bladder epithelium. *Lancet* 2:943, 1968.
71. Koss LG et al: Mapping cancerous and precancerous bladder changes. A study of urothelium in ten surgically removed bladders. *JAMA* 227:281, 1974.
72. Utz DC, Zincke H: The masquerade of bladder carcinoma-in-situ as interstitial cystitis. *Trans Am Assoc Genitourin Surg* 65:64, 1973.
73. Soto EA et al: Bladder cancer as seen in giant histologic sections. *Cancer* 39:447, 1977.
74. Farrow GM et al: Clinical observations on sixty-nine cases of in situ carcinoma of the urinary bladder. *Cancer Res* 37:2794, 1977.
75. van der Werf-Messing B: *Carcinoma Vesicae Treated at the Rotterdam Radiotherapy Institute between 1950 and 1974*. Erasmus University, Rotterdam, 1975.
76. Prout GR Jr et al: The results of conservative treatment in patients with carcinoma in situ of the bladder. Presented to the Annual Meeting of the American Urological Association, Kansas City, May, 1982 (in press).
77. Geraghty JT: Treatment of malignant disease of prostate and bladder. *J Urol* 7:33, 1922.
78. Slack NH, Prout GR Jr: Heterogeneity of invasive bladder carcinoma and different responses to treatment, in WW Bonney, GR Prout Jr (eds): *Bladder Cancer*, AUA Monographs, vol 1, Williams & Wilkins, Baltimore, 1982, p 213.
79. Prout GR Jr et al: Irradiation and 5-fluorouracil as adjuvants in the management of invasive bladder carcinoma.

A cooperative group report after four years. *J Urol* 104:116, 1970.
80. Prout GR Jr et al: Preoperative irradiation as an adjuvant in the surgical management of invasive bladder carcinoma. *J Urol* 105:223, 1971.
81. Prout GR Jr et al: Preoperative irradiation and cystectomy for bladder carcinoma. IV. Results in a selected population, in *Proc 7th Nat Cancer Conf,* Lippincott, Philadelphia, 1973, p 783.
82. Scott R et al: Preoperative irradiation in the surgical treatment of transitional cell cancer of the bladder: Preliminary report based on 12 years of experience. *J Urol* 109:405, 1973.
83. Prout GR Jr: The surgical management of bladder carcinoma. *Urol Clin North Am* 3:149, 1976.
84. Miller LS: Bladder cancer: Superiority of preoperative irradiation and cystectomy in clinical stages B2 and C. *Cancer* 39:973, 1977.
85. Whitmore WF Jr et al: Radical cystectomy with or without prior irradiation in the treatment of bladder cancer. *J Urol* 118:184, 1977.
86. Radwin HM: Invasive transitional cell carcinoma of the bladder: Is there a place for preoperative radiotherapy? *Urol Clin North Am* 7:551, 1980.
87. van der Werf-Messing B: Carcinoma of the bladder treated by preoperative irradiation followed by cystectomy: The second report. *Cancer* 32:1084, 1973.
88. Heney NM et al: Invasive bladder cancer: Tumor configuration, lymphatic invasion and survival (in press).
89. Whitmore WF Jr: Integrated irradiation and cystectomy for bladder cancer. *Br J Urol* 52:1, 1980.
90. Swanson DA et al: Salvage cystectomy for bladder carcinoma. *Cancer* 47:2275, 1981.
91. Daly JJ: Carcinoma in situ of the urothelium. *Urol Clin North Am* 3:87, 1976.
92. Bredin HC et al: Lactic dehydrogenase isoenzymes in human bladder cancer. *J Urol* 113:487, 1975.
93. Shipley WU: Radiation therapy for patients with bladder carcinoma: Rationale, results, techniques, and possible innovations, in WW Bonney, GR Prout Jr (eds): *Bladder cancer,* AUA Monographs, vol 1, Williams & Wilkins, Baltimore, 1982, p 243.
94. Miller LS, Johnson, DD: Megavoltage radiation for bladder carcinoma; alone, postoperative, or pre-operative, in *Proc 7th Natl Cancer Conf,* Lippincott, Philadelphia, 1973, p 771.
95. Goffinet DR et al: Bladder cancer: Results of radiation therapy in 384 patients. *Radiology* 117:149, 1975.
96. Wallace DN, BloomnHJG: The management of deeply infiltrating bladder carcinoma: Control trial of radical radiotherapy vs. pre-operative radiotherpay in radical cystectomy. *Br J Urol* 48:587, 1976.
97. Prout GR Jr et al: Carcinoma in situ of the urinary bladder with and without associated vesical neoplasms. *Cancer* (in press).
98. Edsmyr F et al: Carcinoma of the bladder. Cystectomy after supervoltage therapy. *Scand J Urol Nephrol* 5:215, 1971.
99. Hecker GN et al: Radical cystectomy after supervoltage radiotherapy. *J Urol* 91:256, 1964.
100. Riches E: Surgery and radiotherapy in urology: The bladder. *J Urol* 90:339, 1963.
101. Whitmore WF Jr: Total cystectomy, in EH Cooper, RE Williams (eds): *The Biology and Clinical Management of Bladder Cancer,* Blackwell, London, 1975, p 193.
102. Stump DC, Corder MP: Chemotherapeutic approaches to transitional cell carcinoma of the bladder, Part III, Invasive and metastatic disease, in WW Bonney, GR Prout Jr (eds.): *Bladder Cancer,* AUA Monographs, vol 1, Williams & Wilkins, Baltimore, 1982, p 305.
103. Yagoda A et al: Cis-dichlorodiammine platinum (II) in advanced bladder cancer. *Cancer Treat Rep* 60:917, 1976.
104. Flocks RH: Treatment of patients with carcinoma of the bladder. *JAMA* 145:295, 1951.
105. Milner WA: The role of conservative surgery in the treatment of bladder tumors. *Brit J Urol* 26:275, 1954.
106. Nichols JA, Marshall VF: The treatment of bladder carcinoma by local excision and fulguration. *Cancer* 9:559, 1956.
107. Barnes RW et al: Control of bladder tumors by endoscopic surgery. *J Urol* 97:864, 1967.
108. Marshall VF et al: Survival of patients with bladder carcinoma treated by simple segmental resection. *Cancer* 9:26, 1956.
109. Jewett HJ: Simple cystectomy and segmental resection for cancer of the bladder. *J Urol* 70:620, 1953.
110. Riches E: Choice of treatment in carcinoma of the bladder. *J Urol* 84:472, 1960.
111. Resnick MI, O'Conor VJ Jr: Segmental resection for carcinoma of the bladder: Review of 102 patients. *J Urol* 109:1007, 1973.
112. Utz DC et al: A clinico-pathologic evaluation of partial cystectomy for carcinoma of the urinary bladder. *Cancer* 32:1075, 1973.
113. Brice MH et al: Simple total cystectomy for carcinoma of the urinary bladder: 156 cases for five years later. *Cancer* 9:576, 1956.
114. Bowles WT, Cordonnier JJ: Total cystectomy for carcinoma of the bladder. *J Urol* 90:731, 1963.
115. Wajsman Z et al: Current results from treatment of bladder tumors with total cystectomy at Roswell Park Memorial Institute. *J Urol* 113:806, 1975.

34
TUMORS OF THE PROSTATE

Jeffrey J. Pollen *Joseph D. Schmidt*

HISTORY

Langstaff, who in 1817 described the condition *mycosis haematodes*, is credited with being the first to recognize prostatic cancer. In 1858 Thompson reported several cases in his textbook. The basis for endocrine therapy was established in 1895 when White eloquently presented his experiences of the effects of bilateral orchiectomy in shrinking the hypertrophic prostate. In 1900 Albarran and Hallé were able to separate 14 cases of malignancy by histologic study of 100 surgical specimens of enlarged prostates. A milestone was reached in 1905 when Young, emphasizing the importance of early diagnosis, described the now firmly established procedure of total perineal prostatectomy for cure of the disease.[1]

In 1910 Pachkis and Tittinger and in 1909 Pasteau using intracavitary radium pioneered radiation therapy for the control of prostatic cancer. Kütscher and Wolbergs made the significant biochemical discovery of high phosphatase activity in acidified extracts of prostatic tissue and ejaculate in 1935, and, in the following year, Gutman and others found increased phosphatase activity at the site of osteoblastic metastases from prostatic cancer.[2] It was the publications of Huggins and Hodges in 1941 on the effects of castration and of estrogens in metastatic prostatic cancer that paved the way for effective, albeit temporary, palliation for the many men who present with advanced disease.[3] In 1952 Flocks developed interstitial irradiation of the prostate by injecting radioactive colloidal gold solution. An important contribution to the study of the disease was made by Whitmore in 1956 when he proposed a working clinical staging classification.[4] The long-term results of Jewett, published in 1968, proved that total prostatectomy can cure early prostatic cancer.[5]

EPIDEMIOLOGY

In the United States, prostatic cancer accounts for 16 percent of all malignancies in males, being exceeded in frequency only by lung cancer. It is currently estimated that 64,000 new cases will be diagnosed each year and that 21,000 men will succumb to this disease annually. Prostatic cancer is a disease of older men. The incidence rate increases from age 65 years to age 90 and declines thereafter. Between ages 75 and 79 years, it is responsible for approximately 25 percent of all male cancers, increasing to more than 33 percent of all tumors in the late nineties. Negroid American males are somewhat more prone to develop prostatic cancer than Caucasians.

Prostatic cancer is the third leading cause of cancer-related death in males. It is responsible for 10 percent of all male cancer deaths, being exceeded in frequency only by lung and colorectal tumors. The death rate from cancer of the prostate increases with each decade of life. Over the age of 75 years prostate cancer is second only to gastrointestinal cancer in incidence and as a cause of death.

The age-adjusted death rate for cancer of the prostate of 14.4 per 100,000 United States males is not much different from figures in European countries. However, death from prostatic cancer in Orientals is comparatively unusual, around 2 per 100,000.

Substantial increases in the probabilities of eventually developing or dying of prostatic cancer have occurred due to increases in incidence rates as well as gains in life expectancy.

ETIOLOGY

Carcinoma of the prostate and benign hyperplasia, being common disorders of the elderly, frequently coexist. The etiology of both diseases is unknown, however. They are not believed to be causally related. Similarly, chronic prostatitis and prostatic calculi are frequently noted prior to the clinical and histologic diagnosis of prostatic cancer, but these two benign disorders have not been shown to be precursors of malignancy. A viral etiology of prostatic cancer has been purported to exist, but initial reports have not been verified.

PATHOLOGY

Of primary tumors of the prostate 95 percent are adenocarcinomas arising from the glandular acini. They originate from the peripheral group of glands located in the posterior and posterolateral regions of the prostate. Only 12 percent appear to originate more centrally. Benign hyperplasia begins in a small group of glands situated periurethrally. Tumor differentiation is used to indicate the ability of the cancer to reproduce glandular acini. Those tumors that reproduce glands are graded well-differentiated or moderately well differentiated, and are further subclassified by the type and size of glands present.

There are several features that distinguish well-differentiated adenocarcinoma from benign prostatic hyperplasia. The acini, which are smaller, have a back-to-back arrangement with little intervening stroma. The cells lining the acini are usually in a single layer, the basal layer of cells being absent. Prostatic acini may appear as linear infiltrates in the fibromuscular stroma. Nuclear hyperchromatism, prominent large eosinophilic nucleoli, and mitotic figures may be present. The frequency of intraprostatic perineural invasion makes this a helpful feature in placing a well-differentiated glandular pattern into a malignant category. Spread of cells along the perineural space, which is not a lymphatic channel, takes place early in the natural history. Its occurrence reflects the tendency of tumors of low malignant potential to follow existing tissue planes rather than their ability to produce metastases.

Undifferentiated tumors lose the ability to reproduce a glandular pattern. The cells may occur as sheets, cords, or rows of individual cells. The amount or composition of the stroma as well as the presence or absence of perineural or vascular invasion should be noted.

Complete histological evaluation of prostatic cancer takes into account the cytologic characteristics of individual cells as well as the glandular pattern. Cellular anaplasia is evaluated in terms of nuclear atypia and may be graded 1 to 3. Grade 1 implies slight anaplasia; grade 2, moderate anaplasia; and grade 3, marked anaplasia. In cancers showing multiple histologic grades the area of greatest anaplasia should be emphasized. Both the amount of nuclear atypism and the degree of differentiation may be important indicators of the invasive properties of the tumor, and therefore function as determinants of ultimate prognosis.

Only 5 percent of primary tumors arising in the prostate gland differ from the usual acinar variety. Of these, primary transitional-cell carcinomas which arise in the periurethral prostatic ducts account for 2 to 4 percent. Mucin-secreting elements are not uncommonly seen in prostatic adenocarcinoma; however, the pure mucin-positive variety is rare. Adenoid cystic or salivary gland prostatic carcinomas represent less than 0.01 percent of all carcinomas of the prostate. As a group, these tumors do not produce acid phosphatase, are biologically aggressive, are unresponsive to antiandrogen treatment, and carry a poor prognosis. With these features in mind, staging and management are similar to primary adenocarcinoma.

Endometrial tumors, ectophytic or intraductal, present in the region of the verumontanum. The histological features are indicative of a nonmetastasizing neoplasm, and their management revolves around the management of the more aggressive, commonly associated adenocarcinoma.

Occasionally adenocarcinomas of the prostate show areas of sarcomatoid change. The mesenchymal elements may resemble smooth or striated muscle. These tumors may behave clinically as typical carcinoma of the prostate and metastasize to lymph nodes, liver, lungs, and the skeleton, where they are extensively osteoblastic. Both elements of the tumor may respond to estrogen therapy.

The malignant sarcomas constitute approximately 0.1 percent of all primary neoplasms of the prostate gland. One-third of these tumors appear in childhood and are usually of the rhabdomyosarcoma type. Other soft-tissue tumors occurring in various age groups are leiomyosarcoma, fibrosarcoma, and lymphosarcoma. The tumors grow rapidly, produce obstructive uropathy, and encroach on the rectum and neighboring structures. There is early lymphatic and vascular invasion with resulting lymphatic and visceral metastases. The bony metastases are mostly osteolytic.

SPREAD OF PROSTATIC CANCER

Local Spread

Several degrees of involvement of the laminated capsule are possible. The tumor may extend to, but not invade, the capsule. With further growth the tumor invades the inner layers of the prostatic capsule and finally will penetrate or extend beyond the capsule. Invasion of the capsule may be seen when the tumor consists of a single focus, multiple foci, or is extensive; however, the incidence of penetration increases as the tumor progresses from a single focus to multiple foci to an extensive solid mass. Invasion of the capsule occurs early, but only after the tumor has enlarged and spread within the gland is the capsule finally penetrated. It seems that the tumors arise peripherally, spread centrally toward the urethra, and then finally penetrate the capsule. A similar relationship exists between seminal vesicle invasion and the location and extent of the tumor. As with penetration of the capsule, invasion of the seminal vesicles is a late event in the local growth pattern. Although capsular penetration or invasion of the seminal vesicles may occur separately, they are frequently associated events. Involvement of the seminal vesicles is almost always confined to the muscularis, spread to the lumen occurring only when the whole wall is involved. This suggests that carcinoma of the prostate does not spread by way of ejaculatory ducts but rather by direct extension in the tissue planes of the fibromuscular stroma.

Regional Spread

The lymphatics of the prostate drain into a periprostatic network. Most efferent lymph vessels emerge from the posterior aspect. One group follows the inferior vesical artery to join the external iliac nodes. Another drains posteriorly into the lateral sacral nodes communicating freely with lymphatics from the seminal vesicles and rectum, and finally draining to the common iliac chain. The third pathway of lymphatic drainage, and probably the one most frequently involved by prostatic cancer is to the paravesical obturator-hypogastric chain of nodes (Fig. 34-1).

Involvement of the lymphatic system by prostatic cancer is an early and frequent event in the natural history of this disease[8] and may occur when the primary is quite small. The regional lymph nodes may contain metastasis before there are any abnormalities detectable by routine radioisotopic bone scans, skeletal x-rays, or elevation of the serum acid phosphatase level.

The obturator and hypogastric groups of nodes, which are the most medial of the pelvic lymph nodes, are the first to become involved. These are followed by the external iliac, common iliac, and paraaortic groups of glands. While it is possible for the tumor to skip the pelvic nodes and spread directly to the paraaortic lymph nodes, such skipped areas are rare.[9]

There is no correlation between nodal metastases and the presence of perineural or vascular invasion. The combination of tumor undifferentiation, advanced nuclear anaplasia, and extension of tumor through the prostatic capsule are high-risk circumstances that strongly correlate with lymph node metastases. Nonetheless, well-differentiated primary tumors are not infrequently associated with multinodal metastases. In general, the histologic pattern of metastases in the lymph nodes corresponds closely with that found in the primary tumor. Well-differentiated tumors provide well-differentiated metastatic deposits, and poorly differentiated tumors reproduce themselves in the lymph nodes. Exceptions in both directions may be, but are not necessarily, due to errors inherent in sampling the primary tumor. The more poorly differentiated portion of a neoplasm is likely to metastasize rather than the well-differentiated portion.[9]

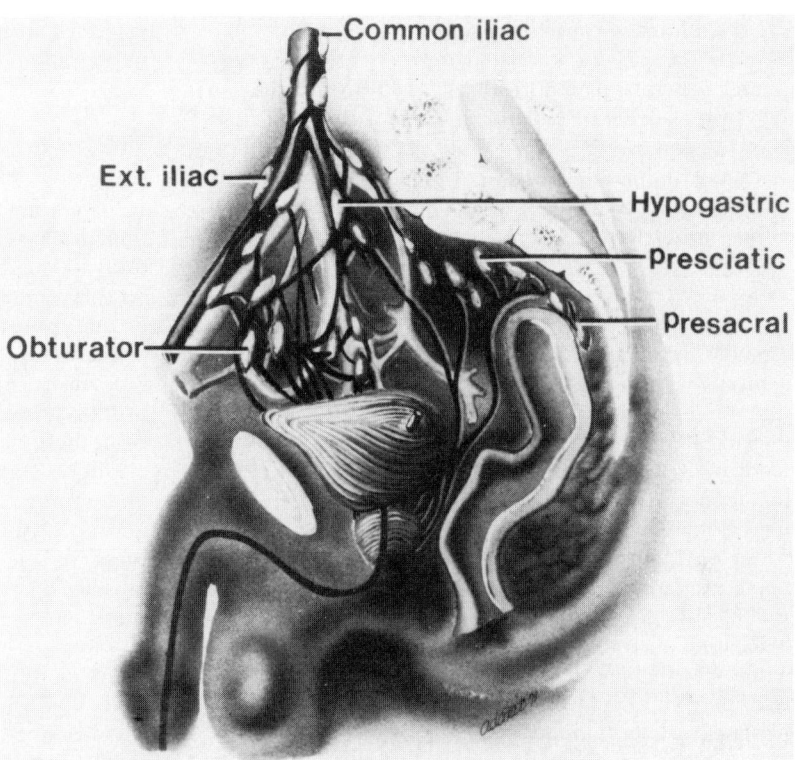

FIGURE 34-1 Lymphatic drainage of prostate.

The incidence of lymph node metastases rises sharply with increasing size of the primary. About 90 percent of patients with local lesions larger than 150 g and a similar number with microscopically demonstrable seminal vesicle invasion have positive regional lymph nodes.[8]

Hematogenous Spread

Blood-borne metastases appear early or late in the course of the disease. Hematogenous spread is most frequently to the bones of the axial skeleton, although no bone is immune. Initially, tumor emboli travel via the periprostatic veins which communicate with the extensive perivertebral network of veins to involve the lumbosacral spine, pelvis, and upper femurs. Bone marrow involvement usually accompanies bony spread but may occur independently. Visceral metastases appear late in the clinical course and may not be detected. At autopsy, metastases in the lungs, liver, and suprarenals are frequently found.

NATURAL HISTORY

The extreme variability of the growth characteristics of prostatic cancer makes a simple discussion of the natural history impossible. The primary tumor may remain dormant for many years without ever showing signs of spread. In other patients, the tumor pursues a rapid downhill course. Prostatic carcinoma is the principal cause of death in 14 percent of patients with stage A (see "Clinical Staging" later in this chapter), 25 percent with stage B, 48 percent with stage C, and 84 percent of patients with stage D disease. The mean survival period for all patients with prostatic cancer, taking into account all causes of death, is 2.6 years. Of patients with generally advanced prostatic cancer, 73 to 82 percent succumb from their disease.[10,11]

An important aspect of prostatic cancer is that the disease occurs in elderly men; 39 to 55 percent of the patients succumb to unrelated diseases. Cardiovascular disorders are common in this age group and frequently are the ultimate cause of death in the patient with prostatic cancer. An unrelated death is a significantly greater threat to patients with localized disease than to those with advanced carcinoma. This is an important consideration in the selection of patients for radical treatment and complicates the evaluation of the results of different modalities of treatment for cancer in an elderly population.

Latent Cancer of the Prostate

Less than 12 percent of all cancers of the prostate found at autopsy are known to have existed during the patient's lifetime. This leaves 90 percent or more that are first detected at postmortem examination. The overwhelming majority of autopsy cases are latent cancers that were not clinically apparent, produced no symptoms, and are not evident on gross inspection of the organ. Latent cancer of the prostate can only be discovered by microscopic examination and in this respect is the equivalent of clinical stage A disease.

Routine microscopy of the prostate from autopsies of males over the age of 40 years reveals carcinoma in 10 to 20 percent of subjects. A more detailed search of the prostate, such as by step-section microscopy, will disclose latent cancer in 20 to 40 percent of all adult male autopsies over age 40 years. The frequency of latent cancer rises with age. Over the age of 80 years, 40 to 80 percent of patients may have microscopic malignancy. The incidence of latent carcinoma in Japan is about the same as in Europe and America in spite of the lower death rate from prostatic carcinoma.

Usually foci of latent carcinoma are small, and most of them show a picture of well-differentiated adenocarcinoma. The tumor may exist as multiple, separate foci. This variety of latent cancer, occurring in some 25 percent of specimens, is termed *multifocal*. It appears as though the tumor has a *multicentric* origin when two or more malignant foci are found some distance apart.[12] Frequently, however, there is continuity of growth between cancer in different sections. The term *diffuse prostatic carcinoma* has been adopted by usage to describe both histological subdivisions. Both focal and multifocal lesions are generally well differentiated and reproduce an acinar pattern, while diffuse prostatic cancer is generally poorly differentiated.

The incidence is generally much lower in surgical specimens of benign hypertrophy, about 10 percent. This is easily understood because the surgical capsule where latent carcinoma originates is usually not removed in operations for benign hypertrophy.

CLINICAL PRESENTATION

In its earliest stages, prostatic cancer is entirely asymptomatic. A small peripheral nodule produces no symptoms to suggest to the patient that something is amiss. As the primary tumor enlarges, it encroaches upon the prostatic urethra or its rigidity effectively splints the prostatic urethra to produce symptoms of bladder outflow obstruction or irritation. Symptoms of prostatism produced by cancer of the prostate are indistinguishable from those of benign prostatic hyperplasia. Initially, the bladder compensates for the outflow obstruction by undergoing compensatory hypertrophy. Irritative symptoms consisting of urgency, frequency, and nocturia occur as the bladder wall thickens and the urinary capacity drops. When the bladder decompensates, irritative symptoms are replaced by obstructive symptoms of a weak stream, intermittency, and postvoid dribbling. Residual volumes increase with time until finally acute or chronic retention of urine develops. Gross hematuria, initial or total, from a friable tumor bleeding into the urethra, is a presenting complaint in only a small percentage of patients with prostatic cancer. Microscopic hematuria is much more frequent.

The patient may present with symptoms or signs of chronic renal failure due to bilateral hydronephrosis, the result of retention of urine in the bladder, or direct invasion of the lower ureters by the primary growth. Stasis of urine in the bladder or upper collecting systems poses a constant threat of superimposed urinary infection. The onset of frequency and dysuria suggests acute cystitis while flank pain, fever, and shaking chills signify pyelonephritis.

Enlarged lymph nodes in the groin usually mean extensive pelvic lymphadenopathy with retrograde spread of metastatis. Palpation of the supraclavicular areas for lymphadenopathy is an important aspect of the examination of any patient with prostatic cancer for metastatic disease. Rarely, gross abdominal lymphadenopathy may produce an abdominal mass. Pressure on the inferior vena cava or deep veins of the pelvis may produce venous occlusion or thrombosis. Anasarca of the lower half of the body may be the result of lymphedema from obstructed lymph flow, edema from venous occlusion, or both. A superior vena caval syndrome from mediastinal lymphadenopathy compressing the superior vena cava may occur.

Skeletal metastasis causing low back pain radiating into the hips is a frequent presenting symptom, while pain in the shoulders, ribs, and legs is not uncommon. Initially, pain may be slight in intensity, and its migratory pattern and diurnal variation may suggest an arthritic condition. As the disease progresses, pain becomes more severe and constant. Replacement of normal bone marrow by metastatic cancer results in a myelophthisic type of anemia. Nutritional deficiency, renal insufficiency, and more rarely acute or chronic blood loss from the primary tumor contribute to the development of anemia, which may be aggravated by radiation therapy or chemotherapy.

Pathologic fractures occur with minimal trauma when osteolytic metastases produce extensive cortical destruction of vertebrae or long bones. Tumors growing in vertebral bodies may encroach upon the extradural space to produce nerve root compression or, even more significantly, spinal cord compression with paraplegia. Constant severe pain in a segmental distribution or persistent severe back pain, particularly when associated with symptoms or signs of weakness in lower extremities, should alert the physician to a possible neurologic complication.

DIAGNOSIS

Rectal Examination

Clinical diagnosis of prostatic cancer depends on careful digital palpation of the posterior aspect of the prostate through the anterior wall of the rectum. A stony hard, irregular, nodular, fixed, enlarged prostate with ill-defined margins leaves little doubt as to the diagnosis.

Detection of the early cancer of the prostate requires a lot more skill and attention to detail. Any area of abnormal induration or the presence of a firm nodule is sufficient for suspecting the diagnosis. Uniform involvement of the prostate gland by carcinomatous infiltration may result in symmetric, smooth enlargement; however, its hardness should suggest malignancy. Rectal examination should include careful evaluation of the seminal vesicles as well as the bladder base for signs of thickening suggestive of periprostatic carcinomatous infiltration.

Spontaneous ulceration through the rectal mucosa in the absence of previous surgical intervention is distinctly unusual. Prostatic cancer tends to project into the rectum or to grow around it in circumferential fashion. An ulcerating lesion of the rectal mucosa is more likely to be a primary rectal carcinoma.

Acid Phosphatase

Serum acid phosphatase is an enzyme capable of hydrolyzing orthophosphoric esters exhibiting maximum activity in the pH range of 4.8 to 6.0. Several molecular variants of acid phosphatase, called isoenzymes, are found in erythrocytes, leukocytes, platelets, reticuloendothelial cells, as well as the liver, spleen, and kidneys. However, the richest sources of acid phosphatase activity are the epithelial cells and secretions of the adult prostate.

Routine measurement of acid phosphatase in the laboratory employs a spectrophotometric analysis of the inorganic phosphate or organic moieties released from the particular substrate added to the serum. Several sources contribute to the total serum acid phosphatase activity measured indirectly in this way. The addition of tartrate to the serum inhibits over 90 percent of the prostatic contribution to acid phosphatase activity and largely separates the prostatic contribution from the total level. β-Glycerol phosphate is a more specific substrate for prostatic acid phosphatase.

An elevated level of serum acid phosphatase is most commonly a sign of metastatic cancer of the prostate, or at least a large local lesion that has grown beyond the bounds of the prostatic capsule. Raised serum levels can also be found in Gaucher's and Paget's disease, hyperparathyroidism, other malignancies with bone metastases, diseases of kidneys, liver, and primary hematologic disorders. False-positive assays occur in sera from hemolyzed blood samples. Transient elevations lasting less than 24 h may follow manipulation of the prostate or instrumentation of the urethra.

Radiographs

Sometimes prostatic cancer is diagnosed by the chance finding of characteristic osteoblastic metastases on radiographs of the chest or abdomen taken for another reason (Fig. 34-2). The combination of osteoblastic bone metastases and raised levels of serum acid phosphatase is virtually pathognomonic for metastatic cancer of the prostate.

Biopsy

The most important diagnostic maneuver is biopsy. A histopathologic diagnosis should be obtained prior to the

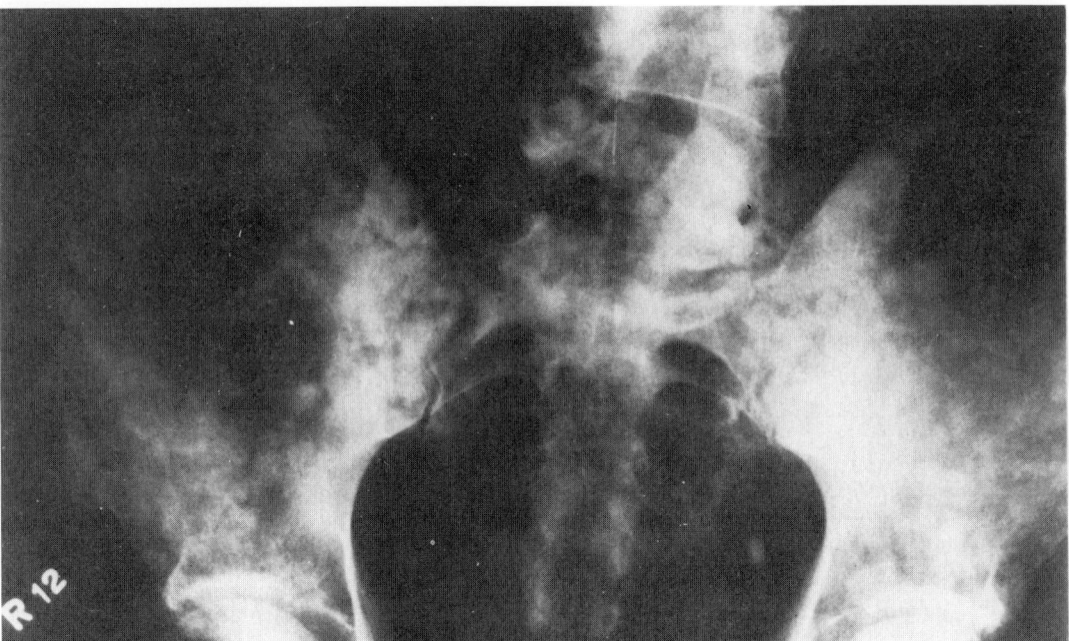

FIGURE 34-2 Plain radiograph of pelvis and lumbar spine showing typical osteoblastic metastases from prostatic cancer.

administration of specific treatment, and biopsy is essential before curative therapy is directed at the primary growth. Tissue from the prostate for histological examination is most easily obtained with a Franklin-Vim-Silverman or Travenol disposable biopsy needle. The transperineal route is the approach of choice for needle biopsy of the prostate. The perineum is infiltrated in the midline with local anesthetic solution. With one finger in the rectum, the biopsy needle is guided through the perineum toward the prostate. A core of tissue is obtained from the suspicious area as well as from the opposite lobe. Transrectal needle biopsy, though a simpler and sometimes more accurate procedure, carries with it the risk of introducing bacteria from the rectal lumen into the bloodstream. A cleansing enema the night before and the introduction of a small-volume retention enema of antibiotic solution just prior to the procedure greatly minimize this risk. A brief course of oral or parenteral antibiotics beginning just prior to, and continuing for a day or two beyond, the procedure is recommended.

Needle biopsy offers the advantage of reaching the periphery of the gland which is the site of origin of most prostatic carcinomas. If the initial biopsy is negative in the face of a palpably suspicious gland, the biopsy should be repeated. A correct diagnosis, positive or negative, should be reached in at least 90 percent of cases. If the procedure is repeated on one or two occasions, the diagnostic accuracy will be enhanced beyond 95 percent.

Transurethral biopsy of the prostate with a cold punch or hot diathermy loop is less satisfactory. If the primary tumor is extensive, there will be no problem obtaining a representative specimen. However, since most prostatic carcinomas begin peripherally in the prostate, transurethral biopsy is subject to greater sampling error. Transrectal fine-needle aspiration biopsy with cytologic examination has not enjoyed widespread usage in the United States as a diagnostic procedure.

There are always a few patients in whom none of the above techniques yields a satisfactory result. In such instances, one must resort to the most accurate biopsy procedure, namely open perineal exposure of the posterior aspect of the prostate and incision biopsy of the suspicious area. When facilities for frozen-section diagnosis are available, the surgeon may proceed with total prostatectomy at the same sitting.

In about 10 percent of patients with cancer of the prostate, the diagnosis is discovered at the time of histological examination of tissue removed by transurethral resection or suprapubic enucleation of the prostate for the clinical diagnosis of benign hyperplasia.

Excision of an enlarged peripheral lymph node may reveal a diagnosis of metastatic adenocarcinoma, though the pathologist may have difficulty indicating the primary source.

CLINICAL STAGING

Once the histological diagnosis of primary carcinoma of the prostate has been established, the next step is to stage the disease as accurately as possible so that a rational plan of management can be instituted. A traditional staging schema is compared to the TNM system in Table 34-1.[4,13,14]

The TNM classification is recommended for usage in all scientific articles discussing management of carcinoma of the prostate. In this way, useful comparative evaluations of different forms of treatment can be made. For purposes of discussion, the older and simpler classification will be used.

Clinical stage A cancer of the prostate is undetected by rectal examination. Patients present with symptoms and signs of benign prostatic hyperplasia, and the diagnosis is made by histological examination of the obstructive tissue removed by surgery. The majority of stage A lesions are focal, showing microfoci of tumor occupying only one to three low-power fields. The prostate contains a great proportion of benign hyperplastic tissue relative to the small bulk of tumor present.[15]

Most focal cancers are well differentiated histologically, and are placed in the stage A_1 category. If a greater

TABLE 34-1 Clinical Staging Classification of Prostatic Cancer

Standard	TNM system—American Joint Committee		
		Primary tumor (T)	Nodal involvement (N), or distant metastases (M)
Stage A: incidental; clinically undetectable	T_X	Minimum requirement not met	N_X Minimum requirements not met
A_1 Focal and well-differentiated	T_0	No tumor palpable; includes incidental findings of cancer in a biopsy or operative specimen	N_0 No involvement of regional lymph nodes
A_2 Diffuse or undifferentiated			N_1 Involvement of a single regional lymph node
Stage B: confined; within the capsule	T_1	Tumor intracapsular surrounded by normal gland	N_2 Involvement of multiple regional lymph nodes
B_1 <1.5 cm in one lobe			
B_2 >1.5 cm or more than one lobe	T_2	Tumor confined to gland, deforming contour, and invading capsule, but lateral sulci and seminal vesicles not involved	N_3 Free space between tumor and fixed pelvic wall mass
			N_4 Involvement of juxtaregional lymph nodes
Stage C: localized; with extracapsular extension	T_3	Tumor extending beyond capsule with or without involvement of lateral sulci and/or seminal vesicles	
C_1 <60 g			M_X Not assessed
C_2 >60 g or involving bladder neck, trigone, or seminal vesicles			M_0 No (known) distant metastases
			M_1 Distant metastases present, site specified as follows: pulmonary, PUL; osseous, OSS; hepatic, HEP; brain, BRA; lymph nodes, LYM; bone marrow, MAR; pleura, PLE; skin, SKI; eye, EYE; other, OTH
Stage D: advanced; extensive	T_4	Tumor fixed or involving neighboring structures; adding suffix (m) after T for multiple tumors (e.g., T2m)	
D_1 Invasion of bladder, ureters, rectum, or lymph nodes below common iliac vessels			
D_2 Nodal involvement at or above common iliac vessels or distant metastases			

proportion of the specimen or the entire specimen is involved by cancer, then the lesion is termed *diffuse*. The multifocal variety with normal intervening tissue is generally well differentiated, whereas diffuse lesions are mostly poorly differentiated. Tumors which are more than focal in their microscopic extent and those of any size which are undifferentiated are categorized as stage A_2. The relative incidences of A lesions, subdivided by extent and degree of differentiation, are presented in Table 34-2.

Stage B prostatic cancer is completely confined within the capsule. While the capsule may be elevated by the tumor, it should be smooth. Any irregularity of the capsule suggests tumor penetration. The seminal vesicles should not be palpable, or if so, should have a normal soft consistency. The intervesicular plateau should be normal and the margins of the prostate well defined. The earliest stage of cancer of the prostate that can be detected clinically is the so-called B_1 nodule. This refers to a palpable hard nodule, 1.5 cm or less in diameter, or occupying less than one lobe of the prostate. Compressible prostatic tissue is present on at least two sides of the nodule. This is the stage of prostatic cancer that is most suitable for consideration for curative total prostatectomy. Any tumor greater in size than 1.5 cm or which occupies one lobe or more of the prostate but yet is palpably confined within the prostatic capsule is placed in the B_2 category.

Stage C carcinoma of the prostate refers to a growth which has penetrated the capsule to become locally invasive, yet the tumor is limited in its extent. Depending on its size and the presence or absence of seminal vesicle invasion, stage C disease can be further subdivided. The smaller C_1 lesion is less than 35 g in estimated weight with no clinical evidence of invasion of the seminal vesicles or bladder base. Tumors which are larger or demonstrate invasion of the seminal vesicles, bladder base, or trigone are classified as stage C_2.

When the primary growth becomes so large that it extends to the lateral wall of the pelvis as determined by bimanual examination, it is called stage D_1. Metastatic involvement of regional pelvic lymph nodes below the level of the bifurcation of the common iliac vessels is also regarded as in category D_1. Lymph node metastasis beyond the confines of the true pelvis, or hematogenous spread to any site, places the tumor in category D_2, irrespective of the extent of the primary growth.

Staging Techniques

LOCAL

Careful clinical examination remains the only practical means for determining the local extent of prostatic cancer. Gray-scale ultrasonography may prove a valuable adjunct in the local evaluation of prostatic cancer in the future (Fig. 34-3). Computerized axial tomography (CAT) may turn out to be the most accurate method for defining the local extent of the primary tumor. For now, we must content ourselves with thorough digital examination. Any opportunity to perform a bimanual examination under general anesthesia should not be missed.

Excretory urography may reveal unilateral or bilateral hydronephrosis caused by direct invasion of the lower ureters by the primary growth. Careful cystoscopic examination is necessary to detect edema or irregularity of the bladder neck or trigone indicative of extensive submucosal spread of the tumor.

REGIONAL

There are major limitations to bipedal lymphangiography for the detection of lymphatic spread in clinically localized malignancy. The lymphangiogram outlines the external iliac, common iliac, and paraaortic nodes, but the medially placed hypogastric, obturator, and sacral nodes are not always opacified unless there is obstruction to lymph flow higher up. It may be difficult to distinguish abnormalities due to benign processes such as fibrosis, fatty infiltration, or hyperplasia from those of metastatic tumor. Lymphangiograms lack the sensitivity to detect microscopic foci of tumors which do not alter the architectural appearances sufficiently to permit detection. A false-positive rate of 59 percent and false-negative rate of 36 percent on radiographs compared with the findings at subsequent pelvic node dissection or biopsy make pedal lymphangiography unreliable for an accurate assessment of the regional lymph node status.[16]

To improve the diagnostic accuracy of lymphangiography it may be combined with percutaneous trans-

TABLE 34-2 Incidence of Stage A Disease by Extent and Degree of Differentiation

	Focal	*Diffuse*
Well-differentiated	75% (A_1)	5% (A_2)
Poorly differentiated	5% (A_2)	15% (A_2)

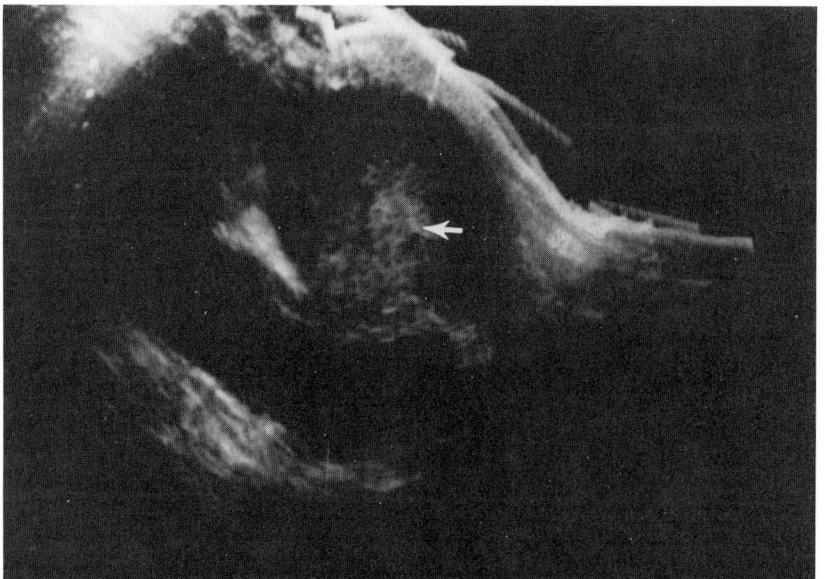

a

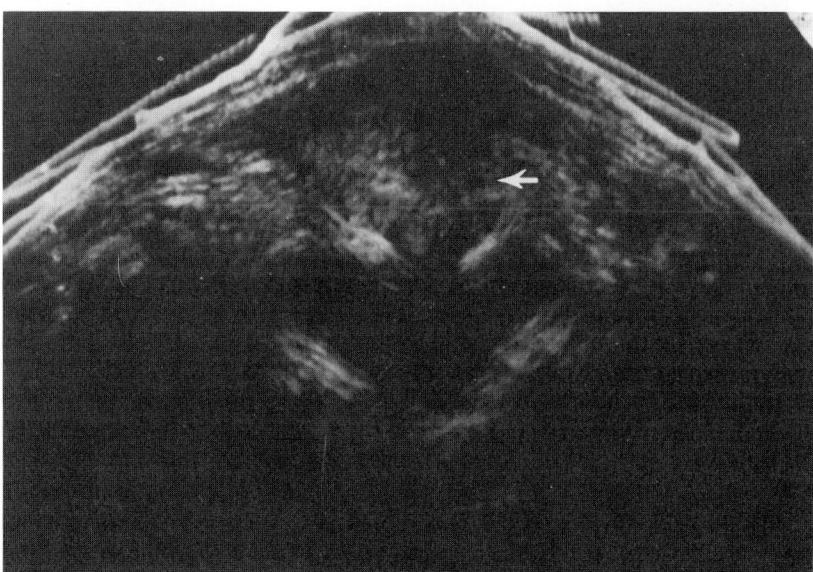

b

FIGURE 34-3 (*a*) Longitudinal and (*b*) transverse ultrasound films showing large soft tissue extension (*arrow*) from prostatic cancer compressing the bladder anteriorly.

peritoneal fine-needle aspiration of suspicious nodes. Positive cytologic evidence of metastatic tumor eliminates the need for exploratory surgery. One indication for lymphangiography is the man with symptomatic primary carcinoma of the prostate who refuses surgery but is thought to be a suitable candidate for curative external beam radiation therapy. If grossly positive, systemic treatment might be instituted rather than external beam radiation. Ultrasound and computerized axial tomography are excellent noninvasive techniques for detection of gross abdominal lymphadenopathy (see Fig. 34-4).

One of the major advances in staging prostatic cancer has been the widespread usage of pelvic lymphadenectomy to detect early lymph node involvement.[17] Undoubtedly in the past a large number of curative attempts directed at the prostate itself failed because of the presence of undetected regional lymph node metastasis. Table 34-3 lists the incidence of positive lymph node metastasis in the pelvis, revealed by lymphadenectomy, in the various clinical stages. Pelvic lymphadenectomy involves a retroperitoneal exploration and a bilateral dissection that completely removes the lymphatic chains along the common and external iliac vessels down to the inguinal ligament as well as along the hypogastric vessels down to the obturator fossa, which is cleared. Generally the dissection does not include the presacral nodes lying behind the rectum, a known site for metastasis. The specimens are carefully labeled and submitted for histological examination. At exploration enlarged or suspicious lymph nodes should be submitted individually for immediate frozen section examination. If positive, the highest accessible involved nodes should be recorded and the procedure terminated. Random sampling of lymph nodes is no substitute for complete lymphadenectomy. Only detailed microscopic search of the permanent paraffin sections from the entire lymphadenectomy specimen can exclude microscopic metastases. There is significant morbidity attached to lymphadenectomy. Some 10 percent of patients develop deep-venous thrombosis, and potentially fatal pulmonary embolism. Despite all attempts at lymphostasis, lymphoceles, which may require aspiration or drainage, develop in 10 percent of cases.

DISTANT

An integral part of the staging process is to exclude the presence of hematogenous spread. By itself, determination of serum acid phosphatase levels cannot be used as a staging procedure, although there is a correlation between serum levels and the stage of disease. Routine enzymatic assays are elevated in 5 percent of patients with disease confined to the prostate, 20 percent where there is extracapsular extension, and up to 80 percent of cases with metastasis to bone.[18] A normal acid phosphatase level does not rule out the presence of metastasis because there may be insufficient production by the tumor or even a complete failure of production.

Recently, specific prostatic acid phosphatase (PAP) was characterized by immunochemical processes. An antibody to PAP can be raised so that precise radioimmunoassay determination of the serum levels can be made.[19] Very small increases in serum PAP can be measured, but whether this means that we can now detect early cancer of the prostate while it is still confined within the prostatic capsule needs to be confirmed. Until the precise meaning of a minimally raised serum PAP is determined, it should not by itself be construed as evidence for metastatic disease. Rather, the patient should be given the benefit of the doubt and every effort made to determine the exact extent of the local disease as well as to exclude distant metastases. In prostatic cancer with high levels of serum acid phosphatase, the overwhelming contribution is from the prostatic fraction. This allows serial measurements by routine enzymatic methods to be a valuable aid in monitoring the patient's course. A precipitous drop in serum activity may occur within 24 h following bilateral orchiectomy. Rising levels in previously stable disease herald clinical relapse.

The most sensitive method for detection of skeletal metastases is a total-body bone scan using a bone-seeking radionuclide such as [^{99}Tc]-pyrophosphate or diphosphonate (see Fig. 34-5). The scan is superior to radiographs for the detection of metastatic disease in that 12 to 60 percent of patients with positive scans have normal radiographs. However, the increased sensitivity of bone scans is slightly counterbalanced by reduced specificity. Isolated areas of increased activity require radiographic correlation, by special views. Finding an old fracture or degenerative conditions is helpful, but cannot entirely rule out dual pathology. Normal radiographs or the presence of sclerotic or lytic lesions point toward metastasis. When curative treatment of the primary is under consideration, it may be necessary to resort to needle or open biopsy of isolated areas of increased activity. For staging purposes, the presence of typical osteoblastic lesions on plain radiographs eliminates the need for a nuclear scan.

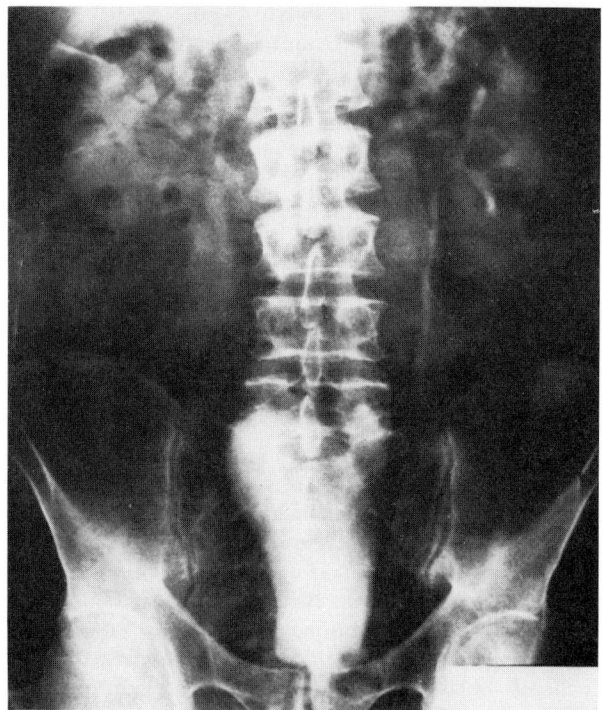
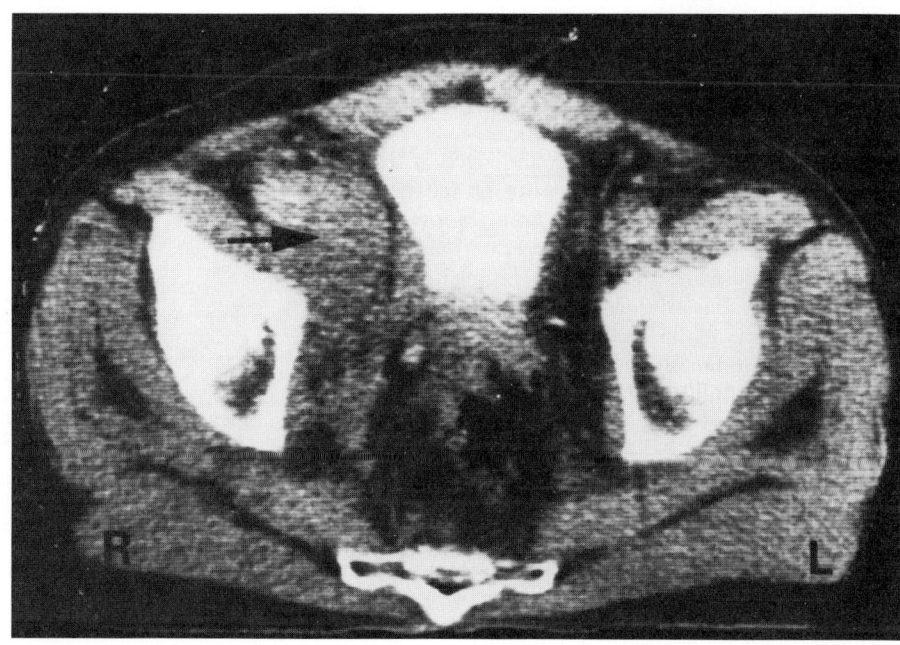

FIGURE 34-4 (*a*) Excretory urogram of 74-year-old male with prostatic cancer showing bilateral compression of the bladder caused by extensive pelvic lymph nodal metastases. (*b*) CT scan with contrast enhancement of same patient demonstrating massive nodal metastases on the right (*arrow*) and lesser involvment on the left.

TABLE 34-3 Incidence of Pelvic Lymph Node Metastases Revealed by Lymphadenectomy*

Stage	Incidence of positive nodes, %
A_1	0–4
A_2	22–37
B_1	8–24
B_2	25–62
C_1C_2	28–82
D_1D_2	≤ 100

* Synthesized from multiple sources.

Widespread availability of nuclear scans has made routine radiographic skeletal surveys unnecessary. A plain film of the abdomen, including the upper femurs and a chest x-ray is all that is required in most circumstances. Metastases from prostatic cancer produce disorganization of the trabecular pattern. New bone formation in response to an osteoblastic factor produced by the tumor gives the dense white appearance characteristic of the osteoblastic metastases, the type most frequently seen in prostatic cancer. Expansion of bone as seen in Paget's disease is almost never a feature. Mixed osteoblastic and osteolytic metastases are seen in 15 percent, whereas pure lytic lesions occur in only 5 percent, of patients with radiographic evidence of spread. Radiographs may be entirely normal in the face of widespread metastases revealed by bone scanning.

Bone marrow metastases may be present in the absence of any changes on bone scan or radiographs. Marrow aspiration and trephine bone biopsy of the posterior superior iliac spine is indicated in patients whose metastatic work-up is otherwise negative. While it is understood that a large sampling error is inherent in this method, it will turn up a few patients with metastases who otherwise would be missed.

Increased acid phosphatase activity is present in bone metastases from prostatic cancer as well as in the bone marrow of patients with positive biopsies. Estimation of bone marrow acid phosphatase may be of value in staging carcinoma of the prostate by detecting early bone metastasis. Comparison with skeletal surveys and isotope bone scans suggests that determination of bone marrow acid phosphatase may provide earlier evidence of metastasis. Considerable controversy exists over the source of such enzyme activity as well as the optimal method for measuring it. Falsely raised results are found in patients with primary hematologic disorders which should be ruled out by microscopic analysis of the bone marrow and peripheral blood smear. Measurement of immune-specific prostatic acid phosphatase in bone marrow should enhance the value of this test.

Clinically evident visceral metastases appear late in the course of the disease. Chest radiographs may reveal lung metastases usually of the lymphangitic variety. Ultrasound examination and liver-spleen nuclear scans capable of detecting space-occupying lesions as small as 2 cm in diameter in these organs should be requested in patients with hepatosplenomegaly or deranged liver function tests.

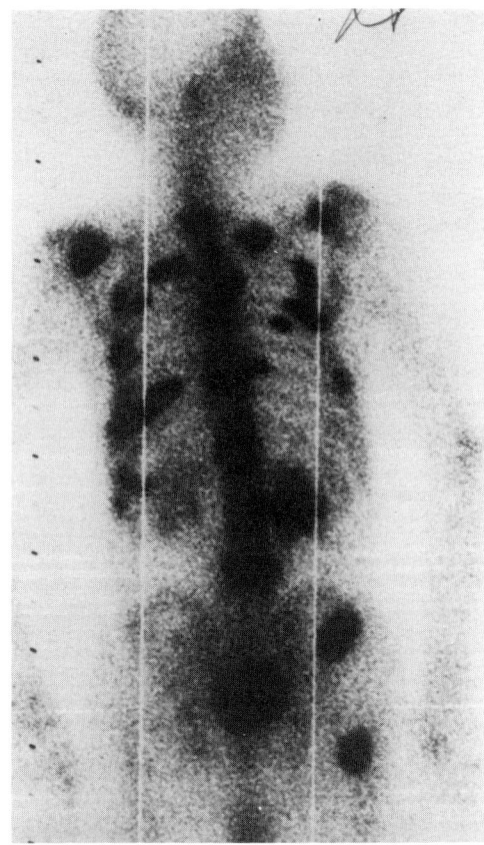

FIGURE 34-5 Nuclear bone scan of 63-year-old male with prostatic cancer and bony metastases in the pelvis, spine, and ribs (posterior view).

PROGNOSTIC DETERMINANTS

Symptomatic prostatic cancer is more frequently associated with high-grade tumors and advanced disease. Irritative or obstructive urinary complaints suggest locally advanced disease while bone pain is even more ominous, suggesting metastasis. When a patient presents with symptoms, the prognosis is worse than when the disease is discovered as a result of routine physical examination.

A direct relationship exists between the size of the primary tumor and the incidence of positive regional lymph nodes and of subsequent metastases.[9] Patients demonstrating seminal vesicle invasion are at greater risk of developing subsequent metastases than those without seminal vesicle invasion. Patients with poorly differentiated tumors have a significantly higher incidence of positive regional nodes and of subsequent metastases than do patients with better differentiated tumors. Within each clinical stage, histological grading shows a strong correlation with mortality rate. Patients with poorly differentiated tumors are at higher risk than those with well-differentiated tumors.

Earlier-staged patients with poorly differentiated cancers have a higher cancer-related death rate than do patients in the next stage with well-differentiated tumors. When the histological grade of the tumor as determined by the glandular pattern is combined with the stage, there is a strong correlation with the mortality rate. The combination of low stage and low grade identifies the group of patients with favorable survival rates.

There is a progressive increase in the probability of metastasis related to the height of the pretreatment level of acid phosphatase. In the absence of demonstrable metastases, patients with elevated prostatic acid phosphatase levels have a definitely higher risk of dying from cancer than do those with local disease and normal acid phosphatase levels. The prognosis for patients with an elevated acid phosphatase without metastasis is better than that for patients with bony metastases. Survival of patients with bony metastases and normal acid phosphatase is better than that for patients with both osseous metastases and elevated acid phosphatase.[20] Determination of bone marrow acid phosphatase may have prognostic importance. Of patients with elevated bone marrow levels and normal serum values, treated by total prostatectomy for clinically early disease, one-third develop evidence of metastasis within 1 to 4 years.

When death from prostatic cancer is taken as the end point, there is no difference in the length of survival between young men and older men with comparably staged and graded disease. However, when a comparison is made between the life expectancy curves, there is a marked discrepancy between the two age groups. Life expectancy is much reduced in young people with the disease compared to the population of the same age. In older men the difference is less marked as the poorer life expectancy curve of the population approaches that of patients with the disease. There would seem to be no evidence for the statement that the disease is biologically more dangerous in younger men.

By far the most important determinant of prognosis is the stage of the disease at the time of diagnosis.

SCREENING FOR PROSTATIC CANCER

Ultrasound has been adapted for the diagnosis of prostatic disorders. Transrectal prostatic ultrasonography involves passing a rotatable transrectal transmitting and receiving ultrasonic probe into the rectum in order to obtain serial sonograms of the prostate and surrounding structures. Malignant nodules are viewed as focally dense asymmetric areas that do not fade with increased instrument attenuation. Transrectal ultrasonography can diagnose prostatic cancer with an accuracy of 77 percent, and is also highly accurate in the differentiation of benign and malignant nodules. Ultrasonar tomography can be adapted for use in a mass screening program for the detection of diseases of the prostate and holds promise as a relatively noninvasive technique for the early detection of prostatic cancer.

As a screening test for the early detection of prostatic cancer, the measurement of serum prostatic acid phosphatase (PAP) holds some promise. In order to be useful, such a test should be simple to perform and able to detect accurately slight elevations of specific PAP. Highly specific immunologic assays for PAP have been developed. The most sensitive are radioimmunoassays, including a solid-phase immunofluorometric method, that are capable of measuring PAP levels in the normal range.[19] Such assays are complex, time-consuming, and expensive. By contrast, the method of counterimmunoelectrophoresis offers simplicity, rapidity of performance, and low cost, at the expense of slightly reduced sensitivity. Raised levels of PAP have been found in 38 percent of stage A_2, 35 percent of stage B, 4 percent of stage C and 69 percent of stage D patients.[21] Added to routine annual rectal examination, sensitive and specific methods for the detection of raised levels of serum PAP may add to effectiveness of a screening program for the detection of early prostate cancer.

So far no test can replace annual digital rectal palpation of the prostate in men over 45 years of age to discover the early nodule of prostatic cancer that is amenable to cure.

MANAGEMENT OF CARCINOMA OF THE PROSTATE

The selection of treatment for patients with prostatic cancer depends primarily on the stage of disease. Natural life expectancy, taking account of age and general health of the patient at the time of presentation, must be considered. Underlying metabolic or degenerative diseases may be more important factors limiting life expectancy than the prostatic cancer. These factors must be weighed against the natural history of the tumor at the stage of diagnosis in terms of ultimate morbidity if the prostatic cancer remains untreated. Almost every form of treatment for prostatic cancer may produce potentially serious and even fatal side reactions. The risks of treatment must be balanced against any potential benefit.

Combinations of radiotherapy and chemotherapy are appropriate for lymphomas and sarcomas. For sarcomas still confined to the prostate, radical cystoprostatectomy is the treatment of choice, though advances in radiation and chemotherapy are changing this approach.[6,7] The remainder of the discussion will be concerned with the treatment of adenocarcinoma of the prostate.

Stage A

Of patients with prostatic cancer, 10 to 15 percent are diagnosed in stage A. The diagnosis of stage A disease is made by the pathologist examining the histologic sections of tissue removed for what clinically was believed to be benign hyperplasia. The mean age of patients at the time of diagnosis is 71 years.

The clinical outcome of incidental prostatic cancer depends both on the size of the tumor and the degree of differentiation.[10,22–24] Only 7 to 10 percent of small or focal tumors show evidence of progression during a period of follow-up. Larger tumors have a generally unfavorable course. Up to 60 percent of diffusely infiltrating lesions show progression, and 25 percent of patients with such lesions may die of prostatic cancer.[15]

Of patients with well-differentiated occult carcinoma, 10 to 20 percent develop symptoms of recurrence after transurethral resection and about 10 percent die of prostatic cancer. Even so, the latter group has a good average survival of 6 to 8 years. For the most part, patients with well-differentiated cancers do well, and sometimes better than a comparable population of the same age group: 61 to 94 percent can be expected to survive 5 years, 38 to 56 percent 10 years, and about one-third of the patients to survive 15 years.

Life expectancy drops sharply for patients with poorly differentiated lesions: 14 to 50 percent of patients with poorly differentiated lesions die of cancer. The 5-year survival is 33 to 60 percent; 10-year survival is 14 to 44 percent; and 15-year survival is 0 to 25 percent.

Stage A_1 carcinoma consisting of occasional microscopic foci of well-differentiated cancer is remarkably unaggressive and rarely presents a threat to life. Only 2 to 4 percent of patients with focal, well-differentiated tumors die of their disease. Autopsy studies confirm that many of these cancers were completely removed by the transurethral resection or enucleation procedure. The clinical course of stage A prostatic cancer is summarized in Table 34-4.

Management of stage A_1 disease, at least initially, is conservative. In order to more clearly define the extent of the disease, patients with focal tumor should have a repeat transurethral biopsy done routinely 3 months after the initial resection. An attempt should be made to remove all remaining prostatic tissue, particularly from the posterior portion of the gland. At the same sitting, transrectal or preferably transperineal needle biopsies are taken from the peripheral zone of each residual lobe. Both the transurethral and needle biopsy

TABLE 34-4 Clinical Course of Stage A Prostatic Cancer*

Type	Disease progression, %	Death from cancer, %
Focal	7–10	0–10
Diffuse	60	25
Well-differentiated	6–20	2–14
Poorly differentiated	26–66	14–50

* Synthesized from multiple sources.

specimens are submitted for histology. If significant residual carcinoma is detected, the disease is reclassified as stage A_2 and treated accordingly. If no cancer is found, the patient is reassured and asked to report back at intervals of 6 months to 1 year for clinical examination.

One out of every three clinically unapparent prostatic carcinomas is stage A_2, either because it is diffuse or not well differentiated. Clinical stage A_2 prostatic carcinoma is more aggressive than stage B_1 cancer when judged by the degree of differentiation, incidence of lymph node metastases, and survival rates. With A_2 lesions, 60 to 70 percent demonstrate a poorly differentiated pattern, whereas most B_1 nodules are well differentiated. Pelvic lymph node metastases can be demonstrated in one-fourth to one-third of all clinical stage A_2 carcinomas at the time of diagnosis, in contrast to the 8 to 24 percent incidence in stage B_1 tumors (Table 34-3). The survival of patients with stage A_2 prostatic carcinoma is substantially lower than that of patients with B_1 disease and may be less than that of patients with stage B_2 disease. Biologically, stage A_2 disease is more advanced than stage B_1, and placing it closer to stage B_2 better reflects its true nature and behavior.

Large and poorly differentiated lesions compete effectively with other causes of death in elderly men. Further treatment is recommended for all those patients in good general health. The primary options are a second operation, total prostatovesiculectomy, or a curative course of external beam radiation therapy.

Secondary total prostatectomy, perineal or retropubic, may be a much more difficult procedure following previous prostatic surgery.[25] There is a 3 percent operative mortality, 15 percent have total incontinence, and some 40 percent have stress incontinence postoperatively. Although previous transurethral resection may not greatly increase the difficulty of later total prostatectomy, these patients have a greater risk of total incontinence postoperatively and are more likely to suffer rectal injury. The greatest operative difficulties are encountered after previous open enucleation. Postponement of the total prostatectomy by at least 4 to 6 weeks after the primary surgery minimizes the complication rate. Residual carcinoma is found in 80 percent of the total prostatectomy specimens.

Because of the difficulties involved in secondary prostatectomy, most patients with stage A_2 carcinoma of the prostate are treated with external beam radiation therapy. The substantial incidence of lymph node metastases points to the need for staging pelvic lymphadenectomy in those patients whose metastatic work-up is otherwise negative, prior to instituting definitive local treatment.

Stage B

Ten to fifteen percent of patients present in clinical stage B. Stage B carcinoma of the prostate refers to the early growth which, by careful digital rectal palpation, appears to be completely confined within the capsule. The natural history of the stage B_1 nodule is extremely variable. Local or distant recurrences occurring 15 years or more after total prostatectomy are an indication of the very slow growth rate of some of these neoplasms, although most recurrences are evident within 2 to 5 years. Treated conservatively with endocrine therapy and transurethral resection, 71 percent of patients can be expected to survive 5 years, 58 percent for 10 years, and 28 percent for 15 years.

In the absence of metastasis, any form of treatment that entirely eliminates prostatic cancer confined by the capsule will effect a cure. Several modalities of treatment have been developed that can achieve local control of prostate cancer. The frequency with which they achieve cure depends on the accuracy of local clinical staging, the efficiency with which distant metastases can be excluded, and the reliability of the treatment modality.

Total prostatovesiculectomy is widely accepted as the treatment of choice for the B_1 lesion.[26-33] The average age of patients undergoing total prostatectomy for early prostatic cancer is 61 years. The indications for total prostatectomy are well defined. The nodule of cancer discovered by rectal examination should be 1.5 cm or less in diameter, and be shown by biopsy to be well-differentiated adenocarcinoma. The patient should be no more than 70 years of age, be in good general health, and have no obstructive symptoms. Naturally, a metastatic work-up including serum acid phosphatase level should be normal.[5] Provided that the strict guidelines for selection of nodules for curative excision are followed, staging pelvic lymphadenectomy is unnecessary, since less than 10 percent of patients will have lymph node metastases. Patients that have tumors larger than 1.5 cm, have obstructive urinary symptoms, or have lesions that are not well differentiated require the additional therapeutic considerations of stage B_2 disease and C_1 disease.

The structures removed during total prostatectomy

are illustrated in Fig. 34-6. Perineal prostatectomy is performed with the patient in the dorsal lithotomy position. The prostate is exposed through an inverted U-shaped perineal incision. After transection of the supramembranous urethra just distal to the apex of the prostate, the bladder neck is circumferentially incised. The vascular pedicles and both vasa are ligated and cut so the prostate and seminal vesicles with their surrounding fascial investments can be removed. A watertight anastomosis of the bladder neck, narrowed as necessary, to the urethra is made under direct vision.

The retropubic operation is performed through a lower abdominal midline or transverse incision. The prostate is mobilized by dividing the endopelvic fascia on either side as well as the puboprostatic ligaments. The urethra is transected immediately beyond the apex, and the prostate is retracted anteriorly to display the seminal vesicles. Thereafter, the vasa and vessels are ligated and the bladder neck transected. A direct suture anastomosis is made between the bladder neck, narrowed if necessary, and the membranous urethra. The main advantage of the retropubic approach, other than possible greater familiarity with suprapubic anatomy, is ready access to the regional pelvic lymph nodes. Disadvantages are greater blood loss during surgery and greater patient discomfort postoperatively.

Most patients have varying degrees of stress incontinence following total prostatectomy. Usually this is temporary, disappearing in 1 to 3 months, although in 10 to 20 percent of patients, stress incontinence may persist. Total incontinence occurs in 10 percent of patients, though with meticulous technique the incidence can be reduced to 1 percent. Those who remain incontinent more than 6 to 9 months postoperatively rarely improve thereafter. Stricture at the site of the vesicourethral anastomosis occurring in some 10 percent of patients

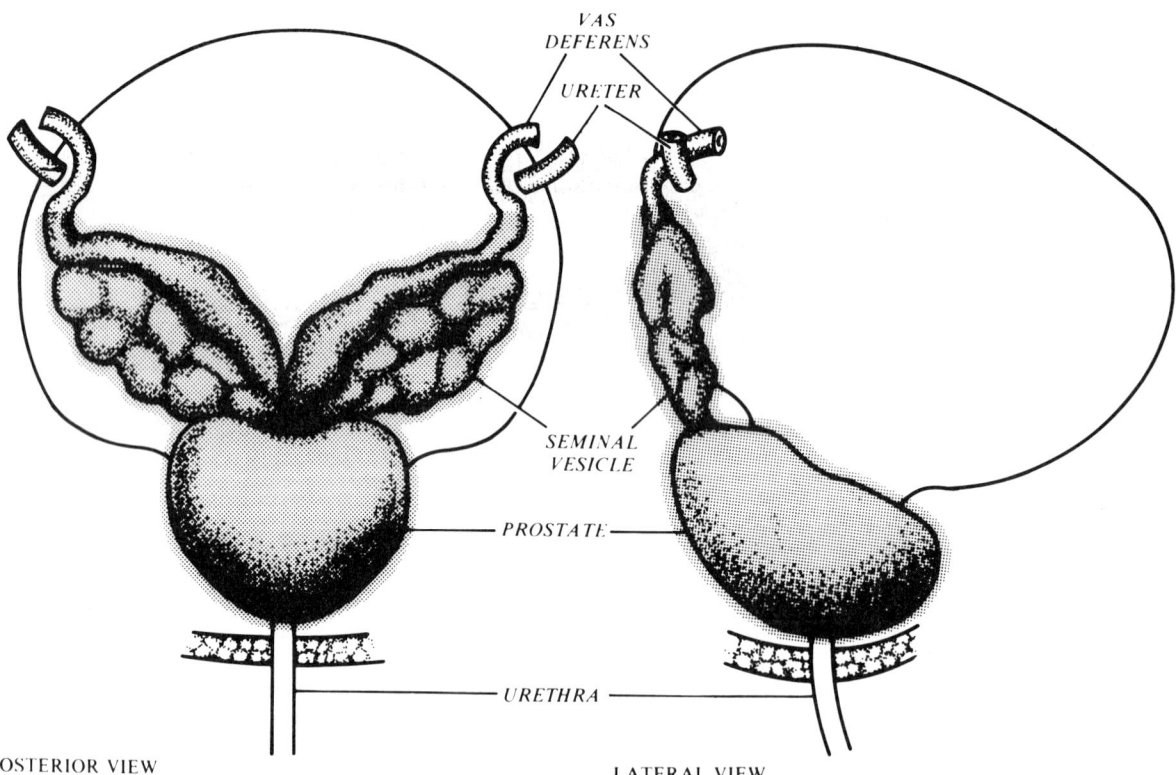

FIGURE 34-6 The shaded areas represent the structures removed during total prostatectomy. (*From JD Schmidt, JJ Pollen: Prostatic Cancer, GP Murphy, ed, PSG Publishing Co., 1979*).

may respond to urethral dilatation. Impotence following total prostatectomy is almost invariable, occurring in over 95 percent of cases.

Of patients treated with total prostatectomy for early cancer of prostate, approximately 60 to 90 percent survive 5 years; 40 to 75 percent survive 10 years; and 30 to 60 percent survive 15 years; 27 to 51 percent can be expected to survive 15 years without evidence of recurrent disease. The results of total prostatectomy by retrospective analysis of those patients whose tumors were histologically confined within the prostatic capsule are obviously superior. Of these patients, 75 to 90 percent survive for 5 years, 50 to 60 percent survive for 10 years, and 30 to 40 percent survive for 15 years. These statistics show that better preoperative selection of patients would improve the results of curative surgery.

During a follow-up period of 15 years or more, 30 percent of patients die of other diseases without evidence of recurrent cancers while 43 percent die with or of prostatic cancer.[22] Local recurrence will occur if the lesion is not completely excised, this being much more likely when histological examination reveals tumor penetrating the capsule or invading the seminal vesicles. Undetected lymphatic or hematogenous spread will inevitably result in failure of total prostatectomy to cure the patient.

The most important determinant of survival after total prostatectomy is the microscopic extent of the tumor. About 60 percent of surgical specimens show the disease to be microscopically more diffuse than was apparent by palpation alone. Nevertheless, with meticulous selection of small nodules, 84 percent are localized to the prostate. Once microscopic size reaches 2 cm or more, survival drops to a plateau, shared with involvement of the seminal vesicles.[34]

Microscopic invasion of the seminal vesicles demonstrated in 16 to 23 percent of total prostatectomy specimens is associated with a poor prognosis in terms of recurrent disease.[8] Unsuspected lymph node metastases may be the source of many of these recurrences. Microscopically demonstrable cancer in the seminal vesicles, even when clinically undetected, is associated with regional lymph node metastases in 80 to 90 percent of cases, in contrast to a 12 percent incidence of lymph node involvement when the seminal vesicles are free of tumor.[8] Microscopic invasion of the laminated capsule without penetration is not commonly associated with regional lymph node involvement, and therefore does not have the same prognostic significance.[35] Only 5.9 percent of patients with growths that extend beyond the prostate are alive at the end of 15 years, and none lives 15 years free of disease.[5] The grade of malignancy is an important determinant of survival. Although patients harboring well-differentiated cancerous nodules are not immune from recurrence and metastases, those with high-grade tumors have significantly shorter survivals. Very few patients with poorly differentiated carcinoma will survive 10 to 15 years.

The rationale of adjuvant treatment to prevent local and distant recurrence from undetectable micrometastasis present at the time of radical treatment of the primary is sound. It is, however, unlikely that endocrine treatment reliably achieves this end. The addition of bilateral orchiectomy with or without estrogens to total prostatectomy gives results comparable to prostatectomy alone. Supplementary estrogens should not be added to patients treated with total prostatectomy for stage A or B disease. Survival is significantly poorer in patients receiving 5 mg of diethylstilbestrol daily due to an excess of cardiovascular complications.[36]

Adjuvant hormonal therapy, if considered at all, should be limited to bilateral orchiectomy in those patients whose surgical specimen shows extraprostatic spread and who are willing to undergo the procedure.

Since hormone treatment selectively kills androgen-dependent malignant cells, the use of chemotherapeutic agents which are nonselective would seem more logical. For effective adjuvant treatment, the cytotoxic agents selected should be highly active against the cancer and safe in long-term usage. Currently cyclophosphamide* and estramustine phosphate* are being tested individually for their effectiveness as adjuvant chemotherapy following definitive external irradiation or total prostatectomy by the National Prostatic Cancer Project. Outside the strict conditions of a prospective clinical trial, adjuvant chemotherapy cannot yet be recommended for treatment of early-stage prostate cancer.

External beam or interstitial radiation therapy may be as efficient as surgery in eradicating the local lesion. If long-term results confirm this promise, then they offer an attractive alternative to radical surgery. In the meantime, they should be reserved for those patients who are not suitable candidates for surgery, refuse operation, or are unwilling to accept the complications of total prostatectomy.

* These drugs have not been approved for this purpose by the Food and Drug Administration at the time of publication.

About 80 percent of B lesions respond to endocrine treatment. When transurethral resection to relieve outflow obstruction is combined with early or delayed endocrine treatment, 28 percent of patients survive 15 years, 15 percent without evidence of cancer. Of the patients that die, one-third die of prostatic cancer and 64 percent of other causes.

Endocrine therapy, particularly estrogens, for stages A and B_1 prostatic cancer should be withheld until there are symptoms of recurrence. The 10- and 15-year survival rates of 47 percent and 24 percent for immediate endocrine treatment are inferior to the 55 percent and 37 percent survivals for delayed hormonal manipulation. The differences in survival between early and delayed treatment are most evident in men less than 70 years old.[37] No further treatment after transurethral resection is a consideration in patients with reduced life expectancy due to associated diseases.

Stage B_2

The importance of size as a reflection of the biologic behavior of a tumor is vividly apparent when the survival of patients with B_1 disease is compared to that of patients with larger B_2 lesions. Treated by transurethral resection of the prostate only, 19 percent live for 5 years, 4 percent for 10 years, and less than 1 percent for 15 years.[10] The prognosis is adversely affected by high-grade lesions. Histologically, 50 percent of B_2 cancers show evidence of penetration through the capsule or invasion of seminal vesicles. Between 25 and 62 percent of patients have lymph node metastases determined by pelvic lymphadenectomy. Treatment of stage B_2 prostatic cancer should proceed along the same lines as treatment for stage C_1 disease.

Stage C

At the time of diagnosis, 30 to 35 percent of patients demonstrate clinical spread through the capsule. Clinical stage C carcinoma of the prostate is diagnosed by the presence of limited periprostatic spread and no evidence of metastasis. The average duration of symptoms prior to diagnosis is 33 months. Survival from the onset of symptoms until death averages 5 years, the median being 38 months. Survival following diagnosis averages 2 years, while one-half of the patients live less than 1 year. Without the benefit of endocrine treatment, 10 to 15 percent of patients survive 5 years and only 5 percent live for 10 years.[11]

Discussion of treatment is confined to B_2 disease and smaller C_1 lesions rather than large tumors, which carry an excessively poor prognosis because of the high incidence of metastases. An aggressive approach to treatment may be adopted for strictly limited disease with no evidence of seminal vesicle involvement. Various therapeutic options, none of which have been clearly shown to be superior to any other, are available, including total prostatovesiculectomy and external beam and interstitial radiation.

The presence of positive lymph nodes is almost always a harbinger of distant metastases. Within 1 to 2 years, many of these patients develop signs of hematogenous spread. When it is considered that, in the presence of locally advanced disease, positive lymph nodes may be detected in from 30 to 90 percent of cases, enthusiasm for major surgery should be tempered by the knowledge that the ultimate prognosis for survival is limited. Whenever possible, staging pelvic lymphadenectomy to exclude lymph node metastases should be carried out prior to definitive treatment of the primary lesion, preferably as a separate procedure.

At least some patients with early local disease can be cured by total prostatovesiculectomy. The 5-year survival rates for stages B_2 and C_1 range from 35 to 74 percent, 10-year survival is 12 to 60 percent, and 15-year survival is 20 percent. Since there is a substantial incidence of pelvic lymph node metastasis, staging lymphadenectomy is mandatory. Once the permanent sections from the lymphadenectomy specimens return negative for tumor, the operation is carried out within 1 to 2 weeks, preferably by the perineal route. At times pressure from the patient who does not wish to have two operations makes it expedient to proceed with total prostatectomy at the time of lymph node dissection if the results of frozen section are negative. This may be accomplished through the suprapubic incision or through a separate perineal approach. It is understood that under these circumstances a few patients will undergo radical prostatectomy in the face of positive lymph nodes.

The local recurrence rate after total prostatectomy of stage B_2 and C_1 disease may exceed 25 percent. Cystoprostatectomy, while more likely to achieve local control, is also associated with a high recurrence rate and is not generally advised.

It seems unlikely that endocrine therapy can downstage the tumor. Such treatment does not completely destroy malignant cells situated in the extraprostatic tissues. Pathological examination of specimens removed by radical excision after estrogen administration discloses persistent cancer in periprostatic structures. Careful histologic study shows no tendency for increased cell destruction in peripheral areas as compared with the center of the neoplasm. Nevertheless, the results of total prostatectomy in carefully selected cases of early prostatic extension can be improved by pretreatment with estrogens or orchiectomy, perhaps by facilitating the surgery. Patients excluded from this combined therapeutic approach are those that have a poorly defined intervesicular plateau, extension beyond the apex, or persistent elevation of acid or alkaline phosphatase levels. Only those who demonstrate excellent regression following endocrine manipulation are considered for surgery. Of patients treated by this regimen 29 percent survive 15 years without evidence of cancer.[38] Results might be further improved by insisting on prior negative staging lymphadenectomy.

External beam radiation offers a potentially curative noninvasive modality in the treatment of localized prostatic cancer. Ideally radiation is administered with a linear accelerator although cobalt 60 is also effective. The approach is to irradiate homogeneously a field limited to the prostatic region, including the prostate, periprostatic tissues, seminal vesicles, and bladder neck. A radiation field of 6 to 8 cm^2, as measured through the axis of rotation, is treated with either 360° rotational therapy or 120° rotational left and right lateral arc therapy. The dose ranges between 7000 rads at the isocenter delivered in 7 weeks to 7600 rads delivered in $7\frac{1}{2}$ weeks.[39]

The routine administration of extended-field ^{60}Co teletherapy, consisting of 7000 rads to the prostate and 5000 rads to the pelvic nodes, without the benefit of surgical staging is associated with a high incidence of radiation morbidity and 5-year survivals no greater than that with small-field radiation. This form of treatment cannot be recommended.

It is difficult to achieve adequate and uniform irradiation of bulky tumors by radiation techniques. Large tumors can be reduced in size by pretreatment with endocrine manipulation. This approach, however, does not permit any compromise in proper staging of the tumor prior to therapy.

In order to avoid failures of treatment due to undetected regional lymph node metastasis, a formal extraperitoneal pelvic lymphadenectomy is recommended prior to treatment. As a rule, the presence of nodal metastasis is a contraindication to unassisted curative radiation therapy to the prostate because of the high risk of early distant metastasis. Also, there is some doubt whether 5000 rads, a limit set by bowel tolerance, delivered to the pelvis is sufficient to sterilize the regional nodes. The argument that minimal metastasis to the pelvic nodes may be controlled by the lymphadenectomy and extension of the field of irradiation to encompass the entire pelvis with possible sparing of the rectum is plausible but has not been subjected to critical trial. Extending the field of irradiation to include metastases in the pelvis and paraaortic areas, as determined by lymphangiography and staging laparotomy, has been followed by severe small-bowel reactions sometimes requiring resection, and appearance of distant metastases within a short time.

It has been found that 59 percent of glands do not change in size immediately following radiation therapy. However, 6 months later 90 percent of glands are smaller and only 7 percent remain the same size. Although 30 percent of glands show significant regression at the completion of therapy, in 11 percent the gland size may actually increase, presumably due to radiation-induced edema.[39]

Rectal palpation alone is inaccurate as a method of following the local effects of treatment. Glands that feel benign may be found to have active carcinoma on biopsy, whereas radiation fibrosis will result in a hard, fibrous prostate that on histological examination is benign. Biopsies performed soon after radiation may be positive in up to 80 percent of cases. Positive biopsies may revert to negative within 12 months of radiotherapy. After 12 months, and certainly after 18 months, positive biopsies rarely revert without further treatment. Between 50 and 60 percent of patients treated by external radiotherapy have biopsy evidence of residual tumor in the prostate 18 to 36 months after therapy. Negative biopsies show a large amount of fibrous tissue in most cases with little residual adenomatous tissue.[40,41]

Among treatment failures, 70 percent are recognized within 24 months. Of those who fail the treatment, 35 percent present with local and disseminated disease, 60 percent with metastasis and apparent local control, and 5 percent with local failure only. Irradiation creates impotence in 40 to 50 percent of patients who were potent before and who do not receive endocrine intervention. Severe symptoms consisting of blood-streaked stools, tenesmus, rectal urgency, and dysuria may persist for 1 year in 12 percent of patients. Transient radiation cystitis and radiation proctitis occur in up to 40 percent of patients.[42] Lymphadenectomy added to pelvic irradiation compounds the incidence of indolent lymphedema of the genitalia and extremities. Approximately

40 to 85 percent of patients receiving definitive radiation therapy for stages B and C prostatic cancer survive 5 years. The 10-year survival rate is 35 to 48 percent.

A variety of interstitial irradiation techniques are available for the treatment of prostatic cancer, including the use of radioactive gold and iodine. Interstitial irradiation of the prostate has certain advantages over external radiation therapy. High tumoricidal doses of radiation are concentrated in the tumor-bearing area. The 100 percent tumor dose represents the maximum dose if given by rotation or multiple small fields, whereas it represents the minimum effective dose by implantation. Localization of the tumor is more precise, and the dose distribution can be more readily adapted to an irregular tumor shape. Interstitial irradiation offers the benefits of highly concentrated tumoricidal doses of irradiation with a relatively low incidence of side effects. The dose falls rapidly outside the implanted volume; thus, radiation effects on the bladder and rectum are kept to a minimum. The incidence of impotence in patients who were sexually potent before radiotherapy is less than 10 percent. The time saved by combining the surgical staging with treatment is also attractive. Interstitial implantation requires a single procedure and a hospital stay of 7 to 10 days as opposed to 6 to 7 weeks of treatment with external beam radiaton therapy.

Radioactive gold (^{198}Au) in colloidal solution has a half-life of 2.7 days. Most of the energy released is in the form of β rays with a fairly good emission of moderately strong γ rays. Intense irradiation occurs in the area injected with the coolest spots ranging from 8000 to 9000 rads. Because the radiation penetrates only about 3 mm in tissue, the rectum and bladder receive relatively small amounts of energy and severe radiation reactions do not occur. About 97 percent of the radiation is delivered over a period of $1\frac{1}{2}$ weeks.

^{198}Au may be most useful in the treatment of earlier stages of prostatic cancer in patients who refuse or are unable to undergo total prostatectomy. The technique calls for perineal exposure of the prostate which is infiltrated with 50 mCi of ^{198}Au in about 2 mL of diluent. Of 10 patients so treated and followed for 10 years or more, 9 survived without evidence of local or distant recurrence of disease. Because of problems related to distribution of the radioisotope, interstitial ^{198}Au in patients with extraprostatic extension is best used as an adjuvant to total prostatectomy.[43] The surgical procedure consists of an extended radical perineal or retropubic prostatectomy. In addition to the removal of as much of the malignant prostate and seminal vesicles as possible, any remaining tissue which seems indurated is thoroughly electrocoagulated and then irradiated by the interstitial injection of 100 mCi ^{198}Au in 2 mL diluent. When this combination of techniques is used, there is a less than 5 percent incidence of local recurrence. The only common complication is delayed wound healing, which can be expected in 80 percent of cases. Again, the best survivals are obtained in patients who have been determined to have no lymph node involvement.

Interstitial ^{198}Au may be combined with external beam irradiation.[40] Initially an extraperitoneal bilateral pelvic lymphadenectomy is performed through a lower abdominal incision. Thereafter, the prostate is mobilized sufficiently to allow the radiotherapist access to the tumor. The radiotherapist implants the prostate with radioactive gold seeds to achieve a tumor dose of 2500 to 3500 rads. When the wound heals, usually about 8 to 10 days postoperatively, external beam radiotherapy is begun from a linear accelerator source; 4000 to 5000 rads are delivered to the prostate and the periprostatic areas through rotational or opposing fields. The average total tumor dose is 7500 rads. Doses less than 6000 rads seldom result in ablation of prostatic carcinoma. Five-year survivals similar to those with external beam irradiation have been achieved with combined interstitial gold and external beam radiotherapy in treatment of smaller stage C neoplasms.[40]

Interstitial radioactive iodine (^{125}I) is currently enjoying popularity.[44] ^{125}I has a 27 keV γ emission and a half-life of 60 days. Irradiation from the ^{125}I seeds decreases exponentially so that its half value layer is 2 cm. The initial step prior to implantation is a formal extraperitoneal pelvic lymphadenectomy through a lower abdominal incision. Next, the prostate gland is exposed retropubically on its anterior and lateral surfaces, with incision of endopelvic fascia on either side to improve exposure.

Hollow 16-gauge stainless steel needles, 15 cm in length, are inserted at right angles to the exposed surface of the prostate until their tips can be sensed by a palpating finger in the rectum. The needles are placed in parallel rows 0.5 to 1 cm apart beginning at the superior border and working down toward the apex. The volume to be implanted is calculated by measuring the length and width of the gland directly and the depth by subtracting the average length of the needles projecting outside the prostate from the overall length of these needles. The average of the three dimensions multiplied by 5 has been empirically determined to yield a value which indicates the amount in microcuries of ^{125}I required to obtain the optimal dose in the implanted volumes. This is divided by the average activity of the available seeds to give the number of seeds to be implanted, and this in turn is divided by the number of needles to estimate the number of seeds available per needle.

A specially designed instrument (Fig. 34-7) with a magazine which automatically delivers the seeds and a ratchet mechanism is used to insert the seeds successively into the tissue at the desired levels as the needle is withdrawn. Seeds are placed no less than 0.5 cm and not more than 1 cm apart.

Following the implantation, adjunctive endocrine therapy can be used to shrink the prostate and increase the effectiveness of the exponentially declining irradiation by bringing the ^{125}I seeds closer together. Patients who present with significant bladder-outlet-obstructive symptoms are best managed by a conservative transurethral resection 6 weeks to 3 months before implantation. Sufficient tissue is removed to relieve the obstruction, but enough is left behind to support the implant.

The procedure is well tolerated with only transient urinary symptoms following the implantation. In the weeks immediately following the operation some prostates increase in size and induration due to edema. Involvement of the pelvic lymph nodes by metastatic cancer is the most significant prognostic factor following this procedure. Distant metastases develop in about 50 percent of patients after 12 to 18 months whether or not supplementary external irradiation is given to the involved nodes.

There is some evidence that patients with limited lymph node metastases, less than 3 cm³ in volume, have as good an outlook as those without nodal metastases.[40] Until this is established, pelvic lymphadenectomy must be regarded simply as a diagnostic maneuver. In the presence of obvious nodal involvement, the plan to insert the seeds should be abandoned. Frequently one proceeds as planned on the argument that by insuring local control, one can prevent future complications. Also the complications of inserting the seeds are minimal.

If the long-term results can match those for linear accelerator treatment, interstitial or combined interstitial and external beam irradiation may become the treatment of choice for localized prostatic carcinoma not amenable to extirpative surgery. An important consideration in younger men is that the incidence of impotence following interstitial irradiation is only 7 percent in those who are potent preoperatively. Interstitial irradiation may be even more effective in the treatment of stage B cancers before periprostatic spread has occurred. If this is true, the prospect of avoiding the morbidity of total prostatectomy for disease confined to the prostate is most welcome.

Poor-risk patients with stage C disease may be treated electively by palliative endocrine therapy, which may delay progression to stage D. With rare exceptions, large stage C_0 lesions, and those that show obvious invasion of seminal vesicles and trigone, are unworthy of consideration for curative management. Even if they are technically removable by radical surgery, there is a high risk, 40 percent or greater, of local recurrence. Lymph node metastases, always a poor prognostic sign, may be demonstrated in up to 90 percent of patients. In any case, modern staging techniques, particularly bone scanning,

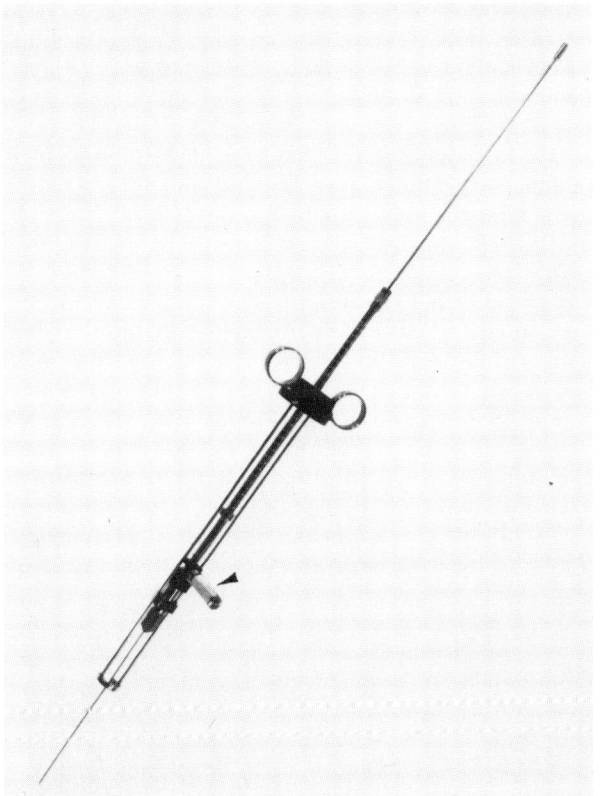

FIGURE 34-7 Mick applicator designed for interstitial implantation of radioactive seeds loaded in the cartridge (*arrow*).

frequently demonstrate osseous metastasis, which immediately places the lesion in stage D. External beam radiation therapy, the only other modality that is potentially curative under the circumstances, has demonstrated little success in the control of large, solid growths. The same arguments apply, with even greater emphasis, to the management of stage D_1 growths which have extended to involve bladder, ureters, rectum, or lateral pelvic walls. These malignancies should be treated palliatively. The 1-year survival rate for patients with stage C prostatic cancer treated with hormone therapy is approximately 85 percent; 3-year survival ranges from 50 to 65 percent; 5-year survival from 30 to 55 percent; and 10-year survival from 5 to 25 percent.

Stage D

A large number of patients with prostatic cancer (32 to 45 percent) are diagnosed at a stage when clinical metastases are present. About 80 percent of patients with advanced prostatic cancer die of their disease. The average duration of symptoms prior to diagnosis is 25 months, and 50 percent of patients have symptoms for 1 year or less. When metastases are present, the duration of survival is short, on the average 16 months, with a median of 9 months from diagnosis. Only 11 percent survive 5 years, although rare survivals as long as 15 years in duration are recorded.

Currently there is no reliable means available for the cure of advanced prostatic cancer. All treatment for this stage of the disease must be regarded as palliative. Those patients with earlier stages of the disease who are over the age of 70 years, or unfit for the anesthesia that goes along with definitive treatment, or refuse to undergo surgery may be considered for treatment along the same lines.

If symptoms are truly absent, no therapy except regular follow-up is in order. However, this situation is relatively unusual, and most patients are offered treatment even when the tumor load is light. Any form of treatment should be instituted only after due consideration has been given to the risks involved.

The mainstay of palliative treatment for the control of prostatic cancer is endocrine manipulation. The growth and function of both the normal adult prostate and most prostatic cancers is supported by androgenic hormones.[45] Testosterone, produced almost exclusively by the Leydig cells of the testes, is the most potent of the major circulating androgenic steroids. Testosterone enters the prostatic cell by diffusion, where it is reduced to dihydrotestosterone by the enzyme 5α-reductase in the cytoplasm. Thereafter, dihydrotestosterone attaches to a macromolecular receptor protein in the cytoplasm. The steroid-receptor complex translocates into the nucleus where it binds to chromatin to direct the formation of messenger RNA. In this way, androgens regulate protein synthesis and cell reproduction. The adrenal androgens dehydroepiandrosterone and androstenedione are also converted to dihydrotestosterone, though to a much lesser extent. The anterior pituitary hormone prolactin increases the accumulation of both testosterone and dihydrotestosterone in prostatic tissue, and acts synergistically with testosterone to increase the growth and function of the prostate gland.

Bilateral orchiectomy or estrogens are the current standard forms of endocrine manipulation. Bilateral orchiectomy is recommended as the initial step in endocrine control of prostatic cancer. More than 95 percent of plasma testosterone in men originates from the testes. Bilateral orchiectomy reduces plasma testosterone levels from a normal of 300 to 900 ng per 100 mL to castrate levels of 50 ng per 100 mL or less.[45]

The operation may be performed through a single midline scrotal incision, each testis being approached in turn. After the tunica vaginalis is opened, the coverings of the testis and spermatic cord are swept upward. Each cord is doubly ligated, the testis removed, and the scrotum closed. The subcapsular technique of removing the contents of each testis from within the tunica albuginea, while probably effective, is not recommended because there is a chance that Leydig cells may remain behind to be reactivated at a later date. Silicone gel prostheses can be inserted in the scrotum, though most elderly men are not concerned with the cosmetic aspects of orchiectomy.

Initial clinical responses to bilateral orchiectomy appear no different from that achieved with diethylstilbestrol. The patient does not have to concern himself with taking daily estrogens; thus, the need for patient compliance to take medication is eliminated. Furthermore, the possibility of thromboembolic complications associated with estrogens, particularly in patients who have underlying cardiovascular disease, is avoided. If subsequent administration of estrogens or chemotherapy becomes necessary, they are given against a background of castrate levels of testosterone, thus eliminating any doubt that the patient in relapse is compromised by his testicular secretions.

As initial hormone therapy, diethylstilbestrol may be reserved for those patients with symptomatic disease who refuse orchiectomy. The main action of estrogens in the control of prostatic cancer is via the negative feedback effect on the hypothalamus. By suppressing gonadotropin releasing factor, luteinizing hormone is not released from the pituitary. Since the testicular Leydig cells only secrete testosterone in response to luteinizing hormone, testosterone levels are effectively suppressed. Estrogen may directly depress testicular steroidogenesis, and suppress prostatic cell function. High doses inhibit DNA-polymerase and 5α-reductase activity in the nucleus.

Estrogens are most commonly prescribed as diethylstilbestrol (DES) 1 mg three times daily by mouth. From a clinical standpoint, 1 mg of diethylstilbestrol is as effective as 5 mg in controlling prostatic cancer, but does not carry the excess hazard of cardiovascular deaths associated with the higher dosage.[46,47] However, doses of 1 mg/day or less do not reliably reduce plasma testosterone levels around the clock, whereas 3 mg/day of diethylstilbestrol suppresses plasma testosterone levels to the castrate range. Conjugated estrogens (Premarin) 2.5 mg three times a day and ethinyl estradiol 0.05 mg twice daily produce effects equivalent to that of 3 mg of diethylstilbestrol per day. Chlorotrianisene (TACE) does not reliably suppress plasma testosterone levels and clinically does not appear to be as active as diethylstilbestrol. Of patients with stage D prostatic cancer treated with endocrine manipulation 70 to 90 percent survive for 1 year. Three-year survival ranges approximately from 20 to 50 percent, 5-year survival from 10 to 30 percent, and 10-year survival less than 10 percent.

The histological effects of treatment with estrogen are seen both in the tumor cells and in normal tissue. Affected malignant cells develop small intracytoplasmic basal vacuoles which coalesce and push the nucleus to one side. The swollen cells are often desquamated and fill the alveolar lumens. The nucleus becomes condensed, hyperchromatic, and pyknotic. Finally, the swollen cells rupture, and the cell and alveolar contents diffuse into the stroma. These changes may be followed by replacement fibrosis.

The most striking estrogenic effect on the nonmalignant tissue is squamous metaplasia of the transitional epithelium of the prostatic urethra extending into the prostatic ducts. Estrogenic changes in the tumor may appear within a very short time after beginning treatment. Clinical regression of the primary is associated with histologic evidence of cell destruction in the prostate. However, even in tumors which show severe degenerative changes, some cells survive without any sign of damage. Hormonal sensitivity is not a property of the tumor as a whole. The term is more accurately applied to those cells which succumb to antiandrogen treatment. Grading is of little value in predicting response to treatment, as estrogen sensitivity of the tumor cells is independent of the degree of differentiation. All grades of tumor cell, from the differentiated to the most anaplastic, seem to respond similarly.[48]

About 70 to 80 percent of patients respond favorably to castration or diethylstilbestrol. The clinical response is frequently dramatic. The prostate may shrink until it is barely palpable, with marked improvement of voiding function. Renal function improves as hydronephrosis resolves. Lymph nodal masses may melt away, relieving lymphedema or venous obstruction. Patients are most grateful for the relief of bone pain they experience, often within a few days. Destruction of tumor in the bone marrow is reflected in a rising hemoglobin and hematocrit. Improved appetite results in weight gain, and most men report a sense of well-being.

Serial bone scans show improvement. There may be a reduction in the number, size, and intensity of areas of increased uptake of the radionuclide. Radiographically, lytic lesions, when present, recalcify. Blastic areas, which rarely resolve, remain unchanged or increase in density and extent as part of the healing response. The serum alkaline phosphatase level may show an immediate sharp increase, sometimes accompanied by hypocalcemia, then a steady decline to normal in keeping with the osteoblastic response. Acid phosphatase levels decline steadily towards normal. Overall survival is improved inasmuch as 20 to 30 percent of patients survive 5 years or more.

When deaths from cancer only are considered, survival curves suggest that estrogen therapy is superior to orchiectomy in retarding the course of prostatic cancer [36,46,47] and improves survival by decreasing cancer-related mortality. However, the decrease may be offset by a significantly increased risk of cardiovascular deaths when diethylstilbestrol at a dose of 5 mg daily or more is prescribed. Included among the cardiovascular deaths associated with estrogen therapy are those due to myocardial infarctions, cerebrovascular accidents, congestive heart failure, arteriosclerotic heart disease, and pulmonary embolism.

The higher mortality rate with estrogens is a true

increase or acceleration of noncancer mortality and is not simply the result of reducing deaths from cancer.[36] The greatest risk of cardiovascular death occurs within the first year; thereafter, there is little increased risk. As the cancer progresses, the risk of dying from the disease greatly outweighs that of dying from cardiovascular problems. Low-dose diethylstilbestrol, 1 mg daily or less, is not associated with excess cardiovascular toxicity. Aspirin 300 mg twice a day, by interfering with platelet aggregation, may possibly reduce the incidence of estrogen-related cardiovascular complications.

Progestational agents show activity in advanced prostatic cancer. Short-term studies show that megestrol acetate* (Megace) in doses of 160 mg daily, decreases prostatic dihydrotestosterone concentrations to castrate levels by competing for cytosol receptor, blocking 5α-reductase and decreasing plasma testosterone. In addition, megestrol acetate produces significant suppression of the adrenal cortical plasma androgen dehydroepiandrosterone sulfate. Unlike DES, megestrol acetate does not increase serum prolactin. Within 1 to 2 months of megestrol acetate treatment, plasma testosterone falls almost to castrate levels. By 2 to 6 months there is an escape of plasma testosterone suppression, associated with a rise in previously suppressed gonadotropins.[49]

Medroxyprogesterone acetate* (Provera) 30 mg daily is not as effective as DES in reducing acid phosphatase levels, and shows little effect on the size of the primary lesion. Progestagens, like estrogens, decrease libido in a significant number of patients, but salt retention, gynecomastia, and thromboembolic disease are less common.

Of patients with advanced neoplasia 20 to 30 percent fail to respond to castration or estrogen therapy, presumably because their growths are androgen independent. The majority of those who respond relapse within 2 to 3 years. Prostatic cancer probably consists of two or more clones of cells, some androgen-dependent and the remainder able to grow without androgen support. Endocrine treatment may selectively destroy the androgen-dependent clones, leaving the remainder to cause relapse.

It seems reasonable to treat advanced prostatic cancer with antiandrogen therapy to destroy the androgen-dependent cells, supplemented by chemotherapy to attack nonandrogen-dependent cancer cells. The management and follow-up of all stages of prostatic cancer are summarized in Table 34-5.

* This drug has not been approved for this purpose by the Food and Drug Administration at the time of publication.

RELAPSING DISEASE

A return of bone pain or symptoms of urinary obstruction signifies further tumor growth. There may be an increase in the extent or number of roentgenographic bone lesions. Serial bone scans may show additional or expanded areas of increased uptake of the radionuclide. A pulmonary infiltrate on chest radiographs suggests lymphangitic metastases, an ominous finding. Peripheral lymphadenopathy, and rarely skin nodules, may appear quite suddenly. Abdominal palpation may reveal lymph nodal masses in the epigastrium or along the pelvic vessels. Enlargement of the liver, particularly if tender or irregular, suggests metastasis which can be confirmed by ultrasound examination and liver-spleen scintiscan. Genital and peripheral edema may develop from lymphatic or venous obstruction. Excretion urography may show progressive hydronephrosis as renal function deteriorates. When anorexia, weight loss, debility, and anemia set in, death follows in a few weeks.

Sometimes the primary tumor remains small while there is obvious evidence of spread of the disease. In other instances, metastases may remain quiescent while the local lesion gradually enlarges and extends. A rising serum acid or alkaline phosphatase level is a predictor of clinical relapse. On the average, patients survive 9 months after the onset of relapse. Approximately 50 percent die within 7 months and 80 percent before 18 months.

Endocrine Treatment

Although the activated disease is frequently resistant to further endocrine manipulation, between 17 and 36 percent of patients may experience some symptomatic relief by the addition of orchiectomy or estrogens for a limited period of time.[50]

It would be most useful at the time of relapse to have a reliable test available for residual androgen dependence of the tumor. Further efforts at endocrine manipulation could then be limited to those patients who might predictably respond to such treatment. Remaining patients would be treated with alternative methods such as chemotherapy. At this time the identification and significance of androgen receptors to determine estrogen sensitivity in prostatic cancer cells is still investigational.

Subjective clinical testing of residual endocrine sensitivity can be done in two ways. Estrogens may be temporarily withdrawn for several days and any increase in pain noted. Pain relief by the reintroduction of estrogens suggests they ought to be continued, supple-

TABLE 34-5 Summary of Management of Prostatic Cancer

Stage	Treatment	Follow-up*	Frequency
A_1	Observation	Rebiopsy	In 3–6 months
		Clinical evaluation	Every 12 months
B_1	Prostatovesiculectomy	Clinical evaluation; creatinine, SAP, alk phos, IVP, CXR, bone scan	Every 12 months
A_2	External irradiation	Same	Every 6–12 months
$B_2 C_1$	External irradiation, interstitial irradiation	Same	Every 6–12 months
$C_2 D_1 D_2$	Endocrine, chemotherapy	Clinical evaluation; creatinine, SAP, alk phos	Every 6 weeks–6 months
		IVP, CXR, bone scan	Every 3–12 months

* SAP = Serum acid phosphatase; IVP = intravenous pyelogram; CXR = chest x-ray.

mented by other treatment as necessary. Alternatively, a course of high-dosage diethylstilbestrol diphosphate (Stilphostrol) 0.5 to 1.0 g IV daily for 5 to 7 days can be administered. Responders may be well maintained on diethylstilbestrol by mouth at increased dosages of 15 to 20 mg daily.

Further endocrine manipulation for patients in relapse is based on the premise that the tumor remains at least partially androgen dependent, being stimulated by adrenal androgens. Androgenic action may be countered at various levels. Ablation of the hypophysis removes the trophic hormones to the adrenals, while bilateral adrenalectomy removes the site of steroid production. The synthesis of androgens may be interfered with by compounds that inhibit steroidogenesis in either the testis or the adrenal. Antiandrogenic agents block the effect of androgens at the level of the tumor cell by interfering with the intracellular events that mediate androgenic action.

Destruction of the hypophysis is utilized in treatment of severe pain refractory to standard endocrine treatment. The rationale for ablation of the pituitary has been the removal of all extratesticular sources of stimuli to the prostate, namely androgen secreted by the adrenal and prolactin secreted by the pituitary. However, the clinical response of patients to hypophysectomy does not correlate well with deficiency of pituitary hormones. Total pituitary ablation is not always necessary for clinical remission. A mechanism related to the interruption of hypothalamic nerve pathways may be the explanation for the immediate and profound pain relief experienced by up to 75 percent of patients.[51]

A variety of ablative techniques, including open hypophysectomy and cryohypophysectomy, are available. The pituitary fossa can be irradiated by the introduction of two or three pellets of yttrium 90, each consisting of 3 to 4 mCi, by the perinasal transsphenoidal route using a cannulated needle introducer. Chemical hypophysectomy can be simply performed by the injection of 5 to 6 mL of absolute alcohol within the sella by a stereotactically guided needle passed transnasally through the floor of the sphenoid sinus. About 50 percent of patients undergoing hypophysectomy experience subjective or objective improvement. The mean survival after hypophysectomy is 5 to 10 months.[52] All patients require hormonal support with cortisone and thyroxine starting on the second postoperative day. Significant diabetes insipidus requires treatment with vasopressin administered by injection, nasal spray, or as a snuff.

Bilateral adrenalectomy produces subjective or objective improvement in about 50 percent of patients who have failed standard endocrine treatment.[52] The operation further reduces serum testosterone below castrate levels. However, cortisone given as replacement is partially converted to androgenic compounds in the liver, so that a completely androgen-free environment is not achieved. Because of the magnitude of the operation and the brevity of the responses, adrenalectomy is infrequently performed.

Antiandrogenic compounds are potent inhibitors of testosterone-stimulated DNA synthesis. They do not block the uptake of androgen into the prostatic cytoplasm. Cyproterone acetate* (SH-714) suppresses pitui-

* This drug has not been approved for this purpose by the Food and Drug Administration at the time of publication.

tary gonadotropin activity, inhibits adrenal androgen synthesis, and prevents the formation of the dihydrotestosterone-protein-chromatin complex in the nucleus of the prostatic cell. Cyproterone, the free alcohol, does not suppress gonadotropin secretion, and like the acetate, does not inhibit formation of dihydrotestosterone.[45]

Flutamide* (SCH-13521) is a nonsteroidal antiandrogen which neither inhibits gonadotropin secretion nor suppresses plasma testosterone levels. By interfering with the complexing of dihydrotestosterone to the cytosol receptor protein, flutamide prevents translocation of the androgen into the nucleus. Serum luteinizing hormone does not decrease, and plasma testosterone levels in noncastrates rise to high normal with flutamide treatment. The dose of flutamide is 250 mg three times a day. As primary treatment, this drug produces clinical responses no different from those to diethylstilbestrol. Gynecomastia develops later than with DES, though sexual potency is not altered. Flutamide is devoid of the metabolic and vascular side effects observed with estrogenic compounds.[53]

There is as yet no established role for inhibitors of steroidogenesis or antiandrogens in the primary treatment of prostatic cancer. In treatment of relapse they might be used to suppress the adrenal production of androgens or block the effects of androgens on prostatic tissue, in place of ablative surgery.

Chemotherapy

Ideally, patients with widespread progressive or relapsing disease should be managed by systemic chemotherapy. Controlled studies have confirmed that several chemotherapeutic agents are active, to a modest degree, in advanced disease no longer responsive to endocrine treatment.[54] Among those studied are 5-fluorouracil,* streptozotocin, dacarbazine,* and estramustine phosphate* (Estracyt). Approximately one-third of patients treated with these agents show a response, mainly in the form of stabilization of the disease process. Estramustine phosphate, a chemical combination of estradiol and nitrogen mustard, owes much of its activity to the estrogenic component. This is manifested clinically by slight gynecomastia and in the laboratory by low levels of luteinizing hormone and castrate levels of testosterone in nonorchiectomized males. Estracyt is taken by mouth 600 mg/m² per day in three divided doses and is fairly well tolerated. Additional side effects are mainly gastrointestinal and rarely hepatotoxicity is observed.

The most promising chemotherapeutic agents tested so far in patients with progressive, estrogen-resistant stage D carcinoma of the prostate are cyclophosphamide and cis-diamminedichloroplatinum* (cis-platinum, DDP, Platinol). Cyclophosphamide in doses of 1000 mg/m² IV every 3 weeks induces stabilization in 39 percent and partial objective remission in 7 percent of patients for a 46 percent response rate. Major side effects include vomiting, hemorrhagic cystitis, and myelosuppression.

cis-Platinum is given by slow intravenous infusion over 1 h in a dose of 60 mg/m² every 3 or 4 weeks. Care is taken to promote an adequate diuresis before, during, and for 12 h following the infusion. In patients treated once a week for 6 weeks and every 3 weeks thereafter, partial objective response was observed in 29 percent, pain relief in 40 percent, and stabilization of disease in 13 percent. Our own experience with this drug has not borne out these favorable results. Major dose-limiting side effects are irreversible auditotoxicity and nephrotoxicity.[55]

Responses to chemotherapy, although no different to endocrine treatment, are less predictable and shorter lived. Patients who respond to chemotherapy survive longer than nonresponders and those who continue on standard treatment. It is predicted that effective chemotherapeutic combinations will be designed for a concerted attack on advanced disease.

Pain Management

Bone pain is one of the most distressing symptoms that patients with disseminated prostatic cancer have to face. Ideally, management consists of specific systemic treatment aimed at inducing tumor regression. However, many patients are in progression or are only partially responsive to specific measures and require additional treatment. A 5- to 7-day course of intravenous diethylstilbestrol diphosphate (Stilphostrol) frequently brings about at least partial relief. Most patients require supplemental analgesic medication. Aspirin or compounds of aspirin with codeine appear more effective than opiates alone.[56] Aspirin and indomethacin,* both powerful prostaglandin synthetase inhibitors, are frequently remarkably effective in relieving bone pain. Some patients report adequate pain control from acetaminophen

---

* This drug has not been approved for this purpose by the Food and Drug Administration at the time of publication.

with codeine. Brompton's solution, a mixture compounded from choloroform, alcohol, cocaine, and morphine sulfate, 20 to 40 mg in 20 mL, is useful. Ingestion of smaller volumes at more frequent intervals reduces the incidence of gastrointestinal effects and provides a background of analgesia which can be supplemented with lower doses of standard analgesics.

Systemic irradiation of bone by the intravenous injection of radioactive phosphorus (^{32}P) has been used as a specific measure to destroy bone metastases.[57] Patients selected for radiophosphorus treatment are those with diffuse bone pain from widespread osseous metastases unresponsive to endocrine therapy or chemotherapy and not controlled by moderate doses of powerful analgesics. Radiophosphorus is administered in a dosage of 1 to 2 mCi of ^{32}P intravenously over a 7- to 12-day period up to a total dose of 10 to 12 mCi. Pretreatment with parenteral testosterone may cause serious effects from stimulation of the cancer, including the development of paraplegia, and should not be used. A course of parathormone injections and subsequent withdrawal may be used to stimulate uptake of ^{32}P by bone. Serum calcium levels must be carefully monitored. Excellent relief of bone pain may be achieved by ^{32}P; however, severe marrow depression may be long-lasting. Marrow reserves may be compromised to the point where subsequent administration of chemotherapy becomes impossible. ^{32}P treatment is not commonly prescribed.

Of much greater use is the deployment of palliative external beam irradiation therapy to localized areas of severe pain. The area of clinical involvement is mapped out with the aid of radionuclide imaging as well as appropriate radiographs. A dose of 2000 rads in 1 week beamed at the appropriate area frequently produces dramatic relief of pain within a few days or weeks of completion of treatment and may sharply reduce the requirement for analgesics. Two or more areas may be irradiated simultaneously or successively as the clinical condition demands. Total-body irradiation, 800 rads single dose to the lower half of the body, can be given to patients with diffuse pain. After an interval of at least 4 weeks to allow recovery of the bone marrow, an additional 800 rads to the upper half of the body may be considered. Patients with extreme myelosuppression may be rescued by autotransfusion of previously banked bone marrow.

Obstructive Uropathy

Symptoms of bladder neck obstruction are often relieved by hormonal therapy or chemotherapy. Transurethral resection of the prostate is the most common surgical means employed for the relief of symptoms due to bladder neck obstruction. It is recommended early in the management of patients who require catheterization for the relief of acute or chronic retention of urine. By rapidly establishing a normal voiding pattern the use of this procedure removes the risks of catheter-induced infection and facilitates patient rehabilitation. The resection entails adequate removal of obstructive tissue, leaving the bladder neck wide open down to the level of the verumontanum. It is neither necessary nor possible to completely remove the primary tumor, though simply cutting a narrow channel is frequently inadequate, because the rigid splinting effect of the surrounding tumor does not permit funneling of the urethra necessary for normal voiding during detrusor contraction. Urinary incontinence occurs more frequently after resection for cancer than after resection for benign disease.

Cryosurgery offers a means of palliation of the primary lesion in clinical stage C and D prostatic cancer. It is a useful alternative to transurethral resection or external radiation therapy for the relief of persistent outflow obstruction. The perineal route provides excellent access to the primary lesion, is well tolerated, and assists in the avoidance of cold injury to the rectum, trigone, and ureters.[58] For large prostates, a pointed probe is inserted into the interstices of the gland. A flat-ended probe is preferred for smaller glands. The probe temperature is reduced to -180 to $-190°C$ for 3 to 5 min as an ice ball forms in the prostate. The probe is then rewarmed to facilitate removal. Further applications of cold are made depending on the size of the gland. The wound is closed about a Penrose drain and an indwelling urethral catheter left for 2 weeks.

The complication rate of perineal cryosurgery is acceptable. Some 14 percent of patients develop a urethrocutaneous fistula which generally closes within 4 weeks on continuous catheter drainage. A fecal fistula may develop if the cryoprobe is directly applied to tumor on the anterior rectal wall. Persistent retention of urine following removal of the catheter in 5 percent of patients requires an additional transurethral prostatic resection which is generally easier and less bloody than if performed primarily. Total incontinence of urine is a risk only in those patients who have invasion of the external sphincter mechanism, and only 1 percent of patients have permanent stress incontinence.

Transurethral prostatic cryosurgery is less precise, and there is an appreciable incidence of significant complications, including incontinence, fistula formation, and bladder contraction.[58] A significant number of patients require a second operation for persistent retention of urine caused by slough. Although it has not replaced palliative transurethral resection, perurethral cryosurgery should be considered for the very poor risk patient in whom only local anesthesia can be contemplated.

Sequential transurethral cryosurgery and open perineal cryosurgery frequently produces relief of bone pain from metastases refractory to hormonal treatment and radiotherapy.[58] This effect is temporary, the average duraton of relief being 4 months. Radiological evidence of regression of osseous metastases, a decrease in pulmonary metastases, or regression of supraclavicular lymph node metastases is seen in 1 to 16 percent of cases treated. Since spontaneous regression of prostatic cancer has not been reported, the regression in these cases has been attributed to cryotherapy. The possibility of an immune response to the release of large amounts of tumor antigen has been raised, but the precise mechanism remains to be defined.

External beam irradiation occasionally shrinks the prostate sufficiently to improve voiding. In frail patients a silastic urethral or suprapubic catheter, changed at regular intervals, may be the most appropriate form of urinary drainage.

Ureteral obstruction is most commonly caused by tumor invasion of the distal ureters. Unilateral obstruction, if asymptomatic, may be treated expectantly with intervention reserved for symptoms of pain or superimposed infection. A cystoscopically placed ureteral catheter or percutaneous nephrostomy may provide adequate drainage and return of renal function. Symptomatic obstruction of the distal ureter may be managed definitively by reimplantation in the bladder, by transureteroureterostomy, or by nephrectomy.

In cases of bilateral ureteral obstruction, management depends on a consideration of several factors. If bone pain is severe and intractable, the patient's recent performance status is poor, and the estimated survival time is less than 3 months, surgical intervention is inappropriate, and uremia should be allowed to supervene. However, if these negative prognostic indicators are absent, and particularly if further modes of systemic control of the disease are available, then management should be more aggressive.

Dangerous electrolyte disturbances should initially be controlled by dialysis. Cystoscopic ureteral catheterization should be attempted, but frequently the orifices cannot be visualized or negotiated because of tumor. Percutaneous nephrostomy under fluoroscopic or ultrasound control is useful in these circumstances. Treatment thereafter by systemic chemotherapy or external beam irradiation directed to the pelvis may relieve the obstruction. Many patients remain comfortable with tube diversion in the form of inlying ureteral catheters, or nephrostomy. If problems arise, permanent diversion can be performed.

Provided that bladder outlet obstruction is controlled, reimplantation of the ureters into the dome of the bladder is sometimes possible. Supravasical diversion can be achieved by ureteroileal conduit. A transverse colon conduit is preferable in those patients who have had extensive pelvic irradiation in order to avoid the use of irradiated small intestine. Cutaneous transureteroureterostomy bringing the more dilated ureter to the skin surface is another alternative.

By itself, bilateral ureteral obstruction does not uniformly imply a hopeless prognosis. Undoubtedly, aggressive treatment in selected cases can increase survival without an associated increase in morbidity.

Spinal Cord Compression

Spinal cord compression from extradural metastases may develop insidiously or present as an acute emergency. The patient may present with progressive weakness of the legs, acute retention of urine, or full-blown paraplegia. At the first indication of possible impending cord compression, the patient should be admitted for an intensive course of intravenous Stilphostrol and dexamethasone. If there is no definite clinical improvement within 24 h, management should proceed as though the patient presented with paraplegia. Immediate neurosurgical consultation should be obtained with a view to performing a myelogram to delineate the site of compression prior to decompressive laminectomy. Postoperatively, a course of external radiation therapy should be administered to the involved area. The development of spinal cord compression is a poor prognostic sign, only because it generally occurs late in the course of the disease process.

Pathologic Fracture

Occasionally patients suffer pathologic fracture of a long bone, such as the humerus or femur. Treatment is by intramedullary fixation followed by a course of external beam irradiation. If such an event can be predicted by symptoms of severe pain in a limb or a radiographic appearance that suggests impending fracture of an osteolytic lesion, prophylactic internal fixation and external radiation therapy are indicated.

DISSEMINATED INTRAVASCULAR COAGULATION

The primary intravascular coagulation and secondary accelerated fibrinolysis seen in widespread malignancy occurs most frequently in prostatic cancer. Usually hemostasis is not much impaired, and clinical bleeding is mild or absent. Sometimes spontaneous hemorrhage from the skin, gastrointestinal tract, or urinary tract is catastrophic. Bleeding from biopsy sites or after surgery may be uncontrollable. Ideally, treatment should be directed against the underlying disease. Previously untreated patients respond favorably to estrogens or orchiectomy. Symptomatic treatment of major hemorrhage consists of heparin to prevent further intravascular coagulation, given alone, or in combination with ϵ-aminocaproic acid to counteract fibrinolysis.

CONCLUSION

The ability of sensitive radioimmunoassays for prostatic acid phosphatase to detect elevated serum levels when the disease is confined to the prostate needs to be confirmed by long-term studies. For now, the opportunity to cure prostatic cancer comes from detection of early disease by regular, routine, careful digital rectal exam of susceptible males.

Ultrasonic techniques and computerized axial tomography have improved the definition of the local extent of prostatic cancer. Pelvic lymphadenectomy has contributed a great deal to our knowledge of the mechanisms of spread. It is unkown whether this operation removes an important barrier to spread of disease. Distant micrometastasis to bone, which cannot be readily detected by any means, remains an uncontrollable source of failure of radical curative efforts directed at the primary tumor.

The high death rate from prostatic cancer is evidence enough that treatment needs to be improved. Total prostatectomy cures disease confined within the capsule. Whether irradiation techniques that avoid much of the surgical morbidity can match the surgical results remains to be proved. Endocrine manipulation has not been superceded by any other form of treatment in the management of advanced disease, although advances in chemotherapy appear to offer hope for the control of endocrine-resistant disease.

REFERENCES

1. Young HH: The early diagnosis and radical cure of carcinoma of the prostate. *Bull Johns Hopkins Hosp* 16:315, 1905.
2. Gutman EB et al: Significance of increased phosphatase activity of bone at the site of osteoblastic metastases secondary to carcinoma of the prostate gland. *Am J Cancer* 28:485, 1936.
3. Huggins C, Hodges CV: Studies on prostatic cancer: I. The effect of castration, of estrogen and of androgen injection on serum phosphatases in metastatic carcinoma of the prostate. *Cancer Res* 1:293, 1941.
4. Whitmore WF Jr: Hormone therapy in prostatic cancer. *Am J Med* 21:697, 1956.
5. Jewett HJ et al: The palpable nodule of prostatic cancer: Results 15 years after radical excision. *JAMA* 203:115, 1968.
6. Mostofi FK, Price EB Jr: Tumors of the male genital system, in *Atlas of Tumor Pathology*, Armed Forces Institute of Pathology, Washington, DC, 1973.
7. Tannenbaum M: *Urologic Pathology: The Prostate*, Lea & Febiger, Philadelphia, 1977.
8. Arduino LJ, Glucksman MA: Lymph node metastases in early carcinoma of the prostate. *J Urol* 88:91, 1962.
9. McLaughlin AP et al: Prostatic carcinoma: Incidence and location of unsuspected lymphatic metastases. *J Urol* 115:89, 1976.
10. Hanash KA et al: Carcinoma of the prostate: A 15-year followup. *J Urol* 107:450, 1972.
11. Nesbit RM, Plumb RT: Prostatic carcinoma: A follow-up on 795 patients treated prior to the endocrine era and a comparison of survival rates between these and patients treated by endocrine therapy. *Surgery* 20:263, 1946.
12. Edwards CN et al: An autopsy study of latent prostatic cancer. *Cancer* 6:531, 1953.
13. Boxer RJ: Adenocarcinoma of the prostate gland. *Urol Surv* 27:75, 1977.
14. American Joint Committee for Cancer Staging and End-Results Reporting: *Manual for Staging of Cancer* Whiting Press, Chicago, 1977, pp 119–124.
15. Correa RJ Jr et al: Latent carcinoma of the prostate: Why the controversy? *J Urol* 111:644, 1974.
16. Loening SA et al: A comparison between lymphangiography and pelvic node dissection in the staging of prostatic cancer. *J Urol* 117:752, 1977.
17. Wilson CS et al: Pelvic lymphadenectomy for the staging of apparently localized prostatic cancer. *J Urol* 117:197, 1977.
18. Woodard HQ: The clinical significance of serum acid phosphatase. *Am J Med* 27:902, 1959.
19. Cooper JF et al: A solid phase radioimmunoassay for prostatic acid phosphatase. *J Urol* 119:388, 1978.
20. Gleason DF and Veterans Administration Cooperative Urological Research Group: Histologic grading and clinical staging of prostatic carcinoma, in M Tannenbaum, (ed): *Urologic Pathology*, Lea & Febiger, Philadelphia, 1977.
21. Chu TM et al: Immunochemical detection of serum prostatic

acid phosphatase: Methodology and clinical evaluation. *Invest Urol* 15:319, 1978.
22. Jewett HJ: The present status of radical prostatectomy for stages A and B prostatic cancer. *Urol Clin North Am* 2:105, 1975.
23. Barnes R et al: Early carcinoma of the prostate: Comparison of stages A and B. *J Urol* 115:401, 1976.
24. Emmett JL et al: Endocrine therapy in carcinoma of the prostate gland: 10-year survival studies. *J. Urol* 83:471, 1960.
25. Goodwin WE: Radical prostatectomy after previous prostatic surgery: Technical problems encountered in treatment of occult prostatic carcinoma. *JAMA* 148:799, 1952.
26. Turner RD, Belt E: A study of 229 consecutive cases of total perineal prostatectomy for cancer of the prostate. *J Urol* 77:62, 1957.
27. De Vere White R et al: The clinical spectrum of prostatic cancer. *J Urol* 117:323, 1977.
28. Schroeder FH, Belt E: Carcinoma of the prostate: A study of 213 patients with stage C tumors helped by total perineal prostatectomy. *J Urol* 114:257, 1975.
29. Dees JE: Radical perineal prostatectomy for carcinoma. *J Urol* 104:160, 1970.
30. Correa RJ Jr et al: Total prostatectomy for stage B carcinoma of the prostate. *J Urol* 117:328, 1977.
31. Belt E, Schroeder FH: Total perineal prostatectomy for carcinoma of the prostate. *J Urol* 107:91, 1972.
32. Boxer RJ et al: Radical prostatectomy for carcinoma of the prostate, 1951–1976: A review of 329 patients. *J Urol* 117:208, 1977.
33. Jewett HJ: Radical perineal prostatectomy for carcinoma: An analysis of cases at Johns Hopkins Hospital, 1904–1954. *JAMA* 156:1039, 1954
34. Culp DS, Meyer JJ: Radical prostatectomy in the treatment of prostatic cancer. *Cancer* 32:1113, 1973.
35. Jewett HJ et al: Radical prostatectomy in the management of carcinoma of the prostate: Probable causes of some therapeutic failures. *J Urol* 107:1034, 1972.
36. The Veterans Administration Cooperative Urological Research Group: Treatment and survival of patients with cancer of the prostate. *Surg Gynecol Obstet* 124:1011, 1967.
37. Barnes R et al: Conservative treatment of early carcinoma of prostate: Comparison of patients less than 70 years old with those over 70 years of age. *Urology* 14:359, 1979.
38. Scott WW, Boyd HL: Combined hormone control therapy and radical prostatectomy in the treatment of selected cases of advanced carcinoma of the prostate: A retrospective study based upon 25 years of experience. *J Urol* 101:86, 1969.
39. Ray GR et al: Definitive radiation therapy of carcinoma of the prostate: A report on 15 years of experience. *Radiology* 106:407, 1973.
40. Carlton CE Jr et al: Radiotherapy in the management of stage C carcinoma of the prostate. *J Urol* 116:206, 1976.
41. Nachtsheim DA Jr et al: Latent residual tumor following external radiotherapy for prostate adenocarcinoma. *J Urol* 120:312, 1978.
42. Bagshaw MA et al: External beam radiation therapy of primary carcinoma of the prostate. *Cancer* 36:723, 1975.
43. Flocks RH: The treatment of stage C prostatic cancer with special reference to combined surgical and radiation therapy. *J Urol* 109:461, 1973.
44. Whitmore WF Jr et al: Retropubic implantation of Iodine 125 in the treatment of prostatic cancer. *J Urol* 108:918, 1972.
45. Walsh PC: Physiologic basis for hormonal therapy in carcinoma of the prostate. *Urol Clin North Am* 2:125, 1975.
46. Bailar JC III et al: Estrogen treatment for cancer of the prostate: Early results with 3 doses of diethylstilbestrol and placebo. *Cancer* 26:257, 1970.
47. Byar DP: The Veterans Administration Cooperative Urological Research Group's studies of cancer of the prostate. *Cancer* 32:1126, 1973.
48. Franks LM: Some comments on the long-term results of endocrine treatment of prostatic cancer. *Br J Urol* 30:383, 1958.
49. Geller J et al: Treatment of advanced cancer of prostate with megestrol acetate. *Urology* 12:537, 1978.
50. Nesbit RM, Baum WC: Endocrine control of prostatic carcinoma: Clinical and statistical survey of 1,818 cases. *JAMA* 143:1317, 1950.
51. Levin AB et al: Chemical hypophysectomy for relief of bone pain in carcinoma of the prostate. *J Urol* 119:517, 1978.
52. Resnick MI, Grayhack JT: Treatment of stage IV carcinoma of the prostate. *Urol Clin North Am* 2:141, 1975.
53. Jacobo E et al: Comparison of flutamide (SCH-13521) and diethylstilbestrol in untreated advanced prostatic cancer. *Urology* 8:231, 1976.
54. Murphy GP: Management of disseminated prostatic carcinoma, in GP Murphy (ed): *Prostatic Cancer*, PSG Pub Co, Littleton, Mass, 1979.
55. Merrin CE, Beckley S: Treatment of estrogen-resistant stage D carcinoma of prostate with cis diamminedichloroplatinum. *Urology* 8:267, 1979.
56. Pollen JJ, Schmidt JD: Bone pain in metastatic cancer of prostate. *Urology* 8:129, 1979.
57. Kaplan E: Historical development of ^{32}P in bone therapy, in RP Spencer, (ed): *Therapy in Nuclear Medicine*, Grune & Stratton, New York, 1978.
58. O'Donoghue EPN et al: Cryosurgery for carcinoma of prostate. *Urology* 5:308, 1975.

SELECTED BIBLIOGRAPHY

Elder JS et al: Radical perineal prostatectomy for clinical stage B2 carcinoma of the prostate. *J Urol* 127:704, 1982.
Middleton RG, Smith JA Jr: Radical prostatectomy for stage B2 prostatic cancer. *J Urol* 127:702, 1982.
Paulson DF et al: Extended field radiation therapy versus delayed hormonal therapy in node positive prostatic adenocarcinoma. *J Urol* 127:935, 1982.

35
TESTICULAR CANCER
Nasser Javadpour

HISTORIC LANDMARKS

Perhaps the most outstanding contribution to the understanding of testicular cancer was Friedman and Moore's proposal and comprehensive histopathologic classification of germ-cell tumors of the testis in 1946. Based on about 1000 cases collected almost entirely from the U.S. Army, these authors classified the germinal tumor of the testis into seminoma, embryonal carcinoma, teratoma, and choriocarcinoma.[1] In 1952 Dixon and Moore, in correlating this classification with survival rate, grouped germ-cell tumors into five categories[2]: (1) seminoma alone; (2) embryonal carcinoma alone or with seminoma; (3) teratoma alone or with seminoma; (4) teratoma with either embryonal carcinoma or choriocarcinoma or both, and with or without seminoma; (5) choriocarcinoma alone or with either embryonal carcinoma or seminoma or both. Although these authors clearly stated that this grouping was merely for correlating survival rate utilizing Friedman and Moore's classification, many physicians make the mistake of regarding these five groupings as a histological classification. More recently, based on a study of over 7000 testicular tumors, Mostofi classified these tumors into those of a single histological type and those of more than one histological type.[3] Finally, in 1977, the World Health Organization (WHO) accepted Mostoffi's classification with some modifications.[3]

Another important contribution to the field of testicular tumors was Patton's demonstration of improvement in survival of patients with embryonal carcinoma with or without teratoma utilizing a transabdominal retroperitoneal lymphadenectomy.[4] Finally, the last two contributions in the area of testicular tumor have made these tumors potentially curable. The contributions are (1) finding effective combination chemotherapy, and (2) developments of specific and sensitive immunochemical techniques to detect small amounts of human chorionic gonadotropin (HCG) and α-fetoprotein (AFP) in the sera and in the cancer cells of these patients, thereby making the diagnosis and monitoring of these tumors more effective.[5-9] The application of computed tomography and meticulous regional lymphadenectomy have also played an important role in accurate staging and designing of appropriate therapeutic strategies.[12-15]

It is the objective of this chapter to discuss the contributions of these advances in early diagnosis and management of testicular cancer.

EPIDEMIOLOGY, ETIOLOGY, AND NATURAL HISTORY

Epidemiologically, testicular cancer is extremely rare in the black populaton when compared with the nonblack population in the United States. The incidence of testicular cancer in these various populations strongly favors the role of genetic rather than environmental factors in the etiology of testicular cancer. There are either lymphatic disseminations or distant metastases in 35 percent of patients when first seen. The natural history usually begins with a small intratesticular lesion. It generally metastasizes to the retroperitoneal lymph nodes and the lungs. The mode of death is almost always secondary to pulmonary mestastes.

The etiology of testicular cancer is not known. Age, genetic factors, trauma, repeated infection, and possible endocrine abnormalities have been incriminated. The incidence of tumor has been reported to be higher in cryptochidism (Table 35-1). Although only 2 percent of cancers in males occur in the testis, nearly 60 percent of these are found in men between 25 and 44 years of age. Testicular tumors are the most common malignancy in men between the ages of 29 and 35, with an estimated 2500 new cases annually. This cancer constitutes the fourth most common genitourinary tumor. Since testicular tumors are not common, it has been difficult to obtain sufficient clinical and pathological experience in one institution. Therefore, there has been considerable controversy concerning the histogenesis, pathological classification, and the roles of surgery, radiation, and chemotherapy.

RECENT DEVELOPMENTS IN HISTOPATHOGENIC CLASSIFICATION

The pathological classification utilized at the National Cancer Institute (NCI) is based on the classification proposed by Friedman and Moore, then modified by Dixon, Moore, Mostofi, and WHO (Table 35-2). These

TABLE 35-1 Testicular Tumors Associated with Cryptorchism

Series	No. of cases	No. of patients with cryptorchidism
Collins and Pugh	995	58
Field	135	9
Hope	282	17
Schwartz and Reed	167	15
Thurzo and Pinter	139	9
Johnson	147	12
Total cases	1865	120 (6.5%)

TABLE 35-2 Histopathologic Classification of Testicular Cancer

GERMINAL-CELL ORIGIN

1. Seminoma
   a. Spermatocytic
   b. Anaplastic
   c. Typical
2. Embryonal carcinoma
   a. Adult type
   b. Infantile type (yolk sac tumor or endodermal sinus tumor)
   c. Polyembryoma
3. Teratoma
   a. Mature
   b. Immature
   c. With malignant transformation
4. Choriocarcinoma
5. Compound tumors
   a. Embryonal carcinoma with teratoma (teratocarcinoma)
   b. Any other combination of the above elements (14 possible combinations)

NONGERMINAL-CELL ORIGIN

1. Interstitial-cell tumor
2. Sertoli-cell tumor
3. Gonadal-stromal tumors
4. Compound tumors (four possible combinations)

investigators proposed that the vast majority of testicular tumors originate from totipotential germ cells and give rise to seminoma, teratoma, embryonal carcinoma, and choriocarcinoma. A relatively common combination is that of embryonal carcinoma with teratoma (teratocarcinoma). However, 10 other combinations of these four elements are possible. About 6 percent of testicular tumors are categorized as specialized gonadal-stromal tumors. These include tumors of interstitial cells, Sertoli cells, and tumors of gonadal-stromal elements. There may be four other possible combinations of these three basic elements. Tumors of the ductal system, the fibrovascular stroma, and the capsule are nongerminal and nonspecialized gonadal-stromal cell tumors, and comprise about 1 percent of all testicular tumors. This classification was accepted by the American Testicular Tumor Registry located at the AFIP.

In 1964, Collins et al. reviewed the British Testicular Tumor Registry containing 774 patients with testicular tumors and proposed a new classification known as the British Testicular Tumor Classification. They originally divided the common testicular tumors into seminoma and teratoma. Under teratoma they group teratoma differentiated (TD) and teratoma malignant (TM) and have further divided teratoma into malignant teratoma intermediate A (MTIA), malignant teratoma intermediate B (MTIB), malignant teratoma anaplastic (MTA), and malignant teratoma trophoblastic (MTT) (Table 35-3). In 1976, they combined the MTIA and MTIB into teratoma malignant undifferentiated (MTU); tumors that contain any of the four of these components and/or seminoma were classified as combined tumors. This classification is compared with the American Classifica-

TABLE 35-3 Comparison of Various Classifications of Testicular Tumors

WHO	Friedman and Moore	Mostofi	Pugh-Cameron
Tumors of one histological type	Not used	Tumors of one histological type	Not used
Seminoma	Seminoma	Seminoma	Seminoma
Spermatocytic seminoma	Not listed	Spermatocytic seminoma	Spermatocytic seminoma
Embryonal carcinoma	Embryonal carcinoma	Embryonal carcinoma, adult type	Malignant teratoma undifferentiated (MTU) (includes yolk sac tumor in adults and some embryonal carcinomas and teratomas)
Yolk sac tumor (infantile embryonal carcinoma)	Not listed	Infantile embryonal carcinoma	Yolk sac tumor in children MTU in adults
Polyembryoma	Not listed	Polyembryoma	Not listed
Choriocarcinoma, pure	Choriocarcinoma	Pure choriocarcinoma	Not listed
Teratoma	Teratoma	Teratoma	Teratoma (includes WHO embryonal carcinomas, yolk sac tumor in adults, teratoma and choriocarcinoma)
Mature	Teratoma	Mature	Teratoma, differentiated
Immature	Teratoma	Immature	Teratoma, differentiated
Teratoma with malignant transformation	Teratocarcinoma	Teratoma with malignant areas other than seminoma, embryonal carcinoma, choriocarcinoma	Malignant teratoma, intermediate (MTI)
Tumors of more than one histological type	Not used	Tumors of more than one histological type	Not used
Embryonal cancer and teratoma (teratocarcinoma)	Teratocarcinoma (also includes teratoma ± seminoma + embryonal cancer ± choriocarcinoma)	Embryonal carcinoma + teratoma (teratocarcinoma)	Malignant teratoma intermediate (MTI) Some MTU
Choriocarcinoma and any other type	Teratocarcinoma	Specify tumor types	Malignant teratoma trophoblastic
Other combinations—specify	Teratocarcinoma	Specify tumor types	MTI, MTU, combined tumors for those with seminoma

tion in Table 35-4. The problems with this classification have been the complexity of the histological diagnoses for those urologic surgeons and pathologists who see only a limited number of such cases. Also, clinically mature teratoma (TD) with a favorable prognosis and pure choriocarcinoma (MTT) with an extremely grave prognosis have been lumped into one group, which is not helpful in understanding the natural history and application of therapeutic modalities to these tumors. A recent change in the histopathologic classification is the addition of intratubular carcinoma in situ and elimination of anaplastic seminoma and adpation of seminoma with syncytiotrophoblostic giant cell (STGC).

Immunocytochemistry of Testicular Tumors

The histopathologic classification currently applied at the NCI is based on intracellular localization of the tumor markers, HCG and AFP, in various tumor cells by the indirect immunoperoxidase technique. One of the major advantages of this technique is that it can be applied to tissue fixed in formalin, thus allowing a prospective or retrospective study.

Testicular germ-cell tumors may contain multiple cellular components with variable growth and metastatic patterns. Intracellular localization of these markers in various cancer cells has improved the diagnosis and understanding of the histopathology of this tumor. To correlate various types of neoplasms with the presence of these tumor markers in tissue sections and serum, a study was undertaken in 40 patients with germ-cell tumors of the testis, all of whom had measurements of serum levels of HCG and AFP. AFP was found within the cells of embryonal carcinoma and endodermal sinus tumors but not in the syncytiotrophoblastic giant cells

TABLE 35-4 Immunohistologic Classification of Germ-Cell Tumor

Type	AFP	HCG	SP_1
Seminoma	−	−	−
Embryonal carcinoma	+	−	−
Embryonal carcinoma with STGC*	+	+	+
Teratocarcinoma with STGC	+	+	+
Choriocarcinoma	−	+	+

* Syncytiotrophoblastic giant cell.

(STGC) occasionally found in seminomas, nor in syncytiotrophoblastic components of choriocarcinoma. In contrast, human HGC was found in syncytiotrophoblastic components of choriocarcinoma and in some cells of some cases of embryonal carcinoma, but only rarely in endodermal sinus tumors or in seminomas. Thus, adult-type embryonal carcinoma is frequently associated with both AFP and HCG; endodermal sinus tumor is associated with AFP; and choriocarcinoma is associated with HCG (Table 35-4). We have prospectively studied 130 patients with pure seminoma in whom we had made serial quantitative measurements of HCG and AFP using specific radioimmunoassays: 10 of the 130 (7.7 percent) patients had elevated serum HCG levels, but with serial sectioning of the tumor specimens, 1 of the 10 patients had an element of choriocarcinoma in the tissue obtained at the time of a retroperitoneal lymph node dissection. After surgery and chemotherapy, the serum HCG level dropped to normal. All but one of the patients had normal levels of AFP. In this patient the serum AFP level was 152 ng/mL. Serial sectioning of the original testicular tumor showed an element of embryonal carcinoma, and this patient subsequently was proven to have metastatic embryonal carcinoma involving the aortocaval lymph nodes. The incidence of elevated levels of HCG was 7 of 18 (40 percent) in patients with proven stage II seminomas.

Clinical Features

History and physical examination constitutes the most important clinical feature in the diagnosis of testicular cancer. The finding of a testicular mass, gynecomastia, or a palpable left supraclavicular or abdominal mass, especially in a young male, should raise the question of ruling out a testicular cancer. In a few patients, mostly those with choriocarcinoma, the course is rapidly fatal. They present with pulmonary metastases from hematogenous spread to the lung.

Staging of Testicular Tumors

The staging of testicular tumors, as for other tumors, must accurately reflect the extent of the patient's disease and should equally reflect the natural history of disease progression. The physician can then make an accurate assessment of the disease, select the appropriate treatment, and gain some insight as to the patient's prognosis. Although the conventional method of staging of testicular tumor does allow prognostication and reflects tumor extent to some degree, it does not provide a precise evaluation of the extent of dissemination, or tumor volume and resectability of this disease. The major problems with the conventional staging method include lack of discrimination between varying degress of local and metastatic spread within the category of stage I disease. This lack of discrimination results in lumping patients with disease localized within the testis with those having microscopic retroperitoneal disease, with or without documented spermatic lymphatic involvement. The stage II designation also does not adequately reflect the variable degree of regional lymphatic involvement, thus combining patients with minimal, potentially surgically curable disease with patients who have massive, surgically incurable disease. The stage III category lacks the provision for describing single or multiple metastases, and does not distinguish between pulmonary and other sites of parenchymal metastases. In view of these observations, in 1978 we proposed a new staging classification;[10] although somewhat more complex, it has the potential to define more accurately the extent of disease, assist in determining appropriate therapy, and improve our prognostic skills. This staging method for testicular cancers more fully takes into consideration the factors that are essential in modern therapy and prognosis of this disease[10] (Table 35-5).

In addition to the conventional laboratory and radiological procedures used in staging of patients with testicular tumors, we have investigated the efficacy of chest tomograms, computerized tomography of the retroperitoneum, tumor markers, inferior venacavography, and lymphangiography. By using such procedures, one can more reliably distinguish between the various stages and substages of disease. A persistently elevated serum AFP or HCG level, or both, in a patient with testicular tumor treated by inguinal orchiectomy indicates stage II or stage III disease. Similarly, inferior venacavography, computerized tomography, and lymphangiography can be used to distinguish patients with minimal stage II (A to D) disease from other characterized by obstruction or invasion, or both, of the inferior vena cava and the ureters (stage II, C,D). Using these diagnostic modalities for testicular carcinomas, we have reduced our staging error to 14 percent. We have studied 118 cases of nonseminomatous testicular tumor with lymphangiogram, excretory urogram, inferior venacavogram, chest tomograms, and serial serum levels of HCG and AFP. The 118 cases underwent surgical ex-

TABLE 35-5 A Comprehensive Staging for Testicular Cancer

Stage	Description of tumor
1	Local
A_1	Confined to the testis
B_1	Invading testicular adnexa
C_1	Invading scrotal wall
2	Confined to the retroperitoneal lymph nodes
A_2	Microscopic
B_2	Grossly confined to the lymph nodes
C_2	Invading the capsule of lymph nodes and all visible tumor resectable
D_2	Bulky grossly nonresectable tumor
3	Disseminated beyond the retroperitoneum
A_3	Solitary metastasis
B_3	Multiple metastases

SOURCE: From N Javadpour, SM Bergman,[10] with permission.

ploration with retroperitoneal lymphadenectomy. All these cases had a minimum of 18 months' follow-up. Of these 118 patients, 72 were staged and classified as stage 1 after orchiectomy; 20 of these 72 had positive lymph nodes at the time of retroperitoneal lymphadenectomy; and an additional 3 had negative nodes but manifested distant metastases within 3 months. On the basis of persistently elevated postorchiectomy markers in 15 patients, only 57 would have been classified as stage I. With markers, therefore, the clinical staging error is cut down from a range of 28 to 32 percent to a range of 9 to 14 percent based on whether one considers "true" stage I status to have been represented by 49 or 52 patients.

By clinical and radiological criteria, 46 patients were considered to be stage II. Surgicopathologic sectioning of the nodes was positive for tumor in 40 of these patients eventually confirmed as having stage II disease and in 2 patients with negative lymph node status. In addition, of the 6 patients with negative markers, 2 had positive retroperitoneal lymphadenectomy for tumor. The staging error without markers, therefore, is 13 percent, while with markers it ranges from 5 to 10 percent based on whether one includes only marker-producing tumors or both marker- and nonmarker-producing tumors. Relapse in distal sites ensued in patients with persistently positive markers after retroperitoneal lymphadenectomy. However, the lack of accuracy of these methods in patients with microscopic or minimal disease remains a problem.

CHEST TOMOGRAPHY

Conventional and computed tomography of the chest is more sensitive than chest x-ray in that it can detect lesions as small as 2 to 5 mm and distinguish these lesions from blood vessels. However, computed tomography is apparently too sensitive and may pick up small benign lesions.

INFERIOR VENACAVOGRAPHY (IVC)

Although IVC is not helpful in detection of early retroperitoneal metastases, it may be valuable in bulky stage II or III testicular cancer, when detection of partial or complete caval obstruction is essential in management of the patient.

LYMPHANGIOGRAM (LA)

LA has been a time-honored conventional radiological technique in staging of testicular tumor; its role, however, has been diminished with the advent of CT and sonography of the retroperitoneum. The role of supraclavicular node biopsy for all testicular tumor patients has also been diminished because of the low yield of positives in node patients with clinically nonpalpable supraclavicular lymph nodes.

COMPUTED TOMOGRAPHY (CT)

CT has had some contribution in diagnosis and follow-up of patients with retroperitoneal and liver metastases. However, its role in early diagnosis or detection of early tumor recurrence is limited.

Testicular Tumor Markers

The development of sensitive and specific radioimmunoassay by Vaitukaitis et al.[5] for HCG and by Waldmann and McIntire[6] for AFP has proved to be valuable in the detection and subsequent management of testicular tumors. These two proteins have been localized in trophoblastic and nontrophoblastic cells of testicular tumors in our laboratory at the NCI, and this cellular localization has helped in our histological diagnosis and understanding of the natural history of these heterogeneous tumors.

HCG

HCG is made up of α and β subunits. The β subunit has been isolated, purified, and utilized to immunize rabbits to produce an antibody specific for HCG. This highly specific antibody does not cross-react with physiologic concentrations of the other glycoprotein hormones such as luteinizing hormone (LH). In our study of this marker in patients with germ-cell tumors of the testis, HCG was elevated in the serum (7.7 percent) in 10 of 130 patients with seminoma (39 percent of patients with stage II seminoma), in 87 of 145 (60 percent) patients with embryonal carcinoma with or without teratoma, and in all patients (100 percent) with choriocarcinoma (Table 35-3). Elevated levels of HCG usually decrease to normal when effective therapy gives a complete response. When elevated levels persisted or the initial normal level increased after therapy, recurrent tumor was invariably found[11] (Table 35-6).

AFP

AFP is produced in the liver, yolk sac, and gastrointestinal tract of the fetus as the predominant circulating protein. The previously utilized technique of immunoprecipitation has a sensitivity of about 3000 ng/mL, and thus about 30 percent of AFP-producing tumors had detectable serum levels of this marker. The development of sensitive and specific radioimunoassay by Waldmann and McIntire has yielded more reliable detection. In our series of 130, none of the patients with seminoma and 102 of 145 (70 percent) patients with embryonal carcinoma, with or without teratoma, had elevated levels of this marker (Table 35-6). The decline of serum AFP correlated directly with the metabolic decay of this marker after effective therapy. If an elevated level persisted, recurrent metastatic tumor generally was found.

Radioimmunoassay of Urinary HCG

This highly sensitive urinary HCG radioimmunoassay has improved the detection of persistent tumor burden

TABLE 35-6 Frequency of HCG and AFP in Patients with Testicular Cancer

Type	AFP	%	HCG	%	AFP and HCG	%
Seminoma	$\frac{0}{130}$	0	$\frac{10}{130}$	7.5*	$\frac{10}{130}$	7.7
Teratoma	$\frac{6}{16}$	37.5	$\frac{4}{16}$	25.0	$\frac{7}{16}$	43.7
Embryonal carcinoma	$\frac{102}{145}$	70.3	$\frac{87}{145}$	60.0	$\frac{127}{145}$	87.5
Embryonal carcinoma with teratoma	$\frac{36}{56}$	64.2	$\frac{32}{56}$	57.0	$\frac{48}{56}$	85.7
Choriocarcinoma	$\frac{0}{5}$	0	$\frac{5}{5}$	100.0	$\frac{5}{5}$	100.0
Yolk sac tumor	$\frac{3}{4}$	75.0	$\frac{1}{4}$	25.0	$\frac{3}{4}$	75.0

* 40 percent in patients with stage II tumors.

and has been rewarding in selecting the patients in whom further therapy is warranted.

It has been shown that concentrating HCG in urine specimens and utilizing an antibody directed at the carboxyl terminal of the HCG molecule offers the potential for more sensitively monitoring the tumor burden and guiding the therapy of patients with testicular cancer.[12]

Simultaneous serum and urinary HCG levels were measured in 15 patients with disseminated testicular cancer. Initially, these 12 patients, who had either seminoma, embryonal carcinoma, teratocarcinoma, or choriocarcinoma of the testis, had elevated levels of serum HCG. After these patients were treated with intensive chemotherapy and/or surgery, the elevated serum HCG levels decreased to conventionally undetectable levels. The 24-h urinary HCG level, measured by carboxyl-terminal radioimmunoassay of urine concentrates, was elevated in these 12 patients despite undetectable levels of HCG in the serum, indicating the persistence of tumor producing this marker. Indeed, in 5 initial patients serum HCG was undetectable but elevated levels of urinary HCG were found. These 5 patients were proved to have persistent tumor.

Pregnancy-Specific β_1-Glycoprotein (SP$_1$)

In the past few years, a new placental protein has been purified, and we have utilized this protein as a tumor marker in our laboratory. Specific radioimmunoassay (RIA) and IP techniques have been developed to identify SP$_1$ in the sera and tumor cells of 97 men with testicular cancer. SP$_1$ was elevated at 11 to 440 (ng/mL) in 3 of 6 with choriocarcinoma, 5 of 17 with embryonal carcinoma and teratoma, and 5 of 50 with embryonal carcinoma. None of 24 sera from men with seminoma and none of 5 men with orchitis had elevated SP$_1$. The highest value in a group of patients with nonmalignant disease was 9.1 ng/mL.[13] The new biologic marker was identified in the syncytiotrophoblastic giant cell (STGC). The STGC are seen occasionally in patients with embryonal carcinoma, teratoma, and seminoma.

It remains to be determined whether SP$_1$ concentrations correlate with tumor burden, prognosis, or therapy, or whether other tumor cell(s) can also produce this marker.

Lactic Dehydrogenase (LDH)

Electrophoretically in human beings there are five heterogenous isoenzymes of LDH. During the past several years it has become apparent that cancer cells have increased glycolysis leading to increased synthesis of lactate. Therefore, LDH may be utilized as a nonspecific tumor marker in several cancers, including that of testicular germ cells. We have utilized LDH as a tumor marker in testicular tumor for the following reasons: (1) availability and simplicity of the assay when compared with RIA, (2) lack of frequency of other markers in seminoma, (3) in bulky nonseminomatous testicular cancer with normalization of serum AFP and HCG while patients are on intensive chemotherapy, the serum LDH may monitor the therapy, and (4) to monitor the therapy of bulky seminomatous tumor. The correlation of LDH with tumor bulk and serum levels of HCG and AFP is under investigation in our laboratory at the present time.

LOCALIZATION OF METASTATIC TESTICULAR CANCER

Localization and subsequnt treatment of metastatic testicular cancer plays an important role in prolonging the survival of patients with testicular cancer. Although utilizing the conventional modalities such as computed tomography and ultrasonography have helped to detect and localize metastatic testicular cancer, these modalities are neither specific nor quantitative. In this presentation we would like to discuss three newer modalities that have been useful in detection and localization of metastatic testicular cancer.

Selective Venous Catheterization

The veins draining a tissue that produces a special substance (tumor marker or hormone) should contain a significantly higher level of this substance than the veins peripheral to this tissue. The ability to measure this gradient depends on five general factors: (1) an assay sensitive and specific enough to measure the difference (or step-up); (2) sampling that is close enough to the source and done before the substance of interest is diluted to or close to the concentration of the peripheral blood; (3) a rate of blood flow slow enough that will not further dilute out the substance of interest; (4) the rate of production of the substance; and (5) the half-life of the substance. All of these factors are interrelated and all hinge on the sensitivity of the assay. The closer one is to the source, the slower the blood flow from the source, the greater the rate of production, and the shorter the half-life; therefore, the greater will be the step-up and the higher the likelihood that the assay will be able to detect a significant increase in the draining venous blood over the peripheral blood level.[10,14]

HCG and AFP Scans

Utilizing specific antisera to AFP and HCG labeled with a γ-emitting radionuclide such as ^{131}I, one may localize a solitary testicular metastasis by external scintography. This noninvasive technique appears to be helpful in detection and localization of tumors that are not clinically detectable using the conventional diagnostic modalities. Clinical applications of HCG and AFP scans have been utilized in actual management of several patients with testicular cancer at the NCI. However, the false-positive and false-negative rates remain to be determined.

Hepatic Localization of Metastatic Testicular Cancer Utilizing Liposoluble Contrast Material

It appears that liver metastases from testicular cancer are a poor prognostic indicator and require aggressive treatment in nonseminomatous testicular tumor and a change of therapy from radiation to chemotherapy in seminomatous testicular cancer. The conventional modalities of detection of liver metastases including nonspecific radionuclide liver scan are not satisfactory. Over the past few years we have utilized a liposoluble contrast material administered intravenously. This contrast material is picked up by the hepatic reticuloendothelial system and enhances the computed tomography image of metastases. The clinical applications of this enhancing modality still needs further study in terms of its reliability in management of patients with testicular cancer.

THERAPY—GENERAL CONSIDERATIONS

When a suspicious scrotal mass is discovered, an exploration is advisable. The high inguinal incision allows delivery of the testis and its tunica after gently clamping the spermatic cord with a noncrushing vascular clamp. The specimen, after a radical orchiectomy, can be examined by the surgeon and the pathologist, and subsequent treatment depends on the cell type and clinical stage of tumor.[15]

Retroperitoneal Lymph Node Dissection

Retroperitoneal lymph node dissection has a unique role in the treatment of nonseminomatous testicular tumor. Patton has reported a significant improvement in survival of patients with nonseminomatous testicular tumor undergoing bilateral retroperitoneal lymph node dissection. He demonstrated that 65 percent of 125 patients with positive retroperitoneal lymph node survived 5 years or better after surgical lymphadenectomy.[4] This was in contrast to only 13 percent of 5-year survival after irradiation alone. This experience has been confirmed by other authors. To our knowledge, in no other cancer is lymphadenectomy so effective as in testicular tumor. At the NCI we perform a bilateral lymphadenectomy, including both renal lymphatics as well as aortic, caval, ipsilateral iliac, and obturator lymphatics as we will now describe. Patients undergoing the retroperitoneal lymph node dissection are explored through a midline vertical incision from the xyphoid process to the pubis. An incision is made over the posterior peritoneum from the ligament of Treitz to the aortic bifurcation and then extended over the common iliac arteries. The inferior mesenteric artery is clamped with a noncrushing vascular clamp to ensure the adequacy of collateral circulation to the sigmoid colon and rectum before it is ligated. Both gonadal arteries and veins are ligated and included in the specimen. The lateral borders of the dissection are the ureters. The superior border of dissection is the superior mesenteric artery, and inferiorly the border is the proximal portion of the common iliac artery on the contralateral side but is the distal part of the external iliac artery on the ipsilateral side.

Radiotherapy in Testicular Tumors

Radiotherapy is the treatment of choice for stage I and early stage II seminoma since this tumor is radiosensitive, having a 90 to 95 percent 5-year survival. A retroperitoneal lymphadenectomy is rarely indicated. Also, radiotherapy for metastatic lesions produces about a 28 percent 5-year survival rate. Maier and Sulak have treated 336 patients with seminoma of the testis with cobalt 60 megavoltage x-ray. The 5- and 10-year survival rates were identical at 90 percent and remained unchanged when the analysis was done 14 years after treatment. Results of this analysis indicate that the treatment of choice for stage I and II testicular seminoma is inguinal orchiectomy followed by postoperative irradiation to the lymphatic drainage of the testis. These areas include the inguinal, aortic, and caval lymph nodes in stage I and many include mediastinal and supraclavicular lymph nodes in stage II disease. Therapeutic doses of 3000 rads in 3 weeks and prophylactic doses of 2000 rads in 2 weeks with supervoltage equipment are recommended. Maier and Sulak have reported minimal complications from this dose of irradiation. However, if serum HCG is elevated, one should search for nonseminomous elements by serially sectioning the orchiectomy specimen.

Whether lymph node dissection is superior to irradiation in anaplastic seminoma and seminoma with elevated marker (IICG) is not clear. Prospective randomized studies to evaluate these problems are needed. Although radiotherapy is established as the treatment of choice in stage I and II seminoma, its role is becoming more controversial in stage III seminoma. The 5-year survival for stage II seminoma is about 28 percent with radiotherapy alone. However, there is some evidence that chemotherapy should be utilized in stage III seminoma. Since the 2-year survival for stage III nonseminomatous testicular tumor has been reported to be over 70 percent, with intensive chemotherapy one can also obtain improved survival for stage III seminomatous tumors.

The treatment for a nonseminomatous testicular tumor (NSTT) with radiotherapy is controversial and is not universally accepted as the treatment of choice in the United States. The major reasons for lymphadenectomy in NSTT are to stage the tumor, and in resectable tumors, the removal of lymphatics containing tumor serve as therapy. Whether radiotherapy alone is adequate or superior to lymphadenectomy in stage I and II NSTT is not clear. Prospective randomized clinical trials are needed to answer this dilemma with certainty.

Chemotherapy

The natural history of testicular tumor has demonstrated that the majority of patients with this disease die of pulmonary metastases. The rationale behind systemic therapy needs no elaboration. In the long and checkered history of searching for effective chemotherapy in testicular cancer, it has been only in the last few years that chemotherapists and surgeons have found effective chemotherapeutic regimens for this cancer. In 1958 Li, while working at the NCI, reported his findings of the dramatic effect of methotrexate on gestational choriocarcinoma. In 1960 Li et al. reported the first successful chemotherapeutic regimens in testicular tumor by combining actinomycin D, chlorambucil, and methotrexate as a triple agent therapy.[16] The findings of Samuels et al. that vinblastine and bleomycin had a synergistic effect was the first major thrust of the current chemotherapeutic regimens.[17] In the last several years there have been increasing trials of different chemotherapeutic agents, including Adriamycin, cyclophosphamide, and cis-platinum. A combination of vinblastine, actinomycin D, bleomycin, cyclophosphamide, and cis-platinum (VAB VI) has been reported to be effective with an acceptable toxicity. The data from Golbey et al. have indicated a 70 percent 2-year survival in nonbulky stage III testicular cancer. Einhorn and Donohue have treated 66 disseminated NSTT with vinblastine, bleomycin, and cis-platinum and have reported 74 percent (49 of 66) of patients being free of disease with adequate follow-up.[18]

A final assessment comparing these two regimens is not possible due to the lack of a randomized study.[20,21] The advent of both regimens has marked a significant contribution in the treatment of NSTT during the past several years. However, a significant toxicity, including septicemia, has been attributed to vinblastine. For this reason Einhorn and Donohue have decreased the dosage of vinblastine from the original 0.4 mg/kg to 0.3 mg/kg and this has decreased the life-threatening toxicity with the same results.

In spite of effective chemotherapy in testicular tumor, the results of treatment in bulky testicular tumor are still unsatisfactory. The standard treatment of stage III bulky tumor has been chemotherapy. In view of the relatively poor survival we have an ongoing prospective randomized study at the NCI evaluating the role and timing of cytoreductive surgery in NSTT. With the advent of these new combinations it appears that disseminated testicular cancer is being considered a more potentially curable disease in solid tumors.

Cytoreductive Surgery in Management of Advanced Testicular Cancer

Chemotherapy has been shown to be more effective in experimental animal tumors when the size of the tumor is small. In spite of available effective chemotherapeutic agents, the prognosis of patients with massive bulky disseminated testicular cancer is not favorable. In human beings cytoreductive surgery has been advocated in testicular cancer, Wilms's tumor, rhabdomyosarcoma, and Burkitt's lymphoma. The features of bulky testicular cancer rendering it a suitable model for cytoreductive surgery include the availability of effective chemotherapeutic agents and reliable markers. These tumors become bulky and occur in young men, who can tolerate intensive surgery and chemotherapy. There is no randomized clinical trial to answer the important question as to whether cytoreductive surgery has any effect on prolonging the survival of patients with massive bulky accessible tumor.

The next important question is the timing of cytoreductive surgery in relation to the chemotherapy. To answer the first question we have designed a protocol to randomize patients with disseminated bulky NSTT to chemotherapy alone or to cytoreductive surgery first followed by intensive chemotherapy. This protocol has been in operation since December, 1976. The final results indicates that cytoreductive surgery preceeding chemotherapy is not superior to chemotherapy followed by cytoreductive surgery. Patients with bulky disease should be treated by intensive chemotherapy followed by cytoreductive surgery for residual disease or teratomatous conversions.

Testicular Tumors in Children

The incidence of testicular tumors in children less than 15 years old is less than 2 per 100,000. Most of these tumors are from primitive germ cells, and most are embryonal carcinomas or teratomas. Seminoma and pure choriocarcinoma have not been reported in infants or prepubertal adolescents, and no prospective randomized study of testicular tumors in children exists.

Some of the cell types of testicular cancer in children have a different natural history than those in adults. We have studied 15 children with testicular cancer with serial quantitative serum AFP and HCG levels utilizing sensitive and specific RIA at the NCI for the past 7 years. Our data show that yolk sac tumor presented exclusively as stage I or III in these patients. Since yolk sac tumor synthesizes AFP, and presents as stage I or III, the role of lymphadenectomy is questionable. The disease can be easily followed by AFP and chest tomograms as an indicator of the need for adjuvant chemotherapy after orchiectomy.

Follow-up

The vast majority of patients with testicular tumor who are going to die of their tumors do so within 18 to 24 months. Therefore, the follow-up after the initial therapy plays an important role in overall management of these patients. The follow-up consists of monthly physical examinations, chest x-rays, tomogram if necessary, and tumor markers for the first year. This follow-up should then be every 3 months for another 12 months and then yearly.

Therapy of Recurrence

The recurrences are treated according to the number, location, and cell type. A solitary nonseminomatous tumor located in the retroperitoneal area is best treated by surgical resection and in the chest best treated by chemotherapy. Multiple tumors and nonresectable tumors are to be treated by chemotherapy. Recurrences of seminoma are treated by radiation unless multiple sites are involved and/or are located in an area which precludes radiotherapy. Such recurrences are best treated by conventional chemotherapeutic regimens.

CURRENT AND FUTURE PROBLEMS AND RESEARCH IN TESTICULAR TUMOR

Early diagnosis and proper therapy of testicular tumor are desirable. It is also essential to measure the tumor markers prior to the initial radical inguinal orchiectomy. The main current problems are lack of prospective randomized studies and comparing different therapeutic modalities in different stages of nonseminomatous testicular cancer. Also, the need for improved chemotherapeutic agents with maximal efficacy and minimal toxicity needs no elaboration The use of computed tomography in non-marker-producing testicular tumors may determine the improvement in better staging and earlier detection of metastatic or recurrent testis tumor. The role of positive or negative markers in testicular tumor must be evaluated preferably by prospective randomized studies with careful control to avoid any bias. Also, the role of immunotherapy as an adjuvant therapeutic modality should be investigated. The significance of a positive serum marker (HCG) in seminoma should be clarified in a controlled study.

The discovery and development of sensitive and specific RIAs to measure the testicular tumor markers, coupled with effective chemotherapeutic agents, has helped the understanding of the testicular tumor. The advent of tumor markers has had a significant impact in management and will have an even more important role in the future management of testicular tumors. It also must be emphasized that in using the testicular tumor markers one should consider the metabolic decay rate (half-lives are for HCG 24 h and for AFP 5 days) in interpretation of these markers. The decisions regarding an operation, chemotherapy, and radiation therapy should not be based on a single elevated value of HCG and AFP unless the half-lives of these markers are taken into consideration. Obviously, this precaution is necessary to avoid the erroneous interpretation of elevated HCG or AFP because of residual serum AFP or HCG secreted by primary testicular or metastatic tumor which has already been removed.

Since about 10 to 20 percent of nonseminomatous and 80 to 90 percent of seminomatous testicular tumors do not produce these markers, their value in differential diagnosis of scrotal masses is limited. Secondly, one should consider the other causes of elevated serum HCG and/or AFP, such as hepatocellular and pancreatic carcinoma. However, with routine studies these causes of elevated HCG or AFP should rarely pose a problem. The major problem in evaluating the survival in patients with testicular cancer has been lack of prospective randomized clinical trials. The majority of the reported series evaluating the different treatments in testicular cancer are either retrospective and/or lack control. Therefore, one cannot interpret the data with certainty. In an ongoing prospective randomized clinical trial at the NCI, we are attempting to assess the role and timing of cytoreductive surgery in a prospective randomized study, and this protocol is accepting patients with disseminated bulky stage III nonseminomatous testicular cancer.

Recently the NCI has collaborated in an intergroup comprehensive prospective randomized protocol treating stage II nonseminoma, nonchoriocarcinoma testicular cancer with or without chemotherapy after inguinal orchiectomy, extended retroperitoneal node dissection, and marker monitoring. Hopefully, the successful execution of these protocols will answer a number of essential questions in reliable fashion, thereby eliminating the serious doubts to the validity of the retrospective studies.

REHABILITATION AND SOCIOECONOMIC IMPACTS

Testicular cancer occurs mainly in young men at the prime of life; therefore, it has economical, emotional, and social implications. Although the recent advances in the therapeutic modalities of these patients have been encouraging, these treatments, including orchiectomy, lymphadenectomy, intensive chemotherapy, and radiotherapy, have some adverse physical and emotional impacts on these young men in terms of sexual activity, masculinity, and infertility. Further adverse effects such as nausea, vomiting, loss of hair, and physical weakness result from their intensive chemotherapy. These patients should be assured that acquiring this cancer is not a punishment and that with the exception of infertility, the remainder of their sexual activity should not suffer a permanent damage. Also, infertility resulting from therapy may be discussed with the patient prior to such therapy. The availability of sperm banks and adopting children may also be suggested to these patients. The necessity of marriage counseling, psychiatric consultations, and frequent assurance in certain patients must be a part of the overall objective of cancer cure and improvement of quality of life resulting in a socially productive and happy individual.

REFERENCES

1. Friedman NB, Moore RA: Tumors of the testis: A report on 922 cases. *Milit Surg* 99:573, 1946.
2. Dixon FJ, Moore RA: Tumors of the male sex organs, in *Atlas of Tumor Pathology,* Armed Forces Institute of Pathology, Washington, DC, fascs 31, 32, 1952.
3. Mostofi FK: Pathology of germ cell tumors of testis: A progress report. *Cancer* 45:1735, 1980.
4. Patton JF et al: Diagnosis and treatment of tumors of the testes. *JAMA* 171:2194, 1959.
5. Vaitukaitis JL et al: A radioimmunoassay which specifically measures human chorionic gonadotropin in the presence of human luteinizing hormone. *Am J Obstet Gynecol* 113:751, 1972.
6. Waldmann TA, McIntire KR: The use of a radioimmunoassay for alpha-fetoprotein in the diagnosis of malignancy. *Cancer* 34:1510, 1974.
7. Kurman RJ et al: Cellular localization of alpha-fetoprotein and human chorionic gonadotropin in germ cell tumors of the testes using an indirect immunoperoxidase technique: A new approach to classification utilizing tumor markers. *Cancer* 40:2136, 1977.
8. Scardino PT et al: The value of serum tumor markers in the staging and prognosis of germ cell tumors of the testes. *J Urol* 118:994, 1977.
9. Javadpour N, Scardino PT: Recent advances in immunobiology of genitourinary cancer. *Urology* 9:377, 1977.
10. Javadpour N, Bergman SM: Recent advances in testicular cancer. *Curr Probl Surg* 6:1–64, 1978.
11. Javadpour N: The role of biologic tumor markers in testicular cancer. 45:1755, 1980.
12. Javadpour N: The National Cancer Institute's experience with testicular cancer. *Urology* 9:377, 1977.
13. Rosen SW et al: Pregnancy-specific B_1-glycoprotein (SP_1) is increased in certain nonseminomatous germ cell tumors. *J Natl Cancer Inst* 62:1439, 1979.
14. Javadpour N: The value of biologic markers in diagnosis and treatment of testicular cancer. *Sem in Oncol* 6:37, 1979.
15. Whitmore WF Jr: Surgical treatment of adult germinal testis tumors. *Sem in Oncol* 6:37, 1979.
16. Li MC: Management of choriocarcinoma and related tumors of uterus and testis. *Med Clin North Am* 45:661, 1966.
17. Samuels ML et al: Stage III testicular cancer: Complete response by substage to velban plus continuous bleomycin infusion (VB-3). *Proc Am Assoc Cancer Res* 18:146, 1977.
18. Einhorn LH, Donohue JP: *cis*-Diamminedichloroplatinum, vinblastine, and bleomycin combination chemotherapy in disseminated testicular cancer. *Ann Intern Med* 87:293, 1977.
19. Golbey RB et al: Chemotherapy of metastatic germ cell tumors. *Sem in Oncol* 6:82, 1979.
20. Jacobs EM et al: Chemotherapy of testicular cancer: From palliation to curative adjuvant therapy. *Sem in Oncol* 6:14, 1979.

SELECTED BIBLIOGRAPHY

Einhorn LH, Williams SD: Chemotherapy of disseminated testicular cancer: A random prospective study. *Cancer* 46:1339, 1980.

Paulson DF: Testicular carcinoma. *Curr Prob Cancer,* vol 6, no 11, 1982.

Paulson DF et al: Cancer of the testis, in DeVita VT Jr et al (eds): *Cancer Principles and Practice of Oncology.* Lippincott, Philadelphia, 1982, pp 786–822.

36
TUMORS OF THE PENIS AND URETHRA

David F. Paulson

CARCINOMA OF THE PENIS

Squamous-cell carcinoma accounts for less than 1 percent of male malignancies on the United States; however, in populations where circumcision is not a common practice and personal hygiene is not well maintained, squamous-cell caricinoma of the penis accounts for 10 to 12 percent of all malignancies of males.[1,2] Prognosis correlates well with the stage of disease at the time of initial diagnosis. Unfortunately, although the penis is readily visible, the lesion frequently is ignored when it first appears. This presumably results from patients' reluctance to admit the possibility of disease in such a psychologically charged organ site. The most common presenting symptoms are phimosis, the presence of mass, or a nonhealing ulcer.

Many staging systems have been proposed for classification of the disease. The most commonly accepted staging system is that recommended by Jackson: stage I refers to tumors limited to the glans and/or prepuce; stage II, to invasion involving the shaft or corpora, but without nodal or distant node metastases; stage III, to tumor confined to the shaft, but with proven regional node metastases; and stage IV, to tumor invasive from the shaft with inoperable regional node metastases or with distant metaseases.[3] It is estimated that 50 to 65 percent of patients are diagnosed as at clinical stage I at the time of presentation; however, some isolated series report an incidence figure as low as 39 percent for stage I disease.[3-6]

It is important to recognize the areas of nodal drainage of the penile skin and of the corpora in order that adequate monitoring of the primary areas of nodal extension be established.[7-9] The cutaneous lymphatics of the foreskin and the shaft drain initially to the superficial inginal nodal areas and subsequently to the deep inguinal and external iliac nodes. However, once the corpus spongiosum or corpus cavernosum is involved, lymphatic drainage resembles the lymphatic drainage of the urethra with early involvement of the hypogastric and obturator nodes (Fig. 36-1). In addition, once there is involvement of the vascular channels of the corpus cavernosum, the probability of early vascular spread increases rapidly, as indicated by the progressive decline in survivorship among patients with stage II and stage III disease.[1,4,10,11]

Two primary problem areas exist in the treatment of this disease. The first is selection of the appropriate form of treatment for the primary lesion; the second is the evaluation of noda extension and the appropriate treatment for patients with identified noda disease.

This work was supported in part by the Medical Research Service of the Veterans Administration.

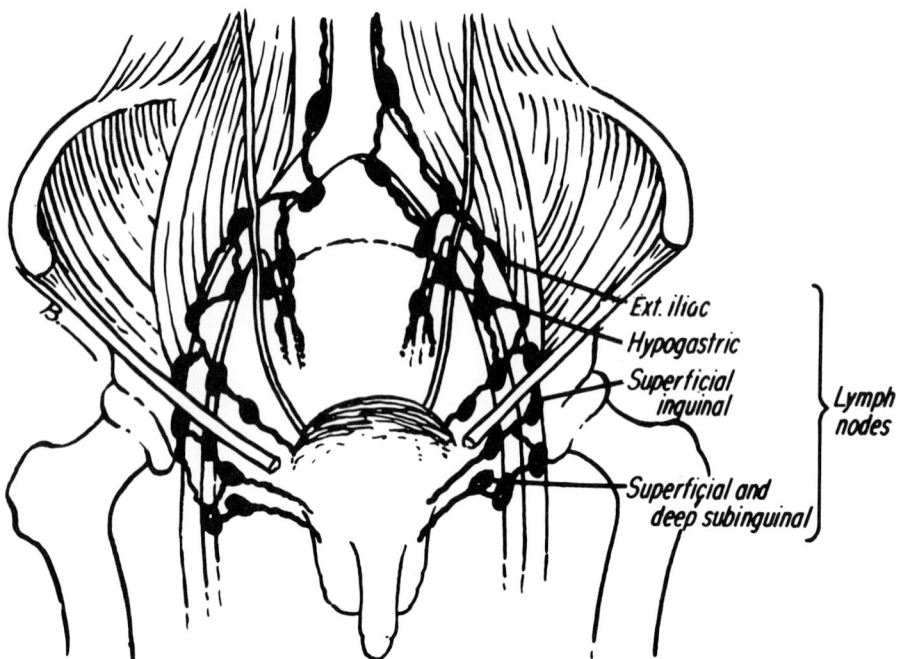

FIGURE 36-1 Lymphatic drainage of the penis and urethra.

Treatment of the Primary Lesion

If a cure is to be expected, adequate control of the primary tumor must be accomplished. Therapeutic modalities available for primary control are radiotherapy and/or surgery. It seems reasonable to select that form of therapy which would provide preservation of functional integrity while guaranteeing survivorship. Radiation therapy, either external or interstitial, offers the promise of maintaining organ integrity at no risk or decreased survivorship.[11–15]

Radiation therapy is applicable in the management of both superficial and invasive lesions even though approximately 50 percent of all lesions will be refractory or will recur. Patients with low-stage disease may anticipate control rates of 70 to 80 percent, with the control rates dropping to 40 to 60 percent with invasive disease. The identification of radiation failure, either through resistence of the lesion or recurrence after completion of radiotherapy, does not compromise subsequent surgical intervention, nor does it seem to impact adversely upon the control rates achieved for that given stage of the disease should salvage surgery be necessary.[16,17] Controversy does exist, however, as to the form of radiotherapy which should be chosen and as to the type of lesion optimally responsive to radiotherapy. Interstitial implantation, using iridium 192, produces control rates similar to those obtained with either radium molds or with external beam cobalt.[13,14] However, functional preservation is reported higher in patients receiving interstitial therapy with a reduced incidence of tumor necrosis after ^{192}I treatment. Radiation therapy has the potential to produce tumor necrosis, and, in lesions which involve the corpus cavernosum, to result in severe urethral stricture after treatment. Nonetheless, radiation therapy should be considered as a mode of primary therapy for patients in whom there is a definite desire to maintain functional integrity.

Surgical therapy involves excision of the lesion with adequate margins to ensure failure of local recurrence (Fig. 36-2). Small tumors which are limited to the prepuce are best treated by circumcision alone. When the nature of the lesion demands amputation, partial penectomy should be performed with the amputation being conducted 2 cm proximal to visible tumor. The margin of excision must be monitored by frozen section.

Local recurrence is rare in patients treated by these methods. As recorded by deKernion et al., there were no recurrences in 48 cases of penile carcinoma treated by partial penectomy or adequate local extension.[4]

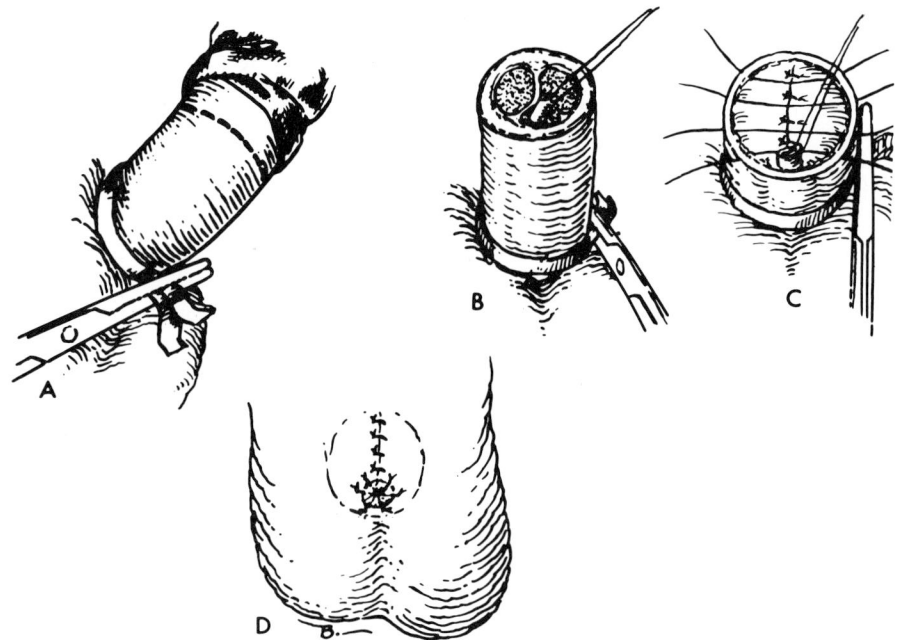

FIGURE 36-2 Partial penectomy. (*a*) The lesion is covered with a sterile dressing to prevent spread by contact and a tourniquet is applied at the base for hemostasis. (*b*) The lesion is amputated with histologically controlled margins. (*c*) The proximal margin is closed in two layers, the inner layer being the fascia of the corpora, the outer layer being the skin margins. (*d*) A spatulated mucocutaneous anastomosis is established at the urethral margin.

Tumors of the glans penis itself should not be locally excised, as malignancies in this area tend to have broad local spread due to early involvement of the vascular plexus of the glans. Of locally excised lesions 40 percent may be anticipated to recur, and either partial penectomy or radiation should be considered for lesions of this area.

Treatment of the Regional Lymph Nodes

Clinical assessment of regional nodes is particularly perplexing in penile carcinoma, The incidence of palpable nodes in patients presenting with carcinoma of the penis ranges between 35 percent and 60 percent.[4,10] Approximately 35 percent of these patients will fail to demonstrate positive nodes when node dissection is undertaken.[4,18] The staging error also is compounded when one examines that population of patients with clinically positive nodes who after a negative node biopsy subsequently develop regional nodal metastases. Approximately 10 percent of patients with clinically positive nodes that are negative on node biopsy will subsequently demonstrate regional disease.[4,11,19,20] This data would argue that biopsy alone of a clinically positive node is not sufficient but that the patient should have, as a minimun, a superficial inguinal node dissection. When the nodes are clinically positive, node dissection is advised. Approximately 40 to 55 percent of patients with positive nodes have disease control after node dissection, whereas progressive disease with death occurs at approximately 2 to 3 years in those patients who fail to undergo treatment.[10,14,21–23] The present controversy concerns the issue of early node dissection for patients with clinically negative nodes versus the recommendation of surgery only after identification of clinically positive nodes. Regional metastatic disease is seldom seen in lesions which fail to invade the corpora;[4,18] however, the presence of inguinal adenopathy is common and usually reflects inflammation at the site of the primary tumor. Only nodes which are enlarged 3 to 5 weeks following adequate local excision should be condidered clinically positive.[4,21,22] As reported by deKernion and by Hardner et al., only 32 percent and 26 percent, respectively, of those patients with pathologic stage I primary lesions had persistent adenopathy 3 weeks following surgical treatment of their primary lesions.[4,11]

Late development of nodal extension to the groin after adequate excision of noninvasive primaries occurs in 5 to 11 percent of patients. The low incidence of metastatic nodal disease makes routine ilioinguinal node dissection difficult to justify for stage I tumors.[4,11] However, pathologic invasion of the corpus cavernosum is associated with a higher probability of nodal extension. Two-thirds of patients with invasive of primary disease will have proven nodal extension at some time during their follow-up period.[4,11,21] When the primary tumor invades the corpus, 70 to 75 percent of clinically positive nodes maintained 3 to 5 weeks after primary surgery will be pathologically positive. There is no evidence that prophylactic node dissection in the presence of clinically negative disease produces enhanced survival. Although some reports indicate that with invasive disease, 16 to 20 percent of patients with surgically negative nodes will develop positive nodes, other reports give incidence figures as low as 2 percent.[1,10,11,19]

There is evidence to indicate that delaying surgery until regional metastases are clinically palpable does not decrease the chance for surgical control.[23,24] Ekstrom and Elsmyr identified a 50 percent disease control rate in patients who had node dissection delayed until adenopathy was evident on follow-up.[23]

Frew et al., identified no cancer deaths in patients in whom lymph node dissection was deferred until the presence of clinical nodal extension was evident.[24] Finally, the controversial report of Beggs and Spratt indicated that the mortality rate of lymphadenectomy of 1 percent was approximately equal to that of patients who died of cancer due to delayed nodal excision.[10]

Given this background, it seems appropriate to establish a reasonable policy for the management of penile carcinoma. Patients with pathologic stage I disease, i.e., those who do not show evidence of invasion and who have no clinically palpable disease 3 to 5 weeks after primary resection, can be safely monitored with careful clinical evaluation for nodal extension with initiation of delayed resection.

Patients who demonstrate invasion of the corpora at presentation are at greater risk for developing nodal extension. However, it seems reasonable to delay dissection 3 to 5 weeks to permit inflammatory changes to resolve. The clinically positive node should be biopsied to determine the presence or absence of nodal disease. The incision should be chosen so as not to compromise formal nodal dissection. In the presence of nodal disease, attention should then be turned immediately to the external and internal iliac node-bearing chains. This can be accomplished through a midline incision with bilateral pelvic node dissection. In the absence of massive pelvic adenopathy, bilateral superficial and deep inguinal node dissection should then be conducted.

Queyrat's Erythroplasia

Queyrat's erythroplasia manifests itself by single or multiple asymptomatic papules or palques on the glans penis, or around the urethral metus, and is seen predominantly in uncircumcised males between 20 and 80 years of age.[26-29] The bright red lesions may be ulcerated. The disease progresses slowly, and the interval between onset and diagnosis may be years. The cause of the disorder is unknown, and the diagnosis confirmed only by histological examination. The disease seems to be well controlled with topical 5-fluorouracil with normal histology and recurrence-free follow-up up to 70 months after treatment.[27,28]

URETHRAL CARCINOMA IN MEN AND WOMEN

The Male Urethra

Tumors of the male urethra may be categorized according to the histology of the cells lining the various anatomic regions (Fig. 36-3).[30,31] Tumors of the lining of the prostatic urethra should be separated from those of the posterior and anterior urethra as the cell type is different. The transitional epithelium of the prostatic urethra produces transitional-cell malignancies which are histologically and clinically distinct from the adenocarcinoma commonly associated with prostatic disease. Squamous-cell cancers arise from the bulbous and membranous urethra with distal penile urethra, the meatus, and perimeatal regions harboring condyloma acuminatum and benign papilloma.

Tumors of the Prostatic Urethra

Primary transitional-cell carcinomas of the prostatic urethra do occur; however, when transitional-cell tumors of the prostatic urethra are seen in association with histologically similar bladder carcinomas, they are felt to result from implantation following transurethral resection of the primary vesical malignancy or to reflect direct extension of the primary tumor. Transitional lesions of the prostatic urethra are thought to begin as carcinoma in situ of the ductal epithelium with subsequent invasion into the substance of the prostate itself.[21-23] No characteristic symptomatology heralds this lesion at a clinical level. In patients with infiltrating transitional-cell carcinoma, the prostate frequently has palpably hard areas.

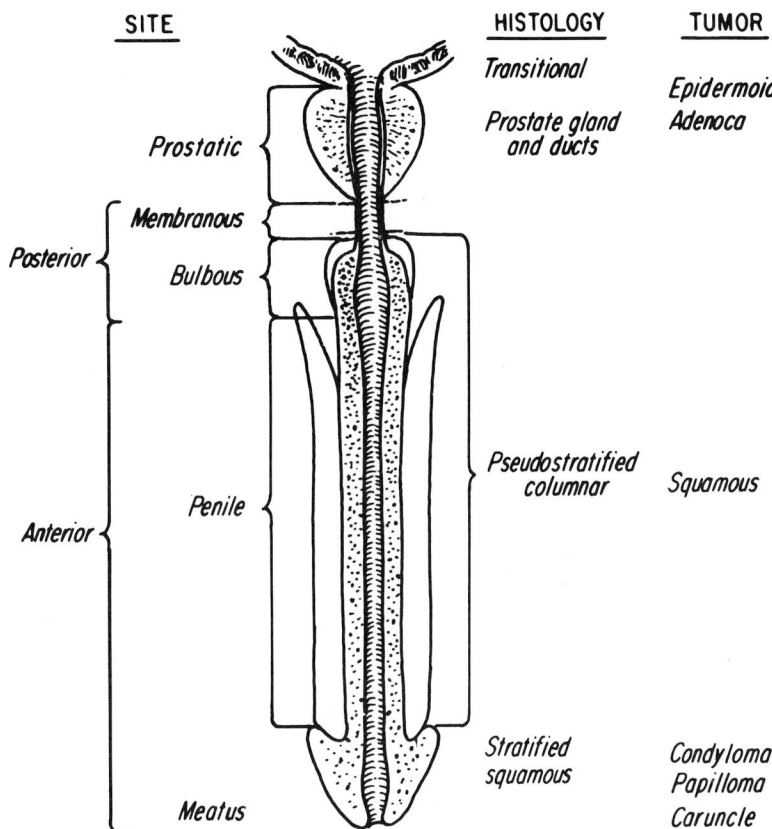

FIGURE 36-3 Cell type within the male urethra.

The age range of affected patients is between 60 and 78 years.[30,32] The serum acid phosphatase level is normal. These tumors feature complete resistance to endocrine therapy with poor response to radiation therapy and a poor response to surgery once the disease has invaded the prostatic stroma. If the tumor is superficially infiltrating, transitional-cell tumors of the prostatic urethra can be controlled in over 50 percent of the patients by transurethral resection alone.[30,35] However, in most instances, the primary prostatic transitional tumors involve the bulk of the prostate, so that one must consider radical prostatectomy or radical cystoprostatectomy with simultaneous pelvic lymph node dissection as an appropriate form of aggressive therapy. The frequency of lymph node involvement is not known. It is likely that if deep pelvic nodes are involved, the prognosis is extremely poor.

Aggressive radiation therapy to the prostate at dose levels between 4000 and 7000 rads has produced an occasional long-term survival.[30,32] One might therefore consider aggressive external beam radiation therapy as the initial form of treatment, with biopsy monitoring for up to 6 months following completion of radiotherapy. Patients failing to have tumor-free biopsies at that time could then be considered for radical cystoprostatectomy. Absolute recommendations regarding therapy are not possible due to the small series which are available and the multiple treatment regimens which have been applied to various recorded experiences. However, the experience with transitional-cell tumors of the bladder would indicate that a course of aggressive radiotherapy might very well produce some modification of tumor biology, and therefore either immediate or delayed radical surgery in conjunction with pelvic node dissection could be deemed appropriate.

Epidermoid carcinoma of the bulbomembraneous urethra is the most common urethral malignancy, comprising about 75 percent of carcinomas of the male urethra.[30,36,37] The association of chronic urethral infection, urethral stricture, and malignancy has long been recognized. In many individuals, an antecedent history of gonorrhea can be established. In a large series published by Kaplin, 37 percent of the patients had antecedent venereal disease, 35 percent had strictures, and 7 percent had antecedent urethral trauma. Of all patients with urethral malignancy who are able to provide an adequate history, 76 percent have an antecedent history of stricture.[36]

Therefore, it is not uncommon to have an antecedent history of urethral infection with stricture felt to be benign and a long-standing history of intermittent urethral sounding. The duration of the symptoms is variable. The most common presenting symptom complex is obstruction, seen in up to 47 percent of patients, with 39 percent of patients presenting with a palpable mass, 31 percent with a periurethral abscess, 20 percent with a fistula, and 22 percent urethral discharge.[38] A predominant characteristic is suspicion of malignancy without confirmation of diagnosis, as biopsies of this involved area usually reveal only chronic inflammatory disease until deep-tissue bites are secured.[30,39] Differentiation between malignancy and periurethral abscess may be difficult, and the physician is aided most by a high index of suspicion. Retrograde urethrography may define the extent of the disease and indicate spread into the surrounding tissues should there be fistulization.

The lymphatic drainage of the male urethra defines the potential areas of spread.[40] The drainage of the glans penis is via a plexus that anastomoses at the symphysis pubis and empties directly into deep inguinal and external iliac nodes. The penile urethra is drained by lymphatics which accompany those of the glans. Therefore, lesions of the glans or of the penile urethra may extend to superficial as well as to deep inguinal nodes. Two lymphatic channels drain the bulbous urethra, one draining to the external iliac nodes along the dorsal vein of the penis beneath the infrapubic ligament, the second level of drainage to the hypogastric nodes via the pudendal artery. Direct extension to adjacent structures is the primary mode of spread of urethral malignancies. Involvement of the vascular spaces, both of the corpus and the periurethral tissues, is common. Tumors of the bulbomembranous urethra can involve the deep structures of the perineum, including the penile and scrotal skin and urogenital diaphragm, and can extend into the prostate. The posterior urethral tumors metastasize via the above-identified lymphatic channels to hypogastric and common iliac nodes. If there is no involvement of penile skin, superficial inguinal nodes also can be involved. In general, tumors involving the anterior urethra metastasize primarily through the inguinal nodes, those of the posterior urethra drain into the pelvic and deep inguinal nodes.

Untreated patients can anticipate a median survivorship of 3 months with a range between 1 week to 15 months.[38] Only 16 percent will survive more than 5 years.[30] The extent of the disease at the time of identification is such that even extensive radical surgery rarely effects long-term survivorship.

The Female Urethra

The female urethra may be considered pathologically as being separated into two segments, the distal third, and the proximal two-thirds (Fig. 36-4).[30,41,42] Tumors have been traditionally classified as anterior when they are limited to the distal third of the urethra, and entire when more than the anterior third is involved.

Urethral tumors are more common in women than in men, being reported at a female-to-male ratio of 5:1.[30,41,52] The age range is variable, with the majority of patients being between 50 and 60 years of age.[30,41,42]

The predominant cell type is squamous-cell carcinoma, with adenocarcinoma ranking second, and a scattering of patients having myeloma, lymphosarcoma, or miscellaneous other tumor types. Tumor grade is not identified in most series; however, the accumulated experience would indicate that the tumors are predominantly of low grade when the anterior urethra is involved, with a slightly higher grade when the entire urethra is involved. The presentation is usually one of

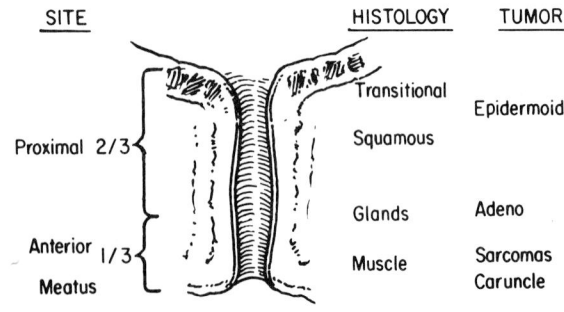

FIGURE 36-4 Cell type within the female urethra.

local swelling, with painful urination, frequency, and bleeding.

Lymph node involvement is not uncommon: 35 to 50 percent of patients may have clinically involved nodes at the time of presentation with an additional 15 percent subsequently developing nodes during the follow-up.[30,41,42,44,45]

Grabstald et al., reported clinical evidence of lymph node involvement in 25 of 79 patients during the course of their disease with pathologic examination of the clinically suspicious node confirming disease in 24 of 25 patients. In contradistinction to penile carcinoma, all palpable nodes are abnormal. In this original series, 22 of 79 patients, or 38 percent, had histological identification of inguinal lymph node involvement.[30,41] Pelvic node involvement is less readily identified, as node dissection in this area is not routinely conducted. In 26 of 79 patients explored by Grabstald et al., metastatic pelvic nodes were found in 13 patients.[41]

Treatment of tumors of the female urethra should be based primarily on the tumor stage and to a lesser extent on the pathology. Squamous-cell carcinoma limited to the anterior urethra is best treated by partial urethrectomy. The incidence of lymph node metastases with distal urethral tumors is low, and partial urethrectomy alone often is sufficient for cure. However, equally good results can be obtained with interstitial radiation, supplemented by intracavitory or external beam therapy.[30,41]

Squamous-cell carcinomas of the entire urethra have an exceedingly poor prognosis irrespective of the form of treatment, whether surgery, radiotherapy, or combination of both. Treatment of patients with adenocarcinoma involving the entire urethra is similarly dismal. In a series reported by Ziggerman 27 patients were cured of carcinoma involving the entire urethra.[46] Of this group of 27 patients, 14 had radiation therapy of various types and were reported alive at least 5 years after treatment; 13 were treated by various surgical methods, including simple excision, partial urethrectomy, or radical hysterectomy. The average survival rate was 8 years in the radiation treatment group, and 11.6 years for those receiving surgical therapy. Bracken et al. reported 81 cases of carcinoma of the female urethra, with the overall 5- and 10-year survival range for the entire group being 32 percent. The survival expectations for patients with squamous carcinoma, transitional-cell carcinoma, and adenocarcinoma were similar when analyzed according to stage, and all cell types appear to respond equally well to radiation.[47] The high incidence of local recurrence as noted for all forms of single modality therapy, ranging from 46 to 64 percent, suggests the need for combination preoperative radiotherapy followed by definitive surgical removal.[47] Based on the accumulated series, it would appear that when epidermoid carcinoma involves the entire urethra, careful preoperative radiation therapy followed with exenterative surgery is the treatment of choice.[30,41,47] In tumors of either epidermoid or squamous nature involving the urethra, treatment of the regional nodes should be reserved for the demonstration of disease. These nodes should be identified by either clinical examination or lymphangiography. It is felt that groin dissection should be conducted only when there is palpable disease.[30,41]

In conclusion, carcinoma of the penis or urethra is controlled optimally by judicious selection of treatment prior to systemic dissemination. Chemotherapeutic programs, at present, offer little disease control. The stage of the tumor at initial presentation appears to be the single most important item in assessing the biologic hazard of the disease.

REFERENCES

1. Kursivilla JT et al: Results of surgical treatment of carcinoma of the penis. *Aust NZ J Surg* 41:157–159, 1971.
2. Kyolwazi SK: Carcinoma of the penis: A review of 153 patients admitted to Mulago Hospital, Kanysala, Uganda. *East Afr Med J* 43:415–421, 1966.
3. Jackson SM: The treatment of carcinoma of the penis. *Br J Surg* 53:33–35, 1966.
4. deKernion JB et al: Carcinoma of the penis. *Cancer* 32:1256–1262, 1973.
5. Dean AL Jr: Epithelioma of the penis. *J Urol* 33:252–283, 1935.
6. Furlong JH, Uhle RA: Cancer of the penis: A report of eighty-eight cases. *J Urol* 69:550–555, 1953.
7. Havnanian AP: The evaluation and present status of pelvi-inguinal lymphatic excision. *Surg Gynecol Obstet* 124:851–862, 1967.
8. Mathe G: Study of the clinical efficacy of Bleomycin in human cancer. *Br Med J* 2:643–645, 1970.
9. Young HH: A radical operation for the cure of cancer of the penis. *J Urol* 26:285–294, 1931.
10. Beggs JH, Spratt JS: Epidermoid carcinoma of the penis. *J Urol* 91:166–172, 1964.
11. Hardner GJ et al: Carcinoma of the penis: Analysis of therapy in 100 consecutive cases. *J Urol* 428–430, 1972.
12. Green JP et al: Carcinoma of the penis: Radiotherapeutic approach for the primary lesion. *Radiol Clin Biol* 39:1–8, 1970.

13. Pierquin B et al: Consistent local control of certain malignant tumors. *Radiology* 99:661–667, 1971.
14. Da'nczak-Ginalska Z: Treatment of penis carcinoma with interstitially administered iridium: Comparison with radium therapy. *Recent Results Cancer Res* 60:127–134, 1977.
15. L'utolf UM et al: Radiotherapy of penile carcinoma: Indications and results. Strahlentherapie 152:333–337, 1976.
16. Marcial VA et al: Carcinoma of the penis. *Radiology* 79: 209–220, 1962.
17. Orr PS et al: Carcinoma of the penis: A review of 42 cases. *Br J Urol* 49:733–738, 1977.
18. Gregl A et al: Life expectancy in penile carcinoma: Statistical evaluation of 150 penile carcinomas in the period 1912–1970. *Urologe [A]* 16:107–109, 1977.
19. Hanash K et al: Carcinoma of the penis: A clinicopathologic study. *J Urol* 104:291–297, 1970.
20. Whitmore WF Jr: Tumors of the penis, urethra, scrotum, and testis, in MF Campbell, JH Harrison (eds): *Urology*, Saunders, Philadelphia, 1190–1229, 1970.
21. Skinner D, Leadbetter WF: The surgical management of squamous cell carcinoma of the penis. *J Urol* 107:273–277, 1972.
22. Doeven JJ et al: Penile cancer. *Arch Chir Neerl* 27:41–52, 1975.
23. Ekstrom T, Elsmyr F: Cancer of the penis. *Acta Chir Scand.* 115:25–45, 1958.
24. Frew JD et al: Carcinoma of the penis. *Br J Urol* 39:398–404, 1967.
25. Cabanas RM: An approach for the treatment of penile carcinoma. *Cancer* 39:456–466, 1977.
26. Merino MJ et al: Penile Paget's disease and prostatic carcinoma. *J Urol* 120:121–123, 1978.
27. Goette DK, Carson TE: Erythroplasia of Queyrat: Treatment with topical 5-fluorouracil. *Cancer* 38:1498–1502, 1976.
28. Gotte DK et al: Erythroplasia of Queyrat: Treatment with topically applied fluorouracil. *JAMA* 232:934–937, 1975.
29. Goette DK: Review of erythroplasia of Queyrat and its treatment. *Urology* 8:311–315, 1976.
30. Grabstald H: Tumors of the urethra in men and women. *Cancer* 32:1236–1255, 1973.
31. Mullin EM, Paulson DF: Carcinoma of the male urethra. *J Urol* 112:610–613, 1974.
32. Johnson DE et al: Transitional cell carcinoma of the prostate: A clinical morphological study. *Cancer* 29:287–293, 1972.
33. Melicow MM, Hollowell JW: Intra-urothelial cancer, carcinoma *in situ*, Bowen's Disease of the urinary systems: Discussion of 30 cases. *J Urol* 68:763–772, 1952.
34. Ortega LG et al: *In situ* carcinoma of the prostate with intraepithelial extension into the urethra and bladder. *Cancer* 6:892–923, 1953.
35. Shenasky JH, Gillenwater JY: Management of transitional cell carcinoma of the prostate. *J Urol* 108:462–465, 1972.
36. Dixson FJ, Moore RA: Tumors of the urethra, in *Atlas of Tumor Pathology*, fasc 32, Armed Forces Institute of Pathology, Washington, DC, pp 143–147, 1952.
37. Zaslow J, Priestly JT: Primary carcinoma of the male urethra. *J Urol* 98:365–371, 1967.
38. Kaplan GW et al: Carcinoma of the male urethra. *J Urol* 98: 365–371, 1967.
39. Mandler JI, Pool TL: Primary carcinoma of the male urethra. *J Urol* 96:67–72, 1966.
40. Hand JR: Surgery of the penis and urethra, in MF Campbell, JH Harrison (eds): *Urology*, Saunders, Philadelphia, 3: sec. 16, pp 2541–2647, 1970.
41. Grabstald H et al: Cancer of the female urethra. *JAMA* 197: 835–842, 1966.
42. Roberts TW, Melicow MM: Pathology and natural history of urethra tumors in females: Review of 65 cases. *Urology* 10:583–589, 1977.
43. Pointon RC, Poole-Wilson DS: Primary carcinoma of the urethra. *Br J Urol* 40:682–693, 1968.
44. Simon N: Iridium 192 as a radium substitute. *Am J Roentgenol Radium Ther Nucl Med* 93:170–178, 1965.
45. Riches EW, Cullen TH: Carcinoma of the urethra. *Br J Urol* 23:209–221, 1951.
46. Zeigerman JH, Gordon SF: Cancer of the female urethra: A curable disease. *Obstet Gynecol* 36:785–789, 1970.
47. Bracken RB et al: Primary carcinoma of the female urethra. *J Urol* 116:188–192, 1976.

SELECTED BIBLIOGRAPHY

Cartwright RA, Sisson JD: Carcinoma of the penis and cervix. *Lancet* 1:97, 1980.

Haile K, Declos L: The place of radiation therapy in the treatment of carcinoma of the distal end of the penis. *Cancer* 46:1980, 1980.

MacGregor JE, Innes G: Carcinoma of penis and cervix. *Lancet* 1:1247, 1980.

PART SEVEN

GYNECOLOGIC NEOPLASMS

37

CERVICAL CANCER

J. R. van Nagell, Jr.

Cervical cancer is perhaps the best example of a tumor in which early detection has significantly reduced patient mortality rates. Routine cervical cytologic examination has enabled the majority of patients with cervical neoplasia to be diagnosed when the lesion is in the preinvasive stage and therefore curable. However, there remains a significant number of patients, most of whom have not had regular cytologic examinations, who present with invasive cervical cancer. It is estimated that over 15,000 such patients will develop cervical cancer annually in the United States, and that over 7000 patients will die of this disease each year. Furthermore, data from the end results section of the National Cancer Institute indicate that the 5-year survival rate for patients with invasive cervical cancer has not changed significantly over the past 15 years. Recent investigations have suggested that there are a number of histologic and anatomic variants of cervical cancer which are prognostically significant. In this regard, it is essential that every patient with cervical cancer undergo a thorough and uniform evaluation so that adequate data is available that can be used to determine optimal therapy. The best treatment results have generally been achieved in centers where there is a coordinated program by gynecologic and radiation oncologists to individualize therapy to the needs of each patient.

This chapter will present a discussion of (1) the historical advances in the diagnosis and treatment of patients with cervical cancer, (2) the etiology and epidemiology of cervical cancer, (3) the evaluation of cervical cancer patients prior to treatment, (4) the therapy for cervical cancer, (5) survival and follow-up, and (6) experimental approaches to current therapeutic problems.

HISTORICAL ADVANCES IN THE DIAGNOSIS OF AND THERAPY FOR CERVICAL CANCER

Although considerable knowledge concerning the anatomic sites of spread of cervical cancer was gained during the early nineteenth century, the majority of significant advances in the diagnosis of and therapy for cervical cancer have occurred during the past 100 years. Vaginal and abdominal operations were performed in patients with cervical tumors as early as 1825 (Meigs[1]), but surgical procedures designed specifically for the treatment of cervical cancer were developed much later. Radical hysterectomy with pelvic lymphadenectomy was first described in 1895 by Ries[2] and Clark[3], but its practical use can be attributed to Wertheim,[4] who performed the operation extensively in Europe. At approximately the same time, the technique of radical vaginal hysterectomy was described by Schuchardt[5] and Schauta.[6] Unfortunately the mortality rate of these radical surgical procedures was in excess of 10 percent, and even more patients died of postoperative infections. Wertheim,[4] for example, reported that 63 of 250 patients (25 percent) undergoing radical hysterectomy died from the operation. An additional 78 patients (31 percent) developed tumor recurrence, whereas 106 patients (42 percent) were free of disease 5 years after treatment.

Roentgen rays were discovered in 1895, and radium was first used in the treatment of cervical cancer 8 years later (Cleaves[7]). In 1913, Abbe[8] reported the cure of a patient with cervical cancer by intravaginal radium application. Because of the relatively low mortality rate and comparable cure rate associated with it, radiation therapy soon became the treatment of choice for cervical cancer in most centers throughout the world. The efficacy of radiation therapy was further strengthened by Regaud,[9] who developed the concept of time-dose relationships for radium. These concepts were used to determine tumoricidal doses to the cervix while minimizing the dose to adjacent normal structures. Similarly, the discovery of induced radioactivity by Frederic and Irene Joliot-Curie in 1934 served as the basis for the later use of high-activity cobalt 60 in the therapy of cervical cancer. Several major schools of radiation therapy developed, one at the Curie Foundation in Paris, a second in Manchester, England, and a third at the Radiumhemmet in Stockholm. Therapists at the Curie Foundation recommended delivery of low-intensity radium to the cervix over a prolonged period of time, whereas those at the Radiumhemmet utilized a short application of higher-intensity radiation 2 or 3 times each week. Investigators at Manchester emphasized the combination of external therapy and intracavitary radium in the treatment of cervical cancer, and defined anatomic reference points at which to measure paracervical radiation. The techniques of radiation therapy developed at these centers were used throughout the world and form the basis for modern methods of pelvic irradiation.

The development of high-energy accelerators and their use in the treatment of cervical cancer was also a major therapeutic advance. The first betatron was constructed by Kerst[10] in 1943, and linear accelerators were first used in the treatment of cervical cancer two decades later (Miller[11]). These high-intensity sources made it possible to treat extensive cervical tumors with tumoricidal doses of radiation deep within the pelvis.

The renaissance of the surgical treatment of cervical cancer occurred with the work of Meigs.[11a] In 1944, this outstanding surgeon published a report of 47 cervical cancer patients on whom he performed radical hysterectomy with bilateral pelvic lymph node dissection. The operative mortality rate was zero, and the survival time in patients with early-stage disease was superior to that obtained with radiation therapy. Concomitant advances in anesthesia, blood transfusion techniques, and antibiotic synthesis greatly facilitated the use of radical surgery as a therapeutic method in patients with cervical cancer. In a subsequent series of 139 patients with stage I disease treated by radical hysterectomy, Liu and Meigs[12] reported a 5-year survival rate of 75 percent. Although modifications of this operation have been made (Symmonds and Pratt,[13] van Nagell and Schiwietz[14]), the basic surgical techniques advocated by Meigs have persisted to the present.

The use of pelvic exenteration as a surgical method in the treatment of extensive primary and recurrent cervical cancer was first advocated by Brunschwig in 1948.[15] The design of the operation was based on the observation that certain cases of locally extensive cancer produced death while remaining confined to the pelvis. Consequently, it was reasoned that surgical excision of all pelvic viscera with the creation of an ileal urinary conduit and a colostomy would be curative in these patients. Although the indications for this operation have been considerably refined (Barber and Jones,[16] Creasman and Rutledge[17]), pelvic exenteration has been curative in selected patients with recurrent cervical cancer when all other therapeutic measures have failed.

The modern era of individualized cervical cancer therapy began with the work of Kottmeier[18-20] at the Radiumhemmet and Fletcher and Rutledge[21] at the M. D. Anderson Hospital in the United States. These investigators and their colleagues published numerous papers concerning the recurrence rate, incidence of complications, and survival times of patients receiving various methods of therapy for cervical cancer. Their knowledge of the biology of cervical cancer, meticulous attention to detail, and insistence on adequate long-term follow-up provided objective data which could be used to determine optimal therapy for patients with varying stages of disease.

Advances in the diagnosis and evaluation of patients with cervical cancer have also been of major significance. It is generally accepted that effective cervical cytologic screening has been the single most important factor in reducing mortality rates due to cervical cancer. The cytologic diagnosis of cervical cancer was reported independently in 1928 by Babes[22] in Hungary and Papanicolaou[23] in the United States. Some 13 years later, Papanicolaou and Traut[24] reported their classic paper concerning the diagnostic value of vaginal smears in carcinoma of the uterus. Although these investigators demonstrated the accuracy of cervical cytology in the diagnosis of early carcinoma of the cervix, this technique was not accepted by practicing physicians until much later. Erickson et al.,[25] in reporting the results of mass cervical cytologic screening programs in the United States, noted that significant numbers of patients with early cervical cancer diagnosed cytologically were entirely asymptomatic. Subsequently, Christopherson[26] and Fidler et al.[27] showed that cervical cytologic screening decreased mortality rates due to cervical cancer by early diagnosis. At present, it is estimated that cervical cytologic screening saves tens of thousands of lives annually.

A second diagnostic method utilized in cervical cancer detection is colposcopy. In 1925, Hinselmann designed the first colposcope and began reporting its use in the diagnosis of cervical epithelial abnormalities. His original idea was that vascular abnormalities present in early cervical cancer could be recognized by appropriate illumination and magnification provided by the colposcope. Hinselmann found that all cervical cancers demonstrated characteristic changes in surface vascular patterns. He believed this so-called adoptive vascular hypertrophy resulted from increased perfusion requirements of the rapidly cycling neoplastic epithelium. The technique of colposcopy was utilized extensively throughout Europe, but was not practiced in much of the English-speaking parts of the world until the 1960s. This was because Hinselmann's publications[28] were exclusively in German and also because colposcopy was viewed by some as a screening method competing with cytology. In fact, colposcopy and cytology are complementary disciplines, and colposcopy is now recommended in all patients with abnormal cervical cytology. Colposcopy is presently the most reliable method for localizing the site and extent of a cervical epithelial abnormality, and greatly facilitates identification of the optimal area for biopsy.

Any discussion of advances in the diagnosis and treatment of cervical cancer would be incomplete without mentioning the importance of histologic classification and clinical staging. A uniform classification and staging system is essential in order to properly evaluate various treatment modalities and to predict clinical outcome for the individual patient. Although there have been numerous systems for the histologic classification of cervical cancer, the one proposed by Reagan et al.[29] has been the most significant prognostically. These investigators divided all cervical cancers into keratinizing squamous cell cancer, large-cell nonkeratinizing cancer, small-cell cancer, and adenocarcinoma. Since the initial descriptions of this classification were made, a number of investigators have shown that the different cell types of cervical cancer have varying biologic characteristics which are often clinically important. For example, keratinizing squamous cell cancers have been shown to have a poorer prognosis than nonkeratinizing cancers of the same size and configuration when treated by radiation therapy (Wentz and Lewis,[30] Swan and Roddick[31]). Similarly, small-cell carcinomas of the cervix have been reported to have a significantly higher incidence of lymph node metastases than the other cell types of cervical cancer independent of lesion size (van Nagell et al.[32,33]).

Prior to 1950, there was no uniform staging system for cervical cancer. Clinical staging systems had been proposed by Schmitz[34] in the United States and by Winter and Doderlein[35] in Germany. In these systems each case was designated as operable or inoperable, but the criteria for placing a patient in either category were not clearly defined. In 1929, the original League of Nations classification was adopted. According to this system, four stages of cervical carcinoma were described, with ascending stages corresponding to greater tumor involvement. The League of Nations classification subsequently underwent a number of revisions and became the basis for the present International Federation of Gynecology and Obstetrics (FIGO) staging system. The final evolution of a unified staging system for cervical cancer came in 1976 when the American Joint Committee and the International Union against cancer formally adopted the FIGO staging system. For the first time, there was a universally accepted staging system which allowed evaluation of varying methods of therapy for cervical cancer patients with comparable tumors.

ETIOLOGY AND EPIDEMIOLOGY

Presently available data support the concept that cervical cancer is related to a venereally transmitted agent. Women with cervical cancer typically begin intercourse at an earlier age and with a larger number of sexual partners than those without cervical cancer. Also, squamous cell carcinoma of the cervix is extremely rare in virginal females. Recent evidence also suggests that the incidence of cervical cancer is increased in the wives of men who previously had been married to women with cervical cancer.

The infectious agent most commonly implicated in the genesis of cervical cancer is genital herpes simplex virus, type 2 (HSV-2). Evidence to support the association between HSV-2 infection and cervical cancer is illustrated in Table 37-1 and includes (1) seroepidemiologic studies, (2) data establishing the venereal transmission of HSV-2, (3) ability of HSV-2 to cause neoplastic transformation, (4) identification of HSV-2 genetic information in cervical tumor cells, and (5) prospective studies demonstrating an increased risk of developing cervical neoplasia following infection with HSV-2.

Numerous seroepidemiologic studies have indicated that antibodies to herpes nonvirion antigens are present in a significantly higher percentage of women with cervical cancer than in age-matched control populations without cervical cancer. For example, Hollinshead et al.[36] reported that the sera of 88 percent of patients with invasive carcinoma of the cervix contained complement-fixing antibodies to herpesvirus tumor-associated antigens as opposed to 4 percent in normal control patients. In a similar study, Rawls and Adam[37] noted that only 2 percent of patients with cervical cancer did not have elevated HSV-2 antibody titers regardless of the population studied.

The propensity of HSV-2 to be spread venereally is also consistent with the observed epidemiology of cervical cancer. Clinical evidence for venereal transmission of HSV-2 is derived largely from virus isolation studies as well as from the observed viral cytopathic effects in cervical epithelial cells from sexual contacts of males with confirmed HSV-2 penile infections. Nahmias et al.,[38] for example, examined eight female sexual contacts of seven males with confirmed HSV-2 genital infections within 1 week of the initial detection of penile herpetic lesions. Seven of these eight contacts had clinically demonstrable HSV-2 infections of the vulva or cervix, and genital herpesvirus was isolated from each of them. Similarly, Rawls et al.[39] examined 30 female contacts of males with confirmed HSV-2 penile infections. Genital herpesvirus was isolated in 33 percent of these women, compared with 2 percent in a control population examined at the same clinic.

A prerequisite for the etiologic association of any virus with cancer is that it have the capability of inducing neoplastic transformation. Genital herpesvirus has been shown to induce neoplastic transformation of hamster embryo cells (Rapp and Duff[40]). When transplanted into newborn hamsters, these transformed cells produce both fibrosarcomas and adenocarcinomas. Recently, the transforming sequences of HSV-2 have been identified, and the cells transformed by these sequences have been reported to express specific viral antigens (Aurelian et al.[41]). Cervical tumor induction has also been demonstrated in mice inoculated intravaginally with HSV-2. Wentz et al.[42] reported that 60 percent of mice developed carcinomas of the cervix or vagina after inoculation with inactivated HSV-2. In approximately one-third of the animals intraepithelial neoplasia progressed to invasive cancer. Likewise, intravaginal infection with HSV-2 in Cebus monkeys has been shown to produce irreversible severe dysplasia in 35 percent of the cases (Palmer et al.[43]).

Recent immunohistochemical and electron microscopic studies have also demonstrated the presence of HSV-2 viral antigens and genetic material in cervical tumor cells. Viral DNA sequences and messenger RNA have been expressed by cervical tumor cells in culture (McDougal et al.,[44] Frenkel et al.[45]). Similarly, Notter et al.[46] have been able to localize HSV-2 tumor-associated antigens in biopsies of cervical cancer by using a sensitive peroxidase-antiperoxidase system.

Perhaps the most convincing bit of evidence suggesting a relationship between HSV-2 infection and cervical cancer is the observation from prospective studies that exposure to genital herpesvirus places a woman at higher risk for the subsequent development of cervical neopla-

TABLE 37-1 Evidence to Support Association between Genital Herpesvirus (HSV-2) Infection and Cervical Cancer

Seroepidemiologic studies indicating significantly higher incidence of HSV-2 exposure in cervical cancer patients than in matched control groups

Venereal transmission of HSV-2

Ability of HSV-2 to cause neoplastic transformation

Identification of HSV-2 genetic information in cervical tumor cells

Prospective studies demonstrating an increased incidence of both carcinoma in situ (CIS) and invasive squamous cell carcinoma in patients with HSV-2 infection

sia. Naib et al.[47] followed 44 women with cytologic evidence of HSV-2 infection for over 4 years. Twenty-five percent of the women exposed to HSV-2 developed cervical intraepithelial neoplasia as opposed to only two percent of the age-matched control group. In a more recent review of case-control data, Thomas and Rawls[48] reported that the relative risk of invasive cancer increased from 2- to 17-fold in patients with documented HSV-2 infection. These data are also supported by the findings of Naib et al.[49] that the mean age of exposure to HSV-2 is approximately 10 years prior to the peak age of patients with carcinoma in situ and 20 years prior to the mean age of patients with invasive cervical cancer.

Although the above data strongly imply that HSV-2 infection plays an etiologic role in the genesis of cervical cancer in some patients, it is also true that the majority of patients exposed to genital herpesvirus will not develop epithelial abnormalities of the cervix. Therefore, it is quite likely that there may be other causative factors or cofactors involved in the development of cervical neoplasia. In certain patients, HSV-2 infection may initiate a multistep process which results in cervical epithelial abnormalities. However, the promotion of these abnormalities to invasive cancer probably depends upon additional factors which have yet to be identified.

A second theory of the etiology of cervical cancer is that spermatozoa itself may be the source of abnormal DNA. Certain spermatozoa contain high concentrations of arginine-rich histones which have been identified as possible carcinogens (Singer et al.[50]). During the dynamic phase of metaphasia, this abnormal DNA from the heterochromatin fraction is incorporated into the host epithelial genome, causing cellular neoplasia (Coppleson[51]). The intracellular degradation of this abnormal sperm would then place the host at high risk for the development of cancer. Reid[52] injected radiolabeled sperm intravaginally in the mouse and was able to identify the radioactive label in the nucleus of regenerating stromal cells within 17 hours following injection. Further studies by these investigators (Reid and Blackwell[53]) demonstrated an altered pattern of DNA in the host epithelial cell following incorporation of spermatic DNA. According to this theory, variation in the genetic content of DNA in the heterochromatin of different sperm populations would explain the observations by Singer[54] that certain males are more prone than others to have associated cervical neoplasia in their spouse.

Chemical carcinogens have also been implicated in the genesis of cervical epithelial neoplasia. Christopherson and Broghamer[55] were able to produce carcinoma in situ of the cervix in mice by the local application of methylcholanthrene. The incidence of epithelial neoplasia depended upon the frequency and duration of methylcholanthrene application. However, no cases of invasive cancer were noted. Similarly, Patten et al.[56] were able to produce cervical dysplasia by the intravaginal injection of *Trichomonas vaginalis*. This histologic abnormality disappeared when *Trichomonas* inoculation was discontinued.

The relationship of circumcision to the etiology of cervical cancer is presently uncertain. Early observations that Jewish and Moslem women had an unusually low incidence of cervical cancer (Wynder[57]) were interpreted as indicating a protective effect of circumcision on cervical cancer induction. Furthermore, smegma was reported to be carcinogenic in experimental animals despite the fact that it did not contain any known chemical carcinogen (Pratt-Thomas et al.[58]). More recent studies, however, have not confirmed the protective effect of circumcision on the incidence of cervical cancer (Terris et al.,[59] Megafu[60]).

As has been mentioned previously, the major reduction in cervical cancer mortality rates has been achieved through the use of effective cervical cytologic screening. In the United States, the annual death rate from cervical cancer has decreased from over 20 per 100,000 in 1930 to less than 7 per 100,000 at the present time (Silverberg[61]). Although the precise temporal relationship between carcinoma in situ and invasive cervical cancer is not known, it is quite likely that the majority of invasive cervical cancer was preceded by carcinoma in situ. Cytologic screening has facilitated detection of cervical neoplasia at an intraepithelial stage when it is curable, thereby preventing the subsequent development of invasive cancer. The annual rate of cervical cytologic screening of the at-risk population varies from 5 to 25 percent depending upon socioeconomic status and geographic location. A number of epidemiologic studies (Fidler et al.[27], and Cramer[62]) have shown that the death rate from cervical cancer is inversely related to the annual percentage of the population screened. It is quite disturbing to note that 10 percent of women in the United States have never had a Pap smear. This figure increases to 25 percent in black women of low socioeconomic status who live in rural areas (Rochat[63]). It is apparent, therefore, that regular cervical cytologic screening is often not obtained by precisely those women who are at highest risk to develop cervical cancer. Although recently there have been modifications in the recommended frequency of cervical cytologic screening, it is strongly advised that all women obtain a yearly Pap smear and pelvic examination beginning at the onset of sexual activity.

EVALUATION

One of the most serious deficiencies in the management of patients with invasive cervical cancer is the lack of a detailed evaluation system which can be uniformly applied to all patients. Too often, patients are treated on the basis of stage alone without adequate knowledge concerning such histomorphologic variables as cell type, lesion size, or lymph-vascular space invasion by tumor cells. These variables are prognostically important and play an important role in determining optimal therapy for each patient.

Although cervical cytology is an effective screening method for cervical epithelial abnormalities, therapy should not be instituted prior to histologic confirmation of invasive cancer. A cervical biopsy or conization specimen should include enough tissue to accurately establish depth of stromal invasion, histologic type, and lymph-vascular space invasion by tumor cells.

Before discussing the histologic classification of invasive cervical cancer, it is necessary to define microinvasive cancer. There have been numerous definitions of microinvasion in the recent literature, with the reported incidence of lymph node metastases varying from 0 to 4.8 percent (Boronow,[64] Hasumi et al.[65]). It should be emphasized, however, that the definition of microinvasive carcinoma is clinically meaningful only if it precludes the presence of regional lymph node metastases. In 1974, the Society of Gynecologic Oncologists adopted a definition of *microinvasive cervical cancer* that included tumors with invasion limited to 3 mm of the cervical stroma without lymph-vascular space invasion. This diagnosis could be made only from a cervical conization specimen in which an adequate number of sections had been taken to rule out the presence of coexisting invasive cancer. Using this definition, Boronow[64] reported that there were no lymph node metastases in 35 patients with microinvasive cancer. In contrast, 21 percent of patients with more extensive stromal invasion had pelvic lymph node metastases. In more recent study, Hasumi et al.[65] noted that only 1 of 106 patients with stromal invasion limited to 3 mm had lymph node metastases, and no patient demonstrated microscopic tumor metastasis in the parametria. At the present time, the aforementioned definition of microinvasive cancer is recommended.

The diagnosis of invasive cervical cancer is established when there is unequivocal stromal invasion to a depth greater than 3 mm or when there is lymph-vascular space invasion by tumor cells. As has been mentioned previously, there are numerous systems for histologic classification of cervical tumors. However, the most clinically useful has been that proposed by Reagan et al.[29] According to this classification, cervical cancer is divided into large-cell nonkeratinizing cancer, keratinizing squamous cell cancer, small-cell cancer, and adenocarcinoma. Patients with keratinizing squamous cell cancers have been reported to have poorer survival rates than those with large-cell nonkeratinizing cancer when treated with radiation (Wentz and Lewis,[30] Swan and Roddick[31]). However, no such difference in survival rates was noted when patients with these cell types were treated by radical surgery (van Nagell et al.[32]). Therefore, it appears that the prognostic difference noted is due to differential radiation sensitivity rather than an inherent biologic aggressiveness of keratinizing tumors. In contrast, patients with small-cell carcinomas have been shown to have the highest incidence of lymph node metastases and the poorest survival rates irrespective of the method of therapy used (van Nagell et al.[33]).

The difference in survival rates of patients with adenocarcinoma and squamous cell carcinoma noted by several investigators is more related to anatomic configuration and tumor volume than to an increased metastatic potential of endocervical adenocarcinomas.

Additional histologic criteria of prognostic significance are lymph-vascular space invasion and the degree of lymphoplasmacytic infiltration around tumor cells. Barber et al.,[66] for example, reported that the presence of lymph-vascular space invasion decreased the survival rates of patients with stage IB cervical cancer from 90 percent to 60 percent. Lymphoplasmacytic infiltration around tumor cells has been correlated with host immune response in patients with cervical cancer, and the lack of lymphocytic infiltration around cervical cancer cells has been associated with decreased patient survival rates. Both lymph-vascular space invasion and lymphocytic infiltration are therefore of potential clinical significance and should be evaluated in all patients with cervical cancer.

Once the histologic diagnosis of invasive cancer has

been established, each lesion should be staged. *Staging* is defined as the clinical estimation of the extent of disease, and is based on a thorough understanding of the anatomic pathways of spread of cervical cancer.

Basically, the lymphatic drainage within the cervix is arranged in three layers. Subepithelial lymphatics drain into stromal lymphatic trunks which course laterally to anastomose in a network beneath the serosa of the cervix. Lymphatic drainage from the cervix occurs along three major anatomic pathways (Fig. 37-1).

1. Superiorly, cervical cancer cells spread in the stromal lymphatics to involve the lower uterine segment and myometrium. This type of spread has not been recognized in present staging systems for cervical cancer. However, this finding is usually indicative of increased tumor volume and has been noted in 4 to 17 percent of the cases (Wentz and Jaffe,[67] Perez et al.[68]).

2. Inferiorly, cervical cancer spreads to the vagina through a rich network of lymphatics. The lymphatics from the anterior wall of the upper and middle portions of the vagina anastomose with the paracervical and vesical lymphatics to empty into the internal iliac and external iliac lymph nodes. In contrast, lymphatics from the posterior vagina drain to the obturator, pararectal, and aortic lymph nodes. Further extension of a cervical tumor into the lower one-third of the vagina is clinically significant since the lymphatics from this area drain primarily to the inguinal lymph nodes.

3. Laterally, cervical cancer spreads in the paracervical and parametrial lymphatics to involve the ureter and lateral pelvic wall structures. This is the most common pathway of spread of cervical cancer (Plentyl and Friedman[69]). The four primary regional lymph node groups to which cervical cancer most often metastasizes

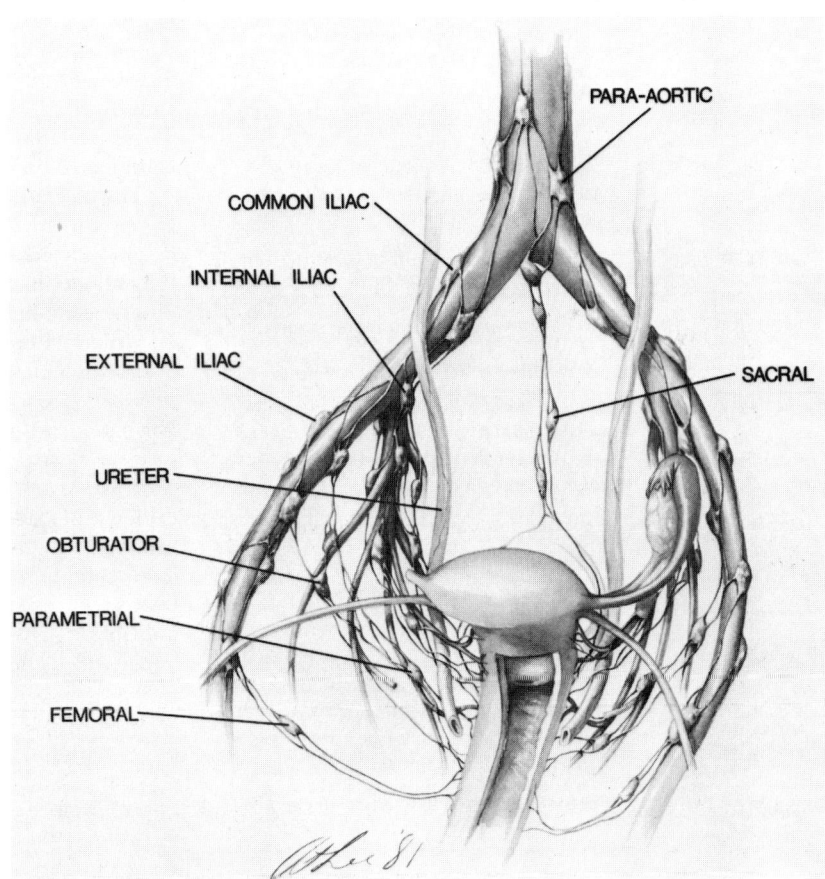

FIGURE 37-1 Lymphatic drainage of the cervix.

are the (1) internal iliac, (2) obturator, (3) external iliac, and (4) common iliac lymph nodes. In a review of the specific sites of lymph node spread in over 700 patients with cervical cancer, Plentyl and Friedman[69] reported that metastases were present in the external iliac group in 23 percent of cases, the obturator nodes in 19 percent, the internal iliac nodes in 17 percent, and the common iliac group in 12 percent.

Although numerous staging systems for cervical cancer have been advocated, the most useful has been the International Federation of Gynecology and Obstetrics (FIGO) staging system (Table 37-2). It is important to note that stage is determined prior to therapy and cannot be changed should more extensive disease be noted at the time of surgery. Therefore, staging allows for an objective comparison of different treatment methods in the therapy of clinically similar lesions. In addition to clinical examination, intravenous pyelography, chest x-ray, radiocolloid scans, cytoscopy, and sigmoidoscopy can be used in determining stage.

The anatomic proximity of the ureters to the cervix makes examination of the lower urinary tract essential in evaluating patients with cervical cancer. Bilateral ureteral obstruction and consequent renal failure is still the most common cause of death in patients with cervical cancer, and the presence of unilateral ureteral obstruction is also of prognostic significance. For example, Bosch et al.[70] noted that patients with advanced-stage disease and ureteral obstruction had a 5-year survival rate of 33 percent, compared with 51 percent in those without this finding. For this reason, the presence of ureteral obstruction automatically places a patient into FIGO stage IIIB. The incidence of ureteral obstruction is directly related to tumor volume, but may occur in patients with clinical evidence of early-stage disease. In a review of intravenous pyelographic findings related to clinical extent of disease, van Nagell et al.[71] reported that 4 out of 181 patients whose tumors were clinically confined to the cervix actually had ureteral obstruction.

The indications for cystoscopy in the evaluation of patients with cervical cancer are less clear. Some investigators have advocated the routine use of cystoscopy in the evaluation of all patients with cervical cancer, whereas others recommend its use only in patients with palpable or visible extension of the tumor toward the bladder. Van Nagell et al.[71] reported the results of cystoscopy in 583 patients with previously unstaged cervical cancer. No patient with stage I or II disease had extension of invasive cervical cancer into the bladder mucosa. In contrast, over 20 percent of patients with palpable evidence of stage IIIB disease had biopsy-proven bladder invasion. At the present time, it is recommended that cystoscopy be performed on all patients with stage IIB disease or greater, or in any case in which there is palpable extension toward the bladder. Histologic evidence of bladder mucosal invasion is necessary for inclusion into stage IVA.

In addition to staging each cervical cancer, every effort should be made to accurately describe the size and anatomic location of each tumor. This is particularly important in stage IB lesions, which may vary extensively in size and configuration. Piver and Chung[72] noted that the 5-year survival rate of patients with stage IB lesions

TABLE 37-2 International Federation of Gynecology and Obstetrics Staging System for Invasive Cervical Cancer

Stage I	Carcinoma strictly confined to the cervix (extension to the corpus should be disregarded).
Stage IA	Microinvasive carcinoma (early stromal invasion).
Stage IB	All other cases of stage I. Occult cancer should be marked "occ."
Stage II	The carcinoma extends beyond the cervix, but not the lower third.
Stage IIA	No obvious parametrial involvement.
Stage IIB	Obvious parametrial involvement.
Stage III	The carcinoma has extended on to the pelvic wall. On rectal examination there is no cancer-free space between the tumor and the pelvic wall.
Stage IIIA	No extension on to the pelvic wall.
Stage IIIB	Extension on to the pelvic wall and/or hydronephrosis or nonfunctioning kidney.
Stage IV	The carcinoma has extended beyond the true pelvis or has clinically involved the mucosa of the bladder or rectum. A bullous edema as such does not permit a case to be allotted to stage IV.
Stage IVA	Spread of the growth to adjacent organs.
Stage IVB	Spread to distant organs.

less than 3 cm in diameter was 88 percent, compared with 65 percent in patients having tumors greater than 3 cm in diameter. Similarly, van Nagell et al.[73] reported a recurrence rate of 9 percent in patients with stage IB cervical cancer and a lesion size of 2 cm or less in diameter. In contrast, patients with the same-stage disease but with lesions greater than 2 cm experienced a recurrence rate of 44 percent. Recent evidence would suggest that tumor regression during radiation therapy is a most reliable parameter for monitoring tumor response and patient outcome. For example, Marcial and Bosch[74] found that patients whose tumors demonstrated significant regression by the end of external therapy had a 96 percent 3-year survival rate as opposed to a 2 percent survival rate for patients whose tumors never regressed during therapy. For this reason, an accurate description of tumor dimensions prior to treatment is essential.

The correlation between clinical staging and surgical findings is approximately 70 percent, with the majority of patients having more extensive disease than is clinically apparent. For this reason, certain investigators (Bernadino and Dodd[75]) have advocated the use of CT scanning as an adjunct to clinical staging. Computed tomography is very accurate in detecting the extension of cervical cancer into the structures of the lateral pelvic walls. Also, it can be used to determine response to treatment and to diagnose persistent cervical cancer. Pelvic fibrosis occurring after radiation therapy may mimic tumor recurrence, but, unlike recurrent cancer, is usually symmetrical. An asymmetrical area of pelvic soft-tissue density diagnosed after radiation therapy by computed tomography is highly suspicious for recurrent cancer and should be biopsied by fine-needle aspiration.

Another area of tumor spread which is often undiagnosed is the paraaortic lymph nodes. The incidence of extrapelvic lymph node metastases may be as high as 30 percent in patients with bulky advanced-stage disease (Averette et al.,[76] Buchsbaum[77]), and these metastases would not be included in the traditional pelvic fields of radiation therapy. Consequently, it has been recommended that patients with bulky stage IB and IIB tumors as well as all patients with more advanced stage disease should have lymphangiography and CT scans to identify lymph node metastases. The accuracy of lymphangiography in determining the presence of lymph node disease has varied widely in the literature. Piver and Barlow[78] reported that 23 of 24 cervical cancer patients with abnormal lymphangiographic findings actually had histologic evidence of tumor metastases in the paraaortic nodes. Nevertheless, small foci of metastatic disease may not be detected by lymphangiography (Brown et al.[79]). Patients with suspicious or positive findings on lymphangiogram and computed tomography should have further evaluation, such as selective lymph node biopsy or fine-needle biopsy. Although an intraperitoneal approach to pretherapy selective lymph node biopsy was once advocated (Buchsbaum[80]), this method has been associated with a significant incidence of complications when followed by radiation therapy. Consequently, a retroperitoneal approach to the paraaortic lymph nodes has recently been recommended (Schellhas,[81] LaGasse et al.[82]). This method does not allow for as extensive an exploration of the lower pelvic lymph nodes as does the intraperitoneal approach. However, it has been associated with extremely few postradiation complications.

Percutaneous transperitoneal lymph node biopsy using a small-gauge needle has been utilized successfully in a small number of cervical cancer patients with suspected extrapelvic lymph node metastases (Zornoza et al.,[83,84] Wallace et al.[85]). Fine-needle biopsy is directed by fluoroscopy or ultrasound and has been effective in confirming the presence of metastases in the iliac and paraaortic lymph nodes. This technique can be performed using local anesthesia, and has been associated with very few complications (Holm et al.[86]). Nevertheless, the accuracy of this technique in detecting microscopic metastases in a small area of a lymph node must be questioned.

In addition to those studies related to tumor biology, there are a number of clinical variables which should be evaluated in patients undergoing radiation therapy. All patients should be questioned concerning a history of prior abdominal surgery. Previous surgery is often associated with intraperitoneal adhesions and fixation of the bowel within the pelvis. Consequently, radiation therapy following surgery is often associated with an increased incidence of enteric complications, including small-bowel obstruction and fistula formation. Similarly, pelvic inflammatory disease has been shown to produce reactive vasculitis and fibrin thrombosis in the small arterioles of the bowel and bladder (van Nagell et al.[87]). Radiation-induced capillary endothelial proliferation and lumenal narrowing often causes localized tissue hypoperfusion and hypoxia, and the combination of radiation and pelvic inflammation has been associated with an increased incidence of bowel or urinary tract injury. For the same reason, patients with underlying vascular disease such as diabetes mellitis or hypertension are also at high risk to develop radiation-related enteric complications (van Nagell et al.,[88,89] Maruyama et al.[90]). Several investigators (van Nagell et al.[91]) have shown a direct correlation between retinal and pelvic vessel status. Patients with a history of vascular disease should undergo a complete evaluation including fundoscopic examination in an effort to quantitate the severity of arteriolar narrowing.

Finally, nutritional status is very important in cervical cancer patients being treated either with radiation therapy or radical surgery. The incidence of radiation complications has been shown to be higher in patients who prior to therapy are underweight according to standard height and weight charts (van Nagell et al.[88,89]). Also, Copeland[92] has reported that patients who are malnourished have delayed wound healing and increased morbidity rates following surgery. Therefore, a careful nutritional history including recent weight change should be documented in all patients prior to treatment.

THERAPY

Microinvasive Cancer

The optimal treatment of microinvasive carcinoma of the cervix has been somewhat controversial since a variety of definitions of this entity have been adopted. In addition, a number of these definitions have been associated with a low but appreciable incidence of lymph node metastases (Christopherson et al.[93], Ruch[94]). In order for patients with microinvasive cervical cancer to be adequately treated by conservative hysterectomy alone, a definition must be accepted which precludes the possibility of metastatic cancer being present in pelvic lymph nodes. As previously stated, the recommended definition of microinvasion was first proposed in 1974 by the Society of Gynecologic Oncology, namely, cervical carcinoma in which stromal invasion is limited to a depth of less than 3 mm without lymph-vascular space invasion. This diagnosis can be made only from a conization specimen which has been sectioned adequately and examined with an ocular micrometer to accurately establish the depth of invasion. By these histologic criteria, the optimal therapy for microinvasive carcinoma is total abdominal hysterectomy. Abdominal hysterectomy is preferable to vaginal hysterectomy in that it enables any palpably enlarged lymph nodes to be biopsied and sent for pathologic examination. Colposcopy should be performed prior to surgery on all patients with microinvasive carcinoma in order to adequately define the presence of any areas of vaginal extension. Should there be any question as to whether the depth of stromal invasion extends beyond 3 mm or whether lymph-vascular space invasion by tumor cells exists, then a radical hysterectomy with pelvic lymphadenectomy should be performed.

Invasive Cervical Cancer

The major prerequisite of any therapeutic method in the treatment of invasive cervical cancer is that it treat not only the primary tumor but also the regional lymph nodes to which the primary tumor might spread. Both radical hysterectomy with pelvic lymphadenectomy and radiation therapy have been advocated in the treatment of cervical cancer. However, there have been few prospective randomized clinical trials which establish the specific indications for the use of one therapeutic method or the other. There are a number of studies that provide meaningful data concerning optimal treatment for varying stages of disease. In a randomized study of 100 patients with all stages of invasive cervical cancer, Roddick and Greenlaw[95] reported that survival rates were generally higher in the radiation therapy group. However, prognosis was virtually the same in patients with stage I disease treated by either method. Similarly, Masubuchi et al.[96] noted no significant difference in the survival rates of patients with stage I invasive cancer treated by radical hysterectomy either with pelvic lymphadenectomy or with radiation therapy.

More recently, certain investigators have proposed a more individualized approach to determine optimal therapy based on the analysis of a number of factors including stage, lesion size and configuration, and cell type. This approach is also based on the general concept that the efficacy of radical surgery decreases markedly when cervical cancer has spread to regional pelvic lymph nodes. Brunschwig and Barber,[97] in a study of 273 patients undergoing radical hysterectomy and pelvic lymphadenectomy for stage IB cervical cancer, reported that the 5-year survival rate of patients with pelvic lymph node metastases was 50 percent, compared with 83 percent when the lymph nodes were free of tumor. Similarly, Webb and Symmonds[98] reported that the 5-year survival rate of patients with stage IB cervical cancer and lymph node metastases treated with radical surgery was only 57 percent. It is reasonable to assume that radical hysterectomy is most effective in the treatment of cervical cancer when the incidence of positive pelvic lymph nodes does not exceed 20 percent. As has been mentioned previously, it is not always possible to diagnose preoperatively which patients have microscopic pelvic lymph node metastases. Lymphangiography is quite accurate if the lymph node is replaced by tumor. However, microscopic metastases to these lymph nodes are often missed by this technique (Averette et al.[99]). In this regard, analysis of the relationship between cervical lesion size and lymph node metastases is helpful. Piver and Chung[72] reported a direct correlation between lesion size and the incidence of pelvic lymph node metastases. Thirty-five percent of patients with stage IB lesions greater than 3 cm in diameter had pelvic lymph node metastases, compared with only 21 percent in lesions less than 3 cm in diameter. The 5-year survival rate of patients with stage IB cervical cancer and lesions less than 3 cm in diameter was 88 percent, but fell to 66 percent in patients with larger lesions. These investigators concluded that radical surgery was the indicated method of therapy in patients with stage IB disease and a lesion size of less than 3 cm, whereas radiation therapy was preferable in larger or more advanced stage lesions. These results were confirmed by van Nagell et al.,[32] who noted a survival rate in excess of 90 percent when patients with stage IB cervical cancer and a lesion size 2 cm or less in diameter were treated with radical hysterectomy and pelvic lymphadenectomy.

Finally, the cell type of cervical cancer has also been related to metastatic potential. Small-cell carcinomas of the cervix have been shown to have a significantly higher incidence of lymph node metastases than large-cell tumors. For example, van Nagell et al.[33] reported that lymph node metastases were present in over 50 percent of patients with stage IB small-cell cancers as opposed to less than 20 percent in patients with stage IB large-cell cancers. Recurrent carcinomas developed in 54 percent of small-cell carcinomas treated with radical surgery compared with 31 percent in patients treated with radiation therapy. This difference in recurrence rate occurred despite the fact that the larger cervical lesions were generally treated by radiation therapy.

Based on a thorough analysis of the previously mentioned data, this author believes that radical hysterectomy with pelvic lymphadenectomy is the treatment of choice in young women with stage IB large-cell squamous carcinomas of the cervix less than 3 cm in diameter. In addition, radical surgery may be preferable when the patient has pelvic inflammatory disease or when benign pathology has distorted pelvic anatomy in such a way as to prevent the proper application of intracavitary radiation. The advantage of radical surgery over radiation therapy, particularly in the younger patient, is that ovarian and vaginal function is preserved, while major radiation-related complications, such as pelvic fibrosis and fistulas of the bowel or bladder, are avoided. Although there is no data from controlled trials establishing the beneficial effect of postoperative radiation on the survival rates of patients found to have pelvic lymph node metastases at the time of surgery, its use is recommended. Theoretically, a certain number of patients with positive pelvic lymph nodes will have microscopic metastases in the intervening lymphatics. These microscopic lymphatics should be susceptible to radiation therapy given in doses within the tolerance of normal lateral pelvic wall structures. For this reason, it is recommended that all patients with lymph node metastases receive postoperative external therapy to the pelvis. A dose of 5000 to 6000 rads is given to a field size including the area from which positive lymph nodes were removed. Dose fractionation is increased following surgery owing to the decreased radiation tolerance of tissues previously devascularized by operative intervention, and external therapy is given at a dose rate of 150 to 180 rads/day. In patients with paraaortic metastases, every effort should be made to biopsy the scalene lymph nodes. Buchsbaum et al.[77] reported that up to 30 percent of patients with paraaortic lymph node metastases had scalene nodal spread. Should metastatic cervical cancer be present in mediastinal or scalene nodes, then it is necessary to treat the patient with primary adjunctive chemotherapy.

Recently, tumor cell invasion of lymph-vascular spaces within the surgical specimen has been shown to significantly increase the incidence of tumor recurrence (Barber et al.[66]). Van Nagell et al. noted that lymph-vascular space invasion was associated with a 30 percent increase in the recurrence rate of patients with stage IB disease. Over one-half of these patients had recurrences confined to the pelvis. For this reason, it is also suggested that patients with histologic evidence of lymphvascular space invasion in the surgical specimen receive postoperative radiation therapy.

The operation of radical hysterectomy with pelvic lymphadenectomy has undergone numerous modifications since its original description (Clark,[3] Ries[2]). The purpose of this procedure is the en bloc removal of the cervix, uterus, parametria, and upper vagina, together with the obturator, internal iliac, external iliac, and common iliac lymph nodes (Fig. 37-2). The uterine artery is ligated near its origin on the internal iliac artery, and the ureters are dissected free of parametrial lymphatic tissue until their entrance into the bladder. The pubovesical ligament and superior vesical artery are preserved in order to maintain the blood supply to the distal ureter and to decrease the incidence of fistula formation. The uterosacral ligaments are resected at the pelvic sidewall, and the upper one-third of the vagina is removed. Every effort should be made to meticulously remove all lymph nodes in the obturator and iliac groups. Kolbenstveldt and Kolstad,[102] utilizing preoperative and postoperative lymphangiography, noted that pelvic lymphadenectomy was often incomplete. Specifically, the lateral sacral nodes of the internal iliac group were the lymph nodes most often missed.

Medical advances such as the perfection of methods for rapid blood transfusion, improved anesthesia, and the use of prophylactic antibiotics have significantly reduced the operative morbidity and mortality rates of radical hysterectomy. In addition, there have been technical improvements in the operation itself. These include (1) vaginal vault closure with peritonealization of the bladder base, rectum, and ureters; (2) retroperitoneal suction drainage; and (3) suprapubic bladder drainage. Symmonds and Pratt[13] first advocated the technique of vaginal cuff closure and retroperitoneal suction drainage in radical hysterectomy and pelvic lymphadenectomy. Hemovac drains are placed in both iliac fossae and are brought out through the lower quadrants of the abdomen (Fig. 37-3). These investigators reported that the use of vaginal vault closure and retroperitoneal suction drainage caused a significant reduction in the incidence of vesicovaginal fistulae, ureterovaginal fistulae, and lymphocysts following radical hysterectomy with pelvic lymphadenectomy. With proper placement of drains the volume of retroperitoneal drainage can be measured, and the specific protein and electrolyte losses replaced. The drainage volume usually is 300 to 400 mL on the first postoperative day and declines to 50 mL by the sixth day following surgery.

The extensive dissection of the bladder base and lateral parametrium in radical hysterectomy with pelvic lymphadenectomy often results in interruption of autonomic nerve fibers, initially causing bladder hypertonicity and decreased vesical capacity. This phase is followed by bladder hypotonicity and increased residual volume, which increases the risk of urinary tract fistulae. For this reason, Green et al.[103] postulated that constant catheter drainage of the bladder for up to 6 weeks following surgery would decrease fistula formation. These investigators reported that postoperative bladder drainage following radical hysterectomy reduced major ureteral

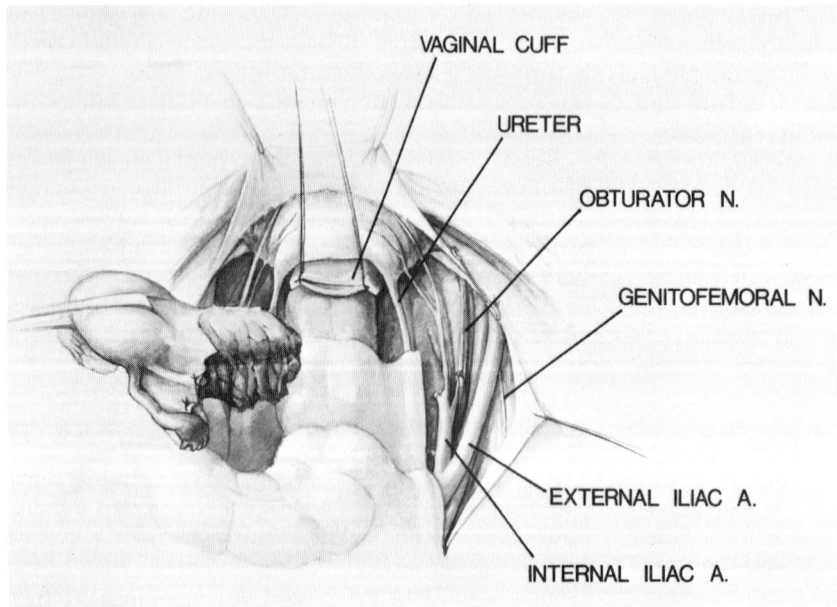

FIGURE 37-2 Schematic illustration of radical hysterectomy and pelvic lymphadenectomy. The surgical specimen including the uterus, parametrial tissue, and pelvic lymph nodes is reflected to the left.

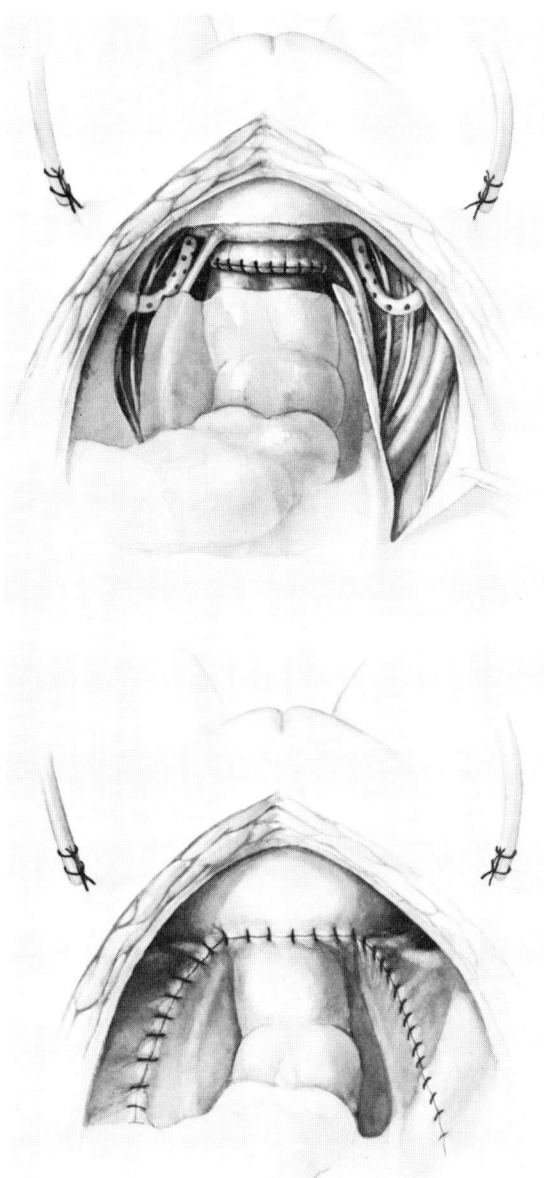

FIGURE 37-3 Illustration of proper placement of Hemovac drains in the retroperitoneal space following radical hysterectomy and pelvic lymphadenectomy. Reperitonealization of the pelvis is performed after these drains are in place.

complication by over 50 percent. More recently, van Nagell et al.[104] reported the use of suprapubic bladder drainage in patients undergoing radical hysterectomy. A Foley catheter is placed in the bladder under direct vision at the time of surgery and brought out suprapubically through the anterior vesical space (Fig. 37-4). The catheter is removed only when the postvoiding bladder residual is less than 50 mL. This method of catheter drainage is associated with a lower incidence of urinary tract infection than urethral catheterization, and is more comfortable for the patient.

The most common complications following radical hysterectomy and pelvic lymph node dissection involve the urinary tract. Bladder hypotonicity and the resultant increase in residual volume predispose the patient to the development of infection. Webb and Symmonds,[98] for example, reported that 15 percent of patients undergoing radical hysterectomy developed a urinary tract infection during the postoperative period. For this reason, patients should be maintained on a urinary antibacterial agent as long as a catheter remains in the bladder. The incidence of urinary tract fistulae following radical hysterectomy and pelvic lymphadenectomy is presented in Table 37-3. The incidence of ureterovaginal fistulae is generally higher than that of vesicovaginal fistulae, but both have decreased in frequency over the past decade. Underwood et al.[105] reported no ureteral fistulae following 92 radical hysterectomies performed since 1967. Similar findings have been reported by Sall et al.[106] and Averette.[99]

Ureterovaginal fistulae occur most commonly in the distal ureter where the ureter has been dissected from the parametrial tunnel. These fistulae should be repaired as soon as possible after diagnosis in order to prevent damage to the upper urinary tract. In most cases, extensive surgical dissection of the distal ureter makes ureteral anastomosis impractical, and resection of the fistula with ureteroneocystotomy is the procedure of choice. Should the ureter be injured above the pelvic brim, primary reanastomosis or transureteroureterostomy is indicated. Ureteral stenosis following radical hysterectomy is quite rare, being reported in less than 1 percent of patients. However, it may cause impairment of renal function without producing any symptoms. Therefore, patients undergoing radical hysterectomy with pelvic lymphadenectomy should have postoperative intravenous pyelography to rule out the presence of occult ureteral stenosis, and should have repeat intravenous pyelography each year following surgery. Patients

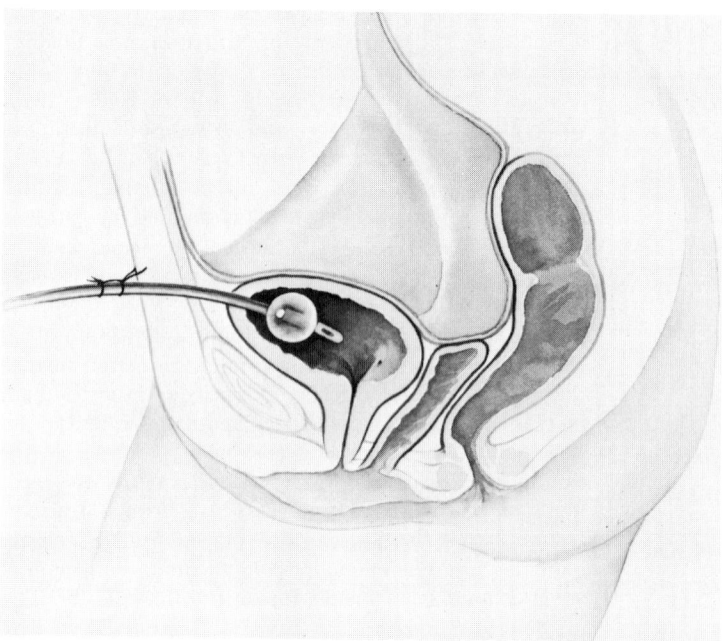

FIGURE 37-4 Suprapubic bladder drainage utilized in patients undergoing radical hysterectomy and pelvic lymphadenectomy. Catheter is brought out through a suprapubic skin incision.

with ureteral stenosis may respond to periodic ureteral dilatation, but in selected cases ureteral resection with ureteroneocystotomy is necessary.

Vesicovaginal fistulae are less common than ureterovaginal fistulae since bladder injury is often recognized and repaired intraoperatively. It is suggested that the bladder be filled with 300 mL of saline following completion of radical hysterectomy and node dissection. This allows detection of defects in the bladder wall, which can be surgically corrected prior to fistula formation. Should a vesicovaginal fistula be diagnosed, the patient should undergo cystoscopy to fully define the size and location of the injury. The patient should be placed on antibiotics and the fistula site free of necrosis prior to attempting surgical repair. Vesicovaginal fistulae can be repaired either vaginally or from an intracystic approach, and a new source of blood supply such as the omentum should be transposed to the operative site when possible. In the absence of previous radiation therapy, vesicovaginal fistula repair is almost always successful, and urinary diversion can be avoided.

A major life-threatening medical complication, parti-

TABLE 37-3 Incidence of Ureterovaginal and Vesicovaginal Fistulae Following Radical Hysterectomy with Pelvic Lymphadenectomy

Investigator	Number of patients	Uretero-vaginal fistula	Vesico-vaginal fistula
Liu and Meigs[12]	473	28 (5.9%)	3 (0.6%)
Green et al.[103]	623	53 (8.5%)	14 (2.2%)
Green	65	1 (1.5%)	0 (0.0%)
Averette[99]	44	0 (0.0%)	0 (0.0%)
Park et al.[153]	189	0 (0.0%)	0 (0.0%)
Sall et al.[106]	349	7 (2.0%)	3 (0.9%)
Webb and Symmonds[98]	564	15 (2.6%)	13 (2.3%)
Underwood et al.[105]	92	0 (0%)	0 (0%)

cularly in older patients undergoing radical hysterectomy, is pulmonary embolism. Webb and Symmonds[98] reported that 29 of 564 patients (5.1 percent) experienced phlebitis following radical hysterectomy, and 1 patient died of pulmonary embolus in the immediate postoperative period. For this reason, it is recommended that patients undergoing radical hysterectomy be given "minidose" heparin subcutaneously in doses of 5000 units beginning 2 h prior to surgery and every 12 h thereafter until full ambulation. This regimen has reduced the incidence of phlebitis and has not been associated with postoperative bleeding or hematoma formation.

Although several investigators have advocated the use of radical hysterectomy and pelvic lymphadenectomy following radiation therapy, (Surwit et al.,[107] Rampone[108]), the combination of two radical therapeutic methods is generally associated with an increased incidence of major enteric or urinary tract complications without increasing patient survival rates. The effect of radiation on the microcirculation causes devascularization of normal pelvic organs, which are often further damaged by the extensive dissection necessary for complete lymphadenectomy. Underwood et al.,[105] for example, reported that 8 of 12 patients given radiation therapy prior to radical hysterectomy developed vaginal fistulae, and concluded that the increased morbidity and mortality rates associated with combined therapy did not justify its use.

There is more evidence to support the use of extrafascial hysterectomy following radiation therapy in patients with barrel-shaped stage IB and IIB lesions, and in selected cases of stage IB tumors that do not respond to radiation therapy. Barrel-shaped lesions characteristically contain a large volume of hypoxic, noncycling cells, and their anatomic configuration is such that the endocervical component of the tumor is often outside the isodose curve of curative radiation therapy. Consequently, there is a high incidence of central recurrence when these lesions are treated by radiation alone (Jampolis et al.[109]). In order to reduce the high central recurrence rate in patients with bulky endocervical tumors, Fletcher and Rutledge[91] proposed the addition of extrafascial hysterectomy following radiation therapy. External therapy was reduced to 4000 rads and followed by one intracavitary implant providing a dose of 4000 to 5000 milligram-hours. Extrafascial hysterectomy was then performed 4 to 6 weeks later. Using this technique, Durrance et al.[110] reported a reduction in central recurrence from 15 percent to 3 percent. In a later study from the same institution, Nelson et al.[111] reported that the use of postradiation hysterectomy increased the 5-year survival rate of patients with bulky stage IB lesions to that of patients with nonbulky stage IB tumors. The incidence of localized pelvic recurrence in patients treated with combination therapy was reduced to only 2 percent. In a similar study, van Nagell et al.[73] reported that the addition of extrafascial hysterectomy to radiation therapy significantly reduced the recurrence rate of stage IB cervical cancers greater than 5 cm in diameter.

A second indication for the use of adjunctive extrafascial hysterectomy is the presence of persistent cervical disease in patients with stage IB lesions treated initially by irradiation. Marcial et al.[74] carefully studied the regression patterns of cervical cancers during radiation therapy and related them to prognosis. Those patients with tumors demonstrating significant regression by the end of external therapy (4500 rads) had a 96 percent 3-year survival rate, whereas only 2 percent of patients whose cervical tumors did not regress during radiation therapy survived 3 years. Likewise, Hardt et al.[112] noted that cervical cancer patients having no palpable or visible evidence of disease 1 month following completion of therapy had a 95 percent 5-year survival rate. Patients with residual gross tumor at this time had a recurrence rate of 80 percent. In general, the response rate of tumors to radiation was directly related to the extent of disease prior to treatment. However, the recurrence rate of stage IB lesions not regressing during radiation therapy was 60 percent. At present, the benefit of extrafascial hysterectomy has not been confirmed in a prospective randomized study. Such studies are in progress, however, and it is recommended that patients with stage IB lesions not responding to radiation should be considered for adjunctive hysterectomy.

Radiation therapy is presently the therapeutic method of choice in most patients with (1) stage IB lesions greater than 3 cm in diameter, (2) small-cell carcinomas, and (3) stages II to IV lesions. This assertion is based generally on the assumption that radiation therapy is superior to radical surgery when cervical cancer has metastasized to pelvic lymph nodes. In patients with lymph node spread, there is a high probability that microscopic tumor metastases that are not visible are present in the intervening lymphatics. Therefore, it is extremely difficult, if not impossible, to surgically remove these microscopic metastases. The higher the frequency of lymph node metastases, the lower the efficacy of radical surgery as a treatment method in cervical cancer. The validity of this assumption is strengthened by the reported low survival rate of patients with advanced-stage disease treated primarily with radical surgery (Brunschwig and Daniel,[113] Roddick and Greenlaw[95]). However, it must be emphasized that the optimal treatment method must be selected individually for each patient. In a patient with pelvic inflammatory disease or a specific anatomic abnormality precluding proper intracavitary therapy, radical surgery either alone or in combination with external radiation may be preferable.

A concept essential to effective radiotherapy is that the radiation dose should be given in such a way as to obtain the maximum tumor control with a minimum of normal tissue complications. Most treatment plans are designed to give doses which will produce no more than a 5 percent normal tissue complication rate. Radiation therapy for cervical cancer is usually given as a combination of external therapy and one or two intracavitary implants. The primary purpose of external therapy is to decrease tumor volume and to reduce the gross anatomic distortion produced by invasion of normal pelvic structures. In patients with stage IB and IIA disease, 4000 rads external therapy is given from a linear accelerator or a cobalt-60 source at a dose rate of 200 rads/day. Patients with more advanced stage disease are treated with 4000 to 5000 rads external therapy given over 5 to 7 weeks. Any patient with prior abdominal surgery, extremely poor nutritional status, or severe vascular disease is treated at a reduced dose rate of 160 rads/day since this group is at high risk for the development of radiation-related complications. The field size for pelvic irradiation is individualized but is generally 16 by 16 cm with the top of the field being at the L4-L5 interspace. Patients who have a small anterior-posterior (AP) diameter (< 20 cm) are usually treated with two AP ports, whereas larger patients are often treated with an arrangement of two AP and two lateral ports to obtain optimal dosimetry. Midline shielding is employed, with the width of the shielded area varying from 3 to 6 cm depending upon the implant isodose pattern. A pelvic sidewall boost of 500 to 1000 rads is given in selected patients, depending upon the stage and anatomic configuration of the tumor. Intracavitary therapy, usually in the form of an intrauterine tandem and vaginal ovoids, is given after completion of external radiation. Most often, two radionuclide implants are given 14 to 21 days apart. Through a combination of intracavitary and external therapy, the tumor is given 12,000 to 15,000 rads, the paracervical area (point A) 8000 rads, and the lateral pelvic wall 5500 to 6000 rads. The major limiting factor to the amount of radiation given to the tumor is the radiation tolerance of normal adjacent structures. In general, the bladder should be given no more than 7000 rads, the ureters no more than 7500 rads, the rectum and sigmoid colon no more than 6000 rads, and the small bowel no more than 4500 rads.

As has been previously discussed, the incidence of paraaortic metastases in patients with cervical cancer may be as high as 40 percent in advanced-stage disease (Nelson et al.,[111] Piver and Barlow[114]). The diagnosis of extrapelvic lymph node metastases is usually made by lymphangiography or computed tomography, but must be confirmed histologically by fine-needle aspiration or retroperitoneal lymph node sampling prior to therapy. When paraaortic metastases are documented, the radiation field is reduced in width and extended upward from the pelvic field (L4-L5 interspace) to the level of the T12 vertebral body. A total dose of 5000 to 5500 rads is given to this extended field at a dose rate of 150 to 200 rads/day (Fletcher et al.,[21] Piver and Barlow[114]). Although long-term survival data on significant numbers of patients undergoing extended-field radiation for paraaortic metastases are unavailable, preliminary results suggest that the 5-year survival rate of these patients may be as high as 20 percent (Hughes et al.[115]).

Radiation-related complications in cervical cancer patients are generally dose-related. Kottmeier and Gray,[116] in a study of 500 patients treated at the Radiumhemmet, reported that there was a direct correlation between measured bladder and rectal doses and complications. The incidence of radiation-induced complications was also related to the dose of external therapy and to the volume of tissue irradiated. There were no radiation injuries when the dose of external radiation was less than 4000 rads.

Patients at high risk to develop major radiation complications are those with (1) poor nutritional status, (2) previous abdominal surgery, (3) severe vascular disease, (4) pelvic inflammatory disease, or (5) radiation reactions during therapy. As has been previously stated, patients who are underweight and malnourished have a decreased tissue response to all forms of injury and have an increased incidence of radiation complications (van Nagell et al.[88,89]). Every effort should be made to improve protein intake, including intravenous hyperalimentation, in a malnourished patient undergoing radiation therapy for cervical cancer. Likewise, a patient with previous abdominal surgery may have fixation of small bowel in the pelvis and be at high risk to develop enteric complications following radiation. Buchler et al.[117,118] have reported that patients experiencing severe radiation reactions during therapy are more likely to experience subsequent enteric or urinary tract injuries. The majority of complications from radiation therapy are related to the vascular damage caused by ionizing radiation. Radiation causes capillary endothelial and intimal thickening with lumenal narrowing and decreased tissue perfusion. The superimposed systemic microangiopathy present in patients with diabetes mellitus or hypertension further accentuates lumenal narrowing in the arterioles of the bowel and bladder, and the resultant tissue hypoxia may cause local necrosis and fistula formation. Likewise, pelvic inflammatory disease causes a reactive vasculitis of the small vessels of the bowel and bladder, which are then particularly susceptible to radiation damage (van Nagell et al.[87]).

The incidence of specific radiation complications as summarized from selected large series in the literature is illustrated in Table 37-4. Severe radiation complications including enteric or urinary tract fistulae and small-bowel obstruction are fortunately quite rare, being reported in less than 5 percent of patients. The most common complication in cervical cancer patients undergoing radiation therapy is vaginal stenosis. It has been reported that vaginal stenosis occurs in over 70 percent of patients. Although this complication is usually not associated with significant morbidity, it can impair sexual function. Therefore, it is recommended that patients continue vaginal activity during radiation therapy, and that vaginal dilators be used in specific cases.

The three most severe radiation-related complications in cervical cancer patients are rectovaginal fistulae, vesicovaginal fistulae, and small-bowel obstruction. The rectum is more susceptible to radiation than any other organ because of its anatomic proximity to the vagina and cervix. Sigmoiditis or proctitis occurs in approximately 10 to 15 percent of patients, and should be treated by a low-residue diet, antispasmodics, and cortisone enemas in severe cases. Rectovaginal fistula occurs in approximately 1 percent of patients undergoing therapy for cervical cancer and is caused by radiation necrosis of the anterior rectal wall. Barium enema and proctoscopy should be performed in order to rule out the presence of recurrent cancer. Generally, a diverting colostomy is performed to facilitate healing at the fistula site. Once the fistula is clean and the necrotic tissue has been removed, fistula repair can be attempted. Adequate blood supply is extremely important to successful healing, and transposition of the omentum to the operative site is often routinely performed at the time of fistula repair.

Vesicovaginal fistula also occurs in approximately 1 percent of cervical cancer patients undergoing radiation therapy. Patients with radiation-induced vaginal vault necrosis are particularly susceptible to the subsequent development of vesicovaginal fistulae, and should be treated with peroxide douches. The principles of vesicovaginal fistula repair are similar to those used in the management of rectovaginal fistulae. Surgical repair of small vesicovaginal fistulae may be successful provided that the fistula site is clean and has a good vascular supply.

Perhaps the most severe radiation injury in cervical cancer patients is small-bowel obstruction. The mucosa of the small bowel is quite sensitive to radiation, the incidence of small-bowel complications is highest in patients with previous surgery and underlying vascular

TABLE 37-4 Radiation-Related Complications in Patients Treated for Cervical Cancer

Investigator	Number of patients	Sigmoiditis	Rectovaginal fistula	Small-bowel obstruction	Ureteral stricture	Hemorrhagic cystitis	Vesicovaginal fistula
Chau et al.[154]	741	42 (5.7%)	8 (1.0%)	6 (0.8%)	11 (1.5%)	18 (2.4%)	4 (0.2%)
Peckham et al.[155]	346	18 (5.2%)	4 (1.2%)	16 (1.7%)	6 (1.7%)	16 (4.6%)	1 (0.2%)
Stockbine et al.[156]	831	76 (9.1%)	18 (2.2%)	36 (4.3%)		6 (0.7%)	16 (1.9%)
Villasanta et al.[157]	641	61 (9.5%)	18 (2.8%)	10 (1.6%)	13 (2.0%)	35 (5.6%)	6 (0.9%)
Bosch et al.[70]	1139	86 (7.5%)	9 (0.8%)	5 (0.4%)	1 (0.1%)	25 (2.2%)	3 (0.3%)
Total	3698	283 (7.6%)	51 (1.4%)	73 (2.0%)	31 (0.8%)	100 (2.7%)	30 (0.8%)

768 GYNECOLOGIC NEOPLASMS

disease who have received high doses (approximately 5000 rads) of whole-pelvis or extended-field irradiation. The patient with partial small-bowel obstruction usually presents with a history of crampy abdominal pain and progressive weight loss. The diagnosis of bowel obstruction is confirmed by flat and upright abdominal radiograms. Patients with mild degrees of intermittent obstruction should be treated by conservative measures and nutritional support. However, if complete small-bowel obstruction is present, surgical intervention is required as soon as possible to prevent perforation. The terminal ileum is the most common site of small-bowel obstruction because it is fixed at the ileocecal junction and has a relatively poor blood supply. At present, there is controversy concerning the optimal surgical therapy for radiation-related small-bowel obstruction. Wheeless[119] has advocated bypassing the involved segment with the creation of mucous fistulas (Fig. 37-5). Conversely, Schmitt and Symmonds[120] favor excision of the localized area of obstruction with primary anastomosis of the ileum to the cecum or the ascending colon. In patients having widespread necrosis of the bowel wall with perforation, excision may be impractical. However, in cases of isolated small-bowel obstruction, primary resection with side-to-side anastomosis of the ileum to the ascending colon is indicated.

Recently, there has been increased interest in the possible role of chemotherapy in the primary treatment of cervical cancer. Data concerning the efficacy of single-agent chemotherapy in cervical cancer is summarized in

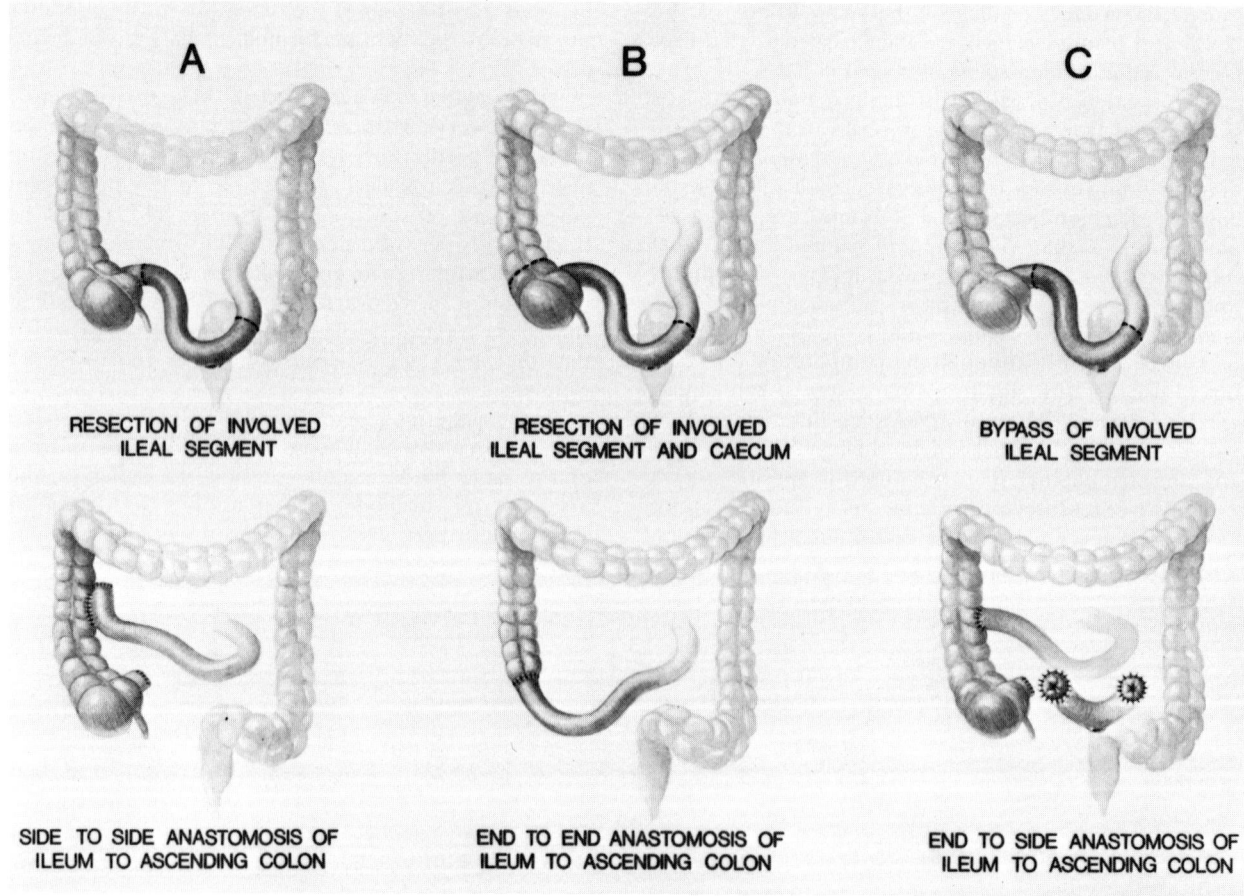

FIGURE 37-5 Surgical procedures used in the treatment of postradiation small-bowel obstruction. Site of obstruction is either bypassed or excised.

Table 37-5. A response was defined as reduction in measurable tumor dimensions of at least 50 percent for a time period of 1 month or more. Most of these agents induce objective responses in 10 to 25 percent of cases. However, the majority of these responses are not complete and are of relatively short duration. Although the number of patients evaluated is small, cis-platinum appears to be a relatively effective drug, with over 25 percent of treated cases achieving partial remission and 12 percent reporting complete tumor disappearance (Thigpen et al.[121]). Combination chemotherapy has been evaluated by a number of cooperative oncology groups. Combinations of bleomycin and mitomycin C or cis-platinum have been particularly effective, producing remission rates in excess of 27 percent (Table 37-6). Nevertheless, the majority of responses have been observed in extrapelvic metastatic disease, and the median response duration has been less than 4 months. Importantly, the use of combination chemotherapy has had a minimal effect on survival rates despite apparently increased response frequency. There remains a definite need for the implementation of clinical trials to evaluate the efficacy of chemotherapy as an adjunct to radiation and surgery in the primary therapy of certain types of cervical cancer at high risk for extrapelvic recurrence. Two such groups are (1) patients with stages IIB to IV small-cell carcinoma of the cervix and (2) patients with histologically confirmed paraaortic lymph node metastases.

TABLE 37-5 Single-Agent Chemotherapy in Cervical Cancer

Drug	Patients evaluated	Response
Alkylating Agents		
Cyclophosphamide	188	29 (15%)
Chlorambucil	44	11 (25%)
Melphalan	20	4 (20%)
Antibiotics		
Adriamycin	82	14 (17%)
Bleomycin	172	17 (10%)
Mitomycin C	18	4 (22%)
Porfiromycin	78	17 (22%)
Miscellaneous Agents		
Piperazinedione	33	2 (6%)
cis-Platinum	34	13 (38%)
Dianhydrogalactitol	36	7 (19%)
ICRF-159	28	5 (18%)
Baker's Antifol	32	5 (16%)

SOURCE: Devita et al.,[158] Wasserman and Carter,[159] and Thigpen et al.[140]

TABLE 37-6 Multiple-Agent Chemotherapy in Cervical Cancer

Drug combination	Patients evaluated	Response
Methotrexate, vincristine	29	5 (17%)
Methotrexate, cyclophosphamide	23	10 (43%)
Methotrexate, bleomycin	20	12 (60%)
Vincristine, cyclophosphamide	19	2 (10%)
Mitomycin C, bleomycin	15	14 (93%)
Adriamycin, cis-platinum	19	6 (32%)
Adriamycin, vincristine	54	9 (17%)
Methotrexate, bleomycin, cis-platinum	9	8 (89%)
Mitomycin C, cis-platinum, vincristine, bleomycin	13	10 (77%)

SOURCE: Devita et al.,[158] Wasserman and Carter,[159] Wallace et al.,[160] and Thigpen et al.[140]

Cervical Cancer in Pregnancy

Pregnant patients with early-stage invasive cervical cancer traditionally have been treated with radical surgery (Ulfelder et al.,[122] Dudan[123]). There have been few clinical trials indicating that the prognosis of cervical cancer is actually changed by pregnancy. Therefore, the same histologic and clinical variables should be considered when determining optimal therapy for both pregnant and nonpregnant patients. In the first two trimesters of pregnancy, therapy for cervical cancer should be instituted as soon as possible without considering fetal outcome. In patients with stage IB large-cell squamous carcinomas less than 3 cm in diameter, radical hysterectomy with pelvic lymphadenectomy is the treatment of choice. Patients with more advanced stage disease should be treated with a combination of 4000 to 5000 rads external therapy to the pelvis followed by one or two intracavitary implants. Radiation therapy usually causes spontaneous abortion within 1 to 2 months (Bosch and Marcial[124]). After 32 weeks of gestation, therapy may be delayed until fetal lung maturation has occurred. It is recommended that placental function and fetal maturation studies be obtained at 2-week intervals until fetal maturity. Cesarean section followed by radical hysterectomy with pelvic lymphadenectomy is then performed in patients with stage IB disease. In more advanced disease cesarean section is performed, and the patient is treated postoperatively by a combination of external and intracavitary radiation therapy.

Approximately 30 percent of patients with invasive cervical cancer will have recurrent or persistent disease following primary therapy (van Nagell et al.[73]). The diagnosis of recurrent cancer may be difficult because the majority of patients have been treated with radiation and it is often impossible to differentiate between pelvic fibrosis and recurrent cancer on clinical examination. Also, radiation-related cytologic change may be confused with changes suspicious for malignancy if the cervical smear is obtained within 4 months following completion of radiation therapy. Although the presence of abnormal cells in a cervical cytologic sample is highly suggestive of tumor recurrence, histologic confirmation of carcinoma is essential. One of the most reliable methods to obtain histologic verification of recurrent cancer is fine-needle biopsy. In a recent study, Nordqvist et al.[125] reported that aspiration biopsies taken transvaginally or transrectally with a 22-gauge spinal needle correlated precisely with open biopsy findings in all patients with pelvic recurrences of squamous cell carcinoma of the cervix. This method is obviously less useful in the diagnosis of upper abdominal recurrences (El-Minawa and Perez-Mesa[126]). The development of ureteral obstruction following therapy in a patient with cervical cancer is also highly suggestive of tumor recurrence. Radiation-induced ureteral stricture can occur in patients receiving high-dose external therapy (Slater and Fletcher[127]), but this complication is extremely rare (Table 37-4). Consequently, a patient developing unilateral ureteral obstruction following treatment should be considered as having recurrent cancer until proved otherwise, and should undergo a thorough evaluation to obtain histologic confirmation of recurrence. Van Nagell et al.,[73] for example, noted the development of unilateral ureteral obstruction in 36 patients, and tumor recurrence was documented in all of them.

The incidence of recurrent cervical cancer is directly related to cell type, lesion size, and stage of disease. Consequently, the majority of patients who develop recurrence have had extensive disease treated initially with a full course of radiation therapy. In selected cases where recurrent cervical cancer is confined to the central pelvis, radical surgery may be curative. The specific surgical procedure utilized depends upon the extent and location of tumor recurrence. Radical hysterectomy modified to include the complete removal of all periureteral tissue and excision of up to three-fourths of the vagina (class IV radical hysterectomy) has been utilized for recurrent cervical cancer confined to the cervix and upper vagina (Piver et al.[128]). With extension of recurrent cancer to a localized area of the bladder or distal ureter, the operation is extended to include partial resection of these structures with ureteroneocystotomy (class V radical hysterectomy). Using these operative techniques, Piver et al.[129] reported a 5-year survival rate of 50 percent in selected patients with recurrent cervical cancer. In patients with more extensive central recurrence, the operative procedure of choice is pelvic exenteration, initially described by Brunschwig in 1948.[15] The purpose of this operation is the en bloc dissection of the pelvic viscera that contain or could contain recurrent cervical cancer. In total pelvic exenteration, the bladder, rectum, distal ureters; and entire female reproductive tract are excised, and urinary and gastrointestinal diversions are performed (Fig. 37-6). Anterior pelvic exenteration, in which the rectosigmoid colon is preserved, may be used when recurrent carcinoma is confined to the anterior vagina or bladder. Since its initial description, numerous technical advances have been made in the operation. These include (1) the use of the ileum as a urinary conduit (Bricker[130]), (2) the use of an omental lid to cover the denuded pelvis (Buchsbaum and White[131]), and (3) the use of myocutaneous pedicle grafts for vaginal reconstruction (Rutledge et al.[132]).

Even when perfomed by an experienced surgeon, pelvic exenteration is a complex operation associated with a significant incidence of complications. Karlen and Piver[133] reported that 25 percent of patients died of complications during or following pelvic exenteration. The most common complications were urinary tract infection or obstruction followed by small-bowel obstruction and enteroperineal fistulae. Complications were most common in patients who had received more than 4000 rads external radiation therapy prior to surgery and in those who had pelvic lymphadenectomy at the time of exenteration. Nevertheless, the cumulative 5-year survival rate of patients undergoing pelvic exenteration for cervical cancer is as high as 34 percent (Symmonds et al.[134]). A most important factor in the treatment of recurrent cancer is the proper selection of patients for radical surgery. Both Barber[135] and Creas-

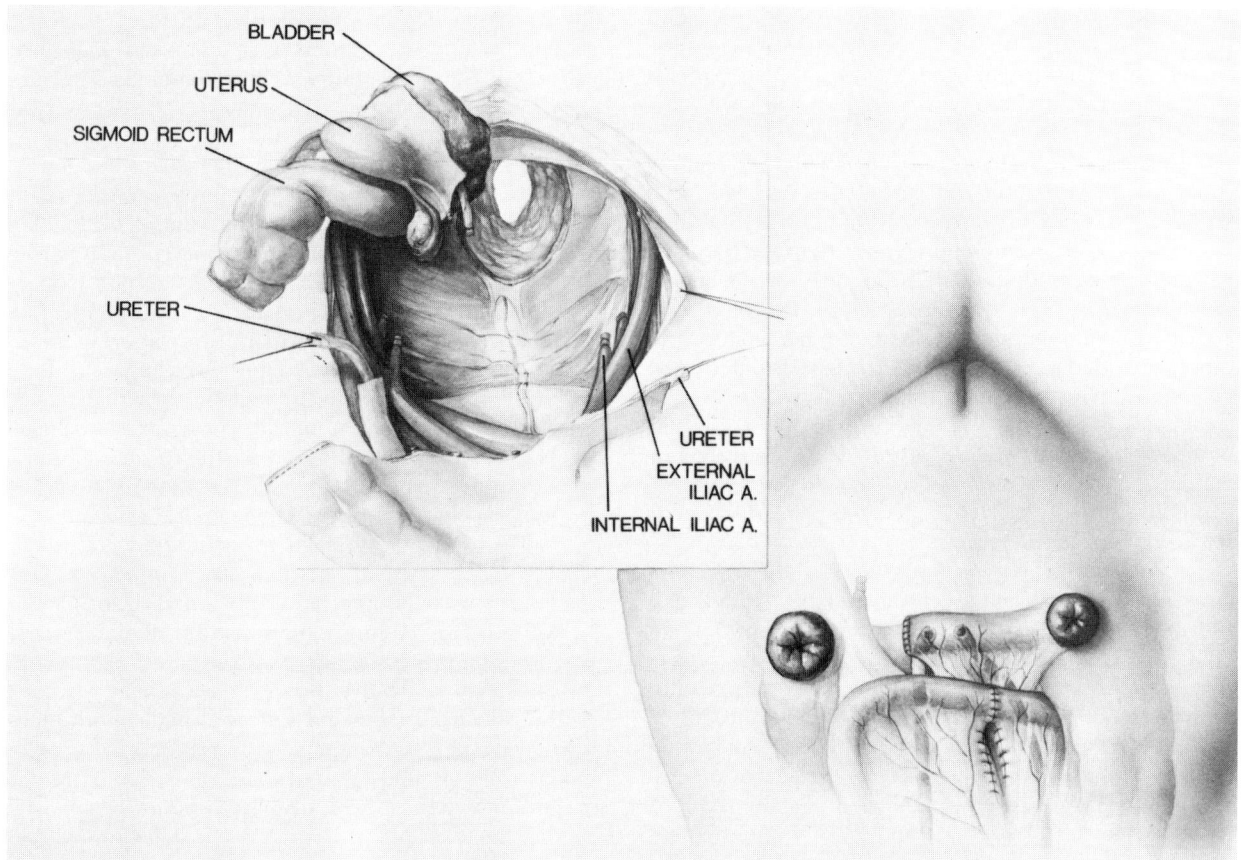

FIGURE 37-6 Total pelvic exenteration showing removal of the bladder, rectum, and reproductive organs. Ileal conduit and a colostomy are then constructed.

man and Rutledge[17] have reported uniform evaluation systems to determine which patients can benefit most from exenterative surgery. Included in this evaluation are (1) the presence or absence of symptoms, (2) the location and extent of recurrent cancer, (3) the time from primary treatment to the diagnosis of recurrence, and (4) findings on intravenous pyelography. Patients with symptoms including back pain, weight loss, and leg swelling generally had extensive inoperable cancer and a low survival rate. In fact, unilateral leg swelling associated with sciatic nerve pain is usually considered a contraindication to the operation. Over 80 percent of central pelvic lesions were resectable as opposed to less than 40 percent of lateral pelvic wall recurrences. The presence of paraaortic lymph node metastases was also interpreted as a contraindication to pelvic exenteration. The time from primary treatment to recurrent cancer often reflected the biologic activity of the tumor. Survival time of patients undergoing pelvic exenteration more than 2 years after initial therapy was nearly double that of patients in whom recurrence was noted less than 2 years after primary therapy. Finally, the findings on intravenous pyelography were also directly related to patient survival rates. Barber et al.,[136] for example, noted that only 10 percent of patients with recurrent cervical cancer producing unilateral ureteral obstruction survived for 5 years following exenteration. Likewise, van Dyke and van Nagell[137] reported that no patient with obstructive uropathy undergoing pelvic exenteration survived more than 2 years after surgery. Finally, the presence of pelvic lymph node metastases in patients with recurrent cervical cancer is associated with extremely limited chances for survival. Karlen and Piver[133] reported that only 5 percent of patients with histologically confirmed pelvic lymph node metastases survived for 5 years. For this reason, enlarged lymph nodes should be biopsied prior to exenteration, and if they are found to contain metastatic disease the procedure should be terminated. Pelvic exenteration, therefore, can be a very effective operation in the treatment of recurrent cervical cancer provided its use is limited to patients with localized recurrence. With the present use of modern supervoltage techniques of radiation therapy, it is highly likely that pelvic exenteration will be indicated in relatively few patients. However, every effort should be made to surgically explore selected patients who might benefit from this operation.

Patients developing recurrent cancer after primary treatment with radical surgery should be treated with radiation therapy. External therapy in a dose of 5500 to 6000 rads is given to a pelvic field, the size of which is determined by the site of recurrence and the presence of lymph node metastases. Extended-field therapy is indicated in patients having histologically confirmed spread to the high common iliac or paraaortic nodes. The dose rate of external radiation is usually reduced to 150 to 160 rads/day in order to avoid enteric complications. Following completion of external radiation the patient is treated with one intravaginal implant providing approximately 10,000 to 12,000 rads surface dose to the vaginal vault. The 5-year survival rate of patients treated with radiation therapy for recurrent cervical cancer depends upon the site and extent of tumor recurrence, but has varied between 15 and 20 percent (Deutsch and Parsons,[138] Evans et al.[139]).

The most common sites of extrapelvic recurrence from cervical cancer are the lungs, paraaortic and supraclavicular lymph nodes, bone, and liver. In a study of 526 cervical cancer patients followed for a mean of 6 years after treatment, van Nagell et al.[73] reported that 22 (4.1 percent) developed lung metastases. An additional 18 patients (3.4 percent) developed paraaortic or supraclavicular lymph node metastases, and spread to the liver was noted in 5 patients (1 percent). Extrapelvic metastases are best treated by chemotherapy. The response rate of cervical cancer to various chemotherapeutic agents has been previously presented (Tables 37-5 and 37-6). The highest response rates have been achieved with cis-platinum usually combined with bleomycin or mitomycin C. Thigpen et al.[140] reported that cis-platinum, in a dose of 50 mg/m^2 intravenously every 3 weeks, produced a 50 percent objective response rate of metastatic cervical cancer. A complete response, defined as the disappearance of all clinical evidence of disease for at least 1 month, was achieved in 15 percent of patients. The median duration of response was 6 months, and the median survival time of responders was 9 months, compared with 6 months for nonresponders. Although the median increase in survival time produced by cis-platinum was relatively small, selected patients had significant prolongation of life. Combination chemotherapy with cis-platinum and bleomycin or mitomycin C is therefore advocated in the treatment of patients with extrapelvic metastases from cervical cancer.

Palliative therapy for patients with recurrent cervical cancer is indicated in specific clinical situations. Bony metastases occur in approximately 2 percent of patients (Carlson et al.[141]) and are often painful. Radiation therapy in doses of 2000 to 3000 rads over a 2-week period is usually quite effective in reducing this pain. Similarly, pelvic pain from recurrent cancer in patients who have had inadequate radiation may be relieved by an additional 1000 to 2000 rads. In these cases, it is extremely important that the dose of primary radiation be recorded so that the tolerance of normal pelvic structures will not be exceeded by additional palliative therapy. Certain patients with debilitating pelvic or lower-extremity pain refractory to analgesics will benefit from percutaneous chordotomy. This procedure has been effective in providing immediate pain relief in over 80 percent of cases (Rosomoff,[142]). The most common side effects of percutaneous chordotomy have been lower-extremity paresis and bladder dysfunction, but these complications have been reported in less than 5 percent of patients.

Palliative urinary diversion in a patient with ureteral obstruction from recurrent cervical cancer is generally contraindicated. These patients have usually had a full course of radiation therapy, and further treatment is not possible. The high incidence of surgical complications generally outweigh the possible symptomatic benefits of the procedure. Also, several investigators (Chau et al.[143]) have reported no significant difference in the survival rate of patients with ureteral obstruction from recurrent cervical cancer who were treated with urinary diversion and those who were not so treated. Nephrostomy tube drainage may provide symptomatic relief to patients with extensive recurrent cancer and urinary tract fistulae (Meyer et al.[144]).

SURVIVAL AND FOLLOW-UP

The 5-year survival rate of patients with invasive cervical cancer recently treated at various centers throughout the world is summarized in Table 37-7. Prognosis is directly related to extent of disease and varies from over 80 percent in patients with stage I disease to less than 10 percent in patients with stage IV cancer. It should be emphasized that the best cure rates have been achieved in institutions where there is excellent radiation therapy, radical surgery, and pathology, and where treatment is individualized after thorough review of pertinent clinical and histopathologic variables.

Approximately one-half of patients who develop recurrent cervical cancer do so within 1 year following therapy, and an additional 25 percent within the second year after treatment (van Nagell et al.[73]). Only 5 percent of patients develop tumor recurrence more than 5 years after therapy. For this reason, it is recommended that patients be seen at monthly intervals during the first year following treatment, every 2 months for the next year, and every 6 months thereafter. Careful pelvic examination including a cervical cytologic sample should be performed at each visit. In addition, intravenous pyelography and a chest x-ray should be obtained at yearly intervals for the first 5 years after treatment.

FUTURE ADVANCES

In assessing future diagnostic and therapeutic approaches in patients with cervical cancer, none would seem more important than the continued development of educational and health care delivery systems which allow all women of reproductive age or older to receive adequate cervical cytologic screening. Numerous studies have shown convincingly that the rate from cervical cancer is inversely related to the annual percentage of the population screened. Yet, up to 25 percent of certain lower socioeconomic rural populations in the United States have never had a Pap smear. The necessity of developing a program providing annual cervical cytologic screening for high-risk populations is evident. Should these women obtain annual cytologic screening, it is quite likely that cervical cancer would no longer be a major cause of mortality in this country.

In the therapy for cervical cancer patients, two major problems remain. The first is the diagnosis and treatment of extrapelvic metastases. Extrapelvic lymph node metastases may be present in any patient with invasive cervical cancer, but are particularly common in patients with advanced-stage disease. Unfortunately, there is no truly reliable method for the diagnosis of lymph node metastases. Lymphangiography is quite accurate if a significant portion of the lymph node is replaced by metastatic tumor. However, microscopic lymph node metastases are virtually impossible to detect with present methodology. Computed tomography adds little to this diagnostic accuracy unless the involved lymph node is markedly enlarged. Recently, Deland et al.[145] reported the successful detection of lymph node metastases from breast cancer by axillary lymphoscintigraphy using ^{131}I-labeled antibodies to carcinoembryonic antigen (CEA). Since cervical cancer spreads most often through the lymphatics, such an approach using radiolabeled antibodies to cervical tumor–associated antigens may prove beneficial.

At present, the treatment of extrapelvic lymph node metastases has met with only limited success. Extended-field radiation may cure 10 to 20 percent of these patients. However, the treatment of systemic disease with

TABLE 37-7 Five-Year Survival Rate of Treated Patients with Cervical Cancer According to Stage

Location of treatment facility	Number of patients	Percent survival by stage			
		I	II	III	IV
Norwegian Radium Hospital	1429	83	59	30	7
Radiumhemmet (Sweden)	924	88	59	27	11
Munich (Germany)	415	91	76	38	13
Tokyo (Japan)	973	92	74	51	11
Manchester (England)	1501	73	55	35	7
Massachusetts General Hospital (United States)	803	82	56	19	10
M. D. Anderson Hospital (United States)	2281	84	61	29	14

SOURCE: *Annual Report on the Results of Treatment in Gynecological Cancer*, vols. 16, 17, Stockholm, Sweden, 1973, 1976.

a local therapeutic modality has inherent limitations. Clearly, randomized trials testing the efficacy of various chemotherapy regimens in the treatment of metastatic cervical cancer are needed. Although agents such as *cis*-platinum and bleomycin have been shown to have a therapeutic effect on cervical cancer, the survival chances of patients treated with these agents has not improved significantly. Considerable effort must be given to the synthesis and testing of new drugs which will be more effective against squamous cell carcinoma of the cervix. In vitro chemotherapy testing may prove helpful in the initial evaluation of such drugs. Recently, a number of preliminary investigations have used tumor markers as targets for antibody-directed therapy. These antibodies are tagged with radioactive labels or chemotherapeutic agents, both of which are capable of producing cell death. These trials are still experimental and are limited largely by the specificity of the antibody. However, the potential use of this type of therapy in patients with lymphatic metastases from cervical cancer is great.

A second major problem is the failure of conventional therapeutic modalities to cure bulky, advanced-stage cervical cancer. The 5-year survival rate of patients with stage III and stage IV cervical cancer is 30 percent at best. Advanced-stage cervical cancers contain a high percentage of hypoxic cells, many of which are noncycling and quite resistant to gamma irradiation. In an effort to counteract this oxygen effect in bulky cervical tumors, several experimental approaches have been attempted. The first of these is the use of high-pressure oxygen (HPO) during therapy. In a preliminary clinical trial undertaken by the British Medical Research Council, patients with advanced-stage cervical cancers were given HPO in special lucite chambers while receiving external therapy. Bulky tumors were significantly better controlled when treated in hyberbaric oxygen than when treated in air (Watson et al.[146]). However, normal tissue complications were also higher in patients receiving HPO.

A second experimental approach in the therapy of advanced-stage cervical cancers is the use of high-linear-energy transfer (LET) particles such as fast neutrons or negative pions. Both these particles have a low oxygen-enhancement ratio (OER) and are effective in treating hypoxic cells. A new radiation source which has received much recent attention is californium 252 (^{252}Cf). Californium is a radionuclide which emits both neutrons and gamma photons. This source has been used for the past 3 years in the intracavitary therapy of cervical cancer. In a preliminary clinical study, Maruyama et al.[147] reported that intracavitary californium 252, when combined with conventional external therapy, produced complete local regression of bulky stage IB and IIB cervical tumors in over 90 percent of the cases. The 4-year survival rate of these patients was 80 percent. Although the dosimetry of ^{252}Cf has yet to be fully delineated, presently available data suggest that neutrons are effective in the treatment of bulky hypoxic cervical tumors. It is highly probable that ^{252}Cf will be a valuable source in the future treatment of cervical cancer.

A third area of clinical investigation which shows promise in the treatment of hypoxic tumors is the use of radiation sensitizers. These compounds are generally electron-affinic and sensitize cells to radiation by fixation of free radicals in DNA by oxidation. To date, the most effective radiosensitizing agents have been nitroimidazole compounds such as misonidazole. These compounds have the advantage of diffusing freely into poorly vascularized and hypoxic tumor areas without being metabolized. Preliminary data suggest that the combination of misonidazole and radiation therapy is effective in the treatment of glioblastomas (Urtasun et al.[148]), and clinical trials to test the efficacy of this combination in the therapy of advanced-stage cervical cancer are in progress (Brady et al.[149]).

A final area of recent research interest in cervical cancer is tumor markers. Although oncofetal antigens such as CEA have been useful in predicting occult recurrent cancer in selected patients, the lack of specificity of these antigens has precluded their use in diagnosis. Recently, Kato et al.[150,151] reported a tumor-specific antigen (TA-4) for squamous cell carcinoma of the cervix. A radioimmunoassay for TA-4 has been developed, and elevated serum antigen concentrations have been reported in approximately 50 percent of cervical cancer patients. The specificity of this antigen has yet to be confirmed in a large number of cervical cancer patients. However, the theoretical clinical applications of tumor-specific antigens are obvious. Immunodetection procedures utilizing radiolabeled antibodies to nonspecific tumor-associated antigens have been successful in localizing both primary and metastatic cervical cancer (Goldenberg et al.[152]). Should a truly specific cervical cancer antigen be isolated, this same methodology could be used to develop immunodetection procedures which would be useful in defining the extent of tumor spread.

Furthermore, a tumor-specific marker could act as a target for cytotoxic radiolabeled antibodies which could be used in the therapy of cervical cancer.

REFERENCES

1. Meigs JV: *Surgical Treatment of Cancer of the Cervix,* Grune & Stratton, New York, 1954, pp 1–8.
2. Ries E: Modern treatment of Carcinoma of the Uterus. *Chicago Med Rec* 9:284–289, 1895.
3. Clark JC: A more radical method of performing hysterectomy for cancer of the uterus. *Bull Johns Hopkins Hosp* 6:120, 1895.
4. Wertheim E: The extended abdominal operation for carcinoma. *Am J Obstet Gynecol* 66:169–232, 1912.
5. Schuchardt K: Eine neu methode der gebarmutterextipalton. *Centralbl F Chir* 51, 1893.
6. Schauta F: Die operation des gebarmutterkrebses mittels des schuchartschen paravaginalschnettes. *Monatschr Geburtsh Gynak* 15:133, 1902.
7. Cleaves MA: Radium with a preliminary note on radium rays in the treatment of cancer. *J. Adv Ther* 21:667–682, 1903.
8. Abbe R: The use of radium in malignant disease. *Lancet* 2:524, 1913.
9. Regaud C, Fernoux R: Discordance, des effects des rayons X, d'une part dans lapeau, d'autre dans le testicule, par le fractionnement de la dose: Dimution de l'efficacité dans le peau, maintein de l'efficacité dans le testicule. *CR Soc Biol* 97:431–434, 1927.
10. Kerst DW: The betatron. *Radiology* 40:115–120, 1943.
11. Miller CW: Recent development in linear accelerators for therapy. *Br J Radiol* 35:182–185, 1962.
11a. Meigs JV: Carcinoma of the cervix: The Wertheim operation. *Surg Gynecol Obstet* 78:195–199, 1944.
12. Liu W, Meigs JW: Radical hysterectomy and pelvic lymphadenectomy: A review of 473 cases including 244 for primary invasive carcinoma of the cervix. *Am J Obstet Gynecol* 69:1–32, 1955.
13. Symmonds RE, Pratt JH: Prevention of fistulas and lymphocysts in radical hysterectomy. *Obstet Gynecol* 57:17–21, 1961.
14. Van Nagell JR, Shiwietz DP: Surgical adjuncts in radical hysterectomy and pelvic lymphadenectomy. *Surg Gynecol Obstet* 143:737–739, 1976.
15. Brunschwig A, Pierce V: Necropsy findings in patients with carcinoma of the cervix: Implications for treatment. *Am J Obstet Gynecol* 56:1134–1137, 1948.
16. Barber HRK, Jones W: Lymphadenectomy in pelvic exenteration for recurrent cervix cancer. *JAMA* 215:1945–1969, 1971.
17. Creasman WT, Rutledge FN: Preoperative evaluation of patients with recurrent carcinoma of the cervix. *Gynecol Oncol* 1:111–118, 1972.
18. Kottmeier HL: Ten year end results, radiological treatment of carcinoma of the cervix. *Acta Obstet Gynecol* 111:195–203, 1962.
19. Kottmeier HL: Complications following radiation therapy in carcinoma of the cervix and their treatment. *Am J Obstet Gynecol* 88:854–866, 1964.
20. Kottmeier HL: Surgical and radiation treatment of carcinoma of the uterine cervix. *Acta Obstet Gynecol Scand Suppl* 43, 1964.
21. Fletcher GH, Rutledge FM: Extended field technique in the management of the cancers of the uterine cervix. *Am J Roentgenol* 114:116–122, 1972.
22. Babes A: Diagnosis of cancer of the uterine cervix by smears. *Presse Med* 36:451–454, 1928.
23. Papanicolau GN: *Proceedings of the Third Race Betterment Conference,* Battle Creek, Mich, 1928, p 528.
24. Papanicolaou GN, Traut HG: The diagnostic value of vaginal smears in carcinoma of the uterus. *Am J Obstet Gynecol* 42:193–196, 1941.
25. Erickson CC et al.: Preliminary report of 20,000 women studied by the vaginal smear technique in a general population screening project. *Proc Am Assoc Cancer Res* 1:14, 1953.
26. Christopherson WM: the control of cervix cancer. *Acta Cytol* 10:6–10, 1966.
27. Fidler HK et al: Cervical cancer detection in British Columbia. *J Obstet Gynaecol Br Cwlth* 75:392–404, 1968.
28. Hinselmann H: Verbesserung der inspektronsmoglichkeit von vulva, vagina und portio. *Muench Med Wochenschr* 77:1733–1743, 1945.
29. Reagan JW et al: Analytical study of cells in cervical squamous cell cancer. *Lab Invest* 6:241–250, 1957.
30. Wentz WB, Lewis GC: Correlation of histologic morphology and survival in cervical cancer following radiation therapy. *Obstet Gynecol* 26:228–234, 1965.
31. Swan DS, Roddick JW: A clinical-pathological correlation of cell type classification of cervical cancer. *Am J Obstet Gynecol* 116:666–670, 1973.
32. Van Nagell JR et al: The prognostic significance of cell type and lesion size in patients with cervical cancer treated by radical surgery. *Gynecol Oncol* 5:142–151, 1977.
33. Van Nagell JR et al: Small cell carcinoma of the uterine cervix. *Cancer* 40:2243–2249, 1977.
34. Schmitz B: The classification of uterine carcinoma of the study of the efficacy of radium therapy. *Am J Roentgenol* 7:383–395, 1920.
35. Winter G, Doderlein A: Noch einmal die carcinomstatistik. *Archiv fur Gynak* 120:219–222, 1923.
36. Hollinshead AC et al: In vivo and in vitro measure of the relationship of human squamous carcinomas to herpes

simplex virus tumor-associated antigens. *Cancer Res* 36: 821–828, 1976.
37. Rawls WE, Adam E: Herpes simplex viruses and human malignancies, in HH Hiatt et al (eds): *Origins of Human Cancer,* Book B: *Mechanism of Carcinogenesis, Cold Spring Harbor Conferences on Cell Proliferation,* vol. 4, Cold Spring Harbor, New York, 1979, pp 1133–1155.
38. Nahmias AJ et al: Prospective studies of the association of genital herpes simplex infection and cervical anaplasia. *Cancer Res* 33:1491–1497, 1973.
39. Rawls WE et al: Genital herpes in two social groups. *Am J Obstet Gynecol* 110:682–689, 1971.
40. Rapp R, Duff R: Oncogenic conversion of normal cells by inactivated herpes simplex virus. *Cancer* 34:1353–1362, 1974.
41. Aurelian L et al: Viruses and gynecologic cancers: herpesvirus protein, a cervical tumor antigen that fulfills the criteria for a marker of carcinogenicity. *Cancer* 48:455–471, 1981.
42. Wentz WB et al: Cervical carcinogenesis with herpes simplex virus, type 2. *Obstet Gynecol* 46:117–122, 1975.
43. Palmer AE et al: A preliminary report on investigation of oncogenic potential of herpes simplex virus type 2 in Cebus monkeys. *Cancer Res* 36:807–809, 1976.
44. McDougal JK et al: Cervical carcinoma: Detection of herpes simplex virus RNA in cells undergoing neoplastic change. *Int J Cancer* 25:1–8, 1980.
45. Frenkel N et al: A DNA fragment of herpes simplex 2 and its transcripts in human cervical cancer tissue. *Proc Natl Acad Sci* 69:3784–3789, 1972.
46. Notter MDF et al: Detection of herpes simplex virus tumor-associated antigen in uterine cervical tissue: Five case studies. *Gynecol Oncol* 6:574–581, 1978.
47. Naib Z et al: Genital herpetic infection. *Cancer* 23:940–945, 1969.
48. Thomas DB, Rawls WE: Relationship of herpes simplex virus type 2 antibodies and squamous dysplasia to cervical carcinoma-in-situ. *Cancer* 42:2716–2725, 1978.
49. Naib AM et al: Relation of cystohistopathology of genital herpesvirus infection to cervical anaplasia. *Cancer Res* 33: 1452–1463, 1973.
50. Singer et al: The role of a high risk mole in the etiology of cervical carcinoma—A correlation of epidemiology and molecular biology. *Am J Obstet Gynecol* 1:110–115, 1976.
51. Coppleson M: The etiology of squamous carcinoma of the cervix. *Obstet Gynecol* 32:432–436, 1968.
52. Reid BL: Interaction between homologous sperm and somatic cells of the uterus and peritoneum in the mouse. *Exp Cell Res* 40:679–683, 1965.
53. Reid BL, Blackwell PM: Evidence for the possibility of nuclear uptake of polymerised deoxyribonucleic acid of sperm phagocytosed by macrophages. *Aust J Exp Biol Med Sci* 45:323–326, 1967.
54. Singer A: A male factor in the etiology of cervical cancer. *Oxford Med Sch Gaz* 25:18–21, 1973.
55. Christopherson WM, Broghamer WL: A study of the reversibility of dysplasia of the uterine cervix, *Proceedings of the First International Congress of Exfoliated Cytology,* Lippincott, Philadelphia, Pa, 1962, pp 269–273.
56. Patten SF et al: An experimental study of the relationship between *Trichomonas,* vaginalis, and dysplasia in the uterine cervix. *Acta Cytol* 7:187–195, 1963.
57. Wynder EL: Early cervical neoplasia. *Obstet Gynecol Surv* 34:1697–1711, 1969.
58. Pratt-Thomas HR et al: The carcinogenic effect of human smegma: An experimental study. *Cancer* 9:671–680, 1956.
59. Terris M et al: Relation of circumcision to cancer of the cervix. *Am J Obstet Gynecol* 117:1056–1066, 1973.
60. Megafu U: Cancer of the genital tract among the Ibo women in Nigeria. *Cancer* 44:1875–1878, 1979.
61. Silverberg E: Cancer statistics, 1979. *Cancer* 31:23–28, 1980.
62. Cramer DW: The role of cervical cytology on the declining morbidity and mortality of cervical cancer. *Cancer* 34: 2018–2027, 1974.
63. Rochat R: The prevalence of cervical cancer screening in the United States in 1970. *Am J Obstet Gynecol* 125:478–483, 1976.
64. Boronow RC: Stage I cervix cancer and pelvic node metastasis. *Am J Obstet Gynecol* 127:135–140, 1977.
65. Hasumi K et al: Microinvasive carcinoma of the uterine cervix. *Cancer* 45:928–931, 1980.
66. Barber HRK et al: Vascular invasion as a prognostic factor in stage IB cancer of the cervix. *Obstet Gynecol* 52:343–348, 1978.
67. Wentz WB, Jaffe RM: Squamous cell carcinoma of the cervix with higher uterine involvement. *Obstet Gynecol* 28: 271–272, 1966.
68. Perez CA et al: Prognostic significance of endometrial extension from primary carcinoma of the uterine cervix. *Cancer* 35:1493–1504.
69. Plentyl AA, Friedman E: *The Morphologic Basis of Oncologic Diagnosis and Therapy,* vol. 2: *Lymphatic System of the Female Genitalia,* Saunders, Philadelphia, Pa, 1971.
70. Bosch A et al: Prognostic significance of ureteral obstruction in carcinoma of the cervix uteri. *Acta Radiol* 12:47–56, 1973.
71. Van Nagell JR et al: The effect of intravenous pyelography and cystoscopy on the staging of cervical cancer. *Gynecol Oncol* 3:87–93, 1975.
72. Piver MS, Chung WS: Prognostic significance of cervical lesion size and pelvic node metastases in cervical carcinoma. *Obstet Gynecol* 46:507–512, 1975.
73. Van Nagell JR et al: Therapeutic implications of patterns of recurrence in cancer of the uterine cervix. *Cancer* 44: 2354–2361, 1979.

74. Marcial VA, Bosch A: Radiation-induced tumor regression in carcinoma of the uterine cervix: Prognostic significance. *Cancer* 108:113–123, 1970.
75. Bernardino ME, Dodd GD: Imaging of the pelvic contents in the female oncologic patient. *Cancer* 45:504–510, 1981.
76. Averette HE, et al: Exploratory celiotomy for surgical staging of cervical cancer. *Am J Obstet Gynecol* 113:1090–1093, 1972.
77. Buschbaum HJ: Extrapelvic lymph node metastases in cervical carcinoma. *Am J Obstet Gynecol* 113:814, 821, 1979.
78. Piver MS, Barlow JJ: Para-aortic lymphadenectomy, aortic node biopsy, and aortic lymphangiography in staging patients with advanced cervical cancer. *Cancer* 32:367–370, 1973.
79. Brown RC et al: The accuracy of lymphangiography in the diagnosis of para-aortic lymph node metastases from carcinoma of the cervix. *Obstet Gynecol* 54:571–575, 1979.
80. Buschbaum HJ: Para-aortic lymph node involvement in cervical carcinoma. *Am J Obstet Gynecol* 113:942–947, 1972.
81. Schellhas H: Extraperitoneal para-aortic node dissection through an upper abdominal incision. *Obstet Gynecol* 46:444–447, 1975.
82. LaGasse LD et al: Pre-treatment lymphangiography and operative evaluation in carcinoma of the cervix. *Am J Obstet Gynecol* 134:219–224, 1979.
83. Zornoza J et al: Transperitoneal percutaneous retroperitoneal lymph node aspiration biopsy. *Radiology* 122:111–115, 1977.
84. Zornoza J et al: Percutaneous Retroperitoneal lymph node biopsy in carcinoma of the cervix. *Gynecol Oncol* 5:43–51, 1977.
85. Wallace S et al: Lymphangiography in the determination of the extent of metastatic carcinoma: The potential value of percutaneous lymph node biopsy. *Cancer* 39:709–718, 1977.
86. Holm HH et al: Ultrasonically guided percutaneous puncture. *Radiol Clin North Am* 13:493–503, 1975.
87. Van Nagell JR et al: The effect of pelvic inflammatory disease on enteric complications following radiation therapy for cervical cancer. *Am J Obstet Gynecol* 128:767–771, 1977.
88. Van Nagell JR et al: Small bowel injury following radiation therapy for cervical cancer. *Am J Obstet Gynecol* 118:163–167, 1974.
89. Van Nagell JR et al: Bladder or rectal injury following radiation therapy for cervical cancer. *Am J Obstet Gynecol* 119:727–732, 1974.
90. Maruyama Y et al: Radiation and small bowel complications in cervical carcinoma therapy. *Radiology* 12:699–703, 1974.
91. Van Nagell JR et al: Correlation between retinal and pelvic vascular status: A determinant factor in patients undergoing pelvic irradiation for gynecologic malignancy. *Am J Obstet Gynecol* 134:551–555, 1979.
92. Copeland EM et al: Nutrition as an adjunct to cancer treatment in the adult. *Cancer Res* 37:2451–2456, 1977.
93. Christopherson WM et al: Microinvasive carcinoma in the uterine cervix. *Cancer* 38:629–632, 1976.
94. Ruch RM: Microinvasive carcinoma of the cervix: A confusing dilemma. *South Med J* 63:1123–1126, 1970.
95. Roddick JW, Greenlaw RH: Treatment of cervical cancer. *Am J Obstet Gynecol* 109:754–764, 1971.
96. Masubuchi K et al: Five year cure rate for carcinoma of the cervix uteri. *Am J Obstet Gynecol* 103:566–573, 1969.
97. Brunschwig A, Barber HRK: Surgical treatment of carcinoma of the cervix. *Obstet Gynecol* 27:21–29, 1966.
98. Webb MJ, Symmonds RE: Wertheim hysterectomy: A reappraisal. *Obstet Gynecol* 54:140–145, 1979.
99. Averette HE et al: Current role of radical hysterectomy as primary therapy for invasive carcinoma of the cervix. *Am J Obstet Gynecol* 105:79–89, 1969.
100. Van Nagell JR et al: Evaluation and treatment of patients with invasive cervical cancer. *Surg Clin North Am* 58:67–85, 1978.
101. Van Nagell JR et al: The significance of vascular invasion and lymphocytic infiltration in invasive cervical cancer. *Cancer* 41:228–234, 1978.
102. Kolbenstveldt A, Kolstad P: Pelvic lymph node dissection under pre-operative lymphographic control. *Gynecol Oncol* 2:39–59, 1974.
103. Green TH et al: Urologic complications of radical Wertheim hysterectomy: Incidence, etiology, management and prevention. *Obstet Gynecol* 20:293–312, 1962.
104. Van Nagell JR et al: Suprapubic bladder drainage following radical hysterectomy. *Am J Obstet Gynecol* 113:849–850, 1972.
105. Underwood PB et al: Radical Hysterectomy: A critical review of twenty-two years' experience. *Am J Obstet Gynecol* 134:889–898, 1979.
106. Sall S et al: Surgical treatment of stages IB and IIA invasive carcinoma of the cervix by radical abdominal hysterectomy. *Am J Obstet Gynecol* 135:442–446, 1979.
107. Surwit E et al: Radical hysterectomy with or without preoperative radium for stage IB squamous cell carcinoma of the cervix. *Obstet Gynecol* 48:130–133, 1976.
108. Rampone JF et al: Combined treatment of stage IB carcinoma of the cervix. *Obstet Gynecol* 41:163–167, 1973.
109. Jampolis S et al: Analysis of sites and causes of failures of irradiation in invasive squamous cell carcinoma in the intact uterine cervix. *Radiology* 115:681–685, 1975.
110. Durrance FY et al: Analysis of central recurrent disease in stages I and II squamous cell carcinomas of the cervix on intact uterus. *Am J Roentgenol Radium Ther Nucl Med* 106:831–838, 1969.
111. Nelson AJ et al: Indications for adjunctive conservative extrafascial hysterectomy in selected cases for carcinoma of the uterine cervix. *Am J Roentgenol* 123:91–99, 1975.

112. Hardt N et al: Radiation induced tumor regression as a prognostic factor in patients with invasive cervical cancer. *Cancer* 49:35–39, 1982.
113. Brunschwig A, Daniel W: The surgery of pelvic lymph node metastases from carcinoma of the cervix. *Am J Obstet Gynecol* 83:389–392, 1962.
114. Piver MS, Barlow JJ: High dose irradiation to biopsy confirmed aortic node metastases from carcinoma of the uterine cervix. *Cancer* 38:1234–1236, 1977.
115. Hughes R et al: Extended field irradiation for cervical cancer based on surgical staging. *Oncology* 9:153–161, 1980.
116. Kottmeier HL, Gray MJ: Rectal and bladder injuries in relation to radiation dosage in carcinoma of the cervix. *Am J Obstet Gynecol* 82:74–82, 1961.
117. Buchler DA et al: Radiation reactions in cervical cancer therapy. *Am J Obstet Gynecol* 111:745–750, 1971.
118. Buchler DA et al: The relationship of NSD to reactions and complications following treatment for malignant uterine cervical neoplasms. *Radiat Biol* 110:687–690, 1974.
119. Wheeless CR: Small bowel bypass for complications related to pelvic malignancy. *Obstet Gynecol* 92:661–666, 1973.
120. Schmitt EJ, Symmonds RE: Intestinal radiation injuries: Resection vs bypass. *Obstet Gynecol* (in press).
121. Thigpen T et al: Cis-Dichlorodiammineplatinum (II) in the treatment of gynecologic malignancies: Phase II trials by the Gynecological Oncology Group. *Cancer Treat Rep* 63:1549–1555, 1979.
122. Ulfelder H et al: Invasive Carcinoma of the cervix during pregnancy. *Am J Obstet Gynecol* 93:424–428, 1967.
123. Dudan RC et al: Carcinoma of the cervix and pregnancy. *Gynecol Oncol* 1:283–289, 1973.
124. Bosch A, Marcial VA: Carcinoma of the uterine cervix associated with pregnancy. *Am J Roentgenol Radium Ther Nucl Med* 96:92–99, 1966.
125. Nordqvist S et al: Five-needle aspiration lytology in gynecologic oncology. *Obstet Gynecol* 54:719–723, 1979.
126. El-Minawa MF, Perez-Mesa CM: Parametrial needle biopsy follow-up of cervical cancer. *Int J Obstet Gynecol* 12:1, 1974.
127. Slater JM, Fletcher GH: Ureteral strictures after radiation therapy for carcinoma of the uterine cervix. *Am J Radiol* 61:269, 1971.
128. Piver MS et al: Five classes of extended hysterectomy for women with cervical cancer. *Obstet Gynecol* 44:265–272, 1974.
129. Piver MS et al: Para-aortic lymph node irradiation for carcinoma of the uterine cervix using split course technique. *Gynecol Oncol* 3:168–175, 1975.
130. Bricker EM: Bladder substitution after pelvic evisceration. *Surg Clin North Am* 31:1511–1521, 1950.
131. Buchsbaum HJ, White AJ: Omental sling for management of the pelvic floor following exenteration. *Am J Obstet Gynecol* 117:405–412, 1973.
132. Rutledge FN et al: Clinical studies with adjunctive surgery and irradiation therapy in treatment of carcinoma of the cervix. *Cancer* 38:596–602, 1976.
133. Karlen JR, Piver MS: Reduction of mortality and morbidity associated with pelvic exenteration. *Gynecol Oncol* 3:154–167, 1975.
134. Symmonds RE et al: Exenterative operations: Experience with 198 patients. *Am J Obstet Gynecol* 121:907–915, 1975.
135. Barber HRK: Relative prognostic significance of preoperative and operative findings in pelvic exenteration. *Surg Clin North Am* 49:431–447, 1969.
136. Barber HRK et al: Prognostic significance of preoperative non-visualizing kidney in patients receiving pelvic exenteration. *Cancer* 16:1614–1615, 1963.
137. Van Dyke AJ, Van Nagell JR: The prognostic significance of ureteral obstruction in patients with recurrent carcinoma of the cervix uteri. *Surg Gynecol Obstet* 141:371–373, 1975.
138. Deutsch M, Parsons JA: Radiotherapy for carcinoma of the cervix recurrent after surgery. *Cancer* 34:2051–2055, 1974.
139. Evans SR et al: External vs interstitial irradiation in unresectable recurrent cancer of the cervix. *Cancer* 28:1284–1288, 1971.
140. Thigpen T et al: Chemotherapy in the management of advanced or recurrent cervical and endometrial carcinoma. *Cancer* 48:658–665, 1981.
141. Carlson V et al: Metastases in squamous carcinoma of the uterine cervix. *Radiology* 88:961, 1967.
142. Rosomoff HL: Bilateral percutaneous cervical cordotemy. *J Neurosurg* 31:41–74, 1969.
143. Chau DT et al: Palliative urinary diversion in patients with advanced carcinoma of the cervix. *Cancer* 20:93–97, 1967.
144. Meyer J et al: Palliative urinary diversion in carcinoma of the cervix. *Obstet Gynecol* 55:95–98, 1980.
145. Deland FH et al: Axillary lymphoscintigraphy by radioimmuno-detection of carcinoembryonic antigen in breast cancer. *J Nucl Med* 20:1245–1250, 1979.
146. Watson ER et al: Hyperbaric oxygen and radiotherapy: A Medical Research Council trial in carcinoma of the cervix. *Br J Radiol* 51:879–887, 1978.
147. Maruyama Y et al: Tumor regression and histological clearance after neutron brachytherapy for large localized cervical carcinomas by combined radiation and surgery. *Cancer* (in press).
148. Urtasun RC et al: Metronidazole as a radiosensitizer. *New Engl J Med* 295:901–903, 1976.
149. Brady LW et al: The potential for radiation sensitizers and radiation protectors combined with radiation therapy in gynecologic cancer. *Cancer* 48:650–657, 1981.
150. Kato H, Torigoe T: Radioimmunoassay for tumor antigen of human cervical squamous cell carcinoma. *Cancer* 40:1621–1628, 1977.
151. Kato H et al: Tumor antigen of human cervical squamous cell carcinoma: Correlation of circulating levels with disease progress. *Cancer* 43:585–590, 1979.

152. Goldenberg DM et al: Use of radiolabeled antibodies to carcinoembryonic antigen for the detection and localization of diverse cancers by external photoscanning. *N Engl J Med* 298:1384–1388, 1978.
153. Park RC et al: Treatment of stage I carcinoma of the cervix. *Obstet Gynecol* 41:117–122, 1973.
154. Chau PM et al: Complications in high dose whole pelvis irradiation in female cancer. *Am J Roentgenol Radium Ther Nucl Med* 87:22–40, 1962.
155. Peckham BM et al: Radiation dosage and complications in cervical cancer therapy. *Am J Obstet Gynecol* 104:485–494, 1969.
156. Strockbine MJ et al: Complications in 831 patients with squamous cell carcinoma of the intact uterine cervix treated with 3,000 rads or more whole pelvis irradiation. *Am J Roentgenol Radium Ther Nucl Med* 108:293–304, 1970.
157. Villasanta U: Complications of radiotherapy for carcinoma of the uterine cervix. *Am J Obstet Gynecol* 114:717–726, 1972.
158. Devita VT et al: Perspective on research in gynecologic oncology. *Cancer* 38:509–525, 1976.
159. Wasserman TH, Carter SK: The integration of chemotherapy into combined modality treatment of solid tumors VII cervical cancer. *Cancer Treat Rev* 4:25–46, 1977.
160. Wallace HJ et al: Comparison of the therapeutic effects of Adriamycin versus Adriamycin plus vincristine versus Adriamycin plus cyclophosphamide in the treatment of advanced carcinoma of the cervix. *Cancer Treat Rep* 62:1435–1441, 1978.

SELECTED BIBLIOGRAPHY

Rapp F: Herpes simplex virus type 2 and cervical cancer. *Curr Prob Cancer,* vol 6, no 4, 1981.

Ulfelder H (ed): Carcinoma of the cervix. *Sem Oncol* 9:249–391, 1982.

38
CANCERS OF THE UTERINE CORPUS
William E. Lucas

Cancers of the uterine corpus can be subdivided into adenocarcinomas of endometrial origin and a heterogeneous group of sarcomas which constitute no more than 4 percent of the total. The major emphasis in this chapter will be placed on discussion of the more common adenocarcinomas, although the sarcomas form a sufficiently challenging subgroup to warrant more than passing attention.

ENDOMETRIAL ADENOCARCINOMA

Historical Aspects

In the first two decades of this century, the development of safe techniques for surgical removal of the uterus and its adnexa and the advent of effective irradiation techniques, particularly for the use of intrauterine and intravaginal radium, focused attention on carcinoma of the endometrium as a common cancer afflicting postmenopausal women. It was found to be readily diagnosed by simple techniques and to be curable in a substantial portion of cases by hysterectomy, irradiation, or a combination of the two modalities.

Accumulation of a significant data base has pinpointed a number of areas of particular interest. These will be enumerated now and discussed in greater detail in subsequent sections:

1. The apparently increased incidence of endometrial cancer in the last decade.
2. The relationship of abnormalities of endogenous estrogen production and the therapeutic administration of estrogen to the genesis of endometrial hyperplasia and adenocarcinoma.
3. Recognition of the patient at risk and improved methods for surveillance and early diagnosis.
4. The importance of clinical staging and histological grading to patterns of spread, treatment, and prognosis.
5. The relative importance of surgery and radiotherapy, alone or combined, as primary treatment.
6. The role of adjunctive endocrine and/or cytotoxic chemotherapy.
7. The early recognition and aggressive management of recurrent disease.

Incidence, Epidemiology, and Etiologic Aspects

Intense interest has been generated by an apparent increase in the incidence of endometrial carcinoma since the late 1960s, particularly relative to the possible causal role of the use of exogenous estrogen.[1] Thus, data from the Connecticut Tumor Registry shows an increase from approximately 27 cases per 100,000 women at risk to just over 40 per 100,000 between 1965 and 1975, when the data is adjusted for prior hysterectomy.[2] During this period endometrial cancer has supplanted invasive cervical cancer as the most common malignancy of the female reproductive tract in the United States. In excess of 38,000 new cases of endometrial cancer, compared to less than 20,000 cases of invasive cancers of the cervix, are diagnosed annually (1982). As recently as two decades ago the ratio of invasive cervical cancer to endometrial cancer was in excess of 3:1.

There are several possible explanations for this trend. Over 75 percent of endometrial cancers are diagnosed in women past the menopause, with an average age at diagnosis of 59. With the average life expectancy for women in the United States now approaching 80, the population at risk is expanding. At the same time, improved surveillance, early detection, and prompt treatment of preinvasive cervical cancer has steadily reduced the incidence of invasive cervical cancer. The increased incidence of endometrial cancer parallels a major increase, since 1955, in the use of exogenous estrogen therapy for menopausal symptoms, as well as for less well defined indications.

Although the precise role of exogenous estrogen as a primary etiologic factor in the genesis of endometrial cancer is by no means resolved, several retrospective epidemiologic studies have been published which show a 4- to 14-fold increased risk of development of endometrial cancer among estrogen users, with length of use and dosage the most significant variables.[3-7] Although the case against long-term estrogen therapy has not been proven, the evidence cannot be ignored. There is also an increasing body of evidence that while estrogen may predispose to an increased incidence of endometrial cancer, it appears that such use does not lead to increased mortality from this condition.

Endocrinologic factors in the genesis of a substantial portion of endometrial cancers have been suspected for many years. Following the characterization of estrogen as the primary trophic hormone of the endometrium in the early 1920s, adenomatous hyperplasia and adenocarcinoma of the endometrium was induced in rabbits treated with estrogen. Taylor, and subsequently Gusberg and others, noted the frequent occurrence of adenomatous endometrial hyperplasia in association with and as an apparent precursor to endometrial cancer.[8,9] In a review by Gusberg 19 percent of 562 patients with adenomatous hyperplasia subsequently developed adenocarcinoma.[10]

It was also noted that progesterone could frequently reverse the changes induced by estrogen, leading to the landmark observation by Kelley and Baker in 1959, repeatedly reconfirmed, that pharmacologic doses of progesterone are effective in inducing regression of pulmonary metastases in approximately 30 percent of patients so afflicted.[11]

Recent evidence sheds light on the mechanism of action of estrogen and progesterone on endometrial glandular epithelium. The former binds to specific cytoplasmic receptor protein, and is then transported to the nucleus where an increase in genetically determined DNA-dependent RNA synthesis and protein synthesis occurs, leading to epithelial proliferation. Progesterone may function as an "antiestrogen" in several respects: by decreasing the number of available estrogen receptor sites, by inhibiting estrogen-induced DNA synthesis, and by stimulating the effect of estradiol dehydrogenase in converting estradiol (E_2) to estrone (E_1), a relatively weaker estrogen. Progesterone transforms proliferative endometrium to mature secretory endometrium.

The majority of studies to date indicate more histochemical, ultrastructural, and cytogenetic similarities than differences between proliferative endometrium and well-differentiated endometrial cancer. As the cancer becomes poorly differentiated, these similarities disappear, and the tumor cell becomes aneuploid and loses its quantitative ability to bind estrogen and progesterone.

Several well-established clinical observations support the concept that estrogen unopposed by progesterone is a modulating factor in the genesis of endometrial cancer.[12] Obese women, particularly those who are infertile due to disturbance of ovulation characterized by unopposed (by progesterone) estrogen secretion, are at greater risk to develop endometrial cancer than are fertile, normally ovulating women of normal weight. The prototype is the patient with the polycystic ovary syndrome, long known to predispose to development of adenomatous endometrial hyperplasia. Chamlian and Taylor in a careful study of 97 premenopausal women with ovulatory disorders and endometrial hyperplasia noted progression to endometrial carcinoma in 14 over a period of 1 to 14 years.[13] The studies of obese perimenopausal and postmenopausal women conducted by MacDonald et al. are particularly revealing.[14] These women convert a substantially higher percentage of the adrenal precursor androstenedione to estrone than do their nonobese counterparts, and this conversion occurs peripherally, principally in fat depots.

Because of the long-standing observation that the triad of obesity, infertility, and ovulatory disorders occurs in some 25 to 50 percent of patients destined to develop endometrial cancer, it is reasonable to assume that an underlying endocrinopathy involving the hypothalamic-pituitary-ovarian axis is a common denominator. However, the somewhat fragmentary evidence is conflicting with regard to specific endocrine abnormalities. In a recently completed study Lucas and Yen could find no significant difference in pituitary function or carbohydrate metabolism between a group of patients with endometrial cancer and control subjects matched for age, parity, and weight.[15]

Two other clinical observations are pertinent to consideration of estrogen as an endometrial carcinogen. Although spontaneous endometrial carcinoma in women with dysgenetic gonads (Turner's syndrome) is extremely rare, there are at least 14 reported instances of endometrial carcinoma occurring in patients with dysgenetic gonads who have been treated with estrogen for prolonged periods of time.[16] Also recognized for many years is the increased incidence of endometrial hyperplasia (up to 35 percent) and carcinoma (up to 10 percent) in women with estrogen-secreting granulosa-theca cell ovarian tumors.[12] However, the relative rarity of these tumors makes them an uncommon predisposing factor. Lest one conclude that all women who develop endometrial cancer can be categorized as obese, infertile, or chronic estrogen users, it should be pointed out that a substantial number of women who develop endometrial cancer are not obese, are normally fertile, and have never taken exogenous estrogen. Figure 38-1 is a diagrammatic summary of the "estrogen hypothesis," showing the sources of long-term stimulation of the endometrium.

The role of carcinogens or cocarcinogens other than estrogen is unknown. There does appear to be a clear increase in the late occurrence of uterine cancers, particularly sarcomas, among women who have been irradiated for previous benign or malignant pelvic disease. However, this is a potential factor in only a small percentage of patients who develop endometrial cancer. There is no evidence implicating any known infectious agent.

Pathology and Patterns of Spread

As noted above, there is convincing evidence that adenomatous endometrial hyperplasia may progress, in an unopposed estrogen milieu, to frankly atypical epithelium and finally unequivocal adenocarcinoma. Of all the criteria for diagnosing frank carcinoma, stromal invasion is the most important.[16a] The pathologist is often confronted with curettings showing epithelium with marked proliferation and crowding of glands, cellular atypia, and numerous mitoses, but no frank stromal invasion. It may be impossible to distinguish between atypical adenomatous hyperplasia and early adenocarcinoma (Figs. 38-2 and 38-3). From a therapeutic standpoint, particularly among postmenopausal women, these should be regarded as well-differentiated adenocarcinomas and treated as such. In premenopausal women regression of this type of endometrial abnormality after treatment with synthetic progestins has been described by Kistner and others, and on occasion this may be a justifiable approach where for medical or psychological reasons hysterectomy is undesirable, provided meticulous follow-up with careful periodic endometrial sampling is ensured.[17]

Benign squamous metaplasia is frequently found in association with well-differentiated adenocarcinoma, giving rise to the descriptive term *adenoacanthoma* (Fig. 38-4). This finding is of no particular prognostic significance. On the other hand, Reagan, Julian, and others have reported an increasing incidence during the past decade of adenosquamous carcinoma, where both histological elements are frankly malignant.[18,19] The reasons for this increased occurrence, if real, are unknown, but the prognosis appears to be worse than for pure adenocarcinoma or adenoacanthoma.

Tumor grade of differentiation is a major evaluable pretreatment finding, and a significant factor in determining treatment and estimating prognosis. Grade is directly related to depth of myometrial invasion, which in turn is also related to incidence of metastatic disease and prognosis. It can be shown that a relative, rather than absolute, scale of myometrial penetration is the more valid prognostic indicator. Thus, involvement of only the inner one-third of the myometrium is associated with a significantly better prognosis than is penetration to the outer one-third (Table 38-1). Because of the variability in myometrial width from patient to patient, 5 to 10 mm of penetration may be shallow invasion in one patient and deep in another. Figures 38-5 and 38-6 show, respectively, adenocarcinoma limited to the fundal endometrium and deeply invading the myometrium. Figure 38-7 shows a grade 2 endometrial adenocarcinoma from endometrial curettage.

In addition to direct extension of endometrial cancer to contiguous structures, metastatic spread from endometrial cancer occurs in several ways. Spread via the regional lymphatics is to pelvic, paraaortic, and inguinal lymph nodes and to the vagina. Transtubal spread to intraperitoneal surfaces, including those of the ovary and bowel, probably occurs with greater frequency than to the lungs, liver, and bone (Table 38-2).

Signs, Symptoms, and Early Detection

The cardinal symptom of endometrial cancer is abnormal uterine bleeding. Since 80 percent of endometrial cancers occur in postmenopausal women, any vaginal bleeding in this age group demands immediate and thorough investigation. Persistent intermenstrual bleeding in premenopausal or perimenopausal women requires the same approach, recognizing that the premenopausal patient who develops endometrial cancer is often obese and infertile and has a long history of menstrual disorders associated with infrequent ovulation.

Since approximately 75 percent of endometrial cancers are diagnosed while disease is confined to the corpus, it is apparent that abnormal bleeding brings the patient to seek attention relatively early in the course of her disease (Table 38-3). In recent years a variety of instruments adapted to sampling the endocervix and endometrium as an office procedure have been developed. Two points need emphasis: (1) the endocervix should be sampled separately with a small sharp curette before any instrument is introduced into the uterine cavity, so that clinical staging can be accurately carried out from the outset; (2) if the endocervical-endometrial office biopsy is not diagnostic, formal fractional endocervical and endometrial curettage under anesthesia must be carried out (Fig. 38-8).

The woman who is receiving estrogen for postmenopausal symptoms represents a special circumstance. Since at any given time an estimated 20 percent of women with endometrial cancer will be asymptomatic, an endometrial biopsy to exclude hyperplasia or cancer should be done prior to instituting estrogen therapy. Likewise, prudence dictates endometrial sampling in these women at yearly intervals or whenever irregular bleeding occurs.

Routine cervicovaginal cytological sampling cannot be relied upon as a screening method since 40 to 60 percent of known endometrial cancers will be missed by this technique.

Diagnostic Techniques, Staging, and Work-up

Evaluation of a patient with abnormal uterine bleeding is outlined in Fig. 38-8. The information derived is of crucial importance to consistent clinical staging, and in determining appropriate treatment and prognosis.

The most widely accepted staging system at the present time is that of the International Federation of Gynecology and Obstetrics (FIGO), as shown in Table 38-4. The validity of this system of classification as a prognostic index is indicated in Table 38-3. In fact the gross extent of disease at the time of initial treatment is the chief determinant of 5-year survival.

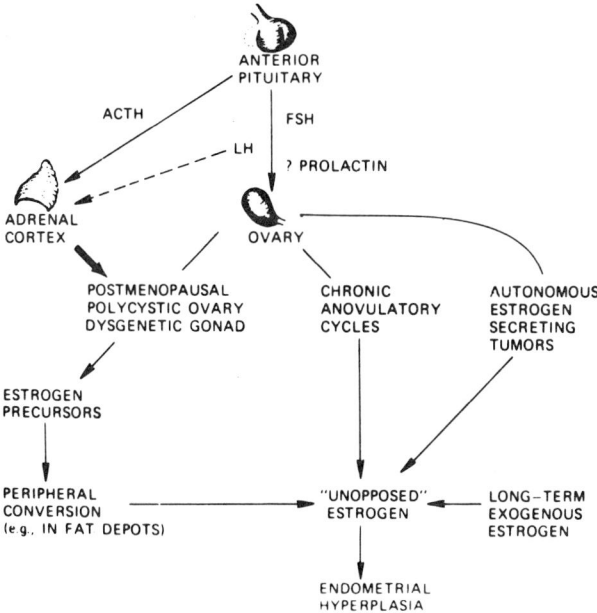

FIGURE 38-1 Sources of estrogen leading to long-term stimulation of the endometrium by estrogen "unopposed" by progesterone.

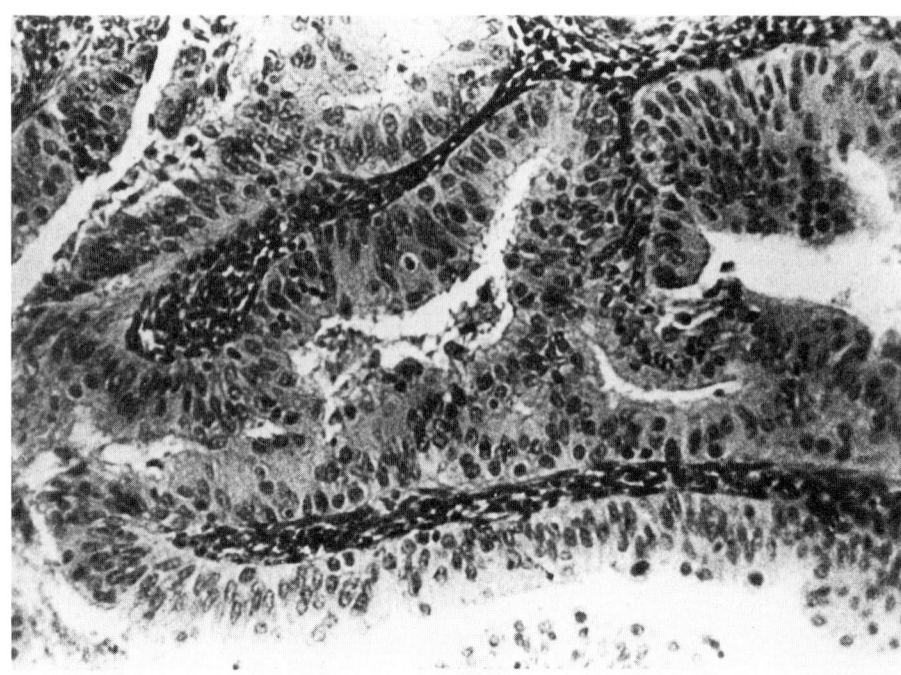

FIGURE 38-2 Well-differentiated endometrial adenocarcinoma (grade 1).

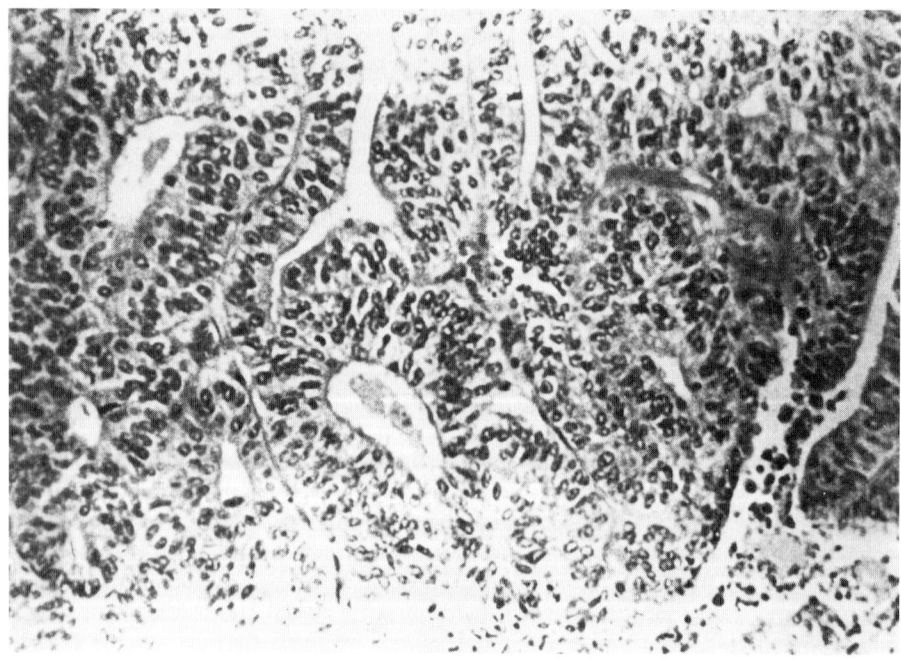

FIGURE 38-3 Well-differentiated endometrial adenocarcinoma.

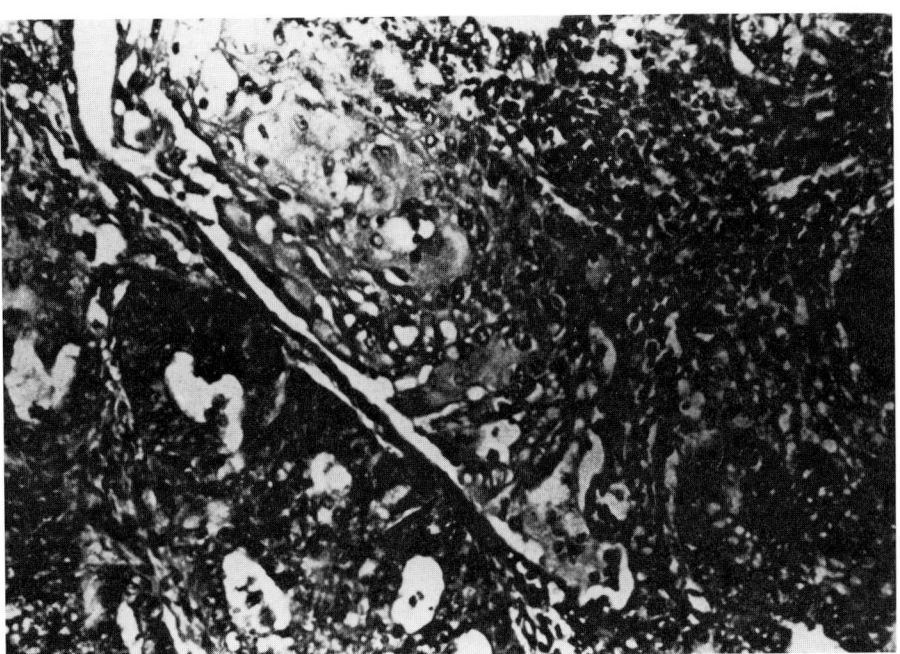

FIGURE 38-4 Adenoacanthoma of the endometrium.

The following areas demand particular attention:

1. Does cancer involve the endocervix? With spread of endometrial cancer to the endocervix the likelihood of extension into paracervical lymphatics and metastasis to regional pelvic lymph nodes increases. Approximately 13 percent of patients with disease confined to the corpus (stage I) have pelvic lymph node metastasis (Table 38-5). In addition, over 6 percent have paraaortic lymph node metastases at the time of diagnosis. Estimates of regional lymph node involvement in patients with stage II disease approach 35 percent.

2. What is the grade of tumor differentiation? The present FIGO system of categorizing differentiation as grade 1 (well-differentiated), grade 2 (moderately well differentiated), and grade 3 (poorly differentiated), although hardly quantitative, is clearly of value in several respects. Tumor grade is directly correlated with the incidence of lymph node metastases (Table 38-6), the depth of invasion of the myometrium by cancer (Table 38-7), and the ultimate prognosis (Table 38-8). Obviously, poorly differentiated tumors demand a more aggressive therapeutic approach.

3. Is depth of the endometrial cavity of prognostic importance? Although the FIGO staging system divides stage I endometrial cancer into IA and IB, subsets based on an endometrial cavity depth of less or more than 8 cm, prognosis based on this parameter does not appear to worsen until a depth of over 10 cm is reached (Table 38-9). However, depth of the uterine cavity is of greater importance than uterine

TABLE 38-1 Endometrial Carcinoma: The Influence of Depth of Myometrial Invasion on 5-Year Survival in Stage I

Depth	Total cases	5-Year survival, %
None	175	88
Superficial	312	83
Deep	121	60
Total cases and average 5-year survival	608	80

SOURCES: Nahhas WA et al: Carcinoma of the corpus uteri. *Obstet Gynecol* 38:564, 1971; and Homesley HD et al: Treatment of adenocarcinoma of the endometrium at Memorial-James Ewing Hospital 1949–1965. *Obstet Gynecol* 47:100, 1975.

size per se, since benign leiomyomas of the uterus are a common cause of uterine enlargement in the patient population at risk.

4. What are the most common sites for metastatic spread, and with what frequency is metastatic disease found? The majority of endometrial cancers are diagnosed while disease is confined to the uterus (Table 38-3). Involvement of the uterine adnexa, adjacent pelvic structures, and extrapelvic peritoneum or spread to the vagina is found in 10 to 20 percent at the time of initial evaluation. Hematogenous spread to distant sites will be found initially in less than 15 percent, and the sites of predilection are the lungs and liver and, less commonly, bone. Isolated intracranial metastases, presumably via the paravertebral plexus of Batson, occur on occasion.

The initial diagnostic work-up, therefore, should be directed toward these sites depending on the initial history, physical examination, and evaluation of the endometrial curettings. The basic work-up for all patients should include the following:

1. History and complete physical examination
2. Fractional endocervical and endometrial uterine curettage
3. Measurement of estrogen and progesterone receptor protein in the carcinomatous tissue
4. Chest x-ray
5. Intravenous urography
6. Barium enema
7. Cystoscopy
8. Proctosigmoidoscopy
9. Liver function studies
10. Peritoneal washings for cytology at the time of surgery

Radionuclide scanning or computerized tomographic studies of lungs, liver, brain, and bone should be reserved for patients with high-grade tumors or other abnormalities in the basic work-up which suggest an increased likelihood of either extensive local disease or distant metastases.

As yet, no biologic tumor markers of an endocrine, enzymatic, or antigenic variety have proved of significant

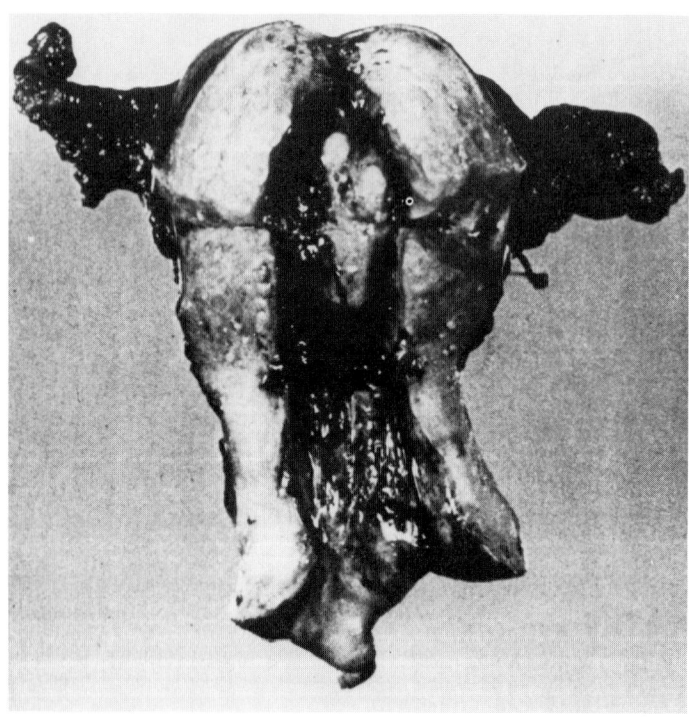

FIGURE 38-5 Adenocarcinoma of the endometrium localized to the fundus, gross.

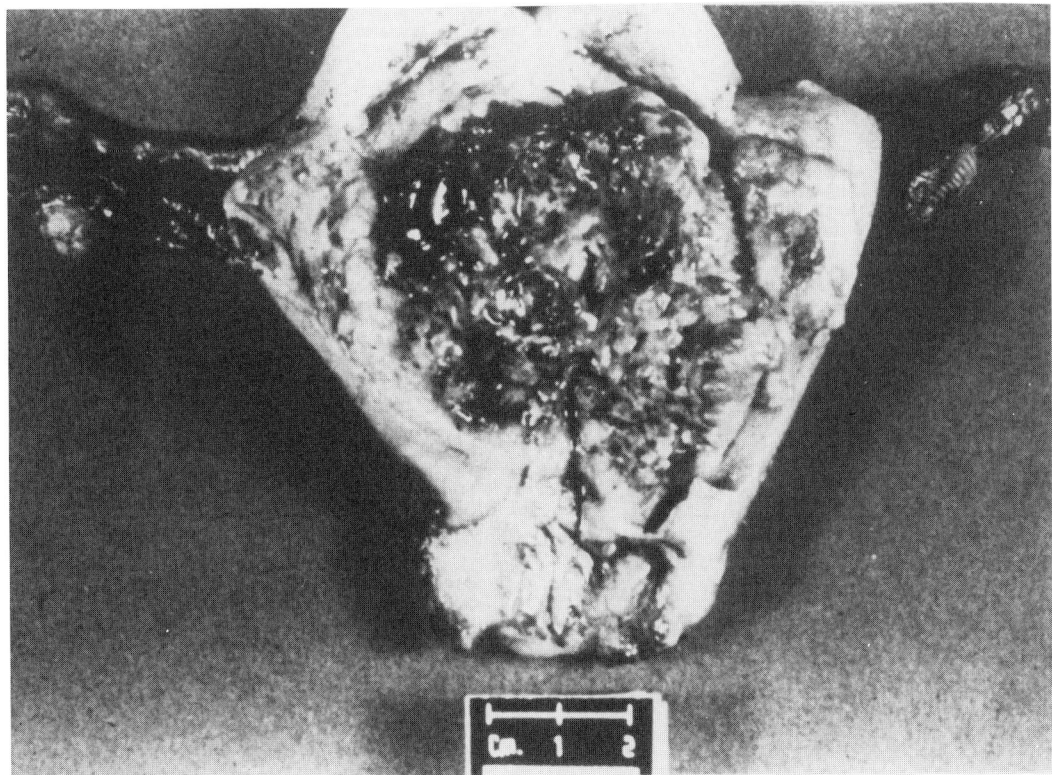

FIGURE 38-6 Deeply invasive, extensive adenocarcinoma of the fundus, gross.

diagnostic or prognostic value in the management of patients with endometrial cancer. Considering the immense potential practical importance of immunologic and other biologic markers and the scope of research now in progress, it is logical to hope that clinically useful diagnostic aids will be available in the not too distant future.

Therapeutic Options for Primary Treatment

The significance of stage and grade of endometrial carcinoma has been discussed in some detail because of their direct bearing on selection of appropriate treatment. With the evolution of total hysterectomy as a safe and relatively simple surgical technique it became apparent that many patients with stage I and a significant number with stage II disease could be cured by surgery. At the same time centers with an emphasis on radiotherapeutic techniques were also able to report a significant degree of success. Although controversies still exist regarding the respective role of these modalities, alone or in combination, a consensus has gradually evolved that most patients with stage I and II endometrial cancer are best treated, when possible, by hysterectomy, with irradiation an important adjunct in specific circumstances to be discussed below. Bickenbach et al. carefully matched two groups of patients with endometrial carcinoma, each with 190 women, on the basis of 35 different variables, and found a 20 percent improvement in 5- and 10-year survival in the surgically treated patients compared to those treated with irradiation alone.[20]

Before outlining treatment on a stage-by-stage basis, it is well to consider specific areas where either a reasonable consensus exists or where there is still considerable debate.

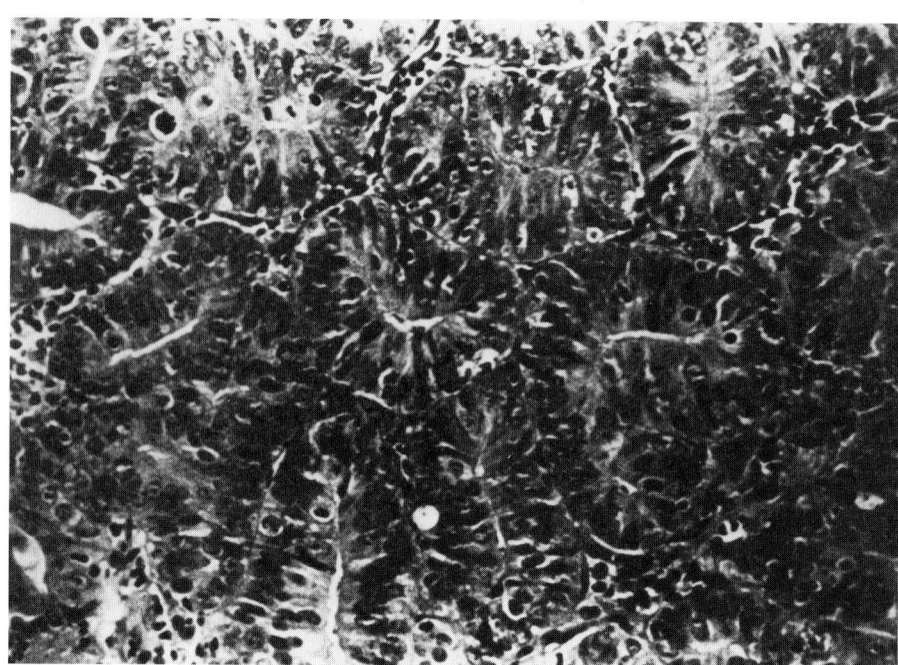

FIGURE 38-7 Moderately well-differentiated (grade 2) adenocarcinoma of the endometrium.

TABLE 38-2 Endometrial Adenocarcinoma: Distribution of Distant Metastases

Site	No.	%
Peritoneum	120	10.9
Lung	91	8.3
Ovary	88	8.0
Vagina	81	7.3
Liver	65	5.9
Bowel	59	5.3
Bone	37	3.4
Total number studied	1103	110.0

SOURCE: Plentl AA, Friedman EA: *Lymphatic System of the Female Genitalia,* Saunders, Philadelphia, 1971.

TABLE 38-3 Endometrial Adenocarcinoma: Stage Distribution at Time of Diagnosis and 5-Year Survival

Stage	Total No.	%	5-Year survival No.	%
I	1692	79	1349	80
II	140	7	81	58
III	180	8	59	33
IV	138	6	10	7
Totals and average 5-year survival	2150	100	1499	70

SOURCES: Boronow RC: Carcinoma of the corpus, in Rutledge F, Boronow RC, Wharton JT: *Cancer of the Uterus and Ovary,* Year Book, Chicago, 1969; Morris JM: The value of preoperative irradiation in carcinoma of the corpus, in *Cancer of the Uterus and Ovary,* Year Book, Chicago, 1969; Frick HC et al: Carcinoma of the endometrium. *Am J Obstet Gynecol* 115: 663, 1973; Homesley HD et al: Treatment of adenocarcinoma of the endometrium at Memorial-James Ewing Hospital 1949–1965. *Obstet Gynecol* 47:100, 1975; and Malkasian GD Jr: Carcinoma of the endometrium; effect of stage and grade on survival. *Cancer* 41:996, 1978

1. Well-differentiated (grade 1) stage IA cancer can be adequately treated by hysterectomy and bilateral salpingo-oophorectomy alone. There is no convincing evidence that either pre- or postoperative irradiation improves the chances for primary cure.

2. Less well differentiated (grades 2 and 3) stage I cancers are better treated by a combination of surgery and irradiation than by either modality alone. The same may apply when the endometrial cavity is over 10 cm in depth.

Controversy exists as to whether irradiation should precede or follow surgery, and whether preoperative irradiation should primarily be teletherapy to the whole pelvis and vagina, or intrauterine irradiation alone, or a combination of both.

Arguments in favor of preoperative irradiation to the whole pelvis include the ability to sterilize micrometastases outside the uterus, within the therapeutic radiation field, and in an area with an undisturbed blood supply and better tissue oxygenation, thereby enhancing radiobiologic effectiveness. In addition, with preoperative irradiation there may be less risk of disseminating viable cancer due to surgical manipulation. Figures 38-9 and 38-10 show a poorly differentiated endometrial adenocarcinoma before irradiation and following 5000 rads of external preoperative irradiation. There is marked necrosis of the tumor. This patient is alive and well more than 5 years after treatment.

The chief argument in favor of postoperative irradiation is that this approach affords the opportunity to surgically stage the extent of cancer including the depth of myometrial invasion by cancer and the presence or absence of extension of cancer to other pelvic structures and regional lymph nodes. This should allow better selection of those patients who may benefit from adjunctive irradiation and reduce the total number of patients subjected to the added hazards and expense of irradiation.

Unfortunately, there are no data to clearly support the superiority of one approach over the other for at least three reasons: the first is the lack of controlled trials comparing these approaches; the second is that because of the relatively favorable prognosis for stage I cancer treated with a variety of combinations of surgery and irradiation, it will be necessary to accumulate large groups of patients in randomized prospective studies and follow them well in excess of 5 years to provide better answers; the third is that many series prepared in the past have compared the results of surgery alone applied to patients with well-differentiated lesions with the results of combinations of surgery and irradiation for patients with grade 2 and grade 3 cancers.

3. Less controversy exists regarding the management of stage II endometrial cancer. The best results reported to date are obtained where treatment has been by a combination of external and intracavitary irradiation followed by hysterectomy.

4. The role of a more radical surgical approach to both stage I and II endometrial cancer has been explored in several centers and largely abandoned. Although this

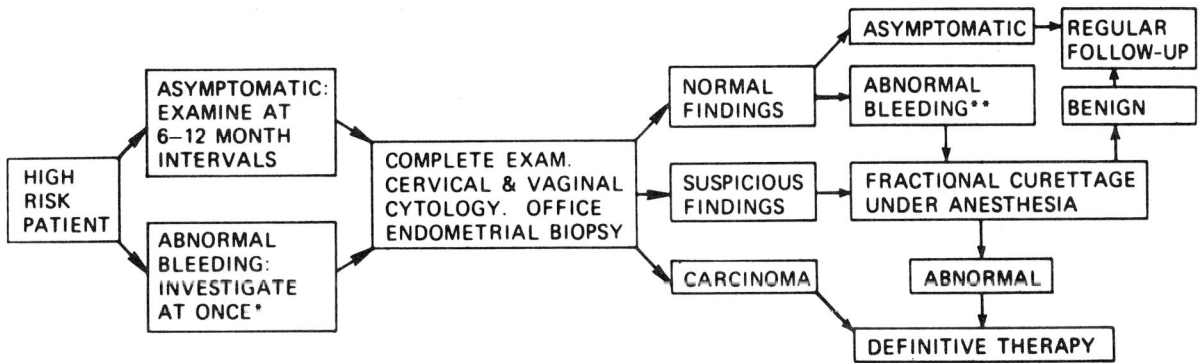

FIGURE 38-8 Diagnostic evaluation of the patient with abnormal uterine bleeding. *All patients, irrespective of risk. **Patient receiving estrogen who has a normal pelvic exam and normal cytology and endometrial biopsy—discontinue estrogen and currette at once if bleeding continues or recurs.

TABLE 38-4 Staging Classification of Endometrial Carcinoma

Stage I	The carcinoma is confined to the corpus.
Stage IA	The length of the uterine cavity is 8 cm or less.
Stage IB	The length of the uterine cavity is more than 8 cm.

Stage I cases should be subgrouped as regards histological grade of carcinoma as follows:

Grade 1	Highly differentiated.
Grade 2	Differentiated with partly solid areas.
Grade 3	Predominantly solid or entirely undifferentiated carcinomas.
Stage II	The carcinoma involves corpus and cervix.
Stage III	The carcinoma extends outside the corpus but not outside the true pelvis (it may involve the vagina or parametrium but not the bladder or rectum).
Stage IV	The carcinoma involves the bladder or rectum (proved by mucosal biopsy) or extends outside the pelvis.

approach has afforded invaluable information regarding the relationship of lymph node metastases to stage and grade, in neither stage I nor stage II has the added risk of radical surgery afforded a cure rate surpassing more conservative surgery combined with irradiation. The majority of patients with endometrial cancer are over age 50 and many are obese and have major medical problems such as diabetes and hypertension, making them relatively unsuitable candidates for radical hysterectomy and regional lymphadenectomy.

TABLE 38-5 Endometrial Adenocarcinoma: Lymph Node Metastases in Stages I and II

Metastases	Total cases evaluated		Node metastases, %	
	Stage I	Stage II	Stage I	Stage II
Pelvic	623	77	13	42
Aortic	290		6	

SOURCES: Davis EW Jr: Carcinoma of the corpus uteri. *Am J Obstet Gynecol* 88:163, 1964; Carmichael JA: Carcinoma of the endometrium in Saskatchewan. *Am J Obstet Gynecol* 9:294, 1967; Lees DH: An evaluation of the treatment of carcinoma of the body of the uterus. *J Obstet Gynecol Brit Commw* 76:615, 1969; Lewis BV et al: Adenocarcinoma of the body of the uterus. *J Obstet Gynaecol Brit Commw* 77:343, 1970; Rutledge F: The role of radical hysterectomy in adenocarcinoma of the endometrium. *Gynecol Oncol* 2:331, 1974; and Creasman WT et al: Adenocarcinoma of the endometrium; its metastatic lymph node potential. *Gynecol Oncol* 4:239, 1976.

TABLE 38-6 Endometrial Adenocarcinoma: Influence of Histological Grade on Lymph Node Metastases in Stage I

Grade	Total cases	Node Metastases	
		Pelvic, %	Aortic, %
Grade 1	65	3	1.5
Grade 2	50	10	4.0
Grade 3	25	36	28.0

SOURCE: Creasman WT et al: Adenocarcinoma of the endometrium: Its metastatic lymph node potential. *Gynecol Oncol* 4:239, 1976.

5. Data now available regarding the incidence of lymph node metastases pose new questions regarding the adequacy of conventional treatment of stage II and less well differentiated stage I cancers. Approximately one-third of patients with poorly differentiated stage I cancers will have metastases to paraaortic lymph nodes at the time of diagnosis and will be doomed to an unsuccessful outcome from the outset unless a more aggressive therapeutic approach is considered. Although there is no evidence at this time that extending radiation fields to include the paraaortic nodes or adding adjunctive chemotherapy will cure any of these patients, it can be argued that paraaortic lymph node biopsy at the time of hysterectomy will at least select out those patients who might benefit from a more aggressive approach. Protocol studies to test this possibility are in progress.

6. The prognostic significance of peritoneal cytology at the time of surgery deserves mention. It is becoming apparent that as many as 15 percent of stage I patients have positive peritoneal cytology at the time of surgical exploration[20a], and that such patients in whom positive cytology is the only evidence of extrauterine spread may benefit from postoperative intraperitoneal instillation of

TABLE 38-7 Endometrial Adenocarcinoma: The Influence of Histological Grade on Myometrial Invasion in Stage I

Grade	None, %	Superficial, %	Deep, %
Grade 1	56	28	16
Grade 2	48	25	27
Grade 3	36	14	50

SOURCES: Gusberg SB et al: Selection of treatment for corpus cancer. *Am J Obstet Gynecol* 80:374, 1960, and Cheon HK: Prognosis of endometrial cancer. *Obstet Gynecol* 34:680, 1969.

TABLE 38-8 Endometrial Carcinoma: The Influence of Histological Grade on 5-Year Survival in Stage I

Grade	Total cases	5-Year survival, %
Grade 1	1023	88
Grade 2	823	87
Grade 3	796	68
Total cases and average 5-year survival	2642	82

SOURCES: Boronow RC: Carcinoma of the corpus, in *Cancer of the Uterus and Ovary*, Year Book, Chicago, 1969; Morris JM: The value of preoperative irradiation in carcinoma of the corpus, in *Cancer of the Uterus and Ovary*, Year Book, Chicago, 1969; Frick HC et al: Carcinoma of the endometrium. *Am J Obstet Gynecol* 115:663, 1973; Homesley HD et al: Treatment of adenocarcinoma of the endometrium at Memorial-James Ewing Hospital 1949–1965. *Obstet Gynecol* 47:100, 1975; and Malkasian GD Jr: Carcinoma of the endometrium: Effect of stage and grade on survival. *Cancer* 41:996, 1978.

TABLE 38-9 Endometrial Adenocarcinoma: Relationship between Depth of Endometrial Cavity and Prognosis

Depth	Total cases	5-Year survival, %
< 7.5 cm	61	85
<10 cm	220	70
≧10 cm	64	64

SOURCE: Cheon HK: Prognosis of endometrial cancer. *Obstet Gynecol* 34:680, 1969.

STAGE I, GRADE 1

1. Total extrafascial abdominal hysterectomy and bilateral salpingo-oophorectomy.
2. Postoperative irradiation where examination of the surgical specimen reveals a less well differentiated cancer, myometrial invasion to greater than one-third of myometrial thickness, or unsuspected involvement of the lower uterine segment or endocervix, including the following options:
   a. Whole-pelvic external irradiation, between 4000 and 5000 rads midpelvic dose.
   b. Vaginal vault irradiation with cesium or radium to deliver a surface dose of 5000 to 6000 rads.

12 to 15 millicuries of radioactive colloidal chromic phosphate (^{32}P).

The following are acceptable therapeutic options stage by stage, for the treatment of endometrial cancer based on current 5- and 10-year survival data.

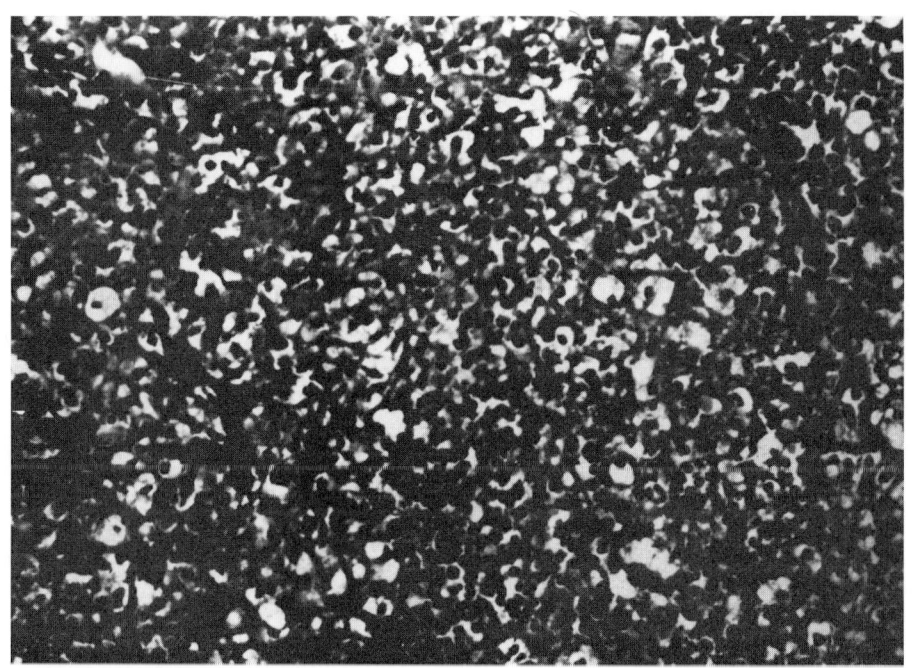

FIGURE 38-9 Poorly differentiated adenocarcinoma of the endometrium prior to irradiation.

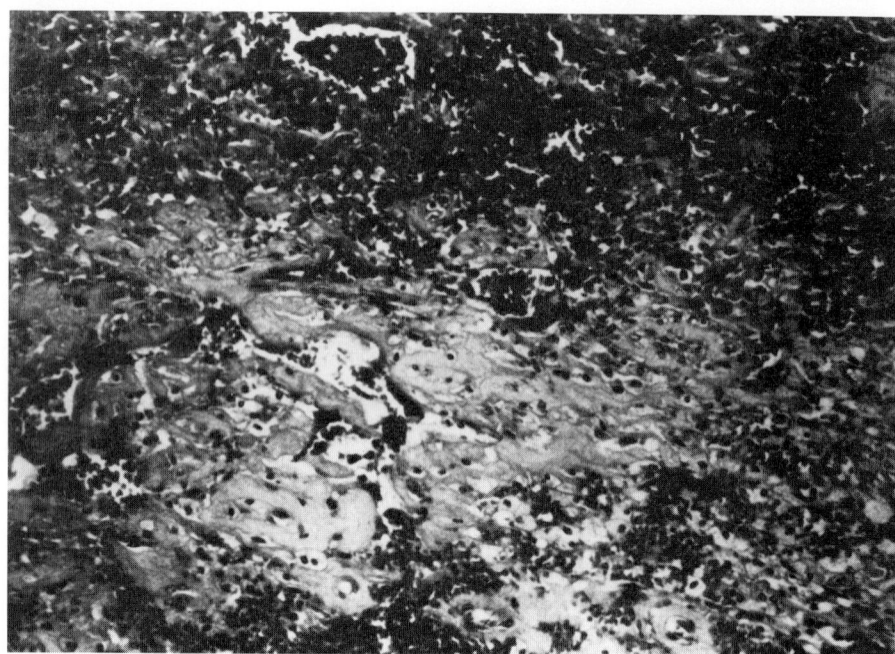

FIGURE 38-10 Same endometrium as in Fig. 38-9 after 5000 rads of external beam irradiation.

    c. Individualized combinations of external and intracavitary irradiation.
3. Intraperitoneal radioactive colloidal chromic phosphate (^{32}P), 12 to 15 millicuries, when peritoneal washings contain tumor cells.
4. Primary irradiation therapy for inoperable patients.

STAGE I, GRADES 2 AND 3, AND/OR
LARGE ENDOMETRIAL CAVITY

1. Preoperative irradiation, followed promptly by total abdominal hysterectomy, bilateral salpingo-oophorectomy, and paraaortic lymph node biopsy.
   a. Endometrial cavity not enlarged: 4000 to 5000 rads whole-pelvic and upper vaginal irradiation via external beam.
   b. Endometrial cavity enlarged (over 10 to 12 cm in depth): 4000 rads whole-pelvic external irradiation, and intracavitary irradiation, a single application using an intrauterine tandem or Heyman capsule and vaginal ovoids to deliver a total dose of approximately 6000 to 7000 rads 2 cm lateral to the midplane of the cervix and 5000 rads 5 cm lateral to the midplane.
2. Surgery followed by postoperative irradiation where myometrial invasion in excess of $\frac{1}{3}$ to $\frac{1}{2}$ of the thickness of the myometrium is present, invasion of vascular spaces within the myometrium is found, or there is involvement of parametrial tissues or lymph nodes in the pelvis or paraaortic area.
3. Intraperitoneal ^{32}P when peritoneal washings are positive (see above).
4. Primary irradiation for inoperable patients.

STAGE II

1. Preoperative irradiation, as described above for stage I, grades 2 and 3, with enlarged endometrial cavity, followed by extrafascial abdominal hysterectomy, bilateral salpingo-oophorectomy, and paraaortic lymph node biopsy.
2. Radical hysterectomy and pelvic lymphadenectomy where adequate preoperative irradiation is not possible.
3. Primary external and intracavitary irradiation for medically inoperable patients.

STAGE III

1. Primary external and intracavitary irradiation.
2. On an individualized basis, combinations of irradiation and surgery may be justified. Even though disease in the lower vagina and parametria may respond well to irradiation, it may be impossible to deliver adequate doses of irradiation to sterilize cancer in the uterine fundus, particularly where appreciable myometrial invasion exists. Therefore post irradiation surgical exploration and hysterectomy if disease appears limited to the uterus may be warranted. Currently implantation of these lesions with iridium needles is being explored as an additional therapeutic option.
3. Postoperative whole-pelvic irradiation where unsuspected spread of cancer, limited to the pelvis, is found at the time of primary surgery.

STAGE IV

1. Primary external and intracavitary irradiation where disease is limited to the pelvis (bladder or rectal involvement).
2. Individualized combinations of pelvic irradiation to achieve local control of tumor for palliation and systemic chemotherapy.

As implied above, compilation of results from various centers over the last two decades supports the following conclusions regarding the treatment of stage I and II endometrial cancers (Tables 38-10 and 38-11).

TABLE 38-10 Endometrial Adenocarcinoma: 5-Year Survival According to Type of Treatment in Stage I (1962–1977 Reports)

Treatment	Total cases	5-Year survival, %
Hysterectomy	2287	81
Hysterectomy and postoperative RT	1336	83
Hysterectomy and preoperative external RT	362	87
Hysterectomy and preoperative intracavitary RT	2190	80
Radical hysterectomy	510	72
Radiation therapy	814	60

NOTE: RT = radiation therapy.
SOURCES: Rutledge F: The role of radical hysterectomy in adenocarcinoma of the endometrium. *Gynecol Oncol* 2:331, 1974, and Salazar OM et al.[21,22]

TABLE 38-11 Endometrial Carcinoma: 5-Year Survival According to Type of Treatment in Stage II

Treatment	No. of patients	5-Year survival, %
Radiation therapy	153	43
Surgery + RT	128	74
Total cases and average 5-year survival	281	57

NOTE: RT = radiation therapy.
SOURCES: Boronow RC: Carcinoma of the corpus, in *Cancer of the Uterus and Ovary*, Year Book, Chicago, 1969; Kottmeier HL: Individualization of therapy in carcinoma of the corpus, in *Cancer of the Uterus and Ovary*, Year Book, Chicago, 1969; Hernandez W et al: Stage II endometrial carcinoma: Two modalities of treatment. *Am J Obstet Gynecol* 131:171, 1978; Bruckman JE et al: Combined irradiation and surgery in the treatment of stage II carcinoma of the endometrium. *Cancer* 42:1146, 1978; and Surwit EA et al: Stage II carcinoma of the endometrium. *Obstet Gynecol* 52:97, 1978.

1. Surgical removal of the uterus is clearly superior to irradiation alone, with 5-year survival in the 70 to 90 percent range (average 80 percent) for surgery versus an average of 60 percent for irradiation.
2. The addition of irradiation to surgery for less favorable stage I and all stage II cases decreases the incidence of vaginal vault recurrence from the average of 7 percent to less than 3 percent (Table 38-12) and increases chances for 5-year survival. The improved survival among patients treated with combination therapy over those treated by surgery alone becomes more apparent as the extent of disease and degree of anaplasia increase. An analysis of survival according to treatment, stratified for grade, by Salazar et al. suggests superiority for preoperative external irradiation (Table 38-13).[21,22]
3. Radical hysterectomy and pelvic lymphadenectomy

TABLE 38-12 Endometrial Carcinoma: Vaginal Recurrences According to Type of Treatment for Stage I

Treatment	No. of patients	Vaginal recurrences, %
Surgery	1289	6.9
Radiation	511	4.1
Surgery + radiation	1595	2.8

SOURCE: Plentl AA, Friedman EA: *Lymphatic System of the Female Genitalia*, Saunders, Philadelphia, 1971.

TABLE 38-13 Endometrial Carcinoma: Grade 3 vs. Total 5-Year Survival According to Treatment of Stage I

Treatment	5-Year survival			
	Grade 3		Total	
	No.	%	No.	%
Hysterectomy	17	71	43	81
Hysterectomy + postoperative RT	10	70	22	73
Hysterectomy + preoperative external RT	59	86	93	90
Hysterectomy + preoperative intracavitary RT	12	75	19	79
Radiotherapy	11	36	16	44
Total	109	76	193	81

NOTE: RT = radiotherapy.
SOURCE: Salazar et al.[21,22]

provides no improvement in chances for cure over simple hysterectomy combined with irradiation. In any event it is not a technique applicable to the frequent type of the elderly and obese patient without unwarranted risk.

Adjuvant Therapies

Significant interest and effort have been directed toward progesterone and its potent synthetic analogues (progestins) as adjuvant therapy for endometrial cancer. Both in vivo and in vitro studies support the ability of progesterone to inhibit DNA synthesis and induce regression of endometrial hyperplasia and well-differentiated adenocarcinoma.[23,24] Concurrent use of progestins with primary therapy therefore has theoretical merit. Unfortunately very little data is available to support this premise. Bonte, in 1970, conducted a controlled study of 40 patients, all treated with intracavitary radium and hysterectomy.[25] Of these 20 received medroxyprogesterone for 4 weeks preoperatively. Of this group only 7 had "viable" cancer still present in the uterus at hysterectomy, whereas 18 of the 20 who did not receive medroxyprogesterone still had viable tumor present. More recently Decoster and Bonte compared the effect of preoperative intrauterine medroxyprogesterone and radium on the incidence of residual cancer in the surgical specimen in a small series of patients with stage I disease.[24] No viable residual tumor could be found in 59 percent after medroxyprogesterone or in 62 percent after intracavitary irradiation. An adjuvant study of medroxyprogesterone versus placebo in the management of stage I endometrial cancer, reported by Lewis in 1974, revealed no difference in survival, but the groups were not sufficiently randomized or stratified to permit any meaningful conclusions.[26] Most recently the estrogen antagonist tamoxifen has been reported to be effective where progestin therapy has failed.

To firmly establish the merits, if any, of adjunctive treatment using progestins will require extended clinical trials. A large patient population will be needed to test this hypothesis since the greatest benefit from progestins can be anticipated in patients with early and well-differentiated cancers, a group with 5-year disease-free survival in the 90 percent range following conventional treatment. In favor of progestin therapy is virtual freedom from serious side effects, particularly when used for limited periods.

Neither adjunctive cytotoxic chemotherapy nor immunotherapy has received any degree of attention in the primary management of endometrial carcinoma. Again, the chief reason is the relatively favorable prognosis with conventional treatment methods. To accumulate meaningful data would be a formidable undertaking in terms of both patient numbers and time required.

The role of adjunctive therapy in high-risk, poor-prognosis patients needs to be explored by means of carefully chosen prospective protocols as more data accumulates regarding the effect of available cytotoxic drugs on recurrent endometrial cancer. A prospective, randomized trial of adjunctive chemotherapy needs to be carried out in patients with poorly differentiated cancers, in those with deep myometrial invasion, and in those with residual viable cancer in the uterus after preoperative irradiation or with local spread outside the uterus which has been completely excised.

Since most patients found to have paraaortic lymph node metastases at the time of primary surgery will also have systemic metastases, the use of adjunctive chemotherapy in this group should be studied. In this group, assay of the primary tumor, as well as metastases, for estrogen- and progesterone-binding receptor protein should be included as part of the protocol to permit selection of those patients most likely to benefit from progestin or Tamoxifen treatment.

Follow-up Techniques

An aggressive approach to the detection of recurrent or metastatic cancer is clearly in the best interest of the patient, since significant objective response rates are now obtainable with appropriate therapy. It should be noted that 80 percent of all treatment failures occur within 3 years.

Among the commonest sites for recurrence of endometrial carcinoma are the lungs and vagina, which are readily evaluable by systematic follow-up. Abdominal and pelvic examinations should be done at 3-month intervals for the first 2 years post treatment, and then at 6-month intervals, and chest x-rays should be obtained at 6-month intervals. Patients in poorer prognostic categories by reason of stage and grade of the primary tumor require particularly meticulous follow-up. The occurrence of abnormal findings or symptoms demands more intensive investigation, including appropriate contrast and scanning techniques.

When there is a question of intraperitoneal recurrence of cancer the use of peritoneoscopy has proved of definite value. Positive peritoneoscopic findings may obviate the need for more extensive work-up, since biopsies and washings for cytological examination can be obtained at the same time.

Transcutaneous or transmucosal needle biopsies may be of aid in defining the nature of isolated pulmonary nodules, as well as hepatic nodules and pelvic masses. This technique can now be carried out with increasing accuracy and safety in conjunction with sonographic and x-ray scanning and tomographic techniques.

The Treatment of Recurrent and/or Metastatic Disease

The most common site for metastatic spread is the peritoneum, which is found to be involved with an average frequency of 10 percent of cases, followed by lung, ovary, and vagina, each averaging a frequency of approximately 8 percent. Metastatic spread to liver, bowel, and bone is found less often, with an average frequency of 3 to 6 percent.

One form of metastatic disease amenable to cure on occasion is isolated posttreatment recurrence in the vaginal vault and adjacent central pelvis. Peritoneoscopy to rule out widespread intraperitoneal disease and a systematic survey for distant metastases should precede definitive therapy. In the nonirradiated posthysterectomy patient the primary approach to this problem should be irradiation, including whole-pelvis external beam therapy and intravaginal therapy with radium or cesium, or transvaginal therapy with iridium needles. Isolated vaginal or central pelvic recurrence in the previously irradiated patient demands an attempt at surgical cure. In general, because of the intimate adherence of bladder and rectum to the area of recurrence, total pelvic exenteration will be required. Surgery of this extent should only be undertaken after careful preoperative survey has excluded distant metastases, and intraoperative evaluation has ruled out spread to peritoneal surfaces, retroperitoneal lymph nodes above the pelvis, or liver.

Disseminated metastatic disease, found either at the time of the original diagnosis or as a recurrence, demands systemic therapy. The longest and most extensive experience is with the use of high doses of synthetic progestins. The efficacy of progestin therapy in producing objective responses in approximately 30 percent of patients with metastatic endometrial cancer has been confirmed by many observers. Several points bear emphasis: Recurrences which appear within 2 years of diagnosis and which follow poorly differentiated primary cancers respond less well than late recurrences which follow well-differentiated primaries. This is consistent with the recent observations of Young and others that the highest concentration of progesterone receptors are found in well-differentiated cancers and the lowest concentration or absence in poorly differentiated cancers.[27] Figures 38-11 to 38-14 show the effect of high-dose progestin therapy on pulmonary metastases over an 8-week period.

With the present availability of progesterone and estrogen receptor assays in many centers, assay of the primary tumor as well as biopsies of recurrences for receptors should be done wherever possible.[27,27a] The information should then be considered as a future guide for choosing cytotoxic chemotherapy (progesterone receptor–negative patient) versus progestin therapy with or without cytotoxic chemotherapy (progesterone receptor–positive patient).

The three synthetic progestins shown in Table 38-14 are currently in use for treatment of metastatic endometrial cancer. Medroxyprogesterone acetate is the most potent of these progestins in accepted test systems and may be the most effective clinically, although no clear superiority for any of these drugs has been demonstrated.[28] Recommended doses and schedules vary

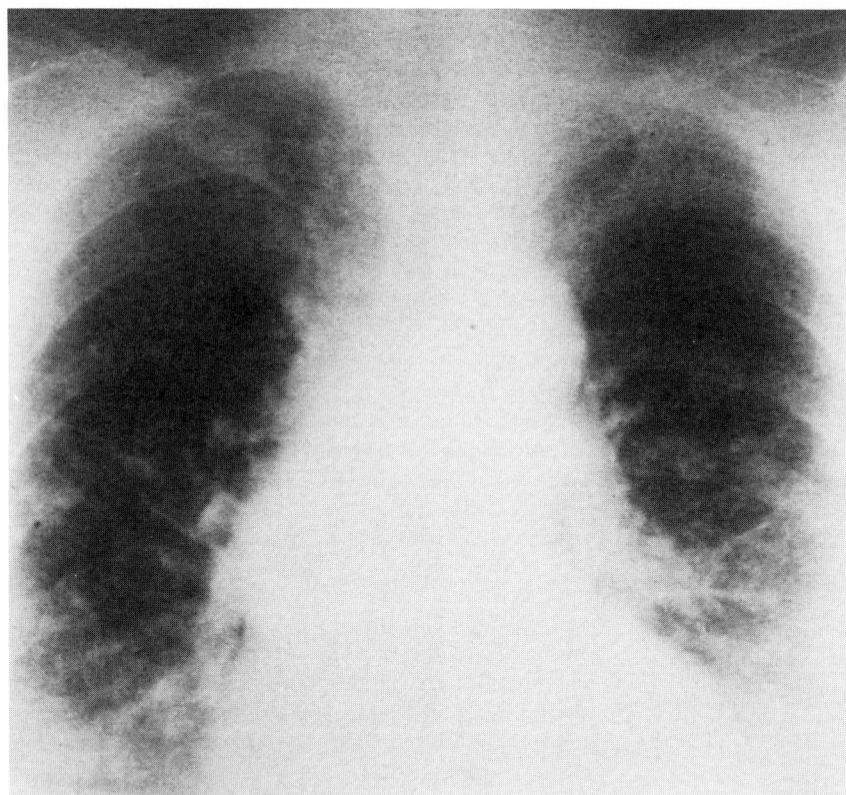

FIGURE 38-11 Pulmonary metastases due to adenocarcinoma of the endometrium.

widely, although the present consensus would seem to be that an initial loading dose should be given for 8 to 10 weeks, followed by maintenance therapy at weekly to biweekly intervals in the case of the injectable preparations, and a daily dose for the oral preparation. Since significant regression of tumor may not be apparent for 8 to 10 weeks, progestin therapy should not be abandoned until at least a 10-week trial has elapsed. The great advantages of progestin therapy are a relative freedom from side effects, compared to cytotoxic agents, and a substantial subjective response rate, above and beyond objective response, reported by many observers. Side effects to be looked for are increased insulin requirement in diabetic patients, fluid retention, and occasional abscesses at injection sites.

Perhaps as a result of the occasional dramatic response of metastatic endometrial cancer to progestin therapy, trials of nonhormonal cytotoxic chemotherapeutic agents have lagged behind those in other forms of cancer. To date no large series of metastatic or recurrent endometrial cancer treated with single-agent nonhormonal chemotherapy or with drug combinations has been reported. However, drugs with reported activity, either alone or in combination, include doxorubicin, cyclophosphamide, 5-fluorouracil, and *cis*-platinum. In preliminary trials with these agents objective response rates of 40 to over 60 percent have been reported.[28a,28b] In order to accumulate valid data patients with recurrent endometrial cancer treated with nonhormonal chemotherapeutic agents or combinations of agents should be placed in protocol studies as often as possible.

Current Areas of Research and Future Prospects

Because of the epidemiologic clues and laboratory evidence supporting the concept of hormonal dependence for many endometrial carcinomas, it is not surprising

CANCERS OF THE UTERINE CORPUS

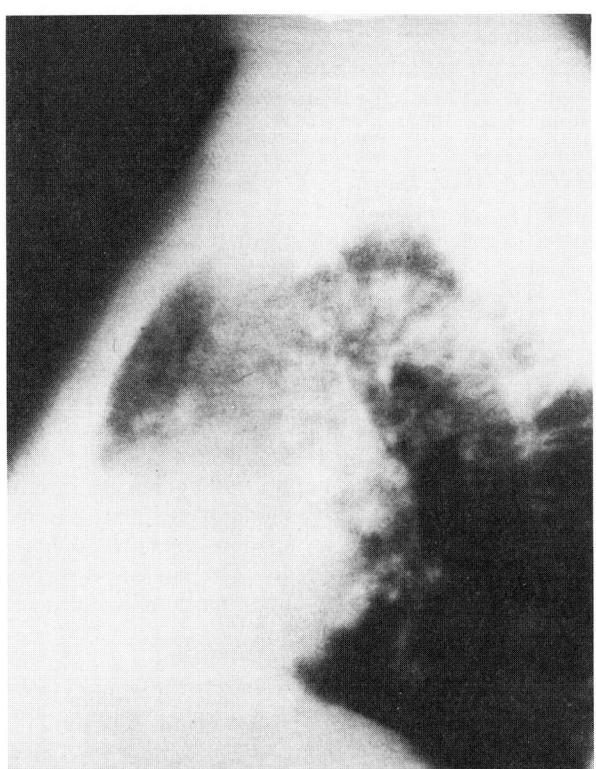

FIGURE 38-12 Pulmonary metastases due to adenocarcinoma of the endometrium.

expanded ability to cure while minimizing undesirable short- and long-term morbidity.

The search for screening methods to permit easy early diagnosis of endometrial cancer and its precursors is by no means ended. Although periodic endometrial sampling is a relatively accurate diagnostic technique, routine use of this method of asymptomatic postmenopausal women is neither cost-effective nor likely to be universally accepted, even if made universally and easily available. Here, as in many other tumor systems, it is to be hoped that specific immunodiagnostic or other biologic diagnostic techniques will be forthcoming from basic research in tumor immunology and cell biology.

Rehabilitation of the Endometrial Cancer Patient

As a rule the physical rehabilitation of a patient subjected to hysterectomy and/or irradiation for endometrial cancer is relatively uncomplicated. In the great majority

that a substantial portion of the research being conducted is endocrinologic. Of particular interest are studies being undertaken to define and elaborate the role of estrogen and progesterone receptors in the origin and evolution of endometrial cancer, and to define the therapeutic implications of the presence or absence of receptors in the cancer cell. As implied above, more rational selection of hormonal versus nonhormonal chemotherapy for recurrent or metastatic disease may well be possible with foreknowledge of receptor status.

The role of adjunctive chemotherapy, hormonal and nonhormonal, as part of primary therapy in high-risk patients deserves careful prospective evaluation. It is unlikely that more extensive surgery or more aggressive conventional radiotherapeutic techniques will improve the outlook for patients with endometrial cancer. It is to be hoped, however, that research into the use of radiosensitizing and radioprotective agents will result in an

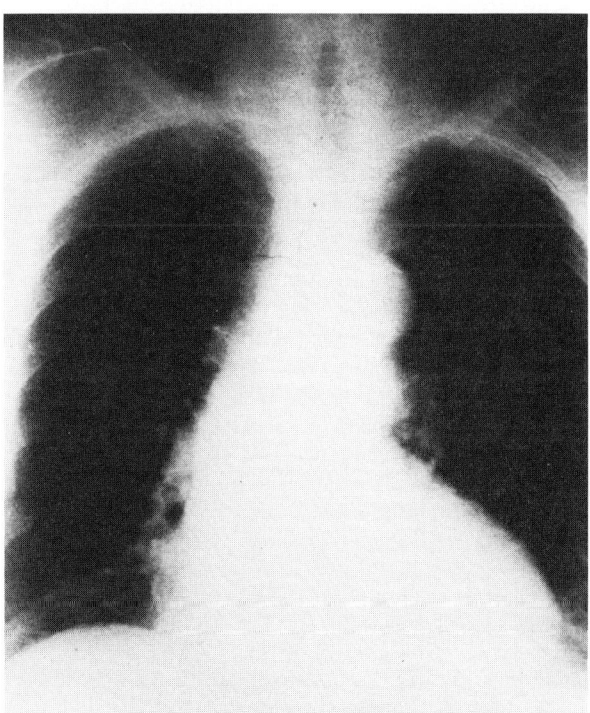

FIGURE 38-13 Complete clearing of pulmonary metastases following progestin therapy.

798 GYNECOLOGIC NEOPLASMS

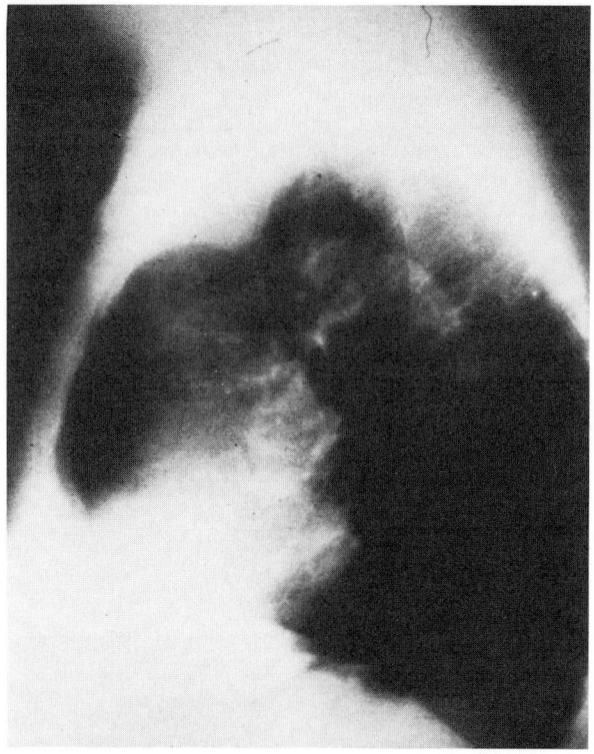

FIGURE 38-14 Complete clearing of pulmonary metastases following progestin therapy.

there is no significant long-term physical disability. The psychological impact of the cancer diagnosis and the subsequent treatment may, on the other hand, be significant. Aside from the fear engendered by the diagnosis, the loss of a woman's reproductive organs, even long after the menopause, may be perceived as a loss of femininity. The already stressful changes suffered by many women as they pass through the menopause may be significantly intensified and prolonged. Depression may originate or worsen as a result of the cumulative stresses. An understanding, reassuring, and supportive family and physician will do much to ease the stress of coping with diagnosis, treatment, and convalescence, and hasten the ultimate goal of complete recovery. Fortunately, the majority of patients with endometrial cancer will, with competent and compassionate professional care, achieve complete physical and emotional recovery.

UTERINE SARCOMAS

Although much less common than endometrial adenocarcinomas, uterine sarcomas have historically exhibited much more aggressive behavior and a relatively poor prognosis. As a group, therefore, they deserve careful study and development of rational plans for aggressive combinations of surgery, irradiation, and chemotherapy based on improved understanding of patterns of spread and of the responsiveness of specific histological types to adjunctive treatment.

The heterogenous nature of these tumors has intrigued and challenged the medical taxonomist. Ober pioneered efforts to introduce a logical and orderly system of classification.[29] A reasonably straightforward and simple classification is one based on Kempson's modification of the Ober classification (Table 38-15).

Homologous tumors contain only cellular elements normally found in the uterus, and heterologous tumors contain cellular elements not normally found in the uterus. The most commonly held concept of the histogenesis of these tumors is that they arise from the least specialized müllerian mesenchyme, which has the pluripotential to develop both sarcomas and carcinomas. From a practical standpoint it is convenient to consider these tumors in four major categories: leiomyosarcomas (LMS), endometrial stromal sarcomas (ESS), mixed mesodermal sarcomas (MMS), and a miscellaneous group of individually uncommon sarcomas.

TABLE 38-14 Endometrial Carcinoma: Progestational Drugs Useful in Treatment of Metastatic Disease

Agent	Route	Loading dose	Maintenance
Medroxyprogesterone acetate	IM	800 mg weekly × 10	800 mg every 2–4 weeks
17-Hydroxyprogesterone caproate	IM	1000 mg weekly × 10	1000 mg every 2–4 weeks
Megestrol	Oral		80–160 mg/day

TABLE 38-15 Classification of Uterine Sarcomas

1. Pure Sarcomas*
    a. Pure homologous
        (1) Leiomyosarcoma
        (2) Endometrial stromal sarcoma
        (3) Fibrosarcoma
    b. Pure heterologous (rhabdomyosarcoma, osteosarcoma, chondrosarcoma, etc.)
2. Mixed sarcomas*
    a. Mixed homologous (leiomyosarcoma plus stromal sarcoma)
    b. Mixed heterologous (with or without homologous elements)

* With or without carcinoma.

Incidence, Epidemiology, and Etiology

A reasonable estimate of the relative occurrence rate of uterine sarcomas is that they constitute no more than 2 to 4 percent of all corpus cancers (Table 38-16). In a review of over 700 uterine sarcomas collected from a variety of sources Ariel and Pack found that 68 percent were leiomyosarcomas and 32 percent mesenchymal endometrial sarcomas of the homologous, heterologous, and mixed varieties.[30] More recent data suggests that mixed mesodermal sarcomas comprise approximately 40 percent of the total, leiomyosarcomas 40 percent, and endometrial stromal sarcomas 10 percent (Table 38-17).

Although little is known regarding the epidemiology of uterine sarcomas, the relationship of leiomyosarcomas to benign leiomyomas is of some interest. The majority of uterine leiomyosarcomas do appear to arise from previously benign myomas. Considering the rarity of sarcomas compared to the frequency of benign leiomyomas, it is apparent that malignant degeneration of a myoma is a rare occurrence. Even so, estimates of the relative incidence vary widely, from 0.13 percent, or 1 in 800, to almost 1 percent among 2500 myomatous uteri studied by Thornton and Carter.[31,32]

Hart and Billman conducted a careful reassessment of a series of 28 uterine neoplasms originally diagnosed as leiomyosarcomas.[33] Of these, 13 (46 percent) were reclassified as cellular myomas rather than sarcomas based on a low mitotic index (less than three mitoses per 10 high-power microscopic fields), lack of nuclear atypism, and a uniformly benign course. These findings suggest that the true incidence of leiomyosarcomas relative to benign uterine myomas is probably closer to 0.1 percent than 1 percent. Figure 38-15 shows the gross picture of a leiomyosarcoma arising in an intramural myoma. Figure 38-16 shows the microscopic appearance of this tumor.

Brief mention should be made of a rare form of smooth-muscle neoplasm which is quite distinct from leiomyosarcoma—intravenous leiomyomatosis. Fourteen instances of this entity, reported by Norris and Parmley from the Armed Forces Institute of Pathology files, were characterized by histologically benign smooth muscle invading uterine and pelvic veins as wormlike projections.[34] The major clinical significance is that with invasion of the vena cava, death due to venous obstruction occurs, and metastases to the lungs and heart have been described.

Two relatively benign forms of homologous endometrial stromal sarcomas also deserve separate mention. The first is the localized stromal nodule with a low

TABLE 38-16 Uterine Sarcomas: Relative Incidence of Uterine Corpus Cancers

Type	No.	%
Carcinomas	2843	96
Sarcomas	111	4

SOURCES: Taylor HC Jr, Becker WF: Carcinoma of the corpus uteri. End results of treatment in 531 cases. *Surg Gynec Obstet* 84:129, 1947; Climie ARW, Rochmaninoff N: A ten-year experience with endometrial carcinoma. *Surg Gynecol Obstet* 120:73, 1965; Dobbie BMW et al: A study of carcinoma of the endometrium. *J Obstet Gynec Brit Commw* 72:659, 1965; Carmichael JA: Carcinoma of the endometrium in Saskatchewan. *Am J Obstet Gynecol* 9:294, 1967; and Badib AO et al: Biologic behavior of adenoacanthoma of the endometrium. *Am J Obstet Gynecol* 106:205, 1970.

TABLE 38-17 Uterine Sarcomas: Relative Incidence of Major Types

Type	No.	%
Mixed mesodermal sarcomas	238	43
Leiomyosarcomas	232	42
Endometrial stromal sarcomas	53	9
Miscellaneous	32	6
Total	555	100

SOURCES: Aaro LA et al: Sarcoma of the uterus. A clinical and pathological study of 177 cases. *Am J Obstet Gynecol* 94:101, 1966; Edwards CL: Undifferentiated tumors, in *Cancer of the Uterus and Ovary*, Year Book, Chicago, 1969; Gilbert HA et al: The value of radiation therapy in uterine sarcoma. *Obstet Gynecol* 45:84, 1975; Vongtama VY et al: Treatment, results, and prognostic factors in Stage I and II sarcomas of the corpus uteri. *Am J Roentgenol* 126:139, 1976; and Salazar OM et al.[21]

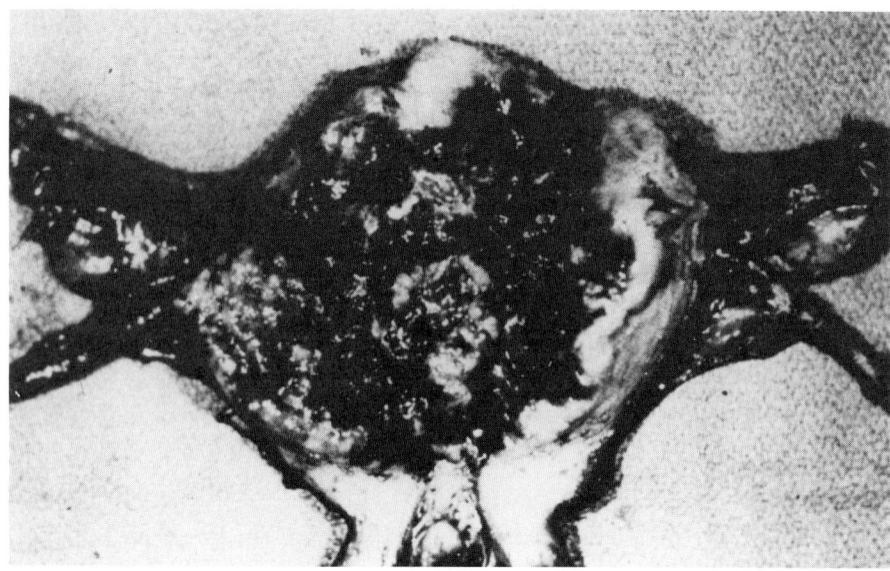

FIGURE 38-15 Infiltrating leiomyosarcoma arising from an intramural leiomyoma.

mitotic index and little or no tendency to invade or to metastasize. The second is stromatosis or endolymphatic stromal myosis, where relatively benign-appearing endometrial stromal extensions into myometrial and parametrial vascular spaces occur. The course tends to be indolent. Local recurrence after hysterectomy, which is refractory to irradiation and chemotherapy, is, at times, the eventual outcome.

A history of prior pelvic irradiation is found in between 5 and 10 percent of patients with uterine

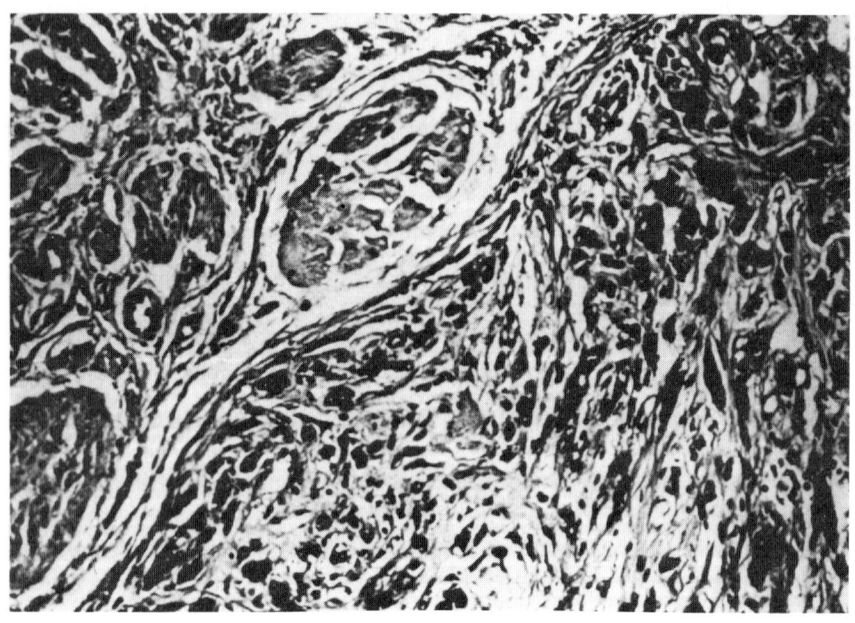

FIGURE 38-16 Microscopic appearance of uterine leiomyosarcoma.

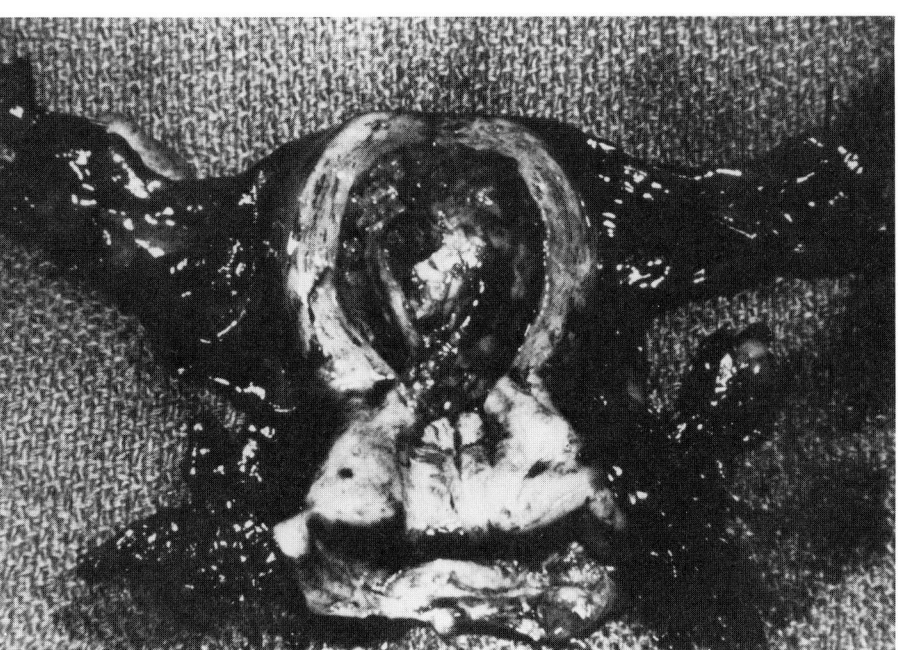

FIGURE 38-17 Endometrial stromal sarcoma.

sarcomas.[21,22,35-38] The latent period of 10 to 20 or more years between radiation exposure and cancer is consistent with reports of radiation-induced cancer in other locations.

Although much attention has been directed toward estrogen as a possible endometrial carcinogen, any causal relationship of estrogen to myometrial and endometrial stromal cancers is based entirely on isolated case reports. Estrogen does exert a trophic effect at both sites, but the rarity of uterine sarcomas has prevented meaningful epidemiologic analysis. Estrogen and progesterone receptors should be studied in these tumors. Figures 38-17 and 38-18 show an endometrial stromal sarcoma arising in a patient who had received estrogen replacement therapy for over 5 years.

Signs, Symptoms, and Early Detection

Although these cancers may occur at any age, the majority occur in women between the ages of 45 and 70. Leiomyosarcomas tend to occur at a somewhat earlier age than the other uterine sarcomas, with a peak age of approximately 50 for the former and 60 for the latter.

Abnormal uterine bleeding is the cardinal symptom. Rapid enlargement of a known myomatous uterus or the presence of a polypoid endocervical mass associated with pain and bleeding should alert the clinician to the possibility of a uterine sarcoma.

There is no useful screening technique other than routine periodic abdominal-pelvic examination and thorough investigation of abnormal uterine bleeding and of any previously undetected or changing uterine enlargement.

An obvious problem is evaluation of the frequently encountered patient with apparently benign uterine leiomyomas. It would be necessary to remove several hundred uteri containing asymptomatic benign leiomyomas to prevent one sarcoma from developing, which is hardly justifiable from the standpoint of morbidity or cost. A reasonable alternative is to remove any myomatous uterus that clearly enlarges over a 3- to 6-month interval of observation, is associated with pain or intractable bleeding, or reaches an arbitrary size in excess of 12 to 15 cm in any dimension. Parenthetically, it is well to bear in mind that detection of discrete ovarian masses becomes increasingly difficult as the uterus enlarges; to misdiagnose an ovarian cancer as a uterine myoma can be a tragic mistake.

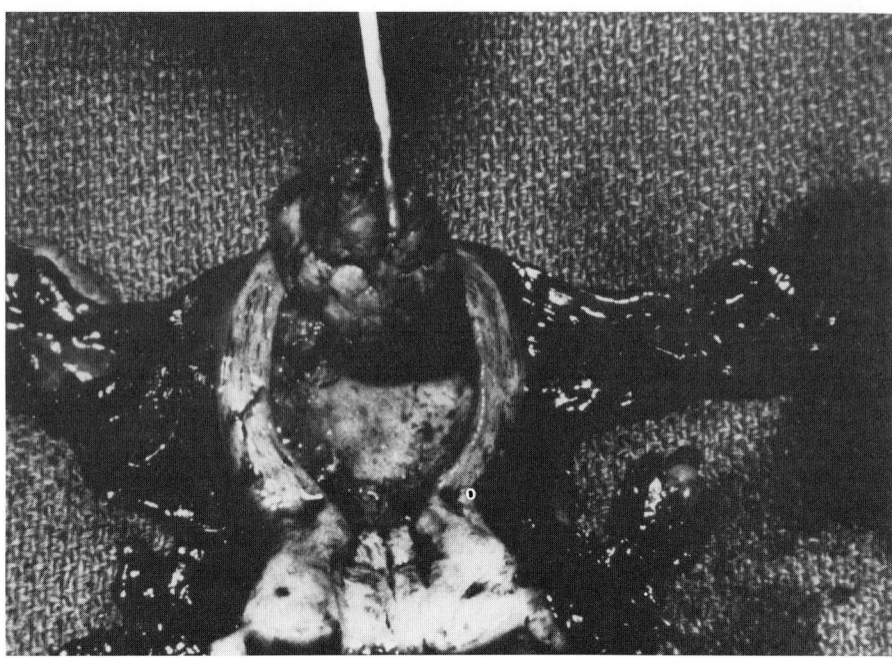

FIGURE 38-18 Endometrial stromal sarcoma.

Diagnostic Techniques, Work-up, and Staging

Since no staging system unique to uterine sarcomas has been developed, the FIGO staging criteria for endometrial carcinomas should be used for the uterine sarcomas. The diagnostic techniques and work-up described for endometrial carcinomas are appropriate or the investigation of suspected uterine sarcomas. Ultrasound or axial tomographic techniques to aid in differentiating uterine from ovarian masses and in evaluating the retroperitoneum may be particularly helpful. Where doubt persists about the differentiation of ovarian and uterine masses, the surgeon should proceed with exploratory laparotomy, although on occasion peritoneoscopy as a preliminary to laparotomy may suffice and spare the patient a major procedure.

In conducting the work-up, and because of its relevance to developing a plan for treatment, pattern of spread must be appreciated. Although the tendency for anaplastic uterine sarcomas to invade blood vessels and undergo hematogenous spread, particularly to the lungs, is well recognized, the tendency for local lymphatic spread is not so well acknowledged. Since a preoperative diagnosis of uterine leiomyosarcoma is rarely possible, systematic surgical evaluation of lymph node involvement has not been carried out. DiSaia et al., under the auspices of the Gynecology Oncology Group, found that of 28 patients with endometrial stromal sarcomas who underwent "extensive" paraaortic and pelvic node sampling, 10 (35.7 percent) had pelvic lymph node metastases.[39] In every instance of nodal involvement there was myometrial invasion to the middle or outer one-third.

As with endometrial adenocarcinomas, the importance of histological characteristics to prognosis deserves particular emphasis. Norris and Taylor, Hart, Kempson, and others have shown that for leiomyosarcomas and endometrial stromal sarcomas mitotic activity is a clear index of virulence.[33,40–42] A mitotic index of over 10 mitoses per 10 high-power microscopic fields (HPF) indicates unequivocal malignancy, 5 to 10 mitoses per 10 HPF a somewhat more favorable prognosis, and less than 5 mitoses per 10 HPF a generally benign course and favorable outcome. It should be clearly recognized that these are by no means absolute or sole criteria for malignancy. For heterologous endometrial sarcomas (e.g., rhabdomyosarcoma) cellular atypism and clinical extent of the neoplasm assume primary prognostic importance. In fact, for all the histological types, extent of disease at the time of diagnosis remains the most significant determinant of curability.

Therapeutic Options

The aggressive, highly lethal nature of most uterine sarcomas has long been recognized, but no clear concensus exists as to the best therapeutic approaches. There is no disagreement about the desirability of a primary surgical attack on localized disease. The extent of surgery and the role of adjunctive irradiation and chemotherapy are the chief areas of debate.

In a collected series of 871 cases of uterine sarcoma, Salazar et al. found survival at 2 years to be 38 percent and at 5 years to be 27 percent.[21,22] Several authors cite improved outcome with adjunctive irradiation for the endometrial sarcomas, but not for leiomyosarcomas, while a few find supplemental irradiation of benefit for all histological types (Table 38-18). It is quite apparent that no systematic attempts have been made to evaluate the benefits of combined surgery and irradiation for leiomyosarcomas.

Because up to 35 percent of patients with endometrial sarcomas have pelvic lymph node metastases when diagnosed, logic dictates a therapeutic approach which treats these nodes either surgically or with irradiation and less extensive surgery.

When the diagnosis of endometrial sarcoma has been made by curettage and careful work-up reveals no evidence of extrapelvic spread, preoperative irradiation is recommended, including 5000 rads to the pelvic midplane via an external megavoltage source. Intrauterine irradiation by cesium or radium application should be added when the endometrial cavity is significantly enlarged (over 10 to 12 cm in depth), the tumor is highly anaplastic, or the cervix is involved, to deliver a total dose of 6500 to 7000 rads to *point A* (2 cm lateral to the midplane of the cervix, 2 cm above external cervical os).

Surgery should include, in addition to routine systematic inspection and palpation of the abdominal cavity and retroperitoneum, sampling of the paraaortic lymph nodes and any grossly suspicious pelvic lymph nodes. Radical hysterectomy with pelvic lymphadenectomy should be considered when there is no evidence of paraaortic lymph node metastases or other local or distant extrauterine spread. Patients of this group, if found to have regional lymph node metastases or compromised surgical margins, would be candidates for postoperative irradiation.

Since leiomyosarcomas will usually be diagnosed as a result of examination of the surgical specimen, these patients become candidates for a meticulous postoperative search for metastases. No good argument can be made for primary postoperative irradiation where all gross tumor has been removed and the surgical margins are clear, or when there are distant metastases. There may be a role for primary or secondary pelvic irradiation when the sarcoma is unresectable or has been incompletely resected and macroscopic disease is still limited to the pelvis.

In view of the modest successes now being obtained with chemotherapy as adjunctive treatment for sarcomas and in the treatment of recurrences and metastases, an

TABLE 38-18 Uterine Sarcomas: 5-Year Survival According to Treatment

| | 5-Year survival | | | | | |
| | MMS | | LMS | | ESS | |
Treatment	No.	%	No.	%	No.	%
Surgery	54	20	42	60	16	56
Surgery + RT	66	44	5	0	11	73
RT	15	20	—		4	25
Total cases and average 5-year survival	135	32	47	53	31	58

NOTE: MMS = Mixed mesodermal sarcoma; LMS = leiomyosarcoma; ESS = endometrial stromal sarcoma; RT = radiotherapy.
SOURCES: Edwards CL: Undifferentiated tumors, in *Cancer of the Uterus and Ovary,* Year Book, Chicago, 1969; Vongtama VY et al: Treatment, results and prognostic factors in Stage I and II sarcomas of the corpus uteri. *Am J Roentgenol* 126:139, 1976; and Salazar OM et al.[22]

aggressive surgical approach is justified. By this is meant wide excision of the primary tumor and removal of involved lymph nodes where possible without unnecessarily compromising function. At times excision of portions of organs adjacent to the uterus may be justified if careful preoperative study and intraoperative evaluation indicate the cancer is limited to the pelvis. Extensive surgical procedures in the presence of known extrapelvic cancer, except to relieve symptomatic bowel or urinary tract obstruction, are ill-advised.

Adjuvant Therapies

The unfortunate fact is that upward of 90 percent of all patients who fail primary treatment do so because of metastases outside the pelvis. Therefore, hope for improved long-term survival and cure rates rests squarely on finding effective systemic adjuvant therapy. Experience to date with the chemotherapy of uterine sarcomas gives modest encouragement. The hopeful early results of combined surgery, irradiation, and chemotherapy in the treatment of childhood rhabdomyosarcomas have lead to similar trials for adult uterine sarcomas. Smith et al, reported early disease-free control in 7 out of 8 patients with recurrent or metastatic leiomyosarcoma for from 10 to 40 months at the time of their report.[43] Unfortunately only 4 of 18 patients with recurrent mixed mesodermal sarcomas remained free of disease for periods from 26 to 56 months, reemphasizing the lethal nature of these tumors. The drugs used were vincristine, actinomycin D, and cyclophosphamide, combined with whole-pelvic, and in some cases, whole-abdominal irradiation. Not surprisingly, complications were severe, and included five drug-related deaths among the 35 patients treated.

Doxorubicin, among other relatively new chemotherapeutic agents, has a significant activity against the sarcomas and is under study alone and in a number of combination drug protocols, with encouraging early results. *cis*-Platinum also appears to be of value in the treatment of carcinosarcomas.

From these results it can be inferred that improvement in long-term results should be anticipated from the adjuvant use of chemotherapy in treating uterine sarcomas, particularly where a high risk of local recurrence and distant spread exists based on known prognostic factors such as a high mitotic index, marked cellular pleomorphism, deep myometrial invasion, and regional lymph node involvement.

Follow-up Techniques

The follow-up should be along the lines outlined for endometrial adenocarcinoma, with particular attention to screening for pulmonary metastases and pelvic recurrence. Patients receiving adjunctive chemotherapy should be considered candidates for baseline abdominal-pelvic sonography or axial tomography which can be repeated at periodic intervals to aid both in early detection of recurrent disease and in evaluating the response of deep-seated masses to therapy.

Treatment of Recurrence and/or Metastases

Because of the multiplicity of variables involved in each case of local recurrence or metastatic spread, treatment must be individualized. Tumor reductive surgery, local irradiation, and chemotherapy are the available options. Alone or in combination they may find application, based on knowledge of extent and location of disease and the known response potential of a given variety of sarcoma to irradiation of chemotherapy. Because of the lack of concrete data to firmly establish the value of one regimen over another it is important that as many patients as possible with these uncommon cancers be entered into well-designed multi-institutional protocol studies.

Current Areas for Research and Future Prospects

In addition to well-designed trials of new drugs as they become available as well as a carefully thought out, aggressive approach to combinations of tumor reductive surgery, irradiation, and chemotherapy, there is need, as in all types of cancer, for continuing research into possible causative factors, basic tumor cell biology, and tumor and host immune mechanisms. It is to be hoped that immunodiagnosis will become a real force in improving our ability to recognize these highly lethal tumors at an early stage of development.

The sensitivity of endometrial stromal tumors to endocrine manipulation should be explored. Endometrial stromal tumors are, to a degree, tumors of müllerian origin which like their parent tissue may respond to estrogen and progesterone. Assays for estrogen- and progesterone-receptor protein need to be done. As with endometrial adenocarcinomas, the therapeutic implications are obvious.

Reconstruction and Rehabilitation

Because of the wide range of patient ages and the many possible therapies, it is apparent once again that the specifics of reconstruction and rehabilitation will depend on and vary widely according to the individual clinical situation. In the present era of increasingly effective combined modality therapy, ultraradical surgical procedures are not often indicated or justifiable as an appropriate option in the risk-benefit equation. However, when procedures such as exenteration with vaginectomy are, on occasion, indicated and carried out, it is incumbent on the surgeon to consider in detail the psychological rehabilitation and anatomic reconstruction of the patient as part of the overall plan of management. Proper adjustment to and care of stomas can almost always be effected. Vaginal reconstruction, even in the irradiated patient, can be accomplished in a satisfactory manner by a variety of techniques, the details of which are beyond the scope of this text. However, the reader should be aware that the use of the labia where present, molds with split thickness skin grafts, and myocutaneous pedicle grafts have all produced satisfactory results in terms of sexual rehabilitation.

REFERENCES

1. Weiss NS et al: Increasing incidence of endometrial cancer in the United States. *N Engl J Med* 293:1164, 1975.
2. Marrett LD et al: Recent trends in the incidence and mortality of cancer of the uterine corpus in Connecticut. *Gynecol Oncol* 6:183, 1978.
3. Smith DC et al: Association of exogenous estrogen and endometrial carcinoma. *N Engl J Med* 293:1164, 1975.
4. Ziel HK, Finkle WD: Increased risk of endometrial carcinoma among users of conjugated estrogens. *N Engl J Med* 293:1167, 1975.
5. Mack TM et al: Estrogens and endometrial cancer in a retirement community. *N Engl J Med* 294:1262, 1976.
6. McDonald TW et al: Exogenous estrogen and endometrial carcinoma: Case-control and incidence study. *Am J Obstet Gynecol* 127:572, 1977.
7. Gray LA Sr et al: Estrogens and endometrial cancer. *Obstet Gynecol* 49:385, 1977.
7a. Chu J et al: Survival among women with endometrial cancer: A comparison of estrogen users and non-users. *Am J Obstet Gynecol* 143:569, 1982.
8. Taylor HC Jr: Endometrial hyperplasia and carcinoma of the body of the uterus. *Am J Obstet Gynecol* 23:309, 1932.
9. Gusberg SB: Hormone dependence of endometrial carcinoma. *Obstet Gynecol* 30:287, 1967.
10. Gusberg SB et al: Endometrial cancer: Factors influencing the choice of treatment. *Gynecol Oncol* 2:308, 1974.
11. Kelley RM, Baker WH: Effects of 17-alpha-hydroxyprogesterone caproate on metastatic endometrial cancer in *Conference on Experimental Clinical Cancer Chemotherapy*, National Cancer Institute, Bethesda, Md, 1959, p 235.
12. Lucas WE: Causal relationships between endocrine-metabolic variables in patients with endometrial carcinoma. *Obstet Gynecol Survey* 29:507, 1974.
13. Chamlian DL, Taylor HB: Endometrial hyperplasia in young women. *Obstet Gynecol* 36:659, 1970.
14. MacDonald PC et al: Effect of obesity on conversion of planus androstenedine to estroin in postmenopausal women with and without endometrial cancer. *Am J Obstet Gynecol* 130:448, 1978.
15. Lucas WE, Yen SSC: A study of endocrine and metabolic variables in postmenopausal women with endometrial carcinoma. *Am J Obstet Gynecol* 134:180, 1979.
16. McCarty, KS Jr et al: Gonadal dysgenesis with adenocarcinoma of the endometrium. *Cancer* 42:512, 1978.
16a. Kurman RJ, Norris HJ: Evaluation of criteria for distinguishing atypical endometrial hyperplasia from well-differentiated carcinoma. *Cancer* 49:2547, 1982
17. Kistner RW: Effects of progestational agents on hyperplasia and carcinoma in situ of the endometrium: 10 year follow-up. *Int J Gynaecol Obstet* 8:561, 1970.
18. Reagan JW: The changing nature of endometrial cancer. *Gynecol Oncol* 2:144, 1974.
19. Julian C et al: Adenoepidermoid and adenosquamous carcinoma of the uterus. *Am J Obstet Gynecol* 128:106, 1977.
20. Bickenbach W et al: Factor analysis in endometrial carcinoma in relation to treatment. *Obstet Gynecol* 29:632, 1967.
20a. Creasman WT et al: Prognostic significance of peritoneal cytology in patients with endometrial cancer and preliminary data concerning therapy with intraperitoneal radiopharmaceuticals. *Am J Obstet Gynecol* 141:921, 1981.
21. Salazar OM et al: Uterine sarcomas. *Cancer* 42:1152, 1978a.
22. Salazar OM et al: Uterine sarcomas. *Cancer* 42:1161, 1978b.
23. Gerulath AH, Bonte R: Effect of progesterone on nucleic acid synthesis in vitro in carcinoma of the endometrium. *Am J Obstet Gynecol* 128:722, 1977.
24. DeCoster JM et al: Medroxyprogesterone acetate release from silastic devices as replacement for local irradiation by radium tubes in preoperative packing for endometrial carcinoma. *Gynecol Oncol* 5:189, 1977.
25. Bonte J et al: Radiosensitization of endometrial adenocarcinoma by means of medroxyprogesterone. *Cancer* 25:907, 1970.
26. Lewis GC Jr et al: Adjuvant progestogen therapy in the primary definitive treatment of endometrial carcinoma. *Gynecol Oncol* 2:368, 1974.
27. Young PCM et al: Progesterone binding in human endometrial tissue. *Am J Obstet Gynecol* 125:376 1976.

27a. Ehrlich CE et al: Cytoplasmic progesterone and estradiol receptors in normal, hyperplastic and carcinomatous endometria: Therapeutic implications. *Am J Obstet Gynecol* 141:539, 1981.
28. Shapiro SS et al: Synthetic progestins: In vitro potency on human endometrium and specific binding to cytosol receptor. *Am J Obstet Gynecol* 132:549, 1978.
28a. Piver MS et al: Melphalan, 5-fluorouracil and medroxyprogesterone acetate in metastatic or recurrent endometrial cancer. *Obstet Gynecol* 56:370, 1980.
28b. Seski JC et al: *Cis*-platin therapy for disseminated endometrial cancer. *Am J Obstet Gynecol* 59:225, 1982.
29. Ober WB, Tovell HMM: Mesenchymal sarcomas of the uterus. *Am J Obstet Gynecol* 77:246, 1959.
30. Ariel IM, Pack GT: Sarcoma of the uterus, Pack in GT Pack, IM Ariel (eds): *Tumors of the Female Genitalia*, Harper & Row, New York, 1962.
31. Corscaden JA, Singh BP: Leiomyosarcoma of the uterus. *Am J Obstet Gynecol* 75:149, 1958.
32. Thornton WN Jr, Carter JP: Sarcoma of the uterus. *Am J Obstet Gynecol* 62:294, 1951.
33. Hart WR, Billman JK: A reassessment of uterine neoplasms originally diagnosed as leiomyosarcomas. *Cancer* 41:1902, 1978.
34. Norris HJ, Parmley T: Mesenchymal tumors of the uterus: V. Intravenous leiomyomatosis. *Cancer* 36:2164, 1975
35. Aaro LA et al: Sarcoma of the uterus: A clinical and pathological study of 177 cases. *Am J Obstet Gynecol* 94:101, 1966.
36. Badib AO et al: Biologic behavior of adenoacanthoma of the endometrium. *Am J Obstet Gynecol* 106:205, 1970.
37. Williamson EO, Christopherson WM: Malignant mixed Müllerian tumors of the uterus. *Cancer* 29:585, 1972.
38. Gilbert HA et al: The value of radiation therapy in uterine sarcoma. *Obstet Gynecol* 45:84, 1975.
39. DiSaia PJ et al: Endometrial sarcoma. Lymphatic spread pattern. *Am J Obstet Gynecol* 130:104, 1975.
40. Norris HJ, Taylor HB: Mesenchymal tumors of the uterus. *Cancer* 19:755, 1966.
41. Hart WR, Yoonessi M: Endometrial stromatosis of the uterus. *Obstet Gynecol* 49:393, 1977.
42. Kempson RL, Bari W: Uterine sarcomas. Classification diagnosis and prognosis. *Hum Pathol* 1:331, 1970.
43. Smith JP et al: Combined irradiation and chemotherapy for sarcomas of the pelvis in females. *Am J Roentgenol* 123:571, 1975.
44. Yoonessi M, Hart WR: Endometrial stromal sarcomas. *Cancer* 40:898, 1977.

39

TUMORS OF THE OVARY

Philip J. DiSaia *William M. Rich*

CLASSIFICATION

Neoplasms of the ovary present an increasing challenge to the physician. They are the cause of more deaths than any other female genital cancer. There are about 18,000 new cases diagnosed each year with about 11,000 deaths annually. In the United States a woman dies from ovarian cancer every 50 min. The gynecologic oncologist is frustrated by the paucity of knowledge of the etiologic factors in ovarian cancer and by the failure to achieve a significant reduction in mortality rates from these neoplasms over the past five decades.

The student of ovarian pathology is often confused by the prodigious variation in histological structure and biologic behavior. Currently the most popular and practical scheme of classification is based on the histogenesis of the ovary (Table 39-1).[1] The early development of the ovary may be divided into four major stages. During the first, undifferentiated germ cells (primordial germ cells) become segregated and migrate from their sites of origin to settle in the genital ridges, which are bilateral thickenings of coelomic epithelium. The second stage occurs after arrival of the germ cells in the genital ridges and consists of a proliferation of the coelomic epithelium and of the underlying mesenchyme. During the third phase, the ovary becomes divided into a peripheral cortex and a central medulla. The fourth stage is characterized by the development of the cortex and the involution of the medulla. The histogenic classification given in Table 39-1 categorizes ovarian neoplasms as to their derivation from coelomic epithelium, germ cells, and mesenchyme, respectively.

BENIGN OVARIAN TUMORS

Since the differentiation between benign and malignant ovarian enlargements is often the exclusive decision of the pathologist, a short discussion of these lesions (Table 39-2) is pertinent even in a textbook of oncology. Although functional ovarian cysts are usually asymptomatic, they on occasion can be accompanied by a minor degree of lower abdominal discomfort, pelvic pain, or dyspareunia. In addition, rupture of one of these fluid-filled structures can result in additional peritoneal irritation and possibly an accompanying hemoperitoneum; however, this is rarely of a serious nature. More intense lower abdominal discomfort will result when these ovarian tumors undergo torsion or infarction. As with functional cysts of the ovary, benign ovarian neoplasms do not produce any symptoms which readily differentiate them from malignant tumors or a variety of other pelvic diseases. Although these tumors are more prone to twist,

TABLE 39-1 Histogenic Classification of Ovarian Neoplasms

I. Neoplasms derived from coelomic epithelium
   A. Serous tumor
   B. Mucinous tumor
   C. Endometroid tumor
   D. Mesonephroid (clear cell) tumor
   E. Brenner tumor
   F. Undifferentiated carcinoma
   G. Carcinosarcoma and mixed mesodermal tumor
II. Neoplasms derived from germ cells
   A. Teratoma
      1. Mature teratoma
         a. Solid adult teratoma
         b. Dermoid cyst
         c. Struma ovarii
         d. Malignant neoplasms secondarily arising from mature cystic teratoma
      2. Immature teratoma (partially differentiated teratoma)
   B. Dysgerminoma
   C. Embryonal carcinoma
   D. Endodermal sinus tumor
   E. Choriocarcinoma
   F. Gonadoblastoma
III. Neoplasms derived from specialized gonadal stroma
   A. Granulosa-theca tumors
      1. Granulosa tumor
      2. Thecoma
   B. Sertoli-Leydig tumors
      1. Arrhenoblastoma
      2. Sertoli tumor
   C. Gynandroblastoma
   D. Lipid cell tumors
IV. Neoplasms derived from nonspecific mesenchyme
   A. Fibroma, hemangioma, leiomyoma, lipoma, etc.
   B. Lymphoma
   C. Sarcoma
V. Neoplasms metastatic to the ovary
   A. GI tract (Krukenberg)
   B. Breast
   C. Endometrium
   D. Lymphoma

resulting in infarction, malignant neoplasms may have the same fate. Indeed, one of the most unfortunate features of benign ovarian neoplasms is that they are *indistinguishable clinically from their malignant counterpart.* While it is not known whether malignant ovarian tumors arise de novo or develop from benign tumors, there is strong inferential evidence that at least some benign tumors will become malignant. All too often cancer in an ovarian tumor presents with increasing abdominal distention as the first symptom, although benign ovarian neoplasms may present with increasing abdominal girth, and indeed the "giant tumors" of the ovary are often benign mucinous cystadenomas. True functional cysts of the ovary will remit in a 6- to 8-week follow-up period of observation. *All persistent adnexal enlargements must be considered malignant until proven otherwise.*

INCIDENCE, EPIDEMIOLOGY, AND ETIOLOGY

Approximately 23 percent of gynecologic cancers are of ovarian origin but 47 percent of all deaths from cancer of the female genital tract are of this source. Cancer of the ovaries is the fourth most frequent fatal cancer in women in the United States. It ranks high as a cause of female deaths in countries of Northern Europe, Canada, New Zealand, and Israel. Approximately 12 out of every 1000 women in the United States over the age of 40 will develop ovarian cancer, but only 2 or 3 will be cured. The remainder will develop repeated bouts of intestinal obstruction as the tumor spreads over the surface of the bowel, develop inanition, malnutrition, and literally starve to death.

Malignant neoplasms of the ovaries occur at all ages including infancy and childhood. Throughout childhood and adolescence, United States death rates for neoplasms of the ovary are exceeded only by those for leukemia, lymphomas, and neoplasms of the central nervous sys-

TABLE 39-2 Benign Ovarian Tumors

1. Nonneoplastic tumors
   a. Germinal inclusion cyst
   b. Follicle cyst
   c. Corpus luteum cyst
   d. Pregnancy luteoma
2. Tumors derived from coelomic epithelium
   a. Cystic
      (1) Serous cystoma
      (2) Endometrioma
      (3) Mucinous cystoma
      (4) Mixed forms
   b. Tumors with stromal overgrowth
      (1) Adenofibroma
      (2) Brenner tumor

tem, kidney, connective tissue, and bone. Overall death rates for neoplasms of the ovary are higher in nonwhite Americans at ages under 39 years; after age 40, however, rates for white women are signficantly higher. The major histological types occur in distinctive age ranges. Malignant germ cell tumors are most commonly seen in females below the age of 20 (Table 39-3), whereas epithelial cancers of the ovary are primarily seen in women over 40. The age-specific incidence rates for ovarian cancer show a steady rise up to age 80 where they drop off slightly in the older ages. The greatest number of cases is found in the age group 50 to 59 years. Studies of the Connecticut Tumor Registry would suggest that the age-adjusted rate for all ages has remained about the same over the last 30 years.

Several reports have described families in which girls and women of the same or succeeding generations develop similar neoplasms of the ovaries. Most of these neoplasms were serous carcinomas, but other types were also observed. Cancers of the breasts, colon, and other sites were also found more commonly in female members of these afflicted families. Investigators at the National Cancer Institute have studied four families in which women of two or three generations developed papillary-serous adenocarcinomas at ages past 35 years. The M. D. Anderson Cancer Institute is presently conducting a large study of the pedigree of patients with ovarian cancer, and preliminary conclusions would suggest that there are definitely family tendencies to this condition. In addition, the dysgenetic gonads of sex chromatin–negative individuals, most of whom are phenotypic females, are prone to develop a distinctive, ordinarily benign neoplasm called *gonadoblastoma*.

In common with other prevalent epithelial cancers, epidemiologic evidence strongly suggests that environmental factors are a major etiologic determinant in cancer of the human ovary. The highest rates are recorded in highly industrial countries, which suggests that physical or chemical products of industry are major causes of epithelial neoplasms. A notable exception is highly industrialized Japan in which rates for malignant neoplasms of the ovary have been among the lowest recorded in the world. Interestingly, one observes higher rates of cancer of the ovary in Japanese migrants in the United States and their offspring, eventually approaching that of Anglo-Saxon whites by the second generation. This suggests strongly that the causative carcinogens can probably be focused on factors in the immediate environment such as food, personal customs, and other influences that change gradually during the cultural transition. To date, there are no clues as to which possible dietary items or other environmental contacts might be specifically carcinogenic for the ovary.

No epidemiologic or experimental evidence exists to incriminate viruses in neoplasms of the human ovary. Attempts to isolate viruses from cultured human ovarian cancer cells have been unsuccessful to date. Because of its gonadotropic properties, mumps virus is an obvious candidate among known viruses for oncogenic activity in the ovary. Case-controlled studies have revealed a possible negative association with mumps parotitis, but these historic accounts were not supported by skin tests or serological evidence of reactivity to mumps virus. The evidence for mumps virus as an etiologic agent in ovarian cancer remains indeed speculative.

Knowledge of the etiologic mechanisms involved in cancer of the ovary is limited to fragments of information. The multi-institutional therapy programs offer an ideal population of women for case control studies. Each patient should be questioned for a history of preexisting gynecologic abnormalities, documented by clinical or laboratory data where possible, and for information about exposure to environmental carcinogens. Many programs of this nature are currently under way.

SIGNS, SYMPTOMS, AND ATTEMPTS AT EARLY DETECTION

Although diverse ovarian tumors generally manifest themselves in a similar manner, the diagnosis of early ovarian cancer is more a matter of chance than a triumph of the scientific method. As enlargement occurs, there is a progressive compression of the surrounding pelvic structures, producing vague abdominal discomfort, dys-

TABLE 39-3 Malignant Ovarian Neoplasms

Tumor	Age distribution in patients under 20 years, %
Germ cell	60
Epithelial	15
Stromal	15
Miscellaneous	10

SOURCE: RL Jensen, AJ Norris: Epithelial tumors of the ovary: Occurrence in children and adolescents less than 20 years of age. *Arch Pathol* 94:20, 1972.

pepsia, urinary frequency, and "pelvic pressure" (Table 39-4). The insidious onset of ovarian cancer needs no elaboration. As the neoplasm gains the diameter of 15 cm, it begins to rise out of the pelvis and may account for abdominal enlargement. It is time, however, to change the generally accepted notion that there are no early symptoms of ovarian cancer. Symptoms often include vague abdominal discomfort, dyspepsia, and other mild digestive disturbances which may be present for several months prior to the diagnosis. Such complaints are usually not recognized as anything more than "middle-age indigestion." A high index of suspicion should exist in all women between the ages of 40 and 69 who present with persistent gastrointestinal symptoms which cannot be diagnosed. Unfortunately, the majority of such nonspecific complaints are often functional in origin, causing the internist or family physician to overlook the possibility of ovarian cancer. Indeed, it is only when the patient presents with gross enlargement of the abdomen marking the occurrence of ascites and extension of the neoplastic process to the abdominal cavity that the patient receives appropriate diagnostic evaluation.

Methods for early diagnosis have been investigated in limited studies utilizing cul-de-sac aspiration for peritoneal cytology and frequent pelvic examinations. All of these endeavors have failed to show a significant impact on early diagnosis of this disease. These ovarian neoplasms grow quickly and painlessly. Any ovarian enlargement should be considered ovarian cancer until proven otherwise, especially in the post menopausal woman where an ovarian enlargement should be an immediate indication for exploratory laparotomy. The diagnosis really rests with the pathologist. Mere size, such as a 100-lb tumor, does not indicate severity of disease. Indeed, some of the largest neoplasms are benign histologically. In addition, many large adnexal masses may be of a nonovarian etiology. Frequently encountered nonovarian causes of an apparent adnexal mass are diverticulitis, tuboovarian abscess, carcinoma of the cecum or sigmoid, pelvic kidney, and uterine or ligamentous myomata. At the time of surgery it may be difficult to discern the malignant potential of a particular ovarian neoplasm. Although there are many characteristics suggestive of a malignant ovarian neoplasm (Table 39-5), there is sufficient overlap of morphological criteria to cause considerable confusion. Again the diagnosis rests with a histological review of the specimen.

DIAGNOSTIC TECHNIQUES AND STAGING

Routine pelvic examinations will detect only one ovarian cancer in 10,000 examinations of asymptomatic women. However, pelvic examination remains the most reliable means of detecting early disease. Pain is usually a late complication and is seen with early disease only when associated with a complication such as torsion, rupture, or infection. Any ovary palpated in a patient 3 to 5 years or more postmenopausal should raise a high index of suspicion for an early ovarian neoplasm. These patients should be considered for immediate laparoscopy and/or laparotomy.

Routine laboratory tests are not of great value in the diagnosis of ovarian tumors. The major value of laboratory tests is in ruling out other pelvic disorders (Table 39-6). Abdominal roentgenograms may reveal calcifications consistent with myomas or toothlike calcifications consistent with benign teratoma. Pyelogram and gastrointestinal series are often helpful in ruling out disease in adjacent pelvic structures. A barium enema is probably advisable with any pelvic mass, but the need for a gastrointestinal series can be individualized based upon

TABLE 39-4 Most Frequent Presenting Symptoms of Ovarian Cancer

Symptom	Relative frequency
Abdominal swelling	++++
Abdominal pain	+++
Dyspepsia	++
Urinary frequency	++
Weight change	+

TABLE 39-5 Surgical Findings

Finding	Benign	Malignant
Surface papilla	Rare	Very common
Intracystic papilla	Infrequent	Very common
Solid areas	Rare	Very common
Bilaterality	Rare	Common
Adhesions	Infrequent	Common
Ascites (100 ml)	Rare	Common
Necrosis	Rare	Common
Peritoneal implants	Rare	Common
Capsule intact	Common	Infrequent
Totally cystic	Common	Rare

TABLE 39-6 Complete Work-up for Ovarian Cancer

Careful history

Physical examination

Pelvic exam and Pap smear

Proctosigmoidoscopy, where indicated

CBC and urinalysis

Blood chemistries

Chest x-ray

IVP

Barium enema

GI series, where indicated

---

the patient's symptoms. A similar comment can be made for proctosigmoidoscopy which is particularly valuable in patients who have lower intestinal symptoms. The outcome in ovarian cancer relies so heavily on early diagnosis that procrastination with numerous diagnostic procedures such as ultrasound is somewhat hazardous. Laparotomy is the ultimate test as to the nature of the disorder. Paracentesis for the purpose of obtaining a cell block and cytological smear of the peritoneal fluid appears unnecessary and is, at times, dangerous. If, indeed, one is dealing with a self-contained malignant cyst, such a procedure can result in a spill of malignant cells into the peritoneal cavity. In addition, whether or not the fluid reveals neoplastic cells, laparotomy is still necessary to either remove the large benign neoplasm or define the extent of the malignant process. In addition, up to 50 percent of ascitic fluid samples from patients with true ovarian malignancy will be negative for malignant cells on cell block analysis. Diagnostic paracentesis in a patient with ascites and a pelvic-abdominal mass is unnecessary and dangerous.

The staging of ovarian cancer is surgical (Table 39-7). A longitudinal midline incision is recommended to facilitate removal of the neoplasm and to permit adequate visualization of the entire abdominal cavity, including the undersurface of the diaphragm. Ovarian cancer is classically a serosal spreading disease, and so all peritoneal surfaces must be carefully inspected, especially where disease is thought to be limited to the pelvis. Any peritoneal fluid encountered on opening the peritoneal cavity should be aspirated and submitted for cytological examination. In the absence of peritoneal fluid "four washings" should be taken by lavaging the peritoneal surfaces of the undersurface of the diaphragms as one specimen, lateral to the ascending and descending colon as the second and third specimens, and the pelvic

TABLE 39-7 FIGO Stage-Grouping for Primary Carcinoma of the Ovary

Stage I		Growth limited to the ovaries.
	Stage IA	Growth limited to one ovary; no ascites.
	1	No tumor on the external surface; capsule intact.
	2	Tumor present on the external surface and/or capsule ruptured.
	Stage IB	Growth limited to both ovaries; no ascites.
	1	No tumor on the external surface; capsule intact.
	2	Tumor present on the external surface and/or capsule(s) ruptured.
	Stage IC	Tumor either stage 1A or stage 1B, but with ascites* present or positive peritoneal washings.
Stage II		Growth involving one or both ovaries with pelvic extension.
	Stage IIA	Extension and/or metastases to the uterus and/or tubes.
	Stage IIB	Extension to other pelvic tissues.
	Stage IIC	Tumor either stage IIA or stage IIB, but with ascites* present or positive peritoneal washings.
Stage III		Growth involving one or both ovaries with intraperitoneal metastases outside the pelvis and/or positive retroperitoneal nodes. Tumor limited to the true pelvis with histologically proven malignant extension to small bowel or omentum.
Stage IV		Growth involving one or both ovaries with distant metastases. If pleural effusion is present, there must be positive cytology to allot a case to stage IV. Parenchymal liver metastases equal to stage IV.
Special category		Unexplored cases which are thought to be ovarian carcinoma.

* Ascites is peritoneal effusion which, in the opinion of the surgeon, is pathological and/or clearly exceeds normal amounts.

peritoneal surfaces themselves as a fourth specimen. These specimens are obtained by lavaging these areas with 50 to 75 ml of saline and retrieving the fluid for cell block analysis. Care should be taken to visualize and palpate all peritoneal surfaces including the underside of the diaphragm, the surface of the liver, and the small- and large-bowel mesentery. Fiberoptic light sources are particularly helpful in properly visualizing the peritoneal surfaces of the upper abdomen through a vertical lower abdominal incision. The omentum should be carefully scrutinized, and any suspicious areas removed by excision or biopsy. If the disease is apparently limited to the pelvis, it is judicious to remove the most dependent portion of the omentum or any portion of the omentum adherent to pelvic structures as a biopsy. Often, microscopic disease will be present in the omentum which is not obvious grossly. Recent data from one institution[2] suggest that routine omentectomy may be of benefit in improving survival, but additional data are needed to confirm this observation. If, indeed, the disease is limited to the pelvis, great care should be taken to avoid rupture of the neoplasm during its removal. All roughened or suspicious surfaces in the peritoneal cavity should be removed as a biopsy. This includes adhesions which should be excised, not incised, since often the adhesions contain microscopic disease. Several studies are under way, investigating the efficacy of "blind" peritoneal biopsies and routine retroperitoneal node dissections in the proper staging of early epithelial cancer of the ovary. These studies are preliminary, and a firm recommendation must await their conclusion. At the present time, it has not been our practice to routinely biopsy normal-appearing peritoneum or diaphragmatic surfaces. A high index of suspicion is always maintained for any abnormal-appearing surface, and biopsies are readily performed.

THERAPEUTIC OPTIONS FOR PRIMARY TREATMENT

Neoplasms Derived from Coelomic Epithelium

BORDERLINE MALIGNANT EPITHELIAL NEOPLASMS

In the last decade clear evidence has been presented for a group of epithelial ovarian tumors that have histological and biologic features occupying a position between those of clearly benign and frankly malignant ovarian neoplasms. These borderline malignancies, which account for approximately 15 percent of all epithelial ovarian cancers, were often referred to as *proliferative cystadenomas*. A 10-year survival rate of approximately 95 percent has been obtained in these borderline neoplasms. However, symptomatic recurrence and death may develop as long as 20 years after therapy in a few patients. These neoplasms can correctly be labeled as being of low malignant potential. On the basis of their almost benign behavior, many gynecologists have advocated conservative therapy, especially in patients who are desirous of further childbearing and have stage IA disease.

MALIGNANT EPITHELIAL NEOPLASMS

Ovarian carcinoma initially grows locally, invading the capsule and mesovarium and then adjacent organs by contiguous growth and lymphatic spread. Once the malignancy has reached the external surface of the capsule, cells may exfoliate into the peritoneal cavity, where they are free to circulate and later to implant. Local and regional lymphatic metastasis may occur which involves the uterus, fallopian tubes, and pelvic lymph nodes. Involvement of the periaortic lymph nodes by way of the infundibulopelvic ligament is also common. Probably the most important variable influencing the prognosis in each case of ovarian cancer is the stage or extent of disease. A staging system has been devised which allows a comparison of treatment results among different institutions. Although staging does not mandate treatment, discussing treatment by stage is often helpful.

Survival depends on the stage of the lesion, the grade of differentiation of the lesion, the amount of residual tumor remaining following surgery, and the additional treatment following surgery. The 5-year survival figures from the *FIGO Annual Report* for the years 1959 to 1963 are stage I, 77 percent, stage II, 56 percent, stage III, 32 percent, and stage IV, 9.1 percent. The overall 5-year survival was 27 percent. There is improved survival stage for stage in those patients with well-differentiated lesions, in those with all or most of the tumor removed at surgery, and in those who received postoperative irradiation and/or chemotherapy.

Stages IA, IB, and IC Total abdominal hysterectomy with bilateral salpingo-oophorectomy is undoubtedly the best therapy for stage I lesions. Many institutions also practice omentectomy for stage I lesions, especially if adjunctive therapy is planned in the form of intraperitoneal instillation of radioactive phosphorous. In addition to being an organ that may harbor microscopic disease in patients with apparent stage I lesions, removal of the omentum also deletes an organ to which radioactive colloidal substances such as ^{32}P have a great affinity and thus theoretically allows a greater amount of radioactive substance to be available for distribution over the visceral and parietal peritoneal surfaces of the abdomen. The value of omentectomy in and of itself as a therapeutic modality for stage I disease is yet to be conclusively established.

Other institutions prefer chemotherapy with alkylating agents such as melphalan or chlorambucil as postoperative therapy. The drug is usually continued for a period of 12 to 18 months after which patients clinically free of disease are usually subjected to a "second-look" procedure. If no evidence of disease is found, therapy is discontinued. If residual disease is uncovered, appropriate radiotherapy or alternate chemotherapy may then be instituted. Not uncommonly, an isolated focus of residual disease is found at second-look laparotomy; a radical excision of this focus is judicious. In the management of low-grade lesions, the physician must balance the possible benefits of adjuvant chemotherapy versus the risks suggested by some preliminary reports linking the development of fatal acute leukemia in patients with ovarian cancer treated with alkylating agents and surviving 10 years or more.

In the young woman with stage IA disease who is desirous of further childbearing, unilateral salpingo-oophorectomy may be associated with minimal increased risk of recurrence provided a careful staging procedure has been performed and due consideration has been given to grade and apparent self-containment of the neoplasm.

Stages IIA and IIB In stages IIA and IIB, too, total abdominal hysterectomy with bilateral salpingo-oophorectomy, omentectomy, and installation of ^{32}P is the treatment of choice in many institutions. Other centers prefer to utilize abdominal plus pelvic irradiation as postoperative therapy. Still other institutions have had reasonable success with a combination of pelvic irradiation and systemic chemotherapy. A fourth and commonly used treatment plan is to follow surgery with 12 to 18 months of chemotherapy, usually with an alkylating agent, and advising a second-look procedure if the patient is clinically free of disease at that time. As with stage I disease, the value of omentectomy remains inconclusive. Here, as in stage I disease, the variety of treatment plans is the reflection of retrospective studies which report acceptable survivals following a number of treatment regimens. One issue appears to be clear; the entire abdomen should be considered at risk, and the treatment plan should include some form of therapy for all peritoneal surfaces. Even very large institutions have low numbers of cases of stage I or stage II disease, making prospective randomized studies difficult. Fortunately, these problems are currently being studied by cooperative groups, and some firm answers concerning optimum therapy may be forthcoming.

Stage III In stage III as with other stages every effort should be made to remove the uterus with both adnexa. Every effort should be made short of major bowel surgery to remove the bulk of the tumor, including the removal of a large omental cake. Retrospective studies have suggested strongly that the survival in patients with stage III disease relates to the residual tumor following surgery, such that those patients with minimal residual appear to have a better prognosis with adjunctive therapy. Adjunctive therapy in the form of abdominal plus pelvic irradiation is utilized in many centers but has found less and less favor in recent years. Unless the residual masses are no larger than 2 cm at any locus in the abdomen, irradiation will not likely be effective. Thus, patients with bulky residual disease should be treated with chemotherapy. Standard chemotherapy at this time would be in the form of a single-drug alkylating agent (Alkeran, chlorambucil, thiotepa, or Cytoxan). The alkylating agent of choice in many institutions is Alkeran, but comparable responses have been reported with these other agents in smaller series. Again, the agent should be continued for at least 12 to 18 months or as long as clinical disease is apparent. Should the patient survive this period of time and have no clinical evidence of disease, a second-look procedure is usually recommended.

Recent evidence suggests that even in the optimum group (patients with residual disease no greater than 2 cm in diameter at any site) the survival and response rate to single-agent chemotherapy is equivalent to that of abdominal and pelvic irradiation. The morbidity of irradiation therapy is, of course, much greater, and therefore this finding may have considerable influence on future postoperative therapy for stage III disease. Several groups have now reported prospective studies randomizing patients between single-agent chemotherapy and multiple-drug regimens, with a similar conclusion by most stating that polychemotherapy had little advantage over single-agent regimens. This issue is quite important since the morbidity of polychemotherapy is considerably greater than that of the single-drug alkylating agent regimen. Several ongoing studies of still other drug combinations may in the future alter this preference for single agent. Preliminary results of combinations including *cis*-platinum, such as Adriamycin, Cytoxan, and *cis*-platinum (CAP), have shown dramatic (80 percent) response rates and significant (30 percent) negative "second look" laparotomy rates in stages III and IV epithelial cancer of the ovary. Subsequent relapse rates and overall survival figures are pending.

Stage IV The ideal management in stage IV is to remove as much cancer as possible and subject the patient to postoperative chemotherapy.

Neoplasma Derived from Primitive Germ Cells

TERATOMAS

The dermoid cyst, or benign cystic teratoma, is one of the most common ovarian neoplasms; it accounts for over 95 percent of all ovarian teratomas. It is composed entirely of mature (adult) tissues, usually representing all three germ layers. Removal either by oophorectomy or by cystectomy appears to be adequate therapy.

About 1 percent of teratomas are composed entirely or partially of incompletely differentiated tissues resembling embryonic rather than adult structures; often these are neural ectodermal derivatives. The malignant potential and subsequent prognosis for these patients appear to be related to the amount and degree of tissue immaturity contained in these neoplasms. Although numerous long-term survivals of individuals with immature or partially differentiated teratomas have been documented, at least one-third of patients of all cases reported in the literature die of their tumor. As with all germ cell tumors, a thorough search of the material should be made for choriocarcinoma or embryonal carcinoma components which would significantly worsen the prognosis. Conservative management of partially differentiated teratomas is often desirable since these neoplasms commonly occur in young women desirous of further childbearing. The risk of conservative management is unknown, but recurrences, in general, may occur in 20 to 80 percent of patients depending on the grade of the neoplasm. The value of postoperative chemotherapy is being assessed in some institutions at present and may offer a diminished recurrence rate, especially in the more wholly undifferentiated or higher grade lesions.

DYSGERMINOMAS

Dysgerminomas histologically resemble the sexually undifferentiated germ cells of the early gonad. They occur predominantly in children and young women, with 80 percent found in females between the ages of 10 and 30 years. Dysgerminoma is the most frequently occurring malignant neoplasm associated with intersex states and often develops in a gonadoblastoma. The tumors are notable by their predilection for lymphatic spread and their acute sensitivity to radiation.

In a patient under the age of 35 years with a tumor which has spread beyond the ovary or in patients with testicular feminization, the ideal treatment is removal of all internal sex organs. In the young woman with a unilateral encapsulated dysgerminoma who wants to retain her childbearing capability, conservative management is indicated. In these patients the treatment of choice is unilateral salpingo-oophorectomy, biopsy of the other ovary, and careful exploration to rule out disseminated disease. The patient should then be followed closely for 2 to 3 years with periodic examinations including liberal use of lymphangiography and second-look procedures for possible recurrences. Fortunately, 75 percent of recurrences can be successfully eradicated with radiotherapy, and they usually occur within 2 years of initial therapy. Only 5 to 10 percent of these lesions are bilateral, and survival rates approach 90 percent.

EMBRYONAL CARCINOMA

Embryonal carcinoma is one of the most malignant cancers arising in the ovary. This neoplasm, only recently described, closely resembles the embryonal carcinoma of the adult testes, where it is relatively common; however, it represents only about 4 percent of malignant ovarian germ cell tumors. Its rarity in the ovary and its confusion with choriocarcinoma and endodermal sinus tumor in the past accounts for its late identification as a distinct entity. It usually presents as an abdominal or pelvic mass in patients with a mean age of 15 years. Over 50 percent of patients have hormonal manifestations, consisting of precocious puberty or abnormal vaginal bleeding. Pregnancy tests may be positive in patients with this malignancy.

Total abdominal hysterectomy with bilateral salpingo-oophorectomy is the usual operative therapy. Most cases are confined to one ovary at the time of diagnosis, and this has suggested that a unilateral salpingo-oophorectomy may be sufficient in the initial operative treatment. Radiotherapy alone has not proved to be of significant value as a postoperative adjuvant. Promising results with improved survivals may lie in the area of multiple-drug chemotherapy. Patients on therapy should be monitored with serial radioimmunoassays for human chorionic gonadotrophin.

ENDODERMAL SINUS TUMOR

The endodermal sinus tumor is the second most frequent form of malignant germ cell tumor of the ovary, accounting for 22 percent of germ cell lesions in one large series. Three-fourths of the patients present with a combination of abdominal pain and an abdominal or pelvic mass; median age of these patients is 19 years. α-Fetoprotein levels are often elevated in patients with any of this group of tumors. The endodermal sinus tumor is characterized by extremely rapid growth and extensive intraabdominal spread; nearly one-half the patients present with symptoms of 1 week's duration or less. Triple-drug chemotherapy, consisting of vincristine, actinomycin D, and cyclophosphamide (VAC), employed immediately after unilateral salpingo-oophorectomy in patients with stage I tumors is presently advocated, and preliminary data would suggest very acceptable survival rates. Patients with lesions other than stage IA should be treated with a total abdominal hysterectomy and bilateral salpingo-oophorectomy followed by triple-drug chemotherapy. Several reports have now established the efficacy of triple-drug chemotherapy in improved progression-free interval and apparent increased cures of this devastating malignancy.

CHORIOCARCINOMA

Nongestational choriocarcinoma arising in the ovary is extremely rare and usually occurs as part of a mixed germ cell tumor. The treatment is much like that described for embryonal carcinoma. The excellent therapeutic achievements with antineoplastic drugs noted in gestational choriocarcinoma has not been realized in choriocarcinoma of germ cell origin. However, polydrug chemotherapy regimens may be of help and usually include methotrexate as one of the components.

GONADOBLASTOMA

Gonadoblastoma, a rare ovarian tumor, is composed of germ cells resembling those of a dysgerminoma and gonadal stromal cells resembling those of a granulosa or Sertoli cell tumor. Sex chromatin studies usually show a negative nuclear pattern (45,XO) or a sex chromosome mosaicism (XO/XY). Most patients are intersex problems with a phenotypical female habitus, amenorrhea, and possibly virilization. The malignancy rate is high with about one-half the reported cases being complicated by dysgerminoma. Occasional cases of choriocarcinoma, embryonal carcinoma, and mixed germ cell tumors have also been reported. With this in mind and with the realization that the gonads are useless, bilateral oophorectomy is recommended.

Neoplasms Derived from Specialized Gonadal Stroma

GRANULOSA AND THECA NEOPLASMS

Granulosa and theca tumors occur with approximately equal frequency, and not uncommonly there is a mixture of granulosa and theca elements. Those cases with mixed components should be classified as malignant. The designation *theca cell tumor* or *thecoma* should be reserved for neoplasms consisting entirely of theca cells which are benign. True granulosa tumors are low-grade malignancies, the great majority of which are confined to one ovary at the time of diagnosis. Only 5 to 10 percent of the stage I cases recur, and they usually appear more than 5 years after initial therapy. The prognosis for these patients is excellent, with long-term survivals of 75 to 90 percent having been reported for all stages. These lesions are adequately managed during the reproductive years by removing the involved ovary and ipsilateral tube. The uterus and the uninvolved adnexa should be removed in the perimenopausal and postmenopausal age groups, as is the practice with other benign or low-malignant-potential tumors.

SERTOLI-LEYDIG NEOPLASMS

Sertoli-Leydig cell tumors are characterized by differentiation toward testicular structures. These lesions were formerly grouped together as *arrhenoblastoma*, but that designation has been criticized since not all these tumors produce masculinization. The tumors are managed in the same manner as the granulosa cell tumors. Total hysterectomy and removal of the remaining ovary are recommended when the patient is no longer interested in childbearing.

GYNANDROBLASTOMA

Rarely a gonadal stromal tumor contains unequivocal granulosa cell elements combined with tubules and Leydig cells characteristic of an arrhenoblastoma. These mixed tumors are designated as gynandroblastomas and may be associated with either androgen or estrogen production. They can be expected to behave as low-grade malignancies similar to the individual components, and conservative surgery is appropriate for the individual desiring preservation of childbearing or ovarian function.

LIPID CELL NEOPLASMS

Lipid cell neoplasms constitute a heterogeneous group of tumors that have in common a parenchyma composed of polygonal cells containing lipid. Included are neoplasms that have been variously designated as hilus cell tumors, Leydig tumors, adrenal rest tumors, stromal luteomas, or musculinovoblastomas. Lipid cell tumors are unilateral and are commonly found in the medulla or hilar region of the ovary. Tumors that have spread to contiguous organs or have a microscopic cellular pleomorphism with a high mitotic activity should be considered malignant. Reincke's crystals, which normally occur in mature Leydig cells of the testes, are often found in these neoplasms, and their presence can be interpreted as signifying a benign lesion. Regardless of the presence or absence of Reincke's crystals, neoplasms less than 8 cm diameter can be expected to behave in a benign fashion.

Neoplasma Derived from Nonspecific Mesenchyme

Benign and malignant tumors may arise in the ovary from nonspecific supporting tissues that are common to most organs. Such tumors include fibromas, hemangiomas, leiomyomas, soft-tissue sarcomas, lymphomas, and other rare neoplasms. The fibroma and the lymphoma are the most common and the most important in this category. Benign lesions are managed with simple excision of the neoplasm, and malignant tumors are usually treated with total abdominal hysterectomy, bilateral salpingo-oophorectomy, a careful staging procedure, and frequently postoperative radiation or chemotherapy.

Neoplasms Metastatic to the Ovary

Approximately 30 percent of women dying of cancer are found to have ovarian metastases at autopsy, and one-fifth of those undergoing palliative oophorectomy for metastatic breast cancer have microscopic evidence of metastases in the ovaries. The most common sources of metastases to the ovary are the gastrointestinal tract, breast, and pelvic organs; however, the last two sites seldom produce clinically significant ovarian metastases. In 75 percent of cases of ovarian secondaries, both ovaries are grossly involved by metastases, and, with rare exception, when metastases are present in the ovary, there is metastatic disease in other parts of the body.

ISSUES IN THERAPY

Maximal Surgical Effort on Initial Laparotomy

The so-called debulking procedure has gained considerable attention in the management of ovarian cancer. The concept is simply to diminish the residual tumor burden to a point where adjuvant therapy will be optimally effective. All forms of adjuvant therapy are most effective when a minimal tumor burden exists. This is particularly true of ovarian carcinoma, which is one of the more sensitive solid tumors to chemotherapy. A careful and persistent surgeon can often remove large tumor masses which on first impression appear to be unresectable. Utilizing the clear retroperitoneal spaces, one can usually identify the infundibulopelvic ligament and ureter, then isolate the vessels of the infundibulopelvic ligament and the blood supply of the ovary. Once this is ligated and transected, a retrograde removal of large ovarian masses is easier and safer. The ureter is, of course, kept under direct vision throughout the dissection, and fear of traumatizing this pelvic structure is minimized. In a like manner, a clear space exists on the transverse colon whereby large omental "cakes" of ovarian carcinoma can be removed after ligating the right and left gastroepiploic vessels. Removal of the large ovarian masses and the omental involvement often reduces the tumor burden by 80 to 90 percent.

The theoretical value of debulking procedures lies in the obvious reduction of cell numbers and the advantage this afford to adjuvant therapy. This is especially relevant in bulky solid tumors such as ovarian cancer where removal of large numbers of cells in the resting phase (G_0) can result in propelling the residual cells into the vulnerable proliferating pool. Several careful retrospective studies have repeatedly demonstrated improved survival in patients who can be surgically brought to a status of minimal tumor burden. A recent report from the very large experience of the M. D. Anderson Hospital and Tumor Institute has illustrated significantly improved salvage in patients with stage II and stage III epithelial cancer of the ovary in whom initial surgery was followed by no gross residual tumor or a reduction where no single tumor mass exceeded 1 cm in diameter. This report boasts of a 70 percent 2-year survival in stage III patients in whom no gross disease was remaining and a 50 percent 2-year survival where residual nodules were limited to 1 cm in diameter. This compares very favorably with the usually quoted overall survivals (Table 39-8).

The Role of Radiation Therapy in Epithelial Ovarian Cancer

As a better understanding of the effects of chemotherapeutic agents in ovarian cancer has been gained, the role of radiation therapy in this disease has diminished in prominence. The spread pattern of ovarian cancer and the normal tissue bed involved in the treatment of this neoplasm makes effective radiation therapy difficult (Table 39-9). When the residual disease following laparotomy is bulky, radiation therapy is particularly ineffectual. The entire abdomen must be considered at risk and therefore the volume which must be irradiated is very large, resulting in multiple limitations for the radiotherapists (Table 39-10).

As long as a decade ago, several institutions abandoned the use of radiation therapy as postoperative therapy in patients with bulky residual epithelial cancer of the ovary. However, these same institutions continued to test the applicability of radiation in the patient with minimal residual disease after surgery. Recently a study was reported by Smith[3] from the M. D. Anderson Hospital which gave the results of a randomized prospective study in patients with minimal residual disease (no nodule greater than 2 cm) who were randomized between single-agent alkylating agent chemotherapy and whole-abdomen irradiation (moving strip technique) with a pelvic boost. This study showed no advantage to the irradiation therapy and a significant increase in morbidity. Based on this study the role of radiation therapy in many institutions has become very limited for stage III and stage IV disease. The Gynecologic Oncology Group tested the feasibility of utilizing radiation therapy in conjunction with chemotherapy. A prospective randomized study utilizing four approaches, assessing (1) radiation therapy alone versus (2) radiation therapy prior to chemotherapy (Alkeran), (3) chemotherapy alone, and (4) chemotherapy prior to radiation therapy, was recently completed with no significant difference being found in any of the four approaches. It thus becomes difficult to justify the morbidity of extensive radiation therapy for this disease process.

The role of radiation therapy in localized disease also

TABLE 39-8 Epithelial Cancer of the Ovary: Survival by Stage

Stage	Survival	
	2-Year, %	5-Year, %
Stage I	80	70
Stage II	40	25
Stage III	18	12
Stage IV	5	0

TABLE 39-9 Special Problems in Ovarian Cancer

1. Limits of tumor spread often unknown.
2. Variability of radiosensitivity.
3. Total tumor burden usually very large.
4. Free mobility of tumor cells within the abdominal cavity.
5. Radiation dosage restricted by neighboring organs.
6. Detection of early disease infrequent.

TABLE 39-10 Dose Restrictions

1. Tolerance of small intestine
2. Limited tolerance of kidneys
3. Bone marrow depression
4. Radiation enteritis due to large volume of intestine irradiated
5. Adhesive peritonitis

needs some discussion. A recent prospective randomized study of stage I epithelial cancer of the ovary conducted by the Gynecologic Oncology Group had the following results. Patients were randomized between three methods of treatment: (1) no further therapy; (2) Alkeran; and (3) pelvic radiation. Preliminary results would indicate that those patients receiving Alkeran did the best with no appreciable benefit being noted from the use of pelvic radiation. On the other hand, the role of pelvic radiation in stage II ovarian cancer has yet to be defined. Indeed, many institutions utilize pelvic radiation in conjunction with systemic chemotherapy as a customary treatment of stage II disease. Retrospective studies would suggest that pelvic radiation improves survival over and above the use of surgery alone. The efficacy of pelvic radiation as compared to chemotherapy in stage II disease in a prospective randomized study has yet to be conducted.

Management of Ovarian Cancer in Young Women

Generally speaking, the management of stage I ovarian cancer, if recognized as being malignant, is radical; that is, bilateral salpingo-oophorectomy and hysterectomy. Occasionally, however, unilateral oophorectomy has been carried out in a young and childless woman whose unilateral tumor later turns out to be malignant. Not proceeding with further therapy is a calculated risk, the justification for which exists in the statements in the literature of many authoritative gynecologists summarized in the comments which follow.

The requirements for conservative management of stage IA ovarian cancer are listed in (Table 39-11). The unilateral salpingo-oophorectomy may be the definitive treatment of a young woman of low parity found to have a well-differentiated serous, mucinous, endometroid, or mesonephric carcinoma of the ovary. The tumor must be unilateral, well encapsulated, free of adhesions, and not associated with ascites or evidence of extragonadal spread. Peritoneal washings for cytology should be taken from the pelvis and upper abdomen, and the opposite ovary should be bivalved for pathological examination. The incidence of microscopic metastases in the opposite ovary has been calculated by Munnell and others to be approximately 12 percent. The periaortic and pelvic wall nodes must be carefully palpated and an adequate sample biopsy of the omentum taken. In addition, the preserved pelvic organs should be reasonably normal since there

TABLE 39-11 Epithelial Ovarian Cancer: Requirements for Conservative Management

1.	Stage IA
2.	Grade 1 or 2 serous, mucinous, endometrioid, or mesonephric histology
3.	Young women of low parity
4.	Otherwise normal pelvis
5.	Encapsulated and free of adhesions
6.	No invasion of capsule, lymphatics, or mesovarium
7.	Peritoneal washings negative
8.	Contralateral bivalved and negative
9.	Omental biopsy negative
10.	Close follow-up
11.	Excision of residual ovary after completion of childbearing

is little to be gained by retaining the opposite ovary in a patient who is not fertile. With the finding of carcinoma in any of these areas conservative surgery must be abandoned. Dysgerminoma, granulosa cell tumor, and arrhenoblastoma may also be managed conservatively under these special circumstances. After the patient has completed her family, some consideration should be given to the removal of the other ovary because of the risk of eventually developing another ovarian malignancy.

The key issue in patients treated conservatively for epithelial tumors of the ovary is the histology. Mucinous lesions fare better than serous lesions; the grade 1 and borderline lesions being the most easily treated conservatively. In a recent study from the Mayo Clinic of 33 women, ages 16 to 29, who had stage IA ovarian cancer, it was shown that unilateral salpingo-oophorectomy or just resection of the ovary was adequate to result in no recurrences in a period of follow-up from 3 to 10 years. These results are encouraging but are not the final answer since many low-grade lesions are prone to late recurrence.

The management of dysgerminoma is frequently singled out as an example of conservative surgery. Table 39-12 reveals the statistics in patients treated in various manners. The exquisite radiosensitivity of dysgerminoma allows us to be somewhat liberal in its management. Although the recurrence rate in this disease is approx-

TABLE 39-12 Dysgerminoma

	Cases	Treatment	Recurrence Rate, %	5-year Survival, %
Radium hem	22	CO + x-ray therapy	18	95
AFIP	46	CO	22	91
AFIP	21	RO	10	90

NOTES: CO = unilateral oophorectomy; RO = total abdominal hysterectomy and bilateral salpingo-oophorectomy; Radium hem = Radium hemmet (Stockholm); AFIP = Armed Forces Institute of Pathology.

imately 20 percent in stage I, the overall survivals approach 95 percent because of this exceptional response to radical irradiation therapy. Note that the incidence of recurrence is approximately the same despite the initial treatment. The treatment of recurrences results in approximately 75 percent 5-year survival. The questions, however, that have not been answered are, What would be the overall 5-year survival if all patients were treated with radical irradiation following conservative or radical surgery? Would we salvage the other 5 percent of patients? It is difficult to answer these questions, but we assume that not all of them would be salvaged since we are convinced that some of these patients who succumb to dysgerminoma have immature embryonal components which were not recognized.

It should be noted that many ovarian neoplasms which have dysgerminoma elements also have immature embryonal components. This presents quite a different problem clinically. Table 39-13 shows the histological classification of the germ cell tumors. Those malignant tumors with embryonal or extraembryonal components formerly invariably resulted in death of the patient within 2 years' time. We feel that these patients should not be treated conservatively today, even when the disease is apparently limited to one ovary. Total abdominal hysterectomy and bilateral salpingo-oophorectomy is the surgical approach of choice. This should be followed by *intensive* chemotherapy. Nine young women with embryonal and extraembryonal malignant neoplasms treated with intensive triple-drug chemotherapy (vincristine, actinomycin D, and Cytoxan) following removal of their malignancy have now come to second-look procedures on our service, and all nine have been free of malignant tumor on second look. Three of these patients initially had more than stage I disease (two stage III and one stage II), and they, too, are surviving without evidence of disease following a negative second look. Similar results were obtained with another five patients with malignant teratomas (Table 39-14). Four additional patients with malignant teratomas were found at second look to have residual disease which was composed entirely of mature elements (like benign teratoma). No further therapy was given these patients, and they are alive and well at 2 to 6 years. Indeed, recent improved survivals with these unusual ovarian malignancies have resulted in the recommendation by some oncologists that stage IA lesions undergo conservative initial surgery with

TABLE 39-13 Germ Cell Tumors

Germinoma (dysgerminoma)

Tumors of totipotent cells

    Extraembryonal
        Choriocarcinoma

      Endodermal sinus tumor

      Embryonal carcinoma

    Embryonal ectoderm
    mesoderm and endoderm

      Teratoma

      Malignant teratoma

TABLE 39-14 Immature (Malignant) Teratomas

Grade	No.	Tumor deaths	%
0	4	0	0
1	18	4	22
2	23	9	39
3	11	7	64

SOURCE: HJ Norris et al: Immature (malignant) teratoma of the ovary: A clinical and pathologic study of 58 cells. *Cancer* 37:2359, 1976.

potential childbearing capacity preserved. All patients are recommended for 6 to 18 months of intensive adjuvant chemotherapy with the potential for retaining adequate ovarian function diminishing as the period of chemotherapy lengthens. Patients receiving 18 months of triple therapy are often not capable of ovulation after the discontinuation of therapy. Unfortunately, the minimal treatment period has not been clearly defined at this time.

Spill of Tumor

This subject has been quite controversial in gynecologic oncology for some time. It is logical to assume that implantation and germination of cancer cells is conceivable and probable when a malignant cyst ruptures at the time of surgery. The question remains only to prove that this is so.

The early studies of Munnell[4] did not support the theoretical possibility that rupture of a malignant ovarian tumor would enhance dissemination. He studied 99 patients with stage I and stage II ovarian cancer and had an overall 5-year survival of 71 percent. In his retrospective study, 27 of the patients had had spill at the time of surgery. Of these patients 22, or 81 percent survived 5 years. Of these 27 patients, postoperative irradiation was administered to 21, and there was 66 percent 5-year survival in this group of 21. Six of the patients did not receive x-ray therapy, and all six survived 5 years. It would appear from this very limited retrospective study that spill eruption does not endanger the patient's prognosis, and that if this occurrence does take place, postoperative irradiation is not necessarily indicated.

It is obvious that the number of patients studied here is very small, and one would have to carefully study the histology in the six patients who did not receive x-ray therapy. One may find that these were highly differentiated lesions, maybe of the borderline quality. There is, in addition, an obvious bias interjected here in that the patients with more malignant lesions probably received the irradiation therapy. There have been very few studies with enough patients to shed further light on this subject. However, recently a report by Decker[5] of the Mayo Clinic involving some 223 stage I cases of ovarian epithelial cancer revealed that rupture during surgery did seem to lower the survival cure. Another study by Grogran[6] from Harvard analyzed 124 patients with ovarian cancer. Rupture of an ovarian tumor cyst during surgery occurred in 16 of 124 patients. For our purposes, however, only nine patients are worthy of consideration since only these patients had stage I lesions. Six of these nine patients survived 5 years or more. One succumbed to a massive myocardial infarction and the other two to their malignancy. The six patients who survived had a well-differentiated grade 1 histological pattern. Both of the patients who died of tumor presented with a poorly differentiated histological picture. The two patients who did die of their tumor had received irradiation therapy following hysterectomy with bilateral salpingo-oophorectomy. However, the irradiation therapy was delivered in very moderate dosages of 2500 to 3000 rads on a 200-kV machine. This is far below optimum irradiation therapy.

The issue is difficult to resolve because one is very prone to treat more vigorously patients who have spill at the time of surgery, and this may equalize the survival rates in the group of patients. In the era when whole-abdomen irradiation and pelvic boost was the only therapy which could be offered these patients, some hesitation in instituting postoperative therapy appeared to be justified. However, we now have comparatively less toxic chemotherapeutic regimens which can be adequately used postoperatively. A reasonable and seemingly adequate recommendation in these instances is a year of chemotherapy administered in the form of Alkeran pulse therapy and then a second-look procedure to verify the absence of disease within the pelvic and abdominal cavity. If rupture does occur, lavage of the peritoneal cavity with sterile water has been recommended to cause lysis of the cells and may be helpful.

Multiple-Drug Chemotherapy versus Single-Agent Chemotherapy

With the improved remission rate demonstrated in childhood leukemia from combination chemotherapy, there came an enthusiastic group of studies investigating the efficacy of multiple agents for epithelial cancer of the ovary. The standard chemotherapy had been the use of single-agent alkylating-type drugs such as Alkeran, Cytoxan, chlorambucil, etc. Over the last decade several prospective randomized studies have been completed alternating patients between single-agent therapy and combination therapy. Some of these studies have identified other active agents in epithelial cancer of the ovary; three of these agents are adriamycin, hexamethylmelamine, and *cis*-platinum. Several studies which were initially performed at large cancer institutes, or by cooperative groups show no advantage of multiple-drug therapy over alkylating agents used alone. Recently, however, several preliminary reports have suggested that combinations such as Adriamycin and *cis*-platinum, Cytoxan and hexamethylmelamine, and *cis*-platinum alone and a combination of hexamethylmelamine, Cytoxan, Adriamycin, and 5-FU (Hexacaf) may have significant improved response rates when studied opposite single-agent therapy. A word of caution has to be inserted here because of the preliminary nature of these studies and rather poor information concerning toxicity. Patients with epithelial cancer of the ovary respond well to many chemotherapeutic agents and have a reasonable life-span in spite of advanced disease. Therefore, they are not good candidates for drugs which are severely dose limited and can only be administered for several months (e.g., Adriamycin and *cis*-platinum). In addition, the toxicity of some drug combinations is so severe that the improved survival (often measured in months) is not justified when compared with outpatient chemotherapy such as Alkeran or chlorambucil. These remarks are particularly pertinent in the adjuvant treatment category where many patients are treated who are free of disease but have a statistical probability of recurrence. Because of this, many institutions have limited the more toxic regimens to patients with bulky postoperative residual tumor and poor prognosis for reasonable survival.

Recently, Creasman et al. have reported a series of patients treated with Alkeran plus *C. parvum* immunotherapy.[7] The immunomodulating agent chosen for this study was a gram-positive bacterium called *Corynebacterium parvum*. This agent has been shown to increase nonspecific tumor resistance, to potentiate specific tumor rejections, to affect bone marrow proliferation, and to have additive antitumor effects when combined with alkylating agents. The pilot study done by Creasman et al. on 45 previously untreated stage III ovarian epithelial cancer patients showed a definite suggestion of improved response with the combination of chemotherapy and immunotherapy. A prospective randomized study in patients with minimal residual following laparotomy is now being conducted by the Gynecologic Oncology Group (Table 39-15).

FOLLOW-UP AND TECHNIQUES FOR EARLY IDENTIFICATION OF RECURRENCE AND/OR METASTASES

As stated above, ovarian cancer is fast-growing and insidious in that it is late to cause symptoms, and thus follow-up examinations are imperative to detect early recurrence. Even then, implants many centimeters in diameter can be hidden in the many crevices of the abdominal cavity and escape physical detection. There is a reasonable limit to the use of such sophisticated techniques as computerized axial tomography in the surveillance of a patient who has had ovarian cancer. The key to the proper assessment of the extent of disease is liberal use of surgical procedures (laparoscopy and laparotomy) to assay the contents of the abdominal and pelvic cavities.

"Second-Look" Operation

The so-called second-look operation was first defined by Owen Wangenstein in the late 1940s with reference to exploratory laparotomy procedures in colon cancer patients from whom he had previously removed all gross tumor but in whom there was a high risk of recurrence. At varying intervals, usually 6 months initially, he would explore these patients in the hope of detecting early recurrence at a time when secondary resection still offered a chance of cure. Since then, the term *second-look*

TABLE 39-15 Gynecologic Oncology Group Protocol 25

Procedure: Exploratory laparotomy, plus total abdominal hysterectomy and bilateral salpingo oophorectomy, plus omentectomy with debulking of tumor

Regimen A	Regimen B
Melphalan alone 7 mg/m² per day × 5 days PO; repeat every 4 weeks	Melphalan alone, 7 mg/m² per day × 5 days PO; repeat every 4 weeks; *plus C. parvum*, 4 mg/m² IV day 7 following chemotherapy

operation has been used to describe many procedures. With reference to ovarian cancer it appears that a second-look procedure may have three main indications: first, to restage a patient who presents with probable localized disease who has not had a proper staging procedure as defined in the text above; second, to evaluate the effect of chemotherapy in patients receiving both standard and investigational regimens. In this regard, some institutions have instituted serial laparoscopic examinations in order to assess the extent of regression or progression of bulk disease several months following commencement of chemotherapy with the option to offer other therapy should a poor response be noted. Lastly, the second-look operation has been utilized in patients who are clinically free of disease after receiving what is considered a sufficient course of chemotherapy (10 to 18 months) and are then eligible for assessment as to possible "cure" and discontinuation of therapy. This latter indication has been the most widely used and, indeed, has resulted in small numbers of patients with even advanced disease who are free of detectable malignant cells at the second procedure. The most difficult second-look procedure is that in which no evidence of disease apparently exists since very extensive and thorough surgery must be performed to establish lack of disease.

These second-look procedures are often begun with a laparoscopic examination to rule out widespread disease. Should this lesser procedure illustrate diffuse miliary studding (which was not clinically detectable), a laparotomy is not necessary. It is obvious that these patients need to continue on therapy of some sort and are not candidates for a second attempt at surgical resection. On the other hand, at the present state of our knowledge, a negative laparoscopic exam is not sufficient evidence for classifying the patient as without evidence of disease, and a laparotomy must be carried out. At the time of laparotomy a detailed exploration of the abdominal cavity must be conducted in a manner quite similar to the initial staging procedures previously described. Should focal residual disease be encountered, it should be surgically resected and the area marked with metal clips for regional radiation therapy. Careful inspection of the entire abdominal cavity, including the undersurface of the diaphragms, the root of the mesentery, and all parietal and visceral peritoneal surfaces must be tediously carried out with liberal use of biopsy for suspicious areas.

With the religious use of an extensive second-look operation one can expect a very low subsequent recurrence rate should the results be negative. In the hands of most individuals, less than 20 percent of these patients will subsequently appear with evidence of recurrent disease. Thus, these procedures can significantly influence the physician's ability to give an accurate prognosis to the patient and allow the patient to approach the future with reasonable expectations. In the absence of reliable tumor markers in epithelial cancer of the ovary, these second-look operations have great value.

On the whole, the germ cell tumors of the ovary and the tumors of specialized gonadal stroma (which are usually of low malignant potential) behave in a similar manner and are followed as outlined above. The exception, of course, would be advanced dysgerminoma, which is usually treated with irradiation therapy, and a second-look operation is not usually advised unless there is strong evidence of recurrence. These patients are best followed with lymphangiography, which is quite helpful in the detection of dysgerminoma in lymph nodes.

The germ cell tumors with embryonal or extraembryonal components behave much like epithelial cancer of the ovary and are usually treated with intensive chemotherapy. Thus, they follow closely the tenets outlined above for epithelial cancers of the ovary.

Radiation therapy is much less effective in this group of tumors, and that should be considered in devising any treatment plan. Many patients with endodermal sinus tumor of the ovary will have detectable α-fetoprotein levels in the serum. In a like manner, patients with embryonal carcinoma of the ovary often have positive human chorionic gonadotropin (HCG) titers. Thus, in these two rare embryonal neoplasms, a tumor marker may exist and can be utilized in monitoring the patients for response to therapy and detection of early recurrence.

THERAPEUTIC OPTIONS FOR THE TREATMENT OF RECURRENCES AND/OR METASTASES

Second-Line Chemotherapy

In all forms of ovarian cancer, second line chemotherapy has, to date, been very disappointing. When effective drug combinations are initially used and fail, there is virtually no chance of inducing a significant response with a second drug or combination of drugs. A partial response and control of malignant infusions can be achieved on occasion, but these are usually short-lived. However, most gynecologic oncologists attempt to treat these drug failure patients, using a reasonable second-line regimen usually consisting of active chemotherapeutic agents which have not been utilized in the first treatment plan. It is hoped that as new agents evolve, a more effective second echelon of drugs will be available for use. Although not generally advocated, every experienced gynecologic oncologist has a group of patients who have responded well to a second surgical attack on local or regional recurrent disease which initially had not responded to chemotherapy. This is especially relevant to the patient who at the time of second-look operation following chemotherapy has what appears to be localized persistent disease.

Malignant Effusions and Ascites

Fortunately, these clinical situations are nowhere near the problem that they were a decade ago. Chemotherapeutic regimens control malignant effusions in a good 90 percent of the cases. The patient who presents with a distended abdomen and probable ascites is the initial problem. There is a tendency to perform a paracentesis for diagnostic purposes when the situation is somewhat doubtful. We would like to make a plea for *not* performing paracentesis in patients who are highly suspect of ovarian malignancy, and the reasons are as follows:

1. Cytological examination of fluid may be negative in the presence of malignancy and laparotomy is still indicated.
2. Even when cytological examination of the fluid is positive, it seldom provides a sufficient clue to the origin of the primary tumor and laparotomy is indicated.
3. If the patient has a large, fluid-filled cyst rather than ascites, rupture of the cyst and seeding into the peritoneal cavity, often long before laparotomy, may occur.
4. Paracentesis may be associated with complications other than seeding such as rupture of an intraabdominal viscus, bleeding, infection, and severe depletion of electrolytes and proteins. We would, therefore, recommend that these patients be investigated short of paracentesis and that the disease be defined at laparotomy where the situation can be controlled with more ease.

Our comments are to discourage paracentesis as a diagnostic tool, but in instances where intraabdominal pressure causes respiratory embarrassment or severe pain the procedure should be performed as therapy. Often, improved gastrointestinal function and relief of nausea, vomiting, and constipation may be seen following such a therapeutic paracentesis.

It is a long-standing practice to instill antineoplastic agents into the peritoneal cavity at the time of exploratory laparotomy if unresectable tumor is found. It has been shown by multiple animal studies and other testing in humans that this topical use or intraperitoneal installation of chemotherapeutic agents is effective primarily by absorption from the peritoneal cavity into the systemic circulation. Since this is the case, it would follow that a much more scientific and controlled situation can be achieved by direct systemic use of the drug. Other agents such as Atabrine and nitrogen mustard have an effect on effusions by producing an adhesive serositis which will partially obliterate the peritoneal or pleural cavity making the accumulation of ascites more difficult. However, these agents also create a situation where further surgical intervention is almost impossible. When ascites reaccumulates following surgery, it is almost always a problem associated with unresectable carcinoma, and patients with this problem usually can be controlled with systemic chemotherapy of one form or the other. Should one drug fail, other combinations should be tried and are sometimes successful. Unfortunately, there are some patients whose ascites cannot be completely controlled by systemic chemotherapy, and often these patients can be kept comfortable with periodic paracentesis. This can be done on an outpatient basis at intervals determined by the patient's symptoms. The site of paracentesis is usually selected at the lateral border of the rectus muscle and at the level of the umbilicus. The midline is avoided since tumor or adhesions are often present, and complications can result. It is advisable to infiltrate the abdominal wall with a small amount of local anesthetic and then using the same syringe and needle explore for a clear spot in the peritoneal cavity. A larger trocar can then be inserted over the exact area of the exploration, and in this way one can avoid the complication of inserting a trocar into an adherent segment of bowel. Measurements of the weight and abdominal girth are recorded before and after paracentesis, and the volume of fluid is also noted. Sometimes fluid will continue to leak out of the trocar sites, and attaching a urostomy bag to the area will provide some comfort for the patient. Irradiation techniques are usually not recommended in the management of ascites because systemic chemotherapy is so effective. Installation of ^{32}P or ^{198}Au is often difficult because of the need to obtain a uniform distribution of the radioactive substance. In addition, one is usually dealing with a situation where large individual tumor masses are present, and even the γ emission of radioactive gold is effective only for 2 to 4 mm. There are situations in which a diffuse miliary spread of disease is suspected, and ascites is only partially controlled with chemotherapy. In these instances radioactive chromium phosphate (a β emitter) may be very beneficial and may provide minimum chance of severe injury to the bowel.

Pleural effusion is another problem confronting the management of ovarian cancer. Approximately one-third of the patients with ascites will have a pleural effusion. This usually responds to systemic chemotherapy along with the ascites. Pleural effusion in the absence of ascites usually indicates involvement of the pleura with disease. The same techniques which have been outlined for the management of ascites can be used. Nitrogen mustard or Atabrine injected into the pleural cavity is associated with a high success rate. Obliteration of the pleural cavity prevents the accumulation of fluid in that space. Nitrogen mustard (10 or 15) mg creates enough pleural reaction to cause obliteration of the potential space resulting in relief of this troublesome symptom for patients who are not responding optimally to systemic chemotherapy. Another method recently employed with some success is the installation of bleomycin (60 to 120 mg) into the pleural cavity after thoracentesis. This drug can be used with systemic chemotherapy because of its minimal myelosuppressive effect.

The etiology of malignant effusions is not known. The most common explanations are that they are the result of (1) an irritant effect of the tumor on normal serous membranes; (2) lymphatic obstruction; and (3) venous obstruction. Graham studied ascites circulating in patients with peritoneal carcinomatosis. He noted a large increase in the production of fluid by *non-cancer-bearing* peritoneal surfaces which was most marked from the omentum and small-bowel surfaces. He also noted a significant elevation of portal pressure in the presence of ovarian cancer with ascites as compared to normal patients and patients with ovarian cancer without ascites.

The surgical approach to recurrent malignant effusions has been somewhat limited. In the instance of pleural effusion, decortication of the lung and pleurectomy have been used with varying results. Installation of nitrogen mustard and similar caustic compounds has essentially replaced these procedures. Other agents have been used to create pleuritis including hypertonic glucose and talc. Again, they are variable in success rates depending upon the investigator. A surgical procedure for uncontrollable ascites called ileoentectropy was promoted by Brunschwig at Memorial Hospital. Some of the patients with ascites due to ovarian cancer had control of their effusion using this method, but it has not proved to be a practical approach.

CURRENT AREAS OF RESEARCH

Most of the advances that have been made in the treatment of cancer of the ovary in the last 10 years have utilized the multimodality approach. A combination of modalities used in a logical and flexible manner can achieve notable successes on an individual basis. This combined with improved chemotherapy agents and possible addition of immunotherapy as a new modality will hopefully result in improved outcome for this devastating group of malignancies.

By far the greatest advance on the horizon is in the area of early detection by immunodiagnostic techniques. Several crude experimental procedures have strongly suggested the presence of commonly shared tumor-associated antigens in epithelial cancers of the ovary. Unfortunately, isolation of these antigens has been more difficult than initially conceived and is essential to the creation of a clinically useful immunodiagnostic tool. Given that there are commonly shared tumor-associated antigens in epithelial cancer of the ovary and that a small amount of this antigen or an antibody to it are detectable in the serums of patients with subclinical disease, all the ingredients for a dramatic improvement in the battle against this disease are at hand.

RECONSTRUCTION AND REHABILITATION

The nature of ovarian cancer is such that the major vital organs such as lung, heart, liver, and kidneys remain unaffected. The disease itself and its therapy appear to attack the gastrointestinal tract primarily. Indeed, the terminal event for most patients who succumb to this disease is electrolyte imbalance from prolonged gastrointestinal obstruction, malnutrition, and significant protein and electrolyte loss from repeated paracentesis and thoracentesis. It is necessary to support these patients with various forms of alimentation during therapy in order to sustain the host sufficiently to tolerate the somewhat vigorous therapy often prescribed. Intermittent episodes of partial small- and large-bowel obstruction are common, and they must be treated conservatively initially and surgically ultimately if the patient is to continue the fight. The issue as to whether a patient with a high-grade small-bowel obstruction from ovarian cancer carcinomatosis should be explored for a possible bypass procedure to reestablish the continuity of the alimentary tract is a subject that has been long debated. Management of these patients is extremely difficult because of the intactness of their vital organs and alert mental status. Although most of these patients will not survive 6 months from the time of the bowel obstruction, surgical intervention should be considered in light of the difficulty that all individuals have observing the slow process of death by starvation. Any procedure which can result in the patient returning to her home and family seems to be worthy of consideration even in these hopeless cases. If nothing else, the performance of a gastrostomy to avoid the uncomfortable nasogastric intubation or persistent agony of constant vomiting is in itself humane and allows more easy return of the patient to a home setting where the gastrostomy can be used to decompress the patient as the need arises.

In general, the most discouraging aspect in the management of ovarian cancer patients is the apathy of many physicians. In all truth these diseases are discouraging but positive attack is both medically sound and reassuring to the patient. Significant numbers of patients referred as unresectable have been debulked and have responded nicely to postoperative therapy. Still other patients have survived, utilizing a complicated combination of multiple surgical and adjuvant therapies. If for no other reason, a positive approach to the disease restores hope in the patient with this devastating illness and is justified on that basis alone.

REFERENCES

1. DiSaia PJ et al: *Synopsis of Gynecologic Oncology*, Wiley, New York, 1975.
2. Parker, RT et al: Cancer of the ovary. *Am J Obstet Gynecol* 108:878, 1970.
3. Smith JP et al: Chemotherapy of ovarian cancer: New approaches to treatment. *Am J Obstet Gynecol* 116:261, 1973.
4. Munnell EW: Is conservative therapy ever justified in Stage I (1a) cancer of the ovary? *Am J Obstet Gynecol* 103:641, 1969.
5. Decker DG et al: Radio gold treatment of epithelial cancer of ovary: Late results. *Am J Obstet Gynecol* 115:751, 1973.
6. Grogan RH: Accidental rupture of malignant ovarian cysts during surgical removal. *Obstet Gynecol* 30:716, 1967.
7. Creasman WT et al: Chemoimmunotherapy in the management of primary stage III carcinoma of the ovary. *Cancer Chemother Rep* 63:319, 1979.

SELECTED BIBLIOGRAPHY

Cohen CJ et al: The results of therapeutic end staging laparotomy (second look surgery) in patients with epithelial cancer of the ovary, stages III and IV treated by surgery and multi-drug chemotherapy containing cis-platin. *Proc Amer Soc Clinical Oncol* 22:392, 1981.

Decker DG et al: A treatment program for stage III and IV ovarian cancer—cyclophosphamide vs cyclophosphamide and cis-platinum. *Abstracts Soc Gynecol Oncol* 10:368, 1980.

Ehrmann RL et al: Distinguishing lymph node metastases from benign grandular inclusions in low grade ovarian carcinoma. *Am J Obstet Gynecol* 136:737, 1980.

Gershenson DM et al: Single-agent cis-platinum therapy for advanced ovarian cancer. *Obstet Gynecol* 58:487, 1981.

Howell S et al: Intraperitoneal cis-platin with systemic thiosulfate protection. *Ann Intern Med* 97:845, 1982.

Katz ME et al: Epithelial carcinoma of the ovary. Current strategies. *Ann Intern Med* 95:98, 1981.

Order SE et al: The integration of new therapies and radiation in the management of ovarian cancer. *Cancer* 48:590, 1981.

Ozols RF et al: Advanced ovarian cancer: Correlation of histologic grade with response to therapy and survival. *Cancer* 45:572, 1980.

Ozols RF et al: Phase I and pharmacological studies of Adriamycin administered intraperitoneally to patients with ovarian cancer. *Cancer Res* 42:4265, 1982.

Ozols RG et al: Peritoneoscopy in the management of ovarian cancer. *Am J Obstet Gynecol* 140:611, 1981.

Parker LM et al: Combination chemotherapy with Adriamycin-cyclophosphamide for advanced ovarian carcinoma. *Cancer* 46:669, 1980.

Smith JP, Schwartz PE: Second look laparotomy and prognosis related to extent of residual disease, in Van Oosterom AJ, Muggia FM (eds): *Therapeutic Progress in Ovarian Cancer, Testicular Cancer and the Sarcomas.* Martinus Nijhoff Publishers, The Hague, 1980.

Vogl SE et al: Combination chemotherapy of advanced ovarian cancer with cyclophosphamide (C), hexamethylmelamine (H), Adriamycin (A) and diamminedichloroplatinum (D)—The "CHAD" regimen. *Abstracts Soc Gynecol Oncol* 10:369, 1980.

Vogl SE et al: Hexamethylmelamine and cis-platin in advanced ovarian cancer after failure of alkylating-agent therapy. *Cancer Treat Rep* 66(6):1285, 1982.

Wharton JT et al: Longterm survival following chemotherapy for advanced epithelial ovarian carcinoma, in Van Oosterom, AJ Muggia FM (eds): *Therapeutic Progress in Ovarian Cancer, Testicular Cancer and the Sarcomas,* pp 95. Martinus Nijhoff Publishers, The Hague, 1980.

Wharton JT, Herson J: Surgery for common epithelial tumors of the ovary. *Cancer* 48:582, 1981.

Williams CJ et al: Chemotherapy of advanced ovarian carcinoma: Initial experience using a platinum-based combination. *Cancer* 49:1778, 1982.

40

TUMORS OF THE VULVA, VAGINA, AND FEMALE URETHRA

Samuel C. Ballon

TUMORS OF THE VULVA

Historical Aspects

The treatment of patients with carcinoma of the vulva by radiation therapy produced cure rates of 0 to 20 percent.[8] These poor results occurred because the tissues of the vulva are intolerant to cancericidal doses of radiation, which produce erythema, edema, pain, and desquamation with secondary infection. Symptomatic, radiation-induced cystitis and proctitis also can occur. Simple excision of the carcinoma in addition to radiation therapy increased cure rates to only 30 percent.

Although radical vulvectomy was described as a standard approach to the treatment of these patients as early as 1912, it remained for Taussig and Way to establish that improved survival related directly to wide, deep removal of the entire vulva with an aggressive operative attack on the regional lymph nodes.[1] Their studies provided a rational basis for the management of invasive carcinoma of the vulva, and little in the past 30 years has altered the now-accepted treatment of this disease.[2]

Incidence, Epidemiology, and Etiology

Carcinoma of the vulva accounts for about 4 percent of malignant tumors of the female genital tract. Although the disease is most common in women over 50 years of age, younger women with intraepithelial neoplasia of the vulva, vagina, and cervix appear at risk to develop squamous carcinoma of the vulva.[3] A possible viral etiology is suggested by the association of some premalignant lesions with condyloma acuminata and a high frequency in these patients of antibodies to herpes simplex type 2 virus. Patients with invasive squamous carcinoma of the vulva tend to be postmenopausal, obese, hypertensive and diabetic. A prior history of lues or other granulomatous venereal disease often is present.[4]

Hypertrophic epithelial dystrophy of the vulva, which appears as a raised, white hyperkeratotic area commonly referred to as *leukoplakia,* is associated with squamous carcinoma. Although it precedes invasive cancer in up to 50 percent of patients, the neoplastic potential of leukoplakia appears to be overemphasized, as less than 10 percent of these lesions become malignant.

Over 85 percent of malignant tumors of the vulva are squamous carcinomas. About 10 percent are malignant melanomas while adenocarcinomas, sarcomas, and other rare tumors make up the remainder. This section deals primarily with squamous carcinoma of the vulva and its precursors. Melanoma, Paget's disease of the vulva, adenocarcinoma, basal cell carcinoma, and sarcoma will be discussed briefly.

Signs, Symptoms, and Early Detection

Patches of skin on the vulva which are red, dark brown, or white and areas which are firm to palpation or in which the patient has noted pruritis or bleeding must undergo biopsy to rule out carcinoma. Excision and histological evaluation of nevi in the genital region is required to exclude melanoma; an enlarged or thickened Bartholin's gland should be sampled to diagnose carcinoma of this structure. A delay in diagnosis and therapy frequently exists on the parts of both the patient and her physician. Although improved treatment modalities have increased survival from carcinoma of the vulva, these delays have not been reduced.

A continuum of disease which includes dysplasia and carcinoma in situ occurs in the vulva as in the cervix. Unlike in situ epidermoid carcinoma of the cervix, however, this preinvasive stage of squamous carcinoma of the vulva often is associated with a visible lesion. The concept of a multifocal origin of dysplasia and carcinoma has been emphasized but does not apply to each patient.

A cytological smear of the vulva, staining with vital dye, and colposcopy are of limited diagnostic use because of the normal keratinization of the skin of the vulva and the hyperkeratotic nature of many premalignant lesions.[5] Biopsy with appropriate histological interpretation is required to diagnose intraepithelial carcinoma of the vulva.

Invasive squamous carcinoma can fungate or ulcerate, and with continued growth can bleed and produce discharge secondary to infection and pain. The tumor originates, in order of decreasing frequency, in the labium majus, labium minus, clitoris, and perineum; however, the advanced presentation of some lesions precludes determination of their precise origin. The histological appearance of these tumors is typical of squamous carcinoma elsewhere with the presence of epithelial pearls, penetration of the malignant epithelial cells into the stroma, and lymphatic and vascular involvement (Fig. 40-1).

Staging and Prognostic Factors

The International Federation of Gynaecology and Obstetrics has adopted the TNM staging system for primary squamous carcinoma of the vulva (Table 40-1). Of the many histological types of cancer of the vulva, this classification is applicable only to squamous carcinoma because of its tendency to invade adjacent structures and its characteristic route of metastases to superficial and deep regional lymph nodes in the groins and then to pelvic and distant nodes.

Survival correlates with the size of the tumor, its location, structures invaded, and metastases to the re-

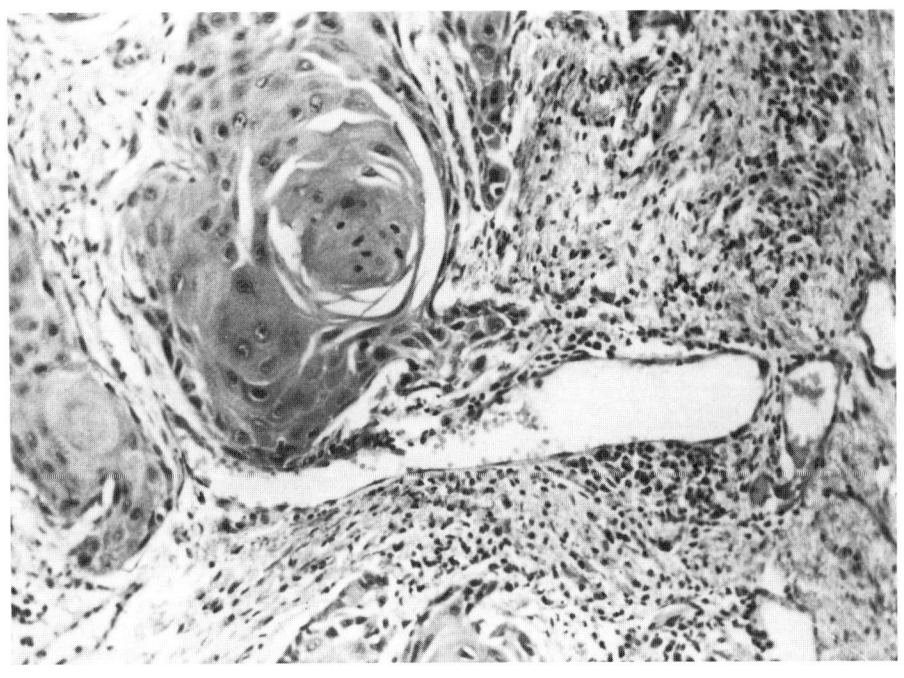

FIGURE 40-1 Invasive squamous carcinoma of the vulva. Well-differentiated tumor with epithelial pearl formation penetrates a blood vessel.

TABLE 40-1 FIGO Staging of Squamous Carcinoma of the Vulva

PRIMARY TUMOR (T)

- T_1 Tumor confined to the vulva, 2 cm or less in largest diameter.
- T_2 Tumor confined to the vulva, > 2 cm in diameter.
- T_3 Tumor of any size with adjacent spread to the urethra and/or vagina and/or anus.
- T_4 Tumor of any size infiltrating the bladder mucosa and/or the rectal mucosa including the upper part of the urethral mucosa and/or fixed to the bone.

REGIONAL LYMPH NODES (N)

- N_0 No nodes palpable.
- N_1 Nodes palpable in either groin, not enlarged, mobile (not clinically suspicious of neoplasm).
- N_2 Nodes palpable in either one or both groins, enlarged, firm, and mobile (clinically suspicious of neoplasm).
- N_3 Fixed or ulcerated nodes.

DISTANT METASTASES (M)

- M_0 No clinical metastases.
- M_{1a} Palpable deep pelvic lymph nodes.
- M_{1b} Other distant metastases.

STAGE	TNM	CLINICAL
I	$T_1N_0M_0$ $T_1N_1M_0$	All lesions confined to the vulva with a maximum diameter of 2 cm or less and no suspicious groin nodes.
II	$T_2N_0M_0$ $T_2N_1M_0$	All lesions confined to the vulva with a diameter > 2 cm and no suspicious groin nodes.
III	$T_3N_0M_0$ $T_3N_1M_0$	Lesions extending beyond the vulva but without grossly positive groin nodes.
	$T_1N_2M_0$ $T_2N_2M_0$ $T_3N_2M_0$	Lesions of any size confined to the vulva and having suspicious groin nodes.
IV	$T_1N_3M_0$ $T_2N_3M_0$ $T_3N_3M_0$ $T_4N_3M_0$	Lesions with grossly positive groin nodes regardless of extent of primary.
	$T_4N_0M_0$ $T_4N_1M_0$ $T_4N_2M_0$	Lesions involving mucosa of rectum, bladder, urethra, or involving bone.
	TNM_{1a} TNM_{1b}	All cases with distant or palpable deep pelvic metastases.

gional and distant lymph nodes.[6] Squamous carcinoma of the vulva usually spreads first to the ipsilateral groin nodes; however, because of abundant anastomoses of the lymphatic channels of the vulva, involvement of the contralateral groin nodes occasionally has been observed in the absence of ipsilateral metastases. Metastases to the groin nodes increase with advanced stage of disease, as does the frequency of bilateral groin node involvement. Metastases to the pelvic or periaortic lymph nodes in the absence of tumor in the groin nodes are unusual but are described in patients in whom the primary tumor involves the clitoris, urethra, or anus. Many investigators now report no patients with positive pelvic lymph nodes in the absence of metastases to the groin nodes.[7]

Poor correlation exists between the clinical and histological status of the groin nodes. Nonpalpable nodes (N0) rarely are involved with tumor while nodes which are matted, fixed, or ulcerated (N$_3$) are diagnosed with assurance. It is difficult to determine, however, if mobile, palpable nodes (N$_1$,N$_2$) contain tumor. Clinical correlation with histological findings in this group of patients is about 50 to 75 percent.[8,9]

In most recent series the 5-year survival of patients with invasive squamous carcinoma treated by radical vulvectomy and groin node dissection is greater than 80 percent in the absence of lymph node metastases and 40 to 50 percent with involvement of unilateral inguinal or femoral nodes. Survival is reduced to 25 percent at 5 years with spread to either bilateral groin nodes or unilateral groin and pelvic lymph nodes. Patients with bilateral involvement of the pelvic lymph nodes have an expected 10 to 20 percent 5-year survival.

Primary Treatment

The standard treatment of intraepithelial carcinoma is wide, complete removal of the skin of the vulva. This approach is based on the documented tendency of the preinvasive lesions to be multifocal and to recur after inadequate excision. A decision not to perform a total vulvectomy requires that the patient accept both frequent examinations and a potential need for multiple local excisions. A subtotal vulvectomy which preserves the clitoris is suitable treatment for selected patients with posterior lesions.

Preoperative evaluation of patients with invasive carcinoma includes chest roentgenogram, intravenous pyelogram, cystoscopy, barium enema, sigmoidoscopy, complete blood count, urinalysis, and tests of hepatic and renal function. A careful pelvic examination is required to assess the status of the vagina, cervix, urethra, base of bladder, and rectovaginal septum with biopsy of these areas as indicated. A radical vulvectomy with removal of the vulva to the external pelvic fascia and an in-continuity dissection of the inguinal and femoral lymph nodes is the standard therapeutic approach (Fig. 40-2). Pelvic lymphadenectomy or irradiation of the pelvic lymph nodes is performed if regional groin node metastases are present, and is advocated by some if the primary tumor involves the clitoris, urethra, or anus.

Complications from this extensive operative procedure occur in virtually all patients. These include break-

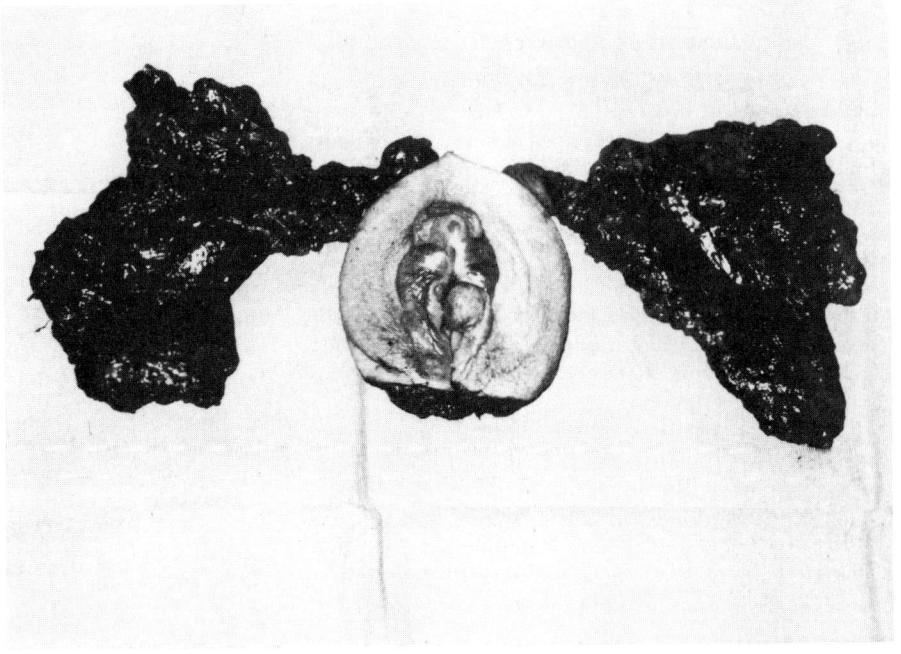

FIGURE 40-2 Radical vulvectomy with in-continuity bilateral inguinal and femoral lymphadenectomy.

down of the incisions over the groins and vulva, local infection, sepsis, thromboembolism, and chronic edema of the lower extremities. Transplantation of the head of the sartorius muscle to cover the denuded femoral vessels and the use of suction catheters to facilitate drainage have decreased morbidity from sepsis and hemorrhage previously encountered with groin node dissection.

Adjuvant Therapy

Patients with metastases to the groin nodes at the time of radical vulvectomy undergo pelvic lymphadenectomy and/or radiation therapy to the whole pelvis. Standard operative approaches to the pelvic and periaortic nodes involve incision of the external and internal oblique fascia parallel to the inguinal ligament or transection of the ligament. If the pelvic lymph nodes contain metastatic tumor, patients receive 4000 to 5000 rads of whole-pelvic irradiation delivered over 4 to 5 weeks. Treatment begins after complete healing, which generally occurs within 3 weeks of operation. No controlled studies exist to demonstrate the benefits of postoperative radiation therapy; however, many investigators report long-term survivors treated by this approach.[2]

Identification of Recurrent Disease

Local recurrence of squamous carcinoma of the vulva should be unusual if care is taken to ensure tumor-free margins at the time of resection. In spite of this, patients who develop a recurrence frequently do so in the area of the vulvectomy deep to the skin or vaginal mucosa. Recurrent tumor can extend posteriorly to involve the ischiorectal fossa, rectovaginal septum, and gluteal region or anteriorly through the subvaginal tissues to the urethra and base of bladder. Concurrent lymphatic dissemination to distant nodes is common in these patients. In addition, metastases by the hematogenous route can involve the lung, liver, or skeleton.

Examination following radical vulvectomy and groin node dissection thus must include a careful inspection and palpation of the surrounding tissues and is performed every 3 months for the first year and semiannually thereafter together with a complete blood count, urinalysis, and tests of hepatic and renal function. A chest roentgenogram is obtained on a yearly basis.

Treatment of Advanced and Recurrent Disease

Patients in whom the primary tumor invades the rectum, urethra, or bladder have disease beyond the limits of a standard radical vulvectomy. Pelvic exenteration in combination with a radical vulvectomy and groin node dissection has not eliminated the problem of local recurrence and has resulted in a 5-year survival of only 15 to 20 percent.[10] Studies are ongoing in such patients to assess the benefits of a combination of radiation therapy followed by operations less extensive than exenteration. Preliminary results in patients so managed at the UCLA Medical Center suggest that the risk of associated distant disease with these advanced tumors is high. In three such patients treated by radiation and radical operation, two achieved local control of their tumor. These two patients died, however, of pulmonary metastases while the third succumbed to a combination of local and distant recurrence.

The available chemotherapy for the treatment of disseminated squamous carcinoma of the vulva has produced no complete, sustained remissions in our patients. An objective response rate of 10 to 15 percent has been observed for up to 4 months in patients receiving bleomycin, an alkylating agent, or *cis*-platinum. Death has been from cachexia or respiratory failure secondary to extensive pulmonary metastases.

Current Research and Prospects for the Future

5-Fluorouracil, dinitrochlorobenzene (DNCB), and bleomycin prepared as hydrophobic ointments have been applied directly to the skin of the vulva in women with carcinoma in situ.[11] DNCB and bleomycin also have been injected intradermally. Several preliminary reports have indicated regression of intraepithelial neoplasia using these drugs; however, in a pilot study performed at UCLA Medical Center, two patients had progression to invasive carcinoma while on topical bleomycin therapy. The use of wide local excision and topical chemotherapy in the treatment of intraepithelial carcinoma of the vulva requires further study. Many affected patients are young and would benefit from efforts designed to minimize the physical and psychosexual aftermath of total vulvectomy. Such studies must be designed carefully to ensure that cure is not sacrificed in favor of a better cosmetic result.

Invasive squamous carcinoma of the vulva, although not preventable, theoretically is detectable at an early stage. A concerted effort toward patient education is required if these early invasive lesions are to be brought to the attention of the physician. Education of the practicing physician will avoid frequent delays in diagnosis. Any suspicious area of the vulva requires biopsy and histological interpretation prior to the institution of treatment such as topical ointment. If these educational efforts are successful, most patients with carcinoma of the vulva will undergo definitive therapy at a time when it is likely to be curative.

The place of radiation in the primary treatment of patients with squamous carcinoma of the vulva deserves further investigation. The ability of external beam therapy to irradiate microscopic foci of metastatic tumor in the groin nodes should be documented, as should the ability of whole-pelvis irradiation to sterilize tumor in the pelvic lymphatics. A combination of radiation and extended operation for advanced local disease, perhaps in conjunction with adjuvant chemotherapy, warrants consideration.

Reconstruction and Rehabilitation

The concept that squamous carcinoma of the vulva metastasizes to the nodes by embolization rather than by direct extension has lead investigators at UCLA Medical Center to use separate incisions in selected patients rather than perform lymphadenectomy in continuity with the radical vulvectomy. Separate incisions have been shown to decrease the early and late postoperative morbidity which is secondary to groin wound breakdown and have not been associated with an increase in local tumor recurrence.[8]

In those patients who require a pelvic lymphadenectomy, an extraperitoneal approach to these node-bearing tissues recently has been favored.[12] Bilateral lymphadenectomy to the level of the third lumbar vertebral body has been performed through a left-sided, J-shaped incision. Improved exposure by this technique permits a more complete lymph node dissection. Absence of morbidity when this operation is combined with subsequent radiation allows for potential therapeutic benefit from lymphadenectomy and extended field radiotherapy in selected patients with advanced carcinoma.

When the size and location of the primary tumor allow the operator to utilize separate incisions, morbidity relates to breakdown of the vulvectomy incision and frequent postoperative difficulty with urination. Attention now has turned to reconstruction of the defect left by radical vulvectomy, and gracilis myocutaneous flaps have been rotated from the legs to cover the defects in the vulva (Fig. 40-3).[13] On occasion, when the radicality of the node dissection has prevented primary closure of the groin wound, a myocutaneous flap also has been used to cover this defect.

Malignant Melanoma

INCIDENCE, EPIDEMIOLOGY, AND ETIOLOGY

Malignant melanoma accounts for up to 10 percent of patients seen in most treatment centers with cancer of the vulva. Although the vulva represents only 1.5 percent of the body surface area and has less than 0.1 percent of nevi, 5 percent of cases of malignant melanoma in the female occur on the vulva. Melanoma can arise de novo, from junctional nevi or the junctional component of compound nevi, and virtually all nevi which occur on the vulva are of the junctional variety.[14]

Patients with melanoma of the vulva average 55 years of age, but its occurrence in younger women is not uncommon. It is three times more prevalent in Caucasian than in black women. The disease is more frequent in warm latitudes and with increased exposure of the skin to ultraviolet light. Some melanomas occur in genetically predisposed individuals. Melanoma is the fourth most common malignant tumor that occurs in pregnancy following breast cancer, the leukemias, and lymphomas. It is the most common tumor to metastasize to the placenta and fetus.

SIGNS AND SYMPTOMS

Eighty percent of melanomas of the vulva arise from the labium minus or clitoris and often extend to involve the urethra and vagina. Malignant change in a flat, hairless nevus is suggested by enlargement, ulceration, weeping, crusting, or bleeding. Melanoma of the vulva can be flat, elevated, or polypoid. Ulceration can occur, and a surrounding flare and satellite metastases are common. On occasion, the overlying epidermis undergoes pseudoepitheliomatous hyperplasia.

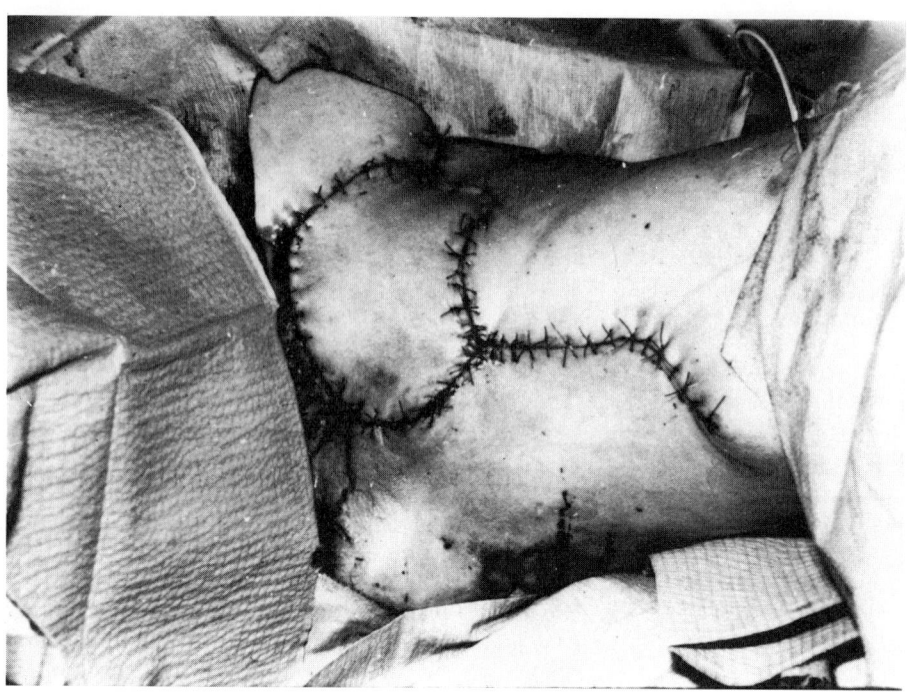

FIGURE 40-3 Gracilis myocutaneous flap rotated to cover defect in left hemivulva.

STAGING AND PROGNOSTIC FACTORS

The TNM staging which is applied to squamous carcinoma has also been shown to reflect prognosis from melanoma of the vulva.[15] In addition to spread by direct extension to adjacent urethra and vagina, metastases to regional and distant lymph nodes are common. Metastatic tumor can be demonstrated in the lymphatics of the tissues over the groins. Hematogenous dissemination is responsible for the presence of distant visceral metastases and accounts for the high rate of recurrence long after diagnosis and treatment of the primary tumor.

In the absence of metastases to regional lymph nodes in the groins, patients have better than a 50 percent 5-year survival. When metastases to the groin nodes are present, survival is less than 15 percent at 5 years. Pelvic lymph node involvement, which is rare in the absence of groin node metastases, carries a virtual 0 percent 5-year survival. Gross 5-year survival is less than 40 percent, and the 10-year survival is under 30 percent. Patients with occult metastases should have a better prognosis than those with clinically positive groin nodes. After treatment of only the primary lesion 25 to 50 percent of patients develop groin node metastases, which suggests a high incidence of occult metastases at diagnosis.

Women tend to have a better survival from malignant melanoma than do men. Survival decreases with advanced age at diagnosis, increased extent of the primary tumor, lymph node metastases, urethral or vaginal involvement, the presence of satellite lesions, and distant metastases (Table 40-2). As with melanoma found elsewhere, depth of invasion of the primary lesion correlates both with the tendency to metastasize and survival. Clark's classification can be applied to melanomas which arise in the vulva.[16] One more specifically related to the unique structure of the vulvar tissues also relates depth of invasion to prognosis (Table 40-3).[17]

PRIMARY TREATMENT

That nevi of the vulva are uncommon and invariably junctional suggests that they should undergo prophylactic removal for histological examination by total excision with a wide margin of normal skin. Minimal acceptable therapy for malignant melanoma of the vulva is radical vulvectomy with in-continuity bilateral removal

TABLE 40-2 Melanoma of the Vulva

Feature associated with poor prognosis	Frequency of occurrence, %*
Lymph node metastases	30
Spread to urethra or vagina	10
Satellite lesions	5
Distant metastases	5

* Percent of all patients affected.

of inguinal and femoral lymph nodes. This is required because of the frequent presence of in-transit metastases and a propensity for bilateral groin node involvement. Removal of the pelvic lymph nodes should be considered in patients with clitoral involvement and performed in all those with groin node metastases. Care should be taken to ensure disease-free margins especially at the junction of the urethra and vaginal mucosa.

TREATMENT OF ADVANCED AND RECURRENT DISEASE

Although melanoma of the vulva has been viewed as a radioresistant tumor, in the absence of clinically apparent metastases radiation therapy has produced up to a 70 percent 5-year survival with melanoma of other sites. This decreases to less than 30 percent when metastases are present. To be effective, however, radiation should include 10 to 15 cm of normal skin around the primary tumor, and this is poorly tolerated by the tissues of the vulva. Palliative therapy has produced about a 50 percent response rate with 2000 to 3000 rads delivered to patients with pain secondary to skeletal metastases or central nervous system symptoms caused by brain metastases.

Survival in patients with disseminated disease is less than 5 percent at 5 years. Transient responses are reported with alkylating agents, vinca alkaloids, procarbazine, DTIC (dimethyl triazeno imidazole carboxamide), and the nitrosoureas (Table 40-4). Combination therapy usually includes a vinca alkaloid and DTIC. Women respond more often than men to chemotherapy of disseminated melanoma and appear to have a longer median survival if a response occurs.

CURRENT RESEARCH AND PROSPECTS FOR THE FUTURE

Spontaneous regression of melanoma has been reported. Cutaneous hypersensitivity to melanoma cells, antibodies to cell surface and cytoplasmic antigens, and lymphocyte cytotoxicity to melanoma cells have been demonstrated in patients with this disease. These phenomena form the basis for immunotherapeutic approaches, which include injection of tumor cells from each of a pair of melanoma patients into the opposite member of the pair and transfusion of thereby activated lymphocytes from the recipient to the donor. A 20 percent response rate has resulted from this technique in selected patients.[18] Bacillus Calmette-Guérin (BCG) and MER, the methanol extraction residue of BCG, when injected into cutaneous lesions have produced regression in up to 90 percent of injected lesions if the patient can mount a delayed

TABLE 40-3 Classification of Melanoma Based on Level of Invasion

Level	Clark[16]	Chung[17]
1	All tumor cells above basement membrane (in situ melanoma)	All tumor cells above basement membrane (in situ melanoma)
2	Penetration of tumor cells into papillary but not reticular dermis	Superficial penetration of tumor into subepithelial tissues to depth of 1 mm or less
3	Penetration of tumor cells to interface between papillary and reticular dermis	Superficial penetration of tumor into subepithelial tissues between 1 and 2 mm
4	Penetration of tumor cells into reticular dermis	Penetration of tumor cells beyond 2 mm but not into subcutaneous fat
5	Penetration of tumor cells into subcutaneous fat	Penetration of tumor cells into subcutaneous fat

TABLE 40-4 Response of Disseminated Melanoma to Chemotherapy

Agent	Response Rate, %
Alkalating agent	15–20
Vinca alkaloids	20
Procarbazine	25
DTIC*	25–35

* Dimethyl triazeno imidazole carboxamide.

hypersensitivity response to DNCB and can react to tuberculin after BCG therapy.[19] A combination of chemotherapy and immunotherapy in patients with advanced or recurrent melanoma now is under investigation in several centers.

Paget's Disease

Paget's disease of the vulva is a distinctive form of intraepithelial carcinoma which causes pruritis with secondary excoriation and bleeding.[20] The characteristic lesion is red with raised, irregular margins (Fig. 40-4). The thickened epithelium is infiltrated with mucin-containing Paget cells which probably arise from adjacent glands (Fig. 40-5). Often, the grossly normal surrounding skin exhibits histological involvement by Paget cells.

For therapeutic purposes the disease is considered as two separate entities.[21] The abnormality is confined to the epidermis in 75 percent of patients, while 25 percent have an underlying invasive adenocarcinoma. This distinction usually can be made clinically; however, on occasion this is not possible. For this reason a radical vulvectomy is recommended in the primary treatment of patients with vulvar Paget's disease. A wide margin of normal skin should be excised.

If no invasive adenocarcinoma is found on examination of the vulvectomy specimen, subsequent management is directed toward the identification of local recurrence. If a coexisting adenocarcinoma is present, the role of bilateral inguinal and femoral lymphadenectomy deserves consideration. In the absence of clinically suspicious nodes, this procedure is of prognostic importance but has not produced a demonstrable improvement in survival. Similarly, the therapeutic value of lymphadenectomy in patients with palpable groin node metastases is questionable.[22] Death in these patients usually results from disseminated disease. Patients with a suspected invasive adenocarcinoma require thorough investigation to rule out metastatic disease prior to the performance of a radical vulvectomy. A less radical

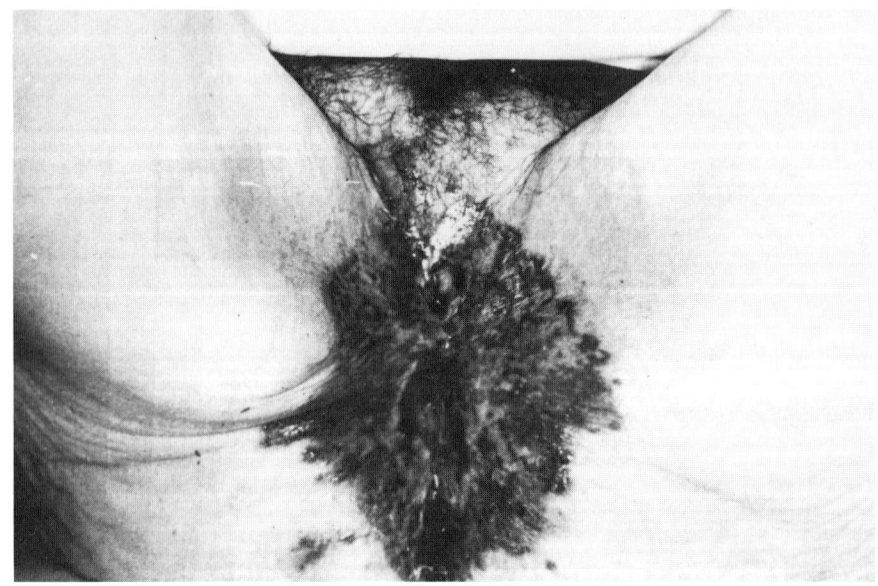

FIGURE 40-4 Raised, irregular margins of recurrent Paget's disease of vulva extend into vagina and rectum.

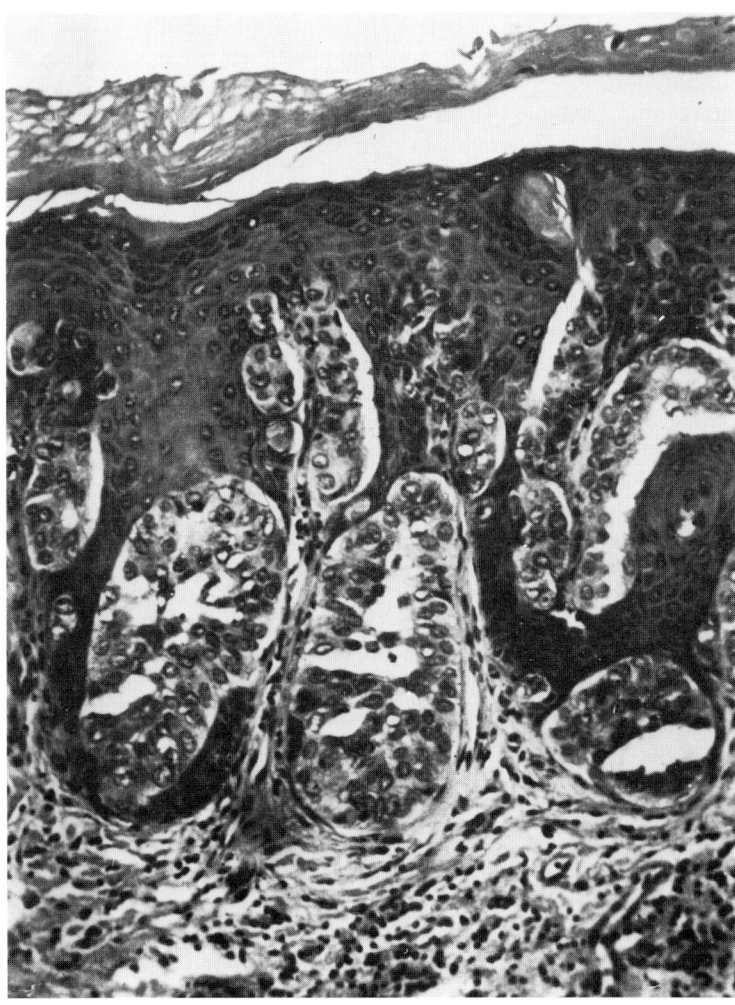

FIGURE 40-5 Mucin-containing Paget's cell infiltrate squamous epithelium of vulva.

procedure designed to achieve local control might be indicated if metastases are found.

Paget's disease of the vulva is associated with a high rate of local recurrence, and many patients have undergone multiple local excisions following a radical vulvectomy. At the UCLA Medical Center, seven patients with recurrent Paget's disease have been treated with topical bleomycin ointment.[23] Of this group, four patients experienced a complete objective response and one of these has responded to the treatment of a subsequent recurrence.

The treatment of intraepithelial Paget's disease with radiation therapy is not warranted; in the presence of invasive adenocarcinoma its value is unproven. However, isolated patients have responded to radiation for local recurrence of their disease.

Patients with this disease appear to be at risk to develop unrelated second primary tumors. The lower genital tract, skin, and gastrointestinal tract most often are affected.

Basal Cell Carcinoma

As with basal cell tumors in extragenital sites, basal cell carcinoma of the vulva most often affects elderly, Caucasian women. Pruritis or a mass can exist for many years prior to diagnosis. The tumor commonly involves the anterior labium majus. Prior irradiation of the vulva has been reported in some patients. This tumor is locally invasive but does not metastasize; therefore, treatment includes wide, deep local excision of the lesion with careful documentation of tumor-free margins. Unlike squamous carcinoma, this tumor is rarely multifocal, and radical vulvectomy is not indicated.[24]

Sarcoma

Primary sarcoma of the vulva accounts for approximately 1 percent of tumors in this area, and usually affects young women. All varieties of sarcoma, both homologous and heterologous, have been identified, with leiomyosarcoma the most frequent.[25]

Treatment of sarcomas must allow for a tendency both to local recurrence and to hematogenous and lymphatic metastases. A radical vulvectomy with bilateral inguinal and femoral lymphadenectomy has been successful in the prevention of local recurrence and on occasion has prolonged survival in patients with groin node metastases.[26] Adjunctive chemotherapy for women at risk to develop widespread disease currently is under investigation with various combinations of chemotherapeutic agents reported successful in the short-term control of disseminated sarcoma.

Adenocarcinoma

Adenocarcinoma of Bartholin's gland is extremely rare and affects women of all age groups.[27] The criteria for diagnosis of this tumor include correct anatomic position, location of the tumor deep in the labium, and the presence of glandular elements. Too few cases exist to permit a definitive statement as to the natural history and biologic behavior of these tumors. The diagnosis often is made late in the course of the disease, and these tumors have a high rate of regional and distant lymph node involvement, secondary to the deep location of Bartholin's gland and a rich supply of lymphatic vessels which drain directly to the pelvic lymph nodes as well as to those in the groin.

The physician should recognize that inflammation of Bartholin's gland is uncommon after the fourth decade and virtually unreported in postmenopausal women. Any swelling in this area should be subjected to biopsy. If adenocarcinoma is found, a radical vulvectomy with groin and pelvic lymphadenectomy probably constitutes minimal acceptable therapy. Survival data suggest that if diagnosed early this tumor can be cured.[28]

TUMORS OF THE VAGINA

Incidence, Epidemiology, and Etiology

In 1939, statistics from the United States Census Bureau indicated that 238 American women died of a primary carcinoma of the vagina. By 1944, a relative increase of 14.3 percent had occurred with 272 reported deaths.[29] With the continued use of cytological techniques more women with preinvasive and early invasive tumors now are being identified.

Primary carcinoma of the vagina at this time accounts for 1 to 2 percent of gynecologic malignancies. Although extension to the vagina from a tumor of the cervix or vulva is seen frequently, those which involve both vagina and cervix are classified as cervical cancers while those which involve the vagina and vulva are considered neoplasms of the vulva. Over 90 percent of vaginal cancers are of the epidermoid variety, and most of the remainder are adenocarcinomas. Primary sarcoma and melanoma of the vagina are so infrequent that they do not warrant separate discussion.

As with carcinoma of the cervix and vulva, invasive epidermoid carcinoma of the vagina is preceded by dysplasia and carcinoma in situ. Unlike carcinoma of the cervix, however, the natural history of this continuum as it applies to the vagina is poorly understood. The factors which influence dysplasia of the vagina to progress to intraepithelial and invasive carcinoma, and the time required for progression from intraepithelial to invasive cancer are not known. That the vagina is involved in a field change which results from exposure to a carcinogen common to both the cervix and vagina is suggested by the frequent association of cancer of the vagina with a previous history of in situ or invasive cancer of the cervix.[5,30] A possible viral etiology in the genesis of epidermoid carcinoma of the vagina is suggested by the presence of circulating antibodies to herpes simplex type 2 virus in some women with this disease.

During the 1940s many physicians prescribed synthetic, nonsteroidal estrogens to pregnant women with a history of prior abortion, diabetes, or toxemia in an attempt to increase fetal salvage. In 1972, an association between maternal nonsteroidal estrogen therapy and the subsequent occurrence of clear cell adenocarcinoma of the vagina in females exposed to this drug in utero was reported.[31] In all cases of malignancy for which precise information is available the drug was initiated before the eighteenth week of gestation. As little as 1.5 mg of diethylstilbestrol (DES) administered daily throughout pregnancy has been associated with subsequent cancer in the female offspring.

The number of pregnant women treated with DES or chemically related compounds has been estimated at over 2 million, but only about 200 cases of adenocarcinoma of the vagina have been reported in the female offspring of these women. The risk of adenocarcinoma under 30 years of age appears to be minimal in view of the large exposed population and the low incidence of the disease. Because women have developed adenocarcinoma of the vagina without exposure in utero to synthetic, nonsteroidal estrogens, other factors must play a role in the etiology of these tumors.

Signs, Symptoms, and Early Detection

Carcinoma of the vagina should readily be detectable on the basis of its accessibility to direct examination and the early onset of symptoms. In spite of these features it is associated with a poor prognosis because of frequent spread to regional lymph nodes and adjacent viscera.[32] This is attributed to a rich supply of lymphatic vessels and the fact that the vaginal mucosa and surrounding areolar tissue offer no effective barrier against invasion of adjacent bladder or rectum.

The diagnosis of dysplasia or intraepithelial carcinoma of the vagina is suspected on the basis of an abnormal cytological smear and confirmed by appropriate biopsies. Symptoms usually are absent at this stage, but a vaginal discharge or irritation occasionally is present. No specific area of the vagina is at increased risk for the development of dysplasia, and as is the case with dysplasia of the vulva the disease often is multifocal. A careful colposcopic examination and the use of vital dyes such as toluidine blue and Lugol's solution assist in the localization of potentially abnormal areas. Biopsy is required to confirm the presence and severity of the dysplastic or neoplastic process; however, on occasion the area responsible for the abnormal cytological smear cannot be identified.

Patients should be advised of the continued need for annual pelvic examination and cytological smear of the vagina after a hysterectomy has been performed for any indication. In women previously treated for in situ or invasive epidermoid carcinoma of the vulva or cervix this is especially true, as an increased tendency to vaginal dysplasia and intraepithelial carcinoma has been demonstrated in these patients.

Most vaginal adenocarcinomas are associated with adenosis, the presence of benign glandular epitheium in the vagina. Adenosis is found histologically in over 97 percent of women with vaginal adenocarcinoma whether or not a history of exposure to nonsteroidal estrogens in utero is confirmed. It occurs in more than one-third of women exposed during the first 4 months of gestation but is rare in unexposed women. Other abnormalities such as vaginal bands and cervical sulci also are associated with intrauterine exposure to synthetic estrogens and suggest the presence of adenosis. Adenosis often can be suspected by the detection of columnar cells and metaplastic squamous cells on a cytological smear from the vaginal wall.[33] Although these patients usually are asymptomatic, on occasion the columnar epithelium on the surface of the vagina produces a watery discharge. No patient has yet demonstrated a transition from benign to malignant glandular epithelium while under observation for a history of in utero exposure to synthetic, nonsteroidal estrogens.

Asymptomatic females with known or suspected exposure to DES in utero should receive a thorough pelvic examination at menarche or age 14. Younger girls should be examined if they develop abnormal bleeding or discharge. If symptoms are present, investigation is imperative regardless of the age of the patient. Inspection and palpation of the entire vagina, cytological smear of the cervix and vagina, and staining of the cervical and vaginal epithelium with a vital dye should be performed. Areas which are nodular, indurated, or hemorrhagic must undergo biopsy.

Invasive epidermoid and adenocarcinoma of the vagina have distinctive features as shown in Table 40-5. Both tend to involve the proximal and middle one-third of the vagina. A location on the posterior wall is most common followed by anterior wall lesions. These areas can be obscured by the blades of a speculum, and the entire vagina must be inspected carefully and palpated in any woman with abnormal bleeding or an atypical cytological smear. The symptoms associated with invasive cancer of the vagina are similar to those seen with carcinoma of the cervix, with bleeding and/or discharge the most frequent. Bladder discomfort and frequency

TABLE 40-5 Comparison of Adenocarcinoma and Epidermoid Carcinoma of the Vagina

Criteria	Adenocarcinoma	Squamous carcinoma
Mean age at diagnosis (years)	20–40	45–65
Coexisting adenosis	++	−
In utero exposure to synthetic nonsteroidal estrogen	++	−
Prior in situ or invasive cancer of the cervix	−	+
Preceded by dysplasia and in situ carcinoma of the vagina	−	++
Prior radiation to the vagina	−	±
Cytology aids in diagnosis	+[33]	++
Frequent presenting symptoms	Bleeding, discharge	Bleeding, discharge

NOTE: −, Not associated; ±, occasionally associated; +, associated. ++, strongly associated.

of urination are more common in patients with vaginal tumors than in those with cancer of the cervix because their more distal location can irritate the base of the bladder and urethra at an earlier stage.

Staging and Prognostic Factors

The staging of invasive carcinoma of the vagina as established by the International Federation of Gynaecology and Obstetrics (FIGO) is shown in Table 40-6. This emphasizes the tendency of these tumors to progressively invade surrounding structures but ignores factors of tumor volume within a given stage and location in the vagina as it relates to lymphatic spread. The vaginal lymphatics are abundant in the mucosa and submucosa and are continuous throughout the entire organ. Despite this continuity the lymphatic drainage of cancers of the vagina generally follows a pattern based on the specific region of the vagina involved.[34] Lymphatic channels in the proximal posterior vagina pass through the rectal septum and uterosacral ligaments to terminate in the rectal nodes. Those from the proximal anterior vagina traverse the cardinal ligaments to involve the internal and external iliac nodes, while those from the distal vagina follow the vaginal artery and turn posteriorly to the inferior gluteal nodes. Anastomoses in the distal vagina with lymphatics of the vestibule also drain to regional nodes in the femoral triangle. All portions of the vagina have lateral lymphatic trunks which travel to the pelvic floor, the superior gluteal region, and occasionally to the common iliac nodes.

The stage of the primary indirectly reflects tumor volume and the risk of lymphatic metastases, both of which relate to prognosis. Unfortunately, the clinical staging of vaginal carcinoma is difficult and is less reliable than with other pelvic malignancies. Patients with tumors confined to the vaginal mucosa have a low incidence of lymph node metastases and about a 70 percent cure rate. Forty to 50 percent of those with involvement of paravaginal tissues and 10 percent of those with invasion into the bladder, urethra, or rectum, all of which are associated with an increased tendency to lymphatic spread, are cured. Investigators who use the FIGO staging system have reported a 55 percent survival in patients with stage I disease, 31 percent with stage II, and no survivors with stage III and IV cancer.[35]

Primary Treatment

An intraepithelial neoplasm of the vagina suspected on the basis of an atypical cytological smear must not be treated as such until an invasive lesion has been excluded by directed biopsy. Effective treatment of carcinoma in situ of the vagina can be accomplished by intravaginal radium or cesium, total vaginectomy, or the application of topical chemotherapeutic agents. Radiation often produces a marked decrease in vaginal function secondary to loss of vaginal caliber and elasticity. Preservation of a functional vagina after a total vaginectomy requires the use of a free split-thickness skin graft obtained from the thigh of the patient to construct a neovagina.

At the UCLA Medical Center 12 patients with intraepithelial neoplasia of the vagina have been treated with topical 5-flourouracil cream.[36] Lugol's solution applied to the vaginal mucosa permitted directed biopsies which revealed carcinoma in situ in six patients, moderate dysplasia in five, and mild dysplasia in one. Colposcopy, performed in eight patients, detected the abnormal vaginal epithelium in four. All patients were asymptomatic at the time of their abnormal cytological smear. 5-Fluorouracil cream was applied twice daily for 10 to 14 days with care to protect the normal skin of the vulva with a barrier ointment. All patients noted intense burning and soreness in the vagina. Cytological smears obtained 3 months after treatment were normal in all patients; however, three patients developed a recurrence after an initial disease-free interval of 11 to 16 months. These patients have been retreated successfully with topical 5-fluorouracil cream.

The appropriate management of patients with asymptomatic vaginal adenosis has not been defined. At present, no patient has been reported in whom vaginal adenosis progressed to cancer under direct observation. Extensive adenosis of the vaginal epithelium associated with a watery discharge can be managed with topical cream designed to acidify the vagina and promote metaplastic squamous transformation of the columnar epithelium. For most women, observation probably is sufficient.

Patients with invasive epidermoid or adenocarcinoma of the vagina require thorough investigation to define the extent of their disease. Pretreatment evaluation includes a complete blood count, urinalysis, determination of blood urea nitrogen and serum creatinine, and tests of hepatic function. Chest roentgenogram, intravenous pyelogram, and barium enema should be performed. Cystoscopy and sigmoidoscopy are important to identify extension into bladder or rectum. Lymphangiography has not been adequate to predict tumor in the pelvic or periaortic lymph nodes. In eight patients with adenocarcinoma of the vagina treated at the UCLA Medical Center, a lymphangiogram accurately reflected the status of the lymph nodes at the time of their operative removal in only three patients.[37]

Radiation therapy and radical pelvic operation both have been advocated in the primary treatment of invasive carcinoma of the vagina, and both have been reported to produce cures. A treatment plan for any patient should take into account her age, childbearing status, desire for preservation of vaginal function, and the extent of her disease. Patients with small, well-differentiated stage I lesions and no demonstrable metastases to the pelvic or periaortic lymph nodes can be managed by a primary operative approach which includes radical removal of the vagina. The placement of a split-thickness skin graft at the time of vaginectomy facilitates follow-up examination and restores the patient to a functional status with minimal delay.[38]

Patients with large, poorly differentiated primary tumors and those in whom lymph node metastases are present should be treated with a combination of external and intravaginal radiation tailored to the extent of the disease. A dose of 5000 rads to the whole pelvis through parallel opposed ports over 5 weeks is tolerated well by

TABLE 40-6 **FIGO Staging of Carcinoma of the Vagina**

Stage 0	Carcinoma in situ; intraepithelial carcinoma.
Stage I	The carcinoma is limited to the vaginal wall.
Stage II	The carcinoma has involved the subvaginal tissue but has not extended to the pelvic wall.
Stage III	The carcinoma has extended to the pelvic wall.
Stage IV	The carcinoma has extended beyond the true pelvis or has involved the mucosa of the bladder or rectum. Bullous edema as such does not permit a case to be allotted to stage IV.
Stage IVA	Spread of the growth to adjacent organs.
Stage IVB	Spread to distant organs.

most patients. An additional 1000-rad boost can be delivered by external beam to a site of known pelvic lymph node involvement. Periaortic irradiation has been given with little morbidity in doses up to 4500 rads over 4 to 5 weeks in patients with metastases to the common iliac or periaortic lymph nodes. Additional radiation can be delivered to the site of the primary tumor by an intrauterine tandem and vaginal ovoids, a mold fitted to the individual patient, or implant techniques utilizing radioactive iodine seeds. The risk of a vesicovaginal and/or rectovaginal fistula is increased with higher doses to the primary tumor.

Many patients are treated best by a combination of radiation therapy and radical pelvic operation. Using these techniques adjunctively the dose of irradiation and extent of the operation can be modified to reduce morbidity and maintain a high rate of cure.

Identification of Recurrent Disease

Most recurrences of epidermoid carcinoma of the vagina occur within 3 years of primary treatment. Occasionally the recurrence is confined to the central pelvis and permits further operative treatment; however, more often it is in the form of regional or distant disease which requires systemic therapy. Adenocarcinoma of the vagina, particularly the clear cell variety, is associated with later recurrences. These patients often present with regional and distant disease and rarely are candidates for additional local treatment.

Intensive follow-up should be maintained for at least 3 years after initial therapy. At the UCLA Medical Center patients are seen every 3 months for the first year and every 4 months for the subsequent 2 years. In addition to a general physical examination, the vagina, vulva, and inguinal regions are carefully evaluated. A cytological smear is obtained at each visit. When radiation therapy has been used, the epithelial cells can assume characteristics difficult to distinguish from those often seen with a malignancy. Care must be exercised in the interpretation of the significance of cells reported to show changes of radiation dysplasia. The presence of recurrent in situ or invasive cancer must be ruled out. Chest roentgenogram and intravenous pyelogram are obtained annually together with a complete blood count, urinalysis, and tests of hepatic and renal function. Cytoscopy or sigmoidoscopy should be performed if symptoms related to bladder or rectal function are present.

Treatment of Advanced and Recurrent Disease

Local recurrence following primary operation can be managed by irradiation tailored to the extent of the disease. A reduction in dose should be considered as previously operated tissues often are less resistant to damage by subsequent radiation. Patients who develop a central recurrence after radiation therapy occasionally can benefit from an exenterative operation. Care must be taken to ensure that all disease is amenable to removal by this extended procedure, which should not be performed with other than curative intent.

Unfortunately, many patients who develop a recurrence do so on the basis of disease beyond the scope of additional local therapy. Systemic chemotherapy in the treatment of disseminated epidermoid carcinoma of the vagina has involved the use of most available agents with few objective responses.[39] Bleomycin, a drug which has been shown effective in squamous lesions of the head and neck and cervix, has been tried in patients with epidermoid carcinoma of the vagina and has produced occasional responses. Recurrent adenocarcinoma of the vagina generally has been treated with a progestational agent and a combination of cytotoxic drugs.[40] Effective control of pulmonary metastases has been obtained in two patients with a combination of radiation therapy and dactinomycin. Tumor regression also has been observed after the administration of 5-fluorouracil, methotrexate, cyclophosphamide, vincristine, and prednisone in a patient whose tumor had been unresponsive to other combinations of chemotherapeutic agents.

Current Research and Prospects for the Future

Pretreatment operation designed to assess the extent of the primary tumor and the status of the pelvic and periaortic lymph nodes has been performed at the UCLA Medical Center by an extraperitoneal approach originally designed for the operative evaluation of patients with carcinoma of the cervix.[41] Applying this technique to patients with vaginal cancer has allowed treatment modification in accordance with the findings at operation.[42] This is especially important in young women with clear cell adenocarcinoma of the vagina in whom menstrual and reproductive function potentially can be preserved by transposition of the ovaries away from the field to be irradiated and a combination of operation and radiation therapy designed to produce cure with minimal sacrifice of normal organs.[43]

The use of topical chemotherapeutic agents in the treatment of intraepithelial carcinoma of the vagina has been encouraging. Disappearance of the lesion has been noted in most patients so treated, and the occasional recurrence has been managed successfully by retreatment.

The natural history of vaginal adenosis and the true incidence of adenocarcinoma in patients exposed to synthetic, nonsteroidal estrogens in utero require definition. The potential for metaplastic transformaton of vaginal adenosis to be associated with an increased incidence of squamous dysplasia and carcinoma in situ of the vagina requires further study. Preliminary reports suggest that this might occur as more exposed women are identified and observed for longer periods of time.

TUMORS OF THE FEMALE URETHRA

Incidence, Epidemiology, and Etiology

Precise incidence figures for tumors of the female urethra are difficult to obtain. This relates, in part, to the fact that tumors which involve the urethra and neck of bladder often are classified as bladder tumors while those which invade the vulva and vagina often are regarded as primary tumors of those sites. In addition, patients with this somewhat uncommon tumor receive care from urologic oncologists, gynecologic oncologists, and radiation therapists, and attempts to combine data from these various sources have been infrequent.

Squamous carcinoma is the usual histological type with occasional transitional cell tumors identified. Adenocarcinoma of the urethra originates from the periurethral ducts and also is uncommon.[44] These tumors frequently are confused with an ectropion, urethral caruncle, polyp, leukoplakia, or erythroplasia. This is based on a gross appearance of these lesions which is similar to carcinoma, and no data exists to establish their premalignant potential. Exposure to aniline dyes and a history of smoking have not been shown to correlate with the subsequent development of urethral carcinoma. Similarly, the obese, hypertensive, and diabetic female with a history of lues or other chronic granulomatous disease of the vulva does not appear to be at increased risk to develop carcinoma of the urethra.

Signs, Symptoms, and Early Detection

The signs and symptoms of these tumors relate to their location along the length of the urethra. Tumors of the distal urethra and meatus can ulcerate, bleed, and cause pain. Hematuria and dysuria also are associated with tumors of the middle third while proximal lesions can cause urinary retention in addition to these other symptoms. That these tumors can be confused with the benign urethral polyp and caruncle has lead, on occasion, to a treatment policy based on watchful neglect. Definitive diagnosis must be obtained by histological interpretation of biopsy material from any patient suspected of having a carcinoma of the urethra. Cytological examination of the urine occasionally can suggest the presence of a malignant process but does not obviate the need for biopsy and histological review.

Staging and Prognostic Factors

Carcinoma of the urethra is described on the basis of its location, as this is of prognostic importance. The lymphatics of the urethra pierce the urogenital diaphragm to anastomose with those which drain the anterior surface of the urinary bladder. Inferior lymphatic trunks drain to the external iliac, hypogastric, and obturator lymph nodes while superior channels terminate in the nodes of the femoral triangle or the external iliac group. Lymphatics from the distal urethra can travel anterior or posterior to the pubic symphysis and enter the pelvic lymph nodes. Those which are anterior emerge between the insertions of the rectus muscles and follow the upper medial edge of the anterior public ramus to the femoral lymph nodes. Those which travel behind the symphysis follow the dorsal vein of the clitoris to terminate in the iliac or obturator lymph nodes.[34]

Survival is related to the size as well as the location of the primary tumor: 75 percent of women with early tumors can be cured while only 10 to 15 percent with advanced lesions survive. Up to 90 percent of patients with tumors of the distal urethra have been cured while survival in those with tumors of the proximal urethra is under 30 percent at 5 years, as carcinoma in this location can spread early to pelvic lymph nodes. A reported decrease in survival with cancers at the meatus is difficult to explain and appears independent of the relative frequency of femoral lymph node metastases.

Primary Treatment

The treatment of carcinoma of the urethra is based on the extent and location of the primary tumor. Women with small tumors confined to the distal urethra can be managed by operative removal of the distal three-fourths of the urethra together with the periurethral tissues.[45,46] Continence has been preserved in patients at the UCLA Medical Center in whom up to 90 percent of the distal urethra has been removed. Routine inguinal and femoral lymphadenectomy in these patients is open to question but should be performed at the time of resection of the primary tumor in all women with palpable groin nodes.

Patients in whom the size or location of the primary tumor does not permit primary operation can be managed by a combination of brachytherapy and external radiation. Radium needles placed as a single-plane, double-plane, or volume implant are combined either with megavoltage therapy to the groins and pelvis or with a transvaginal cone. From 5000 to 8000 rads delivered by implantation is well tolerated by the urethral tissues. A painful slough is an almost constant occurrence but relates in its extent to the precision with which the dosimetry of the implant is calculated. Most women who require implantation of their tumor also should undergo bilateral inguinal and femoral lymphadenectomy. If metastatic tumor is present in the regional lymph nodes, consideration must be given to pelvic lymphadenectomy and/or external radiation therapy.

Treatment of Advanced and Recurrent Disease

The role of exenterative operations in the treatment of advanced and locally recurrent carcinoma of the urethra appears limited. These tumors often are associated with metastases to regional and distant lymph nodes, and the morbidity and mortality of the procedure appears to outweigh its potential therapeutic benefit.

Reconstruction and Rehabilitation

Preservation of urinary continence is an important feature of any treatment plan. Operative approaches to these patients which include the removal of much of the urethra can result in stress incontinence. Aggressive radiation therapy which involves high doses or large volume implants can produce a vesico- or urethrovaginal fistula. The standard approaches to the operative correction of patients with urinary stress incontinence are difficult in heavily irradiated tissues. A fistula which occurs in a radiated bladder or urethra is unlikely to heal spontaneously and often is resistant to operative correction. On occasion, a myocutaneous flap of bulbocavernosus muscle can be applied to the defect with subsequent healing. If this is not possible, patients often will request a diversion of the urinary stream. This should be undertaken with great caution and requires careful consideration of the method of diversion to be used. An indwelling suprapubic catheter, vesicostomy, continent vesicostomy, and ileal conduit all have been performed with relative success in selected patients with complications from intensive therapy of their urethral carcinoma.[47]

REFERENCES

1. Way S: Carcinoma of the vulva. *Am J Obstet Gynecol* 79:692, 1960.
2. DiSaia PJ et al: Cancer of the vulva. *Calif Med* 118:13, 1973.
3. Franklin EW, Rutledge FN: Epidemiology of epidermoid carcinoma of the vulva. *Obstet Gynecol* 39:165, 1972.
4. Green TH et al: Epidermoid carcinoma of the vulva: An analysis of 238 cases. *Am J Obstet Gynecol* 75:834, 1958.
5. Ballon SC: Colposcopy in the follow-up of women with lower genital tract or perianal carcinoma. *Can Med Assoc J* 114:339, 1976.
6. Rutledge F et al: Carcinoma of the vulva. *Am J Obstet Gynecol* 106:1117, 1970.
7. Piver MS, Xynos FP: Pelvic lymphadenectomy in women with carcinoma of the clitoris. *Obstet Gynecol* 49:592, 1977.
8. Ballon SC, Lamb EJ: Separate inguinal incisions in the treatment of carcinoma of the vulva. *Surg Gynecol Obstet* 140:81, 1975.
9. Morley GW: Infiltrative carcinoma of the vulva: Results of surgical treatment. *Am J Obstet Gynecol* 124:874, 1976.
10. Thornton WN Jr, Flanagan WC Jr: Pelvic exenteration in the treatment of advanced malignancy of the vulva. *Am J Obstet Gynecol* 117:774, 1973.
11. Weintraub I, Lagasse LD: Reversibility of vulvar atypia by DNCB-induced delayed hypersensitivity. *Obstet Gynecol* 41:195, 1973.
12. Ballon SC et al: Extraperitoneal pelvic and periaortic lymphadenectomy in patients undergoing radical vulvectomy and groin dissection. Submitted for publication.
13. Ballon SC et al: Reconstruction of the vulva using a myocutaneous graft. *Gynecol Oncol* 7:123, 1979.
14. Morrow CP, DiSaia PJ: Malignant melanoma of the female genitalia: A clinical analysis. *Obstet Gynecol Surv* 31:233, 1976.

15. Morrow CP, Rutledge FN: Melanoma of the vulva. *Obstet Gynecol* 39:745, 1972.
16. Clark WH Jr et al: The histogenesis and biologic behavior of primary human malignant melanoma of the skin. *Cancer Res* 29:705, 1969.
17. Chung AF et al: Malignant melanoma of the vulva: A report of 44 cases. *Obstet Gynecol* 45:638, 1978.
18. Luce JK: Chemotherapy of malignant melanomas. *Cancer* 30:1604, 1972.
19. Morton DL: Immunotherapy of cancer. *Cancer* 30:1647, 1972.
20. Fetherston WC, Friedrich EG Jr: The origin and significance of vulvar Paget's disease. *Obstet Gynecol* 39:735, 1972.
21. Creasman WT et al: Paget's disease of the vulva. *Gynecol Oncol* 3:133, 1975.
22. Boehm F, Morris JM: Paget's disease and apocrine gland carcinoma of the vulva. *Obstet Gynecol* 38:185, 1971.
23. Watring WG et al: Treatment of recurrent Paget's disease of the vulva with topical bleomycin. *Cancer* 41:10, 1978.
24. Breen JL et al: Basal cell carcinoma of the vulva. *Obstet Gynecol* 46:122, 1975.
25. Gallup DG et al: Epithelioid sarcoma of the vulva. *Obstet Gynecol* 48:14S, 1976.
26. DiSaia PJ et al: Sarcoma of the vulva. *Obstet Gynecol* 38:180, 1971.
27. Addison A: Adenocarcinoma of Bartholin's gland in a 14-year-old girl: Report of a case. *Am J Obstet Gynecol* 127:214, 1977.
28. Barclay DL et al: Cancer of Bartholin's gland: A review and report of 8 cases. *Obstet Gynecol* 24:329, 1964.
29. Livingston RG: *Primary Carcinoma of the Vagina*, Charles C Thomas, Springfield, Ill, pp 10, 1950.
30. Rutledge F: Cancer of the vagina. *Am J Obstet Gynecol* 97:635, 1967.
31. Herbst AL et al: Clear-cell adenocarcinoma of the genital tract in young females. *N Engl J Med* 287:1259, 1972.
32. Murad TM et al: The pathologic behavior of primary vaginal carcinoma and its relationship to cervical cancer. *Cancer* 35:787, 1975.
33. Ng ABP et al: Cellular detection of vaginal adenosis. *Obstet Gynecol* 46:323, 1975.
34. Plentl AA, Friedman EA: *Lymphatic System of the Female Genitalia,* Saunders, Philadelphia, p 51, 1971.
35. Frick HC et al: Primary carcinoma of the vagina. *Am J Obstet Gynecol* 101:695, 1968.
36. Ballon SC et al: Topical 5-fluorouracil in the treatment of intraepithelial neoplasia of the vagina. *Obstet Gynecol* 54:163, 1979.
37. Ballon SC et al: Primary adenocarcinoma of the vagina. *Surg Gynecol Obstet* 149:233, 1979.
38. Lagasse LD et al: The gynecologic oncology patient: Restoration of function and preservation of disability, in L McGowan (ed): *Gynecology Oncology,* Appleton-Century-Crofts, New York, 1978.
39. Piver MS et al: Adriamycin alone or in combination in 100 patients with carcinoma of the cervix or vagina. *Am J Obstet Gynecol* 131:311, 1978.
40. Robboy SJ et al: Clear-cell adenocarcinoma of the vagina and cervix in young females: Analysis of 37 tumors that persisted or recurred after primary therapy. *Cancer* 34:606, 1974.
41. Berman ML, et al: The operative evaluation of patients with cervical carcinoma by an extraperitoneal approach. *Obstet Gynecol* 50:658, 1977.
42. Berman ML, et al: Modification of radiation therapy following operative evaluation of patients with cervical carcinoma. *Gynecol Oncol* 6:328, 1978.
43. Nahhas WA et al: Lateral ovarian transposition: Ovarian relocation in patients with Hodgkin's disease. *Obstet Gynecol* 38:785, 1971.
44. Fagan GE, Hertig AT: Carcinoma of the female urethra. *Obstet Gynecol* 6:1, 1955.
45. Taussig FJ: Primary cancer of the vulva, vagina, and female urethra: Five-year results. *Surg Gynecol Obstet* 60:477, 1935.
46. Auer ES: Cancer of the female urethra. *Am J Obstet Gynecol* 30:318, 1935.
47. Smith ML, et al: Continent vesicostomy: Application in a patient. *Obstet Gynecol* 52:247, 1978.

SELECTED BIBLIOGRAPHY

Baker J, Diggory P: Vulva, vagina, ovaries and fallopian tube, in Halman KE (ed): *Treatment of Cancer*, Chapman and Hall, London, pp 529–549, 1982.

Buscema J et al: Carcinoma *in situ* of the vulva. *Obstet Gynecol* 55:255, 1980.

Di Saia PJ, Rich, WM: The management of cancer of the vulva and vagina, in Carter SK, Glatstein E, Livingston RB (eds): *Principles of Cancer Treatment*, McGraw-Hill, New York, pp. 519–525, 1982.

Morley GW: Cancer of the vulva: A review. *Cancer* 48:597, 1981

41
DIAGNOSIS AND TREATMENT OF GESTATIONAL TROPHOBLASTIC NEOPLASIA

Charles B. Hammond *John L. Currie*

The spectrum of diseases currently known as *gestational trophoblastic neoplasia* (GTN), including choriocarcinoma and related tumors, has attracted the sustained interest of oncologists for decades, historically because of the virulence of their malignant component, and, more recently, because of their susceptibility to intensive modern management. Utilizing aggressive treatment with chemotherapy, surgery, and irradiation, the clinician can expect overall cure rates approaching 100 percent.[1]

HISTORICAL ASPECTS

"Dropsy of the uterus," described by Hippocrates in 400 B.C., is the earliest known reference to GTN, and in A.D. 600, Aetius of Armida described "bladderlike" objects filling the uterus. The Countess of Henneberg, on Good Friday in 1276, was delivered of "365 children," undoubtedly a report of hydatidiform mole during the Renaissance.[2] William Smellie in 1700 related the terms *hydatid* and *mole*, and in 1827, Boivin recognized the grapelike swellings as cystic dilatation of chorionic villi.[2,3]

Max Sanger in 1889 described a malignant tumor derived from the decidua of pregnancy and labeled it "sarcoma uteri decidua cellulariae"; 6 years later, Felix Marchand demonstrated these tumors to be sequelae of pregnancy, abortion, or mole, and described the proliferation of the syncytium and cytotrophoblast. Marchand's concepts were confirmed by Teacher in 1903 to further negate Sanger's sarcoma theory.[2,3]

The demonstration in 1929 by Fels, Ehrhart, Reassler, and Zondek that patients with hydatidiform mole excreted high levels of human chorionic gonadotropin (HCG) heralded the modern cornerstone of diagnosis and management of GTN.[4]

In 1947, Hertz demonstrated the high folic acid requirements of fetal tissue, and Thiersch, in 1952, showed fetal death could be induced by the folic acid antagonist, methotrexate.[5] The classic report by Li, Hertz, and Spencer in 1956, documenting the use of methotrexate in the treatment of metastatic choriocarcinoma and the resulting sustained remission of disease in that patient, ushered in a new era in the treatment of GTN.[6] Subsequent reports not only confirmed these results but also demonstrated the effectiveness of actinomycin D in disease resistant to methotrexate and as an initial therapy drug, and also the efficacy of combinations of other drugs for treatment of choriocarcinoma.[7-11,12,13]

More recent advances have included the categorization of GTN into prognostic groups with subsequent improved individualization of therapy[14,15] and the utilization of appropriately vigorous chemotherapeutic regimens with adjunctive use of surgery, irradiation, arterial perfusion, and even immunotherapy.[16,17,18]

DEFINITIONS AND CATEGORIZATION

Benign hydatidiform mole is described as a pregnancy, usually lacking an intact fetus, in which the placental villi are characterized by edema, decreased vasculare, and varying degrees of trophoblastic proliferation.[19] While more than 80 percent of patients with moles spontaneously enter remission after evacuation, 15 to 20 percent will secondarily develop a malignant form of GTN. Hydatidiform mole is the antecedent pregnancy for nearly 80 percent of patients with *malignant* GTN, while the remainder follow term pregnancy, abortion, or ectopic gestation.[1] Malignant GTN comprises persistent mole, invasive mole (chorioadenoma destruens), and choriocarcinoma, with further categorization into nonmetastatic disease—disease confined to the uterus—and metastatic groups. Additionally metastatic GTN is subdivided into good-prognosis and poor-prognosis groups as will be discussed later. Table 41-1 summarizes the classification of GTN. Choriocarcinoma of primary ovarian or testicular origin will not be discussed in this chapter.

INCIDENCE AND EPIDEMIOLOGY

There is marked geographical variation in the occurrence of GTN. In parts of the Orient, the rate of hydatidiform mole has been reported as high as 1 in 125 live births[20,21] and the incidence of choriocarcinoma as high as 1 in 625 pregnancies.[22] The best estimates of the frequency of mole in the United States are 1 in 1000 to 2000 pregnancies,[23] while that of choriocarcinoma is 1 in 20,000 to 40,000 pregnancies. The reported incidence of mole in patients undergoing therapeutic abortion in one U.S. center is 1 in 600, emphasizing the need for careful examination of aborted material.[24] There is a high association between poverty and malnutrition and the development of GTN,[21] and older patients have a greater likelihood of molar pregnancies than teenagers do. Parity does not alter the occurrence rate of molar pregnancies, and does not influence the development of malignant trophoblastic disease.[19] Although Bagshawe[15,25] and others have suggested a relationship between maternal ABO blood type and the development of molar pregnancies, other studies in this country have failed to show any significant correlation.[19,26]

TABLE 41-1 Gestational Trophoblastic Neoplasia (GTN)

I. Benign GTN
  A. Hydatidiform mole
  B. ? Molar degeneration (transitional mole)
  C. ? Hydropic villi in blighted ovum
II. Malignant GTN
  A. Nonmetastatic
   1. Persistent hydatidiform mole
   2. Invasive mole (chorioadenoma destruens)
   3. Choriocarcinoma
  B. Metastatic GTN
   1. Good prognosis, low risk
    a. Initial urinary HCG titer <100,000 IU per 24-h period or serum HCG titer < 40,000 mIU/mL
    b. Duration of symptoms < 4 months
    c. No liver or brain metastasis
    d. No previous chemotherapy
   2. Poor prognosis, high risk
    a. Initial urinary HCG titer > 100,000 IU per 24-h period or serum HCG titer > 40,000 mIU/mL
    b. Duration of symptoms > 4 months
    c. Liver or brain metastasis
    d. Previous chemotherapy
    e. Disease following term pregnancy

PATHOPHYSIOLOGY

Whether in their benign or malignant forms, GTNs exhibit distinct and unique histologic, immunologic, and hormonal properties. Although the pathologic features are quite characteristic in the progression from mole to choriocarcinoma, it is the unique property of all GTNs to secrete HCG, which provides a marker to aid in diagnosis and for monitoring treatment, and has become the key to the modern therapeutic plan. The therapeutic role of immunologic properties is less well defined at this time.

Pathology

HYDATIDIFORM MOLE

The gross appearance of most moles is easily recognizable, with clusters of grapelike vesicles 0.5 to 2 cm in size connected by a thin, hemorrhagic, friable supporting tissue (Fig. 41-1). Occasionally, the vesicles may be only a few millimeters in diameter, and often microscopic analysis of grossly normal-appearing abortal tissue shows evidence of the three classic findings of edema of villous stroma, diminution of villous vasculature, and proliferation of the trophoblast. Without trophoblastic proliferation, differentiation must be made between the "transitional mole," a blighted ovum with simple hydropic change of the villus, and an occasional normal gestation with relatively large villi. Rarely, there can be a coexisting viable fetus,[27] with usually a single placenta with a portion undergoing molar degeneration or a twin gestation in which only one pregnancy is molar.

The predictive role of histologic grade as a determinant to malignant sequelae after molar pregnancy has now been superseded by accurate measurements of serial HCG titers, but many pathologists still apply the grading system originally derived by Hertig and Sheldon.[28] Although their conclusion—that more abundant, varied, and complex the trophoblast surrounding the villus, the worse the prognosis for the patient—holds true for a majority of patients, it lacks predictive specificity for the individual patient. Many moles appearing "benign" proceed to malignant sequelae, while the reciprocal is often seen. In general, increased proliferation and anaplasia of the trophoblast portend a greater likelihood of secondary malignancy, but such grading cannot be relied upon for management of the patient.[4] Therefore, any patient with evidence of molar change should be followed with serial HCG titers, and future management should be determined by the pattern of these values and the patient's clinical course.

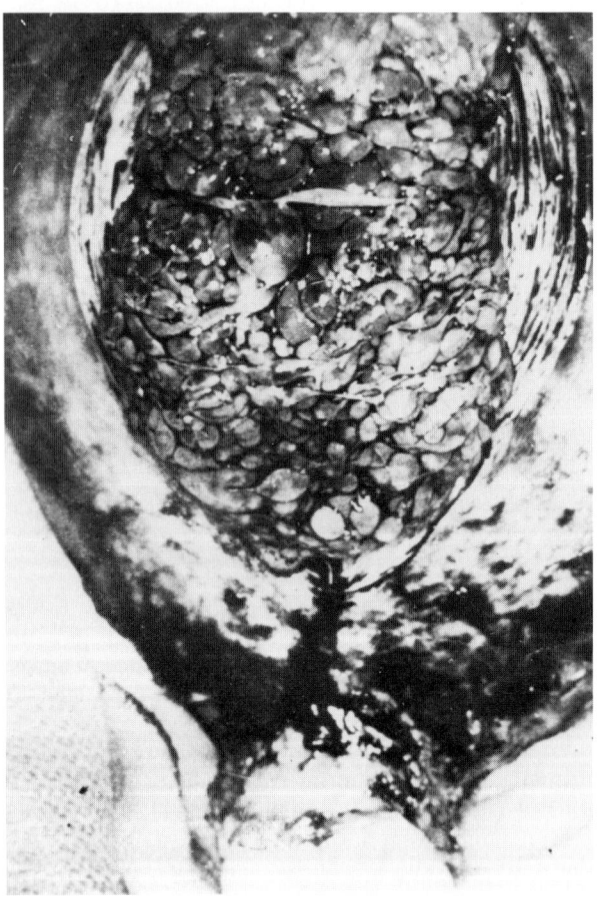

FIGURE 41-1 Hydatidiform mole: Clusters of grape-like vesicles are seen protruding from the uterus—hydatidiform mole treated by total abdominal hysterectomy.

INVASIVE MOLE (CHORIOADENOMA DESTRUENS)

By definition, the villous pattern of hydatidiform mole is maintained in invasive mole, but marked trophoblastic proliferation and invasion of the myomentrium is usually seen. Occasionally metastases are present. Because of the effectiveness chemotherapy, and because a standard curettage specimen is not likely to reveal sufficient myometrium to establish invasion, this diagnosis is made less frequently than in the past. Similarly, the presence of metastatic invasive mole is rarely confirmed because chemotherapy is preferred to surgical extirpation of metastatic lesions. Invasion of the myometrium can extend to the serosal surface of the uterus, and hemoperitoneum may be a presenting clinical feature. The site of myometrial invasion is also weakened by invasive mole, and iatrogenic perforation with hemoperitoneum or retroperitoneal hematoma can easily result from diagnostic curettage.

CHORIOCARCINOMA

A pure epithelial tumor composed of syncytiotrophoblasts and cytotrophoblastic cells, choriocarcinoma can accompany or follow any type of pregnancy.[29] Histologically, there is no persistence of the villous structure, and only sheets or foci of trophoblasts are seen (Fig. 41-2). It may be hazardous to make the diagnosis of choriocarcinoma on curettage specimens since foci of trophoblasts may be dislodged from underlying normal villi which are present and would be identified if the full uterine specimen were available.[4] Similarly, isolated sections of myometrium only millimeters removed from the villous pattern of invasive mole might be falsely interpreted as chorioepithelioma. Thus, the total processing of specimen material, such as curettage specimens following postabortal or postpartum bleeding, is necessary not only to prevent overdiagnosis, but also to help detect a tiny focus of choriocarcinoma.

The histologic similarity of the trophoblastic pattern of very early human pregnancy to that of choriocarcinoma can lead to diagnostic dilemmas. At the placental site, especially if a tangential cut is made, even normal trophoblastic invasion is worrisome, and further study may be necessary to firmly establish the diagnosis. Such differentiation can be even more difficult when there is an ectopic site of implantation in the tube, ovary, or peritoneum. Pathologically, almost all metastatic GTN is choriocarcinoma, and the histologic pattern is usually exuberant, anaplastic growth. Metastatic GTN has been reported in virtually every site in the human body.[30]

Immunology

GTNs are grafts of malignant fetal tissue on a maternal host, and as such provide an intriguing model for immunologic study and research. The therapeutic implications of such immunogenicity have yet to be established.

That pregnancy itself is a state of relative immunosuppression is well known, and certain mechanisms, as yet incompletely understood, prevent the rejection of the fetus by the maternal host. There is circumstantial evidence to suggest that patients with malignant GTN have a persistence of this relative immunosuppression, as is well established for other cancers.[15,31] Patients who show poor response to chemotherapy frequently have evidence of immune incompetence prior to therapy, and exhibit continued immune incompetence as therapy with cytotoxic agents continues.[32] Patients with choriocarcinoma who show poor response to chemotherapy have less inflammatory reactions in their histologic specimens.[33]

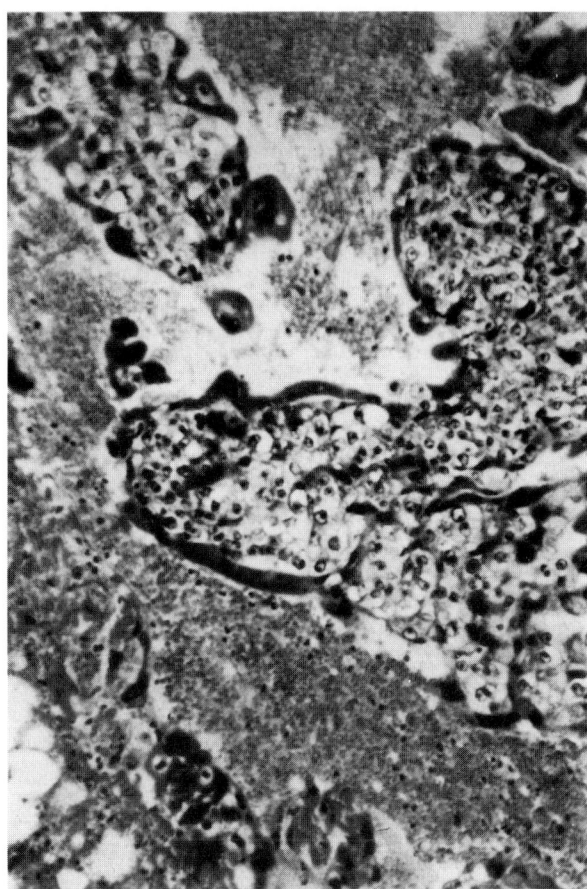

FIGURE 41-2 Choriocarcinoma: There is exuberant growth of the cytotrophoblast and severe nuclear and cellular atypia. The bizarre syncytiotrophoblasts are less numerous. There is a total absence of a villous pattern. (H&E stain; ×40).

The HLA system and trophoblastic tumors have been extensively studied by Bagshawe and others.[15,31] They found that hydatidiform moles are more likely to provoke HLA antibody formations and that patients with choriocarcinoma exhibit more histocompatibility with their offspring than would be expected. Further study is necessary, however, to draw firm conclusions.

Although early trials using immunotherapy in GTN have been disappointing, the antigenic potential of trophoblastic tumors would suggest possible utilization of these properties in diagnosis and therapy. The use of radionucleotide-labeled antigens for both therapy and localization of metastasis is currently under investigation.

Endocrinology

Other than the measurement of HCG, endocrinologic tests have been of only limited use in characterizing gestational trophoblastic disease (GTN). A variety of hormonal determinations (serum or urinary estrogens, serum progesterone or urinary pregnanediol, human placental lactogen, and serum leucine aminopeptidase, etc.) have all been studied, but have been of very limited usefulness. In patients with GTN, although such values often differ somewhat from those seen in the normal pregnant patient, the range of overlap is too great to allow reliance on them for an individual patient.[28,34]

Both normal and neoplastic human trophoblastic tissue produce a gonadotropic hormone which, to date, seems immunologically and biologically indistinguishable. This hormone, human chorionic gonadotropin (HCG), has been shown to be elaborated in essentially all patients with GTN, and the amount produced correlates with the amount of trophoblastic tissue in the patient.[12] In tissue culture, 1000 cells produce approximately 1 mIU/mL HCG per 24-h period,[35] and, thus, quantitation of the serum HCG can provide a rough estimate of tumor burden. Presumably, cells do not have to be in the actively dividing phase of the cell cycle to produce HCG, and this possibly accounts for the gradual decline often seen after evacuation of benign mole.

In normal pregnancy and with sensitive radioimmunoassay, HCG becomes detectable after the 8th to the 10th day after ovulation and rises quite rapidly thereafter, peaking around the 80th day. After a modest decline in the next 7 to 8 weeks, the HCG level plateaus until delivery. A variety of nonneoplastic conditions have been associated with alterations of HCG concentrations or excretion in pregnancy. Such changes associated with increased levels of HCG have included multiple gestation, toxemia, renal disease, and a variety of rare metabolic diseases. Lower levels of HCG have been noted in patients with threatened or inevitable abortion or ectopic pregnancy.[3] Unfortunately, the range of overlap between these groups precludes a single sample from having a high level of correlation for individual patients.

Levels of HCG decline quite rapidly after the termination of normal pregnancy, reaching nondetectable levels (sensitive radioimmunoassay or biologic assay) by 10 to 20 days after term delivery in the normal patient.

Patients with unevacuated hydatidiform mole (or coincident normal pregnancy and GTN) tend to have higher levels of HCG than do women with normal pregnancies, and the secondary decline which usually occurs after 80 days is not observed. In this latter group, a slow but consistent increase of HCG continues until the pregnancy is terminated. Although there is no definite abnormal level for patients with GTN, a value in excess of 100,000 mIU/mL or the failure to note the secondary decline of HCG after 80 days suggests that a primary hydatidiform mole may be present. In general, HCG levels fall more slowly after molar pregnancy than after normal gestation, and there is some variability in the rate of HCG decline depending upon the assay used (radioimmunoassay being the slowest). A plateau or rise of HCG seen in the patient after evacuation of molar pregnancy strongly suggests the development of malignant GTN, and prompt diagnostic and therapeutic intervention should be initiated.

With the development of a highly specific radioimmunoassay for the β subunit of HCG,[36] thus markedly reducing crossover with pituitary luteinizing hormone (LH), accurate assessment of residual disease is possible. Such assays are readily available at regional trophoblastic disease centers, as well as many medical centers and commercial laboratories. The latter facilities should be used with caution since standardization may be a problem. It is important that the clinician have adequate knowledge of the particular type of assay being used, including its level of sensitivity and its accuracy.

HCG is elevated in all patients with malignant GTN, and its level closely mirrors the success or failure of treatment. HCG will remain elevated (using radioimmunoassay for the β subunit) even after clinically apparent tumor has disappeared, and its presence mandates continued therapy.

HYDATIDIFORM MOLE

Diagnosis

The most common symptom of primary hydatidiform mole is bleeding, and although this is a common symptom in complicated nonmolar gestation, molar pregnancy should be included in the differential diagnosis. Other common presenting symptoms are failure of the mother to feel movement or a sudden increase in the size of the uterus. Further progressive size discrepancy, failure to detect fetal heart tones in a uterus of midtrimester size, hyperemesis, symptoms of toxemia, or history of passage of grapelike vesicles suggests the diagnosis of hydatidiform mole.

Physical examination would confirm a size-date discrepancy, and fetal heart tones would not be audible. On pelvic examination, frequently vesicles can be seen protruding from the cervical os. Additionally, the presence of ovarian enlargement suggesting theca lutein cysts may further lead to the suspicion of hydatidiform mole; in one series of 325 patients, significant enlargement of the ovaries (8 cm or greater in diameter) occurred in 1 of 6 patients with in situ molar pregnancy.[19]

Sophisticated ultrasound equipment has provided the most reliable noninvasive method of in utero diagnosis of hydatidiform mole.[28] Because of the safety of this technique, it is an ideal method for distinguishing normal pregnancy from hydatidiform mole and missed or pending abortions (Fig. 41-3). The newer gray scale and real-time ultrasound units provide higher soft tissue resolution, and diagnostic errors, especially in early pregnancy, are unusual. The oval shape of the gravid uterus at the apex of the vagina affords excellent anatomic orientation, and the distended urinary bladder adjacent to the uterus shows optimal scanning through an acoustically homogeneous anterior window and displaces loops of bowel which block the penetration of sound. A normal gestational sac is sonographically identifiable at roughly the same time that the typical urinary pregnancy test turns

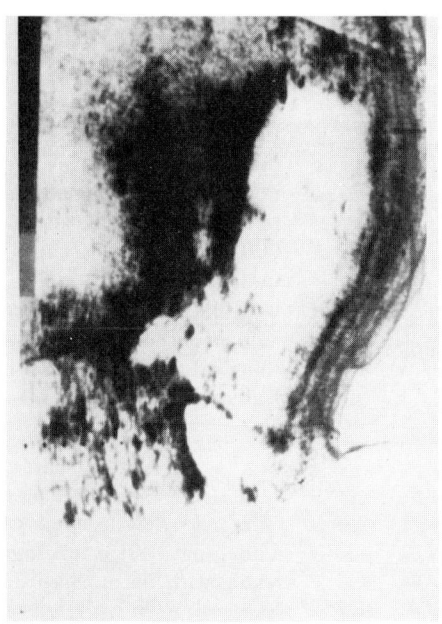 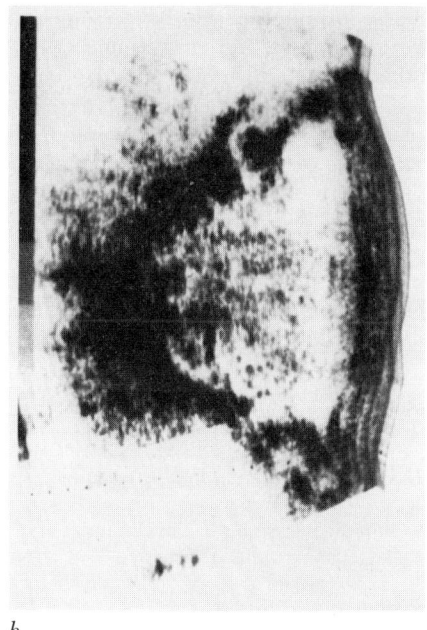

a *b*

FIGURE 41-3 (*a*) Longitudinal and (*b*) transverse ultrasonography of hydatidiform mole: In the longitudinal scan, the distended urinary bladder can be seen in the lower pelvis adjacent to the uterus with classic nonspecificity characterizing the acoustic appearance of a hydatidiform mole. Cephalad to the uterus is a large cystic structure representing large theca lutein cysts. In the transverse scan, the central pattern of hydatidiform mole is distinct; on either side of the uterus are cystic theca lutein ovarian cysts.

positive; and at approximately 8 weeks' gestation, identification of fetal echoes within the sac is routine. By 10 weeks, fetal heart motion can be observed. Occasionally, serial scanning at approximately 2-week intervals is required to distinguish normal pregnancy from hydatidiform mole or missed abortion. The acoustic pattern of hydatidiform mole is relatively specific with echoes being reflected from the surface of hydropic villi and the attendant change in acoustic impedance (Fig. 41-3). The false-positive rate of sonography is approximately 1 percent, and the diagnostic error usually stems from not identifying the uterus separate from a complex echo pattern of the pelvis. The false-negative rate is reported to be approximately 7 percent, but this is probably higher than the current rate since these data include older bistable scanning techniques.[37] The hemorrhage which frequently occurs with hydatidiform mole may result in blood clot within the uterus as well as external bleeding. These intrauterine clots have a somewhat variable acoustic appearance and may mimic cystic areas within an otherwise typical molar pattern. The coexistence of a fetus and hydatidiform mole is rare, but can usually be readily documented by sonography.[27] The acoustic characteristics of placental molar changes are essentially the same as those of hydatidiform mole, and the volume of molar echoes may be as large or larger than a molar pregnancy. Additionally, the ultrasound technique is useful in detecting the ovarian enlargement by theca lutein cysts which occurs in approximately one-sixth to one-fourth of the patients with hydatidiform mole.

TABLE 41-2 Hydatidiform Mole

SIGNS AND SYMPTOMS
1. Uterine bleeding in first or second trimester
2. Size-date discrepancy
3. Rapidly increasing size of fundus
4. Toxemia in the first trimester
5. Hyperemesis
6. Hyperthyroidism
7. Unexplained pelvic pain
8. Rapid ovarian enlargement
9. Passage of vesicles vaginally

DIAGNOSTIC TESTS
1. Urinary HCG > 100,000 or serum β-HCG < 40,000
2. Sonographic evidence of mole
3. Amniography positive
4. Histologic study of curettage material

TABLE 41-3 Hydatidiform Mole: Preoperative Assessment

1. History and physical examination
2. Complete blood count (CBC), platelet count, clotting function studies
3. Chest x-ray, AP and lateral
4. Pelvic ultrasound
5. VDRL
6. Urinalysis
7. Thyroid panel
8. Blood type and cross-match
9. Electrocardiogram
10. 24-hour urine for HCG or serum β-subunit HCG titer
11. Multipanel blood chemistry panel (including LFTs)
12. Indicated consultations

Other useful tests in establishing the diagnosis of hydatidiform mole include amniography, which before the advent of sonography was the most accurate method of establishing this diagnosis. The failure to observe a fetal skeleton in the uterus of midtrimester size on a plane x-ray of the abdomen would also suggest hydatidiform mole, but this is not specific. As noted, urinary HCG determinations greater than 100,000 IU per 24-h period (β-subunit radioimmunoassay greater than 40,000 mIU/mL in serum) are common in hydatidiform mole,[38] but may occur in normal pregnancy, especially with the presence of multiple gestation.

The signs and symptoms and results of common diagnostic tests in hydatidiform mole are summarized in Table 41-2.

Clinical Management

Once the diagnosis of primary hydatidiform mole is made, aggressive management should give excellent results with low morbidity and mortality rates. Immediate hospitalization with full work-up is recommended with vigorous supportive treatment of superimposed medical problems such as anemia, cardiovascular disease, infection, or hyperthyroidism. The preoperative assessment and work-up is summarized in Table 41-3.

Suction curettage is clearly the preferred method of evacuation of the molar gestation when preservation of the uterus is desired. Other methods such as dilatation and sharp curettage; prostaglandin suppositories; or intraamniotic prostaglandin, intraamniotic saline, hysterotomy, or primary use of oxytocins are not recommended. In patients in whom further pregnancy is absolutely not desired, and in whom permanent sterilization is desired, primary total abdominal hysterectomy with the hydatidiform mole in situ is an acceptable choice of treatment. The adnexa can usually be spared. (See Fig. 41-1).

Evacuation of the uterus utilizing suction currettage may be done under local anesthesia, but most physicians prefer general anesthesia with a large-bore intravenous catheter and blood replacement available. Although some prefer to use laminaria tent for initial dilatation, this is usually unnecessary. A small-bore suction curette, usually 8 mm, is sufficient to evacuate the uterus of hydatidiform mole. After evacuation has begun, oxytocic agents may be administered. Blood loss may be quite rapid and severe, and blood for transfusion should be available and used promptly if indicated. Sharp curettage may be performed after the uterus has contracted following initial evacuation.

The presence of systemic signs of hydatidiform mole, such as toxemia, hyperthyroidism, hyperstimulation of the ovaries, or anemia usually resolve with vigorous supportive care after primary evacuation. The patient may be discharged from the hospital when the uterus is well contracted, bleeding is minimal, and the systemic signs have abated. This is usually permissible within 24 to 48 h.

It is *imperative* that patients evacuated of primary hydatidiform mole be followed with serial HCG titers. Serum HCG titers every 1 to 2 weeks until completely negative, followed by a confirmatory titer in 1 month, then followed by titers every 2 to 3 months for 1 year are recommended. Good contraception for 1 year is strongly recommended. Although some reports infer that use of oral contraceptives increases the likelihood of malignant GTN, this has not yet been confirmed, and oral contraceptives will usually prevent any pituitary output of LH which might be confused with HCG on less specific assays. Routine follow-up of patients following hydatidiform mole utilizing commercial pregnancy tests is unwise since the sensitivity of these tests is insufficient.

So long as HCG titers are falling after evacuation of mole, no further therapy is indicated. Previous reports of combining evacuation with prophylactic chemotherapy reported a lower incidence of GTN after molar pregnancy;[39,40,41] however, several deaths have resulted from poorly administered chemotherapy, and its routine use in hydatidiform mole is not recommended. The overall clinical management of hydatidiform mole is summarized in Table 41-4.

Occasionally recurrent or persistent uterine bleeding or other symptoms of hydatidiform mole may herald malignant GTN, and repeat curettage may be necessary to control bleeding. Either recurrence of symptoms or plateauing or elevation of HCG levels after evacuation of a mole demands immediate staging and diagnosis of malignant trophoblastic disease.

MALIGNANT GTN

Diagnosis

Rising or plateauing HCG titers during follow-up after the evacuation of hydatidiform mole are the basis for establishing the diagnosis of malignant trophoblastic disease in a significant percentage of patients. When there is no history of molar pregnancy, the presence of abnormal uterine bleeding in a woman of childbearing age, especially if this is temporally related to pregnancy, should arouse suspicion of malignant GTN. Indeed, hematemesis, hemoptysis, or melena in young women should prompt HCG determination in the diagnostic work-up for such bleeding.[42] Malignant trophoblastic disease has been reported up to 17 years after the last known or possible antecedent pregnancy.[15,22] Measurement of HCG should be performed in any woman with a suspicious mass or x-ray evidence suggesting a neoplasm.

TABLE 41-4 Hydatidiform Mole: Overall Clinical Management and Follow-Up

1. Thorough preoperative evaluation (see Table 41-3)
2. Suction curettage *or* therapeutic hysterectomy
3. Postoperative physical exam and chest x-ray
4. Follow-up HCG titers
   a. Serum HCG titers every 1 to 2 weeks until negative
   b. Confirmatory titer 1 month following first negative
   c. Then titer every 2 to 3 months for 1 year
5. Good contraception for 1 year
6. Pregnancy permissible after negative titers for 1 year
7. Plateauing HGC titer or elevation of HCG titer demands staging and work-up for malignant GTN.

The diagnosis of malignant GTN is also made on diagnostic curettage, but this is often unnecessary, and perhaps even dangerous, if the preceding pregnancy was a molar pregnancy. On physical examination, the uterus is often enlarged and soft, and iatrogenic perforation may easily occur.

Chest x-ray, posteroanterior (PA) and lateral, is the single most important radiological screening test because of the high frequency of metastatic GTN in the lung.[42] Frequent chest x-rays should be obtained during therapy for a patient with nonmetastatic GTN because of the rapidity with which such metastatic foci can appear. Chest tomography is indicated if (1) routine film is inconclusive, (2) high index for suspicion of pulmonary disease needs confirmation, (3) granulomas or infectious disease cloud interpretation, or (4) a persistently elevated HCG titer is present with no clinical evidence of disease in a patient with previous pulmonary metastases.[28] Intravenous pyelography is useful for locating metastases in renal parenchyma; retroperitoneal metastases or parametrial and pelvic sidewall disease may show ureteral deviation or obstruction of ureteral flow. Radionucleotide scanning of the liver and spleen can detect mass lesions and should be part of the initial evaluation of patients with metastatic GTN. Computerized axial tomography (CAT) is of value in search of metastatic trophoblastic disease, particularly in the brain where nodules as small as 6 mm have been identified using this technique. Choriocarcinoma has high-identity characteristics by CAT scanning,[43] and this alone might suggest a diagnosis of trophoblastic disease without other obvious clinical features. Brain metastasis from choriocarcinoma shows high density with a clear gradient to adjacent normal brain tissue, features shared only by metastatic melanoma, colonic carcinoma, and osteogenic sarcoma. This is often further highlighted by surrounding edema.

Patients with normal CAT scans of the brain who exhibit neurological symptoms can further be evaluated with electroencephalogram and examination of the cerebrospinal fluid (CSF). Patients without brain metastasis have a plasma-CSF ratio of HCG titers of greater than 60:1, whereas those with cerebral metastasis are likely to have lower plasma-CSF HCG ratios.[44,45] The use of CSF examination may likewise be helpful when searching for clinically inapparent metastasis.

Arteriography may be helpful in selected individuals to document both pelvic and extrapelvic recurrence of trophoblastic disease. Higher degrees of accuracy may be obtained in identifying uterine persistence utilizing transfemoral pelvic arteriography.[17] The findings of prominent uterine arteries, arteriovenous shunts, hypervascularity of the uterus due to involvement of endometrial vessels, and tumor blush all are important findings. Selective arteriography of other organs, e.g., kidney and lung, may also be of benefit when clinically indicated for identification of isolated metastatic nodules. However, arteriography may be misleading since some patients may demonstrate the apparent changes of trophoblastic malignancy when only "ghost" tumor exists. Such changes may persist years after all active disease has been eradicated.

Although the above-noted sophisticated tests are important in localizing small metastatic foci, a careful physical examination is likewise essential. Careful palpation and inspection of the vagina may detect early metastatic GTN. Fastidious examination of all mucous membranes, skin, fundi, and extremities will occasionally locate a rare focus of metastatic disease.[46] Careful neurologic examination is also essential because of frequency of cerebral metastases.[44] Additionally, complete blood count with clotting parameters, liver function studies, and thyroid testing are all essential for the assessment of the patient and her disease. The overall staging studies for malignant GTN are summarized in Table 41-5.

Clinical Management
NONMETASTATIC GTN

Once the diagnosis of malignant trophoblastic disease has been tendered, hospitalization and complete staging is mandatory, with evaluation of all possible sites of metastases and complete medical consultation and workup as indicated. When staging studies reveal no evidence of metastases outside the uterus, the patient is classified as having nonmetastatic GTN.

Nonmetastatic GTN can be treated either with single-agent chemotherapy, with or without hysterectomy, depending upon the age, parity, and further pregnancy desires of the patient.[3,12] A recent report indicates that early use of hysterectomy will shorten the total number of courses of chemotherapy as well as the total number of hospital days, and this therapeutic option should be considered in patients whose childbearing years are over.[1,47] It is recommended, when hysterectomy is performed, that single-agent therapy with actinomycin D, 10 to 12 μg/kg intravenously, be administered daily for 5 days with the surgery planned for the second or third

TABLE 41-5 Malignant GTN

STAGING STUDIES

1. Thorough history and physical examination
2. Blood studies
   a. CBC, differential, platelet count
   b. APTT, prothrombin time
   c. VDRL
   d. Serum electrolytes, blood urea nitrogen (BUN), glucose, creatinine, bilirubin, transaminases, LDH, proteins, uric acid, cholesterol, alkaline phosphatase, Ca^{2+}, PO_4
   e. Blood type and Rh
   f. HLA typing (optional)
   g. Thyroid panel
3. Urinalysis and urine culture
4. Papanicolaou smear
5. Chest x-ray, AP and lateral; chest tomography, if indicated (see text)
6. Pelvic sonogram
7. Intravenous pyelogram
8. Liver scan (radionucleotide or CAT)
9. Brain CAT scan (or radionucleotide if CAT unavailable)
10. 24-h urine for HCG or serum HCG level
11. Electrocardiogram
12. Indicated medical consultations

OPTIONAL STAGING STUDIES

1. EEG
2. Selective arteriography
3. Lumbar puncture and CSF HCG level

---

day. No problems with wound healing or infections have been noted in two large series utilizing this technique.[1,47] Chemotherapy must be continued in usual fashion in the postoperative interval while HCG monitoring continues. Hysterectomy alone, even under "covering" chemotherapy, will rarely result in cure of the patient.

If further childbearing is desired, or if age and parity are such as to make hysterectomy undesirable, single-agent chemotherapy is the treatment of choice. Currently, three regimens are available for use which have received widespread acceptance. These are summarized in Table 41-6. Single-agent treatment with methotrexate, utilizing relatively high dosages, and with folinic acid rescue[48] has become the treatment of choice in patients with nonmetastatic disease in many centers. Its extremely low toxicity level is one reason for its popularity. Methotrexate, 1 mg/kg, is administered intramuscularly on days 1, 3, 5, and 7; and folinic acid, 0.1 mg/kg, is administered intramuscularly on days 2, 4, 6, and 8. Hematologic, hepatic, and renal parameters are monitored; and treatment courses are repeated at 7-day intervals.

Methotrexate, 0.2 to 0.5 mg/kg alone, may be administered as a single dose, intramuscularly, on days 1, 2, 3, 4, and 5 and is an equally acceptable chemotherapeutic regimen with repeat courses every 7 to 10 days depending upon recovery of hematologic and hepatic enzymes. Actinomcyin D, 10 to 13 $\mu g/kg$ intravenously for 5 days, with repeat courses at 7- to 10-day intervals, is also acceptable treatment for nonmetastatic trophoblastic disease.

Whichever regimen is chosen, treatment should continue until HCG titer, measured by sensitive β-subunit assay, reaches negative levels. Treatment with one course beyond the first negative titer is recommended. A patient is not considered in remission until she has had three consecutive negative weekly HCG titers.

Throughout treatment, weekly HCG determinations are performed to monitor treatment effectiveness. In addition, during therapy, daily measurements of hematopoietic factors as well as hepatic enzymes should be done. Chest x-ray and repeat pelvic examination should be performed every 2 weeks. Once a negative titer is achieved, a single treatment "for the road" is given, and HCG levels are measured every 2 weeks for 3 months, every month for 3 months, every 2 months for 6 months, and then every 6 months for life. Good contraception is mandatory for at least 1 year after treatment; and pregnancy, if desired, may be attempted at that point.

METASTATIC GTN

If initial staging studies of malignant GTN reveal metastatic disease, patients are further subcategorized into good-prognosis metastatic disease and poor-prognosis metastatic disease. If the initial HCG titer is greater than 100,000 IU per 24-h period in urine (or greater than 40,000 mIU/mL in serum), if brain or liver metastases are present, if the duration of symptoms of disease has been greater than 4 months, if significant chemotherapy has been administered previously, or if the disease follows a term pregnancy,[49] the patient is categorized as having poor-prognosis metastatic GTN and probably should be referred to a trophoblastic disease center for more intensive treatment. With vigorous management, patients with low-risk metastatic disease should be curable virtually 100 percent of the time, but intensive combinations of chemotherapeutic agents, radiotherapy, and surgery may be necessary to provide even a 75 percent cure rate in patients with poor-prognosis GTN.

Good-Prognosis Metastatic GTN Most patients with low-risk metastatic GTN can be treated with single-agent therapy, either methotrexate or actinomycin D in regimens similar to nonmetastatic disease. Careful monitoring of HCG titers should be performed; and if levels plateau or rise, treatment should be changed to multi-agent regimens (see below). After a negative titer is obtained, at least one treatment course "for the road" is recommended with follow-up of HCG titers as for nonmetastatic disease. Even with the presence of metastatic disease, it appears that aggressive surgical management of uterine disease may shorten both the number of courses of chemotherapy as well as the days of hospitalization;[1] therefore, the parity and further childbearing desires of the patient should be carefully considered prior to initiation of therapy.

Poor-Prognosis Metastatic GTN Once staging studies have revealed metastatic disease and any one or more of the five criteria of prognosis noted above is present, hospitalization and vigorous treatment, preferably in a trophoblastic disease center, is mandatory for best results in patients with poor-prognosis GTN.[16]

Combination chemotherapy must be used primarily in these patients, since failure to begin intensive treatment portends poor results. Although the triple-therapy combination of methotrexate, actinomycin D, and chlorambucil has been the standard in such patients for many years, recent use of a modified multiagent regimen of Bagshawe has resulted in sustained remission of poor-prognosis patients with reduced toxicity.[18] These regimens are summarized in Tables 41-6 and 41-7. Additionally, selected patients may be treated with vinblastine and actinomycin D, utilizing vinblastine 2 to 3 mg b.i.d. for 3 days, and actinomycin D 0.5 mg IV for 5 days, with repeated courses every 2 to 3 weeks depending upon toxicity. The use of vinblastine, *cis*-platinum, and bleomycin in combinations similar to those used with testicular tumors has been tried with early success, but long-term data are lacking.[16]

TABLE 41-6 Nonmetastatic GTN

TREATMENT REGIMEN OPTIONS

1. Methotrexate 15 to 25 mg IM daily for 5 days
   Monitor toxicity daily
   Repeat on seventh to ninth nontreatment day if toxicity permits

   OR

2. Actinomycin D 10 to 13 μg/kg IV daily for 5 days
   Monitor toxicity daily
   Repeat on seventh to ninth nontreatment day if toxicity permits

   OR

3. Methotrexate 1 mg/kg IM on day 1, 3, 5, 7 at 7 p.m.
   Folinic acid 0.1 mg/kg IM on day 2, 4, 6, 8 at 7 p.m.
   Monitor toxicity daily
   Repeat on nontreatment day 6 or 7 depending on toxicity
   Folinic acid should be available on ward prior to giving previous methotrexate dose

4. Treatment limitations
   No regimen to be started until:
   WBC > 3000
   Segs > 1500
   Platelets > 100,000
   SGPT—WNL
   BUN—WNL

5. All patients followed with weekly HCG determinations

6. Continue treatment until three consecutive negative HCG titers

Patients with brain and liver metastases present special problems and whole-organ irradiation should be considered simultaneously with institution of multiagent chemotherapy to reduce the likelihood of hemorrhage, possibly to potentiate chemotherapy, and to improve chances of tumor kill.[44] The use of hepatic perfusion with methotrexate or actinomycin D or intrathecal methotrexate has met with limited success and is of dubious overall benefit.

As in the management of other malignant trophoblastic disease, weekly measurement of HCG is mandatory. Once remission is obtained, which is defined as three consecutive negative HCG titers, at least 2 to 3 courses of chemotherapy should be given to improve chances of sustained remission. HCG titers should be further monitored every 2 weeks for 3 months, every month for 3 months, every 2 months for 6 months, and every 6 months for life. Good contraception is mandatory after remission, and pregnancy may be achieved after 1 year in complete remission.

Aggressive management may include surgical extirpation of peripheral, accessible metastases, and occasionally irradiation of discrete metastases may be of benefit.[50] Even when further childbearing is desired, secondary hysterectomy may be necessary to eradicate stubborn disease. Localized arterial perfusion of isolated metastases may be of benefit in selected cases.

TABLE 41-7 High-Risk Metastatic GTN

TREATMENT REGIMEN OPTIONS

1. Standard triple therapy (MAC):
    Methotrexate 12 to 15 mg IM
    Actinomycin D 8 to 10 µg/kg IV daily for 5 days
    Chlorambucil 8 to 10 mg PO
   Monitor toxicity daily
   Repeat treatment course as soon as toxicity permits

2. Modified Bagshawe regimen
   Day 1: Hydroxyurea 500 mg PO at 6 a.m., 12 noon, 6 p.m., midnight
    Actinomycin D 0.2 mg IV

   Day 2: Vincristine 1 mg/m² IV at 7 a.m.
    Methotrexate 100 mg/m² IV push at 7 p.m.
    Methotrexate 200 mg/m² infusion over 12 h
    Actinomycin D 0.2 mg IV

   Day 3: Actinomycin D 0.2 mg IV at 7 p.m.
    Cytoxan 500 mg/m² IV
    Folinic acid 14 mg IM

   Day 4: Folinic acid 14 mg IM at 1 a.m.
    Folinic acid 14 mg IM at 7 a.m.
    Folinic acid 14 mg IM at 1 p.m.
    Folinic acid 14 mg IM at 7 p.m.
    Actinomycin D 0.5 mg IV

   Day 5: Folinic acid 14 mg IM at 1 a.m.
    Actinomycin D 0.5 mg IV at 7 p.m.

   Days 6 and 7: No treatment

   Day 8: Cytoxan 500 mg/m²
    Adriamycin 30 mg/m² IV

Repeat treatment course as soon as toxicity permits, usually in 10 to 12 days.
After profound toxicity, reduce dose of actinomycin D, Cytoxan, and Adriamycin by 25 percent.

TABLE 41-8 Common Complications of Therapy of GTN

1. Hydatidiform mole
    a. Hyperstimulation (ovarian) syndrome with or without shock, ascites, peritonitis
    b. Iatrogenic uterine perforation with hematoma or hemoperitoneum
    c. Shock lung (after molar evacuation)
    d. Disseminated intravascular coagulation

2. Malignant GTN
    a. Intracavitary bleeding from metastasis (chest, liver, brain, intraperitoneal)
    b. Arteriovenous fistula with high-output heart failure
    c. Pleurodynia
    d. Agranulocytosis
    e. Septic shock
    f. Thrombocytopenia
    g. Cerebral edema
    h. Cerebrovascular accidents
    i. Iatrogenic uterine perforation with hematoma or hemoperitoneum
    j. Intestinal obstruction
    k. Disseminated intravascular coagulation
    l. Paralysis secondary to spinal metastasis
    m. Pathological fractures (rare)
    n. Stomatitis and ulcerations
    o. Severe malnutrition
    p. Hepatitis and/or nephritis
    q. Alopecia
    r. Dermatological eruptions
    s. Photosensitivity

COMPLICATIONS OF THERAPY

The aggressive use of potent chemotherapeutic agents will necessarily lead to occasional complications, and vigorous supportive care and attention to hematopoietic parameters is essential. With multiagent regimens, agranulocytosis and severe thrombocytopenia are, unfortunately, common, and vigorous antibiotic treatment, isolation, prompt treatment of septic shock, and occasional white cell transfusions may be necessary.[16] Thrombocytopenia may be a severe problem in patients undergoing long-term chemotherapy, and platelet transfusions may be required to prevent serious hemorrhage. Additional less frequent complications of chemotherapy in treatment of trophoblastic disease are listed in Table 41-8.

Patients who undergo long-term intensive chemotherapy are severely nutritionally depleted, and total parenteral nutrition may be of benefit in maintaining weight and assisting in maintaining an optimal overall patient condition. After 2 to 3 courses of intensive chemotherapy, nutritional assessment may be performed utilizing body fat stores, total lymphocyte count, and serum protein determinations. When these indicate nutritional depletion, additional support is needed. Initially, this may be performed with nasogastrostomy tube feeding, but often total parenteral nutrition is necessary.[16]

SUMMARY

Gestational trophoblastic neoplasia, once a feared and usually fatal disease, has evolved into one of the most treatable of malignant diseases. In its benign form, hydatidiform mole, GTN can be managed with surgical therapy, but malignant forms require chemotherapy with the utilization of proper staging and diagnostic techniques, combined with appropriate chemotherapy and surgical intervention. Nearly 100 percent of patients with gestational trophoblastic neoplasms can be cured.

After an appropriate interval of remission, usually 1 year, patients cured of GTN can anticipate normal pregnancy and childbearing if desired. The risk of recurrent GTN is exceedingly small (although slightly greater than the general population), and published reports reveal little, if any, increase in fetal wastage. There has been no apparent increase in fetal anomalies secondary to intensive chemotherapy of prior GTN in the relatively small number of reported cases.

Patients with poor-prognosis GTN remain a challenging problem for the clinician, and long-term, aggressive, intensive chemotherapeutic management with surgical intervention is best performed in a trophoblastic disease center. The success of these centers in managing these patients is well documented; and the availability of such services, not only in assisting in the management of more complex problems, but also in providing sensitive HCG assays, has assisted in the improved survival rates of these patients.

REFERENCES

1. Hammond CB et al: The role of operation in the current therapy of gestational trophoblastic disease. *Am J Obstet Gynecol* 13:844, 1980.
2. Ober WB, Fass FO: The early history of choriocarcinoma. *J Hist Med* 16:49, 1961.
3. Hammond CB, Parker RT: Diagnosis and treatment of trophoblastic disease. *Obstet Gynecol* 35:132, 1970.
4. Hammond CB et al: Gestational trophoblastic disease, in L McGowan (ed): *Gynecologic Oncology*, Appleton-Century-Crofts, New York, 1978, p 287.
5. Li MC: The historical background of successful chemotherapy for advanced gestational trophoblastic tumors. *Am J Obstet Gynecol* 135:266, 1979.
6. Li MC et al: Effects of methotrexate therapy upon choriocarcinoma and chorioadenoma destruens. *Proc Soc Exp Biol Med* 93:361, 1956.
7. Hertz R et al: Five years' experience with the chemotherapy of metastatic choriocarcinoma and related trophoblastic tumors in women. *Am J Obstet Gynecol* 82:631, 1961.
8. Hammond CB et al: Primary chemotherapy for nonmetastatic gestational trophoblastic neoplasms. *Am J Obstet Gynecol* 98:71, 1967.
9. Lewis JL Jr: Chemotherapy for metastatic gestational trophoblastic neoplasms. *Clin. Obstet. Gynecol* 10:330, 1967.
10. Goldstein DP, Reid DE: Recent developments in the management of molar pregnancy. *Clin. Obstet. Gynecol* 10:313, 1967.
11. Ross GT et al: Sequential use of Methotrexate and Actinomycin D in the treatment of metastatic choriocarcinoma and related trophoblastic diseases in women. *Am J Obstet Gynecol* 93:223, 1965.
12. Bagshawe KD: Treatment of trophoblastic tumors. *Ann Acad Med GB* 5:273, 1976.
13. Webster A: Gestational trophoblastic disease—A comparative study of the results of therapy in patients with invasive mole and with choriocarcinoma. *Am J Obstet Gynecol* 109:335–340, 1971.
14. Hammond CB et al: Treatment of metastatic trophoblastic disease: Good and poor prognosis. *Am J Obstet Gynecol* 115:451, 1973.
15. Bagshawe KD: Risk and prognostic factors in trophoblastic neoplasia. *Cancer* 38:1373, 1976.
16. Surwit EA, Hammond CB: Treatment of poor prognosis metastatic trophoblastic disease, *Obstet Gynecol* 55:565, 1980.
17. Maroulis GB et al: Arteriography and infusional chemotherapy in localized trophoblastic disease. *Obstet Gynecol* 45:397, 1975.
18. Surwit EA et al: A new combination chemotherapy for resistant trophoblastic disease. *Gynecol Oncol* 8:110, 1979.
19. Curry SL et al: Hydatidiform mole, diagnosis, management and long term follow up of 347 patients. *Obstet Gynecol* 45:1, 1975.
20. Matalon M, Modan B: Epidemiological aspects of hydatidiform mole in Israel. *Am J Obstet Gynecol* 112:107, 1972.
21. Teoh ES et al: Epidemiology of hydatidiform mole in Singapore. *Am J Obstet Gynecol* 110:415, 1971.
22. Paranjothy D, Samuel I: A rare case of choriocarcinoma recurring twelve years after hysterectomy. *Am J Obstet Gynecol* 110:410, 1971.

23. Hammond CB, Suciu TU: Preferable management of gestational trophoblastic neoplasia, in Zuspan FP, Christian CD (eds): *Reid's Controversy in Ob-Gyn:* III, Saunders, Philadelphia, 1983, pp 325–333.
24. Cohen BA et al: Gestational trophoblastic disease within an elective abortion population. *Am J Obstet Gynecol* 135:452, 1979.
25. Stone J et al: Relationship of oral contraception to development of trophoblastic tumor after evacuation of hydatidiform mole. *Br J Obstet Gynecol* 83:913, 1976.
26. Yen S, MacMahon B: Epidemiologic features of trophoblastic disease. *Am J Obstet Gynecol* 101:126, 1968.
27. Jones WB, Lauersen NH: Hydatidiform mole with coexistent fetus. *Am J Obstet Gynecol* 122:267, 1975.
28. Hertig AT, Sheldon WH: Hydatidiform mole—A pathological-clinical correlation of 200 cases. *Am J Obstet Gynecol* 53:1, 1947.
29. Bagshawe KD: *Choriocarcinoma,* Williams and Wilkins, Baltimore, 1969.
30. Hammond CB et al: Diagnostic problems of choriocarcinoma and related trophoblastic neoplasms. *Obstet Gynecol* 29:224, 1967.
31. Lawler SD: HLA and trophoblastic tumors. *Br Med Bull* 34:305, 1978.
32. DiSaia PJ, Rich WM: Value of immune monitoring in gynecologic cancer patients receiving immunotherapy, *Am J Obstet Gynecol* 135:907, 1979.
33. Deligdisch L et al: Gestational trophoblastic neoplasia: Morphologic correlates of therapeutic response. *Am J Obstet Gynecol* 130:801, 1978.
34. Odell WD et al: Endocrine aspects of trophoblastic neoplasms. *Clin Obstet Gynecol* 10:290, 1967.
35. Patillo RA, Gey GO: The establishment of a cell line of human hormone-synthesizing trophoblastic cells in vitro. *Cancer Res* 28:1231, 1968.
36. Vaitukaitis JL et al: A radioimmunoassay which specifically measures human chorionic gonadotrophin in the presence of human luteinizing hormone. *Am J Obstet Gynecol* 113:751, 1972.
37. Kobayashi, M: D White, RE Brown (eds), in *Ultrasound in Medicine,* Plenum Press, New York, 1977, pp 727–738.
38. Delfs E: Quantitative chorionic gonadotropin; prognostic value in hydatidiform mole and chorionepithelioma. *Obstet Gynecol* 9:1, 1957.
39. Holland JF et al: Controlled clinical trials of Methotrexate in the treatment and prophylaxis of trophoblastic neoplasia. *Abstracts, Tenth International Cancer Congress,* Houston, May 1970, Medical Arts Publishing, Detroit, 1970.
40. Ratnam SS et al: Methotrexate for prophylaxis of choriocarcinoma. *Am J Obstet Gynecol* 111:1021–1027, 1971.
41. Goldstein DP: Prevention of gestational trophoblastic disease by use of Actinomycin D in molar pregnancies. *J Obstet Gynecol* 43:475–479, 1974.
42. Libshitz HI et al: The pulmonary metastasis of choriocarcinoma. *Obstet Gynecol* 49:412, 1977.
43. Deck MOF et al: Computed tomography in metastatic disease of the brain. *Radiology* 119:115, 1976.
44. Weed JC Jr, Hammond CB: Cerebral metastatic choriocarcinoma: Intensive therapy and prognosis. *Obstet Gynecol* 55:89, 1980.
45. Bagshawe KD, Harland S: Immunodiagnosis and monitoring of gonadotrophin-producing metastases in the central nervous system. *Cancer* 38:112, 1976.
46. Salimi R: Metastatic choriocarcinoma of the nasal mucosa. *J Surg Oncol* 9:301, 1977.
47. Lewis J et al: Surgical intervention during chemotherapy of gestational trophoblastic neoplasia. *Cancer* 19:1517, 1966.
48. Goldstein DP et al: Methotrexate with citrovorum factor rescue for gestational trophoblastic neoplasms. *Obstet Gynecol* 51:93, 1978.
49. Miller JM et al: Choriocarcinoma following term pregnancy. *Obstet Gynecol* 53:207, 1979.
50. Jones WB: Gestational trophoblastic neoplasms. *Surg Clin North Am* 58(1):167, 1978.

SELECTED BIBLIOGRAPHY

Berkowitz RS et al: Methotrexate with citrovorum factor rescue: Reduced chemotherapy toxicity in the management of gestational trophoblastic neoplasms. *Cancer* 45:423, 1980.

Berkowitz RS et al: Laparoscopy in the management of gestational trophoblastic neoplasms. *J Reprod Med* 24:261, 1980.

Federschneider JM et al: Natural history of recurrent molar pregnancy. *Int J Gynaecol Obstet* 15:207, 1980.

Goldstein DP, Berkowitz RS: Management of gestational trophoblastic neoplasms. *Curr Prob Obstet Gynecol* 3:1–42, 1980.

Jones WB: Trophoblastic tumors—prognostic factors. *Cancer* 48:602, 1981.

Martinibeau PW (ed): Gestational trophoblastic disease. *Semin in Oncol* 9:155–246, 1982.

Weed JC Jr, Hammond CB: Cerebral metastatic choriocarcinoma: Intensive therapy and prognosis. *Obstet Gynecol* 55:89, 1980.

PART EIGHT

MELANOMA, SARCOMAS, AND LYMPHOMAS

42

MALIGNANT MELANOMA

Yosef H. Pilch

Malignant melanoma, once a rare tumor, has increased in prevalence so rapidly over the past several decades that it is now more common than Hodgkin's disease or thyroid cancer, representing approximately 2 percent of all cancers by incidence. It is estimated that there will be 14,800 new cases of malignant melanoma in the United States in 1982 (based on rates from the NCI SEER program from 1973 to 1978) and 5100 deaths.[1] The overall incidence of melanoma is increasing steadily, having almost doubled in the past decade and increased almost eightfold during the past 40 years.[2] Melanoma is almost twice as prevalent in the southern United States than in the northern states, and in some regions, notably the southwest, the incidence of malignant melanoma has risen to as high as 25 cases per 100,000. It is the fifth leading cause of cancer deaths for American males in the 15 to 34 age group and is responsible for nearly two-thirds of the deaths from skin cancer. Blacks have a much lower age-adjusted annual incidence (0.8 per 100,000) than white (just under 6.0 per 100,00).[2]

Melanomas arise from melanocytes, cells which have the ability to synthesize melanin, the only pigment normally found in human beings. In human skin melanocytes are to be found in the basal layer of the epidermis near the dermal-epidermal junction. Although it can be shown both clinically and histologically that some malignant melanomas arise in association with preexisting melanocytic nevi, it is clear that some melanomas arise de novo from apparently normal intraepithelial melanocytes. There is no good evidence to support the notion that melanomas that arise from nevi are significantly different than melanomas that arise de novo.[3]

There are several lines of demographic evidence implicating exposure to sunlight as an etiologic factor in cutaneous malignant melanoma; however, the relationship of malignant melanoma to sun exposure is by no means clear-cut. Most of the evidence that melanoma may be caused, at least sometimes, by sun exposure is derived from epidemiologic studies. Parts of the world (e.g., Australia and Israel) in which light-skinned individuals are exposed to large amounts of sunlight have high incidences of melanoma.[4] In many countries (e.g., Australia, Norway, and the United States) which extend over many latitudes, the incidence of melanomas among Caucasians is highest in populations residing nearest to the equator. (The high incidence of melanoma in the southern United States has already been mentioned.) In Israel, the incidence of melanoma correlates with the duration of exposure of population subsets to the intense sun of Israel. Several authors have noted the markedly lower incidence of melanoma in non-Caucasians and in Caucasians with deeply pigmented skin.

The role of sunlight as a causative factor in malignant melanoma has been recently reviewed by Kopf et al.[5] These authors enumerate eight observations supporting an association between sun exposure and melanoma:

1. Individuals who develop malignant melanoma are more likely to be fair-skinned, with light-colored eyes and hair, and to sunburn more readily than persons who do not develop melanoma.
2. Patients with xeroderma pigmentosum have a markedly increased risk of developing malignant melanomas, including multiple melanomas.
3. Melanomas occur much less frequently on "doubly clothed" areas of the body (bathing suit area in males and females, and breasts of women).
4. More melanomas develop on the legs of women than on those of men, which are less exposed to sunlight by men's habit of dress. There was a sharp rise in melanomas on the legs of women after World War II, possibly due to the fact that sheer nylon stockings permitted more sunlight to reach the skin than did the prewar stockings, which were more opaque.
5. The geographic incidence of skin cancers, including melanoma, correlates positively with ultraviolet light intensity.
6. Ultraviolet light in combination with a topically applied carcinogen (dimethylbenzanthracene) has induced metastasizing malignant melanomas in hairless mice.
7. The location on the face of most cases of lentigo maligna and lentigo maligna melanoma strongly suggests an association with exposure to sunlight.
8. Ocular melanomas do not show the north-south incidence variation seen with cutaneous malignant melanomas.

CLINICOHISTOLOGIC TYPES OF PRIMARY CUTANEOUS MALIGNANT MELANOMAS

Most primary cutaneous malignant melanomas may be divided into four types on the basis of clinical and histopathologic features. They are (1) lentigo maligna melanoma, (2) superficial spreading melanoma, (3) nodular melanoma, and (4) acral lentiginous melanoma. Primary mucosal melanomas and ocular melanomas will be considered separately.

Lentigo Maligna Melanoma

This type of melanoma accounts for 4 to 10 percent of cutaneous melanomas and is 2 to 3 times more common in females than in males. It arises within a preinvasive lesion known as lentigo maligna or Hutchinson's melanotic freckle. These lesions occur almost exclusively in the elderly (median age of 70), and most occur on the face. However, they occasionally occur on other cutaneous surfaces exposed to considerable sun exposure. Lentigo maligna begins as a small, tan, macular lesion which gradually increases in size over many years. This protracted period of growth is called the *radial growth phase*. During this radial growth phase, margins become irregular and the color modifies so that there are areas of tan and brown and black, or even pink and white. However, the growth remains intraepidermal with an intact basal lamina. After a period of 5 to 20 years of intraepidermal growth, invasion of the papillary dermis occurs, and a *vertical growth phase* begins. This event of dermal invasion is also known as *tumor progression* and tends to evolve very slowly. Clinically, when dermal invasion occurs, the involved area becomes elevated and may become papular or nodular or, at times, even ulcerated. Once tumor progression has occurred, the lesion acquires the capacity to metastasize and is termed *lentigo maligna melanoma*.

Superficial Spreading Melanoma

This is by far the most common type of cutaneous melanoma, making up 70 to 75 percent of all cases. It occurs approximately equally in males and females and commonly occurs throughout adult life and tends to appear in persons younger than those who develop lentigo maligna melanoma. The lesions have somewhat irregular outlines and may exhibit "notched" borders. They tend to exhibit multicolored shades of brown but may contain areas of gray and black and combinations of pink, white, and blue. They are characteristically flat to slightly papular. Superficial spreading melanomas have an initial radial growth phase which is shorter than that of lentigo maligna melanomas. The radial growth phase for superficial spreading melanomas lasts from 2 to 10 years, although 3 to 5 years is most common. During this period, the lesions slowly enlarge at the periphery but remain intraepidermal and do not metastasize. Areas of regression may occur, characterized clinically by pale-gray or whitish areas and histologically by lymphocytic infiltrates, melanophages, and an absence or paucity of tumor cells.

Following the radial growth phase, tumor progression occurs, and the vertical growth phase supervenes. This occurs focally in one or more areas within the preexisting lesion. Clinically, elevated nodules develop which may be either lighter or darker than the surrounding areas and may ulcerate. Occasionally, amelanotic nodules may occur. As dermal invasion occurs, metastatic potential develops.

Nodular Melanoma

These lesions make up about 10 to 15 percent of all melanomas and occur almost twice as frequently in males as in females. They can occur in any location and appear throughout adult life. Nodular melanomas are distinguished by the absence of a radial growth phase. These tumors are in the vertical growth phase from their inception. Consequently, they have a shorter history and, when seen, are usually more deeply invasive. Because they lack a radial growth phase, nodular melanomas lack a so-called surround component. They present as raised plaques or nodules which may be dark brown or black in color, often with a grayish or bluish cast. Occasionally, they are amelanotic.

Acral Lentiginous Melanoma

Acral lentiginous melanoma has been recognized as the fourth clinicopathologic type of cutaneous malignant melanoma since the early 1970s. It accounts for approximately 5 percent of cutaneous melanomas. It occurs on the acral, or peripheral, portions of the limbs, i.e., on the volar surfaces of the hands and feet and the subungual and periungual areas of the fingers and toes and terminal phalanges. Since other types of melanomas may arise in these sites, not all acral melanomas are true acral lentiginous melanomas. In a recent series reported by Krementz et al., 67 of 180 patients with acral melanomas were found to have the specific features of acral lentiginous melanoma.[6]

Acral lentiginous melanoma is characterized by a slow radial growth phase during which the lesions may become quite large. A vertical growth phase then occurs, during which ulceration commonly takes place. These lesions tend to become unusually large and are, in most cases, thick and ulcerated. Unlike the other types of cutaneous melanomas, acral lentiginous melanoma predominates in blacks, Asians, and some dark-skinned Caucasians.

WHICH LESIONS TO BIOPSY AND HOW TO BIOPSY THEM

Since all humans, except albinos, have nevi (estimated by Pade and Davis to average 15 per individual,[7] it is not only inadvisable but logistically impossible to biopsy all pigmented cutaneous lesions. Fortunately, the vast majority of nevi never become suspicious and do not require biopsy. However, since it has been estimated that approximately two-thirds of melanomas arise in preexisting nevi,[8] it is important to recognize and biopsy all pigmented lesions which are clinically suspicious. There is no good evidence that any particular location makes nevi more likely to be harbingers of melanoma and makes routine removal of all nevi arising in such places mandatory (e.g., palms of the hands or soles of the feet).

The clinical signs suggesting melanoma in a pigmented skin lesion are, in order of importance, variegated color, irregular border, a history of increase in size and an irregular papillary, nodular, or ulcerated surface. The colors most suggestive of melanoma are various shades of red, white, and blue (a triad of colors readily remembered by most Americans). White, gray, and pink shades may represent areas of focal regression, which occur commonly in superficial spreading melanomas and occasionally in lentigo maligna melanomas. Although many melanomas contain variations in color distribution, nodular melanomas commonly display a uniform color—bluish gray, bluish red, or bluish black. It is important to remember that melanomas may be entirely or in part amelanotic. Any significant change in color suggests melanoma.

Irregular borders, often notched, are particularly common in melanomas of the superficial spreading and lentigo maligna types.

Increase in size occurs during the radial growth phase of melanomas. A sudden growth spurt in a long-standing nevus should suggest the development of a melanoma. The presence of an irregular surface or the development of nodules or ulcerations in a previously flat lesion suggests melanoma. These events commonly accompany tumor progression, i.e., the development of a vertical growth phase. Obviously, nodular melanomas commonly present as elevated lesions.

Certainly, in all the above criteria, the most important

word is *change*. Goldsmith has enumerated five types of change which suggest the possibility of melanoma[9]:

1. A change in surface area
2. A change in elevation whereby a previously flat lesion becomes raised, papular, nodular, or thickened
3. A change in color
4. A change in surface characteristics whereby a previously smooth lesion becomes scaly or ulcerated, with or without the occurrence of serous discharge or bleeding.
5. A change in sensation, e.g., the development of itching or tingling

Once the decision to biopsy has been made, several principles should be considered in planning the conduct of the biopsy procedure. Since the microstaging of a primary melanoma (see later) requires a full-thickness specimen of skin, biopsies should always consist of a full thickness of skin down to and including a bit of subcutaneous fat. "Shave" biopsies may not reach beyond the maximum depth of the lesion and may make accurate microstaging impossible. Including underlying fascia is neither necessary nor advisable. When a lesion is small, excisional biopsy is both feasible and desirable, since it provides the pathologist with the entire lesion, thereby eliminating sampling error. The biopsy should include only a small margin of normal skin, since the lesion may be benign.

However, excisional biopsy is not necessary and need not be pursued for larger lesions, provided that adequate, representative areas are samples. Either incisional biopsies or biopsies utilizing a "skin punch" are adequate. It is important that incisional or "punch" biopsies sample the margin of the lesion. If the lesion is homogeneous, a single biopsy may suffice. However, if, as often occurs, the lesion contains one or more areas of different color and/or nodular or ulcerated areas, it is advisable to sample each different area. This will maximize the likelihood of sampling the most deeply invasive area and result in specimens which will provide for the most accurate microstaging.

STAGING THE PRIMARY LESION

The first attempt to stage primary malignant melanomas by measuring the microscopic depth of invasion histologically was reported in 1965 by Mehnert and Heard.[10] They described four stages of invasion: stage 0, melanoma in situ, confined to the epidermis without any invasion of the dermis; stage 1, invasion of the papillary dermis superficial to the deepest penetration of the rete pegs; stage 2, invasion of the reticular dermis to any depth superficial to the bases of the deepest sweat glands; and stage 3, invasion of the subcutaneous fat (see Fig. 42-1). This system was later superseded by the method of Clark described below.

There are two different systems for histologic staging. Both yield invaluable information as to the vertical depth to which a melanoma has penetrated through the skin. This degree of vertical penetration correlates with the incidence of lymphogenous and hematogenous dissemination and, therefore, with prognosis. The two systems are complementary rather than mutually exclusive, and therefore both should be employed in the evaluation of each biopsy specimen.

The Method of Clark: Level of Invasion

The method of Clark[11,12] depends on using histologic landmarks in order to describe the depth of invasion in terms of five levels. This method is presented diagrammatically in Fig. 42-2. The skin is divided into four levels: the epidermis is level I, the papillary dermis is level II, the junction of the reticular and papillary dermis is level III, and the reticular dermis proper is level IV. The subcutaneous fat is level V. These morphologic landmarks are readily apparent histologically (see Fig. 42-3). Thus, according to Clark's staging system, a melanoma confined to the epidermis, without penetration through the basal lamina, is designated as level I. (These lesions are essentially in situ or preinvasive melanomas, are rare, and, like other in situ neoplasms, present no danger.) Level II designates invasion of the papillary dermis. Level III describes a lesion which has filled the papillary dermis and abuts upon the junction of the reticular and papillary dermis. Level IV indicates invasion of the reticular dermis. Level V denotes invasion of subcutaneous tissue.

The Method of Breslow: Greatest Thickness

This method of microstaging melanoma measures the greatest thickness of the tumor, and expresses this thickness in millimeters.[13,14] Maximal thickness is measured at right angles to the adjacent normal skin. An

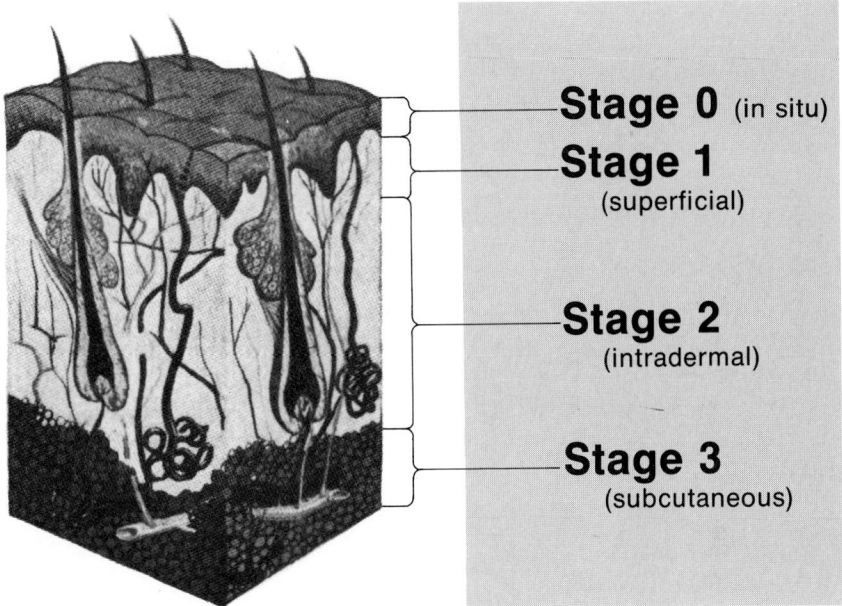

FIGURE 42-1 The microstaging system proposed by Mehnert and Heard in 1965, defining four levels of invasion based on the histologic anatomy of the skin. It was later superseded by the method of Clark. (*From JH Mehnert, JL Heard: Am J Surg 110:168, 1965.*)

ocular micrometer is usually employed, but is not essential. The upper reference point is the top of the granular cell layer of the epidermis of the overlying skin or the base of the ulcer if the lesion is ulcerated. The lower reference point is usually the deepest point of invasion (see Fig. 42-4). However, this is not always true, since the area of maximal thickness depends on the contour of the surface as well as the contour of the invading edge of the tumor mass (see Fig. 42-5). Sometimes the lower reference point is an isolated tumor cell or group of tumor cells deep to the main tumor mass (see Fig. 42-6).

CLINICAL STAGING OF THE PATIENT'S EXTENT OF DISEASE

The American Joint Committee on Cancer published a revised staging system for melanoma in 1980. It is available from The American Joint Committee, 55 East Erie Street, Chicago, Illinois 60611. It utilizes the TNM system, as usual, but bases the classification of the primary tumor (T) on the depth of invasion of the melanoma utilizing both the Clark and Breslow systems of microstaging. The TNM staging criteria are presented in Table 42-1 and the system for grouping various Ts, Ns, and Ms into stages is depicted in Table 42-2.

This staging system recognizes four clinical and histologic types of malignant melanoma: lentigo maligna melanoma, superficial spreading melanoma, nodular melanoma, and malignant melanoma, unclassified. The acral lentiginous variety of malignant melanoma is not

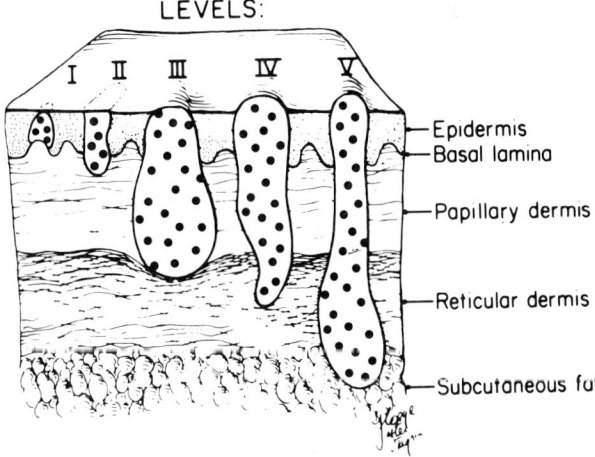

FIGURE 42-2 The microstaging system of Clark, wherein five histologic "levels," indicated by Roman numerals, are utilized to describe the depth of invasion.

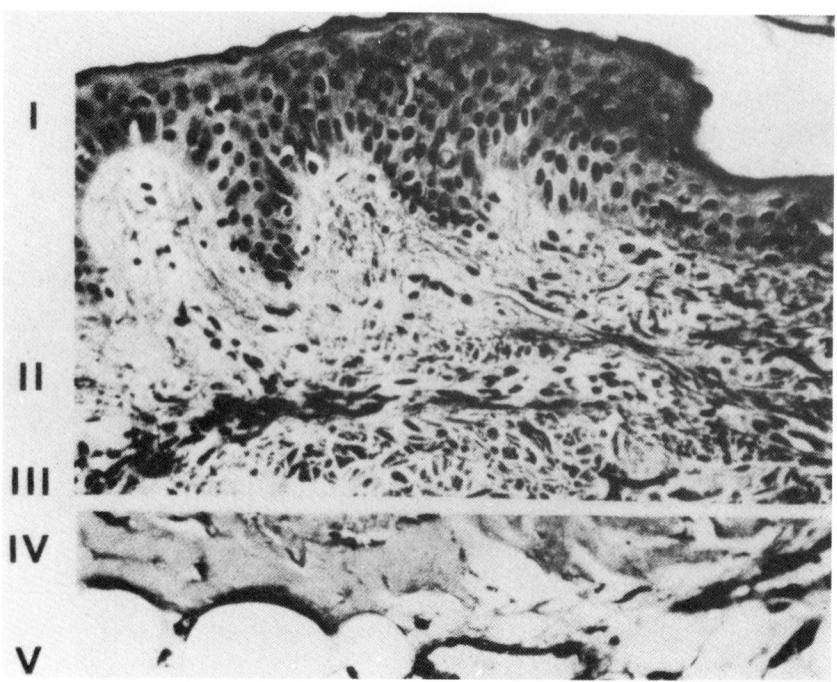

FIGURE 42-3 A composite photomicrograph demonstrating the histologic appearances of normal skin with the five histologic levels of Clark indicated by Roman numerals. The central three-quarters of the reticular dermis have been omitted. (*From A Breslow, SD Macht: Plast Reconstr Surg 61:342, 1978.*)

specifically designated as a separate type. This system replaces an earlier staging system, in use for many years, which was based entirely on the anatomic extent of disease. This earlier clinical staging system is provided in Table 42-3. Since it appears very widely in the literature, even today, it is this staging system which we will employ throughout this chapter.

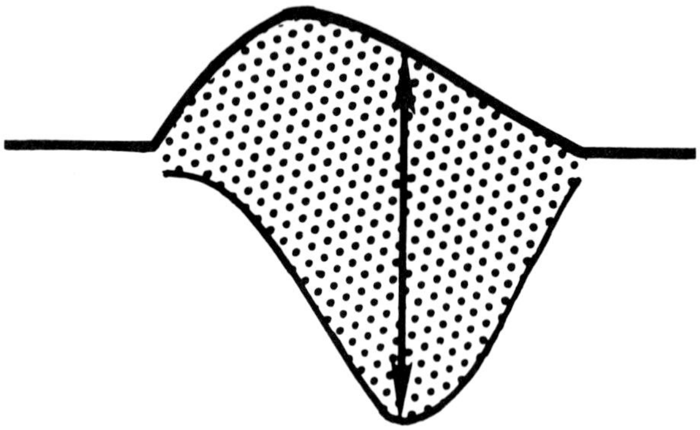

PROGNOSTIC FACTORS

Many factors have been implicated as prognostic variables which influence the clinical course of primary cutaneous malignant melanoma. Breslow[14] provides the list given in Table 42-4. While the significance of some of these factors is questionable, (e.g., amelanosis) sex, age, size, presence of ulceration, anatomic site, and level of invasion have been proved to be of prognostic value, with the last factor, level of invasion, being the single most important variable.[14] In addition, the clinical stage of disease at the time of presentation and diagnosis is, obviously, of major importance.

Sex

Females have a clear survival advantage over males from the time of initial diagnosis. This appears to be true irrespective of whether the stage at the time of diagnosis is local or regional.[15,16] The improved survival in females

FIGURE 42-4 Measurement of maximal thickness by the method of Breslow. In this illustration, the area of maximal thickness coincides with the point of deepest invasion. (*From A Breslow: Pathol Ann Part I 15:1, 1980.*)

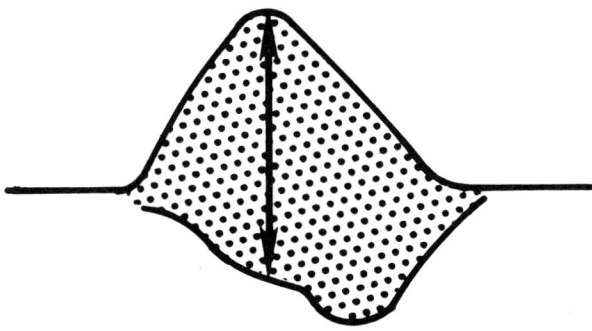

FIGURE 42-5 Measurement of maximal thickness by the method of Breslow. In this illustration, the area of maximal thickness does not coincide with the point of deepest invasion. (*From A Breslow: Pathol Ann Part I 15: 1, 1980.*)

may be related to their hormonal milieu or to earlier diagnosis due to increased cosmetic awareness. Among patients with advanced disease, females have also been reported to survive longer than males following treatment with chemotherapy, despite the fact that no real difference in response rates was observed.[17] Mastrangelo et al. have tabulated the data from seven different series involving 2450 patients (1238 males and 1202 females), and they found a 5-year survival of 42 percent for males and 58 percent for females.[18] This difference was found to be highly statistically significant ($p < .00001$).

Age

Younger patients have a significantly better survival than older patients with reference to age at the time of initial diagnosis. Mastrangelo et al. reported, on the basis of data from several reported series, that 46 percent of individuals who were under 45 years of age at the time of diagnosis survived 5 years, whereas only 35 percent of individuals over 45 years of age survived 5 years.[18] This difference was statistically significant ($p = .022$).

Anatomic Site

Melanomas of the extremities have the best prognosis.[18] There seems to be little difference in outlook between primary tumors of the arm and leg. Head and neck primaries carry an intermediate prognosis, and melanomas originating on the trunk have the worst prognosis.

Size

As is the case with most tumors, patients with smaller tumors fare better than patients with larger tumors. The diameter of primary melanomas correlates inversely with 5-year survival.[18] Diameter correlates with depth of invasion, and this factor may be as important or more important than surface size in determining prognosis.

Ulceration

Ulcerated tumors carry a significantly worse prognosis than do nonulcerated tumors.[18] Ulcerated tumors tend to be larger and more deeply invasive than do nonulcerated tumors; therefore, it is difficult to evaluate the influence of ulceration as an independent prognostic variable.

Histologic Type

It has been commonly believed that the histologic type of melanoma per se was a significant prognostic variable, with lentigo maligna melanoma having the best prognosis, superficial spreading melanoma an intermediate prognosis, and nodular melanoma the worst prognosis.[19]

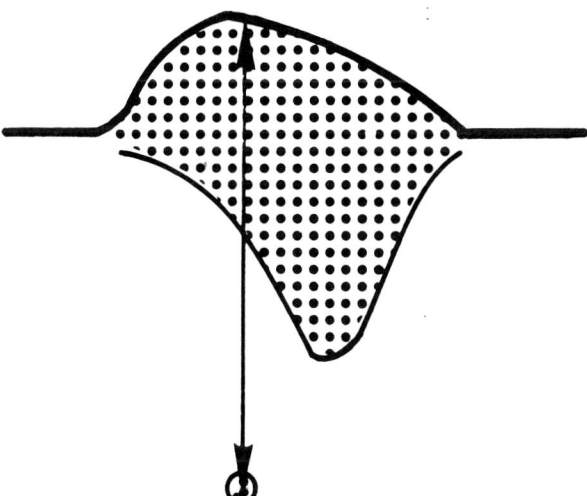

FIGURE 42-6 Measurement of maximal thickness by the method of Breslow. In this illustration, the lower reference point is a small cluster of tumor cells deep to the main tumor mass. (*From A Breslow: Pathol Ann Part I 15:1, 1980.*)

TABLE 42-1 TNM Classification For Malignant Melanoma

Primary tumor (T)

T_X — No evidence of primary tumor (unknown primary or primary tumor removed and not histologically examined).

T_0 — Atypical melanocytic hyperplasia (Clark level I); not a malignant lesion.

T_1 — Invasion of papillary dermis (level II) and/or 0.75 mm thickness or less.

T_2 — Invasion of the papillary-reticular-dermal interface (level III) and/or 0.76 to 1.5 mm thickness.

T_3 — Invasion of the reticular dermis (level IV) and/or 1.51 to 4.0 mm thickness.

T_4 — Invasion of subcutaneous tissue (level V) and/or more than 4.0 mm thickness OR satellite(s) within 2 cm of any primary melanoma.

Nodal involvement (N)

N_X — Nodes cannot be assessed.

N_0 — No regional lymph node involvement

N_1 — Involvement of only one regional lymph node station; node(s) movable and not over 5 cm in diameter OR negative regional lymph nodes and the presence of less than five in-transit metastases.

N_2 — Any one of the following:
Involvement of more than one regional lymph node station.
Regional node(s) over 5 cm in diameter or fixed.
Five or more in-transit metastases or any in-transit metastases with regional lymph node involvement.

Distant metastases (M)

M_X — Not assessed.

M_0 — No known distant metastases.

M_1 — Involvement of skin or subcutaneous tissue beyond the site of primary lymph node drainage.
Specify _____.

M_2 — Visceral metastases (spread to any distant site other than skin or subcutaneous tissues).
Specify _____.

Histopathology
Types of malignant melanoma: lentigo maligna (Hutchinson's) with adjacent intraepidermal component of radial spreading type (superficial spreading), without adjacent intraepidermal component (nodular), unclassified.

Grade
Well-differentiated, moderately well differentiated, poorly to very poorly differentiated, or number 1, 2, 3–4.

Recurrent tumor(r)
Recurrent tumor is not to be considered the same as residual tumor left after biopsy or incomplete resection. Residual tumor calls for no special recognition because it is such a common clinical circumstance. The development of local recurrence at the site of previous surgery calls for specific recognition when staging by using the prefix "r" (rTNM).

However, there is no good evidence to support a difference in prognosis among these types of melanomas *for the same levels of invasion*. The apparent differences in prognosis are probably due to differences in the frequency distribution of various depths of invasion at the time of presentation for each of these three histologic types. These differences are almost certainly due to the different durations of radial growth phase among the three types, lentigo maligna having a very long period of radial growth, superficial spreading melanoma having a much shorter radial growth phase, and nodular melanoma having no radial growth phase at all. Kopf et al.

TABLE 42-2 Stage Grouping

Stage I	T_1 or T_2, N_0, M_0
Stage IIA	T_3, N_0, M_0
IIB	T_4, N_0, M_0
Stage III	Any T, N_1, M_0
Stage IV	Any T, N_2, M_0
	Any T, any N, M_1 or M_2

have provided data from the Malignant Melanoma Clinical Cooperative Group describing the frequency of the various Clark's levels at the time of presentation for melanomas of these three histologic types.[20] These data are presented in Table 42-5.

Depth of Invasion

The depth of invasion, measured by either or both microstaging methods discussed above, correlates well with the incidence of blood vessel and lymphatic invasion, incidence of lymph node metastasis, and survival. The level of invasion is the single most important prognostic factor in primary cutaneous malignant melanoma. Table 42-6 summarizes data from four representative series relating Clark's level of invasion to survival. The series are presented in chronologic order. It is apparent that the two later series indicate a better prognosis, level for level, than do the two earlier series. This may be due to tumor sampling errors in the older studies or to an actual improvement in prognosis in patients treated more recently. Furthermore Wanebo et al.[21,22] and others have shown that the presence of histologically demonstrable metastases in clinically negative (but electively dissected) lymph nodes is related to Clark's level. Wanebo et al. found tumor present in 1 of 19 patients with level II tumors and in 2 of 46 patients with level III tumors but in 11 of 44 patients with level IV tumors and 3 of 4 patients with level V tumors.[21,22]

When the depth of invasion is measured as a function of thickness, several facts emerge. Breslow[13,14] and others[23,24] have shown that primary cutaneous melanomas less than or equal to 0.75 mm in thickness essentially never recur following excision and very rarely metastasize. These tumors are associated with a 98 percent to 100 percent 5-year survival. Melanomas 0.76 to 1.50 mm in thickness also have an excellent prognosis, although it is slightly worse than for lesions less than 0.76 mm thick, with 90 to 94 percent of patients surviving 5 years or more. Lesions greater than 1.50 mm in thickness have a poorer prognosis, and the outlook for patients with melanomas greater than 3.0 mm thick is particularly grave, with only 40 to 45 percent surviving to 5 years.

TABLE 42-4 Prognostic Variables in Cutaneous Melanoma

Clinical History	Satellitosis
Sex	Mitotic rate
Age	Level of invasion
Anatomic site	Size of tumor
Ulceration	Volume
	Diameter
Amelanosis	Thickness
Histologic type	
Inflammatory reaction	

SOURCE: Breslow.[14]

TABLE 42-3 Previous Clinical Staging System of the American Joint Committee

Stage I
Primary lesion or primary lesion with satellite(s) within 5 cm of primary lesion. No other demonstrable disease.

Stage II
Involvement by malignant melanoma of a single draining lymph node basis with or without in-transit metastases.

Stage III
Involvement by malignant melanoma of two or more lymph node groups, disseminated cutaneous disease, or visceral metastases.

TABLE 42-5 Frequency of Clark's Levels in 1117 Melanomas (In Percent)

	Lentigo maligna melanoma	*Superficial spreading melanoma*	*Nodular melanoma*
Level II	46.2	33.2	0.0
Level III	25.0	32.9	33.7
Level IV	17.3	29.6	44.0
Level V	7.7	3.6	20.6
Unknown	3.8	0.6	1.7

TABLE 42-6 Correlation of Level of Invasion of Primary Melanomas with Survival

Level of invasion	Clark et al.[11] 5-yr survival, %	McGovern[20] 5-yr survival, %	Wanegbo et al.[21] 5-yr disease-free survival, %	Sober et al.[2] 5-yr survival, %
II	72.2	82	100	93
III	46.5	65	88	74
IV	31.6	49	66	63
V	12.0	29	15	39

Recently, Day and his colleagues[25,26] have refined the "breakpoints" for tumor thickness originally proposed by Breslow. They have found that "the thickness-survival relation is best characterized as a step-function with the following four natural thickness groups: less than 0.85 mm, 0.85 to 1.69 mm, 1.70 to 3.64 mm, and greater than or equal to 3.65 mm." The 5-year overall survival rate for patients with melanomas less than 0.85 mm thick was 99 percent. For lesions 0.85 to 1.69 mm thick, survival was 94 percent, for lesions 1.70 to 3.64 mm thick, 76 percent, and for patients with melanomas greater than 3.65 mm in thickness, only 41 percent.[25,26] These authors note that tumor thickness is associated not only with the proportion of disease-related fatalities but with the rate of death as well. They also found that anatomic site was a very important prognostic variable.

For convenience, Day's group has devised the acronym BANS to identify those anatomic sites carrying a poorer prognosis. They are as follows: the upper *b*ack, the posterolateral upper *a*rm, the posterolateral *n*eck, and the posterior *s*calp. In the 0.85- to 1.70-mm thickness group, they found that patients with primary melanomas in "non-BANS" locations had a prognosis almost as favorable as patients with melanomas less than 0.85 mm thick, whereas patients with melanomas in the BANS locations had a poorer prognosis (almost 10 percent died within 5 years). For lesions between 1.70 and 3.60 mm of thickness, the prognosis for patients with melanomas of the extremities (excluding BANS sites, hands, and feet) was quite good. Patients with trunk melanomas (excluding BANS sites) had an intermediate prognosis, and patients with melanomas arising in BANS sites, hands and feet, and head and neck had a very poor prognosis. For melanomas greater than 3.60 mm thick, only patients with extremity melanomas on "non-BANS" sites had a relatively favorable prognosis. Patients with thick melanomas at all other sites had a dismal prognosis. Fitzpatrick, of Day's group, using tumor thickness and anatomic site criteria, has described six groups with different risks of fatality from melanoma.[27] These risk groups are presented in Table 42-7.

Stage of Disease

As is the case with most malignancies, the clinical stage of disease at the time of presentation and diagnosis is of major prognostic significance in malignant melanoma. Since virtually all published series employ the former staging system presented in Table 42-3 rather than the new system presented in Tables 42-1 and 42-2, the earlier staging system must be used. Localized melanoma (stage I) has a relatively good prognosis, with 5-year survival rates between 55 and 80 percent commonly reported.[18] The great variability in survival statistics is undoubtedly due to lack of comparability of various series with respect to all of the risk factors pertaining to primary melanomas that were discussed earlier. In ad-

TABLE 42-7 Risk Factors for Patients with Clinical Stage I Malignant Melanoma

Minimum risk (<2% mortality)
All melanomas less than 0.85 mm thick
Melanoma 0.85–1.69 mm thick at non-BANS* sites

Low risk (2–20% mortality)
All extremity melanomas 1.70 mm thick at non-BANS sites, excluding hands and feet

Intermediate risk (20–35% mortality)
Melanomas 0.85–1.69 mm thick at BANS sites
Trunk melanomas 1.70–3.60 mm thick at non-BANS sites

High risk (35–40% mortality)
Head and neck melanomas greater than 1.70 mm thick at non BANS sites
Melanomas of the hands and feet 1.70 mm–3.60 mm thick

Very high risk (40–67% mortality)
Melanomas 1.70–3.60 mm thick at BANS sites

Maximum risk (67–100% mortality)
Melanomas greater than 3.60 mm arising at BANS sites, on the trunk, or on the hands and feet

* BANS = upper back, posterolateral upper arm, posterolateral neck, and posterior scalp.
SOURCE: Fitzpatrick.[27]

dition, some series utilize clinical assessment of regional nodes, and others employ histologic evaluation of regional nodes (following regional lymphadenectomy).

As is true with breast cancer and several other epithelial malignancies, the prognosis of patients with stage II melanoma depends, to a certain extent, on the degree of nodal involvement, patients with a single positive node having a better prognosis than those with two or more involved nodes. Moreover, the prognosis for patients with grossly involved nodes is probably worse than for individuals with microscopically involved nodes, although there is insufficient data to permit a meaningful discussion of this point. Although approximately 30 percent of clinical stage II, pathologic stage II patients are alive at 5 years, 10-year survivors in this group of patients are few (less than 10 percent in some series[28,29]), although Goldsmith has reported a 10-year rate of over 20 percent for clinical stage II patients.[30]

The prognosis for patients with disseminated (stage III) malignant melanoma depends primarily on the anatomic distribution of the metastatic disease, since melanoma has several metastatic patterns. Many patients with stage III melanoma have only nonvisceral metastases (skin, subcutaneous tissue, and, sometimes, lymph nodes). Such patients clearly have a more favorable outlook than those with visceral metastases.[17] Even among patients with visceral metastatic disease, prognosis varies. Patients with pulmonary metastases have a better prognosis than those with extrapulmonary visceral disease (liver, brain, bone, etc.). Because of this variability, the 5-year survival statistics reported by various authors for patients with stage III melanoma range widely, between 0 percent[31] and 18 percent.[32]

Melanoma of Unknown Primary (Occult Melanoma)

At this point, it is important to discuss malignant melanomas presenting initially as metastases to lymph nodes or visceral sites with no apparent primary lesion. Such presentations, while infrequent, are by no means rare. The prevalence of occult primary melanoma has been reported to by 3.7 percent by Das Gupta et al.,[33] 4 percent by Baab and McBride,[34] 6.5 percent by Shaw and Goldsmith,[32] 8.7 percent by Smith and Stehlin,[35] and 15 percent by Einhorn et al.[17] Possible explanations for the absence of a clinically demonstrable primary tumor in such patients include the following: (1) The primary melanoma may have undergone spontaneous regression; (2) the primary may have been removed previously without having been examined histologically or may have been destroyed accidentally; (3) the primary melanoma may be present but inapparent, i.e., indistinguishable from normal-appearing pigmented nevi or located deeply in skin adnexae; (4) the primary may be visceral; or (5) the primary tumor may have originated in nevus cells occasionally found in lymph nodes.

Most authors agree that the prognosis for patients in whom a primary lesion is never found is approximately the same as that for patients with known primary lesions at the same stage of disease.[32,33,36,37] Baab and McBride noted improved 5- and 10-year survival rates for patients with unknown primaries[34] and speculated that this was due to heightened host immunity, which was expressed in the spontaneous regression of the primary tumor. However, Milton et al. have reported that their patients with occult primary melanomas had an inferior prognosis.[38]

METASTASES—LYMPHOGENOUS AND HEMATOGENOUS

In addition to the type of regional lymphogenous dissemination (i.e., to regional lymph nodes) usually associated with epithelial neoplasms, malignant melanoma metastasizes by two unique varieties of lymphogenous spread: satellite formation and the formation of in-transit metastases. Since prevention and/or treatment of satellitosis and in-transit metastases are goals which have determined approaches to the treatment of malignant melanoma, these types of metastases must be mentioned prior to any discussion of therapy.

Satellitosis refers to the occurrence of small cutaneous nodules of melanoma discontiguous with the primary lesion (or surgical scar) but in close proximity to it. It is presumed that this type of circumfugal spread is due to dissemination of melanoma cells via the dermal lymphatics. By definition (based on extremely arbitrary criteria) the term *satellitosis* refers to nodules within 5 cm of the primary site. Since the vast majority of such lesions occur within 3 cm of the primary, some investigators prefer to utilize a 3-cm cutoff point.

In addition, melanoma may disseminate via the lymphatics running between the primary site (or surgical scar) and the regional lymph nodes to form cutaneous or subcutaneous nodules along the course of these lymphatics. These nodules are termed *in-transit metastases* and are defined as "a cutaneous or subcutaneous spread of malignancy more than 5 cm (or 3 cm) beyond the primary site in the direction of, but not beyond the regional lymph nodes."[39]

No malignancy metastasizes hematogenously more widely than malignant melanoma. It can involve virtually every organ in the body, including such rare sites as the spleen, heart, urinary bladder, thyroid, pancreas, and intestine. The lungs, skin, and subcutaneous tissue and the liver are among the most common sites. Moreover, cerebral metastases are common[39,40] and are frequently the cause of death. The patterns of metastasis of malignant melanoma have been recently reviewed by Lee.[40]

TREATMENT OF CUTANEOUS MALIGNANT MELANOMA

We shall consider the treatment of cutaneous malignant melanoma in four phases: (1) treatment of the primary tumor, (2) treatment of the regional lymph nodes, (3) adjuvant therapy, and (4) treatment of metastatic disease.

Treatment of the Primary Tumor: The Extent of Local Excision

The matter of how to treat the primary tumor involves three questions: (1) How much apparently normal skin should be removed around the tumor (or biopsy scar) and how should closure be effected? (2) Should underlying muscle fascia be included in the resection routinely? (3) Should additional skin and subcutaneous tissue be excised between the primary tumor and the regional tumor and the regional lymph nodes in an attempt to encompass the extent of lymphatic drainage?

Since there is very little in the scientific literature concerning the optimal size of resection margins and there have been no prospective studies assessing this issue, it is not surprising that margins ranging from 2 to 15 cm have been suggested. Breslow noted, in 1980,[14] that "the most frequent recommendation is a 5 cm margin, and this has become almost a surgical dogma. It has been attributed to Handley . . ." He was undoubtedly correct, at least at the time he wrote those words for, in 1976, we find the following in a textbook, *Management of the Patient with Cancer:*

The basis of all therapy is the control of the primary melanoma. The principle of management graphically depicted by Handley in 1907 has not been improved upon. A minimal skin margin of 5 cm is resected, with a circumferentially wider dissection of subcutaneous tissue and fascia.[41]

Indeed, it appears likely that the seed of the "5-cm rule" was probably sown by Handley in his Hunterian Lectures of February 25 and 27, 1907.[42,43] In 1977, we read, "The basic principle of wide excision of the primary site is generally accepted as the proper management of the primary lesion.(9)"[44] (Reference number 9 refers to Handley.) Again in 1977, we read, "All patients with Clark levels II, III, IV, and V melanoma, irrespective of the clinical status of the nodes, were treated with excision of the primary tumor with a 5 cm margin on all sides, including the deep fascia."[45] As late as 1979, we again read, "The principle of "wide" surgical removal in a three-dimensional plane was advocated by Sampson-Handley in 1907 because centrifugal, dermal lymphatic permeation was frequent."[46] The author operated accordingly.

Handley's work has already been referred to in Chap. 12. It consisted of a histopathologic study of material obtained from a single necropsy (necropsy no. 186, the Middlesex Hospital, 1905) of a 34-year-old woman who died of metastatic malignant melanoma.[42] The primary tumor had been excised from the skin "at the insertion of the right tendo achillis" where "a small healthy linear scar" remained. The patient has "a considerable mass in the situation of the femoral glands" in the right groin and what were certainly numerous in-transit metastases "occupying an area roughly circular in shape and perhaps eight inches in diameter" overlying this mass. (This may be seen in Fig. 42-7 which is identical to Fig. 12-1 in Chap. 12. This figure was published as Figure 1 in Handley's original paper,[42] and the legend is Handley's original legend.) A strip of "skin, subcutaneous fat, deep fascia, and a thin layer of muscle," measuring 17 cm in length, was removed for examination and formed the basis of Handley's papers.[42,43] Its location is indicated as line *AB* on the figure. This postmortem histopathologic study dealt with the lymphatic distribution of tumor cells and surrounding *metastatic* skin lesions, and did not, in fact, deal with the lymphatic distribution of tumor cells surrounding the primary melanoma. The primary tumor had been removed previously and had not recurred, and Handley did not sample that area. There is no proven relationship between the lymphatic distribution of tumor cells surrounding metastatic deposits of tumor and those surrounding primary lesions.[14] Therefore, it would seem that the evidence in favor of a 5-cm margin is no better than that for any other margin.

Olsen, in 1966, published a study of 302 melanoma patients in which no relationship was found between the

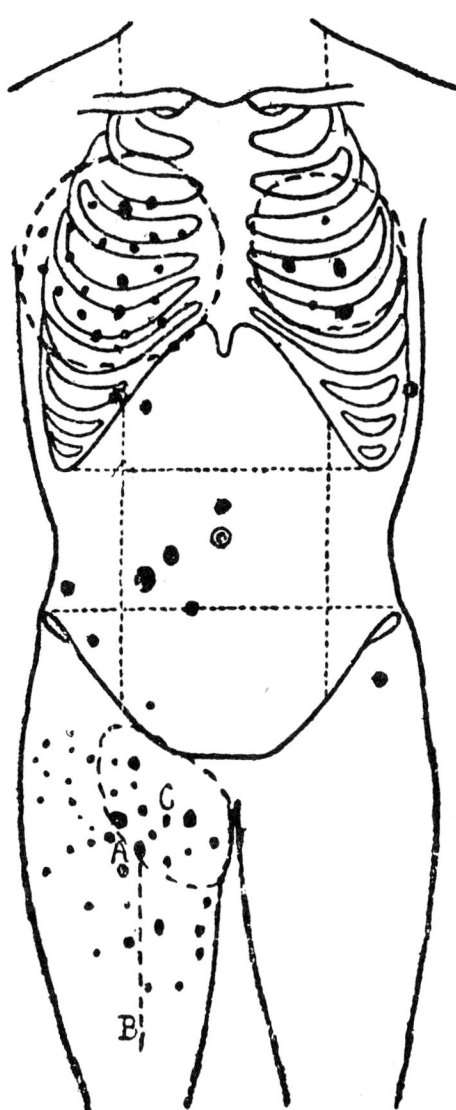

FIGURE 42-7 "Showing all the visible subcutaneous nodules of melanotic growth present in the anterior aspect of the body, except on the face. The dotted line *AB* shows the position and extent of the strip of tissue removed for examination. The dotted circles in the mammary region represent prominent masses of secondary growth in the breasts. Note that the growth was on the right heel and that most of the secondary nodules are situated on the right side of the body." (*From WS Handley: Lancet 1:927, 1907.*)

incidence of local recurrence and the size of resection margins for resection margins ranging from less than 1 cm to greater than 5 cm.[47] Recently, Bagley et al. have reported that among patients with "inadequate resection margins" (adequate margins were defined as being equal to twice the diameter of the primary lesion) local recurrence was slightly higher than in those with "adequate" margins (8 vs. 4 percent).[48] However, this difference was not statistically significant. There were also no significant differences in the incidences of in-transit metastases (4 vs. 6 percent), regional node metastases (6 vs. 11 percent), and systemic metastases (8 vs. 9 percent). In the "inadequate" margins group 5-year survival was slightly *higher* than in the "adequate" margin group (82 vs. 78 percent); but this difference was not significant. Four of six locally recurrent melanomas had margins of 1 cm or less. However, "*no improvement could be demonstrated in survival by increasing the margin of resected free tissue above this minimal figure.*" These authors conclude that "resection of a margin of clinically uninvolved skin measuring twice the diameter of the primary melanoma minimizes local recurrence (2.5 percent or less), does not adversely affect survival, and reduces the need for skin grafting. *Arbitrary wide margins are not justified.*"

It is becoming increasingly clear that the incidence of local recurrence correlates more with the depth of invasion of the primary melanoma than with the extent of surgical excision.[24,48] In the report of Bagley et al.,[48] no significant difference in local recurrence rates was noted in patients with thin melanomas treated with narrow or wide surgical margins. However, in patients with melanomas of moderate or high thickness, a 13 percent incidence of local recurrence was observed in patients treated with narrow margins as opposed to 2.5 percent in patients whose melanomas were more widely excised. It is important to note that although local recurrence was more frequent with narrow margins, this did not appear to significantly affect the clinical course of the disease, since there were no differences between the two groups with respect to the incidence of in-transit metastases (13 vs. 7 percent), regional node metastases (10 vs. 10 percent), or systemic metastases (13 vs. 13 percent), and there was no difference in 5-year survival (79 vs. 76 percent). They concluded that "width of margin does not correlate with survival in any risk (i.e., tumor thickness) group".[48]

Cascinelli et al. on behalf of the WHO melanoma study group reviewed 593 patients with stage II melanoma collected by the WHO Collaborating Centres for

Evaluation of Methods of Diagnosis and Treatment of Melanoma.[49] They reported that although the chances of cure of these patients were reduced with increasing thickness of the primary melanoma ($p < .001$), "survival was not influenced by the size of resection margins ($p = .66$)."

Therefore, it seems appropriate to excise melanomas with surgical margins which vary with the depth of invasion of the primary tumor. A conservative position appears to be supported by the data suggesting that even if local recurrence develops following more limited excision, ultimate clinical course will not be affcted. In the absence of data from prospectively randomized clinical trials (although two are now in progress), one can only discuss the recommendations of individual workers in the field. All agree that narrower margins are appropriate for thinner melanomas. Breslow and Macht, noting no recurrences among 62 melanomas less than 0.76 mm thick despite resection margins which ranged from 0.10 to 5.50 cm with 32 percent being 1.0 cm or less, urge that such melanomas "be treated conservatively, the size of the resection margin being dependent upon the anatomic location of the tumor."[50] They do not recommend a specific excision dimension, but note that "in most instances, skin grafting should not be necessary." Day et al. recommend a 1.5-cm resection margin for all melanomas less than 0.85 mm thick and for melanomas 0.85 to 1.69 mm in thickness which are not located on the upper back, posterolateral arm, posterior and lateral neck, and posterior scalp.[51] For all other melanomas, they recommend an excision margin of 3.0 cm. These authors state that "the 3-cm border probably adds no further beneficial effect on survival when compared with a narrower margin, (but) it is almost certainly as good for local control as a 5-cm border, and it represents a reasonable compromise with contemporary ethics until a proper trial can be done." Bagley et al. advise that "a margin of normal tissue of at least two times the diameter of the melanoma" be used in order to "minimize local recurrence," although they note that "narrower margins may be used in low-risk (i.e., thin) melanomas."[48] Balch recommends that a 1-cm excision margin be employed for "in situ" melanomas (i.e., Clark's level I), a 2-cm excision margin for invasive melanomas less than 0.76 mm in thickness, and a 3- to 4-cm margin for all thicker melanomas.[24,52]

Bagley et al. and several others have shown that the manner of closure is not a factor in success of treatment.[24,38,47,50,51] Many defects can be closed primarily. On the trunk, proximal extremities, or on the head and neck a variety of local flaps may be utilized. Furthermore, there is no good evidence to indicate that it is necessary or advisable to routinely excise the underlying fascia except as a matter of technical convenience.[47]

Treatment of the Regional Lymph Nodes

THERAPEUTIC LYMPH NODE DISSECTION

Therapeutic regional lymphadenectomy is indicated for all or most patients with clinically suspected or histologically proven nodal metastases. Preoperative assessment of the status of regional lymph nodes is approximately 90 percent accurate when the nodes are judged to be clinically positive,[52] although only 75 to 80 percent accurate when nodes are judged to be clinically negative.[9,53]

It is obviously important for surgeons performing lymphadenectomies for melanoma to be aware of the patterns of lymphatic drainage for various areas of the integument. Das Gupta and McNeer, in 1964, published a classic paper on the incidence of metastasis to various nodal basins for cutaneous melanomas of various primary sites on the trunk and extremities.[54] Melanomas of the lower extremities drain to the superficial inguinal nodes primarily, although both the superficial (iliofemoral) and deep (ilioobturator-inguinal) nodes may be involved. It is relatively uncommon for metastasis to "skip" the superficial inguinal nodes and to involve the deep nodes only. In a large series reported by Das Gupta, 40 patients with lower-extremity primary melanomas had inguinal node metastases. Of these, 25 (62.5 percent) had metastases to the superficial inguinal nodes only, 8 (20 percent) had involvement of both the superficial and deep nodes, and only 7 (17.5 percent) had metastases to the deep nodes only.[45] Therefore, it seems appropriate to perform a deep-inguinal (ilioobturator) node dissection only in the presence of histologically proven (preoperatively or intraoperatively by frozen section) involvement of superficial inguinal nodes. Occasionally the superficial nodes may be considered negative at the time of operation, but later may be found to contain melanoma by the pathologist. In such instances, a subsequent deep-inguinal lymph node dissection may be performed through a separate lower abdominal midline incision, although there is no data to support the efficacy of this practice. Popliteal lymph nodes only rarely become involved. When involvement does occur, it is usually in the context of blockage of lymphatic drainage through the groin, nodes due to tumor,[55] or previous node dissection.

Melanomas on the arm drain primarily to the axillary nodes. However, melanomas on the extreme upper arm or anterior shoulder may also drain to cervical lymph nodes.[54]

Melanomas of the trunk have a more complicated drainage pattern due to the greater opportunity to drain to more than one lymph node area. The trunk may be divided into four quadrants by the midline anteriorly and posteriorly, and by a line running transversely between the umbilicus anteriorly, the eighth rib laterally, and the first lumbar vertebra posteriorly. These quadrants describe nodal drainage patterns to the inguinal and axillary nodes on each side. In addition, it is important to remember that melanomas arising high on the back (above the spines of the scapula) or on the anterior shoulders may drain to cervical as well as axillary lymph nodes.

Essentially all melanomas of the head and neck drain into the cervical lymph nodes. Melanomas of the occipital area of the scalp may also drain into lymph nodes in the posterior cervical triangle. Melanomas arising on the psoterior cheek, anterior ear, forehead, eyelids, and frontal and temporal areas of the scalp drain into the preauricular or parotid group of lymph nodes.[56] When lymphadenectomies are performed for melanomas arising in these locations, a superifical parotidectomy should be performed in conjunction with the usual neck dissection. Preservation of the spinal accessory nerve is recommended whenever possible.

ELECTIVE (PROPHYLACTIC) LYMPH NODE DISSECTION

Perhaps the single most important (and controversial) question in the treatment of primary cutaneous melanoma is when, if ever, to perform an elective, i.e., prophylactic, lymphadenectomy in clinically node-negative patients. There is a marked discordance in the results of retrospective and/or historically controlled studies and the results of two recent prospectively randomized clinical trials. There is also a marked discordance between the conclusions reached in studies published prior to 1978 and the recommendations contained in papers published more recently. Breslow asserts that "the literature prior to 1977, including part of (his own) 1975 paper,[57] is worthless."[58] Elsewhere, he calls these studies "difficult if not impossible to evaluate," rather than "worthless."[14] He asserts that "because of the likelihood of bias in patient selection, retrospective studies cannot be used to compare different methods of treatment."[14,58] Certainly, it is difficult to disagree with such a statement.

Prior to the advent of the histologic microstaging systems of Clark and Breslow, most surgical oncologists performed elective lymphadenectomy more or less routinely on most patients with stage I melanoma based on the finding that when elective node dissections are performed, approximately 30 percent of clinically node-negative patients will be found to be histologically node-positive[59] and on the argument that if one waited until nodes became clinically involved, regional disease would usually be extensive and few patients would be salvaged. This argument has been advanced most recently by Fortner et al., who reported on 145 patients treated by wide excision only in whom 18 percent subsequently required therapeutic lymphadenectomy. Of those patients only 6 percent survived 10 years.[60]

Since the advent of microstaging, it has been possible to identify patients in whom all or most workers in the field agree that elective regional node dissection is clearly *not* advisable because of a uniformly good prognosis: (1) patients with in situ (Clark level I) melanoma, (2) patients with melanomas confined to Clark's level II, and (3) all patients with melanomas less than 0.76 mm thick (including some thin level III melanomas). The recent work of Day et al. suggests that the figure of 0.76 mm should be revised upward to 0.85 mm.[25,26] It is possible, therefore, to focus on the question of whether or not elective regional node dissection is of value in patients with more deeply invasive melanomas in whom the risk of occult nodal metastases is higher.

Let us review some of the data, derived from retrospective studies, suggesting that elective lymphadenectomy may be advantageous in certain patients, particularly those with melanomas of at least moderate thickness. In 1972, Hansen and McCarten reported that elective node dissection appeared to double the survival of patients with melanomas of the head and neck which are 1.50 mm thick or greater, but was not advantageous for patients with thinner tumors.[61] Breslow, in 1975, published similar findings in a retrospective study of patients with melanomas of the extremities and trunk.[57] (It is of interest that Breslow later reexamined his data and found that 50 percent of patients with extremity melanomas had undergone node dissections, while only 28 percent of patients with melanoma of the trunk had been treated with node dissection. In addition none of the nine patients with level V melanomas had undergone node dissection. Breslow concluded that his surgeons had inadvertenly "selected for node dissection (those) patients with the best prognosis."[14])

Wanebo et al., in 1975, published a retrospective study of 151 patients with stage I primary cutaneous melanoma of the extremities whose tumors were microstaged by both the Clark and Breslow methods.[21] Of these 151 patients, 113 had undergone wide excision plus elective node dissection and 38 had been treated by wide excision alone. They plotted the 5-year disease-free survival for patients in each treatment group against the depth of invasion (in millimeters) of their primary tumors. These curves are depicted in Fig. 42-8. The survival curves for the two treatment groups began to diverge at a tumor thickness of 1.5 mm, and the difference became quite marked at a thickness of 2.0 mm.

However, these differences were not statistically significant, perhaps due to the small numbers of patients in each group. They then analyzed patients with superficial spreading melanoma and nodular melanoma separately. These data are presented in Figs. 42-9 and 42-10. In patients with superficial spreading melanoma (see Fig. 42-9) the two survival curves diverged at a depth of invasion of 2.75 mm. For patients with nodular melanoma (see Fig. 42-10) the difference between the two curves was more striking, and divergence began at a thickness of only 1.0 mm. Based on these data, Wanebo and his coauthors asserted that "overall, patients with either histologic type had markedly improved results when node dissection was done for any lesion showing greater than 1.0 mm of microinvasion." They recommended that "wide excision alone should suffice for primary stage I melanoma of the extremities classified as Clark level II and measuring less than 0.9 mm in depth" and suggested that "prophylactic node dissection . . . should be done for all primary melanomas classified as Clark level III to V, for lesions showing 0.9 mm of invasion or greater at any Clark level, and for all melanomas typed as nodular melanoma."[21]

In 1977, based on a comparison between patients treated with or without elective node dissection from 1974 to 1964 and patients treated from 1972 to 1976 with elective node dissection in every instance, Fortner concluded that "the infrequency of (nodal) metastases from primary melanomas microstaged at Clark's levels I and II warrants treatment by wide excision only . . . (but) risks for melanomas categorized as levels III, IV, and V are too great to withhold lymphadenectomy."[60] He based this recommendation primarily on the relatively high incidence of occult lymph node metastases found in patients with level III (12.5 percent), level IV (35 percent), and level V (71 percent) melanomas. In the same year, Das Gupta, based, at least in part, on similar findings, advised that elective node dissections be performed on all stage I melanoma patients with thick level III lesions (i.e., greater than 0.75 mm in thickness), and for all melanomas of levels IV and V.[45] He considered wide local excision alone to be "adequate" for level II and probably for thin (less than 0.76 mm) level III. Holmes et al. in another paper published in 1977, advanced a similar argument.[44] They found that patients with Clark's level III melanoma had a 29 percent incidence of regional lymph nodd metastases, Clark's level IV, a 42 percent incidence of metastases, and Clark's level V, a 58 percent incidence of regional lymph node

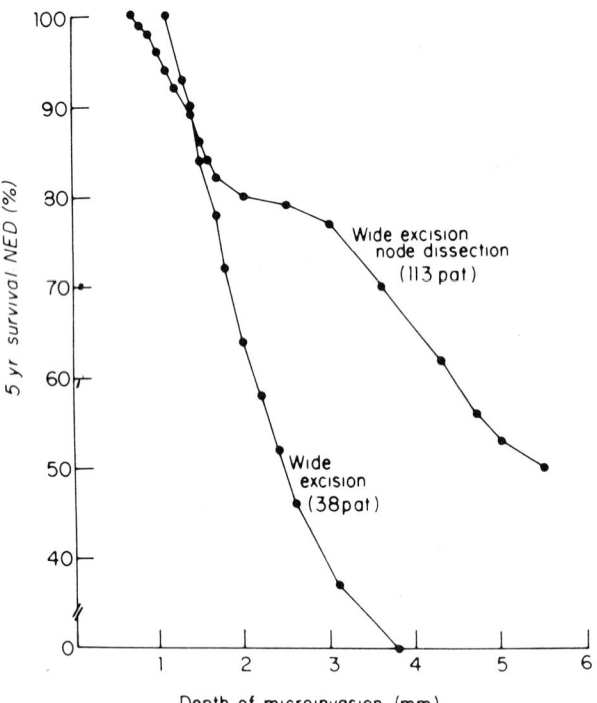

FIGURE 42-8 Disease-free 5-year survival curves obtained by Wanebo et al. for patients with stage I extremity melanomas of various thickness treated by wide excision or wide excision plus elective node dissection. (*From JH Wanebo et al: Ann Surg 182:302, 1975.*)

metastases. Overall, they found a 38 percent incidence of nodal metastases in patients with primary melanomas greater than 1.5 mm in thickness. Based on these findings, they recommended "a regional lymphadenectomy in patients with Clark's levels III, IV, and V and all melanomas that are greater than 1.5 mm in thickness." They emphasized that "iliac obturator (deep-inguinal) lymph node dissections (were) not performed unless the (superficial) inguinal lymph nodes (were) found to be involved by frozen section examination at the time of surgery."[44] Goldman and his colleagues, also relying primarily on the incidence of positive nodes found at elective lymphadenectomy, too recommended elective regional lymphadenectomy in patients with level IV and V primary melanomas and in patients with "thick" level III lesions.[46] They advocated withholding lymphadenectomy in patients with level II and "thin" level III primary melanomas.

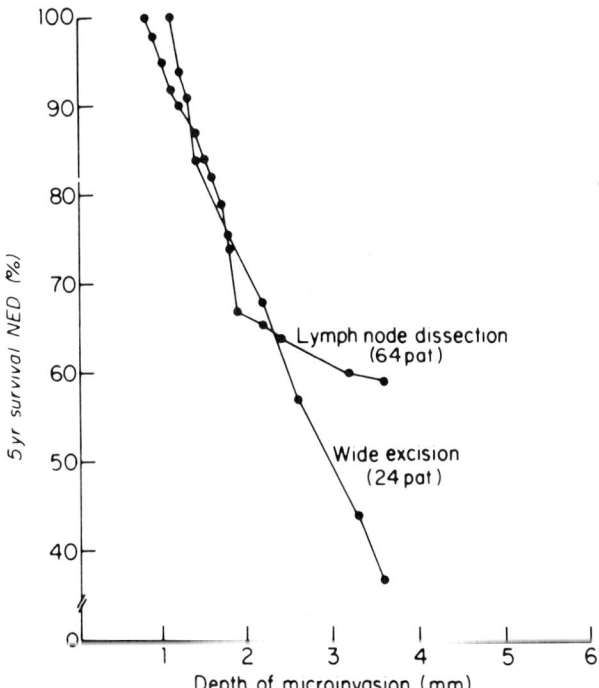

FIGURE 42-9 Disease-free survival curves for patients with superficial spreading melanoma of the extremities treated as indicated and plotted according to the depth of microinvasion. (*From JH Wanebo et al: Ann Surg 182: 302, 1975.*)

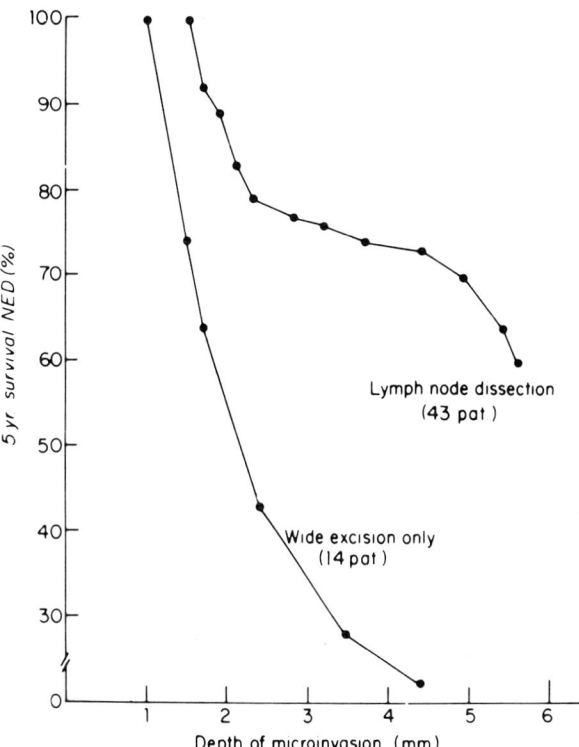

FIGURE 42-10 Disease-free survival curves for patients with nodular melanoma of the extremities. (*From JH Wanebo et al: Ann Surg 182:302, 1975.*)

Balch et al. retrospectively reviewed the records of 284 patients with clinical stage I cutaneous malignant melanoma treated between 1960 and 1977. Original biopsy slides of the primary tumor were not available for 111 patients, and they were excluded from analysis. An additional 17 patients were excluded for other reasons. The remaining 156 patients formed the basis for their report.[24] They then compared the incidence of distant metastases and the 5-year survival in patients treated by wide local excision only (78 patients) and in patients treated by excision plus elective regional node dissections (78 patients). Patients were grouped according to the thickness of their primary melanomas. For patients whose primary melanomas were less than 0.76 mm thick there were no differences between the two groups (incidence of metastases was 0 and survival was 100 percent for both groups). Moreover, for patients whose melanomas were greater than 3.99 mm thick there were no significant differences between the two groups. However, in patients with primary melanomas of intermediate thicknesses differences between the two groups were noted. For patients whose melanomas were 0.77 to 1.49 mm in thickness, those who underwent wide local excision plus elective node dissection appeared to fare better than those who were treated by wide local excision alone; the incidence of metastasis was lower at 5 years (8 vs. 25 percent; $p = .23$), and the 5-year survival was greater (94 vs. 58 percent; $p = .04$). More marked differences were noted among patients with melanomas between 1.50 and 3.99 mm in thickness—once again in favor of patients who underwent elective node dissection, the incidence of metastasis being much lower (15 vs. 78 percent, $p < .001$) and the 5-year survival being significantly better (83 vs. 37 percent; $p = .01$) for patients treated with node dissection.

Based on these data, Balch presently recommends that elective regional node dissection be withheld from patients whose primary melanomas are less than 0.76 mm thick or greater than 4.0 mm thick.[52] He advises elective node dissection in "selected patients" with primary melanomas 0.76 to 1.5 mm thick. (He does not specify which type of patients he would select for elective node dissection other than to state that this may be of value "especially" in male patients.) Balch recommends elective node dissection for all patients whose melanomas are between 1.5 and 4.0 mm thick.

It is important to remember that the conclusions reached in the studies reported above were usually based on one or both of the following findings: (1) patients with more deeply invasive primary melanomas have a higher incidence of occult lymph node metastases when and if the regional lymph nodes are removed; (2) retrospective analysis of the clinical course of such patients (often excluding a sizable proportion of patients for one reason or another) suggests a more favorable outcome for patients undergoing elective regional node dissection. It is usually impossible to determine whether the groups of patients being analyzed were comparable with respect to known risk factors, and, more important, it is usually impossible to determine why some patients were treated with elective node dissection and others were not. The opportunities for bias, therefore, are large, as Breslow found when he reviewed his own data in 1975 (see above).

Two *prospectively randomized clinical trials* and two retrospective studies have been reported recently indicating that elective node dissection may be of no therapeutic value. We shall review the retrospective studies first, since they suffer from all the shortcomings just discussed.

In 1981, Elias et al. reviewed the records of 248 melanoma patients treated in 1965 through 1969 and reported on the results obtained in 70 patients who were found to have primary lesions in the Clark's level IV and V category.[62] (Eight patients who were lost to follow-up were excluded.) Of these 70 patients, 51 presented with wide local excision alone. Of these, 26 never required therapeutic lymphadenectomy while 25 patients did. However, the survival figures at 10 years were not significantly different ($p < .10$) for the two groups.

Bagley et al., in their report of 147 melanoma patients treated at the Lahey Clinic between 1955 and 1979, reviewed the records of 59 patients treated without elective node dissection and 44 patients who underwent elective regional lymphadenectomy.[48] No clear survival advantage to prophylactic lymph node dissection was observed regardless of the depth of invasion of the primary tumor. These authors concluded that "prophylactic regional lymphadenectomy is of no value in low-risk and moderate-risk groups; in high-risk groups prophylactic regional lymphadenectomy may be associated with a cure rate of 60 percent in those patients in whom positive nodes are found but does not increase the overall survival of this group probably because this salvage figure is not different from that achieved by later therapeutic lymphadenectomy."

In 1977, Veronesi et al. reported the results of a prospectively randomized clinical trial carried out between 1967 and 1974 by the WHO Melanoma Group to evaluate the efficacy of elective regional node dissection in the treatment of malignant melanoma of the extremities in patients with clinically uninvolved regional lymph nodes.[63] Patients with T_1, T_2, T_3, N_0 M_0 melanoma of the extremities were prospectively randomized to wide excision plus immediate elective node dissection (267 patients) or to wide excision and regional node dissection only if and when nodal metastases appeared (286 patients). At 8 years of follow-up, no difference in survival was noted between the two groups regardless of how the data were analyzed, i.e., according to sex, site of origin, maximum diameter of the primary tumor, Clark's level, or Breslow's thickness. Presently, this group has published an update of their data with up to 11 years of follow-up.[64] Again the survival curves of the two treatment groups could be superimposed (see Fig. 42-11).

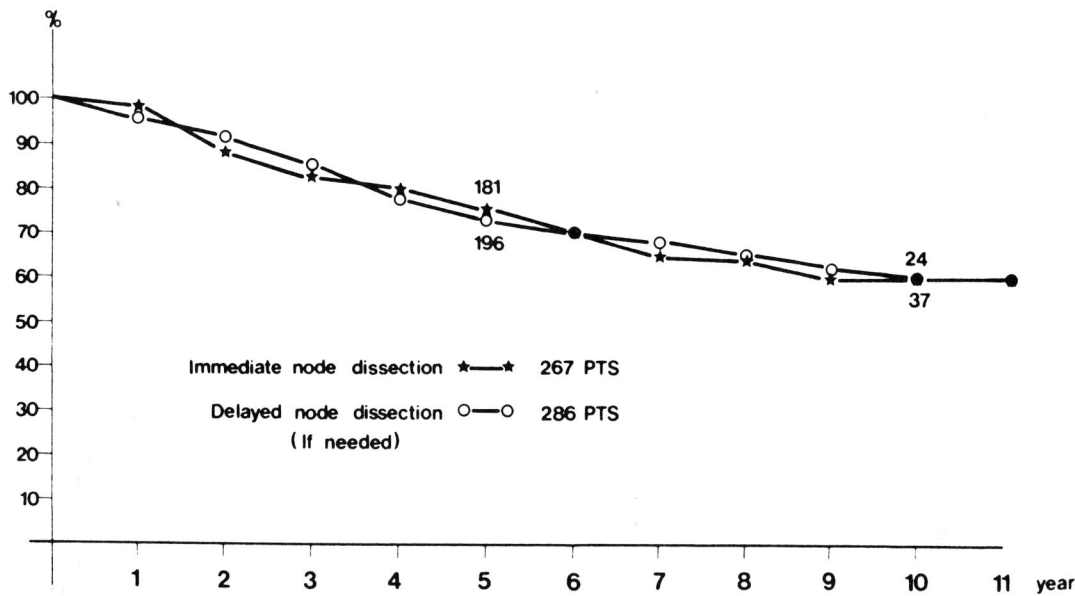

FIGURE 42-11 Overall survival in 553 stage I melanoma patients according to treatment. (*From U Veronesi et al: Cancer 49:2420, 1982.*)

No subsets of patients who appeared to benefit from immediate node dissection could be discerned.

In 1978, Sim et al. reported on a prospectively randomized study initiated at the Mayo Clinic in 1972.[65] Patients with stage I malignant melanoma were stratified by the site of the lesion and then randomized into one of three treatment groups: (1) no lymphadenectomy, (2) delayed lymphadenectomy 2 to 4 months after excision of the primary lesion, and (3) immediate excision of the regional nodes. All patients underwent wide local excision. Patients with primary melanomas of the head and neck or midline trunk were excluded. Of the 173 patients studied, 63 were randomized to no lymphadenectomy, 56 to delayed lymphadenectomy, and 54 to immediate lymphadenectomy. With 5 years of follow-up, none of the regimens differed significantly from the others with respect to disease-free survival (interval to metastasis) or overall survival. This was true even among patients who had primary lesions of the Clark level IV or V category or lesions greater than 1.50 mm thick. In summary, at the present time, the therapeutic value of elective node dissection, even for patients with thick primary melanomas, is in doubt. Final resolution of this question must await the results of additional well-controlled clinical trials. At least two are now in progress.

Finally, there are two questions relating to the performance of lymph node dissections which remain to be discussed: (1) the timing of the lymphadenectomy with relation to excision of the primary tumor, and (2) whether or not lymph node dissection should be performed in continuity with resection of the primary melanoma.

At one time there was some enthusiasm for delaying regional lymph node dissection for 4 to 8 weeks following resection of the primary tumor in order to allow the regional nodes to "filter out" tumor cells within the lymphatics between the primary tumor site and the regional nodes in the hope of thereby reducing the incidence of in-transit metastases. It is now clear from the work of Sim et al.[65] and others that this is not the case. There are no good data to indicate that delayed node dissection is advantageous, and most authors now recommend simultaneous node dissections.

The objective of in-continuity node dissection is also to reduce the incidence of in-transit metastases (by excising the intervening lymphatics). In 1975, Fortner et al. reported a 4 percent incidence of development of in-transit metastases following lymph node dissections performed in discontinuity and only a 2 percent incidence of in-transit metastases after in-continuity lymph node dissections.[66] However, Veronesi[67] has reported no significant difference in the incidence of in-transit metastases between patients treated by en bloc operations (4 of 52) and those treated by operations in discontinuity (1 of 31).[67] In addition, several investigators have reported no difference in survival statistics.[68,69] It would appear that there is no clear benefit to in-continuity node dissection, and the matter is probably more a matter of technical convenience than of oncologic significance.

Adjuvant Therapy

ADJUVANT CHEMOTHERAPY

Trials of adjuvant chemotherapy in malignant melanoma have been few due to the early enthusiasm for adjuvant immunotherapy and chemoimmunotherapy (see below). The most important trial was that conducted by the Central Oncology Group (COG) under the leadership of Hill. In this prospectively randomized clinical trial, patients with stage I, II, or III melanoma, in whom all detectable disease had been surgically excised, were randomly assigned, following surgery, to receive either dimethyltriazeno imidazole carboxamide (DTIC), at a dose of 4.5 mg/kg/per day for 10 days, IV, every 12 to 14 weeks for 1 year, or to have no additional therapy. The treated group fared significantly *worse* than the control group with respect to both disease-free interval and survival.[70] Interestingly, treated patients experiencing thrombocytopenia had significant prolongation of disease-free survival and overall survival when compared to treated patients who had no hematologic toxicity,[71] suggesting that a different dosage schedule might have produced different results.

A study from the M.D. Anderson Hospital, utilizing DTIC at a dose of 2 mg/kg/per day × for 10 days, IV, every 3 months, 5 times as postsurgical adjuvant therapy in 37 melanoma patients with clinically palpable as well as histologically positive regional lymph nodes; demonstrated improved disease-free interval and survival for treated patients compared to *historical* controls.[71]

Because of the disappointing results of the COG trial, studies of adjuvant chemotherapy were largely abandoned in favor of trials of immunotherapy and chemoimmunotherapy.

ADJUVANT IMMUNOTHERAPY AND CHEMOIMMUNOTHERAPY

Malignant melanoma has received a disproportionate degree of attention from tumor immunologists because of observations suggesting that it might be among the most immunogenic of human tumors. Such observations include the spontaneous regression of primary melanomas, the long disease-free intervals frequently observed between the treatment of the primary tumor and the onset of metastases, and the spontaneous regression of metastatic deposits. In addition, melanoma was one of the few human tumors in which unique tumor-associated antigens were demonstrated by rigorously controlled in vitro studies. Immunotherapy seemed particularly suitable for adjuvant therapy since animal studies suggested that immunotherapy might be effective only when the body burden of tumor cells was small, i.e., less than 10^7 or 10^8 cells.

Enthusiasm for adjuvant immunotherapy was greatly stimulated by preliminary reports from UCLA and M.D. Anderson Hospital that intradermal injections of bacillus Calmette-Guérin (BCG) improved disease-free survival and prolonged overall survival when given to patients with stage II or III melanoma following surgical resection of all detectable disease.[72–75] These initial reports utilized historical controls of one sort or another. Unfortunately, subsequent prospectively randomized trials (including one from the UCLA group itself) have failed to reproduce the observations of the original nonrandomized studies.[76–78] The combination of BCG with DTIC chemotherapy was reported by Wood et al. recently to yield results superior to that achieved with either treatment alone.[79] However, preliminary analysis of data from two recent trials, one of which was a large trial coordinated by the World Health Organization, found the same combination to be of no value.[78,80]

Other approaches to adjuvant immunotherapy utilizing levamisole[81] or *Corynebacterium parvum*[82] have also yielded negative results. A very recent study by Blume et al. has reported improved disease-free survival and overall survival in patients with "high risk" stage I melanoma (primary melanomas invasive to Clark's level III or deeper and exceeding 1.0 mm in thickness) treated with transfer factor.[83] However, this study again employed *historical controls* and remains to be confirmed.

Therefore, at the present time, it is fair to say that no form of adjuvant immunotherapy, alone or in combination with chemotherapy, has demonstrated consistent value in the treatment of melanoma. Adjuvant immunotherapy in melanoma patients remains of unproven clinical benefit and should not be recommended outside a research setting.

ISOLATION LIMB PERFUSION AS ADJUVANT THERAPY FOR EXTREMITY MELANOMA

We shall not discuss this subject in detail. Although a number of authors have reported that limb perfusion with Melphalan and/or other agents, sometimes combined with hyperthermia, increases disease-free survival, improves overall survival, and/or diminishes the incidence of regional metastases, there is at present no firm support for its use as an adjuvant in the treatment of primary malignant melanoma. In a recent critical review of this subject Au and Goldman[84] point out that all of the studies reported to date are either uncontrolled or use historical controls. They correctly note that all of the available data suffers from one or more of the following limitations:

1. Most studies "lump" all cases together, including those treated in the adjuvant setting and those treated for recurrent and/or metastatic disease.
2. The extent of associated surgery is often incompletely defined and/or highly variable.
3. The extent of disease is often highly variable.
4. Recent staging criteria (e.g., depth of invasion and tumor thickness) were not available or not utilized.
5. End results are compared to a wide spectrum of historical controls, often at considerable variance with one another.
6. Other potential prognostic variables (e.g., sex, age, etc.) are largely ignored.
7. Considerable variations are present in the perfusion technique (e.g., chemotherapeutic agent, temperature, duration, etc.).

Au and Goldman conclude that "no concrete evidence . . . supports the value of isolation limb perfusion as an adjuvant in the primary treatment of malignant melanoma in the extremity."[84]

Treatment of Recurrent and Metastatic Melanoma

CHEMOTHERAPY OF METASTATIC MALIGNANT MELANOMA

Robert Benjamin points out, in his excellent review of this subject, that "despite extensive study of new chemotherapeutic agents and regimens in the treatment of patients with advanced melanoma, no treatment program has been of significant benefit to more than a small minority of patients, and the disease remains a major challenge to the medical oncologist."[85]

DTIC remains the most important agent in the chemotherapy of melanoma, producing a response rate of about 20 percent when used as a single agent. The only other drugs with response rates comparable to that achieved with DTIC are the nitrosoureas. Comis and carter, in their review, report an overall response rate of 13 percent for CCNU and 18 percent from BCNU and methyl-CCNU.[86] In studies with various nitrosoureas, used alone or in combination with agents other than DTIC, response rates ranging from 6 to 41 percent have been reported, with an average of 24 percent.[85]

The obvious approach to the use of two active agents is to combine them. However, unfortunately, most combinations of DTIC and nitrosoureas have been no more successful than either agent alone, nor has use of combinations of these two agents with other drugs succeeded in improving results. The chemotherapeutic agents which have been combined with DTIC or nitrosoureas include cyclophosphamide, Melphalan, *cis*-platinum, cyclocytidine, vincristine, procarbazine, ICRF-159, and methotrexate. None of these combinations has shown significant additive effect.

High-dose methotrexate with citrovorum rescue had shown considerable promise in phase II trials. Eilber et al. have reported a 36 percent response rate in 22 patients who received the drug on a 3-week schedule[87] and a 50 percent response rate in 12 patients treated weekly in combination with DTIC.[88]

An exhaustive discussion of the results of specific trials is beyond the scope of this chapter, and the reader is referred to the recent reviews by Benjamin,[85] Comis and Carter,[86] and Bellet et al.[89] Bellet et al., and most other authors, presently recommend DTIC, used as a single agent, as the drug of first choice in the treatment of patients with metastatic malignant melanoma. BCNU or methyl CCNU constitutes second-line treatment. Bellet et al. recommend the addition of vincristine to BCNU or methyl CCNU because of data suggesting some improvement in response rate without additive toxicity.[89]

ISOLATION LIMB PERFUSION FOR REGIONAL METASTASES

There is little doubt that regional perfusion plays a role in the treatment of recurrent and/or regionally metastatic melanoma of the extremity. This therapeutic modality is particularly appealing in patients with recurrences and/or metastases clinically confined to a single extremity. The technique for isolation limb perfusion was originally reported in 1959, by Creech et al., who treated six patients with recurrent cutaneous metastases of the extremity.[90] Variable degrees of tumor destruction were noted in all six patients.

In 1970, Krementz reported on 28 patients with satellitosis in whom perfusion was used as the sole treatment.[91] Seven remained free of disease for periods beyond 5 years. In 1967, Stehlin introduced hyperthermic isolation limb perfusion with Melphalan and first reported on its use in 1969.[92] His technique has been employed ever since by the majority of workers in the field. He has recently reported the results of his experience over the previous 11 years.[93] The 5-year survival rate for his 73 patients with recurrences or metastases confined to an extremity was 52.5 pecent. Prior to the introduction of hyperthermic perfusion in 1967, the 5-year survival rate for such patients when treated by Stehlin with normothermic perfusion had been only 22.2 percent,[94] strongly suggesting substantial improvement related directly to hyperthermia.

It would appear that regional isolation limb perfusion (especially hyperthermic perfusion) can induce regression of regionally recurrent melanoma, and can effect cure in some patients. Until such time as the results of systemic chemotherapy improve, this technique appears to be quite valuable in the treatment of those patients with recurrent or metastatic melanoma confined to an extremity.

THE TREATMENT OF CUTANEOUS METASTASES BY LOCAL IMMUNOTHERAPY

Local immunotherapy is accomplished by the intralesional injection or topical application of agents that produce a delayed cutaneous hypersensitivity (DCH) reaction in or around an intradermal, subcutaneous, or other accessible tumor deposit. Although it is essential that the patient mount an immune response to the agent injected, a role for specific antitumor immunity in mediating tumor destruction has not been proved.

The most widely employed agent for local immunotherapy has been BCG. Morton et al. demonstrated that 90 percent of cutaneous metastatic lesions of malignant melanoma regressed following one or multiple intralesional injections of BCG, provided the patient was immunocompetent as measured by skin testing.[73,95] Morton also reported that in 17 percent of patients, uninjected tumor nodules regressed along with the injected lesions. The uninjected lesions which regressed were usually in close proximity to injected nodules, so that this response may have been due to local migration of BCG organisms or other local phenomena. There was no compelling evidence that a systemic antimelanoma immune response was generated. Other investigators then confirmed the regression of cutaneous nodules injected with BCG,[96] although a number failed to confirm the regression of injected nodules.[97] Although Morton and others have reported that up to 20 percent of patients with metastases limited to the skin were brought into complete remission and enjoyed long-term disease-free survival by this treatment, visceral metastases were not affected by the injection of cutaneous nodules. Most patients develop recurrent lesions and ultimately succumb to their disease. Whether intralesional therapy actually prolongs survival has not been established, since this form of treatment has never been tested against a comparable untreated control group of patients. Intralesional BCG is associated with significant side effects, and serious local and systemic toxicity may occur.[98]

The skin-sensitizing organic hapten dinitrochlorobenzene (DNCB) is a strong immunogen, and following sensitization, topical application or intralesional injection elicits a strong DCH response in immunocompetent patients. This agent has been used for local immunotherapy in a manner similar to BCG with roughly comparable results.[96] Toxicity is limited to transient pain upon injection and local inflammation at the injection site. Usually, no systemic toxicity occurs. Because of its substantially lower toxicity, DNCB may be preferable to BCG as an agent for local immunotherapy.

Other agents have been administered intralesionally for local immunotherapy, but have not been widely studied. These include vaccinia virus, transfer factor, *Corynebacterium parvum,* and phytohemagglutinin-activated autologous lymphocytes.

SPECIAL TYPES OF MELANOMA

Amelanotic Melanoma

Much has been written over the years suggesting that amelanotic melanomas constitute a distant subtype of melanoma with an especially poor prognosis, presumably due to the more poorly differentiated nature of such tumors. Several retrospective analyses, such as the series of 28 patients reported in 1972 by Huvos et al.,[99] indicated that overall survival rates at 5, 10, and 15 years were substantially worse for patients with amelanotic melanoma than for patients with pigmented melanomas. It was speculated that this poor survival might be due to a more aggressive biologic behavior related to an "extreme degree of cell undifferentiation, as evidenced by the inability of these melanin-producing cells to make pigment."[55] However, in the same report Huvos et al. demonstrated that amelanotic melanomas tended to come to diagnosis at a more advanced clinical stage than did pigmented melanomas, perhaps because the lack of pigmentation resulted in their initial misdiagnosis as a benign lesion.[99] They pointed out that the apparent biologic aggressiveness of amelanotic melanomas might simply represent diagnostic delay, allowing these tumors to advance significantly prior to biopsy and treatment.

Most papers reporting a poor prognosis associated with amelanotic melanoma were written prior to the introduction of systems for microstaging the depth of invasion of primary melanomas. Therefore, it is entirely possible that more amelanotic melanomas presented with a deeper depth of invasion at the time of initial biopsy, possibly due to delays in diagnosis.

Today, most melanoma pathologists do not recognize amelanotic melanoma as a specific histologic subtype, although Breslow acknowledges that amelanosis may be a prognostic variable.[14,58] Elder et al. point out, in their excellent review of the surgical pathology of cutaneous melanoma, that "even in the so-called amelanotic melanoma, a few flecks of pigment are usual, and the total absence of melanin . . . suggests another diagnosis."[100]

At the present time, there is little reason to treat an amelanotic melanoma any differently than a pigmented melanoma. The same principles of clinical staging and microstaging apply, and treatment should be dictated by the same considerations as those governing the treatment of pigmented melanomas.

Subungual Melanoma

Subungual melanoma is a special type of acral lentiginous melanoma developing in the nail bed beneath a nail. Like amelanotic melanoma, subungual melanomas have been thought to carry a poor prognosis. However, like amelanotic melanoma, this is probably due to diagnostic delay rather than to a particularly or uniquely aggressive biologic behavior. Diagnostic delay is often due to the fact that subungual melanoma may resemble a pyogenic granuloma, fungal infection, or subungual hematoma. In addition, there may be a delay in diagnosis because of hesitation (or inability) on the part of the examining physician to remove the overlying nail in order to obtain an adequate biopsy.

Treatment of subungual melanoma requires amputation of the involved digit. Amputation of the entire involved digit including all or a portion of the corresponding metacarpal or metatarsal bone (ray amputation) is usually recommended.[58,101] However, there is no good data to indicate that ray amputation is necessary, nor are there any studies to indicate what the appropriate level of amputation should be. The value of elective lymphadenectomy, isolation limb perfusions, and other procedures is not established.

Malignant Melanoma of the Female Genital Tract

Malignant melanoma of the female genital tract is rare, constituting only 3 percent of all melanomas afflicting females.[102] Melanoma of the vulva is by far the most common. Vulvar melanoma is usually treated by radical vulvectomy and bilateral radical groin dissections (including both inguinofemoral and ilioobturator nodes) in continuity. Ariel states that "radical vulvectomy and radical groin dissection is the treatment of choice."[102] Rutledge writes that "the optimal treatment for vulvar melanoma is total vulvectomy and bilateral inguinal and pelvic lymphadenectomy in continuity."[103] However, there is little or no data to indicate that lesser procedures are less effective. Rutledge himself admits that although "there is a consensus that the groin (inguinal and femoral) lymph nodes must be removed routinely, . . . the rule with pelvic (iliac) lymphadenectomy has not been precisely defined."[103]

In fact, there is little data to indicate that routine pelvic node dissection is necessary, nor is there good data to indicate that elective (i.e., prophylactic) inguinal node dissections are required.

Five major series of vulvar melanoma have been reported since 1964, with a total of 169 patients, most of whom were treated as described above. The average 5-year survival is approximately 35 percent, with a range of 30 to 50 percent.[102,103] In patients with negative regional lymph nodes 5-year survival is better (approximately 55 percent) than in patients with positive regional lymph nodes (approximately 13 percent).

Only 80 cases of melanoma of the vagina have been reported, and cures are an extreme rarity. Forty cases of melanoma of the female urethra have been reported, with only five survivors.

Anorectal Melanoma

Primary melanomas of the anorectum are extremely rare, accounting for 0.4 to 1.6 pecent of all melanomas,[104] and are associated with an extremely poor prognosis in spite of aggressive therapy. Approximately 220 cases have been reported. Wanebo et al., in a recent review, note that the prognosis of primary anorectal melanoma appears to be directly related to tumor size and thickness.[104] In their review of 51 patients with this disease treated at the Memorial Hospital, only 6 (12 percent) survived 5 years. Although all four of the five survivors had radical surgery, the three whose tumors could be measured had superficial lesions. They report that, in general, radical surgery was no more effective than local excision or cryosurgery. One patient, however, did have a thin lesion but also had nodal metastases and survived over 5 years after radical surgery. They conclude that although radical resection may cure patients with lesions thinner than 3 mm, the possibility that local excision may also be curative cannot be excluded.

Pickard et al. reviewed 16 patients with anorectal melanoma treated at the M.D. Anderson Hospital and reached similar conclusions.[105] They recommend wide local excision as the therapy of choice, although they note that an abdominoperineal resection may be necessary in order to acomplish this. They state that elective inguinal lymphadenectomy has not improved survival rates.

Melanoma Occurring during Pregnancy

The basis for the pessimism associated with melanoma occurring in a pregnant woman is the belief that the gestational process accelerates malignant activity in general, and the fact that the hormonal changes associated with pregnancy have a profound effect on melanoblast activity. In addition, sporatic reports in the literature suggested that survival statistics in pregnant women were lower than those of their nonpregnant counterparts. However, no good evidence has been reported to incriminate pregnancy in the exacerbation of melanoma.

This matter has been addressed in a recent paper by Houghton et al., who conducted a population-based study from the Connecticut Tumor Registry.[106] They found that cutaneous melanomas occurring during pregnancy were diagnosed at a later stage and at prognostically worse sites than those in nonpregnant women, and that, therefore, survival at 3 and 5 years was significantly lower for pregnant women. However, when pregnant patients were matched to nonpregnant patients by anatomic site and stage at diagnosis, 3-year and 5-year survival statistics were not different. They concluded that the lower survival in pregnant women was due to poor prognostic features at the time of initial diagnosis. Once diagnosed, the clinical course of these patients was not worse than that of matched nonpregnant controls.

REFERENCES

1. Silverberg E: Cancer statistics, 1982. *CA* 32:15, 1982.
2. Sober, AJ, Fitzpatrick TB: Melanoma fact sheet. *CA* 29:276, 1979.
3. Clark WH Jr et al: Tumor progression in primary malignant melanomas, in WH Clark Jr et al (eds): *Human Malignant Melanoma*, Grune & Stratton, New York, 1979, pp 15–31.
4. Davis NC: Cutaneous melanoma. *Curr Probl Surg* 13:1, 1976.
5. Kopf AW et al: In *Malignant Melanoma*, Masson, New York, 1979, pp 4–6.
6. Krementz ET et al: Acral lentiginous melanoma: A clinicopathologic entity. *Ann Surg* 195:632, 1982.
7. Pade CT, Davis J: The pigmented mole. *Postgrad Med* 27:370, 1960.
8. McNeer G, Das Gupta TK: Prognosis in malignant melanoma. *Surgery* 56:512, 1964.
9. Goldsmith HS: *Melanoma in Practice of Surgery*, Harper & Row, Hagerstown, Maryland, 1978, pp 1–26.
10. Mehnert JH, Heard JL: Staging of malignant melanoma by depth of invasion. *Am J Surg* 110:168, 1965.
11. Clark WH Jr et al: The histogenesis and biologic behavior of primary human malignant melanoma of the skin. *Cancer Res* 29:705, 1969.
12. Clark WH Jr et al: The developmental biology of primary human malignant melanomas. *Semin Oncol* 2:83, 1975.
13. Breslow A: Thickness, cross-sectional areas and depth of invasion of the prognosis of cutaneous melanoma. *Ann Surg* 172:902, 1970.
14. Breslow A: Prognosis in cutaneous melanoma: Tumor thickness as a guide to treatment. *Pathol Annu* Part I 15:1, 1980.
15. Heise H, Krementz ET: Survival experience of patients with malignant melanoma of the skin, 1950–1957. *Natl Cancer Inst Monogr* 6:69, 1961.
16. Bodenham DC: Basic principles of surgery—malignant, melanoma, in WH McCarthy (ed): *Melanoma and Skin Cancer*, VCN Blight, Sydney, 1972, pp 375–383.

17. Einhorn LH et al: Prognostic correlations and response to treatment in advanced metastatic melanoma. *Cancer Res* 34:1995, 1974.
18. Mastrangelo MJ et al: Prognostic factors, in WH Clark Jr et al (eds): *Human Malignant Melanoma*, Grune & Stratton, New York, 1979, pp 273–282.
19. McGovern VJ: The classification of melanoma and its relationship with prognosis. *Pathology* 2:85, 1970.
20. Kopf AW et al: *Malignant Melanoma*, Masson, New York, 1979, p 13.
21. Wanebo AJ et al: Selection of the optimum surgical treatment of Stage I melanoma by depth of microinvasion: Use of the combined microstage technique (Clark-Breslow). *Ann Surg* 182:302, 1975.
22. Wanebo JH et al: Malignant melanoma of the extremities: A clinicopathologic study using levels of invasion (microstage). *Cancer* 35:666, 1975.
23. Eldh J et al: Prognostic factors in cutaneous malignant melanoma in Stage I: A clinical, morphological, and multivariate analysis. *Scand J Plast Reconstr Surg* 12:243, 1978.
24. Balch CM et al: Tumor thickness as a guide to surgical management of clinical Stage I melanoma patients. *Cancer* 43:883, 1979.
25. Day CL et al: The natural breakpoints for primary tumor thickness in clinical Stage I melanoma. *N Engl J Med* 305: 1155, 1981.
26. Day CL et al: Cutaneous malignant melanoma, Prognostic guidelines for physicians and patients. *CA* 32:113, 1982.
27. Fitzpatrick TB: Early recognition of primary cutaneous melanoma. *Hosp Practice* 17(no 1):67, 1982.
28. Mundth ED et al: Malignant melanoma: A clinical study of 427 cases. *Ann Surg* 162:15, 1965.
29. Balch CM et al: A multifactorial analysis of melanoma. III. Prognostic factors in melanoma patients with lymph node metastases (Stage II). *Ann Surg* 193:377, 1981.
30. Goldsmith HS et al: Prognostic significance of lymph node dissection in the treatment of malignant melanoma. *Cancer* 26:606, 1970.
31. Cochran AJ: Malignant melanoma: Review of 10 years' experience in Glasgow, Scotland. *Cancer* 23:1190, 1969.
32. Shaw JP, Goldsmith HS: Prognosis of malignant melanoma in relation to clinical presentation. *Am J Surg* 123:286, 1972.
33. Das Gupta TK et al: Malignant melanoma of unknown primary origin. *Surg Gynecol Obstet* 117:341, 1963.
34. Baab GH, McBride CM: Malignant melanoma. The patient with an unknown site of primary origin. *Arch Surg* 110: 896, 1975.
35. Smith JL, Stehlin JS: Spontaneous regression of primary malignant melanoma with regional metastases. *Cancer* 18: 1399, 1965.
36. Chang P, Knapper WH: Metastatic melanoma of unknown primary. *Cancer* 49:1106, 1982.
37. Lopez R et al: Malignant melanoma with unknown primary site. *J Surg Oncol* 19:151, 1982.
38. Milton GW et al: *Malignant Melanoma of the Skin and Mucous Membrane*, Churchill Livingstone, Edinburgh, 1977.
39. Kopf AW et al: In *Malignant Melanoma*, Masson, New York, 1979, p 12.
40. Lee Y-TN: Malignant melanoma: Pattern of metastasis. *CA* 30:137, 1982.
41. Booker RJ, McPeak CJ: Melanoma, in TF Nealon Jr (ed): *Management of the Patient with Cancer*, Saunders, Philadelphia, 1976, pp 117–159.
42. Handley WS: The pathology of melanotic growths in relation to their operative treatment. *Lancet* 1:927, 1907.
43. Handley WS: The pathology of melanotic growths in relation to their operative treatment. *Lancet* 1:996, 1907.
44. Holmes EC et al: A rational approach to the surgical management of melanoma. *Ann Surg* 186:481, 1977.
45. Das Gupta TK: Results of treatment of 269 patients with primary cutaneous melanoma. *Ann Surg* 186:201, 1977.
46. Goldman LI: The surgical treatment of malignant melanoma, in WH Clark Jr et al (eds): *Human Malignant Melanoma*, Grune & Stratton, New York, 1979, pp 285–293.
47. Olsen G: The malignant melanoma of the skin. *Acta Clin Scand (Suppl)* 365:140, 1966.
48. Bagley FH et al: Changes in clinical presentation and management of malignant melanoma. *Cancer* 47:2126, 1981.
49. Cascinelli N et al: Stage I melanoma of the skin: The problem of resection margins. *Eur J Cancer* 16:1079, 1980.
50. Breslow A, Macht SD: Optimal size of resection margin for thin cutaneous melanoma. *Surg Gynecol Obstet* 145:691, 1977.
51. Day CL et al: Narrower margins for clinical Stage I malignant melanoma. *N Engl J Med* 306:479, 1982.
52. Balch CM: Pathology, prognostic factors, and surgical treatment of cutaneous melanoma. *Curr Concepts Oncol* 4: 8, 1982.
53. Cohen MH et al: Prognostic factors in patients undergoing lymphadenectomy for melanoma. *Ann Surg* 186:635, 1977.
54. Das Gupta TK, McNeer G: The incidence of metastasis to accessible lymph nodes for melanoma of the trunk and extremities—its therapeutic significance. *Cancer* 17:897, 1964.
55. Goldsmith HS: Melanoma: An overview. *CA* 29:194, 1979.
56. Storm FK et al: A prospective study of parotid metastases from head and neck cancer. *Am J Surg* 134:115, 1977.
57. Breslow A: Tumor thickness, level of invasion and node dissection in Stage I cutaneous melanoma. *Ann Surg* 182: 572, 1975.
58. Breslow A: The surgical treatment of Stage I cutaneous melanoma. *Cancer Treat Rev* 5:195, 1979.
59. Gumport SL, Harris MN: Results of regional lymph node dissection for melanoma. *Ann Surg* 179:150, 1974.

60. Fortner JG: Biostatistical basis of elective node dissection. *Ann Surg* 189:101, 1977.
61. Hansen MG, McCarter AB: Tumor thickness and lymphocytic infiltration in malignant melanoma of the head and neck. *Am J Surg* 128:557, 1972.
62. Elias EG et al: Deeply invasive cutaneous malignant melanoma. *Surg Gynecol Obstet* 153:67, 1981.
63. Veronesi U et al: Inefficacy of immediate node dissection in stage I melanoma of the limbs. *N Engl J Med* 297:627, 1977.
64. Veronesi U et al: Delayed regional lymph node dissection in stage I melanoma of the skin of the lower extremities. *Cancer* 49:2420, 1982.
65. Sim FH et al: A prospective study of the efficacy of routine elective lymphadenectomy in management of malignant melanoma. *Cancer* 41:948, 1978.
66. Fortner JG et al: En block resection of pulmonary melanoma with regional node dissection. *Arch Surg* 110:674, 1975.
67. Veronesi U, Cascinelli N: Surgical treatment of malignant melanoma of the skin. *World J Surg* 3:279, 1979.
68. Shaw JP, Goldsmith HS: Incontinuity versus discontinuous lymph node dissection for malignant melanoma. *Cancer* 26:610, 1970.
69. Papachristou D, Fortner JG: Comparison of lymphedema following in-continuity and discontinuity groin dissection. *Ann Surg* 185:13, 1977.
70. Hill GJ et al: DTIC melanoma adjuvant study: Final report. *Proc Am Assoc Ca Res* 18:309, 1978.
71. Mastrangelo MJ et al: Postsurgical adjuvant therapy, in WH Clark Jr et al (eds): *Human Malignant Melanoma*, Grune & Stratton, New York, 1979, pp 304–324.
72. Eilber FR et al: Adjuvant immunotherapy with BCG in the treatment of regional-lymph-node metastases from malignant melanoma. *N Engl J Med* 294:237, 1976.
73. Morton DL et al: BCG immunotherapy of malignant melanoma: Summary of a seven year experience. *Ann Surg* 180:635, 1974.
74. Gutterman JU et al: Active immunotherapy with BCG for recurrent malignant melanoma. *Lancet* 1:1208, 1973.
75. Gutterman JU et al: Immunoprophylaxis of malignant melanoma with systemic BCG: Study of strain, dose, and schedule. *Natl Cancer Inst Monogr* 39:205, 1973.
76. Pinsky CM et al: Randomized trial of bacillus Calmette-Guérin (percutaneous administration) as surgical adjuvant immunotherapy for patients with stage II melanoma. *Ann NY Acad Sci* 277:187, 1976.
77. Morton DL et al: Multi-modality therapy of malignant melanoma, skeletal and soft tissue sarcomas using immunotherapy, chemotherapy and radiation therapy, in SE Jones, SE Salmon (eds): *Adjuvant Therapy of Cancer II*, Grune & Stratton, New York, pp 497–506.
78. Cunningham TJ et al: A controlled ECOG study of adjuvant therapy in patients with Stage I and II malignant melanoma, in SE Jones, SE Salmon (eds): *Adjuvant Therapy of Cancer II*, Grune & Stratton, New York, pp 507–517.
79. Wood WC et al: Randomized trial of adjuvant therapy for "high risk" primary malignant melanoma. *Surgery* 83:677, 1978.
80. Terry WD: Immunotherapy of malignant melanoma. *N Engl J Med* 303:1174, 1980.
81. Spitler LE, Sagebiel RA: A randomized trial of levamisole versus placebo as adjuvant therapy in malignant melanoma. *N Engl J Med* 303:1143, 1980.
82. Hilal EY et al: Surgical adjuvant therapy of malignant melanoma with *Corynebacterium parvum*. *Cancer* 48:245, 1981.
83. Blume MR et al: Adjuvant immunotherapy of high risk stage I melanoma with transfer factor. *Cancer* 47:882, 1981.
84. Au FC, Goldman LI: Isolation perfusion in limb melanoma: A critical assessment and literature review, in WH Clark Jr et al (eds): *Human Malignant Melanoma*, Grune & Stratton, New York, 1979, pp 295–308.
85. Benjamin RS: Chemotherapy of malignant melanoma. *World J Surg* 3:321, 1979.
86. Comis RL, Carter SK: Integration of chemotherapy into combined modality therapy of solid tumors. IV. Malignant meloma. *Cancer Treat Rev* 1:385, 1974.
87. Eilber FR, Isakoff W: High-dose methotrexate therapy for disseminated malignant melanoma. *Proc Am Assoc Clin Oncol* 17:262, 1976.
88. Dufour FD et al: High-dose methotrexate combined with DTIC for metastatic melanoma. *Proc Am Assoc Cancer Res* 19:360, 1978.
89. Bellet RE et al: Chemotherapy of metastatic malignant melanoma, in WH Clark Jr et al (eds): *Human Malignant Melanoma*, Grune & Stratton, New York, 1979, pp 325–351.
90. Creech OC et al: Treatment of melanoma by isolation-perfusion technique. *JAMA* 169:339, 1959.
91. Krementz ET, Creech OC Jr: Advances in the treatment of malignant melanoma. *Proc Natl Cancer Conf* 6:529, 1970.
92. Stehlin JS Jr: Hyperthermic perfusion with chemotherapy for cancer of the extremities. *Surg Gynecol Obstet* 129:305, 1969.
93. Stehlin JS Jr et al: Eleven years' experience with hyperthermic perfusion for melanoma of the extremities. *World J Surg* 3:305, 1979.
94. Stehlin JS et al: Melanomas of the extremities complicated by in-transit metastases. *Surg Gynecol Obstet* 122:3, 1966.
95. Morton DL et al: Immunological factors which influence response to immunotherapy in malignant melanoma. *Surgery* 68:158, 1970.
96. Goodnight JE, Morton DL: The role of immunotherapy in the management of patients with malignant melanoma. *World J Surg* 3:309, 1979.
97. Israel L et al: Effect of intranodular BCG in 22 melanoma patients. *Panminerva Med* 17: 189, 1975.

98. Sparks FC et al: Complications of BCG immunotherapy in patients with cancer. *N Engl J Med* 289:827, 1973.
99. Huvos AG et al: a clinicopathologic study of amelanotic melanoma. *Surg Gynecol Obstet* 155:917, 1972.
100. Elder DE et al: The surgical pathology of cutaneous malignant melanoma, in WH Clark Jr et al (eds): *Human Malignant Melanoma*, Grune & Stratton, New York, 1979, pp 55–108.
101. Kopf AW et al: *Malignant Melanoma*, Masson, New York, 1979, pp 159–161.
102. Ariel IM: Malignant melanoma of the female genital system: A report of 48 patients and review of the literature. *J Surg Oncol* 16:371, 1981.
103. Rutledge FN: Malignant melanoma of the vulva, in *Neoplasms of the Skin and Malignant Melanoma*, Year Book Medical, Chicago, 1976, pp 401–407.
104. Wanebo HJ et al: Anorectal melanoma. *Cancer* 47:1891, 1981.
105. Pickard LR, McBride CM: Anorectal melanoma, in *Neoplasms of the Skin and Malignant Melanoma*, Year Book Medical, Chicago, 1976, pp 443–451.
106. Houghton AN et al: Malignant melanoma of the skin occurring during pregnancy. *Cancer* 48:407, 1981.

SELECTED BIBLIOGRAPHY

Adam YG, Efron G: Cutaneous malignant melanoma: Current views on pathogenesis, diagnosis, and surgical management. *Surgery* 93:481, 1983.

Guiliano AE et al: Melanoma from unknown primary site and amelanotic melanoma. *Seminars in Oncology* 9:442, 1982.

Lee Y-T N: Noninvasive screening tests for metastatic melanoma: Rationale and results. *Am J Clin Oncol (CCT)* 6:225, 1983.

Petrelli NJ: Opinion: Lymph node dissection for stage I melanoma: The unresolved dilemma. *Cancer* 32:314, 1982.

Seigler HF (ed): *Clinical Management of Melanoma*. Martinus Nijhoff, The Hague, 1982.

Veronesi V, Cascinelli N: Response: Lymph node dissection for stage I melanoma: The unrsolved dilemma. *Cancer* 32:316, 1982.

43
SARCOMAS OF BONE AND SOFT TISSUE

Frederick R. Eilber

MALIGNANT TUMORS OF BONE (OSTEOSARCOMA)

Historical Aspects

Although the first description of osteosarcoma is lost in time, this disease was recognized and described in antiquity. Hug photographed and described the proximal humerus of an iron-age skeleton from Münsingen, Switzerland, which had all the characteristics of osteosarcoma.[1]

In 1786, Hunter clearly described an ossifying tumor of the distal femur of a young person that extended through the cavity of the bone and involved the adjacent musculature. The patient had an amputation, and autopsy 4 weeks later showed bilateral pulmonary metastases.[2] This description was the first convincing evidence of osteosarcoma as it is known today.

It was not until the early nineteenth century that this tumor justified its reputation as one of the most malignant and rapidly fatal neoplasms. Before that time, bone tumor pathology included all tumorous conditions of bone in one category. This confused pathology clearly was a disadvantage in terms of understanding the natural history of primary osteosarcoma, because the classifications included metastatic tumors to bone as well as primary infectious bone conditions. Ewing, in 1923, proposed classifications that separated the various tumorous conditions.[3] Tumors composed of tissues destined to become bone were categorized as primary bone tumors, and metastatic lesions were classified separately. In 1930, Phemister proposed separating chondrosarcoma from the general classification of bone tumors such as osteosarcoma because chondrosarcoma has a relatively benign clinical course.

The local surgical resections of primary osteosarcoma in the early 1900s resulted in failure of local tumor control, and patients quickly died. The dictum of amputation for primary tumor control was adopted and persists to this day.[4] The treatment regimen for osteosarcoma did not change much until the early 1970s, when, for the first time, chemotherapeutic agents were found that not only affected the clinical course but improved survival rates of patients with metastatic disease. These findings prompted many investigators to test the chemotherapeutic agents as adjuvant treatment immediately following amputation and, more recently, to test their use for preoperative treatment in an effort to avoid amputations.

Incidence, Epidemiology, and Etiologic Aspects

The American Cancer Society estimates that there are between 300 and 400 new cases of osteosarcoma diagnosed annually in the United States. The largest series of patients with osteosarcoma described in the literature comes from the Mayo Clinic. After a review of 600 cases, Dahlin clearly characterized the natural history of the disease.[5] Osteosarcoma occurs in the teenage population between the ages of 12 and 20 at the skeletal sites most responsible for growth—the distal femur, proximal tibia, and humerus, in that order of frequency. Even though it has been found in almost every bone in the body, it occurs at least 80 percent of the time at these three sites. In an unusual form, osteosarcoma can be multifocal, where it affects multiple bones simultaneously.[6] There are approximately 39 cases of primary multifocal osteosarcoma, with an average of 18 separate lesions per patient. Following the definitive treatment, or amputation, this disease invariably proceeds to pulmonary metastases in 80 to 90 percent of the patients within 6 months. Several autopsy series have indicated that the majority of these patients die from these pulmonary metastases rather than from metastases at any other site.[7]

Of patients with Paget's disease of bone, 0.9 percent develop osteosarcoma. Approximately 10 percent of those patients who have had advanced polyostotic disease for more than 10 years will develop subsequent osteosarcoma. This form of osteosarcoma appears to be a most virulent type; there are only three known survivors. Osteosarcoma has been described in large dogs, particularly Saint Bernards and Great Danes, but also is known to arise spontaneously in the mouse, cat, fox, reptile, and fish.[8]

There are no known etiologic causes for osteosarcoma. In animal tumor systems, it can be induced by hydrocarbons such as dibenzanthracene and methylcholanthrene. Viruses such as Moloney sarcoma virus can cause osteosarcoma in mice that can be transmitted.[9] However, in humans, the only known predisposing features appear to be Paget's disease and high-dose radiation therapy, probably in excess of 10,000 rads. For example, of 455 luminous dial painters, who are routinely exposed to radioactive substances, 26 developed osteosarcomas from 7 to 43 years after exposure.[10] When thorium was used as a diagnostic agent for tuberculosis, 14 in 53 patients developed osteosarcoma. More recently, studies indicate a 10 to 15 percent incidence of osteosarcoma in patients who received radiation for giant-cell tumors or Ewing's sarcoma, and in children treated with radiotherapy for rhabdomyosarcoma of the orbit. The latency period for development of osteosarcoma in these circumstances was approximately 6 to 8 years following high-dose radiation therapy.

Signs, Symptoms, and Attempts at Early Detection

Unfortunately, patients with these tumors do not present with any systemic symptomatology. Most patients with osteosarcoma present with pain in the affected extremity, and in the majority of patients the pain has been present for at least 3 to 4 months. Early evidence certainly can be obtained by x-ray examination because the radiographic characteristics of this tumor are destruction of bone, tumor bone formation, and periosteal reaction exemplified by Codman's triangle. Although serum alkaline phosphatase is elevated in patients with this disease, this finding is not useful as an early diagnostic technique because many teenagers have an elevated alkaline phosphatase without any sign or symptom of bone disease.

Diagnostic Techniques in Work-Up and Staging

The determining factor for a diagnosis of osteosarcoma is biopsy; either the needle biopsy or the open biopsy will suffice so long as enough uncrushed tissue is obtained for the pathologist to identify and characterize the tumor. The histologic hallmark of osteosarcoma is the malignant spindle cell producing osteoid. There are several histologically different types of osteosarcoma—chondroblastic, fibroblastic, telangiectatic osteosarcoma; parosteal osteosarcoma; and "osteosarcoma ordinaire." However, several studies indicate that although these different histologic patterns exist, they do not imply a difference in prognosis. The only exception would be the parosteal osteosarcoma that originates from the periosteum and/or cortex but does not invade the medullary cavity, and tends to occur in the posterior aspect of the distal femur in young women.[11] This tumor has much less metastatic potential than the other types. Also, recent reports suggest that telangiectatic osteosarcoma may have a worse prognosis.

Some precautions should be taken before the biopsy is performed. Either of the above techniques can be used, but if an incisional biopsy is done, the incision must be placed so that it can be encompassed entirely by the subsequent surgical procedure. In general, a longitudinal biopsy incision is required. Transverse incisions should be avoided. The biopsy should not involve the Codman's triangle, as this tissue is only reactive periosteum adjacent to the tumor, and this area seldom, if ever, contains tumor. The most appropriate place for biopsy is the soft-tissue extramedullary component of the tumor. Because these tumors can be extremely vascular, the biopsy should be performed in the operating room. For a time, physicians at the Mayo Clinic performed biopsies only at the time of the definitive surgical procedure. A tourniquet was placed proximal to the biopsy site to prevent potential dissemination of tumor cells during the biopsy procedure. However, results of these non-controlled trials showed that there was no advantage for patients who had the tourniquet technique, the immediately frozen biopsy section, and amputation over the patients who had a routine biopsy and a subsequent amputation. The incidence of subsequent disseminated disease, pulmonary metastasis, was the same.

Systemic evaluations of patients with osteosarcoma becomes a very important consideration. The recommended systemic evaluation should include routine CBC and blood chemistries for any changes, such as elevated alkaline phosphatase. Very few patients (less than 1 percent) with metastatic osteosarcoma will have metastases to the lymph nodes. But nearly all will have metastases to the chest. Therefore, standard chest x-rays are mandatory. Furthermore, studies in which the more sensitive technique of whole-lung tomography has been used indicated that 20 percent of patients with a normal chest x-ray will have metastatic disease. Additionally, the Mayo Clinic recently reported that whole-lung CAT scans revealed that 10 percent of their patients had nodular metastatic disease of the chest that was not apparent either on chest x-ray or whole-lung tomography.[12] Therefore, the present policy at UCLA includes chest x-rays and CAT scans of the chest for accurate initial staging of the extent of disease.

As far as the extent of the disease at the primary site is concerned, some authors advocate angiography to determine the extent of extramedullary growth. Experience at UCLA has shown that CAT scanning of the extremity provides a very valuable means for determining the extent of extramedullary involvement as well as the potential for examining the intramedullary canal for any evidence of "skip areas." Osteosarcomas originate within the medullary cavity of the long bones and spread longitudinally within the marrow cavity. They also destroy the adjacent cortex and have a propensity for extramedullary extension and direct invasion of adjacent muscles. Originally, the cartilaginous epiphyseal plate was thought to be a barrier to their spread within the bone, but pathologists reported that, in fact, the cartilage in no way prevented extension of the tumor. Enneking et al. demonstrated skip areas of the medullary canal of long bones in approximately 10 percent of patients with osteosarcoma.[13] For example, in longitudinal sections of bone, foci of osteosarcoma cells were found at a distance from the primary tumor with normal intervening marrow. However, several other studies contend that these skip areas occur in less than 6 percent of the patients.

Direct invasion of adjacent nerves and arteries rarely occurs. Bone scans are another useful diagnostic tool for examining the entire skeleton for any evidence of unusual isotope uptake. These scans also provide a means for careful examination of the involved primary bone to determine extramedullary extent and potential skip areas within the bone.

Therapeutic Options for Primary Treatment

Amputation one joint above the area of involved bone has been the treatment of choice for osteosarcoma. In order to encompass all the potential avenues of tumor spread, this surgical treatment includes any extramedullary involvement of adjacent muscles and any potential skip areas within the bone itself. The incidence of local recurrence has been reported to be less than 5 percent with this therapy. However, in a large series of patients, the Mayo Clinic performed transmedullary amputations for distal femoral lesions with the same local recurrence rate (5 percent) as reported for a series of hip disarticulations.[14] With the standard amputation technique, a primary tibial lesion required an above-the-knee (AK) amputation; a distal femoral lesion required a hip disarticulation or a high AK; and proximal femoral lesions resulted in a hip disarticulation or hemipelvectomy. Lesions of the humerus involved a shoulder disarticulation or intrascapular thoracic amputation. Despite these radical surgical procedures, the overall survival rate ranged between 15 and 35 percent. The usual cause for failure was not local recurrence but progressive pulmonary metastases, even with a normal chest x-ray at the time of diagnosis. For these reasons, there always has been considerable pessimism with any type of treatment for these tumors.

Cade et al. reported several trials in the 1940s and 1950s in which high-dose radiation therapy (6000 to 8000 rads) was given 6 months before amputation in an effort to improve these miserable survival rates.[15] They proposed to sterilize the tumor and then determine which patients would develop pulmonary metastases in order to avoid amputation in those who were already destined to die of their distant disease. Allen reported that with less than 10,000 rads, viable tumor cells were present in 10 to 15 percent of the selectively resected specimens.[16] Survival rates in several series in which this theory was applied were approximately the same as those of the primary amputation series, except that amputation was avoided in patients who were going to succumb early to their metastatic disease. The long-term complications of high-dose radiation in those patients who did not develop metastases but who had subsequent amputation were extremely high.

Limb Salvage

With the advent of effective chemotherapy and more aggressive surgical treatment for metastases to the lungs, several investigators began to reevaluate the necessity for amputation. It was evident that not all patients were going to die from their disease, and a more circumspect look at the treatment of the primary tumor was warranted. In 1974, a trial of preoperative therapy for osteosarcomas followed by local en bloc excision was initiated at UCLA. Intraarterial Adriamycin chemotherapy and rapid-fraction radiation preceded the surgical resection. The preoperative treatment was proposed to obtain sufficient tumor kill to allow a local surgical procedure. In a consecutive series of 35 patients treated with this protocol, tumor cell necrosis was observed in approximately 80 percent of the specimens compared with 5 percent necrosis in untreated specimens.[17] Rosen et al., at Memorial Hospital, employed only cycles of chemotherapy preoperatively to achieve approximately 50 percent tumor cell destruction.[18]

Operative procedures in this setting must maintain the basic principles of cancer surgery—wide excision of any previous biopsy scar and dissection of all tumor-involved tissue, including the adjacent muscle. All operations include tissue planes well beyond the reactive tumor capsule. Most investigators remove the bone at least 10 cm proximal to any gross radiographic or scan evidence of disease, but some investigators remove the entire bone. One very important consideration in the operative procedure involves the proximity of the tumor to the adjacent joint. In this instance, the entire joint and its capsule must be removed to prevent or to encompass any spread of tumor along the joint capsule.

Several different materials have been used for replacement of the large segments of resected bone. Basically, these materials fall into two categories: the cadaver allografts and the metallic endoprostheses. Although other investigators have reported fairly successful results with cadaver allograft replacements,[19,20] experience with 22 consecutive allografts at UCLA has been disappointing. Frequent fractures in the lower extremity and loosening of the intramedullary fixation in the upper extremity occurred in approximately 80 percent of the grafts. Repeated bone scans of the patients showed absolutely no incorporation of the nonviable grafts.

The metallic endoprosthesis has been a much more satisfactory replacement for the large bony defects. These prostheses are custom-made of Vitallium alloy, and fixation to contiguous normal bone is achieved with polymethacrylate cement. It is now possible to fabricate complete replacements of the femur and humerus, and to replace the entire knee and shoulder joint. The types of knee replacement include hinge-type joints, such as the Guepar and Waldius, the spherocentric ball-and-socket joint, and, most recently, the Kinomatic total knee design. The failure rate for the metallic endoprostheses has been considerably less than that of the cadaver allografts, even though there has been a major problem with loosening of the metallic segment at its fixation point with normal bone. Occasionally, less than 5 percent of the time, the prosthesis itself fractures. Replacement of bone for proximal tibial defects has been a major problem because it has not been consistently possible to reinsert the patellar tendon into the metallic endoprosthesis. In these instances, the alternative procedure of knee fusion may be performed by sliding bone grafts on long intramedullary rods that are inserted from the trochanter to the distal tibia, as originally described by Enneking and Shirley.[21]

There are defects that require no bony replacement. For example, bony replacement is unnecessary in the forearm, radius, or ulna or after large en bloc excisions of the fibula. Marcove and Rosen have reported an excision of the proximal humerus without replacement (so-called Tickoff-Lindberg procedure),[22] and large portions of the ilium, pubis, and ischium, including the acetabulum, have been removed with no bony replacement.[23] These patients can bear approximately 80 percent of their body weight on the extremity, with excellent knee and ankle motion but marked weakness on flexion against gravity at the hip.

The results of the series of patients who received the limb-salvage operation for their osteosarcomas have been extremely encouraging. Certainly there are considerable functional defects, mainly stiffness at the knee and potential late failure of metallic or cadaver allografts, but the local recurrence rate is less than 5 percent, a rate equal to that achieved by primary amputation (Table 43-1). Therefore, at the present time, the therapeutic options for treatment of primary osteosarcoma include amputation or limb salvage. All reports of successful limb-salvage procedures stress the need for some type

TABLE 43-1 Local Recurrence after Limb Salvage or Amputation for Osteosarcoma

Investigator	Institution	Number of patients	Number of limb salvage	Knee replacement	Number of amputations after replacement	Local recurrence		Follow-up months	Year reported
						Limb salvage	Amputation		
Marcove, Rosen	Memorial	66	64	Guepar	13 (19%)	8 (12.5%)	....	(1–67.5)	1980
Watts, Jaffe	Sidney-Farber	10	8	Guepar	2 (20%)	0 (0)	....		1978
Eilber, Morton	UCLA	36	36	Allograft, spherocentric	2 (5%)	1 (2%)	....	(3–54)	1980
Campanacci	Bologna, Italy	248	....	....	....	....	13 (5.2%)		1980

of preoperative therapy, either chemotherapy alone, or chemotherapy plus radiation.

Adjuvant Therapy

Prior to 1970, numerous chemotherapeutic regimens were prescribed for patients with metastatic osteosarcoma, but none achieved a response rate of more than 10 percent. However, by 1972, two drugs, high-dose Adriamycin and very high dose (200 mg/kg of body weight) methotrexate, were being tested in large-scale phase I clinical trials. Adriamycin, originally investigated by Tan et al.[24] and, in osteosarcoma, by Cortes et al., was administered in doses of 90 mg/m² divided over 3 consecutive days.[25] With an objective response rate of 40 to 50 percent, Cortes et al. were able to show a definite correlation between response and dose when more patients responded to higher doses of Adriamycin than to lesser doses of drug. Jaffe followed very high doses of methotrexate with citrovorum factor rescue and achieved an extremely high (40 to 50 percent) response rate in patients with metastatic osteosarcoma.[26] Although methotrexate had been used in the conventional dose, 50 mg/m², with little response, very large doses, 100 to 200 mg/kg, were successful. However, these high doses were possible only with adequate hydration and alkalization to prevent methotrexate toxicity. With the development of a method to monitor blood levels of methotrexate as it was cleared from the bloodstream, it was possible to determine the proper dosages of citrovorum which were necessary to bypass the metabolic block of methotrexate. With all these maneuvers, the clinical toxicity of methotrexate has been reduced to less than 5 percent.[27]

Combination chemotherapy for osteosarcoma was first reported by Sutow et al.[28] from the M. D. Anderson Hospital. These investigators achieved a very high response rate with the Compadri regimen (Cytoxan, L-PAM, Oncovin, and Adriamycin). Rosen et al. reported that the combination of Adriamycin, high-dose methotrexate, and Cytoxan produced a very high (60 percent) objective response rate for metastatic disease.[29]

With this background of high response rates for established metastatic disease, many investigators were encouraged to use these agents as adjuvants immediately following the primary surgical resection for patients with no evidence of metastatic disease. These various trials began around 1972, and their results are shown in Table 43-2.[30-39] The expected 15 to 20 percent disease-free rate at 3 years was dramatically increased to between 40 and 75 percent. The overall survival rate for these patients was markedly improved, but whether this improvement was due to adjuvant chemotherapy or to more aggressive surgical resections for pulmonary disease is still unclear. However, it is clear that the natural history of the disease has been altered by the early administration of chemotherapeutic agents.

Therefore, over the past 6 years, almost every investigator who treats patients with osteosarcoma has administered adjuvant chemotherapy of some type. No two programs are exactly alike, and very few have been performed as randomized, controlled trials. A review of the results of these numerous clinical trials of adjuvant chemotherapy clearly shows that a wide variety of treatment schemes with the single agents Adriamycin and high-dose methotrexate, as well as combination regimens, have been used. All of the trials, with the exception of the most recent reports from the Mayo Clinic, have relied on "historical controls" in order to evaluate the effectiveness of their adjuvant programs. The most successful clinical trial in terms of disease-free relapse appears to be that of Rosen et al. with the T7 and T10 protocol using high-dose methotrexate, Adriamycin,

TABLE 43-2 Results of Adjuvant Therapy for Osteosarcoma

Investigator	Institution	Drug	Number of patients	Percent disease-free	Follow-up median	Year reported
Sutow	M. D. Anderson	Compadri I Compadri II	36	47	4.0 years	1978[30]
Cortes	ALGB	Adriamycin	88	36	5.0 years	1979[31]
Fossati-Bellani	Milan	Adriamycin	19	47	23.0 months	1979[32]
Rosen	Memorial	T_4, T_5	54	50	4.0 years	1979[18]
		T_7–T_{10}	61	88	27.0 months	
Goorin	Sidney-Farber	MTX (1)	12	42	4.0 years	1980[33]
		MTX (2)	22	59	3.0 years	
		MTX (3)	30	78	19.0 months	
Rosenberg	NIH	MTX	39	38	27.0 months	1979[34]
Eilber	UCLA	Adriamycin, MTX, Cytoxan				1979[36]
		(1)	27	33	24.0 months	
		(2)		50		
Strander	Karolinska	Interferon	33	58	3.0 years	1979[37]
		None	33	37		
Taylor	Mayo	None (1)	29	20	5.0 years	1980[38]
		None (2)	43	40	5.0 years	
		None (3)	41	50	2.5 years	
Edmonson	Mayo	MTX, none	37	54	18.0 months	1980[39]

bleomycin, Cytoxan, and actinomycin D. Again, this trial employed historical controls, but the overall disease-free survival rate of 72 percent is truly impressive.

The reasons for the discrepancies in disease-free rates among these various trials are as diverse as the results. The possibilities include nonuniform staging criteria, differences in administration of total dosages (protocol violations), frequency of administration of the drugs, employment of different drug combinations, total duration of treatment, and, finally, possible variations in tumor histology.

Therefore, several investigators are now trying to answer the question of whether or not adjuvant chemotherapy is indicated in randomized prospective trials with nontreatment controls.

Follow-Up and Techniques for Early Identification of Recurrence or Metastases

Postoperative follow-up for patients with osteosarcoma usually includes monthly chest x-rays for 2 years and a monthly SMA-12 for changes in alkaline phosphatase levels. Whole-lung tomography and x-rays of the primary tumor site are usually performed once every 3 to 6 months and once every 2 months, respectively, if less than amputation has been performed. Clearly, the highest risk period is during the first 2 years. At the present time, with or without adjuvant chemotherapy, fully 80 percent of these patients who will have recurrence of their disease will do so within the first 2 years.

Therapeutic Options for the Treatment of Recurrences and/or Metastases

In the 1960s, several uncontrolled clinical reports suggested that surgical resection of metastatic pulmonary disease was possible for patients with metastatic osteosarcoma. The original reports were based on a 6-month observation period to ascertain if the metastases were truly confined to the chest. Amazingly, these trials showed that approximately 35 percent of the patients could be rendered disease-free by resection of their metastatic deposits. The eligibility criterion for resection included evidence of control of the primary lesion and no new metastases for 6 months. This latter concept was based on autopsy studies that showed that over 80 percent of the patients died from their metastatic disease in the chest.

In 1971, Morton et al. started systematically plotting the growth rates of the metastatic deposits.[40] In a retrospective analysis of 60 pulmonary resections, they observed that approximately 40 percent of the patients whose tumor doubling time was greater than 60 days could be rendered continually free of disease by wedge resection of their pulmonary metastatic deposits. However, those patients whose tumor doubling times were less than 60 days showed no improvement in overall survival rates or quality of life. A recent analysis of these studies revealed that neither bilateral disease nor multiple nodules were major determinants for operative success. However, pleural effusion, disease in hilar nodes, or a tumor doubling time of less than 60 days were contraindications for pulmonary resection. Very few patients who exhibited these signs or symptoms could be salvaged with the pulmonary wedge resections. Several studies have now confirmed a 35 precent disease-free rate after the pulmonary wedge resections for patients who fit these operative criteria. Thus, with a more aggressive attack on pulmonary metastases, the overall survival rate of patients with metastatic osteosarcoma has significantly improved, and pulmonary wedge resection now represents an accepted method of treatment for selected patients.[41,42]

Patients who are not candidates for surgical resection of their metastatic disease receive additional chemotherapeutic agents. For patients who have not received Adriamycin as an adjuvant, this drug is the treatment of choice and appears to be an absolute necessity for successful chemotherapeutic treatment. Different combinations of chemotherapeutic drugs have been tried, with very little success, in patients who were chemotherapy adjuvant failures. Recently, reports indicate that single-agent *cis*-platinum may have response rates as high as 20 to 30 percent, and many centers are now evaluating its use either as a single agent or in combination with Cytoxan and Adriamycin for those patients who failed on other adjuvant chemotherapy. Radiation therapy to symptomatic, localized metastases has been in some reports, effective for alleviating symptoms, but rarely results in long-term disease control.

Current Areas of Research and Prospects for the Future

As stated, there has been an improved overall survival rate for patients with osteosarcoma over the past 10 years. Although the exact reason for this is not yet apparent, the fact that it exists is unquestioned. It may be due to the more aggressive approach to the resection of pulmonary metastases, the early administration of effective adjuvant chemotherapeutic regimens, a combination of these two factors, or, finally, better staging with more sensitive CAT scanning of the chest. Whether because of one or all of these factors, the overall survival rate and disease-free intervals are markedly improved.

In order to answer the question of the efficacy of adjuvant chemotherapy, multiinstitutional trials conducted in a carefully controlled, randomized fashion are absolutely essential. Any one institution is unlikely to see more than 20 to 30 patients with this disease in a single year, certainly an insufficient number for randomized trials. Uniform staging criteria are an absolute necessity, as are uniform pathologic interpretations of the primary tumors. The experience of the Sidney-Farber Cancer Institute attests to this latter requirement.[43] Of the original 11 osteosarcoma patients treated with adjuvant high-dose methotrexate, there was disagreement in pathologic interpretation of the tumor type among the consultants in approximately 30 percent of the patients. Thus, a centralized pathology group who would be responsible for histologic diagnoses would seem to be very important before any further adjuvant trials are undertaken.

From all the available data, it appears that patients who have the limb-salvage-type procedures do as well as the patients who have primary amputations. Although there are complications for patients who have limb salvage, there are certainly complications for patients who have artificial limbs following amputation. Future research must produce better prosthetic replacements, and, hopefully, a porous metal can be developed that would allow for fibrous ingrowth of normal body tissues. At the present time, the surgical principles and techniques for local control with less than amputative surgery can be applied to the majority of patients with this disease. Whether these techniques prove to be advantageous for long-term function remains to be seen.

Future emphasis must be directed toward more sensitive staging techniques. Approximately 70 to 80 percent of the patients with the primary diagnosis of osteosarcoma will survive for at least 3 to 5 years following a surgical procedure. However, it is not yet possible to distinguish between those patients who are at high risk for recurrence and those who can be successfully treated with the surgical procedure alone. In order to prevent potential cardiac toxicity or other unknown problems associated with carcinogenic chemotherapeutic agents, it is highly desirable to be able to select out those patients who can be cured by a surgical procedure alone. The capability for determining the presence of micrometastases has certainly been improved with such imaging techniques as computerized axial tomography. However, even at its best resolution, this technique is limited to a tumor nodule approximately 3 mm or 10^5 cells. With the refinement of immunologic techniques, such as the measurement of circulating antigen in the serum and determination of excretion of urinary antigens as described by Huth et al.,[44] or by the ability to analyze the primary tumor for the presence or degree of production of alkaline phosphatase as reported by Thorpe et al.,[45] the unique markers that will separate those patients who require adjuvant treatment with chemotherapy from those who do not may become apparent.

SOFT-TISSUE SARCOMAS

Historical Aspects

It wasn't until the late 1800s and early 1900s that a clear distinction was made between neoplastic conditions of the soft tissue and other nonneoplastic conditions such as infectious disease. This separation required accurate histopathologic examination of those conditions which were, in fact, infectious and those which were neoplastic. The evolution of the microscopic examination was the determining factor. The several outstanding anatomists and pathologists who contributed to this development included Morgani and Rokatanski.

However, the terminology for describing these diseases was extremely confusing until Stout and Lattes, in 1940, classified the tumors according to their cells of origin.[46] A summary of their observations of 8686 tumors, 1349 of which were malignant, from Columbia University from 1906 to 1951 appears in the Armed Forces Institute of Pathology fasicle of 1966.[47]

At the present time, there are at least 60 different histologic types of soft-tissue sarcoma that apparently are distinct from one another. The most common malignant soft-tissue sarcomas and their benign counterparts are listed in Table 43-3. This extremely varied histologic spectrum may be simplified, since it appears that all of these tumors are derived from primitive mesenchymal cells and neuroectodermal tissue. It should be noted that certain portions of a particular tumor may contain well-differentiated cells and another section may be totally undifferentiated, making classification by origin very difficult when only small tissue samples are available. Furthermore, tissue culture studies show that these tumors have the potential for dedifferentiation into any of the soft-tissue elements—fat, blood vessels, nerves, muscle, or connective tissue. The advent of electron microscopy in the 1950s held great promise for clarifying the cell of origin of the soft-tissue sarcomas, but, unfortunately, only a very few tumor types were identified, usually those involving neurofibrils or cross-striations, leading to the classification of the neurosarcomas or rhabdomyosarcomas, respectively. Finally, the most recent historical event has been the classification of these tumors by histopathologic grading. Basically, this system disregards to a large extent the cell of origin and looks instead at the number of mitoses per high-power field. With this classification system, the ultimate prognosis of these tumors can be assessed more accurately.

Originally, the primary treatment for these tumors was local surgical excision with drainage, a technique that resulted in a high local recurrence rate. Operative procedures were extended to include a radical local excision that reduced the local recurrence rate somewhat and, finally, to the amputative procedures that have been employed since the 1930s.

Incidence, Epidemiology, and Etiologic Aspects

Malignant tumors of the soft parts comprise less than 1 percent of all malignancies diagnosed annually. According to the American Cancer Society, there are approximately 5500 new cases diagnosed per year, and 2500 persons will die of these tumors annually.[48]

Soft-tissue sarcoma can arise in any age group, although it has a peak incidence in children and again in adults between the ages of 45 and 50 years. The majority of the childhood tumors are rhabdomyosarcomas or undifferentiated tumors in the head and neck area. Soft-tissue tumors in the adults tend to arise most frequently in the extremities, with the retroperitoneum

TABLE 43-3 Classification of Tumors of Soft Somatic Tissues *

Type of tissue	Malignant tumors	Benign tumors

1. Fibrous tissue	a. Fibrosarcoma
	b. Dermatofibrosarcoma protuberans
		a. Fibroma
		b. Keloid
		c. Fibromatosis
		   (1) Dupuytren's contracture; plantar fibromatosis
		   (2) Desmoid tumor of the abdominal wall
		d. Dermatofibrosarcoma protuberans
		e. Nodular fasciitis

2. Undifferentiated mesenchyme	a. Myxoma b. Mesenchymoma	a. Myxoma b. Mesenchymoma
3. Adipose tissue	a. Liposarcoma	a. Lipoma (solitary and multiple) b. Congenital diffuse lipomatosis
4. Smooth muscle	a. Leiomyosarcoma	a. Leiomyoma b. Dermatoleiomyoma
5. Striated muscle	a. Rhabdomyosarcoma	a. Rhabdomyoma b. Granular-cell myoblastoma
6. Synovial mesothelium	a. Synovial sarcoma (malignant synovioma)	a. Giant-cell tumor of tendon sheath b. Synovial xanthoma
7. Blood and lymph vessels	a. Angiosarcoma b. Lymphangiosarcoma c. Kaposi's idiopathic sarcoma d. Hemangiopericytoma e. Granulation-cell sarcoma	a. Hemangioma b. Lymphangioma c. Cystic hygroma d. Glomus tumor e. Hemangiopericytoma
8. Peripheral nerves	a. Malignant neurilemmoma b. Malignant schwannoma and malignant neuroepithelioma	a. Neurofibroma b. Schwannoma (neurilemmoma or perineurial fibroblastoma) c. Neurofibromatosis (von Recklinghausen's disease)
9. Heterotopic bone and cartilage	a. Osteogenic sarcoma b. Chondrosarcoma	a. Myositis ossificans
10. Unknown origin	a. Malignant granular-cell myoblastoma b. Alveolar soft-part sarcoma (malignant organoid granular-cell myoblastoma)	a. Granular-cell myoblastoma

* Modified from a classification originally proposed by Stout.[46,47]

affected much less often. The head and neck is the area affected the least. The sex incidence is approximately equal between male and female.

From all available evidence, these tumors develop de novo and not by dedifferentiation from preexisting conditions. A possible exception may be von Recklinghausen's disease; approximately 10 to 12 percent of patients with multiple benign neurofibromas will develop neurofibrosarcomas.[49] There are reports of malignant soft-tissue tumors arising in granulating wounds or burn scars or following high-dose radiation injury. Lymphangiosarcomas have been known to develop in the chronically lymphedematous extremities of some patients, although the exact incidence is well below 10 percent.[50] In animal tumor systems, soft-tissue sarcomas occur spontaneously, but they can be induced by carcinogens such as dibenzanthracene, methylcholanthrene, or Moloney sarcoma virus. The sarcoma virus can be transmitted between animals.[51]

Signs, Symptoms, and Attempts at Early Detection

Malignant soft-tissue tumors often present as very large, asymptomatic local masses. Growth is relatively slow in most patients and very seldom causes any early symptomatology. Often these tumors are detected only when the mass has become very large. If contiguous areas, such as nerves or vascular structures, are compromised, the major symptoms are paresthesia, lymphedema, or venous engorgement. However, most of the symptoms can be related to the effect of the mass with its compression of normal structures. Fully 80 percent of patients seen with soft-tissue sarcomas report its presence for at least 6 months, and almost all patients give a history of injury or trauma to the area in which the subsequent mass either did not resolve or gradually increased in size. These masses are commonly misdiagnosed as chronic hematomas or muscle sprains. Although xerograms, CAT scans, and arteriograms have value in terms of identifying the anatomic site and extent of the mass, their value for establishing diagnosis is unproved. Although neovascularity can be clearly associated with these tumors, it is not pathognomic, as benign conditions such as myositis ossificans can have neovascularity.

Diagnostic Techniques, Work-Up, and Staging

The sine qua non for diagnosis of a large, firm, growing mass is biopsy. The type of biopsy is important because adequate uncrushed tissue must be obtained in order for the pathologist to make a diagnosis of malignancy and to determine the grade of the malignancy and possible tumor type. The preferred biopsy techniques include needle biopsy, "skinny-needle" aspiration, or incisional biopsy. The "excisional" biopsy should be avoided because it disturbs a large number of tissue planes, which compromises additional treatment. If the incisional technique is used, it is very important that the operative scar is placed so that it can be widely excised during the definitive surgical procedure. Transverse biopsy incisions are never indicated in an extremity.

These tumors tend to spread in a three-dimensional fashion—longitudinally, laterally, and penetrating—but their greatest microscopic extension occurs longitudinally along fascial planes up to 6 or 7 cm beyond all gross palpable disease. Metastasis to regional lymph nodes is extremely uncommon, except with childhood rhabdomyosarcoma or adult synovial-cell sarcoma, both of which have an incidence of regional lymph node metastases of approximately 10 to 15 percent. The majority of these tumors metastasize to the lungs, and approximately 80 percent of the patients who die from soft-tissue sarcoma do so from either an uncontrolled primary tumor and/or its metastases in both lungs.[52] The remaining 20 percent of the patients will have metastases to other sites, with the order of decreasing frequency being to liver, bone, additional soft tissue, and, rarely, to the central nervous system.

Therefore, along with the biopsy, the systemic evaluation of all patients with soft-tissue sarcoma must include careful evaluation of regional lymph nodes, a chest x-ray, whole-lung tomograms and/or CAT scans of the chest, and routine SMA-12 for any gross chemistry abnormalities, even though there is no specific enzyme abnormality indicative for soft-tissue sarcomas.

Prognosis for patients with soft-tissue sarcomas is a function of the histopathology and the anatomic site and extent of disease. Because these tumors occur so rarely, an accurate histologic diagnosis has been a problem. A task force, the American Joint Committee on Staging and End Results Reporting, was appointed in an effort to establish some guidelines. This committee evaluated the end results of surgical therapy for 1215 patients treated since 1968.[53] It soon became clear that among the pathologists there was marked disagreement (at least 40 percent of the time) regarding the tissue of origin of many of the tumor specimens. The disagreement was most apparent when the undifferentiated and poorly differentiated tumors were examined. Finally, agreement was achieved if the number of mitoses per high-power field, or grade of the tumor—i.e., grade 1 having the least number of mitosing cells and grade 3 the highest mitotic activity—was used as the basis for histologic diagnosis in approximately 90 percent of the patients. When this system was applied in a retrospective review, it became obvious that the tissue of origin was of less importance for prognosis than was the grade of the tumor (the mitotic figures per high-power field). Therefore, it was reasonably easy to standardize a reproducible system for assessing the grade of the tumor. This staging system was developed based on the TNM system with the addition of G for grade. After classifying the tumors and evaluating the outcome of treatment for all the patients by the surgical procedure, the committee was able to stage these sarcomas as clinical-pathologic stage I through IV. Tumors of stage I have an 80 to 90 percent 10-year survival rate and are the low-grade, low-mitotic-rate tumors; those of stage II, determined by grade 2, have a 60 percent overall survival rate; clinical-pathologic stage III—largely grade 3 tumors or with nodal metastases—have a 25 percent rate; and stage IV—any tumor of any grade if it involves soft tissue and directly invades nerves and blood vessels, or involves distant metastases—has a 3 percent survival rate. Thus, this clinical-pathologic staging system is both useful and reproducible. It should be emphasized that this system obviates the necessity for exact histologic classification of the tumor and substitutes a more objective evaluation of its malignancy using the number of mitoses per high-power field. The only exception to the original grading system has been with the definition of rhabdomyosarcomas and synovial-cell sarcomas as grade 3. An updated classification by the American Joint Committee suggests that there are grade 1 synovial-cell sarcomas which do not carry the dire prognosis of the grade 3 tumors.

Therapeutic Options for Primary Treatment

Surgical excision of soft-tissue sarcomas is the treatment of choice. In order to accomplish the goal of completely eradicating the local tumor, the surgeon must consider all potential three-dimensional avenues of tumor spread. The proximal extension, the microscopic extension of the tumor for 10 cm along the fascial planes, must also be considered. Local excision of gross tumor with narrow margins of less than 1 cm surrounding the tumor cannot be classified as complete excision. A 90 percent local recurrence rate is the result for patients treated with such narrow excisions.[54] Failure in these instances was directly related to the mistaken impression that these tumors are surrounded by a true capsule.

MUSCLE-GROUP EXCISION

Well-differentiated tumors arising in a particular muscle group or fascial plane can be treated successfully if the excision includes the entire soft-tissue part from origin to insertion and encompasses the adjacent fascial planes.[55] For example, when a tumor arises in the sartorious, an operation that completely encompasses this muscle from its origin to insertion is appropriate. However, because 85 percent of these tumors do not arise in a recognizable muscle group or anatomic location, the muscle-group-excision concept is of limited clinical value.

AMPUTATION

Amputative procedures are necessary for tumors that are deep-seated; involve multiple fascial planes, and major blood vessels and nerves; and directly invade bone. The techniques for amputation are well known, but the decision for the level of the amputation is derived from the patterns of tumor spread. Above-the-knee amputations are usually performed for tumors originating in the calf, and below-knee amputations are reserved for more distal tumors in the foot. Hip disarticulations are performed for proximally placed tumors in order to remove the origin of the muscle grouping. Intrascapular thoracic amputations or hemipelvectomy may be required for those tumors that are proximally placed in the axilla, proximal thigh, or groin for the same reason, the removal of muscles.

The overall results for patients treated by surgery alone is a 90 percent local recurrence rate with local excision, approximately 50 percent recurrence rate for muscle-group excision, and a local recurrence rate reduced to 30 percent with amputation or complete en bloc excision.[55,56] For soft-tissue sarcomas that arise in the retroperitoneum, surgical treatment is often difficult and usually results in failure.[57] The principles used for excision of these tumors in the extremity are equally valid for those in the retroperitoneum. Complete excision of the tumor and its soft part from origin to insertion is almost impossible in the retroperitoneum; however, wide surgical excision is still the accepted method of therapy, and best results have been achieved with a margin of at least 3 cm.

HEAD AND NECK SARCOMAS

Malignant sarcomas of the head and neck, although rare, present anatomic problems for complete surgical extirpation similar to those of the retroperitoneum. Complete en bloc excision is seldom possible because of the very narrow space limits associated with the head and neck. In addition, the cosmetic deformities from massive resection in this area often make aggressive surgical therapy of the head and neck untenable. Local recurrence rates, even with radical excision, are between 60 and 70 percent, reemphasizing the fact that a wide surgical excision with adequate surgical margins is not possible in most patients.[58]

RADIATION THERAPY

Radiation therapy by itself is of marginal value for treatment of this group of tumors. When used alone, it results in a local recurrence rate of between 80 and 85 percent and a survival rate of less than 15 percent.[59]

Suit et al. and Lindberg et al. examined the role of modern radiation therapy as an adjunct, either preceding or immediately following, surgical excision of soft-tissue sarcomas.[60] Patients with primary tumors located distal to the elbow or distal to the knee who received complete local excision of all gross tumor with at least 1-cm margins were given high-dose postoperative radiation therapy in the range of 5000 to 6000 rads. With this combination, the local recurrence rate for patients with extremity sarcomas was less than 10 percent, whereas the predicted local recurrence rate after surgery alone was at least 80 percent. These results are believed to be equal to those achieved with muscle-group excision and radical amputation. When those patients with more proximally placed tumors (thigh, upper arm, or head and neck) were treated in an identical fashion, local control was much less, with local recurrence rates of 30 to 40 percent. This combination therapy has not been of benefit for tumors of the retroperitoneum because of the radiotherapy dose limitations to intraabdominal structures.

The rationale for high-dose radiation therapy of the involved extremity was based on the hypothesis that even though gross tumors were radioresistant, microscopic disease was radiosensitive. This reasoning was borne out by the results of the clinical trials. For patients with primary tumors of the forearm or calf, complete excision followed by postoperative radiation therapy appears to be a reasonable alternative to amputative surgery. The advantage of maintaining a potentially functional extremity makes the choice an attractive one.

Reports from Stehlin indicate that isolated limb perfusion with actinomycin D and L-PAM has achieved beneficial responses in selected patients with extremity sarcomas.[61,62] The addition of hyperthermia to this perfusion regimen may augment the activity of the actinomycin D. Even so, this technique cannot be used to perfuse the head and neck, the retroperitoneum, or proximal thigh. The basic concept for this treatment is to perfuse the tumor in situ, wait for a proscribed period of time, and then perform the definitive wide local excision of the perfused area. A summary of these experiences in a nonconsecutive series indicates that again there is a 30 percent local recurrence rate.

Eilber et al. recently described a preoperative treatment regimen in which intraarterial Adriamycin was followed by rapid-fraction radiation and radical en bloc excision.[63] In a consecutive series of 110 patients with high-grade, mostly proximally placed, tumors, they achieved an overall local control rate greater than 95 percent with a follow-up of 36 months. This extremely encouraging local tumor control resulted in a functional extremity for over 90 percent of these patients.[64]

Finally, an excellent local control rate of 90 percent has been achieved in soft-tissue sarcomas of children with vincristine, actinomycin D, Cytoxan, (VAC) and concomitant radiation once the diagnosis is made by biopsy.[65]

A Summary of Appropriate Treatment

EXTREMITY TUMORS

Since the majority of extremity tumors in children are rhabdomyosarcomas, the most appropriate treatment appears to be the chemotherapy with VAC; then complete surgical excision, if possible; followed by postoperative radiation therapy and continuing cycles of chemotherapy.

Adults with extremity tumors present a different set of factors that must be considered before a decision can be made on the appropriate therapy. Patients with well-differentiated localized tumors can be adequately treated by radical en bloc excision or amputation. Clinical-pathologic stage I or II tumors do not appear to require either local radiation or systemic chemotherapy preoperatively because the local recurrence rates for these grades are less than 10 percent and survival rates are higher than 60 percent. However, patients with stage III or IV tumors, or tumors that are well-differentiated but proximally placed where adequate excision is compromised, do require additional therapy following or preceding surgical procedure. These adjunctive therapies include postoperative radiation or preoperative chemotherapy and radiation therapy.

HEAD AND NECK TUMORS

The appropriate therapy for patients with head and neck sarcomas has yet to be defined. The results of surgical treatment alone certainly indicate that a better treatment method needs to be found. Several centers are using preoperative Adriamycin and radiation therapy followed by surgical excision in an effort to improve the local control rate.

RETROPERITONEAL SARCOMAS

Complete radical excision of retroperitoneal sarcomas should be performed where it is technically possible regardless of the histologic grade of the tumor. This aggressive surgical therapy in many instances requires resection of major blood vessels, such as the vena cava and the aorta, in order to achieve adequate tissue margins. Radiation therapy does not seem to be applicable in these areas since the 5000 to 6000 rads required for tumor kill is not possible without significant damage to adjacent bowel, kidney, and liver.

Adjuvant Therapy

Although soft-tissue sarcomas have a history of extreme resistance to chemotherapeutic agents, several new drugs have been used effectively. Adriamycin induces a beneficial response in approximately 30 to 40 percent of patients with disseminated disease.[66] Combination chemotherapy with CYVADIC (Cytoxan, vincristine, Adriamycin, and imidazole carboxymide), as originally described by Gottlieb and Benjamin et al.[67] produces an even higher response rate of approximately 45 percent. Chemotherapy with vincristine, actinomycin D, and Cytoxan (VAC) has achieved a 90 percent response rate for metastatic childhood rhabdomyosarcomas.[65] Recently, cis-platinum or the CAP regimen (cis-platinum, Adriamycin, and Cytoxan) has achieved a response rate of between 35 and 40 percent.

The current trials of adjuvant chemotherapy for soft-tissue sarcomas are extremely limited and the results are preliminary. These reported trials are listed in Table 43-4.[68–73] It must be mentioned that each of the reported trials used a different combination of chemotherapeutic agents and none included a nontreatment control arm. All of the drug regimens contain Adriamycin as the common denominator, and there is no convincing evidence that polychemotherapy is more beneficial. A randomized prospective trial at M. D. Anderson Hospital, in fact, showed that patients treated with the CYVADACT (Cytoxan, vincristine, Adriamycin, actinomycin) regimen fared somewhat worse than patients treated by surgery alone. Recently, the Mayo Clinic reported a trial suggesting that there may be some benefit for patients treated with a polychemotherapy regimen vs. surgery alone in a group of soft-tissue sarcomas in a randomized prospective fashion; however, this trial is very new and it is not clear whether the short-term benefit will be

TABLE 43-4 Soft-Tissue Sarcoma: Adjuvant Chemotherapy Results

Series	Adjuvant	Number of patients	Local recurrence, %	NED*, %	Follow-up, months
1. AJCS	None	439	?	35	60[53]
2. Memorial	ALOMAD	34	25	58	18[68]
3. M. D. Anderson	CYVADACT	27	12	66	24[69]
4. UCLA	Adriamycin, methotrexate	29	0	86	22[70]
5. NIH	Adriamycin, Cytoxan, methotrexate	49	11	88	16[71]
6. Farber	Cytoxan, Adriamycin, DTIC	19	?	79	28[72]
7. Mayo	Vincristine, Cytoxan, DACT	30	10	68	24[73]

* Continued free of disease.

borne out with time. Furthermore, the local recurrence rate in this series was at least 30 percent.

Follow-Up Techniques for Early Identification of Recurrence and/or Metastases

The usual and appropriate method for follow-up includes physical examination once a month for careful assessment of the primary treatment site. CAT scanning of the primary tumor site also may play a role in the search for recurrence of the deep-seated masses. Monthly chest x-rays for 1 year and bimonthly for the second year appear to be indicated, as well as whole-lung tomograms or a CAT scan once every 3 to 6 months. Routine blood chemistry examinations are necessary, but routine bone scans, liver scans, or brain scans are not warranted unless there is physical complaint by the patient or an abnormality in the blood chemistry.

Therapeutic Options for the Treatment of Recurrences and/or Metastases

The metastatic pattern of soft-tissue sarcomas to the lungs is very similar to osteosarcoma. In noncontrolled trials, approximately 35 percent of patients with an isolated metastasis and a disease-free interval of greater than 6 months could be rendered long-term survivors with wedge resection of their pulmonary disease. The criterion of a tumor doubling time greater than 60 days appears to be a valid marker for patients with metastatic soft-tissue sarcomas if the primary tumor is adequately controlled and if pleural effusion and/or hilar adenopathy is absent. The results of a series appear to indicate that approximately 20 percent of the patients can be rendered long-term survivors by pulmonary resection alone.[74]

The usual treatment for patients with nonoperable metastatic disease is chemotherapy. In patients who have not received Adriamycin, either as a single agent or in combination, treatment should be at high dosages, at least 90 mg/m^2 divided over 2 days. The addition of *cis*-platinum, or a *cis*-platinum regimen, appears to provide an additional 20 percent response rate in patients for whom other chemotherapy regimens have failed.

The value of whole-lung irradiation or radiotherapy to pulmonary metastases or isolated bony metastases appears to be beneficial. Although response of these sites to radiation is extremely high, approaching 80 to 90 percent, the duration of remission or improvement in overall survival rate is not much more than 3 to 5 months. However, the quality of life for the patient is certainly improved by local radiation therapy.

Current Areas of Research and Prospects for the Future

The rarity of soft-tissue sarcoma, its confusing histopathology, and the many treatment schemes available tend to obscure which patients should be the subjects of future trials. Those patients with grade III or clinical-pathologic stage III to IV soft-tissue sarcomas who have a very high local recurrence rate, as well as the potential for metastases, appear to be the group in greatest need. Clearly, answering the very important questions of which local treatment method is best for local control and whether an adjuvant regimen is necessary will require a multiinstitutional trial, such as the trial for treatment of rhabdomyosarcoma, and a trial to evaluate the efficacy of single-agent adjuvant Adriamycin chemotherapy for soft-tissue sarcomas. An essential requirement of these trials is the creation of a central pathology review panel to establish a pathologic uniformity that can be applied to patients across the country.

Other determinants of risk for recurrence, other than histopathologic criteria, are under study. The clonogenic assay, in which biopsied tumors are placed into short-term tissue culture and then exposed to various drugs, has great potential for selecting the drug with the greatest activity for each individual tumor. Additionally, it appears that the rapidity of the colony growth may be an indicator of metastatic potential and possibly a more accurate reflection of grade than mitoses per high-power field.

Finally, efforts to define the specific or tumor-associated antigens of these tumors and relate the patient's immunologic response to these antigens is a vital field of study. The presence or absence of circulating immune complexes and the presence of a sarcoma-associated antigen in the urine as reported by Huth et al. appear to hold promise for selecting those patients at high risk for recurrence who could benefit most from adjuvant chemotherapy.[75]

REFERENCES

1. Brothwell D: *Diseases in Antiquity*, 1967.
2. Livingstone E, Livingstone S (eds): *Descriptive Catalogue of the Pathological Series in the Hinterian Museum of the Royal College of Surgeons of England*, pt I, London, 1966, case 78.

3. Coley BL: *Neoplasms of Bone,* Hoeber, New York, 1949.
4. Coley BL, Harrold C: Fifty-nine cases of osteosarcoma with 5 years survival. *J Bone Jt Surg Am Vol* 32:307, 1950.
5. Dahlin DC, Coventry MB: Osteogenic sarcoma: A study of 600 cases. *J Bone Jt Surg Am Vol* 49:101, 1967.
6. Amstutz HC: Multiple osteogenic sarcoma. Metastasis or multicentric? Report of 2 cases and review of the literature. *Cancer* 24:923, 1969.
7. Farrell JT: Pulmonary metastases: A pathological, clinical, roentgenologic study based on 78 cases seen at necropsy. *Radiology* 24:444, 1935.
8. Owen LN: *Bone Tumors in Animals and Man,* Butterworth, London, 1969.
9. Finkel MP et al: Virus induction of osteosarcomas in mice. *Science* 151:698, 1966.
10. Sabanas AO et al: Postradiation sarcoma of bone. *Cancer* 9:528, 1956.
11. Unni KK et al: Parosteal osteogenic sarcoma. *Cancer* 37:2466, 1976.
12. Simm FR, Pritchard DJ: Computer tomography for the detection of pulmonary metastasis in patients with osteogenic sarcoma. *Proc Am Assoc Cancer Res* 21:148, 1980.
13. Enneking WF, Kagan A: "Skip" metastases in osteosarcoma. *Cancer* 36:2192, 1975.
14. Campanacci M, Laus M: Local recurrence after amputation for osteosarcoma. *J Bone Jt Surg Br Vol* 62:201, 1980.
15. Cade S: Osteogenic sarcoma: A study based on 133 patients. *J R Coll Surg Edinburgh* 1:79, 1955.
16. Allen CV, Stevens KR: Preoperative irradiation for osteogenic sarcoma. *Cancer* 31:1364, 1973.
17. Morton DL et al: Limb salvage from a multidisciplinary treatment approach for skeletal and soft tissue sarcomas of the extremity. *Ann Surg* 184:268, 1976.
18. Rosen G et al: Primary osteogenic sarcoma: The rationale for treatment with preoperative chemotherapy and delayed surgery. *Cancer* 43:2163, 1979.
19. Mankin HJ et al: Massive resection and allograft transplantation in the treatment of malignant bone tumors. *N Engl J Med* 294:1247, 1976.
20. Parrish FF: Allograft replacement with all or part of the end of a long bone following the excision of a tumor: Report of 21 cases. *J Bone Jt Surg Am Vol* 55:1, 1973.
21. Enneking WF, Shirley PD: Resection artholesis for malignant and potentially malignant lesions about the knee using an intramedullary rod and local bone grafts. *J Bone Jt Surg Am Vol* 58:223, 1967.
22. Marcove RC, Rosen G: En bloc resections for osteogenic sarcoma. *Cancer* 45:3040, 1980.
23. Eilber FR et al: Internal hemipelvectomy—Excision of the hemipelvis with limb preservation: An alternative to hemipelvectomy. *Cancer* 43:806, 1979.
24. Tan C et al: Adriamycin—An antitumor antibiotic in the treatment of neoplastic disease. *Cancer* 32:9, 1973.
25. Cortes EP et al: Amputation and Adriamycin in primary osteosarcoma: 5-year report. *Proc Am Soc Clin Oncol* 18:297, 1977.
26. Jaffe N: Recent advances in the chemotherapy of metastatic osteosarcoma. *Cancer* 30:1627, 1972.
27. Isacoff WH et al: High-dose methotrexate therapy of solid tumors: Observations relating to clinical toxicity. *Med Pediatr Oncol* 2:319, 1976.
28. Sutow WW et al: Multidrug chemotherapy in primary treatment of osteosarcoma. *J Bone Jt Surg Am Vol* 58:629, 1976.
29. Rosen G et al: High-dose methotrexate with citrovorum factor rescue and Adriamycin in childhood osteosarcoma. *Cancer* 33:1151, 1974.
30. Sutow WW et al: Multidrug adjuvant chemotherapy for osteosarcoma: Interim report of the Southwest Oncology Group Studies. *Cancer Treat Rep* 62:265, 1978.
31. Cortes EP et al: Adjuvant therapy of operable primary osteosarcoma—Cancer and leukemia group B experience. *Recent Results Cancer Res* 68:16, 1979.
32. Fossati-Bellani F et al: Adriamycin in the adjuvant treatment of operable osteosarcoma. *Recent Results Cancer Res* 68:25, 1979.
33. Goorin A et al: Adjuvant chemotherapy and limb salvage procedures for osteosarcoma. A seven-year experience. *Proc Am Assoc Cancer Res* 21:472, 1980.
34. Rosenberg SA et al: Treatment of osteogenic sarcoma, I: Effect of adjuvant Adriamycin and methotrexate after amputation. *Cancer Treat Rep* 63:739, 1979.
35. Eilber FR et al: Is amputation necessary for extremity sarcomas? A seven-year experience with limb salvage. *Ann Surg* 192:431, 1980.
36. Jasmin C: Adjuvant therapy of osteogenic sarcoma: G.T.E.O.R.T.C. Working Party Group, in S Jones, S Salmon (eds): *Adjuvant Therapy of Cancer,* Grune & Stratton, New York, 1979.
37. Strander H et al: Adjuvant interferon treatment of human osteosarcoma. *Recent Results Cancer Res* 68:40, 1979.
38. Taylor WF et al: Osteogenic sarcoma experience at the Mayo Clinic 1963–1974, in W Terry, D Windhort (eds): *Immunotherapy of Cancer—Present Status of Trials in Man,* Raven Press, New York, 1978.
39. Edmonson JH et al: Postsurgical treatment of primary osteosarcoma of bone—Comparison of high-dose methotrexate versus observation: Preliminary report. *Proc Am Assoc Cancer Res* 21:476, 1980.
40. Morton DL et al: Surgical resection and adjunctive immunotherapy for selected patients with multiple pulmonary metastases. *Ann Surg* 178:360, 1973.
41. Holmes EC et al: The surgical management of pulmonary metastasis. *Semin Oncol* 4:165, 1977.
42. Van Dongen JA, van Slooten EA: The surgical treatment of pulmonary metastases. *Cancer Treat Rev* 5:29, 1978.
43. Frei E et al: Adjuvant chemotherapy of osteogenic sarcoma: Progress and perspectives. *J Natl Cancer Inst* 60:3, 1978.

44. Huth JF et al: Development of an enzyme immunoassay to detect and quantitate tumor-associated antigens in the urine of sarcoma patients. *Cancer* 47:2856, 1981.
45. Thorpe WP et al: Prognostic significance of alkaline phosphatase measurements in patients with osteosarcoma receiving chemotherapy. *Cancer* 43:2178, 1979.
46. Stout AP: Sarcomas of the soft tissue. *Cancer* 11:210, 1961.
47. Stout AP, Lattes R: Tumors of the soft tissue, in *Atlas of Tumor Pathology*, 2d ser, fas I, AFIP, Washington, D.C., 1967.
48. *Cancer Statistics*, American Cancer Society, 1976.
49. Wander JV, Das Gupta TK: Neurofibromatosis, in *Current Problems in Surgery* V:XIV, Year Book, Chicago, 1977.
50. McBride CM et al: Angiosarcoma in the lymphedematous limb. *South Med J* 62:378, 1969.
51. Moloney JB: Biological studies on a lymphoid-leukemia virus extracted from Sarcoma 37, I: Origin and introductory investigations. *J Natl Cancer Inst* 24:933, 1960.
52. Farrell JT: Pulmonary metastases: A pathologic, clinical, roentgenologic study based on 78 cases seen at necropsy. *Radiology* 24:444, 1935.
53. Russell WO et al: A clinical and pathological staging system for soft tissue sarcoma. *Cancer* 40:1562, 1977.
54. Bowden L, Booher RJ: The principles and techniques of resection of soft parts for sarcoma. *Surgery* 44:963, 1958.
55. Martin RG et al: Soft tissue tumors: Surgical treatment and results, in *Tumor of Bone and Soft Tissue*, Year Book, Chicago, 1965.
56. Shiu MH et al: Surgical treatment of 297 soft tissue sarcomas of the lower extremity. *Ann Surg* 182:597, 1975.
57. Cody HS et al: The continuing challenge of retroperitoneal sarcomas. *Cancer* (in press).
58. Farr HW: Soft tissue sarcomas of the head and neck. *Am J Surg* 122:714, 1971.
59. Gilbert HA et al: Soft tissue sarcomas of the extremities: Their natural history, treatment and radiation sensitivity. *J Surg Oncol* 7:303, 1975.
60. Suit HD et al: Management of patients with sarcoma of soft tissue in an extremity. *Cancer* 31:1247, 1973.
61. Stehlin J: Isolated limb perfusion. *Surg Gynecol Obstet* 129:305, 1969.
62. Stehlin JS Jr: Regional chemotherapy for soft tissue sarcomas, in *Tumors of Bone and Soft Tissue*, Year Book, Chicago, 1965.
63. Eilber FR et al: Preoperative intraarterial Adriamycin and radiation therapy for extremity soft tissue sarcomas: A clinicopathologic study, in *Management of Primary Bone and Soft Tissue Tumors*, Year Book, Chicago, 1977.
64. Eilber FR et al: Is amputation necessary for sarcomas? A seven-year experience with limb salvage. *Ann Surg* 192:431, 1980.
65. Maurer HM et al: The intergroup rhabdomyosarcoma study: A preliminary report. *Cancer* 40:2015, 1977.
66. Tan C et al: Adriamycin—An antitumor antibiotic in the treatment of neoplastic disease. *Cancer* 32:9, 1973.
67. Gottlieb JA et al: Chemotherapy of sarcoma with a combination of Adriamycin and dimethyltriazeno-imidazole carboxamide. *Cancer* 30:1632, 1972.
68. Sordillo P et al: Adjuvant chemotherapy in adult soft part sarcomas with ALOMAD. *Proc Am Soc Clin Oncol* C-187:353, 1978.
69. Lindberg RD, Murphy WK: Adjuvant chemotherapy in the treatment of primary soft tissue sarcomas, in *Management of Primary Bone and Soft Tissue Tumors*, Year Book, Chicago, 1977.
70. Eilber FR et al: A clinicopathologic study: Preoperative intraarterial Adriamycin and radiation therapy for extremity soft tissue sarcomas, in *Management of Primary Bone and Soft Tissue Tumors*, Year Book, Chicago, 1977.
71. Rosenberg SA et al: Prospective randomized evaluation of the role of limb-sparing surgery, radiation and adjuvant chemoimmunotherapy in the treatment of adult soft tissue sarcomas. *Surgery* 84:62, 1978.
72. Antman KH et al: Effect of adjuvant chemotherapy for localized soft tissue sarcoma. *Proc Am Assoc Cancer Res* 21:141, 1980.
73. Edmonson JH et al: Reduced hematogenous metastasis in patients who receive systemic chemotherapy following excision of soft tissue sarcoma. *Proc Am Assoc Cancer Res* 21:476, 1980.
74. Huth JF et al: Pulmonary resection for metastatic sarcomas. *Am J Surg* 140:9, 1980.
75. Huth JF et al: Development of an enzyme immunoassay to detect and quantitate tumor-associated antigens in the urine of sarcoma patients. *Cancer* 47:2856, 1981.

SELECTED BIBLIOGRAPHY

Rosenberg SA et al: The treatment of soft-tissue sarcomas of the extremities. Prospective randomized evaluations of (1) limb-sparing surgery plus radiation therapy compared with amputation and (2) the role of adjuvant chemotherapy. *Ann Surg* 196:305, 1982.

Sears HF (ed): Soft tissue sarcomas. *Sem Oncol* 8:129–240, 1981.

Suit HD et al: Preoperative radiation therapy for sarcoma of soft tissue. *Cancer* 47:2269, 1981.

Suit HD: Soft tissue sarcomas: The role of radiation therapy. *Hosp Pract* 17:114, 1982.

44

HODGKIN'S DISEASE AND THE NON-HODGKIN'S LYMPHOMAS

Mark R. Green   *Joan F. Kroener*

Hodgkin's disease and the non-Hodgkin's lymphomas constitute about 3 to 4 percent of all newly diagnosed cancers seen in the United States each year. Despite this relatively small percentage, these neoplasms have been the focus of enormous academic interest and extensive investigative research. During the past three decades, our knowledge of the natural history and pathobiology of these lesions has vastly increased. Rigorous staging has led to greater awareness of the possible variations of clinical presentation and pathologic extent of disease. Treatment capabilities have exploded. With major technical advances and sophisticated application in radiation oncology, plus the advent of the entire field of combination chemotherapy, potentially curative therapy is available for a majority of Hodgkin's and non-Hodgkin's lymphoma patients. For those in whom cure is not yet highly likely, significant palliative benefit can be achieved. The promise of further progress in this entire area for the decade to come is high.

HODGKIN'S DISEASE

Historical Perspective

In 1832, Dr. Thomas Hodgkin described clinical data and postmortem findings of seven patients with enlarged lymph nodes and splenomegaly.[1] He was convinced that the process was not inflammatory but rather a proliferation inherent in the nodal tissues themselves. Dr. Hodgkin did not attempt to link his own name with the process he described. However, some 33 years later another English physician, Samuel Wilks, described a series of 10 cases of lymphadenopathy and splenic enlargement. Having become aware of Dr. Hodgkin's earlier writing, Wilks referred to the condition as Hodgkin's disease. In the last third of the nineteenth century, numerous European pathologists described giant, multinucleated cells in the nodal material of Hodgkin's disease patients. These cells were more completely characterized just around the turn of the century by both Sternberg and Reed, whose names have been associated with the pathognomonic cell of Hodgkin's disease since that time. In the 1930s and 1940s Jackson and Parker[2] developed the first widely utilized, all-inclusive, histopathologic classification of Hodgkin's disease, dividing the condition into three pathologic subtypes. Over the ensuing 25 years further contributions to the pathologic description of Hodgkin's disease emphasized the need for major revamping of the Jackson and Parker classification system. In the early 1960s, Lukes and coworkers[3] proposed a six-entity classification for Hodgkin's disease. This system was further modified in 1965 to include the four pathologic categories recognized today.

Epidemiology

The etiology of Hodgkin's disease remains uncertain. Extensive research has been done on a possible infectious etiology. This consideration of an infectious cause for Hodgkin's disease is stimulated by several characteristics of the disorder which are clearly recognized. The clinical and pathologic features are consistent with infection (fever, sweats, adenopathy, splenomegaly, weight loss, elevated sedimentation rate, leukocytosis, reactive infiltrate in involved nodes, granuloma formation). There is alteration of the immune status. Epidemiologic data on social class, age, and geographic distributions of Hodgkin's disease are consistent with an infection-related epidemiologic model.

In developed countries the incidence of Hodgkin's disease is clearly bimodal. In these areas the disease is infrequent in children under age 10. Incidence rises rapidly in later adolescence, and has its first peak in the mid to late twenties. Subsequently the incidence falls until after age 45, when the rate of new cases begins again to rise slowly. This second upslope in incidence then continues into the seventh and eighth decades. In underdeveloped areas of the world, a different distribution of Hodgkin's cases is seen for the younger age groups. There is a markedly increased percentage of all cases seen in children under 15 and only a very modest further increase in incidence in the late teens and twenties. The rising incidence in cases in the older (greater than 45 years of age) segment of the population is similar to the developed-country (e.g., United States) pattern. As geographic areas evolve from underdeveloped to developed, the pattern of incidence of Hodgkin's cases shifts as well: there is an overall increase in cases appearing, and the cases among individuals less than 45 years of age become focused in the early-adult range.

Other characteristics of Hodgkin's populations have been identified which focus on a possible infectious etiology for the disease. Childhood social environment appears to play some role. An only child has a substantially increased statistical risk of Hodgkin's disease, while in children from large sibships, the individual risk per child is below the average. For later children within a large sibship, the risk is particularly low. In developing societies, the general level of home hygiene correlates inversely with Hodgkin's disease incidence—the better the general sanitation, the higher the risk of the disease among children in the household. All these factors appear to have their impact only on the early peak of Hodgkin's disease cases. The late rise in cases after age 45 appears relatively similar across societal groups.[4]

Epidemiologists have drawn parallels between these characteristics of Hodgkin's epidemiology and the patterns previously seen in paralytic polio. It has been suggested that Hodgkin's disease may represent some form of aberrant or exaggerated host response to a common infectious agent. When there is widespread exposure to very young individuals, the host response leading to emergence of clinical Hodgkin's disease is less frequent than when somewhat older children are similarly exposed.[5] Given the differences in histology and clinical presentation of cases in the older age groups, and the failure of the older cases to show major variations across economic, geographic, and social strata, it is possible that the etiology of Hodgkin's cases in the early modal peak may be different than that of those occurring after age 45.

The hypothesis that Hodgkin's disease is related to an infectious agent does not imply direct contagion. The exposure leading to the disease may well have occurred long before the disease process is manifested clinically. In addition, most other individuals may have been exposed to the responsible infectious agent long before and already handled that exposure in the more routine fashion. Some provocative studies have suggested a link between adolescent or early-adult social groupings and a high incidence of Hodgkin's disease. Such a relationship has not been substantiated in large groups carefully studied with appropriate techniques. Specific investigations of high-risk populations of medical professionals fail to reveal any increased incidence of Hodgkin's disease based on a high rate of exposure to Hodgkin's disease patients.[6]

The Epstein-Barr virus, already associated with infectious mononucleosis, Burkitt's lymphoma, and nasopharyngeal carcinoma, has been studied extensively as the possible etiologic agent in Hodgkin's disease. Titers of Epstein-Barr virus–related antibody are higher in Hodgkin's patients than in matched controls. Large populations of patients confirmed to have infectious mononucleosis have shown an increased risk of subsequently developing Hodgkin's disease. Whether these factors reflect a direct causal relation between Epstein-Barr virus infection and later Hodgkin's disease remains to be further pursued.

Pathologic Classification

The variation in microscopic appearance of nodal tissue involved by Hodgkin's disease has been recognized for a century. Once the diagnostic cell was clearly described by both Sternberg and Reed, pathologists began to subdivide Hodgkin's disease into histologic subtypes based both on the frequency and appearance of the diagnostic cells and on the accompanying cellular infiltrate and background stroma. Since Reed-Sternberg–like cells can be seen in entities other than Hodgkin's disease, the presence of both these diagnostic cells and the appropriate cellular surroundings must be confirmed in order to make the diagnosis of Hodgkin's disease.

Jackson and Parker[2] divided Hodgkin's disease cases into three subcategories—granuloma, paragranuloma, and sarcoma—based on histologic appearance (see Table 44-1). Each was correlated to some degree with clinical presentation and subsequent natural history. Paragranuloma cases were characterized as usually of limited extent at diagnosis, with an indolent course and often prolonged survival despite minimal available treatment. Hodgkin's sarcoma, on the other hand, was highly aggressive with a very limited natural history. Hodgkin's granuloma encompassed the middle ground. The most useful aspect of the Jackson-Parker scheme was its ability to define natural history and prognosis for the slowly progressive paragranuloma cases and the highly malignant Hodgkin's sarcoma. Unfortunately, the number of cases fitting the paragranuloma and sarcoma subtypes was small, at most 10 to 20 percent of all Hodgkin's cases, leaving the large majority of patients in the middle ground of Hodgkin's granuloma. This latter group was obviously heterogeneous both clinically and pathologically, limiting the clinical applicability of the Jackson and Parker classification.

In 1965, a large group of experts on Hodgkin's disease met at Rye, New York, to discuss all aspects of the disease. A committee on nomenclature in Hodgkin's disease, chaired by Dr. Robert Lukes,[7] proposed a new histologic classification for Hodgkin's disease, subsequently known as the Rye classification. Four distinct histologic subtypes of Hodgkin's disease were enumerated: lymphocytic predominance, nodular sclerosis, mixed-cellularity, and lymphocytic depletion (see Table

TABLE 44-1 Histopathologic Classifications of Hodgkin's Disease

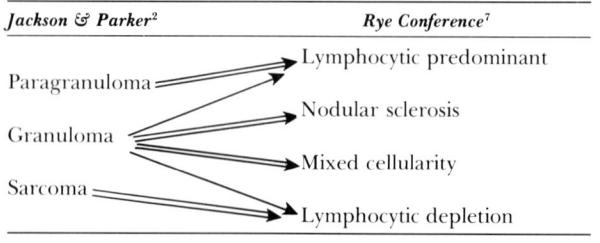

TABLE 44-2 Histologic Characteristics of Hodgkin's Disease Subtypes

Lymphocytic predominant
Obliteration of normal architecture: cellular infiltrates of normal-appearing small lymphocytes and benign histiocytes. Classic Reed-Sternberg cells infrequent. May have subtle nodularity. Variant Hodgkin's cells (L&H variant) may be numerous.

Nodular sclerosis
Nodal tissue divided by frequent bands of mature collagen. Cellular population usually a mixture of eosinophils, plasma cells, lymphocytes. Occasional Reed-Sternberg cells. Lacunar-cell variant characteristic. "Cellular phase" may lack collagen.

Mixed-cellularity
Nodal architecture usually obliterated. Mixed background population of eosinophils and plasma cells. Reed-Sternberg cells frequent. Atypical mononuclear cells seen along with lymphocytes and histiocytes.

Lymphocytic depletion
Nodal architecture effaced. Reed-Sternberg cells abundant. Disorderly fibrosis present. Lymphocyte infiltration minimal.

44-2). Each category had well-defined histologic characteristics and implied certain features of natural history. Prior to the availability of highly curative radiation and chemotherapy, these subcategories implied notable differences in expected survival. In recent years the differences in survival, based on the histologic subtypes, have diminished substantially.

The frequency of the different subtypes of Hodgkin's disease varies widely from series to series. Lymphocytic predominant lesions, including nearly all paragranuloma cases of Jackson and Parker, make up 10 to 15 percent of cases. Lymphocytic depletion, analogous to the Hodgkin's sarcoma category, is responsible for another 5 to 15 percent. The frequency of nodular sclerosis is highly variable, 30 to 70 percent, though review of cases suggests that a true incidence closer to the high side of the range is probably valid. Mixed-cellularity histology is present in 20 to 40 percent of cases.

Reproducibility of the Rye classification has been studied on several occasions; the interpretations made on nodal tissue by individual institutional pathologists and a lymphoma pathology review panel were compared. Overall concurrence in the diagnosis of Hodgkin's disease is high, over 90 percent. However, classification into subtypes is far less congruent, especially in the subcategories other than nodular sclerosis. Part of the difficulty in subclassification of Hodgkin's disease cases has been ascribed to the quality of available pathologic material. Another variable is the failure of Hodgkin's disease to develop strictly "by the book." Tissues with transitional characteristics of more than one subtype are occasionally seen. Evolution of the histologic subtype of Hodgkin's disease has been documented in studies of serial biopsies. Progression of histology almost always moves toward the more malignant subtypes. Nodular sclerosis histology, again distinct from other subtypes, shows less tendency to undergo evolution.[8]

Multiple biopsy specimens obtained essentially concurrently (e.g., diagnostic node biopsy soon followed by exploratory laparotomy) usually show congruence of histologic appearance. In some nodular sclerosis cases, differences in the degree of sclerosis may occur in material from different sites, but one is usually able to classify all the material as belonging to the nodular sclerosis subtype.

Staging

The subdivision of all possible presentations of a given malignancy into a limited number of meaningful specific categories, or stages, is crucial to advancing knowledge about the disease. The widespread use of a single staging system permits investigators to define homogeneous groups for evaluation of natural history and response to therapy. It allows for comparison of different therapies applied to similar populations. Once validated, an effective staging system can at once direct the diagnostic workup, be correlated with the most appropriate type of therapy, and imply prognosis.

In Hodgkin's disease, the currently accepted staging classification was devised in 1971 during a symposium held at the University of Michigan. This staging system, known as the Ann Arbor Classification,[9] represents only a modest evolution of the staging classification agreed to 7 years before during the Rye conference.

The Ann Arbor system for staging Hodgkin's disease includes two subcomponents, one or both of which may be defined. These are the *clinical stage* and the *pathologic stage*. In the era of the staging laparotomy, these are often not the same.

Clinical stage (CS) is the extent of disease as defined by the history, physical examination, roentgenographic and isotope studies, laboratory tests, and the initial diagnostic biopsy. Palpable splenomegaly is sufficient to define clinical spleen involvement. Liver enlargement and an abnormal alkaline phosphatase level, an abnormal liver scan plus one abnormal liver chemistry test, or two or more abnormal liver function studies (in the absence of other obvious cause for such abnormalities) is considered sufficient for clinical liver involvement. In addition to clinical staging, biopsy evaluation of specific tissues utilizing invasive techniques provides information on the pathologic stage (PS) (see Table 44-3). The patient's clinical and pathologic stages are written with a Roman numeral (I to IV) to indicate extent of disease. Subscripts following this number stage define the actual presence or absence of tumor involvement documented by biopsy of specific tissues or organs. An organ or tissue may be listed as involved (+) or not involved (−) in the pathologic stage only if specifically evaluated by biopsy.

Each patient's clinical or pathologic classification is defined further by the presence or absence of specific disease-related symptoms. These symptoms include unexplained fever greater than 38°C, night sweats, and weight loss greater than 10 percent of total body weight in the 6 months preceding the diagnosis. Patients with any or all of these symptomatic complaints are said to have "B" symptoms. Patients without these symptoms are "A."

The concept of "E" lesions (extralymphatic extension) in Hodgkin's disease staging is included in the Ann Arbor classification (see Table 44-4). This refers to situations in which extension of tumor from a lymph node or group of lymph nodes infiltrates a contiguous extralymphatic site to a limited enough degree that both

TABLE 44-3 Tissues Sampled during Pathologic Staging

Abbreviation	Meaning
N +/−	Biopsied node *other than* initial diagnostic tissue is/is not involved.
H +/−	Liver biopsy is/is not involved.
S +/−	Spleen removed and is/is not involved.
M +/−	Marrow aspirate or biopsy is/is not involved.
P +/−	Pleural biopsy or pleural fluid by cytology is/is not involved.
O +/−	Osseous tissue (not marrow cavity) is/is not involved.
D +/−	Skin biopsy is/is not involved.
L +/−	Lung parenchyma is/is not involved.

TABLE 44-4 Ann Arbor Staging Classification for Hodgkin's Disease

Stage	Sites of Disease Involvement
I	Involvement of a single lymph node region (I) or of a single extralymphatic organ or site (I_E)
II	Involvement of two or more lymph node regions on the same side of the diaphragm (II) or localized involvement of an extralymphatic organ or site and of one or more lymph node regions on the same side of the diaphragm (II_E)
III	Involvement of lymph node regions on both sides of the diaphragm (III), which may also be accompanied by localized involvement of extralymphatic organ or site (III_E) or by involvement of the spleen (III_S), or both (III_{SE})
IV	Diffuse or disseminated involvement of one or more extralymphatic organs or tissues with or without associated lymph node enlargement
"B" symptoms	(1) Unexplained weight loss of >10% of body weight in 6 months preceding diagnosis; (2) unexplained fever >38°C; (3) night sweats

SOURCE: Carbone.[9]

the lymph node group and the extralymphatic extension can be included in a single radiation therapy field with curative intent. The decision to define this extranodal extension as E rather than as disseminated disease (stage IV) tests the clinical judgement of the staging physician, since it is not more clearly specified in the Ann Arbor classification. A second use of the E lesion concept is applied to the infrequent occurrence of an isolated extranodal site of Hodgkin's disease (for example, in lung or bone), which is designated I-E. The Ann Arbor system does stipulate that liver and bone marrow disease are never considered E lesions. Any involvement of these organs must be classified as stage IV.

The major groupings within the Ann Arbor classification are based on the extent of nodal disease and the presence or absence of extralymphatic dissemination. Stage I disease involves a single node or group of nodes, while stage II involves two or more nodal groups on the same side of the diaphragm. Stage III disease requires nodal involvement on both sides of the diaphragm without extranodal spread, while in stage IV disease there is diffuse or disseminated involvement of one or more extralymphatic organs, almost always associated with nodal involvement as well. Within the staging system, the spleen is considered lymphatic tissue, and splenic involvement carries the same impact on overall stage as any other subdiaphragmatic nodal site. By the same token, involvement of Waldeyer's ring or the thymus is considered lymphatic involvement. All of Waldeyer's ring is considered one nodal area, while the thymus is considered part of the mediastinal lymphoid tissue.

As a practical example, consider a 43-year-old man with a 3-week history of nightly temperatures of 38.4 to 38.8°C and frequent night sweats. A left cervical node is the only abnormality on physical exam and the chest x-ray is normal. The node biopsy is read as mixed-cellularity Hodgkin's disease. Workup for infradiaphragmatic disease reveals a normal lymphangiogram and normal liver function studies. The patient is then considered a clinical stage CS I-B, because only one site of disease has been identified. The patient then undergoes a laparotomy for more definitive pathologic staging. At surgery, multiple iliac and paraaortic nodes are sampled, all of which are negative. The spleen is removed and found to contain Hodgkin's disease. Wedge biopsies of both lobes of the liver are negative. An intraoperative bone marrow biopsy is also free of tumor. Following surgery the patient's pathologic stage is definable as PS III-$B_{S+\ N-\ H-\ M-}$. Had the entire laparotomy been negative for tumor, the pathologic stage would have been equal to the clinical stage but all the subscripts associated with the pathologic stage (PS I-$B_{S-\ N-\ H-\ M-}$) would have been indicative of the operative staging procedures undertaken.

Recent modifications of the Ann Arbor staging classification have been proposed to further subdivide stage III cases. In this modification, nodal involvement in the "upper abdomen"—spleen, splenic hilum, celiac axis, and porta hepatis—is called III_1 while involvement of nodal tissue elsewhere in the abdomen, with or without upper-abdominal disease, would be considered III_2. The value of this subclassification of stage III cases in terms of directing therapy and reflecting prognosis remains controversial.

Staging Evaluation

A "standard" staging workup in a patient with biopsy-proven Hodgkin's disease was proposed at the Ann Arbor meeting in 1971.[10] New techniques have been developed (e.g., ultrasonography, CT scanning) since that time. However, the final place of this new technology in the evaluation of patients with Hodgkin's disease remains thus far uncertain. Required procedures in every patient include (1) the initial biopsy demonstrating Hodgkin's disease; (2) a careful history specifically identifying the presence or absence of "B" symptoms, and inquiring about possible use of anticonvulsant medications; (3) a detailed physical examination with specific attention to all nodal groups, including Waldeyer's ring, and the presence or absence of hepatosplenomegaly or bone tenderness;(4) laboratory hemogram, sedimentation rate, and chemistry panel including hepatic and renal function studies plus an alkaline phosphatase determination; and (5) radiographic studies including a posteroanterior and lateral chest x-ray and bipedal lymphangiography.

Percutaneous bone marrow biopsy has become part of nearly all Hodgkin's evaluations. However, it is very infrequently positive in early-stage, asymptomatic patients. According to the guidelines from the Ann Arbor meeting, it is required only in patients who manifest (1) an evaluated alkaline phosphatase level; (2) unexplained depression of hemoglobin, white count, or platelet count; (3) x-ray or bone scan evidence of osseous abnormalities; or (4) clinical stage III or IV disease. It is probably warranted as well in all symptomatic patients and in those with mixed-cellularity or lymphocytic depletion histology.

Additional staging procedures are appropriate in specific patients. Whole-lung tomography or chest CT scanning should be considered in any patient whose plain chest film is not *completely* normal. These procedures may help to define the extent of intrathoracic involvement and aid in distinguishing between E lesions or stage IV disease in the pulmonary parenchyma. These techniques appear substantially superior to isotope scanning (i.e., gallium 67) for demonstrating the true character of intrathoracic pathology.

Staging below the diaphragm remains an area of controversy. Clinical evaluation of the spleen by palpation is of limited value. One-quarter to one-third of clinically negative spleens can be pathologically documented to contain tumor on careful sectioning. Similarly, one-third or more of clinically positive (palpable) spleens will be uninvolved pathologically.[10,11] False-positive and false-negative rates for lymphangiography are somewhat less discouraging. The accuracy of carefully performed lymphangiograms is in the area of 80 to 90 percent. Totally normal or grossly positive studies are rarely found to be misleading when evaluated by laparotomy. On the other hand, more subtle abnormalities within normal-sized or minimally enlarged nodes may be due to a variety of reactive changes. These changes can be misinterpreted by the less experienced lymphangiographer and lead to errors in clinical staging.[13]

One clear limitation of lymphangiography is its inability to opacify a number of nodal groups in the abdomen. Mesenteric and porta hepatis nodes are not filled with lymphangiogram dye. This is of limited consequence, however, because these sites are rarely involved by Hodgkin's disease. On the other hand, splenic hilar and high-celiac nodes will also remain invisible following lymphangiography. Unfortunately, these nodes are involved by Hodgkin's disease in a substantial pecentage of all patients with intraabdominal involvement. Obviously the lymphangiogram provides no information about splenic involvement.

Lymphangiography dye will remain present for up to 18 months or longer. The opacified nodes can be easily followed with repetitive KUBs, an accurate technique for measuring responses to therapy when the opacified nodes are initially involved. If the nodes are initially negative, early Hodgkin's relapse may be identified by nodal enlargement. After prolonged intervals, a majority of the dye will be eluted. If further evaluation of these retroperitoneal nodes is required subsequently, a second lymphangiogram may be performed without substantial change in technical difficulty or diagnostic accuracy.

After nearly two decades of experience with lymphangiography, its role as a staging tool in Hodgkin's disease remains secure. Three other imaging procedures have been suggested to complement or supplant lymphangiographic evaluation of retroperitoneal nodes. The first, gallium-67 scanning, has a few strong proponents, but by and large is not considered a useful staging adjunct. Ultrasound and CT scanning may have more utility in this regard. In selected settings such as failure to obtain a technically adequate lymphogram or where high-celiac disease is suspected, these tests may be very helpful. However, since their resolution is low, these tests will not be helpful in deciding whether architecturally abnormal but normal-sized nodes identified by the lymphangiogram contain Hodgkin's disease. Thus far, neither ultrasound nor CT scanning has been shown to be very helpful in demonstrating limited splenic or hepatic involvement. As further technical refinements in these procedures are made, their roles in the routine staging of Hodgkin's disease patients will likely need to be reconsidered.

Pathologic evaluation of Hodgkin's disease involvement below the diaphragm is required whenever treatment decisions may be altered by the findings. Two techniques of obtaining important tissue samples have been utilized in pathologic staging. One is peritoneoscopy with multiple directed liver biopsies. The other is exploratory laparotomy.

Peritoneoscopy has been utilized extensively in some centers to determine the presence of liver involvement when there is already clinical evidence of disease below the diaphragm. Investigators at the National Cancer Institute (NCI) have suggested that peritoneoscopy with multiple directed needle biopsies is as effective as open liver biopsy in demonstrating liver involvement with Hodgkin's disease.[14] The procedure is easier to perform than formal laparotomy and has far less morbidity and essentially no mortality. It is clearly limited in yield, however, providing no information about the retroperitoneal nodes and only a gross description of the size and surface appearance of the spleen. While its accuracy in assessing liver involvement may be high, the overall low yield of peritoneoscopy has been responsible for its failure to gain wide following as a staging procedure in most Hodgkin's disease patients.

The use of exploratory laparotomy as an investigative procedure in Hodgkin's disease staging was initiated in the late 1960s. A major benefit of extensive experience with this procedure has been to define patterns of intraabdominal involvement in Hodgkin's disease and to correlate treatment approaches with outcome in patients in whom the total extent of disease was as fully defined as possible at the time of initiation of therapy. Currently, staging laparotomy has moved from the research setting to an important role in routine staging of certain individuals with Hodgkin's disease. It should be employed whenever the findings at surgery will alter the extent of radiation therapy to be administered or when the findings will make chemotherapy rather than radiation therapy the primary modality of treatment. With more recent movement toward combined-modality treatment in a greater percentage of patients with Hodgkin's disease, especially those with "bulky" stage II disease or stage III_2A disease, the need for staging laparotomy to define possible sites of occult intraabdominal disease has become more limited.

A large laparotomy experience has been reported by the group from Stanford. In one Stanford series,[15] 50 of 272 patients (18.2 percent) had their final pathological stage altered by laparotomy. In 48, the stage was increased, while in only 2 (4 percent) did downstaging result from the surgical procedure. (This rate of downstaging is somewhat lower than that reported in smaller series.) Upstaging to pathologic stage III occurred equally frequently in clinical stage I, stage IIA, and stage IIB (19 to 22 percent) patients. Most of the upstaging occurred because of the demonstration of occult splenic involvement. Falsely negative lymphangiograms were distinctly infrequent. Early data from the Stanford laparotomy experience had suggested that right cervical or right supraclavicular node involvement was much less frequently associated with subdiaphragmatic involvement than left neck or left supraclavicular disease. This correlation has not been confirmed either by subsequent data from Stanford or by other institutions.[16]

Staging laparotomy provides a number of small benefits for subsequent management of Hodgkin's patients apart from an accurate determination of extent of disease. Adequate radiation of the spleen requires a generous port covering the left upper quadrant. This port overlaps the left lung base and also at least the upper pole of the left kidney. Removal of the spleen will obviate radiation damage to these particular structures. Movement of the ovaries toward the midline can be accomplished during laparotomy. Such placement allows protection during subsequent radiation and lessens the risk of sterility following radiation therapy. Whether or not splenectomy is associated with less white count and platelet count toxicity during subsequent chemotherapy remains controversial.

The morbidity of staging laparotomy is modest, and surgical mortality is extremely uncommon. However, episodes of overwhelming sepses from encapsulated organisms are well-recognized in the postsplenectomy period, especially in children and teenagers. The increased risk of this syndrome has led to a rethinking of routine splenectomy in staging for Hodgkin's disease. In most cases, splenectomy has been retained. In some settings, long-term postsurgical prophylactic antibiotics or pneumococcal vaccine have been administered. The true utility of these techniques in controlling this infrequent but often lethal complication remains incompletely defined.

The actual staging operation to be performed in Hodgkin's disease patients has been carefully described.[17] Preoperative review of the lymphangiogram directs attention to suspicious or equivocal areas of nodal involvement. At surgery, all nodal groups are carefully evaluated from the celiac axis to the low paraaortic nodes. Particular scrutiny for tumor spread to mesenteric or porta hepatis nodes is required, since these areas will be missed or underdosed in standard Hodgkin's disease radiation portals. Wedge biopsies of the liver are taken from both lobes. The spleen is removed along with the splenic hilar nodes, and clips are placed on the splenic pedicle.

The amount of nodal dissection required during staging laparotomy depends to some degree on the presence or absence of splenic involvement. Therefore, once the spleen is removed, it should be immediately sectioned by the pathologist using the technique of "bread loafing"—making multiple sections through the entire spleen at intervals of just a few millimeters to define gross pathologic involvement with Hodgkin's disease. If splenic involvement is noted, limited biopsy of paraaortic nodal tissue is sufficient. If the spleen is grossly negative, several of the most suspicious nodes from different nodal groups should be removed. Clips should be placed at all biopsy sites as well as around all masses of involved nodal tissue. The clips aid in radiation field planning and help in following changes in tumor bulk during and after therapy. They may be particularly useful in following large nodal masses not opacified adequately by the lymphangiographic contrast.

At the completion of the staging procedure, most patients undergo an open bone marrow biopsy taken from the anterior iliac crest through a separate incision. This specimen is substantially larger than that obtained through core needle biopsies and will occasionally demonstrate previously unrecognized bone marrow involvement.

Clinical Presentations of Histologic Subtypes

Characteristic clinical patterns at presentation can be identified for each of the histologic subtypes of Hodgkin's disease. While such patterns are not distinct enough to obviate specific aspects of the staging workup, they are constant enough to be reasonably easy to profile.

Lymphocytic predominant patients often present with disease limited to one peripheral node or localized group of nodes. Appropriate staging will reveal disease of stage III extent in a minority of cases. Extranodal involvement or B symptoms are distinctly uncommon with this histology. As for Hodgkin's disease as a whole, there is a moderate male predominance among lymphocytic predominance cases. The age range, while broad, tends to exclude patients over the age of 50. The natural history of lymphocytic predominance disease is usually indolent, with long-term survival the rule even prior to the availability of current therapeutic approaches.

Nodular sclerosis is the most distinct category among the Hodgkin's disease subtypes. Clinical presentations characteristically involve cervical and/or supraclavicular adenopathy combined with chest x-ray evidence of anterior mediastinal tumor, occasionally of massive proportions. Most patients with E (extralymphatic extension) lesions will have nodular sclerosis histology. While a majority of fully staged nodular sclerosis patients will have limited disease (stage I or II) above the diaphragm, a significant minority will have splenic or retroperitoneal node involvement as well. Stage IV involvement, however, is relatively infrequent. Well over one-half the patients will be asymptomatic at presentation. Nodular sclerosis cases, as opposed to all other Hodgkin's subtypes, show a female predominance. In addition, the patients are largely clustered in the early-incidence peak of Hodgkin's cases, between ages 15 and 34, among urban populations in "fully developed" countries. Overall, the natural history of nodular sclerosis is intermediate between the indolence of lymphocytic predominance and the more aggressive behavior of mixed-cellularity and lymphocytic depletion disease.

Mixed-cellularity patients tend to have more advanced disease than those with lymphocytic predominance or nodular sclerosis. Half or more will have stage III or IV disease, and up to half will manifest B symptoms. In contrast to nodular sclerosis, however, a minority will have mediastinal involvement. Mixed-cellularity cases again show the usual male predominance. There is a broad age range within this subtype, with a peak in the 30 to 40 age group. Older series showed mixed-cellularity to have a more aggressive natural history than either lymphocytic predominance or nodular sclerosis, with a median survival for all patients in this category of less than 5 years prior to the advent of effective combination chemotherapy.

Lymphocytic depletion Hodgkin's disease is the most aggressive of the four Rye classification subtypes. Extranodal involvement is common, often with limited evidence of nodal disease. B symptoms are the rule. These patients usually fall into the older age ranges of Hodgkin's cases and were recognized to carry a very limited prognosis prior to the development of effective combination chemotherapy.

Treatment

The management of patients with Hodgkin's disease is directed by the extent of involvement identified by staging. All treatment is approached with curative intent. Modalities used in treatment include radiation and chemotherapy. Depending on the clinical situation, these are applied either separately or in a combined-modality approach.

RADIATION THERAPY

Over the past two decades, the development of megavoltage x-ray treatment units (cobalt 60, linear accelerators of 4 MeV or greater) has permitted the introduction of large-field, high-dose radiation therapy as a curative treatment for patients with all but the most advanced presentations of Hodgkin's disease. Standard patterns of treatment have been defined, based on anatomic considerations of nodal groups and also theoretical considerations about the natural spread of Hodgkin's disease from areas of initial involvement to contiguous nodal groups. The general extent of treatment, utilizing doses of radiation capable of achieving sterilization of Hodgkin's disease in the treated area (4000 to 4400 rads) may be either *involved-field* (IF—radiation limited to sites of macroscopic disease), *extended-field* (EF—treatment of all clinically involved nodal groups plus contiguous nodal areas not demonstrated to contain tumor), or *total-nodal irradiation* (TNI—treatment of all major node-bearing areas). The term *total-lymphoid irradiation* (TLI) is often used interchangeably with *total-nodal irradiation*. The former is perhaps preferred, as it connotes the intentional inclusion of the spleen, thymus, and Waldeyer's ring within the radiation fields.

Radiation treatment planning for previously unirradiated patients with Hodgkin's disease rarely involves treatment of a single nodal site. Rather, standard radiation fields have been defined that include several nodal groups, since these contiguous nodal areas are nearly always all radiated together in any given treatment plan. For treatment planning, the main anatomic division is the diaphragm with the supradiaphragmatic treatment field called the "mantle" port and the subdiaphragmatic field referred to as an "inverted Y." The inverted-Y field may be subdivided into an abdominal field including paraaortic nodes and spleen (plus, on occasion, the liver at lesser dose) and a pelvic field. When the pelvis is excluded from subdiaphragmatic treatment, a somewhat longer abdominal field including the common iliac nodes is treated. This is called a "spade." For certain treatment programs a transdiaphragmatic field called the "extended mantle" has been developed. A less frequently used field, called the "Waldeyer's field," provides treatment to preauricular nodes and the lymphoid tissue of Waldeyer's ring. The lymphoid tissue included in a Waldeyer's field will not receive treatment when the only supradiaphragmatic field utilized is the mantle.[18]

The radiation fields utilized are carefully shaped to treat all the nodal tissue but spare normal structures as much as possible. Individual anatomic variations, e.g., E lesions, are taken into account. Radiation-sensitive areas within the overall field, or normal tissues away from sites of involvement, are "blocked" with thick lead shields to lessen toxicity associated with therapy. Radiation fields may be modified during the course of therapy, with shrinkage of radiotherapy ports as tumor mass regresses or by placement of additional blocks as tissues within the treatment field (e.g., spinal cord, heart) are brought to doses approaching a potentially damaging level.

Effective treatment for a majority of stage I and II Hodgkin's disease patients is accomplished with extended-field or total-nodal radiation therapy. Long-term relapse-free survival will result for approximately 75 percent of all patients who are so treated. Patients who develop recurrent disease after radiation are usually "salvageable" with chemotherapy, so that 10-year survival in such patient groups is often in excess of 80 percent.[18]

Patients with bulky mediastinal disease[19] or E lesions[20] are considered to have a somewhat less favorable prognosis by most investigators. These patients have a somewhat poorer relapse-free survival in many series and require either radiation boosts to sites of bulky disease or, more commonly, treatment with a combined-modality approach. Subdiaphragmatic stage I and II disease occurs most often in older-age patients with histologies other than nodular sclerosis. Most of these patients can be effectively treated with total-nodal irradiation.

Approaches to the management of stage IIIA Hodgkin's disease are currently under intense scrutiny. Low- and high-risk subsets of IIIA disease have been postulated and a substaging of stage III has been proposed to include III_1 (spleen, splenic hilar, celiac axis, porta hepatis nodes) and III_2 (any abdominal or pelvic nodal site other than III_1).[21] The validity of this subclassification as a prognostic indicator and meaningful guide to therapy remains in dispute. Most investigators concur in the treatment of limited upper abdominal stage IIIA presentations with irradiation alone. For more extensive stage IIIA cases the use of combined-modality treatment or chemotherapy alone is often advocated by many centers.[22]

The radiation therapy program involves several weeks of treatment for each field to be irradiated. During mantle therapy, usually lasting 4 to 5 weeks, acute toxicities include some dysphagia with esophagitis, sore throat, and cough. Nausea is rarely significant. Later toxicities include pulmonary fibrosis in treated sites and possible radiation pericarditis or myocarditis. Decreased thyroid function manifested as increased thyroid-stimulating hormone (TSH) or frank hypothyroidism may occur. Subdiaphragmatic therapy is associated with more substantial acute toxicity. Nausea is common, and diarrhea may occur. Fatigue may be prominent. Blood counts during inverted-Y therapy (which usually follows completion of a mantle field) may fall and should be carefully monitored. Delays in treatment ("split") may be required during subdiaphragmatic treatment because of gastrointestinal or blood count tolerance. Fertility can usually be preserved despite pelvis radiation in Hodgkin's patients because of gonadal shields (and midline oophoropexy in females) employed as a routine part of the radiation set-up.

CHEMOTHERAPY

Numerous antineoplastic agents are active in treatment of Hodgkin's disease. Since the mid 1960s, drugs have been routinely used in combination for treatment of advanced-stage Hodgkin's disease with curative intent. Several different combinations (see Table 44-5) have been well studied and are capable of producing durable complete remissions in a majority of patients with initial disease of stage IIIB or IV extent, though the outcome is more often favorable in stage IIIB than in stage IVB patients. The chemotherapy is, for the most part, equally effective in all histologic subtypes and sites of stage IV disease involvement. Increasing age has a significant negative impact on survival following chemotherapy in adult patients with Hodgkin's disease. Asymptomatic patients of advanced stage have an exceedingly high complete response rate to chemotherapy that is significantly superior to that of symptomatic patients of equivalent anatomic extent.

The median duration of complete remission for all previously untreated advanced (IIIB, IV-stage) Hodgkin's patients who initially achieve complete remission should be in excess of 5 years.[23,24] However, when stage IVB patients are considered as a subgroup, median complete remission duration is less impressive, and recurrent disease within 5 years is the rule. The duration of chemotherapy administered is somewhat arbitrary, with six "cycles" over approximately 6 months being standard. In order to ensure that some patients are not undertreated, all clinically complete responses should be pathologically confirmed before chemotherapy is discontinued. This "restaging" is carried out any time after four to six treatment cycles have been administered, and all clinical evidence of disease has cleared. In restaging, all initially abnormal laboratory tests are repeated. Appropriate x-rays and scans are repeated. Initially involved extranodal sites are often rebiopsied. (Repeat laparotomy is rarely undertaken, but bone marrow needle biopsy, closed liver biopsy, or peritoneoscopy with liver biopsies are performed.) Those patients with pathologically evaluated complete responses are removed from therapy. Those found to have microscopic residual disease remain on treatment for several more cycles and then undergo yet another pathologic restaging.

Chemotherapy for Hodgkin's disease following relapse after initial radiation therapy produces complete

TABLE 44-5 Chemotherapy Combinations for Hodgkin's Disease

Author		Regimen	CR rate, %*
DeVita et al.[24]	MOPP	Nitrogen mustard Oncovin Procarbazine Prednisone	80
Bloomfield et al.[33]	CVPP	CCNU Vinblastine Procarbazine Prednisone	74
Cooper et al.[34]	MVPP	Nitrogen mustard Vinblastine Procarbazine Prednisone	73
Bonadonna[35]	ABVD	Adriamycin Bleomycin Vinblastine DTIC	71

* Largely stage IIIB or IV patients with no prior chemotherapy. CR = complete response rate.

disease control in a large majority of patients so treated. Overall response rates are at least equivalent to those achieved with primary chemotherapy in previously untreated cases. This ability to "salvage" patients after radiation therapy failure through use of multiagent chemotherapy has had a major impact on improving overall survival in Hodgkin's disease patients.[25] However, questions still persist about the ultimate *curative* potential for postirradiation chemotherapy applied at relapse for macroscopic disease. These questions contribute to the controversy about single versus multimodal initial treatment in all stages of Hodkin's disease.

Chemotherapy-induced second remissions in Hodgkin's disease, following failure of initial chemotherapy, are of variable frequency depending on two features: (1) disease-free interval after primary chemotherapy, and (2) what second-line drugs are utilized. Of these, the first is far more significant. Failure to achieve complete disease regression with the initial chemotherapy combination or recurrence of disease while still on therapy augurs very poorly for the quality of regression to second-line therapy. While second responses to certain chemotherapy combinations will be frequent in such settings, durable complete remissions should not be anticipated. Compared to patients who never achieve complete remission, patients who enter complete remission (CR) and then fail within the first year after adequate combination chemotherapy are in a middle ground, while individuals who relapse longer than 1 year after achieving CR with chemotherapy have a high likelihood of achieving a second CR with either the initial drug program or a different standard Hodgkin's disease treatment combination.[26]

COMBINED-MODALITY THERAPY

Despite the excellent complete response rates obtained in most early-stage Hodgkin's patients with radiation therapy alone and the proven effectiveness of combination chemotherapy in producing complete response in advanced disease, recurrent Hodgkin's disease will occur in approximately 10 to 60 percent of Hodgkin's disease patients depending on the initial Ann Arbor stage. While most radiotherapy failures can be "salvaged" into a second complete remission with chemotherapy, the appearance of recurrent Hodgkin's disease is disturbing to patient and physician alike. In some settings, the occurrence of disease relapse may presage eventual progressive disease and death. In order to lessen the likelihood of recurrent disease, a variety of combination radiation-chemotherapy treatment programs have been developed. These have included full-dose, extended-field, or total-nodal irradiation followed by adjuvant chemotherapy, full-dose involved-field radiation and then chemotherapy, or primary chemotherapy either interspersed with or followed by "consolidation" radiotherapy (in the range of 2000 to 3000 rads) to sites of initial disease involvement.[27,28]

Combined-modality programs are employed most widely in situations where "bulky" disease is present.[19,20] In such settings (for example, very large mediastinal masses in nodular sclerosis Hodgkin's disease), risk of recurrence after either radiation or chemotherapy alone appears increased in the area of bulky disease. In some studies, more effective long-term control of bulky tumor seems to have been achieved through the use of a combined-modality approach.

Combined-modality treatment has also been employed in the absence of bulky nodal disease or extranodal involvement.[27] In randomized trials of large numbers of patients, combinations of radiation and chemotherapy have usually been associated with a statistically significant increase in relapse-free survival compared to radiation alone. However, because of effective "salvage" chemotherapy in patients relapsing after radiation alone, demonstration of significant improvement in overall survival has remained elusive. In addition, the role of "consolidative" radiotherapy, combined with chemotherapy for stage IIIB and IV disease, remains inconclusive. Major prospective randomized trials to evaluate these questions are underway.

COMPLICATIONS OF CHEMOTHERAPY

Acute toxicities of nearly all the chemotherapy combinations used for Hodgkin's disease include nausea and vomiting, fatigue, and variable amounts of anorexia and alopecia. Acute bone marrow depression occurs regularly with therapy but is rarely severe enough to be life-threatening during primary treatment. Inadvertent local paravenous infiltration of some of the agents administered intravenously may be associated with skin ulceration or deep-tissue necrosis. Other agents may produce neurologic, skin, pulmonary, or cardiac toxicities. Chemotherapy following radiation therapy, however, may be associated with more severe bone marrow compromise. Combined-modality programs may be limited acutely by a decrease in bone marrow reserve. In addition, combined-modality treatment programs (or sequential radiation and later chemotherapy) are associated with a significantly increased incidence of second malignancies—most often acute nonlymphocytic leukemias occurring 2 or more years after completion of therapy—compared to single-modality programs. The recently recognized syndrome of non-Hodgkin's lymphoma developing several years after successful treatment for Hodgkin's disease also seems most prevalent in combined-modality-treated patients.[29]

An increased rate of infection is seen in patients under treatment for Hodgkin's disease. Deficiencies in cell-mediated immunity lead to an increased risk of disease caused by opportunistic agents. These pathogens are most often seen during or after chemotherapy, which has an additional deleterious effect on immunity and may also compromise granulocyte number and diminish epithelial barriers to infecting organisms. In these latter settings, bacterial infections with more conventional pathogens may become prevalent. Herpes zoster occurs with a markedly increased frequency in patients with Hodgkin's disease. It may appear either during or after radiation and/or chemotherapy. There is also a much increased incidence of dissemination of herpes zoster in Hodgkin's disease patients compared to normal hosts. Despite the relatively frequent dissemination of zoster in these patients, with substantial acute and some chronic morbidity, death from disseminated zoster in patients with Hodgkin's disease is uncommon.[30]

The risk of sterility following treatment for Hodgkin's disease is highly variable, depending on the type of treatment administered. In females, radiation therapy alone not including the pelvis is rarely associated with decreased fertility, and with appropriate shielding fertility can usually be retained even with pelvic radiation. Increased fetal wastage should not be anticipated in such women.

Some percentage of men with Hodgkin's disease will be found to be oligospermic prior to any form of therapy. When treated with radiation, men should have a testicular shield applied. This will effectively reduce but not totally eliminate the radiation dose to the testis. Following radiation treatment to a pelvic field, transient aspermia will occur,[31] but spermatogenesis should recover within 2 years. Permanent sterility following treatment is rare.

Chemotherapy affects gonadal function in both sexes. In women, transient loss of menses will occur in a majority of cases. However, menstrual function will usually recover during or following treatment. In a majority of premenopausal women, long-term fertility is retained. Spermatogenesis is far more seriously compromised by chemotherapy, and prolonged azospermia is expected following combination chemotherapy containing alkylating agents. Some males have been documented to recover spermatogenesis several years after combination chemotherapy, but the overall recovery of fertility for males appears to be quite low. Further study will be required to define the very long-term potential for recovery of fertility in these patients.[32]

NON-HODGKIN'S LYMPHOMAS

The non-Hodgkin's lymphomas are a diverse group of diseases whose unifying feature is their origin in lymphoid tissue. Some lymphoid malignancies are excluded from this group: Hodgkin's disease, acute and chronic lymphocytic leukemia, Waldenström's macroglobulinemia, and hairy-cell leukemia. Within the category of non-Hodgkin's lymphomas, there is a remarkable heterogeneity in presentation, natural history, and therapy. Classification of these disorders remains an area of controversy and change, making interpretation of clinical data using different classification systems difficult. Despite these problems, the non-Hodgkin's lymphomas are a group in which rapid progress in immunology and therapy has been made.

Etiology

A number of factors have been implicated in the development of non-Hodgkin's lymphomas, some of which are host-related, some environmental. Familial cases have been reported, most commonly in siblings.[36] Although there has been documentation of immune dysfunction in some of these families, most cannot be classified as primary immunodeficiency syndromes. Patients with primary immunodeficiency disorders (ataxia-telangiectasia and Wiskott-Aldrich and Chediak-Higashi syndromes) have a markedly increased risk of lymphoreticular malignancies. Their propensity to develop lymphomas may be related to both defective immunoregulatory processes and chronic antigenic stimulation due to repeated infections.[37]

Patients with iatrogenic immunosuppression also have an increased incidence of lymphomas. Renal allograft recipients have a 40- to 100-fold increased risk of developing non-Hodgkin's lymphoma, particularly diffuse histiocytic lymphoma involving the central nervous system.[38] Non-Hodgkin's lymphomas, again with a predilection for the central nervous system, have also been reported after cardiac transplantation.[39] Patients receiving immunotherapy for nonmalignant diseases other than organ transplantation also have an increased risk of lymphomas, but this risk is substantially less than that of transplant recipients.[40] Whether the difference in risk is related to the degree of immunosuppression or to antigenic stimulation related to the graft or other factors is unclear.

Patients with diseases involving the immune system who do not receive immunosuppressive therapy may also have an increased incidence of lymphoma. Non-Hodgkin's lymphomas have been reported in patients with diseases such as rheumatoid arthritis, inflammatory bowel disease, and systemic lupus erythematosis. The highest risk has appeared in Sjögren's syndrome, with 5 to 10 percent of patients developing major lymphoproliferative disorders.[41] Sarcoidosis and gluten-sensitive enteropathy are also associated with an excess of lymphoma. Immunoblastic lymphadenopathy, a benign lymphoproliferative disorder associated with a history of drug allergy, polyclonal hypergammaglobulinemia, and Coombs'-positive anemia, may progress to lymphoma.[43]

Environmental factors may also play a role in the etiology of non-Hodgkin's lymphomas. The role of viruses has been suspected for years, based on induction of lymphomas in animals by RNA viruses. However, there is little evidence to implicate viruses in human lymphomas except for Burkitt's lymphoma, with which the Epstein-Barr virus has been closely associated epidemiologically. Radiation exposure is not strongly associated with non-Hodgkin's lymphoma, although an increase in non-Hodgkin's lymphoma has also been reported in patients with Hodgkin's disease following treatment with radiation and chemotherapy.[43]

In summary, a predisposition to development of lymphoma seems to exist (1) after prolonged antigenic stimulation leading to lymphoproliferation, and (2) with impairment of immune regulation due to immune deficiencies secondary to disease (e.g., connective tissue diseases) or therapy (e.g., immunosuppressive drugs).

Incidence

The non-Hodgkin's lymphomas constitute 2.5 percent of all cancers in the United States, with approximately 15,000 new cases per year. The incidence increases exponentially with age. Mortality rates also rise progressively with age, and the mortality in adults over the age of 20 has gradually increased over the last 25 years.

Some lymphomas occur with high incidence in specific geographic areas. These include Burkitt's lymphoma in the west Nile region of Africa, "Mediterranean" intestinal lymphoma in the Middle East, and nasal lymphoma in conjunction with chronic rhinitis in South America.

Pathology and Classification Systems

Prior to the 1960s the non-Hodgkin's lymphomas were classified into three groups: giant follicular cell lymphoma, lymphosarcoma, and reticulum-cell sarcoma. This classification scheme was abandoned because of inadequate reproducibility (particularly a lack of distinction between lymphosarcoma and reticulum-cell sarcoma) and failure to distinguish differences in prognosis or therapy. Rosenberg's review in 1961 showed that the subset of patients classified as giant follicular cell lymphoma did have a better prognosis, but they accounted for only 10 percent of the population.[44] There was no difference in prognosis for the other two groups.

Rappaport proposed a new classification system for the non-Hodgkin's lymphomas in 1956 which was based on two features: nodal architecture (nodular or diffuse) and cytology (lymphocytic, well- or poorly differentiated, histiocytic, or mixed lymphocytic-histiocytic)[45] (see Table 44-6). This classification has proved to be reproducible, with a 90 percent reliability among a panel of pathologists for reading nodular versus diffuse and a 50 to 75 percent reproducibility for cytology.[46] The least reproducible diagnoses are poorly differentiated lymphocytic lymphoma and mixed lymphoma.

The Rappaport classification has been confirmed to have prognostic and therapeutic implications. There appear to be two prognostic groups: the "favorable" lymphomas, which have a prolonged natural history and a high response rate to therapy, and the "unfavorable" lymphomas, which often have a more rapid downhill course. Included in the favorable group are the nodular lymphomas (except nodular histiocytic) plus diffuse well-differentiated lymphocytic lymphoma (DLWD). The median survival in this group is 8 to 10 years. The unfavorable group includes the diffuse lymphomas (except DLWD) plus nodular histiocytic lymphoma and has a median survival of 1 to 2 years. Despite its classification, the "favorable" group appears to have a continuous death rate with time, with no type of therapy clearly

TABLE 44-6 Rappaport Classification of Non-Hodgkin's Lymphoma

Original[45]	Modified[46]
Nodular	**Nodular**
Well-differentiated lymphocytic	Poorly differentiated lymphocytic
Poorly differentiated lymphocytic	Mixed lymphocytic histiocytic
Mixed lymphocytic-histiocytic	Histiocytic
Histiocytic	
Diffuse	**Diffuse**
Well-differentiated lymphocytic	Well-differentiated lymphocytic
Poorly differentiated lymphocytic	Poorly differentiated lymphocytic
Mixed lymphocytic histiocytic	Mixed lymphocytic histiocytic
Histiocytic	Histiocytic
	Lymphoblastic
	Undifferentiated (Burkitt's and non-Burkitt's)

shown to have curative potential. In the unfavorable group, nonresponders or partial responders die early, but survival curves appear to plateau after 2 to 3 years, suggesting curability for a subset of patients in the "unfavorable" group. In general, lymphocytic subtypes have a better overall prognosis than histiocytic, and nodular architecture better than diffuse, according to the Rappaport classification.

Some patients will be found to have a combination of nodular and diffuse patterns in the initial biopsy specimen. Several studies have shown that these patients behave like those with a purely nodular pattern.[47] Whether the degree of nodularity correlates with prognosis remains controversial. The problem of divergent histologies at presentation in patients with multiple biopsies (in contradistinction to those discussed earlier who have different histologies within one biopsy) has recently been reviewed. Patients with both nodular and diffuse patterns (18 of 101 patients) have response rates and survivals intermediate between those with identical nodular biopsies and identical diffuse biopsies.[48] This presence of two distinct histologic patterns in different tissues biopsied at the time of initial diagnosis should not be confused with the occurrence of histologic change in follow-up biopsies after observation or therapy.

"Favorable" lymphomas may evolve to more aggressive histologic subtypes with loss of nodularity and increase in the proportion of large cells. At autopsy, 60 to 70 percent of cases of nodular lymphomas were reported to have changed histology.[49] The NCI reported histologic progression in 37 percent of patients with nodular lymphomas who had a repeat biopsy more than 3 months after initial diagnosis.[50] Some oncologists have proposed deferring therapy until histologic evolution to specific subtypes which may be curable with combination chemotherapy has taken place. Whether such previously untreated disease which evolves from nodular to diffuse subtypes would be curable is not known.

The initial Rappaport classification has subsequently been modified to split out a number of clinically distinctive groups (see Table 44-6). Lymphoblastic lymphoma, originally included in the diffuse poorly differentiated lymphocytic group, is now considered a distinct entity. Classically, it is found in young males with mediastinal masses. These patients have a high rate of bone marrow invasion and central nervous system involvement, and have an unfavorable prognosis.[51] Also added is the subtype Burkitt's lymphoma, initially described in African children with jaw masses, but now also widely recognized outside Africa as well.

As current concepts of immunology have evolved, with subtyping of lymphocytes by cell surface markers and cell function, it has become clear that the cytologic classification proposed by Rappaport is not immunologically accurate. The "histiocyte" of his classification is usually a transformed lymphocyte and only rarely a true product of the monocyte-macrophage line. As a result of attempts to integrate newer concepts of immunology into a workable classification of lymphomas, a multiplicity of other classification schemes have been proposed.[52,53] None of these systems will be reviewed in detail here; however, some of the relevant immunological concepts will be discussed.

The normal lymph node contains B cells, T cells, and

true histiocytes. *B* refers to the bursa of Fabricius in birds where B cells are processed; *T* to the thymus. B cells are capable of immunoglobulin synthesis and are characterized by having surface immunoglobulin, F_c receptors (a surface structure which binds the F_c fragment of IgG), and usually C3 receptors. T lymphocytes are responsible for immune regulation and cellular immunity. They are characterized by forming nonimmune rosettes with sheep red blood cells and, more recently, by various cell surface antigens. True histiocytes are not lymphocytes, but are derived from the macrophage-monocyte series. They function as phagocytes and processors of antigen and can be distinguished by staining for lysosomal enzymes and by the absence of F_c and C3 receptors.

Lymph nodes contain lymphocytes in two major areas: the superficial cortex and the deep cortex. The superficial cortex is composed of collections of lymphocytes in follicles or nodules composed largely of B lymphocytes. The follicles can enlarge in response to immune stimulation and develop a central area of large proliferating cells called *germinal centers*. The deep cortex and the zones between follicles in the superficial cortex are composed of both T and B lymphocytes in a ratio of approximately 3 to 1. The medullary cords contain differentiating B cells.

The majority of lymphomas are B-cell neoplasms.[54,55] These include all nodular lymphomas, Burkitt's lymphomas, and most diffuse well-differentiated lymphomas. T-cell diseases include lymphoblastic lymphoma[56] and mycosis fungoides. Diffuse poorly differentiated lymphocytic lymphoma is most often a B-cell disease, if one excludes lymphoblastic lymphoma, which was originally part of this group. The largest controversy centers about Rappaport's diffuse histiocytic group, which has been subclassified in most of the newer systems. The majority of these lymphomas are composed of transformed lymphocytes rather than histiocytes. In Stein's review of tumors called histiocytic lymphoma of Rappaport, the distribution of cell types included 76 percent B-cell, 8 percent T-cell, 5 percent histiocyte, and 10 percent undefined.[57] There is some evidence that the T-cell and null-cell (undefined) subgroups of Rappaport's large "histiocytic" category have a worse prognosis than the B-cell subgroups.

The newest proposed classification is a formulation based on a multi-institutional study of 1175 cases of non-Hodgkin's lymphomas. The lymphomas are divided into three grades based on the aggressiveness of their clinical behavior: low grade, intermediate grade, and high grade.[58] The actual effectiveness and acceptance of this new working formulation will require several years to determine.

The remainder of the discussion will approach the non-Hodgkin's lymphomas from the Rappaport classification because most of the data available are based on that system. References to immunologic classifications will be made where relevant clinically.

Clinical Presentation

The largest series of non-Hodgkin's lymphoma patients is that published by Rosenberg in 1961, reviewing 1269 cases.[44] These lymphomas occurred in all age groups from childhood through adulthood with a peak in the fifth decade. There was a slight male preponderance with a ratio of 1.7 to 1, males-females. The initial presenting manifestation in the majority of patients (64 percent) was painless peripheral lymphadenopathy of approximately 6 months' duration. The most common site of adenopathy was the neck, followed by the inguinal region. Symptoms other than painless adenopathy at presentation included fever, weight loss, sweating, and malaise. These occurred in 20 percent of Rosenberg's series. Pain occurred in a majority of the patients who presented with bone lesions or intraabdominal disease. Extranodal presentations accounted for approximately one-quarter of patients, with the most frequent sites being nasooropharynx, skin or scalp, bone, and gastrointestinal tract. Other rarer sites of extranodal presentation have included lung, testis, thyroid, meninges, and breast. Compared with Hodgkin's disease, the non-Hodgkin's lymphomas present more commonly with extranodal primaries and are more likely to spread noncontiguously. Non-Hodgkin's lymphoma is more often stage IV at presentation. The great diversity within the rubric of non-Hodgkin's lymphoma makes its behavior less predictable than that of Hodgkin's disease.

Staging

The non-Hodgkin's lymphomas are staged by the same system used in Hodgkin's disease, the Ann Arbor system. The extent of disease is defined by stages I through IV and the absence or presence of systemic symptoms by "A" or "B." Patients are given both a clinical stage based on physical exam and radiologic studies and a pathologic stage based on surgical procedures such as additional node biopsies, bone marrow biopsies, liver biopsy, laparoscopy, or staging laparotomy. This staging system has been proved to have prognostic and therapeutic significance in Hodgkin's disease. Its value in non-Hodgkin's lymphomas is less definite, but no superior system has been proposed.

The non-Hodgkin's lymphomas are more frequently disseminated at presentation than is Hodgkin's disease, often with bone marrow involvement making the disease stage IV. This does not carry the same negative prognosis in all non-Hodgkin's lymphomas as it does in Hodgkin's disease. The distinction between stages III and IV in non-Hodgkin's lymphoma has less importance than in Hodgkin's disease in terms of choosing appropriate therapy, since neither stage of non-Hodgkin's lymphoma can regularly be cured with total-nodal radiotherapy. Systemic symptoms are less frequent in the non-Hodgkin's lymphomas than in Hodgkin's disease but are generally viewed as having the same negative prognostic impact that they do in Hodgkin's disease. Parameters such as histology, bulk of disease, and site of disease, which are not incorporated into the Ann Arbor staging system, are of prognostic significance in the non-Hodgkin's lymphomas. As discussed previously, patients with nodular patterns of disease have a better prognosis than those with diffuse patterns, and those with lymphocytic histology have a better prognosis than those with histiocytic or lymphoblastic histology.

Complete clinical staging should be performed in all patients, including history and physical examination with careful recording of the size and location of all abnormal lymph nodes. Nodal involvement in the epitrochlear and popliteal areas is more common in non-Hodgkin's lymphomas than in Hodgkin's disease. An enlarged spleen on physical examination is highly suggestive of involvement by lymphoma. At laparotomy 96 percent of palpable spleens were positive, whereas 35 percent of nonpalpable spleens were positive. Splenic involvement presages a high likelihood of liver involvement as well. Routine blood counts and chemistries are obtained but may not accurately reflect organ involvement by lymphoma, as lymphomatous infiltration may not affect organ function. Approximately 50 percent of patients with abnormal blood counts will not have bone marrow involvement on biopsy, and the peripheral blood will be normal in 73 percent of those with lymphomatous infiltration of the marrow.[59] Peripheral blood smear examination may show evidence of circulating malignant cells in 15 percent of patients, most commonly in those with small-cell lymphocytic lymphomas.

Chest x-rays should be routinely obtained, although they are positive in only 20 to 30 percent of cases.[60] Abnormalities reported are mediastinal and/or hilar adenopathy, pulmonary parenchymal disease, and pleural effusion. Pulmonary parenchymal lesions which are due to a direct tumor extension from hilar or mediastinal nodes do not change the stage of disease. Full-lung tomograms generally do not add important information, although they may be of value in patients with extensive abnormalities on chest x-ray. In children with non-Hodgkin's lymphoma, mediastinal disease is much more common than in adults.

Bipedal lymphangiography is a valuable staging procedure in non-Hodgkin's lymphoma. The technique is highly accurate, with a 13 percent false-positive rate and a 12 percent false-negative rate in Stanford's series.[60] The rate of positivity varies with the histology of the lymphoma, with 90 percent positivity in nodular lymphomas and 66 percent in diffuse lymphomas.[61] Most patients with positive lymphangiograms will also have palpable iliac, inguinal, or femoral adenopathy so that their staging is not changed; however, one-third of patients classed as stages I or II will be advanced to stage III on the basis of the lymphangiogram. The lymphangiogram has also been shown to be an excellent predictor of other intraabdominal sites of lymphomatous involvement. Of patients with positive lymphangiograms 81 percent also had disease in liver, spleen, or nodes outside the paraaortic chains at laparotomy. This has significant implications for therapy.[62]

The value of gallium scanning in staging is controversial. It appears to be of most value in diffuse histiocytic lymphoma with 60 to 80 percent visualization of involved nodal sites.[63] In lymphocytic or mixed lymphomas the test is unreliable. Gallium scanning is most useful in the neck and thorax and for lesions larger than 2 cm in diameter. The test is often difficult to interpret in the abdomen because of gallium accumulation in the bowel.

Abdominal computer tomographic (CT) scanning appears to be an important new staging technique although the data assessing it are limited by its recent availability. It appears to be valuable in evaluation of the paraaortic nodes as well as mesenteric and high-abdominal nodes not visualized by the lymphangiogram.[64] This technique is increasingly used as the single noninvasive technique for evaluating subdiaphragmatic involvement in patients with non-Hodgkin's lymphomas.

The intravenous pyelogram is a low-yield procedure as a routine screening test, but has been used to evaluate possible renal obstruction or ureteral deviation in patients with known retroperitoneal involvement. Inferior venocavography has been advocated for evaluation of superior right retroperitoneal nodes but is rarely used currently. Gastrointestinal (GI) series are not generally warranted in a patient without symptoms suggesting stomach or intestinal involvement.

Bone scanning is of value in patients with diffuse histiocytic lymphoma, of whom 25 percent may have bone lesions.[65] Liver-spleen scanning is of limited usefulness, with a high incidence of false-positive and false-negative results. The most common abnormalities are hepatomegaly and parenchymal mottling, which are nondiagnostic. Histiocytic lymphoma may cause large tumor nodules which can be seen as focal filling defects on scan. Splenic scanning has a significant false-negative rate.

Bone marrow involvement is common, with a 40 to 100 percent incidence of positivity in lymphocytic histologies.[59] The rate of positivity in histiocytic lymphoma is much lower, about 15 percent.[62] Marrow involvement in diffuse histiocytic lymphoma has an important correlation with later involvement of the central nervous system and indicates a need for lumbar puncture. Because of the focal nature of marrow involvement, bilateral biopsies should be obtained; a second biopsy increases the positive yield by approximately 10 percent. Bone marrow biopsy will advance about 25 percent of patients to stage IV, predominantly stage III patients with nodular lymphomas. Rarely a stage I or II patient will be upstaged by a positive marrow biopsy.[61]

Percutaneous liver biopsy has a positive yield of approximately 20 percent in poorly differentiated lymphocytic lymphoma and 6 percent in histiocytic lymphoma.[60,61] However, 30 percent of those with negative percutaneous biopsies had positive biopsies with peritoneoscopy direction, and an additional 20 percent of patients with both negative percutaneous and peritoneoscopy-directed biopsies will have positive biopsies at laparotomy. In patients with clinical stage I or II disease above the diaphragm, the yield of liver biopsy is less than 5 percent; therefore, liver biopsy need not be done routinely in that group of patients.

The role of staging laparotomy in non-Hodgkin's lymphomas is less clear than in Hodgkin's disease. Reports on large series of laparotomy-staged patients have provided valuable information about the behavior of these lymphomas: the propensity to involve mesenteric lymph nodes, the incidence of multiple histologies, and the frequency of liver involvement. The mortality of staging laparotomy is low (0.5 percent), even in this group of patients, who tend to be older than those with Hodgkin's disease, but the morbidity is significant in published series.[60,61,66] Complications occur in 11 to 40 percent of patients and include pneumonia, pulmonary embolism, GI bleeding, and subdiaphragmatic abscess. Most importantly, staging laparotomy has a limited impact on determining the final stage or altering treatment in this group of patients. After clinical evaluation including bilateral marrow biopsies, more than 80 percent of patients are stage III or IV.[61] These patients are generally treated with chemotherapy, thus obviating the need for laparotomy. The 20 percent of patients who remain in stages I and II could be considered for laparotomy if localized treatment, i.e., radiotherapy alone, is being contemplated. Of these patients 17 to 28 percent will be upstaged at laparotomy, more commonly those with nodular lymphomas.[61,66] Thus, patients most likely to be candidates for laparotomy are those with stage I or II diffuse histiocytic lymphoma after clinical staging who are being considered for therapy with local radiation alone.

In conclusion, clinical staging of the non-Hodgkin's lymphomas, including history, physical exam, routine chemistries, bilateral bone marrow biopsies, and noninvasive assessment of the abdominal nodes (with lymphangiogram or CT scan), will reveal disseminated disease (stages III or IV) in the majority of patients. If the patient has limited disease after clinical staging and localized therapy is contemplated, further invasive staging should be undertaken. Staging laparotomy is needed in a small number of patients.

Treatment

The majority of patients with non-Hodgkin's lymphoma will have disseminated disease at presentation and will require systemic therapy. Occasional patients with localized disease can be treated with curative intent with regional therapy, either surgery or radiotherapy. The discussion of therapy will be divided broadly between the nodular lymphomas and the diffuse lymphomas.

The nodular lymphomas are generally not curable with current therapy. Exceptions to this rule are two rare subgroups, localized nodular lymphoma, which appears curable with radiotherapy, and advanced nodular mixed lymphoma, for which one series reports prolonged disease-free survival after combination chemotherapy.[67]

The most common nodular lymphoma is the poorly differentiated lymphocytic type, NLPD, which is stage III or IV at presentation in 90 percent of patients. Localized disease (stage I) following surgical staging has been treated with involved-field radiotherapy with excellent local control and prolonged disease-free survival. The outcome of stage II patients similarly treated is less favorable.[68] No significant survival difference has been demonstrated for nodular lymphoma patients of limited extent (stages I and II) treated with involved-field versus total-lymphoid irradiation.[69] The addition of adjuvant chemotherapy to radiation therapy in pathologic stage I and II nodular lymphoma has not resulted in improved survival.[70] Thus, the treatment of choice for the 10 percent of patients who appear to have localized disease after staging, including laparotomy, is localized radiotherapy.

The 90 percent of patients with stages III and IV nodular lymphocytic lymphomas can be treated in a variety of ways. A proportion of these patients (10 to 25 percent) may be asymptomatic with a history of indolent disease. Portlock and Rosenberg have published a series of these patients observed without therapy until they developed symptoms.[71] Most patients eventually developed progressive disease or symptoms necessitating therapy, but their actuarial survival did not differ from that of a similar group of patients treated at presentation. A significant number of the untreated patients had spontaneous tumor regressions lasting various intervals of time. With deferred treatment some of the patients show histologic evolution into diffuse lymphomas. It has been suggested that such patients may be curable with combination chemotherapy after this change in histology has occurred.[72]

In patients with stage III disease, total-lymphoid irradiation has been utilized with curative intent, but its true efficacy remains unproven. Relapses occurred frequently in unirradiated nodes known to be involved in non-Hodgkin's lymphomas, such as the epitrochlear nodes, mesenteric nodes, and Waldeyer's ring. Whether cure could be attained by attempting to irradiate these additional sites is unknown. Total-body irradiation has been employed in the treatment of advanced nodular lymphomas at low doses (150 rads over 5 weeks) with a complete remission rate of 60 to 80 percent. This modality has clear palliative effectiveness but is hampered by hematologic toxicity, primarily thrombocytopenia.[73] Again, cure has not been achieved.

Chemotherapy has been used as single-agent treatment, combination-drug therapy, and in combination with radiation therapy. A variety of single agents, including alkylating agents, vinca alkaloids, nitrosoureas, and anthracyclines, have response rates varying from 20 to 80 percent.[74] One-half or more of patients with advanced nodular poorly differentiated lymphocytic lymphoma can attain complete clinical remissions with single-agent therapy, although prolonged treatment may be required.[75]

Combination chemotherapy with cyclophosphamide, vincristine, and prednisone (CVP) is the most commonly used regimen and has been shown to produce 70 to 80 percent complete remissions in patients with nodular poorly differentiated lymphocytic lymphoma (see Table 44-7). The addition of drugs such as Adriamycin or bleomycin has not improved the response rate. It has not been established that combination chemotherapy is superior to single-agent therapy with an alkylating agent. Trials at Stanford comparing single-agent therapy with combination chemotherapy have shown high response rates in both groups (70 to 90 percent).[76] While median survival is in excess of several years in both treatment arms, there is a continuous relapse rate, and neither therapy has been demonstrated to produce a significant survival advantage. At the National Cancer Institute the advanced-stage lymphomas of favorable histology were treated with either CVP or C-MOPP (cyclophosphamide, Oncovin, procarbazine, prednisone). Of note from their data is the subgroup of nodular mixed lymphomas treated with C-MOPP. Several of these nodular mixed patients have attained durable complete remissions, suggesting the possibility of cure.[67] Further follow-up of this group is required. Combined-modality therapy with radiation and combination chemotherapy has not been shown to be superior to chemotherapy alone.

In summary, despite a plethora of approaches to treatment for advanced-stage non-Hodgkin's lymphomas of favorable histology, no one treatment is clearly superior. There is no firm evidence that these diseases can be cured by any of the available treatment modalities, with the possible exception of chemotherapy for nodular mixed lymphoma. If the intent is palliative, the timing of therapy and choice of treatment modality will depend upon the patient's symptoms, sites of disease, and tempo of disease. If there is no indication for immediate treatment and chemotherapy is deferred, the patient will require careful follow-up examinations to ensure intervention when appropriate.

The diffuse lymphomas generally carry a poor prog-

TABLE 44-7 Combination Chemotherapy in Advanced Diffuse Histiocytic Lymphoma

Regimens	Reported CR rate (%)	Comment
COPP (MOPP)[81]	11/27 (41%)	Aggressively restaged after finishing therapy. 10/11 remain with no evidence of disease.
BACOP[89]	12/25 (48%)	Weekly therapy designed to limit tumor regrowth between cycles.
CHOP[90]	35/53 (68%)	Improved CR rate by adding Adriamycin to CVP combination.
CHOP-Bleo[91]	18/26 (69%)	No clear advantage over CHOP alone.
M-BACOD[92]	45/56 (80%)	High-dose methotrexate employed to limit CNS relapses.
COMLA[93]	23/42 (55%)	Sequence of two drug pairs.

nosis without treatment. In contrast to the nodular lymphomas, patients with diffuse lymphomas will have localized disease (stage I or II) in up to 50 percent of cases. The most common histology is diffuse histiocytic lymphoma, with diffuse poorly differentiated lymphocytic and diffuse mixed histologies being less common.

Localized diffuse histiocytic lymphoma (DHL) has traditionally been treated with radiotherapy. A number of reports of treatment with radiotherapy alone have yielded markedly different data. This variability is in large measure explained by differences in the extent of pretreatment staging. Miller and Jones have cited a 50 percent long-term disease-free survival (cure) rate with radiotherapy in stage I DHL when the patients are clinically staged. The cure rate increases substantially in laparotomy-staged patients.[77] In stage II DHL patients, the reported cure rates range from 35 to 78 percent. Involved-field radiation appears as effective as total-lymphoid treatment if the patients are carefully staged. The role of adjuvant chemotherapy after radiation in early-stage diffuse lymphomas remains controversial, although at least one study suggests benefit.[78] Because of the success in treating advanced-stage DHL with combination chemotherapy (see below), some investigators have evaluated combination chemotherapy as primary therapy in small series of patients with early-stage disease with excellent results. In a series of 23 stage I and II DHL patients treated at Arizona, 15 received combination chemotherapy alone. Only one patient has relapsed, with a median follow-up of 31+ months.[79] Further evaluation of combination chemotherapy alone in early-stage patients with DHL is underway.

The treatment of choice for advanced-stage diffuse histiocytic lymphoma is combination chemotherapy. Complete response rates range from 40 to 75 percent with durable disease-free survival (cure) in 40 to 50 percent. There are important prognostic subgroups within the advanced-disease patients. Patients with gastrointestinal involvement (as part of stage IV disease), tumor masses greater than 10 cm in diameter, or bone marrow involvement carry a poorer prognosis than patients without bulky disease or with other sites of stage IV involvement.[80]

A variety of chemotherapeutic regimens have been utilized in diffuse histiocytic lymphoma patients. CVP (cyclophosphamide, vincristine, prednisone) produces responses in about one-third of patients with no improvement in overall median survival. The addition of procarbazine to CVP (COPP) produced a complete response rate of 41 percent with most of the complete responders remaining continuously disease-free for greater than 2 years and presumably cured.[81] Regimens developed more recently have included the anthracycline antibiotic Adriamycin (hydroxydaunomycin) and the antitumor antibiotic bleomycin—the so-called CHOP and BACOP or CHOP-bleo combinations. Incorporation of cycle-active agents such as high-dose methotrexate with leucovorin rescue or arabinosylcytosine produce regimens referred to as COMLA or M-BACOD (dexamethasone rather than prednisone). All of these Adriamycin-containing regimens appear to be of approximately equal efficacy, each curing up to half or more of patients with diffuse histiocytic lymphoma.

Achievement of a complete remission with chemotherapy is critical in patients with DHL. The survival of partial responders is poor, similar to that of nonresponders. However, complete responders who remain in complete remission for 2 years following completion of chemotherapy rarely suffer late relapses and can be considered cured. When relapses do occur, either during ongoing chemotherapy or after completion of treatment, the first site of evident disease is frequently extranodal, including the central nervous system (CNS). The overall risk of CNS involvement in DHL is less than 10 percent,[82] though patients at high risk for CNS involvement have been identified (they have bone or bone marrow involvement, age <35, advanced disease). The most common clinical presentation is leptomeningeal involvement with cranial nerve abnormalities and mental status changes. The diagnosis is established by lumbar puncture. The treatment is intrathecal chemotherapy and/or cranial or craniospinal irradiation, depending on the individual situation. In high-risk patients, consideration should be given to some form of CNS prophylaxis as utilized in acute lymphocytic leukemia. This may be achieved by employing systemic chemotherapy regimens with high-dose methotrexate or ara-C, agents which cross the blood brain barrier, or with intrathecal chemotherapy and/or neuraxis irradiation.

The diffuse lymphomas of small lymphocytes are a diverse group including classic diffuse poorly differentiated lymphocytic (DLPD) lymphoma, the T-lymphocyte disease called lymphoblastic lymphoma, and the small noncleaved B-lymphocytic proliferation called Burkitt's lymphoma. Diffuse poorly differentiated lymphocytic histology has been included in the unfavorable group, but it has characteristics of the more favorable nodular lymphomas as well. Its natural history is somewhat more indolent than DHL, and it remains quite responsive to aggressive combination chemotherapy. However, groups of patients with DLPD, regardless of initial responsiveness to chemotherapy, tend to have a continuous rate of relapse over time, thus showing no evidence of curability.[83]

Lymphoblastic lymphoma has a very unfavorable natural history, with median survivals measured in months. The tendency for rapid dissemination to bone marrow and CNS has led to design of treatment protocols very similar to those used in childhood acute leukemias. The use of CHOP chemotherapy, the addition of L-asparaginase, and early CNS prophylaxis, often including high-dose methotrexate with rescue, has led to a very high complete response rate in lymphoblastic lymphoma.[84] The durability of these remissions remains to be assessed, but in light of this tumor's high turnover rate and by analogy with treatment in other high-grade lymphomas, long-term disease-free survival seems likely for a substantial proportion of these patients.

Burkitt's lymphoma is a B-cell proliferation with exquisite sensitivity to alkylating agent chemotherapy. Combinations of cyclophosphamide, methotrexate, and vincristine with or without prednisone and Adriamycin produce initial complete responses in 90 to 100 percent of non-African Burkitt's lymphoma cases. With attention to CNS prophylaxis as part of an aggressive initial treatment program, well over half of the newly diagnosed Burkitt's patients may be long-term survivors.[85] Two important characteristics of Burkitt's lymphoma therapy are (1) the observation that debulking surgery which removes 80 to 90 percent or more of all intraabdominal tumor prior to chemotherapy has a major favorable impact on long-term survival, and (2) the tumor cells are so sensitive to cytotoxic chemotherapy that potentially lethal metabolic changes may occur immediately following chemotherapy (the so-called acute tumor lysis syndrome).[86] Awareness of this possible complication will permit early recognition of developing metabolic aberrations and effective management.

Gastrointestinal Lymphoma

Extranodal presentations of non-Hodgkin's lymphomas occur in 16 to 24 percent of all cases. The single most common site is the gastrointestinal tract, responsible for 25 to 50 percent of the primary extranodal cases. Within the gastrointestinal tract, stomach involvement accounts for slightly less than half the cases, while the small bowel is the site in about 30 percent. In children, stomach involvement is much less common, and an ileocecal localization is characteristic. In most series, diffuse histiocytic histology is present in nearly two-thirds of cases, with the remaining patients showing different subtypes of lymphocytic disease. Pain is the leading symptomatic complaint in patients with primary gastrointestinal lymphomas; it is seen in 50 to 90 percent of cases. Weight loss, nausea, and vomiting, GI bleeding, anorexia, and diarrhea are other common complaints, but each is seen in only a minority of patients.[87,88]

The outcome of treatment in patients with primary gastrointestinal lymphomas depends to a large extent on the distribution of disease at presentation. Patients with disease limited to one area of the GI tract (stage I_E) tend to do very well with either surgery and radiation therapy or, in some sites, radiation alone. Other patients have been treated with chemotherapy, usually following local management of the primary tumor, again with favorable results. How much therapy is required and which of the available management schemes is optimal has not been submitted to controlled comparative testing.

Patients with a primary gastrointestinal lymphoma and regional node involvement (stage II$_E$) have a less favorable outlook. The extent of nodal involvement appears to be an important prognostic feature in such patients. Those who have several nodal sites involved have a worse prognosis than those in whom strictly regional node involvement is documented. Once again, both radiation therapy alone and surgery plus postoperative radiotherapy have been advocated as useful modes of therapy. In addition, aggressive chemotherapy, especially in patients with diffuse histiocytic or Burkitt's histology, should play an important role in the treatment of these individuals. As mentioned earlier, patients with gastrointestinal involvement as part of stage IV disease tend to do very poorly, even with the most aggressive treatment approaches.

REFERENCES

1. Hodgkin T: On some morbid appearances of the absorbent glands and spleen. *Med Chir Trans* 17:68–114, 1832.
2. Jackson H Jr, Parker R: Hodgkin's disease. II. Pathology. *N Engl J Med* 231:35–44, 1944.
3. Lukes RJ, Butler JJ: The pathology and nomenclature of Hodgkin's disease. *Cancer Res* 26:1063–1081, 1966.
4. Gutensohn N, Cole P: Childhood social environment and Hodgkin's disease. *N Engl J Med* 304:135–140, 1981.
5. Abramson JH: Childhood experience and Hodgkin's disease in adults. *Isr J Med Sci* 10:1365–1370, 1974.
6. MacMahon B: Epidemiology of Hodgkin's disease. *Cancer Res* 26:1189–1200, 1966.
7. Lukes RJ et al: Report of the Nomenclature Committee. *Cancer Res* 26:1311, 1966.
8. Jones SE et al: Histopathologic review of lymphoma cases from the Southwest Oncology Group. *Cancer* 39:1071–1076, 1977.
9. Carbone PP et al: Report of the Committee on Hodgkin's Staging Classification. *Cancer Res* 31:1860–1861, 1971.
10. Rosenberg SA et al: Report of the Committee on Hodgkin's Disease Staging Procedures. *Cancer Res* 31:1862–1863, 1971.
11. Kadin MF et al: Clinicopathologic studies of 117 untreated patients subjected to laparotomy for the staging of Hodgkin's disease. *Cancer* 27:1277–1294, 1971.
12. Desser RK et al: Staging of Hodgkin's disease and lymphoma. *Med Clin North Am* 57:479–498, 1973.
13. Castellino RA et al: Lymphographic accuracy in Hodgkin's disease and malignant lymphoma with a note on the "reactive" lymph node as a cause of most false-positive lymphograms. *Invest Radiol* 9:155–165, 1974.
14. DeVita VT et al: Peritoneoscopy in the staging of Hodgkin's disease. *Cancer Res* 31:1746–1750, 1971.
15. Kaplan HS et al: Staging laparotomy and splenectomy in Hodgkin's disease: Analysis of indications and patterns of involvement in 285 consecutive, unselected patients. *Natl Cancer Inst Monogr* 36:291–301, 1973.
16. Kaplan HS: *Hodgkin's Disease*, Harvard University, Cambridge, 1980.
17. Cannon WB, Nelson TS: Staging of Hodgkin's disease: A surgical perspective. *Am J Surg* 132:224–230, 1976
18. Hoppe RT: Radiation therapy in the treatment of Hodgkin's disease. *Semin Oncol* 7:144–154, 1980.
19. Mauch P et al: The significance of mediastinal involvement in early stage Hodgkin's disease. *Cancer* 42:1039–1045, 1978.
20. Levi JA, Wiernik PH: Limited extranodal Hodgkin's disease. *Am J Med* 63:365–372, 1977.
21. Stein RS et al: Anatomical substages of stage III-A Hodgkin's disease: A collaborative study. *Ann Intern Med* 92:159–165, 1980.
22. Golumb HM et al: Importance of substaging of stage III Hodgkin's disease. *Semin Oncol* 7:136–143, 1980.
23. DeVita VT et al: The chemotherapy of Hodgkin's disease, Past experiences and future directions. *Cancer* 42:979–990, 1978.
24. DeVita VT: The consequences of the chemotherapy of Hodgkin's disease. *Cancer* 47:1–13, 1981.
25. Lukes RJ et al: Report of the Nomenclature Committee. *Cancer Res* 26:1311, 1966.
26. Fisher RI et al: Prolonged disease free survival in Hodgkin's disease with MOPP reinduction after first relapse. *Ann Intern Med* 90:761–763, 1980.
27. Rosenberg SA et al: An overview of the rationale and results of Stanford Randomized Trials of the treatment of Hodgkin's disease, 1967–1980, in SE Salmon, SE Jones (eds): *Adjuvant Therapy of Cancer III*, Grune & Stratton, New York, 1981, pp 65–76.
28. Farber LR et al: Curative potential of combined modality therapy for advanced Hodgkin's disease. *Cancer* 46:1509–1517, 1980.
29. Brody RS, Schottenfeld D: Multiple primary cancers in Hodgkin's disease. *Semin Oncol* 7:187–201, 1980.
30. Reboul F et al: Herpes zoster and varicella infections in children with Hodgkin's disease. *Cancer* 41:95–99, 1978.
31. Speiser B et al: Aspermia following lower truncal irradiation in Hodgkin's disease. *Cancer* 32:692–698, 1973.
32. Horning SJ et al: Female reproductive potential after treatment for Hodgkin's disease. *N Engl J Med* 304:1377–1381, 1981.

33. Bloomfield CD et al: Combined chemotherapy with cyclophosphamide, vinblastine, procarbazine, and prednisone (CVPP) for patients with advanced Hodgkin's disease. *Cancer* 38:42–48, 1976.
34. Cooper MR et al: A new effective 4 drug combination of CCNU, vinblastine, prednisone and procarbazine for the treatment of advanced Hodgkin's disease. *Cancer* 46: 654–662, 1980.
35. Bonadonna G et al: Improved 5-year survival in advanced Hodgkin's disease by combined modality approach. *Cancer Clin Trials* 2:217–226, 1979.
36. Berard C et al: A multidisciplinary approach to non-Hodgkin's lymphomas. *Ann Intern Med* 94:218, 1981.
37. Louie S, Schwartz RS: Immunodeficiency and the pathogenesis of lymphoma and leukemia. *Semin Hematol* 15:117, 1978,
38. Advisory Committee to the Renal Transplant Registry: The Thirteenth Report of the Human Renal Transplant Registry. *Transplant Proc* 9:9, 1977.
39. Krikorian JG et al: Malignant neoplasms following cardiac transplantation. *JAMA* 240:639, 1978.
40. Kinlen LJ et al: A collaborative study of cancer in patients treated with immunosuppressive drugs. *Br Med J* 2:1461, 1979.
41. Anderson LG, Tolal N: The spectrum of benign to malignant lymphoproliferation in Sjögren's syndrome. *Clin Exp Immunol* 10:199, 1972.
42. Nathwani BN et al: Malignant lymphoma arising in angioimmunoblastic lymphadenopathy. *Cancer* 41:578, 1978.
43. Krikorian JG et al: Occurrence of non-Hodgkin's lymphoma after therapy for Hodgkin's disease. *N Engl J Med* 300:452, 1979.
44. Rosenberg SA et al: Lymphosarcoma: A review of 1269 cases. *Medicine* 40:31, 1961.
45. Rappaport H et al: Follicular lymphoma: A re-evaluation of its position in the scheme of malignant lymphoma based on a survey of 253 cases. *Cancer* 9:792, 1956.
46. Byrne GE Jr: Rappaport classification of non-Hodgkin's lymphoma: Histologic features and clinical significance. *Cancer Treat Rep* 61:935, 1977.
47. Colby TV et al: Nodular lymphoma: Clinicopathological correlations of parafollicular small lymphocytes and degree of nodularity. *Cancer* 45:2364, 1980.
48. Fisher RI et al: Natural history of malignant lymphomas with divergent histologies at staging evaluation. *Cancer* 47: 2022, 1981.
49. Risdall R et al: Non-Hodgkin's lymphoma. A study of the evolution of disease based upon 92 autopsied cases. *Cancer* 44:529, 1979.
50. Jones R et al: Histologic progression in non-Hodgkin's lymphoma. Implications for survival and clinical trials. *Proc Am Soc Clin Oncol* 20:353, 1978.
51. Nathwani BN et al: Malignant lymphoma, lymphoblastic. *Cancer* 38:964, 1976.
52. Dorfman RF: Pathology of the non-Hodgkin's lymphomas: New classifications. *Cancer Treat Rep* 61:945, 1977.
53. Nathwani BN: A critical analysis of the classification of non-Hodgkin's lymphomas. *Cancer* 44:347, 1979.
54. Lukes RJ: Immunologic approach to non-Hodgkin's lymphomas and related leukemias, Analysis of the results of multiparameter studies in 425 cases. *Semin Hematol* 15:322, 1978.
55. Bloomfield CD et al: Clinical utility of lymphocyte surface markers combined with the Lukes-Collins histologic classification in adult lymphoma. *N Engl J Med* 301:512, 1979.
56. Nathwani BN et al: Malignant lymphoma, lymphoblastic. *Cancer* 38:964, 1976.
57. Stein RS et al: Correlations between immunologic markers and histopathological classifications: Clinical implications. *Semin Oncol* 7:244, 1980.
58. Dorfman RF et al: A new working formulation of non-Hodgkin's lymphomas, Background, recommendations, histologic criteria and relationships to other classifications, in *Advances in Malignant Lymphomas, Proc. Third Ann. Bristol Meyers Symposium on Cancer Research,* Academic, New York, 1981.
59. Coller BS et al: Frequencies and patterns of bone marrow involvement in the non-Hodgkin's lymphomas: Observations on the value of bilateral biopsies. *Am J Hematol* 3:105, 1977.
60. Goffinet DR et al: Clinical and surgical evaluation of patients with non-Hodgkin's lymphoma. *Cancer Treat Rep* 61:981, 1977.
61. Chabner BA et al: Sequential nonsurgical and surgical staging of non-Hodgkin's lymphoma. *Ann Intern Med* 85: 149–154, 1976.
62. Chabner BA et al: Staging on non-Hodgkin's lymphoma. *Semin Oncol* 7:285, 1980.
63. Turner DA et al: Gallium 67 imaging in the management of Hodgkin's disease and other malignant lymphomas. *Semin Nucl Med* 8:205, 1978.
64. Jones SE et al: Computer tomographic scanning in patients with lymphomas. *Cancer* 41:480, 1978.
65. Schechter JP et al: Bone scanning in lymphoma. *Cancer* 38: 1142, 1976.
66. Castellani R et al: Sequential pathologic staging of untreated non-Hodgkin's lymphoma by laparoscopy and laparotomy combined with marrow biopsy. *Cancer* 40:2322, 1978.
67. Anderson T et al: Combination chemotherapy in non-Hodgkin's lymphoma, Results of long-term follow-up. *Cancer Treat Rep* 61:1057, 1977.
68. Hellman S et al: The place of radiation therapy in the treatment of non-Hodgkin's lymphomas. *Cancer* 39:843, 1977.
69. Glatstein E et al: The potential for combined modality therapy in malignant lymphomas. *Cancer Treat Rep* 61:1199, 1977.
70. Bonadonna G et al: Combined radiotherapy-chemotherapy

in localized NHL, 5-Year results of a randomized study, in SE Jones, SE Salmon (eds): *Adjuvant Therapy of Cancer II*, Grune & Stratton, New York, 1979, pp 145–153.
71. Portlock CS, Rosenberg SA: No initial therapy for stage III & IV NHL of favorable histologic types. *Am J Med* 90:10, 1979.
72. DeVita VT et al: Changing concepts: The lymphomas, in SE Jones, SE Salmon (eds): *Adjuvant Therapy of Cancer II*, Grune & Stratton, New York, 1979, pp 173–190.
73. Chaffey JT et al: Total body irradiation in the treatment of lymphocytic lymphoma. *Cancer Treat Rep* 61:1149, 1977.
74. Bodey GP, Rodriquez V: Approaches to the treatment of acute leukemia and lymphoma in adults. *Semin Hematol* 15:221, 1978.
75. Jones SE et al: Non-Hodgkin's lymphomas. II. Single agent chemotherapy. *Cancer* 30:31, 1972.
76. Portlock CS et al: Treatment of advanced non-Hodgkin's lymphomas with favorable histologies: Preliminary results of a prospective trial. *Blood* 47:747, 1976.
77. Miller TP, Jones SE: Is there a role for radiotherapy in localized diffuse lymphomas? *Cancer Chemother Pharmacol* 4:67, 1980.
78. Bonadonna G et al: Combined radiotherapy-chemotherapy in localized non-Hodgkin's lymphomas: 5-Year results of a randomized study, in SE Jones, SE Salmon (eds): *Adjuvant Therapy of Cancer II*, Grune & Stratton, New York, 1979, pp 145–154.
79. Miller TP, Jones SE: Chemotherapy or chemotherapy with adjuvant radiotherapy for localized diffuse lymphomas, in SE Jones, SE Salmon (eds): *Adjuvant Therapy of Cancer II*, Grune & Stratton, New York, 1979, pp 155–162.
80. Fisher RI, DeVita VT: Prognostic factors for advanced diffuse histiocytic lymphoma following treatment with combination chemotherapy. *Am J Med* 63:177, 1977.
81. DeVita VT et al: Advanced diffuse histiocytic lymphoma, a potentially curable disease. *Lancet* 2:248, 1975.
82. Sweet DL, Golomb HM: The treatment of histiocytic lymphoma. *Semin Oncol* 7:302, 1980.
83. McKelvey EM, Moon TE: Curability of non-Hodgkin's lymphomas. *Cancer Treat Rep* 61:1185, 1977.
84. Coleman CN et al: Adult lymphoblastic lymphoma—results of a pilot therapy protocol. *Proc Am Soc Clin Oncol* 21:466, 1979.
85. Zeigler JL: Burkitt's lymphoma. *N Engl J Med* 305:735, 1981.
86. Cohen LF et al: Acute tumor lysis syndrome. *Am J Med* 68:486, 1980.
87. Herrmann R et al: Gastrointestinal involvement in non-Hodgkin's lymphoma. *Cancer* 46:215, 1980.
88. Lewin KJ et al: Lymphomas of the gastrointestinal tract. *Cancer* 42:693, 1978.
89. Schein PS et al: Bleomycin, Adriamycin, cyclophosphamide, vincristine, and prednisone (BACOP) combination chemotherapy in the treatment of advanced diffuse histiocytic lymphoma. *Ann Intern Med* 85:417, 1976.
90. McKelvey EM et al: Hydroxyldaunomycin (Adriamycin) combination chemotherapy in malignant lymphoma. *Cancer* 38:1484, 1976.
91. Rodriquez V et al: Combination chemotherapy ("CHOP-Bleo") in advanced (non-Hodgkin's) malignant lymphoma. *Blood* 49:325, 1977.
92. Skarin A et al: Therapy of diffuse histiocytic (DH) and undifferentiated lymphoma (DU) with high dose methotrexate and citrovorum factor rescue (MTX/CF), bleomycin (B), Adriamycin (A), cyclophosphamide (C), Oncovin® (O), and Decadron (D). *Proc Am Soc Clin Oncol* 21:463, 1980.
93. Sweet DL et al: Cyclophosphamide, vincristine, methotrexate with leukovorin rescue, and cytarabine (COMLA) combination sequential chemotherapy for advanced diffuse histiocytic lymphoma. *Ann Intern Med* 92:785, 1980.

SELECTED BIBLIOGRAPHY

Anderson T et al: Malignant lymphoma. I: The histology and staging of 473 patients at the National Cancer Institute. *Cancer* 50:2699–2707, 1982.

Anderson T et al: Malignant lymphoma. II: Prognostic factors and response to treatment of 473 patients at the National Cancer Institute. *Cancer* 50:2708–2721, 1982.

Carde P et al: A dose and time response analysis of the treatment of Hodgkin's disease with MOPP chemotherapy. *J Clin Oncol* 1:146–153, 1983.

Hubbard S et al: Histologic progression in Non-Hodgkin's lymphoma. *Blood* 59:258–264, 1982.

Skarin A et al: Improved prognosis of diffuse histiocytic and undifferentiated lymphoma by use of high-dose methotrexate alternating with standard agents (M-BACOD). *J Clin Oncol* 1:91–98, 1983.

PART NINE

NEUROSURGICAL ONCOLOGY

45

PRIMARY TUMORS OF THE CENTRAL NERVOUS SYSTEM

Mark Rosenblum   *Lawrence F. Marshall*

INCIDENCE, EPIDEMIOLOGY, AND ETIOLOGY

General Considerations

In 1975 there were an estimated 365,000 deaths from cancer in the United States. Of these, the number of patients dying of primary tumors of the brain seems comparatively small (approximately 9000); however, another 60,000 patients (15 percent) who die of cancer have intracranial metastases at the time of autopsy.[1] Thus, in about 20 percent of all patients with tumor, the brain and its coverings will be involved by neoplasm at some time in the course of the illness. Furthermore, central nervous system (CNS) tumors constitute about 10 percent of neurologic diseases encountered in a general hospital population. Among intracranial diseases, tumor is exceeded in frequency only by stroke.

It is difficult to obtain accurate statistics regarding the types of intracranial tumors. Most of them have been obtained from university hospitals and specialized neurosurgical centers that attract the more easily diagnosed and treatable forms. From the figures quoted previously secondary tumors of the brain should greatly outnumber primary ones; yet in the large series reported, only 3 to 6 percent are of this type.

Reports of the frequency of different types of tumor are influenced to a significant degree by the source of material. Statistics obtained from histologically verified tumors do not include tumors treated by irradiation without histologic confirmation (e.g., a pontine glioma or a pineal tumor). Although the distribution of various tumor types in larger medical centers is influenced by patterns of referral, generally in adults, glioblastomas account for approximately 60 percent of all intracranial gliomas, astrocytomas 22 percent, ependymomas 6 percent, and oligodendrogliomas 5 percent. The remaining glial tumors are much less frequent. In children, where 70 percent of the tumors are infratentorial in location, astrocytomas account for 48 percent of tumors of glial origin, medulloblastomas 44 percent, and ependymomas 8 percent.

Primary brain tumors account for over 2 percent of all deaths from cancer and are the most common solid tumor in children, the second most common childhood cancer after leukemia. The overall age-adjusted incidence rate in the United States for cancers of the brain reported by the National Cancer Survey was 4.5 cases per 100,000 population.[2] Among the nine areas reporting in that survey, the highest rate was 5.5 per 100,000 for the San Francisco–Oakland standard metropolitan statistical area (SMA), and the lowest was 3.8 per 100,000 in the Pittsburgh SMA. The geographic distribution shows no clear regional variations.[3] International rates vary from 0.7 per 100,000 for the Indians of Singapore to 10.5 per 100,000 among Israeli Jews.[4] Asian rates tend to be low. The incidence rate is bimodal, showing a childhood peak between ages 5 and 9 and an adult peak between ages 50 and 55. Data from the United

Kingdom shows very little variation by social class.[5] In the United States, the rate is higher among whites than blacks.[2]

Historical Aspects

Although once regarded as rare lesions, brain tumors are the most common of all childhood solid tumors and are among the three most frequently encountered tumors in females through the age of 19 and in males through the age of 39.

Although primary brain tumors rarely metastasize outside of the CNS, they eventually cause death by impairing essential functions, by increasing intracranial pressure, or by predisposing the patient to secondary complications, such as pneumonia. Prognosis is related to the nature of the tumor and to its location and size at the time of diagnosis. Brain tumors may mimic other neurologic and psychiatric diseases, particularly cerebrovascular disease and dementia.

The terms *benign* and *malignant* are applied to CNS tumors in a manner that, although useful, is confusing because of obvious inconsistencies. If left untreated, or only subtotally resected and not treated further, brain tumors can kill by their mere growth—every intracranial growth is potentially fatal. For example, benign is applied not only to meningiomas and craniopharyngiomas but also to those gliomas that are characterized by histologic differentiation and slow growth. In relation to Kernohan's four-grade system of classification, tumors of grades I and II are considered benign, and tumors of grades III and IV are considered malignant.[6] Benign is a misnomer: the better-differentiated grade I and II tumors merely have a better prognosis, and many of these tumors become more malignant at the time of recurrence.[7] Primary supratentorial malignant gliomas constitute a continuum of malignancy, beginning with the slowly growing, well-differentiated astrocytomas and ending with the rapidly growing and highly malignant glioblastoma multiforme.[7] Survival is, as would be expected, inversely related to the histologic malignancy of the tumor. Because these tumors are infiltrative and located frequently in vital areas of the brain, surgery has limited value.

Epidemiology

Little epidemiological research has been done on neoplasms of the central nervous system. A number of factors have been suggested by clinical report as possible causes of brain tumors, but most of the evidence from analytical studies is equivocal and contradictory. Suspected risk factors include livestock farming,[8] exposure to farm animals or sick pets,[9] rural farm or urban residence vs. rural nonfarm residence, and prior infection by *Toxoplasma gondii*.[10] Electricians may have an increased risk for brain cancer,[8,11] and residence near high-current electric wiring configurations vs. low configurations has been implicated in childhood brain cancer.[12] Recently, however, a large amount of suggestive evidence on the etiology of brain tumors has come from studies of workers in the rubber, plastics, and petrochemical industries. These studies suggest associations between occupational chemical exposures and CNS tumors of the glioma series.[13-15]

There is some evidence to suggest ionizing radiation as a potential cause of brain tumors. A number of individual case reports attribute meningiomas to irradiation.[16] Insofar as these case reports are corroborated by research, the findings point towards meningioma as the most likely brain tumor to be induced by radiation.

The most significant published study was done in Israel with children who had been irradiated for ringworm of the scalp (tinea capitis).[17] It found a significantly increased risk of both malignant and benign CNS neoplasms in the irradiated group, and the most striking increase in risk was of brain tumors. There were eight malignant tumors in the cases irradiated vs. one in the controls, and an identical excess of benign tumors, eight vs. one. Histologic type is not reported for the malignant tumors. Four of the eight benign tumors were meningiomas.

The differences between males and females and between children and adults in the incidence rates of the different tumor types have suggested possible genetic factors. It is well established that a genetic factor determines the occurrence of retinoblastomas, neurofibromas, and hemangioblastomas. Although there have been case reports of familial aggregations of meningioma and medulloblastoma, there is no good evidence for a genetic factor in the etiology of the more common brain tumors.[18] Only in the gliomas associated with neurofibromatosis and tuberous sclerosis is there significant evidence of a hereditary predisposition.

SIGNS, SYMPTOMS, AND ATTEMPTS AT EARLY DETECTION

When examining a patient believed to harbor an intracranial tumor, the clinician reaches a provisional diagnosis on the basis of history and neurologic findings. Usually this provisional diagnosis is then modified or confirmed by information from radiologic procedures. Clinical data indicate the biologic behavior of a tumor and neuroradiologic data suggest its morphology. Correlation of the clinical behavior of the tumor with its size, location, and effects on adjacent bone, blood vessels, and cerebrospinal fluid (CSF) spaces enables the experienced clinician to determine its probable pathologic nature.

Clinical Manifestations

Clinically there are some general, basic neurologic signs whereby the presence of brain tumor may be recognized or suspected. Fundamentally a brain tumor must be thought of as a single progressive lesion. It may irritate the brain, initiating a convulsion, the initial manifestation of which will be on the side of the body contralateral to the hemisphere involved. It may compress the brain or cranial nerves, gradually producing a progressive, contralateral focal loss of function. Increased intracranial pressure is a relatively late manifestation of intracranial growth, unless the tumor is uniquely situated to obstruct CSF pathways.

Seizures

The unexplained appearance of convulsions after the age of 21 constitutes one of the cardinal signs suggestive of brain tumor affecting the cerebrum. The clinical study of such a patient is incomplete until all reasonable modes of investigation to eliminate the possibility of tumor have been carried out. Even then, the patient with "negative" results must be followed periodically to be sure a small lesion has not escaped detection.

It must be recalled that motor phenomena constitute only one aspect of the convulsive state. Irritation of frontal structures may produce organic hallucinations. Irritation in the postcentral region may result in a sensation of numbness, tingling, "pins and needles," or of electricity. Stimulation by the tumor of the occipital lobe may produce a sensation of lights or of formed objects, usually in motion. The temporoparietal region may respond by producing auditory hallucinations, often music or voices. A lesion in the tip of the temporal lobe may result in a sensation of taste or of odors. Autonomic discharge may indicate a lesion affecting the deep-lying centers near the third ventricle or areas connected with this region. Any of these hallucinations may be isolated experiences or may constitute the aura of a motor attack.

Focal Neurologic Deficits

Focal paralysis of cerebral activity may appear as an initial sign or may follow evidence of irritation. Progressive motor impairment, particularly that which successively involves the two extremities on one side of the body, should always raise the question of brain tumor in the precentral frontal cortex or its connections. The movement of the face is impaired only slightly, if at all. Usually there is spasticity, with increased deep reflexes and the appearance of the Babinski response. Damage in the postcentral or sensory region will produce loss of appreciation of texture, form, weight, and two-point discrimination. Involvement of the optic pathway or cortical center produces a homonymous defect in part or all of the contralateral visual field. Often this defect will have been unnoticed by the patient. A homonymous field defect is one of the most commonly overlooked signs of brain tumor.

Hypofunction of the pituitary gland may result from lesions near the sella turcica. They may involve the structures near the third ventricle, producing somnolence; metabolic disturbance, such as diabetes insipidus and obesity; and sexual dystrophy.

A psychopathic state is not a common diagnostic sign of brain tumor. Invasion of the corpus callosum or of the deeper portions of the temporal lobe may, however, result in a psychosis that may be the presenting evidence of disease.

Speech may be affected by tumors that involve the dominant cerebral hemisphere of the brain, the left hemisphere in right-handed individuals. Transitory aphasia may be associated with convulsive attacks originating from the dominant side.

Increased Intracranial Pressure

GENERAL

The skull contains three normal components: brain, cerebrospinal fluid, and blood. At normal intracranial pressure, or ICP (120 to 180 mmH$_2$O), these three components maintain volumetric equilibrium. Increased volume of one component elevates ICP unless the volume of the other two components decreases proportionately (Monro-Kellie hypothesis).

An intracranial mass, e.g., tumor, introduces a fourth component, and its appearance initiates compensatory adjustments: (1) intracranial veins are compressed to reduce blood volume; (2) the volume of cerebrospinal fluid is reduced by an increased rate of absorption (and, at greatly elevated pressures, by a reduced rate of CSF production); and (3) the brain adjusts by a poorly understood reduction of intracellular and extracellular bulk. Infants and children have an additional compensatory mechanism—an expandable skull—and the younger the child, the greater the capacity of the skull for enlargement, which explains the massive craniomegaly of infantile hydrocephalus.

Increased ICP indicates failure of these compensatory mechanisms. When the rise in pressure is slow, the intracranial contents can accomplish large volumetric shifts with only slight elevation of pressure, but compensatory adjustments are less effective when the rise in pressure is more rapid.

Increased ICP may be caused by the bulk of the tumor itself or by factors related to the nature of the tumor and its location. A relatively small metastatic tumor can cause increased ICP secondary to a disproportionate degree of tumor-induced cerebral edema. Other small tumors may increase ICP by obstructing the CSF pathways. This most often occurs when tumor lies within or adjacent to the third and fourth ventricles. Consequently, intracranial hypertension does not necessarily indicate a large mass. On the other hand, since the central nervous system can accommodate a slowly expanding mass, tumors such as meningiomas that evolve at a very slow rate may not, even when they attain a large size, alter ICP or may elevate it only slightly.

CLINICAL MANIFESTATIONS

The signs of increased ICP are nonspecific. Tumors obstructing the ventricular system are often manifested solely by increased ICP; increased ICP may precede or follow focal neurologic manifestations of tumors in other sites. As a rule, the history, the neurologic examination, or both provide clues to the tumor's location by the time increased ICP is evident.

Headache is a common symptom of increased ICP. The headache is usually generalized and throbbing; it is aggravated by coughing, straining, or sudden movements. Some patients have episodes of vomiting soon after they reach the height of a paroxysmal headache. Malaise, somnolence, and general dulling of the intellect eventually appear in most patients with sustained intracranial hypertension. Poorly explained but common signs are giddiness and a tendency toward unsteadiness.

In young children, increased ICP causes physical signs, such as a tense anterior fontanelle, separation of cranial sutures with a "cracked pot" percussion noise, and enlargement of the head. In older children and in adults, the classic ophthalmoscopic finding is papilledema. Chronic papilledema may lead to blurring of vision, although, unless the tumor involves the optic nerves directly, visual acuity is seldom disturbed until papilledema is far advanced.

Increased ICP, from whatever cause, may be responsible for false localizing signs. The best known of these is lateral rectus palsy because of stretching of the sixth nerve; facial numbness, tinnitus, and mild facial weakness are less frequent.

The physiologic consequences of *acutely* elevated ICP are a rise in systolic blood pressure, bradycardia, and a fall in respiratory rate. This classic triad is seldom observed in patients harboring brain tumors unless a secondary event—e.g., seizure, acute hypoxia, or intratumoral bleeding—abruptly elevates preexisting intracranial hypertension.

Secondary Effects Due to Displacement of Brain

In response to unevenly distributed forces within the skull, semisolid brain tissue is deformed and displaced as a hernia. Herniation may occur at two important sites: (1) the uncus of the medial temporal lobe might herniate through the incisura of the tentorium and compress the midbrain, and (2) the cerebellar tonsils may herniate through the foramen magnum and compress the medulla. The final event leading to herniation may be vomiting or straining at stool. Lumbar puncture generally should not be done in a patient with a depressed level of consciousness, suspected of harboring an intracranial mass, because it lowers intraspinal pressure and thereby encourages the shift of structures from the intracranial cavity through its apertures.

Headaches Associated with Brain Tumors

The large majority of patients who complain of headache do not have a structural intracranial abnormality; those few who do have lesions usually have serious disorders that should be recognized and dealt with promptly. There are patterns of headache that shift the diagnostic probabilities toward an underlying structural disorder, and often aid the physician in sorting out which patients should be subjected to costly and potentially dangerous diagnostic procedures.

The brain, its ependymal linings, and much of its meningeal coverings are pain-insensitive.[19] The vascular pain-sensitive structures located supratentorially are innervated by the trigeminal nerve. Stimulation of these structures produces pain in the anterior portion of the head. Stimulation of the infratentorial pain-sensitive structures results in pain in the posterior portion of the head; innervation is via the ninth and tenth cranial nerves and the upper three cervical nerves. It follows, then, that posterior fossa tumors often result in occipital headache, and supratentorial tumors often produce frontal headache. However, whereas the large majority (80 percent) of cerebellar tumors result in occipital headache, about one-half of the patients with supratentorial tumors also experience occipital headache.[20] Headache is more likely to be the first symptom of a tumor located below the tentorium than of one above it. Headache is often lateralized (80 percent) homolateral to the tumor.[21] An intracranial mass lesion produces headache by displacing vessels; the headache may have a throbbing quality and may be worsened by exertion, sudden movements of the head, or the Valsalva maneuver. Headache of similar type may also occur in other conditions that predispose to vascular headaches, such as fever, giant-cell arteritis, and migraine. The provocation of headache by the ingestion of certain foods (alcohol, chocolate, dairy products, etc.), a previous history of dramatic "ice cream" headache or orthostatic symptoms (vertigo, visual obscuration, or scintillating scotomata), and headache associated with menses point toward the likelihood of migraine.

At least 60 percent of patients with brain tumors complain of headache; one-half of these consider headache to be their primary complaint.[22] The typical brain tumor headache has a dull (nonthrobbing) quality, is of moderate intensity, occurs intermittently, is worsened by exertion or change in posture, and is associated with nausea and vomiting.[22] The headache presented by brain tumor patients is often not distinctive. There are several features of head pain which, although of infrequent occurrence, have diagnostic value.

Although headaches that disturb sleep occur in only 10 percent of patients with brain tumor, this fact is notable. Sleep also may be disturbed in those with cluster headache or glaucoma, but it is a feature that should alert one to the possibility of neoplasm.

A paroxysmal headache that begins quite suddenly in a patient previously free of headache may suggest an intracranial neoplasm. In the course of 1 or 2 sec pain reaches maximal intensity that may persist for minutes to an hour or two, and then disappear as quickly as it came. The pain is most often bifrontal or generalized, of quite high intensity, and may be associated with loss of consciousness, vomiting, transient amaurosis, or sudden weakness of the legs ("drop attacks"). The presence of one or more of these latter features considerably raises the probability of brain tumor. Certain positions or rapid movement of the head may precipitate the paroxysm; conversely, changing the position of the head or lying supine may dramatically relieve the headache.

Diagnostic Techniques, Work-Up, and Staging

ATTEMPTS AT EARLY DETECTION

Tumors of the brain are manifested by focal or generalized signs and symptoms. Because gliomas are infiltrative in character, they are usually 3 to 4 cm in diameter at the time of first presentation in patients, with symptoms related to focal neurologic deficits, generalized increased ICP, and meningeal irritation. Tumor size at diagnosis is usually small if the presenting symptom is a convulsive disorder.

CT SCANNING

The detection of intracerebral neoplasms was dramatically altered with the advent of computerized tomographic (CT) brain scanning in 1973. As the technology of CT scanning continually improves, the resolution of anatomic structures and the detection of abnormalities is improving. A glioma will present as a space-occupying lesion of either decreased, normal, or increased density. Low-grade astrocytomas generally appear as a region of decreased attenuation with an associated mass effect (e.g., ventricular shift) (Fig. 45-1a) without a significant density change upon the intravenous injection of contrast material; a malignant astrocytoma usually appears as a space-occupying mass of variable density that demonstrates some regions of increasing attenuation after the intravenous injection of contrast (Fig. 45-2).

Detection by CT scanning depends upon the size of the lesion, its contrast-enhancing characteristics, and the machine's resolution. At present, the smallest abnormality discernible on a contrast-enhanced CT scan would measure approximately 3 to 5 mm in diameter. Further refinements in CT technology should improve this resolution in the future. In order to most efficiently screen patients suspected of harboring a brain tumor, a contrast-enhanced CT scan is the single study most likely to

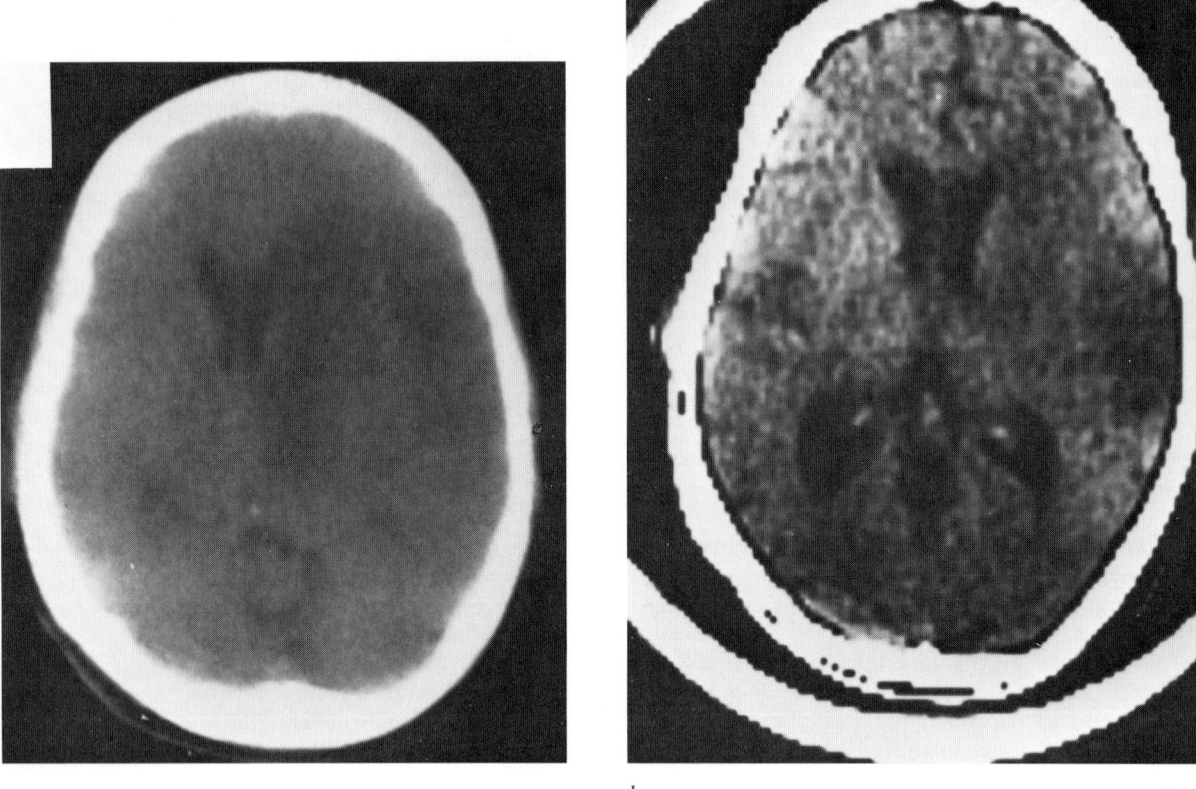

FIGURE 45-1 (*a*) Low-grade astrocytoma of the right hemisphere with significant right-to-left shift of the ventricles. (*b*) Response of low-grade astrocytoma shown in (*a*) to 6000 rads of megavoltage radiation. Note absence of shift.

identify an abnormality. Normal density in the presence of mass effect and a high density suggestive of blood or calcium would dictate the need for non-contrast-enhanced study at a later time. In this manner, patients are subjected to the least radiation exposure and the utility of CT scanners is maximized. The physician is cautioned, however, to select patients for CT scanning carefully since there is a small but definite risk with the injection of contrast material. Reactions to IV contrast material range from nausea and flushing in approximately 50 percent of patients, to vagal and hypersensitivity reactions in less than 2 percent, and death in 0.01 percent.

For detecting tumors and defining their secondary effects, CT scans have high sensitivity and moderate specificity. The CT patterns of a few tumors (i.e., neurinoma of the eighth nerve, meningioma, malignant glioma, etc.) are usually characteristic of the tumor type, and if not characteristic, the scan will be strongly suggestive of the correct diagnosis. It provides information about peritumoral edema (Fig. 45-3), cyst (Fig. 45-4), intracerebral and intratumoral hematoma, and hydrocephalus not obtained with radionuclide (RN) scans. As the initial screening test it is unequaled. To follow patients, it is preferable to have both CT and RN scans, but if circumstances permit only one study, the CT scan, with and without contrast enhancement, is the procedure of choice.

PRIMARY TUMORS OF THE CENTRAL NERVOUS SYSTEM

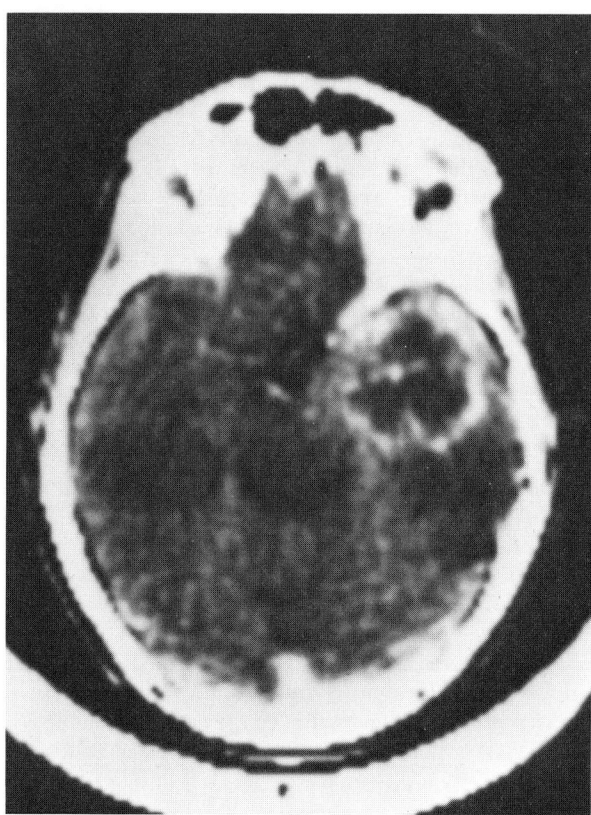

FIGURE 45-2 Typical glioblastoma multiforme with central necrosis and marked irregular enhancement.

RADIONUCLIDE SCINTISCAN (RN SCAN)

Although several radionuclides are available, [^{99}Tc]DPTA is the one widest in use. For demonstrating malignant primary and secondary tumors, the RN scan has a high degree of accuracy. The isotope is excluded by an intact blood-brain barrier (BBB), and while it is nonspecific in revealing transvascular leakage, the RN scan is quite sensitive. The recent wide availability of CT scanners has reduced the importance of the RN scan, but it will continue to have a complementary role; in unpredictable situations it provides information not obtained by CT scanning.

ANGIOGRAPHY

When a preceding CT scan has demonstrated either multiple lesions or a typical lesion in patients known to

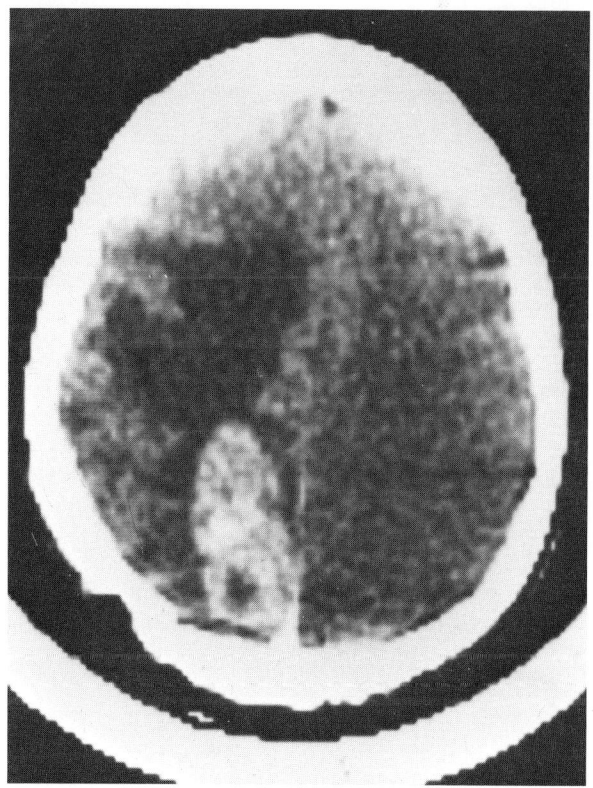

FIGURE 45-3 Anaplastic astrocytoma with marked peritumoral edema.

SKULL FILMS

Plain films of the skull may provide critical information, and without exception they should be obtained when an intracranial tumor is suspected. Findings of diagnostic value include either osteolytic or osteoblastic metastases, evidence of increased ICP displacement or a calcified pineal gland, erosion of the sella turcica, and intracranial calcification.

ELECTROENCEPHALOGRAPHY

Electroencephalography usually demonstrates an abnormality in the presence of a supratentorial intracerebral tumor. However, the localization and diagnostic utility is usually insufficient to aid in the management of patients with suspected tumors.

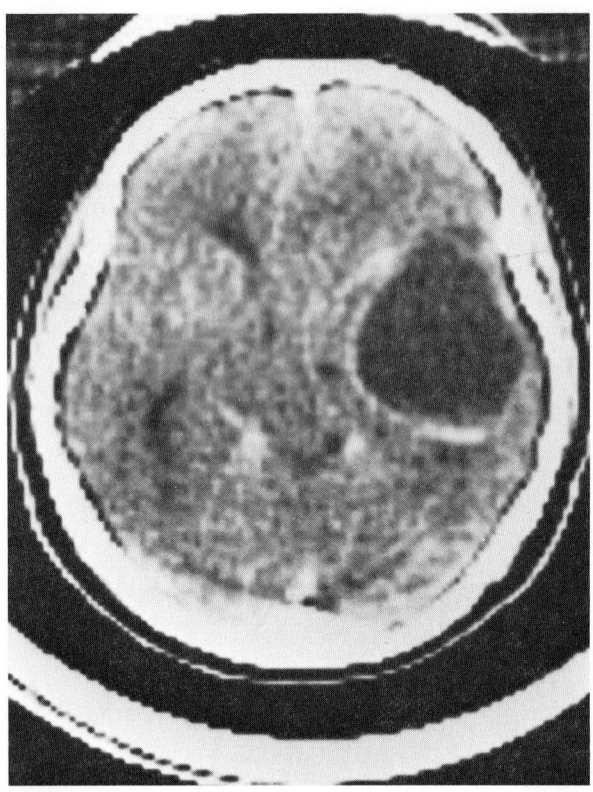

FIGURE 45-4 Anaplastic astrocytoma with large cystic component. Density of cyst is close to cerebrospinal fluid.

have an extracranial malignant primary tumor, angiography will add nothing of value. For the diagnosis of some tumors in the posterior fossa, e.g., fourth ventricle, angiography will contribute little, if anything. In the majority of supratentorial tumors, angiography provides valuable and, at times, essential information, but a decision to perform the study after obtaining a satisfactory CT scan requires the judgement of an expert. Angiography is utilized to delineate the blood supply to intracerebral tumors and to aid in the differential diagnosis of atypical cases.

VENTRICULOGRAPHY AND PNEUMOENCEPHALOGRAPHY

Ventriculography is utilized today only in those cases where an intraventricular low-density, non-contrast-enhancing tumor is suspected. Pneumoencephalography is performed by injection of air into the intrathecal space by spinal puncture.

Except for delineating pituitary and parasellar tumors, air contrast studies are not very useful. Predictably, the forthcoming availability of nontoxic, iodine-containing media that can be introduced directly into the CSF will eliminate the present usefulness of air contrast studies. Since herniation may follow spinal punctures in the presence of an intracranial space-occupying mass and increased ICP, pneumoencephalography should generally not be performed in the work-up of a brain tumor suspect with evidence of intracranial hypertension.

LUMBAR PUNCTURE

Suspicion of a brain tumor constitutes an absolute contraindication to lumbar puncture (LP) prior to examining the optic fundi, obtaining plain skull films, and review of a CT or RN scan. In the presence of a mass and a depressed level of consciousness, LP may cause fatal herniation. The potential danger of LP to a patient with a known or suspected tumor is justified only when knowledge of the nature of the fluid, not its pressure, is essential to management—e.g., when leptomeningeal seeding, subarachnoid hemorrhage, or meningitis are suspected.

NEUROECTODERMAL TUMORS: CLASSIFICATION, MORPHOLOGY, AND MANNER OF GROWTH

Neuroectodermal tumors constitute the majority of primary brain tumors submitted to special diagnostic procedures. Astrocytoma, ependymoma, and medulloblastoma predominate in the younger ages, whereas glioblastoma reaches its peak in later adult life. Gliomas, except for possibly the ependymoma, show a slight predilection for males, being most striking among children with a medulloblastoma.

Bailey and Cushing proposed the first systematic classification of glial tumors based on embryogenesis.[23] A scheme of classification often used in the United States by nonneuropathologists was developed by Kernohan at the Mayo Clinic.[6] For all glial tumors listed, this scheme defined grades of increasing malignancy by numbers I to IV. A critical point relevant to classifying brain tumors relates to morphologic heterogeneity: an opinion based on surgical material is limited to the portion of the tumor that is examined histologically. Probably, more regional differences in histologic morphology are revealed in glial tumors than in tumors elsewhere in the body, and a single tumor commonly contains areas which represent several histologic types.

The classification of tumors is intended to serve two purposes: to advance the knowledge of tumor biology and to serve as a guide to treatment. A classification becomes valuable when the behavior of a tumor and its response to treatment are predictable on the basis of its histologic characteristics. With this principle in mind, the pathologist describes a tumor on the basis of its most malignant component.

In 1972, Rubinstein discussed and offered a classification based on the traditional nomenclature of Bailey and Cushing. The classification employed in this chapter is relatively simple and relates to that of Rubinstein.[24]

The classification of the usual oligodendroglioma and ependymoma offers no problem. When these tumors have histologic features of malignancy (mitotic figures, necrosis, vascular hyperplasia), they may be termed *malignant* or called *oligodendroblastomas* and *ependymoblastomas*. Astrocytomas may be termed in a similar manner: the histologically benign are *astrocytomas;* the histologically malignant tumors *malignant astrocytomas*, or *anaplastic astrocytomas* and *glioblastomas*. The counterpart in Kernohan's classification would be astrocytomas grades I and II (benign) and grades III and IV (malignant).

Some neuropathologists suggest that the term *glioblastoma multiforme* be reserved for an astrocytic tumor with all the histologic features of malignancy described later. They would apply the term *malignant* or *anaplastic* to astrocytomas with some, but not all, of these features.

The astrocytomas can be subdivided according to predominant histologic characteristics. Such terms as *protoplasmic astrocytoma, fibrillary astrocytoma, pilocytic astrocytoma, gemistocytic astrocytoma,* and *polar spongioblastoma* convey precise definitions of particular patterns of neoplastic cells and their glial processes. The validity of this terminology is supported by the consistent location of these tumors in certain portions of the central nervous system.

The term *mixed glioma* describes a tumor that contains nearly equal proportions of more than one tumor type. The term should not be applied to a tumor with small nests or areas of another tumor type (e.g., a small area of olgiodendrocytes in an otherwise homogeneous ependymoma). A common mixed glioma is the mixed astrocytoma and oligodendroglioma in the cerebral hemispheres of children. Pure cultures of any given cell type are, in fact, rare in glioma.

General Considerations

Certain generalizations regarding gliomas are in order. They occur at any period of life from infancy to old age, more often in males than in females. In adults, gliomas are most often found in the cerebrum, whereas those in the cerebellum and brainstem have a greater incidence in childhood. They are always invasive, never being encapsulated in the true sense of the word. They may spread to the meningeal surface and become attached to the dura mater, but they do not advance beyond it.

More than 90 percent of gliomas are localized to a single area of the brain. Occasionally, they have a multicentric origin. Metastases from these tumors within the central nervous system are uncommon,[25] and systemic metastases are rare.[26,27]

Morphology and Manner of Growth

Most gliomas (astrocytoma, glioblastoma, oligodendroglioma, medulloblastoma) are primarily infiltrative; they invade rather than displace surrounding brain. As a consequence, the transition between tumor and normal brain is not distinct, and histologic examination of grossly normal brain obtained from beyond the apparent tumor edge commonly shows microscopic nests of neoplastic cells. A few glioblastomas assume a more or less globular shape and appear sharply circumscribed. The most clearly circumscribed astrocytoma is the cystic tumor of the cerebellar hemisphere; but even here, unless the tumor is confined to a mural nodule, at least some infiltrative growth into grossly uninvolved brain is the rule. Glial tumors may invade the subarachnoid space. Some tumors, especially oligodendroglioma and glioblastoma, may adhere to the dura. They may then derive a portion of their blood supply from the external carotid artery and grossly simulate a meningioma.

Intraventricular tumors are much less common than intracerebral or extracerebral tumors. Gliomas, in particular ependymoma and mixed oligodendroglioma-astrocytoma, may have an intraventricular component but are more often largely intracerebral. Most supratentorial intraventricular tumors involve the lateral ventricles; and in the young, the common types are choroid plexus papilloma, ependymoma, and astrocytoma. The intraventricular tumor most common in adults is a meningioma of the lateral ventricle, but colloid cysts of the third ventricle appear often enough to be considered important.

THERAPEUTIC OPTIONS FOR PRIMARY TREATMENT

Tumors of the central nervous system (CNS) vary, from the relatively benign meningioma or pituitary microadenoma to the exceedingly malignant glioblastoma multiforme. This chapter deals exclusively with primary parenchymal intracranial neoplasms. In addition to the histologic variations, the clinical effects and management of CNS tumors differ according to location: a brainstem astrocytoma presents problems different from those due to a lesion of similar histology in a frontal lobe. Useful therapeutic modalities include surgical resection, radiation therapy, and chemotherapy with single or multiple drugs. Thus, selection of the appropriate treatment for a particular patient requires knowledge of tumor histology, location, extent, and biologic characteristics, as well as the value and limitations of each therapeutic modality used singly or in combination.

Surgery

The primary surgical goals include obtaining the pathological diagnosis; removing mass lesions to decompress adjacent, nonfunctioning cerebral tissue and secondarily decrease patient's symptoms; debulking tumors to improve the response to adjuvant therapeutic maneuvers such as radiotherapy and drugs, and to permit the patient to survive the period required to receive these adjuvant treatments.

Today, as in the recent past, most patients who have a primary brain tumor undergo a neurosurgical procedure. In a few specific cases—for example, when clinical and radiographic evidence is unequivocally diagnostic of a solid brainstem tumor in a child—operation is rarely performed for the sole purpose of confirming the diagnosis.

Morbidity and mortality rates associated with neurosurgical operations have decreased substantially, reflecting more informative diagnostic methods, improved intraoperative and postoperative management of disturbed intracranial physiology, the evolution of microsurgical techniques, and the optimal use of effective agents for combating brain edema—particularly the adrenal corticoids. Steroids are highly effective, and the response to steroids is dose-dependent. When doses once considered maximal are ineffective, a response is often obtained at considerably higher dose levels.

Since the majority of malignant brain tumors are surgically accessible,[28] and particularly in view of the increased response to chemotherapy that can be anticipated after reducing tumor volume, the decision not to biopsy a suspected tumor, or to perform only a needle biopsy, should be discouraged in most circumstances, particularly in younger patients. However, because a malignant brain tumor has never been cured by surgery, the principle of aggressiveness in good *cancer* surgery must be tempered with the principle of preservation of neurologic function in good *brain* surgery. The invasiveness of brain tumors into cerebral areas that subserve such important functions as speech precludes extensive surgical resection of tumor. One does not recklessly pursue infiltrative tumors deep into the dominant hemisphere without the risk of reducing the patient to a vegetative state. Furthermore, if resection has not achieved adequate internal decompression, postoperative edema of the residual tumor and surrounding brain may cause serious complications.

The application of microsurgical techniques to surgery of malignant brain tumors has helped the surgeon to differentiate tumor from normal tissue, and to identify small points of persistent bleeding for coagulation. In addition, some surgeons have relied on the effects of adjuvant radiation and chemotherapy to reduce tumor vascularity, so that additional tumor can be removed at a "second-look" operation.[29]

Shunting for hydrocephalus is used most often for tumors of the posterior fossa. The risk that the procedure may spread tumor cells to extracranial sites such as the peritoneal cavity should be recognized. When indicated, a filter can be inserted into the shunting system. With the recent renewal of interest in intrathecal chemotherapy, neurosurgeons are being called upon to implant ventricular reservoirs. The technical requirements for implanting a functional reservoir seem deceptively simple, but correct placement of the ventricular catheter and its reservoir is not a procedure to be delegated to someone unfamiliar with potential complications.

Perioperative Ancillary Measures

There are several ancillary measures related to surgical removal of brain tumors that should be considered to ensure optimal care of the surgical patient.

PREOPERATIVE

The patient scheduled for elective craniotomy should reach the operating room in optimal condition. The procedure should be postponed in order to correct fluid and electrolyte imbalances, anemia, and active infection. The lungs deserve particular attention, and in the patient with chronic bronchopulmonary disease, a delay of several days is justified for intensive inhalation therapy and supportive measures.

For 1 or preferably 2 days before operation, the patient's scalp and hair are washed with a germicidal soap. To avoid bacterial contamination of razor cuts and abrasions, the scalp is shaved outside of the operating room immediately before induction of anesthesia.

Twenty-four hours before operation, all patients destined for tumor removal receive a priming course of an adrenal corticosteroid. Earlier preoperative administration is advisable if the patient is obtunded as a consequence of increased ICP or compression of midline structures. For patients with tumors that block CSF drainage, external ventricular drainage and shunting have been advocated as a means of reducing ICP and thereby improving the patient's preoperative condition. Because the removal of ventricular fluid can predispose to upward transtentorial herniation of posterior fossa structures, it is preferable, in most instances, to move more quickly to a definitive operation rather than risk this complication.

The patient should reach the operating room after a good night's sleep and as free from apprehension as circumstances permit. The patient's psychological preparation for a life-threatening operation assumes critical importance during the postoperative period when the patient's full cooperation is required.

INTRAOPERATIVE

The patient's position on the operating table can either simplify or complicate the surgeon's task. Attention directed to the details of positioning is time spent wisely.

For approaches to supratentorial tumors, with the exception of biocciptal exposures, the patient's torso is placed in a reclining position, varying from supine to semiprone. The head should never be turned sharply to the side, as angulation of the head can cause venous obstruction. The operating table is elevated 30° above horizontal to assure low intracranial venous pressure, and from this preliminary position, the vertex can be lowered to or below horizontal to assist exposure beneath the frontal or temporal lobe.

Adrenal corticosteroids are more effective in preventing than in treating traumatic brain edema. On this basis a priming dose is administered intravenously at the start of the operation. During the operative procedure, the patient receives maintenance intravenous fluids of 5% dextrose in one-half normal saline.

The surgeon has three means of reducing intracranial bulk to facilitate atraumatic exposure and removal of any brain tumor: removal of cerebrospinal fluid, the use of hypertonic solutions, and hyperventilation.

Removal of cerebrospinal fluid is simple, direct, and generally free of complications. Spinal drainage can be used safely after the dura has been opened. When the surgical exposure permits cannulation of a lateral ventricle, an indwelling catheter may be placed to afford constant or intermittent drainage and provide a means of reexpanding the brain prior to closure.

Hypertonic solutions, usually mannitol, have a well-established role in the operating room; however, because their administration can complicate replacement of fluid and electrolytes and requires a urinary catheter, these agents should not be used unnecessarily. Ventricular drainage often can accomplish the same purpose. Hypertonic solutions are given during the approach to and the removal of tumors in the following circumstances: (1) when elevated ICP cannot be relieved by drainage of CSF, (2) when exposure requires deep retractions, (3) during the approach to a subcortical tumor that one anticipates removing totally, and (4) to minimize retractor pressure on adjacent normal brain.

Moderate hyperventilation, i.e., lowering the Pco_2 to 25 mmHg, can be used during the majority of intracranial procedures for tumor removal. Additional room within the skull can sometimes be obtained by further lowering the Pco_2 to 20 mmHg. Levels below this introduce the possible hazard of ischemic brain injury.

The selection of anesthetic techniques should minimize the use of agents which cause cerebral vasodilation. Sole use of the halogenated agents and ketamine are often contraindicated because they increase the risk of elevating ICP.

POSTOPERATIVE

There is nothing unique about the care of a patient following the removal of an intracranial tumor. The postoperative complications do not differ from those encountered after intracranial operations for nonneoplastic conditions. Two problems may arise: (1) the operation's magnitude often leaves the patient in an obtunded state and particularly susceptible to complications; and (2) when accentuated by delayed edema, a postoperative neurologic deficit may either simulate or mask an intracranial blood clot.

Postoperative management requires meticulous attention to details. Administration of an adrenal corticosteroid is continued during the early postoperative period, the dosage and duration varying according to the patient's course. Water intoxication must be avoided by the administration of only salt-containing fluids and the maintenance of accurate records of serum electrolytes, fluid balance, and body weight is mandatory. Nausea is treated promptly and vigorously by removing stomach contents by suction and administering antiemetics. Codeine effectively relieves headache and pain related to the incision; stronger pain medications should be avoided. The administration of diphenylhydantoin (Dilantin) in therapeutic doses is routine after supratentorial procedures. It is usually initiated in the preoperative period and must be continued indefinitely in almost all patients.

Restlessness may be an indication of hypoxia or of a postoperative hematoma and therefore demands prompt evaluation. Unrelenting headache and restlessness should not be dismissed as components of an uncomplicated postoperative course.

Routine postoperative measures such as body position and pulmonary care are utilized. Intermittent positive-pressure breathing (IPPB), however, and positive end-expiratory pressures (PEEP) greater than 10 mmH$_2$O, both of which may result in increased ICP, should be avoided when possible.

General Principles of Central Nervous System Radiation Therapy

Modern radiation therapy utilizes megavoltage techniques. These are sources with energy greater than 1 MeV. Compared to kilovoltage irradiation, higher-voltage techniques have the advantage of greater penetration, less absorption in bone, decreased side scatter, and reduced dose to skin and subcutaneous tissues. High-dose regimens used for primary brain tumors, especially glioblastoma, carry definite possibilities of radiation injury.

There are a number of factors which are known to influence the degree of risk. The greater the daily dose (individual fraction of treatments if other than daily), the total dose, and the volume irradiated, the greater the risk. The location of radiation injury is dependent upon the site irradiated. The consequences are also dependent on the location. For example, a small lesion in the brainstem could be fatal, but a similar lesion in the frontal lobe might pass undetected. When total doses do not exceed 5000 or 5500 rads, and the individual fractions do not exceed 200 rads, the incidence of clinically significant radiation injury to the brain is low, considerably less than 5 percent. Under circumstances where benign intracranial tumors are being treated, these dose fractions are commonly used. The administration of concurrent chemotherapy appears to increase the likelihood of brain injury secondary to irradiation; however, the data supporting these observations is limited primarily to patients who have received prophylactic irradiation such as in the treatment of acute stem cell leukemia.

Therapy-related changes have been found in children who have received cranial irradiation and chemotherapy. Peylan-Ramu et al. reported CT-scan evidence of ventricular dilatation and wide subarachnoid space, atrophy, and intracerebral calcification after prophylactic treatment of acute lymphocytic leukemia with radiation, which was given in 2400 rads in 12 fractions.[30] These patients also received intrathecal methotrexate. It appears that the changes that occur in patients receiving multiple-modality therapy, including radiation, are more prevalent in those patients who have generalized diseases of the nervous system than in patients who have focal processes such as brain tumors. Nevertheless, there is significant concern about the long-term effects of radiation therapy in patients who have long potential survival times.

Radiation can also produce pituitary dysfunction; growth hormone production is especially sensitive. Pituitary hormone deficiencies have been reported in children and adults after irradiation of the hypothalamic pituitary axis for tumors that were near, but did not involve, the pituitary gland or the hypothalamus.[31-33]

ANATOMIC AND HISTOLOGIC CHARACTERISTICS AND GENERAL PRINCIPLES OF INITIAL TREATMENT FOR DIFFERENT PRIMARY BRAIN TUMORS

Anatomic location and histology influence decisions regarding primary therapy for cancers of all organ systems; however, for primary tumors of the brain, anatomic location exerts an extraordinary influence on operability. There is a correlation between histology and anatomic location. It is important to briefly discuss histology and anatomic location of primary malignant brain tumors, as well as to examine in more detail those characteristics of the most common primary malignant brain tumor, the glioblastoma.

Tumors of Adults

GLIOBLASTOMA MULTIFORME

Glioblastoma multiforme is the most frequent (60 percent of all glial tumors) and most rapidly growing primary brain tumor. It usually occurs in the cerebral hemispheres in direct proportion to the volume that each lobe contributes to the total volume of the brain. Less frequently, glioblastoma multiforme occurs in the brainstem, cerebellum or even in the spinal cord. The peak incidence is in midlife, but no age group is spared.

This tumor is highly malignant and is characterized by extensive infiltration of the brain. The first symptoms, which include increased ICP, focal weakness, speech disturbances, or personality changes, usually occur only a few weeks to a few months prior to diagnosis. Without any intervention the mean survival time for these patients is less than 3 months. At postmortem examination, about half of glioblastomas are bilateral, or occupy more than one lobe of the hemisphere. Between 3 and 6 percent show separate, multicentric foci of growth.

Glioblastoma may present with an abrupt onset or worsening of symptoms as a consequence of intratumoral hemorrhage, and thus mimic vascular catastrophes such as aneurysms, arteriovenous malformations, or stroke.

A less common variant of glioblastoma multiforme is gliomatosis cerebri, in which an entire hemisphere or the entire brain appears to be diffusely infiltrated without a discrete tumor mass. The diagnosis of this condition is extremely difficult, and this particular variant may mimic pseudotumor cerebri, collagen vascular disease, and other disorders which result in diffuse brain swelling, and even slowly progressive degenerative disease.

The term *glioblastoma multiforme* has been used to include all tumors believed to be astrocytic in origin, and which possess histologic characteristics of malignancy. The term should be restricted to those tumors that demonstrate the following abnormalities, characteristic of histologic malignancy in the brain:

1. Glial cellular pleomorphism and hypercellularity
2. Mitotic figures
3. Multinucleated or giant cells
4. Pseudo pallisading of cells among the border and necrotic areas
5. Hemorrhage unrelated to surgical removal
6. Vascular hyperplasia, involving epithelium, endothelium, and adventitia. The neoplastic vessels often form a complex glomerular pattern.

For neoplasms with some but not all of these histologic features, the term *malignant,* or *anaplastic, astrocytoma* may be applied. This separation is somewhat artificial. It is believed that a primary glioblastoma is a tumor malignant from its inception that contains a homogeneous population of malignant cells. The anaplastic astrocytoma, or malignant astrocytoma, has a longer history and contains microscopic evidence of an earlier, more benign state, such as fibrillary astrocytoma.

The sectional surface of the glioblastoma appears variegated, with yellow areas of necrosis and foci of old and recent small hemorrhages. In addition, there are often cysts, which usually are small, less than 1 cm in diameter, but occasionally they are quite large and filled with amber fluid. Some tumors have a firm, rubbery consistency, usually at a site where the tumor is attached to the dura. Glioblastomas can invade the leptomeninges and adhere to the dura; superficial biopsy can reveal fibroblastic and glial components, or, more rarely, frank fibrosarcoma. Occasionally, the neurosurgeon may believe that surface glioblastomas are meningiomas at the time of operation. Usually, however, the deeper portions of the tumor have a distinctly malignant character on and inseparable from the brain, which it deeply infiltrates. On the CT scan, the tumor often appears as an area of central, low attenuation surrounded by irregular areas of contrast enhancement (Fig. 45-2).

Radical resection is usually possible only for polar tumors, i.e., frontal, temporal tip, or occipital lobe. Bulk reduction is of definite value and should be performed when anatomically feasible, guided by the principles elucidated previously.

Postresection radiation therapy has been demonstrated to definitely increase the survivorship of patients with glioblastoma. It is important to recall that the number of 5-year survivors with this tumor is almost nil, regardless of whether or not patients receive radiation therapy. The Brain Tumor Study Group (BTSG), which has been active for more than one decade, found that radiation therapy at a total dose of 6000 rads increased the median survival time from 17 weeks (surgery alone) to 38 weeks.[34] Median survival time can be directly correlated with age and Karnofsky, or general status, rating. Survivorship appears to be dose-related. Irrespective of other variables, median survival time was 28, 36, and 42 weeks for radiation therapy doses of approximately 5000, 5500, and 6000 rads.

Because of the relative failure of radiation therapy to yield long-term control in patients with glioblastoma multiforme, many prospective randomized trials of radiation therapy, in various combinations with adjuvant chemotherapy, have been conducted. Most recent is a report from Walker et al. from the BTSG which demonstrated that the combination of BCNU plus radiation therapy produced a significant, albeit modest, benefit in long-term (18-month and 5-year) survival times compared with radiation therapy alone (5 percent 5-year survival with adjunctive chemotherapy).[35] Patients likely to have a significant response to combination therapy with radiation and BCNU, given in a dose of 80 mg/m^2 for 3 days, every 8 weeks, were those patients under the age of 55 and those with Karnofsky performance scale scores greater than 70. They had significantly improved survival rates compared with patients whose clinical status was worse, or with those who were older at the time therapy was instituted. Thus, although treatment for glioblastoma remains disappointing, radiation and adjuvant chemotherapy can begin to be targeted toward those patients most likely to demonstrate a long-term response, i.e., those whose clinical status is better and those who are younger at the time that they first present. Since this is likely to be the group still most active in a productive capacity in our society, this observation is important.

ASTROCYTOMAS IN THE CEREBRAL HEMISPHERE

Cerebral astrocytomas are generally considered slow-growing tumors of infiltrative character, with a tendency to form large cavities or pseudocysts. Frequently cerebral astrocytomas, particularly in adults, eventually undergo malignant degeneration, so that the term *benign astrocytoma* is, in many instances, inappropriate.

Approximately one-half of the patients with astrocytoma present with focal or generalized seizures, and two-thirds have recurrent seizures during their illness. The onset of focal seizures should always arouse suspicion of a cerebral astrocytoma in individuals between the ages of 20 and 60 years. Subtle changes in personality and in performance occur and often lead to diagnosis. Headaches and symptoms of increased ICP are relatively late occurrences.

In the past, the interval between the initial symptom and the diagnosis was often extremely long. With high-resolution CT scanning, these intervals of 10 years or more are likely to shorten significantly. In contrast to the glioblastoma, the average survival time after the first symptom in patients with astrocytomas is 67 months.

Astrocytoma almost always contains a varying portion of microscopically visible glial fibers. When it contains few glial fibers, it is gray, soft, and similar to other cell-rich, fiber-poor tumors, such as the ependymoma. When it is rich in glial fibers, it is firm and it may be yellow or white, and is easily distinguishable from normal white matter because of its toughness. When the proportion of glial cells is similar to that in normal white matter, the tumor may be extremely difficult to diagnose, both grossly and histologically. Necrosis or hemorrhage are not features of a cerebral astrocytoma. When these features are present, they indicate a malignant, or anaplastic, neoplasm. These neoplasms are frequently cystic, having multiple microcysts or one large macroscopic cyst. The fluid is usually amber in color and characteristically coagulates if left standing.

There have been no randomized controlled studies to evaluate the effectiveness of surgery and radiation in the treatment of better-differentiated astrocytomas, although many of these tumors are radioresponsive (Fig. 45-1a and b). Leibel et al. (1975) reviewed the experience at the University of California at San Francisco (UCSF).[36] Patients underwent craniotomy with biopsy and surgical removal of as much tumor as was consistent with the preservation of satisfactory neurologic status. The patients were separated into three groups for analysis. In the first group, there were 14 patients in whom the surgeon thought he had carried out a gross, complete removal. The second group included 37 patients who had incomplete resections, and who received no radiation therapy. In the third group of 71 patients, radiation therapy followed an incomplete resection.

Group 1 is difficult to evaluate, as 9 of the 14 patients had benign cerebellar astrocytomas of childhood. Radiation therapy is not indicated in this disease unless there are ominous histologic features present at the time of operation, as demonstrated by histopathologic examination. In group 2, the 5-year recurrence-free survival was shorter than for group 3 patients. In patients who had well-differentiated astrocytomas (grade I lesions) the 5-year survival rate with radiation therapy was

58 percent. Without radiation it was 25 percent. In the patients with grade II lesions, there was a 25 percent survival rate in those patients who had been irradiated and no survivors in those who had not received radiation. At 20 years, approximately one-fourth of those irradiated were alive, but all nonirradiated patients had died. Similar results have been reported by Fazekas.[37]

From this data, one can conclude that patients with supratentorial, incompletely excised astrocytomas should receive radiation therapy. Treatment should be initiated when the patient has recovered from surgery and the wound is well healed. Daily fractions of 180 to 200 rads to a total dose of 5500 to 6000 rads is recommended standard therapy. Under circumstances where the pathology is relatively benign, such as a grade I astrocytoma of the hemisphere, dose reduction to 5000 to 5500 rads is considered appropriate by many.

MALIGNANT, OR ANAPLASTIC ASTROCYTOMA OF THE CEREBRAL HEMISPHERES

Anaplastic astrocytomas have characteristically represented the areas of most controversy in clinical neuropathology. These tumors, which by contemporary definition arise from previously identifiable astrocytic cell lines, have some, but not all, of the characteristics of glioblastoma. One unusual feature is their predilection for the temporal lobe. These tumors represent an intermediate stage on the biological continuum of cerebral astrocytoma and glioblastoma multiforme, and thus, the patient's course is usually somewhat intermediate between the two extremes.

Grade III astrocytomas are considered, for the purpose of this discussion, as a single group and will be referred to as either malignant or anaplastic astrocytomas. There have been a variety of studies carried out in patients with anaplastic astrocytomas. It is possible to state with certainty that the 5-year survival rates are improved by irradiation in these patients. If all series are combined, the 5-year survival rate in those who did not receive irradiation was 2 percent vs. 16 percent in those with a resection and irradiation. The average 5-year survival rate for irradiated patients who had received at least 5000 rads was 20 percent. Thus, although the outlook for these patients is poor, it is not hopeless, and aggressive radiation therapy is indicated. Adjunctive chemotherapy exerts a synergistic effect with radiation therapy in approximately one-half of the patients. As in glioblastomas, age and performance states were useful predictors of response.

OLIGODENDROGLIOMAS

Oligodendrogliomas predominate in the cerebral hemispheres of adults. Their growth is generally slow, and calcification of what has been called a "railroad track" type is not infrequent.

The most common sites are the frontal lobes. These tumors are often deep in the white matter with little or no surrounding edema. Occasionally they may occur in the region of the third ventricle. Oligodendrogliomas grow slowly. In the past, the interval between the first symptom and surgical intervention usually varied from 2 to 5 years. More than one-half of the patients present initially with focal and/or generalized seizures.

Histologically, these tumors are soft, gray-pink in color, and are usually clearly demarcated from the adjacent brain. They may spread widely beneath the leptomeninges and not infrequently may intrude above the surrounding surface of the brain, giving an appearance of melted wax as it spreads over the surface of adjacent gyri.

Oligodendrogliomas are rare, and thus it is difficult to assess the absolute value of radiation therapy. Sheline demonstrated, by pooling several series, a 5-year 35 percent survival rate in the nonirradiated patients, with a 63 percent corresponding survival rate for patients who were irradiated.[38] Patients who died shortly after surgery were excluded from this study and there was no attempt to randomize patients. While it appears that irradiation was effective, the pooled data may exaggerate its efficacy.

MICROGLIOMA (RETICULUM-CELL SARCOMA)

Reticulum-cell sarcoma grows as rapidly as a glioblastoma, with the interval between the first symptom and the operation varying between a few weeks to a few months. Headache and signs of increased ICP predominate. This tumor should strongly be suspected in renal transplant patients and other individuals who have been given immunosuppressive drugs for long periods of time. Sometimes it is a complication of obscure medical conditions, such as iridocyclitis and idiopathic parotiditis (Mikulicz's syndrome). This tumor appears to be increasing in frequency. Craniotomy and biopsy are considered necessary for diagnosis. The initial response to radiation therapy is extremely dramatic in this condition, as opposed to its much more moderate effectiveness in the treatment of glioblastoma. The long-term effectiveness of radiation therapy is unclear at the present time, however.

This tumor is the intracranial equivalent of other diseases of the reticuloendothelial (RE) system. Meningeal histiocytes and microgliocytes, which are the representatives of the RE system of the brain, are the source of this tumor. Unlike its systemic counterparts, however, the response rates of this neoplasm to adjuvant chemotherapy or chemotherapy alone have been rather disappointing. This probably represents failure of at least some of the agents to penetrate the blood-brain barrier, a problem discussed in more detail later.

EPENDYMOMA AND EPENDYMOBLASTOMA

Ependymomas arise from the walls of the ventricles and either grow into the ventricle or into adjacent tissue. Approximately 5 percent of all intracranial tumors are ependymal in origin. The percentage is considerably higher in children, approximately 15 percent. About 40 percent of the infratentorial ependymomas occur in the first 10 years of life; a few are seen immediately following birth.

The symptomatology depends on the location of growth. An ependymoma that originates on the floor of the fourth ventricle may invade the subjacent brainstem. Thus, the clinical manifestations of posterior fossa ependymomas almost always include cerebellar dysfunction, and, not infrequently, brainstem dysfunction. In contrast with the brainstem gliomas, these patients almost always have hydrocephalus secondary to obstruction of CSF drainage pathways.

Cerebral ependymomas arise in the lateral ventricle near the trigone and resemble other gliomas in their clinical expression. The time from first symptom to clinical presentation is quite varied because signs and symptoms may be extremely insidious.

On gross examination, ependymomas are usually well demarcated from surrounding brain; most are gray, soft, and moderately vascular. The portion that projects into the ventricle may be nodular or even papillary. The surface of an intracerebral ependymoma is granular, and some of these tumors may occasionally be cystic. Despite its location, an ependymoma seldom spreads through the CSF; consequently, metastasis to the spine is rare either before or after surgery, unless the tumor is of the blastic type. Under those circumstances, its behavior is more similar to the medulloblastoma, where spinal metastasis is relatively common.

For patients treated with postoperative radiation therapy of approximately 4500 rads, 5-year survival rates of between 60 and 87 percent and 10-year recurrence-free survival rates of 50 to 60 percent have been reported.[39,40] These results appear better than the results obtained by surgery alone, and it is recommended that ependymomas be treated with radiation whenever surgical removal is incomplete. There is controversy, however, regarding the extent of the central nervous system that should be irradiated. Although neurosurgeons have the impression that spinal seeding is relatively common with ependymomas, this impression is correct only for infratentorial lesions. In a series of 40 supratentorial lesions, only 1 metastasized to the spine. In patients with infratentorial primaries, there is evidence of seeding in about 25 percent of high-grade and about 4 percent of low-grade tumors. Thus, patients with high-grade, posterior fossa ependymomas should receive craniospinal irradiation. Ependymomas which involve the cerebral hemispheres, on the other hand, appear to be appropriately treated with local irradiation.

SUBEPENDYMAL MIXED GLIOMA

The subependymal mixed glioma, or subependymoma, is a particular type of glioma in which papillary astrocytes dominate the architecture. This tumor is of interest because of its historical association with tuberous sclerosis. The tumor, because of its clearly identifiable ependymal cells, and because of its intraventricular location, is considered by some to be a variant of the ependymoma, although others believe that it is merely a fibrous astrocytoma occurring adjacent to the ventricles. These tumors are very small and often seen in older patients; thus, a considerable number have been coincidental postmortem findings.

Treatment in symptomatic cases is usually excision. If there is any evidence of malignant transformation, radiation therapy is recommended.

CHOROID PLEXUS PAPILLOMA

Although these tumors are relatively rare, accounting for less than 2 percent of all intracranial neoplasms, neurosurgeons have been fascinated with them for many years because of the following characteristics:

1. They may be recognized in newborn infants.
2. There is a striking predilection for males, and for location in the left lateral ventricle.

Furthermore, these tumors may occasionally result in an excessive production of cerebrospinal fluid, a phenomenon which, prior to recent definite recognition, had been hotly debated for many years. These tumors are more frequent in the fourth ventricle in adults and in the lateral ventricle in children, the converse of what is usually the rule for intracranial neoplasms. These tumors have a notorious predilection to seed along the CSF pathways, and occasionally may undergo carcinomatous transformation. The treatment for choroid plexus papilloma is excision. Where carcinomatous change has taken place, radiation therapy has been recommended, but these patients follow a notoriously inexorable course.

Brain Tumors of the Pediatric Age Group

CEREBELLAR ASTROCYTOMA

Cerebellar astrocytomas are the most commonly found intracranial neoplasms in patients under the age of 15 years. In young children, they are more frequently located in the midline, while in the adolescent, they occur more commonly in the lateral hemispheres of the cerebellum. Younger children have signs of obstructive hydrocephalus with gait disturbance and papilledema. In older patients, unilateral hemispheric symptoms and signs predominate with dysmetria and limb ataxia.

As with other neoplasms of the central nervous system, CT scanning has allowed the early recognition of these tumors. When a cystic hemispheric or fourth ventricular mass is seen, which enhances only moderately in the posterior fossa in this age group, cerebellar astrocytoma should be strongly suspected (Fig. 45-5).

Optimal therapy in these children is complete surgical removal if the mass is well circumscribed. Gjerris has demonstrated that children with a specific histologic type, i.e., the juvenile astrocytoma, have a 25-year survival rate of 90 percent.[41] In contrast, where the histology demonstrates a more densely packed tumor, the diffuse astrocytoma of childhood, only one-third of the patients survive over a long period. Thus, in cases where there is dense cellularity and pleomorphism, the likelihood of recurrence and death is very great. Treatment in these patients should be more aggressive than previously proposed, including both radical surgical removal and radiation therapy. There are no trials of radiation therapy from which to draw absolute conclusions, as the recognition of the different biological behaviors related to histology has only recently become apparent.

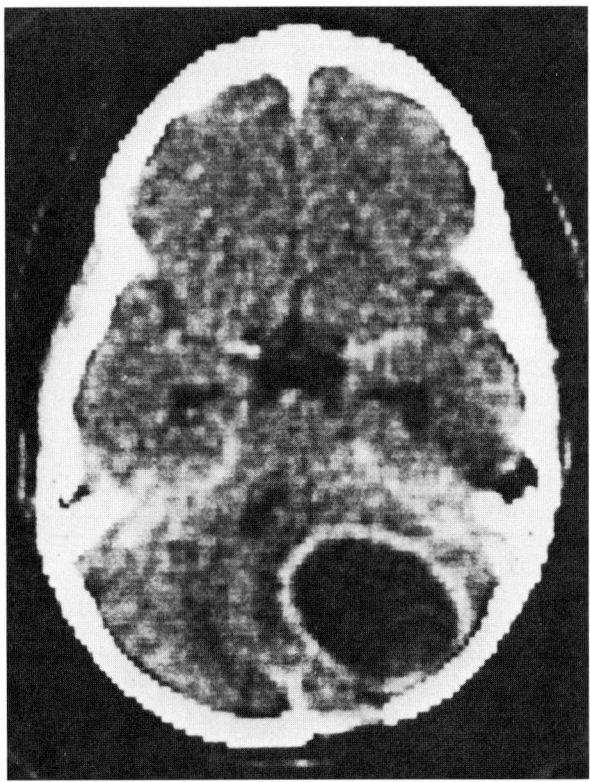

FIGURE 45-5 Cystic cerebellar astrocytoma in the right cerebellar hemisphere. The cyst wall enhances in a uniform fashion.

MEDULLOBLASTOMAS

Medulloblastomas account for approximately 20 percent of all intracranial tumors in children. There is a peak incidence in the first decade of life and a second peak late in the second decade. The tumor occurs with decreasing frequency in older patients. It is twice as common in males as in females. This sex dominance persists, although not to the same degree, throughout life. Historical follow-up of patients in many series demonstrates statistically improved survival rates in females and in patients older than 10 years, indicating a different biological behavior because of sex and age.

Recently, Palmer et al. have hypothesized that medulloblastoma represents a neoplasm arising from a stem cell.[42] They believe that undifferentiated tumors representing the most malignant form are more common in younger children and that tumors of neuronal astrocytic, ependymal, and other cell types occur and can be specifically recognized. Historical evidence which suggests that tumors with desmoplastic features in which there is to be a mesodermal component have an improved survival rate was also supported by their observations.

Medulloblastomas almost always occur in the fourth ventricle. The signs and symptoms of medulloblastoma are generally those of a midline cerebellar lesion. Nausea and vomiting with headache are predominant features, with traumatic gait disturbances following shortly thereafter. Since the majority of these tumors originate from the roof of the fourth ventricle and in the region of the posterior medullary velum, their signs and symptoms depend upon whether the tumor grows upward, downward, or laterally. In most instances, the cerebellar hemispheres are not invaded, but rather separated. Usually the fourth ventricle is obstructed, and this is responsible for the hydrocephalus and its subsequent symptoms. The availability of CT scanning has made the diagnosis of medulloblastoma much easier. The presence of a contrast-enhanced lesion occupying the fourth ventricle, as shown in Fig. 45-6, is strongly suggestive of a medulloblastoma in a patient with a typical history. However, other masses occupying the fourth ventricle, particularly in children, may have a similar appearance, and it is impossible, simply on the basis of a CT scan, to make the diagnosis. In such cases, the children do not require angiography prior to surgery.

In older patients, the signs and symptoms are those of a unilateral hemispheric lesion with incoordination and limb ataxia. These tumors have also been called embryonal sarcomas in adults, but histologically their appearance is identical to that which is seen in children.

The primary goal in the treatment of medulloblastoma is first to establish a diagnosis and second to open up the CSF pathways, if possible. Raimondi and Tomita have argued that patients who have complete resections of their lesions followed by radiation therapy have an improved outcome compared with patients who do not undergo total radical resection.[43] However, in other central nervous system neoplasms, it has been shown that the ease of resection correlates best with specific histologic characteristics of the tumor. In craniopharyngioma, for example, those tumors that grow relatively slowly in tissue culture are those that are most easily removed.[44] The possibility that biologically distinct variants, which grow along tissue planes and are more amenable to surgical removal, may in part explain

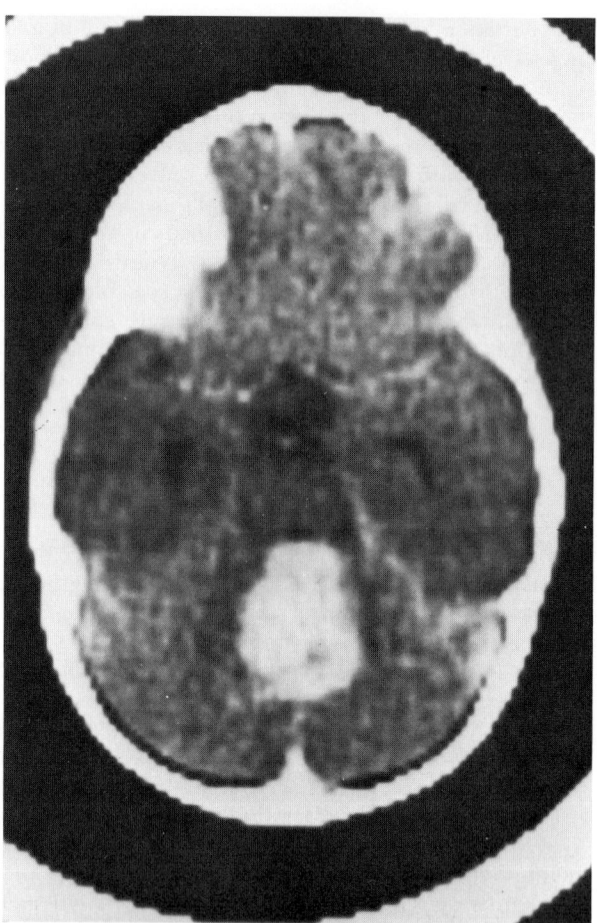

FIGURE 45-6 Large fourth ventricle medulloblastoma. Marked enhancement following contrast strongly suggests this tumor.

Raimondi's observations. The 5-year survival statistics in Raimondi's series are not significantly better than those reported by Mealy and Hall, who recommended biopsy only, followed by radiation therapy.[45] Surgical vigor, therefore, should be tempered by the fact that significant damage can be done to the child by the procedure itself. The primary goal of surgery should be removal of tumor sufficient to allow opening the aqueduct and the fourth ventricle to allow for CSF egress. If this is done, many children who have hydrocephalus preoperatively will not require shunting in the postoperative period. This is an important consideration because approximately 20 percent of the children with medulloblastoma will develop metastases within the subarachnoid space, and some of these, if a shunt is placed, will develop metastasis to the peritoneal cavity. Using the approach outlined here, approximately 40 percent of the children will require shunting following surgical removal of most, if not all, of the tumor. In those children who are shunted, a special millipore filter is inserted in the shunt system in order to prevent dissemination of cells to the peritoneum.

Radiation therapy should be considered the primary mode of postoperative therapy for medulloblastoma. These tumors are among the most radiosensitive of all central nervous system neoplasms. Present treatment schemes usually include a dose of 4400 to 5000 rads to the brain, including the primary site, and approximately 3500 rads to the spinal canal and cord. Subarachnoid metastases are common, making craniospinal irradiation mandatory. Tokars et al., in a recent report, have suggested that intelligent utilization of ports as opposed to conventional means of radiation therapy delivery might improve survivorship of patients.[46] These observations, while optimistic, need to be confirmed by others.

In spite of the fact that radiation therapy is the most important single therapeutic modality for this tumor, it is not without hazard. In young children, retardation of bone growth and, consequently, short stature, as well as deformities of the spine are seen. Suppression of growth hormone and other hormonal secretions from the hypothalamic pituitary access are also noted. Some patients have reduced psychomotor performance following radiation therapy; this must be considered an unacceptable complication of present treatment schemes.

Despite exquisite radiosensitivity and presumed chemosensitivity of the medulloblastoma, there is no evidence to date that adjuvant chemotherapy will improve survival rates. The Children's Brain Tumor Study Group (CBTSG), in their preliminary report on a prospective randomized trial with surgical decompression, followed either by radiation therapy alone or radiation therapy and concurrent multidrug therapy, failed to demonstrate an improved survival rate in children who received chemotherapy with radiation.[47] Other clinical trials utilizing various chemotherapeutic regimens are being studied by other groups, but at present, there is no data that supports the use of chemotherapy with radiation therapy as initial therapy.

In patients who have evidence of recurrence, chemotherapy with BCNU, procarbazine, vincristine, or a combination of these agents often yields dramatic short-term remissions, but the long-term outcome is almost always death. Although the outlook at present for patients with medulloblastoma indicates 10-year survival rates of 30 to 40 percent and must be considered relatively poor, the tumor's exquisite radiosensitivity and chemosensitivity indicates that extensive efforts should be made in an attempt to find regimens that are more satisfactory than those presently utilized. This tumor is likely to be one of the first to yield to combined therapy, and is one of the more encouraging areas of neurooncology.

ASTROCYTOMAS OF THE THIRD VENTRICLE AND ANTERIOR OPTIC PATHWAYS

Astrocytomas that occur in the region of the third ventricle, involving either the optic pathways or the hypothalamus, are common in childhood and adolescence. They may produce visual disturbances; hypothalamic syndromes, including the diencephalic syndrome of infancy; diabetes insipidus; and, occasionally, obstructive hydrocephalus. In contrast to most glial tumors, this tumor is twice as frequent in females and in most instances occurs before the age of 15 years.

The treatment of primary gliomas of the optic nerve, chiasm, and/or hypothalamus is somewhat controversial. Surgical intervention for hypothalamic tumors is illogical, except to establish a diagnosis, since little can be accomplished. In tumors involving one optic nerve, a neoplasm frequently associated with neurofibromatosis, most neurosurgeons advocate surgery for diagnosis, and some suggest tumor excision when the involved optic nerve is no longer functioning and the child is blind. Surgery for tumor excision, when the tumor has already reached the chiasm, usually results in only short-term palliation and may result in diminution of vision in the remaining good eye.

The role of radiation therapy is also not entirely clear. Hoyt and Badhdassarian have noted that some of these tumors have a remarkably benign course and that many patients have no progression.[48] This suggests the possibility that, at least in an occasional patient, these glial-like tumors should be considered hamartomas. However, in a recent review of the experience at the Columbus Children's Hospital, Oxenhandler and Sayers indicated that radiation therapy was beneficial in patients with chiasmal and/or hypothalamic involvement.[49] Each neurosurgeon's experience with these tumors is extremely limited because the disease is relatively rare. It is unlikely that a definitive answer will be forthcoming in the foreseeable future. It is thought that involvement of the optic chiasm and/or hypothalamus requires radiation therapy, although the course can be unusually long in occasional patients who receive no treatment other than surgery. This must be seen as the exception rather than the rule.

BRAINSTEM GLIOMAS

Brainstem gliomas are slow-growing, firm, white infiltrating growths which insinuate themselves between tracts of nuclei. They produce a variable clinical picture, depending upon their exact location in the brainstem. This tumor is most frequent in childhood, with 80 percent occurring in the first two decades. Symptoms are usually insidious in the beginning, and children present 3 to 6 months after first onset. In almost all instances the initial manifestation is a palsy of one or more cranial nerves, most often the sixth and seventh on one side. Long-tract signs follow—hemiplegia, unilateral ataxia, gait disturbances, hemisensory syndromes, gaze disorders, and occasionally hiccups. Occasionally, long-tract signs may precede cranial nerve signs. Obstructive hydrocephalus is unusually rare in these tumors. When hydrocephalus is present on an initial CT scan, another diagnosis should be considered. The course is usually agonizingly slow over several years except under circumstances where the tumor becomes more malignant. The experience at UCSF in the treatment of intrinsic tumors of the brainstem was recently reviewed.[50] Of those patients treated, 71 percent showed distinctive improvement during or shortly after radiation therapy; 10 of 24 (41 percent) and 5 of 15 (33 percent) were living without evidence of recurrence at 5 and 10 years, respectively. The others either had failed to respond or had recurrence, usually within 12 to 18 months, and died shortly thereafter.

Chemotherapy has been disappointingly ineffective despite a variety of extremely aggressive treatment protocols, including high-dose methotrexate with citrovorum rescue. With the exception of those neoplasms where a large exophytic, or extraaxial, component exists, surgical intervention is usually not indicated.

TUMORS OF THE PINEAL REGION

Tumors of the pineal region are relatively rare. The majority are malignant. Over one-half of these tumors are germinomas or atypical teratomas. Less common are the more malignant pineocytoma and pineoblastoma. Teratocarcinomas are found even more rarely.

The symptoms and signs of pineal-region tumors are those of obstructive hydrocephalus—i.e., headache, nausea, and vomiting—and gait disturbance. Occasional Perinaud's sign, or limitation of upward gaze, is seen, and this indicates tectal compression. Precocious puberty, often reported in the literature, is not terribly common.

The CT scan is the best method for establishing the diagnosis. Typically, a mass arising in the posterior portion of the third ventricle is seen. In circumstances where the diagnosis is not clear or localization is not ideal, ventriculography using either water-soluble media or Pantopaque may be useful in further delineating the outlines of the mass. Cerebral panangiography, giving particular attention to the venous phase in order to demonstrate the anatomy of the veins draining the region of the torcular Herophili, is of particular value when surgical intervention is being contemplated.

Stein, in a series of pioneering publications, described surgical techniques which have been utilized and modified by others. These techniques allowed for the biopsy of most, and the surgical removal of some, tumors in the pineal region, with very low morbidity and mortality rates.[51] Most large centers of pediatric neurosurgery that see patients with pineal tumors are now operating on these patients, at least to establish a tissue diagnosis. Some surgeons consider the suboccipital supratentorial approach preferable in most instances, as it allows better access with less morbidity than other approaches. If the tumor is removable, they suggest that complete removal is best accomplished with this technique. The infratentorial supracerebellar approach is relatively easy to carry out, but leaves a much smaller exposure at the end of a deep field, and thus makes removal of potentially curable lesions more difficult. The majority of malignant tumors of the pineal region cannot be removed. The most common tumor, the atypical teratoma, almost always requires other modes of therapy. Many of these patients require ventriculoperitoneal shunting, as previously described, for patients who have medulloblastoma. If, however, the occasional benign lesion can be removed, opening of the CSF pathways may be possible.

Radiation therapy must still be considered to be the primary mode of therapy for the pineal-region tumors that are malignant, i.e., the atypical teratoma, the pineoblastoma, and the teratocarcinoma. In fact, the rapid response of atypical teratomas to irradiation has prompted several surgical centers to suggest that initial treatment of pineal region tumors presenting in the second and third decades is CSF shunting and radiation therapy. Direct surgical attack is then reserved for cases that do not show a radiation response. Present irradiation treatment schemes are similar to those for medulloblastoma. Approximately 4500 rads are delivered to the primary site; however, there is some controversy regarding the need for craniospinal axis irradiation in these patients. The use of spinal irradiation in these patients has been abandoned because it appears that adjuvant chemotherapy offers the probability of long-term control with less morbidity.

Marshall et al. described treatment of three patients with teratocarcinoma of the pineal region with adjuvant chemotherapy.[52] More recently, Neuwelt et al. reported a high response rate to multiagent chemotherapy.[53] Of considerable interest is the fact that the status of the patients can be monitored by serial evaluation both of serum and CSF, and of human chorionic gonadotropin (HCG)—more specifically, the B-polypeptide subunit. This marker is commonly secreted by this neoplasm. Neuwelt et al. have also recently shown that these tumors apparently contain a large number of T lymphocytes, indicating further basis, perhaps, for approaches along the chemotherapeutic and immunotherapeutic routes.[53] The regimen reported was a combination of *cis*-platinum, bleomycin, and vinblastine. Toxicity from this regimen is renal and can usually be avoided by adequate hydration and vigorous diuresis. These results of Neuwelt et al., coupled with other preliminary findings, are encouraging. It appears that the basis for the therapeutic success which has been accomplished with these tumors is the fact that they are histologically identical to certain testicular and ovarian germ-cell tumors. It is important to establish the diagnosis of these teratomatous tumors early on, before bulk is such that chemotherapy is less successful. As improved regimens are developed for testicular carcinoma, their application to this apparent parallel nervous system neoplasm is an exciting area for research.

In the past, treatment of recurrence of malignant pineal tumors usually involved the use of high doses of glucocorticoids. In patients previously untreated with chemotherapy, the use of multiagent therapy with *cis*-platinum, vinblastine, and bleomycin may lead to long-term survival. At UCSF and UCSD, however, it is believed that the present treatment approach to these tumors should be a combination of surgery or radiation therapy and chemotherapy, as this offers the best hope for long-term control of the disease.

DIFFERENTIAL DIAGNOSIS OF RECURRENCE

Symptoms such as headache and lethargy are nonspecific and unreliable as indicators of recurrence. Evidence of increased ICP without accompanying deterioration is an unreliable indication of regrowth. The same is true of CSF cytology and the EEG. Early detection of recurrence is a desirable goal, but present methods and limited experience in discovering the first evidence of regrowth require that physicians adhere to exacting criteria to avoid the pitfalls described in this section on differential diagnosis. An increase in lesion size and increased contrast enhancement on CT-scan examination, or an increase in size on a radionuclide scan, are reliable indicants of tumor progression. If these are coupled with an increase in neurologic deficit, tumor recurrence is established. The need for additional glucocorticoids strongly suggests that tumor recurrence, or progression, is present. Deterioration beginning more than 4 months after operation constitutes presumptive evidence of tumor regrowth if complications, such as hydrocephalus, are excluded. It should be emphasized that no one technique can be relied upon to establish tumor progression. With tumors in neurologically silent areas, such as the frontal pole, neurologic examination may provide little clinical indication of a change in tumor mass. On the other hand, certain neurologic deficits, such as hemianopsia, may be irreversible; and tumor regression may be impossible to demonstrate clinically, despite evidence of shrinkage of neoplasm on radiographic investigation.

In the immediate postoperative period, deterioration raises the surgical problem of cerebral edema or hematoma vs. continued growth of inadequately decompressed tumor. Cerebral edema reaches its peak in the first 2 to 4 days after surgery, and hematomas usually become evident within the first few hours to days after operation. As a rule, improvement following the administration of steroids supports the initial diagnosis of edema, although steroids also benefit the postoperative hematoma. Postoperative impairment of CSF flow or the tumor itself can cause hydrocephalus, which may appear several weeks after surgery or much later. Drowsiness and decreased mentation may develop in the absence of any new abnormality seen on the scan. The CT scan provides a noninvasive means for identifying the problem.

Postoperative radiotherapy can create concern about recurrence and diagnostic confusion in three ways:

1. During radiation, there may be reactive edema with nausea, drowsiness, and worsening of deficit, especially in the poorly decompressed tumor. Ordinarily, this is not a serious diagnostic problem and resolves with a temporary increase in steroids and a lapse of perhaps several days without further radiotherapy.
2. Radiation necrosis, although it is less frequent now owing to the standardization of doses and improving dosimetry, is not infrequent. This condition may develop as early as 4 months or as late a 9 years after irradiation. The occurrence of radiation necrosis is rare if 200-rad fractions are given for a 5600-rad total dose over 5 to 6 weeks. Sheline recently reviewed the literature on radiation necrosis of the CNS.[54] Eighty-four percent of cases with necrosis received fraction sizes of greater than 250 rads. Radiation necrosis has been documented most frequently in the first year (40 percent of cases) and in the second year (33 percent) than subsequently. The symptoms may mimic tumor regrowth.[55] Usually, late studies will show atrophy,[56] but coagulative necrosis can create a mass that, even on gross tissue examination, resembles a tumor. CT scans show findings nearly impossible to differentiate from tumor recurrence. The diagnosis may be suspected from the history of radiotherapy; however, surgery is sometimes required both for definitive diagnosis and to remove the mass. Steroids may help transiently, but the outcome is often fatal.
3. A more difficult and less-known complication is created by transient encephalopathy that may occur 1 to 15 weeks (usually 6 to 10) after the end of x-ray therapy.[57] It can develop after exposure to as little as 2400 rads in children who are receiving CNS prophylaxis for leukemia.[58] The syndrome is manifested by drowsiness, nausea, and malaise, but can include ataxia, dysphasia, and exaggeration or reappearance of previous neurologic deficits. It does not require a preexisting brain lesion and appears related to demyelination, produced either by direct effect on oligodendroglia or by provoking an autoimmune reaction.[59] The tissue is edematous, friable, and vascular, and surgery is usually not helpful. Steroids are effective, but the only way to differentiate this condition from tumor recurrence is to suspect it because of the timing, and to temporize by providing symptomatic care. The patient with radiation encephalopathy will improve without specific treatment, usually within 4 to 6 weeks.

Seizures

The late onset of seizures or the aggravation of preexisting seizures frequently is a consequence of tumor regrowth. Seizures can produce neurologic symptoms suggestive of recurrence, especially in the postictal state. Ordinarily, postconvulsive deficits disappear within a few hours, but they may persist for several days. Uncommonly, deficits may be caused by ongoing seizure, i.e., subclinical status epilepticus. EEG establishes the diagnosis, and neurologic improvement will follow seizure control. The possibility that an unexpected seizure heralds tumor regrowth requires appropriate investigation and treatment.

Cerebral Infarction and Hemorrhage

Cerebral infarction can be spontaneous and unrelated (from arteriosclerosis), can occur as a consequence of postoperative impairment of circulation (for example, surgical occlusion or narrowing of major arteries), or can be a direct result of tumor regrowth. An occasional patient presents with a suddenly increased deficit, an avascular mass near the previous tumor site, a positive scan focus, and stenosis or occlusion of a major artery in the area. In most malignant gliomas, however, the late appearance of a strokelike syndrome is associated with tumor regrowth.

A cerebral hemorrhage can occur within the tumor, occasionally during regrowth but frequently as a complication of effective chemotherapy. If suddenness of onset, angiogram, and CT scan support the diagnosis of hematoma, then treatment, whether surgical or conservative, is directed initially to the hematoma.

Metabolic and Drug-Related Problems

Metabolic and other generalized systemic problems also can cause neurological disorders, including focal deficits, if there is underlying brain damage. Hypoglycemia, acidosis, hypotension, uremia, hepatic failure, anemia, electrolyte imbalance, respiratory insufficiency, fever, and infection can increase focal deficit with or without alteration in consciousness. It is sometimes surprising how much worse a patient with severe deficit can appear even a week after a urinary tract infection. These conditions can be eliminated during the course of a thorough evaluation.

Depressant drugs, e.g., phenobarbital and primidone, can have similar effects, and other compounds such as diphenylhydantoin may have neurologic side effects. In this respect, information regarding serum drug levels may be invaluable. If the patient is receiving anticancer chemotherapy, methotrexate administered intrathecally can cause leukoencephalopathy; procarbazine can cause drowsiness, nausea, and vomiting; and vincristine is occasionally associated with seizures. The patient who is deteriorating and is on maintenance doses of steroids must be checked for irregularity of dosage.

Simple fatigue can intensify a deficit, especially relatively sensitive functions such as speech. Similarly, emotional depression can cause an apparent deterioration, with decreased physical activity and speech, and increased headaches. Understanding the social dynamics of the family can be useful, because they affect the patient's emotional state and possibly the history that the physician obtains.

Infection

Meningitis or abscess in the tumor bed may cause diagnostic difficulty at any time, ordinarily within the first 2 postoperative weeks. Such rapid onset tends to differentiate infection from tumor regrowth, but lumbar puncture, aspiration, or reexploration may be necessary, depending on clinical findings. An abscess developing later, though rare, must be kept in mind, especially if treatment for tumor recurrence will not include more surgery. Angiography, with attention to the pattern of neovascularity and amount of edema, and CT scanning may be helpful in this regard.

Other Neurological Disorders

Finally, the patient known to harbor a brain tumor may contract an independent neurological disease. Collagen diseases, degenerative diseases, multiple sclerosis, viral encephalitis, subdural hematoma, or a different tumor (e.g., meningioma in a patient who has had surgery for astrocytoma) can be overlooked. Most of these diseases cause symptoms atypical for recurrent tumor, and they can be correctly identified by thoughtful and careful neurologic testing.

Unusual Tumor Manifestations

CYST FORMATION

Glioblastoma multiforme and anaplastic astrocytoma may spontaneously develop large cysts that arise from rapidly progressing tissue necrosis and subsequent fluid accumulation. The degree to which intensive radiation therapy and chemotherapy modify this process is unclear.

Afra et al. reported that in 41 patients who were reoperated on for tumor recurrence, 7 (17 percent) harbored tumor cysts.[60] In 4 of the 7 patients with cystic recurrent tumor, the evolution of a cyst was accompanied by clinical signs of acutely increased ICP. Aspiration produced prompt relief. Rapid and pronounced improvement can be expected if the formation or enlargement of the cyst initially causes rapid clinical deterioration. A single aspiration was sufficiently palliative in 5 of the 7 patients. In 2 patients, reaccumulation of cyst fluid necessitated repeated taps and, ultimately, the placement of a reservoir and/or permanent shunt.

The CT appearance of intratumor cyst is that of a relatively well-marginated lesion on its inner aspect with a low-density center (Fig. 45-4). In general, the mean density of a low-density tumor center does not distinguish a cyst from an area of central necrosis, although the latter lesions tend to have more irregular margins.

DISTANT SPREAD

When brains that contain glial tumors are studied carefully, tumor cells are often found distant to the main tumor mass, primarily in perivascular spaces and in the subpial region of the cortex. Infiltration of long white fiber bundles (e.g., of the corticospinal tract) may also occur and may be another mode of distant spread. Up to 5 to 10 percent of glioblastomas may be multicentric. Glial tumors may spread within the central nervous system through the CSF.[61] Leptomeningeal seeding is a behavioral characteristic of medulloblastomas. Uncommonly it results from other suitably situated tumors. Medulloblastomas tend to spread diffusely through the subarachnoid space over the cerebellum to produce the appearance of cake icing and into the spinal subarachnoid space.

Spontaneous metastasis outside the central nervous system is rare.[62] Most intracranial tumors known to have metastasized elsewhere in the body had been subjected to one or more surgical procedures. Among the glial tumors, a tendency to extension beyond the confines of the central nervous system is greatest in ependymoma, which may invade locally and spread distally.⁶³

TREATMENT OPTIONS FOR RECURRENCES

Reoperation

Definitive diagnosis of tumor recurrence will be made based upon changes in neurologic examination, CT scans, or radionuclide scans. A repeat craniotomy and tumor removal is appropriate in a young patient who presents, several years after first diagnosis and initial treatment, with generalized symptoms secondary to increased ICP from neoplastic growth in an accessible, nonvital area of the brain. If the patient still retains good neurologic functioning (high Karnofsky score) at the time of progression, and can receive an "active" chemotherapeutic regimen and/or repeat radiation therapy after repeat tumor debulking, the surgery may result in a prolonged period of useful life. The decision to reoperate, however, is usually not so easily made as in the example. Each patient must be considered individually, with the understanding that the second operation is rarely as efficacious as the first. The theoretical advantage that large amounts of tumor removal will give to the usefulness of subsequent drug and radiation therapy should also be considered. Occasionally, a repeat operation is appropriate to decompress or remove a tumor cyst.

Repeat Radiation Therapy

This is rarely a useful option. Occasionally a patient with a radiation-responsive tumor, such as a medulloblastoma, presents with recurrence several years after initial treatment with irradiation. In those circumstances, the potential usefulness of repeat radiation therapy, with or without a repeat surgical debulking procedure, may outweigh the possible hazards of radiation necrosis, which would follow usually within the following 2 years. The dose of repeat radiation is usually smaller than initial tumor treatment doses (up to 3000 rads over 3 to 4 weeks) and is usually given only to the tumor bed (W. Wara, personal communication). The results of repeat radiation are frequently disappointing and should be reserved only for those patients who have a significant chance of benefiting from it.

Chemotherapy

SPECIFIC DRUGS

Many drugs have been examined in phase II trials. Some have exhibited no activity, and others have not received an adequate trial. Those agents that have been evaluated by an adequate trial or show promising activity will be described.

Nitrosoureas In 1970, two reports introduced BCNU as an effective agent in the treatment of primary and metastatic brain tumors.⁶⁴,⁶⁵ The nitrosoureas, particularly BCNU, remain the most effective agents (Fig. 45-7*a* and *b*).

The nitrosoureas, like most alkylating agents, depress the bone marrow, with peripheral platelet counts decreasing in 3 weeks and white blood cells, principally granulocytes, decreasing a couple of weeks thereafter. The peripheral counts recover 6 to 8 weeks after drug administration, at which time treatment can be repeated but with possible dose modification as indicated by platelet and white cell nadirs during the preceding course. Long-term administration of BCNU frequently leads to chronic erythropoietic depression, although it rarely requires transfusions. More recently, pulmonary fibrosis, occasionally profound and irreversible, has been reported to occur in patients receiving nitrosoureas. Pulmonary toxicity has the characteristic but nonspecific signs of interstitial lung disease, with dyspnea on exertion, a nonproductive cough, and progressive interstitial infiltrates demonstrable on x-ray films of the chest.⁶⁶,⁶⁷ These findings have been associated with decreased lung volume and hypoxemia. Some of the patients have also had pleural fibrosis. The onset of symptoms after the initiation of BCNU treatment has been from a few days to 43 months. Pathological examination of the lungs has shown alveolar-cell dysplasia and interstitial fibrosis. The disease may become apparent several months after termination of the therapy. The pathogenesis of the pulmonary fibrosis is unknown, but it is somewhat dose-related. The frequency of this complication of BCNU therapy is probably about 2 or 3 percent.

Procarbazine Procarbazine (PCB), a methyl hydrazine analogue, is rapidly oxidized to a lipophilic azo derivative and enters the brain. Like the nitrosoureas, it probably functions as a cell-cycle-nonspecific (CCNS) agent. Procarbazine has the advantage of oral administration. Most

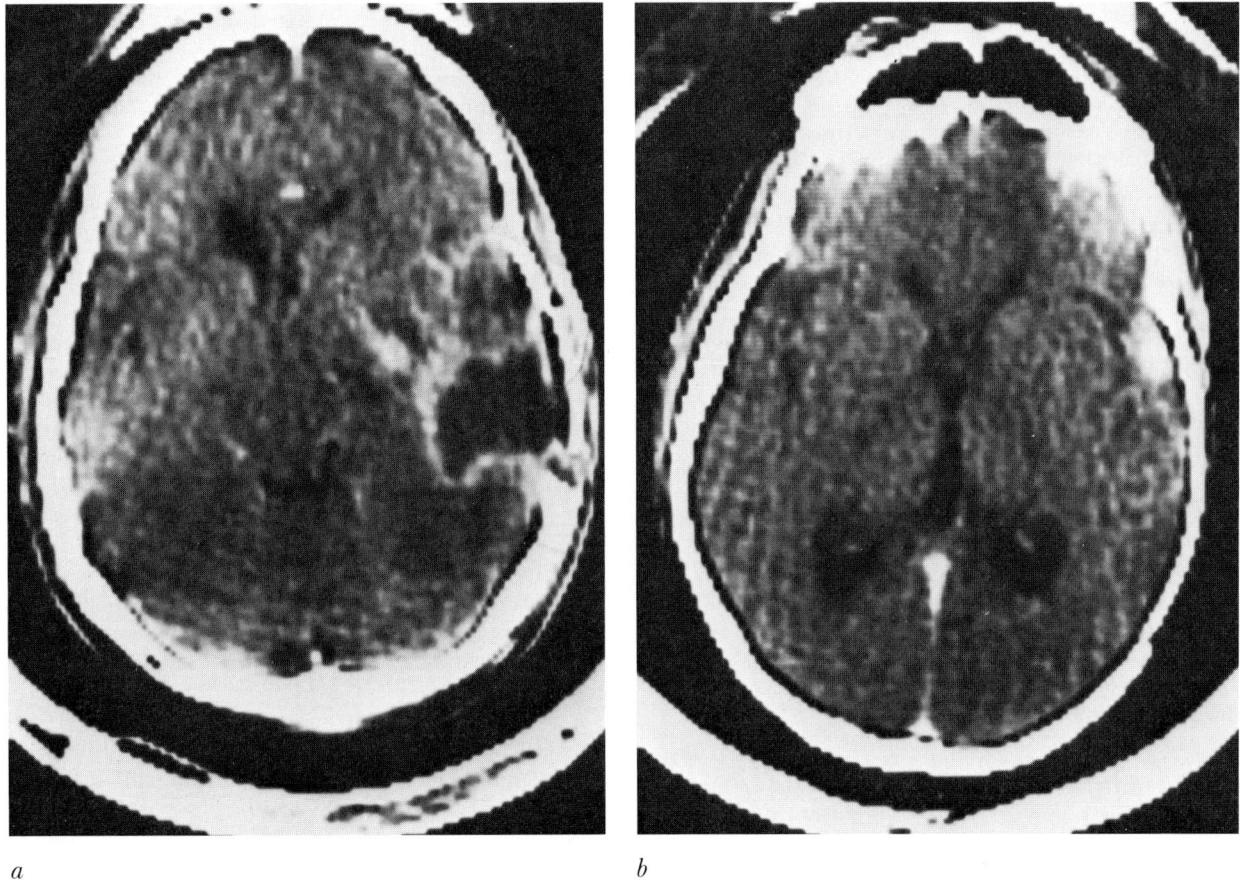

FIGURE 45-7 (*a*) Large recurrent glioblastoma in a previously irradiated patient. (*b*) Objective regression of tumor following 3 cycles of BCNU. Note absence of shift in comparison with (*a*).

patients experience nausea and vomiting during the first few days of each course, but rarely does this require stopping chemotherapy. Like the nitrosoureas, procarbazine depresses the bone marrow, leukopenia being more pronounced than thrombocytopenia. The nadir for white blood cells usually occurs in the latter part of the 30-day period of administration, but low counts may persist for 4 to 6 weeks after the drug is stopped. Because it is a monoamine oxidase inhibitor, procarbazine may produce a psychotic reaction. Among 43 patients receiving the drug, 4 developed a skin rash, but treatment was continued without secondary complications. Other investigators have encountered severe skin reactions requiring that drug treatment be discontinued.

In the one phase II trial reported, the response rate was 52 percent (14 of 27 patients) for a median duration of 6 months. In this study, procarbazine was administered at a single dose of 150 mg/m^2 per day for 30 days.

Procarbazine is an active drug with potential for combination chemotherapy because it has no recognized cross resistance with the nitrosoureas.

Vincristine Vincristine (VCR), has shown limited activity against astrocytomas and medulloblastomas. Rosenstock et al. reported responses in eight of sixteen children harboring recurrent low- and high-grade astrocytomas and medulloblastomas.[68] They encountered minimal toxic effects on a schedule of 1.5 mg/m² weekly for 12 weeks with treatment on alternate weeks thereafter. Vincristine exhibits peripheral neurotoxicity that is monitored easily and has little or no effect on the bone marrow. As a cell-cycle-specific (CCS) agent that spares the bone marrow, vincristine offers some attraction as one component of multiple-drug protocols.

5-Fluorouracil   A cell-cycle-specific agent, 5-fluorouracil (5-FU) has favorable pharmacokinetic characteristics. When given alone, 5-FU has no demonstrable antitumor activity. However, when given in a sequential regimen with BCNU, 5-FU has shown some efficacy.

Hydroxyurea   The cell-cycle-specific agent, hydroxyurea (HU), has been used in conjunction with adjuvant irradiation in the treatment of malignant gliomas. The results of a study by the Western Cooperative Oncology Group suggest some activity, and because of the advantages of oral administration and little toxicity, hydroxyurea has potential as a cell-cycle-specific component of drug combinations.[69]

Epipodophylotoxin (VM 26)   This agent has shown limited activity in one phase II trial, and despite a difficult dose schedule, it may prove to be a useful drug under special circumstances.

Dianhydrogalactitol   Dianhydrogalactitol (DAG) is a remarkably effective drug against the murine ependymoblastoma.[70] Levin has investigated its pharmacokinetic behavior in tumor-bearing animals, and the agent is entering phase II trials. Although it has not shown activity in malignant astrocytomas, one striking response was observed in a patient with recurrent medulloblastoma, suggesting that the drug deserves further consideration.

Glucocorticoids   Certain principles and observations are pertinent to use of steroids in patients undergoing chemotherapy, and briefly, these are as follows:

1. The antiedema effect of steroids is dose-dependent, and high doses (up to and occasionally above 100 mg of Decadron per day) will produce responses not observed at lower dosages.[71]
2. Large doses are well tolerated and associated with few serious complications.
3. In the patient harboring a tumor, maintenance of initial clinical improvement induced by steroids will require continuous administration.
4. In the patient receiving a steroid and an oncolytic drug concurrently, improvement in neurologic function and brain scans (radionuclide and CT) can be considered evidence of drug responsiveness only when improvement occurs while the patient is receiving the same or a smaller dose of steroid.
5. To minimize steroid side effects in a steroid-dependent patient, periodic attempts should be made to reduce the maintenance dose in small decrements. This is true particularly in the early postoperative period, following completion of radiotherapy, and during the course of successful chemotherapy.

COMBINATION CHEMOTHERAPY

The present thrust in the treatment of malignant brain tumors is the concurrent or sequential use of multiple therapeutic modes, i.e., operation, radiotherapy, and chemotherapy.

The results of single and combination drug therapy of recurrent malignant gliomas are presented in Table 45-1. The two most effective chemotherapeutic regimens were BCNU, 5-FU, and PCV (procarbazine, CCNU, and vincristine); the PCV schedule, doses, and precautions appear in Table 45-2.

In both the PCV 3 and BCNU–5-FU studies, patients harboring glioblastoma multiforme did considerably worse (MTP of 23 weeks) than patients who harbored nonglioblastoma malignant gliomas (MTP of 26 to 27 weeks).[72,73] The most important common feature between the BCNU–5-FU and PCV-3 combinations is an ability to halt disease progression; unfortunately, long-term remission was not achieved by the new protocols when the results were compared, respectively, with those with either BCNU alone or PCV 1.[74]

OTHER RECURRENT TUMORS

Oligodendroglioma   Experience with recurrent oligodendroglioma is limited and mostly anecdotal. Levin et al. suggested that PCV 3 is active against these tumors and that, in general, no therapeutic distinctions can currently be drawn between recurrent oligodendrogliomas and recurrent anaplastic astrocytomas.[72]

TABLE 45-1 Responses to Chemotherapy for Recurrent Supratentorial Malignant Gliomas

Agent	All malignant gliomas[a]	GM[b,c]	NGM[c,d]	MTP,[e] weeks
BCNU[65]	20/40 (50%)			38/—[f]
CCNU[79]	10/22 (45%)			24/—[f]
BCNU, PCB[79]	21/52 (40%)	3/3/18	10/5/34	34/20
BCNU, 5-FU[73]	24/29 (83%)	1/2/4	8/13/25	34/26
BCNU, 5-FU, HU, 6MP[9]	10/15 (67%)	1/1/4	4/4/11	38/22
CCNU, PCB, VCR (PCV 1)[74]	18/29 (62%)	1/2/8	11/4/21	30/—
CCNU, PCB, VCR (PCV 3)[72]	16/19 (84%)	0/1/1	8/7/18	31/25
fiCCNU, PCB, VCR (PCV 3)[72]	12/27 (44%)[g]	2/3/11[g]	2/5/16[g]	

[a] Combined GM and NGM groups; responders and stable disease patients combined. No previous chemotherapy given to patients in these studies, with exception of last row.
[b] Glioblastoma multiforme.
[c] Responders/stable disease/total group.
[d] Non-glioblastoma multiforme.
[e] Median time to tumor progression from beginning of treatment for responders/stable disease patients.
[f] These values are overestimated because previous response criteria required clinical deterioration together with RN-scan evidence of tumor enlargement.
[g] Previous chemotherapy failures. Patients failing to receive a second course of chemotherapy excluded.

Ependymoma Levin reviewed his experience with 15 patients harboring recurrent ependymomas who were treated with BCNU, and suggested that palliation is possible with either 3-day or single-dose BCNU therapy administered every 6 to 8 weeks.[72] For either schedule, BCNU slowed tumor progression and improved neurologic signs and symptoms in patients with spinal or fourth ventricular ependymomas. Precise evaluation of the chemotherapeutic efficacy against ependymomas is difficult because of occasional tumor location in the spinal cord, which makes the need for reoperation necessary, and the slow growth of these tumors if they go undetected.

CURRENT AREAS OF RESEARCH AND PROSPECTS FOR THE FUTURE

The location of brain tumors precludes aggressive surgical extirpation or high-dose radiation therapy in most instances because damage to normal brain surrounding the tumor will be excessive, and the resultant quality of the patient's life will be less than satisfactory. While cure of primary malignant gliomas is currently not possible, patients have been seen to improve after a treatment regimen of surgical resection, radiation therapy, and/or chemotherapy. The addition of chemotherapy to radiation therapy and surgery is capable of increasing time to progression or survival time by no more than several months. In most cases, chemotherapy administered at the time of tumor recurrence on the average extends survival 6 months for patients with anaplastic astrocytoma and 4 months for patients with recurrent glioblastoma.

Radiation Therapy

RADIOSENSITIVITY

Radiation therapy provides the most effective adjuvant treatment for patients with malignant brain tumors, but brain intolerance to potentially curative doses of radiation is limiting. Solid tumors are thought to contain a substantial population of cells that are hypoxic; because much of the cell kill caused by ionizing radiation is the result of an oxygen-dependent, free radical–mediated attack on deoxyribonucleic acid, hypoxic tumor cells are

TABLE 45-2 Schedules for Procarbazine, CCNU, and Vincristine (PCV 3)[74]

Pharmaceutical preparation	CCNU: 10-, 40-, and 100-mg capsules are available Vincristine: 1- and 5-mg vials are available with dilutant (90 mg NaCl with 0.9% benzyl alcohol in 10 mL water) Procarbazine is available in 50-mg capsules

Schedules	For glial and metastatic tumors (UCSF PCV 3):
	  CCNU: 110 mg/m² PO on day 1
	  Vincristine: 1.4 mg/m² IV on days 8 and 29
	  Procarbazine: 60 mg/m² PO on days 8 to 21
	The cycle is repeated every 6 weeks.
	For medulloblastomas, neuroblastoma, and primitive neuroectodermal tumors (UCSF PCV 2):
	  CCNU: 75 mg/m² PO on day 1
	  Vincristine: 1.4 mg/m² IV on days 8 and 29
	  Procarbazine: 100 mg/m² PO on days 8 to 21
	The cycle is repeated every 6 weeks.
	Patients having previous spinal irradiation should begin at CCNU and procarbazine doses 60 percent of those above.

Ancillary medication	Foods containing tyramines, such as bananas, aged cheese, wine, etc., should be avoided while procarbazine is being administered. Sedative-hypnotic drugs may also have a prolonged CNS-depressing effect during procarbazine administration. Antiemetics should be administered as needed.

known to be radioresistant and are, therefore, a barrier to cure. Hypoxic cell radiosensitizers are being evaluated. Two nitroimidazoles, metronidazole and misonidazole, have received the most attention. These compounds are thought to mimic oxygen by "fixing" the free radical–induced damage caused by radiation in tumor cells. Toxicities of preliminary results obtained in clinical trials with brain tumor patients are somewhat discouraging; drug toxicity limits the number of radiation treatments with which a sensitizer may be given. The results of ongoing clinical trials with metronidazole and misonidazole and the identification of new, less hypoxic cell sensitizers may improve the potential for this mode of therapy.

HIGH-LET RADIATION

Another effort to improve the therapeutic ratio of brain irradiation is the development of high-linear-energy transfer (LET) modalities (fast neutrons, heavy ions, pions) for use in brain tumor therapy. These modalities provide distinct advantages over conventional photon therapy. Because high-LET radiation depends far less on oxygen for its effectiveness, it is especially useful for treating tumors with a significant percentage of hypoxic cells. In addition, since high-LET-charged particles are subject to the Bragg effect, enormous amounts of energy can be deposited in localized regions of the brain.

Catterall et al. compared the effect of the fast neutrons with conventional megavoltage x-rays (photons) administered to patients immediately after a subtotal removal of malignant gliomas.[75] The results of this controlled study demonstrated that, although neutron therapy did not improve overall survival rates, examination of the histologic material indicated a considerably greater antitumor effect after neutron therapy than after treatment with photons. In the neutron-treated group, at postmortem examination, no tumor or only minimal tumor was found in 10 of 12 patients and in 1 of 4 patients where tissue was obtained from a secondary craniotomy.

In some cases, there was evidence of diffuse damage to normal brain, which was in keeping with a clinical syndrome of progressive dementia without localizing signs. Parker et al.,[76] using a comparable regime in a noncontrolled study of 21 patients with glioblastoma multiforme, published similar findings. A regime is required which will achieve greater local tumor control without incurring serious damage to normal brain tissue.

BRACHYTHERAPY

Brachytherapy, stereotactic interstitial therapy, has been used extensively for palliative and curative treatment of many different malignancies, but the experience with brain tumors is comparatively small. Stereotactic placement of ^{198}Au, ^{192}Ir, ^{125}I seeds into a tumor can deliver very high doses of radiation to a localized volume. In this way, the therapeutic ratio is increased because the surrounding brain can be spared. In addition, there is evidence that hypoxic cells are most sensitive to the lower dose rates delivered by the stereotactic implants.

Stereotactic interstitial radiation, then, combines propitious radiobiology with clinical utility. The technique, in combination with stereotactic biopsy, can be useful for the irradiation of deep, nonresectable tumors, and for localized irradiation of solitary brain metastases. Brachytherapy may be used in combination with external therapy, for a radiation boost to either primary tumors or recurrent, previously irradiated tumors. It may be exceptionally useful when the bone marrow is compromised by previous chemotherapy.

Gutin et al. presented preliminary results from interstitial implantation of radioactive sources in patients with recurrent malignant gliomas.[77] Responses were noted in approximately one-half of the patients, demonstrating the potential utility of this approach. Glioblastomas most frequently (greater than 90 percent) have been noted to recur within 2 cm of the original site, as demonstrated by CT scan. Extending the irradiated field to more adequately cover the 2 cm adjacent to the observed tumor might increase the effectiveness of interstitial radioactive implants.

Chemotherapy

Although we now know many of the major factors responsible for drug therapy failure in malignant brain tumors, we have not effectively developed methods or approaches to overcome them. Still needed are (1) innovative approaches to drug delivery and drug exposure without undue systemic toxicity; (2) better understanding of tumor cell sensitivity to drugs, and ways to prevent the emergence of drug resistance or to overcome its effect; and (3) surgical approaches to improve tumor dead cell removal without excessive morbidity.

PHARMACOLOGIC CONSIDERATIONS

It is well known that the blood-brain barrier (BBB) is defective in many malignant brain tumors and that the extent of BBB "leakiness" is related to malignancy of glial and metastatic tumors. This leakiness results from gaps between adjacent endothelial cells and fenestrae in endothelial walls.

Interestingly, even though malignant brain tumors have "leaky" capillaries capable of allowing entry of even the largest anticancer agents, drugs that can cross the normal BBB seem to be more effective against intracerebral tumor models and human malignant brain tumors than drugs that do not readily cross the BBB.[78-80]

In order for a drug to be effective against a tumor, the drug not only must be capable of killing the tumor cell when it reaches the site in the cell where it exerts its effect, but also must be able to reach this site. For brain tumors, this implies that the drug must cross the tumor and some brain capillaries, diffuse to the cells, and cross the cell membrane if it is to react within the cell. The drug must not be completely metabolized before it reaches the cell, and the drug plasma levels must be at a high enough concentration for a sufficient length of time to achieve some critical cytotoxic level.

Intraarterial Administration Drug delivery can be improved only by increasing the capillary drug level and opening the BBB or increasing the capillary permeability. To achieve higher capillary drug levels without increasing systemic toxicity, intraarterial chemotherapy can be used. Levin and Wilson found intraarterial BCNU resulted in up to a 4 to 5 times increase in the amount of radiolabeled drug found in the area of the brain supplied by the artery injected.[79]

Osmotic opening of the BBB, such as through the use of intraarterial infusions of mannitol or arabinose as advocated by Rapaport,[81] can increase drug delivery to brain tumors and the adjacent peritumoral brain by temporarily increasing capillary permeability. Such transient osmotic opening of the BBB (less than 25 min) results in a greater than fivefold increase in brain capillary permeability by "breaking" the tight junctions between adjacent endothelial cells. Neuwelt et al. studied methotrexate (MTX) uptake into dog brains 1 h after the internal carotid artery infusion of mannitol. They found a 5- to 14-fold increase in MTX levels, depending on the brain region measured; however, MTX levels fell approximately 100-fold in the following 6 h.[82] The possibility that this technique might produce localized increased permeability in tumors with compromised circulation deserves further investigation.

Intraventricular and Intrathecal Administration The ependyma and arachnoid appear to present little restriction to the movement of molecules between cerebrospinal fluid (CSF) and brain extracellular space. Intrathecal and intraventricular routes of administration of chemotherapeutic agents have been advocated for molecules too large to pass the BBB as well as for drugs producing excessive systemic intoxication or drugs that are rapidly inactivated in blood.[83] The obvious advantage of a high level of drug in the CSF, in most instances, is lessened by the tumor's location deep within the brain, at a distance 2 to 4 cm from the CSF.

Intrathecal therapy offers little advantage because the normal fluid dynamics are such that intrathecally administered drugs do not enter the ventricular system to a significant extent.

Intratumoral Administration The implantation of drugs directly into the tumor bed has been of much theoretical interest. The potential problems with such an approach, however, include the following: the manufacture of drug delivery equipment that does not contribute to the tumor mass effect, and one which will stay patent for prolonged periods to permit repeat courses of drug; the binding and chemical degradation of the drug; the diffusion of the drug out of the tumor through "leaky" capillaries in the tumor center; and irregular drug diffusion within the tumor. Nevertheless, preliminary investigations of this approach are underway, utilizing implanted reservoirs for the installation of drug solutions and implanted solid polymers containing a slowly released drug. Future activity with intratumoral therapy will depend upon the results of these studies.

IMPROVING THE THERAPEUTIC INDEX

The tagging of chemotherapeutic agents to tumor-specific antibodies might permit tumor-specific therapy. The development of hybridoma-produced monoclonal antibodies[84] has offered a means to study this approach. Unfortunately, the size of these antibodies with attached drugs may preclude tumor access through an intact BBB.

Studies with animal tumors have suggested that the systemic administration of small, noncytotoxic doses of one chemotherapeutic agent might decrease the host toxicity to a second cytotoxic drug without altering the antitumor activity. The mechanism of this protection is presumably the synchronization of normal host tissues, especially the bone marrow, and the administration of the second drug when the normal tissues are in their least sensitive cell-cycle phase. This approach needs confirmation in other systems.

The therapeutic index can be increased by reducing systemic or normal tissue toxicity. One approach is autologous bone marrow transplantation following high-dose chemotherapy in which BCNU is given at doses up to 1400 mg/m^2.[85,86] This is a form of rescue. In selected patients, the activity of such large doses of BCNU appears to provide surprisingly long tumor remissions. However, because little is known of the possible cellular resistance to BCNU in these patients as well as the possible severe toxicity manifested in the nonrescued host organs such as the liver and the lungs, such an aggressive approach seems premature at this time. The potential usefulness of this technique, in conjunction with measures of cell sensitivity and with other drugs and irradiation, may be very important in the future.

"BIOLOGICAL RESPONSE MODIFIERS"

The use of a new "family" of treatment modalities called *biological response modifiers* is gaining interest. The unifying concept of this approach is the use of methods that are relatively nontoxic by themselves but will selectively potentiate the antitumor activity of other treatment modes. An example is the polyamine inhibitor difluoromethyl ornithine (DFMO), an irreversible inhibitor of the enzyme ornithine decarboxylase, which is required for the production of polyamines, and presumably for tumor cell division. DFMO has no antitumor or host toxicity when given alone to rats with 9L brain tumors, but will potentiate the antitumor activity of simultaneously administered BCNU without additional animal toxicity.

A group of vitamin A analogues, retinols, is gaining attention for its possible modification of carcinogenesis as well as its possible role as a biological response modifier, like DFMO.

Hyperthermia is being investigated in a variety of animal and human tumor systems. Whereas generalized hyperthermia is considered dangerous to brain tumor patients by presumably promoting cerebral edema, selective antitumoral hyperthermia might enhance the activity of systemically or intratumorally administered chemotherapeutic agents. Studies utilizing an antenna implanted intracerebrally to permit tumor heating by microwaves are underway (Salcman, personal communication).

Multimodality Interactions

Studies of the 9L rat brain tumor in vitro have demonstrated that the nitrosoureas BCNU and CCNU will potentiate the activity of radiation therapy only when given in certain sequences and at specific time intervals.[87] Translation of these observations to human tumors seems reasonable. Direct studies of clonogenic human tumor cells and application of the data to patient treatment is required, however, to validate the results and the approach in general.

The possible interaction of chemotherapeutic agents with other drugs commonly administered to patients with brain tumors must be understood. The chronic oral administration of phenobarbital induces a change in liver enzymes, accelerating the clearance of BCNU and reducing the antitumor activity of BCNU. This suggests that phenobarbital should not be used if chemotherapy with nitrosoureas is contemplated; alternate medications, such as diphenylhydantoin, should be used.

Investigations using animal brain tumor models may uncover novel approaches to scheduling of chemotherapy and radiation therapy as an adjunct to surgery. Tel et al. studied the effect of BCNU administered as an adjuvant to the subtotal removal of an established, transplanted 9L rat brain tumor.[88] Compared with control animals not operated on, rats treated with an LD_{10} dose of BCNU 1 h before or 1 or 12 h after surgery on day 16 postimplant had an increased life span of over 200 percent. On the other hand, BCNU administered 12 h before, during, or 24 or 72 h after surgery, did not show any additive effect of surgery on BCNU treatment. If these results could be translated to the clinical setting, a bolus of BCNU administered to tumor patients within 12 h of surgery might increase substantially the total tumor cell kill compared with surgical resection alone.

Two clinical investigations utilizing novel treatment schedules are underway. The Brain Tumor Study Group (BTSG) is presently evaluating the usefulness of preoperative drug or radiation therapy in order to readily decrease the dead cell burden which contributes to tumor bulk in the usual postchemotherapy and postradiotherapy period. The Northern California Oncology Group (NCOG) is studying a regimen that includes preradiation chemotherapy.

Immunotherapy

Both laboratory and clinical studies of immune mechanisms and tumor-specific host responses have shown similarities, as well as striking differences, between tumors existing within and outside the CNS. To date, clinical trials have shown no effectiveness of immunotherapy, but a recent preliminary report of autologous lymphocyte infusion is provocatively encouraging.

Investigations of Tumor Biology

TUMOR CELL KINETICS

The effects of brain tumor chemotherapy are also limited by low growth fractions of these tumors, which limit the activity of cell-cycle-specific (CCS) drugs. CCS drugs will be most effective when the tumor cell burden has been reduced immediately after surgery or following a response to radiotherapy, or during rapid cellular repopulation that follows effective cell-cycle nonspecific (CCNS) chemotherapy. Without significant bulk reduction of tumor, however, delivery of the CCS drug may not achieve significant cell kill of cycling cells.

Present knowledge of the cellular kinetics of human brain tumors was summarized by Hoshino and Wilson.[89] Growth was 0.14 to 0.44 in malignant gliomas (average 0.31 ± 0.10), and cell-cycle time was 75.6 ± 45.7 h. With few exceptions the patients whose tumors showed a labeling index (LI) of 5 percent or more died within 1 year after the onset of disease. In contrast, there was a far better prognosis for patients whose tumors demonstrated an LI of *less* than 1 percent.

CLONOGENIC CELL ANALYSIS

Malignant tumors are composed of tumor cells and normal host cells—e.g., fibroblasts, endothelial cells, macrophages, lymphocytes—within a connective tissue matrix. A change in tumor size can reflect an alteration in any of these three components. Furthermore, tumor cells themselves exist in various states of intactness and have differing capacities for proliferation. As a result of this complexity, it is not surprising that the study of tumor size changes has contributed disappointingly little to our ability to develop more effective treatment methods for patients harboring malignancies. Recently, emphasis has been focused on that group of tumor cells with potential for unlimited proliferation, namely, clonogenic tumor cells. Continuous growth of a malignant tumor reflects multiplication of these cells, and a therapy that would destroy all clonogenic cells should invariably result in tumor cure. The number and types of clonogenic cells within a solid tumor, the kinetics of their growth, and their differential sensitivity to cytotoxic agents probably account for variations in tumor growth and responsiveness described even among tumors of similar histologic appearance.

In vitro colony formation assays have been used to better understand the growth and effects of drugs and irradiation on many established animal and human tumor cell lines. The results of in vitro studies on tumor cell survival following treatment with single agents and multiple modalities have permitted the rational planning of sequential therapy trials with increased activity against animal tumors.[90,91] Extrapolation of this information to human tumors has led to an occasional modification in therapy protocols with improved results.[92]

The ability of this assay to predict tumor resistance to chemotherapy is 95 to 97 percent, whereas the prediction of sensitivity is 50 to 65 percent for heavily pretreated patients. These figures are similar to the predictive efficiency of the estrogen receptor assay, a method considered useful for planning of therapy for patients with breast tumors.[93]

Recently, a clonogenic cell assay for human brain tumors was developed.[94] To date, 12 glioblastomas have been analyzed for in vitro cell sensitivity to BCNU and compared to in situ tumor response with the same agent. Cell survival curves demonstrated a maximum of 90 percent cell kill within the clinically achievable dose range. All seven patients whose cells were resistant in vivo also failed clinically; three of five patients whose cells were sensitive in culture responded in situ. This relationship between in vitro and in situ results implies that the cells disaggregated from a tumor biopsy are representative of the clonogenic cells within the solid tumor. A continued correlation between culture and patient treatments is necessary to validate the assay.

Clonogenic cell assays may explain patient treatment failures. Analysis of cell survival for up to 10 times the clinically achievable BCNU dose demonstrates two distinct patterns of cellular response: (1) essentially no cell kill was noted in six cases for up to 10 times clinically achievable doses of BCNU; (2) modest or no cell kill was noted in six cases at clinically achieveable doses, with a marked increase in cytotoxicity apparent at higher doses. This observation implies that failure of patient response to chemotherapy is caused by inherent tumor cell resistance to drugs in some patients, and to inadequate delivery of BCNU to the tumor in other cases.

TUMOR MARKERS

Investigations of possible tumor markers have included studies of hormonal secretion (e.g., HCG) by teratomatous tumors in an attempt to improve techniques for diagnosis and, more importantly, following the effects of therapy. Recent studies have related the level of polyamines in the CSF and brain tumor growth.

The polyamines putrescine (PU), spermidine (SP), and spermine are low-molecular-weight bases that are ubiquitous in body tissues. Marton et al.[95] showed an absolute correlation between CSF polyamine levels and clinical status determined by neurologic examination, radionuclide and CT scans, myelography, and CSF cytology in 15 of 16 patients with medulloblastoma.

REHABILITATION

Families, as well as the individual patient, are affected and become involved in the rehabilitation process. As with other patients harboring malignant neoplasms, the goals of rehabilitation must be individually adjusted to the degree of deficit and life expectancy.

Visual Disturbances

The brain tumor patient may suffer from visual loss in a particular field of vision. There is frequently a lack of depth perception in addition. Such individuals should be approached by others in a direction consistent with their retained vision in order to avoid startling them. Frequently used objects should be placed within easy reach and within the intact visual field.

Speech Abnormalities

Special considerations must be placed on reducing anxiety and frustration in order to promote success in the rehabilitation of speech abnormalities. The therapist must be calm and objective, use a normal tone of voice, and proceed with conversation in a slow manner. Short, repetitive samples of speech accompanied by visual clues often will be most rewarding in promoting speech training. The substitution of one word for another and the use of written words and pictures may be helpful. Fatigue must be watched for during speech therapy, and encouragement is important. Postoperative speech defects vary with the lesion and procedure performed. If speech centers have not been destroyed, some improvement may be experienced if therapy is successful; improvement begins within weeks and may continue for months.

Musculoskeletal Considerations

Contractures might develop in either flaccid or spastic paralytic states. In both cases, immobility of joints results in contraction of collagen-bearing connective tissue around joints and eventual immobility. These changes might start occurring within 1 week of immobility. Active and passive movements of all involved extremities are necessary to avoid such contractures.

Treatment of the Demented Patient

It should be assumed that a demented person is aware of his or her plight. Emphasis should be placed on maintaining a stable and familiar environment. A schedule of daily events, with fixed times for walking, eating, and visiting should be constructed by the physician in consultation with the family. Advantage should be taken of the remaining cognitive abilities. Reading may have a far more calming effect than drugs. Signs reminding the patient which room he or she is in should be placed in the home. Clocks and calendars that clearly display the year will prevent the anxiety that results from disorientation. Major changes should be avoided. When the patient must finally be transferred to a nursing home, familiar objects from home should be taken along and old friends should be encouraged to visit. A soft light in the evening will allay fears and behavioral outbursts that occur at night.

CONCLUSION

To date, the revolutionary improvement in the ability to diagnose intracranial neoplasms because of CT scanning has not been paralleled by a significant improvement in ability to treat malignant brain tumors. Advances in surgical technique, while of tremendous significance in the treatment of benign intracranial tumors, are likely to have little impact on the treatment of malignant brain tumors. Radiation therapy is the most effective postsurgical modality. Only the availability of better chemotherapeutic agents and strategies to utilize drugs and irradiation in combination are likely to significantly alter the outcome for the majority of these patients. While palliation is improved, particularly due to the availability of high doses of glucocorticoids and because of some modest success in chemotherapy, there is a very great need for innovative approaches, some of which have been discussed here. No new major breakthroughs are likely, except perhaps in the treatment of medulloblastoma. Due to its primitive cell origins, it might be the first to yield to combination chemotherapy, in addition to surgery and radiation therapy. Until more effective drug therapy is available and tumor biology is better understood, significant improvement in patient survival will be difficult to attain.

REFERENCES

1. Posner JB: Management of central nervous system metastases. *Semin Oncol* 4:81, 1977.
2. Third National Cancer Survey: Incidence data, National Cancer Institute Monograph 41, March 1975.
3. Mason T et al (eds): *Atlas of Cancer Mortality for U.S. Counties: 1950–1969*, DHEW Publication No (NIH) 75-780, 1975.
4. Waterhouse J et al (eds): *Cancer in Five Continents*, Springer-Verlag, New York, 1976.
5. *Occupational Mortality: The Registrar General's Dicennial Supplement for England and Wales, 1970–1972*, ser DS, no 1, Office of Population Census and Surveys, London, 1978, p 49.
6. Kernohan JW, Sayer GP: Tumors of the central nervous system, in *Atlas of Tumor Pathology,* fasc 35, Armed Forces Institute of Pathology, Washington DC, 1952.
7. Muller W et al: Supratentorial recurrences of gliomas: Morphological studies in relation to time intervals with astrocytomas. *Acta Neurochir (Wein)* 37:75, 1977.
8. Milham S: *Occupational Mortality in Washington State, 1950–1971*, DHEW PHS Publication No 76, 1976.
9. Gold E et al: Risk factors for brain tumors in children. *Am J Epidemiol* 109:309, 1979.
10. Schuman LM et al: Relationship of central nervous system neoplasms to *Toxoplasma gondii* infection. *Am J Public Health* 57:848, 1967.
11. Guralnick L: Mortality by occupation and cause of death. *Special Rep* 53(3), 1963.
12. Wertheimer N, Leeper E: Electric wiring configurations and childhood cancer. *Am J Epidemiol* 109:273, 1979.

13. Bryen D et al: Mortality and cancer morbidity in a group of Swedish VCM and PVC production workers. *Environ Health Perspect* 17:167, 1976.
14. Monson RR, Fine LF: Cancer mortality and morbidity among rubber workers. *J Clin Neurol* 61:1047, 1978.
15. Thomas TL et al: Mortality among workers employed in petroleum refining and petrochemical plants. *J Occup. Med* 22:97, 1980.
16. Munk J et al: Radiation induced intracranial meningiomas. *J Clin Radiol* 20:90, 1969.
17. Modan B et al: Radiation-induced head and neck tumors. *Lancet* 1:276, 1974.
18. Schoenberg BS: Primary nervous system neoplasms, in BS Schoenberg (ed): *Advances in Neurology*, vol 19, Raven Press, New York, 1978.
19. Ray BS, Wolff HG: Experimental studies on headache: Pain sensitive structures of the head and their significance in headache. *Arch Surg* 41:813, 1940.
20. Northfield DWC: Some observations on headache. *Brain* 61:133, 1938.
21. Kunkle EC et al: Studies on headache: The mechanisms and significance of the headache associated with brain tumor. *Bull NY Acad Med* 18:400, 1942.
22. Rushton JG, Rooke ED: Brain tumor headache. *Headache* 2:147, 1962.
23. Bailey P, Cushing H: *A classification of the tumors of the glioma group on a histogenic basis with a correlated study of prognosis*, Lippincott, Philadelphia, 1926.
24. Rubinstein LJ: Tumors of the central nervous system, in *Atlas of Tumor Pathology*, fas 6, 2d ser, Armed Forces Institute of Pathology, Washington, DC, 1972.
25. Erlich SS, Davis RL: Spinal subarachnoid metastasis from primary intracranial glioblastoma multiforme. *Cancer* 42:2854, 1978.
26. Alvord EC: Why do gliomas not metastasize? *Arch Neurol* 33:73, 1976.
27. Smith DR et al: Metastasizing neurectadermal tumors of the central nervous system. *J Neurosurg* 31:50, 1969.
28. Bartal AD et al: Extensive resection of primary malignant tumors of the left cerebral hemisphere. *Surg Neurol* 1:337, 1973.
29. Balcueva EP et al: Second surgical load (SSL) following adjuvant treatment of glioblastoma. *Proc Am Soc Clin Oncol* 19:371, 1978.
30. Peylan-Ramu N et al: Abnormal CT scans of the brain in asymptomatic children with acute lymphocytic leukemia after prophylactic treatment of the central nervous system with radiation and intrathecal chemotherapy. *N Engl J Med* 298:815, 1978.
31. Tan BC, Kunaratnam N: Hypopituitary dwarfism following radiotherapy for nasopharyngeal carcinoma. *Clin Radiol* 17:302, 1966.
32. Fuks Z et al: Long-term effects of external radiation on the pituitary and thyroid glands. *Cancer* 37:1152, 1976.
33. Shalet SM et al: Pituitary function after treatment of intracranial tumors in children. *Lancet* 2:104, 1975.
34. Walker MD et al: Evaluation of BCNU and/or radiotherapy in the treatment of anaplastic gliomas: A cooperative clinical trial. *J Neurosurg* 48:333, 1978.
35. Walker MD et al: Randomized comparisons of radiotherapy and nitrosoureas for the treatment of malignant glioma after surgery. *New Engl J Med* 303:1323, 1980.
36. Leibel S et al: The role of radiation therapy in the treatment of astrocytomas. *Cancer* 35:1551, 1975.
37. Fazekas JT: Treatment of grades I and II brain astrocytomas: The role of radiation therapy. *Int J Radiat Oncol Biol Phys* 2:661, 1977.
38. Sheline G: Radiation therapy of brain tumors. *Cancer* 39:873, 1977.
39. Bouchard J, Pierce C: Radiation therapy in the management of neoplasms of the central nervous system with a special note in regard to children: Twenty years' experience, 1939–1958. *Am J Roentgenol* 84:610, 1960.
40. Phillips T et al: Therapeutic considerations in tumors affecting the central nervous system: Ependymomas. *Radiology* 83:98, 1964.
41. Gjerris F, Klinken L: Long term prognosis in children with benign cerebellar astrocytoma. *J Neurosurg* 49:179, 1978.
42. Palmer JO et al: Differentiation of medulloblastoma: Studies including immunohistochemical localization of glial fibrillary acidic protein. *J Neurosurg* 55:161, 1981.
43. Raimondi AJ, Tomita T: Medulloblastoma in childhood: Comparative results of partial and total resection. *Child's Brain* 5:310, 1979.
44. Lisczak T et al: Morphological, biochemical, ultrastructural tissue culture and clinical observations of typical and aggressive craniopharyngiomas. *Acta Neuropathol* 43:191, 1978.
45. Mealy J, Hall PV: Medulloblastoma in children: Survival and treatment. *J Neurosurg* 46:56, 1977.
46. Tokars RP et al: Cerebellar medulloblastoma: Results of a new method of radiation treatment. *Cancer* 43:129, 1979.
47. Evans AE et al: Adjuvant chemotherapy for medulloblastoma and ependymoma, *Proceedings of the Symposium on Multidisciplinary Aspects of Brain Tumor Therapy* (in press).
48. Hoyt WF, Badhdassarian SA: Optic gliomas of childhood: Natural history and rationale for conservative management. *Br J Ophthalmol* 53:793, 1969.
49. Oxenhandler DC, Sayers MP: The dilemma of childhood optic gliomas. *J Neurosurg* 48:34, 1978.
50. Sheline GE, Wara WM: Radiation therapy for tumors of the central nervous system, in JT Hoff (ed): *Practice of Surgery, Neurosurgery*, Harper & Row, Hagerstown, Md, 1979.
51. Stein BM: The infratentorial supracerebellar approach to pineal lesions. *J Neurosurg* 35:197, 1979.
52. Marshall LF et al: Teratocarcinoma of the brain: A treatable disease. *Child's Brain* 5:96, 1979.
53. Neuwelt EA et al: Suprasellar germinomas (ectopic pinealomas): Aspects of immunological characterization and suc-

cessful chemotherapeutic responses in recurrent disease. *Neurosurgery* 7:352, 1980.
54. Sheline G: Radiation necrosis (unpublished observations).
55. Verity GL: Tissue tolerance: Central nervous system. *Radiology* 91:1221, 1968.
56. Wilson GH et al: Atrophy following radiation therapy for central nervous system neoplasms. *Acta Radiol Ther (Stockh)* 11:361, 1972.
57. Pool JL: Management of recurrent gliomas, in RG Ojemann (ed): *Clinical Neurosurgery,* vol 15, Williams & Wilkins, Baltimore, 1968.
58. Freeman JE et al: Somnolence after prophylactic cranial irradiation in children with acute lymphoblastic leukemia. *Br Med J* 4:523, 1973.
59. Lampert P et al: Disseminated demyelination of the brain following ^{60}Co (gamma) radiation. *Arch Pathol* 68:322, 1959.
60. Afra D et al: Cysts in malignant gliomas—Identification by computerized tomography. *J Neurosurg* 53:821, 1980.
61. Bryan P: CSF seeding of intra-cranial tumors: A study of 96 cases. *Clin Radiol* 25:355, 1974.
62. Russel DS, Rubinstein LJ: *Pathology of tumors of the nervous system,* 3d ed, Williams & Wilkins, Baltimore, 1971.
63. Fragoyannis S, Yalcin S: Ependymomas with distant metastases: Report of two cases and review of the literature. *Cancer* 19:246, 1966.
64. Walker MD, Hurwitz BS: BCNU (1,3-bis(2-chloroethyl)-1-nitrosourea, NSC 409962) in the treatment of malignant brain tumor: A preliminary report. *Cancer Chemother Rep* 54:263, 1970.
65. Wilson CB et al: 1,3-bis(2-chloroethyl)-1-nitrosourea (NSC-409962) in the treatment of brain tumors. *Cancer Chemother Rep* 54:273, 1970.
66. Holoye PY et al: Pulmonary toxicity in long term administration of BCNU. *Cancer Treat Rep* 60:1691, 1976.
67. Durant JR et al: Pulmonary toxicity associated with bischloroethylnitrosourea (BCNU). *Ann Intern Med* 90:191, 1979.
68. Rosenstock JG et al: Response to vincristine of recurrent brain tumors in children. *J Neurosurg* 45:135, 1976.
69. Levin VA et al: A phase III comparison of BCNU, hydroxyurea and radiation therapy for treatment of primary malignant gliomas. *J Neurosurg* 51:526, 1979a.
70. Levin VA et al: Dianhydrogalactitol (NSC-132313): Pharmacokinetics in normal and tumor-bearing rat brain and antitumor activity against three intracerebral rodent tumors. *J Natl Cancer Inst* 56:535, 1976.
71. Renaudin J et al: Dose dependency of Decadron in patients with partially excised brain tumors. *J Neurosurg* 39:302, 1973.
72. Levin VA et al: Modified procarbazine, CCNU, and vincristine combination chemotherapy (UCSF PCV3) in the treatment of malignant brain tumors. *Cancer Treat Rep* (in press).
73. Levin VA et al: BCNU-5-fluorouracil combination therapy for recurrent malignant brain tumors. *Cancer Treat Rep* 62:2071, 1978.
74. Levin VA: Chemotherapy of recurrent brain tumors, in A Prestayko, S Cooke (eds): *Nitrosoureas,* Academic Press, New York, 1981.
75. Cattarell M et al: Fast neutrons compared with megavoltage x-rays in the treatment of patients with supratentorial glioblastoma: A controlled pilot study. *Int J Radiat Oncol Biol Phys* 6:261, 1980.
76. Parker RG et al: Fast neutron beam radiotherapy of glioblastoma multiforme. *Am J Roentgenol* 127:331, 1976.
77. Gutin PH et al: Stereotactic interstitial irradiation of brain tumors. *Proc ASCO* 21:397, 1980.
78. Levin VA, Kabra PM: Effectiveness of nitrosoureas as a function of their lipid solubility in the chemotherapy of experimental rat brain tumors. *Cancer Chemother Rep* 58:787, 1974.
79. Levin VA, Wilson CB: Chemotherapy: Agents in current use. *Semin Oncol* 2:63, 1975.
80. Geran RI et al: A mouse ependymoblastoma as an experimental model for screening potential antineoplastic drugs. *Cancer Chemother Rep* 4:53, 1974.
81. Rapaport SI: Target organ modification in pharmacology: Reversible osmotic opening of the blood-brain barrier by opening of tight junctions, in T Teorell et al (eds): *Pharmacology and Pharmacokinetics,* Plenum, New York, 1974.
82. Neuwelt EA et al: Osmotic blood-brain barrier disruption: Pharmacodynamic studies in dogs and a clinical phase I trial in patients harboring malignant brain tumors. *Cancer Treat Rep* (in press).
83. Hoshino T: Therapeutic implications of brain tumor cell kinetics, in *Modern Concepts in Brain Tumor Therapy: Proceedings of the National Cancer Symposium, Atlanta, Ga., February 26–28, 1976,* DHEW, 1977.
84. Schnegg JF et al: Human glioma-associated antigens detected by monoclonal antibodies. *Cancer Res* 41:1209, 1981.
85. Fay JW et al: Treatment of neoplastic disease of the central nervous system (CNS) with high-dose 1,3-bis(2-chloroethyl)-1-nitrosourea (BCNU) and autologous marrow transplantation (AMTX). *Proc ASCO* 32:353, 1980.
86. Takvorian T et al: Single high doses of BCNU with autologous bone marrow (ABM): A phase I study. *Proc ASCO* 21:341, 1980.
87. Wheeler KT et al: Modification of the in vitro radiation response of rat 9L brain tumor cell by BCNU. *Int J Radiat Oncol Biol Phys* (submitted for publication).
88. Tel E et al: Effect of surgery on BCNU chemotherapy in a rat brain tumor model. *J Neurosurg* 52:529, 1980.
89. Hoshino T, Wilson CB: Cell kinetic analysis of human malignant brain tumors (gliomas). *Cancer* 44:956, 1979.
90. Valeriote FA et al: Synergistic action of cyclophosphamide and 1,3-bis(2-chloroethyl)-1-nitrosourea on a transplanted murine lymphoma. *J Natl Cancer Inst* 40:935, 1968.
91. Rosenblum ML et al: In vivo clonogenic tumor cell kinetics

following BCNU brain tumor therapy. *Proc AACR* 17:219, 1976.
92. Wilson CB et al: Brain tumor chemotherapy: Translation of laboratory experiments into clinical trials. *Trans Am Nuerol Assoc* 101:1, 1976.
93. McGuire WL et al: Estrogen receptors in human breast cancer: An overview, in SL McGuire et al (eds): *Estrogen Reception in Human Breast Cancer*, Raven Press, New York, 1975.
94. Rosenblum ML et al: Development of a clonogenic cell assay for human brain tumors. *Cancer* 41:2305, 1978.
95. Marton LJ et al: Predictive value of cerebral spinal fluid polyamines in medulloblastoma. *Cancer Res* 39:993, 1979.

46

THE TREATMENT OF METASTATIC DISEASE TO THE CENTRAL NERVOUS SYSTEM AND SPINE

Lawrence F. Marshall

The treatment of metastatic disease to the central nervous system remains a difficult problem for all physicians. Despite the introduction of computerized axial tomographic scanning, a diagnostic tool which has revolutionized the recognition of intracranial mass lesions, the treatment of metastatic disease to the central nervous system remains primarily palliative. The presence of brain or spinal metastases often heralds the presence of more widespread systemic disease, but the diagnosis and treatment of these entities differs so from that of generalized metastases that they are worthy of separate consideration.

INCIDENCE

Each year approximately 700,000 cases of cancer are diagnosed in the United States. Of the 425,000 deaths reported for 1981, approximately 13 percent were directly associated with the spread of a malignancy to the central nervous system (CNS). The incidence of metastatic carcinoma to the CNS appears to be increasing in proportion to the increased diagnosis of cancer in the population as a whole. However, the rather dramatic increase in the incidence of carcinoma to the lung in women in the United States may also be responsible for the apparent trend towards a higher incidence of CNS involvement from cancer in the general population. Previous autopsy data has shown that in patients dying of cancer the incidence of cerebral metastasis has varied from 12 percent to 37 percent.[1] In many instances these reports have come from hospitals where a disproportionate number of patients suffer from carcinoma of the lung, a neoplasm that has a particular predilection for spread to the brain. In a review of cases from the Memorial Hospital in New York, intracranial metastases were present in 18 percent of patients who came to autopsy, and intracerebral metastases were present in 12 percent.[2] These figures are in keeping with those reported nationally and are a truer reflection of the incidence of metastasis to the brain.

Of greater importance to the treating physician than the absolute incidence of metastatic disease to the brain at postmortem is the incidence of solitary or multiple metastases within the brain which cause symptoms leading to diagnosis. The advent of computerized axial tomographic scanning has made available accurate premorbid data regarding the incidence of solitary and multiple metastases. In the experience of most major centers, approximately 60 percent of patients undergoing scanning are found to have multiple lesions, and 40 percent have a single metastasis. Autopsy statistics demonstrate a slightly higher incidence of multiple lesions. If a careful autopsy is performed, a second lesion may be found which is too small to be seen using present scanning techniques. A second metastasis may develop also following treatment of the first lesion and thus is present only at the time of the patient's demise.

While intraparenchymal metastases represent the most common type of intracranial secondary deposits, meningeal carcinomatosis appears to be occurring with increasing frequency. This appears to be particularly true in the case of carcinoma of the breast, and is in our view of reflection of the increased survival times in patients with metastatic breast carcinoma because of the availability of satisfactory chemotherapeutic regimens for organ systems other than the brain. This is analogous to the history of treatment of acute stem cell leukemia in children where development of better chemotherapeutic strategies resulted in the need for prophylactic treatment to the neuroaxis to prevent demise from CNS spread.

METASTASIS TO THE BRAIN

Signs and Symptoms of Intracranial Metastases

The signs and symptoms of metastatic carcinoma to the brain differ little from the signs and symptoms of other intracranial mass lesions. However, the time from onset of symptoms to diagnosis is often relatively short (less than 2 months in 65 percent) because of the suspicion of metastatic disease in patients who have had a previously removed primary lesion. While various reports have emphasized the relative frequency of symptomatology, it is clear that the great majority of patients with metastatic carcinoma to the brain demonstrate either focal neurological deficit, headache, or impairment of intellectual function. The incidence of papilledema varies from series to series but is decreasing. This is almost certainly a reflection of earlier diagnosis. As one would expect, the neurological picture that develops is a reflection of the location of the metastatic lesion. Lesions of the frontal region are more likely to produce disturbances of intellectual function or focal weakness, while lesions in the posterior fossa are much more likely to produce disturbances in gait and coordination.

Other than headache, symptoms such as focal weakness or behavioral and mental changes occur approximately 50 percent of the time. However, a careful neurological examination will often demonstrate a higher incidence of signs particularly if care is taken to perform a careful mental status examination and to look for focal weakness. It should be emphasized that the presence of cranial nerve palsies as a presenting symptom in a patient with a history of carcinoma should always suggest the possibility of spread to the leptomeninges, particularly if the neurological deficit is multifocal and difficult to explain on the basis of one lesion.

Focal and generalized seizures are presenting symptoms in approximately 20 percent of the patients seen in our clinic. No pattern of convulsive disorder is particularly helpful in delineating the etiology of a seizure disorder. It is our view that in patients with a previous history of carcinoma, a computerized axial tomographic scan is indicated following the occurrence of even one focal seizure. It should also be recognized that seizures may accompany other neurological symptoms and that the use of anticonvulsants in patients with metastatic disease, if seizures have occurred, is certainly indicated.

Diagnostic Techniques and Evaluation of Patients with Probable Metastatic Carcinoma of the Brain

The diagnosis of metastatic disease to the brain has been revolutionized by the advent of computerized axial tomographic (CT) scanning. Prior to the availability of scanning devices, neurodiagnosticians were dependent on radionucleotide scanning and angiography to evaluate patients with probable metastatic disease. While these diagnostic techniques were extremely useful in delineating lesions with abnormal vascular patterns and/or those which produced shift or distortion of the cerebral vasculature, they were often misleading in determining the number of metastatic lesions present. In the author's experience, scanning and angiography (when compared with the postmortem findings in a consecutive series of patients) underestimated the incidence of multiple lesions by 30 percent. This represents a critical failure in diagnosis since with the CT scanner multiple lesions have been missed only 15 percent of the time. Surgical intervention for solitary metastases remains conventional and, in most instances, logical therapy, while surgical intervention for multiple deposits is almost always contraindicated because it gives poor palliation.

Each generation of CT scanners has been able to detect progressively smaller and smaller lesions. Metastases of 1 cm or more are now usually recognizable. With further advances in technology even smaller deposits will be recognized. The CT scan is the appropriate initial study because it is both more time- and more cost-efficient. There are specific circumstances where electroencephalography and pneumoencephalography may be useful, but these techniques are generally of limited value in the evaluation of CNS metastases. Lumbar puncture is now very rarely indicated in the evaluation of patients with suspected intracranial mass lesions, with the exception of suspected meningeal carcinomatosis, because the diagnostic yield is low.

Certain features of the CT scan are particularly useful in the evaluation of patients with suspected metastatic disease. The presence of multiple areas of edema with or without enhancement (Fig. 46-1) in patients with a known primary lesion is usually diagnostic of multiple metastases even if only one of the lesions enhances with contrast. In patients presenting with symptoms of neurological disturbance and in whom there is no previous history of cancer, the presence of multiple lesions should always suggest metastatic carcinoma, and a thorough search for a primary lesion should be undertaken. However, multiple lesions on CT scan may represent other diagnostic possibilities such as arteritis, or in the southwestern United States, cysticercosis or *Echinococcus* cysts of the brain. Furthermore, in patients with a previous history of carcinoma, progressive multifocal leukoencephalopathy may yield a CT scan appearance indistinguishable from that of multiple metastases. In instances where this viral entity is a diagnostic possibility, as in patients with altered immune states, and particularly with lymphoma, this diagnosis should always be kept in mind, and appropriate steps taken to obtain a tissue diagnosis.

While angiography has been displaced as the primary diagnostic tool in evaluating patients with probable metastatic carcinoma, angiography is often helpful in further delineating the exact location of a solitary mass. Furthermore, because the CT scan appearance of a relatively vascular metastatic deposit may look identical to a primary glioblastoma of the brain, angiography may be useful in distinguishing the type of intracranial mass.

Under certain circumstances cerebral angiography may differentiate such lesions and eliminate the need for a tissue diagnosis. However, if the diagnosis is in doubt, and a previous primary lesion has not been established, then a tissue diagnosis is absolutely indicated. It should be emphasized that angiography generally is not required in instances where multiple lesions are demonstrated in patients with a previous history of cancer. Under such circumstances the intracranial lesions almost always represent central nervous system spread of the primary tumor. Extremely long free intervals between the diagnosis of the primary lesion and the presence of a secondary deposit can be seen. This is true particularly in breast cancer where metastatic lesions have been demonstrated as long as 20 years following the initial treatment of the breast primary.

Initial Treatment

The initial treatment of a patient with a suspected mass lesion to the central nervous system is dependent on the severity of the patient's neurological deficit. If only mild symptoms such as headache are present, no immediate therapeutic intervention need be taken prior to diagnostic evaluation. However, the presence of focal neurological deficit or severe headache is usually an indication for the initiation of corticosteroid therapy. Although doses utilized vary widely and are determined, at least in part, by the severity of the patient's neurological deficit, a starting dose of 16 mg per day in four divided doses in a patient with moderate dysfunction is usual. This can be increased if symptoms and signs warrant. When rapid deterioration occurs in a patient, more vigorous therapy should be employed to control brain swelling, which is almost always a major factor causing such rapid deterioration. Under such circumstances mannitol, in doses of 1 g/kg, controlled ventilation with hyperventilation, and the judicious use of high doses of corticosteroids, up to 80 mg per day, may be employed. Such aggressive therapy for initial stabilization is indicated particularly if there is a long free interval in a patient with no evidence of other systemic disease, or when the diagnosis is in doubt.

Under circumstances where widespread systemic disease is present, the decision to institute such aggressive therapy is usually inappropriate. Once initial stabilization with either corticosteroids or the above regimen has been obtained and the appropriate diagnostic procedures performed, a rational plan of treatment can be devel-

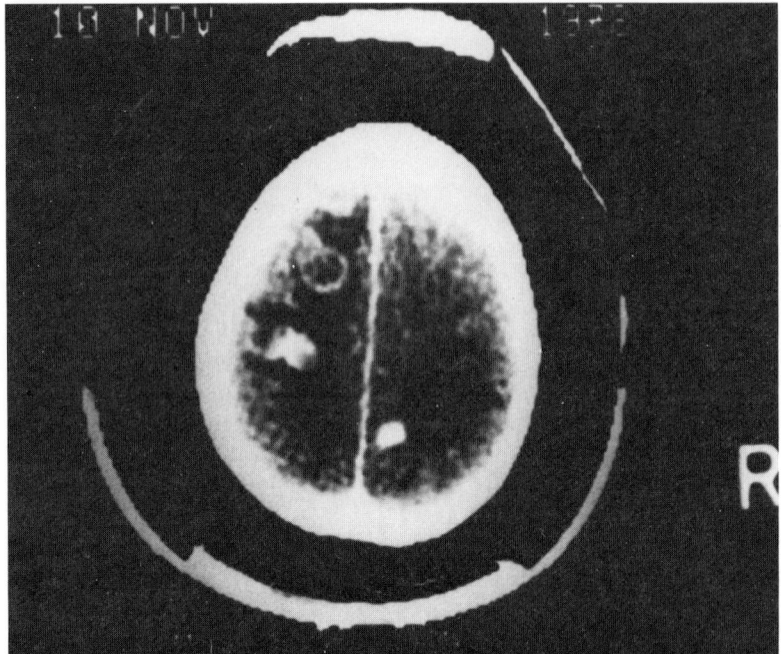

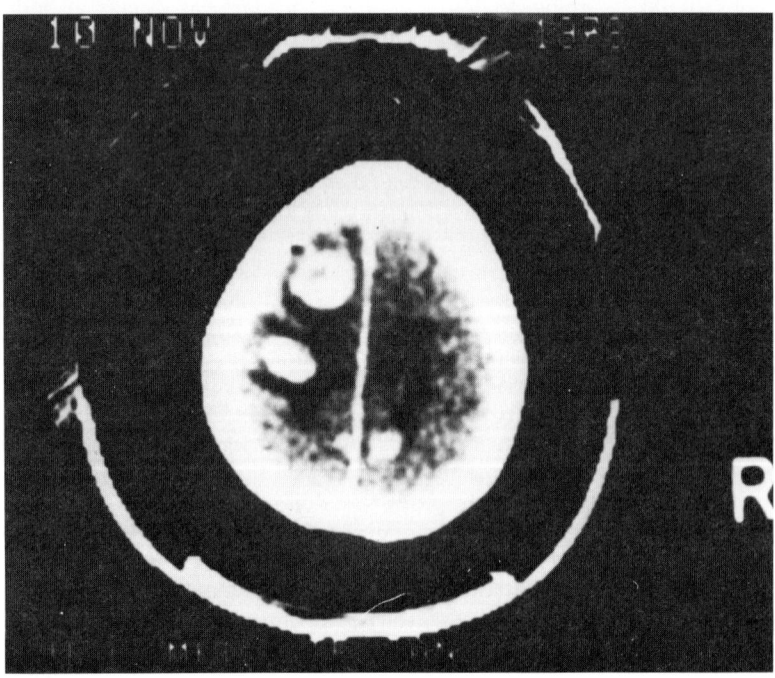

FIGURE 46-1 Multiple lesions in a patient with metastatic breast cancer. (*a*) CT scan without contrast, and (*b*) CT scan with contrast. Note the areas of enhancement in *b*.

oped. Table 46-1 illustrates the usual approach to the treatment of metastatic disease practiced by most neurosurgeons.

Definitive Treatment of a Solitary Metastasis

The presence of a solitary metastasis in a patient with no evidence of other visceral involvement is usually an indication for surgical removal of the metastatic lesion, if the tumor is considered surgically accessible (Table 46-1). In most instances, this approach is both logical and superior to radiation therapy as a single-modality treatment, since under certain circumstances long-term survivals and even cures may be obtained in such cases. Although the long-term salvage rate is low (less than 10 percent), it appears that the small group of patients in this category should not be deprived the possibility of long-term survival or cure when such a possibility exists. The desire for intervention, however, must be tempered with wisdom. If the patient has evidence of involvement of any other organ system which is likely to be determinant of a short survival, it is extremely unlikely that surgical removal of the brain metastasis will lead to long-term quality palliation. A decision must then be made on the best evidence available as to whether a craniotomy, in light of the presence of other metastatic disease, will significantly prolong the patient's life and make that life a good one. Retrospective analysis of patients treated both surgically and with radiation therapy demonstrates that in patients in whom the cerebral lesion commenced primarily with headache and minimal neurological signs, a median survival of approximately 6 months can be expected following either modality of treatment. However, if the patient presents with focal neurological deficit, survival is often considerably shorter. This information can be useful in determining whether or not a patient should be subjected to craniotomy.

While neurosurgeons differ in their opinions of indications for removal of a solitary metastasis, it is accepted by many that the presence of visceral metastasis to the liver or lung should be a relative contraindication to surgical intervention.

The availability of dexamethasone and other cerebrally active corticosteroids for both the pretreatment and posttreatment of patients with solitary metastases has significantly altered both surgical morbidity and mortality. In a consecutive series of 37 patients with intracranial metastasis treated surgically at the University Hospital in San Diego, there was one postoperative death and significant morbidity in two other patients. This reflects the possibility of a minimal operative mortality and morbidity with appropriate patient selection and good neuroanesthesia. The general principles of neurosurgical intervention also must always be kept at the forefront. Deep lesions not considered accessible by craniotomy can be biopsied either through a twist drill under CT scan control or stereotactically if the lesion is small, and no other site is available for establishing the diagnosis. It must be emphasized that when surgical diagnosis by needle biopsy or treatment by craniotomy is undertaken, preoperative preparation of the patients with high doses of corticosteroids appears to significantly improve the operative outcome. We use dexamethasone, 10 mg every 6h for 12 to 24 h prior to needle biopsy and then taper the dose postoperatively. A similar regimen is used prior to and following craniotomy. This preoperative preparation satisfactorily explains the relative infrequency of complications which we encounter following needle biopsy or craniotomy. Needle biopsy does not appear to be indicated when the diagnosis of carcinoma is well established, and systemic disease is

TABLE 46-1 Therapeutic Strategy for Metastatic Carcinoma

USUAL TREATMENT

I. Surgery for *solitary* metastasis if
  A. No liver involvement
  B. No class III risks
  C. Oncologist feels 3-month survival is probable
  D. Long free intervals likely if lesion is operable
  E. EMI shows *only* one lesion

II. Radiation therapy if
  A. More than one lesion
  B. Particularly favorable tumor (reticulum cell sarcoma)
  C. Surgery contraindicated

HERETICAL TREATMENT FOR SOLITARY METASTASIS*
I. High-dose dexamethasone until symptoms break through (80 mg/day)
II. Tumor-specific chemotherapy, e.g., adriamycin, CeeNU, VM 26 for breast; DTIC and CCNU for melanoma
III. Surgery if I and II fail late; no surgery if steroid-unresponsive

* **Rationale:** Avoid craniotomy in patients who will develop systemic metastases within 1 month of surgery (Darwin's law).

present. In such circumstances there is no diagnostic difficulty, and nonsurgical modes of therapy are required.

In any patient in whom there is doubt as to the histology of the mass or in a patient with a previous diagnosis of cancer, in whom there has been a significant free interval, a tissue diagnosis is mandatory. In situations where craniotomy is not thought to be therapeutically useful but a tissue diagnosis is required, needle biopsy will often yield such a diagnosis. In patients with metastatic disease, needle biopsy of the suspected lesion has yielded a diagnosis in approximately 85 percent of the cases. With CT scan localization, it is probable that the percentage yield will be even higher in the future.

Following craniotomy in patients with solitary metastasis, radiation therapy is often employed as an additional treatment modality. There is evidence from one trial that combination therapy is superior to the use of surgery alone. Doses of radiation therapy recommended following craniotomy vary widely. Between 4000 to 5000 rads, a dose higher than that used strictly for palliation, has been employed by several groups. The logic behind radiation therapy, particularly in patients with a long free interval, lies in the belief that sterilization of the surgical field with radiation following surgery can lead to a higher number of long-term survivors. In the series of Ransohoff and his colleagues, almost 40 percent of patients survived for more than 1 year, and 13 percent survived beyond 2 years.[3] This is the strongest evidence to support the use of both modalities. A second argument for the use of radiation therapy following removal of what is thought to be a solitary metastasis is the possibility of a second, undetected, small lesion. Because two-thirds of patients with symptomatic brain metastasis die from recrudescence of initial disease, adjunctive therapy in the patient with a solitary metastasis seems indicated. It is of interest to note that of patients in whom no evidence of disease other than the brain metastasis is present at the time of treatment, two-thirds die of their CNS lesion, while of patients with the presence of other disease at the time of treatment of the CNS metastasis, only one-third succumb to their CNS lesion.

The decision to surgically extirpate a solitary metastasis must always consider the general well-being of the patient. If, for example, a patient has a disabling pain from recurrent disease or failure of control of the primary lesion, a quality survival will not be obtained from surgical therapy, and palliation with corticosteroids and radiation therapy is more appropriate.

Aside from the fact that a metastatic deposit is solitary on CT scanning, the most important single factor in deciding whether surgical extirpation should be carried out is the length of the free interval. In patients, for example, in whom a primary bronchogenic carcinoma has been discovered only 2 to 3 months prior to discovery of the brain metastasis, the likelihood of long-term survival following surgical extirpation of the metastasis is extremely low.

Under these circumstances we have perferred to carry such patients on corticosteroids for as long as possible in order to determine whether evidence of more widespread systemic disease develops (Table 46-1). Tumor-free surgical extirpation can then be carried out at a later date with somewhat more assurance that a quality survival can be obtained.

Adjunctive Chemotherapy of a Solitary Metastasis

At present there is little evidence to support the use of adjunctive chemotherapy in the treatment of solitary brain metastasis. This is a reflection of the diversity of the neoplasms treated in any one center and the unavailability of suitable agents for treatment. The sole exception is metastatic trophoblastic disease. Until centers are capable of collecting large groups of patients with similar disease states and agreeing on controlled trials, the use of chemotherapy will remain an individual and relatively unsupported mode of therapy for solitary brain metastasis.

Treatment of Multiple Metastases

The treatment of multiple metastases to the brain is nonsurgical. With the exception of the patient who requires a biopsy to establish the diagnosis, surgical intervention is usually of no avail and should not be employed. Satisfactory palliation in patients with multiple metastases is best achieved by the use of radiation therapy and the judicious use of corticosteroids. Kramer and his colleagues,[4] reporting for the Radiation Therapy Oncology Group (RTOG), have demonstrated that 3000 rads delivered over 2 weeks is equal to 4000 rads given over a 3-week course and is superior to short-course, high-dose therapy as had been advocated by others.[5] The median survival in patients treated with radiation therapy for multiple brain metastases is directly proportional to the presence or absence of neurological deficit at the time radiation therapy is initiated and is not a product of the number of metastases demonstrated on CT scan. In patients in whom minimal or no symptoms other than headache are present, the median survival time reaches approximately 6 months, while in patients in whom significant symptomatology is present, especially a depressed level of consciousness, radiation therapy yields a much shorter survival. In the RTOG experience, addition of corticosteroids to radiation therapy improved symptoms but did not lengthen survival. This data must be interpreted with caution since the doses of steroids employed concomitantly with radiation therapy were relatively small. Significant palliation of patients once they have broken through radiation therapy can often be achieved with either reirradiation or the utilization of higher doses (up to 100 mg a day) of dexamethasone. This is similar to the experience reported by Renaudin et al., in patients with a glioblastoma multiforme who have become resistant to other therapies.[6]

The value of chemotherapy in prolonging survival of patients with multiple brain metastases also remains to be proved, although there has been some success in palliation of individual tumor types. Poulliart, utilizing a combination of adriamycin, VM 26, and CCNU in repetitive cycles when marrow reconstitution had occurred, was able to produce objective improvement and regression of multiple metastases in six of eight patients with breast metastases.[7] A median survival of 9 months was obtained, and in five of the patients resolution of their radionucleotide abnormality was seen. Two patients are long-term survivors. In a relatively small series of patients with small cell carcinoma of the lung who had broken through radiation therapy and treatment with dexamethasone, 4 of 15 demonstrated objective remissions on a regimen of procarbazine, 150 mg/m² given in 2-week cycles. The efficacy of this agent may be a product of the fact that it does cross the blood-brain barrier. The response in small cell carcinoma to other agents has so far been disappointing; and since in small cell bronchogenic carcinoma a tremendous number of patients die because of their CNS spread, the need for improved treatment regimens for this particular entity is essential. Bunn et al. have recently advocated prophylactic craniospinal irradiation and intrathecal therapy.[8] Bunn reviewed the experience with both randomized and nonrandomized control trials. While prophylactic cranial irradiation resulted in lower instances of CNS parenchymal metastasis in patients with small cell bronchogenic carcinoma, there was a disturbingly high rate of recurrence in the leptomeninges and in the intradural and epidural space of the spine. This suggests that prophylactic cranial irradiation should be expanded to include the spinal axis and that perhaps prophylaxis using intrathecal medication such as methotrexate or cytosine arabinoside would be appropriate not only to treat the meningeal disease once it has been absolutely indentified but also prophylactically. The Ommaya Reservoir, or other external devices which allow direct introduction of medication into the ventricular system, appears to be preferable, particularly in situations where radiation therapy has been delivered to the craniospinal axis. Lumbar puncture is often difficult under those circumstances, and the permanent cannula ensures that the drug is delivered into the subarachnoid space. Regimens of maintenance intrathecal therapy have employed both single and multiple agents in small cell bronchogenic carcinoma, and no advantage of multiple agents for intrathecal administration has been demonstrated. Because the relapse rate remains high in this particular lesion and because multiple metastases are so common, this tumor provides a particularly fruitful area for the use of a combination of radiation therapy with adjunctive chemotherapy. This disease entity serves to emphasize the need for prophylaxis to prevent the development of CNS symptomatology in patients with prolonged survival from neoplasms which have a particular predilection for spread to the CNS.

Metastatic melanoma is a very common CNS metastasis. Because these lesions are often multiple and thus inoperable, a combination of DTIC, 250 mg/m² for 5 days, and CCNU, 100 mg/m², both repeated every 6 weeks, has yielded objective remissions in 10 to 30 percent of patients with a median duration of response of approximately 5 to 7 months. While the response rate is small, it can usually be predicted following the first or second course. If the patient continues to deteriorate, therapy can then be rapidly abandoned.

Although isolated reports of the effectiveness of single or multiple agents in the treatment of multiple metastases continue to surface, we are in the infancy of the use of chemotherapy to control CNS metastases. Some progress has been made in the treatment of breast cancer, and more logical therapeutic strategies are developing for the treatment of small cell bronchogenic carcinoma. Future progress utilizing chemotherapeutic regimens requires new drugs and better strategies, particularly in cases where prolonged survival with an ultimate death from central nervous system involvement can be predicted.

Therapeutic Agents for the Treatment of Recurrent Metastasis

In general, with the exception of the use of reirradiation, the treatment of recurrent intracranial metastasis is unrewarding. If a total dose of under 6000 rads has been delivered to the brain initially, reirradiation to that total dose may induce a remission for a second time in a small group of patients. In patients in whom reirradiation is not possible, the use of high doses of corticosteroids may occasionally prolong quality survival for several weeks, and in rare instances for several months.

Current Areas of Research and Prospects for the Future

The control of central nervous system metastasis is a problem which in the great majority of instances has defied a satisfactory solution. Whether it is blood-brain barrier impenetrability, or the relative ineffectiveness of chemotherapeutic regimens that are effective for other organ systems, or whether other factors are operative is not yet known. However, the difficulty in delivering high enough doses of effective antitumor agents systemically in the great majority of patients is obvious. So far this has limited the effectiveness of chemotherapy for intracranial metastases. Requirements for future strategies for the treatment of intracranial metastasis can be developed along several lines. Pertinent lessons can be learned from the experience of treatment of childhood leukemia with prophylactic craniospinal irradiation, and this approach would appear to be particularly promising in patients with small cell carcinoma of the lung. In view of the fact that many of these tumors recur in the leptomeninges, the prophylactic instillation of intraventricular methotrexate in such patients would also appear to be proper subject for a randomized trial.

The development of carrier molecules such as dexamethasone for active chemotherapeutic agents, thus allowing penetration to the tumor from surrounding edematous brain, remains an attractive idea which is yet to be exploited.

Immunotherapy remains a tantalizing hope, but unanswered questions of a very fundamental nature remain and require scientifically supported evidence, pro or con, about the relative immunologic privilege of the brain. While it appears that immunologic privilege plays some role in the treatment of primary intracranial neoplasms, the evidence to support the concept in metastatic carcinoma to the brain is scanty. It appears that the ineffectiveness of immune therapy is a reflection of the relative failure of this therapy to be effective when applied in other organ systems.

It is clear that surgical extirpation remains a useful means of therapy for only a small number of patients with metastatic disease to the central nervous system. It is absolutely essential to the problem of CNS metastasis that adjunctive chemotherapeutic programs, in conjunction with radiation therapy, be instituted with intelligence and diligence so that better long-term control of neoplastic diseases can be obtained. It is always a tremendous disappointment to the oncologist to have a patient with recurrent CNS disease following successful irradiation of systemic metastasis succumb to brain metastasis. As we have indicated previously, it is likely that as control of metastatic disease to other organ systems improves and survival is prolonged, the problem of the management of brain metastases will become increasingly important. The utilization of prophylactic craniospinal irradiation and intraventricular agents with certain neoplasms, at least those such as small cell bronchogenic carcinoma and perhaps in patients at particular risk with breast carcinoma, are approaches that require controlled application.

METASTASES TO THE LEPTOMENINGES

Although it is usual to discuss metastases to the central nervous system in two broad categories, i.e., metastasis to the brain and to the spinal cord, leptomeningeal metastases have attracted increasing attention in neural oncology. Spread to the leptomeninges is often evident only on postmortem examination, where the only finding may be the presence of an enlarged ventricular system without any apparent explanation. Olsen et al.[9] in a comprehensive review of infiltration of the leptomeninges have emphasized the fact that this complication of systemic cancer is not as rare as previously thought and may well be increasing, particularly since breast cancer, a disease with a particular predilection for spread to the leptomeninges, seems to be coming under better control when spread is to organ systems other than the nervous system.

Leptomeningeal carcinoma should be suspected in

several circumstances in a patient with a previous history of cancer. First, increased intracranial pressure secondary to obstructive hydrocephalus may result in headache and a depressed level of consciousness. More often focal neurological signs not explicable on the basis of one lesion may develop. When widespread and multifocal symptomatology is present in a patient with a previous history of carcinoma, leptomeningeal metastasis must always be considered. Symptomatology from leptomeningeal spread may be secondary either to direct destruction of tissue or from compression ischemia or occlusion of the cortical vasculature.

In general, the diagnosis rests on examination of the cerebrospinal fluid. The CT scanner has been relatively unreliable in identifying leptomeningeal deposits, probably because their small size and closeness to the intracranial vault makes distinction difficult. In most instances, increased intracranial pressure has been present in patients with leptomeningeal metastasis. Examination of the cerebrospinal fluid may be initially unrewarding, but repeat examination may often demonstrate evidence of malignant cells on cytological examination which were not seen on first or second study. As Olsen has noted, the cerebrospinal fluid (CSF) was abnormal in all patients he and his colleagues studied. This is in keeping with the experience of others. Examination usually demonstrates a mild leukocytosis, a slightly elevated to a severely elevated protein, and some depression in spinal fluid glucose. In the great majority of patients, the first and second lumbar puncture will demonstrate malignant cells. However, if the diagnosis is strongly suspected, repeat lumbar puncture is indicated in an attempt to confirm the diagnosis. When CSF cultures are persistently negative in the face of a low CSF glucose, the possibility of leptomeningeal carcinoma is extremely high.

Another clue to the diagnosis of leptomeningeal metastasis is the presence of multiple cranial nerve root or spinal nerve root involvement in an incongruous fashion. For example, patients may present with difficulty of extraocular movement, and at the same time with difficulty with tongue movements, and also pain in the distribution of one or two cervical or thoracic dermatomes. Such signs and the presence of seizures are often confusing initially, until one begins to consider the possibility of leptomeningeal spread.

The treatment of leptomeningeal metastasis must take into account the fact that this is a diffuse disease of the entire craniospinal axis. Radiation to the craniospinal axis up to a dose of 4000 rads has been advocated by some, while others recommend radiation only to areas from which clinical symptoms and signs are emanating. We prefer craniospinal irradiation of 3000 rads followed by the utilization of intraventricular methotrexate in a dose of 10 to 15 mg/m^2 via a ventricular cannula connected to a subcutaneous reservoir. Response rates to this type of therapy are most gratifying in patients with lymphoma and in breast cancer. Our experience in the treatment of leptomeningeal carcinoma secondary to lung cancer has been extremely unrewarding, and, as we have indicated, prophylaxis to the craniospinal axis in that entity appears to be appropriate.

METASTATIC CARCINOMA OF THE SPINE

The presence of metastatic carcinoma involving the spine almost invariably indicates more widespread systemic disease. While a patient will occasionally present with spinal cord compression and a history of cancer, this is a rather rare event in most large series. Because metastatic carcinoma to the spine often yields a paralyzed patient with an intact intellect and months of survival with both fecal and urinary incontinence, the absolute necessity of early diagnosis and treatment of this potentially devastating complication of cancer cannot be overemphasized. It is apparent that a high index of suspicion coupled with an aggressive approach towards the diagnosis and treatment will yield a significantly better outcome for these patients than if one waits, with a negligent eye, until the patient has become paraplegic.

Incidence, Epidemiology, and Etiologic Aspects

Metastatic carcinoma to the spine occurs in approximately 5 percent of patients with a diagnosis of carcinoma. The incidence of this complication of cancer is increasing, particularly in patients with prostatic carcinoma which has a predilection for epidural and vertebral metastases. This increased incidence is a result of the ever-greater length of survival in patients with this disease. The pattern of metastasis in patients with lymphoma also appears to be changing because radiation portals presently in use for initial definitive therapy include the thoracic spine, the site of most frequent metastases in the past. It now appears that disease in the cervical and lumbar regions, areas not included in the initial treatment ports, is becoming more common.

Population-based studies on the incidence of metastatic carcinoma to the spine are few. Many are biased in that they were performed in Veterans Administration hospitals where the incidence of lung carcinoma is high, and the incidence of breast cancer is almost nonexistent. The experience at the Sloan-Kettering Memorial Cancer Center is in general agreement with other series, although the incidence of lung cancer may be slightly underrepresented.[10] In that study, breast carcinoma was equally as common as lung, with prostate and kidney carcinoma and lymphoma also frequent primary neoplasms. Myeloma and melanoma were occasionally represented, while the remaining patients had a variety of primary neoplasms. In some patients the primary lesion is never found. These patients usually have an undifferentiated carcinoma at the time of tissue diagnosis of their spinal lesion.

Metastatic carcinoma spreads to the intervertebral region in a variety of ways. Often there is direct invasion of the vertebral body with subsequent growth into the ventral epidural space, or there may be tumor growth into the paravertebral gutter with compression of the cord. In the latter instance, relatively little may be seen on plain radiographs. Hematogenous spread to bone and soft tissues occurs by the paravertebral plexus of Battson. This is a low-pressure, valvulous system of veins, and probably represents the primary means of spread to the bone and paravertebral space from lung, breast, and prostatic carcinoma. Other tumors appear to spread to the vertebral canal following pulmonary metastasis, and it is postulated that in these patients epidural metastasis is secondary to arterial spread. Tumors such as hypernephroma, whose primary organs lie adjacent to the vertebral bodies, often spread directly to bone and epidural space. It is important to emphasize the fact that the absence of bony changes on plain radiographs does not rule out the possibility of metastatic carcinoma and should not be interpreted as such.

Signs, Symptoms, and Attempts at Early Detection

In patients with a previous diagnosis of carcinoma, particularly primary lesions involving the lung, breast, or prostate, physicians must have an extremely high index of suspicion for the possibility of metastatic disease to the spinal canal. All too often, back pain, which is present in approximately one-half of the patients, is attributed to degenerative arthritic disease or lumbrosacral strain when in fact it is a harbinger of metastatic spread. An additional 30 percent of the patients we see have radicular pain, most commonly in the thoracic region, as a presenting symptom. Again, until proven otherwise, these symptoms should immediately be attributed to the possibility of metastatic carcinoma. Pain in these patients is usually attributable to nerve root compression, which results in radicular symptomatology, or bony invasion, which results in bone pain, and in some instances spinal instability. A significant percentage of patients have pain for weeks or months prior to the development of any neurological deficit.

When the pain is primarily localized, a high percentage of patients will have osteoblastic or osteolytic lesions present on plain radiographs, and an even higher percentage will have positive bone scans. It is imperative that these early symptoms not be ignored because treatment at this stage of the disease, prior to the development of any or significant neurological deficit, is often effective in preventing neurological deterioration.

In the majority of instances, neurological deficit secondary to spinal metastases is a product of vascular compromise. This explains why motor deficits are more common, more severe, and are seen earlier than sensory loss. The larger motor fibers are more sensitive to vascular compromise than are the smaller fibers that carry pain and other sensory modalities. If the lesion is above the conus, myelopathy with weakness, increased tone, and hyperreflexia is the rule, while cauda equina lesions are characterized by decreased reflexes, spotty sensory changes, and less-diffuse weakness.

The location of spinal metastases is thoracic in approximately two-thirds of the cases. This is a reflection of the actual length of the spinal canal and not of a particular predilection for metastasis to this region. However, in reviewing our cases we have found that rapid, devastating neurological deficit is most often associated with spinal metastasis in the region from T4 to T10, an area of the spinal cord that is often dependent on one major feeding vessel, the artery of Adam Kaciez. Thus, the presence of bony changes in a patient with a lesion in this area should be an indication for early therapeutic intervention.

This emphasis on early detection and treatment is based on observations in large groups of patients. In our experience[11] and that of Gilbert et al.[10] response to treatment is directly proportional to the neurological deficit present at the time that treatment was initiated. Patients who could stand by themselves, for example, had a remarkably high incidence of long-term ambulation, while patients in whom paraplegia was present at the time of diagnosis had almost no chance of recovering useful neurological function.

Diagnostic Techniques

The diagnosis of spinal cord compression secondary to metastasis is often supported by plain film changes in patients with a previous history of carcinoma. Furthermore, in patients over 50 years of age in whom no diagnosis of carcinoma has previously been made but in whom localized or radicular pain develops particularly in the thoracic region, in the absence of plain film changes of degenerative disease, the diagnosis of metastatic carcinoma to the epidural space must be considered. Confirmation of the diagnosis rests on myelography, computerized tomography (particularly if this technique is augmented by intrathecal metrizamide), or both. At the present time, the use of CT scanning is limited to those patients in whom the level of involvement can be localized by a combination of plain radiography and/or the presence of a sensory level on neurologic examination which will limit the need to scan the spine to three or four segments. If no such localizing findings exist, myelography must be used. As computerized scanning techniques continue to improve, myelography may eventually be replaced by this technique. However, at the present time, the majority of patients in whom this diagnosis is entertained still require myelography. Myelography may be performed either with an iodinated contrast material such as Pantopaque or with air. In the latter instance the availability of polytomography is absolutely essential. Myelography is important not only in localizing the exact level of spinal cord compression and demonstrating the block for either surgical or radiotherapeutic treatment but it is also extremely useful in detecting occult epidural metastases present at segments that are distant from the lesion causing the patient's neurological signs. Myelography may be performed either by lumbar injection of contrast media or air, preferably at L3 L4, or by cisternal or lateral cervical puncture. Because of the risk of disturbing the dynamics of the cord by puncture below the level of metastases, we have preferred lateral cervical puncture at C2 for the diagnosis and localization of metastatic disease. In rare circumstances, puncture above and below may be required if more than one level of block is present. In almost every instance of patients with significant neurological signs, a complete block will be seen if contrast myelography is employed (Fig. 46-2).

Myelography should not be performed simply as a diagnostic procedure if no therapeutic intervention is planned. It is critical that the patient be told that myelography is a diagnostic procedure to determine the extent and location of the disease in order to plan optimally for therapy. If the patient's general condition is such that a very short survival is likely, or the patient does not wish therapy, myelography is not indicated.

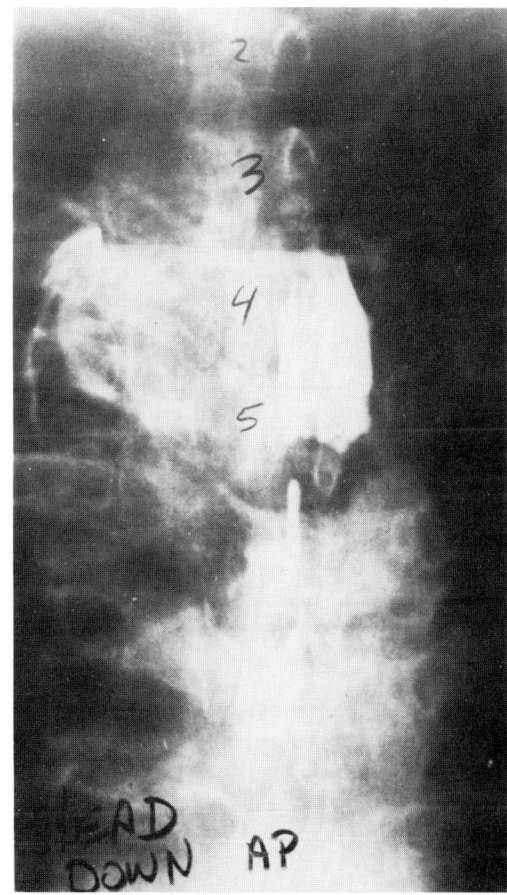

FIGURE 46-2 Myelogram demonstrating classic epidural obstruction of metastatic carcinoma at L4. Lesion has typical "paint brush" appearance.

Therapeutic Options for Treatment

The goals in the treatment of spinal cord metastases are to prevent neurological deterioration in patients who present simply with pain or minimal deficit and to reverse, if possible, neurological deficit that is preventing the patient from being ambulatory. Ambulation must be seen as the major goal of treatment. This means ambulation for months, not days or weeks, and preferably for the entire time of the patient's survival. As we have indicated previously, the neurological status of the patient at the time of presentation is a critical determinant in predicting the response to therapy. Of almost equal importance is the histological type of tumor resulting in cord compression. Interpretation of the results of various therapeutic schemes must take into account these two factors when one attempts to make comparisons between treatment modalities. For example, a patient who presents with back pain and has Hodgkin's disease as the cause of epidural compression is extremely likely to have a gratifying response to radiation therapy. In contrast, a severely paraparetic patient whose symptoms are secondary to metastatic carcinoma from the lung has a relatively poor probability of a response to either radiation therapy or surgical decompression. With these assumptions and general principles in mind, several approaches have been applied in recent years in an attempt to improve the outcome in patients with metastatic spinal cord compression.

Both Posner[2] and this author have advocated a variation from the traditional approach of myelography followed by immediate surgical decompression. Young et al. also found little difference between radiation therapy alone, or surgery followed by radiation therapy.[12] Our present scheme is employed in patients in whom a previous tissue diagnosis of carcinoma has been made and symptoms and signs of spinal cord involvement are present. Dexamethasone is administered in an initial dose of 40 mg intravenously and then 10 mg intravenously every 6 h. Myelography via a C2 puncture is performed for localization of the lesion. Immediate radiation therapy is then instituted, and when appropriate, chemotherapy is also utilized. In patients with prostatic carcinoma, for example, diethylstilbestrol has been used in combination with radiation therapy. The results of this approach are shown in Tables 46-2 and 46-3. As noted previously, response to treatment is a product of both tumor type and the severity of neurological deficit at the time of presentation. As can be seen from the tables, this approach has yielded a satisfactory response in patients with lymphoma, carcinoma of the breast, and carcinoma of the prostate, but has been almost universally unsuccessful in the treatment of carcinoma of the lung. This experience is at variance with that of Posner and his colleagues, who found a response rate to radiation therapy alone of 50 percent.[10] One possibility for this wide divergence in experience is the fact that in our series of 18 patients with metastatic lung cancer, only 3 had a histological type more radiosensitive than epidermoid or adenocarcinoma.

In patients in whom progression occurs despite high doses of corticosteroids, radiation therapy, and appropriate chemotherapy, decompressive laminectomy has

TABLE 46-2 Response to Therapy as a Function of Primary Type

Primary type	Initial dexamethasone response		Sustained response to medical treatment		Response to surgical decompression*	
	Success	Failure	Success	Failure	Success	Failure
Lung	6	12	1	17	3	14
Breast	8	2	6	4	1	3
Hodgkin's disease	7	0	5	2	1	1
Prostate	10	3	18	5	2	3
Kidney	1	1	1	1	1	0
Unknown	1	0	1	0	—	—
Totals	33	18	22	29	8	21

* All failures of medical therapy went on to surgical decompression.

TABLE 46-3 Outcome as a Function of Neurological Status at Start of Therapy

Function	Medical therapy Sustained Success	Medical therapy Failure	Surgical therapy* Success	Surgical therapy* Failure	Total Success	Total Failure
Able to walk with assistance	9	2	1	1	10	1
Able to stand with assistance	7	9	4	5	11	5
Leg movement	6	18	3	15	9	15
Totals	22	29	8	21	30	21

* All failures of medical therapy went on to surgical decompression.

been performed.[10] Table 46-2 shows the outcome in those patients considered failures of medical therapy. These results must be interpreted in light of the fact that such patients are likely to have more rapid progression of their disease, and therefore a less favorable predicted outcome. Secondly, failure to respond to medical therapy predicts a rather poor outcome. The fact that only a small percentage of patients who underwent a laminectomy following failure of medical therapy became ambulatory should not deter the neurosurgeon from decompressive laminectomy. Using such a combined approach to treatment, over one-half of the total patient population treated remained ambulatory for at least 3 months. The conclusion that surgical decompression with radiation therapy offered no advantage over radiation therapy alone, as suggested by Gilbert et al.[11] and Yang et al.[12] is not entirely supported by their own observations and our experience, as well as that of Tang et al.[13] Patients subjected to surgery at the Memorial Hospital were often those with adverse prognostic factors including prior radiation, rapid progression of symptoms, and other factors not explained by the authors. Of course, therapy must be guided by knowledge of the radiosensitivity of the tumor to be treated. Patients with lesions such as lymphoma, myeloma, seminoma, or neuroblastoma are much more likely to respond to radiation therapy than patients with metastatic carcinoma from the lung.

An absolute indication for surgical intervention is the patient who presents with evidence of cord compression, no history of carcinoma, and myelographic demonstration of an extradural block. In this case a tissue diagnosis is mandatory for therapy and thus should be obtained at the time of adequate decompressive laminectomy. An occasional patient with thoracic stenosis of the spinal canal may be mistakenly thought to have metastatic carcinoma to the spine. In this circumstance, radiation therapy can be disastrous, because radiation often results in some cord swelling particularly early; and this, in combination with a narrow spinal canal, can lead to a devastating neurological deficit. For this reason a tissue diagnosis is mandatory in patients in whom a previous carcinoma or lymphoma has not been demonstrated.

Many surgical series have reported a significant incidence of worsening neurological deficit following operation. However, the use of high-dose corticosteroid therapy, either prior to or in concomitance with and following surgical decompression, has limited operative morbidity. In a consecutive series of 29 patients 1 patient underwent laminectomy.

However, morbidity is often associated with operation for spinal compression, particularly when radiation therapy follows a decompressive laminetomy. A 5 percent incidence of wound infection can be expected, and occasionally complete wound dehiscence may occur in patients, particularly if significant debilitation has already taken place secondary to their primary disease. This is a compelling factor in attempting a medical approach to the treatment of metastatic carcinoma since the complications of surgery may often be avoided.

Contraindications to surgical decompression include the presence of physiological transection, i.e., the presence of no motor or sensory function below the level of the lesion, the presence of extensive visceral metastases, and a platelet count of less than 50,000.

Therapy

Adjunctive chemotherapy has beeen used in a limited fashion in the treatment of metastatic carcinoma to the spine. With the exception of prostatic carcinoma, lymphoma, mycloma, and small cell carcinoma of the lung, response to chemotherapy has been uniformly unfavorable. In patients with prostatic carcinoma, we have employed diethylstilbestrol initially as adjunctive therapy in patients receiving radiation therapy, but more recently for breakthrough following treatment with either surgical decompression or radiation therapy, or a combination of these two modalities. There were three patients who were ambulatory for more than 3 months following radiation therapy and surgical decompression who subsequently deteriorated and then were returned to ambulation with hormonal chemotherapy. In patients with small cell carcinoma of the lung, procarbazine has occasionally been effective in alleviating neurological deficit.

Treatment of Recurrent Symptoms

In general, recurrence of symptoms following adequate radiation therapy or surgical decompression of spinal cord metastasis is uncommon. In our experience, approximately 80 percent of the patients remain ambulatory until their death from systemic disease, with approximately 20 percent developing recurrent symptoms. In the great majority, this is secondary to recurrence at adjacent sites, but occasionally metastasis to another level of the spine may be responsible for the symptoms. Although this is not a common occurrence, it is one that merits consideration of further therapy with either radiation or, in those instances where radiation therapy proves to be ineffective, a second surgical decompression. This approach has been applied in 3 of 50 patients managed by the author and his colleagues over the past 5 years. In two patients a second operation yielded a satisfactory result, defined as ambulation for greater than 3 months following surgery. The considerations for deciding whether or not to treat a patient are the same as those used in making initial decisions about therapy at the time of first spinal metastasis; namely, the histology of the tumor, the severity of the neurological deficit, and in addition the general status of the patient. In rare instances, high doses of corticosteroids may be used to carry patients who have spinal metastases and who have had surgical decompression and radiation therapy for several weeks or months but who, for a variety of reasons, are not candidates for a second operation.

It should be emphasized that many patients with spinal metastasis return to their primary physician for follow-up, and that the primary physician caring for the patient, whether a family practitioner, urologist, or pulmonary disease physician, should have clear instructions from the neurosurgeon caring for the patient as to the status at the time of discharge and what symptoms to look for to determine whether recurrent or separate metastasis has occurred to the spine subsequently. Often this type of communication is lacking, and patients return with evidence of physiological cord transection which has developed over several days or weeks because neither the patient nor the primary physician had been educated to have a high index of suspicion of recurrent disease.

Current Areas of Research and Prospects for the Future

The use of adjuvant chemotherapy in the use of spinal cord metastasis is in its infancy. With the rare exception of prostatic carcinoma and also carcinoma of the lung, responses to adjuvant therapies including triple therapy for metastatic breast carcinoma have been unrewarding. Improved treatment of spinal metastases awaits better therapeutic strategies for systemic disease as a whole. In contradistinction to intracranial deposits, spinal cord metastases should be amenable to standard regimes since these metastases occupy the extradural space in most instances. However, it is a necessity in patients with such metastases that the oncolytic effect of the drug be rapid, because the spinal cord is relatively sensitive to compression ischemia, and just a few hours may make the critical difference between ambulation and a permanent bedridden status.

REFERENCES

1. Chason JL, et al: Metastatic carcinoma in the central nervous system and dorsal root ganglia: A prospective autopsy. *Cancer* 16:781, 1963.
2. Posner JB: Management of central nervous system metastases. *Semin Oncol* 4:81, 1977.
3. Ransohoff J: Surgical management of metastatic tumors. *Semin Oncol* 2:21, 1975.
4. Kramer S et al: Therapeutic trials in the management of metastatic brain tumors by different time/dose fraction schemes of radiation therapy. Modern Concepts in Brain Tumor Therapy: Laboratory and Clinical Investigations. *Natl Cancer Inst Monog* 46, 1977.
5. Hindo WA et al: Large dose increment irradiation in treatment of cerebral metastases. *Cancer* 26:138, 1970.
6. Renaudin J et al: Dose dependency of decadron in patients

with partially excised brain tumors. *J Neurosurg* 39:302, 1975.
7. Pouillart P et al: Treatment of malignant gliomas and brain metastases in adults with a combination of adriamycin, VM 26, and CCNU. *Cancer* 38:1909, 1976.
8. Bunn PA et al: Central nervous system metastasis in small cell bronchogenic carcinoma. *Semin Oncol* 5:314, 1978.
9. Olson ME et al: Infiltration of the leptomeninges by systemic cancer: Clinical and pathologic study. *Arch Neurol* 30:122, 1974.
10. Marshall LF, Langfitt TW: Combined therapy for metastatic extradural tumors of the spine. *Cancer* 40:2067, 1977.
11. Gilbert RW et al: Epidural spinal cord compression from metastatic tumor: Diagnosis and treatment. *Ann Neurol* 3:40, 1978.
12. Young RF et al: Treatment of spinal epidural metastases: Randomized prospective comparison of laminectomy and radiation therapy. *J Neurosurg* 53:741, 1980.
13. Tang SG et al: Prognostic factors in the management of metastatic epidural spinal canal compression. *J Neuro Oncol* 1:21, 1983.

PART TEN
MISCELLANEOUS ASPECTS

47

MANAGEMENT OF PAIN IN CANCER

Ronald J. Ignelzi   *J. Hampton Atkinson, Jr.*

Chronic pain associated with cancer is a major therapeutic challenge to nearly every physician at some time; however, until recently little concentrated attention has been directed to this most important national health problem. One of six patients is likely to develop cancer, and painful states will develop in 50 percent of these patients.[1] The incidence of pain in terminal cancer hospitals is 75 percent. In many clinic and hospital settings various modalities of treatment for malignant processes are attempted based upon available resources and the primary physician's experience and personal bias. Even in large cancer clinics there is some evidence that the medical, surgical, and radiation oncologists treating malignant pain have biases which may interfere with effective pain management: for example, the pharmacology of narcotic analgesics may not be known; analgesic dosages may not be individualized; and there may be a marked disagreement between the patient's assessment of the pain and the caretaker's appraisal of it. Today with the notable improvement in the treatment of the primary cancer, long-term survival statistics and even cures are being reported. At times, pain may be the only symptom of cancer preventing many patients from leading a relatively normal existence.

The purpose of this review is (1) to outline basic theory and mechanisms of pain and analgesia; (2) to discuss various therapeutic alternatives to cancer pain management; and (3) to suggest methods for rational evaluation and management.

BASIC MECHANISMS OF PAIN AND ANALGESIA

The word *pain* has its roots in the Greek word for "penalty." It is a negative concept connoting an adverse force affecting an individual and leading to a very disagreeable emotional response. Pain in its simplest definition is a sensory phenomenon which is evoked by stimuli which injure or threaten to injure tissue. Pain as an experience has its neurophysiologic correlate in the term *nociception*. This term implies that there are specific mechanisms associated with anatomic pathways poorly understood at present that respond to noxious stimulation. The mediation and modulation of these mechanisms occurs via neurochemical and neurotransmitter substances whose actions are only recently becoming understood.

This investigation was supported by Grant CA-18866 and by Contract RFP NO1-CN-85417-06 from the National Cancer Institute. It was supported by the Veterans Administration.

Pain often has a diffuse, nonspecific character which is in keeping with its antiquity among phylogenetic mechanisms. For example, its receptors are primitive, naked, free nerve endings. The majority of nerves thought to convey nociceptive information are small in diameter and without myelin, or are poorly myelinated, and therefore are less developed from an evolutionary standpoint than the larger, myelinated, faster-conducting fibers that subserve other modalities. There is a great deal of overlap in the body of dermatomes that subserve pain, suggesting an unsophisticated organizational structure. Furthermore, the poor localization of painful stimuli and the overlap by two or more nerve trunks in most body areas reflects an inefficient and poorly developed mechanism at both the peripheral and central levels.

Pain is an experience and therefore must be received, transmitted, decoded, integrated, and then responded to by the organism. When pain is unrelieved, it leads to an emotional response called *suffering* which over a period of time can lead to *pain behaviors*. Because of the difficulty of correlating complex anatomic, physiological, neurochemical, and psychological aspects of chronic pain, its control has been limited. In addition, most of the basic research on pain has been conducted in acute situations with animal models which do not translate well into chronic human conditions.

Historically, three basic theories have evolved to explain pain perception. The specificity theory of Müller in 1826 proposed that exciting a sensory pathway led to a specific sensation that was characteristic of the pathway and its central connection. This led to a search for specific pain receptors and nerve fibers for pain. Von Frey developed testing techniques for sensory systems and attempted to demonstrate specific anatomic structures in skin for the sensory modalities of pain, cold, warmth, and touch. Von Frey deduced that because pain was experienced following noxious stimulation of almost all areas of the body, free nerve endings were the specific receptors for pain since they were the only receptors so widely distributed. Concomitantly Goldscheider advanced the notion that cutaneous receptors were not specific but rather that stimulus intensity and central nervous system excitability were more important in determining the perceived sensation. His work, however, was largely neglected, and the idea of a specific energy requirement and a specific receptor for that energy held dominance for two centuries.

The second major theory, developed independently by Sinclair and Wollard, has come to be known as the pattern theory of pain perception. This theory denies the existence of specific receptors in the periphery. Instead it implies that when a stimulus is applied to the skin, it produces a nerve impulse pattern in a group of fibers rather than exciting a single fiber or a specific receptor. It is this spatiotemporal pattern in a group of fibers and its interpretation by the central nervous system that provides the basis for the perceived sensation. The pattern theory was influenced in large part by the work of Henry Head, who in 1920 proposed the protopathic and epicritic theory of pain perception based on careful observations he made by cutting a cutaneous nerve in his own forearm. Protopathic sensibility included (1) pain which was strong, nonlocalized, and radiating in nature, (2) sensation in the hairs, and (3) extremes of temperature. Epicritic sensation encompassed all other sensory modalities which require a discriminative ability to detect or distinguish more moderate stimuli. Head proposed that the protopathic pathway, including pain, ended in the thalamus while the epicritic system involved cortical activity.

The gate control hypothesis is the third major concept to be developed and is a more complex proposal which includes aspects of both older theories. The gate control hypothesis acknowledges that there are specific receptors and fibers for pain, but the input of this information is modulated by the numbers and types of fibers activated by different stimuli at the periphery and is dependent on the temporal dispersion with which the impulses reach the spinal cord dorsal horn. The gate theory will be discussed in detail later in this chapter when the dorsal horn is reviewed.

Receptors and Peripheral Nerve Fibers

Pain receptors are coiled, unencapsulated, unmyelinated, free nerve endings. Evidence suggests that substantial numbers of nociceptors exist both in animals and in human beings. Recent electrophysiological studies have shown that receptor units present in the periphery are uniquely responsive to high intensities of cutaneous mechanical deformation. Morphological differentiation of these free nerve ending types cannot yet be made; however, there appears to be a physiological differentiation of receptors: 20 percent innervate either hairy or glabrous skin and conduct centrally via small myelinated fibers at a rate of 5 to 10 m/s. Other receptors convey impulses along small unmyelinated fibers and appear to be of two types. The commonest, a high-threshold receptor, is activated by moderate to intense mechanical stimuli but is more readily activated by heat and irritant chemicals, indicating a broad or polymodal sensitivity. These polymodal elements are characterized by having a lowered threshold to thermal and other stimuli following noxious elevations of skin temperature. Prolonged or repeated noxious stimulation decreases the threshold of these receptors so that they are excited by normally innocuous stimuli, a property which may explain the phenomenon of *hyperalgesia*. It is also true that some terminal endings become less sensitive following injury. Clearly these do not signal the sequelae of injury or contribute to the pain produced at some time after injury. The second most common receptor responds only to intense mechanical stimuli. The discovery of nociceptive fibers is important but does not mean that these fibers convey no other stimuli or that they produce only pain when stimulated. It should be understood that high-frequency discharge in low-threshold fibers of wide dynamic range can play a role in conveying impulses arising from noxious stimuli. Evidence suggests, therefore, that specific receptors can respond to a variety of noxious stimuli but that the spatiotemporal sequence is also very important in determining the message conveyed to the central nervous system by peripheral fibers.

Gasser and Erlinger demonstrated 40 years ago with the oscilloscope the direct relationship between conduction velocity and fiber diameter. They divided the compound action potential into fiber size groups and labeled them A, B, and C. The A fibers were the myelinated nonsympathetic fibers by current convention. These A fibers were subdivided by Gasser and Erlinger into α (12 to 22 μm), β (8 to 14 μm), γ (5 to 10 μm), and δ (1 to 6 μm) fibers according to their diameter. Unmyelinated fibers were classified as C fibers. Another commonly used convention for classifying fibers is the one proposed by Lloyd. He divided the myelinated fibers into groups I, II, and III. The group I fibers have a cross-sectional diameter of 12 to 22 μm; group II fibers, 6 to 12 μm; and group III fibers, 1 to 6 μm. In Lloyd's classification, unmyelinated fibers are termed group IV. Lloyd's system included both afferent and efferent fibers, but modern convention generally reserves the Roman numerals for afferent fibers only, while the major efferent fiber groups are termed α motor, γ motor, B, or preganglionic sympathetic and postganglionic sympathetic fibers.

Present convention uses combinations of these different classifications to describe both size and function. In mixed peripheral nerves, fibers range in size from 1 to 22 μm. Sensory fibers of 2 μ or less are thought to be pain-conducting fibers. Since these fibers are unmyelinated, they conduct impulses very slowly, about 0.5 to 4 m/s. These small unmyelinated fibers constitute what is known as the C and some of the A-delta classification. Occasionally pain impulses may be transmitted over the larger B fibers at a slightly faster rate. The larger IA fibers conduct at rates 300 times faster than these smaller unmyelinated fibers and carry touch as well as proprioceptive information. It is important to remember that no fibers in the large myelinated group have been shown to respond to noxious stimuli.

Dorsal Root and Ganglion

At the beginning of the nineteenth century the important work of Bell and Magendie demonstrated that the ventral spinal roots were limited to efferent (motor) and the dorsal spinal roots to afferent (sensory) function. This led to therapeutic dorsal root section performed originally by Bennett and Abbe for pain relief. It was later shown that some afferent input to the spinal cord occurred through the ventral root, which may partially explain why pain is not always relieved by dorsal rhizotomy. The dorsal root ganglia contain the cell bodies of all sensory nerves, no matter what their size, peripheral distribution, or presumed function. Fibers which mediate pain leave the dorsal root ganglia and enter the spinal cord via the posterior root in the region of Lissauer's tract. Before entering Lissauer's tract, most myelinated and unmyelinated fibers bifurcate. The C fibers bifurcate before entering the dorsal horn, while large myelinated fibers bifurcate after reaching the dorsal columns.

Dorsal Horn of Spinal Cord

Rexed demonstrated that the cytoarchitecture of the dorsal horn of the spinal cord is a well-organized six-lamina structure. The dendritic arborization of the cells in lamina I is dispersed transversely along the dorsal surface of the spinal cord, whereas the dendritic arbors for the cells of laminas II and III are arrayed longitudinally in a tight band. The dendrites of cells in lamina IV are arranged in the form of a cone with the cell body at the apex. Cells of laminas V and VI spread their dendrites vertically in a slender longitudinal field. The architectural structure and interconnections of these laminas are quite complex.

In laminas II and III terminal fields of large, myelinated cutaneous primary afferents form a plexus of continuous sheets of axons which stretch a great distance along the long axis of the cord. Axonal systems originating elsewhere penetrate the bases and apices of these terminal axonal fields, making complex axonoaxonic synapses at each level. The apex of the axonal field is sheathed in a capping plexus derived largely from cells of the substantia gelantinosa of adjacent segments projecting via Lissauer's tract. The base of the axonal field is penetrated by a tract of fibers emerging from the ventral medial part of the dorsal column that is probably derived from the combination of propriospinal axons from laminas IV and V, and from primary afferent collaterals of dorsal roots. The importance of this is that branches of entering dorsal root fibers are influenced by primary afferents, and by propriospinal fibers from the ventral laminas and from rostral and caudal spinal segments, making a complex network of interaction. Furthermore, the dendritic arborization of cells in lamina IV and its inverted cone design suggests the possibility of marked convergence of primary afferent input.

Lamina I axons in the dorsal horn project to the ipsilateral posterolateral column. Lamina II cells have both a short intralaminar axonal system and a somewhat longer propriospinal system projecting in the tract of Lissauer. Lamina III fibers project to a propriospinal system in the ipsilateral dorsolateral fasciculus proprius and may also project to more ventral cellular laminas in the dorsal horn. It appears that cells in lamina IV project in the ipsilateral ascending dorsolateral columns and constitute a portion of the spinal cervical tract to which cells in laminas V and VI contribute. Furthermore, these layers may also contribute to propriospinal projections in the ventromedial portion of the dorsal columns and to commissural and spinothalamic pathways.

Electrophysiological studies demonstrate that lamina I cells fire spontaneously with a slow regular rhythm and respond to proprioceptive and to noxious stimuli except high temperature. Cells in lamina II have not as yet been studied well. Lamina III does not appear to demonstrate spontaneous activity. Single units of lamina III respond to light cutaneous stimuli with brief repetitive bursts. Lamina IV cells are spontaneously active in bursts and characteristically respond to stimulation of hair and of the cutaneous surface. This response does not change with increases in stimulus intensity. Lamina V cells show a decrease in cell responsiveness to stimulation of hair. These cells are spontaneously active in bursts. Increase in stimulus intensity produces a marked increase in the firing rate. Electrical stimulation yields convergence of small myelinated afferents from viscera, muscle, and skin onto cells in layer V. Lamina VI single units respond to proprioceptive stimuli and are essentially unresponsive to noxious stimuli.

In short, of the six laminas in the dorsal horn, only laminas I and V appear to handle information related to intense cutaneous stimuli. Only lamina V cells respond to visceral stimuli and project commissurally. Nitrous oxide facilitates the activity of single units in lamina I and markedly depresses the activity of single units in lamina V, suggesting different functions of their projection pathways.

The above information about the cytoarchitecture of the dorsal horn is important in understanding the gate hypothesis of pain modulation. This hypothesis was promulgated in 1965 by Melzack and Wall. In their original work, they emphasized presynaptic mechanisms of pain inhibition within the dorsal horn of the spinal cord. They observed that activation of large myelinated primary afferent fibers maintains dorsal root negativity while activation of small myelinated and unmyelinated fibers produces dorsal root positivity. They postulated that a continuously maintained afferent barrage from large primary afferents produced a maintained, presynaptically inhibiting dorsal root negativity upon all primary afferents which was decreased or eliminated by the action of small myelinated and unmyelinated primary afferents. The ultimate affect of these reciprocal mechanisms was exerted upon T, or *transmission*, cells in the substantia gelatinosa, the sum of whose activity was directly related to the pain experience. They emphasized that the T cells were affected in a reciprocal manner by the C and A-delta fibers as contrasted to the IA fibers.

The central feature of their hypothesis was that cells excited by injury of afferents could be inhibited by low-threshold afferents. Later it was shown by others that discharge of the lamina I cells, which were excited by noxious heating or by electrical stimulation of A-delta deep cutaneous afferents, was inhibited by electrical stimulation of large cutaneous myelinated afferents. An essential feature of the organization of lamina V cells is that they possess an inhibitory surround receptive field which is activated by the low-threshold afferents. Because of the excitatory nature of the receptive field, low-threshold afferents evoked excitation followed by a prolonged period of inhibition. Inherent in the theory is that the large-diameter fibers as well as the small-diameter fibers project to the substantia gelatinosa as well as to the central transmission T cells. The effect of the large-fiber input on the substantia gelatinosa leads to stimulation of cells in the region which then presynaptically inhibit the transmission of the small fibers to the T-cell synapse. The inhibitory effect exerted by the substantia gelatinosa and the afferent terminals is increased by activity in large fibers and decreased by activity in small fibers. Thus, increased activity in the large fibers "closes the gate," in electrical engineering terms, to transmission of the small fibers at the T cell, and conversely stimulation of the small fibers "opens the gate" by inhibiting the substantia gelatinosa and has a negative effect on T-cell transmission.

A simple clinical correlate may help for remembering these phenomena. If you stub your toe, the first percept is that of a sharp pain (A-delta modality) followed afterwards by a dull aching pain (C-fiber modality). You learn very early that by rubbing the painful toe (stimulating IA fibers), the pain is blocked or lessened. Although the gate theory has been questioned and other investigators have not been able to reproduce Melzack and Wall's experimental results, the importance of the Melzack-Wall gate hypothesis is that it has led clinically to various forms of electrical stimulation to block pain, and has opened a whole new avenue of pain control other than by destroying or interrupting pain pathways per se.

Spinothalamic Tract

Although the exact origin of fibers in the lateral spinothalamic tract in human beings has not been identified, it is assumed that they arise in the substantia gelatinosa as a second-order neuron in the nociceptive pathway. In cats the commissural fibers originate from cells in the lateral portion of Rexed lamina V. As is true of all spinal cord pathways, the second-order neuron crosses the nervous system before it relays centrally. After leaving the dorsal horn, nociceptive fibers cross the longitudinal axis of the spinal cord via the anterior commissure to the contralateral side and form a discrete bundle known as the lateral spinothalamic tract, located directly anterior to the dentate ligament. The decussation of pain fibers occurs over a rather broad area that may extend two to four segments above their point of entry into the spinal cord. Furthermore, some of these pain fibers may ascend or descend in the ipsilateral side of the cord in Lissauer's tract for several centimeters before decussating, allowing a large segmental overlap among themselves in Lissauer's tract. The lateral spinothalamic tract then ascends cephalad with fibers from each higher segment joining it in its ventral medial border so that, in the cervical region, the most posterior lateral fibers come from the sacral segments, while fibers arising from lumbar, thoracic, and cervical areas form successively more anterior and medial layers. Visceral pain is transmitted bilaterally by fibers located deep to the spinothalamic tracts close to the spinal cord gray. It is important to understand this topographical arrangement when one contemplates surgical approaches to destruction of the spinothalamic tract to alleviate specific types and areas of pain.

The spinothalamic tract is composed primarily of small myelinated fibers. Information on the spinothalamic system has been based almost solely on studies after hemisection or anterior spinal cordotomy. Generally speaking, many of these fibers project predominantly to the thalamus in the ventrobasilar complex, the posterior nuclear group, and the medial nuclei, including the intralaminar and some of the midline nuclei. Very few spinothalamic fibers reach the ventral posterior lateral (VPL) nucleus of the thalamus.

From both the physiological and anatomic standpoints, the spinothalamic system has two parts. The lateral component, known as the neospinothalamic tract, projects with a very specific somatotopic arrangement to the ventral posterior nuclear complex and also into the posterior nuclear complex with a less definite somatotopic representation. The other important component is the so-called paleospinothalamic system, which is more medial and projects to the intralaminar area of the thalamus along with the spinoreticulodiencephalic component, which projects into the reticular system at the medulla, pons, and mesencephalon. Eventually it terminates in the intralaminar nuclei of the thalamus, the ventral thalamus, and the hypothalamus. This pathway is particularly important since it projects large numbers of collaterals to the brainstem at all levels, giving the potential for much interaction, integration, and reflex activity. Its importance becomes even more apparent when it is understood that only one-third of all ascending fibers in the anterolateral system reach the thalamus, and only about one-half of these are represented in the lateral, or neospinothalamic, component. Furthermore, it has been shown that the ventral spinothalamic tract in monkeys is an independent entity with fibers distributed in the ventral funiculus, and that as these fibers ascend, they make connections with the brainstem and the thalamus which are analogous but not identical to the connections made by the lateral spinothalamic tract. The fact that the ventral spinothalamic tract projects to areas of the brainstem concerned with nociception lends credence to an anatomic basis for the relay of nociception by pathways outside of the classic lateral spinothalamic tract, and may account in part for the lack of prolonged control of pain after anterolateral cordotomy.

Tracts other than the classic spinothalamic may also be important in pain perception. The spinoreticular tract arises from cells located in the posterior horn, ascends in the anterolateral funiculus uncrossed, and terminates in the medulla, the nucleus reticularis gigantocellularis, and in the lateral reticular nucleus, thus providing another concomitant or alternative pathway for the central transmission of noxious stimuli. The spinocervical tract arises from cells located in the nucleus proprius (laminas III and IV) of the posterior horn. This tract ascends in the most dorsal part of the ipsilateral lateral funiculus to the lateral cervical nucleus located ventrolateral to the dorsal horn at C1 and C2. From this nucleus, the third order axons cross the midline in the upper cervical portion of the cord and ascend in the ventral funiculus. At the level of the medulla, they join the medial lemniscus and proceed to the VPL nucleus of the thalamus. There is anatomic evidence which suggests that the system may convey impulses of painful stimuli and may also be involved in integration of motor functions.

The ascending pathways of the lateral and ventral spinothalamic tracts send collaterals or direct fibers to the nuclei of the reticular formation at the level of the medulla oblongata. Although the lateral component (neospinothalamic tract) of the lateral spinothalamic tract runs directly from the spinal cord to the VPL nucleus of the thalamus, the medial component (medial spinoreticular component, or paleospinothalamic tract) is polysynaptic and distributes to the medullary reticular formation. It has been shown that cells of the reticular nucleus are responsive to noxious stimuli. In the medulla, the ventral spinothalamic tract is just lateral to the inferior olive, where it is intermingled with the lateral spinothalamic tract. A significant number of fibers from the ventral spinothalamic tract terminate in the nucleus gigantocellularis and nucleus paragigantocellularis dorsalis of the medullary reticular formation. The ventral spinothalamic tract separates from the lateral spinothalamic tract at the pontomedullary junction and passes around the medial aspect of the superior olivary complex.

As it passes rostral and lateral, it again comes in close proximity to the lateral spinothalamic tract at its termination in the thalamus.

In the mesencephalon, the ventral and lateral spinothalamic tracts project to specific nuclei in the periaqueductal central gray. The classical concept that in the thalamus the nuclei of the ventral basilar complex, the VPL nucleus and ventral posterior medial nucleus (VPM), are the sole nuclei involved in the sensation of body and facial pain is no longer accepted. It appears that the paleospinothalamic system projects to several thalamic nuclei including the centrum medianum (CN), centralis lateralis (CO), parafasicularis (Pf), the pars magnocellularis, and the medial geniculate body of the posterior complex (PO) of the thalamus. The termination of the more specific neospinothalamic tract appears less diffuse and is confined to the ventral posterior nuclear complex of the thalamus.

Thalamic Cortical Connections

The nuclei of the ventral basilar complex, VPL and VPM, project via the thalamocortical fibers to somatosensory areas SI and SII of the cerebral cortex. The VPL also projects to the orbital cortex. The pricking pain that is conveyed by the neospinothalamic tract relays from the thalamus to the somatosensory cerebral cortex providing somatopy. Burning pain appears to be subserved by the medial components of the system and projects through a more diffuse thalamocortical system with less direct cortical projection. Projections that go to the hypothalamus are subsequently relayed to the frontal lobes and are therefore very important in the affective automatic reactions connected with pain.

NEUROCHEMISTRY OF PAIN AND ANALGESIA

Peripheral Mechanisms

The biochemistry of sensing and transmitting noxious stimuli by peripheral pain receptors is complex. In addition to the classically described mechanoreceptors and thermoreceptors, current evidence suggests there is a polymodal nociceptor which responds to several different noxious stimuli, including mechanical distortion, heat, cold, and chemical irritants. Mammalian nociceptors differ from other somatic sense organs by their (1) high threshold to stimuli and (2) augmented response to repetitive stimuli rather than fatigue. It is apparent that hypersensitization of receptors cannot explain all instances of long-lasting pain of peripheral or central origin. It is possible that altered tissue states secondary to infiltrating tumor, inflammation, or degenerative changes allow normally innocuous stimuli to activate high-threshold pain receptors.

Redness, swelling, and pain are the hallmarks of inflammation. The clinical association of pain with inflammation has led to speculation that a common mechanism not only produces erythema and swelling but also causes pain by activating peripheral receptors. When tissue injury occurs, bradykinin, prostaglandins, histamine, and serotonin are released into tissue fluids—and may activate pain receptors. It is known that bradykinin deactivators, inhibitors of prostaglandin production (such as aspirin), and antihistamines desensitize receptors, and serial addition of these agents to in vitro preparations causes progressive decreases in receptor activity. Bradykinin, serotonin, histamine, and prostaglandin E cause skin and muscle mechano- and thermoreceptors to discharge. From this kind of evidence it has been postulated that a chemical "cascade," similar to the cascade in inflammatory responses, is involved in mediating the effects of noxious stimuli. Bradykinin, a nonapeptide that is formed in plasma and inflammatory exudates, causes skin and muscle receptors to fire and helps modulate vascular responses to inflammation. When injected intraarterially and intraperitoneally in human beings and animals, bradykinin peptides produce pain of relatively long duration. Animal work indicates that bradykinin leads to increased dorsal horn interneuron activity, perhaps by increasing peripheral C-fiber afferent discharge. After tissue injury, histamine is also released, predominantly from mast cells rather than from nerve endings, which lowers the threshold for afferent nociceptor firing. It is of interest that morphine itself releases histamine from mast cells, and that on intravenous injection both histamine and morphine produce hypotension, emesis, tachypnea, and salivation. Serotonin enhances the vascular and noxious effects of bradykinin and prostaglandin E, and potentiates the action of bradykinin and histamine to lower the threshold of sensory nerves. Although the evidence is incomplete, pain may be generated and modified in the periphery by the synergistic or antagonistic action of several agents.

Central Mechanisms

It has long been recognized that central nervous system (CNS) mechanisms can strikingly alter the perception of noxious stimuli. Emotions, behaviors, and psychopharmacologic agents alter pain states, but their CNS mechanisms were largely unknown until recently. Communication in the CNS occurs by chemical transmission of electrical impulses across synapses. The results of this transmission depend on whether the impulse inhibits or facilitates firing in the affected neuron as well as upon which synapses the transmitter substances act.

For the past 20 years the major emphasis in psychobiologic research has been to define the role of neurotransmitters, chemical messengers liberated by presynaptic neurons which bind to receptors on postsynaptic neurons and provide the chemical basis of thoughts, emotions, and behaviors. Several criteria must be met for a substance to qualify as a neurotransmitter: (1) The agent and specific mechanisms for its synthesis and metabolism must be present in neural tissue; (2) neuronal activity in the pathways where the agent is present must release it from nerve endings; (3) specific receptors for the agent must be available on postsynaptic membranes; and (4) specific antagonists of the agent must block synaptic action. Neurotransmitters are thought to be low-molecular-weight substances with a short half-life.[2]

Neuromodulators are larger molecules, such as peptides. They are thought to influence neuronal activity less directly than neurotransmitters and to have a longer half-life, lasting from seconds to days. Neuromodulators may exert their effects *presynaptically*, by modifying the synthesis, release, or activity of neurotransmitters, or *postsynaptically* by effects on receptors.

The brain contains localized concentrations of neurons which liberate specific neurotransmitters. Although at least 20 neurotransmitters have been discovered, two major transmitter systems, named for the type of chemical substance they synthesize and release, dominate current study: (1) the monoamine system [those neurons containing either serotonin, norepinephrine (NE), or dopamine (DA)]; and (2) the cholingeric system (neurons containing acetylcholine). These two major systems are prominent central regulators of mood, motivation, and pain. In the monoamine system serotonin is further classified as an *indoleamine*, and dopamine and norepinephrine are *catecholamines*. None of the group norepinephrine, dopamine, or acetylcholine sensitize peripheral nociceptors or cause them to discharge. Current evidence suggests that some depressive mood disorders may be classified as states of relative serotonin deficiency at the synapse (clinically, patients are anxious, agitated depressives) or of norepinephrine deficiency (patients are withdrawn and apathetic depressives). Therefore, antidepressant medications which increase serotonin at the synapse may be most effective in anxious depressions; those increasing norepinephrine seem to work best on the withdrawn depressions.

Neurotransmitter theory also offers some possible explanation for the affective and motivational accompaniments of pain. Patients with benign pain initially react anxiously to their discomfort ("How can I get relief?"). If pain persists for 3 to 6 months, a depressive mood commonly ensues ("It's hopeless, nothing can be done."). It may be that pain itself alters levels of neurotransmitters and secondarily produces changes in mood and activity. Pharmacologic and neurophysiologic studies imply that pain perception at least partly depends on the *levels* of brain neurotransmitters. A neuropharmacology of pain has developed, with most of the work being done in animal models or on chronic benign pain; the effects of malignancy or other systemic illness on neurotransmitter activity are largely unknown. Three general lines of research in pain modulation by neurotransmitters have been investigated: (1) the analgesic effects of treatments known to alter brain neurotransmitters; (2) the effects of manipulating levels of neurotransmitters on the actions of analgesics, like morphine; and (3) the ability of narcotic analgesics to alter the levels of brain neurotransmitters.

Although some of the findings are contradictory, it appears that increasing brain serotonin produces analgesia. The analgesic effects of changing brain serotonin levels are studied by inhibiting its synthesis with parachlorophenylalanine, a competitive blocker, or by restoring serotonin levels to normal by intracerebral infusions of its immediate precursor, 5-hydroxytryptamine. In rats inhibiting serotonin synthesis increases pain sensitivity, and intraperitoneal injections of 5-hydroxytryptamine restores serotonin levels and returns the pain threshold to normal. Finally, intracerebral infusion of 5-hydroxytryptamine in rats induces an antinociceptive effect. Serotonin may also play a role in the antinociceptive effects of morphine. Lowering the brain serotonin level by inhibiting its synthesis or by destroying serotonin neurons antagonizes morphine analgesia. Lesions in the rat midbrain which deplete forebrain serotonin antagonize morphine analgesia but not the effects of meperidine (Demerol), methadone, or propoxyphene (Darvon). Increasing brain serotonin potentiates morphine. In one preliminary study of human chronic benign pain, Sternbach found chlorimipramine, an investigational antidepressant which increases serotonin availability at the synapse, decreased patients' pain ratings significantly better than both placebo and amitryptilene (Elavil), an antidepressant which predominantly increases norepinephrine activity. Morphine itself increases brain serotonin turnover, but other analgesics like methadone and pentazocine (Talwin) do not. It appears, therefore, that all narcotic analgesics cannot be assumed to affect or work through identical neurochemical mechanisms. It appears that reducing brain or spinal cord serotonin neurotransmission causes either increased sensitivity or behavioral reactivity to noxious stimuli, and decreased analgesic drug potency. Increased serotonin neurotransmission produces analgesia and increased analgesic drug potency.

The role of serotonin in tolerance and in physical dependence on narcotic analgesics remains unclear. Some investigators report that tolerance and dependence cause no change in serotonin turnover rates. Others report that morphine-tolerant and morphine-dependent mice have increased serotonin synthesis, and that blocking serotonin production impedes the development of physical dependence and tolerance.

In the catecholamine subsystem, dopamine has received more attention than norepinephrine or epinephrine, and a growing body of evidence implicates dopamine in pain regulation. Administering L-dopa, a precursor of dopamine, apparently produces analgesia and elevates pain threshold in animals and human beings, perhaps by selectively increasing brain dopamine. In addition, a recent large cooperative study demonstrated that *d*-amphetamine, which releases dopamine, enhances morphine analgesia in postoperative patients. L-Dopa has been used to decrease bone pain from metastatic cancer of breast and prostate. Whether this analgesia occurs by suppressing hormone-dependent tumor growth or via direct effects on central neurotransmitters is unknown. Morphine, pentazocine, and methadone increase dopamine turnover, and pretreatment with narcotic antagonists like naloxone (Narcan) antagonizes this effect. Morphine and pentazocine produce dose-dependent increases in norepinephrine metabolites in the dorsal columns of rat spinal cord, and naloxone blocks this effect. It is possible that narcotic analgesics increase the activity of the postulated bulbospinal inhibitory system, which probably inhibits firing of dorsal horn neurons and transmission of afferent (pain) impulses.

Acetylcholine, the transmitter in the cholinergic system, is not as well-studied as other transmitters. Agents like physostigmine which increase acetylcholine activity at the synapse have analgesic properties in rats, and some of these effects can be attenuated by naloxone. Cholinergic agonists and cholinesterase inhibitors, which increase acetylcholine at the synapse, are analgesics on their own when given systemically or intraventricularly in animals.

The effects of acute and chronic morphine administration on neurotransmitter levels has been studied in many animal systems, and the literature is highly controversial as to whether morphine analgesia increases or decreases with changes in neurotransmitter levels. Some of the apparent discrepancies in the literature can be explained by experimental conditions, animal species, timing and amounts of analgesic doses, and mode of administration. It should be realized that a crucial balance between neurotransmitter activities may be more important than the level or action of any single neurotransmitter. Reserpine and other agents which deplete brain monoamines (serotonin, dopamine, and norepinephrine) antagonize the analgesic action of morphine. Monoamine oxidase inhibitors (MAOI's), agents which raise the level of all three of these biogenic amines by inhibiting their metabolism, enhance morphine analgesia. In rats intracerebral administration of serotonin both enhances morphine analgesia and reverses reserpine-induced antagonism.

Drugs which inhibit norepinephrine and dopamine synthesis may antagonize morphine's effects. The interactions of morphine analgesia and these catecholamines are far from clear, and investigational findings are contradictory. In some animals intraventricular injections of norepinephrine antagonize morphine analgesia; some investigations have found that destroying norepinephrine receptors potentiates morphine's effect. Similar contradictions occur with dopamine. Its intraventricular injection potentiates analgesia, while haloperidol (Haldol), a specific dopamine blocker, antagonizes morphine. Unfortunately, agents which specifically facilitate dopamine transmission (amantadine, Symmetrel) antagonize morphine. From clinical observations it was believed that phenothiazines like promethazine (Phenergan), known to be dopamine blockers, potentiate morphine and meperidine (Demerol) analgesia. More recent evidence suggests phenothiazines may enhance only the narcotic's sedative effects and that promethazine may be antianalgesic.

Morphine itself alters neurotransmitter kinetics. It accelerates total-brain serotonin turnover rates. Morphine increases the production of dopamine metabolites in the cerebrospinal fluid and speeds up the conversion of radiolabeled tyrosine into dopamine. Furthermore, morphine appears to affect the cholinergic system in two directions depending on the dose: initially, it elevates total brain acetylcholine; after large doses, morphine increases acetylcholine release from the brain. When serotonin-rich raphe nuclei are destroyed in rats, morphine neither produces analgesia nor raises brain acetylcholine levels. It is possible that morphine analgesia requires acetylcholine, that morphine and acetylcholine need serotonin to mediate their analgesic action, or that their analgesia depends on an interaction with the endorphins, the endogenous morphinelike peptides.

In summary, norepinephrine, dopamine, serotonin, and acetylcholine all seem to participate in mediating the acute effects of morphine. The site of analgesic action of neurotransmitters may be both at the spinal cord level and at higher centers. Serotonin probably has a prominent role in the development of tolerance and physical dependence, while norepinephrine, dopamine, and acetylcholine are less directly involved. In general morphine inhibits the release of neurotransmitters, perhaps by its ability to decrease intraneuronal calcium, an ion important in the release of neurotransmitters from storage vesicles.

Substance P and somatostatin are peptides, more commonly thought of as neuromodulators in pain perception rather than neurotransmitters. The opioid peptides, or endorphins, are a special class or agent, with more profound effects than those of conventional modulators. Substance P was first isolated from horse brain nearly 50 years ago by von Euler. Substance P is an undecapeptide localized in the substantia nigra, hypothalamus, and dorsal horns of the spinal cord, unmyelinated fibers and afferent pathways. Substance P excites neurons sensitive to nociceptive stimuli in spinal cord and brain and so may have a modulator function in pain pathways. Some of its effects have a slow onset and prolonged action which may be related to the often insidious and persistent quality of pain. Substance P abolishes the narcotic abstinence syndrome in morphine-dependent mice, and tranquilizes hyperaggressive mice.

Although its role remains undefined, development of artificial agonists or antagonists of substance P may herald major advances in understanding its actions.

Somatostatin is a tetradecapeptide which inhibits the output of growth hormone from the anterior pituitary. Its CNS distribution and ability to excite neurons in nociceptive pathways is similar to that of substance P, and it, too, may be a modulator for afferent neurons connecting to spinothalamic pathways.[2]

New Advances in Central Nervous System Mechanisms of Pain Modulation

For many years specificity, pattern, and spinal cord gate theories were of paramount interest, and little attention was given to brain mechanisms of pain modulation. When Reynolds observed that electrical stimulation of the mesencephalon in the central gray matter resulted in sufficient analgesia to perform a laparotomy in rats, a new era in pain theory and modulation began. Mayer, Akil, and Liebeskind demonstrated that electrical stimulation of the periaqueductal gray matter in the midbrains of rats abolished the animal's responsiveness to pain while preserving other sensibility to nonpainful stimuli. It is of considerable importance to realize that analgesia produced by electrical stimulation of the brain can be extremely potent. The magnitude of the effect varies with the intensity, frequency, and duration of the stimulation pulses but has been reported to eliminate totally any overt response to tissue-destructive pinch and pinprick. Extremely high doses of systemically administered morphine (50 mg/kg) can produce effects of comparable magnitude, but severe side effects such as catatonia, ataxia, sedation, and muscular rigidity are present at these doses. Furthermore, stimulation-produced analgesia is not a generalized effect since it often causes analgesia in a restricted anatomic area, while other areas still have an appropriate response to noxious stimuli. It has also been shown that the mechanism of this type of analgesia is not a generalized sensory, motivational, emotional, attentional, or motor effect.

The anatomic substrate for analgesia produced by electrical stimulation appears concentrated in medial brainstem structures extending from the medial diencephalon to the medullary raphe nuclei. Additional active sites have been reported in more rostral periaqueductal regions and sites adjacent to the third ventricle. Involvement of the periaqueductal-periventricular region in analgesia produced by electrical stimulation shows a striking correspondence with the sites now known to be involved in morphine analgesia. It has been shown that morphine injection into these other regions results in behavioral analgesia. In contrast, microinjection of specific narcotic antagonists into the periaqueductal-periventricular regions has been seen to reverse the analgesia produced by morphine microinjection into the same regions. It has been shown that the analgesia is opiate-specific, since inactive stereoisomers are not effective, and local anesthetic agents do not produce analgesia when microinjected into the same areas.

The periaqueductal gray matter has been shown to be high in opiate-binding sites. Neurochemical studies indicate that there is stereospecificity for binding of opiates in the mammalian central nervous system, and even though other areas of the brain have high affinities for opiates, morphine microinjection and electrical stimulation of these areas does not yield analgesia. It has been recently demonstrated that stimulation of the more caudal brain structures, such as the medullary raphe nuclei, results in potent analgesia in experimental animals. The important discovery of medial brainstem regions being involved in a potent pain inhibitory system that can be brought into action by electrical stimulation or the administration of narcotic drugs has obvious theoretical as well as practical therapeutic implications.

It appears that the electrical analgesia produced by stimulation of the medial brainstem is the result of direct activation of neurons. The ultimate result of medial brainstem stimulation is inhibition of transmission of nociceptive information at the level of the dorsal horn and in the trigeminal nucleus caudalis. Evidence has accumulated that a neural system originating in the nucleus raphe magnus in the medulla, descending in the dorsolateral funiculus of the spinal cord, and terminating in the dorsal horn is at least one inhibitory system that is activated by electrical stimulation of the periaqueductal-periventricular regions. Section of the dorsal lateral funiculus in rats blocks the pain inhibition produced by electrical stimulation of the periventricular-periaqueductal regions.

There is evidence to suggest that intracerebral morphine excites neurons in the periaqueductal-periventricular region and that systemic administration of morphine increases neuronal activity in the nucleus raphe magnus. Experiments analogous to those demonstrating that electrical stimulation in the periaqueductal-periventricular regions activates the descending inhibitory pathway have been performed with morphine, showing that morphine also produces its analgesic effect by stimulating this descending inhibitory system. Although there is considerable evidence that both electrical stimulation–produced analgesia and morphine rely on descending pathways to the spinal cord, more rostral sites of analgesic action have not been excluded, and some of these sites have been tested. For example, periaqueductal gray stimulation in the rat has been shown to suppress the nociceptive response of neurons in nucleus gigantocellularis of the medullary reticular formation.

Serotonin, dopamine, and norepinephrine may play important roles in the behavioral expression of analgesia produced by electrical stimulation. Depletion of serotonin has been shown to reduce and the addition of the precursor of serotonin to increase analgesia produced by electrical stimulation. As described above, the involvement of serotonin in morphine analgesia now also seems established. Increasing catecholamine levels with L-dopa potentiates electrical stimulation–produced analgesia. Dopamine and norepinephrine probably play antagonistic roles in the elaboration of such analgesia. Dopamine receptor blockade reduces the analgesia while stimulation of dopamine receptors potentiates it. In contrast selective depletion of norepinephrine potentiates the analgesia. It appears, therefore, that dopamine is necessary for the normal expression of electrical analgesia while norepinephrine reduces the activity of the system.

Evidence suggests that electrical stimulation analgesia and morphine utilize common neurochemical systems. Naloxone, a specific narcotic antagonist, has been shown to anatagonize electrical analgesia from periaqueductal structures in both laboratory animals and humans. It has also been shown that cross-tolerance between these two analgesic manipulations occurs. The most obvious explanation for the striking similarities between electrical stimulation analgesia and morphine analgesia would be that brain stimulation causes the release of a substance endogenous to the central nervous system with opiatelike activity. The extraction of such a substance was first reported by Hughes and has since been confirmed by several other laboratories. The substance has been extracted from the hypothalamus-pituitary region of guinea pig, rat, rabbit, and pig brain and has been termed *enkephalin* by Hughes. *Endorphin*, or endogenous morphinelike substance, refers to all opioid oligopeptides with biologic activity, of which the enkephalins are a member. Distribution of endorphin within the brain shows a good correspondence with opiate-binding sites, and sites where morphine and electrical stimulation exert their analgesic effect contain high concentrations of this substance. There are at least two enkephalins with biologic activity, both pentapeptides different from each other only by the presence of methionine or leucine in the fifth amino acid position. The endorphins are classified in α, β, and γ forms, according to their amino acid sequence. Both extracted and synthesized enkephalin are active in vitro, and synthesized endorphin produces analgesia in both laboratory animals and in human beings. In animals its analgesic activity is relatively short-lived compared to morphine, with a duration of between 5 and 10 min.

The existence of endorphin provides a potentially powerful tool to explain many of the observations of electrical-stimulation–produced analgesia. When injected directly into the brain of experimental animals, endorphin's analgesic activity is more than 48 times as potent on a molar basis than morphine. It appears to have no analgesic activity when given intravenously, presumably because it does not cross the blood-brain barrier well. Mayer, Akil, and Liebeskind demonstrated that electrical analgesia in the periaqueductal region in animals releases β-endorphin. Furthermore, Richardson demonstrated that during chronic brain stimulation for pain in humans, β-endorphin levels increased in cerebrospinal fluid. Hosobuchi has recently demonstrated that intraventricular injections of 200 μg of β-endorphin produced relief of chronic pain in patients often lasting more than 24 h. Foley has also demonstrated the efficacy and safety of intraventricular injection of β-endorphin in humans. Further discussion of the use of electrical stimulation–produced analgesia and the endorphins will be given in the section on neurosurgical alternatives later in this chapter.

In summary, a model of the endorphin–medial brainstem analgesic system has the following major characteristics: (1) the system's effectiveness can be reversed by naloxone or by manipulations which reduce serotonin levels; (2) analgesia persists for a considerable time beyond the period of application; (3) dopamine stimulates, and norepinephrine inhibits, the system; and (4) partial tolerance and tachyphylaxis develop in time. The importance of these exciting discoveries lies in the clinical application which is presently being intensively investigated and may in time alter our perspectives in pain management.

The possibility that other areas of the brain, aside from the medial brainstem, might modulate analgesia has been studied. Stimulation of the medial forebrain bundle and the lateral hypothalamic region in the rat causes analgesia. The analgesia does not outlast the period of stimulation, and stimulation does not inhibit spinal cord nociceptive reflexes, suggesting that the underlying mechanisms of analgesia differ from those in the periaqueductal-periventricular region. It may be that the analgesia resulting from stimulation of the medial forebrain bundle and hypothalamus is related to these areas being reward centers in the brain. There is some evidence to suggest that stimulation of this area can reduce pain in humans. Another region for which analgesic activity is claimed is in the septal region. Both in laboratory animals and in humans stimulation of the septal region has been reported to be effective in relieving pain.

Numerous manipulations have been developed to control pain that have been classified generally as *psychophysical*. Low-frequency electrical stimulation of peripheral nerves at their threshold appears to activate the endorphin system. Although controversy exists as to the clinical efficacy of acupuncture, recent experiments have shown that acupuncture analgesia in humans is reversed by naloxone.

The results of these studies indicate possible involvement of the endorphin system in acupuncture analgesia. In a similar test of hypnosis-induced analgesia in humans, naloxone had no antagonistic effect. This negative result might be due to the complex nature of hypnotic analgesia, which may depend on integrations at higher levels of the nervous system, or upon as yet unknown descending pathways.

SUMMARY

A summary of current knowledge about basic mechanisms of pain and its modulation is as follows: Pain arises from noxious stimuli in the periphery which generate energy in (1) specific and polymodal receptors and then is transmitted along (2) specific peripheral nerve fibers (A-delta and C) and under special circumstances other small fibers, which terminate in their cell bodies located in the (3) dorsal root ganglia and then enter the (4) substantia gelatinosa of the dorsal horn. Complex interactions occur within the substantia gelatinosa which is influenced by local as well as other peripheral nerve input while (5) central descending pathways modulate the information. This integrated information then passes via the (6) anterior commissure to the (7) lateral spinothalamic tract and other polysynaptic pathways which ascend to the (8) brainstem where the message is again modulated by other afferent information as well as ascending and descending pathways in the reticular formation. The brainstem is extremely important in modulating pain and through many nuclei, neurotransmitters, and neuromodulators can inhibit painful input. The third level of integration occurs within the (9) thalamus which appears to be the final conscious seat of pain. From here, (10) thalamocortical projections travel to the (11) cortex for final integration and perception. Neurotransmitters and neuromodulators act at many points along these pathways to either enhance or block impulse transmission. All of these complex factors may act to either stimulate or inhibit pain perception.

THERAPEUTIC ALTERNATIVES

The mechanisms that can lead to pain in cancer include (1) direct mechanical compression of tissue by tumor, (2) infiltration or compression of nerves, (3) obstruction of an organ or viscus leading to distension of pain-sensitive structures, (4) obstruction of vessels leading to ischemia, (5) distension of fascia, and (6) local factors such as the release of histamine or bradykinin which decrease the pain threshold or tolerance. For example cancers of the female genital tract, lower colon, and the rectum often involve the lumbar sacral plexus. The pain may or may not follow a dermatomal pattern. It can occasionally be confused with the pain produced by a herniated intervertebral disk. Pain in malignancy, however, more often is a dull, aching pain that remains constant and does not depend upon the patient's activity or position. It is frequently bilateral. Pain secondary to malignancy in the upper gastrointestinal tract is often vague and refers to the thoracolumbar region of the spine, whereas the pain produced by invasion of the brachial plexus by cancers of the breast or lung is often much more severe and involves the entire upper extremity and occasionally the chest. Constant, sharp, severe pain may be present when the tumor invades and compresses sensory components in the spinal epidural space due to metastasis or in the brachial plexus or even at the base of the skull or in the periosteum of the bone.

Primary and Symptomatic Control

Current methods of management of the pain in cancer may be classified as either primary or symptomatic control. Primary control is therapy directed at the existing disease, such as surgical resection of tumor, radiation therapy, and use of anticancer drugs. When this is not possible, symptomatic control should be sought; for instance, (1) analgesics and narcotics; (2) surgical ablative procedures including dorsal rhizotomy, cordotomy (percutaneous or open), medullary tractotomy, mesencephalic tractotomy, thalamotomy, frontal leukotomy, cingulonotomy, hypophysectomy, and peripheral and cranial neurotomies; (3) neuroaugmentive procedures, including transcutaneous electrical stimulation, or implantation of stimulators on peripheral nerve, dorsal column, or deep brain; (4) anesthetic methods including diagnostic and therapeutic blocks of trigger points, somatic nerves, autonomic nervous system, epidural blocks, or intrathecal blocks; (5) psychotherapy, psychotropic drugs, and hypnosis; and (6) psychophysical techniques including biofeedback, operative conditioning, and relaxation training.

THERAPY DIRECTED AT EXISTING DISEASE

The most satisfactory way of dealing with pain is to remove its cause. That is as true for the pain of neoplasm as it is for the tension headaches. Surgery, chemotherapy, or radiotherapy can often be used to palliate pain, even when the tumor cannot be totally excised. Even in people beyond hope of cure, antitumor treatment may give great pain relief and should be tried before resorting solely to symptomatic control.

Often the pain can be eliminated or at least alleviated by debulking of the tumor, either surgically or with radiation therapy or anticancer drugs. Particularly in diseases where the pain is due to direct compression of adjacent nerves, removal of the mass or reducing its size may be all that is needed to bring at least temporary relief.

MEDICAL ALTERNATIVES

Most people are familiar with the abuse of analgesics and their addictive qualities, but unfortunately few physicians are familiar with their proper use. Some physicians empathetically react to the patient's problem by giving large doses of narcotics early on in the disease without first thoroughly evaluating the complaint. Frequent calls to the doctor's office for more and more narcotics yield additional doses to "help" the patient in terminal disease. Use of narcotic analgesics without adequate diagnosis may only lead to the side effects of nausea, vomiting, mental obtundation, and constipation which obviate the humane goals of the patient's physician and confuse the clinical picture.

The clinical use of analgesic medication is usually passed on by tradition, surrounded by myth, and ruled so rigidly by habit that its premises are never examined. To successfully treat pain, the physician must be free of traditional biases and must understand the basic pharmacology of selected analgesics, the factors influencing their metabolism and distribution, combination drug regimens, equianalgesic doses of drugs administered by different routes, aspects of drug tolerance and dependence, and the use of nondrug treatments. It is the purpose of this section to present a logical approach to analgesic agents, and to review adjunctive analgesic therapies.

Just as in the surgical approach, the physician using analgesics to treat pain must meticulously evaluate the location and cause of the pain, the practicality and desirability of alternative analgesic methods, and the patient's mental and physical condition.

The ideal analgesic is, like the promise of tax relief, often proclaimed but not yet available. This medication would be potent, of duration long enough to allow a full night's sleep, nontoxic and without side effects, lacking addiction potential, and fully effective orally. The ideal analgesic not being available, some clinicians believe that morphine is the only drug choice in terminal cancer pain. Nevertheless, nonnarcotic analgesics can also be very effective. With all analgesics the following principles are important[4-6]:

1. Prevent pain. By far the most important principle in symptomatic control is to *prevent* pain rather than to treat it once it is full-blown. Prevention takes a lower total amount of analgesic than symptom reduction; it diminishes the patient's anxiety and gives confidence that the physician and the therapy can control the pain.

2. Erase pain memory by adequate doses. Analgesics must be given in large enough doses to produce relief. Successful treatment lessens anxious anticipation and the memory of pain. A larger total analgesic dose is often needed in the fearful patient. By far the most common error is to prescribe subtherapeutic amounts of drugs (especially of narcotics) too infrequently—beyond their duration of action. Physicians traditionally overestimate the relief their analgesics confer. In one survey Marks and Sachar,[7] for example, found that meperidine (Demerol) commonly was given in 50- to 75-mg doses spaced nearly 6 h apart, instead of the more analgesic regimen of 100 mg intramuscularly every 4 h, and that 75 percent of patients had inadequate relief. Too frequently no attention is given to response to previous doses when regimens are constructed.

3. Develop a plan. Treatment should proceed from weaker to stronger analgesics, yet no patient should wish for death because of a physician's reluctance to use narcotics. The level of pain intensity and disability should be estimated initially and a logical plan constructed for this degree of impairment.

4. Conduct a clinical trial. The physician should determine the average duration of pain relief produced by one chosen drug over several days of trial. Changing analgesics haphazardly or using several agents simultaneously can obscure the clinical picture. After one drug is chosen, it should be given a fair trial before substitutions or supplements are made. Age may be the most important factor in the degree of initial reported postoperative pain and the amount of relief produced by narcotics, regardless of body weight, height, and sex. Patients over age 55 have the greater relief and higher plasma levels after fixed narcotic doses than younger patients.

5. Consider a fixed schedule. Once the duration of relief is ascertained, the drug can be given at a *fixed* interval [not on pro re nata (prn) basis] just short of the predetermined period of relief. If properly done, this will help prevent pain. A common mistake is to give the analgesics on a prn basis. The difficulty of prn usage is that it leaves the medical judgment in the patient's hands, and by so doing may establish a pattern in which the patient experiences pain and is rewarded with a euphoriant drug. The waning of drug action may be interpreted as "pain" and lead to medication requests. Smaller doses given on an around-the-clock basis require less drug in the long run to relieve the pain, become part of the standard regimen, and thereby are not self-rewarding.

6. Maintain an alert sensorium. Individual regulation of dosage can often give relief without excessive sedation and without producing states of confusion. Some severely ill patients require deep sedation for comfort, but the physician who routinely oversedates cancer patients to ease their struggle with death should examine his or her motives. One may be treating one's own anxiety and not the patient's.

7. Preserve affect. Proper doses often can give relief without euphoria and allow the patient to interact with others as normally as possible.

8. Use oral routes whenever possible. Oral administration gives more even, sustained relief than the parenteral route, and is more convenient for patient and staff.

9. Use one analgesic at a time, and add potentiators or change analgesics only after a trial at adequate doses.

Early in the course of disease the most common cause of pain is surgery, and the management of postoperative pain in malignancy may be more complex than after routine surgery. Born in a setting of anxiety and uncertainty, in a person who is concerned about having cancer, postsurgical pain can be enormous. It is an error to think that some pain is good because it may "take the patient's mind off his problems." On the contrary, every twinge may symbolize the seriousness of the problem and the woe yet to come. Several factors mitigate against effective analgesia. Narcotics in adequate doses inhibit cough and bowel motility. The patient (or the surgeon) may have uninformed fears of drug addiction and may prematurely terminate treatment, thereby perpetuating discomfort. There are also surgeons who refuse to believe that any operation they have performed could be all *that* painful.

Several important studies indicate preoperative psychological support and education have an important effect in reducing postoperative pain and discomfort. Patients who are told to expect pain and that adequate analgesia is available do better than unprepared controls. The patient should be told to expect other discomforts, such as catheters, nasogastric tubes, intravenous lines, and the like. Instruction that it is normal to be confused when awakening from anesthesia, that movement or deep breathing will not reopen the incision, and that addiction to postoperative analgesics need not be feared is very reassuring.[8,9]

In the early stages tumor itself rarely causes pain. Extension or recurrence at the primary site after surgery or radiotherapy may hurt because growth occurs into scarred tissue. Metastasis to bone, nodes, or nerve may be painful, as may be infection or tumor hemorrhage.

Pain in intermediate- or later-stage cancer often signals a worsening in the overall clinical condition from diverse causes—cancer recurrence, local tumor invasion, or secondary complications. Pain at this time should prompt a thorough medical reevaluation. Although some authorities discourage the use of powerful analgesics in patients with a life expectancy of many months or a year, the patient's comfort should be the goal. Adequate amounts of effective analgesics can alleviate pain, and once the pain is stabilized, less potent agents can be used.

Most of the clinical experience in analgesia of late and terminal cancer originates from British hospices and palliative care units, where life expectancy is usually 3 months and where three-fourths of patients have pain as a major problem. Because cancer is so advanced, pain is only one of many symptoms. All symptoms which trouble the patient, not just pain, should be assessed and, if possible, treated, so that misery does not become a disease unto itself. Patients may complain about paresthesias as being "pain," and only careful evaluation will disclose the nature of the symptom. Correcting nausea, vomiting, and dyspnea may relieve discomfort which the patient also interprets as pain and will help develop rapport between patient and doctor and boost the morale of both: the doctor contributes and the patient improves. Once the patient is confident of the physician's interest and competence, pain is rarely overrated.

Palliative care settings generally emphasize independence and activity. Pain medications are given by schedule, so that no patient asks for relief. For the occasional patient who needs medication between the scheduled doses, a mild analgesic may suffice, or at night leaving some medication at the bedside can be a highly psychologically comforting maneuver. Preventing pain by giving scheduled doses allows patients to take the same dose of opiates for weeks or months, apparently without escalating dosages. The patient does depend on medicine for comfort, yet tolerance and addictive behaviors do not appear to develop.

The most difficult part of terminal care—for staff and patient—is mental pain. Few people can accept the fact that their body is letting them down. Patients may become angry or resentful of staff, believing all their troubles derive from treatment. It takes unusual patience and courage to try to understand the patient and to continue to give care.[10]

Nonnarcotic Analgesics

Nonnarcotic analgesics can relieve a good deal of mild to moderate pain. The most frequently used agents are acetylsalicylic acid (aspirin), and acetaminophen (Tylenol). The exact mechanisms of action of nonnarcotic analgesics remain unknown. Aspirin and acetaminophen may act at the periphery, perhaps by inhibiting the release of prostaglandins, thereby blocking prostaglandin-dependent sensitization of afferent nerve endings. Generally aspirin is the drug of first choice for relief of mild to moderate pain. It is versatile and can be combined with other drugs to give additive effects. In a superb double-blind crossover study of 57 ambulatory patients with pain from nonresectable cancer, aspirin 650 mg was equal or superior to oral codeine 65 mg and pentazocine (Talwin) 50 mg. Particularly interesting is that pentazocine produced gastrointestinal and disturbing central nervous system (CNS) side effects in equianalgesic doses. In pain not controlled by aspirin 650 mg, the addition of either codeine 65 mg, oxycodone (Percodan) 10 mg, or pentazocine 25 mg was better than aspirin alone. Single doses of these combinations had equal and quite tolerable side effects. Aspirin combined with phenacetin and caffeine (APC) confers no advantages over aspirin alone. It is possible that overuse of phenacetin combinations for extended periods can produce methemoglobinemia, renal papillary necrosis, and interstitial nephritis. The usual dose of aspirin is 0.3 to 0.6 g every 4 h. Doses of 0.6 to 1.0 g may provide better and more prolonged analgesia without increased side effects. For the cancer patient who does not obtain relief at these doses, it is better to use more potent drugs than to increase the dose.

Salicylates are absorbed in the stomach and small intestine, with onset of analgesia in 30 min and peak action appearing in 2 h. Blood salicylate levels do not correlate well with analgesic effectiveness. The rapidity of absorption depends on gastric emptying time, the rate of dissolutions of the tablet, the mucosal pH, and the amount of non-ionized (absorbable) drug present. Buffered aspirin preparations offer no advantages in analgesic onset, peak effect, or duration, but they may be less irritating to the stomach than regular aspirin. Enteric-coated aspirin, introduced to decrease gastric irritation, is said to have unpredictable rates of absorption and analgesic effect. Sustained-release aspirin, formulated to increase the duration of pain relief, offers no advantages over properly used plain aspirin.

Aspirin's hazards include gastrointestinal hemorrhage, platelet inhibition, and an allergic bronchospasm in susceptible individuals, which can be life-threatening.

Acetaminophen is an effective analgesic without anti-inflammatory action. There is no gastritis or platelet inhibition. In high doses or in patients with compromised hepatic function, it can be hepatotoxic. The usual dose is 0.3 to 1.0 g every 3 to 4 h. It is a good long-term agent if aspirin is contraindicated and is equipotent to aspirin except in conditions where pain is secondary to inflammation.[11]

Narcotic Analgesics

Narcotics is a term which describes the naturally occurring opium alkaloids and the semisynthetic and synthetic opioids which diminish pain, leave the patient conscious, and can produce physical dependence. Changing the parent structure modifies the analgesic, antitussive, and constipating properties of these agents. Their relative properties are summarized in Table 47-1.

Exactly how narcotics produce analgesia is unknown. Microinjection of morphine into primate brain suggests that narcotics block the affective-motivational components of pain by acting on the periventricular-periaqueductal gray region, with additional effects on the dorsal horn. Morphine is the standard by which one should judge all other narcotic analgesics.

MORPHINE

Morphine produces diverse effects on almost all organ systems, as do the other narcotic analgesics. Depending both on the patient's physiology and psychological and social setting, opiates may be sedative euphoriants, or may lead to apprehension, apathy, and mental confusion in therapeutic doses. Acutely they most often dissociate the patient from the searing emotional effects of pain.

Morphine produces respiratory depression by direct action on the brainstem respiratory center and on peripheral chemoreceptors: it decreases respiratory rate, tidal volume, and sensitivity to carbon dioxide tension (PCO_2). Slow, periodic, and irregular respiration ensues. In the severely ill, the additional carbon dioxide retention may produce coma. Administering oxygen to patients in opiate-induced coma may eliminate their hypoxic drive and produce apnea. For these compromised patients, controlled and assisted ventilation may be necessary. Opiate suppression of cough can acutely compromise this protective mechanism, and the cancerous, immunosuppressed patient may become a greater risk for pneumonia. This does not seem to be clinically important in the ambulatory or semiambulatory patient. Narcotics have central and peripheral effects on the gastrointestinal systems. Initial doses stimulate the chemoreceptor trigger zone and produce nausea and emesis. Continued doses suppress the vomiting center and less commonly produce emesis. Unfortunately, narcotics increase vestibular sensitivity, and ambulatory patients may have difficulty walking without dizziness. The invalid patient experiences less difficulty. These agents inhibit gastric, biliary, and pancreatic secretions and reduce gut motility. Increased smooth-muscle tone in the sphincter of Oddi and biliary tree may cause biliary colic and elevated serum amylase levels.

Increased smooth-muscle tone in the urinary tract may cause bladder spasm, urinary hesitancy, urgency, and retention, especially in those patients with prostatic hypertrophy or urethral stricture. Decreased urine out-

TABLE 47-1 Comparative Analgesic Activity and Side Effents

Drug	Equianalgesic dose IM, mg	Average adult dose, mg	Duration of action, h	Side effects			
				Emesis	Sedation	Respiratory depression	Constipation
Codeine	120	30–60	4–5	Low	Low	Low	Low
Hydromorphone (Dilaudid)	1	1–2	4	Low	Low	Moderate	Low
Meperidine (Demerol)	100	50–100	4	Low	Low	Moderate	Low
Methadone (Dolophine)	5–10	5–15	4–6	Low	Low	Moderate	Low
Morphine	10	10–15	4–6	Moderate	Moderate	Moderate	Moderate
Pentazocine (Talwin)	50	31	4	Moderate	Low	Low	Low

put may result from narcotic-stimulated ADH (antidiuretic hormone) secretion or by decreased renal plasma flow. Because of decreased urine output the patient with necrotic tumor or massive postsurgical metabolic demands may develop hyperuricemia.

Narcotics generally decrease heart rate and increase peripheral vasodilation by action on the CNS vasomotor center. The bedridden patient may be unaffected by this, but those who walk or have diminished blood volume may suffer syncope. Initial doses increase cardiac contractility, and larger doses decrease it.

Mild hyperglycemia may occur by narcotic stimulation of epinephrine release, and from narcotics' action on the paraventricular glucostat receptor sites near the foramen of Monroe. ACTH and gonadotropic hormones, as well as plasma and urinary 17OH-corticosteroids and 17-ketosteroids fall. The opiates and their derivatives are absorbed readily from the gastrointestinal tract and after intramuscular injection. With most narcotics the oral route is less potent but of longer duration than an injection. The onset of action is 15 to 30 min and the peak effect is at 1 h. The opiates and their derivates are detoxified in the liver by conjugation with glucuronic acid, and excreted by the kidneys.[4]

OTHER NARCOTICS

Codeine Codeine, a natural opium alkaloid, has been used for over 100 years to treat moderate to moderately severe pain. Orally, 15 mg of codeine is usually ineffective; 30 mg of codeine is roughly equivalent to 650 mg of aspirin, and a dose of 60 mg of codeine outperforms this dose of aspirin. When combined, aspirin and codeine have supraadditive analgesic effects. Because of codeine's wide range of usefulness (it may be given in doses up to 120 mg every 3 to 4 h), it is one of our single most useful analgesics. It has excellent oral efficacy, being about two-thirds as effective orally as parenterally, has limited abuse potential, and has antitussive and sedative effects. Like aspirin for mild pain and morphine for severe pain, it is a standard to which other analgesics for moderate pain must be compared.[12]

Propoxyphene Propoxyphene (Darvon) is less effective than codeine and aspirin for mild pain and may become toxic (nausea, emesis, vertigo) in doses necessary to control moderate to moderately severe pain. It is probably useful only for patients in mild to moderate pain who cannot tolerate aspirin, acetaminophen, or codeine. Some studies find it no better than placebo.

Pentazocine Hydrochloride Pentazocine hydrochloride (Talwin) is a synthetic analgesic and weak narcotic antagonist. It is effective for moderate pain, and its potency is about one-third that of morphine when given parenterally, and equal to codeine orally. Injection produces maximal analgesia in 30 to 60 min and lasts 2 to 3 h. Oral use produces a peak effect in 1 to 3 h, with longer duration than on intramuscular injection. The adverse reactions of pentazocine are similar to those of other strong analgesics. Nausea, emesis, and dizziness are frequent; constipation and urinary retention occur occasionally. Equianalgesic doses give respiratory depression of equal but shorter duration than with morphine; there is less sedation than with morphine or meperidine. Larger doses produce psychotomimetic effects, including visual hallucinations, depersonalization, and severe nightmares. Physical dependence and a mild abstinence syndrome occur after a daily dose of 200 to 400 mg for a month. Like other narcotic antagonists, pentazocine can precipitate an abstinence or withdrawal syndrome in patients dependent on narcotics. Its major disadvantages are its irritative effect at the site of injection, its short duration of action, and its unpredictable oral effectiveness due to poor absorption and complete metabolism. In most cases initial oral doses are at least 50 to 100 mg every 3 to 4 h, with a total daily dose not to exceed 360 mg.[12]

Meperidine Hydrochloride Meperidine hydrochloride (Demerol) is a synthetic phenylpeperidine derivative which resembles morphine in many of its actions. It is less effective than morphine in relieving severe pain. Its maximal analgesic effect occurs 30 to 50 min after intramuscular injection, and its duration of action is about 2 to 4 h. With some exceptions, its side effects are similar to morphine's. It produces less cough reflex depression and constipation than does morphine. It causes biliary tract and intestinal smooth-muscle contraction, and in equianalgesic doses the same degree of respiratory depression as does morphine. The adverse reaction of dizziness, nausea, and vomiting may be lower than with morphine. Convulsions have occurred with large doses, 150 mg or more intramuscularly. Oral doses of less than 100 to 200 mg are often ineffective.

The cautions and contraindications are similar to those for all narcotic analgesics. Since the drug is inactivated in the liver, its dose should be reduced in patients with hepatic insufficiency. In patients receiving sedative-hypnotic and antipsychotic drugs additive CNS depression occurs. The usual dose is 75 to 100 mg intramuscularly or subcutaneously ever 3 h. Oral meperidine is considerably less effective.[12]

Percodan Percodan, a mixture containing oxycodone hydrochloride (a synthetic codeine derivative), homatropine aspirin, phenacetin, and caffeine is useful in moderate to severe pain. Percodan 10 to 15 mg intramuscularly is equivalent to 10 mg morphine and 120 mg codeine. On oral use, its effects begin in 15 min, peak in 45 min, and last 3 to 5 h. The starting oral dose is 50 to 100 mg every 4 h. There are fewer side effects than with morphine. Nausea, emesis, dizziness, constipation, and mild respiratory and cardiac depression occur. It should be regarded as an effective morphinelike agent with equal liability to produce physical dependence.

Methadone Hydrochloride Methadone hydrochloride is a synthetic analgesic whose actions are similar to those of morphine. It is more potent on a milligram basis orally and subcutaneously than morphine. Methadone causes less gastrointestinal tract inhibition but more ventilatory depression than does morphine. It does not produce euphoria as do some other narcotics and so has limited abuse potential. Cautions and contraindications are the same as for morphine. Nausea, vomiting, dizziness, and dry mouth are common side effects. Physical dependence and a mild abstinence syndrome develop on 20 mg per day for 2 weeks. The usual dosage is 2.5 to 10 mg orally every 6 to 8 h, or more frequently for severe pain. Parenteral doses are often one-half the oral dosage. It is a very useful analgesic and deserves more widespread use.

Brompton's Mixture Brompton's mixture was developed by Saunders in the late 1950s and early 1960s and has wide use in British palliative care centers treating patients with terminal cancer. The original mixture contains morphine in varying amounts, from 2.5 to 120 mg, cocaine 10 mg, ethyl alcohol 2.5 mL, and 5 mL of flavoring syrup, brought to a total volume of 20 mL. Prochlorperazine (Compazine), a phenothiazine, 5 mg in 5 mL has been added as an antiemetic and narcotic potentiator. Chlorpromazine (Thorazine) 10 to 25 mg can be added instead to control more severe agitation. The mixture is given every 4 h around the clock, and most patients obtain relief on 5 to 20 mg morphine per dose. For excruciating pain, initial higher doses are used with tapering after 48 to 72 h. At high doses (90 to 120 mg) sedation may persist for 2 to 3 days. If pain has a regular periodicity with specific peaks, increased doses can be scheduled at this time of day as part of the routine. When matching dose to the individual patient, it is better to change only one major variable (either the morphine or the phenothiazine) at a time. Parenteral doses can be given at one-half oral requirements. In Saunders' and Twycross' experience, drug dependence and tolerance has not become a problem.[10] Changes in dosage requirements more often mean a change in the disease's activity, not tolerance. Patients have been maintained in invalid or ambulatory care for 2 to 12 months without dose escalation, a fact that may be surprising to physicians who believe that tolerance and demands for increasing doses invariably accompany the use of narcotics. Some units find oral morphine alone is just as effective as the Brompton mixture.

INTRAVENOUS NARCOTICS

Using narcotics intravenously has short-term advantages for patients resistant or incapable of utilizing other forms of analgesics. In eliminates problems with drug absorption, bioavailability, and latency, and it gives relief to patients who rapidly bind, excrete, metabolize, or otherwise inactivate narcotics. For such patients parenteral injection every 2 h is impractical, time-consuming, and less effective. By intravenous routes, only one-third of the usual intramuscular dose may be used. Meperidine 15 to 30 mg or morphine in 1- to 3-mg doses is given every 20 to 30 min. Some automatic dose dispensing machines have been devised, though they are said to be complicated to use.

Choice of Drug

No single drug is always—even almost always—the best one for every patient. The final arbiter must be the level of comfort balanced against the level of functioning of the patient. In choosing analgesics it is worth reviewing several points:

1. Among both nonnarcotic and narcotic drugs differences in side effects at equianalgesic doses are often insignificant. The notable exceptions to this are pentazocine, which with intramuscular doses of greater than

TABLE 47-2 Addiction Schedule: Estimated Daily Total Intake for 2 Weeks Necessary to Produce Mild Withdrawal Symptoms

Drug	Usual dose, mg	Daily total intake, mg
Codeine	30–60 (PO)	1000
Meperidine	50–100	400
Morphine	10–20	50–100
Methadone	5–10	20–40
Propoxyphene HCl	65–130 (PO)	800

60 mg may produce psychotic symptoms, and meperidine, which at doses greater than 150 mg intramuscularly may cause convulsions. Meperidine may interact with antineoplastic agents, procarbazine, or amphetamines to produce agitated delirium, seizure, or respiratory depression. With drugs of different classes side effects may be important. Morphinelike drugs in general give greater pain relief with fewer side effects than equianalgesic doses of phenothiazines or nonnarcotic analgesics alone.

2. When drugs are given orally, their time curve of action is flatter and more extended than with intramuscular administration. In this regard morphine and (oxymorphine have low oral potency; codeine, oxycodone, and methadone have high oral effect. Appropriate choice of dose and route can make the difference between effective and ineffective use.

3. Tolerance to the respiratory, sedative, and emetic effects develops at roughly the same rate as analgesic tolerance, so increasing doses carries little risk of increased toxicity unless the patient's overall condition changes dramatically.

4. Physical dependence appears at the same rate as does tolerance (see Table 47-2).[4]

Tolerance and Addiction

Tolerance, physical dependence, and addiction are the bane of almost every physician who prescribes psychoactive drugs—stimulants, sedatives, tranquilizers, and analgesics. Tolerance means that with chronic administration larger doses are required to produce effects that were apparent initially at lower doses. Tolerance can develop to stimulants, opiates, and sedatives—but there is no cross-tolerance between them. Physical dependence means that physiological signs appear after the narcotic is withdrawn (see Table 47-3). In formal terms addiction implies (1) tolerance, (2) physical dependence with physical signs of withdrawal upon abstinence, and (3) compulsive abuse. Only those people who have been on very high doses for extended periods of time will develop class IV symptoms. Most physically dependent patients develop a mild flulike syndrome (class I and II) with abstinence. Something other than the fear of withdrawal symptoms motivates the drug abuser. Compulsive abuse means an apparently senseless return to drugs after abstinence. It is important to realize that physical dependence does not necessarily lead to abuse, and that often those individuals who abuse analgesics are not physically dependent. For the cancer patient the physician's fear of causing dependence is not as germane as the goal of providing relief.

Tolerance and dependence develop and disappear in parallel for all psychoactive drugs. Inhibitors of protein synthesis block both phenomena. Mechanisms of tolerance are incompletely known, although the enkephalins (the opioid peptides), and alterations in cellular cyclic AMP (adenosine monophosphate) levels offer some explanations. Enkephalins may be involved by way of feedback loops. In the feedback loop model, giving opiate analgesics adds an "excess" to the system, and endogenous opioid synthesis and release is then decreased, or its degradation increased. With less endogenous opioid available, receptors would then appear "tolerant," and more exogenous opiates would be needed

Table 47-3 Time Course and Symptoms of Narcotic Withdrawal in Physically Dependent Patients

Withdrawal grade	Time after last dose (h)	Symptoms
0	4	Craving, anxiety
I	8	Yawning, lacrimation, rhinorrhea, perspiration
II	12	Above, plus mydriasis, piloerection, remor, myalgia, anorexia
III	18–24	Increased intensity of above symptoms plus insomnia, restlessness, nausea, increased systolic BP, pulse, respiration, fever
IV	24–36	Above, plus emesis, diarrhea, weight loss, leukocytosis, hyperglycemia

to occupy all receptor sites. Although enkephalin turnover cannot yet be measured to test this hypothesis, rats chronically given opiates have increased enkephalin-degrading enzyme activity.

Another possible mechanism comes from observations that in neuroblastoma glioma cells, opiates decrease cyclic AMP and inhibit cyclic AMP–forming enzymes, such as adenylate cyclase. In tolerant cells progressively higher levels of opiates are needed to reduce cyclic AMP levels to previous levels.

Withdrawal symptoms, the evidence of physiological addiction, may be mediated by noradrenergic neurons which have opiate receptors. Many such opiate receptors are concentrated in the locus ceruleus of the medulla. Opiates reduce overall locus ceruleus discharge, and withdrawal causes greatly increased adrenergic firing in this region. This is consistent with the clinical picture of adrenergic hyperactivity—sweating, flushing, tachycardia—in the abstinence syndrome. It appears that adrenergic antagonists, like the antihypertensive medicine clonidine slow locus ceruleus firing and inhibit withdrawal symptoms.

For patients physically dependent on narcotics and needing withdrawal or detoxification, the precedure is relatively straightforward. The patient and physician must agree on withdrawal, and the process must be explained to the patient. The signs of opiate abstinence usually begin 8 to 12 h after the last dose, with more severe symptoms developing over the next 48 to 72 h. Withdrawal symptoms from methadone dependence begin 30 to 48 h after the last dose and last for 2 to 4 weeks. The patient should be observed for physical signs of withdrawal, such as pupillary dilatation, lacrimation, piloerection, or elevated respiratory rate and heart rate. One can generally start by giving 10 mg methadone orally and checking the patient 2 h later. If the patient is symptomatic at this point, another 5 to 10 mg can be given, and the process can be repeated. Few patients require more than 40 mg total per day. Most patients can be stabilized on 10 to 20 mg per day, given once daily, or in a divided dose every 12 h. If the patient appears oversedated, the daily dose can be decreased by 5 or 10 mg. After the patient is stabilized for 2 days, the total daily dose can be decreased by 10 to 20 percent per day. If the patient is dependent on methadone, using more than 20 mg per day, the dose is decreased by 5 mg per day until 20 mg per day is reached. Then every 3 to 4 days the dose can be decreased by 5 mg.

Other Agents
PHENOTHIAZINES

For over 20 years phenothiazines have been used to treat cancer pain, both in acute postoperative states and for unresectable tumor. Phenothiazines block dopamine neurotransmission centrally (the dopaminergic system) and interrupt afferent unput. They may also reduce the affective and motivational response to pain by inhibiting the recticular activating system.

Unfortunately no randomized controlled trials using phenothiazines for cancer pain have been done. Advocates of phenothiazines claim they give a high percentage of success (50 percent), act rapidly, do not cause addiction, and have few unpleasant side effects. Dissenters state that phenothiazines are not real analgesics, that they ablate emotional reactions rather than pain itself, and that they work only by performing a chemical lobotomy. Uncontrolled clinical trials show that while phenothiazines do not eliminate pain, they may be useful against the *disability* and invalidism caused by pain. Spontaneous pain complaints appear to diminish, and activity improves. Those patients who are the most bedridden and have chronic pain respond better than more active patients in acute pain.

It must be remembered that phenothiazines are in most cases of pain best viewed as adjunctive medication. Far too often inadequate doses of narcotics are combined with phenothiazines in hope that potentiation will occur. Many authorities believe that phenothiazines potentiate only the sedative effects of narcotics and that some phenothiazines, like promethazine (Phenergan), are antianalgesic. Until more is known about the potentiating effects of phenothiazines, it is best to use them as adjuncts which increase the physician's flexibility in constructing individual analgesic regimens, diminish agitation, and combat nausea and vomiting. Useful drugs and their side effects are given below.

Chlorpromazine Hydrochloride Chlorpromazine hydrochloride (Thorazine) in 10- to 25-mg increments up to a total of 100 to 300 mg per day, orally, in divided doses or as a single one-time dose at bedtime is effective for severe agitation. Chlorpromazine is quite sedating, long-lasting, and can be given in once daily doses. Single large doses (200 to 300 mg) should be used with care in the elderly or debilitated, and then only after the dose has been gradually increased from very low levels. Side effects include oversedation, urinary retention, constipation, tachycardia, postural hypotension, dyskinesias, and dystonias.

Levomepromazine Levomepromazine (Levoprome) 15 to 900 mg per day orally has been used. This agent is most useful in calming agitated patients; ambulatory patients improved on an average of 300 mg/day, and invalid patients had more activity and fewer pain complaints on an average dose of 150 mg per day. The major side effect appears to be severe postural hypotension.

Haloperidol and Thiothixene Haloperidol (Haldol) and thiothixene (Navane) are nonsedating phenothiazines. They can reduce severe agitation without oversedation, and they may well potentiate the analgesic effects of narcotics. For these reasons they are probably the most useful phenothiazinelike adjuncts for cancer pain, and they are preferable to promethazine. The usual doses are 1 to 5 mg three times a day initially, with careful increases.

TRICYCLIC ANTIDEPRESSANTS

Like the phenothiazines, the structurally similar tricyclics have for 20 years been used against many varieties of pain. Their use alone in cancer pain is not well established, and there are no controlled studies. Tricyclics inhibit the reuptake into neurons of indoleamines and catecholamines (serotonin and norepinephrine) which have been released into the synaptic cleft, thus prolonging and enhancing their action. As discussed earlier, serotonin and norepinephrine may play important roles in depression and in pain transmission and inhibition, with serotonin being especially pain-inhibiting. Sternbach[13] has described the successful utilization of tricyclics in chronic benign pain patients with and without depressive symptoms. Some studies found tricyclics helped decrease pain complaints and activate withdrawn, depressed patients with cancer pain. In cases of depression in patients with malignant or chronic benign pain (such as low back pain), it takes 2 to 3 weeks after therapeutic serum levels are obtained before mood improves and pain complaints decrease. The patient should be informed it may take a week or more to achieve an adequate serum level, and then perhaps another 2 weeks for an effect. Common side effects are dry mouth, postural hypotension, blurred vision, urinary retention, and constipation. At relatively low doses, elderly or debilitated patients may develop an acute confusional state, an anticholinergic organic brain syndrome. Tricyclics should be used with caution in patients with heart disease: they increase heart rate, may cause conduction delays and heart block, and may depress myocardial contractility.

Imipramine hydrochloride (Tofranil) 25 to 250 mg orally per day may be used. In the elderly or debilitated, doses start at 25 mg daily for 3 days, then increase by 25 to 50 mg every 3 days. Most patients respond on 100 to 200 mg per day; again response may be delayed for 2 weeks after therapeutic serum levels are reached. Imipramine is a more "activating" agent than amitriptyline for patients who are withdrawn or hypoactive.

Amitriptyline hydrochloride (Elavil) 25 to 250 mg daily may be used, but in the medically ill most responses occur at less than 200 mg per day. The onset of action may be delayed for 2 weeks. It is best to increase doses slowly as described above. Additionally, amitriptyline and some other tricyclics (but not imipramine) appear to work best at a very specific serum level, which varies with the individual. Levels above or below this level may be ineffectual, and given a standard dose, one-third of individuals will have improper serum levels. Amitriptyline is sedating, and may be useful in patients with agitation.

Because the pharmacokinetics and clinical use of tricyclics can be problematic, it is good to have experienced psychiatric consultation available before the tricyclics are considered for use. These agents can be extremely effective, in patients both with and without obvious mood disorders. They are best reserved for the patient with established pain which has persisted for a month or more and who is unrelieved by analgesics. If these agents are discontinued, pain may return.

COMBINATIONS OF PHENOTHIAZINES AND TRICYCLICS

Taub and others have used a combination of a nonsedating phenothiazine and a tricyclic antidepressant to successfully treat "denervation dysesthesias" like painful diabetic neuropathy, postherpetic neuralgia, traumatic neuropathy, and central pain syndromes. The combination appears to be useful in persistent cancer pain of diverse origin. The Taub regimen combines fluphenazine (Prolixin hydrochloride) 1 mg three times daily and amitriptyline 75 mg at night. Relief usually appears within 1 week, and the degree of relief may continue to increase progressively for a month. Patients can be maintained indefinitely with this regimen. Keeping the total daily dose of Prolixin below 4 mg eliminates postural hypotension and oversedation, and troublesome dyskinesias are avoided. Elderly and very ill patients may need to start on lower doses of both drugs: prolixin at 0.5 to 1.0 mg per day, and amitriptyline 25 mg, with increments added every 2 or 3 days. A combination of haloperidol (Haldol) 1 to 3 mg per day and imipramine up to 100 mg per day in divided doses has also been used.

Psychotropic agents alone or in combination may have a useful role in treating cancer pain patients. More satisfactory controlled trials are needed, and the most responsive clinical syndromes must be defined.

MARIJUANA (CANNABIS SATIVA)

Tincture of hemp came to Western medicine in 1839, advertised as an effective analgesic. Time has not been kind to this view. Although early physicians recommended it for dysmenorrhea, migraine, and the pain of terminal illness, cannabis fell from favor as more potent and predictable drugs were produced. By the turn of this century aspirin and barbiturates were available, and the invention of the hypodermic syringe made injection of soluble opiates possible.

The synthesis of the active ingredient in cannabis, Δ^9-tetrahydrocannabinol (Δ^9-THC) has reawakened medical interest, but Δ-^{9}THC still does not appear to be a useful analgesic. In one study of postoperative pain doses of 10 mg of Δ^9-THC probably had little or no analgesic effect, and doses of 20 mg Δ^9-THC were comparable to 120 mg of codeine. At the 20-mg doses Δ^9-THC was highly sedating and produced adverse mental effects which prohibit its therapeutic use: dreamy withdrawal, feelings of unreality and loss of control, disconnected thinking, lapses in orientation, and recent memory deficits were reported.

Preliminary reports suggest Δ^9-THC may be a useful antiemetic and antinauseant in patients receiving cancer chemotherapy. Δ^9-THC does lower intraocular pressure in patients with glaucoma, and some work is testing its value as a bronchodilator in asthma. Synthetic cannabinoids with improved specific therapeutic activity and fewer undesirable side effects hold some promise for the future. As of now marijuana and Δ^9-THC are not useful agents for the treatment of cancer pain.

PSYCHOPHYSICAL TECHNIQUES AND PSYCHOTHERAPY

Acupuncture

Acupuncture for pain, so enthusiastically introduced into Western medicine almost a decade ago, is of controversial efficacy. Apparently, Chinese medicine traditionally has not held it in high regard for treating the pain of malignancy. Only a few experimental studies in benign pain attend to the role of placebo, hypnotic susceptibility, the type and location of pain, and the patient's psychological and social state as they influence acupuncture analgesia. No studies in malignant pain address these variables. Some authorities believe that the level of pain relief correlates best with the degree of the patient's willingness to report pain rather than true pain sensitivity, and that initially acupuncture may simply distract the patient as would any other counterirritant. In benign pain acupuncture rarely provides relief for over 72 h. Other investigators believe acupuncture stimulates the endorphin system, and that many types of pain may respond to needling. Much more careful work needs to be done to evaluate the usefulness of acupuncture.

Hypnosis

Surgeons coined the word *hypnosis*, ushered in its medical use in the last century, and have by and large lost interest in the technique during this century. Even though there are unfavorable reviews of its effectiveness, hypnosis should be considered a useful adjunct in treating cancer pain. Hypnosislike techniques probably began in India over 3000 years ago, and Egyptian tombs at Thebes depict hypnotists with their patients. Even Aesculapius and Hippocrates apparently knew and used induction techniques. Renaissance surgeons like Paracelsus believed that the body had "magnetic" properties which could induce anesthesia. Mesmer's unscientific theories and exaggerated claims simultaneously popularized and nearly totally discredited hypnosis; but by the 1840s James Esdaile, a British surgeon practicing in India, was using hypnosis for anesthesia in abdominal explorations. James Braid, a Manchester surgeon, devised the name hypnosis, broke away from Mesmer's theories, believed that hypnosis was a physiological state of the brain and spinal cord, and is known as the founder of scientific hypnotism. Since his studies interest in medical hypnosis has waxed and waned, but with a progressively more rational and scientific rigor.

The most important thing to know about hypnosis is that it is a property (or talent) of the patient, not a trance imposed by the hypnotist. If we interpret pain as composed of the sensory stimulus and a distressing emotional reaction, evidence suggests that in individuals with the ability to enter a hypnotic state of analgesia, it works by affecting voluntary and higher level responses to pain rather than involuntary or reflex responses. The hypnotic state may reduce the distress component (motivational-emotional component) leaving the sensory processes intact. An alternative explanation is that hypnosis produces an amnesia, so that pain is momentarily perceived then completely erased from consciousness so quickly that pain recognition does not occur. A formal theory of the neuroanatomical and psychophysiological mechanisms of hypnotic analgesia and hypnotic amnesia is unavailable, and most speculations are premature.

Hypnotic analgesia finds use in burns, dentistry, obstetrics, orthopedics, and in cancer. Its effectiveness depends almost entirely upon the patient's ability to suspend critical judgment and accept a suggestion. Even its adherents believe success in suppressing severe pain requires highly hypnotizable patients, who are a distinct minority, probably less than 25 percent. For patients moderately responsive to hypnosis (perhaps up to 50 percent of patients) it may be a useful supplement to chemical analgesics. Specific techniques include suggestions that (1) the patient displaces the pain to a more comfortable place—for example, to another body part not as threatening, as from the abdomen to the hand; (2) the patient substitutes the unpleasant sensation of pain for more pleasant tingling sensation, like an electric current; (3) the patient relaxes, or relives pleasant experiences through fantasy and thereby is distracted from pain. The therapist's skill involves helping the patient find the most useful technique from a vast list of possibilities.[8]

Autogenic Therapy

In the widest use of the term, autogenic therapy refers to psychophysiologically oriented treatment emphasizing deep muscle relaxation and biofeedback. In autogenic training patients learn to focus selectively on some body state or process such as muscular tension, breathing, or warmth. By focusing on achieving body states incompatible with anxiety and pain, one is said to achieve a certain degree of relief. *Biofeedback* is simply a process wherein monitoring devices electronically display a patient's involuntary biological processes (heart rate, muscle tension, blood pressure, or others), which can then be modified by conscious effort. Of pain states so far investigated, only muscle tension headaches respond to biofeedback. The same level of therapeutic mental and muscle relaxation can probably be achieved by simple relaxation exercises, without the use of electromyographic feedback.

Most studies involving autogenics or biofeedback are uncontrolled. Relaxation instruction may help allay pain or other discomfort. Patients must be able and motivated to concentrate on the task at hand, but probably need no elaborate devices to help this process.

Psychotherapy

Psychiatric consultants should enter early into the evaluation and treatment of cancer pain and be introduced as a regular member of the medical team. If this is done, patients seldom believe their sanity is being questioned.

Five psychiatric disorders can produce pain in cancer patients: depression, hysterical conversion disorder, psychotic states, organic brain syndromes including dementias, and hypochondriasis. Less pathological emotional difficulties can contribute to pain but alone be insufficient to cause it. For example, several weeks after surgery for cancer, as the patient begins to adjust to the full impact of the diagnosis, pain complaints may reappear. Pain at this point may be a combination of postsurgical trauma, anxiety, and the patient's desire to focus on pain rather than upon cancer. Good psychiatric consultation usually can be diagnostic.

In general one should not expect psychotherapy alone to eliminate pain. Adjunctive psychotropics, analgesics, and physical therapy are helpful. Psychotherapy should be directed at understanding the impact pain has on the patient's life, instilling appropriate hope, fortifying the patient's native coping skills, and helping the patient plan useful alternative coping strategies.

NEUROSURGICAL ALTERNATIVES

Neuroablative Procedures

The operative aspects of the control of pain in cancer have been limited largely by a paucity of information concerning exact anatomic and physiological correlates.

Despite this, the various procedures and their indications, which will be discussed in this section, have been developed by the observations of a few and the skill and ingenuity of many. By the time cancer patients are referred to a neurosurgeon, surgical extirpation of the lesion producing pain usually has been attempted on one or several occasions, and/or maximal doses of radiation therapy to various parts of the body have usually been given. Often this means that the patient's lesion is believed to be inoperable or to involve other organs by metastasis or by direct invasion, making a direct attack on the primary lesion no longer possible.

An excellent review has been published detailing the various operations and results.[14] However, these surgical interventions do not always alleviate the patient's complaints. The two major reasons for failure are (1) poor patient selection because the patients are already addicted to narcotics, severely depressed, or severely debilitated, or have developed ingrained pain behaviors because the suffering has gone on too long; or (2) the ablative procedure was inadequate because of variations in anatomy, alternate pain pathways which in time assumed the function of the ablated pathway, or the extent of the disease was not fully appreciated, as in bilateral pain states where one site seems to be the main complaint until after the procedure when the previously minimally involved site becomes as painful as the relieved site was. As with all ablative procedures the patient must trade the loss of the symptom of pain for the gained symptom of loss of sensation of one or more other sensory modalities. Furthermore when dysesthesias or other denervation syndromes may develop after ablation, the altered sensations may be more disturbing to the patient than the original complaints. Fortunately these postoperative dysesthesias occur in only 10 to 15 percent of patients undergoing ablative procedures.

On the other hand patients who are well motivated, in fairly good physical condition, and with life expectancies of less than 2 years in whom the extent of the pain is fully appreciated and the appropriate procedure chosen are some of the most grateful patients the neurosurgeon may treat. The efficacy of various neurosurgical ablative procedures is therefore well-established in the treatment alternatives available for alleviation of symptoms.

NEUROTOMY

The simplest of the neurosurgical ablative procedures for pain relief in cancer involves a neurotomy of either a cranial or peripheral nerve. In the peripheral nervous system this usually entails division of the entire nerve including its somatic, sensory, motor, and autonomic components. The procedure can be performed by section, avulsion, or by using radiofrequency coagulation of the nerve in question. Intercostal nerves lend themselves well to neurotomy for pain of cancer involving the chest wall. Temporary local anesthetic blocks may be performed first to determine the site as well as the extent of the neurotomies. When cancer involves the extremities, neurotomies are of limited usefulness since destruction of a mixed peripheral nerve produces a motor deficit. Even when pure sensory nerves can be divided in an extremity implicated in the pain, their section will produce complete anesthesia involving superficial, deep touch, position, and vibratory sensibilities. If the extent of these sensory neurotomies in an extremity is great, as with brachial or lumbar sacral plexus neurotomies, it is possible that a functioning motor extremity will become useless because of the lack of sensory input. Therefore, plexectomies or other combined extensive sensory nerve denervations of an extremity should not be performed if the extremity is otherwise normal.

Cranial nerve section can give excellent relief for pain from cancer of the face, tongue, nasal pharynx, nasal sinuses, larynx, tonsils, gingiva, parotid gland, and buccal mucosa. However, very often pain involves more than one cranial nerve, and therefore the possibility of multiple sections may have to be entertained. Since the distribution of the trigeminal nerve is fairly constant for the entire face to the vertex suture, peripheral sections or divisions of postganglionic portions of it may bring relief albeit total anesthesia of the involved area. However, in tumors involving the posterior portion of the head and neck and including the ear, very often multiple sections of the ninth, tenth, and eleventh nerves are necessary to achieve relief. Classically, these procedures are done openly, requiring general anesthesia.

With the advent of the radiofrequency lesion generator, partial destruction of the trigeminal nerve and even more recently of cranial nerves IX and XI can be performed percutaneously, which allows a more selective destruction of the pain fibers and possible sparing of other sensory modalities, and is less of a formidable undertaking for the patient.

SYMPATHECTOMY

Sympathectomy and splanchnicectomy can be very useful in the rare patients suffering from pain of purely visceral origin. It must be recalled that visceral trunks are really mixed nerves. The true sympathetic fibers are purely motor. The afferent fibers that conduct pain simply run with the sympathetic nerves rather than in somatic trunks. Sensory fibers in the posterior spinal roots reach the viscera via the sympathetic rami communicantes, paravertebral ganglia, and splanchnic plexus. The vagi contain pain-conducting fibers to the ear, oral pharynx, larynx, trachea, and larger bronchi, and none extend below the diaphragm. In the sacral rami, vesical pain is transmitted almost entirely by the inferior hypogastric plexus and rami from the second, third, and fourth sacral nerves. However, these cannot be cut without causing paralysis of micturition and loss of tone in the sphincter ani. Sensation from the prostate and uterine cervix follows a similar route. In disease of these structures, when the cancer has spread to infiltrate adjacent tissues and thereby involves the lumbar sacral plexus as well as the periosteum of bone, sympathetic denervation is useless. Sympathetic blocks properly done by the anesthesiologist will be very helpful in determining the potential for relief.

DORSAL RHIZOTOMY

In 1889, Abbe and Bennett were the first to attempt posterior rhizotomy for relief of pain in human beings. Forester popularized posterior rhizotomy and outlined dermatomal zones based upon various sections of the roots. Selective preganglionic section of the posterior roots results in destruction of the somatic sensory and visceral sensory fibers. Since posterior rhizotomy, like neurotomy and in contrast to cordotomy, eliminates all forms of sensation, its use is limited to certain areas. For example, total absence of tactile and postural sensation in the extremities leads to a serious loss of function. Muscular power, although intact, is completely uncoordinated. If the second sacral nerve is divided even unilaterally, hemianesthesia of the penis leads to impotence. Furthermore, sacrifice of the second and third sacral nerves is followed by loss of bladder and rectal control, and therefore should be reserved only for those patients who have colostomies and/or loss of bladder function before the contemplated ablative procedure.

Wide areas of the neck, thorax, and abdomen may be made anesthetic with extensive dorsal rhizotomies. However, the extensive sensory overlap that occurs between roots means that section of a single or even two roots may lead to no detectable anesthesia in the individual patient. Therefore, when planning a rhizotomy, one must perform root section at least two levels above and two levels below the distribution of pain as well as specific roots in the area of the pain. The classic neurosurgical approach is via a laminectomy which must be performed at each level that the root section is to be accomplished. Patients must be in fairly good physical condition to undergo the extensive laminectomy. When performing a rhizotomy, care must be taken not to injure important radicular arteries which accompany the root and provide a large part of the blood supply to the spinal cord, particularly in the thoracic and lumbar areas. Postoperative hematoma is a dreaded yet infrequent complication. Previous radiation may retard wound healing. The procedure is not useful in patients with diffuse visceral pain or generalized pain. A 70 percent success rate with a 7 percent mortality is considered acceptable in patients suffering pain from malignant tumor. In malignant disease of the neck and upper thorax, a 58 percent early success rate and a 12 percent late failure rate secondary to extension of the disease has been reported.

Recently the percutaneous surgical approach to the dorsal root and ganglion has been introduced with a radiofrequency lesion technique. It has the advantages of a rhizotomy without the disadvantages of an open procedure in debilitated patients who otherwise would not be considered for major procedures. The technique is relatively simple and definitely less invasive than open surgical rhizotomy. The procedure has the added advantage of being able to be carried out under local anesthesia. However, its success depends heavily upon the availability of good fluoroscopic x-ray monitoring for precise stereotaxic introduction of the probe into the intervertebral foramen. Careful observation of the response to electrical stimulation before the radiofrequency lesion and assessment of the sensory and motor functions during the entire period of the procedure are essential to avoid undesirable complications.

COMMISSURAL MYELOTOMY

Commissural or mediolongitudinal myelotomy was introduced for relief of pain by Armour in 1927. The rationale for the operation was that by cutting the anterior commissure of the spinal cord one would destroy pain fibers of the second-order neuron as they cross to the opposite side of the cord and assume their position in the contralateral spinothalamic tract. By so doing, pain relief can be achieved bilaterally or at the midline. Since it is a single procedure, it has an advantage over a bilateral section of the spinothalamic tracts when the pain is bilateral. Although the operation enjoyed popularity in Europe for years, it was only with the introduction of the operating microscope in the United States that it has become popular here. The operation requires general anesthesia, and a laminectomy is performed over several segments of the spinal cord. In this country it has been used mostly for intractable bilateral pain in the lower abdomen, pelvis, perineum, and lower extremities. Since the pain fibers cross the anterior commissure of the spinal cord at the level of, or up to three segments above, their point of entry into the cord, section of the anterior commissure must take place over several segments. In a series of 24 patients complete relief of pain occurred in 5 patients with carcinoma of the rectum and colon, while 1 obtained partial relief, and 1 obtained none. For cervical and uterine cancer, 3 patients obtained complete and 1 only partial relief. In the remaining 13 patients with bladder, breast, prostate, and lung cancer the results were not as good. In terms of relief related to the anatomic site of pain, the best results are obtained when the rectum, perineum, legs, and hips were involved.

A phenomenon reported by many yet not completely understood is the extremely variable sensory loss following commissural myelotomy. Although often chronic pain in the appropriate segmental areas is alleviated, there is often only a minimal loss of acute pain and temperature sensation. Relief of pain may be due to destruction of the two sensory systems (paleo- as well as neospinothalamic tracts) subserving nociception as discussed earlier in this chapter. It may be that the proposed slow-conducting mediodorsal system and the more rapidly conducting anterolateral system are both involved in the surgical lesion since the sectioning is approached through the posterior commissure and certainly temporary damage is done to the posterior and medial portions of the cord. Hitchcock developed a stereotactically placed small midline lesion in the anterior commissure at the cervical medullary junction and produced profound and extensive analgesia with the procedure.

It is felt that analgesia with the stereotactic technique is due to interruption of both direct and crossed pain pathways close to the gray matter of the spinal cord or due to interruption of fibers of the spinal cervical tract which decussate in the high cervical area. Anterior commissurotomy is often associated with disturbances of proprioception, at least initially. It does, however, avoid the frequent motor and bladder complications of bilateral cervical cordotomy.

SPINOTHALAMIC TRACTOTOMY (CORDOTOMY)

As one moves towards the brain, the next locus of pain-conducting fibers is the lateral spinothalamic tract. Of all the neuroablative procedures on pain pathways, anteriolateral cordotomy has proven the most effective procedure for the relief of pain in cancer. Its advantages over all the procedures discussed thus far is that it preserves the sensations of touch, pressure, position, and vibration while eliminating only pain and temperature appreciation. The procedure is particularly useful when pain is unilateral; however, it also can be useful for midline or bilateral pain when bilateral cordotomies are performed.

The procedure may be done either by the open technique, which requires general anesthesia and laminectomy, or by a closed percutaneous technique under local anesthesia. The open cordotomy may be performed at either the thoracic or cervical levels while the percutaneous cordotomy is performed at the C1 or C2 level. The topographic arrangement of the fibers in the spinothalamic tract is such that the more lateral or superficial fibers come from the lower extremities and the deeper, more medial fibers arise from the upper extremities. In general the majority of sacral and lumbar fibers lie most laterally and dorsally below the dentate ligament, whereas the thoracic and cervical fibers lie more medially and ventrally. A few of the pain-conducting axons from each region may lie far ventral to their usual position. As a result of this mixing of fibers of different areas, it is not possible to obtain segmental zones of equal analgesia without very extensive transection of the anterior quadrant. Also it must be remembered that the higher the level of analgesia desired, the deeper the section must be performed in the cord. In both the upper and lower cordotomy incisions, particularly when the sacral segment must be made analgesic, it is important that the incision is started exactly at the dentate level. In a report of four cases where sacral sparing occurred when the incision was not carried far enough posteriorly, the patients were reoperated and the incision carried 1 mm more posteriorly with resultant analgesia of the saddle area. The open procedures are performed most often in the upper thoracic area. The procedure is quite useful for both somatic and visceral pain and metastasis involving bone or abdominal viscera. It is also useful in pain alleviation when tumor involves neuroplexuses. Once the laminectomy is performed and the dura opened, the dentate ligament is identified, cut, and grasped so the cord may be rotated to put the anterior quadrant under direct visualization. Once this is done, the entire extent of the anterior quadrant is sectioned with a knife. If the procedure is to be bilateral, then the second section is done a few segments above the first.

Perese and Racasso have demonstrated the size of the upper dorsal cord varies from individual to individual. The distance between the anterior root and the anterior spinal artery varies from 2.0 to 3.5 mm at the T3 segment, which is the usual level of the incision. Since the technique usually performed involves a 90° rotation of the spinal cord, the entire extent of the cord incision can be seen. Experience has shown that an incision made 2 mm anterior to the anterior root does not result in damaging the anterior spinal artery, a major risk when extensive incision is performed. Rotating the cord allows direct visualization of the distance from the anterior root to the anterior spinal artery and is important when the distance is unusually small. Obvious care must be taken in rotating the cord to avoid damage to the corticospinal tract and the posterior columns.

When the pain involves areas above the umbilicus, dorsal cordotomy will probably not be effective. In such cases high cervical cordotomy as advocated by Schwartz must be performed to obtain relief. High cervical cordotomy usually is carried out after a laminectomy has been performed on the upper three cervical vertebrae. The procedure is usually combined with cutting of the second, third, and fourth posterior cervical roots bilaterally to minimize pain in the incision and also to raise the level of analgesia. French and others reported considerable variation in the location of the spinothalamic tract in the cervical region and reported incision at the C2 segment produced variable analgesia. Schwartz reported his results with his technique of cervical cordotomy in 120 cases with only short-term follow-up. In 45 survivors of the unilateral section he reported 69 percent success and success in 76 percent with bilateral section. However, there was an overall 8 percent mortality rate and a 20 percent mortality rate when the procedure was done bilaterally. Another author reported on the comparison of 80 cervical and 28 thoracic cordotomies in which there was satisfactory relief of pain in 78 percent in the cervical approach and 64 percent in the thoracic. In most hands the thoracic cordotomy is the safest and most effective for pain relief from the level of the umbilicus downward. However, when the pain is of higher origin the cervical cordotomy must be used.

It must also be remembered that not uncommonly the patient who suffers predominantly from unilateral pain will complain of pain predominantly on the opposite side after unilateral cordotomy. Once the dominant painful side has been rendered analgesic, the other side, which initially had much less pain, may begin to bother the patient as much as the now analgesic side did before the cordotomy. Therefore, one should consider bilateral thoracic cordotomy for patients who complain of pain on both sides of their body even if one side seems much more involved than the other.

When a high open cervical cordotomy is undertaken, reservations must be applied to this bilateral approach since bilateral high cervical cordotomy carries a 20 percent mortality with it. Most of these deaths occurred because of respiratory complications since high cervical cordotomy leads to segmental loss of respiratory reflexes and sleep-induced apnea. *Ondine's curse* is a term often applied to this sleep-induced apnea, which results from the loss of respiratory reflexes, making the patient unable to respond to hypoxic hypercarbia when asleep. When the patient is awake, voluntary control of respiration is usually enough to control ordinary needs. When asleep, the patient is not able to breathe adequately because of the inability to respond to progressive hypercarbia and progressive hypoxia. Therefore the patient may become apneic during sleep and succumb to hypoxia and cardiac arrest. This is particularly a problem in patients with carcinoma of the lung with decreased respiratory reserve following resection or pleural effusions.

Using a microsurgical technique and an anterior approach to the cervical cord through the disk space, Hardy obtained good results in 8 of 10 patients with only one transient complication. The advantages are that this is a lesser procedure for the patient to withstand and allows direct access to the anterior and medial quadrants of the cord. Some problems with spinal fluid leaks have been reported, however.

For debilitated patients the risks of open cordotomy are great. In these cases unilateral high cervical percutaneous cordotomy is an attractive alternative because it is done under local anesthesia, it is no more uncomfortable than a myelogram, and there is no prolonged convalescent period. Percutaneous techniques of cordotomy were developed by Mullen and Rosomoff using the lateral percutaneous approach to the high cervical C1 to C2 spinothalamic tract. Since the patient is awake during the procedure, verification of the electrode position for electrical stimulation prior to lesion making provides a more adequate, more controlled situation.

Once the exact location of the electrode is determined, radiofrequency thermocoagulation is made in increments, and the patient is tested to be sure that the level of analgesia desired is obtained. Since the patient is awake, motor function also can be monitored during the procedure to be sure that the nearby corticospinal motor tracts are not being involved in the lesion. Bilateral percutaneous cordotomy, however, does carry some risk of hypotension, urinary difficulty, and, if the levels are high, respiratory failure. In general patients, a Pa_{O_2} of 70 mmHg or higher assumes little risk. Careful monitoring of blood gases pre- and postoperatively will help to select and protect patients from this very disturbing complication. If bilateral percutaneous cervical cordotomy is entertained, usually the lesions are staged 2 to 3 weeks apart. Rates of success, reported in terms of analgesia are approximately 80 percent, and the failure rate is only 16 percent with this technique. The other serious complication that can develop is urinary incontinence, which occurs in 50 percent of the patients with bilateral cordotomy and in 21 percent after unilateral cordotomy. Urinary tract infection resulting from the incontinence can lead to serious problems in these debilitated patients. It is less frequent in percutaneous techniques and often temporary with either approach.

SPINOTHALAMIC TRACTOTOMY IN THE BRAINSTEM

Because of the variability and multiple sensory nerve overlaps pain relief in the head and upper body is one of the most difficult and challenging problems confronting a neurosurgeon. It is often necessary to perform very high sections of the spinothalamic tract and the descending tract of cranial nerve V to achieve pain relief. Dogliotti and Sjoquist first reported section of these tracts in the brainstem in 1938. Grant and Weinberger modified Sjoquist's original technique of incision into the medulla above the obex to a level 4 mm below the obex, thus avoiding damage to the restiform body. Grant reported that in nine cases of malignant pain, relief was obtained in five patients. It must be noted, however, that there is a very high morbidity and mortality associated with this procedure. Complications include paralysis of the vocal cords, ataxia of the ipsilateral arm and leg, and impairment of postural sensibilities in the ipsilateral limbs.

The operation should be done under local anesthesia with the patient in a sitting position. Exposure is on the side opposite the pain. Care must be used when exposing the area because of minute blood vessels lying near the medulla and also because one must avoid damaging the tenth nerve filaments, which would produce hoarseness.

Trigeminal tractotomy, or section of the descending trigeminal spinal tract, affords an additional procedure for pain in the face. The rationale for effective medullary trigeminal tractotomy is the following: The fibers that conduct pain and most of those that convey temperature for the trigeminal nerve enter the pons and turn caudally as the trigeminal spinal tract. These fibers terminate below the obex and are most accessible in the lower medulla near the surface where the tuberculum cinereum is located. The fibers are arranged in a segmental fashion, with the ophthalmic fibers lying ventrally, the mandibular fibers dorsomedially, and the maxillary fibers in a position between the two. Fibers for the cutaneous components of cranial nerves VII, IX, and X descend in a narrow bundle between the fasciculus cuneatus and the adjacent trigeminal spinal tract. When it is necessary to obtain pain relief in areas of the head and neck extending beyond the trigeminal distribution, one may perform an extension of the incision and obtain ablation of the seventh, ninth, and tenth nerves also. Once the medulla is exposed, the obex is identified, and the tractotomy incision is made about 5 mm below or still farther below if blood vessels are in the way. The incision is approximately 4 mm wide and is carried through the tuberculum cinereum to a depth of 4 mm. To be sure that the total projected area of pain is covered by the ablation, stimulation can be carried out if the patient is under local anesthesia. While still on the operating table the patient can also be tested for sensory loss after the initial lesion to determine if additional section is necessary. Following medullary trigeminal tractotomy, analgesia is obtained with only a slight retention of temperature sense within the distribution of the fifth nerve. Considerable tactile sense is retained since most tactile fibers after entering the pons move cephalad and are therefore spared.

Walker demonstrated that both the spinothalamic and the quintothalamic tracts converge in the mesencephalon deep to the brachium of the inferior colliculus where they are accessible. He also demonstrated that there is a somatopic arrangement of fibers, with pain fibers from the lower portion of the body lying dorsolaterally and those from the upper body, head, and neck lying ventromedially. He therefore devised an operation called *mesencephalic tractotomy*. A common complication of this procedure is a temporary contralateral homonymous hemianopia, probably because of the occipital lobe retraction. The greatest problem with the procedure, however, is the persistent dysesthesias which occur in the majority of cases. These dysesthesias often are worse than the original pain and have made mesencephalic tractotomy undesirable except in the most extreme cases.

In conclusion, spinothalamic tractotomy in the brainstem is an extremely difficult procedure technically which should be done under local anesthesia and carries serious morbidity. Mesencephalic tractotomies have been almost completely abandoned because of the central dysesthesias which develop, and the medullary tractotomies are reserved for severe, intractable pain in the upper chest, neck, or head that does not respond to simpler approaches, such as high cervical cordotomy or multiple cranial or cervical root sections. Often a thalamotomy or limited frontal lobotomy may be indicated when the pain cannot be controlled.

THALAMOTOMY

Clarke's elegant experiments form the basis of stereotaxic surgery. The development of stereotaxic surgery in humans has been intimately associated with the operative therapy of painful disease states. Refinement of techniques has made thalamotomy a technically feasible and operatively safe procedure. The first attempt to relieve pain with a subcortical lesion produced by a guided electrode was made by Spiegel and Wycis in 1947. Using the calcified pineal or the anterior and posterior commissure as intracerebral reference points, they destroyed the dorsal medial nucleus (DM) of the thalamus in addition to interrupting the spinothalamic tract in the midbrain in a patient with atypical facial pain. The patient remained free from pain during the postoperative observation of 17 years. Initially the thalamic targets were based on the experience that prefrontal lobotomy relieved the anxiety associated with pain, and therefore interruption of the thalamofrontal radiation by destroying the dorsal medial nucleus of the thalamus might produce analgesia. The results of the procedure were variable because of the multiple pathways present for the transmission of pain, especially in the reticular formation. Spiegel and Wycis therefore went on to modify the procedure to include not only the then proposed termination of the spinothalamic tract but the medially adjacent reticular formation dorsal to the red nucleus, and labeled their procedure *mesencephalotomy*.

Because of high early recurrence rates with only DM lesions, in other series other target areas in the thalamus were added including the nucleus ventralis posterialis (VPL), nucleus ventralis posterior medialis (VPM), posteromedialis, centromedian (CM), and scattered others in the intralaminary system. The main goal has been to define a correct target in which a lesion could act satisfactorily to produce alleviation of pain. First the targets where concentrated in the VPL, VPM, and intralaminar nuclei, including the CM and sometimes the DM. Currently it appears that lesions made in the reticulothalamic tract and intralaminar nuclear groups give optimum pain relief without sensory disturbances. A further modification has been introduced by Marc, in which chronically implanted electrodes are placed in the thalamus for as long as 9 months. In this way, graded lesions can be made over several months as become necessary to achieve continued pain relief. Satisfactory relief of pain through stereotaxic thalamotomy performed by experienced hands yields 70 to 100 percent relief initially. However, as time goes on pain often returns. The rate of recurrence has been reported to vary from 10 to 50 percent. Complications following thalamotomy are due to the loss of function of the destroyed nuclei themselves as well as to injury to cell groups in close proximity. The lesions are made quite close to vital sensory and motor tracts; therefore, paresthesias, dysesthesias, and hyperesthesias may follow destruction of the sensory nuclei that receive input from the medial lemniscus and spinothalamic tract. Weakness can also develop from involvement of the nearby internal capsule. Destruction of the anterior and dorsal medial nuclei can produce disorientation, confusion, and impairment of recent memory for 48 to 72 h. The mortality rate varies from 0 to 7 percent. Thalamotomy's place today appears to be in patients who are not helped by lesser procedures, whose life expectancy is relatively short, and who are debilitated to the point of not being able to withstand major forms of surgery.

CINGULUMOTOMY

The cingulate gyrus, located directly above the corpus callosum in humans, represents the junction for fibers from the cortex, thalamic nuclei, and probably portions of, or areas connected to, the limbic lobe. The limbic lobe is an ancient part of the brain concerned with expression and emotion. The cingulate area transmits impulses to the hippocampus, mamillary bodies, and anterior thalamic nuclei with projections back to the cingulate to complete the loop. It therefore forms an intricate part of the limbic system. Interruption bilaterally of these pathways may relieve suffering by modifying the patient's reaction to a painful situation. It often results in less intellectual impairment than a frontal lobotomy and less interruption of affective social response, and has been reported to be successful in patients who are addicted to narcotics. The lesion is made stereotaxically with a radiofrequency probe. The target area is 3 cm behind the anterior horn and 1 or 2 cm above the fornix of the lateral ventricle. Foltz and White performed 11 cingulumotomies on patients with cancer of the face, mouth, and neck and reported good to excellent results. The procedure seems particularly useful in cancer patients whose anxiety and affective component of pain seems to be a dominating influence in their suffering.

FRONTAL LOBOTOMY

Frontal lobotomy, introduced originally by Igaz Moniz in the 1930s for psychiatric disorders soon became recognized as useful for problems of intractable pain. With effects based on the interruption of the frontal thalamic projection fibers, it appears to offer relief of the patient's concern and suffering over the pain rather than relief from pain sensation. When the operation is done in its original form and bilaterally, there is often significant alteration in psychological function. This type of lesion is performed under direct vision or stereotaxically with coagulation, freezing, or injection of saline solution. Scarff reported good results with unilateral prefrontal lobotomy in 66 percent of 58 patients, fair results in 20 percent, and poor results in 14 percent. White found that a favorable effect rarely lasted longer than 6 months. This procedure, as well as the more invasive and psychologically more devastating bilateral lobotomy, should be reserved for those patients in whom other procedures have been unsuccessful, and whose life expectancy is short, or in whom profound emotional reactions, agitation, or depression are present.

GYRECTOMY

Linde, Kirsch, and Druckman reported resection of areas of the pre- and postcentral gyrus for facial pain with good response for at least 20 months. The procedure involves destruction of the principal sensory projection area in the cortex from the thalamus, that being the postcentral gyrus of the parietal lobe. Because of the rather extensive craniotomy and sophisticated equipment needed to perform the operation, its use in cancer patients appears to be limited, and it has not found wide acceptance.

HYPOPHYSECTOMY

This procedure has been successfully employed in patients suffering from pain associated with carcinoma of the breast or prostate metastatic to bone who have responded to prior endocrine manipulation. The removal of the pituitary gland appears to change the hormonal balance within the body and actually has an effect directly on the extension of cancer as well as the pain. The procedure can be performed either by subfrontal craniotomy or by the transphenoidal approach. Recently Tindell reported its usefulness in other types of cancer pain. Stereotaxic pituitary ablation has been done with the use of a cold-probe freezing radiofrequency electrocoagulation and isotope implants as well. Direct injection of alcohol into the sella turcica has also been recommended by some anesthesiologists. Although controversy exists around its many uses, in patients suffering from carcinoma of the breast and prostate with metastasis to bone who have previously responded to endocrine manipulations the results are quite dramatic, and have made hypophysectomy the procedure of choice.

Neuroaugmentive Procedures

Within the present decade emphasis has shifted from the classical neuroablative procedures for pain relief to the more physiological techniques of electrical stimulation of neural structures for inhibition of pain. As mentioned earlier, Melzack and Wall's gate theory of pain perception led to the development of many techniques of electrical stimulation for pain relief. The idea that pain perception involves a balance of opposing influences, including an inhibitory system, has led to the belief that inhibiting or augmenting these systems can produce pain relief and the clinical development of electrical analgesia.

Dorsal column stimulation is a direct outgrowth of the gate control theory of pain. It was proposed that if one stimulated the posterior column electrically, the large IA fibers would close the gate to incoming pain signals from C and Aδ fibers. Dorsal column stimulation was employed in several thousand patients with all sorts of pains. Initial results appeared quite promising, with reports of 80 percent of the patients describing pain relief. With time the percentage dropped significantly so that within a few years the success rate was reported only at 50 percent and then only in very selected series. To implant the electrodes required a major operation and often the formidable procedure of total laminectomy in the thoracic or cervical region for most patients. Shelly reported good results in 8 of 17 patients with metastatic carcinoma, and Neilsson reported such results in 10 of 16 patients who had cancer. The major complication in these patients was that a cerebral spinal fluid fistula developed through the tract of the implanted electrode to the subcutaneous receiver. The greatest problem with the procedure, however, was that high failure rates occurred in time. Other problems such as arachnoid scarring and neurological deficit developed in some patients. Because of these complications, the technique of percutaneous placement of one or two wire electrodes within the spinal epidural space was advanced to eliminate the necessity of an extensive laminectomy for electrode placement. Electrode wires are either unipolar or bipolar and are powered by an external pulse generator that is carried and controlled by the patient. Once the electrodes are placed percutaneously and a trial of stimulation reveals that the patient obtains relief, the hardware can be internalized with the subcutaneous receiver similar to the ones used for open dorsal column stimulation. Percutaneous epidural placement of the electrodes is a reasonable alternative since this is a minor surgical procedure even in patients debilitated with cancer. However, the use of dorsal column stimulation is being performed less and less because of the failure rate at long-term intervals.

TRANSCUTANEOUS NEUROSTIMULATION

Placement of electrodes over the skin does not require a surgical procedure and has proven an effective method of pain relief with virtually no risk to the patient. The method involves stimulation through the skin of superficial nerves serving painful areas. Electrodes that are placed on the skin are driven by an electrical pulse generator with voltage pulse width and pulse rate variables controlled by the patient depending upon need and response. The mechanism by which this technique works appears to be direct inhibition of the pain-conducting small, unmyelinated fibers peripherally. The technique has worked well in chronic benign pain problems and is finding wider application at present in cancer pain than it had previously. Since transcutaneous neurostimulation increases the blood supply to the area being stimulated, there is a theoretical—although not practical—danger of causing tumor spread.

DEEP BRAIN STIMULATION

One of the most exciting developments in recent years in understanding the modulation of pain has been the discovery of a brainstem system with a specific and apparently endogenous property of pain inhibition. The theory and proposed mechanisms have been discussed earlier in this chapter. Richardson, Adams, and Hosobuchi extended the concept of central electroanalgesia in humans by implanting electrodes in the region of the periaqueductal gray adjacent to the posterior third ventricle in a number of chronic pain patients—many with cancer—with good results. Concomitant with the above, investigators discovered opiate receptors in various areas of the brain, and isolated a peptide called β-endorphin which is capable of producing analgesia by binding to these sites. It has been further demonstrated that β-endorphin levels increased in cerebral spinal fluid during chronic brain stimulation for pain in humans.

The insertion of electrodes in the periventricular region in human beings is a major neurosurgical procedure requiring expertise in stereotaxic technique as well as expensive equipment.

INTRAVENTRICULAR INJECTION OF β-ENDORPHIN

Hosobuchi demonstrated that intraventricular injections of 200 μ β-endorphin in patients produces prolonged relief of chronic pain, often lasting for more than 24 h. Foley has recently demonstrated the efficacy and safety of intraventricular injection of β-endorphins in humans. It appears that the opiates may act through the endorphin system as well since the analgesic effect of opiates, electrical stimulation analgesia, and β-endorphin itself can be reversed immediately by nalaxone.

ANESTHETIC ALTERNATIVES

In general anesthetic methods for permanent pain relief due to cancer are reserved for those patients who have been found unsuitable for a surgical procedure. On the other hand, the use of conduction anesthesia techniques for diagnosis of the origin of many types of pain can be quite useful in the evaluation of the patient before considering surgical intervention. The types of procedures that can be performed include myofascial trigger point injections, somatic nerve blocks, autonomic plexus blocks, and epidural and intrathecal blocks. Brechner has published an excellent review on the subject.[15]

Myofascial pain frequently accompanies terminal malignancy although it is infrequently diagnosed and treated as such. The patient who has had extensive radical surgery, chemotherapy, and irradiation often becomes emaciated and weakened by a prolonged period in bed; and because of this and the secondary muscular imbalance that develops, myofascial pain is frequent. The cardinal sign of this type of pain is the demonstration of a localized trigger point, which refers pain along nondermatomal but reproducible patterned areas. For example, a trigger point in the trapezius muscle just on the superior medial border of the scapula usually refers pain around the chest, the nipple, and down the inner aspect of the ipsilateral arm. The pain is often misinterpreted as being due to metastasis to the rib or brachial plexus. Once the true identity of the pain is identified by its trigger point, it can be simply treated by injecting the point with 1 or 2 mL of a local anesthetic. If the diagnosis of myofascial pain is correct, pain relief will be achieved and will outlast the usual duration of the local anesthetic. If it returns, it can be treated again by another simple injection as often as necessary. These trigger point injections can be done by a physician at the patient's bedside with ease. The important point to remember is that the possibility of myofascial pain in the patient with malignancy is real and one of the most simply solved pain problems encountered in cancer.

Somatic nerve blocks are useful diagnostically to outline the dermatomal areas involved in pain. If the pain relief occurs after a local block, the patient may then be given the alternatives of definitive surgical or repeat local anesthetic blocks, or of injection of a neurolytic agent either intrathecally or at the appropriate intervertebral foramen for pain relief. Diagnostic block with local anesthetic also has the advantage of giving the patient the experience of anesthesia in the involved area on a temporary basis which permits a decision about whether the anesthesia is worth the analgesia. Analgesia can then be obtained by either a surgical or a neurolytic procedure. It must be remembered that somatic nerve blocks like narcotics often affect the motor as well as the sensory portions of the mixed nerve, and therefore their therapeutic usefulness is often limited when large areas in the limbs covering many dermatomes require pain relief.

Autonomic plexi can be involved in carcinoma and produce pain. The two most important are the stellate ganglion and the celiac plexus. The stellate ganglion is often involved in cancer of the lung or breast, as well as in some head and neck cancers. Celiac plexus involvement occurs particularly with carcinoma of the pancreas. After demonstration of pain relief by the injection of local anesthetics, either alcohol or phenol may be employed to effect a more permanent relief.

Epidural and intrathecal blocks are often useful diagnostically to demonstrate segmental involvement in somatic pain. If temporary relief is attained with local anesthetic, the intrathecal injection of phenol or alcohol into the appropriate dermatomal level may be employed when a surgical procedure is contraindicated.

Patient selection for an anesthetic attempt at pain relief is determined by several factors. First of all, if the diagnosis of the origin of pain is uncertain, diagnostic blocks are very important to delineate the most appropriate anatomic site for a surgical or chemical ablative procedure. Secondly, permanent neurolytic blocks are important alternatives when a more favorable surgical procedure cannot be performed for anatomic reasons or when the general physical condition of the patient is poor enough that the more major surgical approach would not be tolerated. Lastly, an important consideration is the availability of anesthetic and neurosurgical resources.

In deciding if a patient is a candidate for a chemical neurolysis it is important to demonstrate that injection of anesthetics in the appropriate areas relieves the pain. The most conventional way of doing this is by continuous epidural anesthesia. By this technique the dermatomal segments involved in the patient's pain can be demonstrated, a differential between somatic and visceral pain can often be made, the degree of comfort the patient will achieve can be predicted, and the patient can experience the side effects of complications of denervation of the involved neuropathway. Placement of a continuous epidural catheter is a simple procedure and injection of adequate quantities of local anesthetics such as bupivacaine, which produces anesthesia over a period of hours and can be repeated several times over 3 to 4 days, enables the patient to evaluate whether or not the permanent effects of neurolytic agents are tolerable.

One must appreciate, however, the pharmacology, the toxicity, and the low margin of safety of these drugs. In general, the systemic and local adverse reactions are similar for all types of local anesthetics. Systemic reactions occur because of high blood levels due to rapid absorption, overdosage, or accidental intravenous injection. The reactions may involve the cardiovascular and/or central nervous systems. Allergic or idiosyncratic reactions rarely occur. No regional anesthesia should be practiced unless the necessary equipment and drugs are available for cardiopulmonary resuscitation. Aside from the potential hazards mentioned above, specific considerations must be made for the individual patient. For example, if the patient is suffering from perineal pain, it may be a technically simple matter to relieve the pain by denervating the sacral dorsal root ganglia with intrathecal phenol or alcohol; however, this person will also lose bladder and rectal sphincter function, and so if the patient still enjoys an intact bladder and rectum, neurolysis would be contraindicated. If because of previous cancer surgery the patient has had a colostomy or no longer has bladder function, then a sacral neurolytic block might be a good choice for pain relief.

Somatic nerve block with epidural anesthesia also produces a sympathetic nerve block in the involved areas. There are advocates of what is called a *differential diagnostic spinal nerve block*, in which different concentrations of local anesthetic injected intrathecally are relied upon to block the more susceptible sympathetic fibers before blockade of somatic components occurs. In most hands it is not as reliable as an anatomic separation of the sympathetic and somatic systems, which can be achieved by an epidural block of both systems and a separate block on another day of the autonomic ganglia to determine its effect on pain relief in the individual patient. Epidural blocks are accomplished by entering the epidural space in either the lumbar, cervical, or upper or lower thoracic areas. Most commonly the needle is placed somewhere between the T3 and T9 levels and then a postblock area of hypalgesia is used to differentiate the dermatomes involved.

Epidural placement of the needle is accomplished with a 20- or 22-gauge, styletted, 3-in short beveled needle which is inserted into the intraspinous ligament in a manner similar to that employed for intrathecal nerve block. The stylus is removed, and a 2-mL syringe containing either air or liquid local anesthetic is firmly attached to the needle hub. The pressure upon the plunger of the syringe will be met with resistance as long as the needle lies in the muscle or ligaments about the spinal segment. As the needle is advanced slowly with firm pressure continuously applied to the plunger of the syringe, a sudden release of pressure and release of the air or liquid indicates entrance into the epidural space. The stream of air or liquid also has a tendency to create a space in the epidural area convenient for injection of the agent. After careful aspiration, approximately 2 mL of 1% lidocaine is injected as a test dose. If hypotension and other systemic side effects of spinal anesthesia do not appear, 2 mL of anesthetic for each dermatome to be anesthetized is injected. By injecting the anesthetic slowly and maintaining the patient in the lateral position or 30 min following the injection, the ensuing hypalgesia can be confined largely to the dependent side.

If after the diagnostic epidural anesthetic has been employed successfully, both the patient and the physician feel that a chemical neurolysis is indicated rather than a surgical procedure, the chemical neurolysis may be accomplished by the injection of 10% ammonium sulfate, 7% phenol in water, or absolute alcohol at the intravertebral foramen or along the course of the nerve. The use of such neurolytic procedures on a mixed motor and sensory nerve or at the root level should be limited to thoracic or abdominal segments to avoid the expected motor loss to a limb. The agents are exquisitely painful upon injection, so a small quantity of local anesthetic should be injected half an hour before the injection of 1 to 2 mL of the neurolytic agent. Aside from the disadvantage of anesthesia over the area in which the analgesia is obtained, the frequent occurrence of paresthesias and permanent dysesthesias following a neurolytic procedure is significant. It must also be stressed that the dural sheath extends around the nerve root as it leaves the intervertebral foramen. If by accident the needle pierces the sheath, neurolytic agents will be introduced intrathecally, and transverse myelitis may develop. It is extremely important, therefore, to do the procedure in a hospital environment with adequate x-ray facilities and a cooperative radiologist.

The sites of action of the two most commonly used neurolytic agents are different. Phenol in glycerol is markedly hyperbaric and will gravitate to the lowest portion of the spinal canal. In contrast, absolute alcohol is markedly hypobaric and will rise to the uppermost area of the spinal canal. Phenol in glycerol is most often employed to attack the dorsal ganglia which are located at the intervertebral foramen and sacral foramen from which the specific nerve roots emerge. To approach pain originating in the somatic segments T11 to L2 with phenol and glycerol, the patient is positioned with the involved side dependent and in such a posture that T11 to L2 will be the lowest part of the spinal convexity achieved by elevating the pelvis and the shoulders and allowing the remainder of the spinal column to sag. To involve the dorsal elements and hopefully spare the ventral and motor roots, the patient after being positioned is then rotated backwards 45°.

The volume of fluid to be injected varies with the site of the injection. The dural cuffs surrounding cervical roots as they emerge from the intravertebral foramen contain considerably greater volume than dural cuffs in lumbar and thoracic areas. Therefore, 1 to 2 ml of phenol and glycerol can be employed in cervical areas for treatment of pain resulting from invasion of the superior sulcus by carcinoma of the neck; however, in the lumbar area this volume must be reduced to only 0.5 to 1 mL. For the treatment of perineal pain, volumes as high as 2 to 3 mL of phenol and glycerol may be necessary. The action of phenol is associated with the latent period during which reversible local anesthesia develops. It is only at the end of the latent period that an irreversible change will occur. The latent period with phenol may be as long as 20 min, and therefore it is possible to reposition the patient if the initial feeling of warmth which accompanies the injection of phenol is at dermatomal levels other than those desired.

The use of absolute alcohol intrathecally differs in a variety of ways from the use of intrathecal phenol. One marked difference is the hypobaricity of alcohol compared to spinal fluid. The site of action of alcohol is different than that of phenol in that alcohol destroys the sensory or dorsal root as it emerges from the spinal cord. Remembering that the adult's spinal cord is considerably shorter than the adult spinal canal, so that the spinal cord often ends at L1 to L2 vertebral bodies, the placement of the needle must be considerably higher than the dermatomal involvement in the vertebral foramen for lumbar sacral involvement. However, the more one ascends rostrally, the shorter the distance between the dermatome level and the emergence of the dorsal root. In fact in the cervical region the root emerges from the cord at the approximate level of the intervertebral foramen from which it leaves the spinal canal. Injection of absolute alcohol produces paresthesias and discomfort much more severe than a comparable procedure done with phenol. The paresthesias and discomfort are referred along the dermatomes of the involved sensory root. By and large the action of alcohol in contrast to phenol upon the sensory root is instantaneous and not reversible. If the block is successful, the duration and neurolysis last from several weeks to 6 months. Alcohol in 0.5-mL quantities is injected at 2- to 5-min intervals at each site after the patient has been positioned via a 22-gauge spinal needle. The patient remains in place for 45 min following injection.

Neurolysis of various plexuses for pain associated with cancer is limited to injections of the celiac plexus for carcinoma of the pancreas, the stellate ganglion, and the lumbar sacral sympathetic plexuses for pain of causalgic nature or lymphedema. The celiac plexus lies on the celiac axis and aorta anterior to the T12 vertebral body. During laparotomy the surgical oncologist who finds that a tumor of the pancreas is inoperable can do the patient a great service by injecting the plexus itself, which is clearly visualized, with 50 mL of 50% alcohol in water. To perform the celiac plexus block percutaneously the patient is placed on one side, and a 6-gauge needle is advanced to the area of the anterior portion of the vertebral bodies, which must be confirmed by x-ray. If x-ray confirmation is not done, it is quite possible that the proximity of the aorta or the kidney may result in injections into these structures with disastrous results. It is even possible that the needle may be diverted into an intravertebral foramen and injection of a neurolytic agent here will create catastrophic destruction of the spinal cord neural roots. If 50% alcohol is used in the percutaneous injection, the patient must be heavily sedated or the injection must be preceded by 20 mL of 0.5% lidocaine. On the other hand, 7% phenol in water in volumes of 10 to 20 mL injection may be done with the patient conscious and without prior anesthetic. Because vascular dilatation occurs after the block, the patient may develop orthostatic hypotension, particularly if markedly dehydrated or if circulating blood volume is reduced. In order to avoid this complication, proper hydration or replacement of the circulatory volume may be indicated.

Not commonly appreciated is the fact that there are instances in which pain associated with malignancy may be transmitted by the sympathetics because of their connections with somatic nerve trunks. For example, after radical mastectomy an occasional patient may complain of burning dysesthesias at the mastectomy site as well as into the ipsilateral arm. If stellate ganglion block with local anesthesia relieves the pain, the condition may be treated with either a surgical preganglionic sympathectomy or, if the patient is too debilitated to undergo this procedure, the injection of 5 mL of 5% phenol directly into the stellate ganglion itself under x-ray control. Painful lymphedema of the arm following mastectomy or lymphedema of the leg associated with carcinoma of cervix may be treated by sympathetic blocks also.

Although pain relief by nerve blocks is not always complete and often lasts for only several weeks to several months, the combination of blocks along with analgesic drugs can make drug therapy that was often unsatisfactory quite successful in instances where analgesics alone are ineffective or undesirable or where surgical procedures are not indicated.

EVALUATION AND MANAGEMENT

Perhaps more than in any other illness we associate the words pain and suffering with cancer. For whatever reasons pain and suffering are linked with cancer both in the patient's and the physician's mind. While the physician has the task of evaluating and treating pain in cancer, it must be remembered that pain cannot be so readily separated from these diseases, and that the physician who too thoroughly separates pain from patient dooms proper evaluation and treatment. Although the statistical prevalence of pain symptoms in malignancy has been described, it is impossible to estimate the amount of suffering involved. No matter what the cause of pain, suffering is an intensely personal, subjective experience. Even patients who are completely relieved of pain and do not require analgesics may still complain vigorously of the other forms of suffering accompanying early or far-advanced cancer, such as weariness, wakefulness, nausea, stench, and stomatitis. Although pain in cancer is rarely precipitated or perpetuated by psychological forces alone, it is important to weigh the psychological forces in malignant pain both from the patient's and the physician's points of view.

Patient's Response to Pain

It is artificial but practical to describe pain as having two components, the organic and the reactive, or psychological. Most of our noninvasive treatments of pain address or manipulate the emotional component, the fears and anxieties which accompany pain. It appears that the degree of tissue damage does not correlate with the magnitude of the reactive response or the *experience* of pain; nor is there evidence that different personality types, e.g., introverts or extroverts, have different pain thresholds or pain tolerances.

It is also worth dividing pain into its acute and chronic forms, arbitrarily saying that chronic pain has been present for at least 3 to 6 months. The reactive component varies with time. Acute pain, like that after surgery, gunshot accident, or angina, leads to activation of the sympathetic and emotional systems. Acute pain causes a tachycardia, elevated systolic blood pressure, and anxiety. The patient generally wonders what is wrong, what he or she can expect, and when relief will come. Pain which persists for months and becomes chronic evokes different physiological and psychological responses. Heart rate and blood pressure return to baseline. A depressed mood replaces anxious concern. Patients begin to feel helpless, out of control, and unable to plan their lives. They feel unable to handle their pain and fear it will become intolerable, or ruin their job, marriage, or family life.

The patient with pain in the context of established cancer may react with an increased sense of vulnerability, helplessness, disappointment, anger, or depression. Alternatively, intensified complaints may mask underlying emotions, like the fear of cancer, as the patient focuses attention on an apparently more "manageable" problem, the pain. It seems clear that the degree of organic pathology offers few clues to the intensity of pain or the need for medication. Of overriding concern is the personal significance of the disease, its private and social setting.

Physician's Response to Pain

Like it or not physicians bring their own pain psychology—and biases—to the bedside. Hackett has termed this "pain and prejudice," commenting upon the doctor's difficulty in believing that the patient really is in pain. Some documentation of this common attitude even about cancer pain exists. Pilowsky's study of analgesic dispensing practices on a cancer ward revealed that (1) staff frequently withheld analgesics from patients who voiced their sense of illness and who complained loudest of pain; (2) anxious-appearing women were more likely than men to receive analgesics; and (3) the elderly rarely received potent analgesics. The fact that these patients had cancer did not counterbalance the staff's reluctance to give medication. The tendency was for physicians to disagree with the patients' assessment of their plight and discomfort. The common prejudices revealed by this study are worth examining because they may surface in treating the cancer patient with postoperative pain from a staging procedure or the chronically ill patient with far-advanced malignancy.

The most common prejudice is that only pain which has an organic basis can hurt. If no organic pathology appears, the patient is presumed to be lying or faking. The same stance obtains if the magnitude of organic pathology does not match the degree of expressed pain: then the patient is exaggerating. At this point a psychiatrist may be introduced to pursue that fruitless and unanswerable question: How much of the pain is functional and how much is organic? The hard fact remains that there is no satisfactory objective test of pain level and no normal curve of values describing how much one should hurt given specific conditions. In fact psychogenic pain, phantom limb pain, hysterical pain, and pain as a sign of depression all hurt and create suffering. As Wilder Penfield noted, "The patient who says he is in pain must be considered to be in pain until we have proof otherwise."

The second prejudice is that we judge all pain by the behaviors and emotions of acute pain. The physician looks for tears, writhing, and gritted teeth—visible signs of agony. This does not take into account the fact that people adapt to pain over time. When pain persists for weeks or more, most patients adjust to its burden, begin to look relatively untroubled, and carry on limited social interactions. The mood changes to one of quiet stoicism, determination, or disguised resignation. They may shrug off friends' inquiries about their discomfort and try to concentrate on other matters. The physician examining them may find it difficult to believe their relative serenity in the face of so much stated discomfort. The physician naturally doubts they hurt. In fact extensive psychological testing in patients with chronic pain complaints both with and without demonstrable organic pathology detects no emotional differences in their reaction.

The third prejudice, as discussed earlier, is that narcotics should be avoided at all costs, and that they carry with them the inevitable price of tolerance, ever-escalating doses, and addiction. More and more evidence is accumulating that cancer patients on narcotics can obtain pain relief for weeks, months, or years with slight changes in the amount of drug, and without addiction. Furthermore, the addiction–prone person can often be spotted early in treatment, and measures can be taken to correct this.

The fourth prejudice is the view that giving placebos allows one to distinguish real from imagined pain. The idea is that placebos will relieve functional pain but not real pain. Numerous studies in this country and others verify that about one-third of the population reacts to placebo. A positive placebo response is a normal aspect of personality. It is independent of psychopathology, and normals, neurotics, depressives, hysterics, and schizophrenics apparently are equally likely to react to placebo. If an individual is a positive placebo responder, pain will diminish, regardless of whether the cause is cancer, surgical wound, or severe depression. A placebo trial will not separate functional from organic pain. All it determines is whether the patient is a placebo responder. If the physician wishes to conduct a placebo trial it should be done with the patient's full knowledge and cooperation, just as if the patient were entering the trial of an investigational agent and were told that either an active or an inert substance would be administered. The physician should also be blind to the test, and it should be conducted for several days on the active and inactive agents in crossover fashion. To trick patients by slipping them placebos has no scientific merit and may have them feeling manipulated. At this point it is no easy task to regain a patient's rapport and trust.[16]

These prejudices are cited merely to emphasize that the physician's approach is critical for success in a patient with cancer pain. Under the best circumstances treating pain is taxing, and in cancer pain the patient and physician face predicaments apt to bring out the worst in both of them. Patients can easily detect attitudes of helplessness or of defensive apparent lack of concern on the physician's part, and recoil with increased feelings of futility, rejection, or fears of death. Physicians who intend to successfully manage these patients must have the ability to listen, discuss, and gain the patient's confidence. Avoiding the emotional underpinnings of treatment spells doom to the therapy. The goals essential to all cancer treatments include an effort to diminish the patient's feelings of helplessness and to improve functioning whenever possible.

Levels of anxiety, pain expectations, and other psychological variables interact with biologic factors to produce a pain experience. Melzack finds this experience consists of three dimensions: (1) the sensory-discriminative dimension; (2) the unpleasant affect and motivational drive that trigger the person to action; and (3) the evaluative or cognitive component, wherein the patient attaches meaning to the pain. Cancer pain must be understood, evaluated, and treated within this framework.

Measurements of Pain

On a busy oncology service the physician may require a practical and speedy method of evaluating pain and the effectiveness of various therapeutic interventions. In the past clinicians and investigators hesitated to rely upon verbal statements as indicators of what pain patients were feeling. Repeated research indicates, however, the usefulness of verbal reports and shows them often to be more consistent than more "objective" measures, such as galvanic skin responses, cardiovascular responses, or the like.

The most commonly useful subjective scales ask the patient to rate pain by verbal report by choosing a number on a scale corresponding to "average pain these days." Malzack asks patients to rate their "present" pain on a scale of 0 to 5 (0 = none, 1 = mild, 2 = discomforting, 3 = distressing, 4 = horrible, and 5 = excruciating, or "the worst pain I have ever had"). Other investigators ask patients to rate their pain on a 0 to 100 scale, where zero is no pain, and 100 is pain so severe the patient "would immediately go to an emergency room rather than endure it." This is designed to force the patient to make a realistic upper limit to pain, for the person who rates it as "beyond 100" is asked if he or she, in fact, went to an emergency room. There are no adjectives or descriptors attached to the intermediate numbers.

Visual analogue scales use the distance measured in centimeters from 0 to a mark made by the patient on a 20-cm line, the ends of which are marked 0 for "no pain" and 100 for "worst pain ever." Many authors favor visual analogues, believing they more sensitively indicate the patient's condition than verbal estimates.

Quantification of the effectiveness of various therapeutic alternatives can be made by averaging the numbers chosen on each hourly (or less frequent) rating basis. Pain relief from medication can similarly be quantified as follows: 0 = no relief, 1 = slight, 2 = moderate, 3 = a lot, and 4 = complete.

Besides rating pain intensity, it is important to evaluate pain disability. A useful global psychological and social performance scale is the Swiss Cooperative Group Performance scale. This can help the physician stage a patient's emotional and behavioral status just as the extent of disease might be staged. The Swiss scale is a six-point system, where at a score of 0 the patient can maintain normal activity; at 1 he or she can live at home with tolerable illness; at 2 there is disabling illness but the patient spends less than 50 percent of the day in bed; at 3 the patient is bedridden more than 50 percent of each day and is severely disabled; and at 5 the patient is dead.

In a method developed by Fordyce patients themselves keep a daily pain, mood, and activity diary, as in Fig. 47-1, to inform the physician of their performance and to keep track of their response to treatment. Often treatment may greatly relieve pain disability, or enable a patient to become active again, despite little change in pain intensity.

No one claims these instruments measure pain as accurately as one would like. Their value to clinicians exists only in so far as they provide markers or guideposts by which the patient's response to treatment can be followed. In most instances the simpler the measurement, the better it is for all. Once the doctor, staff, and patient launch treatment, it is easy enough for them to lose sight of their starting point and course. The usefulness of simple measures extends beyond intellectual curiosity. It also provides staff and patient with a common language for communication and with a focus on a common goal or measure of improvement, whether it be in terms of activity level, emotional comfort, or analgesia.

Pain Management Team

The cardinal principal of pain control in cancer is to individualize each patient's pain problem by (1) having an appreciation of the disease process, its extent, and probable course, (2) understanding the patient's particular reaction to it, and (3) weighing the risks versus the possible benefits of various therapeutic alternatives. Even in those patients with mild-to-moderate pain impairment in advanced cancer, complaints of discomfort are frequent and often associated with excessive fear. When pain is present, it frequently becomes progressively severe and ultimately develops into relentless suffering, which demoralizes the victim and disrupts almost every activity of life. Physiological and mental deterioration may rapidly ensue, or if the patient lives long enough, negative pain behaviors will be developed that must be dealt with to achieve relief. Cancer pain, therefore, deserves a systematic appraisal directed at relieving and conserving the patient's physical, mental and moral resources, and social usefulness as long as possible.

Selection of appropriate therapy demands wide application of expertise: the type and grade of neoplasm must be identified, the location and mechanisms of pain identified, the physical and mental condition of the

Date

Time	Pain rating	Mood rating	Type and time in activity	Medicine	Relief
12–1 a.m.					
1–2					
2–3					
3–4					
4–5					
5–6					
6–7					
7–8					
8–9					
9–10					
10–11					
11–12 noon					
12–1 p.m.					
1–2					
2–3					
3–4					
4–5					
5–6					
6–7					
7–8					
8–9					
9–10					
10–11					
midnight 11–12					
Totals					

Pain rating
0 = None
1 = Mild
2 = Discomforting
3 = Distressful
4 = Horrible
5 = Excruciating

Mood rating
0 = Very depressed
1, 2, 3, 4 = Normal mood before pain
5 = Very high/good

Activity
S = Sitting
R = Reclining
W = Active, walking, standing, working
P = Recreation, play; reading

Relief scale
0 = No relief
1, 2 = Mild relief
3, 4 = Moderate relief
5 = Complete relief

FIGURE 47-1 Daily diary for pain patient.

patient and family evaluated, the nursing and social needs of the individual attended to properly, and the usefulness and morbidity of the various methods of pain relief measured. A highly trained, coordinated team to perform evaluations, plan interventions, and assess their outcome is essential when addressing such complex problems.

Over 25 years ago Bonica described the necessity for a multidisciplinary approach to pain management.[17] This approach was slow to gain acceptance until recently when clinics for the treatment of chronic benign pain proliferated. By contrast few physicians use a sophisticated team approach specifically designed for cancer patients. From the experiences gained in treating benign pain it is clear that early diagnosis, prompt treatment, and proper management can limit prolonged disability and iatrogenic complications of chronic pain. Bonica's three principles of pain evaluation are as follows: (1) obtain a detailed pain history, (2) perform careful physical and laboratory examinations, and (3) take a social and psychological history. In a busy clinical setting one physician rarely has time for such comprehensive work. It is here that the concerted and coordinated activity of a pain management team (PMT) becomes necessary.

Our multidisciplinary team for cancer pain is organized and coordinated by a single responsible physician, or *patient manager*. In a group practice or institutional setting this can be the patient's primary physician (family practitioner, internist, or general surgeon) or an oncologist. Other core team members include a neurosurgeon, psychiatrist, psychologist, nurse, and social worker. Additional subspecialists such as anesthesiologists or psychiatrists are included as needed. The only requirements for participation are interest and expertise in pain problems and a willingness to cooperate in coordinated care.

The patient manager does the initial examination, estimates prognosis, has the patient seen by other core team members, and coordinates treatment. In addition this person looks for evidence that the pain complaint is a signal of recurrent disease or worsening of the general medical condition. The manager thus acts as liaison between patient, family, and subspecialist consultants.

The neurosurgeon obtains a detailed history of the circumstances incident to the onset of pain, its course and treatment to the present time, and its current characteristics: location, quality, intensity, duration, and accompanying symptoms such as weakness, paresthesias, autonomic dysfunction, muscle spasm, and local tenderness. A careful neurological examination is performed and correlated with the history.

The psychiatrist evaluates the patient's past and present psychological status, the way pain shapes the patient's daily life and mental attitude, and its impact on the patient's family. The patient is examined particularly for depression and evidence of analgesic toxicity or illness-induced organic brain syndromes, and coping strategies are identified. Psychotropic medications (antidepressants, antipsychotics, sedatives or minor tranquilizers), analgesic regimens, hypnosis, or psychotherapy are then recommended.

A psychologist is valuable for the psychological testing needed for diagnosis in treatment, administering pain questionnaires, and formulating behavioral regimens for pain control.

A social worker can be extremely useful in evaluating the impact of cancer and pain on the patient and the patient's family, and the social and economic consequences of the illness. In an outpatient or inpatient setting the social worker and patient manager together can evaluate the family's needs, and provide information, reassurance, empathy, and invaluable support. A family conference at the beginning and end of treatment is a particularly useful format both for obtaining and providing information vital to the patient's care and rehabilitation.

The pain clinic at the University of California at San Diego has a weekly conference to discuss each new patient and others undergoing treatment. All pain management team members, including the oncologist working with the patient, participate. The pain manager presents the history, previous and ongoing treatment, while the other PMT members add their findings. A vigorous discussion of alternative diagnostic or treatment strategies follows. The conference is a useful and efficient method for gathering and analyzing information and arriving at a coordinated treatment plan rather than for individual consultants to communicate by telephone, letter, or consultation note which is far less effective and more time consuming.

Special Units

Specialized nursing units (pain control units, or PCU) analogous to coronary care or intensive care units are recent and useful additions the resources for the treatment of cancer pain. The units may have physician directors, a staff and nurses, a medical social worker, and access to occupational therapists, physical therapists, dieticians, and volunteer services. Nurses trained in pain control are an essential part of a pain control unit, and without them pain management is doomed. They spend far more time with the patient than does the physician; they are an invaluable source of clinical observation and management. Classic nurses' training allots little time to understanding pain psychology and behaviors or to their measurement. Recently, some hospitals have investigated training seminars which cover a complete curriculum of the necessary information: pain psychology, environmental reinforcers and extinguishers in pain; placebos, analgesics and other medications; anatomy and physiology of pain; relaxation training; hypnosis; acupuncture. Nurses are trained to make accurate observations of pain behaviors, administer pain questionnaires, and assess relief by analgesics. Knowledge and training builds enthusiasm and morale which when mingled with dedication produces the *esprit* found in intensive care and coronary care unit nurses.[3] The staff's observations in this setting can be especially useful when combined with a pain management team.

Several hospitals have developed palliative care units to manage the pain and disability of terminal illness. They are the hospital alternative to the hospice: they emphasize family participation in the patient's care and focus on the quality of life sustained; they evaluate and treat only problematic symptoms. They provide follow-up of family needs after admission, and see bereaved families at intervals after the patient's death, say at 2 weeks, 1 month, and 1 year. Some offer home service to terminal patients by way of visiting nurse practitioners.

In these units, too, the value of trained and sensitive nursing staff is immeasurable.

Practical Management Guidelines

Isolated methods of pain management in cancer are limited in scope and efficacy; however, various combinations of treatment modalities within the milieu of a multidisciplinary team approach as outlined above will benefit both the patient and the oncologist. We have found that a useful approach is to determine the degree of pain impairment in an individual patient by using a pain impairment scale. Table 47-4 is an illustration of the three variables that we use to construct the scale and therefore arrive at a score. The life expectancy for each individual patient is given to us by the oncologist. It is a very general estimate, broken down into the categories greater than 5 years, greater than 1 year but less than 5, greater than 6 months but not greater than 1 year, and less than 6 months. These four categories allow us to give a numerical score of 0 to 3 for each category, respectively. The second variable we consider important is the pain severity as related to us by the patient based on a 0 to 100 scale: 0 means no pain, and 100 means more than the patient can possibly bear. We therefore can construct categories of pain severity ranging from none (0) to mild (1 to 30), moderate (31 to 60), and severe (61 to 100). Each category is given a 0 to 3 numerical score, respectively. The third variable we consider important is activity, and this may range from normal (0) to functioning both at home and out of the home with some limitations (1), confined to home but

TABLE 47-4 Pain Impairment Scale*

Criteria	Impairment score			
	0	1	2	3
Life expectancy	>5 yr	>1 yr; <5 yr	<6 mo, <1 yr	<6 mo
Pain severity (0–100)	0	1–30 (mild)	31–60 (moderate)	>60 (severe)
Activity	Normal	Functioning both at home and out of home with some limitations	Confined to home but independent	Bedridden

* Adding individual impairment scores gives a total pain impairment score, i.e., 0 = none; 1–3 = mild; 4–6 = moderate; and 7–9 = severe.

TABLE 47-5 Management based on pain impairment scale*

Mild impairment (score of 1–3)	Moderate impairment (score of 4–6)	Severe impairment (score of 7–9)
Mild analgesics	Stronger analgesics with low abuse potential	Narcotics
Psychotropic drugs	Psychotropic drugs	Psychotropic drugs
Psychophysical and behavior techniques	Psychophysical and behavior techniques	Psychophysical techniques
Counseling	Counseling	Counseling
	Neurosurgical intervention: Deep brain stimulation Ablative techniques	Neurosurgical intervention: Ablative techniques Deep brain stimulation
		Anesthetic blocks if general condition poor

* Management alternatives based on score arrived at from Table 47-3.

independent (2), and bedridden (3). Based on the numerical score in each category we arrive at a total score of 0 to a maximum of 9. Most patients with a score of 0 obviously do not need our help. Those patients whose total score is from 1 to 3 would be classified as being mildly impaired; those with scores from 4 to 6 as moderately impaired; and those from 7 to 9 as being severely impaired. Based on this score, we plan alternative managements based on the category arrived at from the pain scale illustrated in Table 47-5. It must be emphasized that this is only a guide and must be used in the context of the individual patient assessed by a sophisticated team dedicated to pain relief in the patient.

If available resources exclude such a sophisticated approach, the burden of evaluation and treatment of these complex problems falls on the oncologist's shoulders. On the other hand, an interested and dedicated neurosurgeon, neurologist, or anesthesiologist with a similarly oriented psychiatrist may provide sufficient expertise to aid the oncologist and patient in often difficult decisions about alternative treatments for pain control in cancer.

REFERENCES

1. Twycross RG: Measurement of pain in terminal cancer. *J Intern Med Res* 4 [Suppl] 2:58, 1976.
2. Lipton MA et al (eds): *Psychopharmacology: A Generation of Progress*, Raven Books, New York, 1978.
3. Bonica JJ, Albe-Fessard DG (eds): *Advances in Pain Research and Therapy*, Raven Books, New York, vol I, 1976.
4. Catalano RG: The medical approach to management of pain caused by cancer. *Semin Oncol* 2:379, 1975.
5. Mount BM et al: Use of Brompton mixture in treating the chronic pain of malignant disease. *Can Med Assoc J* 115:122, 1976.
6. Mathews GJ et al: Cancer pain and its treatment. *Semin Drug Treat* 3:45, 1973.
7. Marks RM, Sachar EJ: Undertreatment of medical inpatients with narcotic analgesics. *Ann Intern Med* 78:173, 1973.
8. Hackett TP, Cassem NH (eds): *Massachusetts General Hospital Handbook of General Hospital Psychiatry*, Mosby, St Louis, 1978.
9. Egbert LD et al: Reduction of postoperative pain by encouragement and instruction of patient. *N Engl J Med* 270: 825, 1964.
10. Saunders C: Treatment of intractable pain in terminal cancer. *Proc R Soc Med* 56:195, 1963.
11. Halpern LM: Analgesic drugs in the management of pain. *Arch Surg* 112:861, 1977.
12. AMA Department of Drugs: *AMA Drug Evaluations*, Publishing Sciences Group Inc, Littleton, Mass, 1977.
13. Sternbach RA: *Pain Patients Traits and Treatment*, Academic, New York, 1974.
14. White JC, Sweet WH: *Pain and the Neurosurgeon*, Charles C Thomas, Springfield, Ill, 1969.
15. Brechner VL et al: Anesthetic measures in management of pain associated with malignancy. *Semin Oncol* 4:99, 1977.
16. Hackett TP: Pain and prejudice. *Med Times* 99:130, 1971.
17. Bonica JJ: *The Management of Pain*, Lea & Febiger, Philadelphia, 1953.

SELECTED BIBLIOGRAPHY

Black P: Management of cancer pain: An overview. *Neurosurg* 5:507, 1979.

Chung SH, Dickenson A: Pain, enkephalin, and acupuncture. *Nature* 283:243–244, 1980.

Dawson DM, Fischer GF: Pain, in JF Holland, E Frei (eds). *Cancer Medicine,* Lea & Febiger, Philadelphia, 1982, pp 1205–1219.

Glover DD et al: Brompton's mixture in alleviating pain of terminal neoplastic disease: Preliminary results. *South Med J* 73:278–282, 1980.

Ignelzi RJ, Atkinson JH: Pain and its modulation. Part I. Afferent mechanisms. *Neurosurg* 6:577–583, 1980.

Ignelzi RJ, Atkinson JH: Pain and its modulation. Part II. Efferent mechanisms. *Neurosurg* 6:584–590, 1980.

Lathrop JC, Frates RE: Arterial infusion of nitrogen mustard in the treatment of intractable pelvic pain of malignant origin. *Cancer* 45:432, 1980.

Lewis BJ et al: Management of pain, in VT DeVita Jr, S Hellman, SA Rosenberg (eds): *Cancer: Principles and Practice of Oncology,* Lippincott, Philadelphia, 1982, pp 1658–1676.

Maxwell M: How to use methadone for cancer pain management. *Amer J Nurs* September 1980.

Moertel CG: Treatment of cancer pain with orally administered medications. *JAMA* 244:2448, 1980.

Oyama T et al: Profound analgesic effects of β-endorphin in man. *Lancet* 1:122–124, 1980.

Reuler JB et al: The chronic pain syndrome: Misconceptions and management. *Ann Intern Med* 93:588, 1980.

Wang JK et al: Pain relief by intrathecally applied morphine in man. *Anesthesiology* 50:149–151, 1979.

48
PARANEOPLASTIC SYNDROMES
Charles M. Haskell

Systemic or remote regional problems unrelated to physical invasion of organs by primary or metastatic cancer are commonly referred to as *paraneoplastic* in origin. Some of these problems occur together in such predictable patterns that the term *paraneoplastic syndrome* is appropriate. Nathanson[1] has estimated that at least 15 percent of cancer patients develop a paraneoplastic syndrome, and that of these syndromes approximately one-third relate to the elaboration of various hormones, one-third to skin and connective tissue problems, one-sixth to various neuromyopathies, and one-sixth to additional miscellaneous mechanisms.

The term *ectopic hormone production* was coined by Liddle[2] in 1962, based on the demonstration that some patients with classical Cushing's syndrome had a carcinoma that was not in any way directly related to the adrenal glands or the pituitary gland. Subsequently Waldenström[3] drew the distinction between ectopic and topic production of humoral substances to clarify the difference between tissues that produce an unexpected substance and those that produce their usual substances in abnormal amounts. For example, the paraprotein produced in multiple myeloma would be termed a *topic* substance, whereas adrenocorticotropin (ACTH) from a small cell lung cancer would be termed *ectopic*. Although this distinction is of some use, modern methods of molecular endocrinology have been expanding the scope of tissues that normally secrete hormones. Odell and Wolfsen,[4] in an excellent review, identified a wide range of unexpected biologically inactive hormones from nearly all tumor types tested, and postulated that production of inactive peptide hormones may be a universal occurrence with malignancy. They pointed out that the usual sequence for the synthesis of a biologically active hormone is through a "cascade" which starts with a preprohormone that is converted to a prohormone, then converted to a hormone, and finally split into carboxyl and amino fragments. The carboxyl fragment of the hormone is generally inactive, but the amino fragment may be biologically active. They postulated that the critical event that separates tumors with ectopic and nonectopic hormone manifestations is not the elaboration of the hormone but rather the ability of the tumor to convert the hormone or the prohormone into its active constituents. In their model, all tumors produce peptides but only a small percentage manifest the symptoms and signs of a humoral paraneoplastic syndrome.

The biologic basis and pathophysiology of paraneoplastic syndromes are of tremendous theoretical interest, as discussed further in several reviews.[1,3,4] These syndromes are also of great practical importance. Since they usually develop prior to the onset of visible cancer, they may represent an early manifestation of malignancy and possibly can lead to an early diagnosis and, it may be hoped, a cure. Such syndromes may also develop in the presence of well-established, distant metastatic disease. Suffice it to say that a thorough understanding of the biology of these syndromes is essential to make the differential diagnosis between a treatable complication of cancer, an untreatable manifestation of metastatic disease, or a problem totally unrelated to the cancer but caused by another disease process.[5] Nearly every kind of cancer can be associated with such problems (Table 48-1).

Many of the paraneoplastic syndromes listed in Table 48-1 are unusual, and will not be discussed here. Some occur quite frequently, however, and may be confused with other disease processes; these have controversial aspects that deserve comment. Because of the importance of accurate diagnosis and treatment, the more common and controversial paraneoplastic syndromes are discussed individually in this chapter.

SYNDROMES RELATED TO THE ECTOPIC PRODUCTION OF HORMONES AND HORMONE PRECURSORS

Hypercalcemia

Hypercalcemia is one of the most common paraneoplastic syndromes observed in the discipline of oncology.[3-7] It is usually associated with metastatic involvement of the skeletal system, although it may also develop in patients whose bones appear normal on x-ray. It has been related to the elaboration of parathormone (PTH) by tumor cells, to the elaboration of prostaglandin E_2 by some solid tumors, and to a factor thus far found only in multiple myeloma cells called the *osteoclast activating factor*. Hypercalcemia occurs most commonly in patients with carcinoma of the kidney or lung (excluding small cell carcinoma),[8] but it also has been associated with a wide variety of other tumors.

Many benign conditions can also result in hypercalcemia. These include hyperparathyroidism (primary or secondary to previous radiation therapy),[9] hyperthyroidism, the use of thiazide diuretics, sarcoidosis, acute adrenal insufficiency, benign monoclonal gammopathy, acromegaly, vitamin-D intoxication, milk alkali syndrome, myxedema, renal insufficiency related to transplantation, the diuretic phase of acute renal insufficiency, hypervitaminosis A, and Paget's disease.

Hypercalcemia related to the ectopic or topic production of parathyroid hormone (PTH) is generally associated with hyperchloremic acidosis, and, when studied, there is an increase in the ratio of urinary cyclic AMP to creatinine (greater than 4.2 mM/g creatinine).[7] Usually such patients also have a reduced serum phosphorus level, elevated serum alkaline phosphatase, and an inappropriately elevated blood level of PTH.

The treatment of hypercalcemia varies with the etiology and severity of the complication.[6,7] The first consideration is to treat the underlying disease. Secondly, the ancillary factors such as specific drug therapy (estrogen, androgens, or other hormones) or bed rest that increase the level of serum calcium should be changed.

When hypercalcemia results from a tumor that secretes parathyroid hormone, the best treatment is local resection of the tumor, if this is at all possible. Hypercalcemia related to leukemia may abate if the patient achieves a remission, and hormonally induced hypercalcemia in breast cancer usually responds to discontinuing the hormonal therapy and decreasing the time spent in bed.

As an additional consideration, there are many pharmacologic approaches to the temporary control of hypercalcemia. The choice of therapy depends on the severity of the hypercalcemic syndrome. Mild hypercalcemia (serum calcium less than 12 mg/dL) can usually be managed by intravenous hydration with a sodium chloride solution and possibly the use of furosemide diuresis (Lasix). Moderate (12 to 15 mg/dL) or severe (greater than 15 mg/dL) hypercalcemia usually requires a more vigorous therapeutic approach. Detailed reviews of such therapies are available,[6,10] and the precise selection of treatment depends on the basic disease, the clinical situation, the serum inorganic phosphate level, and the baseline renal, hepatic, and bone marrow function.

Hospitalized patients with moderate or severe hypercalcemia and normal cardiopulmonary function should be treated initially with intravenous normal saline enhanced by the use of furosemide. The dosage of furosemide is 40 to 100 mg given intravenously over 1 to 2 h following the administration of 1 or 2L of normal saline solution. Subsequent doses of furosemide and saline are determined by the patient's response. The urinary losses of all electrolytes must be monitored very

TABLE 48-1 Tumors of Various Organs with Ectopic Systemic Manifestations

Location	Tumor	Clinical condition
Bladder	Carcinoma	Fibrinolysis
		Hypercalcemia
		Neuromuscular abnormalities
Bone marrow	Leukemia	Anergy
		Dysproteinemia
		Fever
		Hypercalcemia
		Malabsorption
		Neuromyopathies
Breast	Carcinoma	Acanthosis nigricans
		Cushing's syndrome
		Fibrinolysis
		Hypercalcemia
		Leukemoid reaction
		Neuromuscular abnormalities
Cerebellum	Hemangioblastoma	Polycythemia
Gastrointestinal tract		
Small bowel	Carcinoid	Carcinoid syndrome
		Hypoglycemia
Stomach	Carcinoma	Acanthosis nigricans
		Cushing's syndrome
		Dermatomyositis
		Fibrinolysis
		Leukemoid reaction
		Thrombophlebitis
Colon	Villous adenoma	Dehydration
		Electrolyte imbalance
	Carcinoma	Acanthosis nigricans
		Anemia
		Hypoglycemia
		Leukemoid reaction
		Neuromuscular abnormalities
		Thrombophlebitis and nonbacterial thrombotic endocarditis
Kidney	Renal cell carcinoma	Amyloidosis
		Coagulopathies
		Fever
		? Hepatopathy
		Hypercalcemia
		Hyperglobulinemia (↑ ESR)
		Hyperreninemia
		Hypertension
		Erythrocytosis
		Thrombocytosis, leukemoid reaction
Liver	Hepatoma (hepatoblastoma)	Fever
		Gynecomastia
		Hypercalcemia
		Hypoglycemia
		Erythrocytosis
		Virilization (precocious puberty)

TABLE 48-1 Tumors of Various Organs with Ectopic Systemic Manifestations (*Cont.*)

Location	Tumor	Clinical condition
Lung (bronchogenic cancer)	Adenocarcinoma	Osteoarthropathy
	Bronchial adenoma	Carcinoid syndrome
	Fibroma, fibrosarcoma, endobronchial plasmacytoma	Hypertrophic osteoarthropathy
	Large cell cancer	Gynecomastia
	Oat cell cancer	Carcinoid syndrome
		Cushing's syndrome
		Inappropriate antidiuretic hormone syndrome
		Neuromuscular abnormalities
	Squamous cell carcinoma	Acanthosis nigricans
		Carcinoid syndrome
		Cryofibrinogenemia
		Fibrinolysis
		Hypercalcemia (ectopic PTH)
		Hypoglycemia
		Hypertrophic osteoarthropathy
		Polycythemia
		Scleroderma, dermatomyositis
		Thrombophlebitis
Lymph nodes	Lymphoma	Malabsorption
Mediastinum	Neurolemmoma, neurofibroma, mixed nerve sheath tumor	Hypertrophic osteoarthropathy
Ovary	Carcinoma	Cushing's syndrome
		Hypercalcemia
		Neuromuscular abnormalities
		Thrombophlebitis
	Krukenberg tumor	Androgenic and progestational activity

closely, so that replacement with magnesium, potassium, and sodium can be undertaken. Thiazide diuretics should not be used in this situation since they may aggravate hypercalcemia.

Treatment for patients with cardiopulmonary disease or with persistent hypercalcemia should be with an inorganic phosphate preparation or mithramycin. Mithramycin is usually given in a dose of 25 µg/kg once or twice, followed by one or two doses per week to maintain the normal calcemic state. This drug is particularly useful in patients who cannot tolerate saline-diuretic therapy.

Inorganic phosphate therapy may also be useful. It appears to exert its hypocalcemic effect by precipitating calcium into bone. Soft-tissue calcification may also occur, however, particularly with the intravenous route. Therefore, phosphate should be given orally in the lowest effective dose. Serum inorganic phosphate levels should be kept under 5.5 mg/dL. The usual dose of phosphate to accomplish this task is 1000 to 2000 mg of inorganic phosphorus per day as tolerated. Commercially available preparations include Phos-tabs, Fleet Phospho-Soda, or Neutra-Phos.

Many other pharmacologic approaches to the treatment of hypercalcemia have been recommended, including the use of sulfates, calcitonin, corticosteroids, and hemodialysis.[5] Corticosteroids may be useful in treating an underlying neoplastic disease, but generally the other measures are not worthwhile. Indomethacin is occasionally useful in treating hypercalcemia that results from prostaglandins.[11]

Hypocalcemia

Although an uncommon accompaniment of cancer, hypocalcemia may occur in several situations.[7,12] First, a magnesium deficiency, which is common in cancer pa-

TABLE 48-1 Tumors of Various Organs with Ectopic Systemic Manifestations (*Cont.*)

Location	Tumor	Clinical condition
Pancreas	Non-beta islet cell tumor	Carcinoid syndrome
		Hyperglycemia
		"Pancreatic cholera" syndrome
		Zollinger-Ellison syndrome
	Carcinoma	Cushing's syndrome
Parotid gland	Carcinoma	Cushing's syndrome
Pleura	Fibroma, fibrosarcoma, spindle cell sarcoma, hemangiopericytoma, leiomyosarcoma, mesothelioma	Hypertrophic osteoarthropathy
		Hypoglycemia
Prostate	Carcinoma	Fibrinolysis
		Hypercalcemia
		Neuromuscular abnormalities
Retroperitoneum	Fibrosarcoma	Hypoglycemia
Testis	Choriocarcinoma	Gynecomastia
Thymus	Thymoma	Aregenerative anemia
		Autoimmune disorders: hypogammaglobulinemia, dermatomyositis, disseminated lupus erythematosus, polymyositis, granulomatous myocarditis
		Cushing's syndrome
		Hypertrophic osteoarthropathy
		Myasthenia gravis
		Peptic ulcer
Thyroid	Papillary, follicular tumors	Cushing's syndrome
	Medullary carcinoma	Carcinoid
		Cushing's syndrome
		Hypercalcitonuria
Uterus	Leiomyoma	Erythrocytosis
	Choriocarcinoma	"TSH" syndrome

SOURCE: From Nathanson.[1] Reproduced by permission of the author and W. B. Saunders Company.

tients, may induce this condition. Hypocalcemia may also occur in patients with metastatic breast cancer with widespread lytic bone metastases; they respond to endocrine therapy with rapid bone healing. This produces the so-called hungry bone syndrome, a situation also seen following the removal of parathyroid adenomas. Another extremely rare cause of hypocalcemia is the calcifying chondrosarcoma, where tumor uptake of calcium appears to exceed its capacity to mobilize bone stores. A final cause is oncogenic osteomalacia, in which a tumor product appears to impair production of 1,25-cholecalciferol (1,25-D). It should also be noted that hypocalcemia may result from overly vigorous therapy of hypercalcemia. This may be especially severe in patients treated with calcitonin and mithramycin.[13]

The diagnosis of hypocalcemia is usually suggested by tetany. Patients may also experience paresthesias, muscle cramps, laryngospasms, and even seizures. When hypocalcemia is confirmed by chemical studies, the magnesium level should also be determined.

The treatment of severe hypocalcemia is the intravenous injection of a 10% solution of calcium gluconate or calcium chloride. If hypomagnesemia complicates hypocalcemia, magnesium sulfate, 1 g IV or IM, may be given every 8 to 12 h until the combined defect is corrected.

Patients with healing bone lesions and metastatic breast cancer may receive oral calcium supplements in doses of 2 g of calcium lactate four times daily by mouth. Occasionally, vitamin D must also be administered. Serum calcium level should be carefully followed every 2 to 3 days, and the supplement discontinued when normal serum calcium levels are obtained.

Syndrome of Inappropriate Antidiuretic Hormone (SIADH)

Hypovolemia or hypersmolality, as detected by volume receptors in the body, trigger the release of antidiuretic hormone (ADH) from the hypothalamus.[14] This hormone normally acts on the distal collecting tubule to decrease free water clearance, and results in the reduction of blood-sodium concentration. A variety of neoplasms may be associated with high blood levels of ADH, leading to hyponatremia without concomitant hypervolemia or hyperosmolality (SIADH).[4,7,15] The most common tumor associated with this problem is small cell carcinoma of the lung, and the presence of the hormone both in the tumor and in increased concentration in the blood has been demonstrated by radioimmunoassay. In this situation, hyponatremia develops in the presence of a urine that is not maximally dilute, since normal homeostatic mechanisms are not working. If sodium-containing solutions are administered, the expansion of the intravascular space results in a prompt excretion of sodium in the urine; the sodium is thereby lost, and the syndrome remains uncorrected.

The diagnosis of SIADH in a cancer patient is suggested by the development of lethargy, weakness, confusion, convulsions, or coma. Blood electrolyte and creatinine levels should be determined, and the finding of a low serum sodium concentration with a urine that is not maximally dilute (i.e., specific gravity greater than 1.003 with a normal serum creatinine) suggests the presence of SIADH. Plasma and urine osmolality determinations should be obtained. The urine osmolality need not exceed that of the plasma to establish a diagnosis. Normally, an adult is able to dilute the urine to an osmolality of 50 mosmol/L. If the plasma osmolality is less than 260 to 270, and one finds a urine osmolality of 200, the latter is clearly inappropriately concentrated. In this setting, because of the already expanded extracellular space, the administration of saline is followed by a prompt elimination of sodium in the urine, but there is little change in serum sodium levels. It should be noted that a diagnosis of SIADH cannot be made with certainty in the presence of other fluid-retaining or salt-losing states, an elevated serum creatinine level, or peripheral edema. Some of these considerations are summarized in Table 48-2.

Before assuming that SIADH exists, it is important to rule out the alternative explanations for low serum sodium listed in Table 48-2. Three major groups are of particular concern: "benign" inappropriate ADH syndromes, water-retention states, and sodium-losing states. Of these, heart failure, administration of diuretics with unrestricted fluid intake, and inappropriate intravenous fluid management are perhaps most common. One must also, of course, rule out adrenal insufficiency. Patients with adrenal insufficiency have an impaired ability to excrete a free-water load; however, unlike patients with SIADH, fluid restriction in Addisonian patients will result in an elevation of the blood creatinine level, and hypovolemia will develop with little improvement in sodium concentrations. Nevertheless, if serious doubt exists, baseline and stimulated plasma cortisol determinations may be useful.

The treatment for SIADH is the restriction of fluid to 1L/day. In addition, every effort should be made to control the underlying malignancy, since this may be an even more important long-term mechanism of control. In some patients, demeclocycline in a dose of 800 mg to 1 g/day by mouth may also be useful. In a randomized trial[16] demeclocycline was superior to lithium carbonate; however, both of these measures may cause azotemia

TABLE 48-2 Hyponatremia

INAPPROPRIATE ANTIDIURETIC HORMONE
Malignancies
Chemotherapy—cyclophosphamide; vincristine
Morphine; anesthetics
Pulmonary infections
Repirators
Acute intermittent porphyria
Central nervous system lesions

OTHER CAUSES
With increased total-body sodium (edematous states)
Liver disease
Congestive heart failure
Nephrotic syndrome
With decreased total-body sodium of other types
Addison's disease
Drugs—diuretics, chlorpropamide, acetaminophen
Hypothalamic osmoregulatory defect
Renal salt wasting

SOURCE: From Lowitz.[7] Reproduced by permission of the author and W. B. Saunders Company.

and other undesirable effects. Demeclocycline may also be excessively toxic in patients with liver disease.

Patients who are comatose or those who present with a severe depression of serum sodium concentration (less than 110 meg/L) require aggressive treatment. Normal saline 3% with potassium chloride administered at the rate of 1 L every 6 to 8 h should be initiated. Furosemide (Lasix) should be used to prevent fluid overload, with an initial dose of 40 to 80 mg intravenously and additional doses given as needed. Patients must be monitored frequently for the development of congestive heart failure and hypokalemia.

Ectopic ACTH Syndrome

About two-thirds of all cases of Cushing's syndrome result from disorders of the pituitary gland, with the remainder almost equally divided between lesions of the adrenal cortex and extrapituitary neoplasms producing ectopic ACTH.[17] The clinical ectopic ACTH syndrome is therefore unusual, although recent data suggest that many neoplasms may produce a biologically inactive form of ACTH (proACTH).[4,17] This derives from a precursor that gives rise to many components, including lipotropin (LPH), endorphin, melanocyte-stimulating hormone (MSH), enkaphalin, and corticotropinlike intermediate lobe peptide. The association of ectopic ACTH syndrome with MSH has been known for many years, although the other components have only recently been identified. Indeed, MSH is probably a trivial concomitant, since it is an artifact of some of the methods used in assaying ACTH, and it appears to play no biologically functional role in human beings. Lipotropin, on the other hand, is biologically important, and preliminary studies suggest that it may be an extremely useful marker of the presence of cancer.[4,18]

The ectopic ACTH syndrome is most commonly associated with carcinoma of the lung, particularly of the small cell type. Lung cancer accounts for approximately 50 percent of clinical cases, bronchial carcinoids for about 5 percent, thymomas for about 10 percent, and pancreatic islet cell carcinomas, carcinoids, and adenocarcinomas of other sites for about 10 percent.[4]

Since approximately one-half the patients with the ectopic ACTH syndrome have carcinoma of the lung with a rapidly fatal course, typical signs of Cushing's syndrome may not develop.[4,17] Very high plasma cortisol levels produce weight loss, hypokalemic alkalosis, muscle wasting, edema, hypertension, impaired glucose tolerance, mental changes, and increased pigmentation. Patients with tumors that grow more slowly such as thymomas, bronchial carcinoids, and pheochromocytomas sometimes develop the typical physical findings of Cushing's syndrome many years before the tumor is found. In patients with cancer elaborating bioactive ACTH, hypokalemia is the most common sign suggesting an ectopic ACTH source.

In the clinical ectopic ACTH syndrome, urinary free cortisol, 17-hydroxysteroids, and 17-ketosteroids are markedly increased (Table 48-3).[19] Plasma cortisol is frequently greater than 40 μg/dL, and plasma ACTH is greater than 200 μg/mL in most cases. An ACTH level greater than 200 μg/mL in the appropriate clinical setting is virtually diagnostic of the ectopic ACTH syndrome.[17] When the level is only intermediate, other confirmatory studies may be necessary. Typically, cortisol and ACTH do not become suppressed when 2 mg of dexamethasone are given every 6 h for 2 days to patients with ectopic ACTH syndrome. However, when patients with Cushing's disease related to a pituitary tumor receive this dose of dexamethasone, there is generally a 50 percent suppression or greater of plasma and urinary corticosteroids. In approximately 50 percent of patients with Cushing's syndrome caused by bronchial carcinoids, and in some with thymomas, suppression of cortisol or its metabolites may occur with the administration of dexamethasone. This phenomenon may result from tumor production of corticotropin-releasing hormone (CRH). Hopefully, further studies correlating the ectopic ACTH syndrome with the amount of other hormones such as lipotropin will simplify diagnosis in the future.[17,18]

The treatment of the ectopic ACTH syndrome is the elimination of the ACTH-secreting tumor.[4,17] In unresponsive or unresectable cases, the adrenal corticolytic drug o,p'-DDD (Lysodren) may be used, or metyrapone may be administered as an alternative.

Hypoglycemia

In addition to insulinomas, a variety of neoplasms may be associated with hypoglycemia, and the symptoms may precede a diagnosis by months or even years. Approximately 66 percent of the non-islet cell tumors are of mesenchymal origin, about 21 percent are of hepatic origin, and the remaining 13 percent are of adrenal gland origin or from other miscellaneous sites.[4] In most of the patients with these malignancies, particularly those with mesenchymal tumors, the neoplasms tend to be very large when the hypoglycemia is noted. The range

TABLE 48-3 Differentiation of Hyperadrenocortical Disorders

Disease	Plasma cortisol	Plasma ACTH	Serum potassium	High-dose dexamethasone suppression
Cushing's disease	↑	Normal, ↑	Normal	Yes
Adrenocortical tumors	↑	↓	↓	No
ACTH-producing pituitary adenomas	↑	↑	Normal	No
Ectopic ACTH	↑	↑↑	↓	No
Ectopic CRH	↑	↑	↓	Yes

SOURCE: From Creech.[19] Reproduced by permission of the author and University Park Press.

of tumor size is from 800 to 10,000 g, and the average is about 2400 g. Most of these tumors occur in the abdomen, but some occur in the thorax. The majority of the hypoglycemic cases associated with malignancies of the hematopoietic system are artifactual, produced by the collection of blood in a tube that permits continued glucose metabolism by the many circulating malignant cells. Occasionally, however, a true ectopic humoral syndrome appears to exist.

The etiology of hypoglycemia in most of these patients remains poorly understood. The most likely explanation is tumor elaboration of a somatomedin.[4] The somatomedins comprise a family of peptide hormones normally produced by the liver and believed to be mediated via growth hormone; specifically, growth hormone stimulates hepatic production of one or more somatomedins. The biologic action of somatomedins is identical to insulin, and, in fact, they have been purified with insulin receptor assays. Based on current studies, as summarized by Odell and Wolfsen,[4] substances with identical bioassay properties to insulin and exhibiting full reaction in insulin radioreceptor assays but not in insulin radioimmunoassays are somatomedins. Further studies are needed, however, to establish this firmly as a basis for hypoglycemia in non-β cell cancers.

Treatment of the hypoglycemic syndrome varies with the neoplasm responsible. Surgical resection is preferred if possible, and some tumors associated with hypoglycemia may respond to chemotherapy. Hypoglycemia related to insulin-secreting tumors may respond to diazoxide, streptozotocin,[20] or mithramycin.[21] However, such measures have not been reported to be useful in patients with hypoglycemia related to other ectopic materials.

Gastrointestinal Peptide Hormone Syndromes

There are multiple syndromes caused by tumors that elaborate gastrointestinal peptide hormones.[4,22] Perhaps the best known are the Zollinger-Ellison syndrome and the carcinoid syndrome. Strictly speaking these are topic, rather than ectopic syndromes, since these hormones are derived in abnormal amounts from cells that normally synthesize these peptides. Tumors derived from these cells have synthesized nearly every known gastrointestinal peptide hormone, including gastrin (including big gastrin, little gastrin, and minigastrin), vasoactive intestinal polypeptide (VIP), prostaglandin E, human pancreatic polypeptide, secretin, seratonin, enteroglucagon, pancreatic glucagon, and a "gastric-inhibitory polypeptide." The treatment of these various syndromes is to eradicate the underlying disease, usually by surgical resection. Patients with the carcinoid syndrome may also require other kinds of symptomatic care as discussed elsewhere in this text and in recent reviews.[23,24]

Glycopeptide Hormone Syndromes

Thyrotropin (TSH), luteinizing hormone (LH), follicle-stimulating hormone (FSH), and human chorionic gonadotropin (HCG) are glycopeptides composed of two peptide chains, an α and β chain.[4] The α chain is identical for LH, FSH, and TSH, and differs only slightly for HCG. The β chain of each of these hormones is biochemically and immunologically unique. Either chain alone is inactive, but the α-β chain combination is biologically active. Neoplasms have been shown to elaborate the α chain, the β chain, and/or intact HCG-like gonadotropin. Indeed, there is some evidence suggesting that all cancers synthesize the peptide sequence of HCG, and that its measurable presence in blood as a marker of malignancy depends on the ability of the cancer to add the carbohydrate to the peptide sequence (glycosylation). Currently, these observations have generated a vigorous study of HCG as a possible marker substance in human cancer.[4]

Gonadotropin production or free α chain synthesis by neoplasms produces few or no symptoms. In women no clinical problems have been found, whereas in men gynecomastia may result from intact HCG production. Treatment of the α chain or gonadotropin elevation is not necessary. In the extremely rare situation of ectopic TSH production, treatment is chosen on the basis of the stage and histology of the primary tumor.[25]

Other Hormone Syndromes

PROLACTIN

Prolactin-induced galactorrhea, with or without amenorrhea in women, is frequently associated with microadenomas of the pituitary gland.[26] It has been reported[27] as an ectopic product of lung and renal carcinomas as well, although most oncologists consider this to be an extremely rare event.

GROWTH HORMONE

Sporadic reports of elevated human growth hormone levels have been reported in patients with lung, stomach,[28] and endometrial cancer.[29] The frequency and significance of these observed elevations is currently unclear, although HGH may play a role in the pathogenesis of hypertrophic osteoarthropathy[30] (see below).

CALCITONIN

Calcitonin is commonly elevated in patients with medullary carcinoma of the thyroid. Its measurement is an important part of the preoperative screening and postoperative follow-up of these patients.[31] The specificity of this marker for medullary carcinoma can be challenged, however, since the ectopic production of this material has been reported in diverse carcinomas, including those from the lung (primarily small cell carcinoma)[32,33] and the breast.[33] For now, these measurements are mainly of value as potential tumor markers, since these patients do not have clinical problems with hypocalcemia.

RENIN

Hypertension from the elaboration of renin by malignant tumor is occasionally seen. Such tumors are usually of renal origin, such as Wilms's tumor,[34] but rarely ectopic renin tumors from other sites may be seen. Examples include small cell lung cancer[35] and transitional cell carcinoma of the ureter.[36] Treatment is by extirpation of the primary tumor if feasible.

ERYTHROPOIETIN

Patients with renal tumors (1 to 5 percent) and those with cerebellar hemangioblastomas (9 to 20 percent) may develop polycythemia.[37] Normally, the kidney is a major site of erythropoietin production; however, other tissues, particularly the liver, are able to produce erythropoietin in response to severe hypoxia and anemia in anephric humans or animals. Erythropoietin production by renal or liver tumors thus, strictly speaking, may not represent ectopic hormone production.

Tumor-associated erythrocytosis is diagnosed by an abnormal elevation of red blood cell mass without evidence of splenomegaly, thrombocytosis, or leukocytosis (as occurs in polycythemia rubra vera) and without decreased arterial oxygen saturation or hemoglobinopathy that has increased hemoglobin-oxygen affinity. Demonstration of elevated erythropoietin activity in blood and urine may assist in establishing this diagnosis, and surgical eradication of the tumor will result in the disappearance of erythrocytosis. In symptomatic cases, phlebotomy may be used to control the erythrocytosis.

SYNDROMES RELATED TO THE SKIN, MUSCLE, AND SOFT TISSUES

Internal malignancies may be associated with characteristic skin changes, and some other skin problems may occasionally be considered paraneoplastic in origin. Table 48-4 lists the skin conditions that are frequently and occasionally associated with cancer. Only a few of these will be discussed here. The interested reader should consult the excellent reviews by Waldenström[3] or Curth[38] for more details.

Acanthosis Nigricans

Although rare, this is one of the most classic paraneoplastic skin conditions. It was initially described by two German dermatologists in 1890, and subsequently many

TABLE 48-4 Classification of Dermatoses in Respect to Causal Relationship between Cutaneous Manifestation and Malignant Internal Disease

1. Dermatoses in which the causal relationship between cutaneous manifestations and malignant internal disease is well established. In some dermatoses the association with malignant disease occurs in all instances of the dermatosis; in others, in many instances of the dermatosis:
   a. Malignant acanthosis nigricans
   b. Dermatomyositis of the adult
   c. Flushing
   d. Pachydermoperiostosis
   e. Acquired ichthyosis
   f. Malignant down
   g. Palmar and plantar keratoses
   h. Erythema gyratum repens
   i. Thrombophlebitis migrans
   j. Reticulohistiocytoma
2. Dermatoses in which the association with a malignant internal disease does not occur in all or many instances of the dermatosis:
   a. Pruritus
   b. Urticaria
   c. Dermatitis herpetiformis
   d. Pemphigoid
   e. Erythema annulare centrifugum
   f. Erythema multiforme
   g. Scleroderma (lichen sclerosus et atrophicus)
   h. Herpes zoster
   i. Freckles and seborrheic keratoses
   j. Unilateral epidermal nevi
   k. Hyperpigmentation and Cushing's syndrome
   l. The Peutz-Jeghers-Touraine syndrome
   m. Gardner's syndrome
3. Cutaneous precancerosis
   a. Bowen's disease

SOURCE: From Curth.[38] Reproduced by permission of the author and McGraw-Hill Book Company.

reviews have confirmed the association of the condition with various solid tumors.[4,38] It should be noted that there are two patterns of acanthosis nigricans, one is associated with tumors, and the other is not. The latter is usually seen in young females and is commonly associated with a rare combination of extreme loss of fat and diabetes. The paraneoplastic form of this condition usually presents as symmetrical black skin lesions, predominantly found in flexure creases, especially the axillae, the palms, the soles, and even the mouth. Most of associated tumors are adenocarcinomas, especially of the stomach.

Hypertrophic Pulmonary Osteoarthropathy

This syndrome includes four principal components: (1) clubbing, (2) pulmonary osteoarthropathy, (3) gynecomastia, and (4) pachydermoperiostosis.[1,3] These features may or may not coexist, but clubbing is the most common sign and usually coexists with pulmonary osteoarthropathy or gynecomastia. The causal relationship between these four components is poorly understood, and their etiology is also uncertain.[39] Some people have related it to secretion of various hormones, including luteinizing hormone, follicle-stimulating hormone, human growth hormone, and human chorionic gonadotropin. Other postulated mechanisms invoke abnormal vasomotor reflexes, possibly involving the vagus nerve or the pulmonary circulation. Thus, this can be classified either as an ectopic hormone syndrome or as a paraneoplastic syndrome involving the skin and soft tissues.

Clinical evidence of the onset of clubbing or osteoarthropathy accompanying a tumor is common, but it may also herald the growth of a tumor before actual diagnosis. The most common tumors are adenocarcinoma or epidermoid carcinoma of the lung; however, a variety of benign and malignant diseases and an inherited form of clubbing must be included in the differential diagnosis. Treatment is dependent on the control of the primary malignancy; other measures are rarely worthwhile, although occasional benefit has been reported by thoracotomy or laparotomy without tumor resection.[40] Further discussion of these problems can be pursued in several excellent reviews.[1,39,41]

NEUROMYOPATHIES

The vast majority of neurological problems in cancer patients can be explained by metastatic involvement of the nervous system by cancer or by lesions caused by antineoplastic therapy. Hildebrand[42] has reviewed this general problem carefully, both as a function of the experience at the Institute Jules Bordet, a cancer hospital in Brussels, and by reviewing the medical literature. In his series of 696 cancer patients, neurological disorders related to metastatic disease occurred in 73 percent, lesions related to treatment (including infectious problems) occurred in 6.3 percent, and lesions unrelated to cancer occurred in 10.6 percent. Lesions of undetermined etiology, and therefore classified as carcinomatous neuropathies, developed in 9.5 percent. Based on this experience, as well as the published experience of others,[43] Hildebrand[42] classifies these neuropathies as shown in Table 48-5.

Most, if not all, of the syndromes shown in Table 48-5 may occur in patients without cancer. In most cases there is no correlation between the extent of the neoplasm and the severity of the disorder, and with some exceptions to be discussed, the treatment of the neoplastic disease rarely results in neurological improvement. Frequently the neurological problem precedes the diagnosis of cancer by many months or even by several years. Indeed, the relationship between these neuromyopathies and cancer is largely based on the alleged increased frequency of their association with cancer, even though formal statistical assessments of this inference are generally not made. Because of these factors, one must always be careful to exclude other, possibly more treatable, causes for neurological dysfunction in cancer patients.

An example of a neurological problem that was once widely accepted as a paraneoplastic neurological syndrome is progressive multifocal leukoencephalopathy (PML). This is now recognized as a disease caused by a slow virus infection of the brain, most commonly a papovavirus.[44] It is perhaps more common in patients with cancer than in normal people; nevertheless it should no longer be considered a paraneoplastic syndrome.

A detailed discussion of the paraneoplastic neurological problems listed in Table 48-5 is beyond the scope of this chapter but can be pursued in the excellent review by Hildebrand.[42] A few of these problems will be discussed here briefly because of their relatively greater frequency or because of their responsiveness to specific therapy.

Metabolic Encephalopathies

Neuropsychiatric symptoms are common in cancer patients[42,45]; in one series from Switzerland[45], 20 percent of a group of patients with bronchogenic carcinoma developed such symptoms without autopsy evidence of

TABLE 48-5 Classification of Carcinomatous Neuropathies

Syndrome	Relative frequency	Location of main lesions	Main associated neoplasms
Metabolic encephalopathies	Fairly frequent		Oat cell lung carcinoma when caused by production of active substances by the tumor
Diffuse polyencephalomyelitis	Rare	Limbic system; brainstem; spinal cord	Oat cell lung carcinoma
Subacute cerebellar degeneration	Rare	Degeneration of Purkinje cells	Oat cell lung carcinoma; ovary carcinoma
Opsoclonus	Rare	Cerebellum (?); brainstem (?)	Neuroblastoma
Motor neuron disease	Very rare	Degeneration of spinal motor neurons	Lung and breast carcinomas
Necrotizing myelopathy	Very rare	Spinal (mainly thoracic) cord	Lung carcinoma
Sensory neuropathy	Rare	Root, ganglia, and spinal cord	Lung carcinoma
Sensorimotor peripheral neuropathy	Frequent	Peripheral nerves	Lung and breast carcinomas
Eaton-Lambert syndrome	Fairly rare	Neuromuscular junction	Oat cell lung carcinoma
Muscle lesions			
Neuromyopathy	The most frequent	Proximal muscles and peripheral nerves (?)	Mainly lung and breast carcinomas
Polymyositis and dermatomyositis	Fairly rare	Muscles	Lung, breast, ovary, lymphomas
Carcinoid syndrome myopathy	Very rare	Muscles	Serotonin-secreting tumors

SOURCE: From Hildebrand.[42] Reproduced by permission of the author and Raven Books.

brain metastasis. In a series from Dartmouth[45] involving 100 cancer patients referred for psychiatric evaluation, 56 percent of the patients were diagnosed as depressed and 40 percent as having an organic brain syndrome (OBS). However, only one-third of the patients with OBS were referred with the correct diagnosis. Most of them had been misdiagnosed as depressed, and mental status examinations were commonly lacking in the medical records. Indeed, the authors of this study[45] noted that in many of the patients the status of bowel function had received greater attention than the status of the patient's cognition. This can be a serious error, since OBS may be treatable when related to such things as an ectopic humoral syndrome, electrolyte abnormality, specific drug effect, or other metabolic form of encephalopathy.

In summary,[45] patients with cancer should have a careful mental status examination at regular intervals. Recognition of an organic brain syndrome should result in an immediate search for its cause. Patients with marked behavior abnormalities, such as agitation, panic, severe depression, excitement, or insomnia, may benefit from psychiatric consultation and drug therapy. Haloperidol is particularly useful in the agitated, restless, or delirious patient. Tricyclic antidepressants may be useful for the severely depressed. Treatment of the underlying cancer should not be neglected, nor should it be assumed that the neurological problems of these patients are due to an untreatable paraneoplastic process.

Subacute Cerebellar Degeneration

Cerebellar degeneration may occur alone or in association with diffuse polyencephalitis and/or sensory neuropathy.[42] Cerebellar signs include ataxia in both the upper and lower limbs; dysarthria is also common. The cerebrospinal fluid may be normal or may show a moderately elevated protein concentration (60 to 120 mg/dL).

Histologically the disease is characterized by the diffuse disappearance of Purkinje cells in the cerebellar cortex. This contrasts with the cerebellar degeneration seen with alcoholism, which is usually focal. The mechanism of degeneration is unknown, and there is no known therapy.

Sensorimotor Peripheral Neuropathy

The sensorimotor polyneuritis seen with cancer is clinically similar to neuropathies of other etiologies.[42] Lower extremity symptoms tend to predominate, but rarely an ascending polyneuropathy may be seen (Guillain-Barré syndrome). In myeloma and Waldenström's macroglobulinemia the peripheral neuropathy may be explained on the basis of paraprotein damage of peripheral nerves,[46] either as a direct phenomenon or through amyloid formation. In most other cases of cancer, however, malnutrition is nearly always present, and the neuropathy is indistinguishable from that seen in the malnourished patients without cancer.

Eaton-Lambert Syndrome

Although closely related to myasthenia gravis, the Eaton-Lambert syndrome is best considered to be a separate and distinct paraneoplastic neurological problem.[42] Unlike myasthenia gravis, which is associated with increasing weakness with repetitive muscle contraction, the Eaton-Lambert syndrome starts with marked weakness that eases with repetitive muscle contractions. This can be easily demonstrated by a simple clinical test in which the patient squeezes a partially inflated blood pressure cuff.[46,47]

Table 48-6 summarizes the essential differences between the Eaton-Lambert syndrome and myasthenia gravis. It should also be noted that the Eaton-Lambert syndrome may respond dramatically to therapy of the underlying malignancy, as well as to guanidine hydrochloride (125 to 400 mg, three to four times daily in adults).[7] This fact, plus its very high association with cancer, makes it one of the best-established of the paraneoplastic neurological syndromes.

MISCELLANEOUS PARANEOPLASTIC SYNDROMES

Hematologic and Vascular Abnormalities

ANEMIA

Anemia is a frequent nonspecific event in patients with malignant disease.[1] It may be increased by blood loss, therapy with antineoplastic agents, and a wide variety of nutritional, metabolic, and toxic changes. The degree of anemia ranges from mild to fairly severe. Generally, red blood cells are normocytic and normochromic, although they may become hypochromic. Generally, marrow stores of iron are increased, the plasma iron level is low, and the total plasma iron-binding capacity is decreased. This is in contrast with iron-deficiency anemia, in which case

TABLE 48-6 Comparison between Eaton-Lambert Syndrome and Myasthenia Gravis

Factor	Eaton-Lambert syndrome	Myasthenia gravis
Age and sex	Males over 40 years	Young females
Associated tumors	Malignant tumors in 70% (oat cell lung carcinoma)	Thymoma in 50%
Main location of weakness	Proximal segments of limbs	Oculobulbar muscles
Electromyography (repetitive nerve stimulation, 10–50 cycles/s)	Facilitation: increase of evoked muscle potentials	Fatigue: decrease of evoked muscle potentials
Anomaly of the neuromuscular junction	Impaired release of acetylcholine	Antibodies against acetylcholine receptors
Drug effect Anticholinesterases	Ineffective	Effective
Decamethonium (1.5–2.5 mg)	Produces a more marked weakness in patients with Eaton-Lambert syndrome than in controls	Produces a less marked weakness in patients with myasthenia gravis than in controls
Guanidine	Effective	Poor

SOURCE: From Hildebrand.[42] Reproduced by permission of the author and Raven Books.

the serum iron is low and the iron-binding capacity is increased. Treatment is generally that of the underlying disease, and iron supplementation is rarely helpful. Blood transfusions are occasionally needed.

LEUKEMOID REACTIONS

A leukemoid reaction is defined as a nonleukemic leukocyte response to cancer, with peripheral leukocyte counts occasionally increasing to 50,000 to 100,000 per milliliter. This occurs most frequently in Hodgkin's disease and lung, breast, or gastric cancer, especially if hepatic metastases are present. This syndrome may be difficult to separate from chronic granulocytic leukemia (CML), although the cells in a leukemoid reaction tend to be more mature than those seen in CML. Rarely, prominent eosinophilia may occur due to a tumor-derived eosinophilotactic peptide.[48]

HYPERVISCOSITY SYNDROME

Neoplastic diseases accompanied by dysproteinemia, including cryoglobulinemia, fibrinogenemia, and Waldenström's's macroglobulinemia, may have a tendency toward thrombosis and hemorrhage because of increased viscosity of the blood.[1,3] Plasmapheresis or phlebotomy may be beneficial to such patients.

HYPERCOAGULABLE STATE

A thrombotic diathesis may be observed in some patients with cancer, particularly those with carcinoma of the lung, pancreas,[1,49] liver, or gastrointestinal tract. Clinical features resemble superficial migratory thrombophlebitis, which has little inflammatory reaction and tends to be nonresponsive to anticoagulation. The axillae, neck, and upper extremities may be involved rather than the lower extremities, as in the classic pattern of thrombophlebitis in individuals without cancer. Occasionally, severe, progressive phlegmasia cerulea dolens with development of superficial areas of gangrene may occur. The cardiac valves may be involved in a similar process, leading to a picture of nonbacterial thrombotic endocarditis (marantic endocarditis).[50] Mucin-producing adenocarcinomas of the stomach, lung, or pancreas are the tumors most often associated with this problem.

The mechanisms by which thromboses are produced are unclear, although mucin-secreting tumors have been associated with the production of a factor that can activate factor X.[49] Disseminated intravascular coagulation (DIC) is a related syndrome caused by the release of thromboplastic substances into the bloodstream of patients with tumors. These substances trigger the formation of thrombin, which leads to intravascular clotting with a deficiency of platelets, fibrinogen, factor V, and factor VIII caused by a consumption of these materials. Subsequently, the fibrinolytic system may be activated, producing lysis of local deposits of fibrin and accumulation of fibrinogen-fibrin digestion products in the circulation. Clinical tests in such patients demonstrate these products.

Treatment should be directed toward the primary tumor.[51] Heparin is indicated for DIC, and coumarin anticoagulants may also be useful. Antiplatelet compounds including dipyridamole, aspirin, and fibrolytic agents such as urokinase may also occasionally be beneficial,[52] although in most cases the syndrome is extremely resistant to therapy.

HEMORRHAGE

Hemorrhage may be associated with metastatic cancer from thrombocytopenia or other mechanisms.[53] Platelet agglutinins may occur, particularly as an autoimmune phenomenon, and low platelet counts may also develop from disseminated intravascular coagulation, as described previously.

Metabolic Disorders

FEVER

Fever is a well-established paraneoplastic process in some tumors, particularly those derived from histiocytes or macrophages, Hodgkin's disease, lymphomas, and occasionally carcinomas of the liver or kidney.[54]

When fever is present, infection must be ruled out.[55] Fever is particularly common when infections are associated with tumors that obstruct important organs. This is commonly seen in pelvic tumors, including those of prostate, cervix, bladder, uterus, and ovary. Symptomatic relief of tumor fever usually requires control of the underlying disease. Indomethacin, aspirin, or Tylenol may also be useful.

ANOREXIA AND CACHEXIA

These disorders occur as almost universal features in the natural history of many malignant diseases.[1,3,56] The mechanisms are poorly understood but are generally related to the following: (1) anorexia, (2) hypermetabolism and excessive energy consumption over the available nutritional supply, and (3) wasting resulting from a negative balance of protein and fat in the body. The destruction of muscle protein, impaired cellular respiration, and other multiple complications are responsible for many of the cancer deaths in patients with solid tumors. Attempts to reverse this cycle with careful nutritional support, which occasionally involves hyperalimentation by a parenteral route, is under active study.[57] Of even greater importance, however, is the treatment of the underlying cancer.

ACID-BASE AND ELECTROLYTE DISORDERS

In addition to the acid-base and electrolyte disorders described previously for the ectopic hormone syndromes (SIADH and ectopic ACTH syndrome), cancer patients have other disorders as well. Most of these involve renal function, as reviewed in detail by Fichman and Bethune.[58] Of particular note is the tumor lysis syndrome that may develop in patients with highly drug-sensitive neoplasms, such as Burkitt's lymphoma. A more common variant of this is the uric acid nephropathy syndrome in association with vigorous treatment of malignant lymphomas, leukemia, and rarely carcinomas. In these diseases, the destruction of large amounts of tissue leads to the release of large amounts of purine degradation products, which results in the formation of relatively insoluble urates that precipitate in the kidney and form obstructive lesions. This can largely be prevented by the use of hydration along with alkalinization of the urine and administration of allopurinol to prevent the conversion of the relatively soluble purine precursors to uric acid.[10]

MISCELLANEOUS

Many substances may be produced by malignant neoplasms including various enzymes, fetal products, and other inactive chemicals. Only those known to cause clinical syndromes have been discussed. A variety of other syndromes have been related to abnormal immune states, including the development of various "immune complex" disorders.[59] By and large these disorders are complex, and their relationship to cancer is often obscure. They are discussed further in Chapter 9, "Principles of Immunotherapy."

FINAL COMMENTARY

Physicians must be alert to paraneoplastic syndromes as "biological signals in the diagnosis of cancer."[3] Unravelling the mechanisms involved may improve the understanding of cancer as a biologic process. The protean manifestations of cancer, however, as reflected in this diverse group of paraneoplastic syndromes, should not divert the physician from establishing accurate diagnoses in cancer patients. Nononcologic problems are common in cancer patients, and they should not be confused with an untreatable paraneoplastic process. Lowitz and Benjamin[5] have stated this concern nicely: "With clinical judgment, information, and the eternal question of diagnosticians, 'What else could this be?', a physician can focus not on the inevitability of death but on the quality of life."

REFERENCES

1. Nathanson L: Remote effects of cancer on the host, in J Horton, GJ Hill II (eds): *Clinical Oncology,* Saunders, Philadelphia, 1977.
2. Liddle GW et al: The ectopic ACTH syndrome. *Cancer Res* 25:1057, 1965.
3. Waldenström JG: *Paraneoplasia—Biological Signals in the Diagnosis of Cancer.* Wiley, New York, 1978.
4. Odell WD, Wolfsen AR: Humoral syndromes associated with cancer. *Annu Rev Med* 29:379, 1978.
5. Lowitz BB, Benjamin RS: Nononcologic disease in patients with cancer. *West J Med* 127:5, 1977.
6. Massaferri EL et al: Treatment of hypercalcemia associated with malignancy. *Semin Oncol* 5:141, 1978.
7. Lowitz BB: Paraneoplastic syndromes, in CM Haskell (ed): *Cancer Treatment,* Saunders, Philadelphia, 1980.
8. Bender RA, Hansen H: Hypercalcemia in bronchogenic carcinoma. *Ann Intern Med* 80:205, 1974.
9. Christensson T: Hyperparathyroidism and radiation therapy. *Ann Intern Med* 89:216, 1978.
10. Cline MJ, Haskell CM: *Cancer Chemotherapy,* 3d, Saunders, Philadelphia, 1979.
11. Seyberth HW et al: Prostaglandins and hypercalcemic states. *Annu Rev Med* 29:23, 1978.
12. Raskin P et al: Hypocalcemia associated with metastatic bone disease. *Arch Intern Med* 132:539, 1973.
13. Caro JF et al: Symptomatic hypocalcemia following combined calcitonin and mithramycin therapy for hypercalcemia due to malignancy. *Cancer Treat Rep* 62:1561, 1978
14. Hays RM: Antidiuretic hormone. *N Engl J Med* 295:659, 1976.
15. Bartter FC, Schwartz WB: The syndrome of inappropriate secretion of antidiuretic hormone. *Am J Med* 42:790, 1967.
16. Forrest JN Jr et al: Superiority of demeclocycline over lithium in the treatment of chronic syndrome of inappropriate secretion of antidiuretic hormone. *N Engl J Med* 298:173, 1978.
17. Gold EM: The Cushing syndromes: Changing views of diagnosis and treatment. *Ann Intern Med* 90:829, 1979.
18. Odell WD et al: Ectopic production of lipotropin by cancer. *Am J Med* 66:631, 1979.
19. Creech RH: Paraneoplastic and cancer-associated syndromes, in AI Sutnick, PF Engstrom (eds): *Oncologic Medicine,* University Park Press, Baltimore, 1976.
20. Broder LE, Carter SK: Pancreatic islet cell carcinoma: II. Results of therapy with streptozotocin in 52 patients. *Ann Intern Med* 79:108, 1973.
21. Kiang DT et al: Mithramycin for hypoglycemia in malignant insulinoma. *N Engl J Med* 299:134, 1978.
22. McGuigan JE: Gastrointestinal hormones. *Annu Rev Med* 29:307, 1978.
23. Jager RM, Polk HC Jr: Carcinoid APUDomas, in RC Hickey (ed): *Current Problems in Cancer,* 1:11, 1977.
24. Haskell CM, Tompkins R: Carcinoid tumors, in CM Haskell (ed): *Cancer Treatment,* Saunders, Philadelphia, 1980.
25. Steigbigel NH et al: Metastatic embryonal carcinoma of the testis associated with elevated plasma TSH-like activity and hyperthyroidism. *N Engl J Med* 271:349, 1964.
26. Kleinberg DL et al: Galactorrhea: A study of 235 cases, including 48 with pituitary tumors. *N Engl J Med* 296:589, 1977.
27. Turkington RW: Ectopic production of prolactin. *N Engl J Med* 285:1455, 1971.
28. Beck C, Burger HG: Evidence for the presence of immunoreactive growth hormone in cancers of the lung and stomach. *Cancer* 30:75, 1972.
29. Benjamin F et al: Growth-hormone secretion in patients with endometrial carcinoma. *N Engl J Med* 281:1448, 1969.
30. Steiner H et al: Ectopic growth-hormone production and osteoarthropathy in carcinoma of the bronchus. *Lancet* 1:783, 1968.
31. Goltzman D et al: Calcitonin as a tumor marker. *N Engl J Med* 290:1035, 1974.
32. Silva OL et al: Increased serum calcitonin levels in bronchogenic cancer. *Chest* 69:495, 1976.
33. Coombes RC et al: Plasma-immunoreactive-calcitonin in patients with nonthyroid tumours. *Lancet* 1:1080, 1974.
34. Sheth KJ et al: Polydipsia, polyuria, and hypertension associated with renin-secreting Wilms' tumor. *J Pediatr* 92:921, 1978.
35. Hauger-Klevene JH: High plasma renin activity in an oat cell carcinoma: A renin-secreting carcinoma? *Cancer* 26:1112–1114, 1970.
36. Bruckstein AH et al: Reversible hypertension due to carcinoma of the ureter. *Am J Med* 66:358, 1979.
37. Valentine WN et al: Polycythemia: Erythrocytosis and erythremia. *Ann Intern Med* 69:587, 1968.
38. Curth HO: Cutaneous manifestations associated with malignant internal diseases, in TB Fitzpatrick et al (eds): *Dermatology in General Medicine,* McGraw-Hill, p 1561, 1971.
39. Robinson DR et al: Clinical pathological conference (osteoarthropathy). *N Engl J Med* 299:708, 1978.
40. Greco AF, Kushner I: Loss of symptoms of pulmonary hypertrophic osteoarthropathy after laparotomy (letter). *Ann Intern Med* 81:555, 1974.

41. Fischer DS et al: Clubbing: A review, with emphasis on hereditary acropachy. *Medicine (Baltimore)* 43:459, 1964.
42. Hildebrand J: *Lesions of the Nervous System in Cancer Patients,* European Organization for Research of Treatment of Cancer (EORTC) Monograph Series, Raven Books, New York, vol 5, 1978.
43. Brain WR, Adams RD: Epilogue: A guide to the classification and investigation of neuromuscular disorders with cancer, in L Brain, FH Norris Jr (eds): *The Remote Effects of Cancer on the Nervous System,* Grune & Stratton, New York, p 216, 1965.
44. Van Horn G et al: Progressive multifocal leukoencephalopathy: Failure of response to transfer factor and cytarabin. *Neurology (Minneap)* 28:794, 1978.
45. Levine PM et al: Mental disorders in cancer patients: A study of 100 psychiatric referrals. *Cancer* 42:1385, 1978.
46. Julien J et al: Polyneuropathy in Waldenstrom's macroglobulinemia. *Arch Neurol* 35:423, 1978.
47. Rubinstein MK: Carcinomatous neuromyopathy, the nonmetastatic effects of cancer on the nervous system. *Calif Med* 110:482, 1969.
48. Wasserman SI et al: Tumor-associated eosinophilotactic factor. *N Engl J Med* 290:420, 1974.
49. Pineo GF et al: Tumors, mucus production, and hypercoagulability. *Ann NY Acad Sci* 230:262, 1974.
50. Bedikian A et al: Nonbacterial thrombotic endocarditis in cancer patients: Comparison of characteristics of patients with and without concomitant disseminated intravascular coagulation. *Med Pediatr Oncol* 4:149, 1978.
51. Merskey C: Pathogenesis and treatment of altered blood coagulability in patients with malignant tumors. *Ann NY Acad Sci* 230:289, 1974.
52. Clagett PG, Collins GJ: Platelets, thromboembolism and the clinical utility of antiplatelet drugs. *Surg Gynecol Obstet* 147:257, 1979.
53. Belt RJ et al: Incidence of hemorrhagic complications in patients with cancer. *JAMA* 239:2571, 1978.
54. Bleich HL et al: Pathogenesis of fever in man. *Semin Med Beth Israel Hospital, Boston* 298:607, 1978.
55. Browder AA et al: The significance of fever in neoplastic disease. *Ann Intern Med* 55:932, 1961.
56. Theologides A: The anorexia-cachexia syndrome: A new hypothesis. *Ann NY Acad Sci* 230:14, 1974.
57. Drasin H et al: The importance of nutrition in patients with cancer. *Arch Intern Med* 138:1335, 1978.
58. Fichman M, Bethune J: Effects of neoplasms on renal electrolyte function. *Ann NY Acad Sci* 230:448, 1974.
59. Robins RA, Baldwin RW: Immune complexes in cancer. *Cancer Immunol Immunother* 4:1, 1978.

SELECTED BIBLIOGRAPHY

Becker KL et al: Urine calcitonin levels in patients with bronchogenic carcinoma. *JAMA* 243:670–672, 1980.

Decaux G et al: Treatment of the syndrome of inappropriate secretion of antidiuretic hormone by urea. *Am J Med* 69:99–106, 1980.

Freibush et al: Tumor-associated nephrogenic diabetes insipides. *Ann Intern Med* 92:797–798, 1980.

Gropp C et al: Ectopic hormones in lung cancer patients at diagnosis and during therapy. *Cancer* 46:347–354, 1980.

Hoeg JM, Slatopolsky E: Cervical carcinoma and ectopic hyperparathyroidism. *Arch Intern Med* 140:569–571, 1980.

Krieger DT, Martin JB: Brain peptides. *New Engl J Med* 304:876–944, 1981.

Livingston RB: The management of paraneoplastic syndromes, in Carter SK et al (eds), *Principles of Cancer Treatment,* McGraw-Hill, New York, 1982, pp 233–236.

Lojek MA et al: Cushing's syndrome with small cell carcinoma of the uterine cervix. *Am J Med* 69:140–144, 1980.

Minna JD, Bunn PA Jr: Paraneoplastic syndromes, in DeVita VT Jr et al (eds), *Cancer: Principles and Practice of Oncology,* Lippincott, Philadelphia, 1982, pp 1476–1517.

Odell WD, Wolfson AR: Hormones from tumors: Are they ubiquitous? *Am J Med* 68:317–318, 1980.

Rose DP: Ectopic hormone syndromes, in Kahn SB et al (eds), *Concepts in Cancer Medicine,* Grune & Stratton, New York, 1983, pp 217–226.

Stewart AF et al: Biochemical evaluation of patients with cancer-associated hypercalcemia. *New Engl J Med* 303:1377, 1980.

49
REHABILITATION AND RECONSTRUCTION FOR THE CANCER PATIENT

J. Herbert Dietz, Jr.

Changes in body function, control, and appearance which are caused by the effects of both cancer and its treatment are varied and may be extensive. Cancer patients may also have other, unrelated forms of disease or disability that increase their handicaps and need for care. Appropriate rehabilitation and reconstruction are required to ensure a high quality of treatment for all patients, no matter what the time frame for survival.

It would be a great service to the cancer patient if the basic goal of cancer treatment could be formulated in terms of "control" rather than "cure." With cancer, as with tuberculosis, recurrent disease at the original or another site is always a possibility, but after the disease is controlled, the patient may return to a relatively normal life. Viewing treatment in this way would eliminate the unfortunate problems created in the past by considering cancer patients eligible for a positive rehabilitation program or for vocational rehabilitation only after a disease-free period of, say, from 2 to 5 years. To interpret rehabilitation as the process of readaptation allows coverage for all patients—those who will recover fully, those who will require supportive care, and those who are faced with a relentless progression of disease and will be treated with palliative measures only.

DISABILITIES

Some disabilities presented by the cancer patient represent a general category, and rehabilitation treatment may not differ essentially from that for problems arising from other diagnostic backgrounds. There are, however, disabilities specifically related to cancer or its treatment, such as (1) neuromyopathies secondary to the remote effects of cancer on the nervous system, (2) secondary effects of treatment agents used, (3) changes related to particular surgical procedures, and (4) focal effects, such as pathologic fractures. Treatment for these may require special consideration. It is impossible to make an accurate judgment of future physical ability or length of time before the patient will be able to engage in useful activities. Therefore it is unrealistic and contrary to good rehabilitation practice to defer the provision of rehabilitation services until the status of the disease or the question of its spread is determined. Rather, appropriate measures should be chosen to ensure maximum independence and level of performance.

The physician's first step in the provision of rehabilitation is early recognition of existing or potential disability. The sequelae of scheduled treatments are known, and early measures should be taken to lessen or prevent disabling effects, to reduce complications, to shorten hospital stay, and to improve performance for the patient. Disability without treatment worsens with time.[1]

Initial examination and evaluation of the patient, and provision of the first orders for rehabilitative care, should be made at the bedside. If the physician waits until the patient has no need left except that for disability care, it may be too late.

The disability encountered may be either acute or

chronic. Acute disability is found in the immediate postoperative period, when there may be respiratory problems, enforced immobilization, pain, fear, and confusion. For surgical cases, preoperative as well as postoperative training and counsel are of benefit. Chronic disability is found when there is a long-lasting handicap. In accordance with each patient's needs and findings there should be an individually prescribed program. Provision should be made for physical and occupational therapy, training in the activities of daily living, and psychosocial evaluation and counseling. The patient should be supplied with such orthotic or prosthetic devices as may be required. Reconstructive surgical procedures may be performed early, but are usually done later in the course of care. Planning for hospital discharge should include realistic advice and direction for the patient's training, living, and, if feasible, work.[2]

GOALS

A realistic goal for rehabilitation should be selected for each patient at the onset of care. Suggested are the categories of *restorative,* if the patient can be expected to become able to return to premorbid status without essential residual handicap; *supportive,* if ongoing disease and handicap must persist but can be reduced by proper training and treatment; and *palliative,* if relentless progress of disease and disability are to be expected but appropriate rehabilitation care will reduce complications, dependency, and pain.

It is essential that the therapists have an appropriate goal and approach for each case. If the therapists have an unrealistic outlook, it will be easy for them to feel defeated if the patient fails. It will be hard to keep proficient therapists at work in a cancer setting if they feel destroyed emotionally by the losses they have to face. Prescription for adaptive treatment must have a stated, realistic goal; that is, the goal can be stated in terms of temporary help, of support of general treatment, or of helping provide a restorative end result. This is not a matter of denial to any patient of an all-out effort. Rather, it is a matter of striving for what can be reasonably gained by that all-out effort.

In a hospital for acute diseases the length of time available for provision of a rehabilitation program can range from 1 day to several weeks. Only 1 in 5 patients is hospitalized long enough to receive treatment for over 30 days. Most must be given rehabilitation treatment during the 1 to 2 weeks before discharge. This contrasts sharply with the situation in rehabilitation centers. However, a small number of patients cannot be accepted for treatment with rehabilitation goals because of individual findings or complications, or because of their refusal of care.

Regardless of the goal classification or the type of disability, early availability of care is important. The advantages of early and dynamic assistance and readjustment include prevention of deterioration from disuse and bed rest, support of increased ability to function, development of motivation to comply with the treatment program, and minimization of depression.[1]

The social service worker can make detailed inquiry into the family structure and develop intimate knowledge of the living and working conditions to be faced by the patient after discharge from the hospital. The family must be included in planning and functional assistance, as appropriate. The psychologist or psychiatrist and the vocational counselor may be needed to provide valuable assistance and should be called for guidance and instruction whenever indicated.

Although the majority of patients with a cancer diagnosis are in the employable age group, the ultimate objective of job placement is often difficult to attain. If a change in career must be made, the vocational counselor can direct the patient toward possible reemployment or retraining. For example, amputation of a lower extremity may make little difference in the working life of a person whose job was primarily sedentary. But for those whose work demanded mobility, a complete change in vocation and living arrangements may be necessary. Drastic change will certainly be necessary for patients whose work depended on the use of both hands. All such patients should be referred at the earliest possible moment to a social worker, and then to a vocational rehabilitation counselor for evaluation and aid. Training and job selection, and subsequent acceptance by an employer, often require a great deal of effort.[2] The vocational problems encountered by the patient with cancer are discussed in more detail at the end of this chapter.

Any patient needing further rehabilitation following discharge should be treated as an out-patient or by a physical therapist or visiting nurse at home. Occasionally, patients are candidates for admission to a rehabilitation center for intensive care.

Patient disabilities depend both on the anatomic region or organ system affected by the cancer and on the treatment given. Surgery is ablative or may otherwise interfere with function. Radiation therapy and chemotherapy cause reactions due both to tissue change and to toxicity. These frighten and distress the patients, and so add emotional complications.

CANCERS OF THE BONES AND SOFT TISSUES OF THE EXTREMITIES

Tumors of the bone and soft tissues of the extremities affect individuals of all ages. Rehabilitation of the patient depends on assessment of individual need (see Table 49-1). Historically, amputation was performed in almost all cases, especially in malignant tumors of bone, unless treatment was for a pathological fracture. Adequate resection of soft tissue sarcomas requires wide excision of surrounding soft tissues, including entire muscle groups, nerves, fascia, and overlapping skin cover. In-continuity regional lymph node dissection is a frequent concomitant procedure. Current approaches to bone cancer may include en bloc wide resections of bone or resection of entire long bones and joints, with total replacement procedures.[3] The aim of such extensive regional bone and soft-tissue removal is preservation of the neurovascular bundle leading to end-organ survival and function. Examples of en bloc resection procedures are (1) the Tikhov-Linberg procedure, with removal of the scapula, shoulder joint, and upper humerus, but preservation of the forearm and hand; (2) varied procedures involving total removal of femur, knee, and proximal tibia, with internal prosthetic replacement, and (3) the Van Ness turnoplasty, with knee region resection and attachment of cut ends of femur and tibia at 180 degrees rotation. These lower-extremity procedures allow preservation of the foot, but this salvage is varied and limited in function and cosmetic appearance. Long-term function in comparison to that following classical procedures is under evaluation.[4]

Reconstruction in surgical procedures may involve internal long-bone prosthetic replacement or implants, with use of cement to speed the patient's return to activity. Vascular reconstruction may be required to preserve a functional extremity distal to the level of surgery. Proper splinting and bracing are needed to support skeleton and joints during rehabilitative functional training.[4]

The patient should be told preoperatively of the implications of the surgical procedure and its sequelae, including phantom sensation. A realistic appraisal of the results of rehabilitation should be offered. No unlikely possibilities should be discussed. The level of amputation should be taken into account, as well as the prognosis of the disease and the patient's general physical status, intelligence, athletic ability, and premorbid way of life. In some cases it is helpful to have a rehabilitated amputee with similar problems demonstrate to the patient what can be expected after the amputation. For suitable patients, preoperative discussion of the possibility of providing an artificial limb increases understanding, confidence, and motivation.

Treatment

PREOPERATIVE TREATMENT

Physical therapy for the patient with lower-extremity disease and disability should start preoperatively whenever possible. It should include training in ambulation using crutches and training in stair climbing, with the affected side non-weight-bearing. Instruction should be given for active exercises of both upper extremities, including shoulder depressors, and of the normal opposite lower extremity. These will familiarize the patient with procedures that will help ensure maximum protective function after surgery.

The upper-extremity patient may be scheduled for amputation or for wide soft-tissue or bone resection. Preoperative adaptive training includes early supportive instruction in one-handed proficiency in activities of daily living. Devices which will be of help, such as rocker knives, special nonslip plates and writing board, and Velcro closures for clothes and shoes, should be demonstrated. Preoperative instruction of this kind is especially important for patients who will lose the use of a dominant upper extremity. Preoperative exercises designed to strengthen any muscle groups which will remain in the limb or stump postoperatively will increase the patient's postoperative confidence and performance efficiency.[4]

OPERATIVE PROCEDURES

Adaptive procedures during the actual surgery include the insertion of metal or ceramic devices that will create stability or improve function in the residual limb or stump. These include metal replacements of proximal humeral shaft, the insertion of an Austin-Moore-type femoral head and proximal shaft in a residual soft-tissue

TABLE 49-1 Rehabilitation in Cancer Cases Involving the Extremities

Disability	Adaptive approach
LOWER EXTREMITY	

Radical resection:
  Muscle group (and nerve ?)
  En bloc or total long-bone resection, with endoprosthesis or replacement
Amputation:
  Translumbar (hemicorporectomy)
  Hemipelvectomy
  Hip disarticulation
  Above-knee
  Below-knee
	Preoperative:
	  Crutch or walker ambulation training, including curbs and stairs, non-weight-bearing on operated side
	  Maintenance exercises, normal extremities and also residual musculature (if any) of operated limb
	Operative:
	  For above-knee amputees, adequate surgical myodesis or myoplasty to ensure stump control
	Immediate Prosthesis:
	  As indicated
	Postoperative:
	  Instruction in standing and ambulation with walker, with progression to crutches; PRN bracing for stability
	  Maintenance and strengthening exercises
	  Stump exercises, stump care and conditioning
	  No pillow under above-knee stump—promote extension at hip
	  Prosthesis prescription
	  Training in prosthesis use

UPPER EXTREMITY	

Radical resection:
  Muscle group (and nerve ?)
  En bloc bone resection, with or without endoprosthesis
Amputation:
  Interscapulothoracic
  Shoulder disarticulation
  Above elbow
	Preoperative:
	  One-handed instruction in activities of daily living
	  Exercises for strength maintenance of remaining muscles, and improvement of range of motion
	Postoperative:
	  One-handed instruction in activities of daily living
	    Shoulder cap prosthesis for interscapulothoracic cases
	    Cosmetic arm, on patient demand
	  Upper-extremity prosthesis with training in use, especially if support is adequate or there is residual functional stump

PATHOLOGICAL FRACTURE	
Intramedullary nailing or hip joint replacement	Active exercises and range of motion Ambulation and elevation training with initial limited and gradual increased weight-bearing

stump after hip disarticulation, or proximal or total femoral shaft replacement. For the above-knee amputee, myoplasty, with suture under slight tension of major muscle groups to the drilled femoral end will allow function and control of the stump not otherwise possible, and will help ensure good postoperative tapered shaping of the stump and good prosthetic fit.

Immediate or early fitting of a temporary prosthesis in the operating room will allow earlier return to function of the amputee than will standard prosthetic procedures.

This is of particular value when there is doubt about long-term survival. Immediate application is also useful for the elderly patient, who may become dangerously weakened if allowed to be inactive for a relatively long time. Also benefitted are patients who have preexisting handicaps involving an opposite lower extremity or upper extremities. For example, the patient who already has lost the adductive function of the pectoralis major muscle or muscles following unilateral or bilateral radical mastectomies may have great difficulty in ambulation with crutches because of functional weakness, and immediate application of prosthesis will greatly help such a patient.

For either immediate or early prosthetic fit there is immediate postoperative application of a light, very thin wound dressing covered by a snug cast of elastic plaster conforming exactly to the contour of the stump. This material, in contrast to elastic bandaging, ceases to create any elastic constrictive pressure as soon as it has hardened, and creates sufficient support to prevent edema and swelling of the stump. In cases of immediate fitting, a pylon prosthesis is attached by the surgeon and the prosthetist while the patient is still on the operating table. The prosthesis is in parts that are connected by coupling devices, and can be adjusted both immediately and subsequently for alignment and length.[5] The rigid support of the plaster cast cuts down on postoperative pain, but patients may complain about painful tightness. Removal of the cast may be felt imperative to evaluate circulation. It should be remembered, however, that removal during the initial days postoperatively allows immediate stump swelling, which may interfere with replacement of the cast after 10 to 15 min. Removal should be dictated by such findings as elevated temperature, pulse rate increase, and odor suggesting infection. Immediate replacement should be made if patient intolerance has been the only cause.

In the case of early fitting, the prosthesis is applied 10 to 14 days after surgery, when the operative dressing is first changed and the skin sutures are removed. If no complications are present at that time and the condition of the stump is satisfactory, an elastic plaster mold is immediately taken of the stump for attachment to the pylon, and a tight plaster dressing is applied to maintain stump shape and prevent edema.[5,6]

Use of these and other forms of total-contact prosthesis as soon as possible after amputation creates an increased proprioceptive sense and utilizes the phantom sensation present. The properly snug application of the elastic plaster is essential to either immediate or early fitting. Subsequent treatment for both includes general strengthening exercises for the other extremities, stump conditioning, stump exercises, and training in ambulation with the new prosthesis.[6] Success in immediate or early application of prosthesis depends on the proper and secure attachment, at the time of surgery, of the muscles and fascia to or over the bone end, so as to afford good stump control.

POSTOPERATIVE TREATMENT

Patients who have a stump need an exercise program and instruction in proper positioning of the stump. To prevent flexion contractures at the hip, the above-knee amputee should not be allowed a pillow under the stump, and prolonged sitting should be discouraged. The below-knee amputee should be kept in extension at the knee. This can be helped by the surgical dressing, and some procedures actually include a temporary pin through the joint that keeps it in extension. Isometric exercises for the gluteus and quadriceps muscles repeated throughout the day prevent weakness and instability in later ambulation.[7]

Ambulation training, with an immediate prosthesis or without any prosthesis, should begin as soon postoperatively as the patient's condition and wound healing and stability will allow. Taking chances in this phase of care is not warranted. Initial ambulation training after partial or complete long-bone replacement, with the presence of the distal limb, should be taught non-weight-bearing to toe-touch only. This maximizes the patient's ability to master the techniques that will be necessary for safe mobility. Training in curb mounting and stair climbing during the first 2 to 4 weeks postoperatively will improve the patient's mobility and independence after discharge.

Following amputation most patients have a phantom sensation. If the sensation of the limb is painful or disagreeable, it is referred to as *phantom pain*. Phantom sensation and phantom pain may be constant or intermittent, and the pain may be of varying severity. It is sometimes relieved by simultaneous efforts to "exercise" both the phantom and the normal limb.

Neuromas forming in the amputation stump may be a source of pain. The cut end of every nerve develops a degree of neuroma, which is usually painless if adequately protected. Neuromas subjected to pressure may give great pain and require surgical revision. Capping of the cut nerve ends at surgery has been of benefit in some cases.

PROSTHESIS AND BRACES

Prosthetic evaluation and planning should be made and discussed with each patient. The surgeon, the prosthetist, and the physiatrist or physical therapist make up the team that will guide and instruct the patient.

The weeks of convalescence immediately after surgery are crucial. This is the period during which the patient will or will not develop the attitude that will allow the successful use of any prosthetic device and facilitate the patient's return to society. The question of whether a prosthesis should be prescribed and, if so, what type, comes up for every amputee.[8] A patient's strengths and weaknesses—physical, emotional, vocational, intellectual, and social—must be considered when making a decision. Factors other than the stump or the level of amputation may affect the use of a prosthesis or make it inadvisable to prescribe one. Such factors include severe cardiorespiratory disease, contralateral hemiplegia, prior radical mastectomy, preexisting physical disability, senility, and others. The use of a temporary articulated prosthesis will both answer questions regarding prognosis and help to avoid or to reverse many of the problems of the new amputee.[8] A pneumatic-support prosthesis may be used earlier than one which applies rigid pressure.

In the management of children who are amputees, the restored function and improved appearance afforded by a prosthesis are of practical and psychological value to both the child and the parents. In studies made at New York University a significant percentage of child amputees with malignancies survived 1 to 5 years postoperatively and wore their prosthesis successfully for a year or longer, the majority of them full time. Disease controls have improved since then, and delay in non-contraindicated prosthetic restoration is unjustifiable. The expenditure of time and money involved is justified by the rehabilitation results. If proper prosthesis and training are provided, successful independent ambulation may be accomplished by a 3-year-old child, even after a hemipelvectomy.

Although the cost of an artificial limb is high, it is equivalent to the cost of about a week of hospitalization. Early fitting is important. Changes that may be necessary in socket type and size are also less costly than keeping the patient in the hospital for a prolonged period, waiting for the stump to shrink.[1,7]

Clothing for amputees should be as similar as possible to clothing worn by nonamputees. It should, however, be loose at the point at which it covers the prosthesis to allow room for the sockets and joints, which are frequently bulky.

Psychological adjustment to a prosthesis depends on the realization that the prosthesis is a tool for performing certain activities. Because of the harnessing, the artificial arm cannot be used above the head or behind the back. The upper-extremity amputee must have visual control at all times. The lower-limb prosthesis is effective for one-gait cadence only. Almost all units present difficulties when the patient tries to go up or down steps or inclines, and special instruction is required. It is important to discuss these facts so that the amputee is not deluded into believing that fitting and training with the artificial limb will result in an "almost normal" condition.

The amputee must understand that prostheses have an unstable attachment to the skeletal system, that they feel heavier than the normal limb, that there is a false joint between the prosthesis and the body (leading to socket instability and bell-clapper type of motion that may cause skin irritation), and that perspiration in the socket can result in maceration of the skin. Loss of sensory feedback occurs after all amputations, and this loss is more keenly felt by the upper- than the lower-extremity amputee.

The patient who has had a wide en bloc resection of soft tissue or bone has lost some or all of the power of large muscle groups, as well as control of limb function and support. The lower-extremity patient may, of course, need a knee brace to protect against buckling. The upper-extremity patient may require a static or functional splint for support or motion control. There may be need for a posterior leaf spring ankle brace for foot drop, or a double-bar, short leg brace with a 90 degree dorsiflexion stop to assist toe-off in gait after gastrocnemius function loss.

Bracing is also necessary following long-bone and joint replacement, such as femur and knee or knee and tibia. It should be remembered, however, that the stabilizing forces of rigid bracing create three points of pressure. These may involve a wound area, and in such cases rigid bracing should be avoided until healing permits the patient to wear the brace. Initial bracing is often best provided by soft-material, wrap-around types such as Jordan splints, or by pneumatic splints.

Every patient who has been given a splint, especially for a lower extremity, needs instruction in its application or donning and in its use during transfers, ambulation, and elevation activities such as stair climbing.

Prosthetic arms for the upper-extremity amputee

with a stump or after a shoulder disarticulation can be functional. Prescription and instructions for use depend on the amount of support by the stump and on stump mobility and length.

The patient with an interscapulothoracic ("forequarter") amputation needs a shoulder-cap replacement prosthesis to support clothing and for shoulder symmetry. For a few patients, a cosmetic, nonfunctional arm and hand may be provided on demand. Experiments are being conducted in many centers on fabrication of a functional prosthesis for such patients, either powered by harness or by myoelectric control. Limited success has been reported, but the cost of the prosthesis is greater than most patients can consider. It is hoped that further research will improve the product.

PATHOLOGIC FRACTURES

Primary or metastatic tumors involving bone destroy the bony architecture, and pathologic fractures may threaten or may occur. No passive, or more than gentle, assistance for range of motion is to be given in the presence of metastatic disease of bone, with or without treated or impending pathologic fractures, unless the stability of the bony architecture will permit the associated stress.

The characteristics of an impending fracture include radiographic evidence of a significant lytic area with destruction of 50 percent or more of the bone diameter, or cortical erosion to an extent equal to the diameter, and persistent pain after completion of radiation therapy. Lane recommends evaluation of the patient's prognosis before making decisions regarding management of pathologic fractures.[3] He sets an anticipated life-span of greater than 1 month as the criterion for planning open reduction and fixation. It is also important to consider possible pulmonary involvement or dysfunction, hypercalcemia, and thrombocytopenia or leukopenia, as well as systemic spread of disease.

Appropriate orthopedic surgery, using intramedullary nailing or joint replacement, and radiation therapy will allow physical therapy to include mobilization of the patient. Gentle, active range-of-motion exercises of the involved extremities should be started as soon as the operating surgeon permits.

MASTECTOMY

Currently accepted surgical approaches to breast cancer treatment depend on pathologic findings and clinical variance. There are a variety of procedures, ranging from extended radical, radical, modified radical, and Patey modified radical to occasional simple mastectomies with or without axillary dissection. Involvement of the chest wall entails chest wall resection. Adaptive rehabilitation depends on the disability (Table 49-2).

Radical mastectomy involves removal, along with the breast, of the pectoralis major and pectoralis minor muscles, although some modified procedures preserve the pectoralis major. In almost all cases the long thoracic and thoracodorsal nerves are preserved, but occasional sacrifice of a nerve may occur. Postoperative physical disability is principally related to the loss of the pectoral muscle, and the patient has decreased functional efficiency in horizontal adduction at the shoulder, in abduction and flexion above 90 degrees, and in chopping motion. For example, golfing and tennis will be affected. The muscle that is most effective in substitution is the deltoid in its anterior and middle portions. Some loss of power of shoulder depression will result, which may cause the patient to have a problem in ambulation with crutches, should this need arise. Winging of the scapula will occur when the long thoracic nerve has been divided.

Resections of the chest wall result in local instability and create problems in range of motion and strength in the shoulder on the operated side. Response to physical therapy is slower than after a standard radical mastectomy.

Treatment

PREOPERATIVE TREATMENT

The mastectomy patient is usually dismayed and confused by the impact of the diagnosis and the prospect of hospitalization. These patients are candidates for rehabilitation in both the preventive and restorative areas. If possible, orientation to mastectomy should begin before the surgical procedure. Proper preoperative counsel and instruction can reduce the psychological impact of the postoperative discovery of the mastectomy. Preventive preoperative orientation and support should be started by the operating surgeon and the nurse in the office at the time of finding of a lesion on initial office examination. This can be particularly helpful in reducing the number of unknowns that generate fear and anxiety in the patient. Helpful information for both the patient and her family can be supplied, before admission, by a record or tape which gives advice about the particular hospital's standard procedures of admission. Such in-

TABLE 49-2 Rehabilitation in Mastectomy Cases

Postmastectomy sequelae	Adaptive approach
Psychological	
Fear	Intensive reassurance and support
Anxiety	Recorded and written material for teaching and problem solution
Depression	Psychological and psychiatric therapy, as required
Disappointment	
Severe emotional distress	
Physical	
Decreased range of shoulder motion	Range of motion exercises, individual or class
Weakness	Strengthening exercises, individual or class
Pain and paresthesia	Protective covering, nerve block, reassurance
Lymphedema	Instruction in positioning and preventive self-care
Cosmetic	
Asymmetry	Choice of surgical procedure and placement of incision
Infraclavicular depression	Early prosthetic restoration
Presence of scar and absence of mound	Initial external prosthesis, with subsequent individual prosthesis, according to choice
	Surgical reconstruction, if desired and advisable
Chronic Lymphedema	Preventive: positioning for gravity flow, active exercises, intensive instruction in self-care, avoidance of injections or vaccinations in affected arm, vigorous treatment of slightest infection
	Definitive: positioning, intermittent compression apparatus, elastic sleeve, consideration of possible surgical intervention
	Treatment of infection, if any

formation might include descriptions of what to expect in the way of laboratory work and x-rays, recommendations regarding what clothing and personal items to bring, necessary insurance information, and whatever other instructions may be pertinent.[1]

OPERATIVE PROCEDURES

On rare occasions surgical reconstruction or implant for restoration of breast contour may be performed at the time of mastectomy. Such a surgical procedure is in itself a readaptive approach. Breast reconstruction is discussed in the following pages.

Placement of the incision should be made to avoid as much visibility of the scar as possible. A modified radical mastectomy, when possible, will reduce or eliminate infraclavicular depression and better permit later reconstructive surgery.[3,9] Partial mastectomy with axillary dissection requires consideration only of the disability related to the extent of the axillary surgery.

POSTOPERATIVE TREATMENT

Adjustment after surgery has three main goals: aid in emotional adaptation, maintenance of function and range of motion in the arm and shoulder that have been operated on (including self-care instruction and directions aimed at minimizing chance of development of lymphedema), and restoration of external appearance. The patient's reactions—disappointment, depression, anxiety, fear, and occasional anger—may be severe. She requires credible reassurance and encouragement from the surgeon, the nursing staff, the rehabilitation team, and the family. Indifference from hospital service personnel may be misinterpreted by the patient, and may be regarded as having ominous import. All members of the hospital staff need to maintain a consistent approach in their communication with the patient, and must be tolerant, encouraging, and properly instructive.[1]

The early institution of a rehabilitation program after surgery assures best results in restoring physical function and preventing limitation of motion and pain.

On the first postoperative day the nurse should instruct the patient in the performance of routine movements designed to preserve and restore shoulder, arm, and hand function. Postoperative dressings and positioning should keep the arm in abduction and slight elevation. Early postoperative exercises of the forearm and hand assist in the control of edema and improve general circulation.[9]

EXERCISES

A full program of exercises should start as soon postoperatively as permitted by the surgical procedure. The initial exercise program may depend on what operative procedure has been used. Individual patient effort, and degree of range of motion at the shoulder, may be limited by such factors as skin graft, closures under tension, thoracotomy, chest wall resection, fluid collection, infection, and preexisting disability. The exercises should include gradual efforts in active restoration of range of motion at the shoulder and isotonic and isometric strengthening exercises of the arm, forearm, and hand. The patient can assist her own active performance by properly using a rope and overhead pulley (or substitute). She should avoid substitute movements at the wrist, elbow, and waist or overly vigorous efforts when working toward range of motion at her shoulder. Exercises should be repeated five to six times daily by the patient.[9]

The exercises shown in Figs. 49-1 to 49-7 were chosen and taught at the Rehabilitation Service at Memorial Hospital in New York City, with the support and association of the Reach-to-Recovery section of the New York City Division of the American Cancer Society.[10] At Memorial patients attend postmastectomy classes, but the program is also recommended for the individual patient.

On the first day following surgery and on each additional day as required, the patient is shown how to properly position her arm in bed with elevation and a gauze roll or soft ball. (Figure 49-1 shows three correct arm positions.) Hand-squeezing exercises are begun with the arm elevated as high as is comfortable on pillows to promote lymphatic drainage and reduce or prevent postoperative arm swelling. The patient is instructed to continue this elevation and squeezing combination as long as there is still a tendency for the arm to feel heavy or for the hand to swell.

The exercises shown in Figures 49-2 to 49-7 are

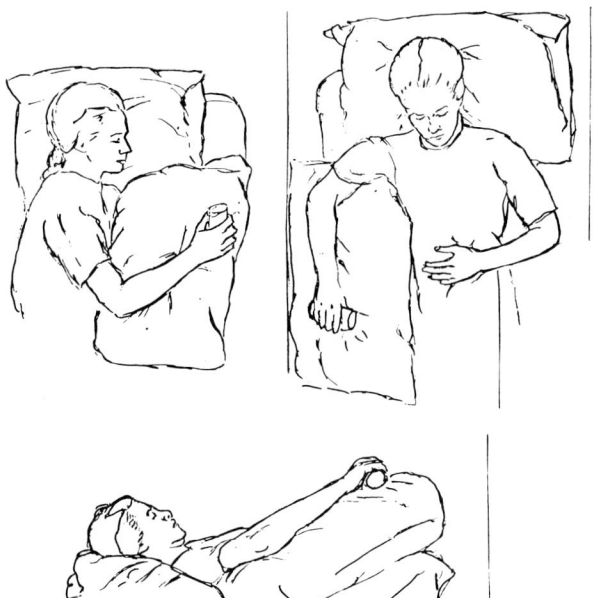

FIGURE 49-1 Arm positions.

designed to restore full range of shoulder motion. The patient is considered to have regained full range of shoulder motion when she is able to reach equally high over her head with *both* hands, with arms held close to her ears.

Exercise 1—Deep Breathing Immediately following surgery the patient is taught breathing exercises to facilitate proper chest wall *excursion* and to produce relaxation when she has discomfort (Fig. 49-2). The patient is instructed to (1) place her uninvolved hand over the center of her chest, (2) take a slow breath in through her nose, feeling her chest expand *fully*, and (3) let all the air out and let her chest and shoulders sag (relaxing fully).

This exercise helps to ease the feeling of tight skin over the chest as well as to relieve the pull and pain that may be caused by reaching in exercise 2. The patient is told to do this breathing exercise by itself frequently during the day.

Exercise 2—Pendulum Swing In this three-part exercise (Fig. 49-3), the uninvolved arm is placed on the back of a chair and the forehead is rested on that arm. The arm on the operated side is allowed to hang loosely until the elbow is straight and the arm and hand are limp. Then:

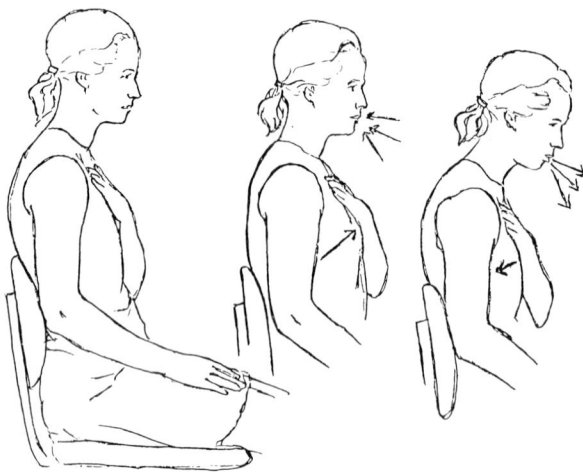

FIGURE 49-2 Breathing exercises.

Part 1. The arm is limply swung from left to right within the comfort range, making sure the motion comes from the shoulder joint and not the elbow. Swing is continued until the arm is relaxed.

Part 2. The arm is swung limply in small circles, again making sure the motion takes place at the shoulder, not the elbow. As the arm relaxes, the size of the circle is increased, staying within comfort range. Circling is then done in the opposite direction.

Part 3. Swing is conducted forward and backward, from the shoulder, within range of comfort.

Exercise 3—Wall Climbing The patient is instructed to face the wall and finger-march her hand up to the level of onset of discomfort. At this point she stops and holds her position, and takes deep breaths to relax tension and discomfort. If she is able, she then proceeds farther. Otherwise she gently finger-marches back down the wall, her point of stance from the wall being dictated by comfort and level of reach. Marked measurements of daily achievement on a wall chart help stimulate her progress. (See Fig. 49-4.)

Exercise 4—Reach and Spread This exercise has four steps (Fig. 49-5); the patient is instructed to do the following:

1. Sit up straight.
2. Clasp her hands together.
3. Slowly raise her hands in the direction of the top of her head. She is instructed that when the incisional area starts to pull slightly, she is to stop, hold that position, and breathe deeply until the pull stops. The hand raising should be repeated until she is able to reach the top of her head. If she has no incisional pain in that position, she can advance to step 4.
4. Advance herself still further by slipping her clasped hands down behind her neck (keeping her head erect). She then gradually spreads her elbows apart, remembering to stop and deep-breathe when pulling or pain occurs. When the pain goes away, she continues to spread her elbows farther apart.

Exercise 5—Pulley exercises In the first part of the pulley exercise the patient is instructed to do the following (Figure 49-6):

1. Place the rope over a secure hook such as a clothes hook. Place the back of a chair under the rope. Sitting up straight, grasp the rope as high as she can, first with her uninvolved hand.

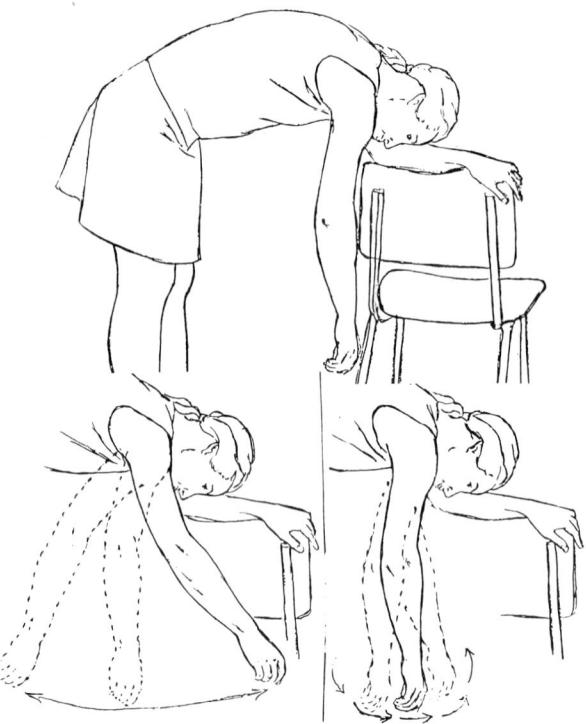

FIGURE 49-3 Limp arm swing.

REHABILITATION AND RECONSTRUCTION FOR THE CANCER PATIENT   1051

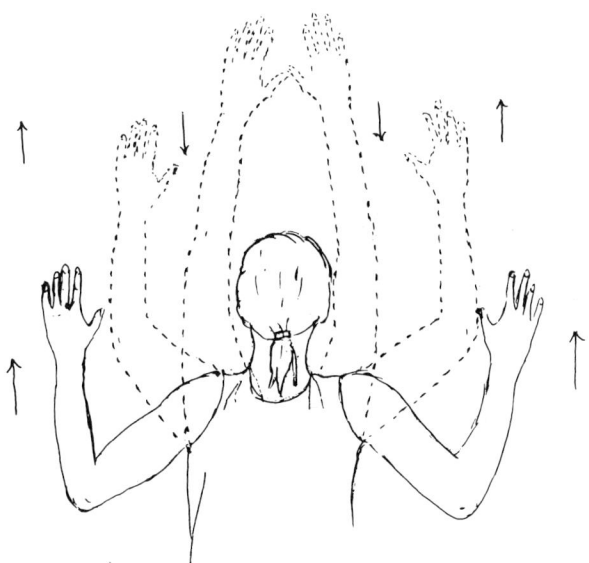

FIGURE 49-4 Wall climbing.

2. With the involved arm, reach or creep up the rope until she starts to feel incisional discomfort. She stops at that level and loops the rope around her hand, letting both arms hang limply while holding the rope.
3. Deep-breathe until all the pulling or pain goes away.

In the second part of the pulley exercise the patient is instructed to (Fig. 49-7):

1. Pull her involved arm upward slowly by pulling down with her good arm, stopping when pulling or pain in the incision occurs.
2. Hang in that position, deep-breathing until all incisional pulling or pain stops. She repeats from step 1 until she is able to get as high with the involved arm as with the uninvolved arm.

TEAM INSTRUCTION

Daily consistent instruction from the immediate postoperative days until time of discharge should be provided for each patient by a team consisting of a physical therapist, a nurse, a social worker, and a lay volunteer from the Reach-to-Recovery program. The fact that there is repetition and overlap in the areas of attention which are divided among the team members is expected.

Such overlap is a valuable part of any program of instruction.

The physical therapist should provide instruction in exercises involving hand and arm use and for increase in range of shoulder motion. All exercises should be tailored to fit the needs of individual cases. The therapist should distribute such informational literature as may be available from the hospital and the American Cancer Society. The nurse who has seen the patient preoperatively and reassured her about care after surgery should then see her at bedside on the first postoperative day and describe the program to follow. The areas covered should include wound and arm care, precautions concerning development of lymphedema, bed and arm

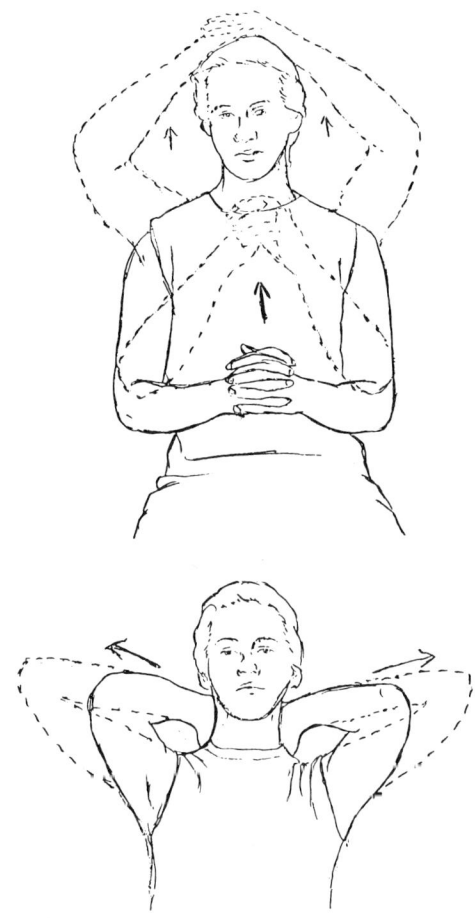

FIGURE 49-5 Reach and spread.

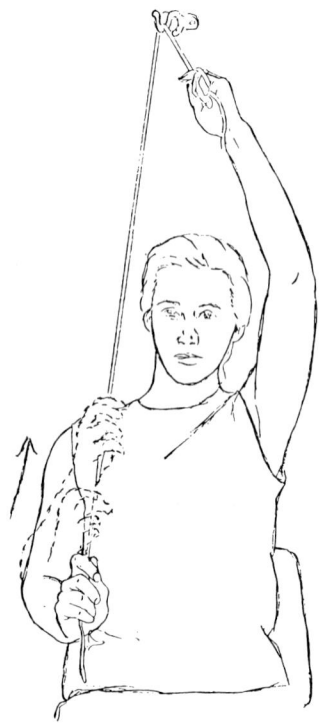

FIGURE 49-6 Pulley exercises.

The patient should be given a temporary prosthesis as soon after surgery as possible in order to provide the psychological support afforded by symmetry of appearance. As early as the first postoperative day a stretch-type "sleep bra" can be provided, which can be filled out with a fluff of gauze or pad of cotton and worn over the patient's dressing. Next, in the early postoperative period, a lightweight air-filled plastic unit placed in the empty brassiere cup can be used as a temporary prosthetic device. A permanent prosthesis can be recommended later. Any member of the team can instruct the patient in use of the prosthesis.

Lymphedema

Approximately 50 percent of mastectomy patients at some point experience a degree of postoperative edema in the arm on the side that has been operated on. There is marked variation in the areas of the arm that become involved, in the time of initial occurrence of the edema, and in its persistence. Slight swelling that may occur in the early postoperative period usually subsides. Swelling

positioning and activity, activities of daily living, clothing, breast prostheses, and home activities and planning. The social worker should direct the rest of the team's attention to the patient's emotional, social, family, community, occupational, and avocational needs, and should provide general as well as personal counseling, at the bedside, in the class, and with the family. The Reach-to-Recovery volunteer fits in well with the team, serving both as an example to the patients of successful physical rehabilitation and personal adjustment and as an experienced source for answers to questions relating to return to family and participation in social functions. The Reach-to-Recovery volunteer can also provide postdischarge contacts and help the patient to cope with personal problems.[10]

All team members should always refer patients to their physicians for answers to those questions which relate to diagnosis, prognosis, differences in surgical technique, medications, radiation therapy, or chemotherapy.

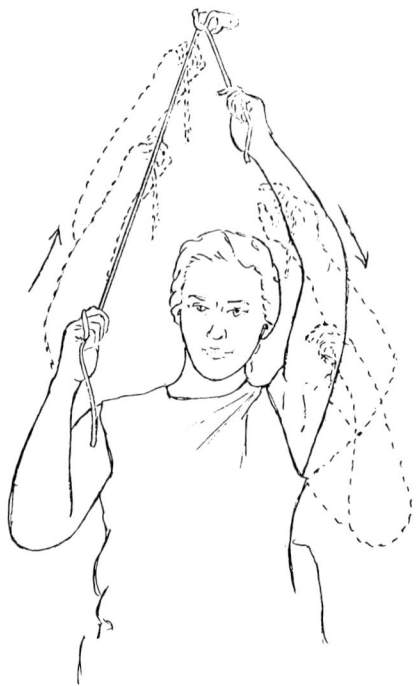

FIGURE 49-7 Pulley exercises.

that occurs weeks or months after surgery is more likely to be persistent or progressive. Disability as a result of lymphedema is proportional to the extent of the edema and the disfigurement it creates. Lymphedema may occur a year or more following institution of supervoltage radiation therapy as a result of fibrosis in subcutaneous tissues. Its actual causes have not been documented, but channel obstruction due to scar tissue and fibrosis is fundamental.[7]

If lymphedema becomes a persistent problem, the patient may require both treatment and continuation of preventive measures to provide protection from factors that may aggravate the condition.

Treatment for lymphedema is varied. The patient should be taught proper attention to elevated positioning of the extremity to promote gravity flow of tissue fluids. Salt-free diets, diuretics, massage, mechanical aids for intermittent compression, elastic sleeves, and various surgical procedures all have value. The intermittent compression must be for frequent short periods daily (20 to 30 min each, five to six times a day) to be effective, and may need the concomitant use of a properly fitted elastic sleeve, often with a separate elastic gauntlet to support the hand. Intermittent compression may be effected by the use of a mechanical apparatus or by a simple pneumatic sleeve with attached blood pressure gauge operated by the patient. Antibiotics may be of value if subclinical infection is suspected, and are mandatory if infection is diagnosed. Compression or massage should not be used where there is potential infection or recurrent carcinoma in the tissues to be handled.

Numerous surgical procedures have been tried. A few have met with some success. Goldsmith has reported success in controlling postmastectomy lymphedema by transposing the partially detached omentum beneath the superficial tissues of the chest wall to the axilla and upper arm.[11] The insertion of nylon threads in the subcutaneous fat has been used to maintain channels to conduct tissue fluids. Amputation occasionally is performed to relieve a patient of a useless and intolerably painful upper extremity. Training in independence in the one-handed performance of activities of daily living will help free the patient from dependence on others, whether she is suffering from disability from lymphedema or has had an amputation performed.

In the prevention of lymphedema, infection must be meticulously avoided and antibiotics used liberally, especially if there is any necrosis of the wound margin, fluid beneath the wound flaps, or a suggestion of infection in the arm on the operated side. Mastectomy patients should not have venipuncture, blood tests, vaccinations, or infusions in the arm on the operated side, and they should be warned about the danger of burns, sunburns, and infection in the fingers or hand. In case of burn or infection, they should seek immediate care. Whenever possible, blood pressure determinations should be taken on the arm opposite the side that has been operated on.

In the postoperative period specific and detailed instructions should be given that are directed at reducing the incidence and severity of lymphedema. The following list of do's and don'ts, covering protection of the patient's hand and arm on the operated side from injury, should be given out and discussed.

1. Avoid possible burns. If smoker, hold cigarette in opposite hand. Wear padded, nonflammable gauntlet gloves when reaching into oven.
2. Leave cuticles alone or use cuticle cream; never cut cuticles.
3. Wear canvas gloves when gardening. Wear rubber gloves when using steel wool for any cleaning.
4. Keep watchband and jewelry loose on operated arm.
5. Keep dress sleeves and underclothing straps loose on operated arm and shoulder. Avoid elastics.
6. Use unaffected arm to carry heavy purse and packages.
7. Use unaffected arm for blood pressure check, injections, vaccinations, blood samples, etc.
8. Wear a thimble when sewing. Avoid pricking fingers with needle.
9. Wash the smallest break in the skin on the operated side immediately with soap and water and cover with a bandage. Check afterward for unusual soreness, which indicates possible infection, and have checked by a physician if suspicious.
10. Use electric razor for shaving underarm. Avoid nicks and scrapes.
11. Never get sunburned. Get tanned very gradually.
12. Call physician if arm on the operated side pains or aches and feels hot, tender, reddened, or swollen.
13. Keep regular appointments for medical checkups. Continue normal activities and hobbies.
14. Avoid using the arm that has been operated on in rapid movements or for heavy work; avoid movement that is circular in nature, since such movement tends to force tissue fluids toward the hand and increase venous pressure.

15. Check with your doctor before using any creams or cosmetics containing hormones.

Convalesence

Most of the exercises that are started in the hospital should be continued at home, and the patient should be appropriately instructed. Dependent-position exercises, for example, Codman's exercises, designed to reduce congestion and prevent edema, are limited to the first two postoperative weeks. Gentle, nonrapid performance at home of all activities of daily living is the ideal goal.

In an attempt to handle efficiently and effectively the many questions and fears which arise postoperatively in the patient's mind, Dr. Guy Robbins, at Memorial Sloan–Kettering Cancer Center, directed both tape and LP recordings of an informal panel discussion between three mastectomy patients, a nurse, and a physician, led by a moderator. This proves helpful if given to the patient a few days after surgery, so that she can play and replay it to herself to obtain reassurance and answers to her own questions. This avoids failure of communication between doctor and patient, and possible embarrassment for the patient, and saves much time for the doctors. This material, or similar material developed by the physician, can also be put on a tape cassette.

During the convalescence period the patient should continue to be visited daily by the rehabilitation team. This consistent support has been found to resolve problems that might otherwise persist. The patient should be encouraged to perform all regular activities of daily living as soon as these activities can be tolerated and will not place undue stress on the area of any specific operative procedure. Normal activities involving use of the arm and hand on the side that has been operated on should be encouraged and repeated frequently each day to maintain strength and range and to help reduce the incidence of lymphedema. Rapid or strenous repetition of circular movement exercises using the arm on the side that has been operated on are discouraged, as they tend to have a centrifugal effect, causing distal circulatory congestion and increased accumulation of interstitial fluid.

Family members—especially teenage daughters—should be given an understanding of the operative procedure and its effects. This can reduce much of the possible shock and distress. Such understanding helps the husband in facing and supporting his wife and contributes to the emotional and physical recovery of the patient. If there are children at home, it improves their relationship with their mother. Printed brochures suggesting approaches in this area have been set up by the American Cancer Society.

Involved staff should frankly encourage the patient to contemplate and expect a return to previous sexual and interpersonal family activities. Avoidance of these subjects may lead to misconceptions and emotional stress. The patient may fear that loss of a breast will mean loss of desirability, and the husband may fear that intercourse will harm his wife. Both may fear a reaction to the sight of the wound. Early postoperative viewing of the wound by the patient and her husband will allow their initial reactions to subside before the patient leaves the protective environment of the hospital. Early acceptance of the surgical procedure and the loss of the breast, together with the desire and need for one another, will advance a healthy return to family and sex life.[9]

Transitional and Posthospital Care

A "couples group" meeting with the social worker and the physical therapist or nurse held one evening each week can serve to air such topics as the wound itself, personal appearance, sexual activities, sports, work, and other related aspects of return to home and society. The couple may be patient and husband or patient and close friend.

External Prosthesis

When considering external prosthetic replacement of the amputated breast, the patient's attitude toward her figure and appearance, her economic status, and her body build must be taken into account.

Satisfactory prostheses can be purchased for reasonable prices in most department stores and at stores that sell women's underclothing. Elaborate, custom-made units are available, but these can be extremely expensive, perhaps costing hundreds of dollars.

There is a prosthesis for any type of figure. Some are simple rubber forms for small-breasted women, and others are weighted with various materials to simulate and balance the light or heavy breast on the opposite side. All patients can obtain an appropriate prosthesis for swimwear.

After a mastectomy, most women are concerned about their wardrobe. They worry about postoperative evidence of deformity, including infraclavicular depression and exposure of scar. Occasionally, there is discomfort caused by cold or by clothing rubbing against an area made sensitive by the operation.

Clothing alterations can usually be minimal. Desired masking can be accomplished with capes, stoles, short jackets, shoulder decorations, and appropriate choice of new garments. Sleeves should be chosen in relatively loose and comfortable styling. Bathing suits with halter-neck fronts are recommended, and slight modifications will make many other styles entirely satisfactory. Discussions between the patient and the nurse and a volunteer from the Reach-to-Recovery program of the American Cancer Society can solve most problems and relieve anxiety.[9]

Postmastectomy Breast Reconstruction

Many patients who have had a mastectomy are candidates for breast reconstruction. Reconstruction is rarely done at the time of initial mastectomy. A minimum waiting period of 3 months is usually necessary, and some surgeons prefer to wait 6 months to 1 year. In fact, some patients lose their desire for reconstructive surgery if they have achieved satisfactory adjustment after 6 to 12 months. There is actually no wait which is surgically "too long."

Reconstruction may be by implant or by plastic rebuilding with free fascia or omental graft.[3,18] If the remaining breast is too large to be easily matched by implant or surface prosthesis, contralateral reduction mammoplasty may be advisable.[9]

Favorable factors for surgical reconstructive procedures are good prognosis, presence of adequate residual skin for coverage of an implant, minimal scarring, preservation of the pectoralis major muscle, and potential for matching breast contour. Consideration must also be made of possible banking of the nipple-areola complex.

Factors that might be contraindications to surgical reconstruction include skin grafts in the closure, surgical defect or loss of contour and integrity of the underlying chest wall, and possible preoperative radiation therapy or ongoing postoperative chemotherapy. Masking of local or chest wall recurrence is not felt to be a risk after reconstruction or implant and is therefore not a contraindication.

Complications in appropriately selected patients occur in about 10 percent of cases and usually can be effectively handled. They include hemorrhage and hematoma, skin breakdown due to stretch and pressure, infection, and firm reactionary scar encapsulation of the prosthesis. Removal of the implant may be needed for control.[3]

The result of most reconstructive procedures is appropriate contour rather than breast likeness-to-normal for any uncovered display. Scarring varies in extent and appearance. Any need for advancing of chest-wall or back skin for defect closures increases the disfigurement.[3]

Complications

If the patient's therapeutic approach has included radiation therapy, the related complications of paresthesia or lymphedema tend to develop late. Skin reactions are seldom seen. Axillary web formation in the scar is also infrequently seen, as current surgical techniques keep the incision line out of the axilla itself. Should such a web develop, the patient may need a plastic repair for release.

Pain in the chest wall or in the pectoralis major muscle following modified radical procedures may respond to moist, warm pack applications followed by range-of-motion exercises for the shoulder (Figures 49-2 to 49-7). These exercises are particularly beneficial when performed in a heated, therapeutic pool. If pain persists, intercostal nerve block may be tried with novocaine. If pain is temporarily relieved, but recurs, permanent block or intercostal nerve section may be considered. Usually the pain eventually subsides to within tolerance levels without radical treatment approaches. The feeling of tightness of the chest wall of which some patients complain also usually subsides without radical intervention.

Occasionally a patient may show evidence of an underlying psychological instability and be unable to face reality. She will require psychiatric advice and therapy. A young patient may be advised to avoid pregnancy and, occasionally, to consider the possibility of sterilization. Such advice must be presented with sympathetic understanding and careful explanation.

Palliative Procedures

To this point consideration has been of rehabilitation of the postmastectomy patient with a restorative goal. Palliative programs, varying according to the needs or disabilities presented, can be offered to the patient who has advanced cancer of the breast with metastases. These patients are candidates for adaptive rehabilitation, with a goal of support, to obtain maximum independence in physical function, comfort, work performance, and emotional stability.

Selected programs should consider the disability in the light of the prognosis, with a realistic attempt at attaining performance levels which can be maintained for the longest period of time. For example, physical therapy for the patient with low cord compression and paraparesis should not be restricted to improving performance in ambulation. Independent ambulation for such patients may be, at best, of short duration, and instruction should be provided in performance of the activities of daily living in a wheelchair. The patient should not be told that use of a wheelchair is inevitable; rather the instruction should be offered as a technique that can be used whenever it may be of benefit.[1,9]

Spine lesions due to metastatic deposits in the vertebrae, at whatever level, can be made less painful with the use of cervical collars or appropriate back braces that limit range of motion. The patient should be taught back-sparing approaches to the activities of daily living. Radiation therapy may also be useful in reducing pain. On occasion, a bivalved, laminated lightweight plastic jacket can be molded to fit the patient's body from chin and occiput to pelvis, to permit mobilization out of bed which would otherwise be impossible because of pain.

Pathologic fractures treated by intramedullary nailing require bracing. Ambulation training and training in upper-extremity active and assistive exercises are also necessary. Patients who have undergone hip and shoulder joint replacement procedures done for the treatment of local bone metastases, with or without pathologic fractures, must be provided with programs of activity and appropriate support as promptly following surgery as tissue healing will allow.

Neurologic deficits, such as paralysis and pain due to brachial plexus involvement by tumor, require sling support, and an assistive exercise program must also be provided. Patients with paraplegia or paralysis from spinal cord compression by a metastatic lesion, whether treated by radiation therapy or decompression laminectomy, should be given training in transfer activities, wheelchair independence, and whatever ambulation is possible using parallel bars, walker, crutches, or canes. Extensive bracing is not recommended for these patients.

Occasionally, patients who have undergone hypophysectomy, or those with intracranial metastatic lesions, may later develop hemiparesis or hemiplegia. These patients will respond to appropriate training with improved function and independence.

Patients with advanced pulmonary complications will benefit from training in adequate voluntary breathing and coughing control, as well as postural drainage.

Walkers, crutches, canes, wheelchairs, and other devices should be provided for the patient as appropriate for reduction of the handicap. The patient who is confined to bed should be trained to achieve self-care in bed, including turning, and attention should be paid to relief of possible pain.

When the patient can be discharged, the medical social worker can assist in outlining plans for improvement in the home setup, particularly the bathroom and the kitchen, to increase independence and patient utilization of facilities. If the patient will need to mount stairs, training should be given in climbing and descending stairs with a stairclimbing walker or with crutches and bannister.[4,9]

CANCER OF THE BOWEL AND URINARY BLADDER

Resection of the rectum and distal sigmoid colon for cancer frequently requires that the patient learn to live with a colostomy. Ileostomy is performed less frequently, but an ileal conduit bladder commonly results from radical bladder and genitopelvic surgery. These stomas result in loss of sphincter control in elimination. Each type of stoma requires different techniques of care and rehabilitation assistance.

Colostomy

PREOPERATIVE TREATMENT

Rehabilitation is of great importance and should start as soon as possible during the preoperative stage. Table 49-3 gives the adaptive approaches used in cancer cases of the bowel following colostomy. If preoperative check of the patient's occupation indicates that intermittent pressure at work will involve repeated stimulation, stoma placement may be recommended preoperatively.

Preoperative examination of the abdomen in standing, sitting, and lying positions with skin marking of the colostomy site will avoid stoma loss into a fold of fat or traction due to position change of dependent tissue.

The shock of finding the artificial stoma is lessened if appropriate advance knowledge and reassurance are provided. The patient may benefit from the visits of a volunteer who has successfully managed a colostomy, known as an "ostomate." Such a visit should be made only with the permission of the operating surgeon. The

TABLE 49-3 Rehabilitation for Cancer Cases Involving the Bowel Following Colostomy

Disability	Adaptive approach
Immediate:	Preoperative:
Depression	Counseling and reassurance
Anxiety	Introduction of volunteer ostomate
Leakage and soiling	Operative:
Odor	Proper placement of stoma
Noisy expulsion of gas	Immediate postoperative dressing to include collecting bag, when stoma open
Social withdrawal	
Loss of sexual potency	Postoperative:
	Early reassurance
	Expert, consistent daily care by same person in irrigation instruction
	Predischarge planning and directions
	Home activities and work planning
	Avoidance of dietary indiscretion
Late:	Regular follow-up
Persistence of immediate problems	Dilation
Stomal stricture	Surgical revision
Bowel loop angulation	Instruction and proper medication
Travel problems	Work and habit adjustment, with inclusion of employer instruction and reassurance
Work interference	

help of an ostomate can be of help both preoperatively, when the patient may be experiencing fear of death, and postoperatively, when the patient is beginning to learn techniques of self-care and needs an example to follow for reassurance that activities of daily life can successfully be resumed. If an "ostomy club" exists in the patient's community, the patient can be encouraged to visit and obtain help from this unit.[1]

OPERATIVE CARE

Attempts should be made to prevent any early distressing postoperative experience for the patient of massive evacuation and soiling. The possibility of soiling can be minimized in the operating room by inclusion in the immediate postoperative dressing of a disposable plastic collecting bag unit when the stoma margins are sutured open to the skin.

POSTOPERATIVE TREATMENT

The presence of a colostomy may create severe adjustment problems for the patient. There may be periods of leakage, noisy expulsion of gas, and odor, with resultant anxiety and embarrassment and often marked social withdrawal. After surgery, bladder control may be lost either temporarily or, in occasional patients, permanently. Impotence occurs about 50 percent of the time in male patients. Perineal area discomfort occasionally results because of the formation of scar tissue.[1]

It is important to select the method of care and the equipment best suited to each patient. Management by irrigation is generally better than management by the less common nonirrigation technique. In management by irrigation a regular enema is given, using a catheter with a special colostomy cover and lead-off apparatus, or a bulb syringe. Commercially made enemas and evacuant suppositories are not consistently satisfactory.

Because of its great impact, the first irrigation should be done in private, under the best circumstances, by an experienced person with ample time and sympathetic understanding. A specially trained nurse or an enterostomal therapist will be of greatest value. The North American Association of Enterostomal Therapists maintains a listing of qualified enterostomal therapists who are available for instruction of patients. Increasing numbers of medical centers are training such therapists.

Continuity of postoperative colostomy care should be provided daily by the same nurse or enterostomal therapist, trained especially in colostomy handling. The patient requires consistent emotional support. Response to training depends on how the patient has been introduced to the diagnosis. Great attention must be paid by the people who care for the patient to provide sympathy and guidance and to avoid any apparent distaste, hostility, or impatience.

Temporary ostomy bags provide early containment of fecal drainage during training in control. They are easier to handle than rubber bags, and they decrease odor. The patient's initial reaction to a colostomy is related to the need for cleanliness, and early bowel control is therefore a primary goal.

A toilet or commode should be used if possible. If the patient must remain lying in bed, a leadoff can be connected to a bedside receptacle. As strength increases, the patient is taught to take over increasing amounts of daily care and, finally, to assume complete care. The patient should have self-administered several irrigations before leaving the hospital. Irrigation equipment appropriate for the method chosen for the individual patient should be provided promptly after the operation. The patient is instructed in the use of this equipment, which becomes the patient's personal property and is taken home for continued use.

The nonirrigation technique is not widely used, but it may have merit when toilet facilities are not satisfactory, when no regulation has been accomplished after trial use of the irrigation method, or when debility, handicap, or old age make any active procedure impossible.

CONVALESCENCE

Choosing the appropriate time for colostomy irrigation involves considering the patient's preoperative living habits and bowel evacuation routine. The best colostomy response to irrigation is about 30 min after a meal, and an hour of uninterrupted time should be available to the patient. Once a time is chosen for a patient for irrigation, that should be the regular hour. If satisfactory control is to be maintained, an effort should be made to adhere to the same time schedule, both in the hospital and later at home.

Usually 7 to 10 days are required to achieve the start of control. Daily irrigation is needed consistently by some patients. Others may be trained to an alternate-day routine.

The amount of water used depends on the method. For catheter equipment, 1 to 2 L is sufficient. Less is needed with the bulb syringe technique. Tepid, plain water is usually adequate, but hard water is helped by addition of 1 teaspoon of bland soap or bicarbonate of soda per liter.

The catheter should be inserted only about 6 in (15 cm). A gentle in-and-out movement of the catheter during irrigation assists the flow into the bowel and also gently stimulates return. Insertion of the catheter should never be done with force. Return of the water may be aided by a slight change of position and also by gentle massage or pressure on the abdomen.[1,7]

The patient should be taught early independence in self-irrigation and proper stoma cleansing, and bag application should be carefully demonstrated. The stoma and surrounding skin should be gently wiped with soft paper to remove feces and mucus, and the surrounding skin should be washed with warm water and soap and gently dried. When there is no irritation, and additional protection is desired, gum Karaya powder may be applied to the skin to enhance the attachment of the adhesive facing about the bag opening. The bag opening should be trimmed to about $\frac{1}{8}$ in (0.3 cm) larger than the colostomy itself to permit adequate adherence and also to prevent bare skin from being irritated by the fecal drainage. Irritated skin about the stoma may be treated with gum Karaya powder, Maalox, or Gelusil. Ointments are not usually recommended.

Ostomy bags are available in many designs. They may be sealed units or openable at the unattached end for emptying purposes. Most are disposable. Many have adhesive applied about the opening. For patients sensitive to adhesive Karaya gum or a Karaya ring can be helpful. Surgical adhesive may also be used. Bags that are not adhesive can be worn with a belt, but these tend to shift position and, therefore, are likely to leak or move away from the stoma. Selection of equipment for the individual patient should include consideration of stoma position, physical limitations and structure, and functional needs in daily living.

Ease of control of the colostomy is related to its level. Sigmoid and descending colon colostomy control are usually gained more promptly and with more dependability than transverse colon colostomy control. Ascending colon colostomy can rarely be controlled with irrigation, and as with ileostomies, there is constant liquid loss. An open-ended disposable plastic bag cover is appreciated by the patient.

Educational materials for the staff and for the patient can be obtained from individual manufacturers of stoma care equipment and from the unit offices of the American Cancer Society.[1,4,9]

TRANSITION AND POSTHOSPITAL CARE

Prior to discharge from the hospital, discussion should cover home plans with the family, so that when the patient reaches home adequate preparations will have been made and needed equipment secured. A visiting nurse may be called in to give a helping hand during the first few days at home to alleviate potential problems.

The time involved in caring for a colostomy, and to a lesser degree the other stomas, may require a change in the patient's and/or family's routine and timetable. Varying degrees of dietary change may be required for a few patients. Many patients report a reduced ability to work. They often change jobs, and some stop work completely.[1,4,7]

The effects of colostomies vary. The patient should be told what might occur and to whom to turn for advice if the problem cannot be simply handled. Control problems include constipation and diarrhea. Constipation usually responds to an increase in fluid intake and ingestion of small amounts of well-diluted milk of magnesia, sipped slowly on an empty stomach about 8 h before irrigation time. Stool softeners are not recommended for colostomy control. Diarrhea may require reduced fluid intake and change of diet. Medication taken for other problems which causes diarrhea as a side effect (diuretics, antibiotics, antihypertensives, and tranquilizers) may have to be discontinued.

Travel or other required changes in daily routine may necessitate changes in type of care of the colostomy. If the patient has to skip irrigation, a bag must be worn as protection against soiling. If the patient travels to a different time zone, the timing of the first irrigation should be based on the time interval since the last irrigation rather than the time of day at the new location. Air travel may require a single dose of paregoric or diphenoxylate with atropine (Lomotil) to reduce the tendency toward increased peristalsis and passage of gas or fecal material stimulated by change in atmospheric pressure, even in pressurized aircraft. The traveler should also be instructed that water in a foreign country that is unsafe to drink is also unsafe to use for irrigation unless it has first been boiled. Mineral waters, bottled or not, often cause diarrhea, at least initially.[1,4]

There may be small amounts of bleeding from the colostomy. These result from minor irritation and do not require specific attention. If bleeding is persistent or greater than spotting, the patient should request medical investigation.

The patient will need family understanding and assistance. However, assistance should be provided only when actually needed. Sexual relations can be maintained according to individual potential. A small cover for the ostomy may be all that is needed during intercourse.

Mutual support and affection between ostomate and family are critical to the success of the patient's tolerance and control of colostomy, and much encouragement and discussion may be needed by the patient.

Regular follow-up facilities should be provided for all patients, since problems may arise and functional changes occur, such as stricture at some level of the stoma. The latter may require local surgical revision to restore adequate functioning, or it may respond to dilation. The patient can be instructed by the surgeon in the technique of dilation of the stoma with a finger covered with a lubricated finger cot. Dilation may be performed daily if necessary, and should be checked regularly by the surgeon.[4]

Ileostomy

PREOPERATIVE TREATMENT

Preoperative care is similar to that required for patients undergoing colostomy.

POSTOPERATIVE TREATMENT

Ileostomy in the cancer patient is usually performed to create a urinary conduit, and drainage is therefore all urinary. Liquid drainage from the ileal urinary conduit is constant, and semiliquid drainage from the functioning ileostomy occurs in spurts. Both forms of drainage are irritating to surrounding skin. This is a particular problem when the drainage contains digestive juices.

An adequate collecting device must be worn at all times both to collect drainage and to protect the skin surfaces surrounding the stoma. The collecting unit may be plastic or rubber. It is part of, or can be detached from, a faceplate. The faceplate attachment to the skin about the stoma must be watertight. Bonding to the skin is effected by a waterproof adhesive. The fit must be exact, and the diameter of the opening, like that of the colostomy, should be no more than a total of $\frac{1}{4}$ in (0.6 cm) greater than that of the stoma (or edges being $\frac{1}{8}$ in (0.3 cm) from the stoma margin). The device should be comfortable and light, and easy to empty, clean, and change.

The faceplate is either plastic or rubber; it is cut to size for the individual stoma. The technique for proper application is first to wash the area about the stoma with mild soap and water, rinse, wipe with alcohol, pat dry, brush a light coat of liquid adhesive both on the skin and faceplate, and then after a short drying period (2 to 3 min) place the faceplate in position. Gum Karaya powder or a Karaya ring washer, creating a double-faced adhesive disk, can be used instead of a liquid adhesive. Removal of the collecting apparatus should be done carefully and slowly, freeing the attachment, a little at a time, with use of surgical cement solvent and a dropper. The pouch should not be simply pulled off. The remaining cement should be removed with cotton soaked in the solvent.

CONVALESCENCE

Irritation of the skin should be treated by careful cleansing with soap and water and dusting with Karaya gum powder. A Karaya gum ring should be used between the appliance and the skin. Such rings dissolve and will require frequent changes of the bag. Emptying of the ileostomy pouch should be done according to individual patient need. When skin irritation is present, careful removal of the ring with adhesive solvent is particularly important.

TRANSITIONAL AND POSTHOSPITAL CARE

Few restrictions in activity or living are necessary for the ileal conduit or ileostomy patient. The ileostomy patient should eat a diet relatively low in residue and should chew all food thoroughly to avoid lumpy residue that may create blockage. Foods poorly tolerated by the individual and gas-forming foods should be avoided. Odor can be controlled by placing a few drops of chlorophyll solution in the pouch and by using vinegar or liquid bleach when cleansing the pouch. Airing each pouch after cleaning and using only a freshly aired pouch also helps.

Thorough cleansing and drying of the skin surrounding the stoma helps prevent and remove the keratotic plaques that form about both ileostomy and ileal conduit openings.

Very occasionally, a patient may be given cutaneous ureterostomies for urinary evacuation. Such patients need a special collecting apparatus, such as devised by Whitmore, and skin care similar to that used for the ileal conduit patient, to prevent inflammatory breakdown.

HEAD AND NECK CANCER

Face, Mouth, and Pharynx

Surgical treatment of cancers of the face and mouth may cause severe cosmetic problems as well as functional defects in speech, mastication, swallowing, salivary control, and vision. It is extremely difficult for the patient to hide the defect, and this can create severe psychological problems, greater in many ways than the problems arising from the physical deficit itself. (See Table 49-4.)

PREOPERATIVE TREATMENT

Adaptive care should start in the preoperative period with counseling of the patient and family, in close communication and cooperation with the surgeon. The patient should be informed of the type of surgery planned and of the expected result. Smoking and alcohol consumption should be stopped, if possible. Both habits are common among these patients, and control is difficult.

Permanent records that should be obtained to facilitate postoperative management include moulage, profile midline template, dental casts, and articulation records and photographs. Good preoperative dental care will help control infection and caries. Nonsalvageable teeth should be extracted. Orthodontic procedures and oral surgery should be performed as needed to support soft tissues, decrease contraction and disfigurement due to scar formation, maintain existing oral structural relationships, protect later surgical areas from trauma, provide scaffolding for grafts, provide pressure, and reduce hemorrhage and improve retention of packs and dressings. Additional benefits of proper preoperative dental care include airway maintenance and facilitation of speech and swallowing.

Radiation therapy may be used in the treatment of head and neck cancer. Oral hygiene and care are necessary before, during, and after radiation therapy to the mouth and face to reduce the incidence of jaw infection and to increase comfort. Dry mouth due to decreased salivation after radiation therapy is relieved by discontinuing smoking and alcohol consumption and by using gelatin and glycerin fruit-flavored pastilles or a mixture of glycerin and mouthwash. Increasing environmental humidity also helps, and fluid intake should be increased when possible. The application of small local quantities of liquid silicone gives effective relief for several hours. Dry, bulky foods should be avoided. When dryness of the nasal cavity is a problem, daily irrigation with corn syrup provides relief. These suggestions apply also in the postoperative period.[1,4,12]

OPERATIVE PROCEDURES

Immediate reconstruction of the surgical defect following major resection for primary carcinomas arising in

TABLE 49-4 Rehabilitation for Cancer Cases Involving the Head and Neck

Disability	Adaptive approach
Facial disfigurement	Plastic and reconstructive surgery by surgical and dental team Prosthetic replacement
Salivation control loss Mastication and swallowing problems	Plastic and reconstructive surgery Prosthetics Food preparation and training in swallowing, tube feeding, temporary medication, and local care

Communication loss or defect	Speech therapy:
	  Initial emotional support and communication assistance; example and help of volunteer patient
	  Use of artificial electrolarynx to initiate communicative effort
	  Esophageal voice training
	  Surgical approaches to improved sound conduction or production

Visual field and depth perception deficit after ocular enucleation	Occupational therapy for improvement in eye-hand coordination, depth perception, and compensation for field deficit
Dropped shoulder	Initial sling and support activities to prevent trapezius overstretch and assist recovery Neck, shoulder, and arm exercises
Withdrawal from community and work	Social service, vocational counseling and rehabilitation, psychological counseling, and employer instruction and involvement

the oral cavity and upper aerodigestive tract can be performed utilizing free skin grafts cervical skin, and forehead skin. Reconstruction of surgical defects of the anterior oral cavity can be performed using skin from the cheek. As pointed out by Shah,[3] immediate reconstruction, when possible, can maintain the anatomic continuity of the patient's alimentary tract. This will not be reestablished for several months, if secondary or staged reconstruction may be necessary. This delay usually results in prolonged or repeated hospitalization, with attendant discomfort and inability to eat by mouth, and thus there should be appropriate selection of patients who are candidates for immediate reconstruction. Other techniques of pharyngoesophageal reconstruction are available to the surgeon for large resections of the pharyngeal wall, hypopharynx, and cervical esophagus. These include staged reconstruction utilizing tubed pedicles, deltopectoral flap, gastric pull-up, use of neck skin, and, finally, free transfer of vascularized intestinal graft using microvascular surgical techniques.[3]

Chaglassian[3] advises that immediate reconstruction of the face and scalp must be performed keeping three factors in mind: function, physiology, and cosmesis. To satisfy the requirements of these three factors, the surgeon should, if possible, use local flap tissue, either from an area close to the defect or from the neck, forehead, posterior auricular area, or chest. Small defects on the face are best closed using geometrical flaps, called Limberg flaps, which are easy to plan and execute.

Chaglassian also favors development of the rotation advancement flap popularized by Mustardé. This flap will close defects around the lower eyelid and can be extended to cover defects of the cheek and nose. Another flap for consideration is the nasolabial flap; this is used primarily for immediate reconstruction of nasal defects and for upper or lower lip defects. Medial canthal area defects, when small, are closed with a glabellar flap. When the facial defect is through and through, that is, when both skin and mucous membrane lining are absent, it is necessary to provide a double coverage, both for lining and skin cover. This means that in most instances two flaps will be used, usually a distant flap and a combination of several local flaps.

Defects of the scalp can be reconstructed in the same

manner as for the face. However, careful attention should be paid to the hairline, and flaps should be designed to ensure (1) viability, (2) primary healing, and (3) closure of the resulting defect. Scalp flaps are difficult to execute because there is very little elasticity and resilience in the scalp.[3]

POSTOPERATIVE TREATMENT

Suctioning should be performed as frequently as necessary to prevent accumulation and aspiration of secretions. It should be gentle, avoiding suture lines. Irrigation of tissue surfaces should be done with a tepid solution of 1 teaspoon salt and 1 teaspoon bicarbonate of soda per liter of water. Stimulation of the gag reflex can be avoided by proper direction of the stream. The patient should exhale through the irrigation phase, and should pinch off tube and flow during inhalation. The stream should be gentle, with the solution container hung about 1 foot above the patient's head. A spray of half-strength peroxide solution used twice daily may precede irrigations. Irrigation should follow all oral feedings and should also be done at bedtime. Prostheses should be removed before irrigating. Use of a toothbrush should be avoided for about 2 weeks following surgery.

CONVALESCENCE

Dental appliances constructed for oral cancer patients should provide maximum coverage, have multiple clasps, permit modification, and be compatible with underlying tissues. Facial prostheses can be constructed as soon as edema has subsided and healing is adequate, usually about 6 weeks after surgery. Provision of dentures may not be possible until 3 to 12 months have elapsed, when tissues that have been irradiated have recovered. Appropriate construction of obturators and other appliances will minimize speech problems associated with palatal defects.[3,4]

Resection of the tongue may result in difficulties in speech and swallowing. The greater the amount of tongue tissue resected, the more serious the difficulties will be. Speech training and instruction in mastication and swallowing can increase proficiency and avoid aspiration problems. Training in swallowing can be accomplished using small amounts of clear water for practice.

Commando procedures involving resection of the jaw create particular difficulties in swallowing and articulation in speech. Normal performance of these functions depends on an intact mandible, and restoration is difficult. Obturators will close resonating cavities and stents can be used to support tissues and restore the contour of the face and oral cavity.

Swallowing difficulty and aspiration pneumonia result when one or both superior laryngeal nerves have had to be sacrificed. Prevention of these problems may be effected by splitting (myotomy) of the cricopharyngeus muscle. The patient can then be taught to exhale while in the process of swallowing, clearing the laryngeal vestibule of material that otherwise would be aspirated.

Enucleation of an eye creates a reduction in total visual field and change in the accuracy of depth perception, as well as need for cosmetic prosthetic replacement. The patient should be given occupational therapy designed to improve eye-hand coordination and accuracy of depth perception.

TRANSITIONAL AND POSTHOSPITAL CARE

Late surgical reconstruction of orofacial defects depends on the extent of functional loss, degree of deformity, patient reaction to the disability, and possible masking of recurrent cancer. Reconstruction procedures include flap closures for fistulas, mobilization or reconstruction of the tongue, bone graft mandibular replacement, muscle transfers for facial nerve palsies, implants, and autografts for correction of contour defects.[3]

Surgical procedures involving several stages are often necessary, and there are tedious waiting periods. Reconstructive plastic surgery requires patience and understanding on the part of both the patient and the team that is providing care and support. The surgical and dental team can supply either a temporary or a permanent maxillofacial prosthesis, functional if possible, to lessen disfigurement and restore all possible useful activity. Either plastic or reconstructive surgery or prosthetic replacement by synthetic materials constitutes an essential part of rehabilitation of the patient. The patient may prefer prosthetic replacement to prolonged multiple surgeries. The cost is also apt to be less.[4]

To some extent, according to Dr. Ronald Spiro, "the importance of reconstruction increases as the prospect for 'cure' decreases. Restoration of speech and swallowing is crucial to the quality of survival when surgery is likely to be palliative at best."[3]

Social service personnel should work extensively with the patient and the family. Vocational counseling should be obtained to encourage the patient and either to arrange for continuation of the job held before surgery or to provide retraining if necessary, in a new field of work.[2] Every effort should be made to prevent the patient from adopting an attitude of social withdrawal.

For patients whose disease is advanced or recurrent, there may be fear and anxiety as well as pain. If there is gradual upper airway obstruction, a tracheostomy may be indicated to relieve choking sensation. If swallowing is blocked, a cervical esophagostomy for feeding is advised in preference to a gastrostomy.

The malnourished patient may develop cachexia. Such a patient becomes anorexic and weak. Although the cachectic patient may appear detached and apathetic, restlessness and anxiety, which represent the mental effects of metabolic disruption, may also be evident.[12]

Replacement of protein loss is difficult. Frequent small meals are better tolerated than large meals. Parenteral feeding can be life-saving and may be used alone or to support supplemental or tube feeding.

Larynx

Cancer of the larynx occasionally can be treated by radiation therapy or hemilaryngectomy. The functional deficits after treatment are slight in comparison to those after total laryngectomy, and the patients need only guidance and suggestions for minor changes in techniques of speech.

Total laryngectomy results in a major loss of communication abilities. Speech training, therefore, becomes the most pressing need in rehabilitation. The development of esophageal speech is the preferred method. It is more satisfactory than use of an artificial larynx insofar as articulation, intelligibility, and phonation are concerned, and it can be successfully taught in the majority of cases. Any form of buccal speech or whispering results in comparatively poor communication. Speech may also be made possible by constructing an independent air tunnel from the tracheostomy to the pharynx. The only remaining methods of communication are by writing or gestures. The greater the amount of tissue removed, particularly when there has been inclusion of musculature of pharynx or esophagus, the smaller the possibility of good esophageal speech production.[1]

PREOPERATIVE TREATMENT

Before surgery, the patient should be advised that the expected loss of speech will be temporary and that there will be a temporary loss of taste. The sense of taste should return when the patient learns to talk. Demonstration can be given of the use of the artificial electrolarynx for the immediate postoperative period, or the patient can be directed only to communicate by writing and signs. This will keep the patient from developing bad communication habits, such as grimacing and whispering. The importance of correct instruction cannot be overemphasized. Only a trained speech therapist or another laryngectomee, a successful speaker, should undertake this training.

Tests of auditory acuity and function should be given to all patients scheduled for esophageal speech training. Hearing loss markedly affects speech efficiency. A hearing aid and auditory training are necessary for proper speech training of patients who have moderate or severe hearing loss.[7]

POSTOPERATIVE TREATMENT

If a trained instructor is not available in the patient's home area, then the patient should travel to the nearest center that offers the appropriate speech training. Preoperative speech training and the ability to "belch" are not related to success in becoming an esophageal speaker. It is generally felt that active speech instruction should start at about the time of discharge from the hospital. It is also valuable at the time of discharge to provide each patient with a postlaryngectomy kit containing the main essentials required for good care, including gauze, a bib, and a shower cover. Instructions and prescriptions should be given to those patients who complain of either dry mouth or drooling.

TRANSITIONAL AND POSTHOSPITAL CARE

The most important period of learning for esophageal speech occurs in the first 2 years after surgery. The longer the time spent in speech training, the more proficient the speaker becomes. It takes at least 4 months, and occasionally as long as a year, for the majority of speakers to achieve sound production and control of articulation and phrasing.

Instructions in esophageal speech production can be obtained at many larger universities and colleges, most medical centers, some private hospitals, private speech clinics, through private instructors, and by arrangement with Lost Chord Clubs. Names and places to contact are readily obtainable from the International Association of Laryngectomees and the American Cancer Society. The American Cancer Society publishes an instruction manual entitled *Your New Voice*, and a booklet entitled *Self-Help for the Laryngectomee* can be obtained from the author, E. Lauder.[13] The International Association of Laryngectomees and the American Cancer Society jointly publish a booklet called *Helping Words for the Laryngectomee*.

The patient should be encouraged to resume as many usual activities as possible. Some things, of course, will be changed. The patient will not be able to hold his or her breath, and thus will be unable to strain or lift heavy loads. Laughter, singing ability, and the ability to have a good cry are lost, and swimming is not safe. Nearly all other regular activities, however, can be enjoyed.

Following laryngectomy the patient benefits from breathing properly humidified air, and should use a humidifier or vaporizer or place open pans of water and plants in living and working quarters.

Vocational training plays a large role in rehabilitation. Training for changes in occupation may be necessary, especially if previous employment required verbal communication, exposure to fumes or dust, or underwater work. The patient and the family require instruction in care of the stoma and use of the bib, and in general hygiene.

Medical indentification and information cards, which must be carried by the laryngectomee, are distributed through the International Association of Laryngectomees, which functions with the service and rehabilitation sections of the state and national offices of the American Cancer Society. These cards provide instruction covering the laryngectomee's individual needs, and include methods for administration of artificial respiration. Detailed first aid manuals covering care for the laryngectomee are published by and obtainable from the same source.

Glossectomy

Intelligible speech is possible for some glossectomized patients. Factors involved in success in speech production and intelligibility include the extent and location of lingual tissue removal, the degree of mobility of the remaining structures, patient-generated compensatory behavior, therapeutic intervention, prosthodontics, and reconstructive surgery. The exact or relative importance of each of these factors has not been conclusively demonstrated. Swallowing behavior is similarly involved.

Disabilities

PAIN

The patient who has developed pain requires special consideration. The causes of pain vary. They include ulceration and infection of the cancer, neoplastic invasion of head and neck structures, and radiation therapy and chemotherapy. Pain may be a result of mouth dryness, drooling, moniliasis, and osteoradionecrosis. Pain may also be caused by contact with irritating substances in foods and fluids, imbibing acid drinks or alcohol, and smoking. Localized soreness, tenderness, and discomfort may be caused by dental prostheses, caries, defective fillings, odontogenic infections, etc., and oral hygiene is of paramount importance in control of such pain. The patient should receive proper instructions in procedures for maintaining dental health and for care of supportive structures, as well as training in corrective measures. Mild inflammation, erosions, and ulcerations may be treated by application of topical protectants, denture adhesive powders, and pastes. Hot or cold applications (warm saline washes, icepacks, heat pads) and topical drugs may be used for mild infections, swellings, and edema. Analgesics, topical anesthetics, antimicrobial agents, astringents, psychopharmacologic agents, and topical corticosteroids may also be useful.

Frank or severe pain may require radiotherapy or surgical decompression. A 5 to 7% phenol injection may be given to alleviate localized pain. Potentiation of effects of mild drugs or small doses may be obtained with Thorazine or Phenergan. Procedures such as peripheral neurotomy and posterior rihizotomy (including trigeminal, vagus, or glossopharyngeal, alone or in combination) may be necessary to control intractable pain. Prefrontal lobotomy changes the patient's reaction to pain and may permit tolerance.

DRY MOUTH

The patient should avoid dry, bulky, or irritating foods and fluids as well as tobacco and alcohol. All sources of mechanical irritation should be eliminated. Lubricating agents are water, a 1 percent saline solution, cocoa butter, vaseline (for the lips), mineral oil, olive oil, glycerine, and solutions of wetting agents. Chewing gum may be useful.[4,12]

DROOLING

Drooling may be controlled by suction, frequent swallowing, tranquilizers, anticholinergic agents, ligation of major salivary ducts, prosthetic appliances, and surgical reconstruction. Reassurance and emotional support are also important.

Radical Neck Dissection

Radical neck dissection frequently results in disability in the shoulder on the side that has been operated on secondary to section of the accessory nerve. The patient may develop varying degrees of trapezius muscle paralysis, with a dropped painful shoulder and a rotated scapula. The degree of paralysis depends on the amount of primary innervation carried to the trapezius by the accessory nerve. The patient with complete trapezius paralysis cannot abduct the arm at the shoulder beyond about 40 degrees and is unable to carry it up and over the head.

Rehabilitative treatment initially requires support of the arm and shoulder with a sling to prevent overstretching of the trapezius. Patients should be taught to practice support of the shoulder and upper arm when seated, by keeping the elbow on a chair arm or pillow, which also prevents stretching of the trapezius. The physical therapy program should include exercises that consciously utilize and strengthen the rhomboid muscles and the levator scapulae for training in movements to facilitate abduction of the arm at the shoulder. Recommended exercises include wall-climbing and pulley exercises similar to those given the postmastectomy patient (see Figures 49-2 to 49-7). Printed instructions for appropriate exercises should be distributed to all patients.[1]

Unfortunately, there is no good substitute muscle for the trapezius. It stabilizes the scapula and elevates the lateral angle. Both the rhomboid muscles and the levator scapulae tip the lateral angle down, while adducting the scapula medially, aggravating the patient's disability. Transplant of the attachment of the levator laterally may help somewhat but is not really satisfactory.

A certain number of patients having primary innervation of the upper trapezius by upper cervical roots retain muscle function lost by the others. In "preventive" surgical rehabilitation of such patients, attempts have been made to use nerve grafts to replace the removed segment of the accessory nerve. The greater auricular nerve can be used for this purpose. Reports of results are varied, but it is considered worthy of trial if the operative opportunity presents easily for the surgeon concerned. During the healing after this procedure, electrical muscle stimulation may be beneficial. Supportive fascial slings in addition to muscle transplant of the levator scapulae have also been used, but this procedure has not proved dependable.

Resection of the sternocleidomastoid muscle causes imbalance in head support and loss of rotation control. Some patients develop a resultant torticollis positioning of the head, which does not respond well to exercises and is not greatly aided by supportive collar devices. Early postoperative instruction in range of motion of the neck and positioning and support of the head, and concomitant instruction in appropriate shoulder exercises, will, however, reduce contracture formation and fixed disability.

Cosmetic help for the radical neck dissection patient can be provided by collars and neck coverings, hair arrangement, and beards. (Men who have had radiation therapy may be unable to grow a beard.) Men should be instructed to use only an electric razor for shaving, since after neck dissection the major neck vessels are covered only by a thin layer of skin.

CANCER OF THE LUNG, ESOPHAGUS, MEDIASTINUM, AND PLEURA

The extent of respiratory disability depends on the combined restrictions created by the site and extent of the surgery (including the postoperative stability of the chest wall) and also on the basic pulmonary preoperative status of the patient. The presence of preexisting chronic obstructive pulmonary disease with emphysema and fibrosis, asthma, chronic infection, old pleural adhesions, etc., decrease the efficiency of the patient's respiratory function. Compensation for disease-related or postoperative decrease in adequate pulmonary function can be provided through instruction in improved voluntary and assisted respiratory performance and through appropriate postural drainage techniques. (See Table 49-5.)

Preoperative Treatment

It is recommended that all patients who are candidates for thoracotomy be given the advantage of preoperative respiratory training in adequate voluntary breathing and coughing control and in nonvigorous exercises of their extremities which maintain general circulation, muscular strength, and function of the arm and shoulder on the side that has been operated on. Training can be resumed as immediately in the postoperative period as is convenient for both the patient and the staff, which facilitates

TABLE 49-5 Rehabilitation for Cancer Cases Involving the Lung, Esophagus, Mediastinum, and Pleura

Disability	Adaptive approach

Preexisting, disease-related:
  Chronic obstructive pulmonary disease
  Emphysema
  Fibrosis
  Asthma
  Bronchiectasis
	Instruction in deep breathing and sighing, voluntary control of adequate cough and "huff," regional costal expansion in breathing control, diaphragmatic breathing, postural drainage

Procedure-related:
  Thoracotomy, with or without radioactive implant or biopsy
  Mediastinotomy
  Sternotomy
  Pleurectomy
  Pulmonary wedge resection
  Lobectomy, with or without chest wall resection
  Pneumonectomy, simple or radical, with or without chest wall resection
	Preoperative:
	  Breathing and coughing training (training in huffing for expected tracheostomy patients)
	  Postural drainage, as indicated
	  Nonvigorous exercises of extremities
	
	Postoperative:
	  Breathing and coughing instruction and assistance (huffing training for tracheostomized patients)
	  Moisturized air
	  Incentive spirometer, with or without mucolytic and/or bronchodilator medication
	  Postural drainage (may be level bed)
	  Nonvigorous exercises of extremities
	  Mobilization, in and out of bed

Postoperative complication:
  Pneumonia
  Atelectasis
  Fistula
	Inclusion of each or all of above, in accordance with both disease and procedure indications and contraindications

maintenance of a clear airway and prevents possible complications. All instructions should be given with the individual patient and the surgery to be performed in mind.

The preoperative program should begin with demonstration and training in breathing control and proper coughing, and, for patients who are to have a tracheostomy, proper "huffing" techniques. "Huffing" is the term used for forceful air expulsion of secretions without closing the glottis. The patient at this point is not distracted by pain or the effects of medication and can better understand directions and become familiar with the chest team. These procedures prior to surgery help clear the tracheobronchial tree of undesirable secretions and make the anesthesiologist's job easier.

Preoperative breathing techniques include regional costal expansion and segmental control, especially of the basal segments. This facilitates maximal ventilatory control and aids in ventilation as well as in expansion. Proper bed position and posture should be stressed. Effective coughing is achieved by correct control of respiration rather than by degree of force or volume of expelled air. To minimize discomfort, activity of the accessory musculature of the chest, neck, and back should be reduced. At this point the patient can also be taught the proper manual techniques for self-splinting of the chest, which will reduce discomfort postoperatively.

These breathing exercises will serve to increase the postoperative control of accessory respiratory muscles and improve lung ventilation and expansion. Effective coughing or, in tracheostomy patients, huffing, assists in clearance of secretions.[14]

Postoperative Treatment

Postoperative treatment should start in the recovery room as soon as the patient is conscious enough to attempt to cooperate. Breathing exercises and coughing while firm support is applied should be encouraged. Full reexpansion of remaining lung tissue is desirable, and elimination of retained secretions promotes reexpansion. Adequately performed deep breathing helps to mobilize bronchial secretions.

Lung resection impairs the residual air space available to the patient. Differences in patient performance and differences in tolerance depend on the extent of the resection, from wedge to radical pneumonectomy. Pain and restrictive dressings add to patients' difficulties. The presence of a postoperative air leak will necessitate the use of more gentle coughing and inhalation techniques, to avoid aggravation.

The patient should be taught proper manual splinting techniques. Active, or patient-controlled, splinting is accomplished when the patient crosses his hand over from the side that has not been operated on to hold the operated side arm against the chest. Passive, or therapist-assisted, splinting may be used if necessary.

The patient should be given pretherapy pain-relief medication necessary to facilitate function. Medication which might depress respiratory function should be avoided, but failure to relieve pain may allow the patient to accumulate secretions and develop atelectasis or pneumonia.

The distal bronchioles dilate on inspiration and collapse on expiration. This tends to trap alveolar air and allow accumulation of CO_2. Improved exchange with alveolar ventilation and CO_2 elimination are promoted by the practice of pursed-lip expiration to create slight positive pressure during the expiratory phase, keeping the distal bronchioles patent.

Postthoracotomy patients who have chronic respiratory disease often perform apical breathing in a relative flutter pattern. Shallow apical breaths and a painful, tightly dressed chest combine to defeat effective coughing. Initially, the patient should be given instructions in deep breathing, with appropriate splinting, and should practice diaphragmatic breathing. Patients should be instructed to relax the accessory muscles of the upper chest and to perform slow diaphragmatic respiration by using their abdominal muscles, relaxing on inspiration and contracting with expiration. Patients should then be taught to take several initial sharp and short diaphragmatic inspirations to "prime" their cough, and follow this with a deep breath and a strong single or, at most, double cough. Spasms of coughing are ineffective and painful, and are to be avoided. They will discourage the patient from attempting appropriate necessary coughing.[13]

Nonvigorous exercises of the arms, trunk, and lower extremities are taught starting on the first postoperative day for the purpose of maintaining free joint motion (especially in the shoulder on the operated side), preserving general strength, and promoting circulatory return in the lower extremities. To prevent stress on the wound area, range of motion in the shoulder on the operated side should be initially limited to 90 degrees in abduction and flexion. The exercises of the upper extremity, neck, shoulders, upper back, and abdominal muscles improve posture and stimulate coughing by mobilizing secretions. Proper posture and arm and shoulder activities help reduce the chance of scoliosis, which can follow thoracotomy.

Postural drainage is an important and effective method of assisting the normal pulmonary clearing mechanisms. The patient is placed in positions which drain the involved bronchial segments by gravity. Most of the lung segments (better than 90 percent) can be drained by rotating the patient on a flat, level bed. Tipping is contraindicated when abdominal surgery has been performed because of the related tendency for peritoneal secretions to run and puddle under the diaphragm, especially on the right side, and develop into a subphrenic abscess. Tipping is also contraindicated in the presence of superior vena cava obstruction; moderate-to-severe hypertension; cerebral hemorrhage, embolism, or thrombosis; prior intracranial surgery; and in patients with low platelet counts. Satisfactory postural drainage for all such patients can be performed by frequent turning of the patient on a level bed.[1,4]

In all positions, the patient should be comfortable and relaxed. Patients should be instructed and assisted in frequent changes of position to be carried out at prescribed intervals. Postural drainage should be performed four to five times daily and for periods of from 10 to 30 min, depending upon tolerance and condition. If postural drainage is ordered, it should be continued until the cough is nonproductive and the patient is ambulatory.

Techniques of chest percussion and shaking or vibration are useful for mobilizing secretions which may be too quick or viscid to flow freely. Such techniques are not used for the early postoperative patient because of the presence of the wound, and are entirely contraindicated in the presence of chest wall defects or reconstructive procedures, the presence of underlying malignancy, when there is a recent history or chance of thoracic bleeding, when platelet counts are low, or when aggravated pain is present. Otherwise percussion is done with a cupped hand over the area being drained, which assists in loosening tenacious material and in moving the secretions into larger bronchi. When wound healing is adequate, two-handed vibration of the chest by the therapist during the patient's exhalation phase in respiration can be used to assist airflow and increase effective coughing. In treating postoperative debilitated patients or small infants, postural drainage can be utilized without associated cupping or vibration.

If the chest wall is secure and the wound healing sufficiently advanced (by the fifth to the seventh postoperative day) and if there are no other contraindications, percussion and cupping can be performed. In cupping, the patient's chest is covered with the hospital gown and the therapist's hands are cupped to provide a cushion of air between the hand and the chest (clapping with a stiff, flat, hand is painful). The breasts, clavicles, vertebrae, and scapular spines are avoided.

Vibration is produced by firmly placing the hands flat on the chest wall and effecting rapid alternating motions of pressure and release on the patient's chest. While the vibration is applied, the patient exhales slowly and completely, which promotes spontaneous coughing. Voluntary coughing and expectoration should be encouraged during the maneuver. Vibration must be gentle, as too-vigorous vibration may cause hemoptysis. Vibration is contraindicated, to repeat, in situations in which there is a recent history or chance of thoracic bleeding.[14]

Inhalation therapy is greatly assisted by proper moisturization of inspired air. Reservoir nebulizers or ultrasonic aerosol generators can be used to create a mist which prevents insipissation of mucus and aids in its liquefication. Nebulization can be combined with bronchodilators or decongestant agents to aid in drainage and ventilation.

An incentive spirometer allows measurement of the volume of inspired air by the patient. Incentive spirometers can have either a fixed flow rate or a variable flow rate, and there are a number of different models available. Variable-flow-rate spirometers are better for children, but both types have wide application. They are disposable and relatively inexpensive. They help motivate patients to cooperate with treatment and attain maximum sustained inspiratory effort.

If the patient has satisfactory voluntary lung expansion, administration of medication and moisturization of inspired air are best provided through the use of a motor nebulizer. Intermittent positive-pressure breathing machines (IPPBs) and mechanical respirators are used primarily for patients unable to control their own functions. The IPPB is not as effective as it was once considered to be.

Patients who have undergone a tracheostomy and who, therefore, cannot perform a regular cough, should be given instruction and practice in proper huffing techniques by the physical therapist. This, when combined with deep breathing, will assist in mobilization of secretions and decrease the frequency of need for tracheobronchial suctioning. Huffing involves the forceful expulsion of air by diaphragmatic, abdominal, and intercostal muscle contraction without vocal cord assistance.

Patients who have had respirator assistance over a period of time require instruction in weaning from the respirator. Such instruction can be provided by the physical therapist, who will give the patient intensive, assisted training in voluntary deep-breathing, techniques of sighing, and coughing, in order to increase the patient's control and conscious utilization of the respiratory apparatus. When the patient is apprehensive, dyspneic, or uncomfortable, the respirator should be reattached, and the instruction repeated later. Frequent, short sessions often work best.

Respiratory assistance of this kind, both preoperatively and postoperatively, has similar value for patients undergoing abdominal surgical procedures, particularly if these are high. It is also useful for patients upon whom diaphragmatic procedures have been performed, for patients who have had phrenic nerve crush or resection, and for patients who have abnormalities involving diaphragmatic function.

The surgical treatment of tumors invading the chest wall involves radical excision. Closure of the wound may include plastic and skeletal reconstruction. Sternal resection is satisfactorily tolerated by the patient if either the upper or lower costal ring is left intact. A total sternectomy requires immediate reconstruction with a rigid replacement to permit normal postoperative respiratory excursions.[3]

Small chest wall defects can be closed with skin and muscle. Bony defects may be filled with a fine steel mesh (Marlex mesh), or, when small, by ox fascia under the skin closure. Large bony defects require supportive closure with Marlex mesh for stability, reduction of paradox, and cosmesis. Molded methylmethacrylate plates make effective replacements also, and McCormack describes use of a molded and shaped "sandwich" of layers of Marlex and methylmethacrylate glue. When there has been extensive skin loss, procedures involving staged, delayed flaps may be necessary to achieve adequate skin coverage. Respiratory function must be supported postoperatively by diligent physical therapy.

CANCER INVOLVING THE NERVOUS SYSTEM

Neoplasms, whether primary or metastatic, involving the brain, spinal cord, and peripheral nerves, directly create motor and sensory deficits and affect coordination. Surgical, medical, and radiation procedures and treatments may directly produce anatomic deficits and toxic or destructive effects. Cancer, particularly when it involves the lung or when it is diffuse, may also have effects on nervous system function. These effects are classified as remote or secondary.[15] Rehabilitation measures should begin as soon as the disability is recognized or can be predicted, in order to minimize weakness due to inactivity or disuse and to maintain proprioceptive and sensory stimuli. (See Table 49-6). As in other regional or system-related disabilities, an appropriate and realistic goal for expected response should be set.

Focal weakness may result from the excision or transection of a major nerve. Treatment consists of prompt range of motion exercises for the affected extremity. If the affected extremity is an arm, a sling should be provided for interval support to limit subluxation and limit pain at the shoulder. Special exercises and practice in the unilateral use of the normal arm and hand are important, especially when the loss of function involves a dominant upper extremity. A functional splint or an ADL splint that facilitates the performance of the activities of daily living may be appropriate for individual patients.

TABLE 49-6 Rehabilitation for Cancer Cases Involving the Nervous System

Disability	Adaptive approach

Central nervous system mono-, hemi-, para-, or quadriplegia or -paresis due to:
  Tumor
  Surgery
  Radiation
Peripheral nerve neuropathy due to:
  Tumor, direct effect
  Steroids
  Chemotherapy
  Radiation therapy
  Remote effects of cancer
Neural section, partial or complete, during surgery
	Full tolerable program of physical therapy, occupational therapy, and activities of daily living
	Sling for upper extremity
	Bracing for lower extremity
	Splinting, prn, static or dynamic

Pain:
  Tractable
  Intractable
  Causalgia
	Analgesics, nerve block, functional training (including proper positioning and sparing)
	Neurosurgery
	  Nerve block
	  Cordotomy
	  Rhizotomy
	  Tractotomy
	  Thalamotomy
	  Alcohol or phenol wash
	Medication—stronger analgesics, narcotics for patients with goal of palliation
	Hypnosis

The entire spectrum of plegias and neuropathies may be encountered. Treatment is usually the standard care program for such disabilities when they are unrelated to cancer, and, unless otherwise contraindicated, should be started on this basis. Early active range-of-motion exercises help prevent pain and deformity.

In lower-extremity unilateral paresis or paralysis, bracing with a long or short leg brace, depending upon the need, may render the patient ambulatory. Muscle reeducation should be carried out when there is any evidence of reinnervation, either functional or suggested by electrodiagnostic testing.

The approaches to rehabilitation of patients who have paralysis secondary to section of the accessory nerve in radical neck dissection are discussed above.

Impairment of coordination may be lessened by giving the patient special exercises in eye-hand coordination and special gait training and practice. Occupational therapy in addition to physical therapy assists the patient with upper-extremity coordination.

Ataxia is found related to tumors involving posterior columns and cerebellum and from cerebellar degeneration secondary to remote effects of cancer. Programs involving ambulation training using the parallel bar, Frenkel's exercises, and mirror self-observation can all be of value for the patient with ataxia.

Tumors which alter cerebellar and hemispheric functions result in bizarre concepts of self-position in space, and require long-term training in ambulation and posture. Problems related to sensory losses involving touch discrimination and sensitivity to pain and temperature are not responsive to direct therapy. The effect of the loss can be minimized, however, by training the patient to use other sensory modalities and to engage in patterns of activity that do not depend on the lost abilities.

Enucleation of an eye creates a reduction in total visual field and a loss of accuracy of depth perception, as well as a need for cosmetic prosthetic replacement. The patient should be given occupational therapy designed to improve eye-hand coordination and accuracy of depth perception.

In a 1965 study involving 1000 autopsies of patients with malignant disease, Vieth and Odom[16] reported brain metastases in 17.6 percent of the cases. The same survey revealed that if no attempt had been made to remove the metastatic tumor, the 2-year survival rate was 4.5 percent, whereas if surgical intervention had been performed, the rate was increased to 12.2 percent.

Cerebral metastasis differs from a cerebrovascular lesion. A metastatic tumor, focal in its effect upon the brain, when removed by the neurosurgeon, may leave behind far less deficit than does a stroke. Therefore, the potential for rehabilitation of the patient with a metastatic tumor is far greater than for a patient with hemiplegia secondary to a vascular lesion.

Remote Effects of Cancer on the Nervous System

The remote effects of cancer on the nervous system produce varying clinical syndromes of neuromyopathy. Symptoms may develop after those of the neoplasm, or they may precede other evidence of the neoplastic disease. Muscular weakness and wasting occur, with weakness most frequently in the limb girdle and in the proximal muscles rather than distally. Pain may accompany the weakness. There is a striking tendency for the symptoms to remit for short or long periods without regard to the course of the tumor or its treatment.[15] Therefore, it is important to teach even asymptomatic patients exercises in order to mitigate the effects of future disuse and range-of-motion disabilities.

Steroids and chemotherapeutic agents used to treat cancer may cause symptoms similar to those produced by the remote effects of cancer on the nervous system. Supervoltage radiation therapy has also been reported to create malfunction in the nervous system. Peripheral nerve dysfunction may not occur until a year or longer after radiation therapy has been administered, whereas reported effects on the central nervous system develop earlier and are directly related to the degree of change within the cells of the central nervous system itself.

Pain

The control of pain is an important factor in rehabilitation. The patients usually experience both pain and anxiety, one serving to reinforce the other, and relief of the anxiety may appreciably decrease the pain.

Eradication of infection may eliminate pain. Pain from nerve compression or invasion by tumor may respond to radiation therapy or surgical decompression. This is worth considering in bone tumor pain, where decompression may be accomplished by removal of the tumor by cryosurgery. Local nerve block with alcohol or an injection of 5 to 7% phenol is useful for focal pain.

Drug treatment should at first consist of nonnarcotic

analgesics and mild sedation. If narcotics are required, they should be given in small doses at first, with attempts made to potentiate their effects by combination with Phenergan or Thorazine. Current studies suggest that there is marked response to the use of diphenylalanine (DPA).

Control of intractable persistent pain may require a neurosurgical approach. Procedures include nerve block, rhizotomy, cordotomy, medullary tractotomy, thalamotomy, and lobotomy. Hypophysectomy or adrenalectomy may be useful, especially in the presence of breast carcinoma with multiple metastases. Unfortunately, after cordotomies, which are usually bilateral when pain is persistent, the pain may recur even in the presence of residual cutaneous anesthesia. Lobotomy procedures are done more for relief of anxiety than for relief of pain per se.

The effectiveness of transcutaneous electrical neurostimulation (TENS) has been evaluated to be no greater than that of a placebo. Pain relief is effected in only 30 percent of patients, and the relief is of varying degree.

Causalgia and paresthesia are occasionally helped by the application of hot packs or cold packs and by gentle massage. Sympathectomy may also help. It has been recommended in some centers that for the persistent uncontrollable cause of pain, or causalgia, the use of hypnosis administered by an accredited hypnotist may be helpful.[16]

LEUKEMIA, THE LYMPHOMAS, AND HODGKIN'S DISEASE

Leukemia and the malignant lymphomas are more apt to be associated with general disability than with focal problems. Anemia may cause generalized weakness, dyspnea on exertion, and physical instability. There may be an increased tendency toward hemorrhage, bone and joint pain, respiratory distress, vision deficits and hearing loss, and focal palsies developing in sequel to primary or secondary involvement of body foci and systems. Subperiosteal infiltration, especially in children, may result in severe foot pain on standing and walking.

Chemotherapy, steroids, and radiation therapy may cause peripheral and steroid neuropathy and myopathy and reversible alopecia.

Freireich wrote that "Supportive therapy for the patient with acute leukemia is of maximal importance to his comfort and well-being and permits more effective use of agents directed at the control of the leukemic process."[17]

Appropriate physical therapy can reduce the severity, duration, and impact of the disability. The program for each patient should be individualized. No activity or training that is painful should be attempted. Gentle exercises, repeated frequently, can preserve function in cases of weakness. A weakened extremity can be supported or assisted by static or dynamic functional bracing, which will either stabilize the extremity or add strength. Splints for foot and wrist drop and cervical and lumbar spine pain will increase the patient's comfort. A wig can improve the patient's appearance and thus acceptance of hair loss.

Mobilization can be increased in the weak patient with training in proper transfer techniques, elevation activities on stairs, and wheelchair activities. Improved function will follow instruction in activities of daily living, especially dressing, toilet use, and bathing. The provision of simple devices for reaching and retrieving small objects and for cutting and eating food will improve function and increase independence for the patient. Such improvements are of value to the patient each day, no matter what the prognosis may be.

Patient reactions to radiation therapy and chemotherapy require the same supportive assistance as in other neoplastic diseases in which these therapeutic modalities are used.

Pathologic fractures may threaten or occur. Multiple myeloma creates particular problems with bone pain and pathologic fractures. These require preventive definitive treatment. Radiation therapy and intramedullary nailing help prevent pathologic fractures and provide relief for existing pain or disability. Treatment depends on the individual disability and tolerance. Initially, the patient should be given training in active range-of-motion exercises. Later, if the patient is able to participate, training and assistance in ambulation should be given, and supports that will facilitate ambulation should be provided as appropriate. If self-ambulation will not be possible, a goal of wheelchair mobilization should be sought.

Spinal cord compression may result in development of paresis or paralysis below the level of the cord lesion. Neuromyopathies, weakness, debility, and the inanition secondary to anemia all respond to supportive care. An active program of bed exercises and training in independence should be followed by training in out-of-bed activities as appropriate.

Back and neck pain may be relieved by the use of a

corset or brace that limits movement. (Such devices do not provide support.) The use of bracing together with training in back-sparing activities of daily living, can reduce the severity of back pain.

Physical therapy involving training in voluntary control of respiratory function may limit or relieve the tendency to develop respiratory insufficiency, congestion, and pneumonia.

Skin problems, including generalized dryness and itching, and the eczematoid changes caused by mycosis fungoides are relieved somewhat by starch baths.

Symptoms of Raynaud's disease and cold urticaria may develop in the presence of cryoglobulinemia associated with multiple myeloma. Patients should use protective gloves and jackets, and avoid exposure to cold.

Immunotherapy

The patient with immunodeficiency, either preexisting or the result of treatment, may exhibit no measurable physical disability or may have a variety of problems. The extent of immunodeficiency-related handicpas varies depending on the individual and the disease complex involved. Susceptibility to infection may necessitate isolation and restriction of activity. If the platelet count is low, the patient may have to be protected from all injury. Treatment and training in activities of daily living must be evaluated for each organ system according to needs and findings.

Mild exercise routines for the restricted and confined patient will slow deterioration of strength and endurance. Specific instruction should be given in performance of bed and bed-area exercises to reduce or circumvent handicaps involving loss of mobility and joint range of movement. Patients with reduced vigor and tolerance will do better with frequently repeated short periods of instruction and performance than they will with prolonged sessions.

The therapist must carefully adhere to the rules and approaches of isolation. The patient must constantly be protected from exposure to infection Therapists must avoid exposing the patient to personal infections which may be transmitted to the patient. These include colds and sore throats and herpes simplex infections, as well as body surface infections, especially of the hands. Physical therapy involving percussion, massage, chest vibration, or any vigorous handling is contraindicted in the presence of coagulopathy and tendency to bleed.

Instruction and support in exercises designed to increase voluntary respiratory function will help promote improved ventilation and mobilization of tracheobronchial secretions. Instruction in appropriate postural drainage techniques will assist patients in maintaining a clear airway. Control of respiratory function is a constant need, and help and instruction should be available to patients throughout the 24-h day. It is essential that the nursing staff provide constant support, and repeat, at regular intervals, instruction given by the rehabilitation staff.

Equipment for use during reverse isolation or in laminar flow units must be sterilized before being given to the patient. The equipment should then be left with the patient rather than shifted for use elsewhere by another patient.

The stress caused by the emotional reactions to the isolation made necessary by immunodeficiency may add to all the patient's other problems. These reactions must be recognized and understood. The patient will need frequent encouragement and empathy, and occasionally a psychiatrist or clinical psychologist will be needed to help the patient cope with stress and to secure the patient's interest in and compliance with the treatment regimen.

Bone Marrow Transplant

The major problem preventing normal functional behavior for the patient undergoing bone marrow transplant is the protective isolation required. Restriction in space and activity is inherent, and associated weakness resulting from disuse, as well as emotional stress, combine to handicap the patient. Table 49-7 outlines the physical therapy program for the patient undergoing bone marrow transplant. Also note immunotherapy section above.

The pretransplant period should include programs of muscle-conditioning exercises, performed without breath-holding, and specific active stretching exercises designed to prevent shortening of hip flexors and hamstrings secondary to long periods of bed rest. Training in voluntary proper deep breathing and coughing should also be provided. The patient should be provided with gel pad and leveling mattress as protection against decubitus pressure lesions.

Following transplant all pretransplant activities and exercises should be continued. In addition, ambulation training should be provided. Suitable physical activity

TABLE 49-7 Rehabilitation in Cases Involving Bone Marrow Transplant

Disability	Adaptive approach
Generalized weakness Decreased endurance	Pretransplant: Conditioning exercises, active and against resistance
Contractures, especially hips and knees	Specific exercises to prevent shortening of hip flexors and hamstrings
Decubitus ulcers, especially sacral	Gel pad and leveling mattress
Respiratory infection	Training in respiratory function
	Posttransplant: Continuation of all pretransplant physical therapy Ambulation training, with or without assistive devices, to increase and maintain endurance

should be encouraged. Emotional support should be provided as necessary. Help in providing emotional support and in maintaining the patient's interest in treatment can be obtained from local therapy services, which can provide crafts and games, and materials and programs for reading, listening, and watching.

DIALYSIS

The problems of patients undergoing dialysis are more likely to be psychological and emotional than physical. Adaptation to their status is aided by giving supportive counseling and training in active exercises, by providing diversional activities, and by evaluating vocational needs. Assistance may be needed in the activities of daily living.

Day-to-day fluctuations in the symptoms of dialysis patients require a daily assessment of each patient's status in order to avoid inappropriate care programs. There will be times when a patient will feel well, and will want to engage in an activity; at other times the same patient may want only to talk, and at others just to sleep.

Bieringer teaches the Memorial Hospital staff that dialysis patients become passive from need to comply with medical orders and should be given an opportunity to act upon something, rather than being acted upon, by working on an activity (which is self-directed and allows emotional satisfying control). Crafts and activities should have some element of aggression, and many must be adaptable for one-handed use. Rug-punching, copper tooling, weaving with raffia, and leather-lacing are examples of these. Games like dart throwing (there are such available in which darts adhere with Velcro rather than sharp pins) are also possible.

Patients who have sore arms for periods and can use only one limb can be taught one-handed techniques for independence in self-care activities.

Performance of an activity in which the patient is interested makes time on the dialysis machine seem shorter and diverts attention from preoccupation with physical symptoms. Individual activities help create a positive self-concept. If the patient is part of a group, positive socialization will promote sharing of common interests other than the illness itself.

Individual activities may also be useful at home during periods of insomnia. Bieringer reports that "some patients have reported that a mechanical repetitive activity lulls them back to sleep, while others have stated that working on a project makes the sleepless night more bearable."

Bieringer also notes:

Patients who take activities home often reveal information about family dynamics when discussing these activities in the Unit. This information can be valuable to the staff;

Home projects may get an entire family working together and sharing a new interest and allowing combined family-patient participation;

Maintaining contact with families and keeping them informed about available rehabilitation equipment, and sources for it, helps ease life at home;

Patients who may at some time return to work can work on projects that have meaning to them and that help overcome self doubts about their disabilities. Vocational possibilities should always be kept in mind and patients encouraged and helped to work in that direction.

PSYCHOSOCIAL AND VOCATIONAL PROBLEMS

The patient with cancer may develop severe psychological problems. Anxiety results from the fear of prolonged suffering, mutilation, and death. Individual patients are likely to relate their problems and their futures to what they have learned from others with a diagnosis of cancer. They may fear being unwanted or considered different by friends or family. Change in the patient's appearance and the ability to perform certain tasks may precipitate strain and tension for the family as well as for the individual, and the patient may be so distressed as to attempt complete withdrawal. The patient may also fear that disability resulting in lack of employment will mean the inability to meet certain expenses, for example, the children's education, recreation, and clothing.

The responsibility for carrying on with rehabilitation programs for the cancer patient frequently rests with the patient's family, but consideration of family involvement is often neglected. Involving the family must be a part of rehabilitation management; the team that plans for the patient must bring the family in and set up a home program. An effort must be made to gain the support of the family in promoting the patient's participation in social activities and work.

The cost of hospital, surgical, and rehabilitation care overburdens most budgets. Available community resources should be fully utilized by families. These should be offered by those concerned with the care of the patient before shortage of funds has created financial hardship and delay in provision of complete care and rehabilitation.[1,6] To return the patient to maximal independence, the advice of social service personnel concerning the best use of home and community agency facilities should be sought. The aid of counselors in vocational rehabilitation should be obtained whenever possible. The full use of social service facilities can remove otherwise insurmountable obstacles. Vocational rehabilitation should be employed even in the case of limited life expectancy, if by so doing the patient may again become temporarily employed or successfully return to a previous family role, such as that of a mother with children. Each patient should be considered on an individual basis, with evaluation of the medical findings, the prognosis, and the maximum eventual gain to the patient, the patient's family, and the community.

A doctor sees cancer patients as people who are ill and in need of medical care. The social worker sees such people as social beings, interacting with their families and with other social groups, who are experiencing stress as a result of illness and are concerned about its effects upon their life situations. The social worker provides help in overcoming anxiety about a medical or surgical procedure. The social worker knows where all affiliated social agencies are located, what they offer, how to contact them, and how to obtain any services that can help the patient in his or her self-family-society relationships.

Our culture permits release from responsibility and work as an accepted response to chronic illness. If a positive attitude toward resumption of employment is to be developed, the physician and social service personnel must work together in motivating the patient to accept optimal rehabilitation goals, including possible employment. The patient with a limited work expectancy may be able to obtain at least temporary employment, and should not automatically be eliminated as ineligible.[2,16] The potential for employment is present both for those cancer patients who can be expected to be cured and for those who must continue to be treated for control of persistent disease. The latter really do not differ from patients with heart disease, diabetes, and many other chronic illnesses.

The problems these patients encounter when they try to reenter the work force often hamper their full potential for rehabilitation and lessen the quality of their lives. No one knows exactly how prevalent the job problem is nationwide, although physicians, vocational counselors, personnel agents, and the government acknowledge that it is commonplace. The American Cancer Society estimates that about 90 percent of patients trying to return to work face serious discrimination. Outdated policies exist in the medical and personnel departments of government agencies, private organizations, and industries. They either flatly reject the job applicant with a cancer history or demand an impossible disease-free waiting period of 5 years before consideration. Doctors know perhaps better than anyone the emotional and physical toll of such a long, needless period of unemployment.

Cancer patients are not only turned away by employers. Employment agencies and even rehabilitation agencies also refuse them. The reasons given include the complexity of the disease; disabilities related to both disease and treatment; mental, social, and cosmetic problems; problems of insurability and expected absenteeism; occasional problems of communication; and the financial burdens presented.

Difficulty in finding employment is demoralizing, and takes its toll not only on the patient but on the patient's family. Help in overcoming these difficulties often can be provided by health and vocational agencies, especially when the patient can be referred to a treatment center that has a social service department.

Preparation of the patient for employment demands adequate goal-oriented rehabilitation measures. The goals selected depend on the individual involved. Age, sex, the extent of disease, possible concomitant disease, education and training, and type and degree of physical disability must all be considered.

If physical disability is present, the patient must accept both the existence of the disability and also the probability of difficulty in obtaining employment. The patient must realize that specialized combinations of services will be needed to overcome any vocational handicap. The physician can play an important role in minimizing the psychological disability associated with physical changes, and can be an important bridge between the patient and the necessary specialized services. The social worker can help to determine rights of reemployment, fringe benefits, job duties, and working conditions. The social worker can also assist in discussions between the physician and a union representative, covering specific job details and recommendations covering discharge of duties. The social worker and the vocational and union counselors can work together to obtain employer acceptance of the worker with a cancer diagnosis, and acceptance, if necessary of the patient's limited ability to use public transportation or need for specialized job placement.

Publicly subsidized vocational rehabilitation services [state department of education, office of vocational rehabilitation (OVR)] are available for patients who have been left with substantial employment handicaps as a result of cancer or its treatment. One of the eligibility requirements is that the person be employable within a reasonable period. The work sought may be competitive employment, self-employment, sheltered employment, or homemaking. Any disability except blindness is covered by OVR services.

The services of OVR personnel include counseling in personal adjustment. Clients may receive services of this agency at a school, college, rehabilitation center, or sheltered workshop. Or the services may be given on a tutorial, corresponding, or on-the-job training basis. Special transportation may be provided.

Individual job placement and followup are provided by the OVR counselor. The counselor assists the client in securing employment that is commensurate with the client's aptitudes, knowledge, and skills. The counselor follows up after job placement to evaluate the appropriateness of the placement.

Physicians must make it their business not only to help their patients return to work but also to use their professional knowledge to help change society's attitudes. This may involve direct contact with employers, with permission of the patient, to explain the facts.[2]

In many communities, public and private agencies are ready to help sick, disabled, or troubled patients. In many cases, information services, such as the information bureau of the local community council or the local offices of the American Cancer Society, are available to help find the appropriate agency for a given problem.[1]

REFERENCES

1. Dietz JH Jr: *Rehabilitation Oncology*, Wiley, New York, 1981.
2. Dietz JH Jr: How doctors can help solve cancer patients' employment problems. *Leg Aspects Med Prac* 6(4):25, 1978.
3. Shah JP (ed): *Current Concepts in Surgical Oncology*, New York, Memorial Sloan-Kettering Cancer Center, 1978.
4. Dietz JH Jr, Rusk HA: Rehabilitation, in Schwartz SI (ed): *Principles of Surgery*, 3d ed, McGraw-Hill, New York, 1979.
5. Burgess EM et al: The management of lower extremity amputations, TR 10-6. US Government Printing Office, Washington, DC, 1969.
6. Russek AS: Investigation of immediate prosthetic fitting and early ambulation following amputation in the lower extremity. Publications Unit, Institute of Rehabilitation Medicine, New York University Medical Center, New York, 1969.
7. Rusk HA: *Rehabilitation Medicine*, 4th ed, Mosby, St. Louis, 1977.
8. Friedmann LW: Rehabilitation of amputees, in Licht S (ed): *Rehabilitation and Medicine*, Elizabeth Licht, New Haven, Conn., 1968.
9. Dietz JH Jr: Rehabilitation and readaptation for the patient with breast cancer, in Gallagher HS et al (eds): *The Breast*, Mosby, St. Louis, 1978.
10. Bobba JP (ed): *Reach to Recovery*, 3d ed., American Cancer Society, New York City Division, and Memorial Cancer Center, New York, 1977.
11. Goldsmith HS et al: Omental transposition in the control of chronic lymphedema. *JAMA* 203:1119, 1968.

12. Zegarelli EV et al: Maintaining the oral and general health of the oral cancer patient. *CA* 19:168, 1969.
13. Lauder E: *Self-Help for the Laryngectomee,* 2d ed. Available from the author at 6334 Dove Hill Drive, San Antonio, Texas 78238.
14. Gaskell DV, Webber BA: *The Brompton Hospital Guide to Chest Physical Therapy,* 2d ed., Blackwells, London, 1973. (Distributed by F. A. Davis Company, Philadelphia.)
15. Brain L, Forbes N Jr, (eds): *Contemporary Neurology Symposia,* vol. 1, *The Remote Effects of Cancer on the Nervous System,* Grune & Stratton, New York, 1965.
16. Healey JE (ed): *Ecology of the Cancer Patient,* The Interdisciplinary Communication Associates, Inc., Washington, DC, 1970.
17. Freireich EJ: Supportive therapy in acute leukemia, in *Clinical Aspects of Acute Leukemia,* American Cancer Society, New York, 1965.
18. Phillips CM: Reconstructive surgery after classical radical mastectomies using omental pedicled grafts and fascia lata. *Breast* 4(2):10, 1978.

SELECTED BIBLIOGRAPHY

Bromley B: Applying Orem's self-care theory in enterostomal therapy. *Am J Nurs* 80:245–249, 1980.

DeLisa JA et al: Rehabilitation of the cancer patient, in DeVita VT Jr et al (eds), *Cancer: Principles and Practice of Oncology,* Lippincott, Philadelphia, 1982, pp 1730–1763.

Dudgeon B et al: Head and neck cancer, a rehabilitation approach. *Am J Occup Ther* 34:243–251, 1980.

Healey JE Jr et al: Principles of rehabilitation, in Holland JF, Frei E (eds), *Cancer Medicine,* Lea & Febiger, Philadelphia, 1982, pp 2221–2236.

Naeve PP, Carter SK: Principles of cancer rehabilitation, in Carter SK et al (eds), *Principles of Cancer Treatment,* McGraw-Hill, New York, 1982, pp 273–280.

INDEX

INDEX

Abdominal tumors:
  adrenal tumors, 610–629
    (*See also* Adrenal tumors)
  carcinoid tumors, 630–642
    (*See also* Carcinoid tumors)
  colorectal cancer, 596–607
    (*See also* Colorectal cancer)
  liver and biliary tract cancer, 559–576
  lymphoma, 923–924
  pancreatic cancer, 580–594
    (*See also* Pancreatic cancer)
  stomach cancer, 543–555
    (*See also* Stomach cancer)
Acanthosis, 278
Acanthosis nigricans, 1033–1034
Acetaminophen as analgesic, 997–998
Acetylcholine and analgesia, 991
Acid-base disorders in cancer, 1038
Acid phosphatase, 703
  bone marrow levels, 710, 711
  prostatic, 708
  in prostatic cancer, 703, 708, 710–712
  in screening, 711–712
Acinic cell carcinoma, 392–393
Acral lentiginous melanoma, 863
ACTH ectopic syndrome, 1031
  differential diagnosis, 1034
  laboratory findings in, 1031
Actinomycin D:
  additive effect with radiotherapy, 193–194
  in gestational trophoblastic tumors, 853
  mechanism of effect, 193
  pharmacology, 127
  skin disease due to, 137

Acupuncture:
  naloxone reversal of analgesia of, 994
  in pain management, 1004
Addiction, 1001–1002
Adenoacanthoma, 782
Adenosis:
  management, 839
  natural history, 841
  vaginal, 837
Adenoviruses, 76–77
Adjuvant chemotherapy (*see* Chemotherapy, adjuvant)
Adrenal gland:
  APUD neurohumoral connection between cortex and medulla, 628
  distinctive hormone excess syndromes, 615, 617
  significance of ablation of, 610–611
  two distinct endocrine organs within, 610
Adrenal hyperplasia, 611
  treatment of hyperfunction in, 619
Adrenal tumors, 610–629
  adrenalectomy in, 614, 616, 618–620
  cortical, 614–621
    adjunctive treatment, 620
    diagnosis, work-up, and staging, 616–619
    Cushing's syndrome, 617–618
    masculinizing-feminizing syndromes, 618–619
    primary aldosteronism, 616–617
    follow-up and detection of recurrence or metastasis, 620

Adrenal tumors, cortical (*Cont.*):
  future prospects, 620–621
  historical aspects, 614–615
  incidence, 615–616
  intravenous extensions from tumor to vena cava, 618
  options for primary treatment, 619–620
  recurrence of metastasis, 620
  signs and symptoms, 616
  cysts, 611
  diagnosis, 613–614
    endocrine studies, 613
    tumor localization studies, 613–614
  functional effects of, 612–613
  hemorrhage, 611
  hyperplasia, 611
  mass effects of, 612
  medulla, 621–628
    (*See also* Pheochromocytoma)
  morphology, 611
  in multiple endocrine adenopathy, 628–629
  structure-function relationships in, 613
  therapy, 614
Adrenal venography, 623, 625
Adrenalectomy:
  for adrenal tumors, 614, 616, 618–620
  corticosteroid requirements after, 620
  pituitary hypersecretion of ACTH after, 619
  in prostatic cancer, 723
Adrenergic blockade in pheochromocytoma, 625–627

Adrenocorticotropic hormone (see ACTH)
Adrenogenital syndrome, 618–619
Adriamycin:
  additive effect with radiotherapy, 194
  in breast cancer, 533
  cardiac toxicity of, 135
  in osteosarcoma, 892
  pharmacology of, 127
  in soft-tissue sarcomas, 899–901
  in thyroid cancer, 420
Aflatoxin, 14
  and liver cancer, 561–563
Age:
  cancer risk related to, 16, 30
  individual and family reactions to cancer related to, 239–241
  and survival in melanoma, 867
Albinism and cancer, 54
Alcohol:
  absolute, in chemical neurolysis, 1016
  cancer risk related to, 17–18
  and carcinoid secretion, 636
  in epidermoid carcinoma of upper aerodigestive tract, 339
  and esophageal cancer, 36, 450
  and laryngeal cancer, 365
  and oral cancer, 276–277
  synergistic effect with tobacco, 339
Aldosteronism:
  diagnosis, 616–617
  differential diagnosis of adrenal lesion in, 617
  distinguishing primary from secondary, 616–617
  prevalance of, 616
Alkeran in ovarian cancer, 813, 820–821
Alkylating agents, 131
  as carcinogens, 13
  mechanism of action of, 130
  in ovarian cancer, 813–814
Alpha-fetoprotein (AFP), 157, 734
  antisera scans to localize metastases, 736
  in liver cancer, 565
  in testicular cancer, 732, 734, 735
Ameloblastoma, 332
Amines, aromatic, 12–13
Aminoglutethimide in adrenal tumors, 620
Amitriptyline, 1003

Amputation:
  management in children, 1046
  neuroma in stump, 1045
  in osteosarcoma, 890
  phantom pain after, 1045
  prosthesis after, 1046
  rehabilitation after, 1043–1047
  in soft-tissue sarcomas, 898
Analgesia:
  acetylcholine effect on, 991
  acupuncture effect on, 1004
  basic mechanisms of, 983–994
  dopamine effect on, 990
  electrical stimulation of brain producing, 992–994, 1012–1013
    deep brain stimulation, 1013
    intraventricular injection of endorphin, 1013
    transcutaneous neurostimulation, 1013
  hypnosis effect, 1004–1005
  neurochemistry of, 988–994
  serotonin effect on, 990
  (See also Pain management)
Analgesic nephropathy, 665–666
Analgesics, 995–1004
  adequate doses, 995–996
  choice of drug, 1000–1001
  clinical trial in use of, 996
  combinations of phenothiazines and tricyclics, 1003–1004
  development of plan in use of, 996
  ideal, 995
  maintaining alert sensorium with, 996
  marijuana, 1004
  narcotic, 998–1002
  (See also Narcotics)
  nonnarcotic, 997–998
  phenothiazines, 1002–1003
  physician errors in use of, 995–996
  preference of oral route for, 996
  principles of use, 995–996
  schedule for use, 996
  tricyclic antidepressants, 1003–1004
Anaphylaxis to chemotherapeutic agents, 137
Anastomotic leak after esophageal surgery, 460
Androgens:
  and prostatic cancer, 720
  receptors in breast cancer, 511
Anemia:
  in cancer, 1036–1037

Anemia (Cont.):
  myelosuppression causing, 130, 132
Anesthesia:
  in carcinoid tumors, 637
  in pain management, 1013–1017
    autonomic plexus blocks, 1014, 1016–1017
    chemical neurolysis, 1014–1016
    epidural and intrathecal block, 1014
    myofascial trigger point injection, 1014
    somatic nerve blocks, 1014
  in pheochromocytoma, 624, 626
Angiofibroma, nasopharyngeal, 328–330
Angiography:
  brain metastases detected by, 966, 967
  in brain tumors, 935–936
  in gestational trophoblastic tumors, 852
  in mediastinal tumors, 474
  in pancreatic cancer, 583–584
  in pheochromocytoma, 623–624
  in renal cell carcinoma, 648
  in renal pelvis and ureteral tumors, 672
  in Wilm's tumor, 659
Angiosarcoma, breast, 534
Aniline dye and bladder cancer, 680
Anorectal lesions:
  melanoma, 884
  (See also Colorectal cancer)
Anorexia in cancer, 1038
Antiandrogens in prostatic cancer, 723–724
Antibodies:
  formation in cancer, 148
  human-human, 171
  monoclonal, 163–172
    in head and neck cancer, 355–356
    (See also Monoclonal antibodies)
  therapeutic use in cancer, 166–171
  (See also Monoclonal antibodies)
Anticoagulation and metastatic spread, 211
Antidepressants:
  phenothiazines combined with, 1003–1004
  tricyclic, 1003
Antidiuretic hormone (ADH), 1030
  (See also Syndrome of inappropriate antidiuretic hormone)

Antigens:
  in breast cancer, 95–104
  carcinoembryonic, 156–157
    (*See also* Carcinoembryonic antigen)
  fetal, 156–157
    in human cancers, 156–157
  sulfaglycoprotein, 546
  tumor-specific transplantation antigens as, 145
  immunoperoxidase procedure for localization of, 96–97
  tumor (T): and cell transformation, 74–75
    in SV40 virus, 74–75
  tumor-associated: adaptive alteration of, 146
    alpha-fetoprotein, 157
    biological significance of, 144–147
    Burkitt's lymphoma, 153
    carcinoembryonic antigen, 156–157
    colon carcinoma, 154
    and concomitant immunity, 146
    herpes simplex antigens in cervical cancer, 754
    in human neoplasms, 152–157
    and immunologic surveillance, 145–147
    and malignant transformation, 144–145
    in melanoma, 154–155
    monoclonal antibodies to, 165–166
    nasopharyngeal carcinoma, 153
    neuroblastoma, 153–154
    oncofetal antigens, 156–157
    questions stimulated by existence of, 145
    sarcomas, 155–156
  tumor-specific transplantation (TSTA): coating by sialomucin, 146
    in experimental animals, 143–144
    and metastasis, 220
    as oncofetal antigens, 145
    in papilloma virus, 76
    of polyoma virus, 144
    tumor immunity related to, 143–144
Antimetabolites, 132–133
  mechanism of action of, 130
Anxiety in early cancer, 243

Apocrine metaplasia, immunoperoxidase staining of, 101–102
Appendix, carcinoid tumors of, 640–641
APUD tumors, 56, 592
  of adrenal medulla, 621–628
  carcinoid tumors, 631
    (*See also* Carcinoid tumors)
  of pancreas, 592–593
    (*See also* Multiple endocrine adenopathy; Pheochromocytoma)
Ara-C (*see* Cytosine arabinoside)
Aromatic amines, 12–13
  and bladder cancer, 680
Arrhenoblastoma, 815
Arsenic as carcinogen, 13
Arteriography (*see* Angiography)
Arylhydrocarbon hydroxylase (AHH) and lung cancer, 434
Asbestos:
  as carcinogen, 13
  tobacco synergism with, 13
Ascites in ovarian cancer, 823–824
Asparaginase:
  anaphylaxis after, 137
  hypofibrinogenemia due to, 137
  mechanism of action of, 130
  methotrexate therapeutic index improved by, 115–116
  nervous system disease due to, 136
  pancreatitis due to, 135
Aspergillus flavus, aflatoxin of, 14
Aspirin:
  as analgesic, 997
  combinations with, 997
  pharmacologic considerations, 997
  for prostatic cancer pain, 724
Astrocytoma:
  anaplastic, 943
  cerebellar, 945
  cerebral, 942–943
    pathology, 942
    seizures in, 942
    symptoms, 942
    treatment, 942–943
  classification, 937
  of third ventricle and anterior optic pathways, 947–948
Atabrine for malignant effusion in ovarian cancer, 823, 824
Ataxia-telangiectasia, 49
Attributable risk, 35
Australia antigen, 78

Autonomic plexus blocks, 1014, 1016–1017
Avian leukosis virus, 69
Avian sarcoma virus, 68–69
Axillary dissection:
  controversy regarding benefit in breast cancer, 519–521
  in intraductal breast carcinoma, 504–505, 507
  in lobular carcinoma in situ, 506
  pectoralis minor muscle preservation in, 518
  and segmental mastectomy, 522–523
Axillary lymph nodes, 514–515
Azygous venography in esophageal cancer, 454–455

Back pain in spine metastases, 974
Balkan nephropathy, 666
Barrett's epithelium, 450
Bartholin's gland, adenocarcinoma, 836
BCG immunotherapy:
  in lung cancer, 439
  in melanoma, 833–834, 880, 882
  vulvar, 833–834
BCNU:
  bone marrow transplantation used with, 958
  in brain tumors, 952, 955
  in glioblastoma multiforme, 942
  pulmonary toxicity of, 952
  (*See also* Nitrosoureas)
Benign lymphoepithelial lesion, 393–394, 397
Benzene as carcinogen, 14
Benzopyrene, 12
Benzpyrine as pancreatic carcinogen, 580–581
Bergman's sign, 670–671
Bilharziasis and bladder cancer, 681
Biliary tract tumors, 559–576
  extrahepatic: associated disorders, 563
    benign, 591–592
    diagnosis, 566, 568
    etiology, 564
    incidence, 563
    prognosis, 575, 576
    treatment, 574–576
  liver cancer (*see* Liver cancer)
    (*See also* Gallbladder cancer)
Biofeedback, 1005

Biological response modifiers in brain tumors, 958–959
Biopsy:
  in bladder cancer, 682
  bone marrow, 909, 911
  in breast cancer, 496–497, 500–501, 503
  brush, 672–673
  kidney, in renal cell carcinoma, 647
  liver (see Liver biopsy)
  in melanoma, 864
  needle (see Needle biopsy)
  in osteosarcoma, 889–890
  in ovarian cancer, 812
  in pancreatic cancer, 584–586
  in prostatic cancer, 703–705
  in renal pelvis and ureteral tumors, 672–673
  of salivary gland neoplasms, 396
  of soft-tissue sarcomas, 897
  in thyroid cancer, 415
Birth-cohort analysis, 29
Black bile theory, 198–199
Bladder:
  anatomy, 683
  drainage after radical hysterectomy, 762–763
  fistula after radical hysterectomy, 764
  outlet obstruction in prostatic cancer, 725–726
Bladder cancer, 679–694
  aromatic amines role in, 12–13
  bilharziasis and, 681
  classification, 683–685
  diagnostic techniques in, 681–686
    bimanual examination under anesthesia, 682
    biopsy, 682
    computerized tomography, 685–686
    cystendoscopy, 682
    evaluation for metastases, 682
    intravenous pyelography, 682
    lymphangiogram, 686
    ultrasonography, 686
  early detection, 681
  epidemiology, 40, 680
  etiology, 680–681
  factors related to occurrence, 21
  historical aspects, 679
  incidence, 679–680
  metastases in, 690

Bladder cancer (Cont.):
  paraneoplastic syndromes associated with, 1027
  radiotherapy with surgery for, 190
  signs and symptoms, 681
  staging of, 682–686
  treatment, 687–694
    carcinoma in situ, 689–690
    chemotherapy, 687–689, 694
    cystectomy, 691–694
    immunotherapy, 688
    invasive carcinoma, 690–694
    radiotherapy, 691–694
    segmental resection, 690
    superficial tumors, 687–689
    surgery, 687, 689–692
    transurethral resection, 682, 690–691
    triethylene thiophosphoramide, 687–688
Bleomycin:
  in esophageal cancer, 463
  in head and neck cancer, 350
  lung damage due to, 135
  for malignant effusion in ovarian cancer, 824
  mechanism of action of, 130
  methotrexate therapeutic index improved by, 116
  mitomycin C synergy with, 117
  pharmacology of, 127
  skin disease due to, 136–137
  as synchronizing agent, 116–117
  in vaginal cancer, 840
  vincristine synergistic effect with, 116
  in vulvar cancer, 830
Blood-brain barrier in brain tumor, 957–958
Bloom's syndrome, 49
Bone grafts in osteosarcoma therapy, 891
Bone marrow biopsy in Hodgkin's disease, 909, 911
Bone marrow failure, 130, 132–134
Bone marrow transplantation:
  rehabilitation in, 1072–1073
  use with BCNU therapy in brain tumors, 958
Bone tumors, 888–895
  of extremities: rehabilitation, 1043–1047
    (See also Extremity cancer, rehabilitation in)
  factors related to occurrence, 21

Bone tumors (Cont.):
  of nose and paranasal sinuses, 331–332
  osteogenic sarcoma of facial bones, 332
  pathologic fractures in, 1047
  (See also Osteosarcoma)
Bowel cancer (see Colorectal cancer)
Braces after long bone and joint replacement, 1046
Brachytherapy (see Interstitial irradiation)
Bracken fern, 14
Bradykinin and pain, 989
Bradykinin shock, 637
Brain:
  deep stimulation in pain control, 1013
  electrical stimulation producing analgesia, 992–994
  herniation of, 932
  injury by radiotherapy, 940
  and pain perception, 992–994
Brain metastases, 965–972
  current areas of research and future prospects, 972
  deficits in, 1070
  diagnostic techniques and evaluation of, 966–967
    angiography, 966, 967
    CT scanning, 966–967
  differential diagnosis of, 967
  incidence, 965–966
  melanoma, 971
  seizures in, 966
  signs and symptoms, 966
  solitary versus multiple, 965–966
  treatment, 967, 969–972
    chemotherapy, 970, 971
    dexamethasone, 969
    immunotherapy, 972
    multiple metastases, 970–972
    radiotherapy, 970–971
    recurrent metastasis, 972
    solitary metastasis, 969–970
    surgery, 969–970
Brain tumors, 929–961
  in adults, 941–945
  astrocytoma, 942–943
    (See also Astrocytoma)
  attempts at early detection, 933
  benign versus malignant, 930
  blood-brain barrier in, 957–958
  brainstem glioma, 948

Brain tumors (*Cont.*):
  cerebellar astrocytoma, 945
  in children, 945–949
  choroid plexus papilloma, 944–945
  clinical manifestations, 931–933
    focal neurologic deficits, 931
    headache, 932–933
    increased intracranial pressure, 931–932
    secondary effects due to displacement of brain, 932
    seizures, 931
  current areas of research and future prospects in, 955–960
    biological response modifiers, 958–959
    brachytherapy, 957
    clonogenic cell analysis, 959–960
    high-LET radiation, 956–957
    hypoxic cell radiosensitizers, 955–956
    immunotherapy, 959
    improving therapeutic index, 958
    intraarterial chemotherapy, 957–958
    intratumoral chemotherapy, 958
    intraventricular and intrathecal chemotherapy, 958
    investigations of tumor biology, 959–960
    multimodality interactions, 959
    tumor markers, 960
  cyst formation in, 951
  diagnostic techniques, work-up, and staging, 933–936
    angiography, 935–936
    CT scanning, 933–934
    electroencephalography, 935
    lumbar puncture, 936
    radionuclide scans, 935
    skull films, 935
    ventriculography and pneumoencephalography, 936
  ependymoma, 944
    (*See also* Ependymoma)
  epidemiology, 930
  etiology, 930
  genetic factors in, 930
  glioblastoma multiforme, 941–942
    (*See also* Glioblastoma multiforme)
  gliomas (*see* Glioma)
  incidence, 929–930
  inherited, 57
  intraventricular, 937–938

Brain tumors (*Cont.*):
  medulloblastoma, 945–947
    (*See also* Medulloblastoma)
  metastases of, 951–952
  metastases to brain, 965–972
    (*See also* Brain metastases)
  neuroectodermal tumors, 936–938
  oligodendrogliomas, 943
    (*See also* Oligodendrogliomas)
  paraneoplastic syndromes associated with, 1027
  pineal tumors, 948–949
  recurrence: cyst formation as sign of, 951
    differential diagnosis of, 949–952
    infection simulating, 951
    metabolic and drug-related problems in, 950–951
    other neurological disorders simulating, 951
    seizures heralding, 950
    strokelike syndrome due to, 950
    treatment, 952–955
  rehabilitation in, 960–961, 1069–1071
    demented patient, 961
    musculoskeletal considerations, 961
    speech abnormalities, 960–961
    visual disturbances, 960
  reticulum-cell sarcoma, 943–944
  subependymal mixed glioma, 944
  third ventricle and anterior optic pathways astrocytoma, 947–948
  treatment, 938–940
    anatomic location and histology influences on, 940–949
    hypertonic solutions, 939
    hyperventilation, 939
    radiotherapy, 940
    recurrent disease, 952–955
      chemotherapy, 952–955
      radiotherapy, 952
      reoperation, 952
    removal of cerebrospinal fluid, 939
    surgery, 938–940
      intraoperative measures, 939
      microsurgical techniques, 938
      postoperative measures, 939–940
      preoperative measures, 939
      shunting for hydrocephalus, 938

Brain tumors (*Cont.*):
  (*See also* Central nervous system tumors)
Brainstem:
  and pain perception, 992
  spinothalamic tractotomy in, 1010–1011
Brainstem glioma, 948
Breast benign neoplasms, immunoperoxidase staining of, 100–102
Breast cancer, 491–536
  antigens involved in, 95–104
    in apocrine metaplasia, 101–102
    differences between mouse and human tumors, 103
    immunoperoxidase staining for, 98–103
    localization in mouse mammary tumors, 96–97
    in malignant breast tissue, 98–100
    in normal and benign breast tissue, 100–101
    role of sugar versus protein moieties, 103–104
  blast transformation after phytohemagglutinin stimulation in, 151–152
  classification, 512–514
  contralateral breast disease: in intraductal carcinoma, 505, 507
    in invasive lobular carcinoma, 508
    in lobular carcinoma in situ, 506–507
  delayed cutaneous hypersensitivity in, 149–150
  diagnosis: biopsy, 496–497, 500–501, 503
    characteristics of malignant mass, 498–499
    mammography, 496–501
    needle biopsy, 500–501, 503
    occult disease, 496–498
    with palpable mass, 498–501, 503
    screening, 491–496
    specimen radiography after biopsy, 497–498, 502
  diet role in etiology, 53
  difficulty in randomization in clinical trials, 263
  epidemiology, 39
  estrogen receptor assays in, 508–512
    as aid in differential diagnosis of metastatic adenocarcinoma, 511

Breast cancer, estrogen receptor assays in (*Cont.*):
  correlation with response to endocrine therapy, 511
  predicting response to chemotherapy, 511–512
  as prognostic factor, 511
  sources and variability in results, 509–511
  and treatment of metastases, 533
  uses for, 511
 etiology, 53
 factors related to occurrence, 21
 familial syndromes, 53–54
  screening for, 60
 histologic types of invasive disease, 507–508
 hydrocortisone levels in, 236–237
 hypocalcemia in, 1029
 immunodeficiency in, 149–150
 intraductal carcinoma, 503–505
  axillary dissection in, 504–505, 507
  mastectomy in, 504, 507
  risk of invasive disease, 504
  treatment of contralateral breast in, 505, 507
 invasive ductal carcinoma, 508
 invasive lobular carcinoma, 508
 lobular carcinoma in situ, 505–507
  mastectomy in, 506–507
  progression to invasive disease, 505–506
  treatment of contralateral breast in, 506–507
 lymphosarcoma, 534
 as major public health problem, 491
 in males, 535–536
 mastectomy (*see* Mastectomy)
 meningeal carcinomatosis in, 966
 mucinous carcinoma, 508
 noninvasive carcinoma, 503–507
 in nuns, 236
 palliative procedures in, 1055–1056
 paraneoplastic syndromes associated with, 1027
 peripheral blood lymphocyte counts in, 150–151
 personality factors in, 236–238
 prognosis: axillary involvement in, 514–515
  estrogen receptors and, 511
  in male, 535
 psychological reactions specific to, 250

Breast cancer (*Cont.*):
 reconstructive surgery after, 1047–1048, 1055
 risk factors for, 39
 sarcomas, 533–535
  angiosarcoma, 534
  cystosarcoma phylloides, 533–534
  lymphosarcoma, 534
  stromal sarcoma, 535
 scirrhous carcinoma, 508
 screening for, 491–496
  breast cancer detection demonstration project, 494–495
  current status of, 495–496
  HIP study, 492–494
 staging of, 512–515
 T and B lymphocytes in, 151
 thymidine labeling index and prediction of response to chemotherapy in, 113
 thymidine labeling index related to estrogen receptor status in, 114
 treatment: adjuvant therapy, 528–531
  chemotherapy, 528–532
   estrogen receptor assay and, 511–512
   local or regional recurrence, 532
   loco-regionally advanced and inflammatory carcinoma, 531–532
   male breast, 535–536
  radiotherapy, 523–528
   in control of subclinical disease, 185
   with surgery, 190–191, 519–521
  skeletal metastases, 532–533
  surgery, 515–523
   in cystosarcoma phylloides, 534
   extended radical mastectomy, 516–517
   in intraductal carcinoma, 504–505
   in lobular carcinoma in situ, 506–507
   lumpectomy, 521–523
   modified radical mastectomy, 517–519
   quadrantectomy, 523
   radical mastectomy, 515–516
   segmental mastectomy, 521–523
   total (simple) mastectomy with and without radiotherapy, 519–521

Breast cancer, treatment, surgery (*Cont.*):
  (*See also* Mastectomy)
  systemic metastases in receptor-negative patients, 533
 tumor-specific particles in, 92–93
 types of, 503–508
 virology, 88–106
  antigenic relationships, 95–104
   (*See also* antigens involved in, *above*)
  sequence homology of RNA, 90–92
  simultaneous detection of reverse transcriptase and high-molecular-weight RNA, 92–94
Breast Cancer Detection Demonstration Project, 494–495
Breast reconstruction, 1055
Brompton's solution, 725, 1000
Bronchogenic carcinoma (*see* Lung cancer)
Bronchogenic cysts, 478, 480
Bronchoscopy in esophageal cancer, 454
Brush biopsy in renal pelvis and ureteral tumors, 672–673
Buccal mucosa cancer, 287–290
 anatomy, 287–288
 clinical presentation, 288–289
 incidence and etiology, 288
 pathology, 288–289
 prognosis, 290
 results of treatment, 290
 and tobacco use, 288
 treatment, 289–290
Burkitt's lymphoma:
 chromosomal abnormality role in, 50
 Epstein-Barr role in, 84–86
 immunopathogenesis of, 57–58
 treatment, 923
 tumor-specific antigens in, 153

Cachexia in cancer, 1038
Calcitonin:
 in cancer, 1033
 in thyroid medullary carcinoma, 411–412, 417
Calcium:
 and carcinoid secretion, 636
 (*See also* Hypercalcemia; Hypocalcemia)
Californium 252 in cervical cancer, 774

CALLA, 165
  monoclonal antibody directed against, 167–168
Cancer:
  cause of (*see* Carcinogenesis; Carcinogens; Epidemiology)
  in childhood (*see* Childhood cancer)
  childhood experiences of patients with, 233–234
  cytologic differences between benign and malignant tumors, 25
  definition, 18, 24
  depression and hopelessness as antecedent to, 232–233
  diabetes and, 581
  effect on family, 238–248
  employment difficulties in, 1074–1075
    (*See also* Vocational rehabilitation)
  factors related to, 9
  family response to, 238–248
  genetic and familial aspects, 41–43, 46–61, 89–90
    breast cancer, 53–54
    central nervous system tumors, 57
    childhood cancers, 46–48
    chromosomes role, 48
    clastogenic syndrome, 49–51
    colon carcinoma, 52–53
    genetic counseling, 61
    multiple endocrine neoplasia, 56–57
    neurofibromatosis, 55–56
    recognition, 51–52
    screening for, 59–61
    skin syndromes, 54–55
    X-linked lymphoproliferative syndrome as model, 57–59
  historical perspectives, 4–5
  host factors in, 210–211
    (*See also* Metastasis, tumor-host factors modulating)
  immunodeficiency related to, 147–152
  metastasis (*see* Metastasis)
  pathologic diagnosis, 18–19
  psychological aspects, 231–251
    (*See also* Psychosocial factors in cancer)
  reactions to diagnosis, 241–243
  registries, 31
  remote effects on nervous system, 1070

Cancer (*Cont.*):
  repressive personality associated with, 234–235
  systemic effects (*see* Paraneoplastic syndromes)
  (*See also* Neoplasms)
Cannabis, 1004
Capillary physiology, metastasis related to, 210–211
Carcinoembryonic antigen (CEA), 156–157
  colorectal cancer followed by, 605
  in human cancers, 156–157
  in liver cancer, 565, 566
  monoclonal antibody to, 166
Carcinogenesis, 7–22
  age, 30
  agents implicated in, 9–16
    aflatoxin and other natural substances, 14
    alkylating agents, 13
    hormones, 14–15
    inorganic chemicals, 13
    nitrosamines, 14
    physical, 10, 12
    polycyclic aromatic hydrocarbons, 12–13
    vinyl chloride and other industrial chemicals, 14
    viruses, 15–16
  classification of agents of, 9–11
  in colorectal cancer, 37–38
  controversy of animal studies on, 19
  historical aspects, 7–9
  host factors involved in, 16–18, 30
    age, 16
    genetic and familial, 30, 46–61
      (*See also* Cancer, genetic and familial aspects)
    heredity, 16
    immune status, 18
    nutrition, 17–18
    sex, 16–17
  hypotheses of, 89
  immunodeficiency related to, 147–152
  immunologic surveillance and, 145–147
  latency period in, 26
  of liver cancer, 559, 561–563
  mechanism of, 19–20
  multistage hypothesis of, 26
  psychosocial factors in, 231–238
  radiation role in thyroid cancer, 419
  sex, 30

Carcinogenesis (*Cont.*):
  threshold for, 9
  tumor-associated antigens related to, 144–145
  unavoidable exposure, 9
  viruses in, 65–87
    (*See also* Oncoviruses)
  (*See also* Epidemiology)
Carcinogens:
  in bladder cancer, 680–681
  in cervical cancer, 755
  in pancreatic cancer, 580–581
  in renal pelvis and ureteral tumors, 665–666
Carcinoid cells:
  characteristics of, 631
  history of, 630–631
Carcinoid syndrome:
  in bronchial tumors, 435, 639–640
  carcinoid tumors causing, 632
  diagnosis, 636–637
    metabolite screening tests, 636–637
    provocative tests, 636
    serum tests, 636
  history, 631
  hormones associated with, 633
  occasional findings in, 633
  and staging carcinoid tumors, 635–636
  treatment, 637–638
  typical features of, 632–633
Carcinoid tumors, 630–642
  appendix, 640–641
  bronchial, 634–635, 639–640
  carcinoid syndrome due to, 632
  diagnosis, 634–635
  early detection of, 633–634
  epidemiology, 632
  follow-up and early identification of metastases, 638–639
  future prospects for, 641–642
  of gastrointestinal tract, 635
  history of, 630–631
  hormones associated with, 633
  incidence, 631–632
  location of, 631–632
  malignant potential of, 633–634
  multicentricity of, 633
  in multiple endocrine adenopathy, 632
  paradoxic response to beta-adrenergic agonists in, 637
  prognosis, 639

Carcinoid tumors (*Cont.*):
  rectal, 641
  signs and symptoms, 633
  small-bowel, 640
  staging, 635–636
  stomach, 640
  tests for associated disorders, 635
  treatment, 637–641
    adjunctive therapy, 637–638
    carcinoid syndrome, 637–638
    chemotherapy, 638
    surgery, 637
Cartilage tumors of nose and paranasal sinuses, 331
CAT scanning (*see* Tomography, computerized)
Catecholamines:
  determination in pheochromocytoma, 622
  morphine interactions with, 991
  reduction in synthesis by alpha-methyl-*p*-tyrosine, 627–628
Celestin tune, 462–463
  in stomach cancer, 553–554
Celiac plexus block, 1014, 1016
Celiacangiography in pancreatic cancer, 583–584
Cell biology and kinetics, 108–119
  chemotherapeutic exploitability, 111–113
  clinical observations and correlations, 113–114
  hormone stimulation, suppression, and response, 114
  in vitro predictive tests, 117–119
    changes in thymidine labeling index and response, 117–118
    direct cloning assays, 118–119
  kinetics of cell kill, 110–111
  proliferation cycle, 108–110
  recruitment and synchronization attempts, 114–117
    experimental tumors, 114–115
    human tumors, 115–117
Cell cycle:
  chemotherapy related to, 109–111
  and radiosensitivity, 179
  stages of, 179
Cell kill:
  cell-cycle specificity of chemotherapy and, 110–111
  kinetics of, 110
Cell loss, 185

Cell-mediated immunity:
  in breast cancer, 149–150
  in cancer, 148
  testing of, 148
Cell transformation by viruses, 66–67
  (*See also* Transformation)
Cells, properties transformed by viruses, 66–67
Cells, tumor:
  adherence, 209–210
  arrest and growth in metastasis, 207–212
    observed morphologic events during, 207
  in circulation, 206–207
    organ arrest pattern by radioactive labeling, 206–207
    transorgan passage of viable cells, 207
  clumping and metastasis efficiency, 207–208
  deformability, 209
  dormancy of, 223–224
  heterogeneity of, 216–219
    demonstration of, 217
    in metastasis formation, 217–218
    and tumor vasculature, 216
  increased detachment from each other, 205
  inefficiency of establishing metastasis, 206–207
  invasive properties, 210
  locomotion in invasion, 204
  lymphatic transport, entrapment, and transnodal passage of, 212
  lytic enzymes facilitating invasion, 204–205
  membrane characteristics important in metastasis, 208–210
    biochemical properties, 210
    deformability or rigidity, 209
    stickiness or adherence, 209–210
    vesicles role, 208
  neovascularization and growth in extravascular space, 211
  relationship to vasculature, 202–203
  rigidity, 209
  selection in metastasis, 224
  stickiness, 209–210
Cellular-embolic theory of metastasis, 199–201
Central nervous system tumors:
  inherited, 57

Central nervous system tumors (*Cont.*):
  metastatic disease, 965–978
    brain, 965–972
    (*See also* Brain metastases)
    leptomeninges, 972–973
    spine, 973–978
  in nasal cavity, 327
  primary, 929–961
  (*See also* Brain tumors)
Centralized cancer patient data system, 31
Cerebellar astrocytoma, 945
Cerebellar degeneration, 1036
Cerebral astrocytoma, 942–943
Cerebral edema after brain surgery, 949–950
Cerebral infarction and recurrence of brain tumor, 950
Cerebrospinal fluid:
  excessive production by choroid plexus papilloma, 945
  in leptomeningeal metastases, 973
  removal in brain surgery, 939
Cervical lymph nodes (*see* Lymph nodes, cervical)
Cervix, cancer of, 751–775
  depression as antecedent to, 232
  diagnostic evaluation, 756–760
    colposcopy, 753
    computerized tomography in, 759
    cystoscopy, 758
    cytology, 752–753
    historical advances in, 752–753
    lower urinary tract, 758
    lymphangiography, 759
    nutritional status, 760
    prior to radiotherapy, 759–760
    recurrent disease, 770
    regional lymph nodes, 757–759
    size and anatomic location of primary lesion, 758–759
  in endometrial adenocarcinoma, 785
  epidemiology, 39–40, 753–756
  etiology, 753–756
  factors related to occurrence, 21
  future advances in, 773–775
  herpes simplex role in, 81–83, 754–755
  histologic classification of, 753, 756
  historical advances in, 751–753
  microinvasive disease, 756
  personality factors in, 235–236, 238
  in pregnancy, 769–770

Cervix, cancer of (*Cont.*):
  prognosis, 773
  prognostic factors in, 756–761
  screening for, 755–756, 773
  spermatozoa role in, 755
  spread of: difficulty in diagnosis, 773
    extrapelvic lymph node metastases, 759, 766
    extrapelvic recurrent metastases, 772
    invasive disease, 760–769
    to regional lymph nodes, 757–758
  staging of, 753, 757–760
  survival in, 773
  treatment, 760–773
    californium 252, 774
    chemotherapy, 768–769, 772
    extrapelvic lymph node metastases, 773–774
    follow-up, 773
    high-pressure oxygen, 774
    historical advances in, 751–752
    invasive disease, 760–769
    linear-energy transfer, 774
    microinvasive disease, 760
    palliation, 772–773
    pelvic exenteration, 770–772
    in pregnancy, 769–770
    radiation sensitizers, 774
    radiotherapy, 187–188, 752, 759–761, 765, 772
    recurrence, 770–773
    surgery, 751–752, 770–773
    tumor markers in, 774–775
Cheek (*see* Buccal mucosa cancer)
Chemical neurolysis, 1014–1016
Chemosurgery in head and neck cancer, 352–355
Chemotherapy, 124–137
  adjuvant: differences between animal and clinical situation, 129
    factors favorable with surgery, 129
    theory, experiment, and practice, 128–130
  in bladder cancer, 687–689, 694
  of brain metastases, 970, 971
  in brain tumors: biological response modifiers, 958–959
    improving therapeutic index, 958
    interaction with other drugs, 959
    pharmacologic considerations, 957–958

Chemotherapy, in brain tumors (*Cont.*):
    recurrent disease, 952–955
      combination, 954
      specific drugs, 952–954
  in breast cancer, 528–532
  in carcinoid tumors, 638
  cell characteristics relating to drug efficacy, 112–113
  cell cycle related to, 109–111
  in cervical cancer, 768–769, 772
  cloning assays in predicting response to, 118–119
  in colorectal cancer, 602–604
  combination, 126–128
  cross-resistance in, 126
  dose response and therapeutic index in, 128
  in endometrial cancer, 796
  in esophageal cancer, 463–464
  factors affecting choice of, 125
  in gestational trophoblastic tumors, 852–855
  in glioblastoma multiforme, 942
  in hard palate cancer, 296
  in head and neck cancer, 348–350
  in Hodgkin's disease, 913–915
  intraarterial infusion: in brain tumors, 957–958
    in liver cancer, 572–573
    in pancreatic cancer, 589–590
  intraperitoneal instillation, 823
  intratumoral administration, 958
  intraventricular and intrathecal administration, 958
    for brain metastases, 971
  kinetics of cell kill by, 110
  in laryngeal cancer, 382
  in liver cancer, 572–573
  in lung cancer, 440–441
  in lymphoma: Burkitt's lymphoma, 923
    diffuse disease, 922–923
    nodular disease, 921
  maintenance rationale, 110
  major classes, 130–134
  marijuana as adjunct in, 1004
  mechanisms of action of, 112, 130
  in medulloblastoma, 947
  in melanoma, 880–881
    vulvar, 833–834
  monoclonal antibody as conjugate in, 170–171

Chemotherapy (*Cont.*):
  in neuroblastoma, 661
  in oral cancer, 284
  in oropharyngeal tumors, 348
  in osteosarcoma, 891–894
  in ovarian cancer, 813–814, 820–824
    second-line, 822–823
  in pancreatic cancer, 589–590
  in paranasal sinus tumors, 326
  pharmacologic principles, 125–127
  of pineal tumors, 949
  prediction of response to, direct cloning assays, 118–119
  in prostatic cancer, 715, 724
  radiotherapy combined with, in head and neck cancer, 348
  in renal pelvis tumors, 676
  resistance developing to, 126
  of salivary gland neoplasms, 403
  sample size requirements for clinical trials related to, 260
  selective antitumor effect of, 124–125
  in soft-tissue sarcomas, 899–901
  in spinal metastases, 977–978
  in stomach cancer, 551–552, 554
  in testicular cancer, 737–738
  thymidine labeling index and prediction of response to, 113–114, 117–118
    in vitro studies, 117–118
    studies in patients, 113–114
  in thyroid cancer, 420
  toxicity of, 130, 132–137
    cardiac damage, 135
    gastrointestinal, 134–135
    myelosuppression, 130, 132–134
    nervous system, 136
    pulmonary damage, 135
    renal damage, 135–136
    skin, 136–137
  treated serum in determining response to, 118
  tumor-specific antibodies used with, 958
  in uterine sarcomas, 804
  in vulvar cancer, 830
  in Wilms's tumor, 660
Chest percussion after thoracotomy, 1067–1068
Chest tumors (*see* Intrathoracic tumors)

Chibba needle, 584, 585
Childhood cancer:
    brain tumors, 945–949
    congenital malformations associated with, 47
    hereditary factors, 46–48
    neuroblastoma, 660–662
    rehabilitation of amputee, 1046
    second neoplasms, 47
    testicular cancer, 738
    Wilms's tumor, 658–660
Chlornaphazin, 13
Chlorpromazine, 1002–1003
Cholangiography, percutaneous transhepatic:
    in jaundice evaluation, 568, 569
    in pancreatic cancer, 584
Cholinergic neurotransmitters, 989–990
Chondroma of nose and paranasal sinuses, 331
Chondrosarcoma, 331
    factors affecting results of treatment, 331
    surgical treatment, 331
Chordoma, 327
    cartilage tumors distinguished from, 331
Chorioadenoma destruens, 846
Choriocarcinoma:
    incidence, 845
    in mediastinum, 481, 483
    in ovary, 815
    pathology, 846–847
    pregnancy confused with, 847
    (See also Gestational trophoblastic tumors)
Choroid plexus papilloma, 944–945
Chromaffin tumors, 621–628
    (See also Pheochromocytoma)
Chromosome abnormalities:
    cancer associated with, 48
    cell transformation causing, 67
    in clastogenic syndromes, 49–51
        ataxia-telangiectasia, 49
        Bloom's syndrome, 49
        chronic myelogenous leukemia, 50, 51
        dyskeratosis congenita, 49–50
        Fanconi's anemia, 49
        Philadelphia chromosome, 50
        solid tumors, 50–51
Cigarettes (see Tobacco)
Cingulumotomy, 1011–1012

Circadian rhythm, disturbance in Cushing's syndrome, 618
Circumcision and cervical cancer, 755
Cirrhosis and liver cancer, 563
Cis-platinum (See Platinum)
Citrovorum rescue, 892
Classification systems, 24–26
    by anatomic site of primary, 24
    by histologic type, 24–26
    by stage of disease, 26
Clastogenic syndromes, 49–51
    screening for, 60
Clinical trials, 254–271
    advantages of patient participation, 269
    blinding and use of placebos in, 265–266
    considerations for protocol planning and experimental design, 256–269
        control group, 264–266
        defining specific aim, 257
        estimating available resources, 257–261
        ethical considerations, 266–269
        preparation of protocol, 261
        randomization process, 261–264
    cost of conducting, 260–261
    data evaluation in, 269–271
        probability values and statistical tests of life tables in, 271
    determining number of patients and length of follow-up in, 257–260
    ethical considerations, 266–269
        consent of participating patient, 267–268
        data integrity, 268–269
        use of control group, 267
    historical background, 255–256
    informed consent in, 267–268
    lack of knowledge about, 254
    randomization process in, 261–264
    rationale for prospective, randomized study, 256
    retrospective studies, 264–265
    three phases in cancer studies, 254–255
Clones, metastatic heterogeneity in, 218–219
Cloning assays in predicting response to chemotherapy, 118–119
Clonogenic assay:
    in brain tumors, 959–960
    in soft-tissue sarcoma, 901

Clubbing in hypertrophic pulmonary osteoarthropathy, 1034
Clumping, 207–208
CMF regimen in breast cancer, 529–531
Codeine, 999
Colon cancer (see Colorectal cancer)
Colon interposition after esophageal resection, 458–459
Colonoscopy in colorectal cancer, 600, 604
Colorectal cancer, 596–607
    brighter outlook in, 596, 597
    carcinoembryonic antigen in, 156–157, 605
    carcinoid tumors, 641
    current research and prospects for future, 606
    diagnosis: colonoscopy in, 600, 604
        in early stages, 599–600
    diet role in etiology of, 17, 37–38
    epidemiology, 37–38, 596–599
    etiology, 596–598
        diet, 596, 598
        genetics, 597
    factors related to occurrence, 21
    familial polyposis and, 597–598
    familial syndromes, 52–53
        screening for, 60
    follow-up for early identification of recurrence or metastasis, 604–605
    historical aspects of, 596, 597
    incidence, 596
    monoclonal antibody in treatment of, 170
    paraneoplastic syndromes associated with, 1027
    psychological reactions specific to, 250
    radiotherapy with surgery for, 190
    reconstruction and rehabilitation in, 606–607
    recurrence, 605–606
    rehabilitation in, 1056–1060
        colostomy, 1056–1059
        ileostomy, 1059–1060
    screening for, 599–600
    staging of, 600–602
    symptoms, 600
    treatment: adjuvant therapy, 602–604
        chemotherapy, 602–604
        liver metastases, 571–572

Colorectal cancer, treatment (*Cont.*):
    options for primary therapy, 601–602
    radiotherapy, 602–603
    recurrence or metastases, 605–606
    surgery, 601–602
  tumor-specific antigens in, 154
  ulcerative colitis and, 598
Colorectal polyposis syndrome, 53
Colostomy:
  control problems with, 1059
  irrigation of, 1058
  ostomy bags for, 1058
  psychological reactions specific to, 250
  rehabilitation after, 1056–1059
    convalescence, 1058
    operative care, 1057
    postoperative treatment, 1057–1058
    preoperative treatment, 1056–1057
    transitional and hospital care, 1058–1059
Colposcopy in cervical cancer, 753
Combined modality therapy, 3
  rationale for, 110–111
Commissural myelotomy, 1007–1008
Common acute lymphoblastic leukemia antigen (*see* CALLA)
Computerized axial tomography (*see* Tomography, computerized)
Confounding variables, 33
Congenital anomalies:
  childhood cancer associated with, 47
  Wilms's tumor associated with, 658–659
Consent in clinical trials, 267–268
Contractures in brain tumors, 961
Control group, 264–266
  ethical considerations, 267
Convulsions:
  in brain metastases, 966
  in brain tumors, 931
  in cerebral astrocytoma, 942
  and recurrence of brain tumor, 950
Cordotomy, 1008–1010
  high cervical, 1009
  percutaneous, 1009–1010
  thoracic, 1008–1009
Corticosteroids:
  for brain metastases, 969
  in brain tumors, 954

Corticosteroids (*Cont.*):
  in carcinoid syndrome, 638
  distinct syndromes of excess of, 615
  hydrocortisone levels in breast cancer, 236–237
  receptors in breast cancer, 511
  requirements after adrenalectomy, 620
  tumor cell kinetics related to, 114
  use with surgery in brain tumors, 939
Corynebacterium parvum immunotherapy in ovarian cancer, 821
Costs of clinical trials, 260–261
Courvoisier's sign, 582
Cranial nerves, neurotomy for pain control, 1006
Craniofacial resection, 323–326
  end results, 326
  morbidity and mortality rates of, 325–326
  reconstruction in, 325
  technique, 323–325
Cryosurgery:
  in head and neck cancer, 350–351
  in prostatic cancer, 725–726
  transurethral, 725–726
Cryptorchidism, testicular cancer association with, 730
CT scanning (*see* Tomography, computerized)
Cushing's disease, hyperplasia therapy causing, 619
Cushing's syndrome:
  adrenal tumors causing, 617–618
  circadian rhythm disturbance in, 618
  clinical features, 616
  diagnosis, 617–618
  ectopic ACTH causing, 1031
  incidence, 616
  recurrent, 620
Cycasin, 14
Cyclamates and bladder cancer, 680–681
Cyclocytidine, sialadenitis due to, 135
Cyclophosphamide:
  hemorrhagic cystitis due to, 136
  mechanism of action of, 130
  pharmacology, 127
  in prostatic cancer, 724
  as synchronizing agent, 116–117
Cylindroma of salivary glands, 392
Cyproheptadine in carcinoid syndrome, 638

Cyproterone acetate in prostatic cancer, 723–724
Cystadenoma, proliferative, 812
Cysteamine as radiation protector, 192–193
Cystectomy in bladder cancer, 691–694
Cystitis, hemorrhagic, chemotherapy-induced, 136
Cystosarcoma phylloides, 533–534
Cystoscopy:
  in bladder cancer, 682
  in cervical cancer, 758
Cysts, mediastinal, 478, 480
Cytology:
  in bladder cancer, 682
  cervical, 752–753
  in lung cancer, 435
  in ovarian cancer, 811–812
  in transitional-cell tumors of upper tract, 672
  urinary, 666, 682
Cytomegalovirus:
  in carcinogenesis, 86
  cell transformation by, 86
Cytosine arabinoside:
  pharmacology, 127
  synchronization effects of, 114–115
    in acute leukemia, 115
  thymidine labeling index and prediction of response to chemotherapy in acute leukemia, 113
Cytoxan (*see* Cyclophosphamide)

Dane particle, 79
Darvon, 999
o,p'-DDD in adrenal tumors, 620
Debulking procedure in ovarian cancer, 816–817
Delayed cutaneous hypersensitivity in cancer, 148–150
Delphian node, laryngeal cancer metastasis to, 364
Dementia in brain tumors, 961
Demerol (*see* Meperidine)
Denial:
  in cancer patient, 234–235
  in terminal phase, 246
Dental tumors, 332
Depression:
  as antecedent to cancer, 232–233
  antidepressant therapy for, 1003
  neurotransmitters in, 990
  in response to cancer, 243–244

Dermoid cyst in mediastinum, 481, 482
DES (*see* Diethylstilbestrol)
Detoxification in physical dependence, 1002
Dexamethasone for brain metastases, 969
Dexamethasone suppression test, 618
Diabetes mellitus:
    and cancer, 581
    after pancreatectomy, 588
    pancreatic cancer and, 38
Diagnosis, patient's response to, 241
Dialysis, rehabilitation in, 1073–1074
Dianhydrogalactitol in brain tumors, 954
Diarrhea in carcinoid syndrome, 633
Diet:
    cancer risk related to, 17–18
    and colorectal cancer, 37–38, 596, 598
    and liver cancer, 562–563
    and stomach cancer, 37
Diethylstilbestrol (DES):
    approach to in utero exposure to, 837
    in prostatic cancer, 721
    use in pregnancy related to cancer in offspring, 15
    vaginal cancer related to maternal use of, 836–837
    (*See also* Estrogen)
Difluoromethyl ornithine, 958
Dinitrochlorobenzene (DNCB), 148–150
    in melanoma, 882
    in vulvar cancer, 830
Disability:
    in extremity cancer, 1044
    in head and neck cancer, 1064–1065
    after mastectomy, 1047–1048
    pain, 1019, 1022
    rehabilitation in cancer, 1041–1042
    (*See also* Rehabilitation)
Disseminated intravascular coagulation in prostatic cancer, 727
DNA:
    base damage in, 184
    halogenated pyrimidines effect on, 193
    repair of radiation damage to, 183–184
    S phase for synthesis of, 108
    in transformed polyoma virus, 74

DNA binders, 131–132
    mechanism of action, 130
DNA viruses (*see* Herpesviruses; Papovaviruses)
DNCB (*see* Dinitrochlorobenzene)
Dopamine:
    and analgesia, 990
    due to electrical stimulation, 993
    interaction with morphine, 991
Dormant cells, 223–224
Dorsal horn of spinal cord and pain perception, 985–987
Dorsal root ganglion and pain perception, 985
Dose response, 128
Down's syndrome, leukemia related to, 48
Doxorubicin:
    in bladder cancer, 688
    in uterine sarcomas, 804
Drooling, 1064–1065
Dry mouth, 1064
DTIC in melanoma, 880, 881
Dying patient:
    psychological stages in, 246–247
    use of imagery and altered states in, 248–250
    (*See also* Terminal illness)
Dysgerminoma:
    ovarian, 814
    in young women, 818–819
Dyskeratosis, 278
Dyskeratosis congenita, 49–50
Dysphagia in esophageal cancer, 452

Eaton-Lambert syndrome, 1036
    myasthenia gravis distinguished from, 1036, 1037
Ectopic hormone production, 1025
    (*See also* Hormones, ectopic production in cancer)
Edema:
    in carcinoid syndrome, 633
    cerebral, 949–950
Effusions:
    ascites, 823–824
    etiology in ovarian cancer, 824
    pleural, 824
    treatment in ovarian cancer, 823–824
Elavil, 1003

Electrical stimulation analgesia, 1012–1013
    deep brain stimulation, 1013
    intraventricular injection of endorphin, 1013
    transcutaneous neurostimulation, 1013
Electroencephalography (EEG) in brain tumors, 935
Electron microscopy in head and neck cancer, 355
Embryonal carcinoma of ovary, 814–815
Employment difficulties for cancer patient, 1074–1075
    (*See also* Vocational rehabilitation)
En bloc resection, cellular-embolic theory as basis of, 199–200
Encephalopathy:
    metabolic, 1035–1036
    radiation-induced, 950
Endocrine disorders:
    in adrenal gland hyperfunction, 615
    in adrenal tumors, 612–613
    in hyperparathyroidism, 425–426
    in mediastinal tumors, 472, 474, 481, 486
    multiple endocrine adenopathy, 628–629
    in pancreatic neoplasms, 592–593
    in thyroid medullary carcinoma, 410–412
    widespread occurrence in cancer, 1025
    (*See also* Hormones; Multiple endocrine adenopathy)
Endodermal sinus tumor of ovary, 815
Endometrial adenocarcinoma, 780–798
    adenoacanthoma, 782
    cervix involvement, 785
    current areas of research and future prospects in, 796–797
    diagnostic evaluation, 785–789
    epidemiology, 780–782
    etiology, 781–782
    exogenous estrogen role in, 781–782
    historical aspects, 780
    increased incidence of, 780–781
    metastases in, 786, 788, 790–791
    pathology, 782
    patterns of spread, 782–783
    progesterone effect on, 781
    screening for, 797

Endometrial adenocarcinoma (*Cont.*):
  signs, symptoms, and early detection, 783, 785
  staging of, 785–790
  treatment, 787–796
    adjuvant therapy, 794
    chemotherapy, 796
    follow-up techniques, 795
    options for primary treatment, 787–791
    progesterone, 794–796, 798
    recurrent or metastatic disease, 795–796
    rehabilitation, 797–798
    stage I, grade 1 disease, 791–793
    stage I, grades 2 and 3 disease, 792
    stage II disease, 792, 793
    stage III disease, 792–793
    stage IV disease, 793
    surgery, 788–794
  (*See also* Uterine cancer)
Endorphin, 993
  and acupuncture analgesia, 994
  and analgesia, 993
  during chronic brain stimulation for pain, 1013
  intraventricular injection for pain control, 1013
Endoscopic retrograde cholangiopancreatography (ERCP):
  in jaundice evaluation, 568
  in pancreatic cancer, 582
Endoscopy:
  colon polyp removal by, 598
  in esophageal cancer, 453–454
  in stomach cancer, 543–544, 547, 553
Enkephalins, 993
  and narcotic dependence, 1001–1002
Environmental factors in cancer, 7–22
  in bladder cancer, 680–681
  in colorectal cancer, 596–599
  in esophageal cancer, 450
  in liver cancer, 563
  in lung cancer, 433
  in lymphoma, 916
  in ovarian cancer, 809
  in renal pelvis and ureteral tumors, 665
  in stomach cancer, 544–545
  (*See also* Carcinogenesis; Carcinogens)

Enzymes:
  and detachability of tumor cells, 205
  increased synthesis in tumors, 112
  key, 112
  replacement after pancreatectomy, 587–588
  role in invasion and metastasis, 204–205
Ependymoma, 944
  chemotherapy of, 955
  classification, 937
  clinical manifestations, 944
  pathology, 944
  treatment, 944
Epidemiology:
  definition, 23
  early applications to cancer, 7–9
  methods and applications in cancer, 23–43
    in bladder cancer, 40
    in breast cancer, 39
    causal inferences from studies, 35
    in cervical cancer, 39–40
    classification, 24–26
    in colorectal cancer, 37–38
    comparing risks, 34–35
    data sources, 30–31
    in esophageal cancer, 36
    familial susceptibility, 41–43
    historical landmarks, 23–24
    in lung cancer, 38
    in lymphoma, 41
    measurement of frequency of occurrence, 26–28
    morbidity data, 31
    mortality data, 31
    multiple primary neoplasms, 41, 42
    in nasopharyngeal cancer, 35–36
    in pancreatic cancer, 38
    prospective studies, 33–34
    in prostate cancer, 40
    retrospective studies, 32–33
    in stomach cancer, 36–37
    time, place, and person determinations, 28–30
  primary considerations in, 23
  rates used in, 26–27
  (*See also* Carcinogenesis *and under specific diseases*)
Epidermoid carcinoma:
  of head and neck (*see* Head and neck cancer, epidermoid carcinoma)

Epidermoid carcinoma (*Cont.*):
  of larynx, 367–368, 372
Epidural block:
  continuous, 1014–1015
  in pain control, 1014
  technique, 1015
Epinephrine:
  and carcinoid secretion, 636
  significance of increased levels of, 622
Epipodophylotoxin in brain tumors, 954
Epstein-Barr virus:
  antigens in cancer, 153
  and Burkitt's lymphoma, 57–58, 84–86
  cancer related to, 15, 153
  cell transformation by, 85
  effect in immunodeficiency, 58–59
  and Hodgkin's disease, 41, 905
  and infectious mononucleosis, 58, 85
  and nasopharyngeal carcinoma, 85–86, 310
  role in carcinogenesis, 84–86
  two types, 85
ERCP (*see* Endoscopic retrograde cholangiopancreatography)
Erythrocytosis:
  in renal cell carcinoma, 646
  tumor-related, 1033
Erythroplasia, Queyrat's, 744
Erythropoietin in cancer, 1033
Esophageal cancer, 448–467
  alcohol and, 36
  brighter outlook in, 448
  carcinoma in situ, 467
  in cervical region: anatomical consideration, 336
    classification, 342, 350–351
    etiology, 337, 339
    incidence, 337, 338
    signs, symptoms, and diagnosis, 340–343
    treatment, 347
  classification, 342, 350–351
  clinical manifestations, 451–452
  current areas of research and prospects for future in, 466–467
  diagnosis, 452–454
    bronchoscopy in, 454
    endoscopy in, 453–454
    in esophagitis, 453–454
    mediastinoscopy in, 454

Esophageal cancer, diagnosis (*Cont.*):
    radiologic examination in, 452–453
  differential diagnosis, 452
  distribution of tumors in, 450–451
  epidemiology, 36, 449–450, 466
  esophagitis developing into, 450
  etiology, 450
    cervical region, 337, 339
  factors related to occurrence, 21
  follow-up considerations in, 465–466
  historical aspects, 448–449
  incidence, 449
    cervical region, 337, 338
  natural history of, 451
  pathology, 450–451
  predisposing conditions, 449–450
  prognosis, 464–465
  rehabilitation in, 1065–1069
  staging of, 451, 454–455
  superficial involvement, 467
  treatment, 455–465
    adjuvant therapy, 463–464
    bypass of lesion without resection, 462
    cervical carcinomas, 347, 455–457
    cervical esophagostomy, 463
    chemotherapy, 463–464
    considerations for primary treatment, 455–461
    fundoplication technique to prevent reflux, 465
    intubation of obstructed esophagus, 462–463
    middle- and lower-third carcinomas, 457–459
    palliation, 461–463
    postoperative complications, 459–461
    radiotherapy, 455–456, 461, 462, 464–465
    results, 464–465
    surgery, 456–461
Esophagitis:
  chemotherapy-induced, 134
  and esophageal cancer, 450
    diagnostic considerations, 453–454
Esophagocoloplasty, 458–459
  anastomotic leak after, 460
Esophagogastrectomy, 457–458
  anastomotic leak after, 460
Esophagostomy, 463

Esophagus, intubation in obstruction, 462–463
Esthesioneuroblastoma, 327
Estramustine in prostatic cancer, 724
Estrogen:
  carcinogenic activity, 15
  cardiovascular disease associated with, 721–722
  effect on nonmalignant prostatic tissue, 721
  and endometrial cancer, 781–782
  receptors for (*see* Estrogen receptors)
  steps in action of, 508–509
  use in prostatic cancer, 716–717, 720–723
  and uterine sarcoma, 801
Estrogen receptors, 508–509
  in breast cancer, 509–512
    assays for, 508–512
    and metastases treatment, 533
    postmenopausal compared to premenopausal levels, 510–511
    in primary versus metastatic tumors, 510
    therapy effects on, 510
    and thymidine labeling index, 114
    variation in content in sequential tumor samples, 510
  and metastasis, 221
  sources of variability in results of assays, 509–511
    hormonal status of patient, 510–511
    obtaining and handling specimen, 509
    specimen, 509–510
    tumor cell density and, 510
  uses of: as aid in differential diagnosis of metastatic adenocarcinoma, 511
    correlation with response to endocrine therapy, 511
    predicting response to chemotherapy, 511–512
    as prognostic factor, 511
Ethics:
  of clinical trials, 266–269
  of control group, 267
  data integrity, 268–269
  patient consent, 267–268
Ethmoid sinus tumors (*see* Paranasal sinus tumors)
Exercises:
  after mastectomy, 1049–1052

Exercises, after mastectomy (*Cont.*):
    deep breathing, 1049
    pendulum swing, 1049–1050
    pulley exercises, 1050–1051
    reach and spread, 1050
    wall climbing, 1050
  for rehabilitation in extremity cancer, 1045
  after thoracotomy, 1067
  (*See also* Physical therapy)
Extremity cancer, rehabilitation in, 1043–1047
  operative, 1043–1045
  pathologic fractures, 1047
  postoperative, 1045
  preoperative, 1043
  prostheses and braces, 1046–1047
Eye, chemotherapy-induced disease of, 137

Facial nerve, injury and repair in parotid tumors, 401–402
Familial cancer syndromes, 46–61
  (*See also* Cancer, genetic and familial aspects)
Familial colorectal polyposis syndrome, 53
  and colorectal cancer, 597–598
Family:
  cancer effect on, 238–248
    age of patient and, 239–241
    in early disease, 243–244
    during no-man's-land, 245–246
    patient and professional problems around diagnosis, 242–243
    in terminal disease, 247–248
  early experiences and development of cancer, 233–234
Fanconi's anemia, 49
Fatal illness (*see* Terminal illness)
Feminizing tumors of adrenal gland, 619
Fetal antigens (*see* Antigens, fetal)
Fetal sulfaglycoprotein antigen, 546
Fetoprotein (*see* Alpha-fetoprotein)
Fever:
  in cancer, 1038
  chemotherapy-induced, 137
Fibrinolysis, role in invasion and metastasis, 205
Fibroma:
  in nasal cavity, 330
  ossifying, 331–332

Fibromatosis, 330
Fibronectin, 205
 and metastasis, 205
Fibrosarcoma in nasal cavity, 330
Fibrous dysplasia of facial bones, 331
Fibrous osteoma of nose and paranasal sinuses, 331–332
Field cancerization, 280
Fistula:
 radiotherapy complicated by, 767
 ureterovaginal and vesicovaginal after hysterectomy, 763–764
Flaps:
 in face and scalp surgery, 1061
 myocutaneous, in head and neck cancer, 356–358
  patterns of blood supply to, 357, 358
   latissimus dorsi, 357
   pectoralis major, 357
   trapezius, 357
Flavonoids and liver cancer, 562
5-Fluorotryptophan in carcinoid syndrome, 638
5-Fluorouracil:
 in brain tumors, 954
 in colorectal cancer, 603
 pharmacology of, 127
 skin disease due to, 136
 in stomach cancer, 551
 use of cream in vaginal cancer, 839
Flush in carcinoid syndrome, 632
Flutamide in prostatic cancer, 724
Follicular carcinoma, 409–410
 surgical management, 416
Fractures:
 pathologic, 1047
  in multiple myeloma, 1071
 in prostatic cancer, 726–727
Free radicals, role in radiation damage, 180
Frontal lobotomy, 1012
Frontal sinus (*see* Paranasal sinuses)
Frozen section, Mohs approach in head and neck cancer, 352–355
Furosemide in hypercalcemia, 1026, 1028

Gallbladder cancer:
 diagnosis, 566
 gallstones role in, 563–564
 long-term survivors in, 574
 surgical treatment, 573–574
 (*See also* Biliary tract tumors)

Gallium scan:
 in Hodgkin's disease, 909
 in lymphoma, 919
Gallstones, role in gallbladder cancer, 563–564
Gardner's syndrome, mutations in, 53
Gastrectomy in stomach cancer, 548–551
Gastric cancer (*see* Stomach cancer)
Gastrinoma, 592–593
Gastrointestinal lymphoma, 923–924
Gastrointestinal peptide hormone syndromes, 1032
Gastrointestinal tract, chemotherapy-induced toxicity in, 134–135
Gate control hypothesis, 984, 986–987
 neuroaugmentive therapeutic procedures based on, 1012–1013
Genetic counseling, 61
Genetics, 46–61
 and brain tumors, 930
 cancer risk related to, 16, 30
 in colorectal cancer, 597
 and lung cancer, 434
 of multiple endocrine adenopathy, 629
 in stomach cancer, 545
 (*See also* Cancer, genetic and familial aspects)
Genitalia:
 melanoma in female, 883–884
 ovarian tumors, 807–825
  (*See also* Ovarian tumors)
 penile cancer, 741–744
  (*See also* Penile cancer)
 testicular cancer, 729–740
  (*See also* Testicular cancer)
 uterine cancer, 780–805
  (*See also* Uterine cancer)
 vaginal cancer, 836–841
  (*See also* Vaginal cancer)
 vulvar cancer, 826–836
  (*See also* Vulvar cancer)
Geographical variations, 29
Germ-cell tumors:
 histologic classification, 819
 immunohistologic classification, 732
 in mediastinum, 481, 484–485
 (*See also* Choriocarcinoma; Ovarian tumors; Testicular cancer)
Gestational trophoblastic tumors, 844–856
 brain and liver metastases, 854
 chorioadenoma destruens, 846

Gestational trophoblastic tumors (*Cont.*):
 clinical management, 852–856
  actinomycin D, 853
  chemotherapy, 852–855
  metastatic disease, 853–855
  methotrexate, 853
  nonmetastatic disease, 852–853
 complications of therapy, 855–856
 definitions and categorization, 845
 diagnosis, 851–853
  HCG levels, 851
  radiologic procedures, 852
 endocrinology, 848
 historical aspects, 844–845
 hydatidiform mole role in, 845
 immunology, 847–848
 incidence and epidemiology, 845
 pathology, 845–847
 pathophysiology, 845–848
 prognostic factors, 854–855
 staging of, 853
 (*See also* Choriocarcinoma; Hydatidiform mole)
Giant cell tumor of paranasal sinuses, 332
Gingiva cancer, 290–294
 anatomy, 290–291
 bone involvement, 291–292
 clinical presentation, 291–292
 incidence and etiology, 291
 pathology, 291
 prognosis, 293
 results of treatment, 293–294
 tobacco and, 291
 treatment, 292–293
Glioblastoma multiforme:
 pathology, 941
 symptoms, 941
 terminology in, 937, 941
 treatment: chemotherapy, 942
  radiotherapy, 941–942
  surgery, 941
Glioma:
 brainstem, 948
 classification, 936–937
 general considerations on, 937
 intranasal, 327
 mixed, 937
 morphology and manner of growth, 937–938
 subependymal mixed, 944
Gliomatosis cerebi, 941
Glomus tumors, 328

Glossectomy:
  difficulties after, 1062
  rehabilitation after, 1064
Glottis, 361–362
  (See also Laryngeal cancer, glottic region; Vocal cords)
Glucagon, danger of use in pheochromocytoma, 624
Glucagonoma, 593
Glucocorticoid receptors in breast cancer, 511
Glucocorticoids (see Corticosteroids)
Glycopeptide hormone syndromes, 1032–1033
Goiter, 405
Gold, radioactive, in prostatic cancer, 718
Gompertzian growth curve, 109–110
Gonadoblastoma, 809
  of ovary, 815
Gonorrhea and urethral cancer, 746
Graft rejection, monoclonal antibody in treatment of, 169
Granulosa-theca cell tumor:
  endometrial cancer associated with, 782
  of ovary, 815
Growth:
  kinetics for tumor cells, 108–119
  metastasis related to primary tumor rate of, 215–216
  radial phase, 862
  vertical phase, 862
Growth fraction, 108–109
Growth hormone in cancer, 1033
Gums (see Gingiva cancer)
Gynandroblastoma, 816
Gynecologic tumors:
  cervical cancer, 751–775
    (See also Cervix, cancer of)
  gestational trophoblastic neoplasia, 844–856
    (See also Gestational trophoblastic tumors)
  ovarian, 807–825
    (See also Ovarian tumors)
  urethral, 841–842
    (See also Urethral cancer)
  uterine cancer, 780–805
    (See also Uterine cancer)
  vaginal, 836–841
    (See also Vaginal cancer)
  vulvar, 826–836
    (See also Vulvar cancer)
Gyrectomy, 1012

Haloperidol, 1003
Halsted, William, role in cancer treatment, 4
Hashimoto's disease, 406–407
HCG (see Human chorionic gonadotropin)
Head and neck cancer:
  chemotherapy in, 284
  classification, 342–343
  combined therapy, 345–348
    failures, 349
  electron microscopy in, 355
  epidermoid carcinoma: anatomy, 335–337
    current ideas and prospects for future, 351–356
    incidence, epidemiology, and etiologic aspects, 337–339
    signs, symptoms, and diagnosis, 340–343
    treatment, 343–351
  esophageal cancer associated with, 449–450
  frozen section examination in, 352–355
  future prospects in, 304–305
  laryngeal cancer, 361–387
    (See also Laryngeal cancer)
  melanoma, 875
    (See also Melanoma)
  metastasis in: distal, 279–280
    regional, 279
  monoclonal antibodies in, 355–356
  multicentric origin, 356, 357
  myocutaneous flaps in, 356–358
  nasal cavity and paranasal sinus tumors, 314–332
    (See also Nose tumors; Paranasal sinus tumors)
  nasopharyngeal tumors, 309–314
    (See also Nasopharyngeal cancer)
  nursing requirements in, 359
  occupational therapy in, 359
  occurrence of, 275
  oral cancer, 275–305
    (See also Oral cancer)
  oropharynx, hypopharynx, and cervical esophagus tumors, 335–360
    anatomical aspects, 335–337
    classifications, 342–343
    current ideas and prospects for future, 351–356
    etiology, 337, 339

Head and neck cancer, oropharynx, hypopharynx, and cervical esophagus tumors (Cont.):
    incidence and epidemiology, 337, 338
    reconstruction and rehabilitation, 356–360
    signs, symptoms, and diagnosis, 340–343
    staging of, 343
    treatment, 343–351
      adjuvant therapy, 347–349
      based on site, 345–347
      evaluation difficulties, 343–344
      factors affecting choice, 344–345
      follow-up, 349–351
      typical case history, 335
  pain control in: cingulumotomy, 1012
    cranial nerve section for, 1006
    trigeminal tractotomy, 1010
  physical therapy in, 359
  prophylactic neck irradiation in subclinical disease, 188
  psychological reactions to, 250
  psychosocial concerns in, 359
  radiotherapy control of, 186–187
  radiotherapy with surgery for metastatic neck nodes, 189
  reconstruction surgery in, 304
  recurrences, 349
  rehabilitation in, 358–359, 1060–1065
    drooling, 1064–1065
    dry mouth, 1064
    face, mouth, and pharynx, 1060–1063
    glossectomy, 1064
    larynx, 1063–1064
    pain, 1064
    radical neck dissection, 1065
  salivary gland tumors, 388–404
    (See also Salivary gland neoplasms)
  sarcomas, 898–900
    (See also Soft-tissue sarcomas)
  second neoplasms in, 349
  staging of, 343
  surgery combined with radiotherapy in, 282–284
  thyroid and parathyroid tumors, 405–427
    (See also Parathyroid tumors; Thyroid cancer)
  treatment, 345–351
    chemotherapy, 348–350

Head and neck cancer, treatment (Cont.):
　cryosurgery, 350–351
　follow-up, 349–351
　immunotherapy, 348–349
　Mohs's chemosurgery, 352–355
　radiotherapy, 186–187
　　failures, 349
　　interstitial implant, 354
　　with surgery for metastatic neck nodes, 189
　reconstruction, 356–359
　　face and scalp, 1061–1062
　　oral cavity, 1060–1061
　surgery: failures, 349
　　radiotherapy combined with, 345–347
　team effort, 359–360
　terminal illness, 359
　unanswered questions, 304
Headache:
　in brain tumors, 932–933
　increased intracranial pressure causing, 932
Health Insurance Plan of New York breast cancer study, 492–494
Heart, chemotherapy-induced toxicity to, 135
Hemangioendothelioma in nasal cavity, 330
Hemangioma of nose, 328
Hemangiopericytoma in nasal cavity, 330
Hemangiosarcoma of breast, 534
Hematopoietic tissue, monoclonal antibodies to, 165
Hematuria:
　in bladder cancer, 681
　in renal pelvis and ureteral tumors, 666
　terminal, 681
Hemoccult test for colorectal cancer, 599–600
Hemorrhage in cancer, 1038
Hepatic resection, 569–572
　complications, 571–572
Hepaticojejunostomy, 575–576
Hepatitis:
　chemotherapy-induced, 135
　different viruses causing, 78
Hepatitis B virus, 77–79
　carrier state, 78, 79
　and liver cancer, 77, 79, 559, 561
　serologic tests associated with, 79
　structure of, 79
　vaccination against, 79

Hepatocellular carcinoma (see Liver cancer)
Hepatoma (see Liver cancer)
Heredity (see Cancer, genetic and familial aspects)
Herniation, brain, 932
Herpes simplex virus:
　cancer related to, 15, 81–84
　cell transformation by, 81, 83–84
　and cervical cancer, 81–83, 754–755
　two subgroups, 81
Herpesviruses, 79–86
　in carcinogenesis, 79–86
　　cytomegalovirus, 86
　　Epstein-Barr virus, 84–86
　　(See also Epstein-Barr virus)
　　herpes simplex, 81–84
　　Lucke frog virus, 80–81
　　Marek's disease virus, 81
　diseases due to, 82
　neoplastic transformation by, 754
Heterogeneity, tumor, 216–219
　demonstration of, 217
　for metastasis formation, 217–218
　origin in primary tumor, 219
　partial retention of maturation gradient in primary epithelial malignancies, 216–217
　and selection for metastasis, 224
　stability of selected high and low metastatic cell lines versus clonal instability of isolated subpopulations, 218–219
　vasculature and intrinsic metabolic variability, 216
　zonal, 217
Hexamethylmelamine, nervous system toxicity of, 136
High-pressure oxygen therapy in cervical cancer, 774
Histamine and pain, 989
Histocompatibility antigen in nasopharyngeal cancer, 310
Hoarseness in laryngeal cancer, 365
Hodgkin's disease, 904–915
　advances in, 904
　clinical presentation of histologic subtypes, 911
　diagnostic evaluation for staging, 908–911
　　bone marrow biopsy, 909, 911
　　below diaphragm, 909–910
　　CT scanning, 909–910
　　gallium scanning, 909
　　laparotomy, 910–911

Hodgkin's disease, diagnostic evaluation for staging (Cont.):
　　lymphangiography, 909
　　peritoneoscopy, 910
　　required procedures, 909
　　splenectomy in, 910–911
　epidemiology, 41, 904–905
　Epstein-Barr virus and, 905
　etiology, 904–905
　frequency of different subtypes, 906
　historical perspective, 904
　incidence, 905
　infection role in etiology, 904–905
　infections in treatment of, 915
　lymphocyte depletion, 906, 911
　lymphocyte predominant, 906, 911
　in mediastinum, 478, 479
　mixed-cellularity, 906, 911
　nodular sclerosis, 906, 911
　non-Hodgkin's lymphoma occurring after cure of, 915
　pathologic classification, 905–907
　recurrence, 914
　staging of, 907–908
　sterility after treatment of, 915
　treatment, 912–915
　　chemotherapy, 913–915
　　combined-modality, 914
　　radiotherapy, 912–913
Hormones:
　as carcinogens, 14–15
　in carcinoid syndrome, 633
　ectopic production in cancer, 1025–1026, 1028–1033
　　calcitonin, 1033
　　ectopic ACTH, 1031
　　erythropoietin, 1033
　　gastrointestinal peptide hormone syndromes, 1032
　　glycopeptide hormone syndromes, 1032–1033
　　growth hormone, 1033
　　hypercalcemia, 1026, 1028
　　hypocalcemia, 1028–1030
　　hypoglycemia, 1031–1032
　　prolactin, 1033
　　renin, 1033
　　SIADH, 1030–1031
　　widespread occurrence, 1025
　in endometrial cancer treatment, 794–796, 798
　in gestational trophoblastic tumors, 848
　kinetics of cell kill by, 110

Hormones (*Cont.*):
  receptor assays in breast cancer, 508–512
  role in endometrial cancer etiology, 781–782, 796–797
  use in prostatic cancer, 715–717, 720–724
  (*See also* Endocrine disorders)
Horner's syndrome in nasopharyngeal carcinoma, 311
Huffing, 1066
Human chorionic gonadotropin (HCG), 734
  antisera scans to localize metastases, 736
  assays for, 734–735, 848
  in gestational trophoblastic tumors, 848, 851
    in follow-up, 854–855
  in hydatidiform mole, 846, 848
  in liver cancer, 565
  in normal pregnancy, 848
  in pineal tumors, 949
  radioimmunoassay for, 734–735
  in testicular cancer, 732, 734, 735
  variety of tumors secreting, 1032–1033
Human-human antibodies, 171
Hurthle cell carcinoma, 412
  surgical management, 417–418
Hybridoma, human-human, 171
Hydatidiform mole, 845, 848–851
  clinical management, 850–851
  diagnosis, 848–850
  HCG titers in, 846
    after evacuation, 851
  incidence, 845
  invasive, 846
  pathology of, 845–846
  predictive role of histologic grade-in, 846
  preoperative assessment, 850
  signs and symptoms, 848–850
  (*See also* Gestational trophoblastic tumors)
Hydrocarbons, polycyclic aromatic, 12
Hydrocephalus, shunting for, 938
Hydrocortisone:
  in breast cancer patients, 236–237
  (*See also* Corticosteroids)
5-Hydroxyindoleacetic acid (5-HIAA) in carcinoid syndrome, 636–637
5-Hydroxytryptophan in gastric carcinoid tumors, 640

Hydroxyurea in brain tumors, 954
Hyperalgesia, mechanism for, 985
Hypercalcemia:
  benign conditions causing, 1026
  in cancer, 1026, 1028
  differential diagnosis, 426–427
  in hyperparathyroidism, 425–426
  in renal cell carcinoma, 646
  treatment, 1026, 1028
Hypercoagulable state, 1037–1038
Hyperglycemia, chemotherapy-induced, 137
Hyperkeratosis, 278
  of larynx, 368
Hypernephroma, 645
Hyperparathyroidism, 424–425
  causes, 424–425
  clinical evaluation, 426
  clinical manifestations, 425–426
  differential diagnosis, 426–427
  primary, secondary, and tertiary, 424
  treatment, 427
  (*See also* Parathyroid tumors)
Hypersensitivity, delayed cutaneous, 148–150
Hypertension:
  in pheochromocytoma, 622
  management, 625–626
  primary aldosteronism causing, 616
Hyperthermia in brain tumors, 959
Hypertonic solutions in brain tumors, 939
Hypertrophic pulmonary osteoarthropathy, 1034
Hyperventilation in brain tumors, 939
Hyperviscosity syndrome, 1037
Hypnosis in pain management, 1004–1005
Hypocalcemia:
  in cancer, 1028–1030
  diagnosis, 1029
  treatment, 1029–1030
Hypoglycemia in cancer, 1031–1032
Hyponatremia:
  causes of, 1030
  in SIADH, 1030
Hypoparathyroidism after thyroidectomy, 415
Hypopharyngeal tumors:
  classification, 342–343
  etiology, 337, 339
  examination for, 340, 341
  incidence, 337, 338
  lymphatic drainage of, 337

Hypopharyngeal tumors (*Cont.*):
  signs, symptoms, and diagnosis of, 340–343
  treatment, 346–347
    difficulty in evaluating, 343–344
  (*See also* Oral cancer)
Hypopharynx, anatomy, 336–337
Hypophysectomy:
  for pain control, 1012
  in prostatic cancer, 723
Hypothalamic tumors, 947–948
Hypoxia, importance in radiotherapy, 180–181
Hypoxic sensitizers, 194
Hysterectomy:
  complications, 762–765
  extrafascial following radiotherapy, 765
  fistulae after, 762–764
  in gestational trophoblastic tumors, 853
  in invasive cervical cancer, 760–765
  in microinvasive cervical cancer, 760
  in ovarian cancer, 812–815
  pulmonary embolism after, 764–765
  technical advances in, 761–762

Ifosfamide, hemorrhagic cystitis due to, 136
Ileoentectropy, 824
Ileostomy, rehabilitation after, 1059–1060
  convalescence, 1060
  pre- and postoperative care, 1059–1060
  transitional and posthospital care, 1060
Imagery use in dying patient, 248–250
Imipramine, 1003
Immunity:
  antigenicity of tumor related to, 143–144
  cancer risk related to, 18
  concomitant, 146
  after tumor transplant, 143–144
  to tumor-specific antigens, 142–143
Immunization against tumors, 142–144
Immunocytochemistry of testicular tumors, 732
Immunodeficiency, 57–59
  cancer related to, 147–152

Immunodeficiency, cancer related to (*Cont.*):
  delayed cutaneous hypersensitivity, 148–150
  Epstein-Barr virus role, 57–59
  lymphocyte function tests, 151–152
  peripheral blood lymphocyte counts, 150–152
  T- and B-cell subpopulations, 151
  rehabilitation in, 1072
  screening for, 61
Immunohistochemical techniques in breast cancer, 95–104
Immunologic disorders:
  evidence in human cancers, 147
  in lung cancer, 439
  and lymphoma, 915–916
  in thymomas, 470, 474
Immunologic surveillance and cancer development, 145–147
Immunology, 142–158
  deficient immune response related to cancer, 147–152
  early studies on, 142–143
  of gestational trophoblastic tumors, 847–848
  host factors and metastasis, 219–221
    immune resistance, 219–220
    immunostimulation, 220–221
    natural resistance and activated macrophage, 221
    therapeutic interventions and injury-repair mechanisms, 221
  immunologic surveillance and tumors, 145–147
  monoclonal antibodies applied to cancer, 163–172
  (*See also* Antigens)
Immunoperoxidase procedure:
  advantages for antigen localization, 96
  for breast cancer, 98–103
  for localization of mouse mammary tumor virus antigens, 96–97
  for non-breast malignancies, 102
Immunoselection, 146
Immunosuppression:
  role in lymphoma, 915–916
  tumor cell substance causing, 146
Immunotherapy:
  in bladder cancer, 688
  for brain metastases, 972
  in breast cancer, 532

Immunotherapy (*Cont.*):
  in gestational trophoblastic tumors, 847–848
  in head and neck cancer, 348–349
  kinetics of cell kill by, 110
  lack of success in cancer, 157–158
  local, 882
  in lung cancer, 440–441
  in melanoma, 880–882
    vulvar, 833–834
  in ovarian cancer, 821
Incidence rates, 27
  calculation of, 28
  relationship to prevalence, 27
  use of, 28
Increased intracranial pressure, 931–932
  clinical manifestations, 932
  pathophysiology, 931–932
  treatment, 939
Infectious mononucleosis:
  Epstein-Barr role in, 85
  immunodeficiency and cancer related to, 58–59
Inferior venacavography:
  in adrenocortical tumor, 618
  in testicular cancer, 734
Inflammation, pain in, 989
Informed consent in clinical trials, 267–268
Inhalation therapy after thoracotomy, 1068
Inorganic chemicals as carcinogens, 13
Insulin:
  pancreatic cancer and, 38
  replacement after pancreatectomy, 588
Insulinoma, 592
  celiacangiography in, 583–584
  (*See also* Pancreatic cancer)
Internal mammary node dissection in breast cancer, 516–517
Interstitial fluid dynamics of tumors, 204
Interstitial implants in breast cancer, 526–527
Interstitial irradiation:
  in brain tumors, 957
  in penile cancer, 742
  in prostatic cancer, 718–719
Interstitial tumor tissue pressures, 203–204
Intracranial tumors (*see* Brain tumors)
Intrathecal block in pain control, 1014

Intrathoracic tumors:
  esophageal cancer, 448–467
  (*See also* Esophageal cancer)
  lung cancer, 433–445
  (*See also* Lung cancer)
  mediastinal tumors, 470–487
  (*See also* Mediastinal tumors)
Intravasation, 202–204
  central-to-peripheral interstitial fluid flow and, 204
  increased interstitial tumor tissue pressures and, 203–204
  location of primary tumor in host and, 204
  tumor vascularization and, 202–203
Intravenous pyelography:
  in bladder cancer, 682
  radiolucent defect in, 669
  in renal pelvis and ureteral tumors, 668, 669
Intubation of obstructed esophagus, 462–463
Invasion, 204–205
  increased detachment of tumor cells from each other in, 205
  locomotion of tumor cells in, 204
  lytic enzymes of tumor cells facilitating, 204–205
  tumor cell properties important in metastasis, 210
Iodine, radioactive:
  complications, 418
  in prostatic cancer, 718–719
  uptake studies in thyroid cancer, 413–414
  use in thyroid cancer, 418–419
Ionizing radiation (*see* Radiation; Radiotherapy)
Iridium-192, 354
  use in radiotherapy, 354
Isolation limb perfusion (*see* Limb perfusion)

Jaundice:
  evaluation of, 566, 568
    CT scanning, 566, 568
    endoscopic retrograde cholangiopancreatography (ERCP) in, 568
    percutaneous transhepatic cholangiography in, 568, 584
    superior mesenteric angiography in, 568
  in pancreatic cancer, 581

Kaposi's sarcoma, cytomegalovirus role in, 86
Kidney, chemotherapy-induced toxicity to, 135–136
Kidney tumors, 645–662
  neuroblastoma, 660–662
    (See also Neuroblastoma)
  paraneoplastic syndromes associated with, 1027
  renal cell carcinoma, 645–658
    (See also Renal cell carcinoma)
  renal pelvis tumors, 664–677
    (See also Renal pelvis tumors)
  Wilms's tumor, 658–660
    (See also Wilms' tumor)
Kinetics, 108–119
  of brain tumors, 959
  of cell kill by chemotherapy, 110
  definitions used in, 108–109
  of micrometastasis growth, 212
  primary tumor growth influence on metastasis, 215–216

Lactic dehydrogenase in testicular cancer, 735
Laminectomy:
  for commissural myelotomy, 1008
  for cordotomy, 1008–1009
  dorsal rhizotomy by, 1007
  in spinal cord compression, 976–977
Laparoscopy prior to second-look operation, 822
Laparotomy:
  in Hodgkin's disease staging, 910–911
  in lymphoma, 920
Laryngeal cancer, 361–387
  classification, 361–363
  clinical presentation in, 365
  diagnosis, 365–367
  factors related to occurrence, 21
  glottic region: anatomic aspects, 362
    cervical lymph node metastasis in, 364
    treatment, 374–375
  incidence and etiology, 365
  metastases in: cervical lymph nodes, 363–365, 371–372
    distant, 365
    regional patterns, 362–363
  pathology of, 367–369
    carcinoma in situ, 368

Laryngeal cancer, pathology of (Cont.):
  epidermoid carcinoma, 367–368, 372
  hyperkeratosis, 368
  malignant tumors other than epidermoid carcinoma, 369
  verrucous, 368–369
prognosis, 382, 387
rehabilitation in, 1063–1064
  postoperative, 1063
  preoperative, 1063
  transitional and posthospital care, 1063–1064
staging of, 367
subglottic region: anatomic aspects, 362
  cervical lymph node metastasis in, 364–365
  lymphatics of, 363
  treatment, 375, 382
supraglottic region: anatomic aspects, 361–362
  cervical lymph node metastasis in, 364, 369–370
  lymphatics of, 363
  treatment, 375
surgical pathology of, 369–372
  cellular differentiation, 370
  histopathologic characteristics, 370–371
  resection margin of primary tumor, 369
  size of primary tumor, 369–370
treatment, 372–382
  chemotherapy, 382
  combined radiotherapy and surgery, 372–373
  laser use, 373
  microlaryngoscopy and vocal cord stripping, 373
  radiotherapy, 187, 372
  surgery, 372–382
Laryngectomy:
  deficits after, 1063
  in laryngeal cancer, 375, 379–380
  rehabilitation after, 1063–1064
Laryngography, 368, 370
Larynx:
  anatomy of, 361–362
  cancer of (see Laryngeal cancer)
  examination of, 367–369
  lymphatics of, 362–363
  radiography of, 368
Laser in laryngeal cancer, 373

Latency period, 26
Latissimus dorsi myocutaneous flaps, 357
Leiomyoma:
  evaluation for uterine leiomyosarcoma, 801
  of nasal cavity, 330
Leiomyomatosis, 799
Leiomyosarcoma:
  benign leiomyoma in uterus related to, 799
  of nasal cavity, 330
  (See also Uterine cancer, sarcomas)
Lentigo maligna melanoma, 862
Leptomeningeal metastases, 972–973
  diagnosis, 973
  treatment, 973
Leukemia:
  acute: chromosomal abnormality in, 50
    synchronization techniques in, 115
    thymidine labeling index and prediction of response to chemotherapy in, 113
  acute lymphoblastic: common antigen to, 165
    monoclonal antibody in treatment, 167–168
  alkylating agents and development of, 13
  avian sarcoma virus in, 68–69
  chromosomal abnormalities and, 49–50
  chronic lymphocytic, monoclonal antibody in treatment of, 169
  chronic myelogenous, chromosomal abnormality in, 50, 51
  depression as antecedent to, 232
  Down's syndrome associated with, 48
  factors related to occurrence, 21
  mammalian sarcoma virus in, 69–71
  paraneoplastic syndromes associated with, 1027
  viruses in humans related to, 72
Leukemoid reactions in cancer, 1037
Leukoencephalopathy, progressive multifocal, 1035
Leukoplakia, 278
  of larynx, 368
  and oral cancer, 278
  and vulvar cancer, 826
Levamisole in lung cancer, 439–440
Levomepromazine, 1003
Leydig cell tumors of ovary, 815–816
Life-table analysis, 34, 269–271

Limb perfusion:
  in melanoma, 881–882
  in soft-tissue sarcomas, 899
Limb salvage in osteosarcoma, 891–892, 894
Limbic system, surgical interruption of, 1011–1012
Linear energy transfer (LET), 178
  in cervical cancer, 774
Lip cancer, 284–287
  anatomy, 284–285
  clinical presentation, 285–286
  herpes simplex role in, 81
  incidence and etiology, 285
  pathology, 285
  prognosis, 287
  recurrence, 287
  results of treatment, 287
  sunlight and, 277
  tobacco related to, 285
  treatment, 286–287
  (See also Oral cancer)
Lipid cell neoplasms of ovary, 816
Lipoma in salivary glands, 393
Lithium for chemotherapy-induced granulocytopenia, 133–134
Liver:
  enlargement in carcinoid syndrome, 633
  function in renal cell carcinoma, 646
  liposoluble contrast material to localize metastases in, 736
  localizing metastases in testicular cancer, 736
  peritoneoscopy in evaluation of, 910
  treatment of metastases in, 571–572
Liver biopsy:
  in liver cancer, 566
  in lymphoma, 920
  peritoneoscopy in Hodgkin's disease for, 910
Liver cancer, 559–573
  alpha-fetoprotein in, 157
  causes, 77–78
  diagnosis, 565–566
    biopsy, 566
    physical examination, 565
    radiological investigations, 565–566
    tumor markers, 565
  etiology, 559, 561–563
    aflatoxin role, 561–563
    alcoholic cirrhosis role, 563
    dietary factors, 562–563

Liver cancer, etiology (Cont.):
    genetic factors, 559, 561
    hepatitis B virus role, 77, 79, 559, 561
  factors related to occurrence, 21
  geographic distribution, 560
  hereditary tyrosinemia and, 561
  incidence, 559, 560
  oral contraceptives and, 15, 563
  paraneoplastic syndromes associated with, 1027
  signs and symptoms, 564–565
  staging in, 571, 572
  treatment, 568–573
    hepatic resection, 569–572
    infusional chemotherapy, 572–573
Liver enzymes in pancreatic cancer, 582
Liver transplantation, 571
Lobotomy, frontal, 1012
Lucke frog virus, 80–81
Lumbar puncture in brain tumors, 936
Lumpectomy, 521–523
  difficulty in randomizing patients in clinical trial for, 263
  ethical considerations in using control group in, 267
Lung, chemotherapy-induced toxicity in, 135
Lung cancer, 433–445
  adenocarcinoma, 434
  brain metastases in, 965
  carcinoid, 435, 634–635, 639–640
  classification, 434–437
  diagnosis, 435
  ectopic ACTH syndrome in, 1031
  epidemiology, 38
  epidermoid carcinoma, 434
  etiology, 433–434
  factors related to occurrence, 21
  histologic types, 25, 434
  immunosuppression in, 439
  mediastinoscopy in, 436
  metastases to lung, 441–445
    surgical management, 441–445
  paraneoplastic syndromes associated with, 1028
  radiocurability versus radioresponsivity of, 185
  rehabilitation in, 1065–1069
    postoperative, 1066–1069
    preoperative, 1065–1066
  risk factors in, 433–434
  screening for, 435

Lung cancer (Cont.):
  second neoplasms in, 435
  SIADH in, 1030
  small-cell carcinoma, 434
  sputum in, 435
  staging of, 435–437
  thymidine labeling index and prediction of response to chemotherapy in, 113–114
  tobacco role in, 12
  treatment, 437–445
    chemotherapy, 440–441
    immunotherapy, 439–440
    radiotherapy, 438–439
    surgery, 437–438
Lymph nodes:
  architecture of, 918
  axillary, as prognostic factor in breast cancer, 514–515
  in bladder cancer, 686
  cell types contained in, 917–918
  cervical: in esophageal cancer, 454
    in floor of mouth cancer, 300
    laryngeal cancer metastasis to, 363–365, 371–372
    in lip cancer, 285, 287
    in oral cancer, 279
    radiotherapy combined with dissection of, 283–284
    in thyroid follicular carcinoma, 416
    in thyroid medullary carcinoma, 417
    in thyroid papillary carcinoma, 416
    in tongue cancer, 301
  in cervical cancer, 757–759, 761, 773–774
  controversy in treatment in head and neck cancer, 345
  in endometrial cancer, 790–791
  epidermoid cancers of head and neck metastasis to, 342
  internal mammary, 516–517
  of larynx, 362–363
  of male urethra, 746
  in melanoma, 874–880
  metastasis to, 212–213
    entrance of tumor cells, 212
    interrelated lymphaticovenous circulation, 212–213
    lymphatic transport, entrapment, and transnodal passage, 212
  parotid gland confused with, 395

Lymph nodes (Cont.):
　in penile cancer, 741, 743–744
　in prostatic cancer, 700–703, 706, 708, 710, 716
　in renal cell carcinoma, 650–651
　in testicular cancer, 736–737
　in urethral cancer, 841
　in vaginal cancer, 838
　in vulvar cancer, 827–829
　(See also Hodgkin's disease; Lymphoma)
Lymphadenectomy:
　in cervical cancer, 760–765
　complications, 762–765
　in melanoma, 874–880
　　prophylactic, 875–880
　　therapeutic, 874–875
　　timing of, 879–880
　in Paget's disease, 834
　in penile cancer, 743–744
　in prostatic cancer, 716, 717, 719
　in testicular cancer, 736–737
　in urethral cancer, 842
　in vulvar cancer, 831
Lymphangiography:
　in cervical cancer, 759
　in Hodgkin's disease, 909
　in lymphoma, 919
　in prostatic cancer, 706, 708
　in testicular cancer, 734
Lymphaticovenous circulation, 212–213
Lymphedema:
　after mastectomy, 1052–1054
　prevention, 1053–1054
　treatment, 1053
Lymphocytes:
　blast transformation after mitogen stimulation, 151–152
　in breast cancer, 150–152
　in vitro tests in cancer, 150–152
　　function tests, 151–152
　　peripheral blood counts, 150–151
　　T- and B-cell subpopulations, 151
Lymphoma, 915–924
　B-cell and T-cell diseases, 918
　Burkitt's (see Burkitt's lymphoma)
　chromosomal abnormalities and, 49–50
　clinical presentation, 918
　cutaneous T-cell, monoclonal antibody in treatment of, 168–170
　epidemiology, 41
　etiology, 915–916

Lymphoma (Cont.):
　factors related to occurrence, 21
　gastrointestinal, 923–924
　Hodgkin's disease, 904–915
　(See also Hodgkin's disease)
　immunologic disorders and, 915–916
　incidence, 916
　of maxillary antrum, 328
　in mediastinum, 478, 479
　metastases in, changing pattern of, 973–974
　monoclonal antibody in treatment of, 168–170
　in nasopharynx, 311
　non-Hodgkin's, 915–924
　occurring after Hodgkin's disease cure, 915
　pathology and classification systems, 916–918
　prognostic factors, 916–917
　of salivary glands, 393
　　treatment, 403
　spleen involvement in, 919
　staging of, 918–920
　　CT scanning in, 919
　　gallium scan in, 919
　　laparotomy, 920
　　liver biopsy, 920
　　lymphangiography in, 919
　　radionuclide studies, 919, 920
　treatment, 920–924
　　Burkitt's, 923
　　chemotherapy, 921–923
　　CNS involvement, 923
　　diffuse histiocytic disease, 921–923
　　diffuse small lymphocyte disease, 923
　　lymphoblastic, 923
　　nodular disease, 920–921
　　radiotherapy, 921, 922
　　total nodal irradiation, 921
　in X-linked lymphoproliferative syndrome, 58–59
Lymphosarcoma of breast, 534

Macrophages and protection against metastasis, 221
Malignant melanoma (see Melanoma)
Mammary stromal sarcoma, 535
Mammography:
　current recommendations in asymptomatic women, 496

Mammography (Cont.):
　findings in breast cancer, 496–501
　localization by needle in, 496, 500
　in screening of breast cancer, 492–496
Mandible, reconstruction surgery on, 300
Mannitol:
　for brain metastases, 969
　in brain primary tumors, 939
Marek's disease virus, 81
Marijuana, 1004
Masculinization, adrenal tumors causing, 618–619
Masseter hypertrophy, 395
Mastectomy:
　breast reconstruction after, 1055
　complications of, 1055
　extended radical, 516–517
　in intraductal breast cancer, 504, 507
　in lobular carcinoma in situ, 506–507
　lymphedema after, 1052–1054
　modified radical, 517–519
　prosthesis after, 1052, 1054–1055
　radical, 515–516
　　disability in, 1047, 1048
　rehabilitation after, 1047–1056
　　convalescence, 1054
　　education and counseling, 1054
　　exercises, 1049–1052
　　goals in, 1048
　　operative, 1048
　　palliation, 1055–1056
　　postoperative, 1048–1049
　　preoperative, 1047–1048
　　prosthesis, 1054–1055
　　team instruction, 1051–1052
　　transitional and posthospital care, 1054
　segmental, 521–523
　total (simple) with and without radiotherapy, 519–521
　variety of procedures, 1047
Maxillary sinus:
　anatomy, 314–315
　lymphoma of, 328
　malignant neoplasms of: classification of, 323
　　clinical course, 317–319
　　staging of, 319–320
　(See also Paranasal sinus tumors)

Maxillectomy, 322–323
  complications, 323
  results in paranasal sinus tumors, 323
Mediastinal tumors, 470–487
  anatomical aspects, 471
  classification, 471
  clinical manifestations, 471–472, 474
  current areas of research and prospects for future, 486–487
  diagnosis, 474–475
    mediastinoscopy, 475
    mediastinotomy, 475
    myelography, 474–475
    radiologic techniques, 472–475
  as examples of functional neoplasms, 470–471
  follow-up techniques, 485
  historical aspects, 470–471
  incidence, 471
  rehabilitation in, 1065–1069
  treatment, 475, 477–478, 481–483, 485, 486
    adjuvant, 483
    ancillary, 483, 485
    cysts, 478, 481
    endocrine tumors, 481
    germ-cell tumors, 481
    lymphoma, 478
    neurogenic tumors, 475, 477
    radiotherapy, 483, 485
    recurrences, 486
    teratoma, 481
    thymomas, 477–478
Mediastinoscopy:
  in esophageal cancer, 454
  in lung cancer, 436
  in mediastinal tumors, 475
Mediastinotomy in mediastinal tumors, 475
Medroxyprogesterone (see Progesterone)
Medullary thyroid carcinoma, 57, 410–412
  (See also Thyroid cancer, medullary carcinoma)
Medulloblastoma, 945–947
  clinical manifestations, 946
  etiology, 945–946
  incidence, 945
  metastasis of, 951
  recurrence of, 952
  treatment, 946–947
    chemotherapy, 947

Medulloblastoma, treatment (Cont.):
    opening aqueduct and fourth ventricle to allow CSF egress, 946–947
    radiotherapy, 947
Megestrol acetate in prostatic cancer, 722
Melanocyte-stimulating hormone (MSH), ectopic ACTH syndrome associated with, 1031
Melanoma, 861–884
  acral lentiginous, 863
  amelanotic, 882–883
  anorectal, 884
  biopsy of skin lesion in, 864
  cells of origin of, 861
  changes in lesions suggesting possibility of, 864
  characteristics of suspicious nevi, 863–864
  clinicohistologic types, 862–863
  decision to biopsy suspicious lesions, 863–864
  etiology, 861–862
  of female genital tract, 883–884
  hereditary, 55
  incidence, 861
  lentigo maligna and, 862
  lymph node involvement in, 874–880
  metastases in, 871–872
    in-transit, 871–872
    satellitosis, 871
    treatment, 881–882
  monoclonal antibody to, 165–166
    in treatment, 170
  of nasal cavity, 326–327
  nodular, 863
  occult, 871
  in pregnancy, 884
  prognostic factors in, 866–871
    age, 867
    anatomic site, 867, 870
    depth of invasion, 869–870
    histologic type, 867–869
    sex, 866–867
    size, 867
    stage of disease, 870–871
    ulceration, 867
    unknown primary, 871
  risk factors for, 870–871
  staging of, 864–866, 868–869
    extent of disease, 865–866
    greatest thickness, 864–865

Melanoma, staging of (Cont.):
    level of invasion, 864
    primary lesion, 864–865
    and prognosis, 870–871
  subungual, 883
  sunlight role in, 861–862
  superficial spreading, 862–863
  thymidine labeling index and prediction of response to chemotherapy in, 113
  treatment, 872–882
    adjuvant therapy, 880–881
    brain metastases, 971
    chemotherapy, 880–881
    controversy regarding prophylactic lymph node dissection, 875–879
    extent of local excision in, 872–874
    immunotherapy, 880–882
    isolation limb perfusion, 881–882
    lymphadenectomy, 874–880
    primary lesion, 872–874
    recurrence or metastases, 881–882
    surgery, 872–880
  tumor cell-endothelial cell bond in metastasis, 222
  tumor-specific antigens in, 154–155
  vaginal, 883–884
  of vulva, 831–834, 883
    classification based on level of invasion, 833
    current research and future prospects, 833–834
    incidence, epidemiology, and etiology, 831
    signs and symptoms, 831
    staging and prognostic factors, 832
    treatment: advanced and recurrent disease, 833
      immunotherapy, 833–834
      primary lesion, 832–833
Melphalan, limb perfusion in melanoma, 881
Membrane, tumor cell characteristics related to metastases, 208–210
Meningeal carcinomatosis, increasing incidence of, 966
Meningioma:
  intranasal, 327
  radiation causing, 930
Meperidine, 999–1000
  cautions and contraindications, 999–1000

Meperidine (Cont.):
  side effects, 999
Mesencephalic tractotomy, 1010–1011
Mesenchephalotomy, 1011
Mesenchymal tumors of salivary glands, 393
Metals as carcinogens, 13
Metastasis:
  arrest of tumor cells and growth of, 207–212
    clumping of tumor cells and, 207–208
    host factors involved in, 210–211
    invasive properties of tumor cell and, 210
    observed morphologic events during, 207
    tumor cell membrane and, 208–210
  in bladder cancer, 690, 694
  to brain, 965–972
    (See also Brain metastases)
  in breast cancer, 532–533
  cellular-embolic theory, 199–201
    en bloc resection of primary tumor and regional lymphatics based on, 199–200
    extensions of surgical perimeter based on, 200
    revisions to include systemic dissemination, 200–201
  to central nervous system, 965–978
  definition, 198
  dormancy of tumor cells in, 223–224
  dose-response relationship in, 206
  in endometrial adenocarcinoma, 786, 788, 790–791
    treatment, 795–796
  entrance of tumor cells into circulation, 202–206
    intravasation in, 202–204
    invasion in, 204–205
    quantitation of, 205–206
  experimental studies of, 201–213
    arrest of tumor cells and growth of metastasis, 207–212
    early data, 201–202
    entrance of tumor cells into circulation, 202–206
    regional lymph node metastasis, 212–213

Metastasis, experimental studies of (Cont.):
    tumor cell circulation and inefficiency of metastasis formation, 206–207
  fibrinolysis role in, 205
  heterogeneity of primary tumor formation, 217–218
  historical perspectives on theories of, 198–201
    black bile theory, 198–199
    cellular-embolic theory, 199–201
    cellular theory, 199
  host factors in (see tumor-host factors modulating, below)
  immunologic factors in, 219–221
  inefficiency of formation, 206–207
  interstitial tissue pressure and fluid dynamics and, 203–204
  kinetics of growth, 212
  leptomeningeal, 972–973
  in lip cancer, 287
  in liver, treatment, 571–572
  locomotion of tumor cells and, 204
  in lungs, surgical management, 441–445
  to lymph nodes, 212–213
    entrance to lymphatics, 212
    interrelated lymphaticovenous circulation, 212–213
    lymphatic transport, entrapment, and transnodal passage, 212
    (See also Lymph nodes)
  lytic enzymes role in, 204–205
  mechanisms of formation, 198–225
  in melanoma, 871–872
    in-transit, 871–872
    satellitosis, 871
    treatment, 881–882
    vulvar, 832
  in oral cancer, 279–280
    distal, 279–280
    regional, 279
  in osteosarcoma, 893–894
  to ovaries, 816
  primary tumor factors modulating, 214–215
    (See also tumor-host factors modulating, below)
  primary tumor growth rate related to, 215
  in prostatic cancer, 700–701, 708, 710
  psychological stress with, 244–245

Metastasis (Cont.):
  in renal cell carcinoma, 649, 656–657
  to salivary glands, 393
  selection process of cells in, 224
  in soft-tissue sarcomas, 897, 901
  to spine, 973–978
    (See also Spine metastases)
  spontaneous regression of, 653
  three phases of, 201
  tumor-host factors modulating, 210–211, 213–224
    capillary physiology, 210–211
    cellular and zonal heterogeneity of primary tumor, 216–219
    effect of therapeutic maneuvers and injury-repair mechanism, 221
    endocrine manipulation of metastasis, 221
    experimental and therapeutic implications of instability of clones separated from primary tumor, 219
    immunoresistance, 219–221
    influence of kinetics of primary tumor growth, 215–216
    interrelationship of growth rate of primary tumor, 215
    natural resistance and activated macrophage, 221
    neovascularization and tumor growth in extravascular space, 211
    organ rejection or selection of metastasis, 221–223
    organ site of primary tumor, 214
    origin of heterogeneity in primary tumor, 219
    role of fibrin, platelets, and anticoagulation, 211
    size of primary tumor and metastatic potential, 214–215
Metastatic potential, 214–215
Methadone, 1000
Methotrexate:
  additive effect with radiotherapy, 194
  asparaginase effect on therapeutic index of, 115–116
  bleomycin effect on therapeutic index of, 116
  citrovorum rescue in use of high doses, 892

Methotrexate (*Cont.*):
  in gestational trophoblastic tumors, 853
  in head and neck cancer, 350
  in laryngeal cancer, 382
  liver disease due to, 135
  in melanoma, 881
  in osteosarcoma, 892
  pharmacology of, 127
  renal disease due to, 136
  skin disease due to, 137
  stomatitis due to, 134
α-Methyl-*p*-tyrosine in pheochromocytoma, 627–628
Methylcholanthrene and cervical cancer, 755
Methyldopa:
  in carcinoid syndrome, 638
  in gastric carcinoid tumors, 640
  in pheochromocytoma, 628
Methysergide in carcinoid syndrome, 638
Metronidazole as hypoxic sensitizer, 194
MGBG:
  hypoglycemia due to, 137
  pharmacology of, 127
  skin disease due to, 137
MIC of chemotherapeutic agents, 125–127
Microglioma, 943–944
Microinvasive cancer, 756
  in cervical cancer, 756, 760
Microlaryngoscopy, 373
Microtubules, chemotherapy related to, 112
Midline malignant reticulosis, 328
Mikulicz's disease, 393–394, 397
Mikulicz's syndrome, 393, 395
Minimal inhibitory concentration, 125–127
Misonidazole:
  in brain tumors, 956
  as hypoxic sensitizer, 194
  use with radiotherapy in cervical cancer, 774
Mithramycin:
  hemorrhagic diathesis due to, 137
  in hypercalcemia, 1028
Mitogens, 151–152
Mitomycin C:
  in bladder cancer, 688
  bleomycin synergy with, 117
  mechanism of action of, 130

Mitomycin C (*Cont.*):
  pharmacology of, 127
  renal disease due to, 136
  in stomach cancer, 551–552
Molar pregnancy (*see* Hydatidiform mole)
Monoamine neurotransmitters, 989–990
Monoclonal antibodies, 163–172
  advantages over antisera, 164–165
  antisera contrasted with, 163, 164
  applications in cancer, 166–171
    in diagnosis, 166
    in treatment, 167–171
  to CALLA, 167–168
  to carcinoembryonic antigen, 166
  in colorectal cancer, 170
  as conjugate to radioisotope, chemotherapeutic drug, or cellular toxin, 170–171
  in graft rejection therapy, 169
  in hematopoietic tissue, 165
  in human-human hybridoma, 171
  to lymphoma antigens, 168–170
  to melanoma, 165–166
  in melanoma treatment, 170
  production and characterization, 163–165
    problems with, 164
  to tumor-associated antigens, 165–166
  in treatment, 167–171
Morbidity rates, data sources, 31
  centralized cancer patient data system, 31
  national cancer surveys for selected cities, 31
  population-based registries, 31
  surveillance, epidemiology, and end results program, 31
Morphine, 998–999
  in Brompton's mixture, 1000
  catecholamine interactions with, 991
  diverse actions of, 998–999
  and neurotransmitter kinetics, 991
  and neurotransmitter levels, 991
  periaqueductal-periventricular region stimulation and analgesia, 992–993
  (*See also* Narcotics)
Mortality rates, 27
  calculation of, 28
  data sources, 31
    international, 31

Mortality rates, data sources (*Cont.*):
    U.S. county, 31
  use of, 28
Mouth:
  anatomy, 336–337
  dry, 1064
  floor of, cancer in, 297–301
    anatomy, 297
    clinical presentation, 298–299
    incidence and etiology, 297
    pathology, 297–298
    prognosis, 300–301
    treatment, 299–300
      results of, 300–301
  (*See also* Oral cancer)
Mucoepidermoid carcinoma of salivary glands, 392
Mucositis, radiation-induced, 184
Multicentric cancer in head and neck cancer, 356
  (*See also* Second neoplasms)
Multiple endocrine adenopathy, 56–57, 628–629
  carcinoid tumor in, 632
  genetics of, 629
  in hyperparathyroidism, 425–426
  importance of follow-up in, 629
  possible danger of disrupting hormonal feedback in, 629
  screening for, 60–61
  Sipple's syndrome, 628, 629
  in thyroid medullary carcinoma, 410–412
  types, 628–629
  Wermer's syndrome, 628–629
Multiple myeloma, pathologic fractures in, 1071
Multiple primary neoplasms (*see* Second neoplasms)
Multistage hypothesis, 26
Mumps and ovarian cancer, 809
Murine mammary tumor virus, immunohistochemical localization in mouse mammary tumors, 96–97
Murine sarcoma virus as model for breast cancer, 90–93
Mutations:
  in familial colorectal polyposis syndrome, 53
  and retinoblastoma, 46–47
  role in carcinogenesis, 19
Myasthenia gravis:
  Eaton-Lambert syndrome distinguished from, 1036, 1037

Myasthenia gravis (*Cont.*):
  thymoma association with, 474
Myelography:
  in mediastinal tumors, 474–475
  in spine metastases, 975
Myelosuppression, 130, 132–134
  lithium treatment of, 133–134
Myelotomy, commissural, 1007–1008
Myocutaneous flaps, 356–358
Myofascial trigger point injection, 1014

Naloxone, reversal of acupuncture analgesia by, 994
Naphthylamine, 12
  and bladder cancer, 680
Narcotics, 998–1002
  Brompton's mixture, 1000
  choice of drug, 1000–1001
  codeine, 999
  dopamine effect on analgesic action of, 990
  intravenous, 1000
  mechanism of analgesia by, 998
  meperidine, 999–1000
  methadone, 1000
  morphine, 998–999
  pentazocine, 999
  percodan, 1000
  phenothiazines interaction with, 991, 1002
  physical dependence related to serotonin levels, 990
  propoxyphene, 999
  serotonin effect on analgesic action of, 990
  tolerance and addiction, 1001–1002
  withdrawal syndrome, 1001–1002
Nasal cavity (*see* Nose)
Nasopharyngeal cancer, 309–314
  anatomical aspects, 309
  chordoma, 327
  clinical manifestations, 311
  diagnosis, 311
  epidemiology, 35–36, 309
  Epstein-Barr virus role in, 85–86, 310
  etiology, 310
  factors related to occurrence, 21
  incidence, 309
  occupational exposures associated with, 36

Nasopharyngeal cancer (*Cont.*):
  pathology, 310–311
  prognosis, 313–314
  risk factors for, 36
  staging of, 311–312
  treatment, 312–313
    complications, 313
    results, 313–314
  tumor-specific antigens in, 153
Nasopharyngeal juvenile angiofibroma, 328–330
  clinical presentation and diagnosis, 328–329
  pathology, 328
  treatment, 329–330
Nasopharynx:
  anatomy of, 309
  examination of, 311
National Cancer Institute as financier of clinical trials, 261
National cancer surveys, 31
Navane, 1003
Neck:
  lymph node enlargement in (*see* Lymph nodes, cervical)
  prophylactic irradiation in subclinical disease, 188
  radical dissection: controversy in head and neck cancer, 345
    in floor of mouth cancer, 300
    in gingiva cancer, 292–293
    in oral cancer, 283–284
    radiotherapy combined with, 283
    rehabilitation after, 1065
    in thyroid cancer, 416, 417, 422–423
    in tongue cancer, 303
Needle biopsy:
  of brain metastases, 969–970
  in breast cancer, 500–501, 503
  in prostatic cancer, 704
  in renal cell carcinoma, 647
Negative pi mesons, 195
Nelson's syndrome, 619
Neoplasms:
  cells of (*see* Cells, tumor)
  characteristics modulating metastasis, 214–215
    (*See also* Metastasis, tumor-host factors modulating)
  classification, 19, 24–26
    based on curability, 186
  definition, 142
  etiology (*see* Carcinogenesis)

Neoplasms (*Cont.*):
  functional, 470–471
  heterogeneity of, 216–219
    (*See also* Heterogeneity, tumor)
  interstitial fluid dynamics in, 204
  interstitial tissue pressures in, 203–204
  metastatic potential of, 214–215
  spontaneous, 9
    (*See also* Cancer; Cells, tumor)
Nephrectomy:
  partial, 654–656
  radical, 650–652
  in renal cell carcinoma, 650–656
  in renal pelvis tumors, 675
  in Wilms's tumor, 659
Nephropathy:
  analgesic, 665–666
  Balkan, 666
Nephroureterectomy in renal pelvis and ureteral tumors, 673–675
Nerve blocks, 1014
Nervous system:
  chemotherapy-induced disease of, 136
  and pain, 984–988
  remote effects of cancer on, 1070
Nervous system tumors (*see* Brain tumors; Central nervous system tumors)
Neurilemmoma in mediastinum, 477
Neuroblastoma, 660–662
  diagnosis, 661
  distribution, 660
  etiology, 660
  maturation to stable benign neoplasm, 613
  in mediastinum, 483
  olfactory, 327
  prognosis, 661–662
  signs and symptoms, 660–661
  staging in, 661
  treatment, 661
  tumor-specific antigens in, 153–154
  Wilms's tumor distinguished from, 659, 661
Neurochemistry of pain and analgesia, 988–994
Neurocristopathies, 55–56
Neurocutaneous syndromes, 56
Neurofibromatosis:
  cancer in, 55–56
  in mediastinum, 477
  soft-tissue sarcomas in, 896

Neurofibrosarcoma in mediastinum, 477
Neurogenic tumors in mediastinum, 475, 477
Neuroma in amputation stump, 1045
Neuromodulators, 989
Neuromyopathies, carcinomatous, 1034–1036
Neurosurgical oncology:
　CNS metastases, 965–978
　　primary central nervous system tumors, 929–961
　　(See also Brain tumors; Central nervous system tumors)
　　procedures in pain management, 1005–1013
Neurotomy for pain control, 1006
Neurotransmitters:
　criteria for qualifying as, 989
　major systems in brain, 989–990
　and mood disorders, 989–990
　morphine effect on kinetics of, 991
　and pain perception, 990
Neutron therapy, 195
Nevi, characteristics suggesting possible melanoma, 863–864
Newborn, factors related to cancer risk in, 18
Nitrates, safety in meat, 14
Nitrites:
　and bladder cancer, 681
　and esophageal cancer, 450
Nitrogen mustard for malignant effusion in ovarian cancer, 823, 824
Nitroprusside in pheochromocytoma, 626
Nitrosamines:
　as carcinogens, 14
　and esophageal cancer, 450
Nitrosoureas, 131
　and bladder cancer, 680, 681
　in brain tumors, 952
　mechanism of action of, 130
　in melanoma, 881
　pharmacology of, 127
　(See also BCNU)
No man's-land, 245–246
Nociception, 983
Norepinephrine:
　and analgesia due to electrical stimulation, 993
　and depression, 990
Nose:
　anatomy, 314

Nose (Cont.):
　polyps, 315
　pathology, 317
Nose tumors:
　benign, 315, 317
　　pathology, 317
　　prognosis, 317
　　treatment, 317
　bone, 331–332
　cartilage tumors, 331
　central nervous system tumors, 327
　fibrous tissue tumors, 330
　glomus tumors, 328
　hemangioendotheliomas and hemangiopericytomas, 330
　juvenile angiofibroma, 328–330
　malignant, 317–326
　　clinical manifestations and course of disease, 317–319
　　diagnostic procedures, 319–320
　　pathology, 317
　melanoma, 326–327
　of mesenchymal origin, 328–332
　midline malignant reticulosis, 328
　olfactory neuroblastoma, 327
　papilloma, 315, 317
　　pathology, 317
　skeletal muscle, 330–331
　smooth muscle tumors, 330
　of vascular origin, 328
Nutrition:
　cancer risk related to, 16
　in cervical cancer, 760
　in gestational trophoblastic tumors, 855–856
　and head and neck cancer, 277, 1063
　and oral cancer prognosis, 304–305
　(See also Diet)
Nutritional therapy:
　in carcinoid syndrome, 638
　in esophageal cancer, 463
　in head and neck cancer, 1063

Occupational cancer, 7–22
　(See also Carcinogenesis)
Odds ratio, 34
Olfactory neuroblastoma, 327
Oligodendrogliomas, 943
　chemotherapy of, 954
　classification, 937
Omentectomy in ovarian cancer, 812–813

Oncocytoma, 391
Oncofetal antigens (see Antigens, fetal)
Oncogene theory, 15
Oncologist (see Physician)
Oncoviruses, 15–16, 65–87
　adenoviruses, 76–77
　animal models, 90
　in breast cancer, 88–106
　　(See also Breast cancer, virology)
　cell properties transformed by, 66–67
　hepatitis B virus, 77–79
　herpesviruses, 79–86
　　cytomegalovirus, 86
　　Epstein-Barr virus, 84–86
　　(See also Epstein-Barr virus)
　　herpes simplex, 81–84
　　Lucké frog virus, 80–81
　　Marek's disease virus, 81
　historical aspects, 65
　papovaviruses, 72–76
　　papilloma subgroup, 75–76
　　polyoma subgroup, 73–75
　retroviruses, 67–72
　　endogenous sequences, 71
　　human and primate, 71–72
　　leukemia/sarcoma virus complexes, 68–71
　RNA containing: reverse transcriptase in, 92–93
　　sequence homology of RNA in, 90–92
　　sequence homologies in nucleic acids of, 90–91
Ondine's curse, 1009
Optic chiasm tumors, 947–948
Oral cancer, 275–305
　alcohol and, 276–277
　buccal mucosa, 287–290
　　(See also Buccal mucosa cancer)
　floor of mouth, 297–301
　future prospects, 304–305
　gingiva, 290–294
　hard palate, 294–297
　history of, 275–276
　incidence, etiology, and epidemiology, 276–277
　metastases: distant, 279–280
　　regional, 279
　lip, 284–287
　　(See also Lip cancer)
　multiple primaries in, 280
　nutrition and, 277
　　influence on prognosis, 304–305

Oral cancer (*Cont.*):
  pathology, 277–279
    gross appearance, 278–279
    microscopic appearance, 279
  poor hygiene and, 277
  premalignant lesions, 277–278
  selection of treatment of, 282–284
    chemotherapy, 284
    surgery and radiotherapy, 282–284
  staging of, 280–282
  sunlight and, 277
  tobacco and, 276
  tongue, 301–304
    (*See also* Tongue cancer)
  verrucous carcinoma, 279
  (*See also* Head and neck cancer; Oropharyngeal tumors)
Oral cavity, anatomy, 336
Oral contraceptives:
  cancer related to use of, 15
  and liver cancer, 563
Orchiectomy:
  in cancer of male breast, 536
  in prostatic cancer, 720–721
Organic brain syndrome in cancer, 1036
Oropharyngeal tumors:
  classification, 336, 342–344
  etiology, 337, 339
  examination for, 340, 341
  factors related to occurrence, 21
  incidence, 337, 338
  lymphatic drainage of, 336–337
  signs, symptoms, and diagnosis of, 340–343
  treatment, 345–346
    difficulty in evaluating, 343–344
    radiotherapy, 186–187
  (*See also* Head and neck cancer; Oral cancer)
Oropharynx, anatomy, 336
Osteoclast activating factor, 1026
Osteoma of nose and paranasal sinuses, 331–332
Osteosarcoma, 888–895
  anatomic distribution, 888–889
  current areas of research and future prospects, 894–895
  diagnostic techniques in work-up and staging, 889–890
    biopsy, 889–890
    CT scanning, 890, 895
    systemic evaluation, 890

Osteosarcoma (*Cont.*):
  epidemiology, 889
  etiology, 889
  of facial bones, 332
  follow-up and early identification of recurrence or metastasis, 893
  historical aspects, 888
  incidence, 888
  multifocal, 889
  signs, symptoms, and early detection, 889
  skip areas of medullary canal in, 890
  treatment: adjuvant therapy, 892–893
    amputation, 890
    bone grafts, 891
    chemotherapy, 891–894
    limb salvage, 891–892
    options for primary lesion, 890–891
    radiotherapy, 890–891
    reconstruction, 891
    recurrence or metastases, 893–894
    resection of pulmonary metastases, 442–443
  tumor doubling time in, 894
Ovarian tumors, 807–825
  benign, 807–808
  classification, 807, 808
  current areas of research in, 824
  danger of paracentesis in, 811, 823
  diagnostic techniques in, 810–812
    biopsy, 812
    cytology, 811–812
    danger of paracentesis, 811, 823
    immunodiagnosis, 824
    pelvic examination, 810
    radiologic procedures, 810–811
  differentiating benign versus malignant, 810
  early diagnosis, 810
  epidemiology, 808–809
  etiology, 809
  familial incidence, 809
  follow-up and early identification of recurrence or metastases, 821–822
  incidence, 808–809
  mumps virus role in, 809
  paraneoplastic syndromes associated with, 1028
  signs and symptoms, 809–810

Ovarian tumors (*Cont.*):
  spillage of tumor during surgery for, 820
  staging of, 811–812
  treatment, 812–824
    borderline malignant epithelial neoplasms, 812
    chemotherapy, 820–824
    choriocarcinoma, 815
    debulking procedure, 816–817
    dysgerminoma, 814, 818–819
    embryonal carcinoma, 814–815
    endodermal sinus tumor, 815
    germ cell tumors, 814–815, 818–820
    gonadoblastoma, 815
    granulosa and theca tumors, 815
    gynandroblastoma, 816
    immunotherapy, 821
    lipid cell neoplasms, 816
    malignant effusions and ascites, 823–824
    malignant epithelial neoplasms, 812–814, 817–818, 820–822
    stage IA, IB, and IC, 812–813
    stage IIA and IIB, 813
    stage III, 813–814
    stage IV, 814
    maximum surgical effort on initial laparotomy, 816–817
    neoplasms derived from coelomic epithelium, 812–814
    neoplasms derived from nonspecific mesenchyme, 816
    neoplasms derived from primitive germ cells, 814–815
    neoplasms derived from specialized gonadal stroma, 81, 815–816
    neoplasms metastatic to ovary, 816
    pleural effusion, 824
    primary treatment, 812–822
    radiotherapy, 817–818
    recurrence or metastases, 822–824
    rehabilitation and reconstruction, 824–825
    second-line chemotherapy, 822–823
    second-look operation, 821–822
    Sertoli-Leydig cell tumors, 815–816
    teratoma, 814, 819–820
    in young women, 818–820
  tumor markers in, 822

Ovary, early development of, 807
Oxycodone, 1000
Oxygen:
   high-pressure in therapy of cervical cancer, 774
   radiosensitivity related to, 180–181
   reoxygenation, 181
Oxygen enhancement ratio, 180

Paget's disease:
   of bone, osteosarcoma associated with, 889
   of vulva, 834–835
Pain:
   basic mechanisms of, 983–994
   brain role in, 992–994
   diary on, 1019, 1020
   disability due to, 1019, 1022
   evaluation of, 1017–1021
   gate control hypothesis of, 984, 986–987
   in head and neck cancer, 1064
   historical perspectives on, 984
   impairment scale, 1022–1023
   in inflammation, 989
   intensity of, 1019
   management in cancer (see Pain management)
   after mastectomy, 1055
   measurement of, 1019, 1022–1023
   mechanisms in cancer, 994
   nervous system and, 984–988
      dorsal horn of spinal cord, 985–987
      dorsal root and ganglion, 985
      peripheral nerve fibers, 984–985
      spinothalamic tract, 987–988
      thalamic cortical connections, 988
   neurochemistry of, 988–994
      central mechanisms, 989–992
      new advances in, 992–994
      peripheral mechanisms, 988–989
   neurotransmitters and, 990
   patient's response to, 1017
   pattern theory of perception, 984
   peripheral nerve fibers and, 984–985
   physician's prejudices about, 1017–1018
   physician's response to, 1017–1018
   receptors for, 984–985
   specificity theory of, 984
Pain behavior, 984

Pain management, 983–1023, 1070–1071
   alternatives in, 995
   analgesics in, 995–1004
      (See also Analgesics)
   anesthetic alternatives, 1013–1017
      autonomic plexus blocks, 1014, 1016, 1017
      chemical neurolysis, 1014–1016
      epidural and intrathecal block, 1014
      myofascial trigger point injection, 1014
      patient selection for, 1014–1015
      somatic nerve blocks, 1014
   biases interfering with, 983
   combinations of phenothiazines and tricyclics, 1003–1004
   erasing pain memory to lessen anxious anticipation, 995–996
   in head and neck cancer, 1064
   marijuana, 1004
   medical alternatives, 995–1004
      (See also Analgesics)
   narcotics, 998–1002
      (See also Narcotics)
   neurosurgical alternatives, 1005–1013
      cingulumotomy, 1011–1012
      commissural myelotomy, 1007–1008
      deep brain stimulation, 1013
      dorsal rhizotomy, 1007
      frontal lobotomy, 1012
      gyrectomy, 1012
      hypophysectomy, 1012
      intraventricular injection of endorphin, 1013
      neuroablative procedures, 1005–1012
      neuroaugmentive procedures, 1012–1013
      neurotomy, 1006
      spinothalamic tractotomy (cordotomy), 1008–1010
      spinothalamic tractotomy in brainstem, 1010–1011
      sympathectomy, 1006–1007
      thalamotomy, 1011
      transcutaneous neurostimulation, 1013
   pectoralis major pain after mastectomy, 1055
   phenothiazines, 1002–1003

Pain management (Cont.):
   physician prejudices in, 1017–1018
   practical guidelines, 1022–1023
   prevention of pain, 995
   primary and symptomatic control, 994–995
   problems in postoperative period, 996
   psychophysical techniques, 1004–1005
      acupuncture, 1004
      biofeedback, 1005
      hypnosis, 1004–1005
      relaxation therapy, 1005
   psychotherapy, 1005
   special units for, 1021–1022
   team approach in, 1019, 1021
   in terminal care, 997
   therapy directed at existing disease, 995
   tricyclic antidepressants, 1003–1004
   (See also Analgesia)
Palate, hard, tumors of, 294–297
   anatomy, 294
   clinical presentation, 294–295
   incidence and etiology, 294
   pathology, 294
   prognosis, 296
   recurrent disease, 296
   treatment, 295–296
      results of, 296–297
Palate, soft, tumors of, 345
Palliation:
   in breast cancer, 1055–1056
   in cervical cancer, 772–773
Pancoast syndrome, 437
   radiotherapy for, 438–439
Pancreatectomy:
   enzyme replacement following, 587–588
   insulin replacement following, 588
   in pancreatic cancer, 586–587
   in periampullary cancer, 576
   regional, 587
Pancreatic benign tumors, 591–592
Pancreatic cancer, 580–594
   body and tail of pancreas, 590–591
   classification, 581
   clinical features, 581–582
   current research and prospects for future, 593–594
   cystoadenocarcinoma, 591
   diagnosis, 582–586
      aspiration biopsy, 584–586

Pancreatic cancer, diagnosis (*Cont.*):
   celiacangiography, 583–584
   CT scanning, 584
   endoscopic retrograde cholangio-
      pancreaticography, 582
   laboratory tests, 582
   percutaneous transhepatic cholan-
      giography, 584
   radiographic procedures, 582
  endocrine, 592–593
   gastrinoma, 592–593
   glucagonoma, 593
   insulinoma, 592
   somatostatinoma, 593
   treatment, 593
   Verner-Morrison, 593
  epidemiology, 38, 581
  etiology, 580–581
  historical aspects, 580
  incidence, 580
  laboratory findings in, 582
  pancreatitis distinguished from, 584
  paraneoplastic syndromes associated
    with, 1029
  physical signs in, 582
  thrombophlebitis in, 582
  treatment, 586–590
   adjuvant therapy, 590
   enzyme replacement following
      pancreatectomy, 587–588
   insulin replacement following pan-
      createctomy, 588
   intraarterial chemotherapy infu-
      sion, 589–590
   radiotherapy, 588–589
   surgery, 586–588
Pancreaticoduodenectomy:
  in extrahepatic biliary tract cancer,
    576
  in pancreatic cancer, 586–587
Pancreatitis:
  asparaginase causing, 135
  pancreatic cancer distinguished
    from, 584
Pap smear:
  history of, 753
  and incidence of cervical cancer, 40
Papillary carcinoma of thyroid gland,
    407–409
  surgical management, 415–416
Papillary cystadenoma lymphomato-
    sum, 390–391
Papilloma virus, 75–76
  in humans, 76

Papovaviruses, 72–76
  in humans, 75
  papilloma subgroup, 75–76
  polyoma subgroup, 73–75
  SV40 virus, 73–74
Paracentesis:
  danger in ovarian cancer, 811, 823
  therapeutic use in ovarian cancer,
    823
Parachlorophenylalanine in carcinoid
    syndrome, 638
Parakeratosis, 278
Paranasal sinus tumors:
  benign, 315, 317
  of bone, 331–332
  cartilage tumors, 331
  chordoma, 327
  lymphoma, 328
  malignant, 317–326
   clinical manifestations and course
      of disease, 317–319
   diagnostic procedures, 319–320
   pathology, 317
   treatment, 320–326
    chemotherapy, 326
    combined radiation and surgery,
      323
    conventional surgery, 322–323
    craniofacial resection, 323–326
    radiotherapy, 320–322
    reconstruction surgery, 325
  olfactory neuroblastoma, 327
  smooth muscle tumors, 330
Paranasal sinuses, anatomy, 314–315
Paraneoplastic syndromes, 1025–
    1039
  acanthosis nigricans, 1033–1034
  acid-base and electrolyte disturb-
    ances, 1038
  anorexia and cachexia, 1038
  biologic basis and pathophysiology
    of, 1025–1026
  cancer types associated with, 1027–
    1029
  definitions in, 1025
  Eaton-Lambert syndrome, 1036
  ectopic hormone production, 1025–
    1026, 1028–1033
   (*See also* Hormones, ectopic pro-
      duction in cancer)
  fever, 1038
  hematologic and vascular abnormal-
    ity, 1036
  hypercoagulable state, 1037–1038

Paraneoplastic syndromes (*Cont.*):
  hypertrophic pulmonary osteoar-
    thropathy, 1034
  hyperviscosity syndrome, 1037
  leukemoid reaction, 1037
  metabolic disorders, 1038
  neuromyopathies, 1034–1036
  related to skin, muscle, and soft tis-
    sues, 1033–1034
  sensorimotor peripheral neuropathy,
    1036
  subacute cerebellar degeneration,
    1036
Parathyroid glands:
  anatomy, 423–424
  surgical removal of, 427
Parathyroid hormone (PTH):
  ectopic production of, 1026
  in hyperparathyroidism, 426
Parathyroid squeeze test, 426
Parathyroid tumors, 423–427
  carcinoma, 425
  historical aspects, 424
  hyperparathyroidism due to, 424–
    425
  in mediastinum, 481
  (*See also* Hyperparathyroidism)
Parotid gland:
  anatomy, 388–389
  differential diagnosis of swelling at,
    395
  tumors of: deep-lobe, 394
   diagnosis, 394–395
   facial nerve injury and repair in,
      401–402
   metastatic carcinoma, 400–401
   prognosis, 403–404
   recurrent, 401–402
   treatment, 398, 400–402
   Warthin's tumor, 391
  (*See also* Salivary gland neoplasms)
Parotidectomy, 398, 400
  facial nerve injury in, 401–
    402
  radical, 400
Parotitis, chronic, 395
Particle therapy:
  fast neutrons, 195
  negative pi mesons, 195
  protons, 196
Pectoralis major:
  myocutaneous flaps, 357
  preservation in modified radical
    mastectomy, 517–518

Pelvic examination, ovarian tumor detected by, 810
Pelvic exenteration:
  in cervical cancer, 770–772
    early use in, 752
  complications of, 770
  in metastatic endometrial cancer, 795
  rehabilitation and reconstruction after, 805
  selection of patients for, 770–772
Penile cancer, 741–744
  incidence, 741
  lymphatic drainage in, 741
  Queyrat's erythroplasia, 744
  staging of, 741
  treatment, 741–744
    primary lesion, 742–743
    radiotherapy, 742
    regional lymph nodes, 743–744
Pentazocine, 997, 999
Percodan, 1000
Periampullary cancer:
  diagnosis of, 566, 568
  treatment, 576
Pericardial cysts, 478, 481
Perinaud's sign, 948
Peripheral nerves:
  blocks in pain control, 1014
  neurotomy for pain control, 1006
  and pain, 984–985
  sensorimotor neuropathy, 1036
Peritoneoscopy:
  in endometrial cancer, 795
  in Hodgkin's disease staging, 910
Person-years analysis, 34
Personality:
  as antecedent to cancer, 232–234
  in breast cancer, 236–238
  in cancer patient, 234–235
  in cervical cancer, 235–236, 238
Pertechnate ion uptake in thyroid cancer, 414
Phacomatoses, 56
Phantom pain, 1045
Pharmacology of chemotherapeutic agents, 125–127
Pharyngeal tumors:
  classification, 346
  treatment, 346
Pharynx, anatomy, 336
Phenacetin:
  complications of, 997
  and renal pelvis tumors, 666

Phenobarbital, chemotherapy interaction with, 959
Phenol in chemical neurolysis, 1015–1016
Phenothiazines:
  in Brompton's mixture, 1000
  for cancer pain, 1002–1003
  interaction with narcotics, 991
  tricyclics combined with, 1003–1004
Phenoxybenzamine:
  in carcinoid syndrome, 638
  in pheochromocytoma, 628
Phenylalanine mustard in breast cancer, 529, 530
Pheochromocytoma, 621–628
  danger of glucagon use in, 624
  diagnosis, 477, 622–624
    catecholamine levels, 622
    radiologic studies, 623–624
    tumor localization studies, 622–624
  follow-up and detection of recurrence or metastasis, 626–627
  history of recognition of, 621
  incidence, epidemiology, and etiology, 621
  induction of anesthesia in, 624, 626
  in mediastinum, 477
  prospects for future, 628
  signs, symptoms, and early detection, 622
  thyroid medullary carcinoma associated with, 410–412
  treatment, 624–626
    adjunctive therapy, 625–626
    adrenergic blockade, 625–627
    hypertension, 625–626
    recurrence or metastasis, 627–628
    surgery, 624–625
Philadelphia chromosome, 50
Phosphate in hypercalcemia treatment, 1028
Phosphorus, radioactive, for prostatic cancer pain, 725
Physical dependence, 1001–1002
Physical therapy:
  for bone marrow transplant patient, 1072–1073
  in head and neck cancer rehabilitation, 359
  for immunodeficient patient, 1072
  in leukemia, lymphoma, and Hodgkin's disease, 1071–1072

Physical therapy (Cont.):
  after mastectomy, 1049–1051
  (See also Exercises; Rehabilitation)
Physician:
  prejudices about cancer pain, 1017–1018
  response to patient's pain, 1017–1018
  role in giving diagnosis to patient and family, 242–244
Phytohemagglutinin, 151–152
Pineal tumors, 948–949
  chemotherapy of, 949
  diagnosis, 948
  radiotherapy of, 948–949
  recurrent disease, 949
  surgery for, 948
  symptoms, 948
  teratocarcinoma, 948–949
Pions, 195
Pituitary gland:
  ablation (see Hypophysectomy)
  dysfunction after radiotherapy, 940
Placebo:
  and pain relief, 1018
  use in clinical studies, 265–266
cis-Platinum:
  in cervical cancer, 769, 772
  in head and neck cancer, 350
  mechanism of action of, 130
  in prostatic cancer, 724
  renal disease due to, 135–136
Pleural effusion in ovarian cancer, 824
Pleural tumors, paraneoplastic syndromes associated with, 1029
Plummer-Vinson syndrome, 450
  nutrition related to, 277
Pneumoencephalography in brain tumors, 936
Polyamines:
  in brain tumors, 960
  chemotherapy related to increased synthesis of, 112
Polycyclic aromatic hydrocarbons, 12
Polyoma virus, 73–75
  DNA synthesis in, 73–74
  structure of, 73
  transformation of, 74
Polyps:
  associated conditions, 597
  and colorectal cancer, 38, 597
  treatment, 598
Postoperative considerations in brain surgery, 939–940

Postural drainage after thoracotomy, 1067
Potentially lethal damage repair, 183
Power of clinical trial, 258
Pregnancy:
 cervical cancer in, 769–770
 choriocarcinoma confused with, 847
 HCG levels in, 848
 immunosuppression in, 847
 melanoma in, 884
 molar (see Hydatidiform mole)
 pheochromocytoma in, 622
Pregnancy-specific glycoprotein (SP_1) in testicular cancer, 735
Prevalence rates, 27
 calculation of, 27–28
 period, 27
 point, 27
 relationship to incidence, 27
 use of, 28
Prevention of carcinogenesis, 20–22
 (See also Screening)
Probability values, 271
Procarbazine in brain tumors, 952–953
Procter-Livingston prosthesis, 463
Proctitis, chemotherapy-induced, 134
Progesterone:
 and endometrial cancer, 781
  in metastatic disease, 795–796, 798
  in treatment, 794–796, 798
 in prostatic cancer, 722
 in renal cell carcinoma, 658
 steps in action of, 508–509
Progesterone receptors, 508–509
 in breast cancer, 509–512
  postmenopausal compared to premenopausal levels, 510–511
  and treatment of metastases, 533
Progressive multifocal leukoencephalopathy, 1035
Prolactin in cancer, 1033
Proliferative ovarian cystadenomas, 812
Prolixin, 1003–1004
Propoxyphene, 999
Propranolol in pheochromocytoma, 626
Prospective studies, 32–34
 comparison with retrospective studies, 32
 concept of, 33

Prospective studies (Cont.):
 concurrent versus nonconcurrent types, 33–34
 methods for analysis of, 34
Prostaglandins and pain, 989
Prostatectomy:
 complications after, 714–715
 after previous prostatic surgery, 713
 in prostatic cancer, 713–716
 in prostatic urethra tumors, 745
Prostatic acid phosphatase, 708
Prostatic cancer, 698–727
 adenocarcinoma, 699
 benign prostatic hyperplasia differentiated from adenocarcinoma, 699
 classification, 705–706
 clinical presentation, 702–703
 cytomegalovirus role in, 86
 diagnosis, 703–705
  acid phosphatase, 703, 711–712
  biopsy, 703–705
  lymphangiography, 706, 708
  radiographs, 703, 704, 708
  rectal examination, 703, 706
  ultrasound, 711
 disseminated intravascular coagulation in, 727
 epidemiology, 40, 698–699
 etiology, 699
 history, 698
 incidence, 698–699
 latent disease, 702
 metastases in: acid phosphatase and, 708, 710, 711
  in bone, 708, 710
  in bone marrow, 710
  distant spread, 708, 710
  in lymph nodes, 706, 708, 710
 multifocal, 702
 natural history, 701–702
 pathology, 699–700
 prognostic determinants, 711
 radiocurability versus radioresponsivity of, 185
 sarcomas, 700
 screening for, 711–712
 seminal vesicle invasion in, 715
 spread of, 700–701
  hematogenous, 701
  local, 700
  regional, 700–701
 staging of, 705–710
 treatment, 712–727

Prostatic cancer, treatment (Cont.):
 adrenalectomy, 723
 chemotherapy, 715, 724
 cryosurgery, 725–726
 disseminated intravascular coagulation, 727
 hormonal therapy, 715–717, 720–724
 hypophysectomy, 723
 interstitial irradiation, 718–719
 lymphadenectomy, 716, 717, 719
 obstructive uropathy, 725–726
 orchiectomy, 720–721
 pain management, 724–725
 palliation, 720–722
 pathologic fracture, 726–727
 prostatectomy, 713–716
 radioactive gold, 718
 radioactive iodine, 718–719
 radiophosphorus, 725
 radiotherapy, 715, 717–718, 725
 relapsing disease, 722–727
 spinal cord compression, 726
 stage A disease, 712–713
 stage B disease, 713–716
 stage B_2 disease, 716
 stage C disease, 716–720
 stage D disease, 720–722
 transurethral surgery, 725–726
 tumors of prostatic urethra, 744–746
Prosthesis:
 in children, 1046
 in extremity cancer, 1044–1047
  decisions on use after amputation, 1046
  early fitting, 1044
 in head and neck cancer rehabilitation, 358
 limb salvage in osteosarcoma using, 891
 for lower extremity, 1046
 after mastectomy, 1052, 1054–1055
 psychological adjustments to, 1046
 for upper extremity, 1046–1047
Protocols, information contained in, 261, 262
 (See also Clinical trials)
Proton therapy, 196
Psychosocial factors in cancer, 231–251, 1074–1075
 age effect on reactions, 239–241
 in brain tumors, 931
 in breast cancer, 236–238

Psychosocial factors in cancer (*Cont.*):
　in cervical cancer, 235–236, 238
　childhood experiences, 233–234
　depression and hopelessness as antecedent states, 232–233
　emotional states early in disease, 243–244
　in endometrial cancer, 798
　epistemological problem in study of, 231–232
　familial aspects, 238–239
　general and specific factors, 235–238
　in head and neck cancer rehabilitation, 359
　historical background, 231
　at no-man's-land phase, 245–246
　pain, 1005
　patient's response to diagnosis and treatment, 241
　problems of patient, family, and professionals around diagnosis, 242–243
　repressive personality, 234–235
　site of disease and special reactions, 250–251
　stress of recurrence and metastasis, 244–245
　in terminal phase, 246–248
　use of imagery and altered states in therapy, 248–250
Psychotherapy for cancer pain, 1005
Pulmonary embolism, radical hysterectomy complicated by, 764–765
Putrescine, 960
Pyelography:
　intravenous (*see* Intravenous pyelography)
　in renal pelvis and ureteral tumors, 668–672
　retrograde, 668–671

Quadrantectomy, 523
Queyrat's erythroplasia, 744

Radial growth phase, 862
Radiation:
　acute effects, 184
　as carcinogen, 10, 12
　chronic effects, 184
　indirect effects of, 178
　management after exposure to thyroid gland, 419–420

Radiation (*Cont.*):
　and meningioma, 930
　osteosarcoma due to, 889
　physics and biology of, 176–185
　　interaction with matter, 177–178
　　linear energy transfer, 178
　　molecular DNA repair, 183–184
　　oxygen and radiosensitivity, 180
　　relative biologic effect, 178
　　repair of damage after, 181–184
　　　molecular DNA, 183–184
　　　potentially lethal damage, 182–183
　　　sublethal damage, 182
　salivary gland neoplasms due to, 389
　thyroid cancer associated with, 419
　ultraviolet (*see* Ultraviolet radiation)
　uterine sarcoma related to, 800–801
　(*See also* Radiotherapy)
Radioactive iodine (*see* Iodine, radioactive)
Radiocurability, 185
Radiofrequency lesion generator:
　for cordotomy, 1010
　dorsal rhizotomy by, 1007
　neurotomy by, 1006
Radioisotopes, monoclonal antibody as conjugate to, 170–171
Radiology:
　in esophageal cancer, 452–453
　in gestational trophoblastic tumors, 852
　in liver cancer, 565–567
　in mediastinal tumors, 472–475
　in pancreatic cancer, 582
　in paranasal sinus tumors, 319
　in pheochromocytoma, 623–624
　in prostatic cancer, 703, 704, 708–710
　in renal cell carcinoma, 648–649
　of salivary gland neoplasms, 396–397
　in stomach cancer, 546–547
Radionuclide scans:
　of adrenal medulla, 623
　brain metastases detected by, 966
　in brain tumor primaries, 935
　in lymphoma, 919, 920
　in mediastinal tumors, 475
　in prostatic cancer, 708, 710
　in renal cell carcinoma, 649
Radioresponsive, 185

Radiosensitivity, 179
　and cell cycle, 179
　and oxygen, 180–181
Radiosensitizers in brain tumors, 955–956
Radiotherapy:
　in bladder cancer, 691–694
　of brain metastases, 970–971
　in brain primary tumors, 940
　　brachytherapy, 957
　　differential diagnosis of recurrence after, 950
　　high-LET, 956–957
　　hypoxic cell radiosensitizers used with, 955–956
　　necrosis after, 950
　　recurrent disease, 952
　　transient encephalopathy after, 950
　in breast cancer, 523–528
　in buccal mucosa cancer, 289–290
　cell cycle and sensitivity to, 179
　in cerebral astrocytoma, 942–943
　in cervical cancer, 765–768
　　complications, 766–768
　　early use, 752
　　evaluation prior to, 759–760
　　extrafascial hysterectomy after, 765
　　in invasive disease, 761
　　for paraaortic metastases, 766
　　in recurrent disease, 772
　　sensitizers used in, 774
　chemotherapy combined with, in head and neck cancer, 348
　classification of, 176–177
　clinical radiocurability in, 185
　in colorectal cancer, 602–603
　complications of, 913
　　in children, 947
　　factors increasing risk, 766–767
　　in nasopharyngeal carcinoma, 313
　control of subclinical disease by, 185
　in endometrial cancer, 788–789, 792–794
　of ependymoma, 944
　in esophageal cancer, 455–456, 461, 462, 464–465
　fistula after, 767
　in floor of mouth cancer, 299–300
　future developments in, 192–196
　　biologic modifiers: radiation protectors, 192–193
　　negative pi mesons, 195

Radiotherapy, future developments in (*Cont.*):
  particle therapy, 195
  protons, 196
  sensitizers, 193–194
 in glioblastoma multiforme, 941–942
 in hard palate cancer, 296
 in head and neck cancer, 344–345, 348
  interstitial implants, 354
 historical aspects, 176
 in Hodgkin's disease, 912–913
 in hypopharyngeal tumors, 346–347
 importance of hypoxic cells in, 180–181
 injury to brain due to, 940
 interstitial, 177
  (*See also* Interstitial irradiation)
 intracavitary, 177
 inverted-Y field, 912
 kinetics of cell kill by, 110
 in laryngeal cancer, 372–373
 for leptomeningeal metastases, 973
 in lip cancer, 286
 in lung cancer, 438–439
 in lymphoma: diffuse histiocytic disease, 922
  nodular disease, 921
 in mediastinal tumors, 483, 485
 of medulloblastoma, 947
 in melanoma of vulva, 833
 in nasopharyngeal angiofibroma, 330
 in nasopharyngeal carcinoma, 312–313
 normal tissue reactions, 184
 of oligodendroglioma, 943
 in oral cancer: factors involved in selection of, 282
  new developments, 305
  surgery combined with, 282–284
 in oropharyngeal tumors, 345–346
 orthovoltage, 177
 in osteosarcoma, 890–891
 in ovarian cancer, 817
 in pancreatic cancer, 588–589
 of paranasal sinus tumors, 320–322
  complications, 321–322
  results, 322
  technique, 320–321
 of pineal tumors, 948–949
 pituitary dysfunction due to, 940
 postoperative, 188
 in pregnancy, 769

Radiotherapy (*Cont.*):
 preoperative, 188
 in prostatic cancer, 715, 717–718, 725
 in prostatic urethra tumors, 745, 747
 protector substances, 192–193
 radical versus palliative, 186
 in renal cell carcinoma, 652
 in renal pelvis tumors, 675–676
 reoxygenation, 181
 of reticulum-cell sarcoma of brain, 943–944
 risk versus gain in, 186
 of salivary gland neoplasms, 403
 small-bowel obstruction after, 767–768
 in soft-tissue sarcomas, 899
 in stomach cancer, 552
 subclinical disease treated by, 188
  prophylactic irradiation of neck, 188
 supervoltage, 177
 surgery combined with: in bladder cancer, 190, 691–694
  in breast cancer, 190–191, 519–521
  in endometrial cancer, 788–789, 792–794
  in esophageal cancer, 461, 464–465
  in laryngeal cancer, 372–373
  for metastatic neck nodes, 189
  in oral cancer, 282–284
  in paranasal sinus tumors, 323
  in rectum-rectosigmoid tumors, 190
  in salivary gland tumors, 189–190
 survival curve reproductive integrity in, 178–179
 in testicular cancer, 737
 in thyroid cancer, 418–419
  external, 418
  radioactive iodine, 418–419
 time/dose relationships in, 184–185
 in tongue cancer, 303
 total nodal irradiation, 912
 treatment philosophy in, 186
 treatment planning in, 177
 tumors cured primarily with, 186–188
  head and neck cancer, 186–187
  laryngeal cancer, 187
  uterine cervix cancer, 187–188
 in urethral cancer, 842

Radiotherapy (*Cont.*):
 in uterine sarcomas, 803
 vaginal stenosis after, 767
 in vulvar cancer, 831
  melanoma, 833
 in Wilms's tumor, 659–660
 (*See also* Radiation)
Randomization:
 dilemmas in, 263–264
 prerandomization process in, 263–264
 process in clinical trial, 261–264
Receptors:
 androgen, 511
 assays in breast cancer, 508–512
  sources and variability in results, 509–511
  and treatment of metastases, 533
  uses for, 511
 estrogen, 508–509
 (*See also* Estrogen receptors)
 glucocorticoid, 511
 pain, 984–985
 progesterone, 508–509
 (*See also* Progesterone receptors)
Reconstructive surgery:
 in buccal mucosa cancer, 289
 after chest wall tumor excision, 1068–1069
 in craniofacial resection in paranasal sinus tumors, 325
 in extremity cancer, 1043–1047
 of face and scalp, 1061–1062
 in floor of mouth cancer, 300
 in gingival cancer, 292–293
 in hard palate cancer, 296, 297
 in head and neck cancer, 304, 356–359
  bony defects, 358
  myocutaneous flaps in, 357–358
  prosthetics, 358
 of mandible, 300
 after mastectomy, 1047–1048, 1055
 of oral cavity, 1060–1061
 in osteosarcoma, 891
 after pelvic exenteration, 805
 rehabilitation associated with, 1041–1065
 in tongue cancer, 303
 in urethral cancer, 842
 after vulvectomy, 831
Rectal cancer (*see* Colorectal cancer)
Rectal carcinoid tumors, 641

Rectal examination in prostatic cancer, 703, 706
Rectovaginal fistula, radiotherapy complicated by, 767
Recurrence:
 psychological stress with, 244–245
 sample size requirements for clinical trial based on, 258–260
Rehabilitation, 1041–1075
 in acute hospitals, 1042
 in bone and soft tissue cancers of extremities, 1043–1047
 in brain tumors, 960–961
 in colorectal cancer, 606–607, 1056–1060
  after colostomy, 1056–1059
   convalescence, 1058
   ileostomy, 1059–1060
   operative care, 1057
   postoperative treatment, 1057–1058
   preoperative treatment, 1056–1057
   transitional and hospital care, 1058–1059
 in dialysis, 1073–1074
 in disabilities, 1041–1042
 in endometrial cancer, 797–798
 in extremity cancer, 1043–1047
  operative, 1043–1045
  pathologic fractures, 1047
  postoperative, 1045
  preoperative, 1043
  prostheses and braces, 1046–1047
 after glossectomy, 1064
 goals, 1042–1043
 in head and neck cancer, 358–359, 1060–1065
  drooling, 1064–1065
  dry mouth, 1064
  face, mouth, and pharynx, 1060–1063
  glossectomy, 1064
  larynx, 1063–1064
  pain, 1064
  radical neck dissection, 1065
 after ileostomy, 1059–1060
  convalescence, 1060
  pre- and postoperative care, 1059–1060
  transitional and posthospital care, 1060
 in laryngeal cancer, 1063–1064
  postoperative, 1063

Rehabilitation, in laryngeal cancer (*Cont.*):
  preoperative, 1063
  transitional and posthospital care, 1063–1064
 in leukemia, lymphoma, and Hodgkin's disease, 1071–1073
  bone marrow transplantation, 1072–1073
  immunodeficiency, 1072
 in lung cancer, 1065–1069
  postoperative, 1066–1069
  preoperative, 1065–1066
 after mastectomy, 1047–1056
  convalescence, 1054
  education and counseling, 1054
  exercises, 1049–1052
  goals in, 1048
  operative, 1048
  palliation, 1055–1056
  postoperative, 1048–1049
  preoperative, 1047–1048
  prosthesis, 1054–1055
  team instruction, 1051–1052
  transitional and posthospital care, 1054
 in nervous system tumors, 1069–1071
  pain management in, 1070–1071
  (*See also* Pain management)
 after pelvic exenteration, 805
 of psychosocial disorders, 1074–1075
 after radical neck dissection, 1065
 in testicular cancer, 739–740
 after thoracotomy, 1065–1069
 vocational, 1042
 (*See also* Vocational rehabilitation)
Rejection, organ, role in preventing metastasis, 221–223
Relative biologic effect (RBE), 178
Relative risk, 34
Relaxation therapy, 1005
Renal artery occlusion in renal cell carcinoma, 652
Renal cell carcinoma, 645–658
 biopsy of, 647
 in contralateral kidney, 657
 diagnostic methods in, 646–647
 epidemiology, 645–646
 etiology, 645–646
 historical aspects, 645
 incidence, 646
 liver dysfunction in, 646

Renal cell carcinoma (*Cont.*):
 metastases in, 649, 654
 paraneoplastic syndromes associated with, 646, 1027
 prognosis, 649–650
 prognostic factors in, 647
 signs and symptoms, 646
 spontaneous regression of, 649, 653
 staging of, 647–649
 treatment, 650–658
  follow-up care, 656–657
  invasion of adjacent structures, 652–654
  localized disease, 650–652
  palliative surgery, 652–654
  radiotherapy, 652
  recurrence, 657–658
  renal artery occlusion, 652
  simultaneous bilateral involvement, 656
  solitary kidney involvement, 654–656
  surgery, 650–656
Renal pelvis tumors, 664–677
 associated nephropathy, 665–666
 carcinogens involved in, 665
 classification, 666–667
 diagnostic techniques in, 668–673
  angiography, 672
  brush biopsy, 672–673
  cytology, 672
  excretory urography, 668
  retrograde pyelography, 668–669
 epidemiology, 665
 etiology, 665
 historical aspects, 664
 incidence, 664–665
 papilloma, 666
 pathologic grading of, 666–667
  adenocarcinoma, 667
  squamous cell carcinoma, 667
  transitional-cell tumors, 666–667
 signs and symptoms, 666
 staging in, 666–667
 treatment, 673–676
  chemotherapy, 676
  conservative surgery, 674–675
  current areas of research, 677
  follow-up and early detection of recurrence, 676
  radical surgery, 673–675
  radiotherapy, 675–676
  recurrence, 676
 viruses causing, 665

Renin:
  in cancer, 1033
  in primary versus secondary aldosteronism, 617
  in renal cell carcinoma, 646
Reoxygenation, 181
Repair:
  of potentially lethal damage, 182–183
  of sublethal damage, 182
Repression in cancer patient, 234–235
Reproductive integrity, 178–179
Research (see Clinical trials)
Resistance:
  to chemotherapy, 126
  cross, 126
  mechanisms of, 126
Reticulum-cell sarcoma of brain, 943–944
Retinoblastoma:
  chromosome abnormalities in, 48
  pathogenetic model, 46–47
Retrograde pyelography in renal pelvis and ureteral tumors, 668–671
Retroperitoneal tumors, sarcomas, 900
Retrospective studies, 32–33, 264–265
  assumptions of, 32–33
  basic design of, 32
  comparison with prospective studies, 32
  confounding variables in, 33
  selection of cases and control in, 33
Retroviruses, 67–72
  biologic properties of, 68
  endogenous sequences in, 71
  human and primate, 71–72
  leukemia/sarcoma virus complexes in, 68–71
  RNA replication in, 68, 69
  structure of, 68
Reverse transcriptase:
  in RNA oncoviruses, 92–93
  simultaneous detection with high-molecular-weight RNA, 91–94
Rhabdomyoma of nasal cavity, 330
Rhabdomyosarcoma:
  of nasal cavity, 330–331
  treatment, 899
  (See also Soft-tissue sarcomas)
Rhizotomy, dorsal, 1007
Riedel's struma, 405–406
Risk:
  attributable, 35
  relative, 34

Risk factors:
  for breast cancer, 39
  in lung cancer, 433–434
  for nasopharyngeal cancer, 36
RNA:
  homologous sequences in cancers, 90–92
  in retroviruses, 68
  (See also Retroviruses)
  simultaneous detection of reverse transcriptase and high-molecular-weight RNA, 91–94
  in tumor-specific particles, 92–95

S phase, 108
Saccharin and bladder cancer, 680–681
Salivary gland neoplasms, 388–404
  acinic cell carcinoma, 392–393
  adenocarcinomas, 393
  adenoid cystic carcinoma, 392
  anatomical considerations, 388–389
  benign lymphoepithelial lesion, 393–394
  benign mixed tumor, 390
  biopsy of, 396
  classification of, 189, 389–390
  data collection in, 397, 399
  diagnosis, 394–397
    minor gland tumors, 396
    parotid tumors, 394–395
    radiologic aids, 396–397
    sublingual tumors, 395–396
    submaxillary tumors, 395
  etiology of, 389
  lymphoma, 393
  malignant mixed tumor, 391–392
  mesenchymal tumors, 393
  metastatic carcinoma, 393
  mucoepidermoid carcinoma, 392
  oncocytoma, 391
  papillary cystadenoma lymphomatosum, 390–391
  pathology and natural history, 389–394
  prognosis, 403–404
  squamous cell carcinoma, 393
  staging of, 397, 398
  treatment, 398, 400–403
    chemotherapy, 403
    minor glands, 403
    parotid gland, 398, 400–402
    radiotherapy, 403
    with surgery, 189–190

Salivary gland neoplasms, treatment (Cont.):
    sublingual gland, 403
    submaxillary gland, 402–403
    (See also Parotid gland; Sublingual gland; Submaxillary gland)
Salivary glands, minor:
  anatomy, 389
  tumors of, 285–286
    clinical presentation, 294–295, 298–299
    diagnosis, 396
    distribution, 299, 300
    in hard palate, 294
    prognosis, 296, 300–301
    treatment, 299–300, 403
Sarcoma virus:
  leukemia related to, 68–71
  murine, 90–93
Sarcomas:
  of bone, 888–895
    (See also Osteosarcoma)
  of larynx, 369
  reticulum-cell in brain, 943–944
  of soft tissue, 895–901
    (See also Soft-tissue sarcomas)
  tumor-specific antigens in, 155–156
  uterine, 798–805
    (See also Uterine cancer, sarcomas)
  vulvar, 836
Satellitosis, 871
Schistosomiasis, role in cancer, 13
Schizophasia, 237–238
Scirrhous carcinoma, 508
Screening:
  for bladder cancer, 681
  for breast cancer, 491–496
  for cervical cancer, 755–756, 773
  for colorectal cancer, 599–600
  for endometrial cancer, 785, 797
  for inherited cancer syndrome, 59–61
  for lung cancer, 435
  for pheochromocytoma, 622
  for prostatic cancer, 711–712
  for stomach cancer, 546
  for upper respiratory tract tumors, 666
  for uterine sarcoma, 801
Second-look operation in ovarian cancer, 821–822
Second neoplasms, 41–42
  in buccal mucosa cancer, 290
  in esophageal cancer, 449–450
  etiologic factors, 42

Second neoplasms (*Cont.*):
  in head and neck cancer, 349, 356, 357
  in laryngeal cancer, 365
  in lip cancer, 287
  in lung cancer, 435
  multicentric cancer, 356
  multiple primaries in oral cancer, 280
  in Paget's disease of vulva, 835
  retinoblastoma associated with, 47
  site pairs occurring with unusually high frequency, 41, 42
Seminal vesicles, invasion in prostatic cancer, 715
Seminoma:
  classification, 731–732
  in mediastinum, 481, 483
  radiotherapy for, 483, 737
  (*See also* Testicular cancer)
Sensitizers, 193–194
  halogenated pyrimidines, 193
  of hypoxic cells, 194
Serotonin:
  and analgesia, 990
  due to electrical stimulation, 993
  antagonists in carcinoid syndrome therapy, 637–638
  and depression, 990
  metabolites in carcinoid syndrome, 636–637
  and pain, 989
  and tolerance to narcotics, 990
Sertoli-Leydig cell tumors of ovary, 815–816
Sex:
  cancer risk related to, 16–17, 30
  and survival in melanoma, 866–867
Sexual activity and cervical cancer, 753–754
Sexuality, psychological reactions in cancer patients related to, 250–251
Shope papilloma virus, 75–76
SIADH (*see* Syndrome of inappropriate antidiuretic hormone)
Sialadenitis, 395
  diagnosis, 397
Sialography, 397
Simian virus, 40
  cell transformation of, 66
Simiansarcoma virus, 72
Sinuses (*see* Paranasal sinus tumors)
Sipple's syndrome, 628, 629

Site, psychological reactions specific to, 250–251
Sjogren's syndrome, 394
  lymphoma in, 916
Skin:
  cancer syndromes related to, 1033–1034
  chemotherapy-induced disease of, 136–137
  familial cancers suggested by disorder in, 54–55
Skin cancer:
  factors related to occurrence, 21
  melanoma (*see* Melanoma)
Skull films in brain tumors, 935
Sleep, disturbance due to headache in brain tumors, 933
Small-bowel neoplasms:
  carcinoid tumors, 640
  paraneoplastic syndromes asociated with, 1027
Small-bowel obstruction:
  radiotherapy complicated by, 767–768
  surgical treatment of, 768
Smoking (*see* Tobacco)
Sodium (*see* Hyponatremia)
Sodium nitroprusside in pheochromocytoma, 626
Soft-tissue sarcomas, 895–901
  anatomic sites of, 895–896
  classification, 895, 896
  clonogenic assay used in, 901
  current research and future prospects, 901
  diagnosis, 897–898
    biopsy, 897
    systemic evaluation, 897
  epidemiology, 895–897
  etiology, 896–897
  of extremities: rehabilitation, 1043–1047
  (*See also* Extremity cancer)
  follow-up and early identification of recurrence or metastases, 901
  historical aspects, 895
  incidence, 895
  metastases in, 897, 901
  in neurofibromatosis, 896
  prognostic factors in, 897–898
  signs, symptoms, and early detection, 897
  staging of, 897–898
  treatment, 898–901

Soft-tissue sarcomas, treatment (*Cont.*):
  adjuvant therapy, 900–901
  amputation, 898
  chemotherapy, 899–901
  extremity tumors, 899
  head and neck disease, 898–900
  isolated limb perfusion, 899
  muscle-group excision, 898
  radiotherapy, 899
  recurrence of metastases, 901
  retroperitoneal disease, 900
Somatic nerve blocks, 1014
  differential diagnosis block, 1015
Somatomedin, role in cancer hypoglycemia, 1032
Somatostatin and pain, 992
Somatostatinoma, 593
Speech:
  in brain tumor, 931, 960–961
  esophageal, 1063–1064
  rehabilitation in laryngeal cancer, 1063
  therapy in head and neck cancer rehabilitation, 358
Spermatogenesis in Hodgkin's disease, 915
Spermatozoa, role in cervical cancer, 755
Spermidine, 960
Sphenoid sinus (*see* Paranasal sinus tumors)
Spinal cord:
  dorsal horn role in pain perception, 985–987
  spinothalamic tract role in pain perception, 987–988
Spinal cord compression:
  diagnosis, 975
  in prostatic cancer, 726
  treatment, 976–977
Spindle-cell carcinoma of larynx, 369
Spine metastases, 973–978
  back pain in, 974
  current areas of research and future prospects in, 978
  diagnosis, 975
  early detection, 974–975
  epidemiology, 974
  incidence, 973–974
  manner of primary tumor spread, 974
  myelography in, 975
  palliation for, 1056
  primary lesions associated with, 974

Spine metastases (*Cont.*):
 signs and symptoms, 974
 spinal cord compression in (*see* Spinal cord compression)
 treatment, 976–978
  chemotherapy, 977–978
  decompressive laminectomy, 976–977
  primary tumor influence on, 976
  recurrent symptoms, 978
Spinothalamic tract and pain perception, 987–988
Spinothalamic tractotomy:
 in brainstem, 1010–1011
 cervical, 1009–1010
 in thoracic spine, 1008–1010
Spironolactone in aldosteronism, 617
Splanchnicectomy, 1006–1007
Spleen in lymphoma, 919
Splenectomy in Hodgkin's disease, 910–911
Spontaneous regression, 147
 of metastases, 653
 of renal cell carcinoma, 649, 653
Sputum in lung cancer, 435
Staging, 280–281
 of bladder cancer, 682–686
 of breast cancer, 512–515
 of carcinoid tumors, 635–636
 in cervical cancer, 753, 757–760
 in classification, 26
 of colorectal cancer, 600–602
 in endometrial adenocarcinoma, 785–790
 of esophageal cancer, 451, 454–455
 of gestational trophoblastic tumors, 853
 of head and neck tumors, 343
 of Hodgkin's disease, 907–908
  work-up, 908–911
 of laryngeal cancer, 367, 370–371
 in liver cancer, 571, 572
 of lung cancer, 435–437
 of lymphoma, 918–920
 of melanoma, 864–866, 868–869
  vulvar, 832
 in nasopharyngeal carcinoma, 312
 in neuroblastoma, 661
 of oral cancer, 280–282
 in ovarian cancer, 811–812
 of paranasal sinus tumors, 319–320
 of penile cancer, 741
 in prostatic cancer, 705–710
 of renal cell carcinoma, 647–649

Staging (*Cont.*):
 of renal pelvis and ureteral tumors, 666–667
 of salivary gland neoplasms, 397, 398
 of soft-tissue sarcomas, 897–898
 of stomach cancer, 548
 of testicular cancer, 732–734
 of thyroid cancer, 412–414
 of urethral tumors, 841
 of uterine sarcoma, 802
 of vaginal cancer, 838, 839
 of vulvar cancer, 827–829
  melanoma, 832
 in Wilms's tumor, 659
Stellate ganglion block, 1014, 1016–1017
Stereotaxic surgery:
 cingulumotomy, 1011–1012
 frontal lobotomy, 1012
 pituitary ablation, 1012
 thalamotomy, 1011
Sterility after Hodgkin's disease therapy, 915
Sternocleidomastoid, disability after radical neck dissection, 1065
Steroid hormone receptor assays in breast cancer, 508–512
 (*See also* Corticosteroids)
Stomach cancer, 543–555
 carcinoid, 640
 classification, 547–548
 current areas of research and prospects for future, 554–555
 diagnosis, 546–548
  endoscopy, 547
  immunodiagnostic assay, 547
  radiology, 546–547
 diet and, 37
 endoscopy in, 547
  difference between Japanese and U.S. experience, 543–544
  as follow-up after surgery, 553
 epidemiology, 36–37, 544–545
 etiology, 545
 factors related to occurrence, 21
 fetal sulfaglycoprotein in, 546
 genetics of, 545
 geographical variation in, 29
 histologic subtypes, 24–25, 36
 historical aspects, 543–544
 incidence, 544–545
 lymphoma, 923
 metastatic spread in, 553

Stomach cancer (*Cont.*):
 paraneoplastic syndromes associated with, 1027
 reconstruction and rehabilitation, 555
 recurrence rate in, 552–553
 screening for, 546
 staging of, 548
 symptoms, 545–546
 treatment, 548–554
  adjuvant therapy, 551–552
  Celestin tube in, 553–554
  chemotherapy, 551–552, 554
  difference between Japanese and U.S. experience, 543
  follow-up and early identification of recurrence or metastasis, 552–553
  options for primary treatment, 548–551
  palliation, 551
  radiotherapy, 552, 554
  recurrence and metastasis, 553–554
Stomatitis, chemotherapy-induced, 134
Streptozotocin:
 in carcinoid tumors, 638
 renal disease due to, 136
Subependymal mixed glioma, 944
Subglottis, 361–362
 (*See also* Laryngeal cancer, subglottic region)
Sublethal damage repair, 182
Sublingual gland:
 anatomy, 389
 tumors: diagnosis, 395–396
  prognosis, 403–404
  treatment, 403
 (*See also* Salivary gland neoplasms)
Submandibular gland (*see* Salivary gland neoplasms; Submaxillary gland)
Submaxillary gland:
 anatomy, 389
 swelling of, 395
 tumors: diagnosis, 395
  prognosis, 403–404
  treatment, 402–403
 (*See also* Salivary gland neoplasm)
Substance P and pain, 991–992
Substantia gelatinosa, role in pain perception, 986–987
Suction curettage for hydatidiform mole, 850–851

Suffering, 984
Sunlight:
    and lip cancer, 277
    and melanoma, 861–862
Superior mesenteric angiography in jaundice evaluation, 568
Suppressor cells, 219
Supraglottis, 361–362
    (*See also* Laryngeal cancer, supraglottic region)
Surgery, 3–5
    in adrenocortical tumors, 618–620
    in bladder cancer, 687, 689–692
    for brain metastases, 969–970
    in brain primary tumors, 938–940
        cerebral edema after, 949–950
        microsurgical techniques, 938
        recurrent disease, 952
        shunting for hydrocephalus, 938
    in breast cancer, 515–523
        (*See also* Mastectomy)
    in buccal mucosa cancer, 289
    in carcinoid tumors, 637
    in cervical cancer: early use, 751–752
        invasive disease, 760–765
        microinvasive disease, 760
        as palliation, 772–773
        pelvic exenteration, 770–772
        recurrent disease, 770–772
    in cervical esophagus tumors, 347
    in chondrosarcoma, 331
    in colorectal cancer, 601–602
    comparison with other treatments, 3
    debulking procedure in ovarian cancer, 816–817
    in endometrial cancer, 788–794
    in esophageal cancer, 456–464
        cervical carcinomas, 347, 456–457
        middle- and lower-third carcinomas, 457–459
    in extrahepatic biliary tract cancer, 574–576
    in floor of mouth cancer, 299–300
    in gallbladder cancer, 573–574
    in gingiva cancer, 292–293
    in hard palate cancer, 295–296
    in head and neck cancer, 344–345
    in hyperparathyroidism, 427
    in hypopharyngeal tumors, 347
    kinetics of cell kill by, 110
    in lip cancer, 286–287
    in liver cancer, 569–572
    in lung cancer, 437–438

Surgery (*Cont.*):
    for lymphedema, 1053
    in medulloblastoma, 946–947
    in melanoma, 872–880
        local excision, 872–874
        lymphadenectomy, 874–880
        vulvar, 832–833
    in nasopharyngeal angiofibroma, 329–300
    in neuroblastoma, 661
    for nose tumors, benign, 317
    in oropharyngeal tumors, 345–346
    in osteosarcoma, 890–891
    in ovarian cancer, 812–822
    in pain management, 995, 1005–1013
        neuroablative procedures, 1005–1012
        neuroaugmentive procedures, 1012–1013
        (*See also* Pain management, neurosurgical alternatives)
    in pancreatic cancer, 586–588
    in paranasal sinus tumors, 322–326
        conventional management, 322–323
        craniofacial resection, 323–326
        radiotherapy combined with, 323
    in penile cancer, 742–744
    in pheochromocytoma, 624–625
    in pineal tumors, 948
    in prostatic cancer, 713–720, 725–726
    for pulmonary metastases, 441–445
    radical operations, 4–5
    radiotherapy combined with: in bladder cancer, 691–694
        in breast cancer, 190–191, 519–521
        in endometrial cancer, 788–789, 792–794
        in esophageal cancer, 461, 464–465
        in laryngeal cancer, 372–373
        in oral cancer, 282–284
        in paranasal sinus tumors, 323
    reconstruction (*see* Reconstruction surgery)
    in renal cell carcinoma, 650–656
    in renal pelvis and ureteral tumors, 673–675
    in salivary gland neoplasms, 189–190, 398, 400–403

Surgery (*Cont.*):
    second-look operation in ovarian cancer, 821–822
    in soft-tissue sarcomas, 898–900
    in spinal cord compression, 976–977
    stereotaxic (*see* Stereotaxic surgery)
    in stomach cancer, 548–551
    in testicular cancer, 736–738
    in thymoma, 478
    in thyroid cancer, 415–418
    in tongue cancer, 303
    in urethral cancer, 747, 842
    in uterine sarcomas, 803–804
    in vaginal cancer, 838–839
    in vulvar cancer, 829–831
        melanoma, 832–833
    in Wilms's tumor, 659
Surgical oncologist, 5–6
Surgical oncology:
    definition, 4
    development of, 4–6
Surveillance, epidemiology, and end results program, 31
Survival rates, 269–271
SV40 virus, 73–75
Swallowing, prevention of difficulty after excising laryngeal nerves, 1062
Sympathectomy, 1006–1007
Synchronization, 114–117
Syndrome of inappropriate antidiuretic hormone (SIADH), 1030–1031
    diagnosis, 1030
    treatment, 1030–1031
Syphilis and tongue cancer, 277

T lymphocytes in breast cancer, 151
TA-4 in cervical cancer, 774
Talwin (*see* Pentazocine)
Tamoxifen:
    in breast cancer, 530–531, 533
    clinical trial evaluation in breast cancer, 266
Teratoma:
    in mediastinum, 481
    ovarian, 814
    pineal, 948–949
    testicular: classification, 731–732
        (*See also* Testicular cancer)
    in young women, 819–820
Terminal illness:
    age of patient and response to, 239–241, 247

Terminal illness (*Cont.*):
  family's problems in, 247–248
  in head and neck cancer, 359
  pain management in, 997
  patient response in, 246–247
  special hospital units for, 1022
  use of imagery and altered states in, 248–250
Testicular cancer, 729–740
  alpha-fetoprotein in, 732, 734, 735
  in children, 738
  clinical features, 732
  cryptorchidism associated with, 730
  current and future problems and research in, 739
  early classification, 729
  epidemiology, 729–730
  etiology, 730
  factors related to occurrence, 21
  histopathogenic classification, 730–732
  historic landmarks in, 729
  human chorionic gonadotropin in, 732, 734, 735
  immunocytochemistry in, 732
  localizing metastases in, 736
    HCG and AFP scans in, 736
    in liver, 736
    selective venous catheterization in, 736
  pregnancy-specific glycoprotein in, 735
  rehabilitation and socioeconomic impact, 739–740
  resection of pulmonary metastases in, 443
  staging of, 732–734
    computed tomography in, 734
    inferior venacavography in, 734
    lymphangiography in, 734
  treatment, 736–740
    chemotherapy, 737–738
    cytoreductive surgery in advanced disease, 738
    follow-up, 738
    radiotherapy, 737
    recurrence, 738–739
    retroperitoneal lymph node dissection, 736–737
  tumor markers in, 732, 739
Testosterone and prostatic cancer, 720
Thalamocortical connections and pain, 988

Thalamotomy:
  complications, 1011
  in pain control, 1011
Thallium scan in thyroid cancer, 414
Theca cell tumors, 815
Therapeutic index, 128
Thioguanine, thymidine labeling index and prediction of response to chemotherapy in acute leukemia, 113
Thiopurines, pharmacology of, 127
Thiotepa in renal pelvis tumors, 676
Thiothixene, 1003
Thoracotomy:
  breathing exercises prior to, 1066
  breathing problems after, 1067
  chest percussion after, 1067–1068
  exercises after, 1067
  inhalation therapy after, 1068
  postural drainage after, 1067
  rehabilitation after, 1065–1069
Thorazine, 1002–1003
Thrombocytopenia, myelosuppression causing, 132–133
Thrombophlebitis in pancreatic cancer, 582
Thrombosis and cancer, 1037–1038
Thymidine labeling index, 108
  estrogen receptor status related to, 114
  and prediction of chemotherapy response, 113–114, 117–118
  in vitro studies, 117–118
  studies in patients, 113–114
Thymoma, 477–448
  anatomical aspects, 477–478
  diagnosis, 477
  distinguishing benign from malignant, 477
  and immunologic function, 470, 474
  paraneoplastic syndromes associated with, 1029
  surgical approaches to, 478
Thyroid adenomas, 405
Thyroid cancer, 405–423
  anaplastic carcinoma, 410
    surgical management, 416–417
  aspiration biopsy in, 415
  classification of malignancy, 407–412
  diagnosis, 413–415
  echography in, 415
  factors related to occurrence, 21

Thyroid cancer (*Cont.*):
  follicular carcinoma, 409–410
    surgical management, 416
  histologic subtypes, 25
  Hurthle cell carcinoma, 412
    surgical management, 417–418
  incidence, 405
  intrathoracic, 481, 486
  iodine uptake studies in, 413–414
  medullary carcinoma, 410–412
    calcitonin secretion in, 1033
    surgical management, 417
  minimal cancer, 409
  in multiple endocrine neoplastic syndromes, 56–57
  papillary carcinoma, 407–409
    surgical management, 415–416
  paraneoplastic syndromes associated with, 1029
  physical examination in, 413
  postoperative complications, 422
  radiation associated with, 419
  recurrent disease, 421
  staging of, 412–414
  survival in, 421
  thyroid scan in, 413–414
  thyroid suppression tests in, 414–415
  treatment: cervical lymph node management, 416–417
    chemotherapy, 420
    external radiotherapy, 418
    radioactive iodine, 418–419
    surgical, 415–418, 422–423
    types of operations used in, 420
Thyroid function tests, 414–415
Thyroid gland:
  benign enlargements, 405–407
  cancer statistics, 405
  classification of malignant tumors, 407–412
  goiter, 405
  management after radiation exposure to, 419–420
  tumors, 405–423
  (*See also* Thyroid cancer)
Thyroid scan, 413–414
Thyroidectomy:
  hypoparathyroidism after, 415
  in papillary carcinoma, 415
  postoperative complications, 422, 424
Thyroiditis, 405–406
Time trends, 28–29

Tobacco:
　asbestos synergism with, 13
　and bladder cancer, 680
　and buccal mucosa cancer, 288
　as carcinogen, 12
　in epidermoid carcinoma of upper aerodigestive tract, 339
　and esophageal cancer, 450
　and gingiva cancer, 291
　and hard palate cancer, 294
　and laryngeal cancer, 365
　and lip cancer, 285
　lung cancer related to, 38, 433
　and oral cancer, 276
　prevention of cancers related to, 20
　and renal cell carcinoma, 645, 646
　strategies for reduction of, 351
　synergistic effect with alcohol, 339
　and upper urinary tract tumors, 665
Tofranil, 1003
Tolerance, 1001–1002
Tomography, computerized:
　in bladder cancer, 685–686
　brain metastases detected by, 966–967
　in brain primary tumors, 933–934
　in cervical cancer, 759
　complications, 934
　in gestational trophoblastic tumors, 852
　in Hodgkin's disease, 909–910
　in jaundice evaluation, 566, 568
　of larynx, 368, 371
　in lymphoma, 919
　in mediastinal tumors, 475, 476
　in osteosarcoma, 890, 895
　in pancreatic cancer, 584
　in pheochromocytoma, 624
　in pineal tumors, 948
　in renal cell carcinoma, 648–649
　in spine metastases, 975
　in testicular cancer, 734
Tongue cancer, 301–304
　anatomy, 301
　clinical presentation, 302
　incidence and etiology, 301
　lymphatic drainage considerations, 301
　pathology, 301–302
　prognosis, 304
　recurrence, 304
　results of treatment, 303–304
　syphilis and, 277

Tongue cancer (*Cont.*):
　treatment, 303, 346
　radiotherapy control of, 186–187
　(*See also* Oral cancer)
Tonsil tumors, treatment, 345
Torticollis after radical neck dissection, 1065
Toxins, monoclonal antibody as conjugate to, 171
Transcriptase, reverse (*see* Reverse transcriptase)
Transcutaneous neurostimulation, 1013
Transformation, 66
　abortive, 66
　in adenoviruses, 77
　by cytomegalovirus, 86
　by Epstein-Barr virus, 85
　by herpes simplex, 81, 83–84
　in polyoma virus, 74–75
　tumor antigens related to, 74–75
　virus role, 66–67
Transitional-cell carcinoma:
　metastasis in, 667
　pathologic grading of, 666–667
　of prostatic urethra, 744–745
　of upper urinary tract, 664–677
Transplantable tumors:
　lack of rejection in early studies, 142–143
　resistance in humans, 147
Transplantation, liver, 571
Transurethral surgery:
　cryosurgery, 725–726
　resection of bladder cancer, 682, 690–691
　resection of prostate, 725
Trapezius:
　disability after radical neck dissection, 1065
　myocutaneous flaps, 357
Treatment, patient's response to, 241
Tricyclic antidepressants, 1003–1004
Triethylene thiophosphoramide (*see* TTPA)
Trigeminal tractotomy, 1010
Trigger point injection, 1014
Trophoblastic tumors (*see* Gestational trophoblastic tumors)
Tryptophan and bladder cancer, 680
TTPA in bladder cancer, 687–688
Tumor antigen (T antigen):
　and cell transformation, 74–75
　in SV40 virus, 74–75

Tumor doubling time:
　calculation of, 441
　in osteosarcoma, 894
　and resection of pulmonary metastases, 442, 443
Tumor lysis syndrome, 1038
Tumor markers:
　acid phosphatase, 703
　(*See also* Acid phosphatase)
　alpha-fetoprotein, 734
　(*See also* Alpha-fetoprotein)
　in brain tumors, 960
　carcinoembryonic antigen, 156–157
　(*See also* Carcinoembryonic antigen)
　in carcinoid tumors, 633–634
　in cervical cancer, 774–775
　human chorionic gonadotropin, 734–735
　lactic dehydrogenase, 735
　in liver cancer, 565
　in ovarian cancer, 822
　pregnancy-specific glycoprotein, 735
　in testicular cancer, 732, 734–736, 739
　in treatment of cervical cancer, 774
Tumor progression, 862
Tumor registries, 31
Tumor-specific antigens (*see* Antigens, tumor-associated)
Tumor-specific particles:
　implication of presence of, 94–95
　in murine mammary tumors, 92–93
Tumor-specific transplantation antigens (*see* Antigens, tumor-specific transplantation)
Tumor viruses (*see* Oncoviruses)
Tumors (*see* Cells, tumor; Neoplasms)
Turcot's syndrome, 52
Two-mutation model, 46–47
Tylosis and esophageal cancer, 450
Tyrosinemia and liver cancer, 561

Ulcerative colitis and colorectal cancer, 598
Ultrasound:
　in bladder cancer, 686
　for hydatidiform mole, 849–850
　in pheochromocytoma, 623
　in prostatic cancer, 711
　in thyroid cancer, 415
Ultraviolet radiation:
　as carcinogen, 10
　and melanoma, 861–862

Ureter:
  obstruction in prostatic cancer, 725–726
  stenosis after radical hysterectomy, 763–764
Ureteral tumors, 664–677
  carcinogens involved in, 665
  classification, 666–667
  diagnostic techniques in, 668–673
    angiography, 672
    antegrade pyelography, 671–672
    brush biopsy, 672–673
    cytology, 672
    excretory urography, 668
    retrograde pyelography, 668–671
  epidemiology, 665
  etiology, 665
  historical aspects, 664
  incidence, 664–665
  pathologic grading of, 666–667
    squamous cell carcinoma, 667
    transitional-cell tumors, 666–667
  signs and symptoms, 666
  staging in, 666–667
  treatment, 673–676
    chemotherapy, 676
    conservative surgery, 674–675
    current areas of research, 677
    follow-up and early detection of recurrence, 676
    radical surgery, 673–675
    radiotherapy, 675–676
    recurrence, 676
Ureterovaginal fistula after radical hysterectomy, 763
Urethral cancer, 744–747
  in female, 746–747, 841–842
    advanced and recurrent disease, 842
    incidence, epidemiology, and etiology, 841
    reconstruction and rehabilitation in, 842
    signs, symptoms, and early detection, 841
    staging and prognostic factors, 841
    treatment, 842
  lymph nodes in, 746, 747
  in male, 744–746
    bulbomembranous urethra, 745–746
    prostatic urethra, 744–745
  radiotherapy for, 745, 747

Uric acid nephropathy, 1038
Urologic tumors:
  bladder cancer, 679–694
    (See also Bladder cancer)
  kidney tumors, 645–662
    (See also Kidney tumors)
  penile cancer, 741–744
    (See also Penile cancer)
  prostatic cancer, 698–727
    (See also Prostatic cancer)
  renal pelvis and ureteral tumors, 664–677
    (See also Renal pelvis tumors; Ureteral tumors)
  testicular cancer, 729–740
    (See also Testicular cancer)
  urethral cancer, 744–747
    (See also Urethral cancer)
Urothelial cancer, 665
  (See also Bladder cancer; Renal pelvis tumors; Ureteral tumors)
Urothelium, 665
Uterine cancer, 780–805
  cervix, 751–775
    (See also Cervix, cancer of)
  endometrial adenocarcinoma, 780–798
    (See also Endometrial adenocarcinoma)
  factors related to occurrence, 21
  paraneoplastic syndromes associated with, 1029
  sarcomas, 798–805
    adjuvant therapies, 804
    classification, 798, 799
    current areas for research and future prospects in, 804
    diagnostic techniques in, 802–803
    epidemiology, 799–801
    estrogen role in, 801
    etiology, 800–801
    follow-up techniques in, 804
    histogenesis of, 798
    incidence, 799
    leiomyosarcoma, 799
    prognostic factors, 802–803
    radiation-induced, 800–801
    reconstruction and rehabilitation in, 805
    recurrences and metastases, 804
    screening for, 801
    signs and symptoms, 801
    staging of, 802

Uterine cancer, sarcomas (Cont.):
  stromal sarcoma, 799–800
  therapeutic options, 803–804

Vaccine for hepatitis B virus, 79
Vaginal adenosis, 837
Vaginal bleeding in endometrial cancer, 783
Vaginal cancer, 836–841
  current research and future prospects, 840–841
  identification of recurrent disease, 840
  incidence, epidemiology, and etiology, 836–837
  maternal use of diethylstilbestrol and, 15, 836–837
  melanoma, 883–884
  signs, symptoms, and early detection, 837–838
  staging and prognostic factors, 838, 839
  treatment, 838–840
    advanced and recurrent disease, 840
    5-fluorouracil cream, 839
    primary lesion, 838–840
    radiotherapy, 839–840
    reconstruction after pelvic exenteration, 805
    surgery, 838–839
Vaginal stenosis, radiotherapy complicated by, 767
Vanillymandelic acid in neuroblastoma, 661
Vascularization of tumors, 202–203
Venography:
  in adrenocortical tumor, 618
  in pheochromocytoma, 623, 625
Venous catheterization in localizing metastases, 736
Ventriculography in brain tumors, 936
Verner-Morrison tumors, 593
Verrucous cancer:
  of larynx, 368–369
  in oral cavity, 279
Vertical growth phase, 862
Vesicovaginal fistula:
  after radical hysterectomy, 764
  radiotherapy complicated by, 767
Vinca alkaloids:
  constipation due to, 134
  mechanism of action of, 130

Vinca alkaloids (*Cont.*):
  nervous system toxicity of, 136
  in renal cell carcinoma, 658
  in testicular cancer, 737–738
Vincristine:
  bleomycin synergistic effect with, 116
  in brain tumors, 953–954
  pharmacology of, 127
  synchronization effects, 115
Vinyl chloride as carcinogen, 14
Virilization, adrenal tumors causing, 618–619
Virogenes, 71
Viruses:
  cancer related to, 15–16
  in carcinogenesis, 65–87
    antigenic evidence for, 156
    herpes simplex role in cervical cancer, 754–755
    (*See also* Oncoviruses)
  and transitional-cell carcinoma, 665
  tumor-specific transplantation antigens of, 143–145
Vision disturbances in brain tumors, 960
VM-26 in brain tumors, 954
Vocal cords:
  cancer of (*see* Laryngeal cancer)
  lymphatics of, 363
  striping in laryngeal cancer, 373
Vocational rehabilitation, 1042, 1074–1075
  in laryngeal cancer, 1064
Von Recklinghausen's syndrome (*see* Neurofibromatosis)
VP-16:
  mechanism of action of, 130
  pharmacology of, 127

Vulvar cancer, 826–836
  adenocarcinoma, 836
  basal cell carcinoma, 835–836
  current research and future prospects, 830
  historical aspects, 826
  identification of recurrent disease, 830
  incidence, epidemiology, and etiology, 826
  luekoplakia and, 826
  melanoma, 831–834, 883
    (*See also* Melanoma, of vulva)
  metastases in, 827–829
  Paget's disease, 834–835
  pathologic types, 826
  preinvasive stage, 827
  sarcoma, 836
  signs and symptoms, 826–827
  staging and prognostic factors, 827–829
  treatment: adjuvant therapy, 830
    advanced and recurrent disease, 830
    chemotherapy, 830
    primary lesion, 829–830
    radiotherapy, 831
    vulvectomy, 829–831
  viruses role in, 826
Vulvectomy, 829–830
  in melanoma of vulva, 832–833
  in Paget's disease, 834

Warthin's tumor, 390–391
  natural history, 391
  pathology, 391
  radiologic diagnosis of, 397

Warts, 75–76
Wermer's syndrome, 628–629
WHDA tumors, 593
Whipple procedure, 586–587
Wilms's tumor, 658–660
  bilateral disease, 660
  congenital anomalies associated with, 47, 658–659
  diagnostic methods in, 659
  historical aspects, 658
  incidence, 658
  neuroblastoma distinguished from, 659, 661
  signs and symptoms, 658–659
  staging in, 659
  treatment, 659–660
    chemotherapy, 660
    follow-up care, 660
    radiotherapy, 659–660
    recurrence, 660
    results, 660
    surgery, 659
Withdrawal syndrome, 1001–1002

X-linked lymphoproliferative syndrome, 57–59
  immunopathogenesis, 57–59
  screening for, 61
X-rays, 177
  (*See also* Radiation)
Xeroderma pigmentosum and cancer, 54–55
Xylocaine, viscous, in drug-induced stomatitis, 134